Volume 1

RADIOLOGY Exam Made Easy

A Comprehensive Case Based Approach to Radiologic Examination

- A complete stepwise aid for radiology board examinations
- Precise structured guidelines for radiology case presentation
- Illustrative system-wise radiological anatomy
- Comprehensive coverage of over 200 examination cases with an all-inclusive list of possible differential diagnoses
- 70+ OSCE/CORE exercises explained with high quality images and original illustrations
- An overview of the international certifying examinations such as FICR, MICR, EDiR
- A complete handbook and reference for residents and young radiologists to guide them in their day-to-day radiological investigations and diagnoses

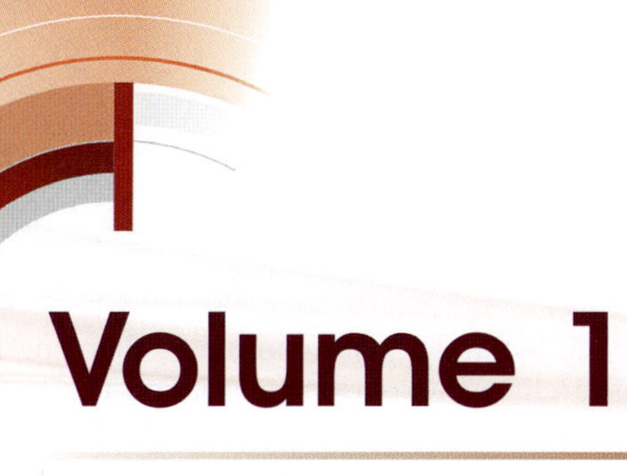

Volume 1

RADIOLOGY
Exam Made Easy

A Comprehensive Case Based Approach to Radiologic Examination

C Amarnath

MD, DNB, MNAMS, FRCR, FICR, FIMSA, MBA, PhD, EDiR, MICR, DiICRI

Professor and Head, Department of Radiodiagnosis
Stanley Medical College, Chennai
Senior Consultant, Scans World and Scans Point, Chennai

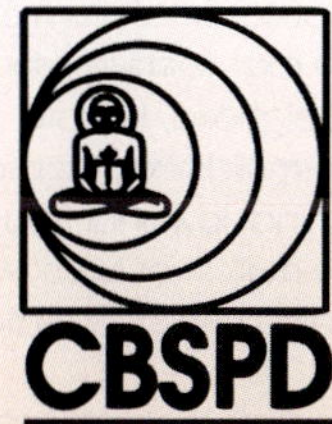

CBSPD

CBS Publishers & Distributors Pvt Ltd

New Delhi • Bengaluru • Chennai • Kochi • Kolkata • Lucknow • Mumbai
Gujarat • Hyderabad • Jharkhand • Nagpur • Patna • Pune • Uttarakhand

Disclaimer

Science and technology are constantly changing fields. New research and experience broaden the scope of information and knowledge. The author has tried his best in giving information available to him while preparing the material for this book. Although all efforts have been made to ensure optimum accuracy of the material, yet it is quite possible some errors might have been left uncorrected. The publisher, the printer and the author will not be held responsible for any inadvertent errors, omissions or inaccuracies.

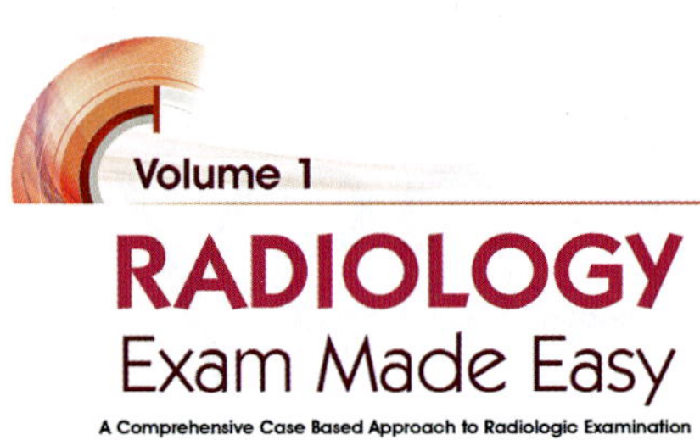

ISBN: 978-93-5466-604-9 (Set ISBN)

First Edition 2024
Reprint: 2026

Published by Satish Kumar Jain and produced by Varun Jain for

CBS Publishers & Distributors Pvt Ltd

4819/XI Prahlad Street, 24 Ansari Road, Daryaganj, New Delhi 110 002, India
Ph: 011-23266838, 23289259 Website: www.cbspd.com
e-mail: delhi@cbspd.com

Corporate Office: 204 FIE, Industrial Area, Patparganj, Delhi 110 092, India
Ph: 011-4934 4934 Fax: 011-4934 4935 e-mail: publishing@cbspd.com; publicity@cbspd.com

Branches

- **Bengaluru:** Seema House 2975, 17th Cross, K.R. Road, Banasankari 2nd Stage, Bengaluru 560 070, Karnataka, India
  Ph: +91-80-26771678/79 Fax: +91-80-26771680 e-mail: bangalore@cbspd.com
- **Chennai:** 7, Subbaraya Street, Shenoy Nagar, Chennai 600 030, Tamil Nadu, India
  Ph: +91-44-26680620, 26681266 Fax: +91-44-42032115 e-mail: chennai@cbspd.com
- **Kochi:** 42/1325, 1326, Power House Road, Opposite KSEB, Power House, Ernakulum 682018, Kochi, Kerala, India
  Ph: +91-484-4059061–67 Fax: +91-484-4059065 e-mail: kochi@cbspd.com
- **Kolkata:** 147, Hind Ceramics Compound, 1st Floor, Nilgunj Road, Belghoria, Kolkata 700056, West Bengal, India
  Ph: +91-33-25633055/56 e-mail: kolkata@cbspd.com
- **Lucknow:** Basement, Khushnuma Complex, 7 Meerabai Marg (behind Jawahar Bhawan), Lucknow 226001, UP, India
  Ph: +91-522-4000032 e-mail: tiwari.lucknow@cbspd.com
- **Mumbai:** PWD Shed, Gala No. 25/26, Ramchandra Bhatt Marg, Next JJ Hospital Gate No. 2, Opp. Union Bank of India, Noorbaug, Mumbai 400009, Maharashtra, India
  Ph: +91-22-66661880/89 e-mail: mumbai@cbspd.com

Representatives

- **Gujarat** • **Hyderabad** • **Jharkhand** • **Nagpur** • **Patna** • **Pune** • **Uttarakhand**

For trade terms please contact customercare@cbspd.com

For general enquiries please contact info@cbspd.com

Printed in Thomson Press India Ltd., Faridabad, Haryana, India

to
my beloved teachers

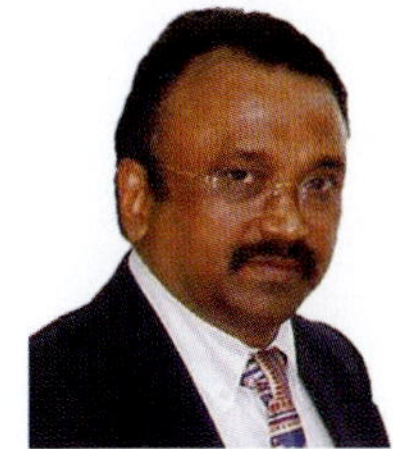

Prof TS Swaminathan
Former Director
Barnard Institute of Radiology
Madras Medical College, Chennai

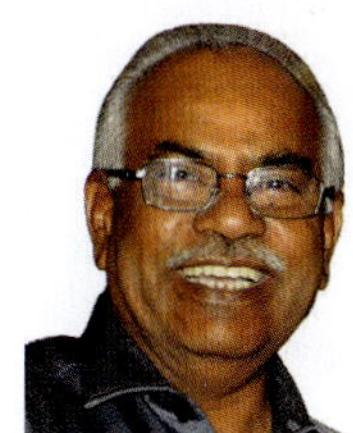

Prof N Kulasekaran
Former Director
Barnard Institute of Radiology
Madras Medical College, Chennai

Contributors

Abubacker Sulaiman
Professor and Head
Department of Radiology
Bhaarath Medical College
Selaiyur, Chennai

Amandeep Singh
Professor, Department of Radiodiagnosis
SGRD Institute of Medical Sciences and Research
Amritsar, Punjab

Anand N
Fortis Hospital
Chennai

Anbarasu A
Aran Diagnostic Imaging
Coimbatore

Ankur Shah
Gujarat Imaging Centre
Ahmedabad

Bagyam Raghavan
Apollo Hospitals
Chennai

Bindu Srinivasan
Research Volunteering
Department of Material Science and Engineering
University of North Texas, Texas

C Amarnath
Professor and Head, Department of Radiodiagnosis
Stanley Medical College
Chennai

Chirtrarasan P
Professor, Department of Radiodiagnosis
Stanley Medical College
Chennai

Devimeenal J
Professor, Department of Radiodiagnosis
Govt Kilpauk Medical College
Chennai

Emaneul R
Senior Consultant Radiologist, Bharat Scans
Chennai

Flora Nelson
Professor, Department of Radiodiagnosis
Govt Thoothukudi Medical College
Chennai

Gaurang Raval
Consultant Radiologist
NM Virani Wockhardt Hospital
Rajkot

Gaurav Shivgiri Goswami
Zydus Hospital
Ahmedabad

I Gurubarath
Professor, Department of Radiodiagnosis
Chettinad Medical College
Chennai

J Chezhian
Associate Professor, Department of Radiodiagnosis
Stanley Medical College
Chennai

Jayaraj Govindaraj
Apollo Hospitals
Chennai

K Gopinathan
Professor, Department of Radiodiagnosis
Govt Kilpauk Medical College
Chennai

K Sudha
Consultant Radiologist
Roentgen Scans World
Chennai

L Kayal
Professor, Department of Dental Surgery
Stanley Medical College
Chennai

M Indrani
Senior Consultant in Nuclear Medicine
Apollo Hospitals
Chennai

Muralikrishna L
Fortis Hospital
Chennai

N Chidambaranathan
Apollo Hospital
Chennai

Parveen Sulthana
Associate Consultant
Perth Radiological Clinic
Western Australia

Periyakaruppan AL
Govt Multi-Specialty Hospital
Omandurar Estate
Chennai

Philson J Mukkada
Associate Professor, Department of Radiology, ACS Medical College
Consultant Radiologist, Roentgen Scans World
Chennai

Rajendra N Solanki
Suyog imaging Center
Mehsana-Radiscan Diagnostics
Ahmedabad

Ravindran
Assistant Professor, Department of Radiodiagnosis
Institute of Child Health, Egmore
Chennai

S Babupeter
Professor, Department of Radiodiagnosis
Madras Medical College

Shelley Simon
Senior Consultant in Nuclear Medicine
Apollo Hospitals
Chennai

S Rajasekaran
Senior Consultant Radiologist
Chennai

V Sivakumar
Consultant Radiologist
Scansworld, Chamiers Road,
Chennai

Yuvabalakumaran
Professor, Department of Radiodiagnosis
Vinayaka Mission's Kirupananda Variyar Medical College and Hospital, Salem

Foreword

I am pleased to write the Foreword to *Radiology Exam Made Easy*, a book that I believe will significantly contribute to the world of radiology. This project has been initiated and compiled by Dr C Amarnath, who has laboriously poured his heart, soul, and knowledge into this textbook with the sole purpose of imparting radiology knowledge to the upcoming generation.

Prof C Amarnath is well known in the radiology fraternity for his flair for teaching and a thoughtful approach to case reading sessions, and is dedicated to making them immensely exciting. He is not only a good teacher but also an able administrator. He was instrumental in leading the Department of Radiodiagnosis in Govt Stanley Medical College to great heights.

This book can be used religiously by residents as they enter the beautiful world of radiology to help them master the art and science of a perfect radiology reporting. The book is designed to make adding annotations, which could facilitate ready reckoning of cases and concepts. The book begins with the basic and most important overview of the radiology examination, and ultraprecise structured guidelines for radiology case presentation. This is followed by basic reporting templates, and a section on illustrated radiological anatomy including X-ray, CT scan, MRI and ultrasound of all the systems. It then moves on to to a comprehensive coverage of more than 220 exam cases with an all-inclusive list of possible differential diagnoses. I am sure this book would serve as a strong stimulus and a useful guide to master the art of radiology case presentation.

My favourite section of the book is the OSCE/CORE exercises, explained with high quality images and original illustrations. Cases discussed in Question and Answer format throughout this book will provide an excellent arena for readers to test out their unique ideas and differentials. High yield *viva voce* materials covering radiological procedures, contrast agents, equipments, physics principles, etc., are described in such detail that these will surely widen the horizons of diagnostic capabilities of the readers. The indispensable and ever important field of emergency radiology is covered with a proactive approach. Keeping up with the role of international certifying exams in enhancing a radiologist's skillset today, an overview of FICR, MICR, EDiR has been presented along with sample papers to complete a perfect book.

I anticipate that this book will be used as a self-testing aid during examinations, and also as a revision tool. It contains a huge arsenal of cases, with an extensive reference collection of full interpreted images, addressed to students as well as consultants. It sets out to be an effective *learning catalyst* as it contains high yield cases and questions that a postgraduate could expect in an examination. With bulk of diagnoses today being made in radiology department, this book will definitely help you narrow down the differentials. We also hope this book would serve as an integral assistant in your daily practice.

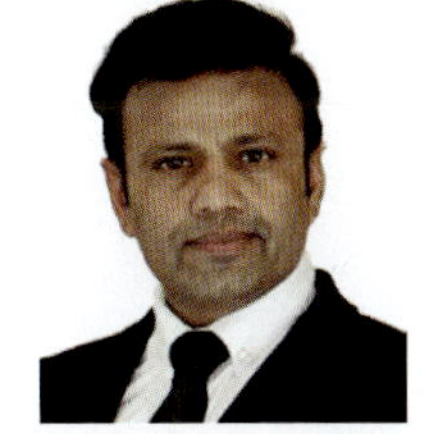

Dr Hemant Patel
Past President, Indian Radiological and Imaging Association
Director, Gujarat Imaging Centre, Ahmedabad

Foreword

Preface

Radiology Exam Made Easy—an exam preparatory manual focuses on crystal clear explanations about the various differential diagnoses from all systems with simple charts, tables, and classical cases to tide over the challenging phase of final year exams.

The content is derived from standard articles, textbooks, and the Stanley Radiology Museum's famed archives with inputs from experienced professors and consultants of radiology—all pieced together in a comprehensive, easy to read format. This book will supplement the information already learned, and enable that information to be used logically while approaching a case in clinical exams. I hope this book provides the sort of information that clinical radiologists will also find useful in their day-to-day practice.

The radiology curriculum consists of: 1. Basic radiology—the radiological anatomy, relevant clinical examination, physics relevant to radiology, and radiological techniques including protocols, 2. Essential radiology—accident and emergency imaging and 3. Core radiology—integrity of various systems in the body. The biggest strength of this project is the massive collection of cases curated diligently for the past 20 years. It is seen that a resident or young consultant radiologist refers to radiological anatomy 2–3 times in a day on an average. In this regard, this book will be really helpful as a one stop reference point.

Fear is nothing more than an obstacle that stands in the way of progress. With the view of vanquishing the fears of residents, this book will provide an easy and holistic approach to theory and practical board exams. Radiological anatomy is where our knowledge of human anatomy meets clinical practice. The third chapter of the book discusses and illustrates radiological anatomy as seen across all imaging modalities.

Case discussion section provides specific and realistic solutions that are needed to improve our practical skills in diagnostic radiology. It features over 220+ cases across all modalities from X-ray to PET CT/SPECT CT. In addition, self-test questions and guidelines on case presentation are included to assess and to boost confidence.

The rapidly growing field of interventional radiology may be intimidating for residents. To tackle this, the section on radiological procedures is specially drafted and is bound to spark an interest in interventional procedures.

Emergency radiology forms an integral part of any hospital's emergency team. To empower the radiologist to make rapid fire diagnoses, thus making huge impact on outcomes in emergency care. A section on international certifying exams provides an overview of design of EDiR, MICR and FRCR exams along with sample questions.

The key motive behind the creation of this book is to *replace the fear of unknown with curiosity*.

We hope this book will serve as a quick primary reference for residents to prepare for their examination and particularly useful in our clinical practice. We are always happy to hear your comments and suggestions.

The only thing to do with good knowledge is to pass it on; It's never of use to oneself.

C Amarnath

Acknowledgements

I extend my thanks to all the people who have worked so diligently and faithfully in shaping up this book. I would like to recognize all the professors and residents who have spent so much of their precious time in contributing their chapters to this book.

My sincere gratitude and respect go to my beloved teachers Prof TS Swaminathan, Prof N Kulasekaran, Prof JR Daniel, Prof K Manoharan, Prof S Vinayagam and Dr R Emmanuel. I would also like to thank my friends Dr AL Periyakaruppan, Dr K Gopinathan, Dr Philson J Mukkada and Dr V Sivakumar.

My colleagues in Stanley Medical College and Scans World have extended their valuable input and support throughout the period it took to bring out this book. I especially thank my colleagues Prof C Nellaiappan, Prof G Sathyan, Prof P Chirtrarasan, Prof J Chezhian, Prof V Sudhakar and Assistant Professors Dr K Sivakumar, Dr G Sakthivel Raja, Dr M Priya, Dr R Jayavarma and Dr S Usha.

I also thank my residents Dr K Arun Alex, Dr G Karthick Kiran, Dr R Karthick Rajan, Dr R Kiruthika, Dr A Ponshankar, Dr M Resnick Banu, Dr X Sebastian Antony, Dr G Anushya, Dr JS Krishnan, Dr Pragadesh Pandian, Dr Manasa, Dr Joel Kevin Raj, Dr Kharat Pandit Jeeja, Dr V Shilpa, Dr Sowmiya PK, Dr G Suresh, Dr T Pradeeba, Dr Thivakaran, Dr A Abdul Salam, Dr D Benin Reejan, Dr M Bharathiraja, Dr P Dineshbabu, Dr AS Kannan, Dr P Lavanya, Dr R Mythili, Dr V Prithviraj, Dr R Rajashree, Dr A Renita, Dr K Sadhana, Dr J Samkamel Sen, Dr TJ Vanathi, Dr P Lenin Prabhu, Dr Hariharan, Dr M Shyamala, Dr V Ramalakshmi, Dr V Dhanalakshmi, Dr R Kadalarasi, Dr R Raghavi, Dr S Sanjeev Prasad, Dr R Manikandan, Dr I Kittu, Dr M Rajkumar, Dr A Sahila Devi, Dr A Ameer Hussain, Dr CS Nischith, Dr K Roopini, Dr Hariharan S, Dr Hariharan M, Dr Vidhyalakshmi, GK, Dr Naveen S, Dr Logamani PK, Dr Magesh P, Dr Tamilselvi S, and Dr Kanchana J who helped me in compiling the cases and publishing my book. Not enough words would capture the part my son A. Anirudh has in being the driving force behind my achievements.

I will be failing in my duty if I do not place on record my sincerest thanks to all of my patients. Finally, I thank Dr M Nanda Kumar, Dr RS Satiish, and Dr RV Guhan for compiling and bringing the entire book together.

C Amarnath

Contents

Approach to Clinical Radiology Board Exams

INTRODUCTION

'Rome was not built in a day'

We always look for shortcuts for success, but real success can be achieved only by hard work and true dedication to our work. At the same time, we should study smart and invest the available time wisely such that we could cover the vast syllabus. Understanding concept is worth the time instead of just cramming facts. Revision plays a key role so that all our valuable efforts may not be wasted. Presentation plays an important role as preparation so that we could effectively communicate our knowledge to the examiner.

1. Study Smart and Hard

A "strategy" for taking the exam was to simply revise everything before the big day. We spent hours upon hours highlighting everything in exam prep book. In retrospect, we could have saved tons of time by simply identifying the key subjects we did not really understand. The best advice usually comes from your seniors (every one of them—don't be happy with just asking one person) who recently took the exam.

Preparation involves

- Knowledge of the subject.
- Technique or approach.
- Knowledge of the exam itself.

Knowledge of the subject: This comes from your hard work of reading books, seeing more cases, attending various courses. Knowledge to pass is one aspect and knowledge to go out and practice is another aspect—both need to be acquired.

Technique or approach: This consists of various skills you need to tackle each component of the exams.

a. **Spotters:** The success in this component is entirely based on your knowledge, seeing more and more 'Aunt Minnie' type of cases.
b. **Cases writing:** Follow the standard case presentation proforma. Time is very important. Do not get bogged down by a difficult case, resulting in below par performance in an easy case due to lack of time. Unknown diagnoses can be handled by giving appropriate differential diagnosis.
c. **Viva:** FRCR Viva is a case presentation, using standard case presentation proforma. For MD/DNB exam viva, we have equipment/instruments.
d. **OSCE:** Some universities are introducing objective structured clinical examination (OSCE) components or in the process—don't be alarmed and in fact, these are easier components and more objective assessment is done and the examiners are silent observers.

Knowledge of the exam itself: Every university/national board exams are slightly different and you need to understand that; again the exams can vary slightly depending on the examiners as well. It is important that you need to look for information about the exams and be updated with the latest information from the university.

Studying for the exam is undoubtedly a daunting task. Not only can the sheer amount of material that one needs to learn seem overwhelming, but also the vast amount of resources available can be more of a burden than an asset. Residents often scramble to make time to go over every single review book out there, in an effort to have all of their bases covered. This strategy is not only nearly impossible but is likely to be counterproductive. Rather, one should focus on one comprehensive textbook while supplementing with question banks.

It seems daunting with all the resources out there. Don't be afraid to use many, but use them wisely. Ideally you should have read the standard textbooks once or twice during the first two and half years itself. Below is a rough plan:

4 months before the exam (first revision of the following books you have read before)

- Review standard textbooks of radiology
- Go through question banks.

- Make notes on what to write for each question, for a quick last minute revision
- Make small study groups among yourself and start doing case discussion/case presentation.

2 months before the Exam

- Continue above
- Review standard textbooks of radiology physics
- Case atlas for spotters
- Exercise spotter bank—you can practise spotter sets in exam pattern on daily basis/2–3 spotter sets per day.
- Case presentation practice in any radiology museum—you may present each case for 15 minutes without any break, others will help to improve the presentation, likewise practise 10 cases per day.
- Stanley Radiology Museum—permits all eager radiology postgraduates to utilise the radiology museum throughout the year for learning purpose.

< 1 month before the exam

- Final revision of standard textbooks
- Review facts/notes.
- Review questions.
- Practise drawing simple self-explanatory diagrams.

2. Stop Freaking Out!

Seriously, even though this seems like the biggest single moment of your life, it really isn't. This is just a test. Stress decreases your memory. To reduce stress, we recommended that students should just put things into perspective. Like I mentioned earlier, this is just a test! Even if you do not pass the first round, you still have family who loves you, friends that support you, and hopefully a roof over your head. Since passing a test will not affect any of these things, you need not make it gigantic impending thing. Take a few deep breaths in and out and begin to look at the exam as simply the culmination of your radiology education. Look, you have made it far so obviously you are capable of passing a test.

3. You Are What You Eat

Avoid foods with high amounts of sugar (including sugar soft drinks), fried foods, sugar substitutes and heavily processed foods (like white bread, pasta, and pizza). The effect these foods have on your brain is they can cause a condition commonly known as brain fog. Brain fog is best described as those times where everything in your head just seems muddy like you are trying to remember a word and no matter how hard you try you just cannot think of it. Avoid excess caffeine intake. Take fresh fruits and vegetables. For best results, don't just clean up your diet the night before the big test but instead try a month or at least the week before.

4. Sleep

This is a huge one as well. What you might not realize is that if you are getting less than 7–8 hours of sleep a night, then your brain is probably not functioning optimally. We recommend trying to stick to a consistent bedtime schedule. Good sleep will improve you memory and concentrating capability. On the day before the exam, you must sleep for 7–8 hours, only then you can concentrate, recollect and perform well in exam. After a night of good sleep, go to the examination hall with a clear and fresh mind without any anxiety or over expectation.

5. Believe in Yourself

In this final step, we simply want you to stop for a second and take a moment to do a heart check. As I mentioned, you have made it this far. You put up with all the mean, unhelpful scenario of a medical curriculum, you passed all the required tests at your school, and you most of all put your life on hold for your radiology education. You can do this! Ok, so maybe you are not the best test taker in the world, or maybe you have zero confidence. We simply want you to take a few moments to reflect on all that you have achieved so far and begin to believe that you can do it!

1.1 APPROACH TO PRACTICAL EXAM WITHOUT TEARS

The practical examination system is different for MD, DNB, FRCR, EDiR and MICR candidates who often have to attend it in a different institution. Staying confident and not getting stressed is important for success. Feel confident about the portion of the syllabus you have covered instead of worrying about the things you didn't cover.

Before the Examination

Prepare answers to potential viva voce questions in advance and practice interactive sessions with seniors who have previously succeeded in the examination. It is imperative to study the viva voce books and actively participate in online radiology forums offering an extensive repository of radiology cases. The residents may participate in small study groups. It is advisable to present a case to senior faculty members, especially those who have been previous examiners; this will improve your presentation skills and confidence. It will reduce your exam phobia. Utilise the local/neighbouring institutions, and their radiology museums.

In the Examination Hall

The candidate is expected to be well groomed and formally dressed to create a good first impression on the examiner and the candidate should reach the examination hall one hour before the exam which will calm the unnecessary nervousness. Avoid nervousness while presenting cases, to convey the content effectively to the examiner.

If a film is given for discussion, begin by describing the film without delay. Start with the modality, anatomical region, radiographic view, etc., and avoid staring at the film in silence. While describing a case, the candidate should, preferably, face the film instead of looking at the examiner. Only after completion of the case description and concluding the case, candidate should turn to face the examiners for further remarks and questions.

Always maintain eye to eye contact with examiner while answering questions. First start describing baseline modality, then proceed to higher modalities, so don't jump into higher diagnostic modalities, without describing the findings in the baseline modality. Choose the modality based on relevant clinical history provided.

During the discussion, listen keenly and understand the examiner's line of questioning. During the course of the examination, the examiner may drop hints if the candidate seems to be going down a wrong path. It is vital to catch such 'lifelines' and change one's line of thought, and answer accordingly.

Do not criticize the quality of film given. Avoid touching the film or using the tip of a pen as a pointer while describing findings of a case. When necessary, use a pointer (like a plastic ruler) rather than the finger. Never contradict/argue with the examiner.

Use correct terminology and definitions during case presentation and while answering specific questions. If the examiner says "plain radiograph", the candidate may use the same terminology. Use of the phrase "I don't remember" is preferable to "I do not know" when the candidate does not know the answer to a certain question. If the question was not clearly heard, politely request the examiner to repeat the question. Listen carefully; answer appropriately to the questions asked especially when the examiners are giving clues.

When the diagnosis is not known/when stuck in a case: In situations when one fails to arrive at a diagnosis it may be useful to start thinking aloud, saying that one is looking at certain parts, e.g. I am now looking at the lung, I am now looking at the cardiac shadow, etc. Try to pick up the findings while talking, instead of waiting to get the diagnosis. Even if you cannot come up with an aetiological diagnosis, it is possible that, while discussing with the examiner and listening intently to the guiding question, one will strike upon the diagnosis.

Checklist before attending practical exams:

- White over coat.
- Radiology exam kit.
- Hall ticket.
- Number badge and TLD badge.
- Dissertation/Logbook

Come relax and attend the exam.

1.2 TIPS FOR WRITING THEORY EXAM

Theory exams form an important part of the assessment of a candidate's knowledge (as well as imagination!). Expect the best, plan for the worst and prepare to be surprised... and to be prepared is half the victory. The other half depends on your presentation style and the evaluator.

Time Management

Totally we have 180 minutes, the first 5 minutes to be allotted to writing the registration number, page number and drawing margins in the answer sheet, then use the next five minutes for reading the questions and make sure to keep the last 15 minutes for verification of the answer sheet.

In MD exam pattern, there will be 25 min for each essay and 10 min for each short note, whereas for DNB (Diplomate in National Board) examinations there will be 15 mins for each short structured question. For each mark spend 1½ minutes writing, plan accordingly.

Question Type

Varies on a course and university basis. In most of the university examinations (MD) they have 2 long questions and 10 short notes, while in DNB examinations they have 10 short structured questions, each carrying 10 marks (Table 1.1). It is vital not to spend more time on the initial questions; otherwise you will run short of time for attempting rest of the questions.

Different universities have different marking schemes. Some universities allot 20 marks for each long note and 6 marks for each short note so that you have to spend 35 minutes for each long note and 8 minutes for each short note.

Table 1.1: Pattern of various examinations and sample for planning the exams

Exam type		*Pattern*	*Marks*	*No. of questions*	*Pages*	*Duration (marks × 1.6)*
DNB		Long notes	10	10	6–7	15 minutes each
MD		Long notes	15	2	10–12	25 minutes each
		Short notes	7	10	3–4	10 minutes each
FRCR 1	Anatomy module	MCQs	200	100	–	90 minutes
	Physics module	MCQs	200	40 × 5 (true or false)	–	2 hours
FRCR 2A		Single best answer questions (2 sets)	–	120	–	3 hours (for each paper)
FRCR 2B		Rapid reporting	–	30	–	35 minutes
		Long cases	–	6 cases	–	60 minutes
		Viva (2 sessions)	16 marks for each session	–	–	30 minutes (each session)

Answer Contents

For long answers, it is necessary to write 10 to 12 pages each with **diagrams/tables/boxes/classification** minimum of 2 to 3 per essay. For short notes—3 to 4 pages each, diagrams/tables minimum 1 per short note. Pay attention to writing the page number in the top and write 15–18 lines per page. Use spacing between words and underline important key points/sentences. Using **bullets, flow diagrams, diagrams, boxes/squares for highlighting the key points** is more vital if handwriting is not good (or) if you run out of time.

Use colour pens and sketches for diagrams, headings and **underlining important key points** and subtitles. **Answer all the questions and in the order** given in question paper. Write in medium size letters. There must be logical organization of the contents or the key points with one or two points in one paragraph. Writing more will not fetch more marks. The examiner looks for key points. If they are covered, you will get marks irrespective of the number of pages written. Writing controversial points is better avoided.

Good presentation in the examination is a skill and this differentiates a topper from a mediocre student (Table 1.2).

Some model theory exam answer papers given as follows for use of colour pencils/charts/diagrams (Fig. 1.1A to D).

Table 1.2: Sample answer outline for theory questions

1. Definition
2. Demography
3. Incidence
4. Causes/anatomy/types /embryology
5. Clinical features
6. Location
7. Pathophysiology
8. Stages/manifestations
9. Radiology: Plain X-ray, barium, USG, CT, MRI, DSA, intervention, PET/SPECT
10. Diagnostic test
11. Associated conditions/manifestations in other systems
12. Differential diagnosis
13. Complications
14. Prognosis
15. Management—further investigations and treatment.

Scurvy Radiological Findings

- Generalized osteopenia
- **Cortical thinning:** "Pencil-point" cortex.
- Periosteal reaction due to subperiosteal hemorrhage
- **Scorbutic rosary:** Expansion of the costochondral junctions, may relate to the fracturing of the zone of provisional calcification during normal respiration. Similar to the rachitic rosary appearance seen in rickets.
- Haemarthrosis
- **Wimberger's ring sign:** Circular, opaque radiologic shadow surrounding epiphyseal centers of ossification, which may result from bleeding.
- **Frankel's line:** Dense zone of provisional calcification
- **Trümmerfeld zone:** Lucent metaphyseal band underlying Frankel's line.

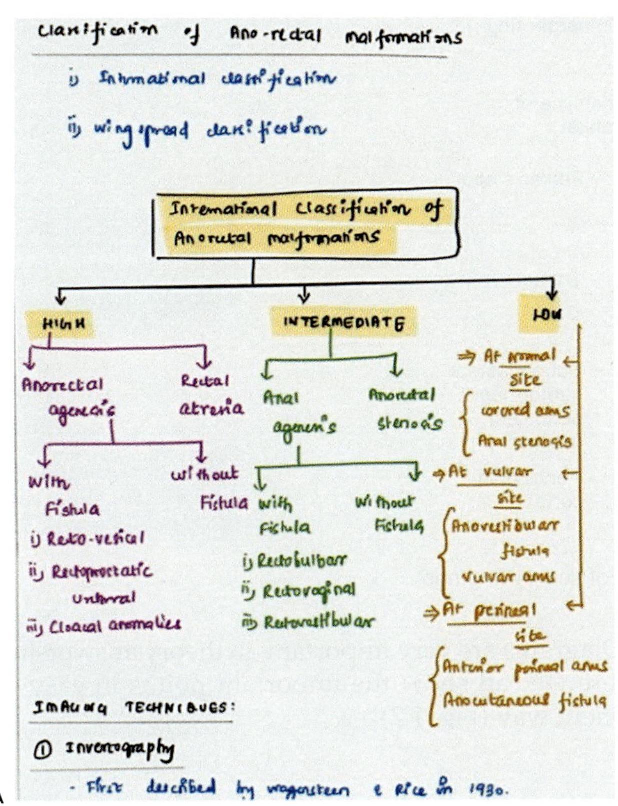

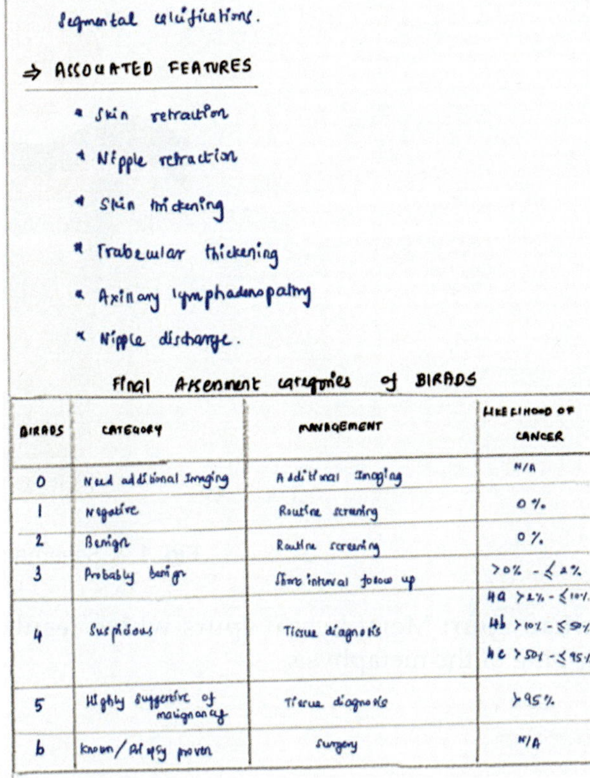
segmental calcifications.

⇒ ASSOCIATED FEATURES

* Skin retraction
* Nipple retraction
* Skin thickening
* Trabecular thickening
* Axillary lymphadenopathy
* Nipple discharge.

Final Assessment categories of BIRADS

BIRADS	CATEGORY	MANAGEMENT	LIKELIHOOD OF CANCER
0	Need additional Imaging	Additional Imaging	N/A
1	Negative	Routine screening	0 %
2	Benign	Routine screening	0 %
3	Probably benign	Short interval follow up	> 0% - ≤ 2%
4	Suspicious	Tissue diagnosis	4a > 2% - ≤ 10% 4b > 10% - ≤ 50% 4c > 50% - ≤ 95%
5	Highly suggestive of malignancy	Tissue diagnosis	> 95%
6	Known / Biopsy proven	Surgery	N/A

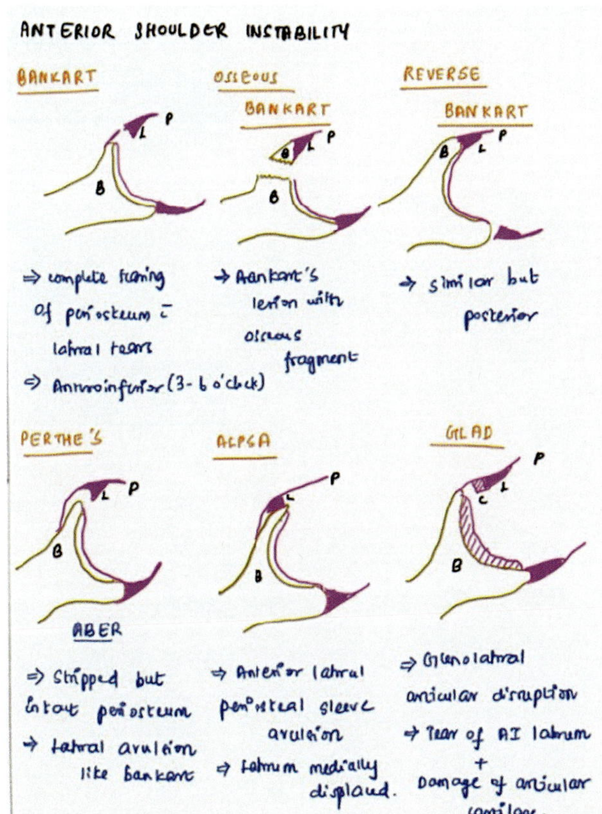

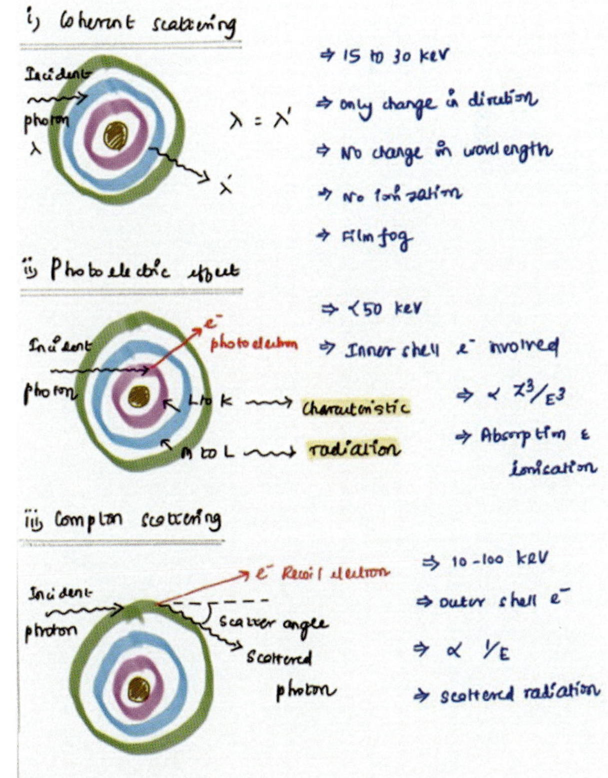

Fig. 1.1A to D: Sample answer sheets

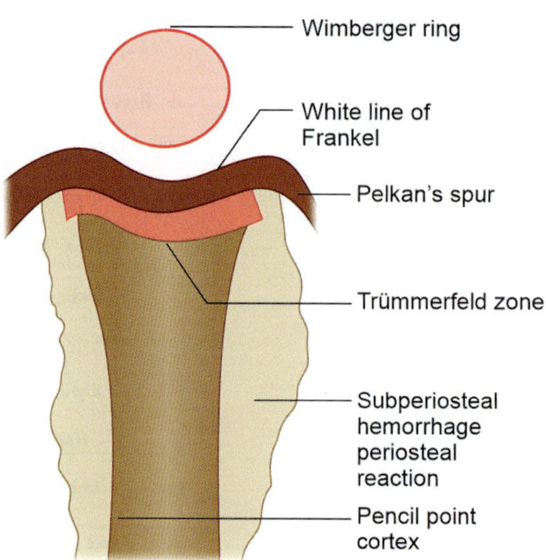

Fig. 1.2: Schematic diagram of scurvy findings

- **Pelkan spur:** Metaphyseal spurs which result in cupping of the metaphysis.

Diagrams are very important, in theory answersheets where we can show the important points in easy and efficient way (Fig. 1.2).

2 Radiology Case Presentation—General Guidelines

Radiology case presentation guidelines followed by the Stanley Medical College is similar to case presentations in various exams and FRCR Viva. It includes short cases and long cases. These guidelines will aid in the structuring of the radiological report and also its evaluation by the examiners. The report should be succinct and relevant. The examination includes X-ray, CT, ultrasound, radionuclide and MR scans. Candidates will be provided with a double viewing box/monitor, a magnifying glass and a ruler. A brief case history and other relevant clinical data will be provided. Each case may comprise up to four modalities in films or dicom images depending on spotter, short or long case. These vary in complexity and difficulty; some require more time for analysis and reporting than others. It should be ensured that sufficient time is allocated to report each case adequately.

Candidates are expected to start reading the films with a little delay as soon as the films are mounted on the viewing box. There is no need to list dates of investigations or to list all sequences unless these factors are of direct relevance. Similarly, there is no need to repeat the clinical information that has been given, but should use the clinical information in interpreting the observations.

A better performance will be expected in the interpretation of common and routine investigations rather than highly specialised investigations. Examiners mostly will show examples from the major clinical radiology sub-specialties. Candidate's power of observation and deduction will be assessed. A logical and informed approach to film interpretation, as well as a clear ability to debate the merits, relevance and role of further investigative modalities, will be expected. Examiners may ask supplementary questions to assess the understanding of the given clinical problem.

In reaching a conclusion, diagnoses should be given in the order of probability. Long lists regurgitated indiscriminately make it difficult for the faculty to assess the true acumen of candidate. In some cases, the correct diagnosis can be directly arrived at. In others, further views or investigations will be helpful and it is important that the candidate clearly substantiates the reasons for wanting the additional data.

During presentation, the faculty will attempt to assist the candidate to perform to the best of his/her ability. Do not stop the discussion unless the examiner interrupts in between. The candidate has to discuss all the positive findings and points relevant to his/her diagnosis. The candidate should not stop presenting a case unless he does not get the answer for a **"What Next"** question. Listen carefully for any clues provided and must not be afraid to ask for clarification regarding questions asked and doubts regarding the patient's clinical presentation. The examiner will point out any incorrect statements, inappropriate further investigations and management made by the candidate.

The amount of discussion that takes place on each case will vary and is at the discretion of the individual examiner. The actual number of cases shown is immaterial. It is more important that a meaningful interaction is taking place with the faculty. Patient confidentiality must be respected.

It is strongly advised to follow a standard format (Stanley Medical College Radiology resident reporting format), i.e. approach to **diagnosis first, followed by management and discussion** about the condition (Table 2.1).

Table 2.1: Sample presentation template

	Stanley Medical College—radiology resident presentation template–**what next?**
1	**Name:** **Age/Sex:** **Occupation:** **Date and time:** **Interval imaging:** **Referred from:** Emergency/OPD/IPD (if relevant and provided)
2	**Clinical presentation:** **Clinical examination:** **Biochemical results:** (if relevant)
3	**Radiological techniques, part in the study, and observations (positive and negative findings, associated findings, complications related to the condition, other organs)** In this section, the candidate should record his/her observations of all the imaging studies available on the films/monitor, including detailed description on positive findings as well as relevant negative findings and brief note on remaining organ systems. Image description of lesion includes site, size, shape, margins, extent, characterisation, skip lesions, nodal involvement/ metastasis and enhancement pattern as appropriate.
4	**Structured analysis and interpretation through logical approach (A-C-B-D-E-F approach)**—there is interpretation of the observed findings which can provide explanation regarding the etiology and complications. For example, description whether lesion being observed is benign or malignant, infective rather than neoplastic, giving your reasons for the same. There is reanalysis with patient data, clinical findings, previous images and biochemical values to arrive at the final diagnosis. **A-C-B-D-E-F approach:** **A**natomy (epicenter) and age **C**haracteristics (size, shape, margins, extents, diffusivity, necrosis, vascularity) **B**ehavior and extension (skip lesions, adjacent organs, enhancement pattern, regional and distal spread) **D**ifferential work up and diagnosis: Substantiate with positive and negative findings. (Further elaborated in the latter part of the section) The steps A-C-B-D should happen in the Radiologist's thought process (Not a part of Reporting template) **E**valuation further and **F**ollow-up imaging
5	**Principal diagnosis (substantiate with positive and negative findings):** Based on the candidate's interpretation he/she should attempt to come to a single diagnosis especially in cases where the findings are classical (e.g. tuberous sclerosis). **Relevant differential diagnosis—balance of probability:** In classical cases, there is no differential diagnosis. If the case is complex, then he should state which diagnosis he/she feels is most likely and then list other possibilities in order of likelihood, in the differential diagnosis section which should be limited to relevant 2–3 conditions. However, in this book we have also added some rarer differential diagnosis for the purpose of elaborate discussion and to enlighten students.
6	**Management (recommended further investigations—treatment goals)/applied radiology in treatment** A. *Critical cases*–immediately inform the referring/appropriate clinician (e.g. acute infarct, EDH with brain herniation, pulmonary embolism, encephalitis, pneumothorax, cardiac tamponade, pseudoaneurysm, acute abdomen) B. *Noncritical cases:* Relevant further investigations—laboratory, radiological and nuclear medicine, HPE (reasons for wanting additional data) to confirm the diagnosis. C. *For tumours:* Confirmatory HPE examinations followed by local and locoregional staging by MRI/CT scan. PET scan for systemic staging. Treatment depends on the stages/cellular type of disease. Final decision on treatment is based on discussion in multidisciplinary tumour board. Similarly, if the candidate makes a diagnosis of an abscess or tumour, he should indicate if a drainage or biopsy is appropriate.
7	**Brief discussion about the condition in viva:** Here the candidate should discuss about the diagnosis of his case and briefly discuss the etiopathology, clinical presentation, treatment options and some note on differential diagnoses.

SPECIMEN REPORTS

Case 1: A six months old child seen unconscious in the emergency department.

Case history: Age—6 months/female child

Clinical presentation: Unconscious/no history of trauma.

Radiological Techniques and Observations

1. Non-contrast CT scan brain (Fig. 2.1)
2. X-ray chest (Fig. 2.2)/X-ray thigh (Fig. 2.3)/X-ray knee (Fig. 2.4)

Observations (*see* Figs 2.1 to 2.4): A non-contrast head CT shows chronic subdural hematoma in bilateral frontal convexity and new subdural haemorrhage in right frontal convexity and posterior interhemispheric SDH. Minimal midline shift is seen to the left side. No skull fracture is seen on these images. X-ray thigh AP view shows displaced spiral midshaft fracture in right femur. X-ray left knee shows corner fracture in upper end of tibia. Chest X-ray shows fractures of the right first to eighth ribs in posterior aspect with evidence of callus formation indicating healing. There are also fractures of the left fourth to ninth ribs posteriorly but no associated

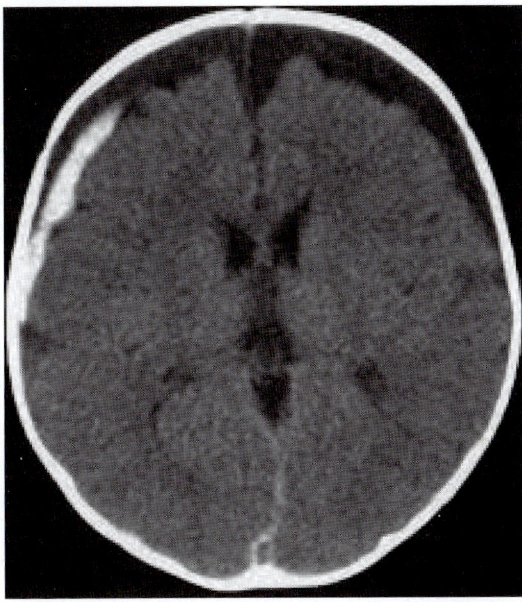

Fig. 2.1

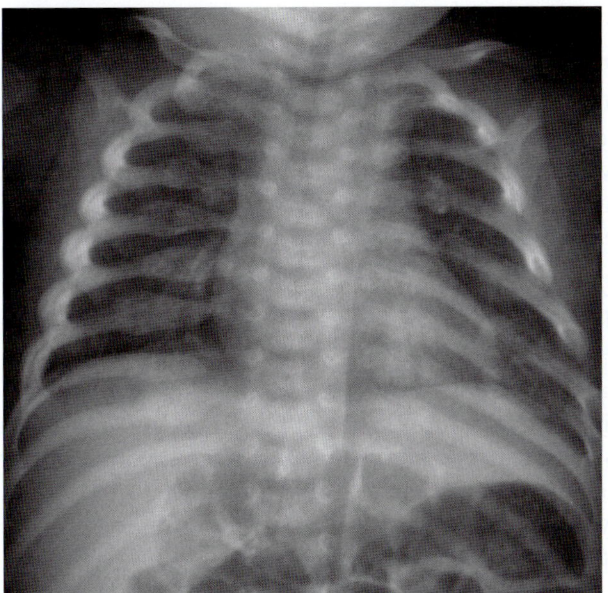

Fig. 2.2

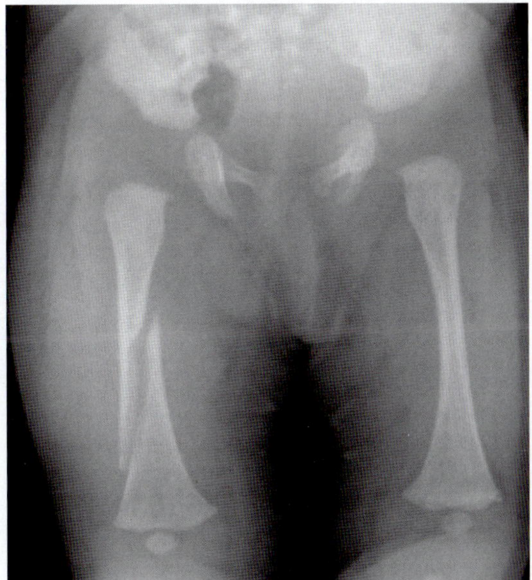

Fig. 2.3

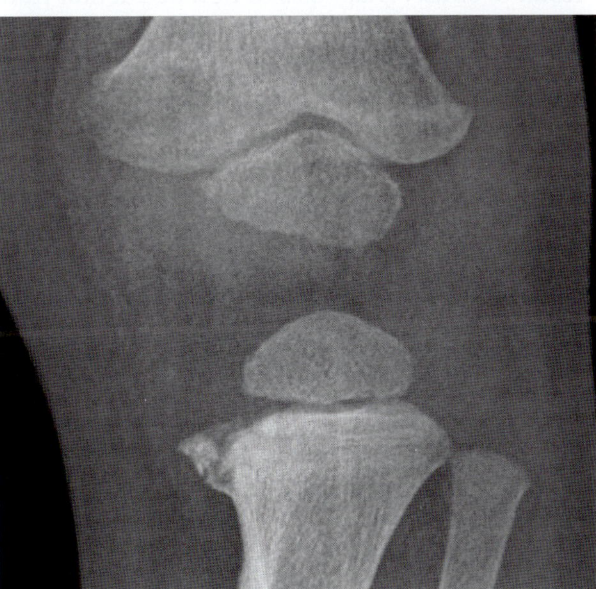

Fig. 2.4

callus or periosteal new bone, suggesting that these fractures have occurred very recently. The lung fields are clear.

Analysis and Interpretation

CT brain: Extra axial fluid collection lies within the sub-dural rather than the sub-arachnoid space. It contains both high and low attenuation material indicating that it is likely to represent an acute or chronic sub-dural haematoma.

Chest X-ray: Shows multiple rib fractures in different stages of healing.

X-ray thigh: Spiral midshaft fracture in right femur

X-ray knee: Corner fracture in upper end of left tibia.

Principal diagnosis: Non-accidental trauma, since the fractures are at different stages of healing and some new fractures also seen and acute on chronic subdural hematoma in brain in absence of skull fracture adds to the diagnosis of non-accidental trauma.

Differential diagnosis: Consider accidental trauma. This appears unlikely in view of the posterior rib fractures of different ages.

Management: The patient needs an urgent neurosurgical opinion and the child protection service must be alerted. A skeletal survey should be performed to look for other fractures and to ensure that there is no evidence of any other skeletal abnormality, such as osteogenesis imperfecta.

Brief discussion about the condition: Non-accidental trauma is a complex injury in infants and young children as a result of abuse. Diagnosis of non-accidental trauma has direct impact on medical, social and legal outcomes of children and families. The classical metaphyseal corner or bucket handle fracture is virtually pathognomonic for abuse. Lateral and posterior rib fractures are highly specific for abuse. Patterns of skull fracture that suggest child abuse are multiple 'eggshell' fractures, occipital impression fractures, fractures crossing sutures. CNS injury especially subdural hematoma is common in child abuse. Visceral injuries include liver, pancreatic laceration and adrenal bleeding are specific for child abuse.

Case 2: A 12 months old child with abdominal distension and seizure.

Case history: 12 months/male child

Clinical presentation: Complaints of abdominal distension for 2 months with 1 episode of seizure.

Radiological investigations and observations: CT brain, MRI brain and CT abdomen.

Observations on CT brain (Fig. 2.5)**:** Hyperdense extra-axial mass lesion noted in right fronto-parietal convexity and left parietal convexity.

Observations on MRI brain (Fig. 2.6): TI post-contrast image shows heterogeneously enhancing extra-axial dural mass noted in bilateral parietal convexity.

Observations on CECT abdomen (Fig. 2.7): Large heterogeneous mass soft-tissue dense mass in left suprarenal fossa extending into midline with coarse stippled calcifications.

Analysis and Interpretation

CT/MRI brain: Diffuse dural mass lesion involving bilateral parietal and right frontal convexity in a 12 months old child.

CT abdomen: Soft-tissue mass in left suprarenal fossa with coarse stippled **calcifications,** this is likely to relate to a malignancy in the adrenal gland.

Principal diagnosis: Neuroblastoma in left adrenal region with cranial metastasis as my principal diagnosis considering the age of the child.

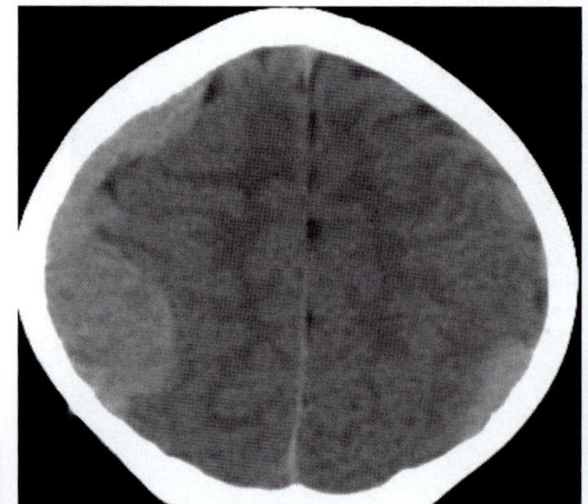

Fig. 2.5

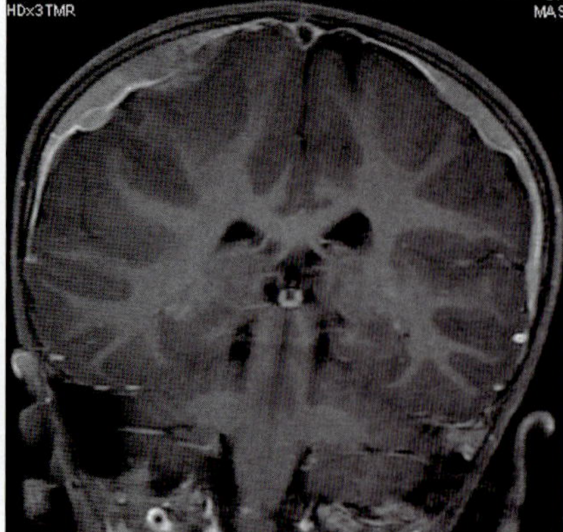

Fig. 2.6

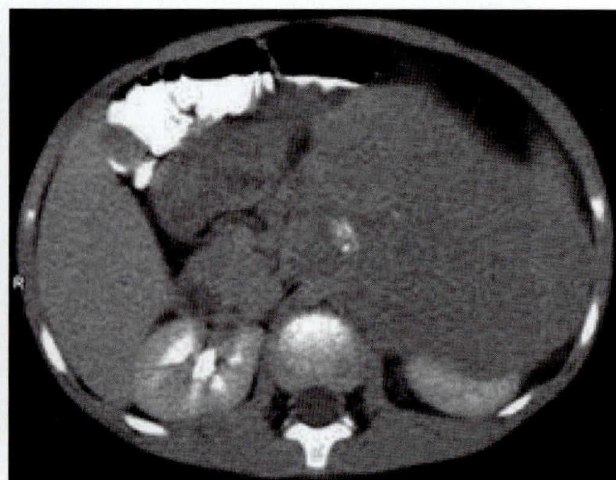

Fig. 2.7

Differential diagnosis: Adrenal carcinoma can rarely occur in this age group and may calcify but is unlikely to extend intraspinally. Wilms' tumor is intrarenal, only occasionally calcifies and rarely metastases to bone so should not give these appearances.

Management: **Further investigations required**—ultrasound, MRI, bone/MIBG scan, PET.

An ultrasound scan would confirm whether the calcified mass lies within the adrenal gland.

Bone scan/I^{131} MIBG scan: Nuclear scintigraphy with areas of increased activity suggests skeletal metastases. An MRI scan and PET scan would be required for staging and monitoring response to treatment. Bone marrow aspiration and catecholamine estimation are usually also performed. A biopsy may also be required.

Brief discussion about the condition: Neuroblastomas are tumors of neuroblastic origin. They represent the most common extracranial solid childhood malignancy. Common metastatic sites are bone, liver, lung, pleura and brain.

SAMPLE REPORTING TEMPLATES

There is no specific standardized reporting template available, here we provided some sample pathological reporting templates used in our department, and reporting templates need constant revision based on recent updates.

Central Nervous System

Arachnoid cyst: Left anterior temporal arachnoid cyst compressing adjacent anterior and medial temporal lobe with adjacent bony scalloping. It measures 40 (TR) × 39 (CC) × 47 (AP) mm. It elevates and displaces left middle cerebral artery medially. There is significant mass effect on the left lateral ventricle with midline shift to right (7 mm)—Galassi type-III.

Medulloblastoma: Evidence of well-defined large heterogeneously enhancing mass lesion measuring about 3.5 × 4.5 × 5.3 cm (AP × TR × CC) arising from the vermis (roof of fourth ventricle) within the 4th ventricle causing moderate obstructive hydrocephalus and transependymal seepage of CSF and cerebellar tonsil herniating 6 mm below the foramen magnum. Fourth ventricle CSF is seen anteriorly as cleft. There is significant compression on the brain stem. No intra-axial edema. The lesion is highly cellular showing T2 hypo/isointense signal with restricted diffusion, areas of necrosis and calcifications. MR spectroscopy shows reduction of NAA, elevation of choline, elevated lipid lactate peak and taurine peak. Entire neuraxis imaging shows no leptomeningeal enhancement or drop metastasis. Mass is extending into the foramen of Luschka on left side and foramen of Magendie (in cases of ependymoma)–medulloblastoma–group 4.

Ectopic posterior pituitary gland: Ectopic posterior pituitary gland along the median eminence of hypothalamus with absent pituitary stalk. Thin anterior pituitary—hypoplastic.

Choroidal fissural cyst: Choroidal fissural cyst measuring about 15 × 7 mm causing mild mass effect over the left hippocampus.

High grade glioma: 2.8 (TRANS) × 5.7 (AP) × 3.6 (CC) cm size hypointense lesion in T1w, hyperintense in T2W sequences seen at the peritrigonal, left parieto-occipital lobe compressing the trigone and posterior horn of left lateral ventricles. There is surrounding perilesional oedema extending to the left optic tract. The lesion extending along the splenium of corpus callosum to the right peritrigonal parietal white matter. It shows peripheral diffusion restriction. There is mild midline shift to the right (5.6 mm). The lesion shows increased vascularity with areas of hemorrhage. MR spectroscopy shows significant elevation of choline, lactate and lipid. On contrast administration the lesion shows heterogeneous enhancement with increased regional CBF and CBV in perfusion imaging. On tractography no significant reduction in the density of the corticospinal tracts and other white matter fibers. Left arcuate fibers are compressed and displaced medially. On finger tapping in the right hand, cortical activation was observed along the superior and lateral aspect of left precentral gyrus. The lesion is well away from the hand motor area.

On word generation (language) fMRI, activation noted in left inferior frontal gyrus and left superior temporal gyrus, left supramarginal gyrus along antero-superolateral aspect of the lesion and parietal opercula anterior to the lesion. Minimal activation also noted in the right supramarginal gyrus and right angular gyrus.

Low grade glioma: Well-defined heterogeneous mass lesion in the left supramarginal gyrus, left angular gyrus and indenting on the posterosuperior aspect of left superior temporal gyrus. The lesion shows areas of hemorrhage. No evidence of mass effect/prominent arterial feeder/contrast enhancement. MR spectroscopy shows mild elevation of choline, lactate and lipid.

DNET: Well-defined T2 hyperintense lobulated expansile, cortical based 42 mm (AP) × 35 mm (transverse) × 38 mm (craniocaudal) size lesion in the left frontal parasagittal region (left paracentral lobule) with facilitated diffusion and partial suppression in FLAIR. No evidence of surrounding perilesional vasogenic oedema/midline shift. On spectroscopy the lesion shows elevated choline, lactate and decreased NAA. No evidence of any other T2/FLAIR grey matter hyperintensity. Above MR features favours dysembryoplastic neuroepithelial tumor (DNET) than low grade glioma.

Functional MRI: Activation of right motor cortex (right precentral gyrus) observed, during finger tapping with left hand. On finger tapping with right hand, cortical activation was observed along the superior and medial aspect of left precentral gyrus and adjacent paracentral lobule and also along the posterior rim of the left paracentral lobule lesion. On bilateral finger tapping, bilateral motor cortex, supplementary motor cortex activation was noted (left > right). No evidence of plasticity.

Tractography: Shows displacement of the corticospinal tract posteriorly. No evidence of infiltration/destruction of corticospinal tract. Corticobulbar fibres are displaced anteriorly and inferiorly. A few posterior fibres were destroyed. Superior longitudinal fasciculus is displaced laterally. Superior fronto-occipital fasciculus appears normal.

Atypical teratoid rhabdoid tumor (ATRT): Evidence of large solid and cystic mass lesion measuring about 7.1 × 6.4 × 7.5 cm (AP × TR × CC) in left side of posterior fossa with significant mass effect over the cerebellum and brainstem. Enhancing solid nodules with hemorrhagic areas seen along the medial aspect of mass. There is compression and narrowing of the 4th ventricle and aqueduct with moderate obstructive triventricular hydrocephalus and periventricular seepage of CSF. Mass is pushing the brainstem and cerebellum to right side. No extension to IAC. Superomedially cystic component is extending up to the pineal region/posterior 3rd ventricular region. Features favour the possibility of atypical teratoid rhabdoid tumor (ATRT) in left side posterior fossa with significant mass effect.

Brainstem glioma: 29 × 28 × 27 mm (AP × TR × CC) size expansile exophytic lesion in the left side of pontomedullary junction and left middle cerebellar peduncle with areas of hemorrhage in the inferior aspect. There is expansion of left middle cerebellar peduncle with compression on the left side of fourth ventricle. There is significant surrounding edema in the medulla, left cerebellum, bilateral thalamus and posterior capsular regions. MR spectroscopy shows marked elevation of choline, marked reduction of NAA peak and presence of lactate. Features favour brainstem glioma. DTI shows displacement of pontocerebellar fibers laterally and corticospinal tract fibres medially. Mass effect noted in the left corticospinal tract without significant white matter loss. Leptomeningeal enhancement seen in/around the spinal cord in the cervicodorsolumbar region—**suggestive of drop metastasis.**

Pineoblastoma: 22 mm (AP) × 19 mm (TR) × 23 mm (CC) size well-defined heterogeneously enhancing lobulated mass lesion with peripherally dispersed calcification in the pineal region extending to the upper part of the aqueduct with areas of haemorrhage causing dilatation of third and lateral ventricles. Tectal plate and suprasellar region appear intact. No evidence of leptomeningeal metastasis. On spectroscopy the lesion shows mildly elevated choline and decrease NAA. The lesion shows diffusion restriction—above features favours pineoblastoma than germinoma.

Choroid plexus papilloma: Large T2 heterogeneous mass with frond-like pattern in the trigone of left lateral ventricle. It measures 6.8 × 4.8 × 6.7 cm. No demonstrable calcification or hemorrhage is seen at present. Both lateral, third and fourth ventricle are dilated. No evidence of acute infarct. Mild midline shift to the right measuring 4 mm. There is moderate dilation of right lateral ventricle and gross dilatation of left lateral ventricle. The lesion shows homogeneous enhancement with cauliflower-like appearance. No obvious evidence of intraparenchymal extension/parenchymal edema. There is prominent arterial supply from the lateral posterior choroidal artery, anterior choroidal artery and the prominent choroidal vein drains into the thalamostriate vein. No obvious evidence of leptomeningeal/drop metastasis. MR spectroscopy shows elevated choline significantly decreased NAA and creatine.

Hypothalamic hamartoma: Well-defined non-enhancing T1 hypointense long TR mild hyperintense lesion in the tuber cinereum/hypothalamus region causing partial narrowing of the third ventricle and abutting the optic tract. MR spectroscopy of the lesion shows mildly decreased NAA peak.

Diffuse cerebral atrophy (children)—Grey matter neurodegeneration: GM gangliosidosis and neuronal ceroid lipofuscinosis. Suggested clinical/biochemical correlation. Other possibilities include: Glycogen storage disorder. Mucolipidosis, multiple sulfatase deficiency, post-encephalitis sequelae.

Cerebellar atrophy (children): Moderate to severe cerebellar atrophy with ex-vacuo dilatation of 4th ventricle. FLAIR hyperintense cerebellar cortex (INAD, Marinesco-Sjögren, late onset GM2 gangliosidosis, late infantile NCL).

Moderate to severe **cerebral and cerebellar atrophy** with increased T2W signal intensity in the white matter and excess iron deposition in the basal ganglia. Possibilities include: Neuro degeneration with brain iron accumulation–pantothenate kinase associated neurodegeneration (Hallervorden-Spatz disease), oculodigital dental dysplasia, Kufor-Rakeb syndrome (pallido-pyramidal degeneration), neuronal ceroid lipofuscinosis, glycogen storage disease.

Severe cerebellar atrophy (children): Severe cerebellar atrophy with T2W/FLAIR increased cerebellar cortex signal intensity. Evidence of flat pons. Clava hypertrophy noted. No evidence of basal ganglia atrophy/basal ganglia T2 hyperintensity/supratentorial hypomyelination. Mild increased iron deposition in globus pallidus. MR spectroscopy of the brain parenchyma shows normal spectral pattern. No significant reduction of NAA/elevation of choline. No abnormal metabolites seen. Possibilities include: Infantile neuraxonal dystrophy, congenital disorder of glycosylation (Pmm2-CDG)—no evidence of flat pons seen, Marinesco-Sjögren SIL1, ceroid lipofuscinosis (late), juvenile GM2 (late).

Arteriovenous malformation (AVM): Abnormal cluster of vessels (arteriovenous malformation nidus) measuring about 27 × 19 mm in the inferolateral aspect of the left inferior parietal gyrus in the angular gyrus and adjacent parieto-occipital region. No acute hemorrhage/surrounding edema. No obvious evidence of infarct/atrophy. Lesion is fed by cortical branches of left MCA and left PCA. Venous drainage to superior sagittal sinus. No adjacent gliosis. Spetzler-Martin grade-I.

Aneurysm: 7.3 × 6 × 8.5 mm size multilobulated saccular aneurysm seen arising from the M1 bifurcation of right middle cerebral artery/anterior communicating artery. The aneurysm is arising from the posterior aspect and pointing posterosuperiorly. Neck of the aneurysm measures 2.3 mm. No obvious evidence of any other aneurysm, wall irregularity/thrombus/vasospasm/subarachnoid hemorrhage/infarct/bleb/lobulation.

Giant cavernous malformation: 37 (TR) × 22 (AP) × 28 (CC) mm size T2W multilobulated lesion in the right inferior frontal gyrus, frontal central white matter extending near the anterior body of right lateral ventricle with minimal surrounding oedema. It shows hyperintense signal with popcorn appearance. The lesion blooms in SWI sequence in the periphery. Mild midline shift to left (2 mm). No obvious dilated feeding artery/draining vein seen. Multiple cavernomas—**familial multiple cavernous malformation syndrome.**

Developmental venous anomaly: Abnormal dilated venous channels draining into the collector subependymal vein in the right frontal region.

Molar tooth malformation—Joubert syndrome: Abnormal configuration of the midbrain with typical "molar tooth" appearance. Enlarged 4th ventricle with "bat-wing" configuration and enlarged cisterna magna. Absent cerebellar primary fissure and fastigial point. Hypoplasia of the vermis with apposition (not fusion) of cerebellar hemispheres and clefting of the superior cerebellar vermis. High riding 4th ventricle with deep pontomesencephalic junction.

Dorsal tegmental tract hyperintensity: Abnormal T2W/FLAIR hyperintensity in the midbrain and upper pons and dorsal tegmental tract—usually seen in cerebral palsy.

Creatine deficiency syndromes: Minimal hyperintensity noted in the dentate nucleus, medial portion of middle cerebellar peduncle and nucleus accumbens. MR spectroscopy of the brain shows markedly decreased creatine—**creatine deficiency syndromes** can be considered (guanidinoacetate methyltransferase (GAMT) deficiency, deficiency of L-arginine: Glycine amidinotransferase (AGAT), defect in a creatine transporter protein).

Parecho virus encephalitis: Evidence of restricted diffusion in bilateral frontoparietal and temporal subcortical white matter and corpus callosum. Punctate T1W hyperintensities seen in bilateral frontoparietal subcortical white matter. MR spectroscopy of the brain parenchyma shows normal spectral pattern. No abnormal metabolites seen. Features favour the possibility of Parecho virus/dengue/chikungunya encephalitis.

Craniosynostosis: Altered shape of the skull. Premature fusion of bilateral coronal suture leading to craniosynostosis with increased convolutional markings in the frontal bone (anterior plagiocephaly). Increased convolutional markings secondary to craniosynostosis. Sagittal, metopic, lambdoid and squamosal sutures are normal.

Microcephaly: Microcephaly with simplified gyral pattern in frontal and temporal region.

CT Cisternogram: **CSF leak:** 1.6 × 3.2 mm size bony defect in the left cribrifrom plate of ethmoid bone with CSF leak into the left nasal cavity.

Pontine tegmental cap dysplasia: Abnormal brainstem with hypoplastic pons and flattened ventral surface. Shrunken cerebellum and focal bulging of the pontine tegmentum projecting into the fourth ventricle—pontine tegmental cap dysplasia.

Hippocampal malrotation/vertical hippocampus/hippocampal inversion: Vertical orientation and medial positioning of head and body of left hippocampus with round hippocampal head—hippocampal malrotation, above features show association with malformations of cortical development and temporal lobe epilepsy.

van der Knaap disease (megalencephalic leukoencephalopathy with subcortical cysts): Diffuse T2 W and FLAIR hyperintensities, not showing restricted diffusion in bilateral cerebral deep and subcortical white matter and external capsule. Multiple subcortical cysts in bilateral temporal lobes and high frontal regions.

Metachromatic leukodystrophy: Confluent bilateral symmetrical periventricular white matter hyperintensity with gliosis and mild ex-vacuo dilatation of both lateral ventricles. Bilateral symmetrical white matter hyperintensity also involves subcortical U fibers, external capsule, posterior limb of internal capsule, dorsal aspect of pons, middle cerebellar peduncles and bilateral cerebellar white matter.

Metachromatic leukodystrophy (early changes): Confluent periventricular white matter hyperintensities on T2 W/FLAIR sequence with no significant restricted diffusion. Both thalami and basal ganglia are preserved. No significant involvement of brainstem/subcortical U fibers. MRS shows mild reduction of NAA, rise in choline with no significant changes in other metabolite peaks.

Krabbe disease: Diffuse T2 W/Flair hyperintensity involving the periventricular, subcortical cerebral white matter, internal capsule, corpus callosum, dorsal brain stem, deep cerebellar white matter with high myelin edema. T2 hypointense signal noted in the bilateral thalamus which is hyperdense in CT. MR spectroscopy shows no significant abnormal metabolite—above features favour Krabbe disease. Suggested clinical/lab parameter correlation.

Hypomyelination: Severe hypomyelination/demyelination (myelination of only perirolandic white matter and central white matter).

Hypomyelination/leukodystrophy with diffuse thinning of corpus callosum: Possibilities include: 1. Hypomyelinating leukodystrophy–III, 2. hypomyelination and congenital cataract, 3. HSP60 chapernopathy, 4. Salla disease.

Canavan's disease: Bilateral cerebral subcortical and periventricular white matter, internal capsule, external capsule, globus pallidus, dentate nucleus, extreme capsule, cerebral peduncle, dorsal brainstem, deep cerebellar white matter shows T2W diffuse hyperintensities and hypointense in T1W FLAIR images. These changes appear bright in diffusion weighted images. Caudate and putamen appear normal. On spectroscopy, the lesion shows increased NAA compounds. Suggested urinary and plasma N-Aspartyl acetic acid/clinical correlation.

Alexander disease: T2W/FLAIR hyperintensity in the bilateral frontal, temporal white matter, external capsule, extreme capsule, basal ganglia, thalamus, brainstem and periventricular white matter garlands in the peritrigonal occipital region without diffusion restriction. On contrast administration mild enhancement noted along the ventricular lining and periventricular white matter in the frontal white matter. On spectroscopy, the lesion shows mildly decreased NAA peak.

Glutaric aciduria type I: Arachnoid cyst in bilateral anterior temporal regions (middle cranial fossa) with hypoplasia of the underlying temporal lobes—Bat wing shape with widened sylvian fissures. Hyperintensity involving caudate and lentiform nucleus, white matter, dorsal brain stem with diffusion restriction.

Anterior temporal pole cyst with calcification: Leukoencephalopathy with calcifications and cysts (LCC), TORCH (congenital CMV infection)/pseudo-TORCH (Aicardi–Goutières syndrome), cystic leukoencephalopathy without megalencephaly (RNASET 2-deficient cystic leukoencephalopathy), Cockaye syndrome (no basal ganglia calcification/cerebral atrophy).

Anterior temporal pole cyst without calcification: Abnormal T2W/FLAIR hyperintensities in bilateral peritrigonal and perilateral white matter, which does not show diffusion restriction. Bilateral anterior temporal pole cyst seen. No obvious evidence of basal ganglia and cerebral calcification seen. MR spectroscopy of the brain parenchyma shows normal spectral pattern. No significant reduction of NAA/elevation of choline. No abnormal metabolites seen. Possibilities include, TORCH (congenital CMV infection)/pseudo-TORCH (Aicardi–Goutières syndrome)—no evidence of calcification seen. Megaloencephalic leucoencephalopathy with subcortical cysts (no obvious megalencephaly). Leukoencephalopathy with calcifications and cyst—no evidence of calcification seen. Congenital muscular dystrophy.

Excessive T2W hyperintense changes noted in the bilateral deep white matter region. No evidence of PVL. No abnormal diffusion restriction. Diffuse and excessive high signal intensity (DEHSI)—**suggestive of normal finding in preterm infant. Mild elevated lactate peak—normal for age.**

Hypoglycemic (hypoxic) ischemic brain injury sequelae: Bilateral parieto-occipital gliosis with ex-vacuo dilatation of occipital horn of lateral ventricles.

Hypoxic ischemic encephalopathy **(HIE):** Diffuse bilateral periventricular white matter hyperintensity with white matter loss, ex-vacuo dilatation of both lateral ventricles with undulated margins. Mild diffuse thinning of the corpus callosum. Features favour the possibility of **periventricular leucomalacia** (hypoxic ischemic encephalopathy).

Abnormal T2W/FLAIR hyperintensity in the bilateral thalamus and posterior putamen—**profound hypoxic ischemic brain injury sequelae.**

Diffusion restricting T2 hypointense lesion seen throughout the cerebral parenchyma involving the deep grey matter and thalamus. Diffusion restricting lesion noted in the entire corpus callosum and internal capsule and extension along the corticospinal tract. Cerebellum and posterior brainstem relatively appear normal. MR spectroscopy of the brain parenchyma shows significantly elevated lactate peak seen throughout the brain parenchyma. **Features are suggestive of severe hypoxic ischemic encephalopathy changes.**

T2W hyperintensity in bilateral posterior lentiform nucleus, thalami, perirolandic frontoparietal regions, bilateral periventricular and deep white matter. Diffuse thinning of corpus callosum. Mild ex-vacuo dilatation of both lateral ventricles. MR spectroscopy shows reduction of NAA and presence of lactate in affected areas: **Features are suggestive of sequelae of perinatal hypoxic ischemic encephalopathy.**

Gliosis in left frontal, temporal, parietal and occipital cortex and white matter with ex-vacuo dilatation of left lateral ventricle, secondary hypoplasia of brainstem on left side and reduced volume of skull. Milder gliosis in right frontal and parietal cortex and white matter. Features are suggestive of sequelae of hypoxic ischemic encephalopathy (**multicystic encephalomalacia).**

Benign enlargement of subarachnoid space: Prominent bilateral frontotemporal arachnoid spaces—benign enlargement of subarachnoid spaces (normal variant). **Or** Widening of bifrontal subarachnoid spaces (craniocortical diameter >5 mm)—suggestive of benign physiologic enlargement of subarachnoid spaces (otherwise known as benign macrocephaly of infancy/external hydrocephalus/physiologic extraventricular obstructive hydrocephalus). It is a self-limited condition with spontaneous resolution of CSF spaces between 12–24 months.

Iron deposition (children): Abnormal T2W/FLAIR hyperintensity in the caudate nucleus, anterior aspect of putamen with bilateral globus pallidus. MR spectroscopy of the basal ganglia shows decreased NAA and mildly increased lactate. Bilateral optic atrophy. Moderate to severe atrophy of cerebellum and pons. Mild diffuse cerebral atrophy. Above feature favour metabolic/neurodegeneration. Possibilities include: Mitochondrial disorder/fatty acid associated neurodegeneration suggested clinical/lab parameter correlation.

Methylmalonic acidemia: Bilateral symmetric altered signal intensity appearing hypointense on T1W and hyperintense on T2W noted in globus pallidus without diffusion restriction/contrast enhancement. MR spectroscopy shows no significant abnormal metabolite. Possibilities include: Methylmalonic Acidemia, Kernicterus (less likely—no history of neonatal jaundice), Succinate semialdehyde dehydrogenase deficiency, L-2-hydroxy glutaric aciduria, isovaleric acidemia, neonatal hypoxia.

Bilateral putaminal T2W/FLAIR hyperintensity (putaminal necrosis): With diffusion hyperintensity and elevated lactate in MR spectroscopy. SWI shows no increased iron deposition. Possibilities include: Mitochondrial disease—including G14459A mutation, SUCLA-2 gene mutation. Pediatric autoimmune neuropsychiatric disorder associated with streptococcal infection (PANDAS). Propionic acidemia. Neuroacanthocytosis—additional features like cerebellar atrophy is absent. No evidence of thalamus, midbrain, pons involvement to suggest Wilson disease. No evidence of T1 hyperintensity in globus pallidus. Methanol intoxication/hypoxic ischemic changes—no supportive clinical history. Juvenile Huntington's disease—no evidence of caudate nucleus involvement. Molybdenum cofactor deficiency—no evidence of caudate nucleus, white matter involvement. Glutaric aciduria—no other white matter/bilateral sylvian arachnoid cyst **(refer to case 4.28).**

Bilateral globus pallidus T2W/FLAIR hyperintensity (adult): Bilateral globus pallidus T2W/FLAIR hyperintensity with diffusion restriction—possibilities include: 1. Poisoning (carbon monoxide), 2. Hypoglycemia/hypoxia, 3. Cocaine/heroine abuse. Neuro degeneration with brain iron accumulation less likely.

Caudate and putamen: Abnormal T2W/FLAIR/diffusion weighted hyperintensities in the caudate and putamen. MR spectroscopy shows elevated lactate—features favours Leigh's disease. Other possibilities include: Propionic academia, molybdenum cofactor deficiency, Wilson's disease, juvenile Huntington's disease, osmotic myelinolysis, hemolytic uremic syndrome, hypoxia—less likely, carbon monoxide poisoning **(refer to case 4.27).**

Prominent Virchow-Robin spaces: In bilateral cerebral hemisphere—possibilities include Lowe syndrome, mucopolysachridoses, hypomelanosis of Ito and velocardiofacial syndrome.

Bilateral thalamus without haemorrhage: Non-diffusion restricting long TR hyperintense lesions noted in the both thalamus, bilateral outer putamen and caudate nucleus and bilateral patchy supratentorial subcortical and deep white matter and pons, midbrain central white matter. Possibilities include: Japanese encephalitis. Cerebral malaria/acute disseminated encephalomyelitis (rare).

Bilateral thalamus with haemorrhage: Bilateral thalamic hyperintensities with/without diffusion restriction and haemorrhages. Normal deep venous system noted. Possibilities to be considered: Flavi virus encephalitis like Japanese encephalitis, cerebral malaria, H3N2 influenza encephalitis with vasculitis (acute necrotizing encephalitis), herpes simplex encephalitis (no involvement of temporal lobe in this patient), dengue fever (haemorrhage less likely).

Reversible splenial lesion: Focal lesion in the splenium of corpus callosum which shows diffusion restriction without hemorrhage—reversible splenial lesion syndrome (RESLES) probably due to encephalitis/encephalopathy of varied etiology.

Tubulinopathy: Diffuse thinning of corpus callosum. Thin anterior commissure. Irregular prominent bilateral lateral ventricles—moderate ventriculomegaly. Enlarged caudate nucleus and fused striatum (absent diminutive internal capsule dividing the caudate from putamen): Dysmorphic basal ganglia—above features favour tubulinopathy (DYNC1H1 mutation).

Arnold-Chiari malformation Type 1: Small posterior fossa with cerebellar tonsilar herniation 8 mm below the foramen magnum line causing crowding of the foramen magnum. Evidence of syringomyelia in the cervical cord from C2 to C5 vertebrae level—Arnold-Chiari malformation Type 1. CSF flow shows pulsatile flow in the syringomyelia. No flow noted in the posterior subarachnoid space. Anterior cervical subarachnoid space and pre-pontine and pre-medullary cisterns show normal CSF flow.

Posterior fossa is smaller than normal. Herniation of the cerebellar tonsil below the foramen magnum up to the lower C2 level. 4th ventricle is elongated and slit-like with moderate triventricular hydrocephalus. There is medullary kink, beaking of tectum, large massa intermedia, scalloped posterior petrous pyramids and clivus, large funnel-shaped foramen magnum. Cerebellum wraps around the medulla. Low lying tentorium and torcula.

Pantothenate kinase associated neurodegeneration (Hallervorden-Spatz disease): Mild diffuse cerebral and cerebellar atrophy with increased signal intensity in the globus pallidus giving eye of the tiger appearance. Bilateral basal ganglia calcification seen. MR spectroscopy shows no abnormal metabolite seen. No evidence of altered signal intensity in the cerebellum. Possibilities include: Neurodegeneration with brain iron accumulation—pantothenate kinase associated neurodegeneration (Hallervorden-Spatz disease). Kearns-Sayre syndrome and other mitochondrial disorder NARP (neuropathy, ataxia and retitis pigmentosa).

Table 2.2: MR parkinsonism index-2 (MRPI 2)

	AP diameter	*Width*	*Volume (mm^3)*	*Interpretation*
Midbrain	14 mm			
Superior colliculus	3 mm			
Midbrain (midline) M			1.17	
Pons (midline) P			5.46	
Pons /midbrain area ratio P/M			5.46/1.17 = 4.67	
Superior cerebellar peduncle in coronal plane SCP		4.8 mm		
Middle cerebellar peduncle in sagittal plane MCP		11.1 mm		
MCP/SCP ratio			2.31	
MRI parkinsonism index = (P/M) × (MCP/SCP)		10.79		PSP >13.55
Third ventricular width (V3): Average width (from three measurements) of the 3rd ventricle on axial image at the level of anterior and posterior commissures	9.5 mm			
Frontal horn (FH) (maximal left to right frontal horn width on axial image in AC-PC plane)		37.7 mm		
MRPI 2.0 = MRPI × (V3/FH)		10.79 × 0.251 = 2.70		PSP-P ≥2.18 PSP-R ≥2.5 PD <2

Fukuyama's congenital muscular dystrophy: Cerebellar hypoplasia noted with tiny cortical cysts. Pontine hypoplasia with Z-shaped deformity. Bilateral lissencephaly with cortical polymicrogyria. Periventricular white matter long TR hyperintense lesion. Absent septum pellusidum noted. Bilateral lateral ventricles dilatation. Thickened tectal plate noted. Basal ganglia and thalamus appear normal.

Progressive supranuclear palsy: Diffuse cerebral and cerebellar atrophy. Disproportionate atrophy of midbrain. AP diameter of midbrain measures 11.9 mm, width of middle cerebellar peduncle 6.6 mm, width of superior cerebellar peduncle 1.7 mm on right side and 2.7 mm on left side. Area of midbrain measures 0.68 sq. cm and area of pons measures 3.4 sq cm.

Pituitary macroadenoma: Dumbbell-shaped well-defined enhancing mass lesion with cystic areas of size 36 (CC) × 26 (AP) × 28 (Trans) mm in the sella-suprasellar region compressing and elevating the distal intracranial optic nerves and optic chiasma. Expansion of sella noted. There is extension to right cavernous sinus, reaching up to the lateral venous compartment. Cavernous segment of right internal carotid artery is mildly pushed laterally without stenosis. Sphenoid sinus is well pneumatised. Normal pituitary gland and infundibulum are not made out separately. Tubercinerium, mamillary body, floor of the IIIrd ventricle are normal: Features are suggestive of pituitary macroadenoma. Post-sellar pneumatisation of the sphenoid sinus with prominent sellae bulge and plannum sphenoidale, dorsum sella pneumatisation. Sphenoid sinus show single midline septum anteriorly and multiple septae posteriorly. Inter-carotid distance—20 mm. Optic chiasma is seen over the pituitary and dorsal sellae—normal/post-fixed chiasma.

Viral encephalitis: Diffusion restricting long TR hyperintense lesion in the both putamen, right thalamus, right posterior parietal cortex and right inferior frontal gyri and right amygdala. Possible viral encephalitis.

Rasmussen's encephalitis: Diffuse gyral thickening and T2 hyperintensity noted involving the left cerebral hemisphere (left temporal, frontal and parietal regions). T2 hyperintensity noted in the left thalamus and caudate part of left basal ganglia and left substantia nigra. Focal T2 hyperintensity noted in the subcortical region with left frontal region. No evidence of restricted diffusion. Mass effect noted on the left cerebral sulci and left lateral ventricle with mild effacement. Mild midline shift to right of 2.0 mm noted. Mild leptomeningeal enhancement noted in the left cerebral hemisphere. The different diagnoses are Rasmussen's encephalitis/viral encephalitis/postictal change associated with status epilepticus.

Acoustic schwannoma: Evidence of a large heterointense extra-axial avidly enhancing mass lesion measuring 5.2 (AP) × 3.6 (TR) × 4.1 (CC) cm noted in the left CP angle region. There is extension into the left internal auditory meatus with intrameatal component measuring 5.1 × 5 mm. Distal 3.4 mm of the internal auditory canal appear normal. Fundus of internal auditory canal and cochlear aperture appear normal. Areas of multiple microhaemorrhages within the mass. The lesion is highly vascular with multiple feeders from the left vertebral artery which is hypoplastic. Left VII-VIII nerve complex in the CP angle cistern and proximal IAM are not visualised separately from the mass. There is compression of the pons, lower midbrain, left middle cerebellar peduncle and adjacent cerebellar hemisphere without intra-axial edema. Effacement of aqueduct and fourth ventricle with early obstructive hydrocephalus (dilatation of third and both lateral ventricles). Increased intracranial tension with bilateral prominent perioptic CSF sheath and tortuous optic nerves, flattening of posterior sclera and partial empty sella. Evidence of tonsillar herniation of 12 mm below the foramen magnum.

Eosinophilic granuloma: Evidence of well-defined lytic lesion in the right parietal bone measuring 37 mm (AP) × 15 mm (TR) × 53 mm (CC) with extra-axial and subgaleal soft tissue components. There is destruction of both inner and outer tables. The lesion intracranially abuts the dura which is thickened and demonstrates increased enhancement. No other calvarial lesions are seen. No definite intra-axial abnormality. The infundibulum and cavernous sinuses have a normal appearance.

Tuberous sclerosis: Multiple subependymal nodules along the lateral ventricles predominantly along the caudothalamic groove, cortical tubers in the left postcentral gyrus and right superior frontal gyrus. No evidence of subependymal giant cell astrocytoma/ocular lesions/white matter changes/vascular lesions.

PRES (posterior reversible encephalopathy syndrome): Bilateral frontoparietal, parietal, occipital and left cerebellar subcortical and cortical T2W FLAIR hyperintensity with/without diffusion restriction.

Colloid cyst: Well-defined T1 hyperintense lesion measuring 12.5 mm (AP) × 10.5 mm (TR) × 10 mm (CC) in anterior third ventricle at the foramen of Monro, more towards left side causing mild asymmetric prominence of left lateral ventricle.

Normal pressure hydrocephalus: Age related diffuse cerebral atrophy with prominent cortical sulci and both lateral ventricles. There is mild disproportionate dilatation of both lateral ventricles compared to sulcal prominence with minimal periventricular hyperintensity along the frontal and occipital horns of both lateral ventricles. Accentuated flow void noted across the aqueduct and adjacent posterior third ventricular region and proximal 4th ventricle. MR spectroscopy of the ventricle shows lactate peak—finding favouring the possibility of normal pressure hydrocephalus over other dementia. No dilatation of IIIrd and IVth ventricle. No ballooning of optic and infundibular recess of third ventricle. No disproportionate dilatation of sylvian fissure.

Alzheimer's disease: Cerebral sulcal spaces, basal cisterns, cerebellar foliae and ventricular system appear prominent. Suggestive of moderate diffuse parenchymal atrophy. Global cortical atrophy scale: score 2. The hippocampus volumes measures 1.30 cm^3 on right side and 1.29 cm^3 on left side—decreased. MTA-scale for Medial Temporal lobe Atrophy: score 3. The interuncal distance at the level of anterior commissure is 31 mm—more than 30 mm is considered as abnormal.

Wilson disease: Bilateral symmetrical FLAIR/T2 hyperintensities in the putamen, thalami, pallidum and tegmentum of midbrain and periaqueductal grey matter. T1 hyperintensity noted in the globius pallidus. Midbrain lesion shows characteristic 'face of the giant panda'—Wilson disease.

Tolosa-Hunt syndrome: Ill-defined hypointense lesion in the right orbital apex and right cavernous sinus, which shows homogeneous enhancement. The lesion measures 20 (AP) × 10 (CC) × 6 (TR) mm. No obvious evidence of dural tail.

Aberrant course of the right anterior inferior cerebellar artery indenting on the right facial nerve at the root entry zone with mild deviation of 7th nerve course. No evidence of **neurovascular conflict at the nerve root entry zone** of left trigeminal nerve.

Mesial temporal sclerosis: Body of the right hippocampus appears small with loss of internal architecture (striations) and loss of hippocampal digitation with increased signal intensity and dilated temporal horn of right lateral ventricle. Right fornix and mamillary body atrophy—right mesial temporal sclerosis. Right hippocampus volume ~1.89 cc. Left hippocampus volume ~2.09 cc.

Acute intracerebral hemorrhage: [60 mm (AP) × 39 mm (TR) × 38 mm (CC)] in the left para sagittal frontal region inter-hemispheric fissure and adjacent sulcal spaces. There is extension to all ventricle more in the left lateral ventricle. Significant mass effect on left lateral ventricle with midline shift to the right (14 mm) anterior body of the corpus callosum is displaced downwards. Mildly prominent right lateral ventricle. Haemorrhage also noted in the sylvian fissure and basal cisterns.

Extra dural haemorrhage: Maximum thickness measuring 18 mm in the left lateral convexity along the parietotemporal region, causing mild mass effect with local sulcal effacement and midline shift of 4 mm to the right. No evidence of hydrocephalus. Basal cisterns appears normal. Linear undisplaced Fracture noted in the squamous part of left temporal bone.

Comment about space of the haemorrhage, size, intraventricular extension, obstructive hydrocephalus, edema, midline shift, herniation, any area of infarction, vessel injury, old gliosis, if any.

Small vessel ischemic changes: Multiple focal discrete and confluence T2W/FLAIR hyperintensities in the periventricular and central white matter which does not show diffusion restriction—small vessel ischemic changes. Fazekas scale for WM lesions—score 2.

Acute disseminated encephalomyelitis (ADEM): Altered signal intensity appearing hyperintense on T2 and FLAIR, not showing restriction of diffusion in bilateral basal ganglia, thalamus, brain stem and deep cerebellar white matter. No abnormal enhancement on contrast administration—features favours acute disseminated encephalomyelitis (ADEM).

Acute infarct in the left middle frontal gyrus, inferior frontal gyrus, pre central gyrus, postcentral gyrus, left centrum semiovale, left superior, inferior parietal gyrus, insula, head of left caudate nucleus, left temporoparietal region. Minimal haemorrhagic transformation in the left parietal region. No evidence of significant mass effect.

Demyelination: Abnormal T2W/FLAIR hyperintensity in the right superior cerebellar subcortical white matter which does not show diffusion restriction/contrast enhancement—demyelination.

Vasculitis/chronic demyelination plaque: Multiple small T2W and FLAIR hyperintensities, not showing restricted diffusion seen scattered in bilateral fronto parietal subcortical white matter and parieto-occipital periventricular white matter. Normal callososeptal interface. No evidence of Dawson's fingers. No evidence of haemorrhage. No optic nerve demyelination.

Multiple sclerosis: Multiple nondiffusion restricting nonenhancing linear, ovoid and globular long TR hypointensity lesions involving the callososeptal interface, perilateral ventricular regions, bilateral frontal, temporal, parietal, subcortical regions and right internal capsule, left cerebellar white matter, superior cerebellar

Table 2.3: Neuroimaging radiological interpretation system (NIRIS)

Category	*Definition*	*Patient management/actions*
NIRIS 0	No abnormal finding	Discharge from the ED
NIRIS 1	Fracture ±	Follow-up neuroimaging and/or admit for observation.
	Extra-axial hematoma, intraparenchymal hematoma/contusion <0.5 mL±	
	Subarachnoid haemorrhage.	
NIRIS 2	Extra-axial hematoma, intraparenchymal hematoma/contusion >0.5 mL±	Admit to a more advanced care unit.
	Diffusion axonal injury ±	
	Intraventricular haemorrhage ±	
	Mild hydrocephalus ±	
	Midline shift 0–5 mm	
NIRIS 3	Extra-axial hematoma, intraparenchymal hematoma/contusion >5 mL±	Consider neurosurgical procedure (ventricular drain, burr hole, craniotomy/craniectomy, surgical drainage/evacuation of hematoma)
	Moderate hydrocephalus ±	
	Midline shift >5 mm ±	
	Focal herniation	
NIRIS 4	Extra-axial hematoma, intraparenchymal hematoma/contusion >25 mL±	High risk traumatic brain injury-related death
	Severe hydrocephalus ±	
	Diffuse herniation/duret haemorrhage	

vermis, pons—right middle cerebellar peduncle junction. Multiple patchy focal lesions in the entire spinal cord involving lateral, central and posterior columns at variable levels. Features favour multiple sclerosis—suggested clinical/CSF of analysis correlation. **Restricted diffusion noted in bilateral central part of the centrum semiovale more on the right side. Patchy peripheral diffusion restriction in the left centrum semiovale lesions (Table 2.4).**

Bilateral T1 hyperintensity in globus pallidus: Bilateral T1 hyperintensity in globus pallidus—possible basal ganglia calcification/hepatocellular—renal dysfunction, manganese deposition (in patients with chronic renal disease on hemodialysis).

Idiopathic intracranial hypertension: Partial empty sella seen. Prominent bilateral perioptic sheath fluid with posterior scleral flattening. Moderate luminal narrowing in bilateral distal transverse sinuses.

Hydrocephalus with post-op status: Post-operative burr hole defect in the frontal and right parietal bone. Moderate dilatation of third and both lateral ventricles with collapsed fourth ventricle–obstructive hydrocephalus. VP shunt tube *in situ* one through the right parieto-occipital and other through the right

Table 2.4: Multiple sclerosis sample reporting

Region	*Location*	*No of lesions*	*Size*	*Diffusion restriction (+/–)*	*Contrast enhancement (+/–) type of enhancement*	*Comparison with previous MRI New lesions/T1 Black Holes*
Periventricular and callososeptal interface						
Juxtacortical/ cortical						
Infratentorial						
Spinal cord						
Lobar-vloume						Volume loss
Corpus callosum-volume						
Other findings (optic nerve)						

frontal lobe with tip in the body of right lateral ventricle. Bifronto-temporal encephalomalacic gliosis. Paucity of subcortical white matter in the frontotemporal region. Right parieto-occipital loculated fluid collection measuring 46 × 18 mm along the shunt tract near the reservoir.

Head and Neck

CA tongue: 19 (AP) × 10 (TR) × 18 (CC) mm size ill-defined mass lesion in the right anterolateral border of the anterior third of tongue with minimal infiltration of the intrinsic muscles. Mylohyoid, hyoglossus and genioglossus, stylopharyngeus appears normal. No evidence of extension into the mandible/retromolar trigone/lingual septum/floor of mouth/midline/posterior third of tongue—features suggestive of carcinoma tongue. **(T2M0N0).**

Ca tongue reporting checklist: **Laterality**: **Right or left, Size: ....× .... × ... cm.** Depth of invasion: (Previous depth of invasion:)

T Stage: To comment on whether the tumor crosses the midline or abuts lingual raphe, involvement of extrinsic muscles like genioglossus, hyoglossus, geniohyoid, involvement of lingual neurovascular bundle (grade: 0/I/II/III) and uni/bilateral involvement.

To comment on whether the tumor extends to posterior one-third of the tongue, RMT, tonsillo-lingual sulcus and tonsil extension of tumor to sublingual space/submandibular space, infiltration of mylohyoid and involvement of floor of mouth, comment on extension to masticator space, infratemporal fossa (ITF), high infratemporal fossa. Inferior extent: Look up to vallecular/epiglottis/PFS, also comment on involvement of hyoid, if not involved—comment on distance from hyoid bone. Look for any bony erosion—mandibular involvement, cortical breach, marrow signal abnormality.

N: Presence of nodal disease: Metastatic/benign (reactive)/indeterminate, if indeterminate/suspicious: Need for additional imaging, laterality: Ipsilateral/contralateral/bilateral levels: Level: IA and IB/II, III, IV, V, VI and retropharyngeal. Size of the largest node: Right side: ..... mm and level, Left side: ..... mm and level, presence of necrosis if any, perinodal extension/extracapsular spread: Absent/present, vascular involvement by the nodes: IJV: involved/compressed; CCA, ICA, ECA abutment: Absent/ Present, If present angle of contact for CCA and ICA: <90, 90–179, 180–269; >270. Strap muscles involvement, Prevertebral fascia invasion. M: Lung, hepatic, adrenal and skeletal metastasis.

Juvenile nasopharyngeal angiofibroma (JNA): Large well-defined lobulated highly vascular enhancing mass lesion measuring about 5 × 4.1 × 4.4 cm (AP × TR × CC) noted in the right spheno palatine foramen, posterior nasal cavity, posterior ethmoidal sinus and right sphenoid sinus. Lesion is highly vascular with multiple flow voids within. Main arterial supply of the mass is seen from the hypertrophied right internal maxillary artery. There is widening of the right pterygopalatine fossa and extension of the soft tissue into the infratemporal fossa. Erosion of the medial and lateral pterygoid plate on right side. There is involvement of right foramen rotundum and vidian canal. There is erosion of the anterior wall of the foramen ovale. Erosion of floor of right middle cranial fossa (greater wing of sphenoid) without intracranial extension. No involvement of the ICA. There is extension into the inferior aspect of the orbital apex on right side through the widened inferior orbital fissure. No involvement of the extraocular muscles/optic nerve. Nasal septum is pushed to left. The mass is extending into the nasopharynx—features are consistent with juvenile nasopharyngeal angiofibroma–stage IIc: (staging system proposed by Sessions, modified by Radkowski).

Multinodular goiter: Thyroid appears diffusely enlarged showing heterogeneous enhancement, right lobe measures ....left lobe measures ....with mild mass effect over trachea, no retrosternal extension of thyroid lobes noted. No significant cervical lymph nodes noted. TIRADS-II.

Post-cricoid carcinoma: An ill-defined soft tissue dense lesion measuring 2 × 1 cm noted in post-cricoid region at the level of C5–C6, the lesion does not extend to bilateral pyriform fossa, the lesion appears to erode cricoid and cricoarytenoid joint, arytenoid appears sclerosed, the lesion infiltrates posterior aspect of larynx with marked narrowing of airways, lesion appears to involve the anterior wall of proximal cervical esophagus for a length of 1 cm causing luminal narrowing of esophagus, recurrent laryngeal nerve appears normal. The parapharyngeal fat planes are infiltrated, no cervical lymphadenopathy.

Glottic growth: Ill-defined soft tissue density lesion measuring about 19 × 11 mm in the right vocal cord. No subglottic extension of the lesion. Minimal infiltration of the right supraglottic fat. No obvious extra laryngeal extension. There is sclerosis of the right arytenoid cartilage - ? Infiltrated.

Supraglottic growth: Soft tissue density lesion measuring about 2.2 × 1.5 cm in the right side of the larynx involving

Table 2.5: Lymphoma reporting tool			
No.	Size (mm) (long-axis diameter) × (short-axis diameter)	FDG uptake (SUVmax)	Location (lymph node location/location within the affected organ)
1.			
2.			

the supraglottic and glottic space. No subglottic extension. There is mild sclerosis of the right aretynoid cartilage and thickening of the right aryepiglottic fold. No involvement of the left vocal cord. A few small subcentimetric lymph nodes in bilateral cervical region.

Lymphoma: Multiple lobulated enlarged lymph nodes noted in the bilateral preauricular, cervical infra-clavicular, hilar, mediastinal lymph nodes. There is no evidence of splenomegaly. With PET scan avid uptake **(SUV 3.0)** noted in the lymph nodes and in the right iliac bone (recommended site for biopsy). No evidence of other lesions in the stomach, liver, lung/pleura, kidney, CNS and skin (Table 2.5).

Vocal cord palsy: Paramedian position of the right vocal cord. Prominent right pyriform sinus with thickened aryepiglottic fold—right vocal cord palsy. No obvious mass lesion in the neck/visualised mediastinum.

Post-radiation status of larynx: Partially abducted left vocal cord with mild effacement of left pyriform fossa and vallecula with thickened (17 × 9 × 17 mm) false cord, supraglottic and glottic region extending to involving the posterior aspect of the pharynx with narrowing of laryngeal inlet. Diffuse non-enhancing edema of the pyriform fossa, Aryepiglottic folds and post-cricoid pharynx. Mild irregularity in the right lateral border of tongue-radiation induced changes

Vagal schwannoma: Evidence of a large extraaxial intra and extracranial dumb bell-shaped heterointense enhancing mass lesion with cystic areas and hemorrhage noted in left jugular foramen, cerebello medullary cistern and CP angle. Extracranially, lesion extends to the upper carotid space. Intracranial component measures 3.9 (AP) × 2.8 (trans) × 3.4 (CC) cm, the component in jugular foramen measures 2 × 1.2 cm, extracranial component in upper carotid space measures 4.5 (trans) × 2.69 (AP) × 3.9 (CC) cm. The left internal carotid artery is displaced anteromedially by the mass and internal jugular vein is compressed posterolaterally and not visualised in the region the mass in carotid space. Medulla and left middle cerebellar peduncle are indented by the mass. No intra-axial edema. No obstructive hydrocephalus. Smooth widening of left jugular foramen. No extension to internal auditory meatus. No extension to hypoglossal canal. Left vocal cord palsy changes seen.

Branchial fistula: 6 mm length linear fistulous tract extending from skin in the left paramedian lower neck extending up to the sternocleidomastoid muscle. No evidence of extension into the left lobe of thyroid/pyriform fossa.

Lower cranial nerve/jugular schwannoma: Large intra- and extra-cranial dumb bell-shaped heterointense enhancing mass lesion with cystic areas and hemorrhage in left upper carotid space, jugular foramen, cerebello medullary cistern and CP angle.

Suppurative lymphadenitis: Conglomerate enlarged left upper and mid cervical lymph nodes and upper posterior triangle lymph nodes with areas of necrosis. No evidence of vertebral, bone or deep neck space involvement.

Carotid body tumor: Well-defined intensely enhancing highly vascular soft tissue density mass lesion measuring 3.6 × 3.7 × 5.2 cm (AP × TR × CC) in the left carotid space at CCA bifurcation level with splaying of the internal carotid and external carotid arteries. The lesion shows salt and pepper appearance in T1/T2 images. Mass is extending superomedially to lower para pharyngeal space. Left internal jugular vein is compressed and pushed laterally without thrombus. There is no encasement of ICA and ECA. No e/o luminal narrowing/thrombus formation. Multiple arterial feeders seen arising directly from proximal external carotid artery, ascending pharyngeal artery and occipital artery. No supply from the ICA.

Chronic otomastoiditis without cholestatoma: Soft tissue noted filling the right middle ear cavity, right external auditory canal, mastoid antrum and mastoid air cells. Soft tissue noted in right facial nerve recess and sinus

Table 2.6: Cochlear implant workup on HRCT	
1	Mastoid cellularity—non-pneumatised / hypo/ normal
2	Middle ear cavity—ossicles integrity and round window
3	Position of genu and descending mastoid segment of facial nerve—any aberrant course
4	Jugular bulb (if high riding)
5	Bony labyrinth structure with special focus on cochlea size, turns, interscalar septum, modiolus, cochlear aperture, cochlear duct length
6	Internal auditory canal
7	Cochlear and vestibular aqueduct

Table 2.7: Cochlear implant workup in MRI	
Signal of fluid in labyrinth	Hypointense in case of labyrinthitis: Balkany classification of labyrinthitis
Inner ear structures with special focus on cochlea. Scalar anatomy, osseous spiral lamina, outlines of modiolus, cochlear aperture size	Inner ear anomalies
Internal auditory canal with 7–8th nerve complex evaluation	Absence of 8th nerve/ undivided 8th nerve, hyoplastic 8th nerve
Lateral bulbopontine and cerebellopontine angle	For evaluation of any mass lesion
Brain stem (fascicular segment of 8th nerve, cochlear nerve nuclei)	For evaluation of any mass lesion in brain stem
Fascicular segment of 8th nerve-course along lateral aspect of pons, cochlear nuclei-hypointense structure along dorsolateral aspect of inferior cerebellar peduncle	
Auditory pathway and brain survey	Any lesion/ hypoxic changes, demyelination in superior olivary nucleus, lateral leminiscus, medial geniculate body, superior temporal gyrus, Heschl gyrus

Table 2.8: Cochlear implantation work up (measurements)		
Cochlea	2.5–2.75 turns, 29.5–32 mm in length, 8–10 mm height	Cochlear anomalies—aplasia/ hypoplasia
Cochlear aperture	Length: 0.8–1.2 mm, diameter: 1.8–2.5 mm	Diameter <1.4 mm—indicative of cochlear nerve deficiency
Cochlear duct length	CDL = (4.16 * A) – 3.98, A: Largest distance from round window to the lateral wall of cochlea	Electrode array of optimal length to be chosen
IAC diameter		<2.5 mm—absent/ hypoplastic 8th nerve
Cochlear aqueduct		>3 mm—dilated, risk of transmission of ear infection to meninges
Vestibular aqueduct	At midpoint between crus and external aperture	>1.5 mm/calibre is more than half of posterior semicircular canal

Table 2.9: CT reporting and staging system of acquired cholesteatoma		
Tympanic cavity involvement (T)	*Mastoid cavity involvement (M)*	*Complications (C)*
T1: Attic cholesteatoma	M0: No mastoid cavity involvement	C0: Uncomplicated cholesteatoma
T2: Tympanic cholesteatoma	M1: Cholesteatoma extending into mastoid antrum	C1: Temporal complications
T3: Attico-tympanic cholesteatoma	M2: Cholesteatoma extending to mastoid cavity and cells	C2: Cranial and intracranial complications
T4: Holotympanic cholesteatoma		

tympani. No evidence of erosion of scutum/widening of Prussak's space, erosion of malleus and incus on both sides. No erosion of tegmen tympani, lateral semicircular canal or facial nerve canal/sinus plate/inner ear.

Chronic left otomastoiditis with cholesteatoma: Soft tissue noted filling the left middle ear cavity, mastoid antrum and mastoid air cells. Soft tissue noted in left facial nerve recess and sinus tympani. There is erosion of scutum, malleus, incus with widening of Prussak's space. Middle ear soft tissue component measures 12 × 9 mm with extension of soft tissue into the left external auditory canal. No erosion of tegmen tympani, lateral semicircular canal or facial nerve canal/sinus plate/inner ear. No evidence of widening/block of left eustachian tube. Partial sclerosis of left mastoid air cells. No obvious evidence of jugular vein, left sigmoid sinus thrombosis. No obvious evidence of intracranial abscess/ meningeal component. Nonecho planar diffusion shows restricted diffusion.

Temporomandibular joint dislocation: Abnormal anterior displacement of articular disc of left temporomandibular joint with inter position of the posterior band between the condyle and the eminence. It remains anteriorly displaced at all times during jaw opening—**anterior displacement without reduction.**

Abnormal anterior displacement of articular disc of right temporomandibular joint with interposition of the posterior band between the condyle and the eminence. It reduces during jaw opening. **Anterior displacement with reduction.**

Right temporomandibular joint articular disc posterior band is located at 12 o'clock position related to condyle in closed mouth and 'bowtie' appearance in between articular eminence and condylar head in open mouth—**normal**.

Obstructive sleep apnoea in dynamic sleep MRI: Severe dynamic airway narrowing with complete obliteration of the lumen at the naso-oropharyngeal junction due to apposition of the posterior margin of the soft plate and the posterior pharyngeal wall during sleep.

Eagle's syndrome: Mildly elongated bilateral styloid process (36 mm in length).

Sinonasalpolyposis: Extensive polypoidal mucosal thickening completely filling the left maxillary, ethmoid, frontal and sphenoid sinuses and nasal cavity. OMU complex is completely blocked on left side. There is extension of the polyp into the nasopharynx through the choana. There is mild sclerosis of the walls of the sinuses—secondary to chronic inflammation. Small mucosal polyp in the right maxillary sinus. Deviation of the nasal septum to right, mild mucosal thickening in right frontal, ethmoid and sphenoidal sinuses. DD: Allergic fungal sinusitis.

Sinusitis: Minimal mucosal thickening in left maxillary sinus. Kero's type I skull base. Bilateral partial concha bullosa. Hypertrophy of both inferior turbinate.

Os terminale–Os odontoideum: Hypoplastic dens with wide gap between the os terminale–os odontoideum complex, which is seen near the basi occiput (dystrophic). Enlarged anterior arch of atlas. Evidence of atlanto-axial instability along with prominent retro os odontoideum soft tissue causing myelomalacic changes in the cervical cord at C1–C2 vertebrae level.

Anteriorly displaced C2 body and posteriorly pointing os odontoideum compromising the spinal canal. T2 W hyperintense/T1 W isointense lesions noted in upper cervical cord at C2 level measuring about 8 mm in length—suggestive of cord edema/contusion.

Os odontoideum: A well-corticated round area of ossification measuring 7 × 7.5 mm articulating with the anterior arch of atlas. Os odontoideum is seen subluxated to right side in relation to body of the C2 with left lateral angulation at C1–C2 level. No canal compromise. Clivus is short. Evidence of mild basilar invagination without canal compromise. Tip of the dens is just below the McRae line, 5 mm above the Chamberlain and 8 mm above the McGregor line.

Evidence of mild **basilar invagination** with tip of the dens minimally indenting the cervico medullary junction without intra-axial edema. Tip of the dens is 2 mm below the McRae line, 4 mm above the Chamberlain and 8 mm above the McGregor line.

Persistent hyperplastic vitreous: Small right eyeball with retrolental soft tissue lesion and hypoplastic vitreous. Hyaloid remnant of cloquets canal visualised. No evidence of calcifications—features favour persistent hypoplastic primary vitreous. Evidence of vitreous hemorrhage with thin subchoroidal collection.

Spine

Scoliosis: Dorsolumbar scoliosis with convexity to the left. Apical vertebrae is L1. Upper end vertebra is D8. Lower end vertebra is L3. Cobb's angle measures 22°. No structural abnormality in the vertebrae.

Sacral agenesis: High bulbous ending cord at upper border of D12 vertebrae level (distal spinal cord hypoplasia). Sacral agenesis involving the lower sacral vertebrae–group I caudal regression syndrome.

Sacroiliitis: Bilateral symmetric sacroiliitis with subchondral erosions, marrow oedema and sclerosis. No evidence of ankylosis—features favour seronegative spondyloarthropathy. Suggested clinical/lab parameter correlation.

Sacroiliitis with ankylosis: Bilateral symmetric sacroiliitis with subchondral erosions, marrow oedema and sclerosis, partial ankylosis in the both sacroiliac joint—features favour seronegative spondyloarthropathy—possible ankylosing spondylitis. Suggested clinical/lab parameter correlation.

Osteitis condensans ilii: Sclerosis of iliac side of bilateral sacroiliac joint without edema/erosion–osteitis condensans ilii.

Dorsal dermal sinus with cutaneous opening in the S1–S2 region coursing anteroinferiorly and extends into the spinal canal at upper part of S1 vertebrae level. Intradural sinus ascends superiorly within the spinal canal through an heterogeneous peripherally enhancing ill-defined intraspinal canal lesion from S1 to L2 levels and attached posterior to the conus at L2 vertebrae level. The intraspinal lesion measures 45 (CC) × 4 (TR) × 6.4 (AP) mm. There is areas of well-defined lobulated cyst (12 × 6 mm) at L5 vertebrae level within the lesion and shows areas of diffusion restriction—suggestive of epidermoid. The lesion does not show peripheral enhancement and leptomeningeal enhancement. 24 × 3 mm size peripherally enhancing infected subcutaneous dorsal dermal sinus at L5, S1 level. Conus ends at L2 vertebrae level.

Myelomeningocele: Evidence of large lumbosacral myelomeningocele with herniation of meninges and the neural elements through the wide posterior osseous spinal defect at L3 to lower sacrum. Myelomeningocele sac measures 9.5 × 9 cm. Neural elements are seen dangling from the myelomeningocele sac. Mild prominence of the central canal of the cord. There is tethering of the cord. No filum terminale lipoma. No sacral hypoplasia. No vertebral segmentation anomalies. No evidence of cerebellar tonsillar herniation.

Meningocele/terminal myelocystocele: Evidence of large lumbosacral meningocele with herniation of meninges through the wide posterior osseous spinal defect at L3 to lower sacrum. Meningocele sac measures 9.5 × 9 cm. Mild prominence of the central canal of the cord. There is tethering of the cord. No filum terminale lipoma. No sacral hypoplasia. No vertebral segmentation anomalies. Terminal end of cord noted at L3 vertebral level. The sac is covered with skin. Cord ends above the L3 vertebra.

Ventral cord herniation: Anterior herniation of the cord at D5 vertebral level with prominent subarachnoid space in the posterior aspect—suggestive of idiopathic ventral cord herniation.

Diastematomyelia: Evidence of diastematomyelia from D9 to upper border of L3 vertebra and tethering of the cord, with conus ending at L3-L4 level. Bony spur seen at D12–L1 vertebrae level measuring 79 mm (AP) × 6.4 mm (width) × 7.8 mm (CC). Two hemicords unite inferiorly at L3 vertebrae level. Focal syringomyelia of the left hemicord at D12 to L2 vertebrae level.

Lipomyelocele: 41 mm (CC) × 20 mm (TRANS) × 13 mm (AP) size transitional lipoma in the dorsal aspect of the conus extending from L1 to S1 vertebrae level with tethering of cord. Conus ends at lower border of L5 vertebrae level. Transitional lipoma continuous up to the subcutaneous fat through the posterior spinal defect at L4, L5 vertebrae level. Focal syringomyelia (16 × 7 mm) at D12, L1 vertebrae level. No evidence of cerebellar tonsilar herniation.

LDM (limited dorsal myeloschisis): Linear fibro neural tract extending from the dorsal aspect of the conus at upper L2 level and connected to the skin through the small posterior spinal defect at L3–L4 level. There is herniation of the CSF through the same posterior spinal defect with CSF sac surrounding the fibro neural tract in the subcutaneous plane. CSF sac measuring about 20 × 10 mm (saccular type).

2

Mucopolysaccharidosis: J-shaped sella seen. Multiple prominent VR space noted along the corpus callosum and white matter. Acute kyphosis (Gibbus) at the thoracolumbar junction due to wedging of L1 vertebral body. Platyspondyly. Prominent—postdens soft tissue thickening and posterior ligamentous thickening (thickened dural ring at the foramen magnum) causing narrowing of postdens space and cervical cord compression. No evidence of altered signal intensity in the cervical cord.

Spinal dural arteriovenous fistula (Type I spinal AVM): Prominent dilated serpiginous vessels in the posterior spinal canal of thoracic region, more prominent in the lower dorsal region from D8 to D12 and in the anterior spinal canal from D5 to D11 level. MR angiography shows feeding vessel from D9 to D10 left radicular artery. Cord hyperintensity noted from D8 vertebral level to conus with mild expansion of cord and heterogeneous enhancement—features favour cord edema/ischemia (venous hypertensive congestive myelopathy).

Grade I spondylolisthesis of L5 over S1 with bilateral spondylolysis of L5 pars interarticularis.

Spondylolysis: Defect in the bilateral pars articularis of the L5 vertebra causing grade 1 anterolisthesis of L5 over the S1 vertebra. Sclerosis and degenerative changes noted in the posterior elements of the L5 vertebra. Associated with pseudodisc bulge and mild bilateral neural foramen narrowing.

Hirayama disease: Moderate localized lower cervical cord atrophy at C3 to C6–C7 with cord hyperintensity predominantly involving central, anterior gray matter (C3 on right hemicord and C4 on the left hemicord to C6–C7). Cervical abnormal curvature and symmetric cord flattening noted. Loss of attachment of dorsal dural sac, anterior displacement of the dorsal dura on flexion (from C3 to D1) and a prominent posterior epidural space with a prominent epidural veins which appears as flow void in space sequence. On contrast administration contrast enhancement noted in the posterior epidural component.

Burst fracture: Burst fracture noted involving body of D9 vertebra with fracture fragment causing mild narrowing of spinal canal and mild injury to the posterior ligamentous complex (PLC). No evidence of any injury to nerve roots and spinal cord compression—**TLICS-4** (Table 2.10).

Spine trauma: Jefferson fracture: Linear fracture noted on the left and right sides of the anterior and posterior arches of the atlas. Minimal displacement of the posterior arch noted. Atlantodental interval is increased measuring 6 mm.

Locked facet: Dislocation of the left facet joint of C6 behind C7 noted resulting in a unilateral locked facet causing grade 2 anterolisthesis of C6 on C7. Associated rotatory subluxation without dislocation of the right facet joint. No associated fracture is seen on the right side.

Table 2.10: Thoracolumbar injury classification and severity score (TLICS) calculation					
Injury morphology	*Point value*	*PLC status*	*Point value*	*Neurological status*	*Point value*
Compression	1	Intact	0	Intact	0
Burst	2	Injury suspected or intermediate	2	Nerve root involvement	2
Translation or rotation	3	Injured	3	Spinal cord or conus medullaris injury Incomplete Complete	 2 2
Distraction	4			Cauda equina syndrome	3

Alignment and articulation of the rest of the cervical vertebra appears normal.

Spinal TB: Altered T2 signal intensity noted involving the body of D6 to D8 vertebrae with collapse and anterior wedging of the D7 vertebra. Loss of intervertebral disc height noted. There is a prevertebral, paravertebral and epidural collection extending from the D5 to L3 vertebral levels. Epidural collection causes narrowing of the spinal canal with compression of the spinal cord at the D6 level. Anterior subligamentous spread noted. Left psoas appears enlarged with a T2 hyperintense collection noted from L2 to L4 levels. On contrast, the collection shows thick, peripheral enhancement. Visualized lung fields show multiple miliary nodules.

Infective spondylodiscitis: D5–D6 disc signal alteration adjacent vertebral marrow signal changes with epidural soft tissue collection causing mild cord compression without significant cord signal abnormality. Lytic destruction of D11 and D12 vertebral bodies with partial collapse of D12. There is involvement of the D11–D12 disc space. Anterior epidural soft tissue thickening at D11–D12 level indenting the cord and extending to the right D11–D12 neural foramina. There is adjacent pre and paravertebral abscess and large right psoas abscess (7 × 6.6 × 20 cm). Right kidney is pushed laterally by the psoas abscess.There is involvement of the adjacent D10 and L1 vertebral bodies. There is marrow edema of pedicles of D11 and D12. Mild scoliosis of lower dorsal spine with convexity to left.

Transverse myelitis: Long segment T2 hyperintensity noted in the cord extending from the C5 to D2 levels. Predominantly central cord involvement noted in the T2 axial images. Cord appears mildly expanded with associated oedema. The rest of the cord appears normal. There is no enhancement on contrast. There is no associated syrinx.

Disc bulge: Disc dessication with diffuse disc bulge noted at the L4–L5 level causing spinal canal narrowing with compression of the ventral thecal sac without causing any significant compression of the nerve roots.

Disc protrusion: Disc dessication with focal right paracentral disc protrusion noted at the L4–L5 level along with facetal arthrosis causing spinal canal narrowing and compression of the right exiting L5 nerve root. No evidence of synovial cyst.

Intramedullary ependymoma: Evidence of intramedullary heterogeneously enhancing mass lesion with cystic areas and hemosiderin rim measuring about 10 × 14 × 62 mm (AP × TR × CC) at lower C2 to upper C7 level. Expanding the cord with cord edema extending up to the lower medulla superiorly and D3 level inferiorly.

Chest

COVID-19: Multiple focal patchy ground-glass opacities with interstitial thickening in bilateral lung fields predominately lower lobe and peripheral involvement—likely viral pneumonitis (CT chest severity score: 10/25), lung involvement 40% (moderate).

Percentage of lobe involved:

1. <5% involvement,
2. 5–25% involvement,
3. 26 to 50% involvement,
4. 51 to 75% involvement,
5. 76 to 100% involvement.

CT severity score: Severe: 16–25, moderate: 9–15, mild: 0–8.

Interstitial pneumonitis: Extensive intralobular and interlobular septal thickening, ground glass opacities in both lungs and minimal traction bronchiolectasis noted in the subpleural interstitium more severe in the basal segments of both lower lobes. Features favour interstitial pneumonitis.

Usual interstitial pneumonia pattern: Subpleural interstitial thickening with early honey combing in both lungs with predominant involvement of the bases.

Hypersensitive pneumonitis: Crazy paving pattern of ground glass opacities with interstitial thickening in bilateral lower lobe lung with mosaic attenuation in bilateral upper lobe lung with sparing of basal segment—possible **hypersensitive pneumonitis.**

Fibrotic lung disease checklist: Zonal distribution, honeycombing, traction bronchiectasis, reticulations, ground-glass opacities, air trapping, cyst, consolidation, emphysema, lymph node, oesophageal dilatation, pulmonary artery size, aorta size, coronary calcification, cardiac chambers, pericardium (thickening/effusion), pleura.

Neuroendocrine cell hyperplasia (children): There is extensive ground-glass opacities with areas of nodules in the central part of bilateral lung with peripheral air trapping—features favour neuroendocrine cell hyperplasia of infancy.

Lobar consolidation: Consolidation with air bronchogram noted in the right upper lobe. Right minimal pleural effusion. No significant mediastinal lymph nodes

Metastasis: Multiple well-defined circumscribed soft tissue dense lesion of varying size with basal predominance noted in the bilateral lung fields. Largest lesion measuring 5 × 6 cm right upper lobe posterior segment and smallest measuring 2 × 1 cm in the superior segment of left lower lobe.

Septic emboli: Multiple well-defined cavitating soft tissue dense nodules with peripheral and basal predominance noted in the bilateral lung fields.

Multifocal pneumonitis: Subsegmental atelectasis with consolidation involving the right middle lobe medial, both lower lobes apical, posterior basal segment with air bronchogram and patchy air space opacities.

Tuberculosis: Centrilobular nodules in tree in bud pattern noted in the apical and anterior segment of right upper lobe. Cavitation with surrounding consolidation measuring 3 × 4 cm noted in the left upper lobe. Right minimal pleural effusion noted. A few enlarged necrotic lymph nodes noted in the right paratracheal region and bilateral hilar region.

Achalasia cardia–post-POEM status: Post-surgical clips noted in the right lateral wall of lower thoracic oesophagus and GE junction. No oral contrast extravasation. No evidence of mediastinal collection/ hematoma. Mild dilatation of esophagus. Minimal air seen in the mediastinum and peritoneal cavity. Bilateral minimal pleural effusion with plate atelectasis changes in both bases.

Lung mass: An ill-defined heterogeneously enhancing mass lesion approximately measuring 4.5 × 4 cm noted in the right upper lobe anterior segment with collapse of upper lobe lung parenchyma. Abrupt cut-off of right upper lobe bronchus. No satellite lesion/ interstitial thickening/pleural effusion/mediastinal lymphadenoapthy noted, the lesion shows no contact with mediastinum and pleura. Chest wall appears normal.Visualized skeleton appears normal. A few enlarged lymph nodes noted in the right paratracheal region. Visualised supraclavicular region, liver and adrenals appear normal (staging T3N0M0).

Checklist: Location, appearance (solid, part solid, ground glass), size, infiltration of adjacent structures (aorta, pericardium, heart, bronchus, carina, diaphragm, pleura, mediastinal fat), lymph nodes, intra and extra thoracic metastases.

Mediastinal lymphoma: Evidence of soft tissue density lesion in the right lower neck and superior mediastinum measuring about 4.9 × 4 × 9 cm encasing the right common carotid artery, IJV, subclavian and brachiocephalic artery and vein, vertebral artery, superior vena cava , ascending aorta and arch of aorta. Trachea is mildly pushed to left side without significant compromise of the airway.

Scimitar syndrome (pulmonary venolobar syndrome): There is volume loss of right lung with mediastinal shift to the right and dextro position of heart. Right superior pulmonary vein is seen draining abnormally into the azygos vein, SVC and another abnormal right inferior pulmonary vein is seen draining into the IVC giving scimitar-like appearance. There is an abnormal arterial feeding vessel to the right lung parenchyma which is arising from the coeliac trunk. Left superior and inferior pulmonary veins are draining into the left atrium. Main pulmonary and left pulmonary arteries appear normal. Measurements (diameter in mm): Scimitar vein; Proximal–7.0, Distal–7.8. Right pulmonary artery: Proximal–8.9, Distal–8.0. Left single pulmonary venous trunk: Proximal–5.4, Distal–2.6. Left pulmonary artery: Proximal–7.3, Distal–6.2.

Acute pulmonary thromboembolism: Main pulmonary artery and its bifurcation appear normal. There is evidence of multiple embolism in right main pulmonary artery, interlobar right lower lobe segmental arteries, left main, left upper lobes and right lower lobe segmental arteries with irregular surface. Size of thrombus measures from 3 to 16 mm. No evidence of total occlusion. Most of thrombus in right lower lobe segmental artery lies freely within the lumen with contrast medium seen surrounding thrombus. Main, right and left pulmonary artery dimensions are within normal limits. No CT evidence of pulmonary arterial hypertension. No evidence of pulmonary infarction. No evidence of consolidation.

Comment about caliber of pulmonary arteries (main trunk, left main branch, right main branch), right heart strain, pulmonary infarction, patency of airways, pleura, pericardium, upper abdomen.

Cardiovascular System

Major aortopulmonary collateral arteries (MAPCAs): Multiple MAPCAs from left subclavian artery. Proximal MAPCA is large and descends down vertically supplying the left lung. Right subclavian artery proximal segment shows a moderate sized MAPCA looping up and descending down. Large MAPCA supplying the confluence arising from the distal arch of aorta. Moderate sized MAPCA arising from descending thoracic aorta at D7 level. Right pulmonary artery measures 11.4 mm. Left pulmonary artery measures 9.8 mm. Main pulmonary artery measures 9.1 mm. Ascending aorta measures 29 mm.

Ascending aortic aneurysm: Ascending aorta measures 4.1 cm with eccentric thrombus suggestive of fusiform aneurysm for a length of 7.6 cm till the origin of brachiocephalic artery. Patent lumen measures 3.1 cm. Arch measures 3.7 cm. Descending thoracic aorta measures 3.7 cm. Abdominal aorta at hiatus measures 3.9 cm. Infrarenal aorta measures 2.3 cm (Table 2.11).

Coronary arteriovenous fistula: Right coronary artery co-dominant and normal. Right posterior descending artery is normal. Separate origin of large conal branch with ectatic segment and communicating with MPA suggestive of coronary to pulmonary AV fistula. The fistula also communicates with first septal from LAD.

Anomalous coronary artery: Left anterior descending coronary artery: Arises from right coronary trunk courses anterior to aorta and pulmonary artery to enter interventricular groove (Type I course). It gives off two diagonals and septals. Type III vessel with 50–60% ostial stenosis and 20–30% stenosis in mid segment. Diagonals are normal. Left circumflex coronary artery: Nondominant; courses posterior to aorta and pulmonary artery. It is small and normal. Right coronary artery: Dominant with mild midsegment irregularities.RV branch continues as PDA and is normal. Large PLV is normal.

Aortic dissection: Dissecting aneurysm involving the distal arch of aorta, distal to the left subclavian artery with intimal flap extending up to the infrarenal abdominal aorta, 3 cm prior to bifurcation. Aortic bifurcation appears normal: Type B Stanford classification. No evidence of aortic wall irregularity/pleural and pericardial hyperdense haematoma to suggest rupture. No evidence of thrombus. SMA, inferior mesenteric artery, right main and accessory renal artery arising from the false lumen. Dissection intimal flap extending to the proximal left renal artery. No evidence of altered perfusion in the kidneys. Tortuous course of descending thoracic aorta seen.

Coarctation of aorta: Ascending aorta measures 26 mm. Arch measures 19 mm. Coarctation noted at D4 level measuring 8.2 mm proximal to the PDA, PDA measures 8 mm in length with 6.8 mm in diameter. Pre-ductal segment of aorta measures 14.8 mm. Post-ductal aorta measures 14.6 mm. Prominent D4, D5, D6 intercostal vessels noted. MPA measures 36 mm. RPA measures 18 mm. LPA measures 15.4 mm. Origin of innominate artery, left common carotid artery and left subclavian artery appear normal.

Transposition of great arteries: Concordant veno arterial connection. Discordant atrioventricular and ventriculo-arterial connection. Aorta is seen anterior and to the left of main pulmonary artery: Levo transposition of the great arteries (L-TGA). Left and right ventricles with their corresponding anteroventricular valves are also transposed. Atrial septal defect measuring about 10.1 mm. Ascending aorta measures 23 mm. Dilated left atrium and appendage. Mildly dilated IVC (24 mm). Right atrium is small. Morphologic right ventricle seen in the left side with prominent trabeculations. Mild hypokinesia of the apical and apex of the left side of ventricle. Altered signal intensity in the myometrium of the left ventricle predominantly involving the anterior wall. No evidence of delayed enhancement. Pulmonary infundibulum hypertrophy with lumen measuring ~2 cm. Main pulmonary artery measures 33 mm. Left pulmonary artery measures 20 mm. Right pulmonary artery measures 13 mm. Main pulmonary artery partly overrides the left ventricular outflow.

Trans catheter aortic valve implantation workup: Cuspidity of native valves, leaflet calcifications, subvalvular calcifications, Agatston score of leaflet calcification, aortic

Table 2.11: The aortic measurements at various levels—sample reporting format

Level	*Dimensions*	*Level*	*Dimensions*
Aortic sinus	42 mm	Descending thoracic aorta	40 mm
Ascending aorta	38 mm	Suprarenal abdominal aorta	32 mm
Proximal to aortic arch	29 mm	At the level of renal arteries	25 mm
Midaortic arch	29 mm	Infrarenal abdominal aorta	22 mm
Just distal to left subclavian artery	50 mm		

anulus measurements both in systole and diastole, annular short and long axis diameter in mm, annular perimeter in mm, annular area in mm^2, inner diameter of degenerative prosthetic valve in mm (for valve in valve procedure), aortic sinus height, width, distance from annular plane to left and right coronary ostium, diameter of sinotubular junction, maximum cross sectional diameter of ascending aorta, comment about patency and luminal diameter of brachiocephalic, subclavian, common iliac, external iliac and common femoral artery.

Concentric left ventricular hypertrophy: The left ventricular myocardium shows concentric hypertrophy. The observed LV mass is 245 gm and the BSA indexed mass (119 gm/m^2) qualifies for hypertrophy as per echo guidelines (>114 gm/m^2). The LV posterior wall and inter-ventricular septum each measure 16 mm in thickness in diastole. There is no dyskinesia/failure to thicken of any of the LV myocardial segments. And all the LV cardiac segments contract well. The inter-ventricular septum is intact.

Conclusions

1. Significant concentric left ventricular hypertrophy suggesting long standing systemic hypertension.
2. Normal cardiac anatomy and myocardial function.

Noncompaction cardiomyopathy: Mild dilatation of left ventricle. Moderate dilatation of left atrium. Global hypokinesis of the left ventricle. Prominent trabeculation noted in the endomyocardium of apex and mild left ventricular cavity. Basal left ventricle is relatively spared. Mild delayed enhancement of the endocardium. Minimal mitral regurgitations seen.

MRI analysis shows: End diastolic (ED) volume–78.2 (ml/m^2). End systolic volume–54 (ml/m^2). Stroke volume–23.3 (ml/m^2). Cardiac index–1.86 (min/m^2).

Table 2.12: Measurements from SSFP images acquired during diastole

Diameter in mm	*Proximal*	*Distal*
Main pulmonary artery	18 × 20	
Aortic annulus	24 × 28	
Aortic sinus	39 × 40	
Sino-aortic Jn	30 × 32	
Ascending aorta	32 × 33	

Myocardial mass at ED–67.2 (gm/m^2). Myocardial mass average–68.2 + 5.5 (gm/m^2). Ejection fraction–29.8%.

Arrythomogenic right ventricular dysplasial cardiomyopathy: Some regions of the **anterior wall of the right ventricle is thinned** out. The RVOT is dilated (31 mm × 34 mm), **dyskinetic and shows systolic anterior bulge**. Apart from the RVOT, there is an area in the **sub-tricuspid region which is also dyskinetic.** The BSA indexed RV end diastolic volume is increased to more than the normal, the end-systolic volume to about twice the normal. **There is global index of RV contractility (RVEF = 23–26%).** The right atrium is mild dilated. The interatrial septum is intact. There is mild tricuspid regurgitation (about 6–9 ml/heart beat, difference in the stroke volumes). The venous drainage, atrio-ventricular and the ventriculo-arterial connections are concordant. The atrio-ventricular valves and the semilunar valves function normally without any stenosis or regurgitation. The inter-atrial and the inter-ventricular septae are intact. The aortic arch is left sided and has normal branching pattern. The main pulmonary artery and its branches have normal caliber. The left atrium is not dilated. The left ventricle has upper limits of normal body surface area indexed end diastolic volume. The indexed LV end systolic volume is about 1 and ½ times the upper limits of normal due to global hypokinesia and IVS dyskinesia.

Table 2.13: Ventricular volume measurements (Heart rate: 77 /min)

	EDV (ml)	*ESV (ml)*	*SV (ml/beat)*	*EF%*	*Ventricular CO (L/min)*
LV	80	28	52	65	4.03
RV	80	26	54	68	4.22
Indexed ventricular volume measurements					
Male standards	*EDV (ml/ m^2)*	*Normal EDV*	*ESV (ml/m^2)*	*Normal ESV*	*Ventricular CI (L/min/m^2)*
LV	39	47–92	14	13–30	1.95
RV	39	55–105	13	15–45	2.05
Great vessel flow (Heart rate: 77/min)					
	FF (ml/beat)	*BF (ml/beat)*	*Net FF (ml/beat)*	*RF%*	*Arterial flow (L/min)*
Aorta	63	4	59	7	4.62
MPA	62	2	59	4	4.60

CO–cardiac output, CI–cardiac index

The IVS is thinned out. The IVS is also dyskinetic. The index of systolic function is significantly depressed (LV EF = 26%). Some areas of the septum also show delayed enhancement suggesting myocardial fibrosis. **The features will fit in with a major criteria for ARVD/C from MRI point of view as per 2010 revised guidelines (regional wall movement abnormalities and RV dysfunction).**

Endocardial myofibrosis: Endocavitatory filling defect in the apex of right ventricle obliterating the ventricular apex with no enhancement consistent with thrombus/ fibrosed soft tissue. Systolic dysfunction in SSFP and gradient sequences of the right ventricular apex noted. Moderate dilatation of both atrium (Right > Left). Thickened soft tissue in the apex of right ventricle with compromised right ventricular cavity. Thin rim of enhancement along the endocardial aspect of right ventricle in the delayed images.

Situs solitus with levocardia. Mild to moderate mitral and tricuspid regurgitation. Dilated IVC and hepatic vein. Global hypokinesia of the left ventricle. No evidence of perfusion defect. RV and LV appear smaller in size. RV apex and LV apex obliterated due to focal thickening.

Ejection fraction of LV is 29%. 16 × 8 mm size non enhancing hypointense lesion ventricular cavity at the anterior wall of left ventricle near the apex with perfusion defect—thrombus. Delayed contrast enhancement study shows mild endocardial enhancement along the basal and mid-LV cavity and intense enhancement along the endocardium in the apical and apex of RV and LV. Patchy transmural enhancement of the apical, anterior and anterolateral wall of left ventricle.

Infarct/scar in the basal inferolateral, basal anterolateral, mid anterior, mid inferoseptal, mid inferolateral, mid anterolateral, apical septal, apical lateral segments of left ventricle with more than 50% of thickness involvement—non-viable myocardium. Rest of the LV is to be assessed for reversible perfusion defects in stress perfusion if indicated (Table 2.14).

Hypokinesia/akinesia with perfusion defect and delayed contrast enhancement involving subendocardial region (>50%) of basal inferoseptal, basal inferior, basal inferolateral, mid anterior, anteroseptal, inferior, apical anterior, septal, lateral and apex suggestive of infarct (nonviable myocardium). Aneurysmal dilatation of left ventricular apex. Situs solitus with levocardia.

Mammogram

Breast mass: **X-ray mammogram:** Ill-defined radio-dense lesions with spiculated margins and internal micro calcifications noted in UOQ of right breast at 11 o'clock position zone II 4 cm depth from skin . Diffuse dermal thickening noted. Nipple and subareolar tissues are normal on the left side.The pectroralis and retro mammary space appears normal. Rounded dense right axillary lymph nodes are seen. **Ultrasound screening:** Irregular hypoechoic mass lesion with internal micro calcifications measuring 4.1 × 3.8 × 2.8 cm noted predominantly in UOQ of right breast. There is extension of the lesion to subcutaneous tissue. With Doppler there is internal vascularity. The left breast shows normal fibrogandular tissues. Enlarged rounded lymph nodes with thickened cortex largest measuring 22 × 15 mm noted in right axilla-**BIRADS V.**

Fibroadenoma: Well-defined hypoechoic lesion measuring about 33 × 20 mm in size seen in the UOQ of the right breast at 10–11 o'clock position. Minimal intralesional vascularity noted. **This lesion is characterized as probable benign (BIRADS category –III)-Fibroadenoma to be considered.**

Gynecomastia: **X-ray mammogram:** Asymmetric increased glandular tissue noted in right breast. **Ultrasound screening:** Retroareolar diffuse hypoechoic tissue noted in both breast (R > L)—findings consistent with glandular tissue. No focal lesions noted. No abnormal vascularity seen.

Breast imaging reporting and data system (BIRADS): Grade 1–Negative. Grade 2–Benign. Grade 3–Probably benign. Grade 4–Suspicious abnormality. Grade 5–Highly suggestive of malignancy. Grade 6–Known biopsy proven malignancy.

Abdomen

Acute edematous pancreatitis: Pancreas appears bulky with peripancreatic inflammation extending to the gastro colic ligament, lesser omentum and left Gerota's fascia. No evidence of pancreatic necrosis/pseudocyst/ pancreatic calcification/pancreatic duct dilatation/ CBD, GB, pancreatic duct calculus/pseudoaneurysm in adjacent vessels/thrombosis of splenic and portal vein/ pancreatic divisum. No biliary dilatation/radiodense CBD calculus.

Mild ascites. Bilateral mild pleural effusion (left >right) with underlying lung parenchymal changes. Above features favour acute edematous pancreatitis. Modified CT severity index 2/10.

Modified CT severity index: Scores are generated by estimating pancreatic inflammation and necrosis to give a score out of 10.

Pancreatic inflammation: 0–normal pancreas, 2–intrinsic pancreatic abnormalities with or without

Table 2.14: Structural and morphology left ventricle on cardiac MRI								
Lateral ventricle segments	*Trabeculation*	*End diastolic (mm)*	*Endsystolic (m)*	*Wall motion*	*Dynamic perfusion*	*Delayed hyper-enhancement*	*Stress perfu-sion*	*Impression*
Basal anterior	P	6.9	11.3	Normal	Normal	No	Not done	Normal/RPD
Basal anteroseptal	A	10.4	13.8	Hypokinesia	MPD	<25 % thickness		Infarct/scar
Basal inferoseptal	A	8.2	8.2	Akinesia	MPD	Transmural		Infarct/scar
Basal inferior	A	5.9	5.8	Akinesia	MPD	Transmural		Infarct/scar
Basal inferolateral	A	3.4	4	Akinesia	MPD	Transmural		Infarct/scar
Basal anterolateral	P	6.3	7.5	Normal	Normal	No		Normal/ reversible perfusion defect
Mid anterior	P	7.9	9.2	Normal	Normal	No		Normal/ reversible perfusion defect
Mid anteroseptal	T	6.9	9.2	Hypokinesia	Mild	25–50%		Infarct/scar
Mid inferoseptal	A	5.7	5.2	Akinesia	PD	Transmural		Infarct/scar
Mid inferior	A	2	2.2	Akinesia	PD	Transmural		Infarct/scar
Mid inferolateral	A	2.2	2.1	Akinesia	PD	Transmural		Infarct/scar
Mid anterolateral	P	6.8	15	Normal	Normal	Normal		Normal/RPD
Apical anterior	P	6.7	13	Normal	Normal	Subendocardial		Infarct/scar
Apical septal	A	4.8	10	Hypokinesia	MPD	50% thickness		Infarct/scar
Apical inferior	A	3.1	3.2	Akinesia	PD	Transmural		Infarct/scar
Apical lateral	P	7.8	10.3	Hypokinesia	MPD	Transmural		Infarct/scar
Apex	T	2.3	4.3	Hypokinesia	--------	Transmural		Infarct/scar

A–absent, P–present, MPD–mild to moderate perfusion defect, RPD–reversible perfusion defect; PD–perfusion defect

*Normal/reversible perfusion defects are assessed with stress perfusion.

*Segmental wall thickness = ES–ED/ED × 100

*Patterns of delayed enhancement–subendocardial/transmural/patchy/linear midwall/epicardial zone. 1 to 25% thickness enhancement (subendocardial). 25 to 50% thickness enhancement. 50 to 70% thickness enhancement. More than 70% thickness enhancement (transmural).

inflammatory changes in peripancreatic fat, 4–pancreatic or peripancreatic fluid collection or peripancreatic fat necrosis.

Pancreatic necrosis: 0–none, 2–30% or less, 4–more than 30%.

Extrapancreatic complications: 2–one or more of pleural effusion, ascites, vascular complications, parenchymal complications and/or gastrointestinal involvement.

Total score: Total points are given out of 10 to determine the grade of pancreatitis and aid treatment. 0–2: mild, 4–6: moderate, 8–10: severe.

USG–acute pancreatitis: Altered echoes in the pancreas with peripancreatic inflammation and left Gerota's fascia thickening. No evidence of pancreatic calcification/calculi/pancreatic duct dilatation—features favours acute pancreatitis.

Chronic calcific pancreatitis: The parenchyma of the neck, body and tail of the pancreas is completely atrophied with dilated and tortuous pancreatic duct. Main pancreatic duct and its branches are dilated with maximum diameter of......mm. Multiple irregular calculi noted within the dilated main pancreatic duct and side branches. Calculus in the neck of pancreas measures ....mm. No parenchymal calcification noted. The pancreatic parenchyma of head and uncinate process are preserved. No altered signals noted within the head and uncinate process. The peripancreatic fat is preserved. The peripancreatic vascular system appears normal. No perivascular cuff noted. No peripancreatic collections.

No stricture of CBD/ IHBRD. No vascular complications like venous thrombosis, pseudoaneurysm formation or splenic infarcts.

Pancreatic divisum variant: Persistent communication between the ventral and dorsal pancreatic ducts.

Pancreatic divisum with mild dilatation of dorsal moiety duct maximum measuring mm. Ventral moiety duct narrowing with focal ductal dilatation measuring mm. Presence/absence of intraductal calculus with/ without intrapancreatic and peripancreatic fluid collection measuring about cm and inflammation extending into the portion of duodenum.

Carcinoma pancreas: Ill-defined heterogeneously enhancing mass lesion approximately measuring 2.4 × 2.3 × 3 cm (AP × TR × CC) noted in the head of the pancreas. The lesion causes abutment of superior mesenteric, splenic, portal vein confluence. No evidence of regional lymph node enlargement, peritoneal deposit, liver lesions, ascites. Celiac artery, superior mesenteric artery, portal vein shows normal opacification. No evidence of distant metastatic nodules in the spleen, adrenals, visualized lung fields, vertebra and pelvic bones.

Carcinoma pancreas–reporting checklist: **Morphology:** Appearance (in pancreatic parenchymal phase): Hypo/ iso/hyper attenuating; Size: Maximal diameters in axial and transverse; Location: Head, uncinated, body or tail; Pancreatic duct status: Presence of abrupt narrowing/ cut off. Presence or absence of upstream dilatation, ductal calculus if any with maximum diameter of the duct. Biliary tree: Cut off/ dilatation, perineural spread. **Arterial evaluation (SMA, celiac axis, common hepatic artery, variant vessel):** Degree of vessel soft-tissue contact (<180 or >180 degrees), degree of haziness/stranding contact (<180 or >180 degrees), focal narrowing/contour irregularity (+/–), extension to branches/bifurcation (+/–). **Venous evaluation:** Vessel degree of solid soft tissue contact (<180 or >180 degrees), Degree of haziness/stranding contact (<180 or >180 degrees), Focal narrowing/contour irregularity (+/–), extension to branches/bifurcation (+/–), extension to first draining vein, thrombus within vein. **Extra pancreatic evaluation:** Liver lesions, peritoneal/omental lesions, ascites, suspicious lymph nodes, extra pancreatic adjacent structure involvement.

Serous cystadenoma pancreas....mm size measuring multilobular cystic lesion with central scar and calcification in the head and uncinate process of pancreas. The lesion causes mass effect on MPD resulting in dilatation (mm in the body of pancreas) of main pancreatic duct.

Mucinous cystadenoma: Evidence of well-defined exophytic cystic lesion measuring about 5.5 × 3.9 × 3.5 cm in the anterior aspect of the head/neck of the pancreas. Thin septa with calcification seen within. No evidence of solid areas/surrounding inflammation. Lesion is communicating with the main pancreatic duct (a rare feature in mucinous cystadenoma). (Even though cyst is communicating with the MPD, possibility of IPMN is less likely due to the presence of calcification.)

Insulinoma: A well-defined strongly enhancing lesion measuring 4 × 6 mm noted in the body of pancreas. No calcification noted within the lesion. Strongly enhancing small lesion in pancreas—to rule out insulionoma.

Extra pancreatic evaluation: Liver lesions, peritoneal/ omental lesions, ascites, suspicious lymph nodes, extra pancreatic adjacent structure involvement.

Cirrhosis liver: Liver is shrunken in size measures 8.5 cm with atrophy of the anterior segment of the right lobe and hypertrophy of the caudate lobe and lateral segment of left lobe. The caudate lobe to right lobe ratio is 0.87 (more than 0.65 definite sign of cirrhosis). There is widening of the fissures for ligamentum teres and ligamentum venosum. There is evidence of posterior hepatic notch noted in segment VI. Diffuse heterodense liver parenchyma with surface nodularity. No evidence of intra or extra hepatic biliary radicle dilatation. No arterial phase enhancing mass lesion to suggest hepatocellular carcinoma. Partial thrombosis of the main portal vein extending into the right and left intrahepatic branches. Main portal vein is enlarged and measures in mm. The superior mesenteric vein appears dilated, measures in mm. The splenic vein appears dilated measures in mm. Portosystemic collaterals noted in splenic hilum, lienorenal ligament and around the GE junction. Left renal vein is normal. Features are suggestive of cirrhosis liver with portal hypertension and portosystemic collaterals. No arterial phase enhancing mass lesion to suggest hepatocellular carcinoma.

Portal hypertension (Doppler): Liver appears shrunken with coarse echoes, irregular surface blunted margins, portal vein measures 12 mm at hilum, no evidence of filling defect in the main portal vein. Portal vein velocity 12 cm/s hepatopetal flow, multiple dilated tortuous splenohilar and splenorenal collaterals. Hepatic veins patent shows monophasic flow. Free fluid noted in the pelvis.

Hepatocellular carcinoma: A round T2 hyperintense lesion, showing restricted diffusion measuring 21 × 40 mm noted in segment VI of liver. The lesion shows significant nonrim arterial phase enhancement with washout in portal venous phase, it shows capsular enhancement in equilibrium phase, the size of the lesion has doubled compared to previous imaging taken 6 months back-**LI-RADS: LR-5 (definite HCC).**

Checklist for HCC: Location (mention the segment), size, tumoral thrombus, nonrim arterial phase hyper enhancement, threshold growth, nonperipheral washout appearance, enhancing capsule appearance, lymph node status, remaining abdomen for extrahepatic mass.

Cholelithiasis: Multiple small GB calculi without diffuse gall bladder wall thickening. No evidence of CBD calculus/CBD, IHBR dilatation/pancreatitis/pericholecystic fluid collection. Features favour cholelithiasis.

Calculus cholecystitis: Multiple small GB calculi with diffuse gall bladder wall thickening (4.2 mm). No evidence of CBD calculus/CBD, IHBR dilatation/pancreatitis/pericholecystic fluid collection. Features favour acute calculus cholecystitis.

Klatskin's tumor: Soft tissue lesion in the confluence of hepatic ducts and proximal CHD causing dilatation of right hepatic duct (... mm in diameter), left hepatic duct (.... mm in diameter) and IHBR. No evidence of periportal/paraaortic lymphadenopathy/focal liver mass lesion. The mass lesion encasing the left hepatic artery and left branch of portal vein causing moderate to severe luminal narrowing. Total length of RHD, LHD and CHD involvement is ....mm. Features favour Klatskin's tumor (Type IV).

Mass forming intrahepatic cholangiocarcinoma: Evidence of well-defined irregular infiltrating heterointense mass lesion measuring about 7.2 × 5.7 × 7.8 cm in segment VIII of right lobe of liver. Lesion is mildly extending to segment IVA and VII of liver. It is indenting right hepatic vein and middle hepatic vein without infiltration. It is Infiltrating and narrowing hepatic duct confluence, RHD and its divisions, proximal LHD and CHD with bilobar intrahepatic biliary dilatation. CBD is not dilated. Tumor is extending to right branch of portal vein. Main portal vein and left branch are normal. It is encasing the right branch of hepatic artery. On contrast administration, mass shows thick irregular peripheral rim enhancement in arterioportal phase with peripheral wash out, central enhancement in delayed images and hepatobiliary phase. Features are consistent with mass forming intrahepatic cholangiocarcinoma (MF-ICC) in right lobe of liver with biliary and portal vein invasion.

Cholangiocarcinoma checklist: Size (maximal axial dimensions in cm), location (upper/mid/lower third of bile duct), hepatic duct involvement (right/left/both). Second-order ductal branch involved and side: (yes/no; right/left), arterial evaluation: Common/hepatic artery proper involvement, portal vein involvement, solid soft tissue contacts, focal vessel narrowing or contour irregularity, aberrant/accessory arterial anatomy: (yes/no—specify), venous variants. Lymph nodal enlargement (>1 cm short axis), bile duct variants, remnant liver volume and distant metastases.

Mirizzi syndrome: ....mm calculus in the cystic duct –CBD junction causing dilatation of CHD (...mm in diameter). Right hepatic duct (...mm in diameter) left hepatic duct (...mm in diameter) and IHBR—possible Mirizzi syndrome.

Type I choledochal cyst: Disproportionate diffusely dilated CHD, CBD, and distal hepatic ducts with multiple hypointense filling defects in the mid and distal CBD suggestive of calculi (largest measuring 7 mm). Mild dilatation of cystic duct and IHBR—features suggestive of Type 1 Choledochal cyst.

Type IVA choledochal cyst: Moderate dilatation of CBD, CHD, proximal right and left hepatic ducts (left > right) with abrupt change to normal calibre of the biliary radicles. Another focal cystic dilatation of segment II intrahepatic bile duct: Type IVA choledochal cyst.

Protein losing enteropathy: Mild dilatation of long segment midsmall bowel loops (jejunoileal region, predominantly involving jejunum) in the left lumbar and left iliac fossa with mild increased vascularity. It shows increased contrast enhancement and thickening of the bowel wall, with the clinical presentation of hypoproteinemia and above radiological features, the following protein losing enteropathy to be considered. Intestinal lymphangiectasia/malabsorption syndromes like celiac disease, tropical sprue/eosinophilic gastroenteritis/food-induced enteropathy. Imaging, however, cannot differentiate these conditions.

Ileocecal TB: Diffuse thickening of terminal ileum (9.1 cm length, 1.4 cm thickness), ileocecal junction, caecum (5.4 cm in length) with pericaecal mesentery fat stranding and multiple pericolic lymph nodes predominantly in the ileocolic mesentery. Diffuse narrowing of the lumen. No focal collection in the adjacent mesentry. Ileocecal junction appears pulled up. Appendix is distended with fluid. Few enlarged lymph nodes seen in the ileocolic mesentery. **Possibilities include:** 1. Tuberculosis, 2. Inflammatory bowel disease.

Active inflammatory bowel disease: Diffuse thickening of terminal ileum (9.1 cm length, 1.4 cm thickness), ileocecal junction, caecum (5.4 cm in length), proximal jejunum, transverse colon and midileum with pericaecal mesentery fat stranding and multiple pericolic lymph nodes predominantly in the ileocolic mesentery. Ileocecal junction appears normal in position. Appendix is distended with fluid and shows heterogeneous enhancement. On contrast administration shows prominent mucosa and submucosa enhancement with prominent vasa recta. No obvious evidence of stricture/sinus tract/fistulous tract/submucosal fat halo seen. No obvious evidence of perianal fistula/sacroilitis—features favour active inflammatory bowel disease—possible Crohn's disease.

Mesenteric panniculitis: A marginally defined subtle increased fat density lesion noted involving the root of the small bowel mesentery encasing the superior mesenteric vessel and its branches. No narrowing or infiltration of the vessels noted. No fibrosing component noted. The above features are suggestive of mesenteric panniculitis.

Umbilical sinus: Umbilical sinus seen measuring .... No significant abscess formation. No obvious evidence of intraperitoneal extension. No evidence of persistent uracus/vitellointestinal duct. **Omphalitis:** Focal thickening of the umbilicus measuring 12 × 10 mm. No evidence of intraperitoneal extension. No evidence of urachal remnant seen—features favour infection (omphalitis). **Urachal remnant:** Tubular channel extending from the dome of bladder along the anterior abdominal wall in the midline toward the umbilicus, representing a urachal remnant.

Incisional hernia: Left para-umbilical incisional hernia with omentum and bowel as content. No evidence of bowel obstruction/strangulation. **M3W2.**

Hirschsprung disease: Reversal of recto sigmoid ratio with more dilatation of sigmoid compared to rectum. No transitional zone identified—possibility of Hirschsprung disease to be considered.

Table 2.15: Incisional hernia reporting format

Midline	Subxiphoid	M1	
	Epigastric	M2	
	Umbilical	M3	
	Infraumbilical	M4	
	Suprapubic	M5	
Lateral	Subcostal	L1	
	Flank	L2	
	Iliac	L3	
	Lumbar	L4	
Recurrent incisional hernia—YES or NO			
Length: ....cm		Width :........cm	
Width (cm)	W1 (<4 cm), W2 (≥4–10 cm), W3 (≥10 cm)		

Appendicitis (USG): Probe tenderness noted in the right iliac fossa. Tubular, blind ending, nonperistaltic bowel loop with maximum diameter of .....mm with significant surrounding inflammation noted in the right iliac fossa suggestive of inflamed appendix.

Acute appendicitis (CT): Thickened oedematous appendix (....cm thickness) with minimal periappendiceal inflammation—features favour retrocecal acute appendicitis. No evidence of periappendicular abscess/mass lesion/appendicolith.

Carcinoma stomach: Abnormal wall thickening with luminal narrowing in distal body and antropyloric canal of stomach with maximum thickness measures 3.8 cm. There is gastric outlet obstruction with retained food particles in the overdistended stomach. No periserosal infiltration. No infiltration of the pancreas/liver. A few adjacent perigastric lymph nodes seen, largest measuring about 12 × 10 mm. No significant enlarged celiac, para aortic lymph nodes. A few tiny oval-shaped lymph nodes in the portocaval and paracaval regions. Diffuse omental fat stranding noted. (**Stage T2N1 Mx**).

CA rectum growth: Circumferential wall thickening (10 mm in thickness) in rectum for a length of 28 mm, about 6.5 cm from the anal verge. The lesion involves predominantly in the anterior rectal wall from 3 o' clock to 9 o' clock position. Lower end of the lesion is 2 mm from the horizontal portion of levator ani and 13 mm from the funnelled portion of levator ani. 7 × 5 mm size solitary enlarged lymph node in the right mesorectal fat at 8 o'clock position. Puborectalis muscle appears normal without infiltration. Internal and external anal sphincters appear normal. No infiltration of the seminal vesicles/prostate/bladder. Mesorectal fascia/Denonvilliers fascia/Waldeyer's fascia appear intact. **(colonic rads–C4/staging work up T3aN1) M staging cannot be ascertained due to limited study).**

Carcinoma rectum check list: Morphology (solid polypoid/solid annular/mucinous), in case of circumferential tumor mention the involvement in clock position. The distance of lesion from the anal verge and anorectal junction, location of lesion with respect to anterior peritoneal reflection (tumors located above the anterior peritoneal reflection in the peritonealised anterior wall do not need surgical resection unless it has invaded adjacent structures), circumferential resection margin, extramural venous invasion (>3 mm), longitudinal, cranio-caudal and largest lesion diameters, perirectal fat invasion and spiculation. Involvement of anal sphincters, presacral fascia and mesorectal fascia (a distance of the tumor to the mesorectal fascia of <1 mm is regarded unsuitable for total mesorectal excision). Extramural invasion depth (based on the depth of invasion <1 mm, 1 to 5 mm, 5 to 15 mm and >15 mm T3 stage divided into T3a, b, c and d respectively) determines the need for neoadjuvant radiation >5 mm consistent with poor prognosis, nodal spread. **Post-neoadjuvant treatment**: Look for residual tumor mass in the T2W-MR images and give **yTNM** staging.

Carcinoma of anal canal: Eccentric wall thickening (14 mm in thickness) in the anal canal for a length of 31 mm, about 31 mm from the anal verge. The lesion predominantly from 11 o'clock to 7 o'clock position. Lower end of the lesion is well below the horizontal portion of levator ani. Involvement of intersphincteric plane/mass is infiltrating the left obturator internus muscle. Presence/absence of post-operative changes with fibrosis seen in the presacral region/rectal bed.

Pilonidal sinus: Evidence of a subcutaneous fluid filled sinus tract noted in the midline in the intergluteal cleft (at the level of lower sacrum at S3–S4) extending inferiorly for about 4 cm and end blindly posterior to the sacrococcygeal junction. No evidence of fistulas communication with the spinal canal. No evidence of enteric (anus and rectum) communication or extension to the ischiorectal or ischioanal fossa. No evidence of secondary tract.

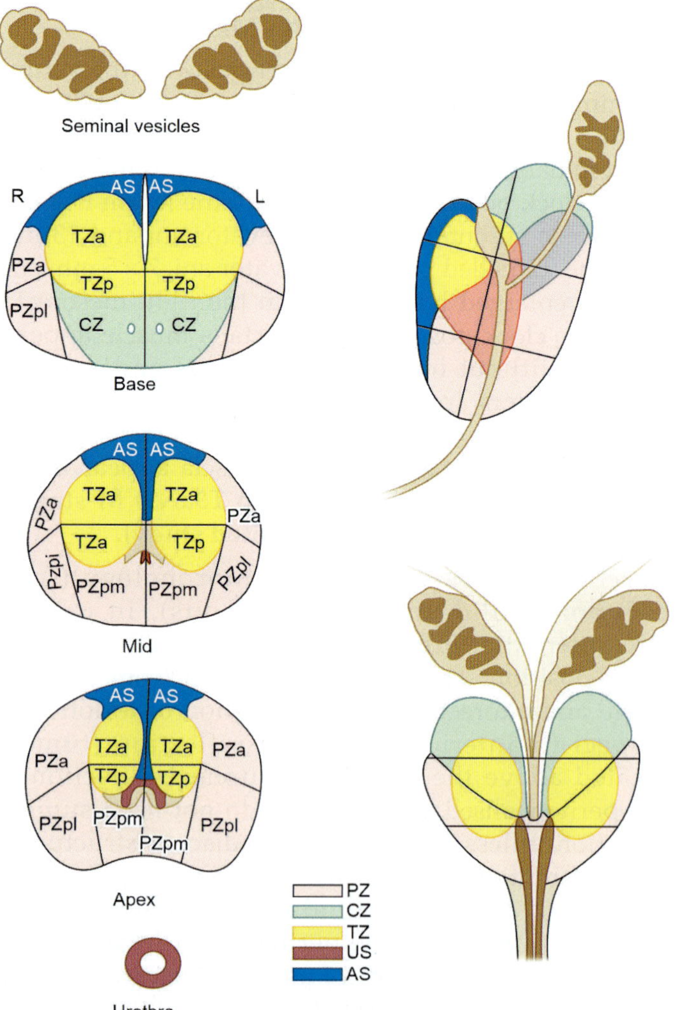

Fig. 2 8: Prostate anatomical zones for reporting

Perianal fistula: Fluid-filled left low perianal intersphincteric fistula with external opening 3 cm from the anal verge and internal opening at 12 o' clock position 1 cm from the anal verge. Total length of the fistulous tract is 38 mm. No evidence of horseshoe tract/secondary tracts/translevator and supralevator extension/ischiorectal and ischioanal abscess—**Grade I** low left perianal fistula (St. James Hospital MR classification).

Fluid-filled left low perianal trans-sphincteric fistula with external opening 12 mm from the anal verge and internal opening at 5 to 6 o' clock position 24 mm from the anal verge. Total length of the fistulous tract is 34 mm. No evidence of horseshoe tract/secondary tracts/translevator and supralevator extension/ischiorectal and ischioanal abscess—**Grade III** low left perianal fistula (St. James Hospital MR classification).

Complex fluid-filled right low perianal trans-sphincteric fistula with external opening 25 mm from the anal verge in the right posterior perineum at 7 o'clock position. The tract extends anterosuperiorly and pierce the external sphincter at 6 to 7 o'clock position and internal opening 6 o'clock position and 24 mm from the anal verge. There is another right lower intersphincteric tract coursing at 6 o'clock position joints with the upper trans-sphincteric tract in the intersphincteric plain at 6 o'clock position 24 mm from the anal verge. Then the common tract extending to the bilateral intersphincteric plain. Right intersphincteric plain tract pierces the external sphincter at 10 o'clock position no significant collection in the right ischioanal abscess. Left intersphincteric tract ends at 3 o'clock position. No evidence of translevator and supralevator extension/ischiorectal and **Grade IV** low right perianal fistula (St. James Hospital MR classification).

Checklist: Number of fistula openings, internal opening clock position, distance between internal opening and anal verge, maximum track diameter, type of fistula (inter/trans/extra/supra sphincteric and superficial), presence of secondary branches, exit site location (gluteal, scrotal, vaginal, labial, urethral, blind ending with comment about right or left side), hyperintensity in T2W images, enhancement of tract, presence of abscess and any other specific additional findings (anovaginal fistula, rectal or sigmoid wall inflammation, Crohn's disease and prior surgeries).

Superior mesenteric artery syndrome (SMA syndrome) **Aorta: SMA distance** is reduced and measures ….. mm. **Aorta: SMA angle** measures …..°, reduced. Compression of the D3 segment of duodenum between the aorta and SMA with over distension of the proximal duodenum and stomach. Left renal vein is compressed between the aorta and SMA. (Normal aorto-mesenteric angle measures 38–65 degrees. The normal distance from the aorta to the SMA at the duodenal crossing is 13–34 mm.)

Carcinoma prostate: Diffusion restricting T2 hypointense mass lesion in the bilateral mid and inferior, left lateral superior aspect of prostate with exophytic component noted on the left lateral aspect with infiltration of the left neurovascular bundles and bilateral seminal vesicles. On contrast, the lesion shows enhancement. Spectroscopy of the lesion shows elevated choline and decreased citrate. Multiple lymph nodes noted in the bilateral obturator and internal iliac regions. Bladder wall thickening—suggestive of chronic bladder outlet obstruction. Prostate measures 6 × 5 × 7 cm (vol 105 cc) enlarged in size. PSA density is 0.106 ng/ml/cm^3. Soft tissue lesion noted in the left superior pubic ramus—suggestive of secondaries: Features are suggestive of carcinoma prostate with extracapsular spread and bony and lymph node metastasis—PIRADS 5 (staging T4N2M1).

Benign prostatic hyperplasia: Prostate measures 5.6 × 5.4 × 5.2 cm (vol ~78 cc) enlarged in size, elevating the bladder base. Diffuse hyperintense central/transitional zone of prostate with multiple nodules. MR spectroscopy shows no elevation of choline/reduction of citrate. Diffusion weighted MRI imaging shows no abnormal restricted diffusion. Peripheral zone is uniformly hyperintense on T2 W images with no focal T2 hypointense lesion detected within. Peripheral zone is compressed. The T2 hypointense capsule is intact. No breech or focal bulge seen. The neurovascular bundle at 5 and 7 o'clock positions are normal. The angle between the seminal vesicle and prostate is maintained. The periprostatic fat plane is preserved. No stranding or infiltration seen. Seminal vesicles are normal in size. No T2 hypointense lesion noted within. No significant enlarged lymph nodes in the pelvis. No free fluid in the pelvis: Grade III prostatomegaly with benign prostatic hyperplasia.

Posterior urethral valve: High grade reflux into the right kidney with distended irregularly thickened bladder and marked dilatation of posterior urethra. Abrupt transition of dilated posterior urethra to small bulbous urethra with thin valve tissue extending from the ventral surface of the urethra—posterior urethral valve (Type I). No significant postvoid residual urine is seen. **Disproportionately dilated posterior urethra with an abrupt transition into a narrow anterior urethra—features could represent posterior urethral valve.**

Liver donor: Normal liver intensity with no focal/diffuse liver disease. Triple confluence pattern of the intraductal biliary anatomy (Type 2 pattern). Biliary ducts of segment IV joints the left hepatic duct 14 mm from the confluence of hepatic ducts. Conventional branching pattern of portal vein and hepatic vein.

Pelvic floor: Posthysterectomy status.There is widening of levator hiatus (transverse diameter), measuring 5.0 cm. H line (AP width of the levator hiatus) measures 7 cm at rest and 8.2 cm on straining—increased. Normal (<5 cm). M line (vertical descent of the levator hiatus) measures 1.1 cm at rest and 3.1 cm on straining—increased (normal<2 cm). Large cystocele noted: Part of the bladder is seen 3.1 cm below the PC line and 2.8 cm below the H line at rest, and 7.2 cm below the PC line on straining. Vaginal vault prolapse noted: Vaginal vault is seen 1.8 cm below the PC line at rest, 3 cm below the PC line on straining. The distance of the pubococcygeal line to the anorectal junction on rest is 1.1 cm below PC line at rest and 3.2 cm on straining—mild rectal prolapse. Herniation of fat between the vagina and rectum at rest and exaggerated on straining. No evidence of descent of small bowel loop between vagina and rectum to suggest enterocele. There is significant caudal inclination of the levator plate on rest (19°) and exaggerated on straining—63 to PC line (anorectal angle normal 90° to 110°). The levator ani muscle is mildly thinned and show normal signal intensities.

There is significant posterior perineal descend on straining and during defecation. M line (vertical descent of the levator hiatus) measures 4 cm at rest and 6.5 cm on straining— significant increased descent (normal <2 cm). Moderate descent of rectum through the levator hiatus. There is anterior rotation of urethra into horizontal plane in the dynamic images—anterior hypermobile urethra. Mild anterior rectocele, measures 2.1 cm anterior to the expected location. Significant caudal inclination of the levator plate on straining—61 degrees to PC line (normal <10 degrees). Transient rectal intussusception on straining. Anorectal angle on straining at rest measures 110°, squeezing 85° and on straining 140°.

Defecogram: Moderate anterior rectocele, measures 4.3 cm anterior to the expected location. No evidence of rectoanal intussusception. Anorectal angle at rest is 90°. During straining 130°.

Patient not able to empty the rectal jelly on evacuation phase. No evidence of rectocele, abnormal descent/rectal intussusception/enterocele. However, possible milder form of pelvic dyssynergia cannot be ruled out.

Anterior rectocele noted on straining and evacuation stage, measures about 2.4 cm. Defecography done at rest, during maximal sphincter contraction (squeezing), during straining, and during defecation. Anorectal angle (ARA), the angle between the two lines that intersect at the ARJ, 121°. During squeezing (maximal pelvic floor contraction), there is elevation of the pelvic organs in relationship to the PCL and sharpening of the ARA (due to contraction of the puborectal muscle) by 15–20. During straining and defecation, the pelvic floor muscles relaxes and, therefore, a mild descent (<2 cm) of the pelvic organs is noted. In addition, the anorectal angle becomes more obtuse, typically 15–20 more than when measured at rest. During defecation, the anal canal opens and the contrast material is evacuated. No e/o rectal intussusception/ prolapse. The levator ani muscle focal thinning on right side.

Renal

Autosomal dominant polycystic kidney disease: Multiple simple bilateral renal cortical cysts are seen. There are multiple (~…) cysts of varying sizes in left kidney (largest measuring ……..cm). There are ~ … cysts of varying size in the right kidney, the largest one measuring ….cm. The right kidney measures ….cm. The left kidney measures ….cm. Both kidneys are enlarged in size. No calculus or caliectasis is seen on either side. Ureters are not dilated. Multiple cysts in liver predominantly in the left lobe of liver. Above features favor autosomal dominant polycystic kidney disease.

Vesicoureteric junction calculus: 6 mm calculus in the left vesicoureteric junction causing mild hydroureteronephrosis. Mild delayed excretion noted. Another 3 mm seen calculus just above the calculus. CT attenuation value of the calculus is + 565 HU.

Pelvic ureteric junction obstruction: Grossly dilated left renal pelvis [6.6 cm (AP)] and mild dilatation of left calyces with partial left pelvic ureteric junction obstruction. Accessory left renal artery indenting on the posterior aspect of left PUJ. Delayed imaging shows contrast in the left renal pelvis. Narrowed segment of left PUJ and upper ureter measures 12 mm in length contrast noted in the left ureter in delayed images.

Wilms tumor:…..size well-defined mass lesion in the anterior aspect of lower pole and interpolar region of right kidney. The lesion is supplied by a prominent arterial feeder from the right renal artery. The right main renal artery courses above the mass. There is a non-occluding tumor thrombus involving the right renal vein and extending to the infrahepatic suprarenal portion of IVC for a length of …. mm. Delayed images show persistent nephrogram with non-opacified dilated right renal pelvic calyx cyst.

Table 2.16: Renal measurements reporting format

Cortical thickness	*Right kidney*	*Left kidney*
Upper pole	25 mm	19 mm
Interpolar region	18 mm	16 mm
Lower pole	18 mm	18 mm

Pyelonephritis: Right kidney appears enlarged and globular with perinephric fat stranding and thickening of anterior and posterior pararenal fascia noted. No focal collection/air pockets/calculi.

Emphysematous pyelopheritis: Right kidney measures cms, normal size. Left kidney measures cm, mildly bulky. Urothelial thickening on left side with perinephric and periureteric fat stranding. Minimal air seen in upper pole/ interpole calyx of left/right kidney. No intraparenchymal air. Presence/absence hydroureteronephrosis. No renal/ perirenal abscess on plain scan. Bladder is partially distended with mild diffuse wall thickening. Minimal air seen in nondependent bladder lumen.

Renal cell carcinoma: Well-defined heterogeneously enhancing >50% exophytic mass lesion measuring 3.4 × 5 cm noted in the posterior surface of lower pole of right kidney which is 10 mm away from the hilum. The lesion shows no contact with renal vessels. No evidence of renal vein thrombosis/para aortic lymphadenopathy/ perinephric extension. Visualised bones appear normal. Areas of non-enhancing hypodensity noted within the mass suggestive of necrosis. **Renal nephrometry score-4. (T1bN0M0).**

Renal carcinoma checklist: Mass size, growth rate (interval scan), type of mass (cystic/solid/indeterminate), presence of fat, enhancement pattern, location, mass margins, capsular location (50% exophytic, <50% exophytic, endophytic), distance to the sinus fat or collecting system. Tumor thrombus (distal extent) [no tumor thrombus/ ipsilateral renal vein (no IVC extension)/IVC below diaphragm/IVC above diaphragm/into right atrium], bland venous thrombus, lymph nodes and metastases in field of view.

Adrenal lesion: Table 2.17.

Renal Donor Angiogram

Right side: Right kidney is normal size, shape position and axis. It measures 10.4 × 5.2 cm. **Moderate perinephric fat seen.** No evidence of mass lesion or hypoperfusion is visualized. No evidence of tumor/cyst/calculus/ angiomyolipoma. Right ureter is normal.

Table 2.17: Adrenal lesion metrics reporting format		
Parameter	*Right adrenal lesion*	*Left adrenal lesion*
Size	52 (CC) × 31 (TR) × 31 (AP) mm	36 (CC) × 21 (TR) × 18 (AP) mm
Morphology	Irregular, heterogeneous enhancement	Heterogeneous enhancement with central necrosis
Unenhanced CT HU	27 HU	27 HU
Enhanced CT HU value (60 sec, portal venous phase)	80 HU	60 HU
Delayed enhancement CT HU value (10 to 15 mins)	58	35
Absolute washout: (enhanced CT-delayed CT)/(enhanced–unenhanced CT) × 100		
>60% suggestive of adenoma	22/53 = 41%	25/33 = 75%
Relative washout: (enhanced CT-delayed CT)/(enhanced CT) × 100		
>40% suggestive of adenoma	22/80 = 27%	25/60 = 41%

Left side: Left kidney is normal size, shape position and axis. It measures 9.1 × 5 cm. **Moderate perinephric fat seen.** No evidence of mass lesion or hypoperfusion is visualized. No evidence of tumor/cyst/calculus/angiomyolipoma. Left ureter is normal.

Single ureters on both sides. Adrenals are normal. No evidence of congenital anomalies noted in both the kidneys and ureter.

Abdominal angiogram and both lower limb angiogram: ***Right side:*** Eccentric thrombus with filling defect in the distal right common iliac extending to external iliac artery of approximate length 4.7 cm (narrowing by 70–80%) with peripheral flow. Common iliac artery diameter above occlusion is 8 mm. Common femoral artery below occlusion is 7 mm. Total occlusion of popliteal artery of approximate length is 12.5 cm with minimal reformation of mid anterior tibial and peroneal artery through collaterals. Popliteal artery above the occlusion measures 4.3 mm in diameter. Narrowing and occlusion of distal anterior tibial artery. No flow in the posterior tibial artery.

Left side: Common iliac, common femoral, superficial femoral, deep femoral and popliteal arteries appear normal. Popliteal trifurcation, anterior, posterior tibial and peroneal artery appear normal.

Infrarenal abdominal aorta aneurysm: There is large infrarenal fusiform aortic aneurysm [55 (TR) × 55 (AP) × 83 mm (length)] with peripheral eccentric thrombus, measuring about 21 mm (AP) × 49 mm (ML) in maximum dimension and 92 mm (CC) in the inferior and lateral walls, distal 1.5 cm of infrarenal abdominal aorta and aortic bifurcation appear normal. Peripheral calcification noted. Renal arteries origin seen just above the upper end of aneurysm and appear normal. No evidence of dissection/intramural hematoma noted. No periaortic inflammation/hematoma noted. Maximum diameter of contrast filled lumen measures 46 × 34 mm. Focal complete occlusion of inferior mesenteric artery. Both common iliac arteries appear normal except mild atherosclerotic changes. Mild osteal and juxtaosteal segment narrowing of left accessory renal artery.

Musculoskeletal System (MSK)

Dislocation of AC joint: Grade 3 injury of right acromioclavicular joint (complete dislocation of AC joint) with complete tear of superior and inferior acromioclavicular ligaments, complete tear of conoid and trapezoid components of coracoclavicular ligament, grade 1 sprain of deltoid and trapezius muscles.

Brachial plexus palsy: Muscles atrophy with increase signal intensity noted in the entire right arm and shoulder muscles. Complete preganglionic avulsion of the right C8 nerve root with pseudomeningocele formation. Retracted thickened C8 nerve root is seen just lateral to the neural foramina. Thickened extra neural foramen portion of right C5, C6 and C7 nerve roots upper and middle trunk forming a ill-defined soft tissue in the right interscalene triangle and minimally extending to the right costoclavicular space (retraction ball). Ill-defined lobulated soft tissue is at the level of divisions and possibility of neuroma formation with adjacent soft tissue fibrosis. Division and cords of the right brachial plexus appear normal. T1 nerve root relatively appears normal (Table 2.20).

Glenohumeral dysplasia following obstetric brachial plexus injury: Posterior subluxation of left shoulder joint (percentage humeral head anterior to the scapular line is 28.5%). Hypoplasia of the mid and inferior glenoid especially posteroinferior part of the glenoid. Glenoid is convex and showing posterior sloping. Glenoscapular angle is 12 degrees. Glenoid retroversion noted (13 degrees). Left scapular width measures 43.0 mm. Right scapular

Table 2.18: Donor renal artery measurements sample format

Renal artery	*Right*		*Left*	
Number	Single		Single	
	Main	*Accessory*	*Main*	*Accessory*
Length—distance between origin and 1st segmental bifurcation	33 mm			17 mm
Distance between the IVC margin and the 1st segmental bifurcation	9.8 mm		NA	NA
Orthogonal diameter	4.2 mm		5.0 mm	
Origin at the level of	D12-L1 vertebrae level		Upper border of L1	
Branching (hilar/polar/capsular)	Superior polar		Hilar	
Stenosis or aneurysm				
	Evidence of early branching like branching occurs < 1 cm from the right IVC margin		No evidence of left early segmentary arterial branching (segmental branching <1.5 cm from the origin of left renal artery.)	

Table 2.19: Donor renal vein measurements sample format

Renal vein	Right		Left	
	Main	Accessory	Main	Accessory
Length—segmental confluence to IVC	mm	mm	mm	
Segmental confluence of left renal vein to left margin of aorta	NA	NA	mm	
			No evidence of retroaortic/circum aortic renal vein	
	No evidence of late segmental confluent (<2 cm from the right side of IVC)		No evidence of late segmental confluent (<2 cm from the left margin of aorta)	
Diameter	mm	mm	mm	
Origin at the level of	L1–L2		L1 vertebrae	
Aneurysm				
Renal vein tributaries	No tributaries		Left adrenal vein Inferior phrenic Left gonadal vein (<5 mm) Lumbar vein (< 5 mm)	
			No abnormal venous drainage of segmental renal veins into lumbar, hemiazygous veins.	
Thrombosis				

width measures 42.3 mm. Left scapular length measures 77.6 mm Right scapular length measures 58.7 mm. Left humeral head appears smaller and flattened.

Hill-Sachs and bony Bankart lesion: Moderate Hill-Sachs impaction fracture of the posteriosuperolateral humeral head measuring 21 (AP) mm × 6 (depth) mm.Tear of the anteroinferior labrum from 3 to 6 o'clock position with fracture of the underlying glenoid—bony Bankart lesion. There is avulsion of IGHL labral complex from the glenoid (2–6 o'clock position) with periosteal stripping (soft tissue Bankart variant—ALPSA: Anterior labroligamentous periosteal sleeve avulsion). Small bony fragment measuring 10 × 4 mm adherent to the inferior glenoid at 6 o'clock position. No significant bony loss in the anteroinferior glenoid.

1. Hill-Sachs interval ...... mm
2. Nonengaging, on track Hill-Sachs defect/engaging, off track Hill-Sachs defect.

<table>
<tr><th colspan="4">Table 2.20: Brachial plexus reporting format</th></tr>
<tr><td></td><td>Pre-ganglionic nerve root</td><td colspan="2">Post-ganglionic</td></tr>
<tr><td></td><td></td><td>Nerve roots and trunk</td><td>Divisions and cords</td></tr>
<tr><td>C5</td><td>Intact. No evidence of nerve root avulsion of pseudo-meningocele</td><td rowspan="2">Thickened proximal C5 and C6 nerve roots with and retracted upper trunk suggestive of rupture.</td><td rowspan="3">Ill-defined lobulated soft tissue is at the level of divisions and possibility of neuroma formation with adjacent soft tissue fibrosis.</td></tr>
<tr><td>C6</td><td>Intact. No evidence of nerve root avulsion or pseudo-meningocele</td></tr>
<tr><td>C7</td><td>Rupture with evidence of nerve root avulsion/pseudo-meningocele</td><td>Middle trunk could not be traced separately from the abnormal soft tissue at the level of divisions and proximal cords</td></tr>
<tr><td>C8</td><td>Intact. No evidence of nerve root avulsion or pseudo-meningocele</td><td rowspan="2">Post-ganglionic nerve root appear normal. Lower trunk could not be traced separately from the abnormal soft tissue at the level of divisions and proximal cords</td><td rowspan="2"></td></tr>
<tr><td>D1</td><td>Intact. No evidence of nerve root avulsion or pseudo-meningocele</td></tr>
</table>

Adhesive capsulitis: Thickened oedematous inferior glenohumeral ligament, axillary pouch of inferior capsule and rotator interval. Fluid distension of biceps tendon sheath—features suggestive of adhesive capsulitis.

Comminuted impacted fracture neck of humerus extending into head with displaced superiorly migrated greater tubercle and inferomedially rotated humeral head. Greater tubercle containing the insertion of the supra and infraspinatus tendon. Displaced inferior aspect of lesser tubercle. Tiny displaced bony fragment noted in subscapularis bursa.

Rotator cuff tear: Irregular partial thickness tear of foot print of supraspinatus tendon involving ~70% thickness, anteroposterior extend of 18 mm, maximum retraction of ~8 mm extending to bursal surface. No muscle atrophy.

Bursal surface partial thickness tear of the foot print of anterior supraspinatus tendon measuring about 7 mm (Trans) × 10 mm (AP) involving ~ 70% thickness. No evidence of musculotendinous retraction/atrophy noted.

Linear intrasubstance partial thickness tear (~60% thickness) of anterior foot print of the supraspinatus tendon measuring about 6 mm (Trans) × 13 mm (AP). No evidence of musculotendinous retraction/atrophy noted.

Full thickness tear of supraspinatus tendon measuring about 15 mm (Trans) × 20 mm (AP) with moderate fatty atrophy of supraspinatus muscle. Full width, full thickness tear of the supraspinatus tendon with significant retraction of ~3.5 cm. Retracted end is irregular and seen at medial humeral head level. Mild fatty atrophy of supraspinatus muscle.

TFCC tear on the ulnar styloid attachment with fluid extending along the base of the TFCC and surrounding the styloid. Evidence of well-defined elongated cystic lesion measuring about 30 × 12 × 16 mm along the dorsal aspect of the distal ulna, extending into the ulnar side of the TFCC.

Ganglion cyst: Well-defined lobulated cystic lesion (1.8 × 0.5 × 0.7 cm) noted in the palmar aspect of the wrist ulnar side, seen behind the flexor carpi ulnaris tendon and communicating to the ulnotriquetteral joint space. No e/o ulnar artery/nerve compression.

Full thickness tear of the ulnar collateral ligament (UCL) of the 1st meta carpophalangeal joint with cortical irregularity of the proximal phalanx. Complete tear of the ulnar collateral ligament of the first metacarpophalangeal joint with proximal retraction and displacement—**Stener lesion.**

Carpal tunnel syndrome: Mild cross sectional enlargement and hyperintensity of median nerve deep to flexor retinaculum. Flattening of the median nerve at the level of hamate with oedema. Palmar bowing of flexor retinaculum at the level of hamate. No evidence of flexor tendon tenosynovitis. Mild hyperintensity in thenar muscles.

de Quervain tenosynovitis: Mild thickening and increase signal intensity of abductor pollicis longus and extensor pollicis brevis and fluid distension of tendon sheath.

AV fistula: Left radiocephalic AV fistula noted with intact anastomosis, flow across AVF measures more than 500 ml/min. Thrombotic occlusion noted in the cephalic vein in the upper forearm with reversal of venous flow towards the wrist. Deep veins appear normal. A few tiny veins in the palmar aspect of the forearm draining into the deep veins. Cephalic and basilic veins around the cubital fossa contracted on both sides. Deep veins and arteries of the both upper limbs appear normal.

Osteoarthritis: Patellofemoral and medial tibiofemoral osteoarthrosis with reduction of medial tibiofemoral joint space, full thickness loss of patellar facet, trochlea and medial condylar cartilage, subchondral sclerosis with marrow oedema in the patellar, trochlea medial femoral condyle and medial tibial plateau. Degenerative changes of the medial meniscus. Tear of posterior root attachment of medial meniscus with extrusion of body into the medial joint recess, 3.5 mm beyond the margin of medial tibial plateau. Moderate mucoid degeneration of anterior cruciate ligament. No tear. Degenerative subchondral marrow changes in the median, tibial eminence.

Chondrosarcoma: Lytic destructive lesion with irregular sclerosis in the medial aspect of left iliac bone with adjacent soft tissue. It measures ~6.1 × 7.1 cm. Destruction involves the iliac articular surface of the left SI joint. There is mild smooth erosion of the adjacent sacrum with minimal marrow edema.

Ewing's sarcoma: X-ray: Irregular cortical thickening with areas of minimal cortical destruction and lamellated periosteal reaction with mild soft tissue component noted in the diaphysis of right humerus.

Osteosarcoma: **X-ray**—ill-defined lytic lesion approximately measuring noted in the metaphysis of distal femur with osteoid matrix, wide zone of transition with aggressive periosteal reaction, adjacent large soft tissue component noted with multiple specs of calcification/ossification noted. An ill-defined lucent lesion involves the metaphysis and distal diaphysis of the femur. It does not appear to reach the growth plate. Laterally the mass elevates the cortex with periosteal reaction.

Osteosarcoma MRI: A right lower femoral shaft metadiaphyseal osteolytic exophytic lesion is seen showing a wide zone of transition with the adjacent normal bone marrow and encasing the posterolateral circumference of the distal femoral shaft. The lesion elicits inhomogeneous isointense T1/T2 and high STIR signals with internal break-down foci of fluid signal. The lesion causes cortical destruction with and extraosseous eccentric soft tissue component measuring 9.1 × 8 × 7.7 cm in orthogonal dimensions. The lesion and the soft tissue component show heterogeneous contrast enhancement. The quadriceps femoris muscle (mainly the vastus lateralis muscle) shows signal changes and post-contrast enhancement similar to the lesion and appears stretched over the lesion/edema of the popliteus, proximal tibialis anterior and posterior muscles. No other lesions in the scanned bones or invasion of the popliteal neurovascular bundle. No obvious extension of the lesion to the physis/epiphysis.There is mild overlying soft tissue thickening. No soft tissue abscess collection.

Ill-defined mass lesion noted in the intramedullary aspect of the lower end of femur in metaphyseal-diaphyseal region with cortical breach in the medial aspect, interrupted periosteal reactions, minimal extra osseous soft tissue component and areas of hemorrhages. The lesion appears to involve the growth plate with minimal involvement of epiphysis. On dynamic contrast, the soft tissue component showing well enhancement in arterial phase with washout on delayed imaging—consistent with high grade neoplasm. Minimal surrounding nonenhancing edema seen. Coronal height of lesion measures 10 cm. Upper limit of lesion seen 13 cm from the femoral articular surface. No evidence of joint effusion. No other skip lesion in the rest of the femur. No evidence of neurovascular bundle involvement.

Femoroacetabular impingement (pincer type): Ossification of superolateral acetabular labrum on both sides, leading to over coverage of femoral head. No acetabular retroversion. Herniation pit noted in anterior femoral head-neck junction on left side. The femoral head neck junction is smooth and concave on both sides. No evidence of any dysplastic bump in the femoral head. No marrow edema. Alpha angle measures 41 degrees on left side, normal.

Femoroacetabular impingement (pincer type): Loss of weight bearing articular cartilage of left hip with subchondral cyst in the acetabulum. Mild left hip joint effusion. Decreased extrusion index –9% (25% in normal subjects). Decreased extrusion index suggests femoral head becomes "more covered". No evidence of femoral head, neck junction offset/bump. α angle measures about 45 (abnormal - >50 degrees).

Femoroacetabular impingement (cam type): Alpha angle on the right and left side measures about 64 and 54 degrees, respectively (normal <60 degrees). Lateral capsular thickening with irregularity noted in the right side. A bump in noted head and neck junction.

Perthes' disease: Left capital femoral epiphysis appears flattened with altered signals and subchondral fractures. Overlying the femoral head, articular cartilage appears intact. Altered marrow signal abnormality extending to the femoral neck. Acetabulum appears normal.

Developmental dysplasia of hip: Bilateral developmental dysplasia of hip with superior dislocation. Bilateral shallow acetabulum with deficient posterior and superior acetabular rim (Table 2.21).

Post-DDH reduction hip joint: Right DDH. Right femoral head is seen within the acetabular cavity.

Table 2.21: DDH sample reporting format

Structure	*Size*	
	Right	*Left*
Femoral head (bone) epiphysis	10 × 12 × 6 mm	10 × 10 × 7 mm
Femoral head (cartilage) epiphysis	25 × 10 mm	21 × 9 mm
Greater trochanter (bone)	8.5 × 10.8 mm	8 × 10.9 mm
Greater trochanter (cartilage)	20 × 19 mm	21 × 20 mm

Acetabulum is shallow and femoral head is small on right side. Edema of soft tissue around right hip joint. No evidence of bony destruction identified. Remaining underlying bones including the neck and upper shaft of the femur appear normal bilaterally. Right femoral head ossified epiphysis appears mildly smaller in size. Post-surgical changes in the right inguinal region and upper medial aspect of thigh.

Avascular necrosis: Avascular necrosis with multiple subchondral crescent fractures leading to minimal collapse of articular surface of femur head on right side. It involves about 60–70% of femur head. No secondary osteoarthritis. No right hip joint effusion. Avascular necrosis with multiple subchondral crescent fractures leading to significant collapse and deformity of femur head on left side. There is secondary osteoarthritis with articular margin irregularity of the acetabulum and marginal osteophytes. Mild left hip joint effusion. Avascular necrosis of bilateral femoral heads—modified Ficat Arlet stage III on right side and stage IV on left side.

Idiopathic chondrolysis of hip: Geometric T1 hypo T2 hyperintense signal intensity alteration in the mid one-third of proximal right femoral head. No obvious evidence of hip joint effusion/synovial thickening/ acetabular oedema—features suggestive of idiopathic chondrolysis of hip.

Odelberg disease: Oedema in the left inferior pubic ramus—van Neck-Odelberg disease.

Anterior cruciate ligament graft: The tibia tunnel is in the anterior third of the tibial plateau mildly anterior to the Blumensaat's line on sagittal images with the tunnel opening through the medial tibial eminence in the coronal images.The distal tibial tunnel measures 13 mm and the tibial opening measures 7 mm. The graft in the tibial tunnel shows hyperintense amorphous signals—suggestive of mucoid degeneration.

Graft in the intercondylar notch: The graft in the intercondylar notch shows hyperintense amorphous signals and buckling—suggestive of graft degeneration. No spurs along the intercondylar roof. T2 dark soft tissue noted in the anterior intercondylar notch anterior to the ACL fibres. Post-operative scar in the Hoffa's fat pad leads to this above-mentioned lesion. Ill-defined synovial soft tissue noted in the intercondylar notch with a metallic artefact (suture material) in the proximal intercondylar notch.

Femoral tunnel: The femoral tunnel is at the intersection of the physeal scar and the Blumensaat's line posterior to the line along the posterior femoral cortex. The femoral tunnel is at the 1 o'clock on coronal images. Femoral tunnel measures 10 mm. The graft in the femoral tunnel shows mild hyperintensity on T2-weighted sequence.

Intrameniscal degeneration of medial meniscus with radial tear of the posterior root attachment and partial extrusion of the body into the medial joint recess, 3 mm beyond the margin of medial tibial plateau.

Meniscal contusion in the posterior horn–posterior body junction of medial meniscus with tiny vertical tear in the peripheral third (red zone) of tibial articular surface.

Chondromalacia patella: Patella shows fraying of articular cartilage with multiple defects that involves less than 50% surface. Increased signal intensity in cartilage is noted, no evidence of edema in bone—chondromalacia patella grade 2.

Osgood-Schlatter disease: T2/ PD shows thickening and edema in distal patellar tendon. Bone marrow edema is noted in patellar tuberosity. Distended deep infrapatellar bursa noted. Soft tissue swelling noted anterior to tibial tuberosity.

Neurofibroma: Multilobulated solid lesion in the left forearm in the upper third, mid-third junction. The lesion shows continuity with the median nerve. The lesion is extending up to the subcutaneous plane in the upper forearm. The lesion shows a few fibrous septa. The lesion shows diffusion restriction—**features favours neurofibroma in the left median nerve.**

Exostosis: Pedunculated exostosis arising from the lower end of femur medial aspect measuring about 2.1 × 2.2 × 4 cm. Cartilage cap thickness measuring about 9 mm. No evidence of bursitis/no evidence of fracture/ no significant muscle altered signal intensity.

Blount's disease: Absent medial most bony epiphysis with adjacent depressed metaphysis which has beak-like protuberance. There is tibial varus deformity. No evidence of bony physeal bar—features favour Blount's disease.

Transient lateral patellar subluxation with bone marrow oedema in the medical patella and lateral condyle of femur. Grade I sprain of medial patellar retinaculum at patellar attachment and grade I strain of vastus medialis oblique muscle. No evidence of osteochondral injury/bone marrow oedema in the inferomedial aspect of patella. Complete tear of medial patellofemoral ligament and medial patellar retinaculum at the femoral attachment. Grade I strain of vastus medialis oblique muscle and tendon.

Insall–Salvati ratio = patellar tendon/patellar length: 4.5/3.9 = 1.44 (patella alta).

Patellar tilt: Lateral patellofemoral angle opens medially (70) – abnormal (positive for patellar tilt). Suggest patellofemoral malalignment. Patellar apex lying lateral to the plane of trochlear apex—patellar subluxation. Patellar congruence angle is positive suggestive of patellar subluxation. **Congruence angle:** Angle of congruence is an index of subluxation but does not assess tilt. If congruence angle is lateral to congruence line, then angle is positive.

If congruence angle is medial to congruence line, then angle is negative. Normal angle is ≤16°. Sulcus angle: **Establish a zero reference line. Normal sulcus angle is** ≤135 ± 10°.

Q angle – normal <15°, abnormal >20–25°

Patellofemoral malalignment

Type I—Patellar subluxation (displacement) without tilt.

Type II—Patellar subluxation with tilt.

Type III—Patellar tilt without subluxation.

Tibial tuberosity—trochlear groove distance is 20 mm. (>20 suggest lateralized tibial tubercle).

Femoral ante version—measurement.

Bump (nipple) in the anterosuperior femoral trochlea–suggestive of femoral trochlear dysplasia. No evidence of crossing sign in X-ray lateral view.

Trochlear articular facet asymmetry. Medial to lateral facet ratio—(0.67, normal) <0.4, abnormal. Degree of patellar lateralization (patellar lateralization more than 6 mm is significant).

Patellar Wiberg morphology

Wiberg I: Medial and lateral facets are concave and identical. Wiberg II: Medial facet is concave and narrow. Lateral facet in concave. Wiberg III: Medial facet is convex and narrow. Lateral facet is concave. Wiberg IV: Medial facet is flat and narrowed.

Patellar tracking; Comparison of static and dynamic study of the knee joint to assess the change in patella related to the femur during knee flexion and extension known case of **patellofemoral instability,** CT and MRI screening shows, avulsion fracture of the medial patellar retinaculum at patellar attachment and grade 2 strain at medial attachment.Widely placed tibial tubercle (TT distance measures about 2.1 cm on left, 2.4 cm on right). Borderline patellar alta. No significant trochlear dysplasia except tiny bony hump in midline.

Patellar tendon lateral femoral condyle friction syndrome: Focal area of high T2 signal (oedema) at the inferolateral aspect of the patellofemoral joint, within the superolateral portion of the infrapatellar (Hoffa's) fat pad—patellar tendon lateral femoral condyle friction syndrome. No evidence of patella alta.

Ligament injury: Proximal medial collateral ligament appears thickened and hyperintense with bone marrow edema noted in medial femoral epicondyle. Posterior oblique ligament, ACL, medial and lateral meniscus and other ligament appears normal—grade 2 **medial collateral ligament injury**.

ACL: Anterior cruciate ligament appears hyperintense with a fluid signal noted at the femoral intercondylar notch. ACL angle appears normal and measures 12°. Hyperintensity noted in the lateral femoral condyle. Proximal MCL appears hyperintense—partial tear of medial collateral ligament.

Post-operative ACL reconstruction: ACL reconstruction status intact without tear. Increased signal intensity noted in the ACL graft.

Lateral collateral ligament: Hyperintensity noted in the lateral collateral ligament, the distal continuity of the ligament not maintained, chip fracture involving fibular head noted. Hyperintensity in popliteus tendon and popliteofibular ligament noted. Other posterolateral corner structures appear uninjured, no meniscal tear, medial collateral and cruciate ligament appear to be intact—**chip fracture in fibular head with a complete tear of lateral collateral ligament.**

Posterior cruciate ligament: Hyperintense posterior cruciate ligament noted with AP diameter on sagittal T2 weigted images measures 12 mm. Bony contusion in tibial plateau noted. Medial collateral ligament appears hyperintense–grade 1 strain. Joint effusion noted—posterior cruciate ligament tear with grade 1 strain on posterior cruciate ligament.

Meniscal tear: Longitudinal tear of the body and posterior horn of medial meniscus, no extrusion or parameniscal disc formation. Lateral meniscus appears intact. Collateral and cruciate ligaments appear normal, no bone marrow edema.

*Bucket handle tear of medial meniscus***,** with flipped fragment in intercondylar notch anterior to posterior cruciate ligament giving double PCL appearance.

The flipped fragment is attached to parent meniscus anteriorly and posteriorly.

Congenital talipes equinovarus (CTEV): Talipes varus deformity noted. No obvious tarsal coalition. No evidence of vertical talus. Mild laterally angulated talus. Muscle mass appears small. Increased subcutaneous fat noted (OR) Mild fatty atrophy of the distal leg and plantar muscles. Mild reduction of tibiotalar joint space.

Plantar fasciitis: Thickening with increased signal intensity of the medial cord of the plantar aponeurosis with marrow edema of the underlying calcaneum and significant perifascial inflammation. Moderate size plantar calcaneal spur noted.

Morton's neuroma: Ill-defined T1 hypointense lesion measuring about 8 × 4 mm noted in the plantar soft tissues in between 2nd and 3rd metatarsal head with surrounding areas of T2 hyperintensity with edema extending into the dorsal aspect of the foot.

Os calcaneus secundarius: Well-defined ossification adjacent to the anterior process of calcaneum without marrow edema.

Bilateral congenital vertical talus: Bilateral congenital vertical talus. No obvious evidence of talo calcaneal/ calcaneo navicular coalition.

Haglund's deformity: Increased thickness of distal Achilles tendon with altered signal intensity at the insertion (Insertional Achilles tendinitis) with calcaneal bony prominence, adjacent Calcaneal oedema and retro calcaneal bursitis.

Mechanical axis of the right lower limb (genu valgum) measuring about 10 degrees.

Obstetrics and Gynaecology

Follicular Study (TVS)

Baseline study on the day of first examination (Table 2.22):

- *Uterus:* Measures 6.7 × 4.3 × 3.1 cm. Uterus is anteverted and anteflexed in position. It appears normal in size and echotexture. Its surface appears normal without any contour abnormality. No myometrial focal lesion is seen. Cervix also appears normal.
- *Right ovary:* 3.1 × 1.5 cm
- *Left ovary:* 2.9 × 1.7 cm. Both ovaries are normal in size, shape and echotexture. Uterine artery PI measures 2.6 on right and 2.3 on left side, suggesting favourable outcome (<3 favourable outcome, >3 less favourable outcome, even with PCOD) (Uterine PI reduces up to 1, near ovulation).
- *Adnexae:* No adnexal mass lesion is seen.

Common measurements in lower limb

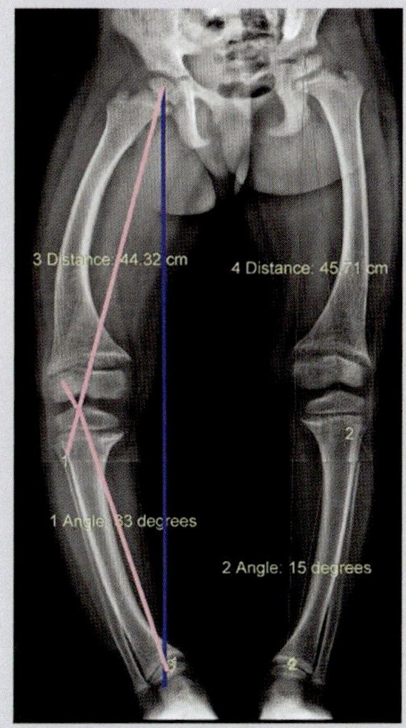

Fig. 2.9: Mechanical axis–varus deformity
The mechanical axis should pass just medial to the center point of the knee joint. If the line passes more medially to the knee center, a varus deformity is present; if the line passes laterally to the knee center or center of the distal femur, a valgus deformity exists

1. The mechanical axis of the lower limb (blue line) is determined on the full-length AP standing radiograph. The axis passes through the center point of the hip joint (center of the femoral head) and through the center point of the ankle joint (midpoint of the tibial plafond).
2. Mechanical axis of the femur (MAF): A line from the center of the femoral head to the center of the distal femur or center of the knee (upper pink line)
3. Tibial shaft axis and mechanical axis of the tibia: A line extending from the center of the proximal tibia to the center of the ankle (lower pink line)
4. Mechanical axis of femur and tibia forms the lower limb valgus / varus angle

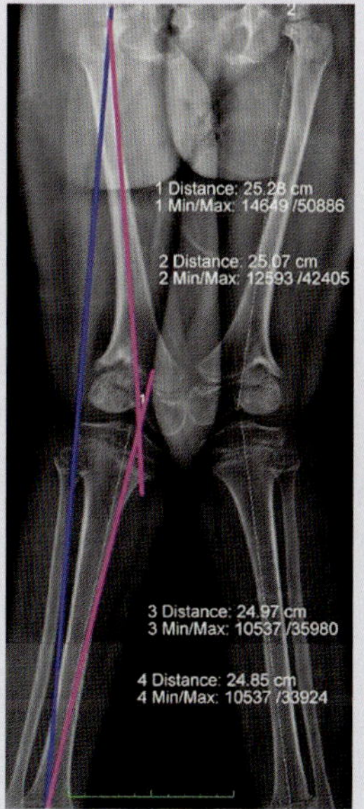

Fig. 2.10: Mechanical axis—valgus deformity

1. Insall–Salvati Index: The Insall–Salvati index is used for measuring the vertical position of the patella. The greatest diagonal length of the patella (LP) is measured from its posterosuperior corner to the apex. The length of the patellar tendon (LT) is measured from the patellar apex to the tibial tuberosity. The ratio of these two measurements (LP/LT) is the Insall–Salvati index

- Normal range: LP/LT = 0.8–1.2
- High-riding patella (patella alta): LP/LT <0.8
- Low-riding patella (patella baja): LP/LT >1.2

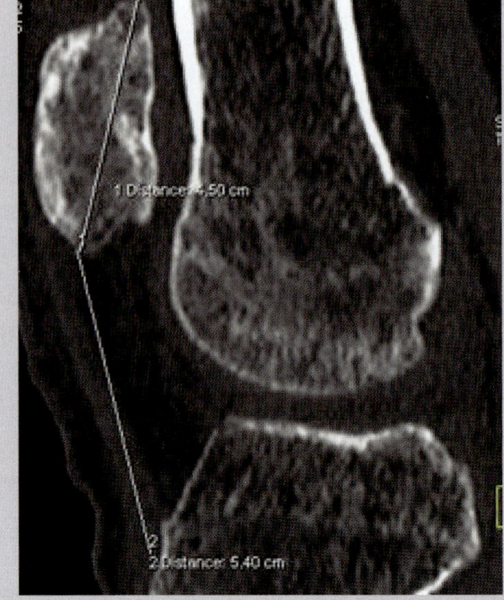

Fig. 2.11: Insall–Salvati index

2. Lateral patellofemoral angle of Laurin: The lateral patellofemoral angle is determined by drawing a line tangent to the highest points on the medial and lateral femoral condyles (A) and drawing a second line (B) across the lateral patellar facet. In a normal joint, these lines will typically form an acute angle that opens on the lateral side. In patients with patellar instability, the lines will often be parallel or may even form an angle that opens on the medial side. Figure 2.12 shows lateral patellofemoral angle opens medially (7°)—abnormal (positive for patellar tilt).

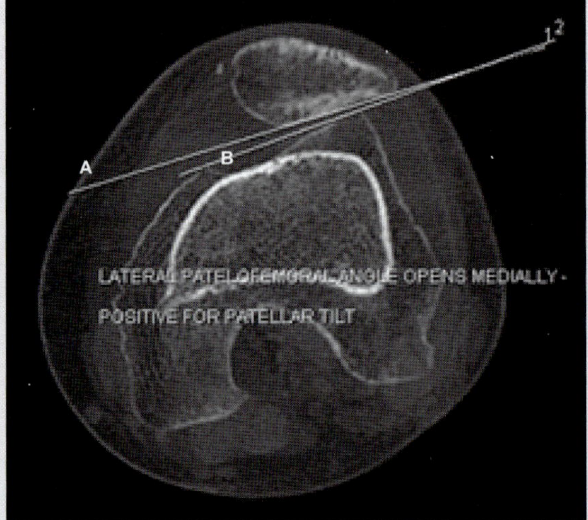

Fig. 2.12: Lateral patellofemoral angle of Laurin

3. Sulcus angle—measured by drawing the following lines. The deepest point of the trochlea is identified (A), and the highest points on the medial (B) and lateral femoral condyles (C) are marked. The angle formed by lines AB and AC is the sulcus angle. Normal sulcus angle is <– 137 degrees

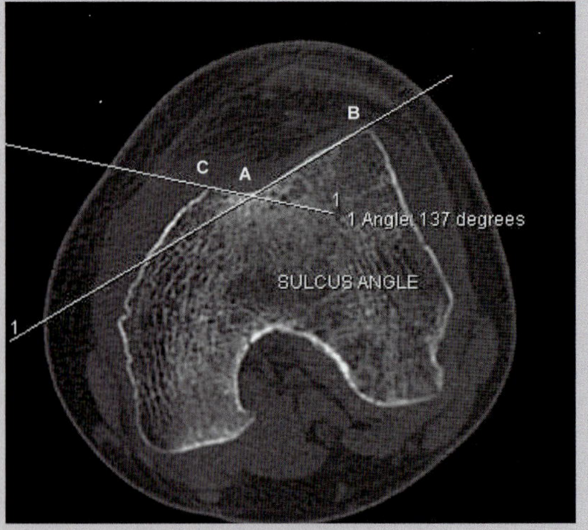

Fig. 2.13: Sulcus angle

4. The congruence angle of the patellofemoral joint—first identify the sulcus angle. The bisector of that angle is drawn as reference line. Another line drawn by joining sulcus and lowest point of patellar articulating surface. The angle between these two is the patellofemoral congruence angle. If second line is medial to first line, the angle has a negative value; if second line is lateral to first line, the angle is positive. Angle of congruence is an index of subluxation but does not assess tilt. Normal angle is <–16 degrees. Angles greater than +16° denote lateral subluxation of the patella.

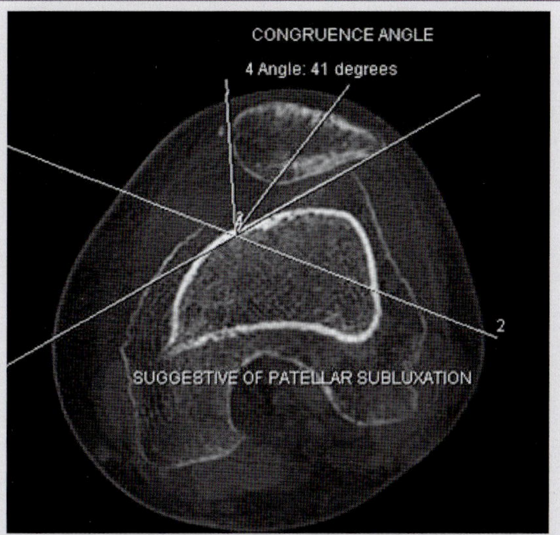

Fig. 2.14: Congruence angle of the patellofemoral joint

5. Trochlear depth: This measures the inset depth of the trochlear groove (sulcus) relative to the average of the maximum anteroposterior distance of the medial and lateral femoral condyles (it is determined on axial images at the same level as trochlear facet asymmetry). Trochlear groove depth < or = 4 mm is normal.

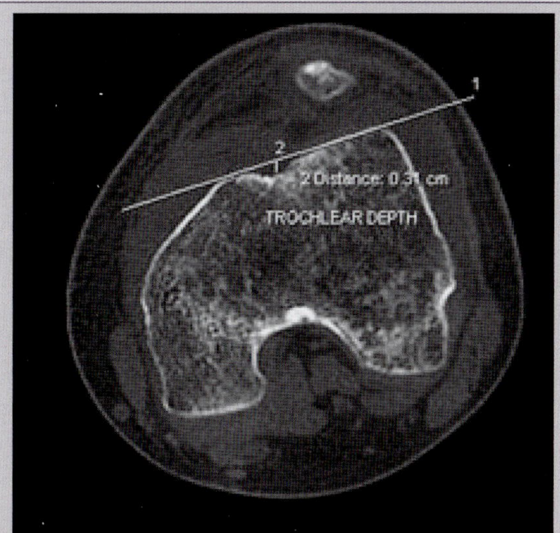

Fig. 2.15: Trochlear facet asymmetry

6. Medial to lateral facet ratio: The ratio of the medial facet length divided by the lateral facet length. <0.4 is abnormal indicates trochlear dysplasia.

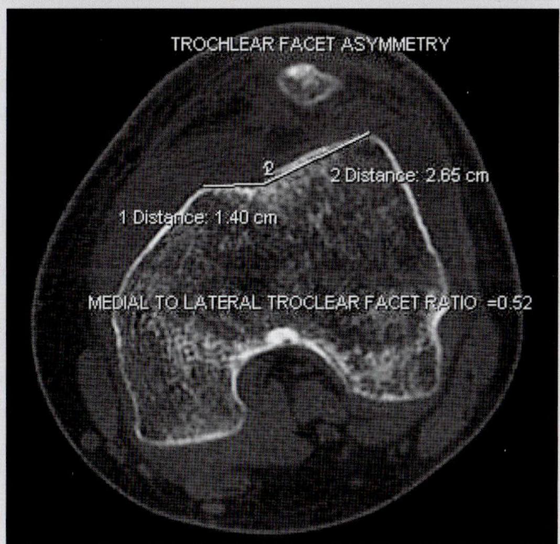

Fig. 2.16: Trochlear dysplasia

7. Lateralization of the patella: This evaluates the lateral patellar displacement, measuring the distance between the lateral margin of the trochlea and the most lateral point of the patella. A distance greater than 6 mm is indicative of trochlear dysplasia.

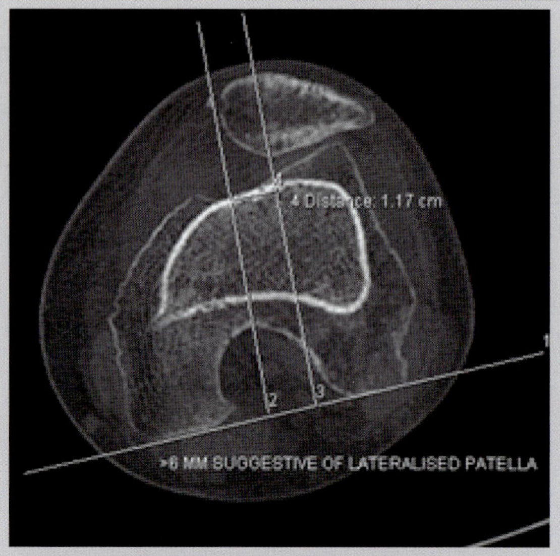

Fig. 2.17: Trochlear dysplasia

8. Lateralization of the tibial tuberosity: The position of the tibial tubercle is crucial for the inferolateral force vector of the patella. If there is excessive lateralization of the tibial tuberosity, the patella is pulled laterally during flexion. Therefore, excessive lateral displacement of the tibial tuberosity is a risk factor for lateral patellar dislocation. Imaging techniques are the only accurate way to measure the tibial tuberosity to the trochlear groove (TT-TG) distance. The distance from the tibial tuberosity to the trochlear groove (TT-TG) is measured parallel to the tangential line through posterior femoral condyles by superimposing transverse images through the apex of the intercondylar notch and the tibial tuberosity. TT-TG distance of more than 20 mm is nearly always associated with patellar instability, and is a measure for lateralization of tibial tuberosity. Values of 15–20 mm are considered borderline and distances less than 15 mm are considered normal.

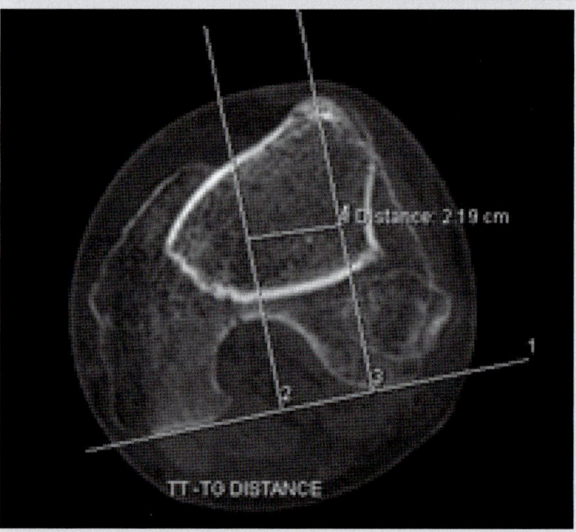

Fig. 2.18: Distance from the tibial tuberosity to the trochlear groove (TT-TG)

9. Femoral anteversion angle: Femoral anteversion refers to the orientation of the femoral neck in relation to the femoral condyles at the level of the knee. Femoral anteversion can be determined by measuring the angle formed between the long axis of the femoral neck and a line parallel to the dorsal aspect of the femoral condyles (posterior condylar axis, or PCA) on axial slices at MRI or CT. Femoral anteversion averages between 30–40° at birth, and between 8–14° in adults. An increased femoral anteversion is often seen in patients with developmental dysplasia of the hip. Moreover, it has been shown that abnormal femoral anteversion can contribute to the development of femoroacetabular impingement (FAI). Reduced femoral anteversion is associated with cam-type FAI.

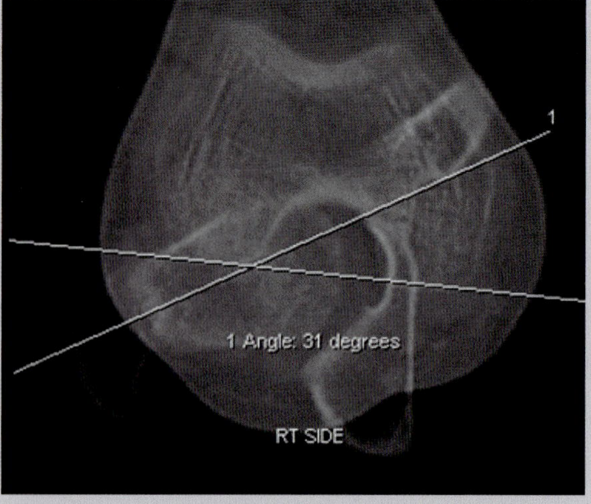

Fig. 2.19: Femoral anteversion angle

- No free fluid is seen in pouch of Douglas
- LMP: 16/02/2022

Polycystic ovary: Multiple peripherally arranged follicles measuring about 3–4 mm in sizes noted in the bilateral ovaries with echogenic stroma. Right ovary volume 15 ml, left ovary volume 17 ml. No evidence of dominant follicle in both ovaries.

Ovarian simple cyst: A large abdominopelvic cystic mass with fluid attenuation measuring 14 × 12 × 15 cm. No obvious solid area, septations or calcifications are noted within. The mass appears to be intraperitoneal and seen to displace retroperitoneal structures, like pancreas and kidneys posteriorly. Right ovary could not be visualized separately. However, the left ovary is seen separate from the lesion (ORADS-3).

Torsion ovary: Right ovary appears enlarged measuring 4.5 × 3.8 cm with heteroechoic central stroma and peripherally displaced follicles, the ovary appears to be in minimal, the ovarian pedicle appears to be twisted with minimal flow through the pedicle, free fluid noted in pelvis. Left ovary appears normal.

Placenta accreta: placenta anterior with absence of placental myometral interface noted, the uterine wall being undistinguishable from the placenta, and the presence of multiple vascular intraplacental lacunae on Doppler ultrasound revealed an extensive vascularity along the anterior portion of the lower uterine segment and appears to extend up to and around the bladder.

Ectopic pregnancy: No evidence of intrauterine gestational sac noted. endometrium appears thickened measuring 10 mm. Complex right adnexal cyst measuring 3 × 4.2 cm which on Doppler ultrasound shows ring of fire appearance—possibly right adnexal ectopic, suggested beta-HCG correlation.

IUGR: All fetal biometric parameters falling below the 3rd percentile, EFW-670 g, average gestation age 21 weeks, LMP gestation age 28 weeks. On Doppler ultrasound umbilical artery shows reversal of diastolic flow. Middle cerebral artery Doppler remained normal, cerebroplacental ratio <1—**features suggestive of Type-I (symmetric) intra-uterine growth restriction.**

Abdominal circumference and estimated fetal weight falls below the 3rd percentile with Doppler ultrasound umbilical artery shows pulsatility index above 95 percentile and reversal of cerebroplacental ratio and oligohydramnios noted—**features suggestive of Type-II (asymmetric) intrauterine growth restriction.**

Ovarian malignancy: Large complex pelvic mass arising from the right adnexa measures about 11.5 × 13.4 × 10.9 cm. The mass compresses the uterus inferiorly and significant compression in the urinary bladder. The lesion shows multiple lobulations with solid, cystic and hemorrhagic component. Both ovaries are not made out separately. Features favour ovarian malignancy with bilateral iliac and paraaortic lymphadenopathy-ORADS 5.

Checklist: Side, component of lesion, invasion to bladder colorectal, pelvic side wall, anterioal abdominal wall, vessels, ascites (none/small/moderate/large), peritoneal metastases, lymphadenopathy (none/only below renal arteries/above and below renal arteries) in the region of internal iliac/external iliac/common iliac/retro-peritoneal/mesentric root/porta hepatis/splenic hilum. Any intra-abdominal organ, bone involvement. Look for any thoracic involvement in the form of parenchymal nodules, pleural effusion, lymphadenopathy.

Endometrial carcinoma: Irregular heteroechoic endometrial thickening measuring 2.5 × 4 cm showing myometrial invasion and minimal fluid collection, on

Table 2.22: Follicular study serial examination

Date	Day	Right ovary	Left ovary	Endometrium			Prefollicular Flow*2	Ov art RI*3		Ov art PSV*4		POD	Remark	Sign
				Width	Type	Flow*1		Right	Left	Right	Left			

*MSF-Multiple small follicles

1. No flow, ±Minimal sparse flow, +±Moderate flow,++±Good flow
2. 25% perifollicular flow—poor prognosis, 25–50% flow—intermediate prognosis, >50% perifollicular flow-good prognosis of conception, on the day of ovulation. However, complete peripheral follicular flow in preovulatory phase of cycle suggest poor outcome.
3. Ovarian artery RI<0.5—better prognosis (just before ovulation), >0.5 poor prognosis (in post-ovulation corpus luteal cyst.)
4. Ovarian artery PSV in cm/s—if >10 cm/sec good prognosis, favourable outcome
5. Endometrial thickness <8 mm is associated with poor pregnancy rates. Uterine artery S/D,RI and PI could not be used alone to predict endometrial receptivity.

Table 2.23: Types of endometrium with respect to normal menstrual cycle

Type	*Days*	*Endometrium description*	*Stages*	*Hormonal levels*
1	1–4	Hyperechoic with irregular borders	Menstruation	Low E2 and P
2	5–8	Linear and thin	Early proliferation	Low E2 and P
3	9–11	Leaf shaped, hypoechoic spongy layer with ill-defined basal layer	Mid proliferation	Increasing E2, ↑↑↑low P
4	12–14	Triple line appearance with well-defined basal layer (6–12 mm)	Late proliferation	E2 surge: E2, low ↑P
5	15–22	Echogenicity of spongy layer, gradual loss of middle inner layer	Early secretory	E2-minor peak, P to peak
6	23–28	Hyperechoic lumpy pattern with regular outline	Late secretory	↓E2, ↓P

Doppler study prominent feeding artery noted—possibly endometrial carcinoma suggested HPE correlation.

Checklist: Myometrial and serosal, presents of other benign lesion (adenomyosis, leiomyomas), cervical stroma, parametrial, bladder, rectal invasion. Comment about vagina and overies. Check for lymph nodes, ascites and peritoneal involvement.

Adenomyosis: Uterus appears bulky measuring 16 × 8 cm, with loss of endometrial and myometrial junction, junctional zone appears thickened measuring 15 mm with multiple small T2 hyperintense cystic areas noted.

Endometriosis: Focal T2 dark well-defined lesion in the torus uterinus extending to the posterior uterine wall with areas of T1 hyperintensity—endometriosis.

Checklist: Uterus size, junctional zone thickness, fibroids, cervix endometrium, ovaries (volume in ml) bladder, ureter, uterine ligaments, rectovaginal septum, anterior rectal wall, sigmoid colon, adjacent small bowl loops, lymph nodes and osseous structures.

Ca cervix: A large infiltrating soft tissue density mass lesion measuring 7.3 × 6.6 × 6.6 cm (CC × AP × TR) noted involving the cervix and lower uterine segment. The lesion shows moderate enhancement on contrast administration. Anteriorly, there is loss of fat plane between the mass and the posterior bladder wall with infiltration of the same. No significant intraluminal extension seen. Anteroinferiorly, mass infiltrates the anterior vaginal wall. Posterior vaginal wall is relatively normal. There is no infiltration of lower 1/3rd of vagina. There is significant parametrial invasion more on the left side with involvement of parametrial venous plexus on left side. There is infiltration of left distal ureter by the mass causing moderate hydroureteronephrosis. There is significant delay in excretion of contrast into the pelvicalyceal system. No pelvic side wall infiltration. Both obturator internus muscles are normal.There is no infiltration of the rectal wall seen. Multiple round soft tissue density deposits are noted along the surface of uterus. No hydrometra/pyometra (T3bN1M0).

Hydrosalpinx: Tubular-shaped anechoic structure with incomplete septation noted in the right adnexa, right ovary visualized separately, uterus and left ovary appears normal.

RADS—Reporting and Data System (Refer OSCE/core for detailed explanation)

TIRADS: A well-defined mixed hypoechoic solid and cystic lesion measuring 1.2 × 1.8 cm in size with the lesion appearing wider than taller and irregular margin containing a few areas of macro calcifications. No evidence of any extra thyroidal extension and punctate echogenic foci or peripheral rim calcifications seen—TIRADS 4 (4–6 points/moderately suspicious of malignancy). Suggested FNAC thyroid and follow-up.

LIRADS—reflect the probability of observation being a HCC and ranges from LR1 (definitely benign) to LR5 (definitely HCC).

Multiple well-defined new small (7 mm) nodular lesions are noted in the right hepatic lobe which are hypervascular on the arterial phase and mildly fades on portal venous phase, compared to background liver enhancement. There is no capsule around any lesion. There is no restricted diffusion and nodular liver surface is compatible with cirrhosis. There is no washout, no presence of an enhancing capsule (pseudocapsule) and no interval growth seen-features favours LIRADS III (intermediate probability for HCC). Suggested follow-up imaging in 3–6 months.

LIRADS can be used only in cirrhosis, Hep B, current/prior HCC. Not to use LIRADS in 18 years, cirrhosis due to congenital hepatic fibrosis, cirrhosis due to vascular disorders (Budd-Chiari, portal vein occlusion, diffuse nodular regenerative hyperplasia, cardiac congestion).

2

PIRADS: A well-defined lenticular shaped homogeneous, moderately T2 hypointense lesion with diffusion restriction noted in transition zone at the apex of the prostate gland noted measuring 9 mm (<1.5 cm in greatest dimension) with surrounding normal peripheral zone. There is no definite extra prostatic extension/invasive behaviour. The surrounding seminal vesicles appears normal. No pelvic nodes and bone involvement noted. Features favours PIRADS IV (high clinically significant cancer is likely to be present).

ORADS: An ill-defined large multi-locular abdomino pelvic cystic mass measuring 23.7 × 10.7 × 19.6 cm with no solid or papillary projections noted. Left ovary not visualised separately. A normal right ovary visualised separate from the mass. Uterus appears normal with endometrial thickness of 4 mm. There is no ascites and no evidence of visceral, peritoneal or nodal metastases noted. Features favour O RADS IV (intermediate risk of malignancy) (10% to <50%).

BIRADS: Refer to Table 4.118.2, page 1038; Table 5.20, page 1575.

An ill-defined isoechoic lesion measuring 3.9 × 3 cm with indistinct margin and posterior acoustic shadowing and architectural distortion of surrounding breast parenchymal tissues noted at 11–12 o'clock position in zone II of right breast. No axillary nodal involvement noted. Features favour BIRADS V (95% probability of malignancy). Suggested FNAC of right breast mass.

Lung RADS: Refer to Table 5.21, page 1576.

A well-defined ground-glass nodule with a mean diameter of 34 mm noted subpleural in location in inferior lingula segment of left lung with the nodule showing spiculated borders. There is double the increase in the size of the nodule compared to previous images taken 1 year back (16 mm in size). There are no enlarged regional lymph nodes noted. Features favour LUNG RADS IV-X (suspicious, >15% chance of malignancy).

Oncoimaging

Renal cell carcinoma: FDG avid partially exophytic soft tissue density mass noted in the upper pole of the left kidney measuring ~59 × 62 × 83 mm (AP × TR × CC). The lesion shows heterogeneous enhancement on arterial phase (HU ~112) and washout on delayed phase (HU~ 59). Pelvicalyceal system is not infiltrated. Perinephric fat plane is not infiltrated. Preserved fat plane noted between the mass and spleen superiorly and descending colon anteriorly. Left renal vein is distended with thrombus, showing heterogeneous enhancement and mild FDG uptake. The thrombus is extending into the infrahepatic IVC. No extension noted into the suprahepatic IVC/right atrium. Left gonadal vein is distended. Dual left renal artery noted and the mass is predominantly supplied by the accessory branch. No other focal lesion noted in the left kidney. Right kidney appears normal. Multiple FDG avid enlarged paraaortic, pericaval and left retrocrural lymph nodes noted, largest measuring ~28 × 23 mm. Left adrenal gland appears normal. No evidence of pulmonary metastasis. No FDG avid skeletal lesions. (T3bN1M0)

Hilar cholangiocarcinoma: Ill-defined isodense soft tissue density lesion with mild FDG uptake is noted at the level of confluence of left and right hepatic ducts, measuring ~44 × 35 mm.The lesion is involving the entire length of common hepatic duct, hepatic duct confluence and left hepatic duct with extension up to the bifurcation. Moderate bilateral intrahepatic biliary radical dilatation noted. Common bile duct is not involved. Parenchymal atrophy noted in the left lobe. Proximal right and left branches of hepatic artery are encased by the lesion. Proper hepatic artery is normal. Left portal vein is infiltrated. Main portal vein and right branch are uninvolved. A few FDG avid periportal, portacaval, coeliac and left gastric lymph nodes noted, largest measuring ~18 × 12 mm. Enlarged left paracardiac lymph node is noted showing mild, FDG uptake, measuring ~12 × 10 mm. Multiple ill-defined hypodense lesions with mild FDG uptake noted in both lobes of liver, largest measuring ~23 × 18 mm in segment VII. **Features suggestive of biliary malignancy involving common hepatic duct, hepatic confluence, and left hepatic duct (Bismuth-Corlette-Type III b) with lymph nodal and hepatic metastases.**

Lymphoma–interim PET: Significant reduction in size and resolution of FDG uptake noted in left level III, level IV and supraclavicular lymph nodes noted, largest measuring ~ 17 × 9 mm, previously measured ~ 33 × 26 mm. Resolution of right hilar and subcarinal lymph nodes noted. Significant reduction in size with resolution of FDG uptake noted in bilateral subcentimetre axillary lymph nodes. Significant reduction in size and resolution of FDG uptake noted in paraaortic, bilateral common iliac and external iliac and inguinal lymph nodes noted, largest measuring ~21 × 7 mm, previously measured ~53 × 28 mm. Resolution of mesenteric lymph nodal mass noted. Mild reduction in size of the spleen noted with resolution of FDG avid hypodense lesions. Resolution of FDG uptake noted in both iliac bones with appearance of subtle sclerosis. **Deauville 2—complete metabolic response.**

Carcinoma lung—Follow-up PET-CT: Mild increase in size and FDG uptake noted in the soft tissue density mass with spiculated margins in apicoposterior segment of left upper lobe, measuring ~47 × 39 mm, previously measured ~40 × 21 mm. Abrupt cut off of the segmental bronchus noted with distal collapse. The mass is infiltrating the mediastinal fat plane. Mild increase in size and FDG uptake noted in right hilar, aortopulmonary and right upper paratracheal lymph nodes, largest measuring ~29 × 17 mm, previously measured ~20 × 13 mm. Appearance of a few subpleural nodules in left lower lobe. Appearance of moderate left pleural effusion. Mild increase in size and FDG uptake noted in ill-defined hypodense lesions in both lobes of liver, largest measuring ~36 × 24 mm, previously measured ~23 × 21 mm. Appearance of FDG avid nodule in left adrenal gland measuring ~20 × 11 mm. Appearance of FDG avid lytic lesions noted in multiple vertebrae, multiple ribs, sternum and left acetabulum. D7 vertebral collapse noted causing moderate spinal canal narrowing. Appearance of nodular enhancement noted in left frontal and temporal lobes. No significant edema/mass effect noted. **Features are suggestive of disease progression (T2bN3M1c).**

Neuroendocrine tumor–68Ga DOTANOC PET-CT; Jejuno-jejunal intussusception noted with a small submucosal lesion in the lead point showing significant 68Ga DOTANOC uptake, measuring ~39 × 14 mm. No evidence of bowel obstruction. Another tiny the mucosal nodular lesion with increased 68Ga DOTANOC uptake noted in the first part of the duodenum in the anterior wall, measuring ~9 × 7 mm. The nodules showing intense enhancement on arterial phase. No periserosal extension noted. Rest of the small bowel loops appear normal. Multiple enlarged 68Ga DOTANOC avid peripancreatic lymph nodes noted, largest measuring ~21 × 17 mm. No significant retroperitoneal lymphadenopathy. Multiple 68Ga DOTANOC avid lesions noted in both lobes of liver, more conspicuous on arterial phase, largest measuring ~21 × 23 mm. **Suggestive of neuroendocrine tumors in first part of the duodenum and the proximal jejunum with jejuno-jejunal intussusception, lymph nodal and hepatic metastases.**

Soft tissue sarcoma–right thigh: FDG avid heterogeneously enhancing mass noted in the anteromedial aspect of the right upper thigh in the muscular plane of right adductor longus and brevis muscles, measuring ~10.7 × 12.1 × 14.5 cm (AP × TR × CC). Enhancing thin capsule noted in the mass. Multiple nonenhancing cystic areas noted along the periphery of mass, predominantly near the inferior margin. Right adductor longus muscle is stretched and noted in the anterolateral aspect of the mass. Atrophic changes noted in the distal muscle fibres. Adductor brevis muscle is not separately visualized. Rest of the adductor compartment muscles appear normal. Neurovascular structures in the right adductor canal displaced anterolateraly. Branches of right profunda femoris are noted along the inferior margin of the mass. Right femur appears normal. No cortical erosion noted. No significant right ilio-inguinal lymphadenopathy. No pulmonary metastasis **(T3N0M0).**

Adenoid cystic carcinoma of sphenoid sinus: Heterogeneously enhancing lesion with mild FDG uptake noted in bilateral sphenoid sinuses, measuring ~68 × 42 × 35 mm. Anteriorly the lesion extending into bilateral posterior ethmoid air cells. Posteriorly the lesion is eroding the posterior wall of the sphenoid sinus. No extension noted into the prepontine cistern. Laterally, the lesion extending into the right pterygopalatine fossa. Further extension noted into the right foramen rotundum and inferior orbital fissure. Remodelling of posterior wall of the right maxillary sinus noted. Erosion and sclerosis noted in the right pterygoid bone. On the left side, the lesion encroaching the left sphenopalatine foramen with no further extension. Minimal erosion noted in the medial wall of the right orbit. No intraorbital extension noted. Superiorly erosion noted in the floor of the sella, planum sphenoidale and ethmoidale. The pituitary gland is displaced upwards. No intracranial extension. No obvious extension noted into the cavernous sinus. No significant cervical lymphadenopathy.

Right adrenal neuroblastoma: Large FDG avid lobulated heterodense mass with moderate enhancement noted in the right suprarenal region, measuring ~11.3 × 13.1 × 16.6 cm (AP × TR × CC). Right adrenal gland is not separately visualized. No calcification noted within the mass. Superiorly the mass is indenting the inferior surface of the liver with no evidence of infiltration. Superior extension noted up to the OG junction. Inferiorly the mass is displacing the right kidney. Inferior extension noted to the level of right common iliac vessels. Medially the mass is displacing the abdominal aorta anteriorly and extending across the midline. Inferior vena cava is encased and compressed by the mass. Laterally the mass abutting the right lateral chest wall. Anteriorly the mass is displacing the pancreas. Posteriorly the mass is extending up to the level of right D12–L1 neural foramen. However, no neural foraminal/intraspinal extension noted. Multiple FDG avid mesenteric lymph nodes noted, largest measuring ~18 × 14 mm. A few FDG avid lymph nodes noted in the paraaortic region, largest measuring ~12 × 12 mm. Moderate ascites noted. No metabolically active focal lesion noted in the liver. Multiple FDG avid bilateral upper paratracheal and prevascular lymph nodes noted, largest measuring ~13 × 11 mm. Multiple FDG avid left supraclavicular lymph nodes noted. No evidence of pulmonary metastasis. No FDG avid skeletal lesions noted. International Neuroblastoma Staging System Committee (INSS) system—**stage 4 disease**.

Radiological Anatomy

3.1 CRANIAL VAULT AND BRAIN

3.1.A Scalp and Cranial Vault

Scalp: The scalp is a soft-tissue envelope that surrounds the cranial vault from the external occipital protuberance and superior nuchal line of occipital bone to the orbital margins of frontal bone and is laterally anchored to zygoma. It has five layers—**S**kin, Sub**C**utaneous tissue, **A**poneurotic layer, **L**oose areolar connective tissue, **P**ericranium (mnemonic–**scalp**). **Skin:** It has thin epidermis and inner layer of thick dermis. It has hair follicles, sebaceous glands, sweat glands, apocrine glands. **SubCutaneous tissue/dense connective tissue**—has nerves, lymphatics, and vessels. **Galea aponeurotica, or epicranial aponeurosis**—it allows attachment for muscles of the scalp, paired occipitofrontalis, tempero-parietal muscles. **Loose connective tissue/subgaleal layer**—also known as "danger zone" because infections can spread into intracranial compartment via emissary veins. This layer being so loose it is a potential space for collections and haematomas. It is the plane of separation of neurosurgical procedures and traumatic avulsions. **Pericranium**—has periosteum of skull bones, firmly attached to skull bones and extends into the cranial sutures. **Three layers are distinguishable radiologically** on MRI and CT images (Figs 3.1.1 and 3.1.2)—**the skin layer, the subcutaneous layer, and the galea-subgaleal-periosteum complex.** Skin appears as high dense structure in CT and low intensity in both T1 and T2 images. Subcutaneous layer because of fat content appears as low dense in CT, high intensity in T1, T2 images. The galea-subgaleal-periosteum complex sometimes become indistinguishable from the high-attenuating calvaria on CT images and from the low signal intensity of the outer table on MR images. Importance of identifying these layers are scalp lesions can be characterized based on their locations in scalp, involving skin or connective tissue, subgaleal layer (between the galea aponeurotica and the skull periosteum), or involving several or all layers of the scalp.

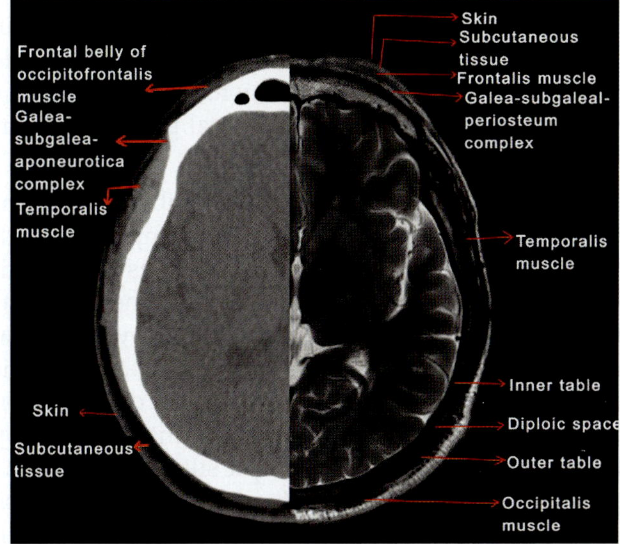

Fig. 3.1.1: Axial image showing scalp layers in CT and MRI

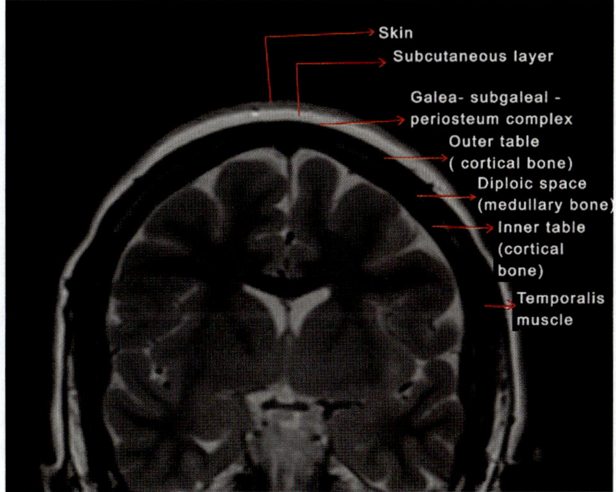

Fig. 3.1.2: Coronal MR images of scalp

Skull: Has 28 separate bones, mostly connected by fibrous sutures. Cranium is divided into calvarial

Table 3.1.1: Skull bones	
Cranium—14 bones include 7 bones in vault and 7 bones in base	
Paired (2 each)	*Unpaired (1 each)*
Parietal, temporal, ear ossicles—malleus, incus and stapes	Frontal, occipital, sphenoid, ethmoid
The facial skeleton is composed of 14 bones	
Paired (2 each)	*Unpaired (1 each)*
Maxilla, zygomatic, nasal, inferior nasal concha, lacrimal, palatine	Mandible, vomer

vault, facial bones, cranial base. Cranial vault is made of frontal bone, paired parietal bones, occipital bone, paired temporal bones. It has outer and inner table separated by diploic space. Outer and inner table being a compact cortical bone, has low signal intensity on MR and is more dense on CT. Diploic space filled with fatty marrow, has high signal intensity. This space contains many thin walled diploic veins, providing cranio-cerebral anastomosis and pathway for route of spread of infection, and also provides collateral pathway during venous sinus occlusion.

Sutures of skull: Sutures are a type of fibrous joint that are unique to the skull. These joints are important in the context of trauma, as they represent points of potential weakness in the skull. The main sutures in the adult skull are: Coronal suture—fuses the frontal bone with the two parietal bones. Sagittal suture—fuses both parietal bones to each other. Lambdoid suture—fuses the occipital bone to the two parietal bones. Frontal bone intially develops as two halves, separated by metopic suture, later fuses to single bone usually at 5 years of age. Occasionally, persist into adult life in 5–10% of individuals. In neonates, the incompletely fused suture joints give rise to membranous gaps between the bones, known as fontanelles. Anterior fontanelle (bregma) closes by 18 months, mastoid fontanelle by 12 months, posterior fontanelle (lambda) by 2–3 months and sphenoidal fontanelle also by 2–3 months.The greater wing of sphenoid and the squamous part of the temporal bone form the side of the skull vault below the frontal and parietal bones. The sutures formed here are: (i) the sphenosquamosal suture between the sphenoid and temporal bones; (ii) the sphenofrontal and sphenoparietal sutures between greater wing of sphenoid and frontal and parietal bones; and (iii) the squamosal suture between temporal and parietal bones. The sphenofrontal, sphenoparietal and squamosal sutures form a continuous curved line. The intersection of the sutures between the frontal, sphenoidal, parietal and temporal bones is termed the pterion and provides a surface marking for the anterior branch of the middle meningeal artery on the lateral skull radiograph. The asterion is the point where the squamosal suture meets the lambdoid suture (Figs 3.1.3 to 3.1.8).

Meninges: Surface of brain is covered by three membranes; Pia, arachnoid (collectively known as **leptomeninges**) and dura **(pachymeninges)**. **Dura** has two layers, **outer periosteal layer** which lines the inner surface of skull, tightly attached to sutures and **inner meningeal layer** which is closely apposed to the arachnoid. Dural venous sinuses are located between these two layers. Dural capillaries lack endothelial tight junctions, hence dura

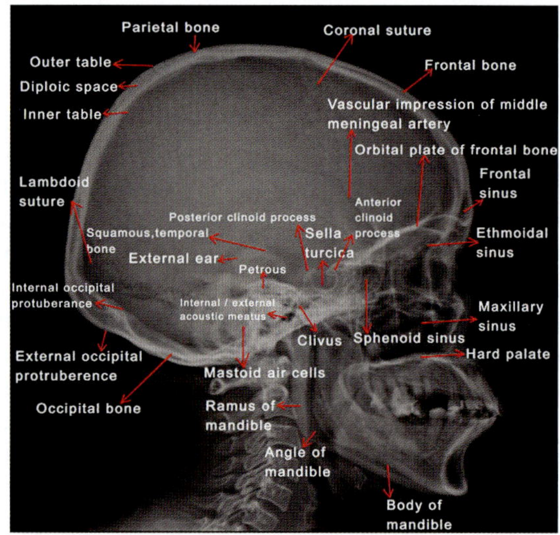

Fig. 3.1.3: Skull radiograph lateral view

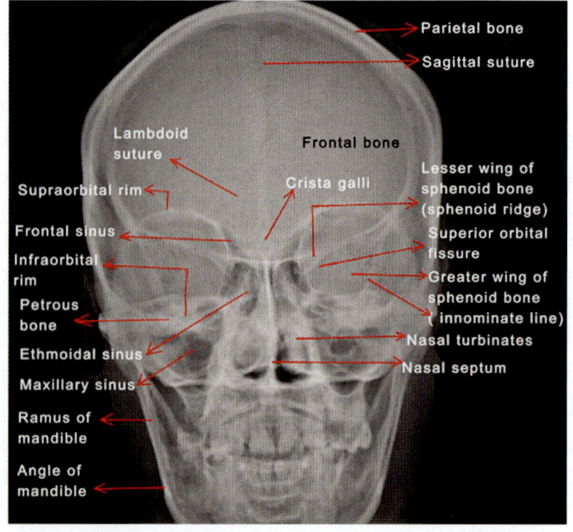

Fig. 3.1.4: Skull radiograph AP view

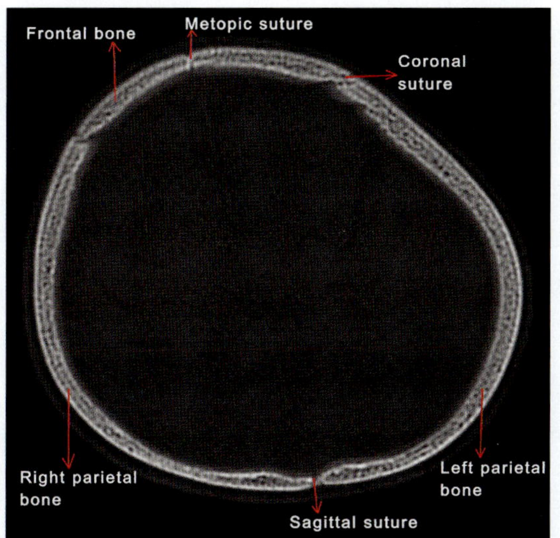

Fig. 3.1.5: CT axial image of skull bones and sutures

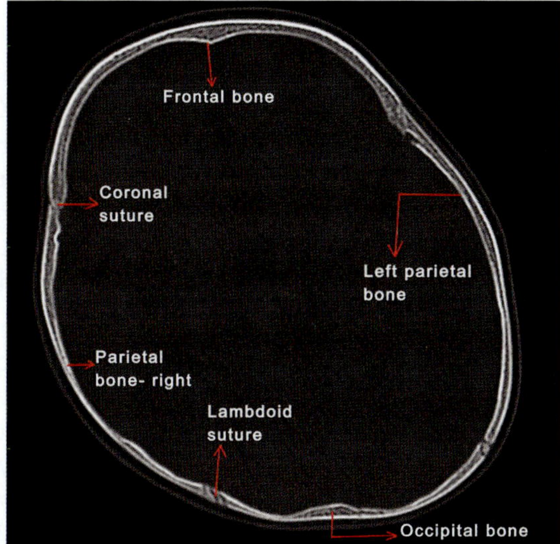

Fig. 3.1.6: CT axial image of skull bones and sutures

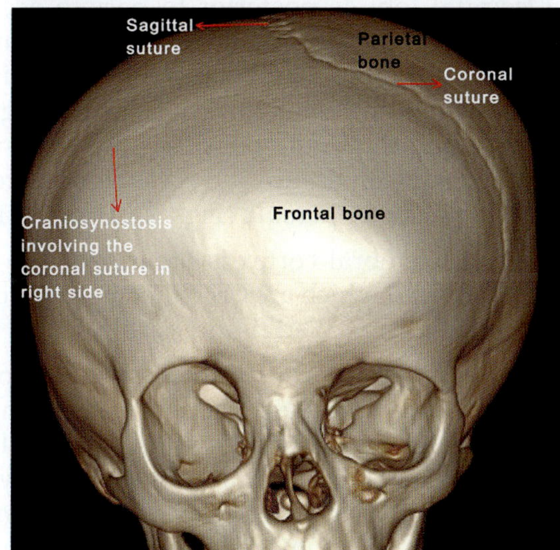

Fig. 3.1.7: VRT image of skull

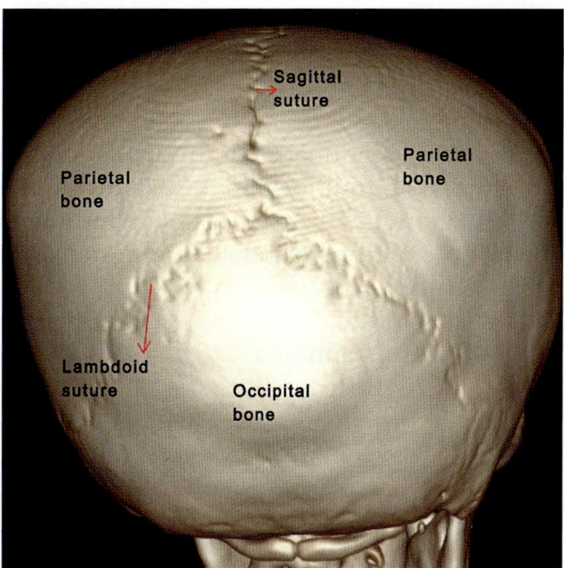

Fig. 3.1.8: VRT image of skull

enhance well with contrast, which is of 1–2 mm thick. **Arachnoid** is a thin layer, which is adherent to dura. Inner layer of dura and arachnoid forms **dural septa** (falx cerebri , tentorium cerebelli, falx cerebelli and diaphragma sellae). Falx extends from crista galli to internal occipital protuberance, where it joins with the tentorium. Tentorium cerebelli separates the supratentorial from the infratentorial compartment. It is attached from the posterior clinoid process along the petrous ridges to the internal occipital protuberance. The two compartments communicate via the tentorial incisura, through which the midbrain passes. **Pia (innermost layer)** covers the entire brain surface and extends into sulci, fissures and fossae. Pia also extends into penetrating cortical arteries into brain, forming perivascular space (Virchow-Robin spaces), which are pial lined interstitial fluid filled spaces along penetrating arteries. They are normally seen as linear/ovoid fluid filled areas in basal ganglia around anterior commissure, midbrain, deep cerebral white matter. **Extradural space** is between dura and skull. Since outer dural layer is firmly attached to sutures, collection in extradural space can cross the midline and is limited by sutures. **Subdural space** is between inner dura and arachnoid. Bridging veins that connect the cortical veins to the overlying dural venous sinuses pass through the arachnoid and inner dural layer, i.e. subdural space. Collection in subdural space can extend into interhemispheric fissure and will not cross the midline. **Subarachnoid space** between arachnoid and pia contains CSF. These subarachnoid spaces are wider in some areas, forming subarachnoid cisterns (e.g. cisterna magna, prepontine cistern). Subarachnoid space contains much of cerebral arterial vasculature, therefore rupture or leakage from these arteries results in subarachnoid hemorrhages. **Arachnoid granulations** (arachnoid villi grouped together) are located in superior sagittal sinus, in posterior fossa near the transverse sinus, near the torcular herophili (confluence of dural venous sinuses) and along floor of middle cranial fossa near sphenoid sinus. These granulations can result in bony erosion/ remodelling of inner table and should not be mistaken for bony destructive process.

3.1.B Cerebral Hemispheres

Consists of gray matter and white matter. Gray matter is mainly composed of neuronal cell bodies and located on superficial surface of cerebral and cerebellar cortex and also in deep gray matter structures like basal nuclei, diencephalon, brain stem nuclei and deep cerebellar nuclei. In T1W images grey matter appears as low signal intensity than white matter, T2/FLAIR images reverse occurs, i.e. grey matter has high signal intensity than white matter. CT, white matter is darker than grey matter, due to its high lipid content in myelin.

Planning of CT, MRI: On CT, the **orbitomeatal line** is the standard reference line. It passes through the outer canthus and the center of the external auditory meatus (Fig. 3.1.9). On MRI, **AC-PC line** is most commonly used in brain axial imaging. It passes through anterior commissure (AC) to posterior commissure (PC) (Fig. 3.1.10). The plane of the angle of the sagittal image is parallel to the interhemispheric fissure. The angle

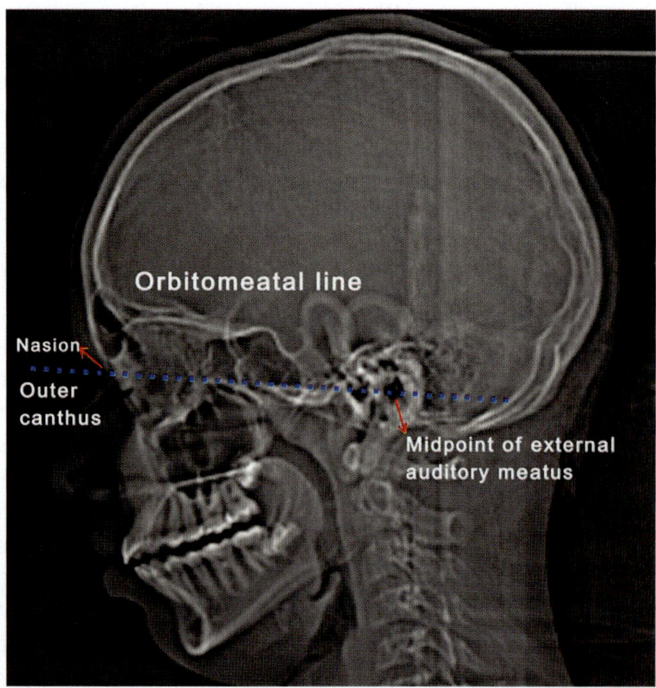

Fig. 3.1.9: Planning of CT (orbitomeatal line)

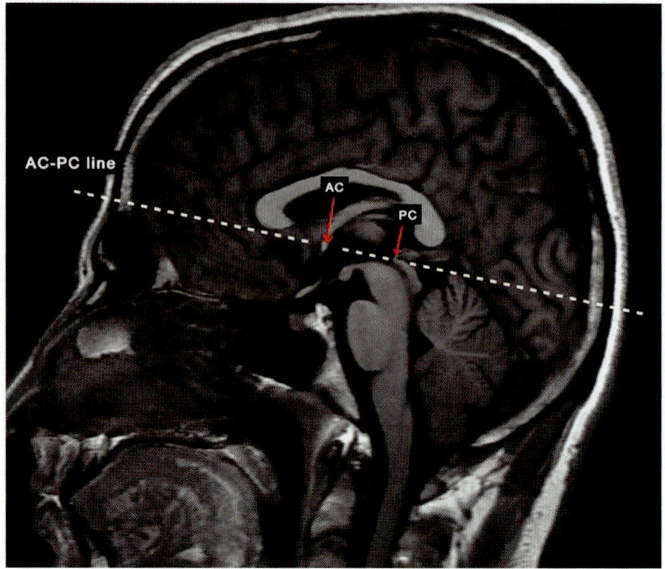

Fig. 3.1.10: Planning of MRI (AC-PC line)

of the coronal image is usually parallel to the bed of the MR equipment or parallel to the brainstem. Other lines—supraorbito-meatal line which passes through the superior orbital wall to external auditory meatus and is recommended for avoiding irradiation to the orbit, subcallosal line (recommended for multiple sclerosis), Reid's baseline (lesions of orbital cavity, PNS, skull base), brainstem vertical line (for brainstem lesions).

Cerebral lobes: Cerebral hemispheres are divided into frontal, parietal, temporal and occipital lobe. In addition to these are insular lobe and limbic lobe. Frontal lobe is seen anterior to central sulcus and superior to sylvian fissure. Parietal lobe is seen posterior to central sulcus and anterior to parieto-occipital sulcus. Temporal lobe is inferior to sylvian fissure and anterior to angular gyrus. Occipital lobe is posterior to parieto-occipital sulcus on the medial surface and on the lateral surface, an imaginary line (lateral parieto-temporal line) divides the occipital lobe from the temporal lobe extending from preoccipital notch to parieto-occipital sulcus. Insula is located deep to sylvian fissure and is covered by frontal, temporal and parietal opercula (Figs 3.1.11 to 3.1.14).

Sulci and gyri: Cerebral cortex is organised into folds called gyri, between which are CSF filled grooves called sulci. Deeper sulci are called fissure (Table 3.1.2).

Sylvian fissure/lateral fissure: Deep fissure seen on the lateral surface of cerebral hemisphere, separating the frontal and parietal lobes above from temporal lobe below. It has stem and many branches. Stem of sylvian fissure also known as sylvian cistern, which contains the M1 segment of MCA (middle cerebral artery) (Fig. 3.1.37). The three main branches are **anterior**

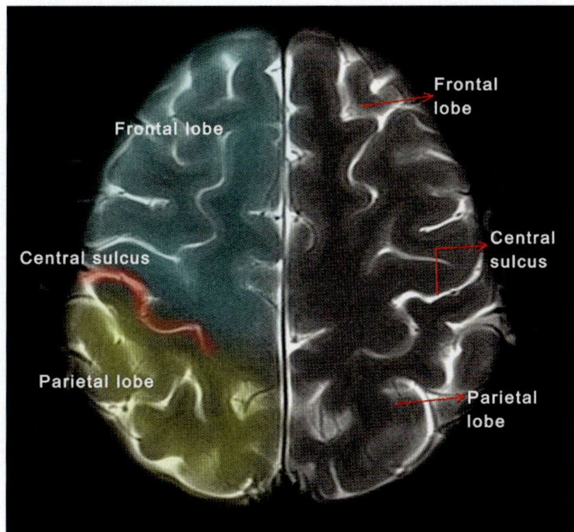

Fig. 3.1.11: Cerebral lobes in MR axial image

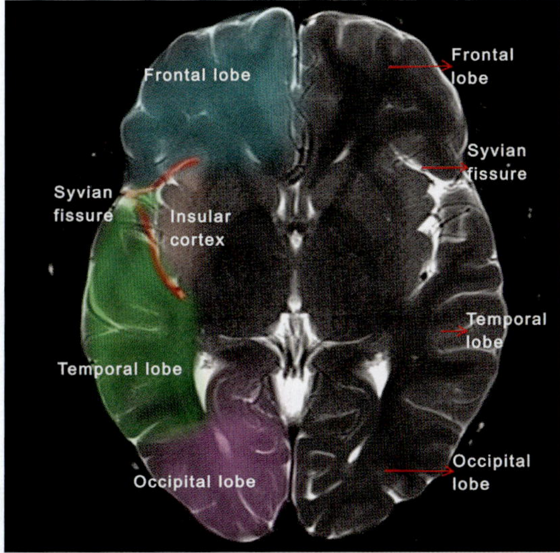

Fig. 3.1.12: Cerebral lobes in MR axial image

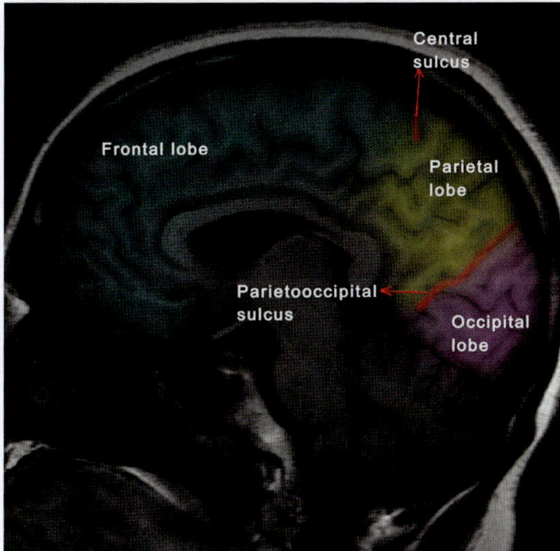

Fig. 3.1.13: Cerebral lobes in MR sagittal image

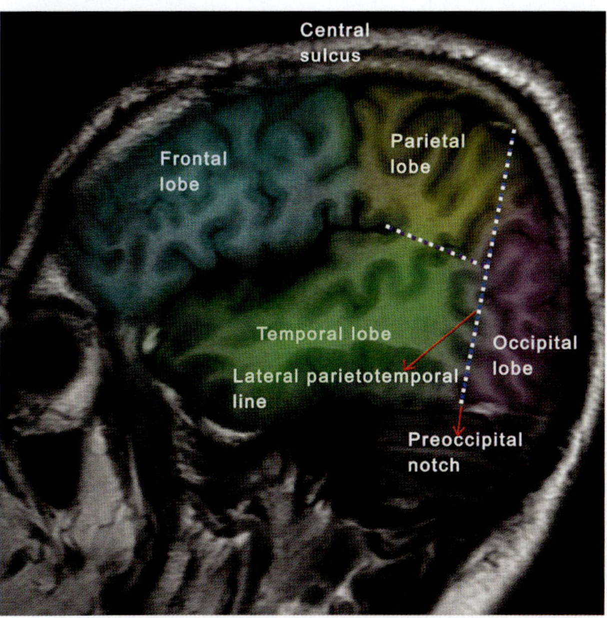

Fig. 3.1.14: Cerebral lobes in MR sagittal image

horizontal rami, anterior ascending rami, posterior ascending rami (Figs 3.1.28 and 3.1.29). Anterior horizontal rami separates pars orbitalis from pars triangularis and anterior ascending rami separates pars triangularis from pars opercularis of inferior frontal gyrus. Posterior ascending ramus ends within the superior marginal gyrus of inferior parietal lobule. Posterior descending rami of sylvian fissure extends into superior temporal gyrus, which is limited anteriorly by the transverse supratemporal sulcus separating planum temporale from Heschl gyrus. Superiorly the lateral sulcus continues as circular sulcus, surrounding the insular cortex (Fig. 3.1.25). Insular cortex is located deep to the sylvian fissure. Deep part of sylvian fissure is made of operculoinsular compartment and sphenoidal compartment. Insular compartment of sylvian fissure is located on the lateral surface of insula and contains M2 segment of MCA. Opercular compartment of sylvian fissure has M3 segment of MCA.

Identifying central sulcus (limiting sulcus): Key anatomic landmark which separates frontal and parietal lobes, primary motor cortex (precentral gyrus) from primary sensory cortex (postcentral gyrus). **Signs for identification of central sulcus:** ***Midline sulcus sign***—central sulcus is the longest sulcus to reach midline and intersect interhemispheric fissure in higher axial sections (Fig. 3.1.16). ***Upper T sign***—superior frontal sulcus intersects the precentral sulcus in a "T" junction. The central sulcus is the next posterior sulcus. ***L sign***—superior frontal gyrus intersects precentral gyrus in "L" junction with the central sulcus lying immediately posterior. ***Omega/sigmoid hook sign***—the precentral

Table 3.1.2: Cerebral fissures and lobes	
Name	*Structures separated from one another*
Longitudinal fissure (Interhemispheric fissure)	Cerebral hemispheres
Central sulcus	Frontal and parietal lobes
Lateral sulcus/Sylvian fissure	Refer to text
Superior frontal sulcus	Superior frontal gyrus and middle frontal gyrus
Inferior frontal sulcus	Middle and inferior frontal gyrus
Precentral sulcus	Precentral gyrus and frontal gyri
Cingulate sulcus	Cingulate gyrus and medial frontal gyrus
Callosal sulcus	Corpus callosum and cingulate gyrus
Olfactory sulcus	Gyrus recti and medial orbital gyrus
Orbital sulcus	Orbital gyri
Post-central sulcus	Post-central gyrus, from remainder parietal lobe
Intraparietal sulcus	Superior and inferior parietal lobules
Subparietal sulcus	Precuneus and cingulate gyrus
Parieto-occipital sulcus	Parietal and occipital lobes
Pars marginalis (marginal sulcus)	Paracentral lobule and precuneus
Superior temporal sulcus	Superior and middle temporal gyrus
Inferior temporal sulcus	Middle and inferior temporal gyrus
Lateral occipitotemporal sulcus	Inferior temporal gyrus and medial occipitotemporal gyri (fusiform gyri)
Collateral sulcus	Parahippocampal gyrus and medial occipitotemporal gyri (lingual/fusiform gyri). Continues as rhinal sulcus medially.
Calcarine sulcus	(Lingual gyrus) Infracalcrine region and cuneus
Lateral (or inferior) occipital sulcus	Middle and inferior occipital gyrus
Intraoccipital sulcus (also known as superior occipital sulcus)	Superior and middle occipital gyrus

gyrus bulges posteriorly shaped like omega at the hand motor area. ***Thin post-central gyrus sign***—the precentral gyrus is roughly 1.5 times thicker than the post-central gyrus. ***M sign***—the inferior frontal gyrus has a characteristic "M" configuration and terminates posteriorly in the precentral gyrus posterior to which lies central sulcus. ***IPS-post CS sign:*** The IPS (intraparietal sulcus) will join with post-central sulcus.

Bracket sign—in sagittal paramedial sections the marginal sulcus is visible posterior to the central sulcus as the continuation of cingulate sulcus. ***Bifid post-central gyrus sign***—the postcentral gyrus is split medially by the pars marginalis of the cingulate sulcus. **Lower T sign**—the inferior frontal sulcus terminates posteriorly in the pre-central sulcus in a 'T' junction. The central sulcus lies posteriorly. ***White gray sign***—this sign is useful for identifying central sulcus on MRI images. Since primary motor cortex and sensory cortex have more myelin than other cortices this causes whitening of the cortex on T1WI especially well appreciated in higher field strengths (Figs 3.1.15 and 3.1.16).

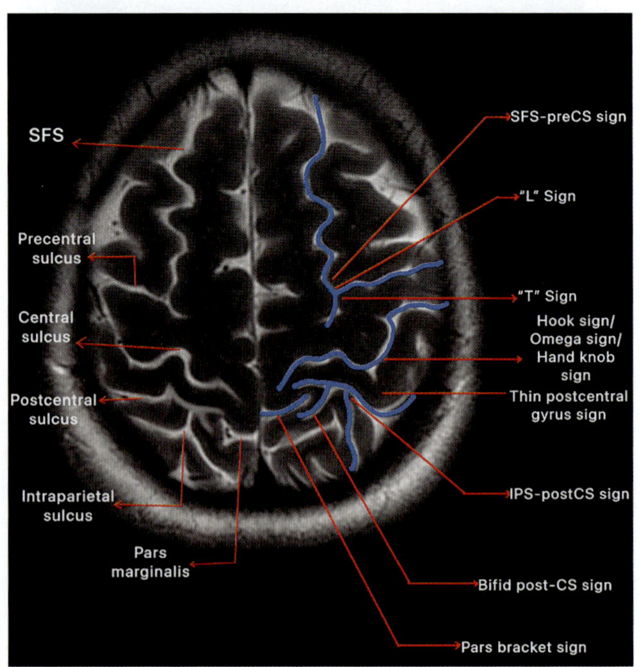

Fig. 3.1.15: Central sulcus identification in axial section

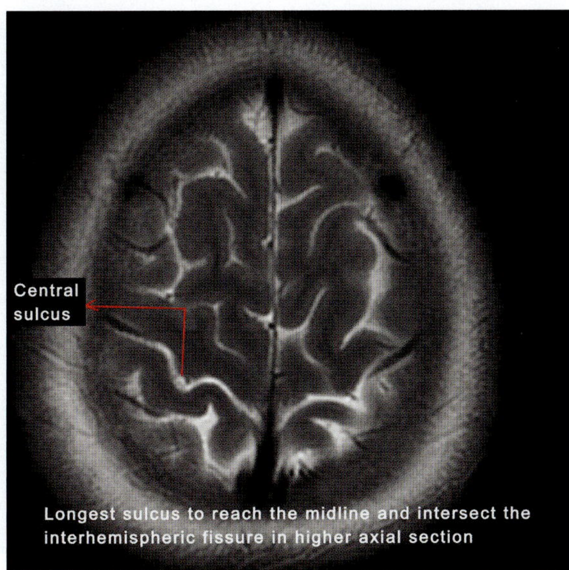

Fig. 3.1.16: Central sulcus identification in axial section

Identification on sagittal sections: Midline sagittal images (Fig. 3.1.20)—sulcus which is immediately anterior to marginal ramus of cingulate sulcus is central sulcus. On lateral sagittal sections—anterior horizontal rami and anterior ascending rami of sylvian fissure forms 'Y' shaped appearance (Fig. 3.1.17), posterior to this is precentral sulcus and a sulcus which is running parallel and posterior to precentral sulcus is central sulcus. Inferior frontal sulcus intersects with precentral sulcus in sagittal section (Fig. 3.1.18). Precentral knob, in sagittal plane the knob has the shape of a posteriorly directed hook facing the postcentral gyrus (Fig. 3.1.19).

Frontal lobe: Supero-lateral surface—has **superior (SFG), middle (MFG) and inferior frontal gyri (IFG) separated by superior (SFS) and inferior frontal sulci (IFS).** Superior frontal sulci is identified as it runs longitudinally and parallel to SFG and terminates posteriorly into precentral sulci which runs horizontally oblique in front of central sulci. Inferior frontal sulcus runs parallel to sylvian fissure separating MFG from IFG. Posterior to **precentral sulcus** is **precentral gyrus** (anterior to central sulcus) (Figs 3.1.21–3.1.24). Inferior frontal gyrus has 3 gyri from anterior to posterior are **pars orbitalis, pars triangularis, pars opercularis** separated by anterior horizontal ramus and anterior ascending ramus of sylvian fissure (Fig. 3.1.29). Medial surface—medial aspect of superior frontal gyrus (medial frontal gyrus), gyrus recti, rostral gyrus. Gyrus recti is located paramedial to either side of midline. It is separated from the rostral gyrus located above by inferior rostral sulcus (Figs 3.1.33 and 3.1.36). Superior rostral sulcus separates rostral gyrus from SFG (medial aspect). **Septal area** is located in front of lamina terminalis (Fig. 3.1.25), inferior

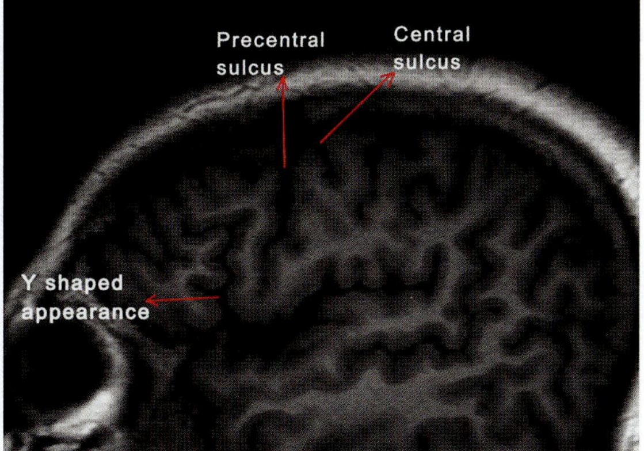

Fig. 3.1.17: Central sulcus in sagittal section

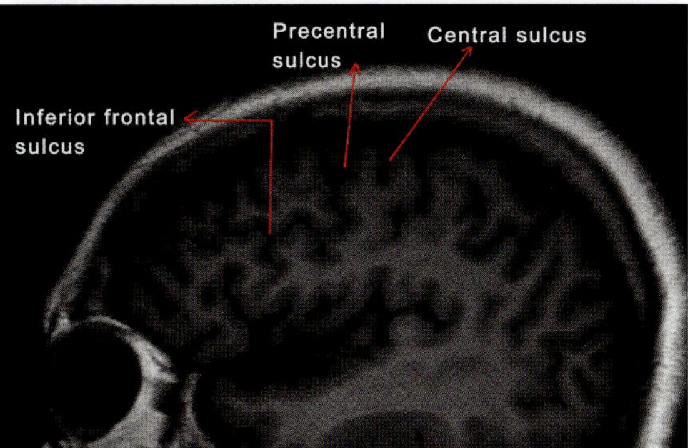

Fig. 3.1.18: Central sulcus in sagittal section

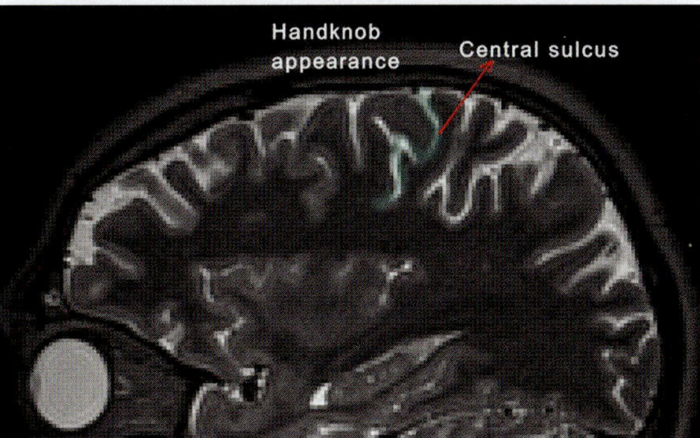

Fig. 3.1.19: Central sulcus in sagittal section

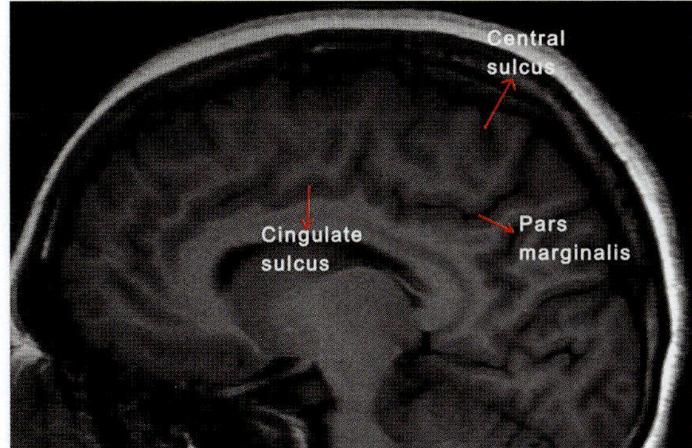

Fig. 3.1.20: Central sulcus in sagittal section

3

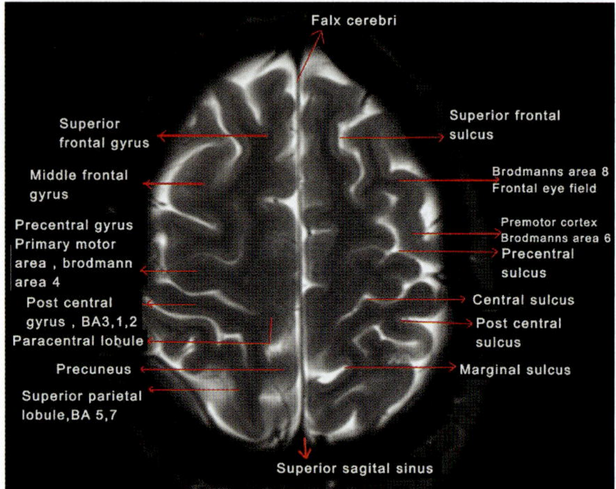

Fig. 3.1.21

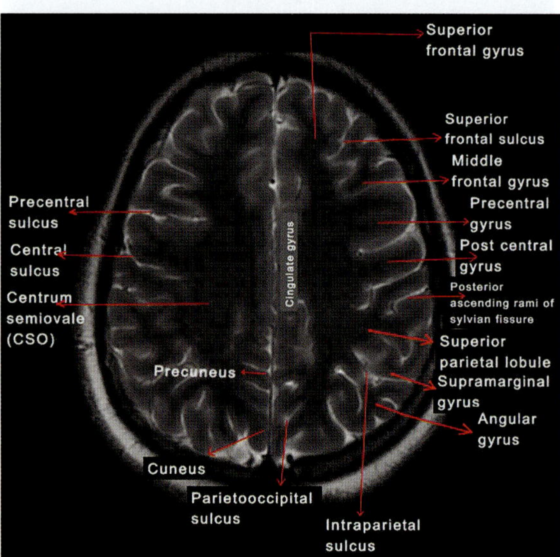

Fig. 3.1.22

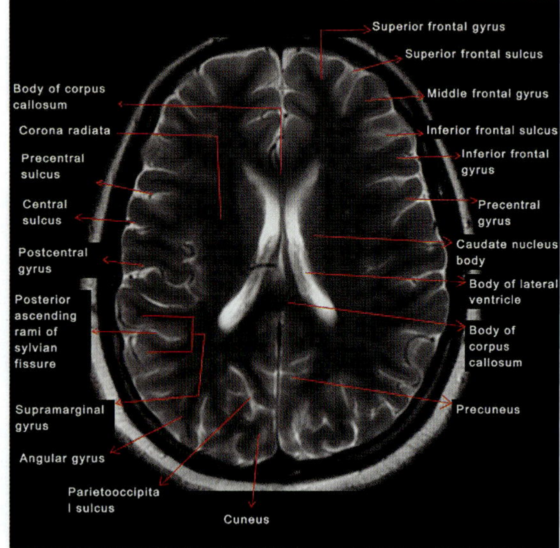

Fig. 3.1.23

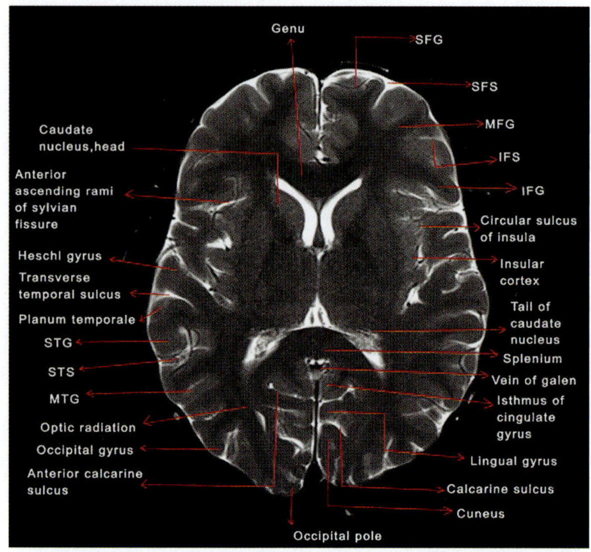

Fig. 3.1.24

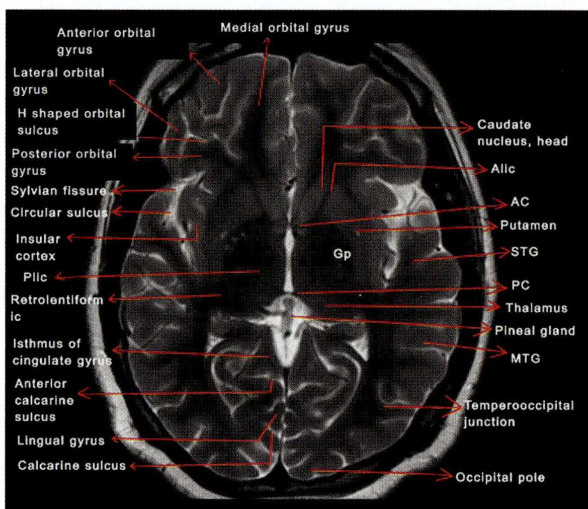

Fig. 3.1.25

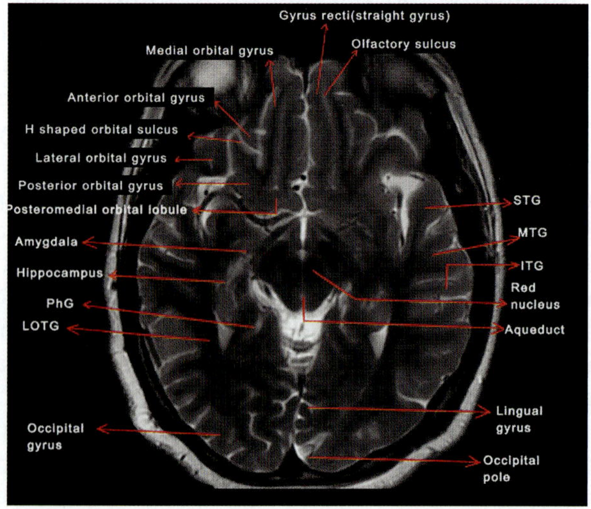

Fig. 3.1.26

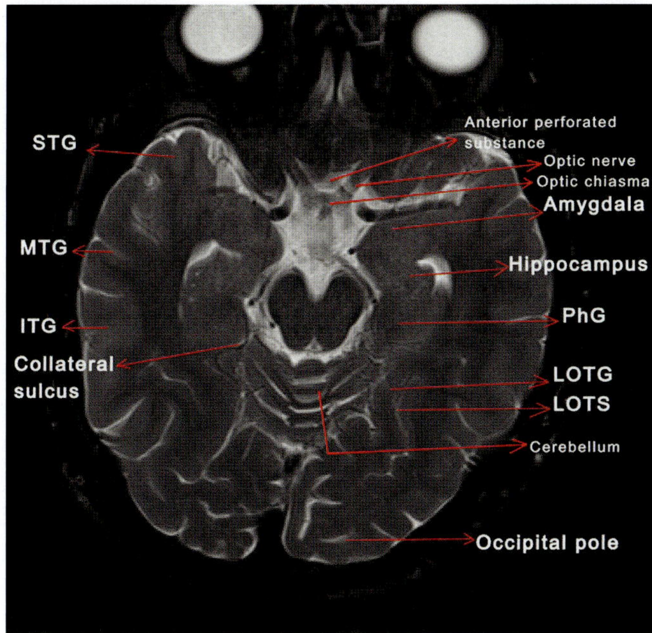

Fig. 3.1.27

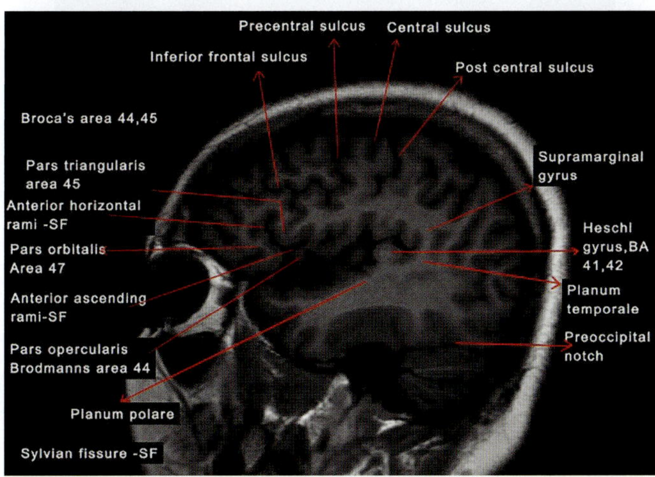

Fig. 3.1.28

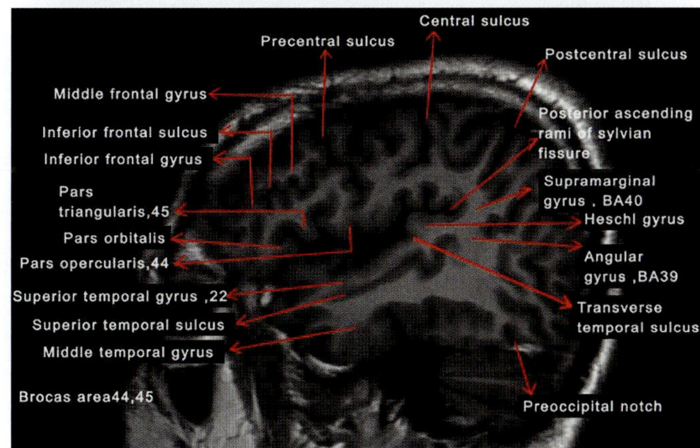

Fig. 3.1.29

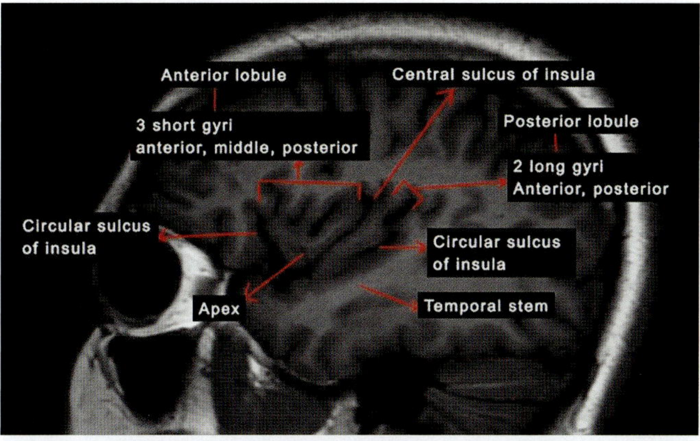

Fig. 3.1.30

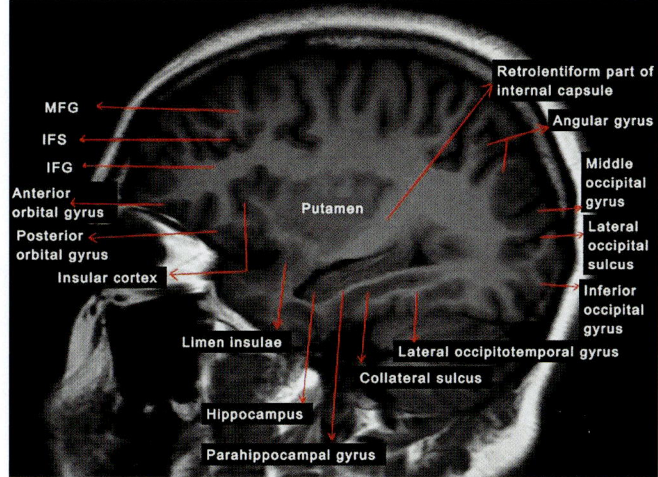

Fig. 3.1.31

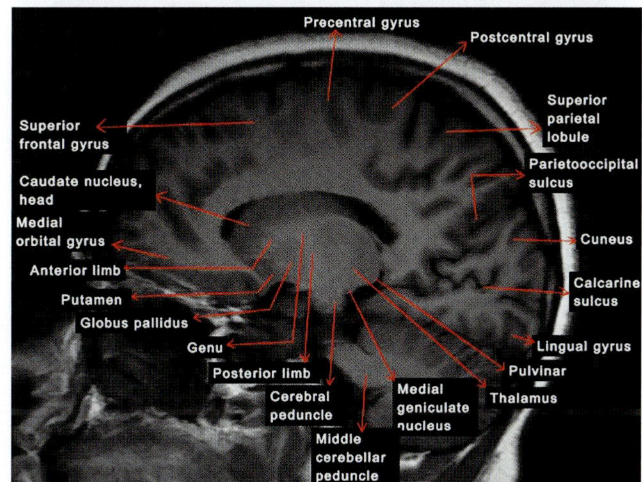

Fig. 3.1.32

to rostrum of corpus callosum and posterior to gyrus recti and rostral gyrus. It has paraolfactory gyrus (subcallosal area) and paraterminal gyrus (just anterior to lamina terminalis) separated by posterior paraolfactory sulcus. Anterior paraolfactory sulcus separates paraolfactory

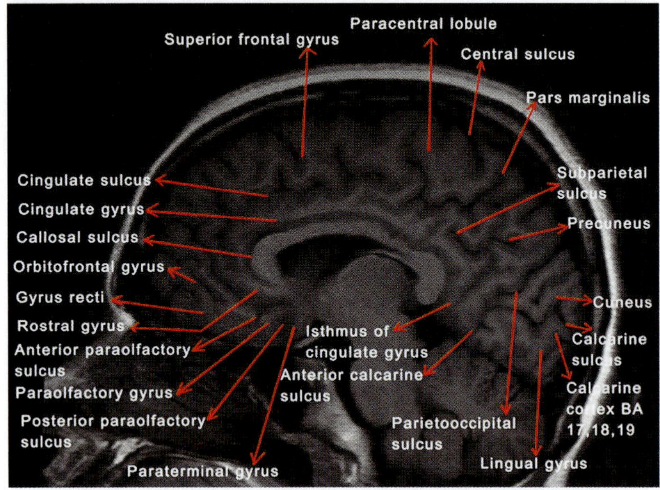

Fig. 3.1.33

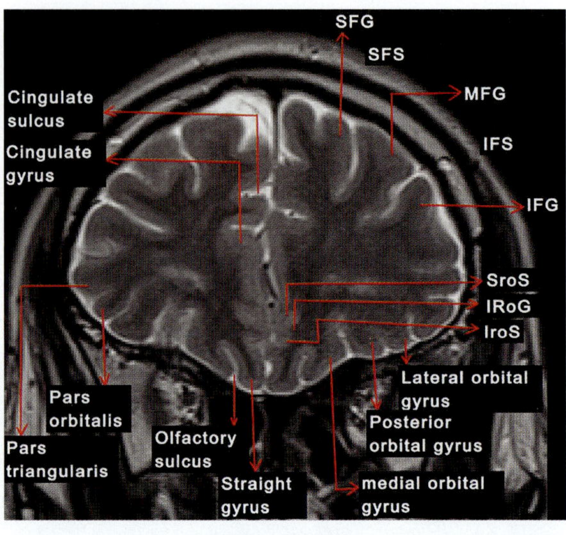

Fig. 3.1.36

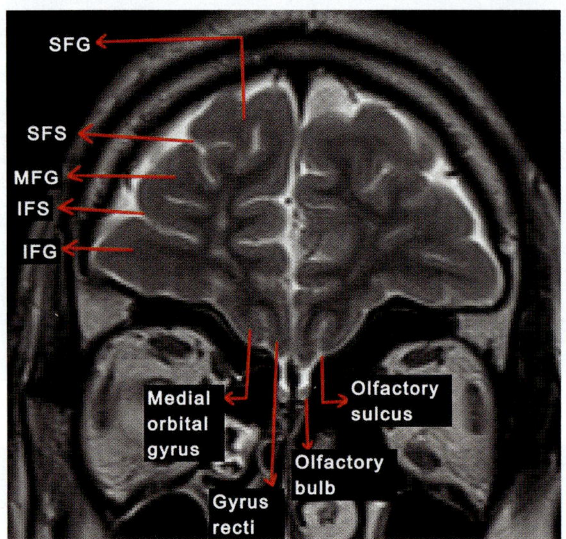

Fig. 3.1.34

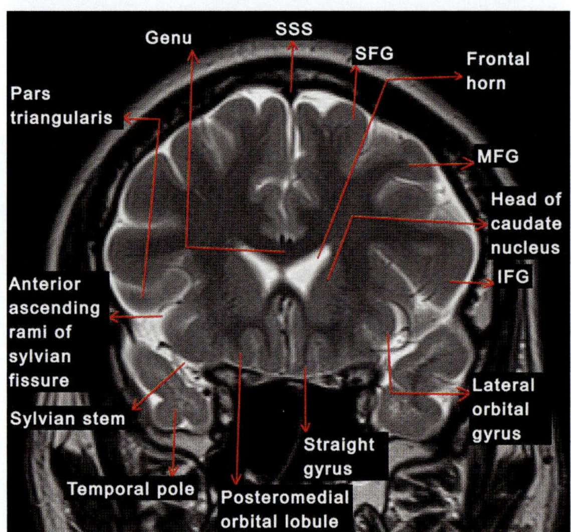

Fig. 3.1.37

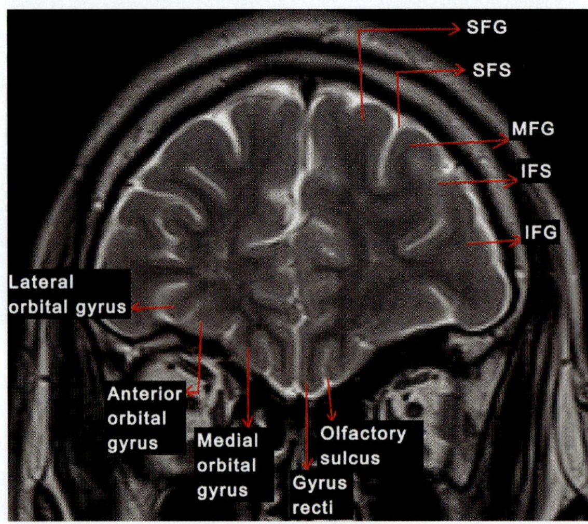

Fig. 3.1.35

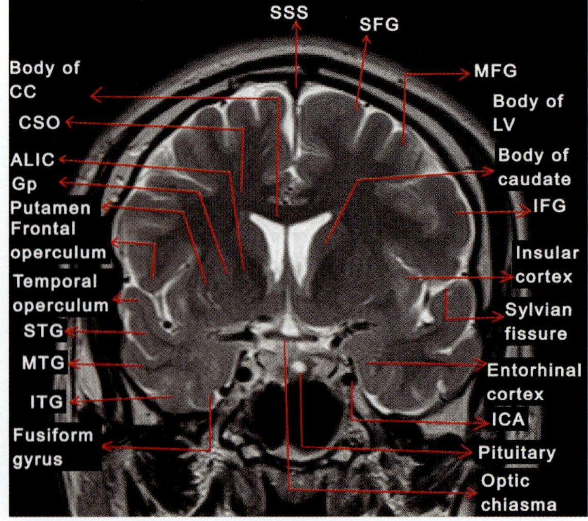

Fig. 3.1.38

gyrus from gyrus recti and rostral gyrus anteriorly (Fig. 3.1.33). Inferior to paraterminal gyrus and subcallosal area is a triangular area known as anterior perforated substance. Inferior surface: **Gyrus recti (straight gyrus)** located on either side of midline, just above the cribriform plate. **Olfactory sulcus** separates **medial orbital gyrus** from gyrus recti. Olfactory tract and bulb is seen in olfactory sulcus. **Orbital gyrus** is seen around the **H-shaped orbital sulcus,** which separates it into **medial, lateral, anterior** and **posterior orbital gyrus** (Figs 3.1.25 and 3.1.26).

Parietal lobe: Superolateral surface—consists of post-central gyrus, superior parietal lobule and inferior parietal lobule (supramarginal gyrus and angular gyrus). **Post-central gyrus** located posterior to central sulcus and anterior to post-central sulcus. **Superior parietal lobule** extends from postcentral sulcus to parietoccipital sulcus posteriorly. Superior parietal lobule is separated from **inferior parietal lobule** by **intraparietal sulcus. Supramarginal gyrus** is seen surrounding the posterior ascending ramus of sylvian fissure. **Angular gyrus** is located posterior to supramarginal gyrus surrounding the distal portion of superior temporal sulcus. Medial surface: **Precuneus** is the medial extension of superior parietal lobule extends from **pars marginalis (marginal branch of cingulate sulcus)** to **parieto-occipital sulcus. Paracentral lobule** is medial aspect of precentral and postcentral gyrus (part of both frontal and parietal lobe). Paracentral sulcus—separates paracentral lobule and medial frontal gyrus (Figs 3.1.21, 3.1.22, 3.1.29 and 3.1.33).

Temporal lobe: Superolateral surface—has **superior (STG), middle (MTG)** and **inferior temporal gyri (ITG)** separated by **superior (STS) and inferior temporal sulci (ITS). Heschl gyrus (transverse temporal gyrus)** is located in STG projecting into the lateral fissure, limited posteriorly by **transverse temporal sulcus,** thus separating it from **palnum temporale** posteriorly. Anterior to Heschl gyrus is **planum polare**. Inferior surface, from lateral to medial, consists of **inferior temporal gyrus, fusiform gyrus (lateral occipito-temporal gyrus), parahippocampal gyrus. Collateral sulcus** separates parahippocampal gyrus from fusiform gyrus, which in turn is separated from inferior temporal gyrus by **lateral occipitotemporal sulcus** (LOTS) (Figs 3.1.28. 3.1.29, 3.1.38, 3.1.39 and 3.1.52).

Occipital lobe: Superolateral surface—occipital lobe has inconsistent arrangement of sulci and gyri. Superior occipital gyrus is located more medially along interhemispheric fissure, which is separated from middle occipital gyrus located laterally by intraoccipital sulcus, which is a continuation of intraparietal sulcus. Inferior

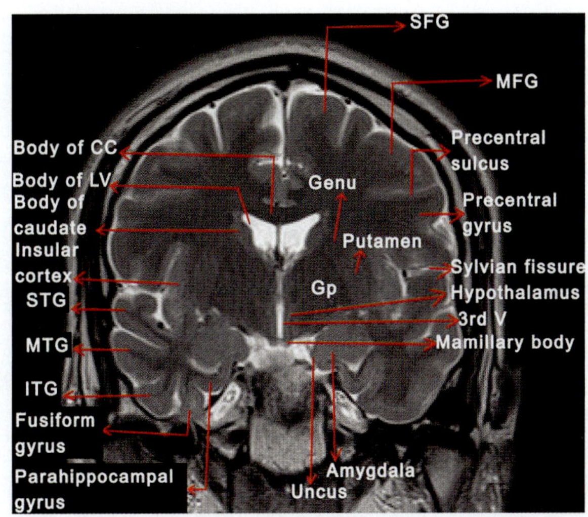

Fig. 3.1.39

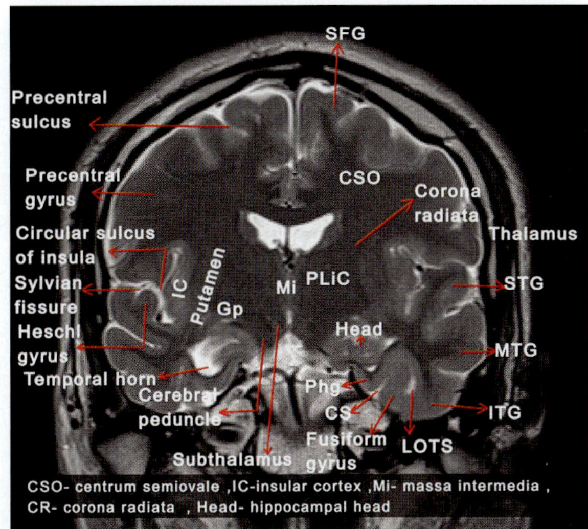

Fig. 3.1.40

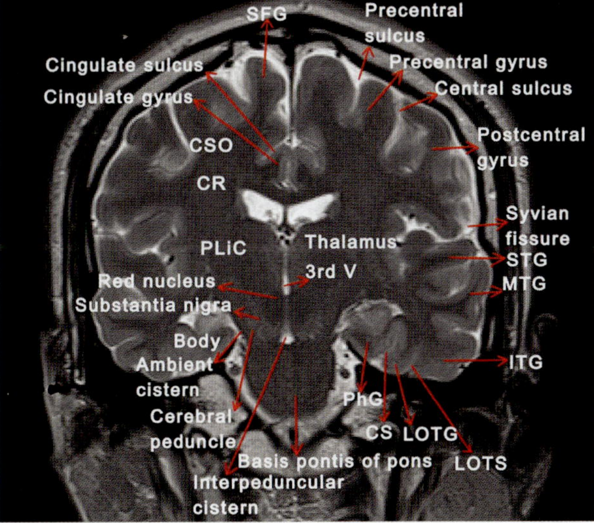

Fig. 3.1.41

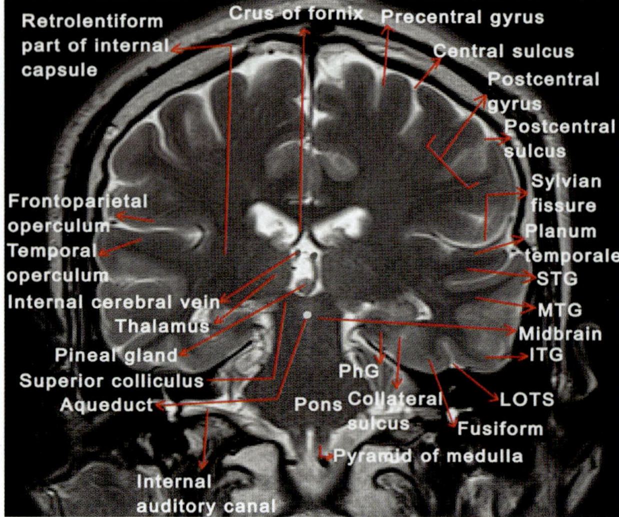

Fig. 3.1.42

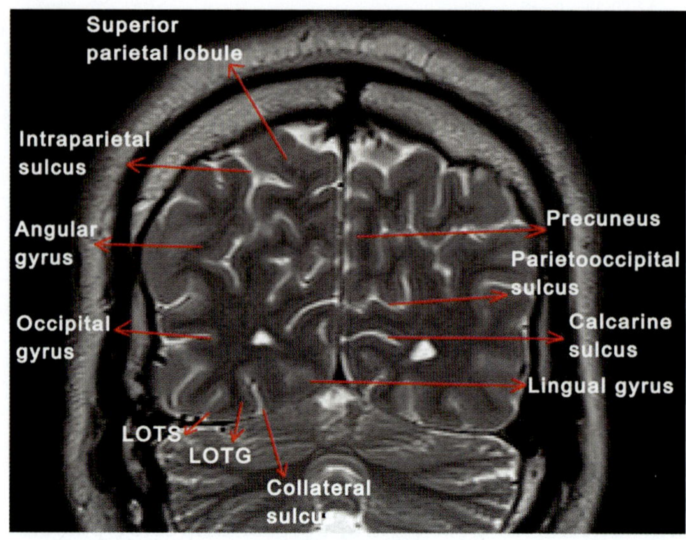

Fig. 3.1.45

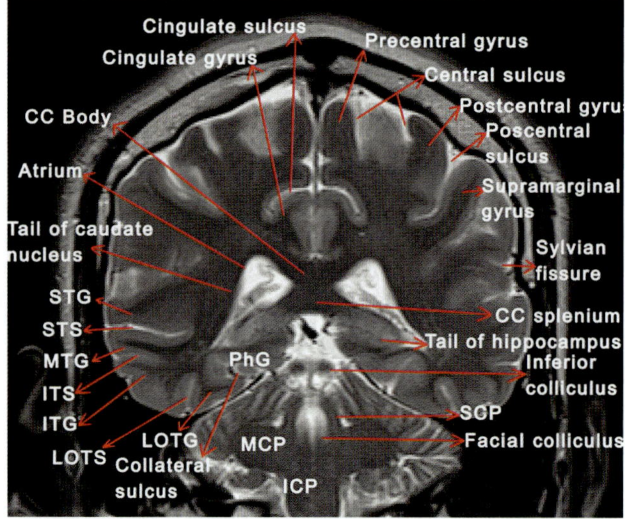

Fig. 3.1.43

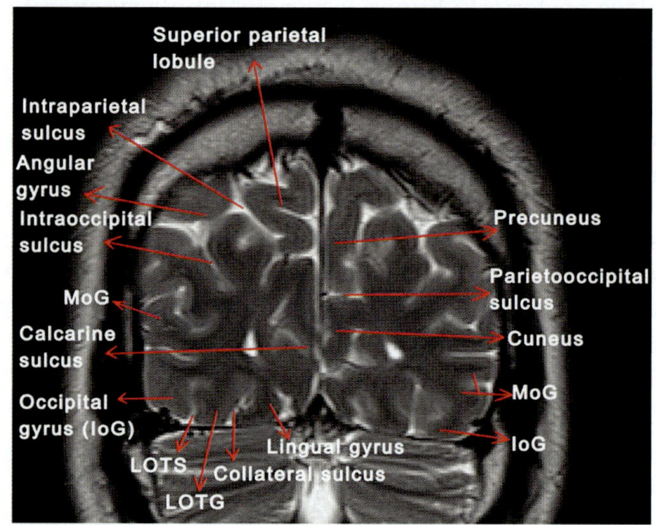

Fig. 3.1.46

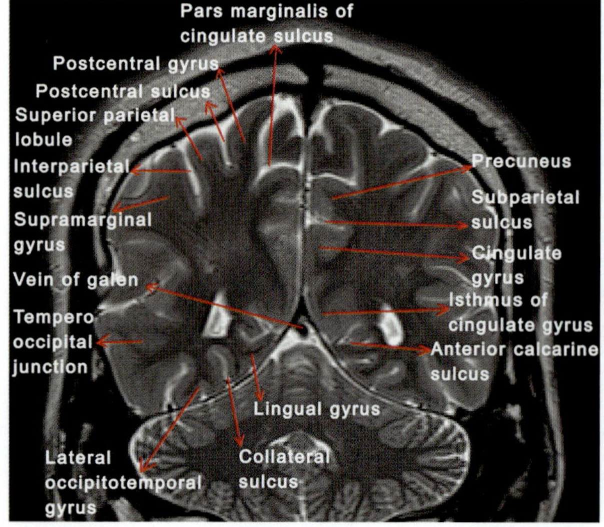

Fig. 3.1.44

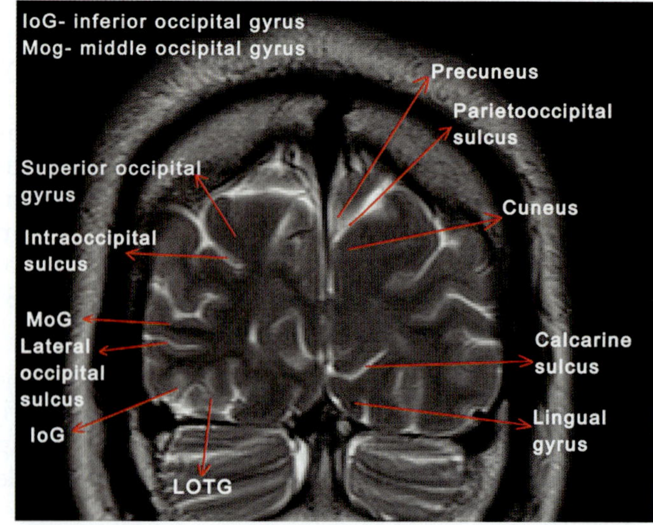

Fig. 3.1.47

occipital sulcus separates middle and inferior occipital gyri. Middle occipital gyrus is largest and sometimes separated by lateral or middle occipital sulcus into superior and inferior portion. Transverse occipital sulcus separates parietal lobe from middle occipital gyrus. Medial surface—**parieto-occipital fissure** separates occipital lobe from parietal lobe. **Calcarine sulcus** separates **cuneus** above from **lingual gyrus** below. **Calcarine cortex (medial occipital lobe)/striate gyrus** is located along calcarine sulcus is the primary visual cortex area (Figs 3.1.21 and 3.1.27).

MR axial sections of brain (Figs 3.1.21 to 3.1.27)

Sagittal sections (Figs 3.1.28 to 3.1.33)

Coronal sections (Figs 3.1.34 to 3.1.47)

3.1.C Basal Forebrain

Anterior perforated substance: Bounded anteriorly by olfactory tigone, posteriorly by optic tracts, medially by interhemispheric fissure, lateraly by uncus of temporal lobe and limen insulae (the transition between insular lobe and basal forebrain) (Figs 3.1.27, 3.1.31 and 3.1.65). Anterior perforated substance is located above the bifurcation of ICA and proximal A1, M1 segments of ACA and MCA. Lenticulostriate arteries (perforating arteries) arise from the A1, M1 segments and penetrate the anterior perforated substance to enter the basal brain. Site of penetration is represented by Virchow-Robin spaces (perivascular spaces). Along the posterior aspect of the anterior perforated substance lies the ventral striatum, which includes the substantia innominata. Ventral striatum, region of basal forebrain, extends from the anterior perforated substance to the anterior commissure. It is bounded laterally by stem of temporal lobe, superiorly the anterobasal portion of anterior limb of internal capsule (ALIC), medially septal region and hypothalamus. **Ventral striatum** (Figs 3.1.48 to 3.1.50) includes **nucleus accumbens**, which is located at the caudal connection of caudate nucleus with putamen and globus pallidus) and **basal nucleus of Meynert** (group of cells that lies in substantia innominata, which is located in posterior part of anterior perforated substance, directly below the subcommisural part of globus pallidus). Olfactory cortical area includes olfactory nerve, bulb, tract, trigone, striae, anterior perforated substance, the diagonal band of broca and piriform lobe. Olfactory tract is located in olfactory sulcus, which is called olfactory trigone before dividing into medial and lateral olfactory striae. Medial olfactory striae projects to septal nuclei in paraolfactory gyrus and then to hypothalamus (Fig. 3.1.137). Lateral olfactory striae projects into

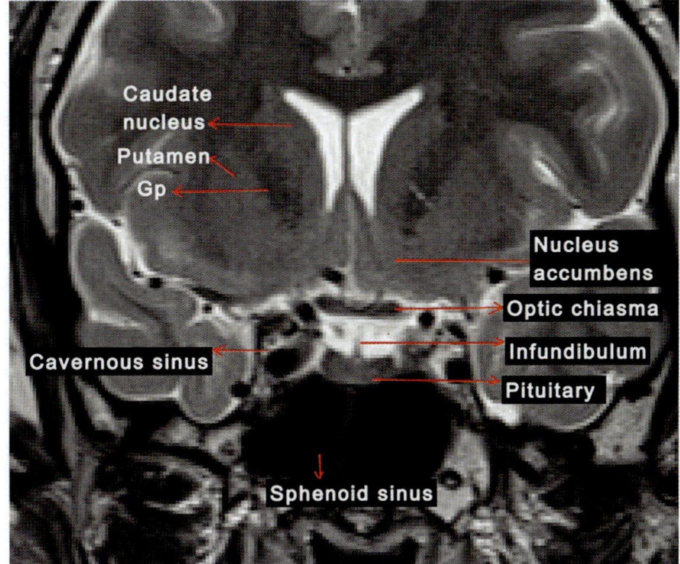

Fig. 3.1.48: Basal forebrain

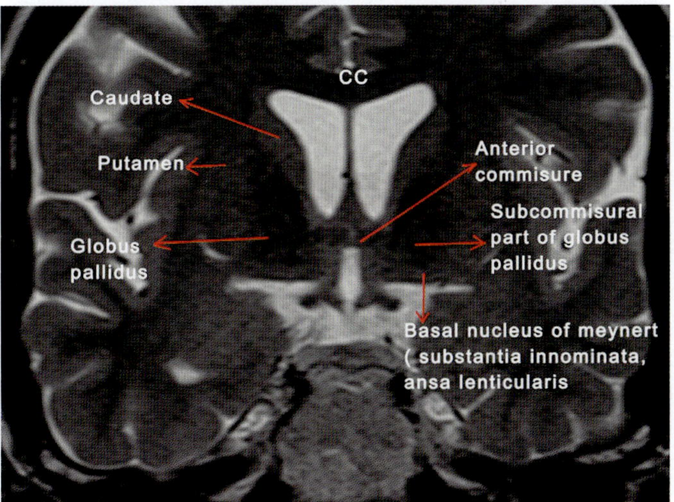

Fig. 3.1.49: Basal forebrain

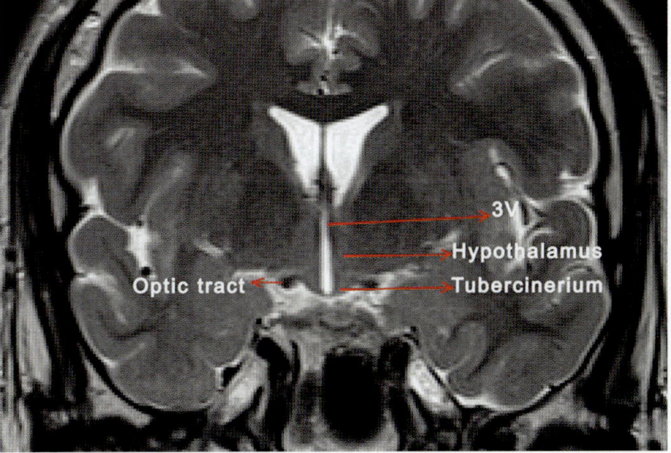

Fig. 3.1.50: Basal forebrain

olfactory cortex (piriform cortex—located at the junction of temporal and frontal lobes, medial to temporal stem), amygdala, entorhinal cortex. **Diagonal band of Broca** is located posterior to anterior perforated substance and continues with paraterminal gyrus on the medial surface. **Septum pellucidum:** Thin translucent membrane between the frontal horn and body of lateral ventricle. It bridges the gap between corpus callosum (rostrum, genu, anteri or body) to fornix. It contains glial cells, some scattered neurons, veins. It is lined by ependyma on ventricular side. Developement of septum pellucidum is linked with developement of corpus callosum, anterior commissure and hippocampal commissure. **Stria terminalis** is a narrow bundle of white matter situated between caudate and thalamus.

3.1.D Functional Areas of Cerebral Cortex

A Brodmann area is a region of the cerebral cortex defined by its cytoarchitecture, or histological structure and organization of cells. There are around 200 areas, which can be grouped under three basic functional divisions: Motor areas, sensory areas and association areas. Some important areas are discussed here (Table 3.1.3).

3.1.E Insula

The insular cortex, lies deep to the lateral surface of the brain (sylvian fissure), completely covered by the frontal, parietal, and temporal opercula (meaning lids) (Figs 3.1.38 and 3.1.51). It has an anterior lobule containing 3–4 short gyri separated from the posterior lobule containing 2 long gyri, by the deep central insular sulcus which passes obliquely from posterosuperior to anteroinferior. Limen insulae is the transitional cortex at which insula continues with the cortex over amygdala and superior temporal gyrus (Fig. 3.1.31).

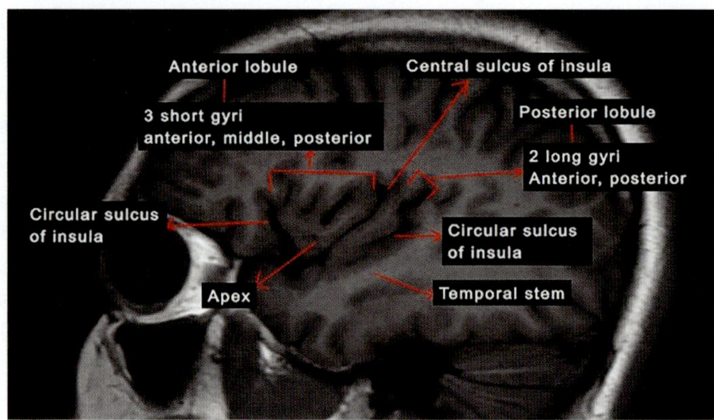

Fig. 3.1.51: Insula

3.1.F Limbic System and Hippocampus

Limbic system is a complex intercalated arrangement of cortical (limbic lobe) and some subcortical structures (e.g. amygdala, mamillary bodies, septal nuclei). The main components of limbic system includes hippocampus, parahippocampal gyrus, amygdala, hypothalamus. Limbic lobe forms border (limbus) around the diancephalon and midbrain, which is arranged in three arches (Fig. 3.1.53). **Outer arch** is comprised of parahippocampal gyrus, cingulate gyrus, subcallosal gyrus. It extends from temporal lobe to frontal lobe. **Middle arch** includes hippocampus proper (cornu ammonis), dentate gyrus, indusium griseum (supracallosal gyrus), paraterminal gyrus. It extends from temporal lobe to frontal lobe. **Inner arch**

Table 3.1.3: Functional areas of cerebral cortex (Brodmann area)

Lobe	*Location*	*Area*	*Area no*
Frontal	Precentral gyrus and paracentral lobule	Primary Motor area	4
	Posterior parts of frontal gyri, just anterior to precentral gyrus	Premotor cortex	6
	Posterior part of middle frontal gyrus, anterior to premotor area	Frontal eye field	8
	Pars triangularis and pars opercularis	Motor speech (Broca's area)	44, 45
	Large anterior portion of frontal lobe	Prefrontal cortex	9, 10, 11, 12, 46
Parietal	Postcentral gyrus and paracentral lobule	Primary sensory area	3, 1, 2
	Superior parietal lobule	Sensory association	5, 7
	Angular gyrus	Speech association	39
	Supramarginal gyrus	Speech association	40
Occipital	In and around the calcarine sulcus (striate cortex)	Primary visual cortex	17
	Surround the striate area	Associative visual cortex	18,19
Temporal	Posterior part of superior temporal gyrus and anterior transverse temporal gyrus (Heschl gyrus)	Primary auditory cortex	41,42
	Rest of the superior temporal gyrus	Wernicke's area	22

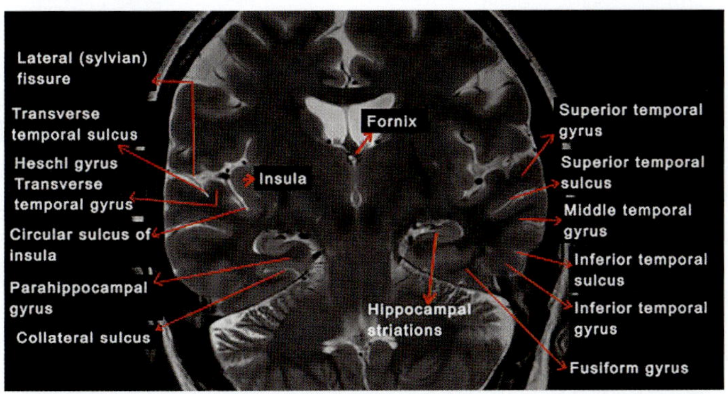

Fig. 3.1.52: Temporal lobe

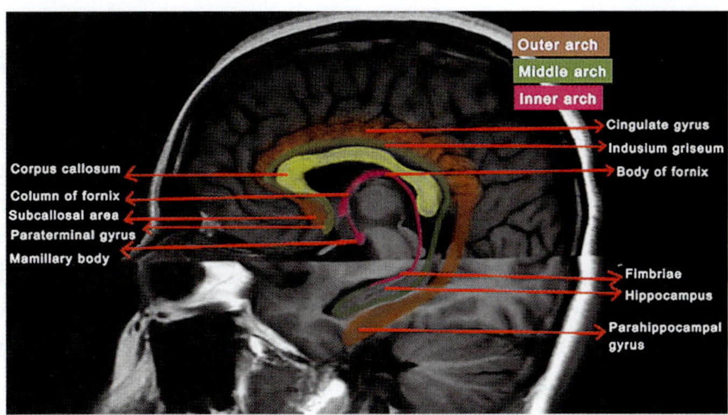

Fig. 3.1.53: Fused sagittal MR sections of limbic system

is comprised of fimbria and fornix. It extends from temporal lobe to mamillary bodies.

Anatomy of hippocampus (Fig. 3.1.54): The hippocampus is a bilaminar gray matter structure located medially in the temporal lobe that protrudes over the temporal horn of the lateral ventricle and occupies the medial region of its floor. MRI anatomy is best appreciated in **oblique coronal plane** perpendicular to the long axis of hippocampal body. The hippocampus consists of **two interlocking C-shaped gray matter folds, the cornu ammonis (or hippocampus proper) and the dentate gyrus.** Ammon horn forms more superolateral C and dentate gyrus forms inferomedial C. In the axial plane, the hippocampus resembles a seahorse (Fig. 3.1.27) (hence, its name) and it arches around the mesencephalon (hence, the term "mesiotemporal"). In the axial and sagittal plane, it can be divided into three parts: (1) The **head** or anterior segment; it has digitations in superior surface (Fig. 3.1.40), (2) the **body** or intermediate segment; it is bordered medially by ambient

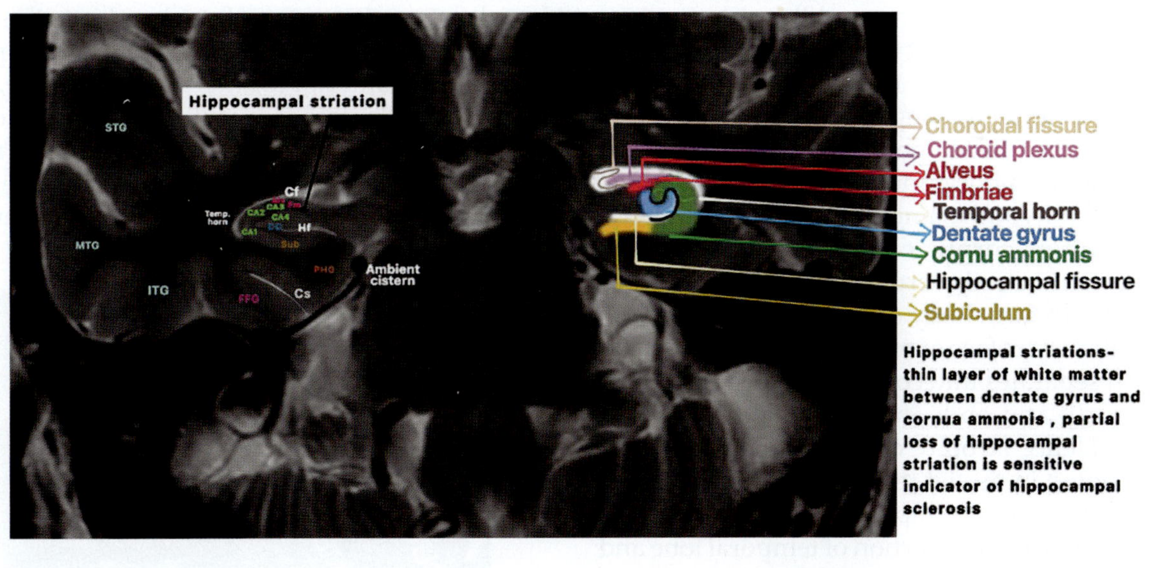

STG- Superior temporal gyrus
MTG- Middle temporal gyrus
ITG- Inferior temporal gyrus
Cf- Choroidal fissure
Hf- Hippocampal fissure
Cs- Collateral sulcus
CA- Cornu ammonis (1,2,3,4)
DG- Dentate gyrus
Sub- Subiculum
Alv- Alveus
Fim- Fimbriae
FFG- Fusiform gyrus
PHG- Parahippocampal gyrus

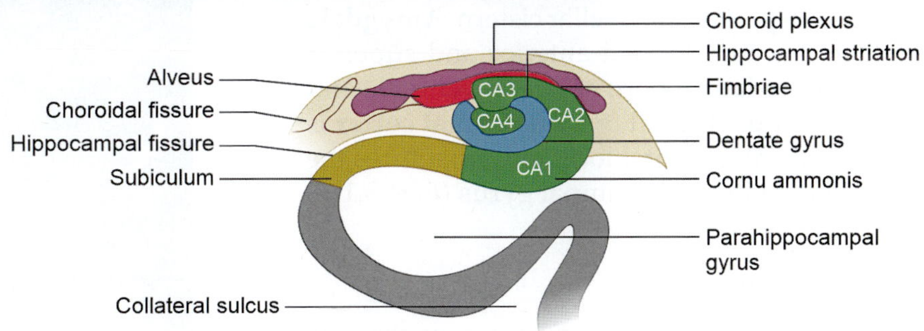

Fig. 3.1.54: Hippocampus

cistern and laterally by temporal horn of lateral ventricle and (3) the **tail or posterior segment** (Fig. 3.1.52). Tail of hippocampus narrows then curves around splenium to form indusium griseum above hippocampus. Indusium griseum ends in paraterminal gyrus (thus completing the middle arch) (Fig. 3.1.53). **Hippocampus proper (cornua ammonis-CA)** is subdivided into four zones CA1, CA2, CA3, CA4 (Fig. 3.1.54). CA4 is enveloped by dentate gyrus. **CA1 is most vulnerable** to injury CA blends laterally into subiculum, which then blends into adjacent parahippocampal gyrus.

Stratum radiata is white matter between CA and dentate gyrus. Loss of this normal **hippocampal striations** is the major earliest finding in mesial temporal sclerosis.Parahippocampal gyrus is separated from adjacent fusiform gyrus by collateral sulcus. Hippocampal fissure, is sulcus within the hippocampal formation, appears as shallow groove on the medial surface of the hippocampus, between the dentate gyrus and subiculum. Most medial portion of fissure is obliterated due to fusion of CA and dentate gyrus. Failure of normal involution results in hippocampal fissural cyst (normal variant). Usually, three arteries arising from the main or branches of the posterior cerebral artery vascularize the hippocampus—the anterior, middle and posterior hippocampal arteries. Efferent fibres from hippocampal pyramidal cells course on the ventral surface as alveus. Alveus is located along the superior surface of hippocampus within the temporal horn. Alveus bundles to form fimbria of hippocampus which enters the crus of fornix to reach hypothalamus. Crus of fornix arches under splenium of corpus callosum. Hippocampal commissure connects the crura of both sides, both crura converges to form body of fornix, where they are attached to inferior surface of septum pellucidum. Body of fornix then separates into columns of fornices which curves inferiorly and ends in mamillary bodies and septal nuclei. Hence atrophy of fornix and mamillary body is also noted in mesial temporal sclerosis. **Uncus** includes part of amygdala, hippocampus and piriform cortex. It is the most medial portion of temporal lobe and forms the lateral aspect of suprasellar cistern. **Amygdala** is grey matter structure located anterior and superior to temporal horn of lateral horn of lateral ventricle and head of hippocampus (Fig. 3.1.39). **Entorhinal cortex** is located in the medial temporal lobe and constitutes the anterior portion of parahippocampal gyrus (Figs 3.1.38 and 3.1.52).

3

3.1.G Basal Ganglia

The basal ganglia (misnomer, since it is a nuclei) are subcortical structures, a group of grey matter nuclei in the deep aspects of the brain, that is interconnected with the cerebral cortex, thalami and brainstem.

It contains mainly three paired nuclei: **Caudate nucleus, putamen, globus pallidus (internal and externa).** Functionally, two additional nuclei are also part of the basal ganglia—subthalamic nuclei and substantia nigra (Figs 3.1.40 and 3.1.41). The corpus striatum includes caudate nucleus, putamen and nucleus accumbens (Fig. 3.1.48). Globus pallidus along with putamen are collectively referred to as lentiform nucleus (Figs. 3.1.32, 3.1.37). Caudate nucleus consists of head, body and tail. Head of caudate nucleus indents the frontal horn of lateral ventricle (Figs 3.1.32, 3.1.37, 3.1.38). Its body curves upwards and posteriorly from the head, following the body of lateral ventricle, and tail is located immediately superior to temporal horn of lateral ventricle (Figs 3.1.24 and 3.1.43). Putamen is located between caudate nucleus and anterior limb of internal capsule. Globus pallidus is located medial to putamen (separated from it by external medullary lamina) and has lateral part, i.e. externa and more medial part, i.e. interna, these two parts are separated by internal medullary lamina. Claustrum is a linear gray matter band, located between external and extreme capsule. Now claustrum is removed from basal ganglia structures. Nucleus accumbens is a symmetric structure, parallel to midline, lying anterior to anterior commissure, caudal to anterior limb of internal capsule and medial to claustrum and piriform cortex (Fig. 3.1.48). Subthalamic nucleus is grey matter that lies medial to internal capsule, lateral to hypothalamus and superolateral to red nucleus, dorsal to substantia nigra (Figs 3.1.55 and 3.1.67).

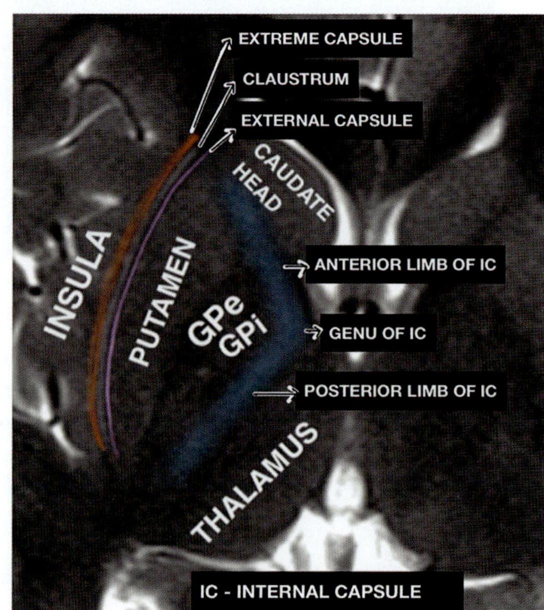

Fig. 3.1.55: Basal ganglia

3.1.H Sella

The pituitary fossa or sella turcica is a midline, dural lined depression in the sphenoid bone, which houses the pituitary gland. Anterior border is formed by tuberculum sella. Dorsum sella forms the posterior wall of sella, it continues inferiorly with the upper portion of clivus (basisphenoid). Laterally related to paired cavernous sinus and its contents. Inferiorly related to sphenoid sinus (Figs 3.1.56, 3.1.57). **Posterior pituitary bright spot** (PPBS) in T1 is due to vasopressin/oxytocin. In order from anterior to posterior parasellar bony structures are planum sphenoidale, limbus, chiasmatic sulcus, tuberculum sellae, lamina dura (forms floor of sella turcica) and dorsum sellae (Fig. 3.1.58).

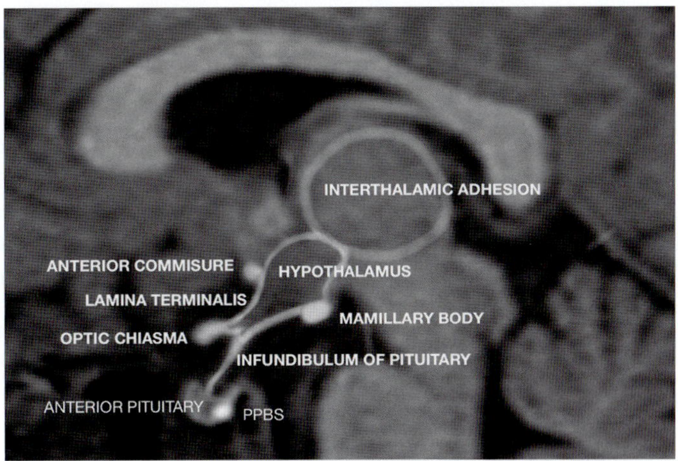

Fig. 3.1.56: Pituitary

3.1.I Cavernous Sinus

Paired interconnected venous sinuses situated on either side of sella turcica and sphenoidal sinus in floor of middle cranial fossa. Internal carotid artery with sympathetic plexus around it and abducens nerve travel within the cavernous sinus. Occulomotor nerve (III), trochlear nerve (IV) and ophthalmic division of trigeminal nerve (V1) travels in lateral wall of cavernous sinus (Figs 3.1.59 and 3.1.60). The maxillary nerve (cranial nerve V2) courses just inferior to the junction of the lateral and medial walls of the cavernous sinus. Cavernous sinus also contains variable amount of fat and fibrous tissue. The cavernous sinus extends from the superior orbital fissure anteriorly to the petrous apex and the dorsum sellae posteriorly. It is bounded by dura and has five walls—lateral, medial, superior, or roof, anterior, and posterior wall. The medial wall is the weakest one and separates the cavernous sinus from the lateral wall of the sphenoid sinus inferiorly and the pituitary gland superiorly (Figs 3.1.61 and 3.1.62). Each cavernous sinus communicates by way of intercavernous communications—anterior, inferior, and posterior intercavernous communications and the basilar venous plexus (Figs 3.1.63 and 3.1.64). Cavernous sinus receives tributaries from superior and inferior ophthalmic veins, central retinal vein, middle and inferior cerebral veins, middle meningeal veins. It also communicates with superior and inferior petrosal sinus, pterygoid plexus. Multiple foramina and fissures act as a conduit of structures from the cavernous sinus to the surrounding spaces, including the orbits (superior orbital fissure and inferior orbital fissure), the face, the pterygopalatine fossa (inferior orbital fissure, foramen rotundum), the nasopharynx (foramen lacerum and carotid canal), the infratemporal fossa (foramen ovale), and the middle and posterior cranial fossae (Meckel's cave). On MR imaging ICA appears as hypointense

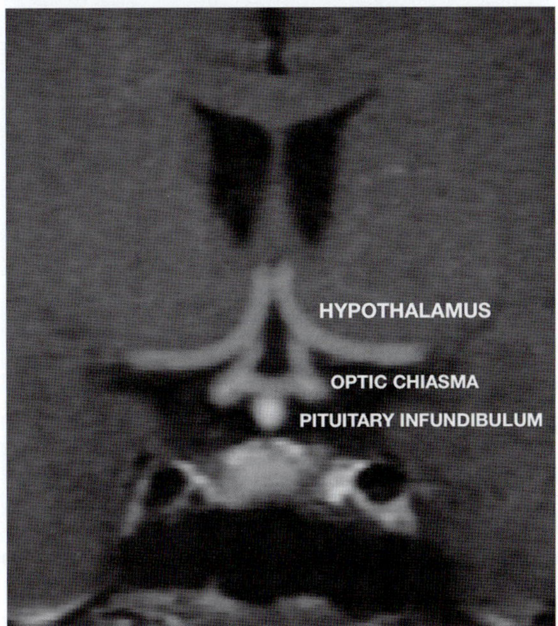

Fig. 3.1.57: Coronal image—infundibulum

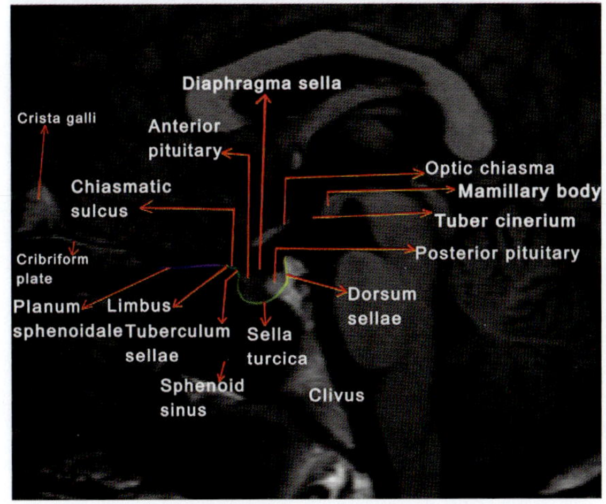

Fig. 3.1.58: Sagittal image

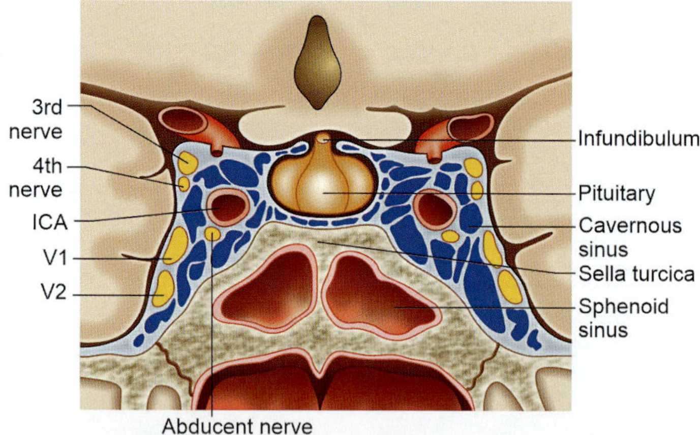

Fig. 3.1.59: Schematic diagram of cavernous sinus

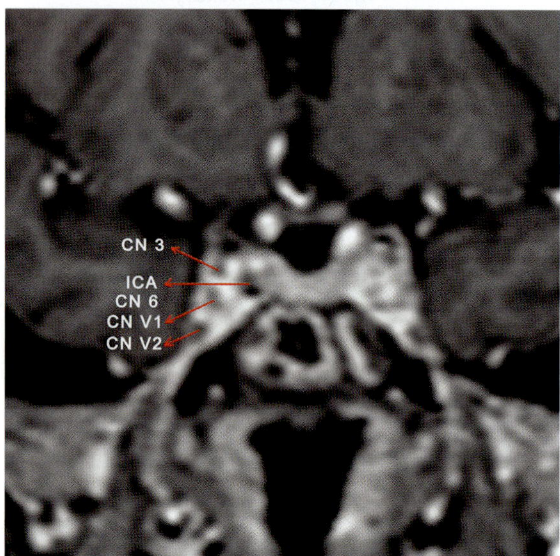

Fig. 3.1.60: Coronal contrast MR image of cavernous sinus with its contents

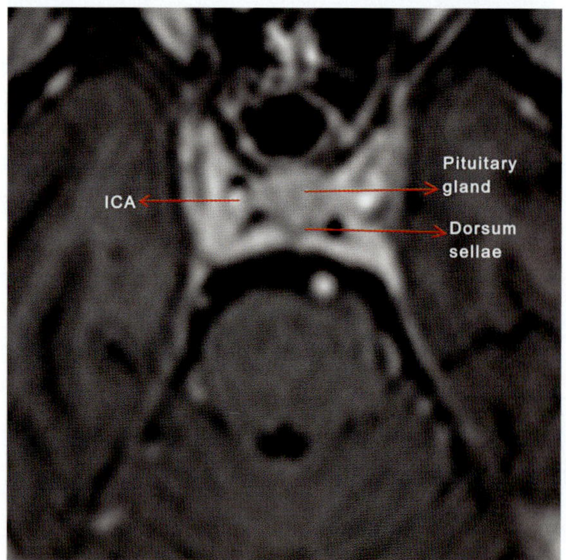

Fig. 3.1.61: Axial contrast MR image

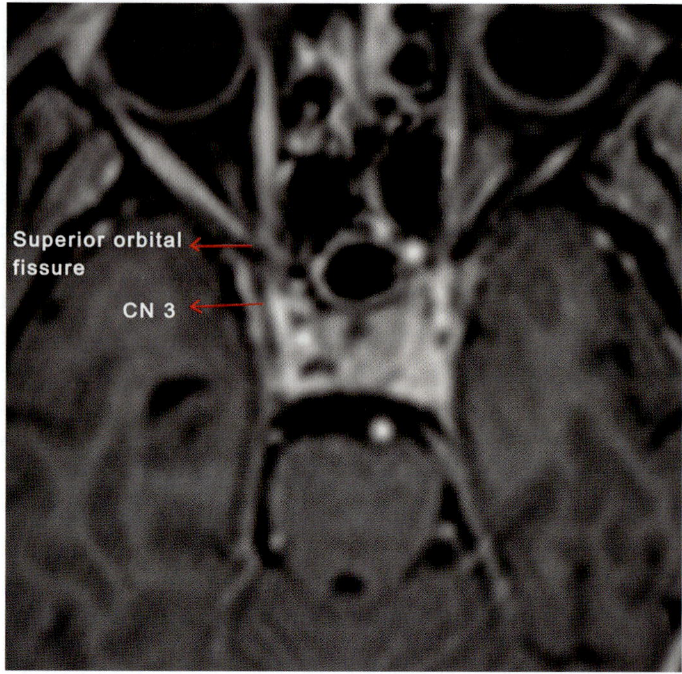

Fig. 3.1.62: Axial contrast MR image—3rd cranial nerve from cavernous sinus entering into superior orbital fissure

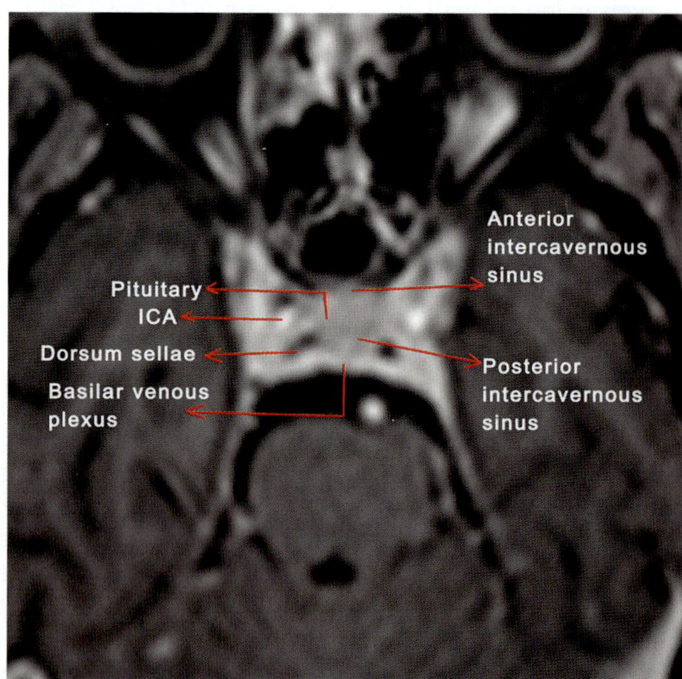

Fig. 3.1.63: Axial contrast MR image—intercavernous connections

structure due to flow void and as hyperintense on MRA sequences. Venous plexus has varied signal and they are homogenously enhanced after contrast injection. Cranial nerves appear as same intensity as of white matter and not enhance after contrast injection. Lateral wall should

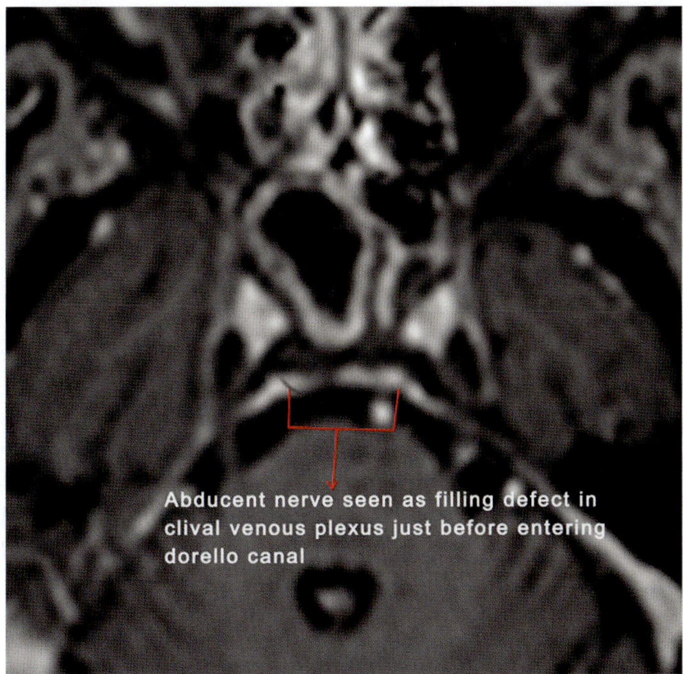

Fig. 3.1.64: Axial contrast MR image—abducent nerve

be **concave or flat**, any bulging or asymmetry indicates pathological involvement of cavernous sinus.

3.1.J Diencephalon

It is located between the telencephalon and midbrain, includes **thalamus, metathalamus, epithalamus, hypothalamus and subthalamus** (Figs 3.1.65 to 3.1.68).

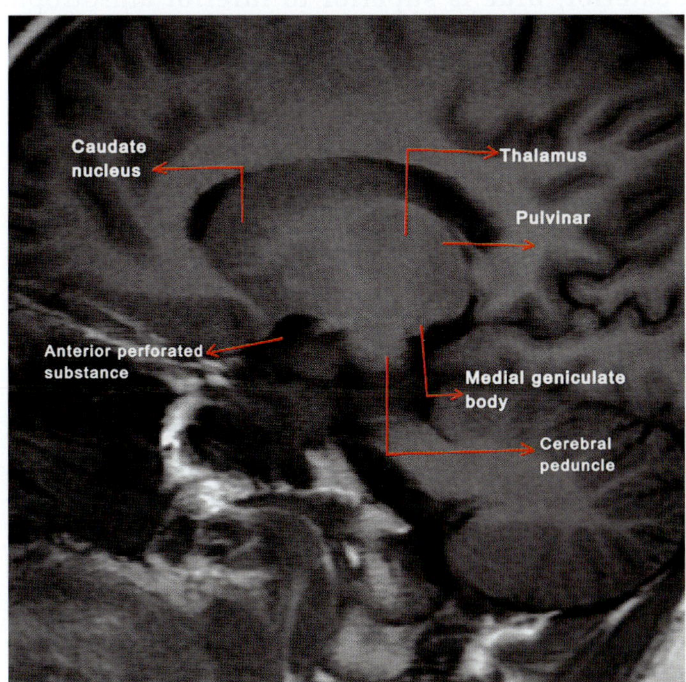

Fig. 3.1.65: Sagittal MR image—diencephalon

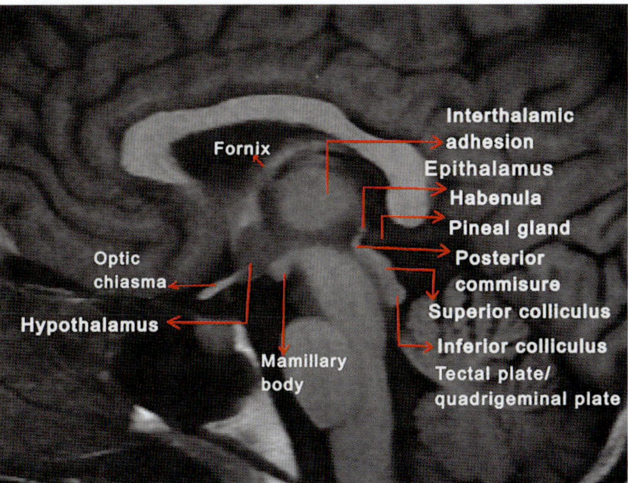

Fig. 3.1.66: Sagittal MR image—diencephalon

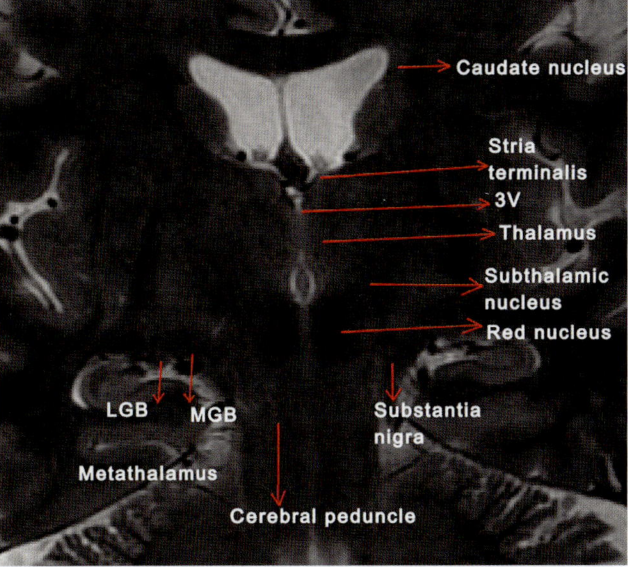

Fig. 3.1.67: Coronal MR image—diencephalon

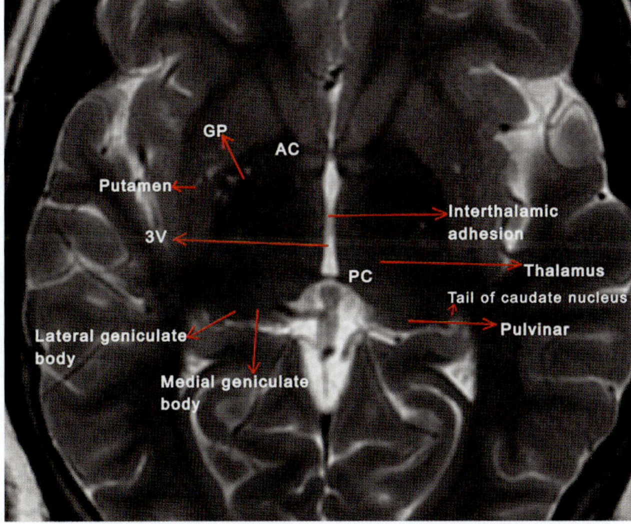

Fig. 3.1.68: Axial MR image—diencephalon

Thalamus: It is a paired ovoid gray matter structure of the diencephalon located on either side of third ventricle, extends from foramen of monro to quadrigeminal plate of midbrain. Medially it forms lateral border of third ventricle and laterally it is separated from putamen by posterior limb of internal capsule. The thalamus is made up of a series of nuclei which are responsible for the relay of the different sensory signals. The internal medullary lamina divides the thalamus into three parts—anterior, medial and lateral nuclear groups. These are further divided into several additional nuclei. The external medullary lamina covers the lateral surface. **Pulvinar** is the most posterior part of thalamus, which is in close proximity to the superior and inferior colliculi (tectal plate). Medial and lateral geniculate bodies are located caudal to pulvinar nucleus. **Massa intermedia/ interthalamic adhesion**—connects two thalami across the third ventricle. Inferior to thalamus lies the hypothalamus ventrally and subthalamus dorsally.

Metathalamus: It includes medial and lateral geniculate nuclei and are considered to be part of thalamus. Medial geniculate body (MGB) (part of auditory pathway) is an oval elevation situated just below the pulvinar of the thalamus and lateral to the superior colliculus. Lateral geniculate body (LGB) (part of visual pathway) is a small oval elevation situated anterolateral to the medial geniculate body, below the thalamus. It is overlapped by the medial part of the temporal lobe, and is connected to the superior colliculus by the superior brachium.

Epithalamus: Dorsal portion of diencephalon, which includes habenula, stria medullaris, pineal gland, posterior commissure.

Subthalamus: Located superolateral to red nucleus. Venous drainage is through the deep venous system into the internal cerebral vein and the basal veins of rosenthal.

Hypothalamus: As the name indicates, hypothalamus is a part of diencephalon that is located below the thalamus. It develops from the neuroectoderm of floor of brain, along with posterior pituitary. Anterior pituitary has a separate developement from Rathke pouch (roof of mouth). The anterior boundary of the hypothalamus is indicated by a "line" that extends from the anterior commissure to the optic chiasm and corresponds to the lamina terminalis. The posterior boundary of the hypothalamus is indicated by a line that extends from the mamillary bodies to the posterior commissure. The lateral boundary of the hypothalamus is the medial thalamus, and the hypothalamic sulcus separates the hypothalamus from the thalamus superiorly. Inferiorly, the hypothalamus forms the **tuber cinereum**, a tubular structure that is composed of gray matter and lies between the mamillary bodies posteriorly and the optic chiasm anteriorly. Hypothalamus forms the roof of interpeduncular fossa and floor of third ventricle. Median eminence is small bulge in tuber cinereum that continues downward to form infundibular stalk, which is attached to posterior lobe of pituitary. Normal infundibulum is 3 mm wide at its origin and 2 mm wide near its insertion. On contrast enhanced MR, infundibular stalk and pituitary show homogenous enhancement, since they lack blood–brain barrier.

Hypothalamus has many nuclei and fiber tracts. The majority of hypothalamic nuclei are located medially. The lateral area contains a heterogeneous group of axons called the medial forebrain bundle, which connects the forebrain and the brainstem. There are two major white matter tracts in the hypothalamus—the postcommissural fornix and the mamillothalamic tract (MT). Individual nuclei cannot be identified with MR images.

3.1.K White Matter of Cerebrum

White matter tracts of brain are of three types: 1. Association tracts—connect distinct cortical regions within the same hemisphere; 2. Projection tracts—interconnect cortical regions in craniocaudal direction; 3. Commissural tracts—connect cortical regions between two cerebral hemsipheres (Table 3.1.4).

Diffuse tensor imaging (DTI): FA (fractional anisotropy) maps are usually color coded with **red** indicating a predominant **left to right, green** indicating **anterior–posterior, blue is superior to inferior** anisotropic diffusion (Figs 3.1.69 to 3.1.74).

3.1.L Arterial Anatomy of Brain

The brain receives arterial blood from the bilateral internal carotid artery (ICA) and vertebral artery (VA).

ICA is divided into seven segments (Bouthillier classification), C1–C7 (Fig. 3.1.84). No branches arise from cervical (C1) segment. Then ICA enters the cranial cavity through the carotid canal in petrous bone. Petrous C2 segment of ICA is within the carotid canal, it has short vertical segment, genu and long horizontal segment. It exits the carotid canal at petrous apex. Branches from C2 segment are vidian artery (artery of pterygoid canal) and caroticotympnaic artery (which supplies the middle ear). Short C3 segment is between petrous apex and cavernous sinus above the foramen lacerum. It is closely related to trigeminal ganglion in Meckel's cave. No branches arise from C3 segment. C4 is the cavernous segment, which turns forwards, then upwards and has posterior ascending portion, posterior genu, horizontal

Table 3.1.4: Cerebral white matter		
Tracts		*Interconnects*
Association tracts		
1. Short association fibers—subcortical U fibers		Connects cortical areas on adjacent gyri
2. Long association fibers		
a. Superior longitudinal fasciculus (SLF) (Fig. 3.1.75) **4 subcomponents**	SLF-I	Superior parietal lobe to frontal and opercular areas
Connecting parietal, occipital, temporal lobes with ipsilateral frontal cortices	SLF-II	Angular gyrus
	SLF-III	Supramarginal gyrus
	SLF-IV	Prefrontal cortex to superior temporal gyrus **(arcuate fasciculus)** (AF)—Broca's area to Wernicke's area
b. Inferior longitudinal fasciculus (ILF) (Figs 3.1.76, 3.1.77)		Connects temporal and occipital lobes (more laterally located)
c. Middle longitudinal fasciculus (MdLF)		Superior temporal gyrus to parietal lobe
d. Superior fronto-occipital fasciculus (SFOF)		Frontal to occipital lobe (lateral to ventricular ependyma below the corpus callosum—**subcallosal fasciculus**)
e. Inferior fronto-occipital fasciculus		Prefrontal cortex with posterior temporal cortex and occipital lobe (runs medial to ILF)
f. Uncinate fasciculus (Fig. 3.1.78)		Inferior frontal gyrus with anterior temporal pole.
g. Cingulum		Connects septal area to uncus (C-shaped fiber that lies immediately beneath the cingulate gyrus, draping over the corpus callosum)
h. External capsule		Connecting cerebral cortex to striatum (loacted lateral to putamen and medial to claustrum)
i. Extreme capsule		From inferior frontal cortex (Broca's area) through middle part of superior temporal gyrus into the inferior parietal lobule (between claustrum medially and insula laterally)
Projection tracts		
a. Internal capsule (Fig. 3.1.81)		
Anterior limb (anterior thalamic radiation, medial forebrain bundle, frontopontine motor tracts, anterior thalamic fibers) **Genu (corticobulbar tracts)** **Posterior limb (corticospinal tract)** **Retrolenticular (optic radiation)** **Sublenticular portion (acoustic radiation)**		Corticospinal tract (primary motor cortex to spinal cord) Optic radiation (from superio colliculi and lateral genciulate body of thalamus to occpital cortex, superior fibers runs posteriorly to visual cortex, inferior fibers wraps around temporal horn of lateral ventricle to reach visual cortex—Meyer's loop) Acoustic radiation—from lateral lemnisci, inferior colliculus, to medial geniculate body
b. Fornix (Figs 3.1.76 and 3.1.77)		Connects hippocampal efferents **(fimbriae)** to anterior septal nuclei, hypothalamus, mammillary body
Commissural tracts		
a. Corpus callosum (rostrum, genu, body, isthmus, splenium) (Figs 3.1.79 and 3.1.80)		**Rostrum** connects frontobasal cortices. **Genu** contains fibers **(forceps minor)** that connect the anterior frontal lobes and anterior cingulate cortices. Fibers in the **body** interconnect the premotor and supplementary motor areas. Isthmus contains fibers from pre- and post-central gyri, Heschl gyri (connects primary motor cortices and primary somatosensory cortices). Fibers in **splenium (forceps major)** connect parietal, temporal and occipital cortices
b. Anterior commissure (Fig. 3.1.80)		Below septum pellucidum just anterior to third ventricle Interconnects olfactory bulbs, orbitofrontal cortex, temporal lobe
c. Posterior commissure (Fig. 3.1.80)		Located in dorsal upper end of cerebral aqueduct Connects the pretectal nuclei, interstitial nuclei of Cajal, nuclei of Darkschewitsch, Edinger-Westphal nuclei
d. Hippocampal commissure (commissure of fornix)		Lies under the splenium of corpus callosum, unites the crura of fornices. Connects the subicular and parahippocampal cortices
e. Habenular commissure (Fig. 3.1.80)		Situated just in front of pineal gland, interconnects the Habenular nuclei

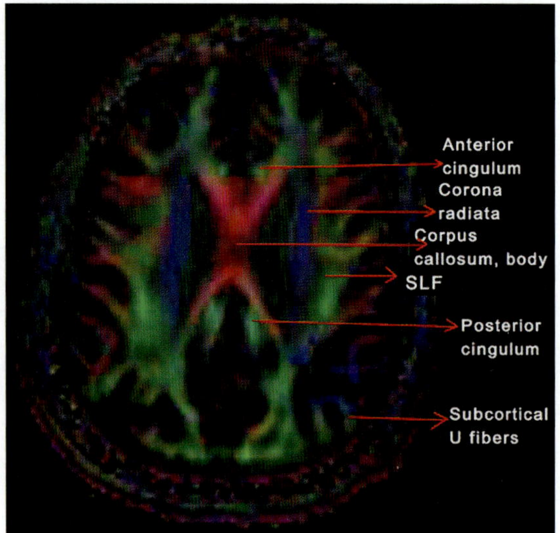

Fig. 3.1.69: DTI

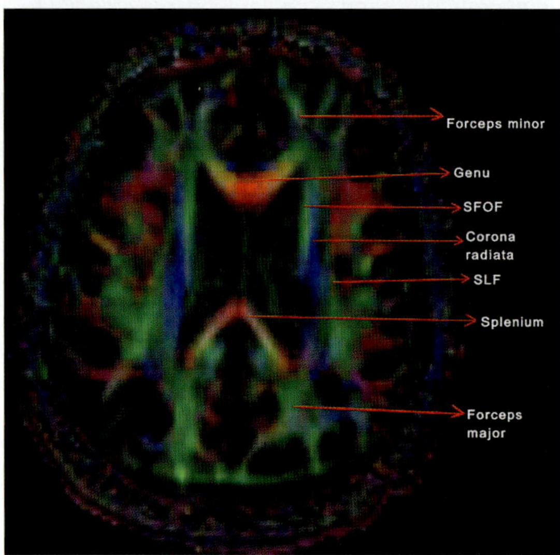

Fig. 3.1.70: DTI

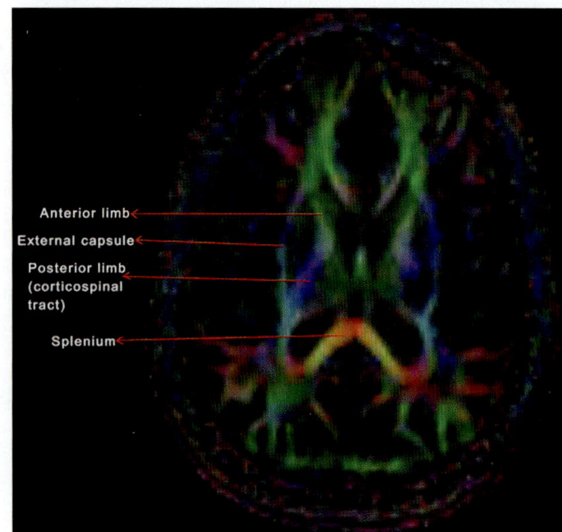

Fig. 3.1.71: DTI

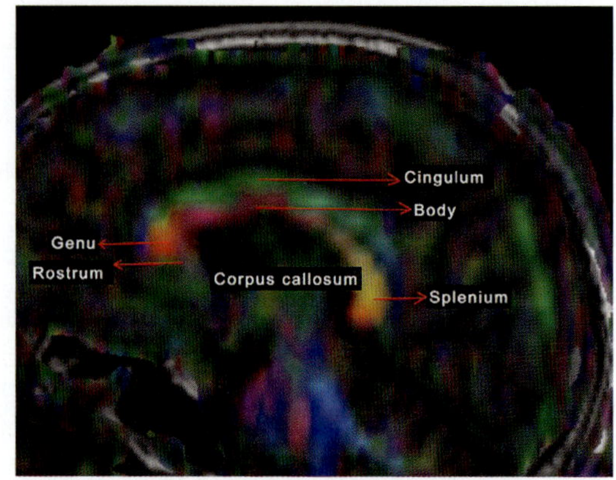

Fig. 3.1.72: DTI corpus callosum

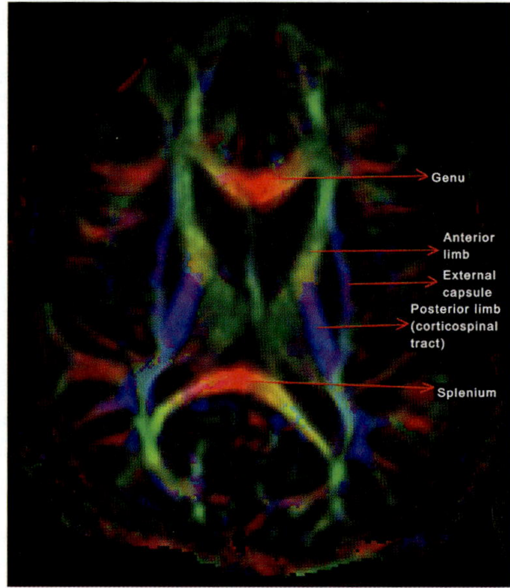

Fig. 3.1.73: DTI

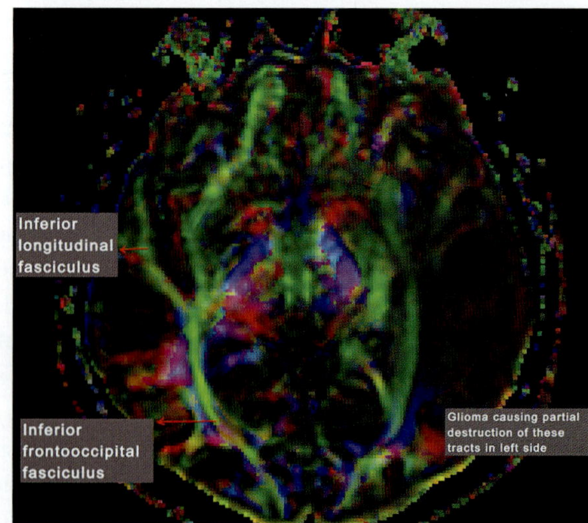

Fig. 3.1.74: DTI normal inferior longitudinal and inferior fronto-occipital fasciculus right side and glioma with destruction of tracts in left side

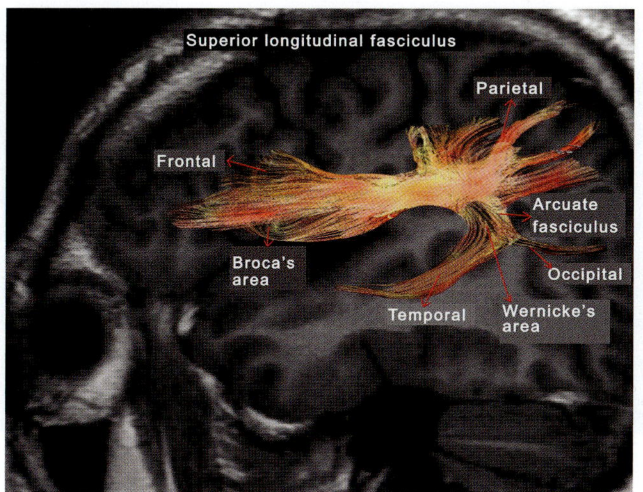

Fig. 3.1.75: DTI superior longitudinal fasciculus

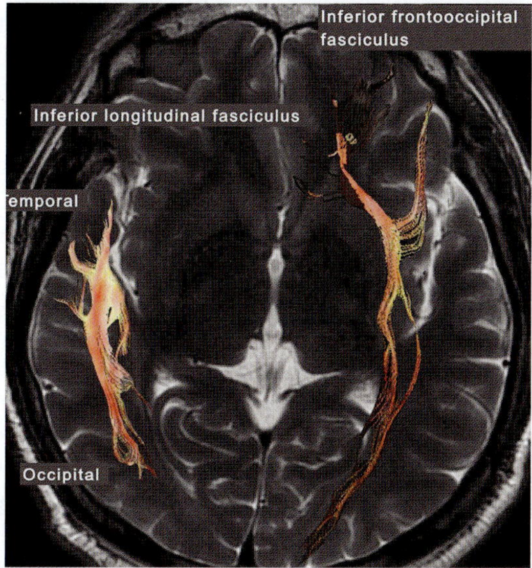

Fig. 3.1.76: DTI inferior longitudinal and inferior fronto-occipital fasciculus

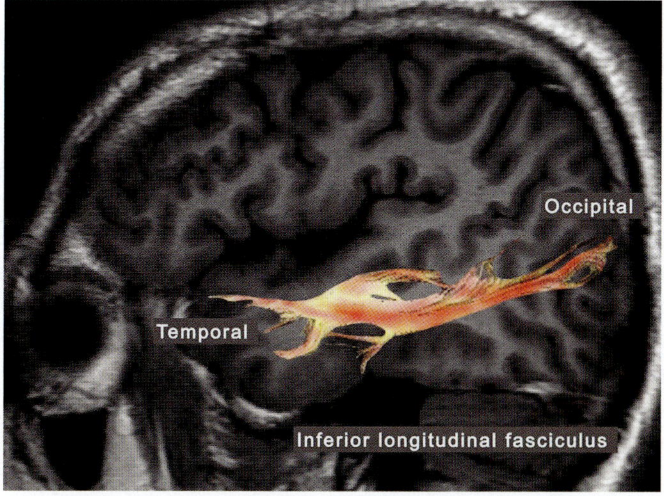

Fig. 3.1.77: DTI inferior longitudinal fasciculus

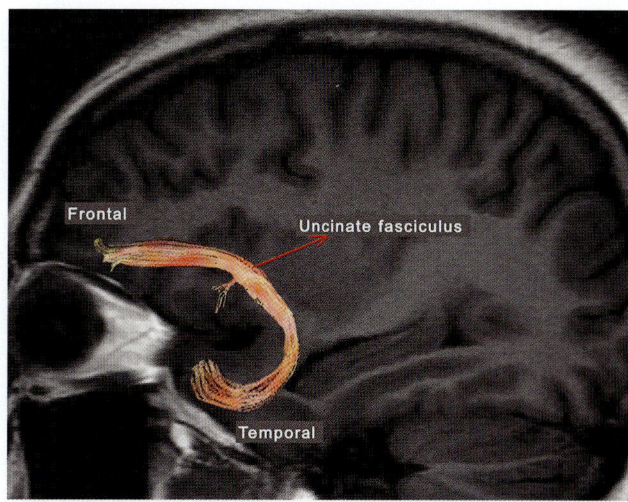

Fig. 3.1.78: DTI uncinate fasciculus

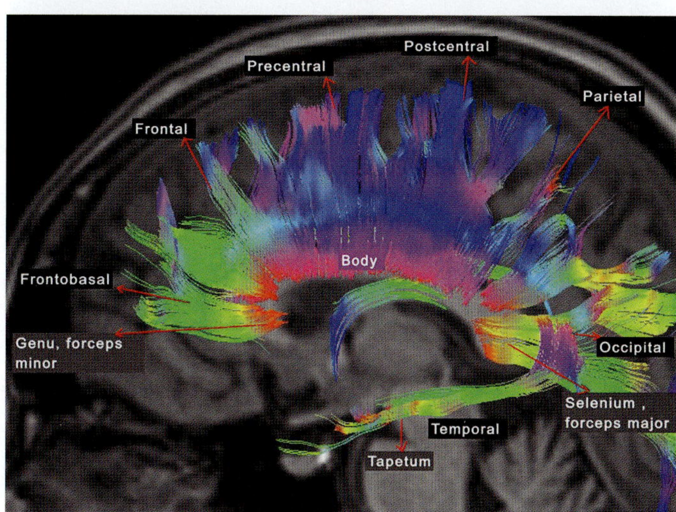

Fig. 3.1.79: DTI corpus callosum

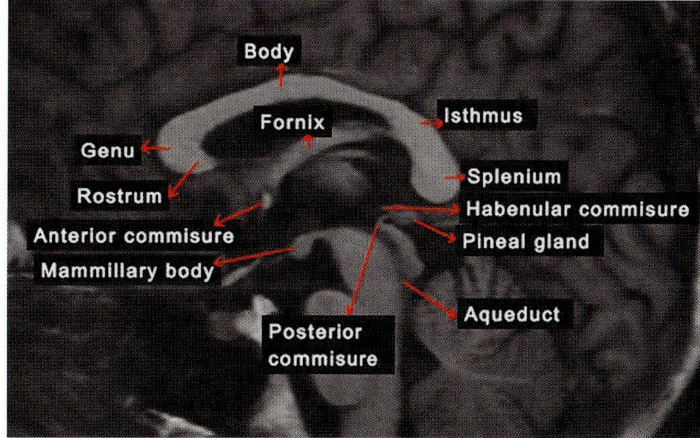

Fig. 3.1.80: MR sagittal image commissural fibers

segment, anterior genu, anterior vertical segment. Major branches from C4 segment are meningohypophyseal trunk (supplies the pituitary, tentorium and clival dura)

3

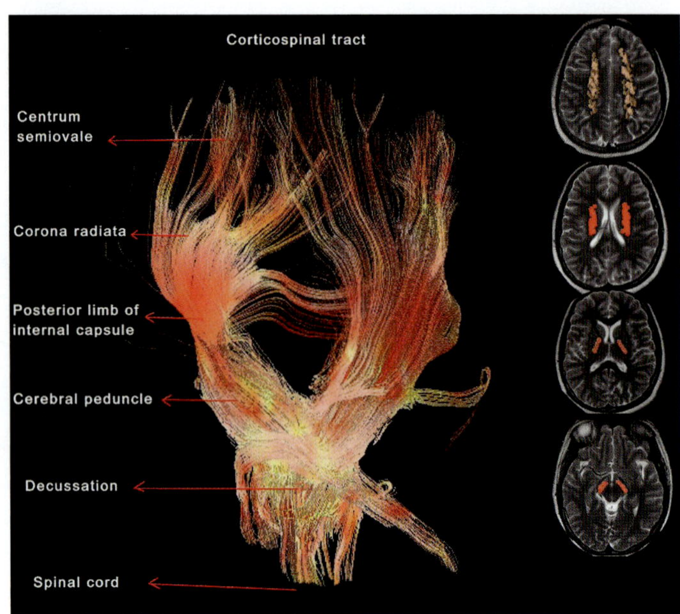

Fig. 3.1.81: Corticospinal tract DTI image

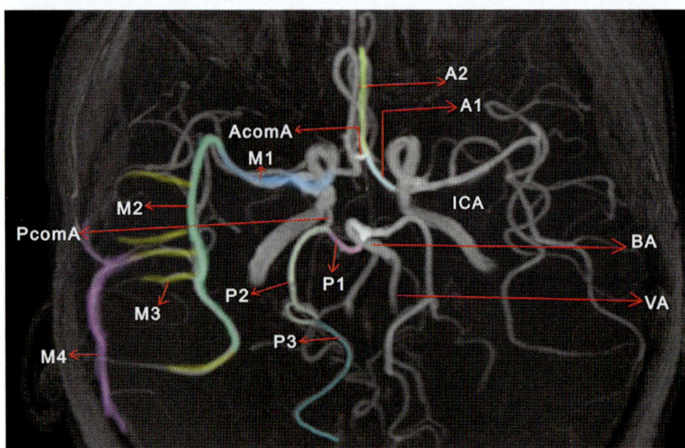

Fig. 3.1.82: MRA

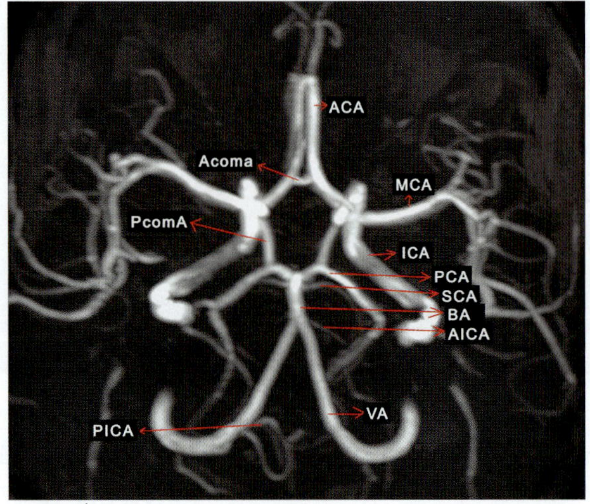

Fig. 3.1.83: MRA circle of Willis

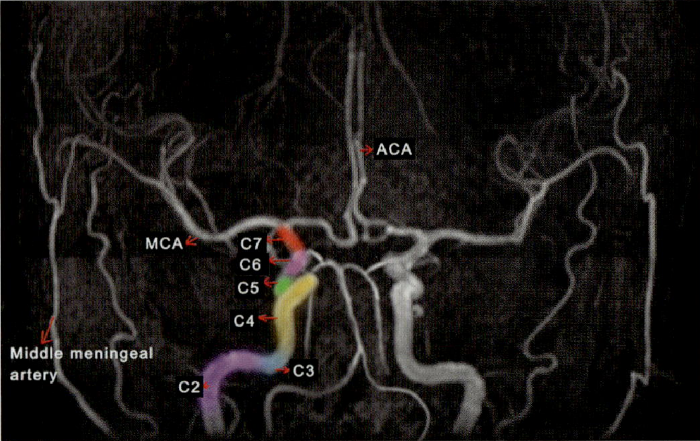

Fig. 3.1.84: ICA-MRA

and inferolateral trunk which supplies cavernous sinus dura and cranial nerves. C5 is the clinoid segment. C6 is ophthalmic segment from superior clinoid to just before the origin of posterior communicating artery (PComA). Ophthalmic artery and superior hypophyseal artery arises from C6 segment. C7 is communicating segment, from PComA origin to terminal bifurcation of ICA into anterior cerebral artery (ACA) and middle cerebral artery (MCA). Posterior communicating artery and anterior choroidal artery are branches from C7 segment (Figs 3.1.85 and 3.1.86).

Anterior cerebral artery (ACA): Medial terminal branch of ICA. Three segment are seen, A1 is horizontal or precommunicating segment, A2 is vertical or postcommunicating segment, A3 is distal segment and cortical branches. Branches are orbitofrontal artery and frontopolar artery, pericallosal artery and callosomarginal artery. Perforating branches are medial lenticulostriate arteries including recurrent artery of Heubner (Figs 3.1.91 and 3.1.92).

Middle cerebral artery (MCA) (Figs 3.1.87 to 3.1.89)***:*** Terminal branch of ICA and has 4 segments. Horizontal M1 segment is seen in sylvian cistern, it usually bifurcates or trifurcates before sylvian fissure. M2 is insular segment, here 6 to 8 stem arteries arise from the postbifurcation trunk and courses over the surface of insula. M3 is opercular segment, along the circular sulcus of insula/operculum up to the cortical surface. M4 is cortical segment, along the convex cortical surface. Branches are lateral frontobasal artery, prefrontal, prerolandic (precentral), rolandic artery, postcentral sulcus artery (anterior parietal artery), posterior parietal artery, angular artery, anterior temporal artery, temporo-occipital artery, posterior temporal and medial temporal

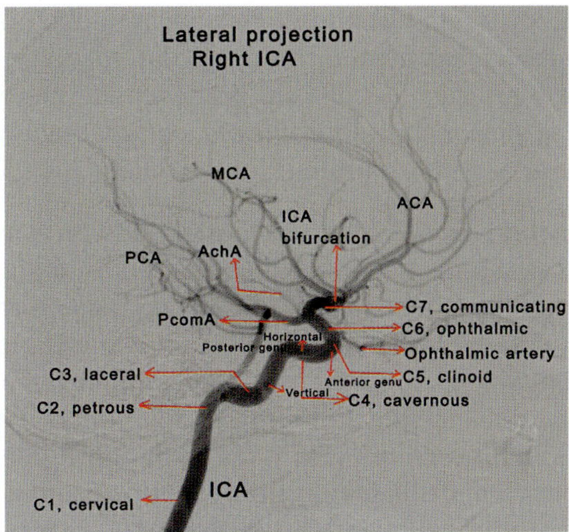

Fig. 3.1.85: DSA lateral view—right ICA

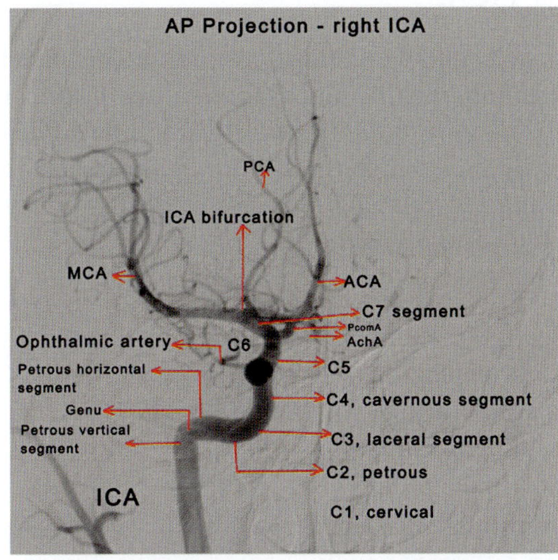

Fig. 3.1.86: DSA AP view—right ICA

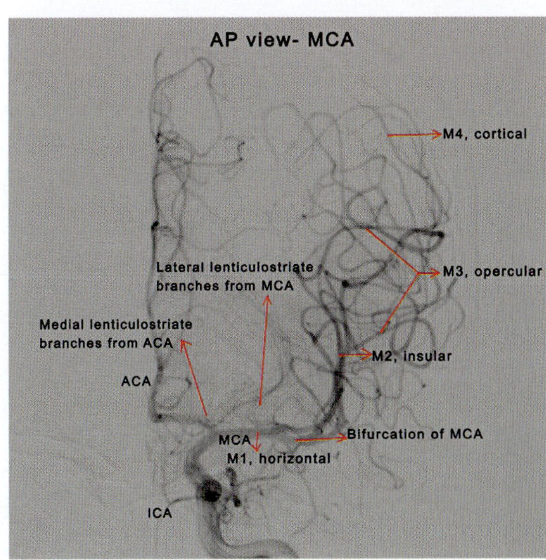

Fig. 3.1.87: DSA AP view—MCA

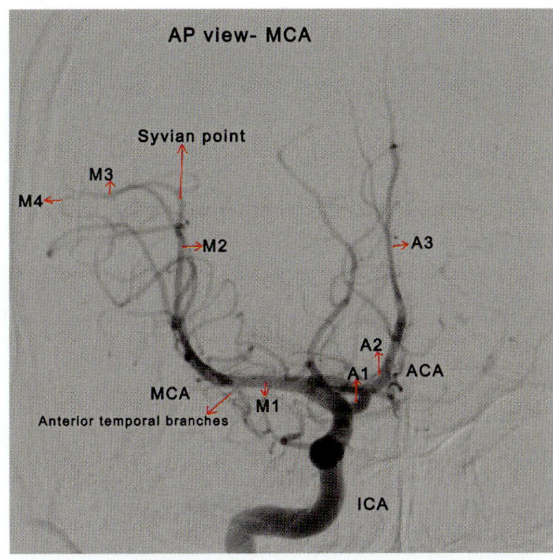

Fig. 3.1.88: DSA AP view—MCA, sylvian point

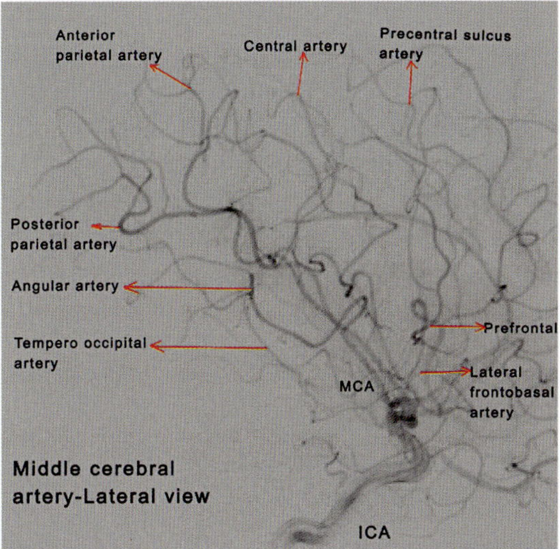

Fig. 3.1.89: DSA middle cerebral artery lateral view

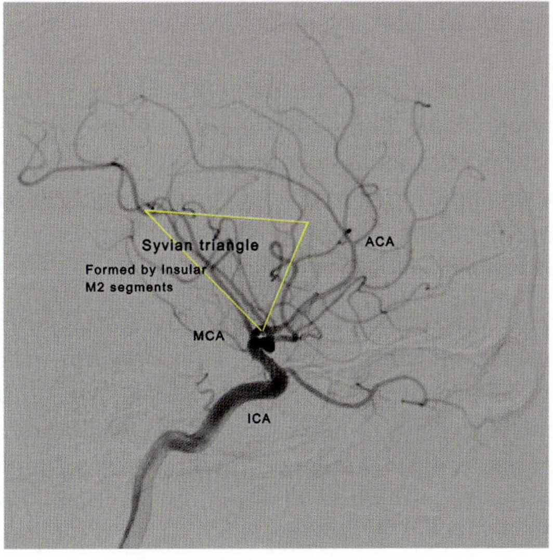

Fig. 3.1.90: Sylvian triangle

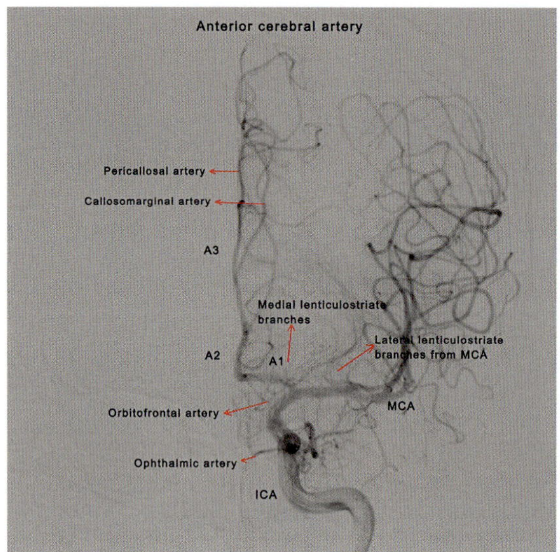

Fig. 3.1.91: DSA AP view anterior cerebral artery

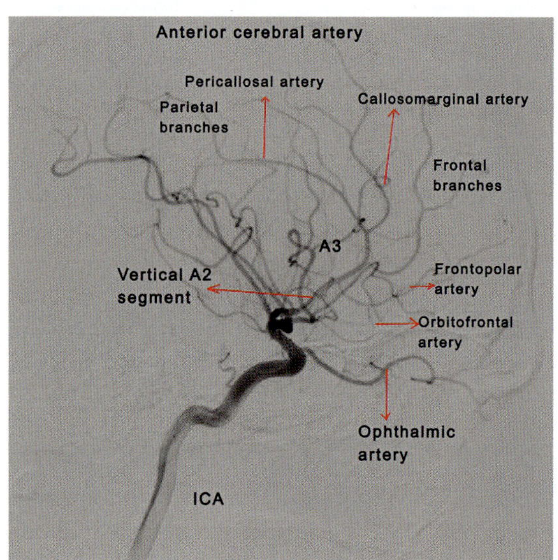

Fig. 3.1.92: DSA anterior cerebral artery lateral view

artery, lateral lenticulostriate arteries. **Sylvian triangle**—represents insula being delineated by middle cerebral artery and its branches, forming the sylvian triangle. Any shift of this landmark by mass lesions is easily identified. The angiographic sylvian point is the highest and most medial insular loop of MCA (Figs 3.1.88 and 3.1.90).

Posterior cerebral artery (PCA): Terminal branch of basilar artery. It has 4 segments, P1 is precommunicating segment, from origin of PCA to PComA, P2 (ambient segment) is around the ambient cistern, P3 (quadrigeminal segment) is within quadrigeminal cistern, P4 (calcarine segment) in calcarine fissure. Branches—cortical branches are anterior temporal artery and posterior temporal artery, terminal trunks—medial branches (medial occipital, parieto-occipital, calcarine and posterior splenial artery) and lateral branches (lateral occipital and temporal arteries). Choroidal branches are medial and lateral posterior choroidal arteries, perforating branches to thalamus and midbrain (Figs 3.1.82 and 3.1.93).

Vertebral artery (VA): Arises from subclavian artery and has 4 segments, V1 (extraosseous) from origin to C6 transverse foramen. V2 (foraminal segment) is through C6–C3 transverse foramina. V3 (extraspinal segment) after exiting from C2 transverse foramen to foramen magnum. V4 (intradural) through foramen magnum courses behind clivus and joins with contralateral VA near pontomedullary junction to form basilar artery. Major branches from V4 segment are anterior and posterior spinal arteries, direct perforating branches to medulla, PICA.

Basilar artery (BA): Courses in prepontine cistern and bifurcates into its terminal branches, posterior cereberal artery (PCA) in interpeduncular cistern. Branches are pontine perforating branches, anterior inferior cerebellar artery (AICA), superior cerebellar artery (SCA) (Figs 3.1.93 and 3.1.94).

Circle of Willis: It is arterial anastomotic ring providing major collateral blood flow to brain, formed by ICA, both A1 segment of ACA, AComA, bilateral PComA, basilar artery and P1 segment of PCA on both sides (Figs 3.1.82 and 3.1.84).

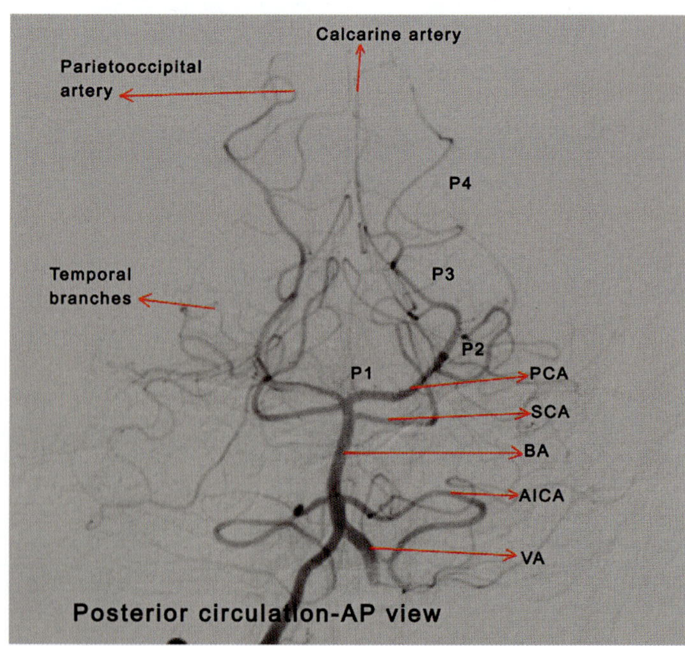

Fig. 3.1.93: DSA posterior circulation AP view

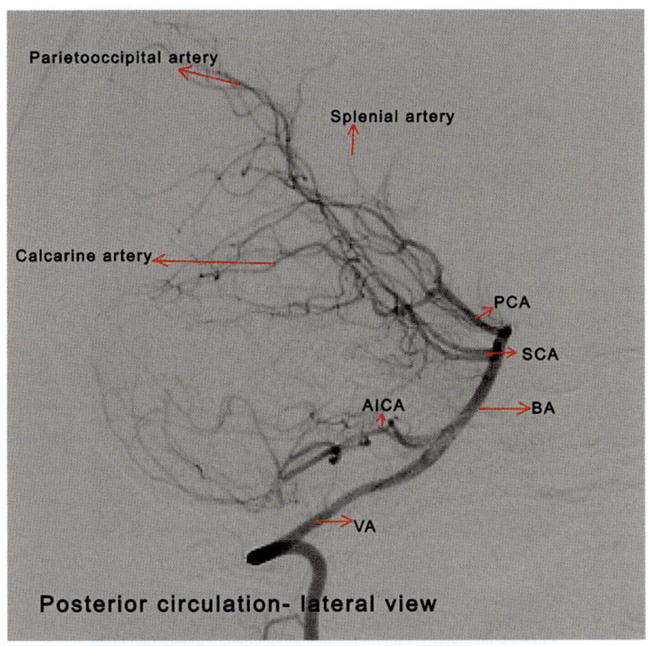

Fig. 3.1.94: DSA posterior circulation lateral view

3.1.M Brain Arterial Territories

Anterior cerebral artery (ACA): Supplies the medial part of frontal and parietal lobe, anterior portion of corpus callosum. **Medial lenticulostriate branches** from A1 segment of ACA supply the anteroinferior parts of basal ganglia (including globus pallidus and medial portion of putamen) and the anterior limb of internal capsule. Heubner's artery, largest medial lenticulostriate branch, supplies the anteromedial portion of head of caudate nucleus and anterior inferior part of internal capsule.

Middle cerebral artery (MCA): Cortical branches supplies the lateral surface of hemisphere, except for the medial part of frontal and parietal lobe (which is supplied by anterior cerebral artery), and inferior part of temporal lobe (which inturn is supplied by posterior cerebral artery). **Lateral lenticulostriate** perfortaing branches from MCA supply the lateral portion of putamen, external capsule, upper portion of internal capsule.

Posterior cerebral artery (PCA): Cortical branches supply the inferomedial part of temporal lobe, hippocampus, occipital pole, visual cortex, splenium of corpus callosum. Posterior thalamoperforating branches from the P1 segment supply the midbrain and thalamus. Midbrain also receives blood supply from superior cerebellar artery and perforating branches from basilar artery.

Anterior choroidal artery: Supplies the part of hippocampus and amygdala, posterior limb of internal capsule, retrolenticular part of internal capsule (optic radiation), lateral thalamus, optic tract, globus pallidus internus and also choroid plexus of lateral ventricle.

Basilar artery (BA): Pontine branches supply pons. Pons also receives blood supply from superior cerebellar artery (SCA) and AICA (lower and lateral pons).

Anterior inferior cerebellar artery (AICA): Supplies the anteroinferior surface of cerebellum.

Superior cerebellar artery (SCA): Supplies the superior surface of cerebellum, superior vermis, superior and middle cerebellar peduncle.

Posterior inferior cerebellar artery (PICA): Supplies the posteroinferior surface of the cerebellum up to horizontal fissure, tonsil, inferior portion of vermis, inferior cerebellar peduncle, lateral part of medulla. Larger the PICA territory, the smaller the AICA and vice versa (AICA-PICA dominance). Medulla also receives blood supply from the anterior spinal artery (medial aspect) and also direct penetrating branches from vertebral artery (Figs 3.1.95 to 3.1.105).

Thalamus blood supply: Thalamus has four vascular territories—anterior, paramedian, inferolateral and posterior territory. Artery of Percheron—variant in paramedian artery, in which single arterial trunk supplies the paramedian thalami and rostral midbrain bilaterally. Hence occlusion results in bilateral thalamic infarct (Fig. 3.1.106).

Border zones: Watershed or border zones are areas that lie at the junction of two different vascular territories. These can be classified into two categories; external (or cortical) and internal (or subcortical) border zones. The **external border zones** are located at the junction of anterior, middle and posterior cerebral artery territories—(1) frontal cortex (between ACA and MCA), (2) parieto-occipital cortex (between MCA and PCA), (3) paramedian white matter (between ACA and MCA). Internal border zones are located at the junction of anterior, middle, posterior cerebral artery territories with the Heubner, lenticulostriate and anterior choroidal artery territories—(1) between lenticulostriate and MCA territory, (2) between lenticulostriate and ACA territory, (3) between Heubner and ACA territory, (4) between anterior choroidal and MCA territory, (5) between anterior choroidal and PCA territory (Figs 3.1.107 to 3.1.109).

3.1.N Venous Anatomy of Brain

The intracranial venous system has two major components, **the dural venous sinuses and the cerebral veins.** These exhibit a wide range of normal variations. **Dural sinuses** are endothelium-lined channels that

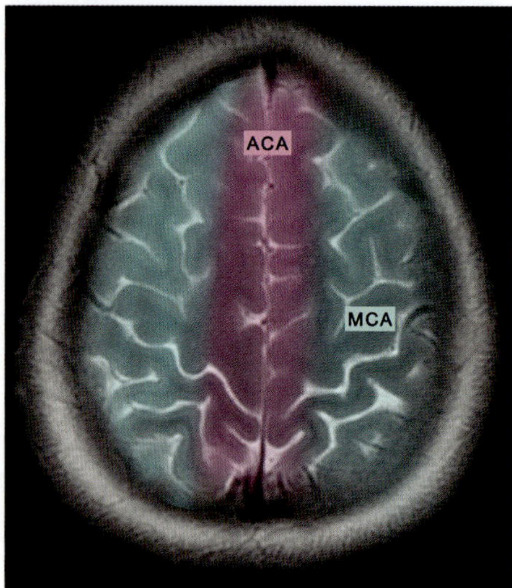

Fig. 3.1.95: Brain arterial territory

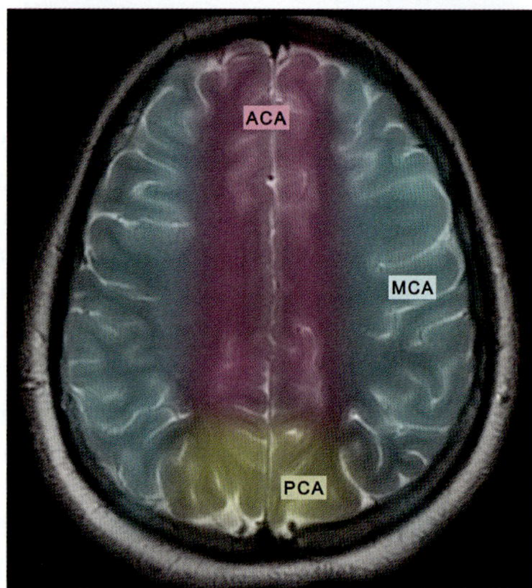

Fig. 3.1.96: Brain arterial territory

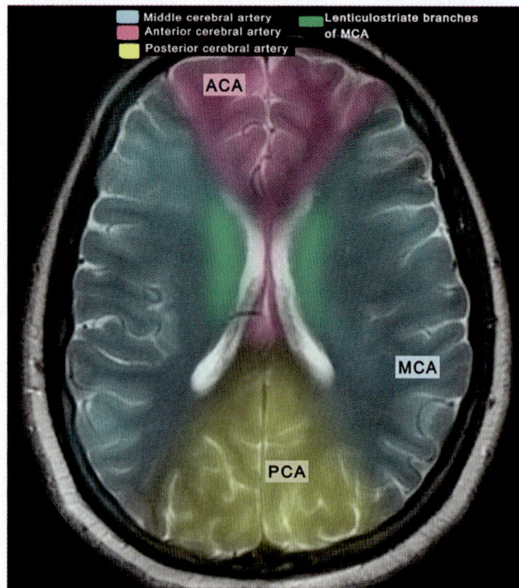

Fig. 3.1.97: Brain arterial territory

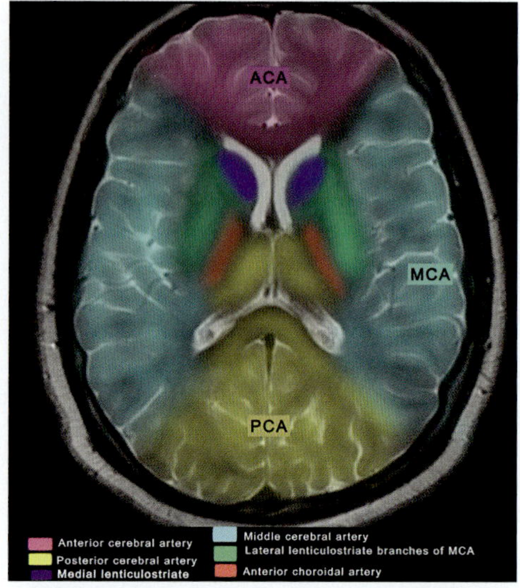

Fig. 3.1.98: Brain arterial territory

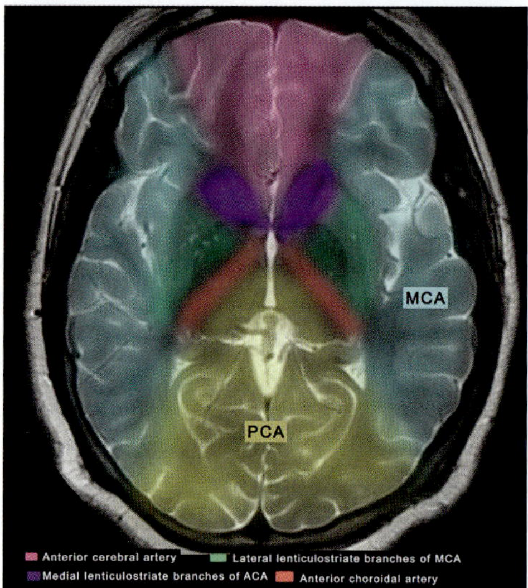

Fig. 3.1.99: Brain arterial territory

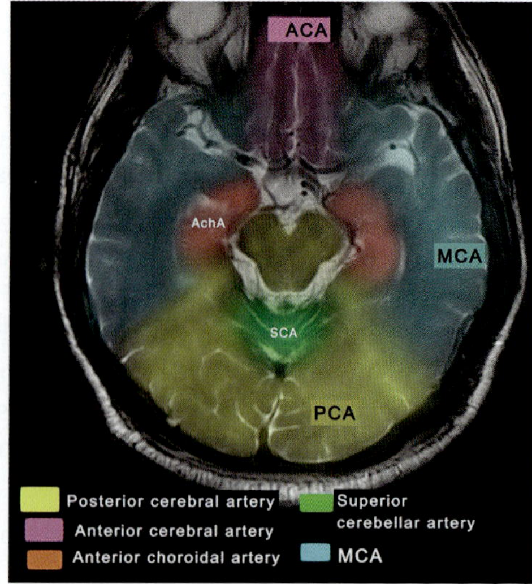

Fig. 3.1.100: Brain arterial territory

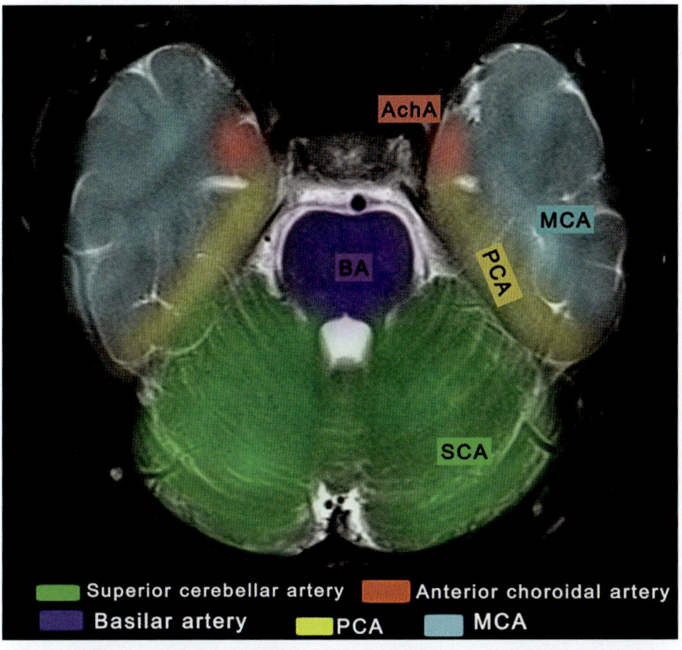

Fig. 3.1.101: Brain arterial territory

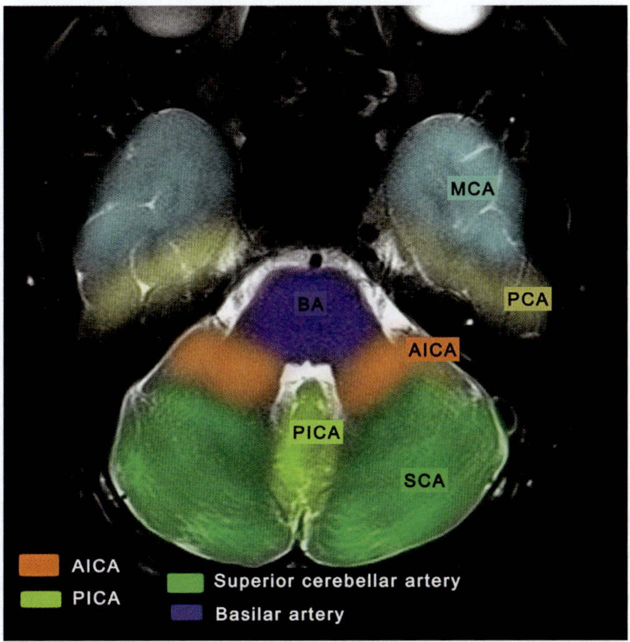

Fig. 3.1.102: Brain arterial territory

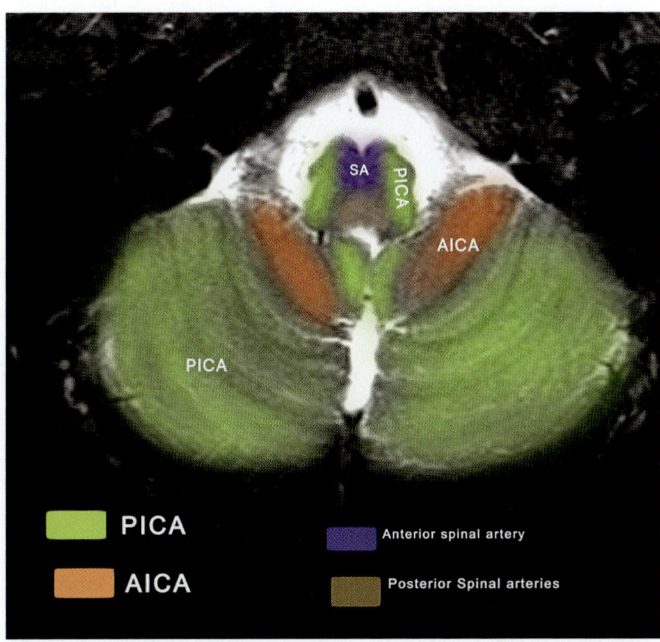

Fig. 3.1.103: Brain arterial territory

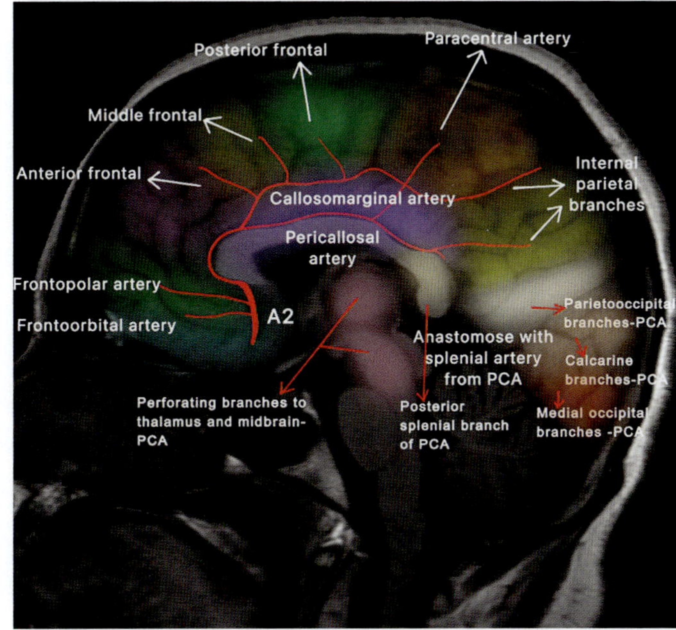

Fig. 3.1.104: Brain arterial territory ACA

are contained between the outer (periosteal) and inner (meningeal) dural layers and are often fenestrated and multichanneled. The dural venous sinuses are subdivided into an anteroinferior group and a posterosuperior group. The posterosuperior group is the more prominent and consists of the superior sagittal sinus (SSS), inferior sagittal sinus (ISS), straight sinus (SS), sinus confluence (torcular herophili), transverse sinuses (TS), sigmoid sinuses, and jugular bulbs. The anteroinferior group consists of the cavernous sinus (CS), superior and inferior petrosal sinuses (SPSs, IPSs), clival venous plexus (CVP), and sphenoparietal sinus (SphPS). **Superior sagittal sinus** starts anteriorly and courses posteriorly in the midline up to the internal occipital protuberance. Posteriorly the sinus turns to one side—usually to the right to become the transverse sinus. The **inferior sagittal sinus** runs in the lower free edge of the falx cerebri. Posteriorly it joins with the great cerebral

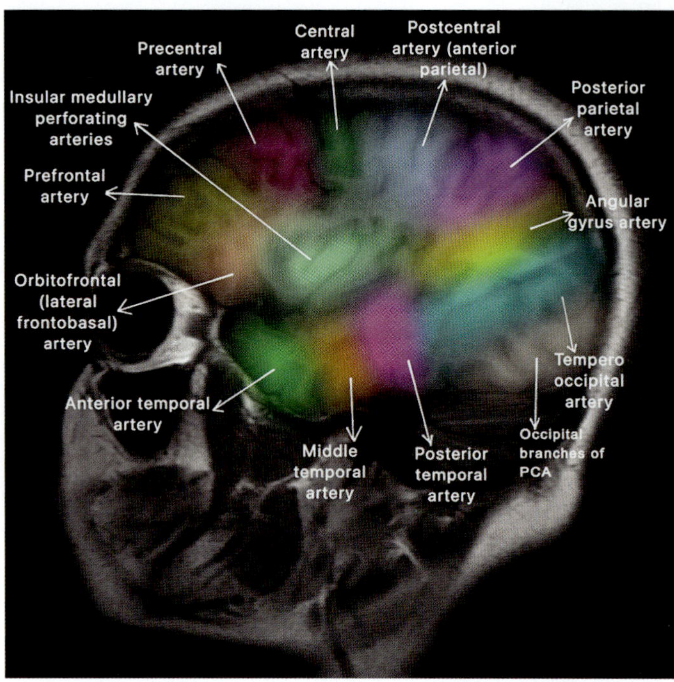

Fig. 3.1.105: Brain arterial territory MCA and PCA

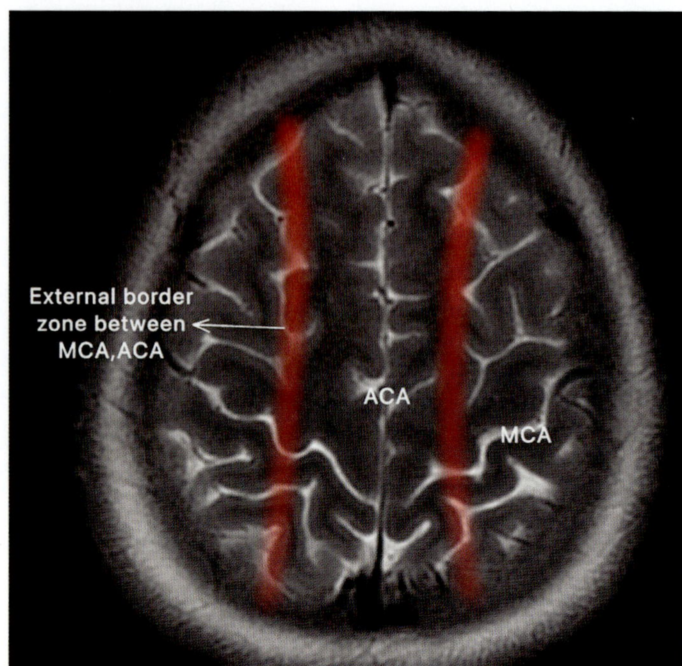

Fig. 3.1.107: External watershed zone

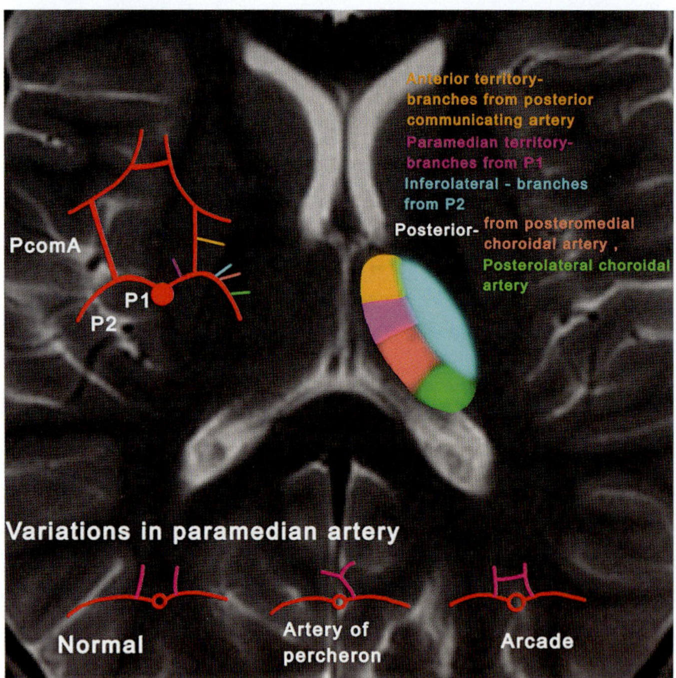

Fig. 3.1.106: Thalamus blood supply

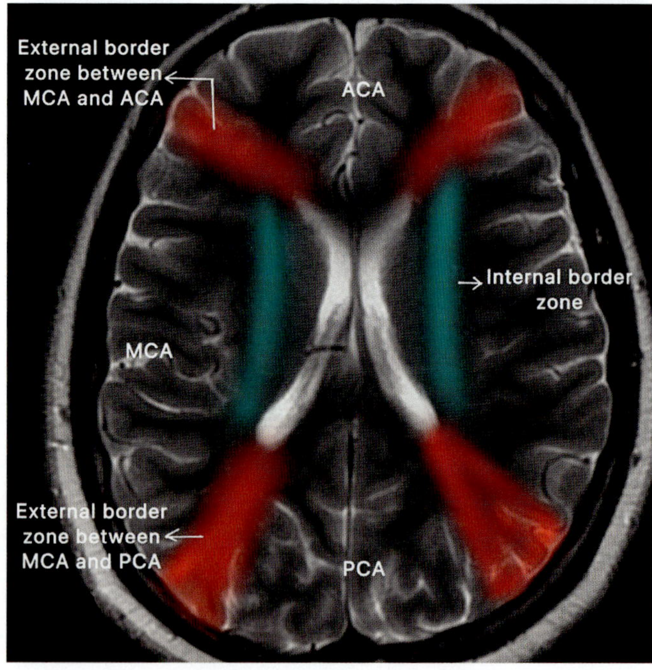

Fig. 3.1.108: Watershed zones

vein of Galen (VOG) to form the straight sinus. The **straight sinus** courses in the tentorium where the falx is attached to it up to the internal occipital protuberance and then to the confluence of sinuses also called torcula herophili. Then it turns to one side, usually to the left to become the transverse sinus. The transverse sinuses run right and left from the confluence of sinuses. They then turn inferiorly to become the sigmoid sinus. The sigmoid sinus courses towards the jugular foramen and at the level of the jugular foramen, becomes the internal jugular vein which further courses downwards and drains into the superior vena cava. There is a focal dilatation of the internal jugular vein within the jugular foramen called jugular bulb (Figs 3.1.110 to 3.1.112, 3.1.115 to 3.1.117).

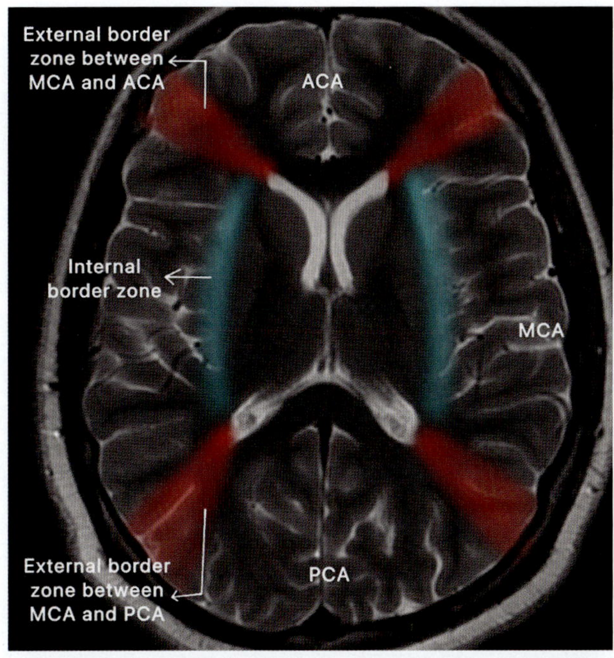

Fig. 3.1.109: Watershed zones

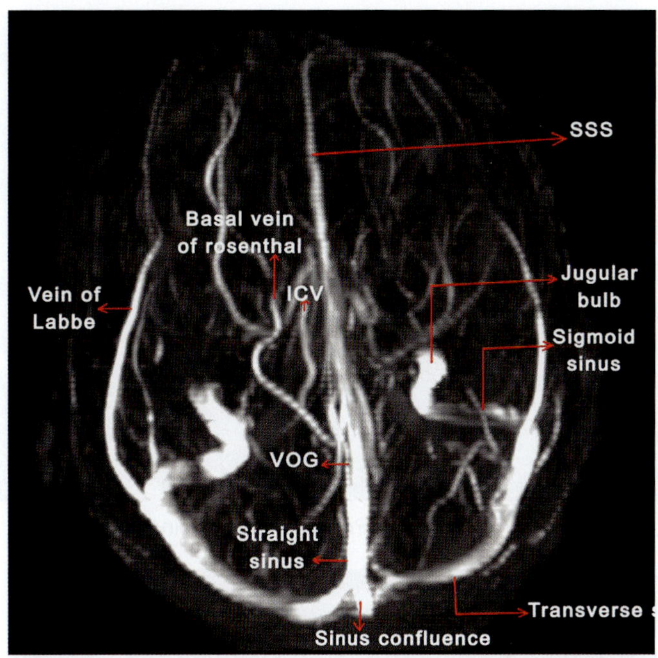

Fig. 3.1.111: MRV

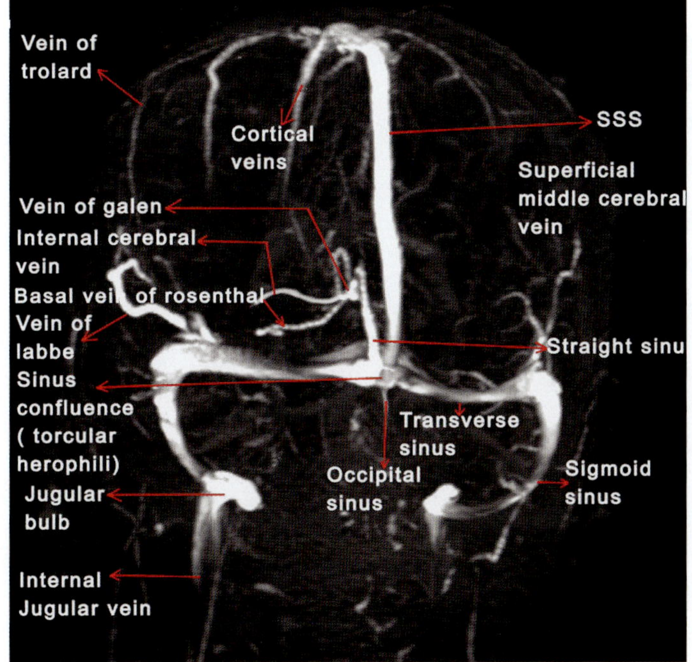

Fig. 3.1.110: MRV

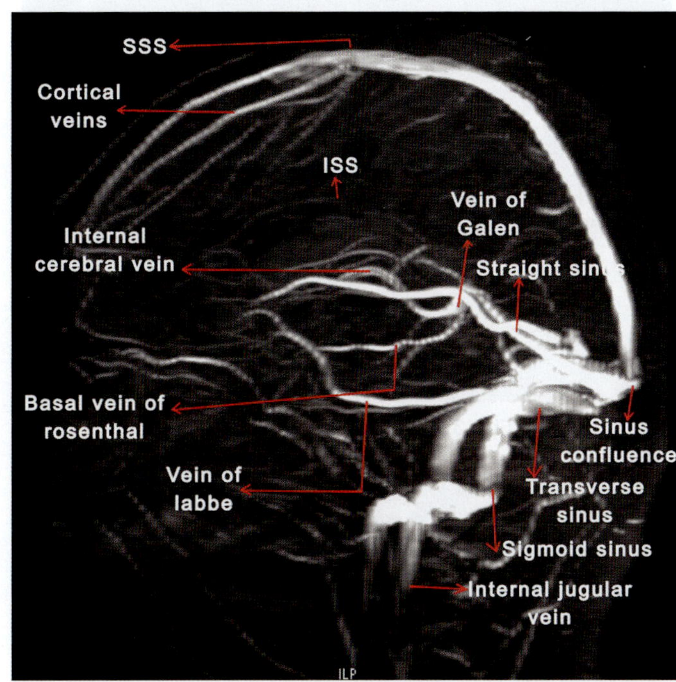

Fig. 3.1.112: MRV

The **cerebral veins** are subdivided into three groups: (1) Superficial ("cortical" or "external") veins, (2) deep cerebral ("internal") veins, and (3) brainstem/posterior fossa veins. Superficial veins of cerebrum empty into dural sinuses. The **superficial cortical veins** consist of a superior group, a middle group, and an inferior group. They are named for the area of cortex that they drain. A dominant anastomotic superior cortical vein, the **vein of Trolard**, receives the superficial middle cerebral vein and courses upward from the sylvian fissure to join the SSS. A prominent posterior anastomotic vein, the **vein of Labbé**, courses inferolaterally over the temporal lobe to drain into the TS (Fig. 3.1.114). **Superficial cortical venous drainage territories**—most of the superior cerebrum is primarily drained into superior sagittal sinus, and also receives drainage from parasagittal cortical regions

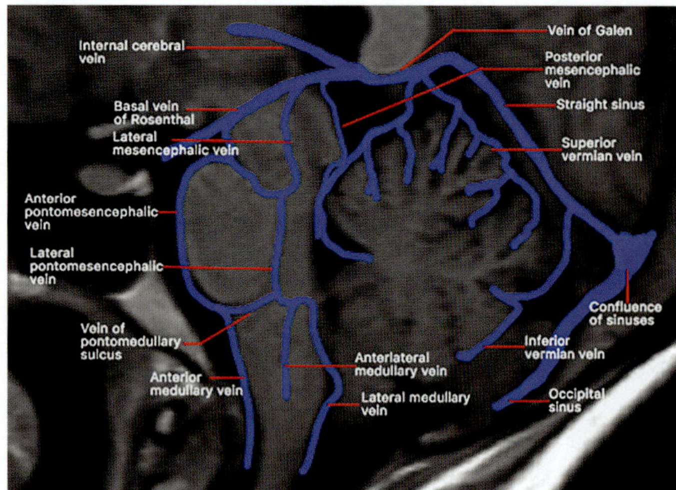

Fig. 3.1.113: Posterior fossa veins

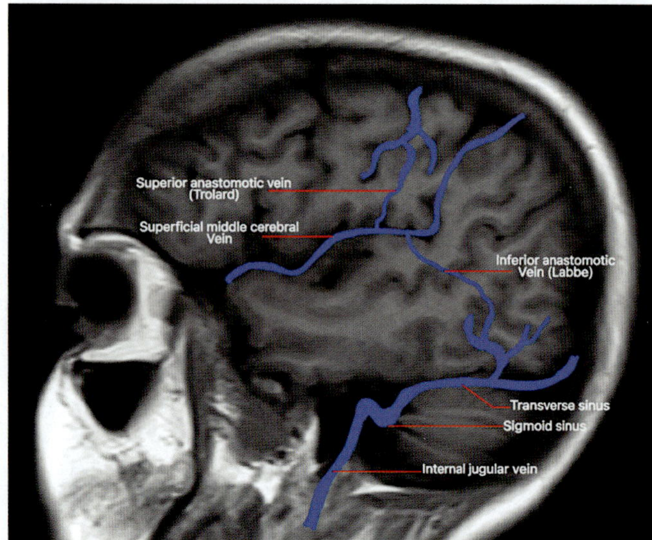

Fig. 3.1.114: Anastomotic veins

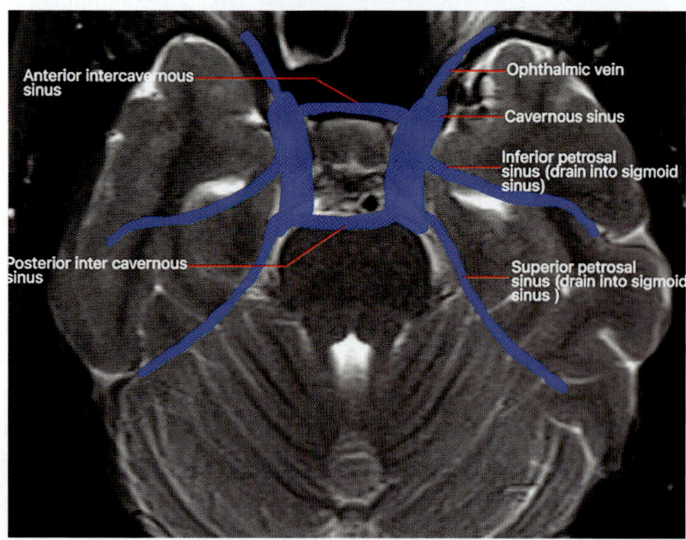

Fig. 3.1.115: Cavernous sinus

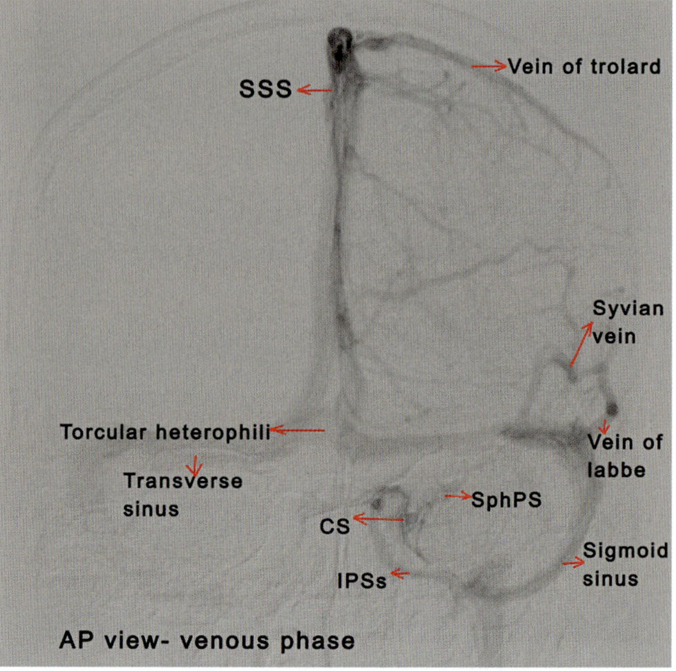

Fig. 3.1.116: DSA AP view

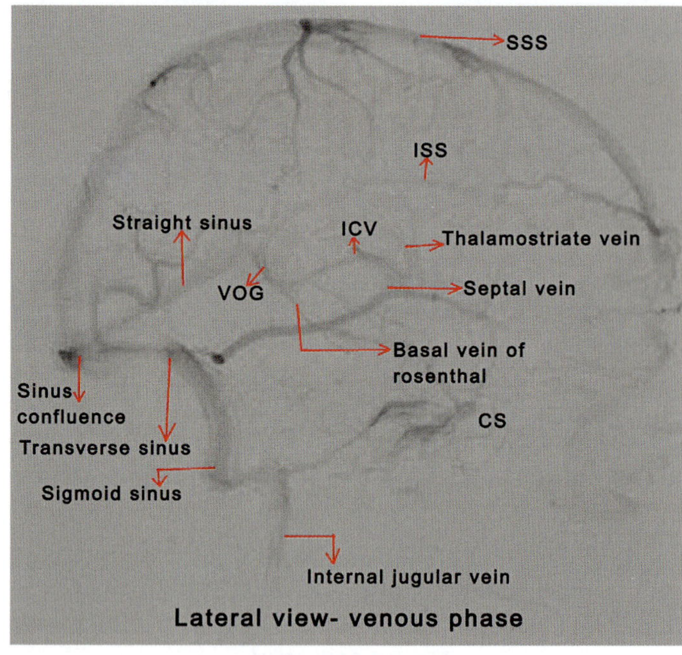

Fig. 3.1.117: DSA lateral view

at lower levels. The sylvian veins (superficial middle crebral vein) drain blood from peri-insular region into the basal dural sinuses (sphenoparietal or cavrnous sinus). The transverse sinuses receive blood from the temporal, parietal, occipital lobes. The Labbe's vein, if dominant, may drain much of this territory (Figs 3.1.118 to 3.1.123).

The deep cerebral ("internal") veins include vein of Galen (VOG), internal cerebral vein and their tributaries,

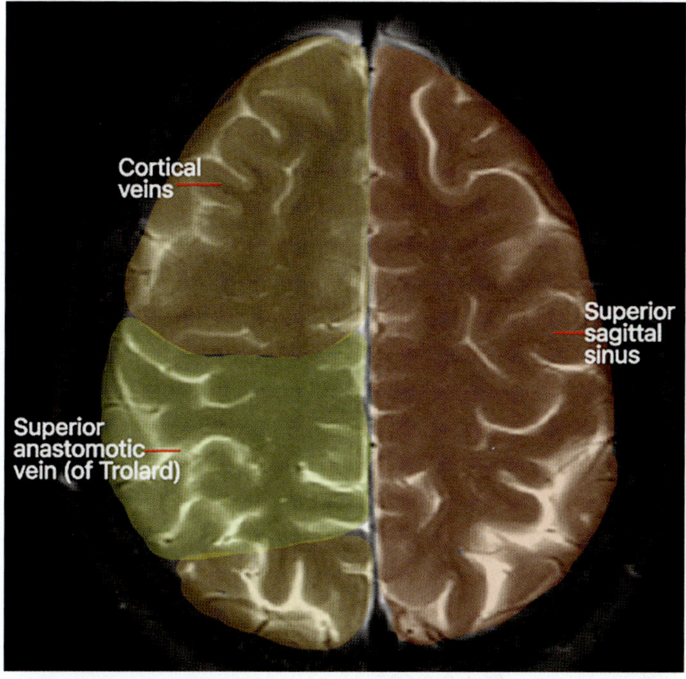

Fig. 3.1.118: Venous territory

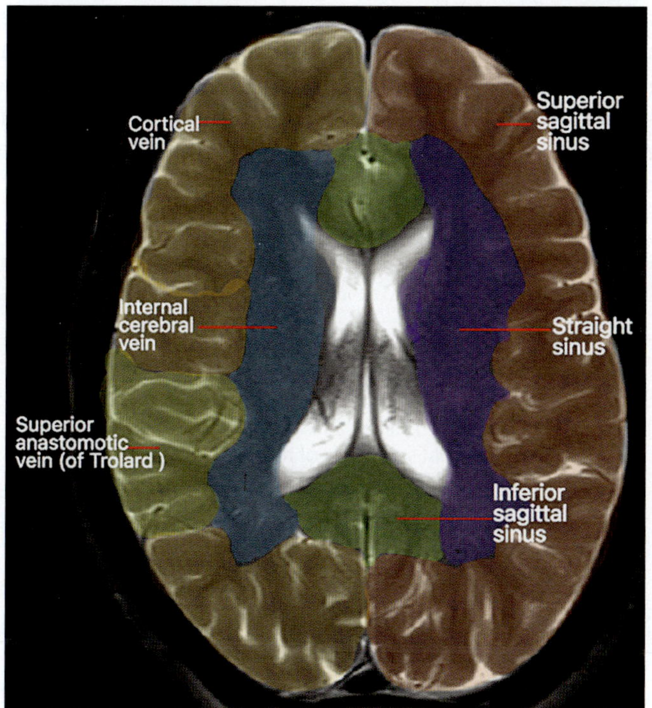

Fig. 3.1.119: Venous territory

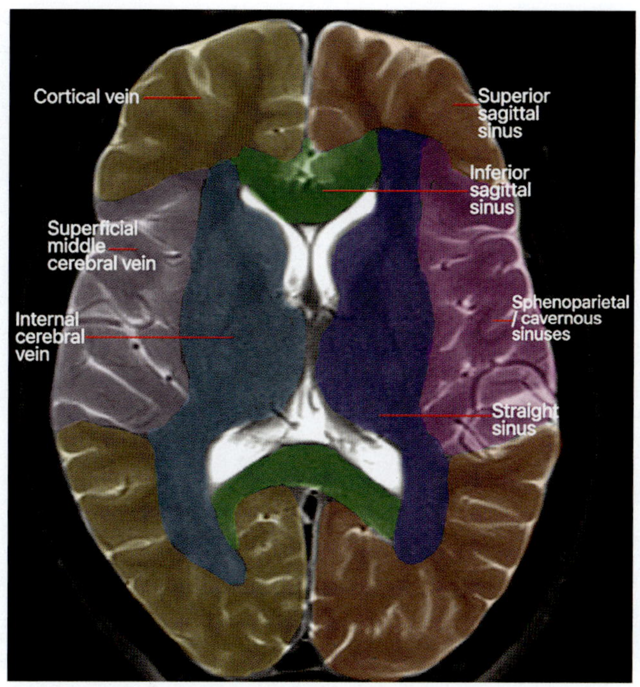

Fig. 3.1.120: Venous territory

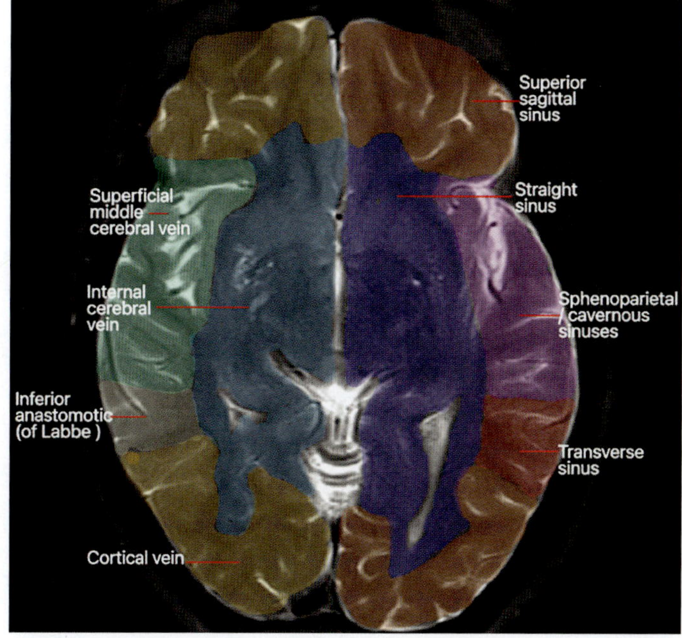

Fig. 3.1.121: Venous territory

Rosenthal's vein (basal vein) and its tributaries, medullary vein and subependymal veins, which drain the hemispheric white matter. The deep system drains the inferior frontal lobe, most of the deep white matter of frontal, temporal and parietal lobes, corpus callosum, upper brainstem, basal ganglia and thalamus.

Thalamostriate + septal veins → ICV (internal cerebral vein) + basal vein of Rosenthal → VOG + ISS → straight sinus. The **brainstem and posterior fossa veins** are likewise divided into three groups: (1) A superior ("galenic") group, (2) an anterior (petrosal) group, and (3) a posterior group. These include—anterior pontomesencephalic vein, posterior mesencephalic vein, precentral cerebellar vein, superior and inferior

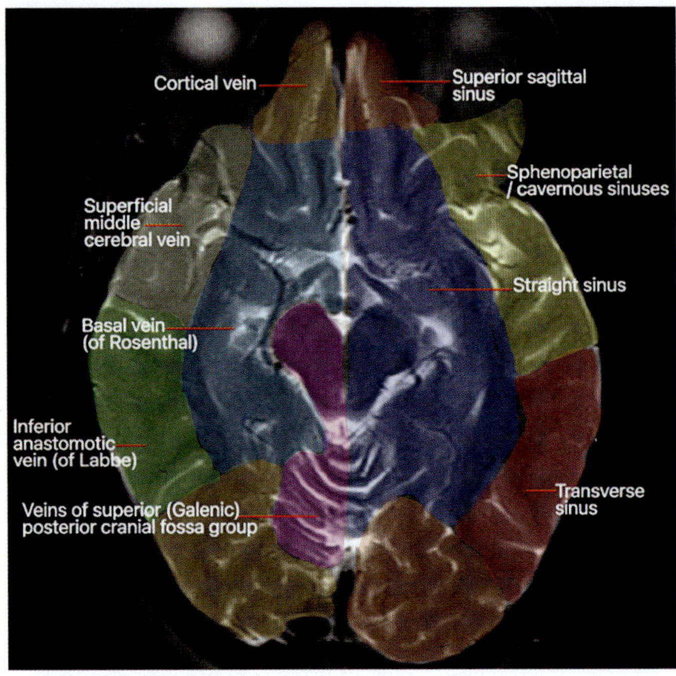

Fig. 3.1.122: Venous territory

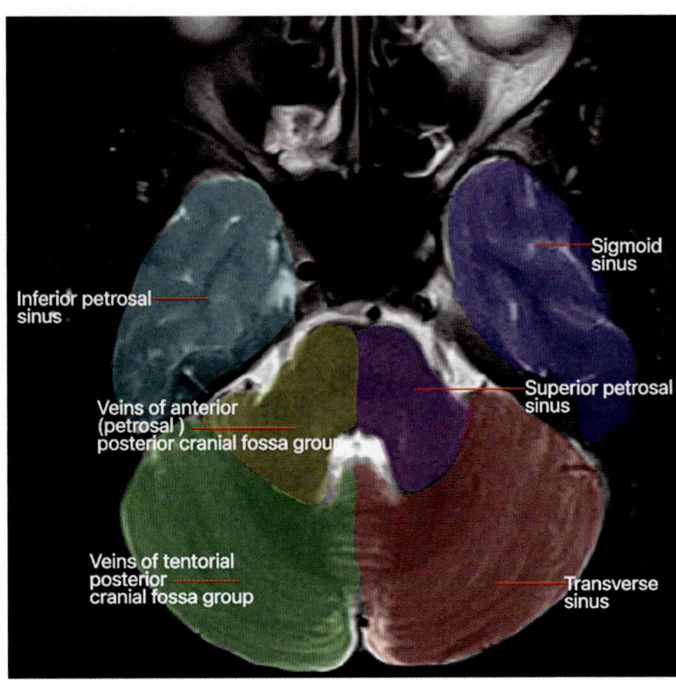

Fig. 3.1.123: Venous territory

vermian veins, pontine veins, inferior medullary veins (Fig. 3.1.113).

3.1.O Cisterns

Focal expansions of the subarachnoid spaces (SASs) form the brain CSF cisterns. These cisterns are found at the base of the brain around the brainstem, tentorial incisura, and foramen magnum. The brain cisterns are conveniently grouped into supra-, peri-, and infratentorial cisterns (Table 3.1.5). All contain numerous important critical structures, such as vessels and cranial nerves (Figs 3.1.124 to 3.1.128).

Table 3.1.5: Cerebral cisterns

Cistern	*Location*	*Contents*
Suprasellar cistern	Between the diaphragma sellae and the hypothalamus	Infundibulum, optic chiasm, and circle of Willis
Interpeduncular cistern	Posterior continuation of the suprasellar cistern	Oculomotor nerves as well as the distal basilar artery and proximal segments of the posterior cerebral arteries.
Perimesencephalic (ambient, crural) cisterns	Wrap around the midbrain	Trochlear nerves, P2 PCA segments, superior cerebellar arteries, and basal vein of Rosenthal.
Quadrigeminal cistern	Connects with the ambient cisterns laterally and the superior cerebellar cistern inferiorly	Pineal gland, trochlear nerves, P3 PCA segments, proximal choroidal arteries, and vein of Galen.
Prepontine cistern	Lie in the midline behind the clivus and anterior to the pons.	Basilar artery and some of its branches, abducent nerve
Premedullary cistern	Lie in the midline behind the clivus and anterior to the medulla.	Vertebrobasilar confluence, anterior spinal artery, PICA hypoglossal nerve (CN 12)
Cerebellopontine angle cisterns	Between the anterior surface of the cerebellum and the lateral surface of the pons.	CN 7,8, AICA, flocculus of cerebellum
Superior cerebellar cisterns	Posterior to the quadrigeminal cistern, between the superior surface of cerebellum and tentorium	—
Cisterna magna	Between the cerebellum and the dorsal surface of the medulla oblongata at and above the level of the foramen magnum	Vertebral arteries, PICA, cranial nerves—9,10,11

Table 3.1.6: Recess of third and fourth ventricle	
Recesses of third ventricle	*Recesses of fourth ventricle*
Inferior—optic and infundibular recesses	Posterior superior recesses
Posterosuperior—pineal and suprapineal recesses	Two lateral recesses (of Luschka) connecting to cerebellopontine cistern

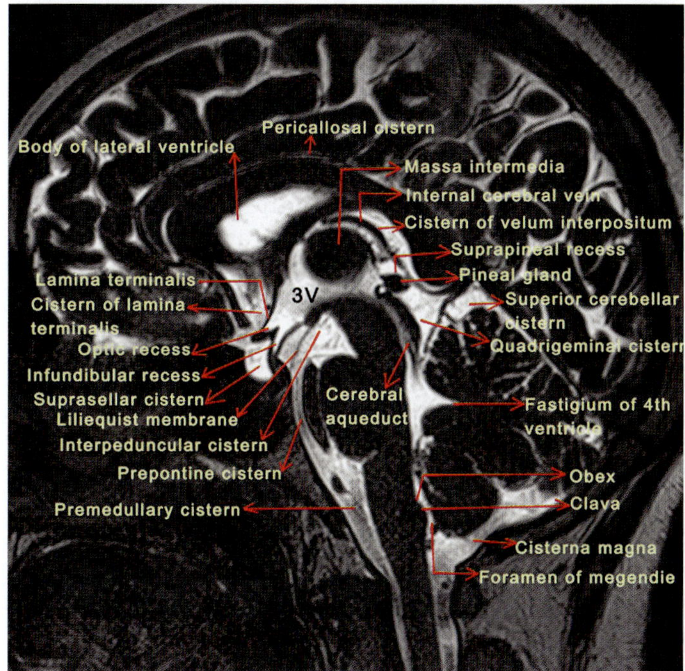

Fig. 3.1.124: Cisterns and recess MR sagittal view

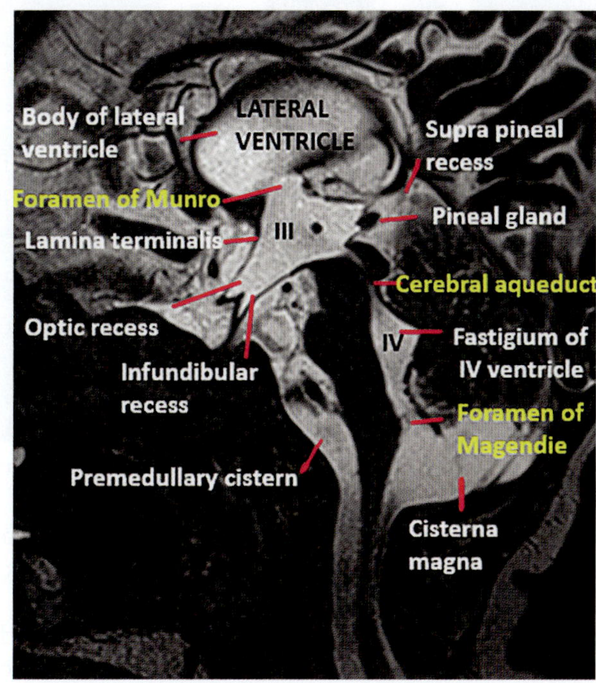

Fig. 3.1.125: MR image sagittal view

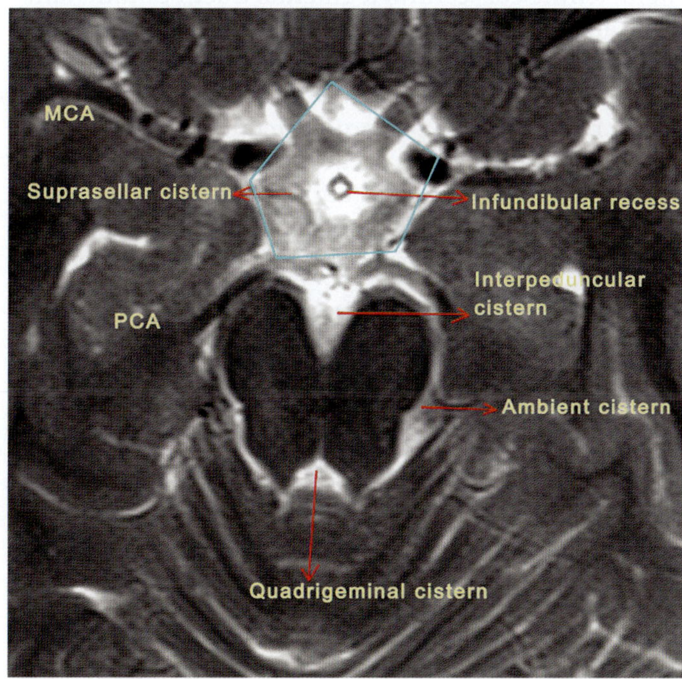

Fig. 3.1.126: Basal cisterns

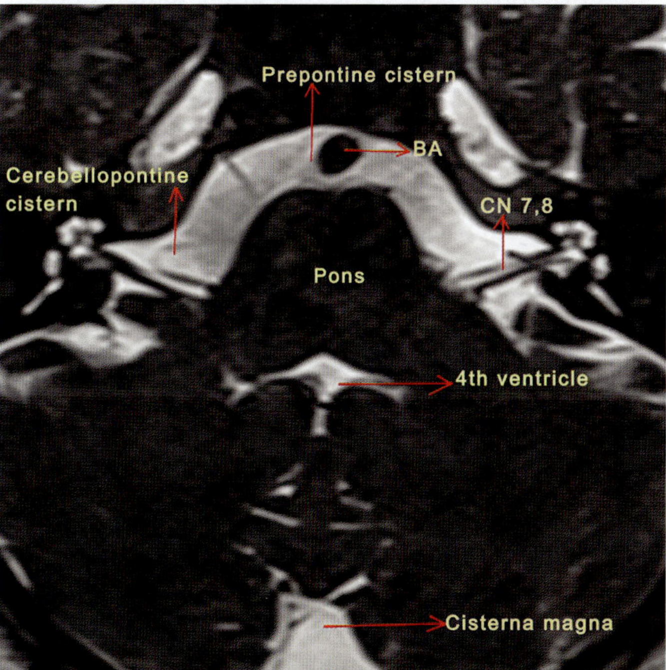

Fig. 3.1.127: Prepontine and cerebellopontine cistern

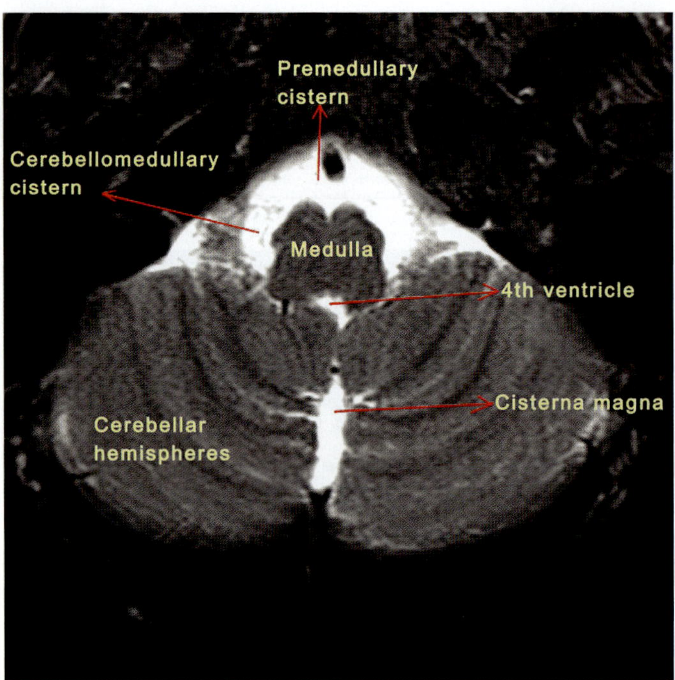

Fig. 3.1.128: Premedullary and cerebellomedullary cistern

Ventricles: The ventricular system in the brain is composed of cerebrospinal fluid (CSF)-filled ventricles and their connecting foramina. CSF is produced by choroid plexus ependymal cells which line the ventricles. They are continuous with the central canal. Ventricles contain around 20% of the total average adult CSF volume, around 20–25 ml.

Sites of choroid plexus: The roof of the temporal horns of the lateral ventricles, extending along the floor of the body of the lateral ventricles, through the interventricular foramen of Monro, and along the roof of the third ventricle, the medullary part of the fourth ventricle, extending into the lateral apertures (of Luschka).

The ventricular system consists of two lateral ventricles, each consisting of frontal horn, body, trigone/atrium, occipital and temporal horns. A midline third ventricle—single, slit-like, midline, vertically oriented cavity that lies between the thalami. A fourth ventricle—diamond-shaped in sagittal cross-section and located dorsal to the lower pons and upper part of the medulla oblongata. The roof is formed by the superior medullary velum and inferior medullary velum overlying the cerebellum.The fourth ventricle gradually narrows as it courses inferiorly, forming the obex which continuous as the central canal of the spinal cord near the cervicomedullary junction.

The interconnections between the ventricles occur through the following: Interventricular foramina (of Monro)—lateral to third ventricle, cerebral aqueduct (of Sylvius)—third to fourth ventricle, median aperture (of Magendie)—fourth to cisterna magna. **Liliequist membrane** is a thin arachnoid membrane, separates suprasellar, interpeduncular and prepontine cisterns. Sellar segment of this membrane extends from dorsum sella and divides into superior diencephalic membrane which attaches to mamillary bodies and inferior mesencephalic membrane (Fig. 3.1.125).

3.1.P Brainstem

It is the most caudal portion of brain and consists of midbrain, pons and medulla, continues as spinal cord.

Midbrain: The midbrain connects the pons and cerebellum with the forebrain and can be divided into a **ventral part, the tegmentum,** and a dorsal part, **the tectal or quadrigeminal** plate (dorsal to cerebral aqeuduct). Ventral part contains crus cerebri (cerebral peduncle) pyramidal and corticopontine tracts. **Dorsal tegmentum** is ventral to aqueduct and contains substantia nigra, red nucleus, nuclei of 3rd, 4th cranial nerve, white matter tracts. Tectal plate includes superior and inferior colliculi. Superior colliculus is part of visual pathway and inferior colliculus is auditory pathway. The cerebral **aqueduct** of Sylvius is located in the midbrain and joins the third and fourth ventricles, surrounded by periaqueductal gray matter. Signal of cerebral aqueduct varies due to flow artefact. The white matter tracts pass through the entire length of the brainstem and include the medial longitudinal fasciculus, medial lemniscus, lateral lemniscus, central tegmental tract, spinothalamic tract, and rubro-olivary tract. Cerebral peduncle (crus cerebri) separated in midline by interpeduncular fossa. Gray matter formations in brainstem are **substantia nigra, red nucleus, periaqueductal gray matter**. 3rd cranial nerve nuclei is located at superior colliculus level, anterior to cerebral aqueduct (Figs 3.1.129 and 3.1.131). 4th cranial nerve nuclei is at inferior colliculus level, anterior to cerebral aqueduct and dorsal to MLF. Edinger-Westphal nuclei is located dorsal to 3rd CN nuclei in periaqueductal gray matter.

The medial longitudinal fasciculus (MLF) is the main central connection for the oculomotor nerve and coordinates conjugate gaze. It is found on each side of the brainstem near the midline, ventral to the periaqueductal grey matter, and ascends to the interstitial nucleus (of Cajal). It links the nuclei of the vestibulocochlear nerve (CN VIII) and the three cranial nerves (3, 4, 6) controlling the movements of the eye.

Superior cerebellar peduncle (brachium conjunctivum) that connects cerebellum with midbrain.They decussate centrally in ventral midbrain at the level of inferior

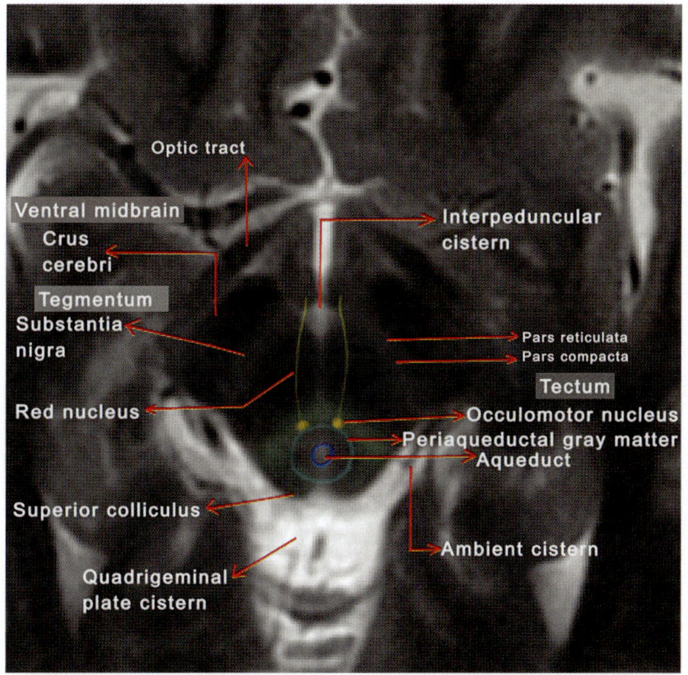

Fig. 3.1.129: Upper midbrain

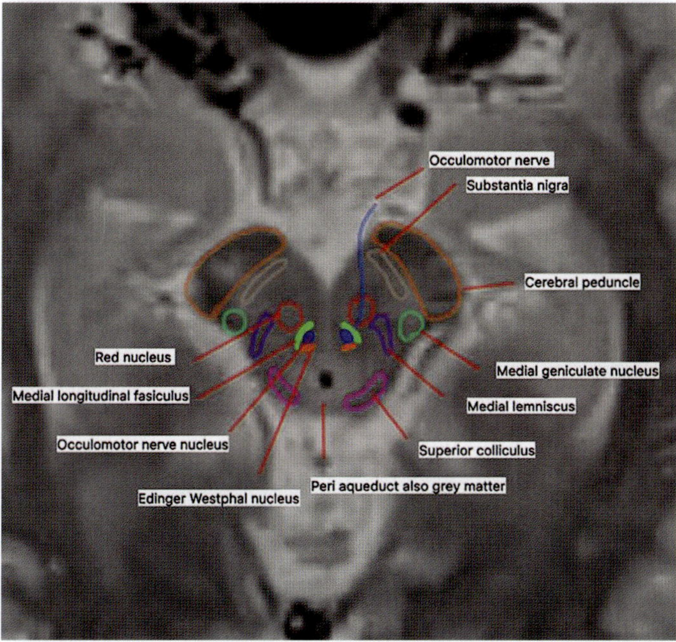

Fig. 3.1.130: Midbrain nucleus

colliculus (Figs 3.1.130 and 3.1.131). **Nigrosome imaging**—substantia nigra has two parts: Pars reticulata ventrally and pars compacta dorsally. Normal substantia nigra in T2 gradient images, has bilateral hyperintensity seen as pocket like indentation at the level of red nucleus and at caudal level they appear as linear hyperintensity (corresponds to substantia nigra pars compacta) between two layers of substantia nigra hypointensity (known as swallow tail sign, nigral hyperintensity, dorsal

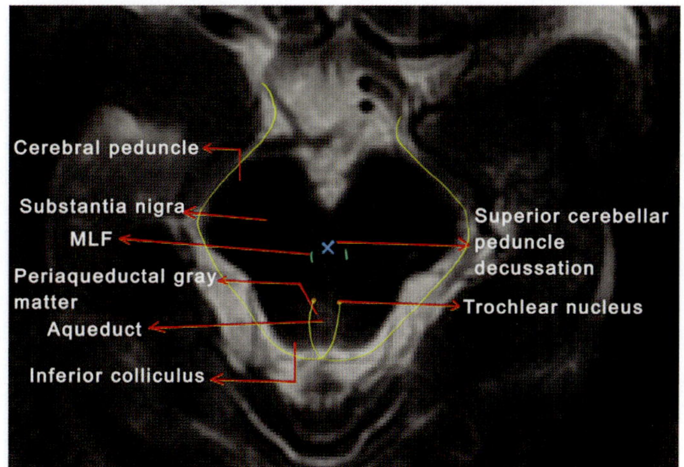

Fig. 3.1.131: Lower midbrain

hyperintensity). Loss of this nigral hyperintensity reflects signal hypointensity due to iron deposition associated with dopaminergic neuronal loss.

Pons: Connects the brain to the cerebellum and can be divided into a **ventral part** and a dorsal tegmentum. The ventral part contains longitudinal fibers primarily from the corticospinal, corticobulbar, and corticopontine tracts and multiple transverse fibers. Ventral part is known as **pontine bulb or belly**. The **dorsal tegmentum** contains the nuclei of the trigeminal (V), abducens (VI), facial (VII), and vestibulocochlear (VIII) cranial nerves, in addition to white matter tracts. **Facial colliculus** (located at the level of middle cerebellar peduncle) is a bulge in floor of 4th ventricle, formed by axons of 7th nerve around abducent nucleus. CPA (cerebellopontine angle) is junction between pons and cerebellum. CN5 root entry zone is at midlateral pons, CN6 exit anteriorly at pontomedullary junction. CN7, 8 root exit zone at pontomedullary junction in lateral brainstem. Middle cerebellar peduncle (brachium pontis) connects cerebellum to pons (Figs 3.1.132 and 3.1.133).

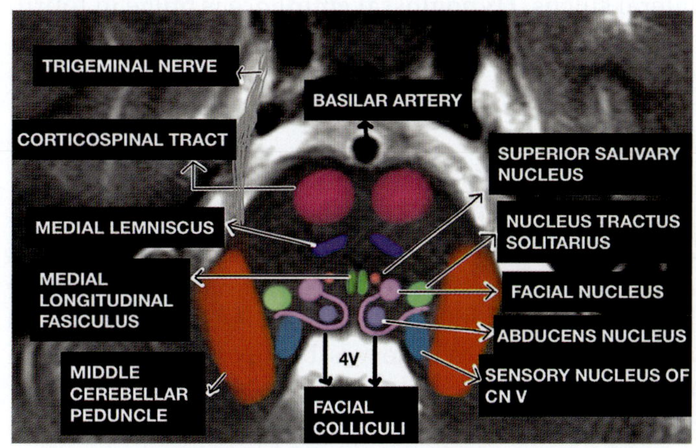

Fig. 3.1.132: Pons nucleus

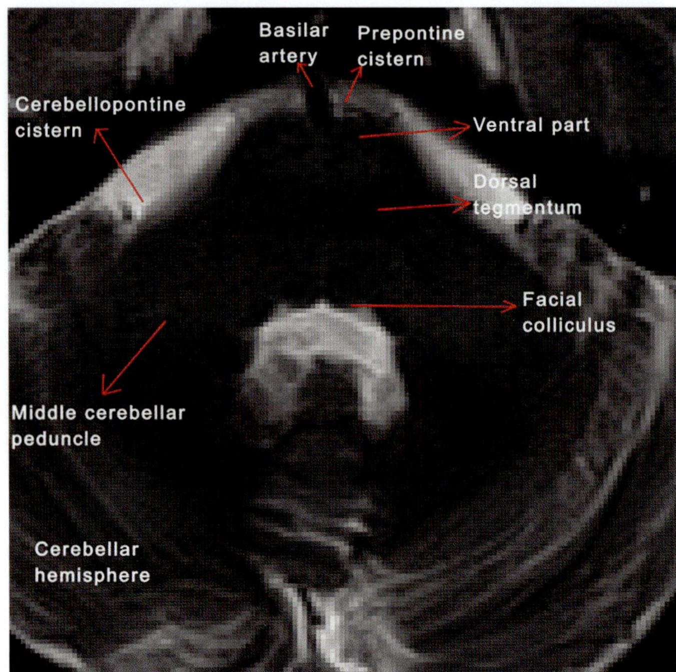

Fig. 3.1.133: Pons

Medulla oblongata: The medulla oblongata relays information from the spinal cord to the brain. The **ventral part** includes the pyramids and the olives. The **dorsal tegmentum** contains the nuclei of the glossopharyngeal (IX), vagus (X), accessory (XI), and hypoglossal (XII) cranial nerves, as well as the continuation of the white matter tracts. Pyramid is paired structure on ventral surface, separated by midline ventral median fissure contains pyramidal tract. **Medullary olives** are lateral to pyramids, separated by preolivary sulcus (ventrolateral sulcus). Posterolateral sulcus (postolivary sulcus) is lateral to olives. **Gracile (medial-clava) and cuneate (lateral) tubercles** form lower aspect of dorsal medulla, produced by nuclei gracilis and cuneatus respectively and separated by dorsal median sulcus and dorsal lateral sulcus. **Hypoglossal eminence** is bulge in fourth ventricle formed by 12th nerve nuclei in dorsal aspect of mid-medulla. Inferior cerebellar peduncle connects medulla to cerebellum (Figs 3.1.134 and 3.1.135).

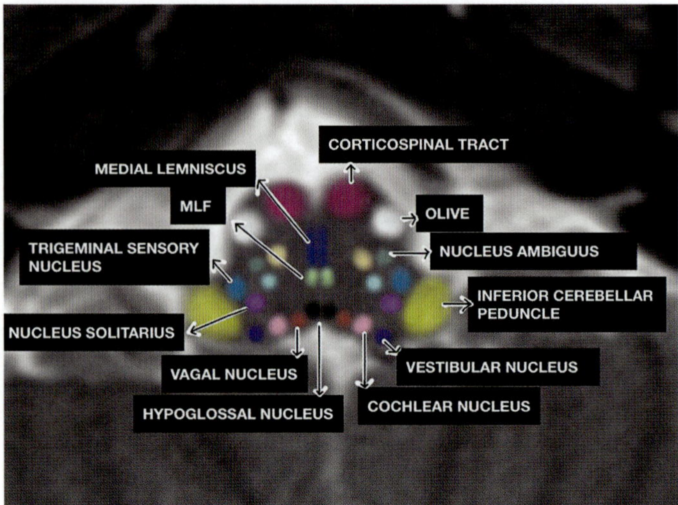

Fig. 3.1.134: Nucleus in medulla

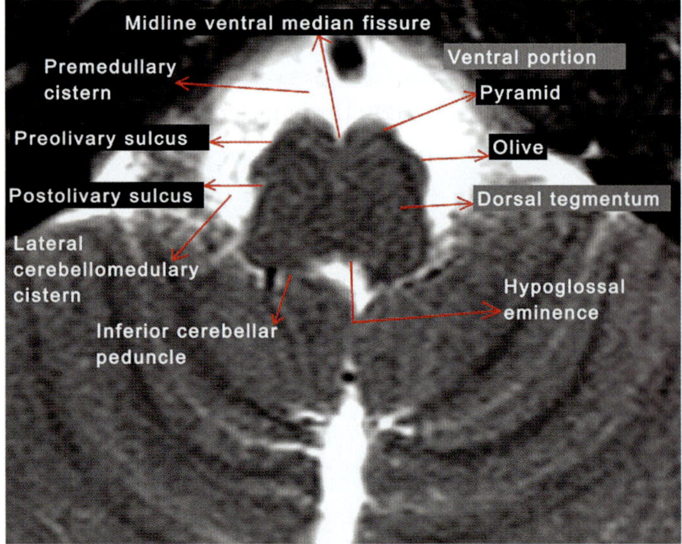

Fig. 3.1.135: Medulla

3.1.Q Cranial Nerves

The anatomy of the cranial nerves is complex, and the evaluation of patients with cranial neuropathies requires an in-depth understanding of the normal course of these important structures. First two pairs of cranial nerves are not truly cranial nerves but extensions of brain (Fig. 3.1.136).

CN1: The olfactory nerve consists of white-matter tracts and is not surrounded by Schwann cells. The

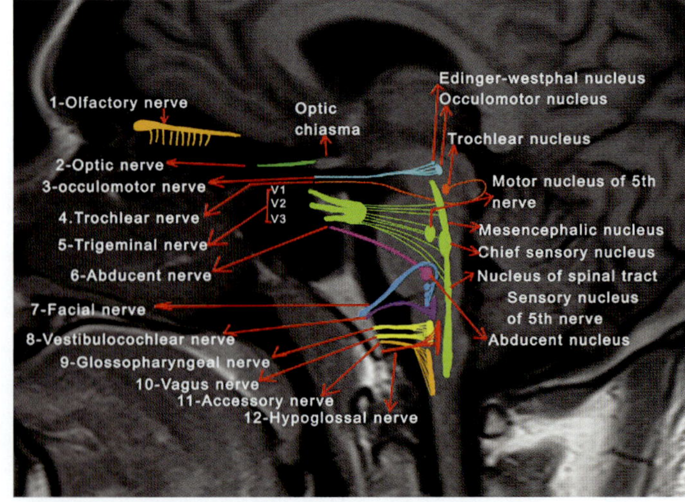

Fig. 3.1.136: Cranial nerves overview

neurosensory cells for smell reside in the olfactory epithelium along the roof of the nasal cavity. The axons of these cells extend through the cribriform plate of the ethmoid bone into the **olfactory bulb**, which gives rise to olfactory tracts. **Olfactory tracts** course posteriorly along olfactory sulcus and terminate opposite to the anterior perforated substance at the olfactory trigone. At this point, olfactory nerve divides into **three striae**, lateral, intermediate and medial olfactory striae. Lateral olfactory striae terminates at medial temporal lobe (olfactory cortex). Medial olfactory striae reach the subcallosal gyrus, intermediate striae terminate at the anterior perforated substance, forming slight elevation called olfactory tubercle (Figs 3.1.137 and 3.1.138).

CN 2: The optic nerve is also a white-matter tract without surrounding Schwann cells. It includes four anatomic segments: Retinal, orbital, canalicular, and cisternal. The **retinal segment**, which consists of axons of ganglion cells of retina, leaves the ocular globe through the lamina cribrosa. The **orbital segment,** which is surrounded by a dural sheath containing CSF, travels through the center of the fat-filled orbit. The **canalicular segment** is the portion that lies in the optic canal, below the ophthalmic artery, which then becomes intracranial. Finally, the **cisternal segment** or prechiasmatic segment of the nerve can be visualized in the suprasellar cistern, where the nerve leads to the **optic chiasm**, in which medial fibers cross to the contralateral side. The **optic tract** extends posteriorly from optic chiasm, projects into lateral geniculate body of thalamus. Efferent axons from the lateral geniculate body form the **optic radiations**, which projects into calcarine (visual) cortex (Figs 3.1.139 and 3.1.140).

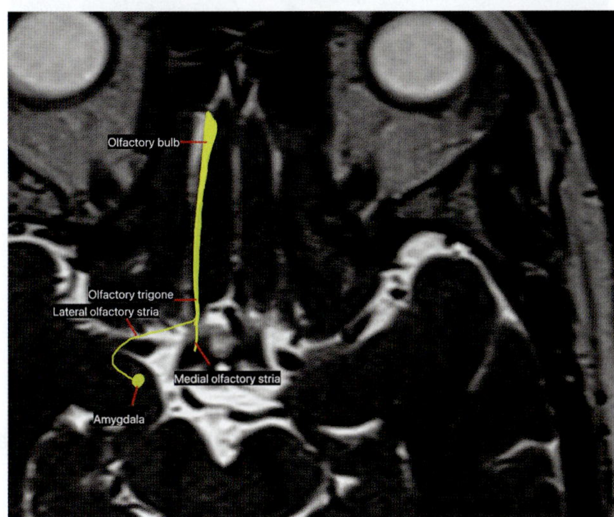

Fig. 3.1.137: Olfactory bulb and tract

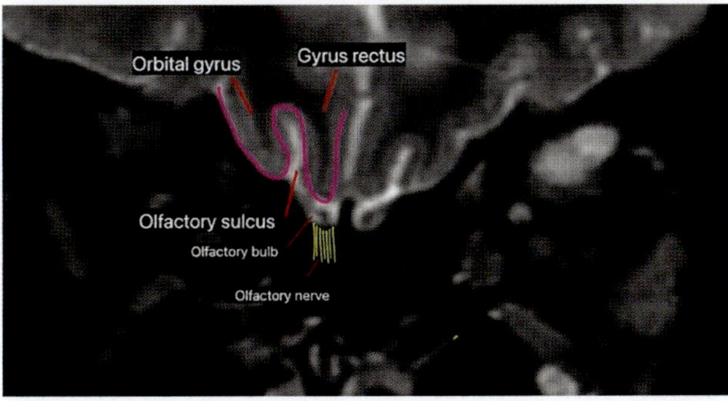

Fig. 3.1.138: Olfactory nerve

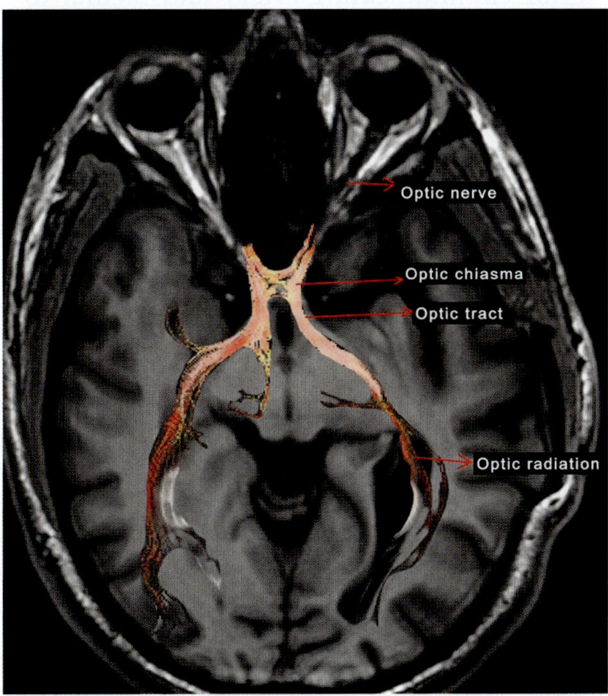

Fig. 3.1.139: Optic pathway DTI

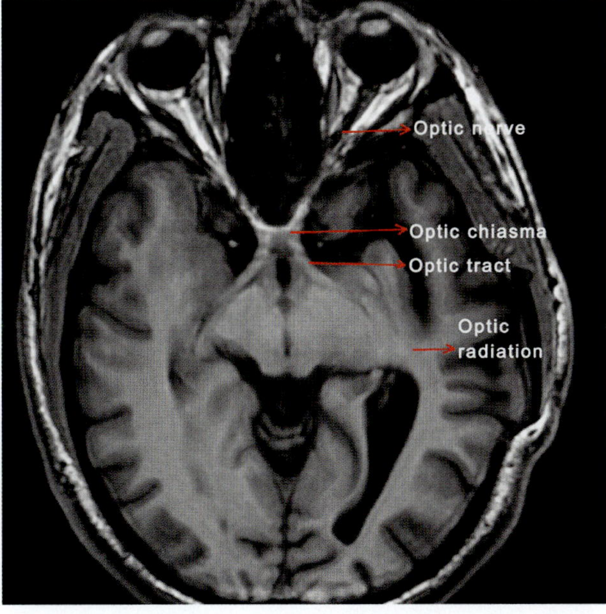

Fig. 3.1.140: Optic nerve

CN 3: The oculomotor nerve originates from **midbrain** nuclei deep to the superior colliculus, ventral to the cerebral aqueduct, and inferior to the pineal gland. The nerve then travels across the midbrain from posterior to anterior to emerges into the lateral aspect of interpeduncular cistern. In the prepontine cistern, the nerve travels between the superior cerebellar and posterior cerebral arteries (Fig. 3.1.143), medial to 4th cranial nerves. Their course extends inferior to posterior communicating artery and medial to free edge of tentorium cerebelli (Fig. 3.1.144). After crossing the petroclinoid segment (Gruber's ligament), enter the cavernous sinus via the occulomotor cistern (Fig. 3.1.142). The cavernous segment of the oculomotor nerve runs along the **lateral wall of the cavernous sinus** and is the most superior of the nerves in this sinus. The oculomotor nerve then enters the orbit through the **superior orbital fissure,** before splitting into superior and inferior divisions lateral to the optic nerve (Fig. 3.1.141).

CN 4: The trochlear nerve is the smallest and has the longest intracranial course (7.5 cm), only nerve to cross the midline (each superior oblique muscle is innervated by contralateral 4th nerve nucleus) and exit on dorsal aspect of brainstem. The nucleus is located just anterior to periaqueductal gray matter at the level of inferior colliculus. The fascicular segment passes posteriorly and caudally in the periaqueductal gray matter, then decussating in superior medullary velum. It emerges from dorsal midbrain just inferior to level of inferior colliculus and then enters into quadrigeminal cistern, ambient cistern, which then passes anteriorly between edges of tentorial incisura adjacent to midbrain. It passes between posterior cerebral and superior cerebellar artery lateral and inferior to occulomotor nerve and then passes through lateral wall of cavernous sinus and then to orbit via superior orbital fissure, and above annulus of Zinn (3rd and 6th pass through the annulus) (Fig. 3.1.145).

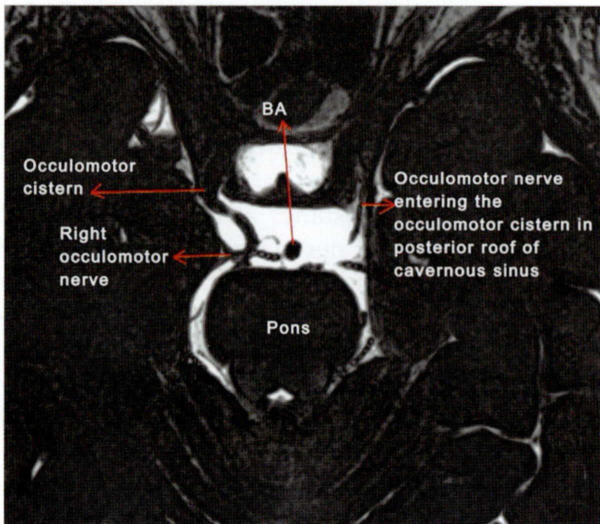

Fig. 3.1.142: Occulomotor cistern

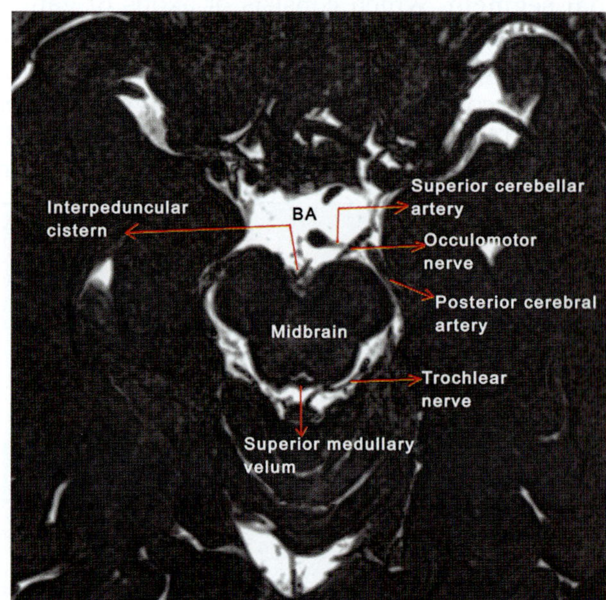

Fig. 3.1.143: 3rd nerve in prepontine cistern between PCA and SCA

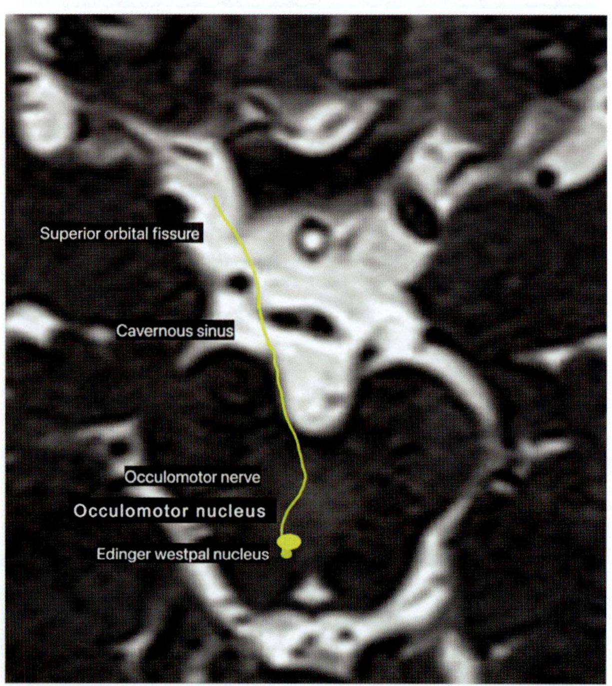

Fig. 3.1.141: Occulomotor nerve pathway

CN 5: The trigeminal nerve is the largest cranial nerve. It is composed of a large sensory root that runs medial to a smaller motor root. Nuclei of trigeminal nerve (3 sensory and 1 motor) are located at various levels of brainstem along its entire length (Fig. 3.1.136). The roots

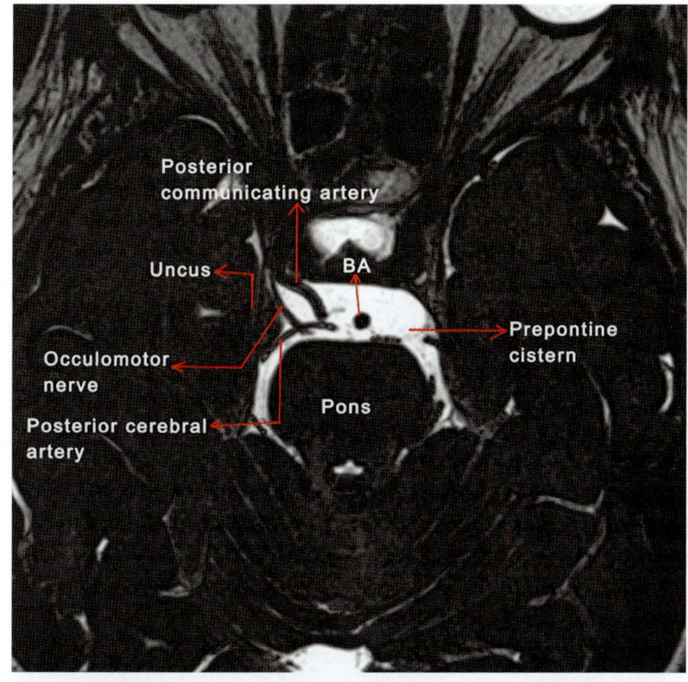

Fig. 3.1.144: 3rd nerve in prepontine cistern

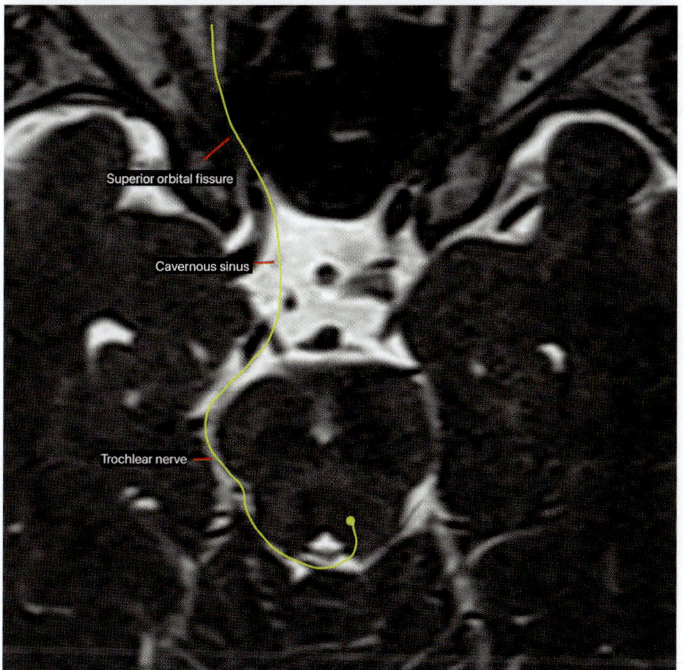

Fig. 3.1.145: Trochlear nerve

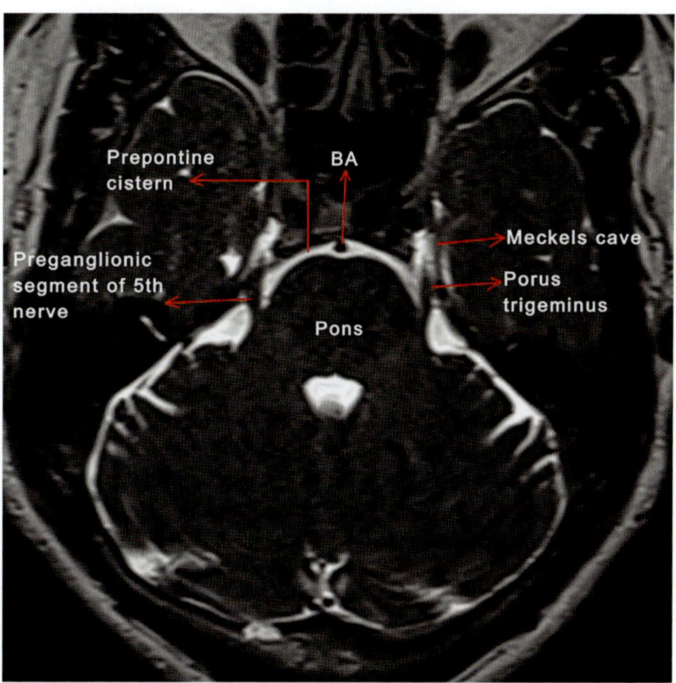

Fig. 3.1.146: Axial MR 5th cranial nerve

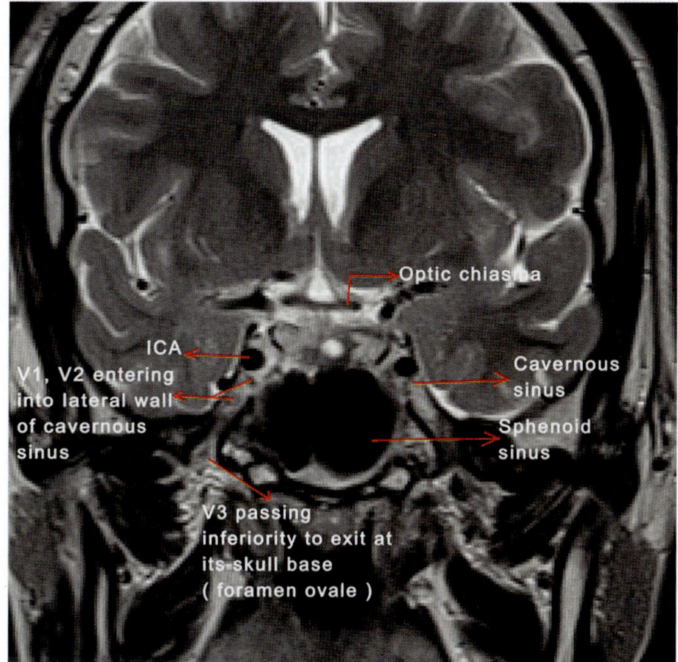

Fig. 3.1.147: Trigeminal nerve divisions

emerge from the lateral midpons and travel anteriorly through the prepontine cistern and the porus trigeminus (opening in dura mater) to the Meckel (trigeminal) cave (Figs 3.1.146 and 3.1.149). The nerve roots are arranged in the same order as V1 (cranial), V2 (medial), V3 (caudal) from superior to inferior. The trigeminal (gasserian ganglion) is located within CSF in Meckel's cave (note—trigeminal ganglion lacks blood–nerve barrier, therefore normally enhances with contrast) (Figs 3.1.147, 3.1.148, 3.1.150). The ophthalmic (V_1) and maxillary (V_2) divisions of the nerve pass within lateral wall of cavernous sinus and exit the skull through the superior orbital fissure and foramen rotundum (to enter pterygopalatine fossa) respectively. The mandibular division (V_3), which includes the motor branches, exits the skull inferiorly through the foramen ovale and reaches the infratemporal fossa.

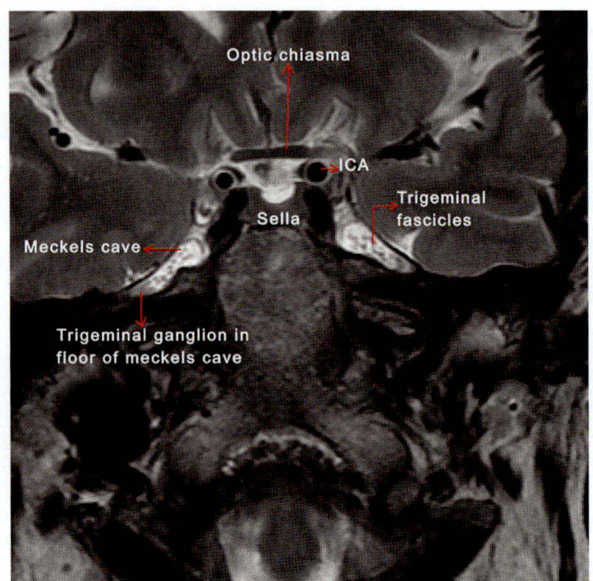

Fig. 3.1.148: Meckel's cave

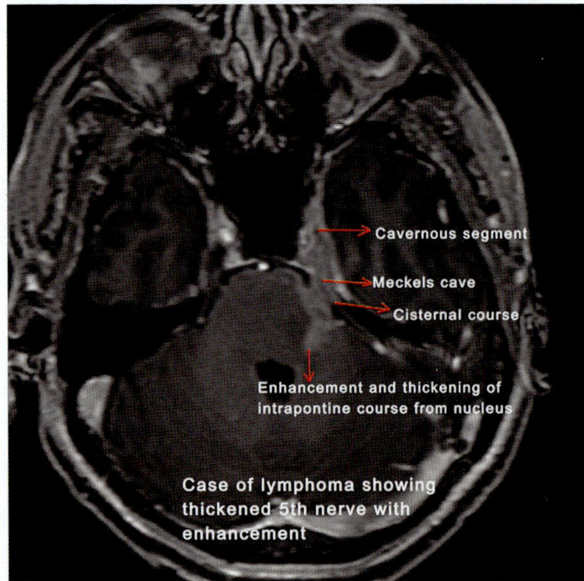

Fig. 3.1.149: Case of lymphoma with thickened 5th nerve

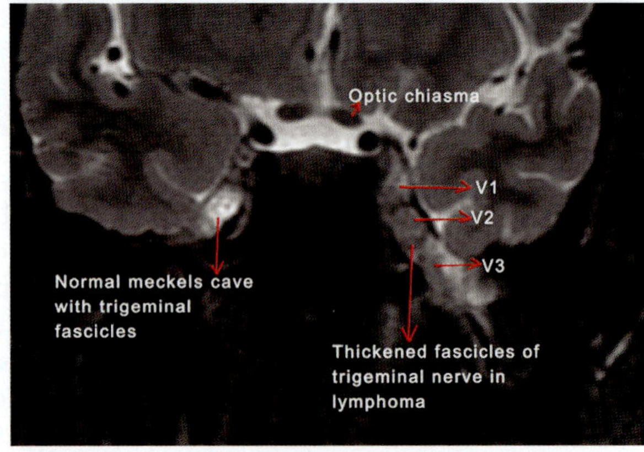

Fig. 3.1.150: 5th nerve in Meckel's cave

CN 6: The abducens nerve emerges from nuclei anterior to the fourth ventricle (at facial colliculus), then courses anteriorly through the pons to exit at the ventral pons at the level of the pontomedullary junction and into the prepontine cistern, then runs vertically along the posterior aspect of the clivus, within a fibrous sheath called the **Dorello canal** (Figs 3.1.151 and 3.1.152). The nerve then continues over the medial petrous apex

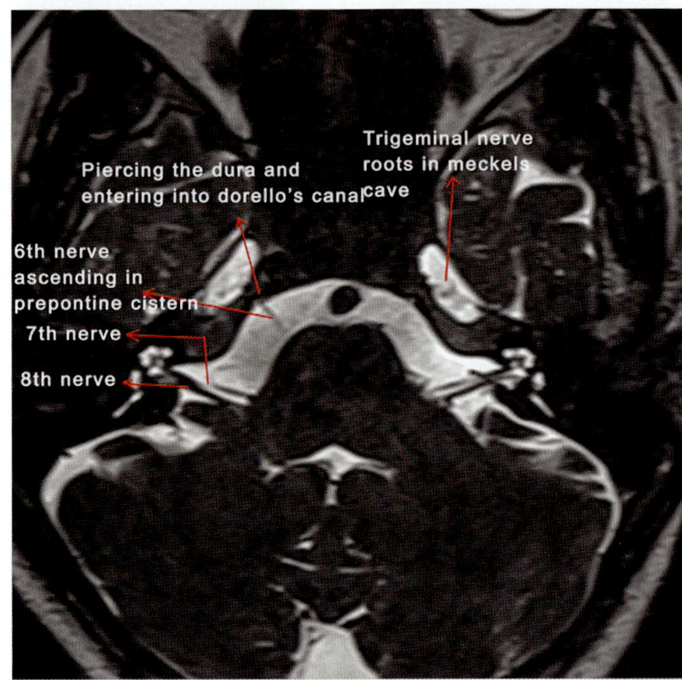

Fig. 3.1.151: Abducent nerve

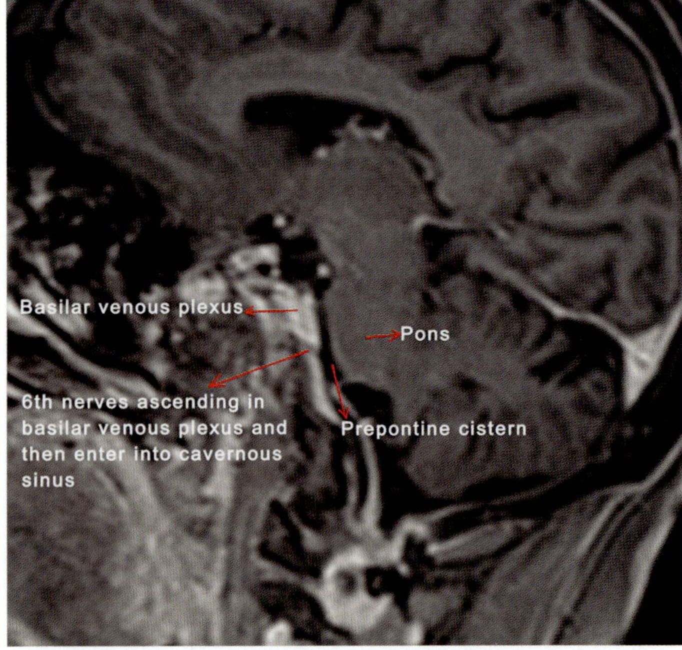

Fig. 3.1.152: 6th nerve in sagittal contrast MR image

and through the medial cavernous sinus, entering the orbit through the superior orbital fissure to innervate the lateral rectus muscle.

CN 7, 8: The facial and vestibulocochlear nerves have similar cisternal and canalicular courses. They both emerge from the lateral aspect of the lower border of the pons and traverse the cerebellopontine angle cistern at an oblique angle. Next, the nerves cross the **porus acusticus** (an opening between the cerebellopontine angle cistern and the internal auditory canal; also known as the **internal acoustic meatus**) and traverse the length of the internal auditory canal. Fundus of IAC has been divided by crista falciformis (horizontal crest) and Bill's bar (vertical crest) into anterosuperior, anteroinferior, posterosuperior and posteroinferior parts. Facial nerve is anterosuperior, cochlear nerve is anteroinferior, superior vestibular nerve is posterosuperior and inferior vestibular nerve is posteroinferior **(Mnemonic: 7UP and COKE DOWN)** (Fig. 3.1.154).

Facial nerve has four segments, namely—**intra-axial, cisternal, intratemporal and extracranial segments**. It is a mixed nerve—containing three nuclei, namely motor nucleus from which motor root arises and winds around the CN 6 nucleus forming **facial colliculus** in the floor of fourth ventricle, **superior salivatory nucleus** from which efferent parasympathetic fibres arise to innervate submandibular, sublingual and lacrimal gland, the third nucleus is **nucleus tractus solitarius** which receives the taste sensation from anterior 2/3rd of tongue. Sensory nerve of facial nerve is called **nervus intermedius** as it travels between the motor component of facial nerve and vestibulocochlear nerve. The facial nerve exits the internal auditory canal and enters the facial canal via the fallopian aqueduct on the anterior aspect of the Bill bar. After a complex course within the petrous bone, the facial nerve exits the skull base through the stylomastoid foramen and enters the substance of the parotid gland. Facial nerve gives off the following branches, namely greater superficial petrosal nerve, nerve to stapedius, chorda tympani nerve and terminal motor branches.

Vestibulocochlear nerve is a **sensory nerve** consisting of cochlear and vestibular parts. Cochlear part arises from bipolar neurons in spiral ganglion which is located within the modiolus of cochlea. The nerve then enters IAC through the cochlear aperture and joins with vestibular nerve near porus acusticus to form vestibulocochlear nerve. Then the nerve traverses in CP angle cistern posterior to facial nerve to terminate in dorsal and ventral cochlear nuclei located on lateral surface of inferior cerebellar peduncle. Vestibular nerve arises from the scarpa ganglion located within the fundus of IAC, and traverse medially to porus acusticus to join cochlear nerve forming vestibulocochlear nerve and terminate in vestibular nuclei complex (4 nuclei—superior, medial, lateral and inferior) which is located

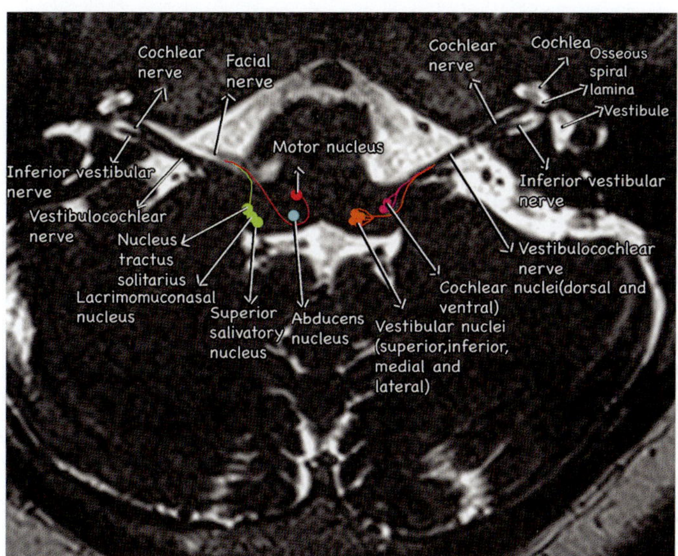

Fig. 3.1.153: 7th, 8th nerve

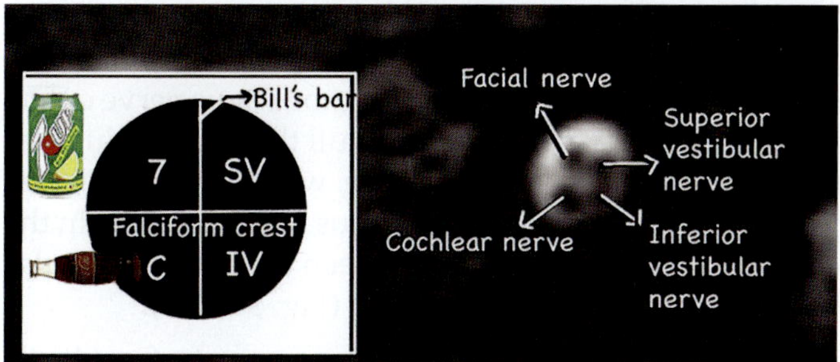

Fig. 3.1.154: Internal auditory canal

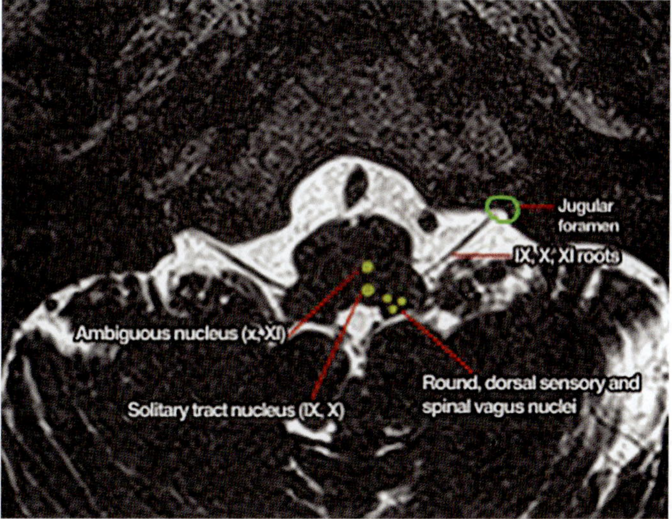

Fig. 3.1.155: 9, 10, 11th cranial nerve

beneath the lateral recess along floor of fourth ventricle in lower pons (rhomboid fossa) (Fig. 3.1.153).

CN 9: The glossopharyngeal nerve nuclei is located in upper and mid-medulla, then emerges from the lateral medulla (postolivary sulcus) into the lateral cerebellomedullary cistern, then the nerve plunges into the jugular fossa and exits the skull through the jugular foramen (pars nervosa along with inferior petrosal sinus) where it is surrounded by its own dural sheath (the glossopharyngeal canal) and then enters into anterior nasopharyngeal carotid space, passes lateral to ICA and stylophargeus muscle and terminates in posterior sublingual space in floor of mouth (Fig. 3.1.155).

CN 10: The vagus nerve nuclei is located in upper and mid-medulla, nerve comprises two roots that emerge from the lateral medulla (in postolivary sulcus between 9th nerve and bulbar portion of 11th nerve), then enter the lateral cerebellomedullary cistern in a position inferior to the glossopharyngeal nerve and run parallel to it through the cistern. After obliquely traversing the lateral cerebellomedullary cistern, the vagus nerve enters the jugular fossa and exits the skull through the jugular foramen (pars vascularis) along with acessory nerve, jugular bulb. In the neck, the vagus nerve lies within the carotid sheath, behind and between the internal jugular vein and common carotid artery (Fig. 3.1.155).

CN 11: The accessory nerve is composed of multiple cranial and spinal rootlets. The cranial rootlets (bulbar portion) exit lateral medulla in postolivary sulcus inferior to 9, 10th nerve and emerge into the lateral cerebellomedullary cistern below the vagus nerve. The spinal rootlets emerge from upper cervical segments of the spinal cord, pass superiorly through the foramen magnum into the cisterna magna (i.e. the posterior cerebellomedullary cistern), in a position posterior to the vertebral artery, and join the cranial rootlets in the lateral cerebellomedullary cistern. The conjoined nerve fibers then leave the skull through the jugular foramen (pars vascularis) (Fig. 3.1.155).

CN 12: The hypoglossal nerve arises from nuclei in front of the fourth ventricle within the mid-medulla, and exits the brainstem at the preolivary nucleus (between olive and pyramid), emerges into the lateral cerebellomedullary cistern and crosses it, where the nerve is surrounded anteriorly by the vertebral artery and posteriorly by the posterior inferior cerebellar artery. The hypoglossal nerve then exits the skull via the hypoglossal canal (within the occipital condyle), then runs medial to the glossopharyngeal, vagus, and accessory nerves and deep to the digastric muscle, looping over the hyoid bone to innervate a large part of

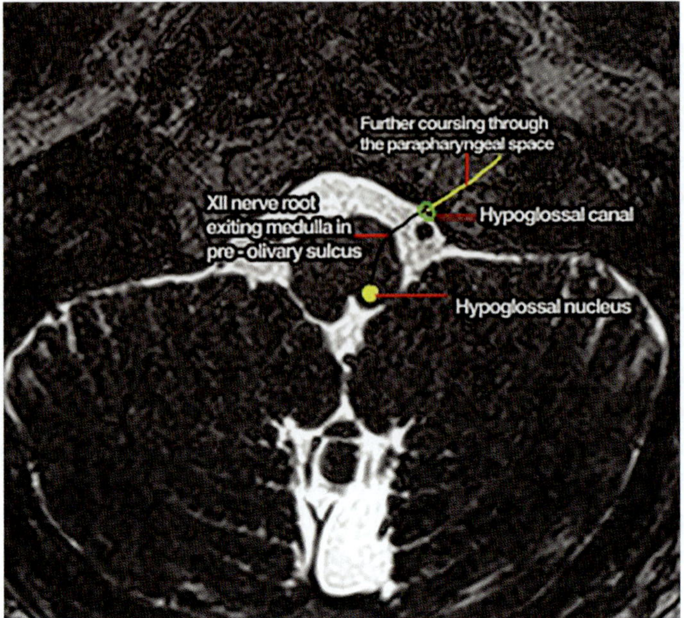

Fig. 3.1.156: Hypoglossal nerve

the tongue. (All tongue muscles except palatoglossus, which is innervated by vagus) (Fig. 3.1.156).

Transition zone: Junction between central myelin (by oligodendrocytes) and peripheral myelin (by Schwann cells). These are the most vulnerable site for nerve injury by neurovascular conflict. For trigeminal—4 mm from root entry (medial—1.1 mm, lateral side—2.5 mm, motor nerve root—4.2 mm), facial nerve—2 mm from root entry, 8th nerve—10 mm from root entry and 9th nerve 1.5 mm from root entry. Root entry/exit zone includes transition zone and adjacent brainstem surface. Sometimes used interchangeably with transition zone.

3.1.R Cerebellum

The cerebellum consists of two cerebellar hemispheres that are united to each other through a median vermis. The cortical mantle overlies the white matter core as in the cerebral hemispheres but the cerebellar cortical ridges, known as the folia, and the intervening sulci are approximately parallel to one another. The flocculus lies posterior to the porus acousticus and separates from the rest of the cerebellum and extends laterally just inferior to the vestibulocochlear (VIIIth) cranial nerve. The nodule is the most ventral structure on the inferior vermian surface and is identified on axial scans indenting the fourth ventricle. On the inferior surface of the cerebellar hemispheres are the tonsils. Posterior and lateral to the tonsils are the biventral lobules. There are three cerebellar peduncles arising from the whitematter core of the cerebellum on each side. The inferior cerebellar peduncle joins the medulla, the middle cerebellar peduncle (the

Table 3.1.7: Cerebellum lobes and fissures

Lobes	*Fissures*
Anterior lobe	Primary fissure between anterior and middle lobes.
Middle lobe	Posterolateral fissure between middle and flocculonodular lobes.
Flocculonodular lobe	

largest), the pons and the superior, the midbrain. Their relationship is best seen on coronal MRI.

The cerebellar nuclei comprise 4 paired deep grey matter nuclei deep within the cerebellum near the fourth ventricle. They are arranged in the following order, from lateral to medial: Mnemonic—(DONT EAT GOOSE FAT)—**D**entate nuclei (the largest and most lateral), **E**mboliform nuclei, **G**lobose nuclei, **F**astigial nuclei (most medial) (Figs 3.1.157 to 3.1.159).

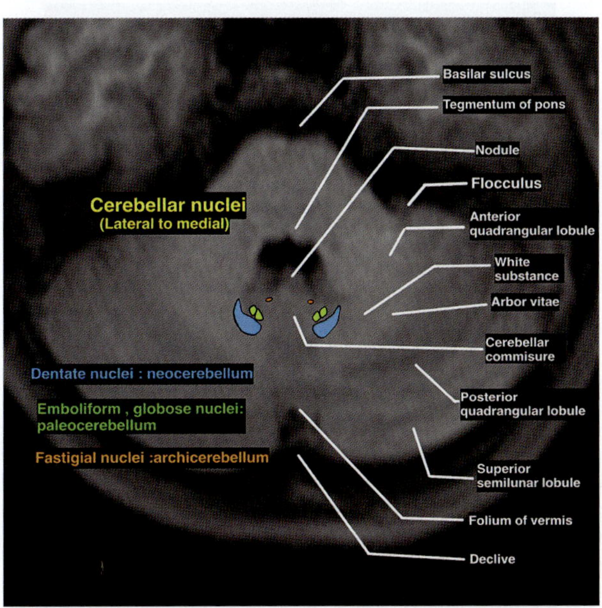

Fig. 3.1.157: Nuclei in cerebellum

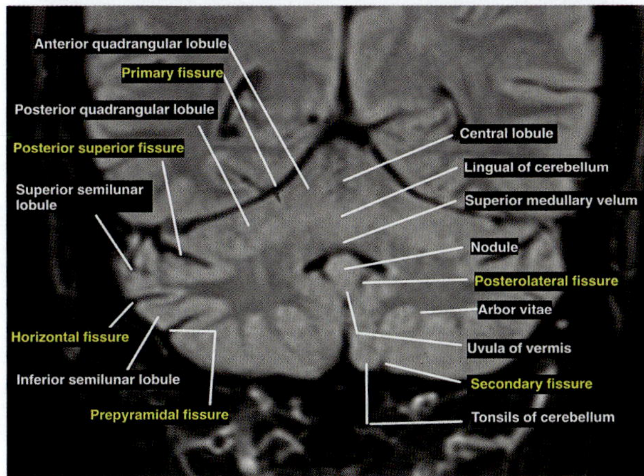

Fig. 3.1.158: Cerebellum

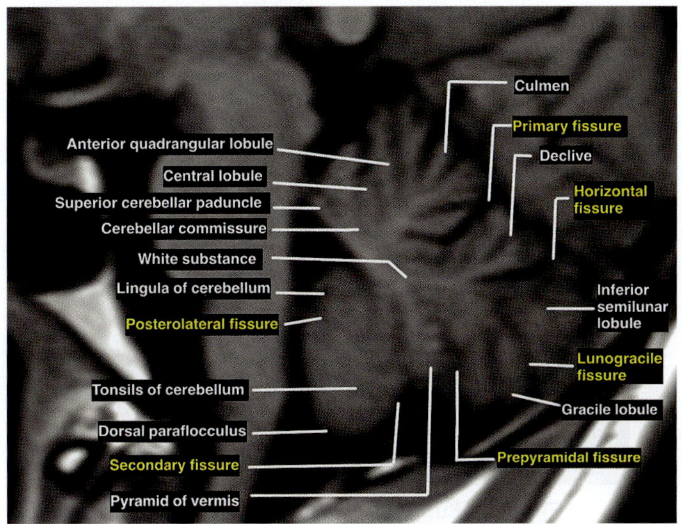

Fig. 3.1.159: Cerebellum

3.1.S Neonatal Cranial Ultrasound

Neurosonography is the noninvasive, widely used technique for intracranial assessment of neonate.

Common indications: Detection of an intracranial hemorrhage, HIE, follow-up of intraventricular hemorrhage and antenatally detected abnormality, screening for congenital structural anomalies, large head, seizures, clinical suspicion of TORCH, intracranial vascular lesions, meningitis and its sequelae.

Technique: High frequency phased array transducer (5–8 MHz), best when small foot prints with wide angle of insonation is used. Acoustic window for cranial ultrasound: Traditional approach—through anterior fontanelle, others—posterior fontanelle imaging and mastoid imaging, temporal window, foramen magnum approach. Anterior fontanelle—it is located at the junction of coronal and sagittal sutures and fuses by about 18 months of age. 3 planes—coronal, sagittal, parasagittal. Coronal view—generally 6 to 8 coronal images are obtained by placing the transducer transversely across the anterior fontanelle and sweeping the plane in anterior to posterior direction, beginning at the anterior frontal lobes and extending to the occipital lobes posterior to the trigone of lateral ventricle (Fig. 3.1.160). Planes may be obtained at the level of frontal lobes (Fig. 3.1.161) (able to visualise the frontal lobes with orbits deep to the floor of skull base), frontal horns (Fig. 3.1.162), foramen of Monro (Fig. 3.1.163), mid-ventricle (Fig. 3.1.164), trigone (Fig. 3.1.165), most posterior (Fig. 3.1.166). The transducer is then rotated 90° (placing the transducer longitudinally across the anterior fontanelle and angling it to each side) and five sagittal images are obtained, including mid-sagittal view

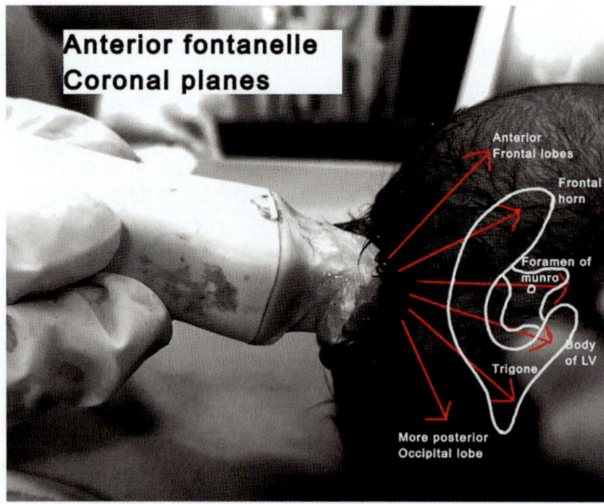

Fig. 3.1.160: Anterior fontanelle approach

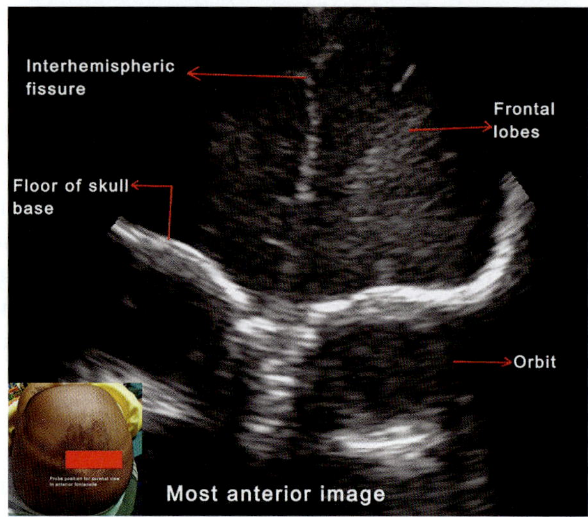

Fig. 3.1.161: Coronal image—anterior most section

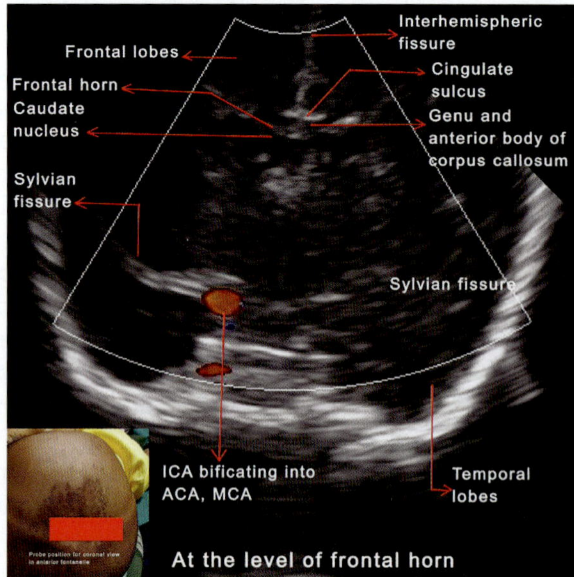

Fig. 3.1.162: Coronal image at the level of frontal horn

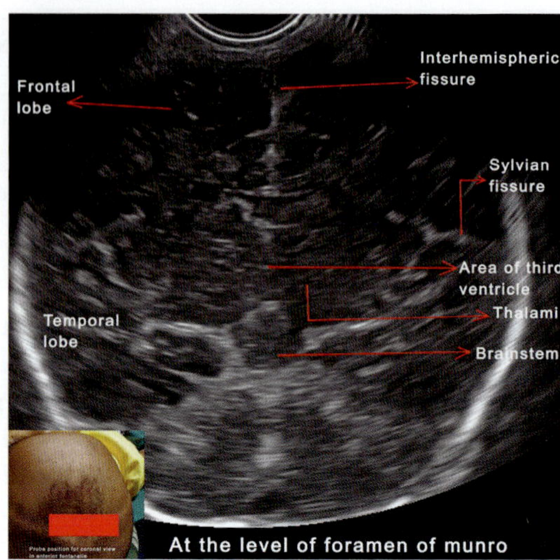

Fig. 3.1.163: Coronal image at the level of foramen of Monro

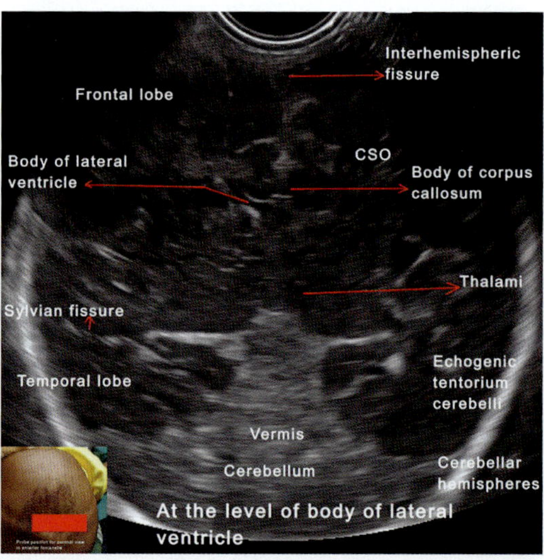

Fig. 3.1.164: Coronal image at the level of body of lateral ventricle

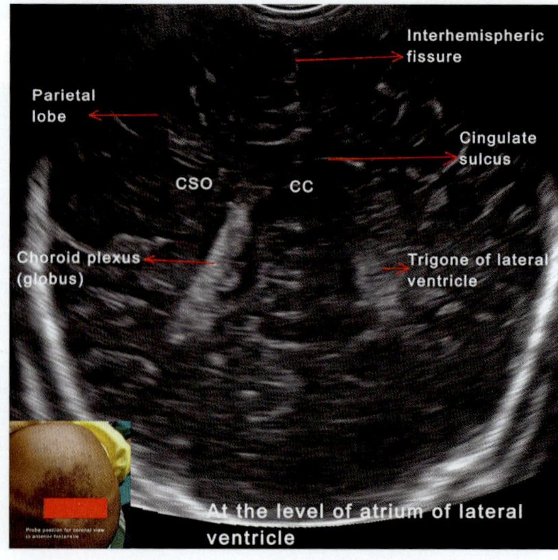

Fig. 3.1.165: Coronal image at the level of atrium of lateral ventricle

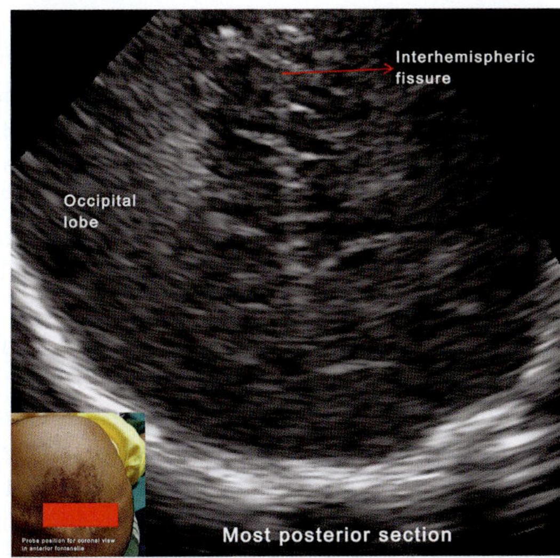

Fig. 3.1.166: Coronal image most posterior section

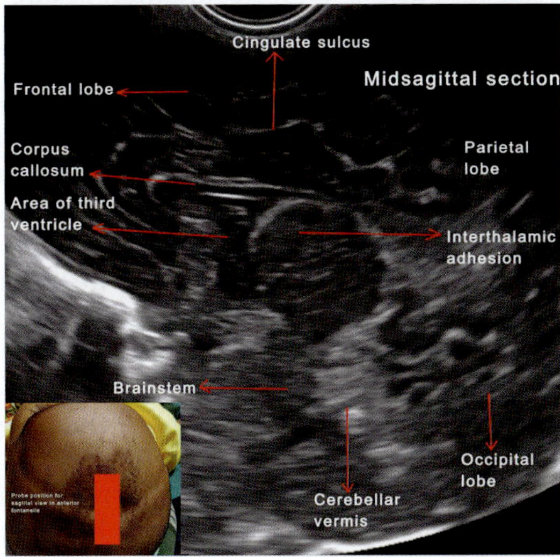

Fig. 3.1.167: Sagittal image

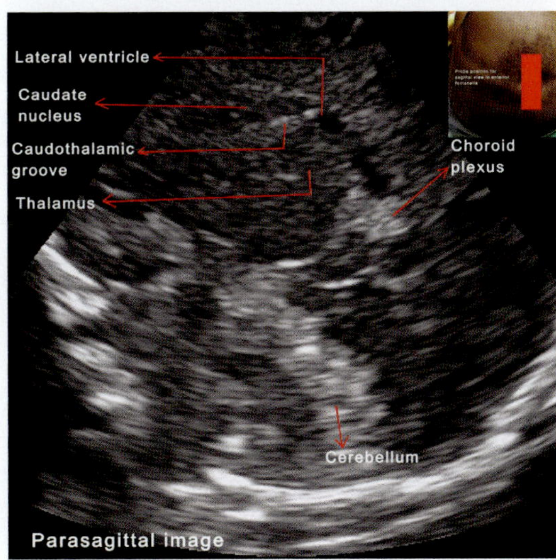

Fig. 3.1.168: Parasagittal image

(Fig. 3.1.167) and two parasagittal views of right and left cerebral hemispheres (Figs 3.1.168 and 3.1.169).

Images through the posterior and mastoid fontanelle is facilitated by placing the infant in lateral decubitus position. **Posterior fontanelle** is located at the junction of the lambdoid and sagittal sutures and it closes by about 3 months of age. Planes obtained are sagittal (Fig. 3.1.170) and axial views (Fig. 3.1.171). It is the best

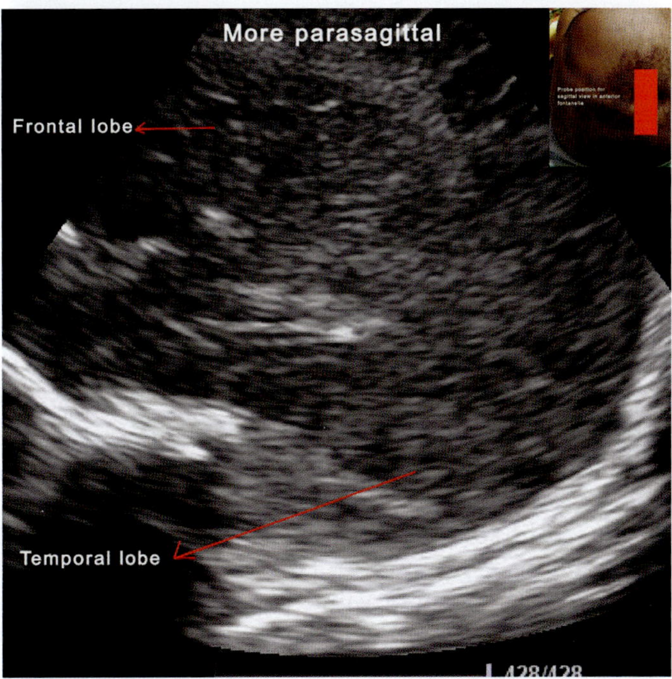

Fig. 3.1.169: Lateral parasagittal image

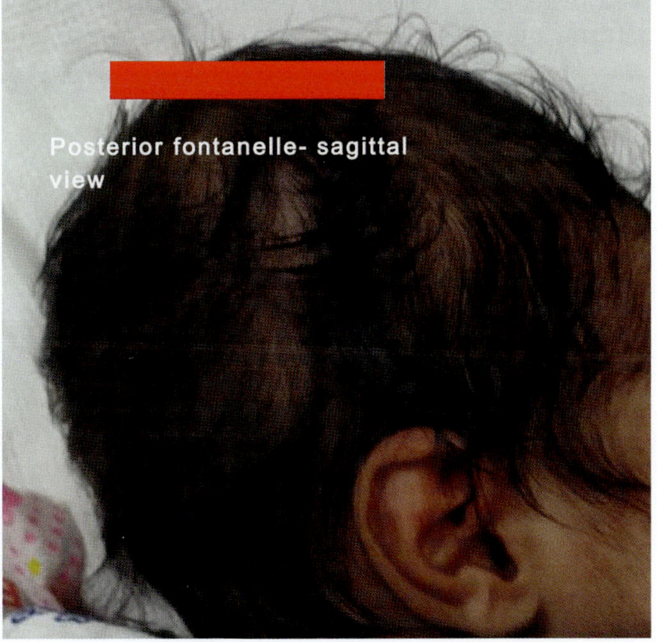

Fig. 3.1.170: Posterior fontanelle—sagittal view

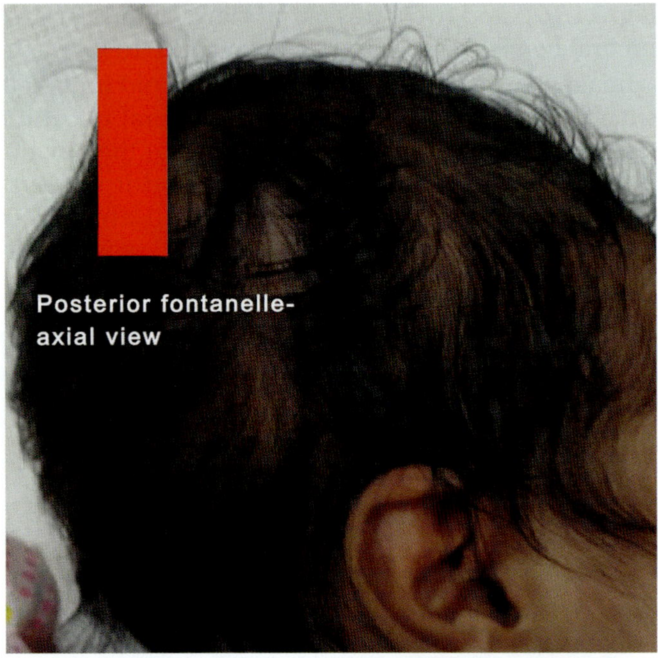

Fig. 3.1.171: Posterior fontanelle—axial view

approach to evaluate occipital horns for ventricular clot. Remember—occipital horn does not contain choroid plexus and is completely anechoic normally. The **mastoid fontanelle** (posterolateral) is located at the junction of squamosal, lambdoidal and occipital sutures. This may not fuse until 2 years of age. The probe is placed about 1 cm behind the helix of ear and 1 cm above the tragus (Fig. 3.1.172). Mastoid imaging depicts clearly brainstem (Thalami, midbrain, third ventricle, aqueduct and perimesencephalic cistern) and posterior fossa (cerebellar hemisphere, vermis, fourth ventricle, cisterna magna and tentorium). These approaches help to detect small intraventricular hemorrhages, subarachnoid hemorrhage, brainstem hemorrhage, structural abnormalities of brainstem and cerebellum. Foramen magnum approach is used in evaluation of upper spinal canal. Temporal bone approach is obtained by placing the transducer about 1 cm anterior and superior to tragus of ear. This approach also clearly depicts brain stem structures mentioned above (Fig. 3.1.173).

Color Doppler images for arterial and venous structures may be obtained for screening of vascular structures, especially imaging of **circle of Willis** (coronal scans by anterior fontanelle, axial scans through temporal bone approach) and **vein of Galen** (midline sagittal view by anterior fontanelle approach) is essential. It helps to diagnose vascular lesions (differential diagnosis for cystic lesions) and also to separate normal structure from clot. It is also used in case of dural venous sinus thrombosis and also used for evaluation of aqueductal patency in case of hydrocephalus.

On USG gray matter is hypoechoic, white matter is hyperechoic, CSF anechoic and choroid plexus as well as small hemorrhages, areas of infarction appear hyperechoic. Comparing structures on both sides and looking for symmetry helps to diagnose certain pathologies. Visible normal layers in cerebral cortex are, superficial pia mater which appears as thin well-defined hyperechoeic layer, which overlies the hypoechoic cortical gray matter, which inturn overlies the hyperechoic white mater. Failure to visualize these normal layers is indicative of any focal pathology like hemorrhage or infarct. Importantly, periventricular white matter normally appears homogenous in echogenicity, which is equally or less echogenic than adjacent choroid

Mastoid view

Fig. 3.1.172: Mastoid view

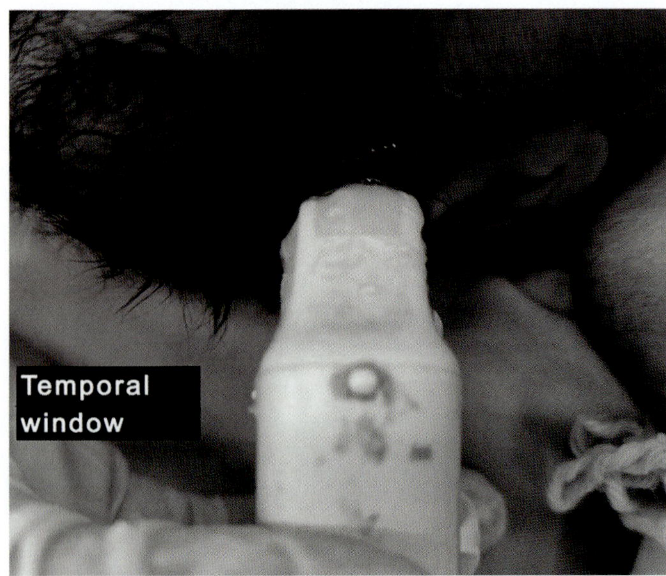

Fig. 3.1.173: Axial view through temporal window

plexus. Asymmetry or heterogeneity of periventricular white matter indicates periventricular leukomalacia.

Image assessment should include anatomy (mainly presence of corpus callosum, cerebellar vermis), maturation (degree of cortical folding along the cortical surfaces and interhemsipheric fissure, echogenicity of basal ganglia and thalami), distinction of cortex and white matter, echogenicity of cortex and white matter and deep grey matter, caudothalamic groove, assessment of ventricular system—size, width, lining, echogenicity, subarachnoid spaces, any midline shift, color Doppler image for circle of Willis, superior sagittal sinus, vein of Galen.

Normal variants: **Cavum septum pellucidum, cavum vergae, cavum velum interpositum,** minor asymmetry of frontal horns or body of ventricles, variations in size of massa intermedia, **choroid plexus cyst, connatal cyst (frontal horn cyst), peritrigonal blush** (normal hyperechogenicity just posterior and superior to ventricular trigone on parasagittal view), **prominent calcar avis** (calcar avis is the paramedial protrusion of the calcarine gyrus into the medial aspect of lateral ventricle at the junction of the trigone with the occipital horn. It is differentiated from the clot by the characteristic location, contiguity with the calcarine gyrus and presence of sulcus, color Doppler showing normal perfusion in contradiction to absence of flow in a clot) and **lobulated glomus of choroid, foramen of Magendie** (normal posteromedian midline outlet of fourth ventricle) especially in posterior approach.

3.2 FACE, SKULL BASE AND NECK

The face is the anterior aspect of the head and contains a unique group of muscles that helps in mastication and facial expressions. **The neck** extends from the mandible above to the shoulders, thorax below. Its superior boundary is formed by the inferior margins of the mandible and bone on the posterior aspect of the skull and inferior boundary is formed by the superior border of sternum, clavicle, adjacent acromion and bony projection of the scapula. A line drawn between the acromion and the spinous process of vertebra C7 can be used to approximate the neck's inferior limit, posteriorly.

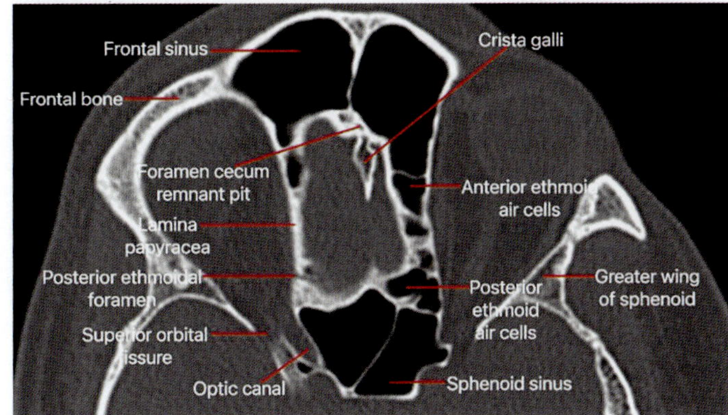

Fig. 3.2.1: CT axial section in bone window shows anterior cranial fossa structures

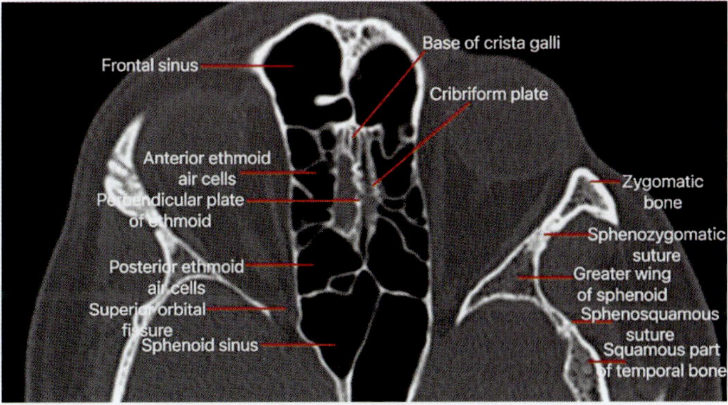

Fig. 3.2.2: CT axial section in bone window shows anterior cranial fossa structures

3.2.A Skull Base

Skull base is a bony surface that delimits the inferior boundary of cranial vault. Paired frontal, temporal bones and unpaired ethmoid, sphenoid and occipital bones form the skull base. Skull base is divided into anterior, middle and posterior cranial bases (Fig. 3.2.7) as described below.

Anterior skull base (ASB): The anterior border is formed by the posterior wall of the frontal sinus and posterior border is formed by the lesser wing of the sphenoid bone and anterior clinoid processes. Roof of the nasal cavity and ethmoid sinuses medially forms the floor. It has multiple foramina, namely cribriform foramina, anterior and posterior ethmoidal foramina, foramen cecum (Figs 3.2.1–3.2.6).

Middle skull base (MSB): Anterior border is formed by the tuberculum sellae, anterior clinoid processes, posterior margin of the lesser sphenoid wings, and the anterior and superior rim of the greater sphenoid wings. Posterior border is formed by superior borders of the petrous part of the temporal bone and the dorsum sellae of the sphenoid. The central part of middle cranial fossa is formed by the body of sphenoid.

Posterior skull base (PSB): The anterior margin is formed by the posterior surface of the clivus.

3

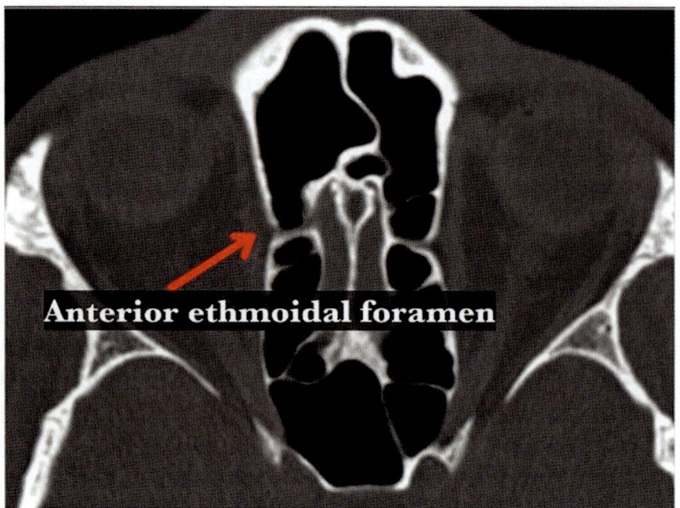

Fig. 3.2.3: CT axial image in bone window shows anterior ethmoidal foramen

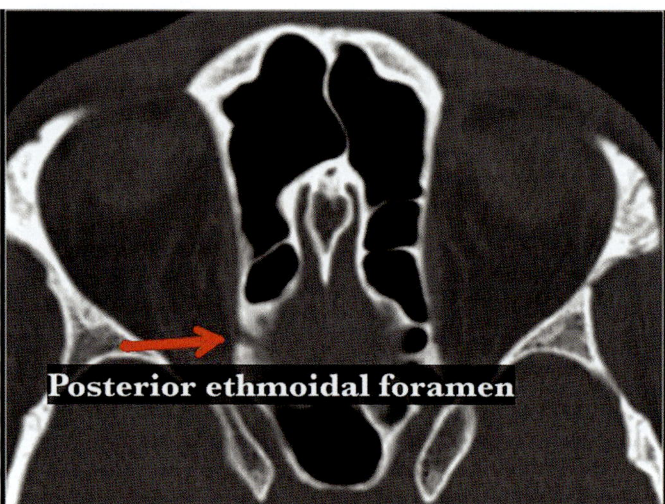

Fig. 3.2.4: CT axial image in bone window shows posterior ethmoidal foramen

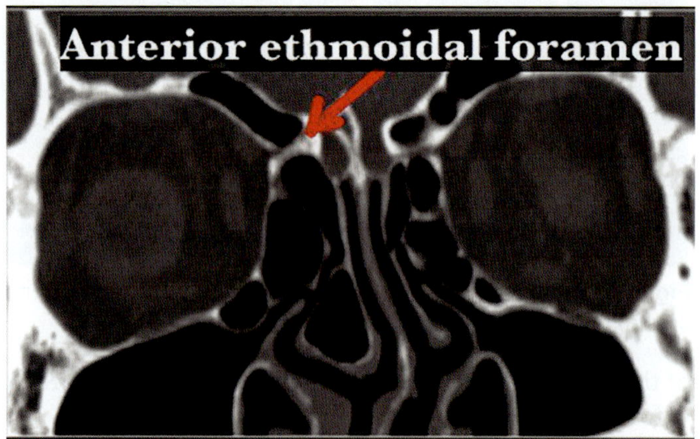

Fig. 3.2.5: CT coronal image in bone window shows anterior ethmoidal foramen

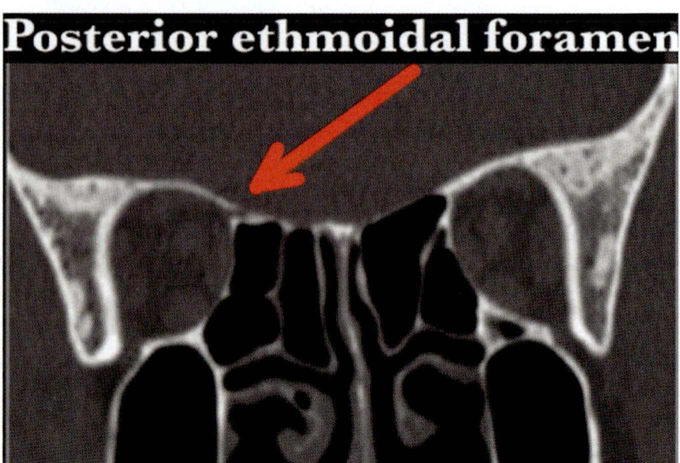

Fig. 3.2.6: CT coronal image in bone window shows posterior ethmoidal foramen

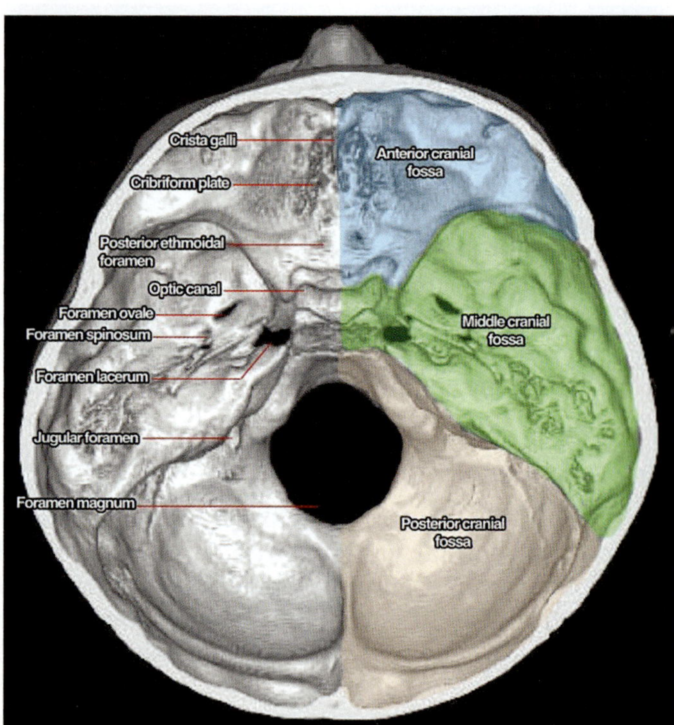

Fig. 3.2.7: Base of skull

The lateral portion of posterior skull base is formed by the posterior surface of the petrous temporal bone superiorly and the condylar part of the occipital bone inferiorly. The mastoid temporal bone and the squamous occipital bone form the posterior portion. It has opening likes jugular foramen, hypoglossal canal, condylar candal and foramen magnum.

The sphenoid bone, which forms the central skull base, resembles a bird with its wings extended when viewed from the front. It has a central body and paired lateral greater and lesser wings. The paired pterygoid projections emerge inferiorly at the ventral junction of the body and wings, mimicking the outstretched limbs of a bird. Body, greater wing, lesser wing, pterygoid processes, and plates are the parts of the sphenoid bone. The sphenoid sinuses and the pituitary fossa (sella turcica), a deep saddle-shaped depression containing the pituitary gland, are located in the sphenoid body (hypophysis). The planum sphenoidale is the smooth superior surface of the sphenoid that continues anteriorly as the anterior boundary of the pituitary fossa (tuberculum sellae). This connects to the cribriform plate of the ethmoid bone, which transmits tiny olfactory nerve fibres, to form the anterior roof of the sphenoid sinuses. The basisphenoid articulates with the basiocciput to generate the clivus (Latin for "slope"). The posterior boundary of the pituitary fossa (dorsum sellae) extends inferiorly as the basisphenoid, which articulates with the basiocciput to form the clivus. The petroclival fissures define the lateral margins of the clivus, which continues posteroinferiorly to the foramen magnum. The bony roof of the nasopharynx is formed by the inferior clivus. The paired sphenoid sinuses are located anterior to the sella turcica. At the sphenoidal crest, the thin anterior wall of the sinuses and the face of the sphenoid body connect with the nasal septum. The sphenoid sinus ostia are located on either side of the crest, allowing secretions to drain into the sphenoethmoidal recesses and ultimately into the superior nasal cavity. The medial cavernous sinus walls are formed by the lateral borders of the sphenoid bone/sinuses, which are typically depressed by the carotid arteries. The anterior clivus, which can be of varying thickness, depending on the level of sinus pneumatisation, forms the posterior walls of the sinuses. This series of CT images highlights the anatomy of the sphenoid bone and its various parts (Figs 3.2.8 to 3.2.14).

The lesser wings or orbitosphenoids are paired thin triangular plates that extend laterally from the planum sphenoidale. Medially they arise from the anterior and superior sphenoid body at two roots. These roots define the optic canal, which transmits the optic nerve and ophthalmic artery. **It is the only canal passing through the lesser wing** and is separated from the superior orbital fissure inferolaterally by the optic strut (lower root). Figures 3.2.9 to 3.2.14 highlights parts of spenoid bone and sella. The superior orbital fissure is a comma-shaped gap between the lesser and greater wings of the sphenoid bone appearing thin superolaterally and bulbous inferiorly. It transmits cranial nerves (CNs) III, IV and VI (oculomotor, trochlear, and abducens), branches of the ophthalmic division of the trigeminal nerve (CN V1), and several vessels including the ophthalmic veins (Fig. 3.2.15). In addition, the annulus of Zinn, common tendinous origin of the four rectus muscles, straddles the

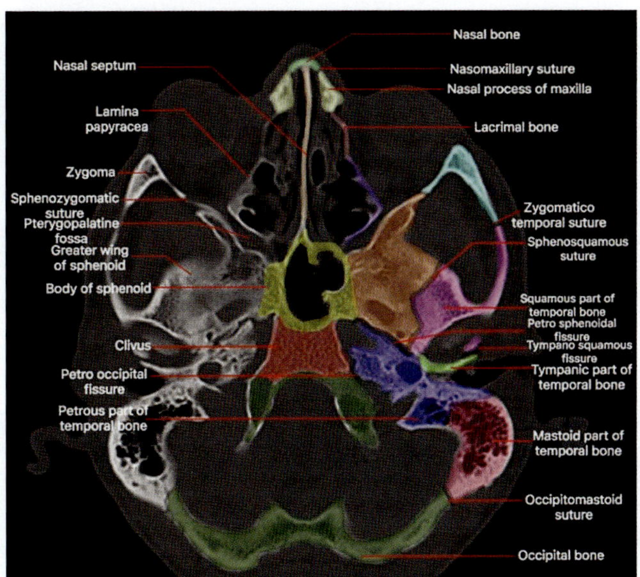

Fig. 3.2.8: Parts of sphenoid bone

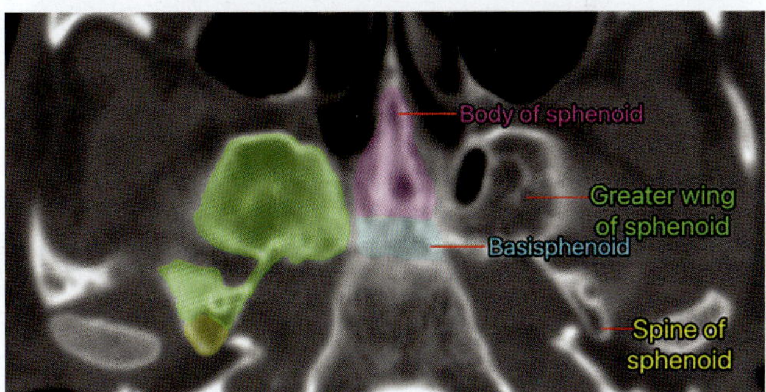

Fig. 3.2.9: CT axial section: Parts of sphenoid bone

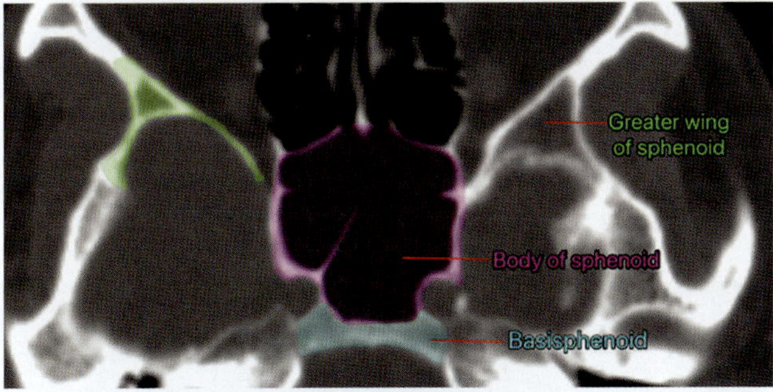

Fig. 3.2.10: Body of sphenoid bone

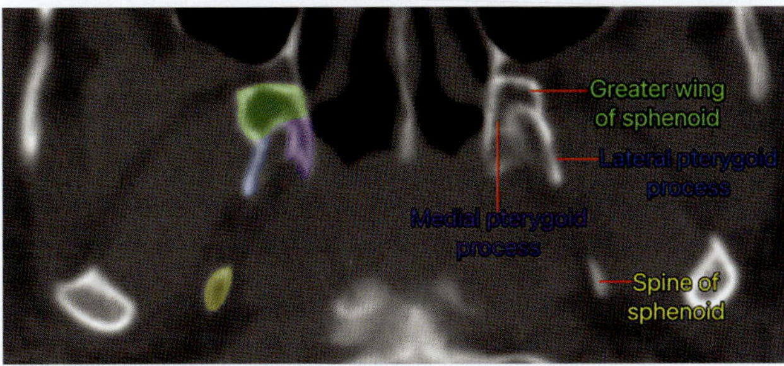

Fig. 3.2.11: Pterygoid bones

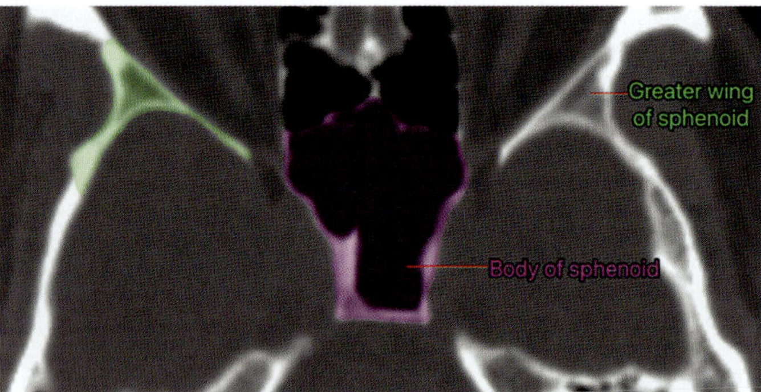

Fig. 3.2.12: Sphenoid sinus

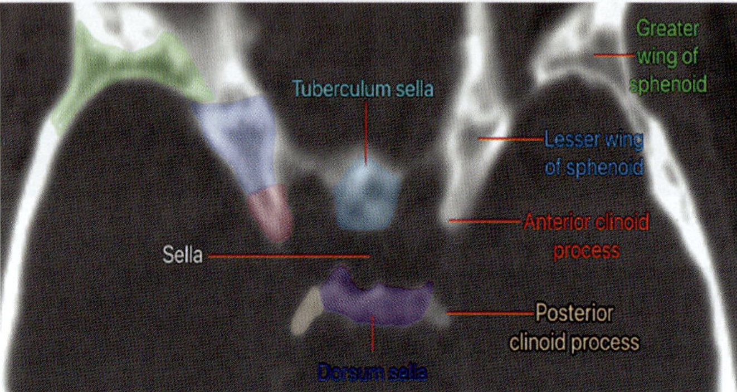

Fig. 3.2.13: CT axial section: Anterior cranial fossa

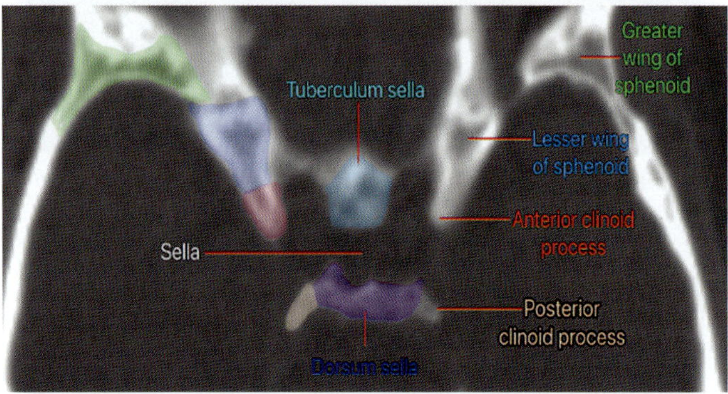

Fig. 3.2.14: CT axial section: Pituitary fossa

superior orbital fissure centrally and encircles the optic canal (Figs 3.2.15 and 3.2.16). The inferior surface of the lesser wing forms the upper boundary of the superior orbital fissure and the posterior orbital roof. The flat superior surface serves as a platform for the basifrontal lobe and posteromedial extensions form the anterior clinoid processes, which are the attachment sites of the tentorium cerebelli. The superior and laterally curved larger sphenoid wings emerge from the sphenoid's body medially. The orbit and middle cranial fossa are formed in part by the larger wings. The lower margin of the superior orbital fissure and the posterolateral margin of the inferior orbital fissure, which transmits the zygomatic branch of the maxillary nerve, are formed by the medial margin of the greater wing at the orbit (CN V2). The orbital part of the greater wing also serves as the orbit's posterolateral wall. A number of foramina pass through the cerebral or superior surface of the larger wing, which makes up the majority of the concave middle cranial fossa.

The foramen rotundum is a circular aperture seen at the base of the greater wing anteromedially, just inferior to the superior orbital fissure. It transmits the maxillary nerve (CN V2) from the middle cranial fossa to the pterygopalatine fossa. The **foramen ovale** arises posterolateral to the rotundum and transmits the mandibular nerve (CN V3) from the middle cranial fossa to the masticator space. The size of the foramina ovale can differ from side to side. Asymmetry of up to 4 mm can be within normal limits. The **foramen spinosum** is located further posterolateral to the foramen ovale and transmits the middle meningeal artery and a recurrent branch of the mandibular nerve (CN V3). Posterior and medial to the foramen spinosum, each greater wing projects as a triangular process articulating with the squamous and petrous portions of the temporal bone. At the apex of

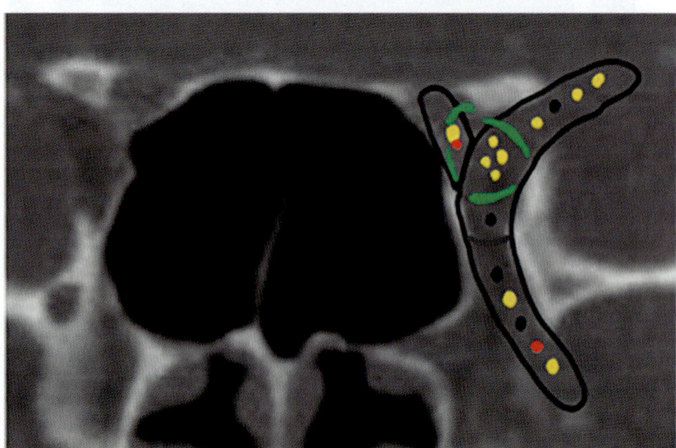
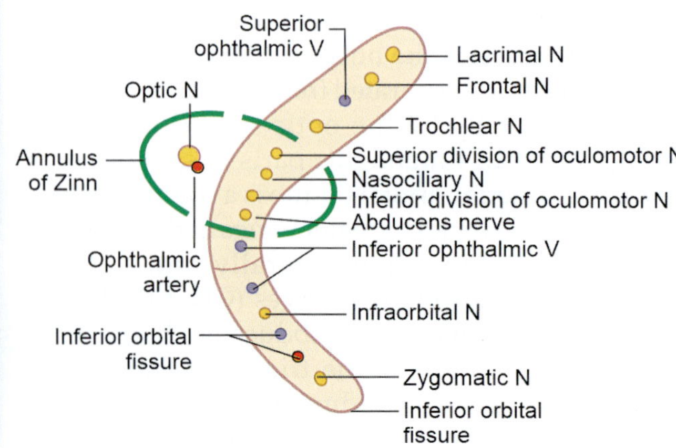

Fig. 3.2.15: Superior orbital fissure and annulus of Zinn

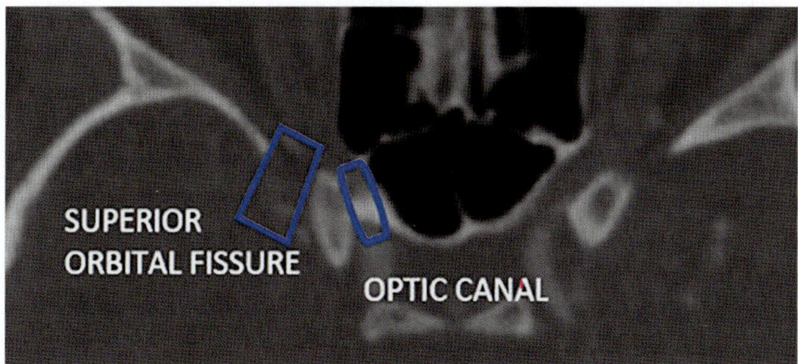

Fig. 3.2.16: CT axial section in bone window highlights superior orbital fissure and optic canal

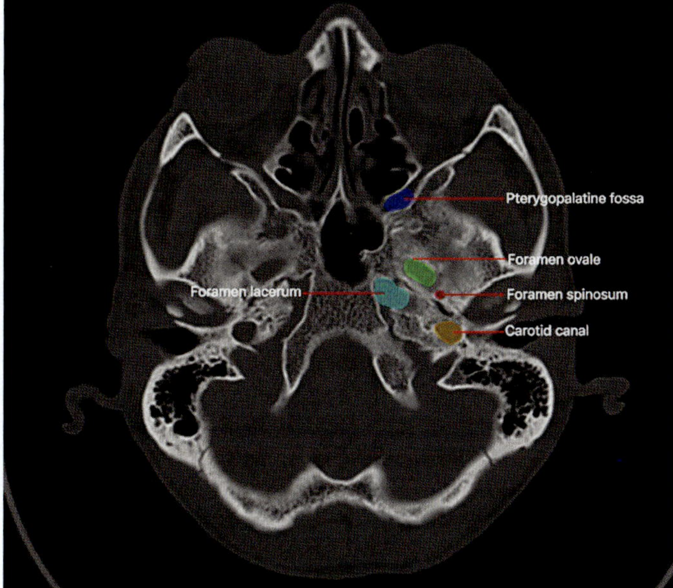

Fig. 3.2.17: CT axial section in bone window shows foramens of middle cranial fossa

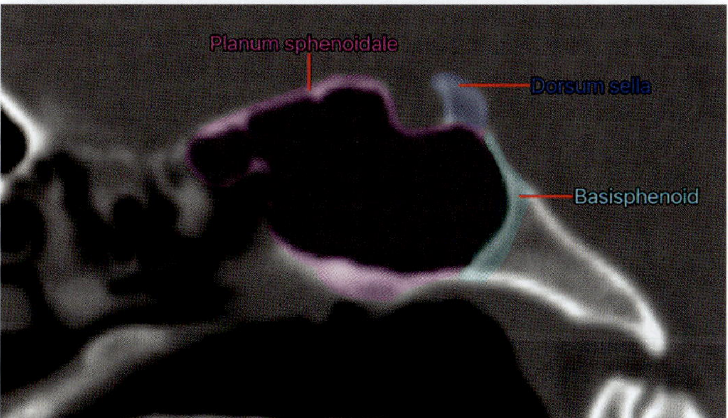

Fig. 3.2.18: Body of sphenoid

this triangle is the inferiorly projected sphenoid spine (spina angularis). This serves as an attachment site of the tensor veli palatini muscle and the sphenomandibular ligament. The anterior margin of the foramen lacerum is formed by the greater wing's posterior margin. This is yet additional route for disease transmission via the nasopharynx. The masticator muscles, including the temporalis (superiorly) and lateral pterygoid (inferiorly), attach to the lateral temporal surface of the greater wing.

The pterygoid processes, which resemble fins, extend inferiorly from the sphenoid's greater wing and body junction. Two plates, lateral and medial, join superiorly and anteriorly to produce each pterygoid process. The posterior wall of the pterygopalatine fossa, which divides the pterygoid processes from the maxillary sinus anteriorly, acts as the fusion site. The **pterygopalatine fossa** is an important neurovascular crossroad of the head and neck, communicating with numerous foramina, including the inferior orbital fissure, foramen rotundum, and the vidian canal. The vidian (pterygoid) canal connects the foramen lacerum posteriorly with the pterygopalatine fossa anteriorly through the medial plate of the pterygoid. The canal is located inferomedial to the foramen rotundum, and the distance between them is determined by the degree of sphenoid sinus pneumatization. The canal houses the vidian artery, vein, and nerve (which is made up of the greater superficial and deep petrosal nerves). The lateral and medial processes diverge posteriorly, and the V-shaped pterygoid fossa is between them.The tensor veli palatini and medial pterygoid muscles are located here. The medial and lateral pterygoid muscles of mastication both originate from the lateral pterygoid process. The tensor veil palatini arises superiorly at the scaphoid fossa, an oval depression at the base of the medial pterygoid plate. The muscle also has an additional attachment place at the scaphoid spine, as previously described. The series of coronal CT images of the skull base highlight the anatomy of the sphenoid bone (Figs 3.2.19 and 3.2.20).

The **pterygopalatine fossa (PPF)**, is a small but complex space in the deep face that is formed by the maxillary bone anteriorly, the pterygoid process posteriorly, and the orbital apex superiorly. Because it can be affected by a variety of infective, inflammatory, and neoplastic disorders, the pterygopalatine fossa (PPF) is an inconspicuous but significant region in the deep face that needs to be studied very carefully in the area of head and neck imaging. The PPF's various contacts with the deep neck spaces provide convenient channels for disease loco-regional dissemination. To improve diagnostic accuracy and patient care, familiarity with its complicated anatomy and a detailed comprehension of the imaging aspects of its prevalent diseases is required. High-resolution computed tomography (HRCT) is the modality of choice for evaluating the various bony communications of the PPF. Typically, very thin axial sections are obtained on a multidetector CT scanner, parallel to the lower borders of the upper teeth, starting

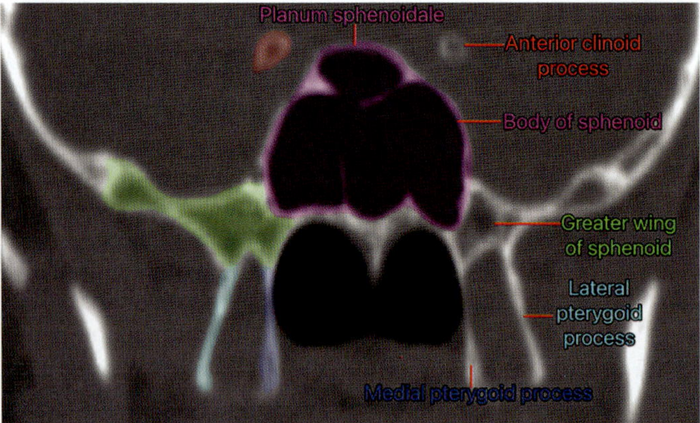

Fig. 3.2.19: CT coronal section: Parts of sphenoid bone

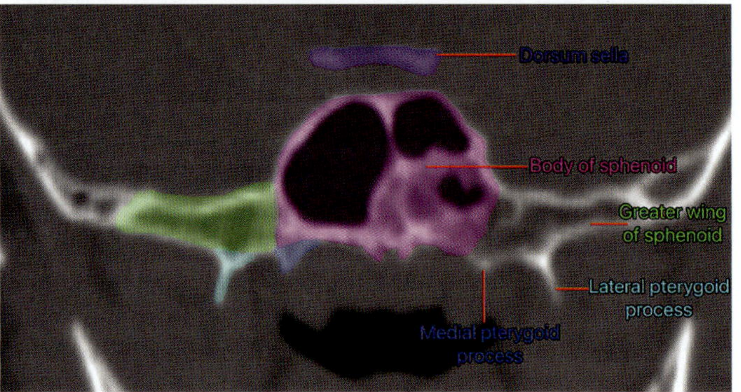

Fig. 3.2.20: CT coronal section: Parts of sphenoid bone

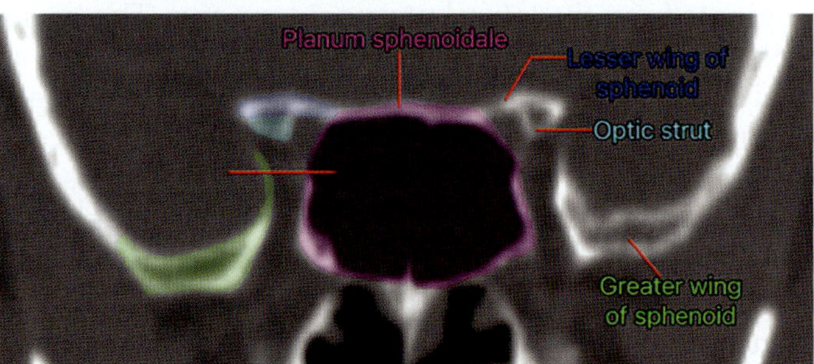

Fig. 3.2.21: CT coronal section: Parts of sphenoid bone

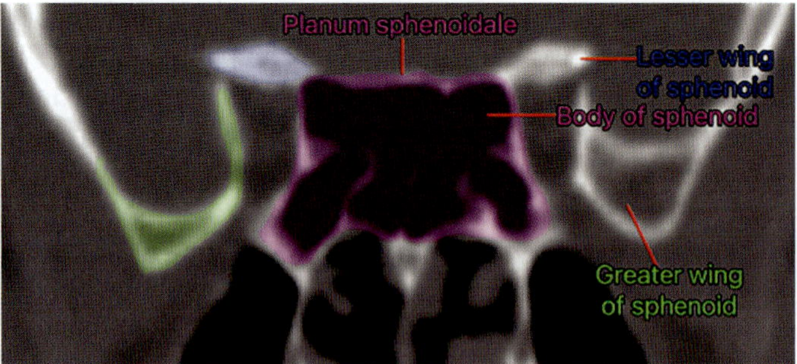

Fig. 3.2.22: CT coronal section: Parts of sphenoid bone

3

from the hard-palate to the mid-hypophyseal fossa. Coronal reformats are obtained parallel to the posterior wall of the maxillary sinus back to the level of the posterior clinoids. Borders are formed medially by perpendicular plate of the palatine bone, laterally narrowing to the pterygomaxillary fissure, anteriorly posterior wall of the maxillary sinus, posteriorly sphenoid bone (pterygoid process and inferior aspect of the greater wing), roof completely formed by the greater wing of the sphenoid bone; inferior orbital fissure, floor narrowing to palatine canals; pyramidal process of the palatine bone. PPF via the sphenopalatine foramen it communicates with the nasal cavity medially and via the pterygomaxillary fissure it communicates with infratemporal fossa laterally, anteriorly communicates with the orbit via the inferior orbital fissure (superiorly), posteriorly and superiorly it communicates with the Meckel cave and cavernous sinus (of the middle cranial fossa) via the foramen rotundum, posteriorly and inferiorly it communicates with the middle cranial fossa via the vidian canal, posteriorly and medially it communicates with the nasopharynx via the palatovaginal canal, inferiorly it communicates with the palate via the greater and lesser palatine canals. PPF contents include pterygopalatine ganglion, maxillary artery and its branches, including the descending palatine artery, emissary veins, maxillary division of trigeminal nerve, nerve of the pterygoid canal. This series of CT images shows the anatomy and communications of the pterygopalatine fossa in axial, coronal and sagittal sections (Figs 3.2.23–3.2.31).

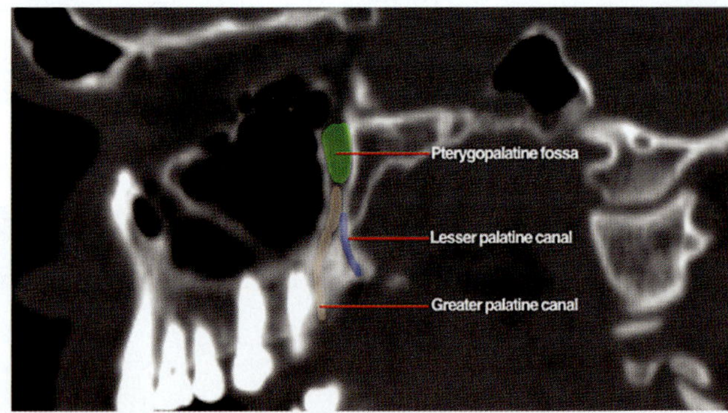

Fig. 3.2.23: CT sagittal section: Pterygopalatine fossa

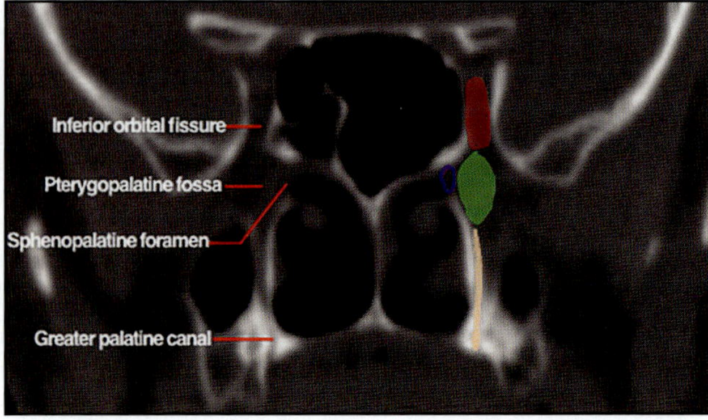

Fig. 3.2.24: CT coronal section: Pterygopalatine fossa

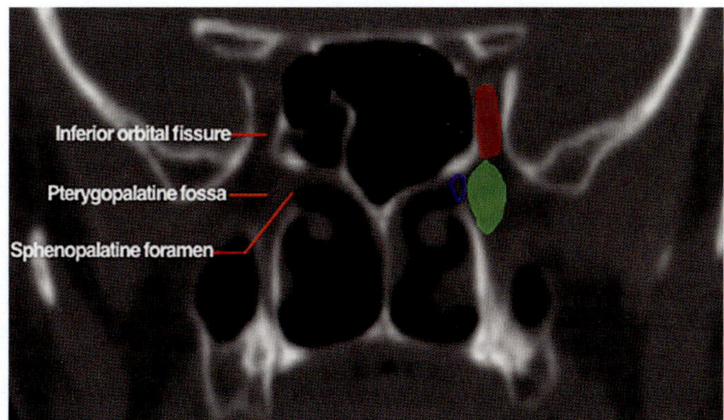

Fig. 3.2.25: CT coronal section: Pterygopalatine fossa

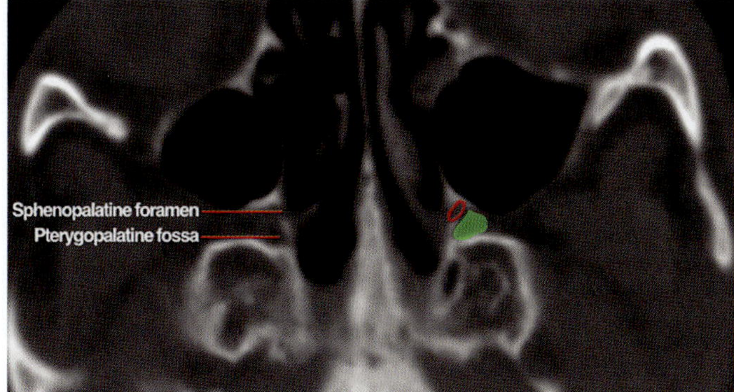

Fig. 3.2.26: CT axial section: Sphenopalatine foramen

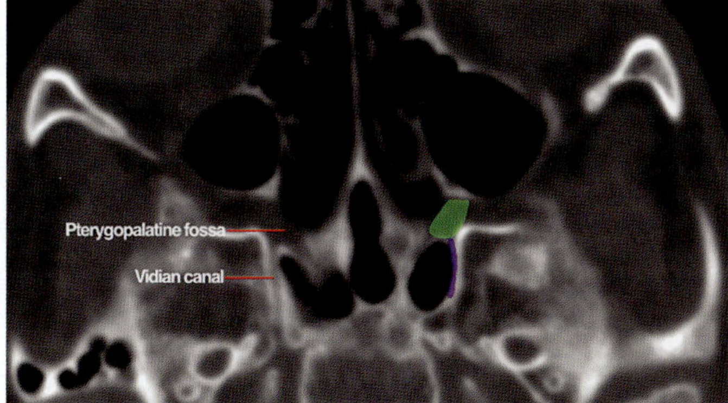

Fig. 3.2.27: CT axial section: Vidian canal

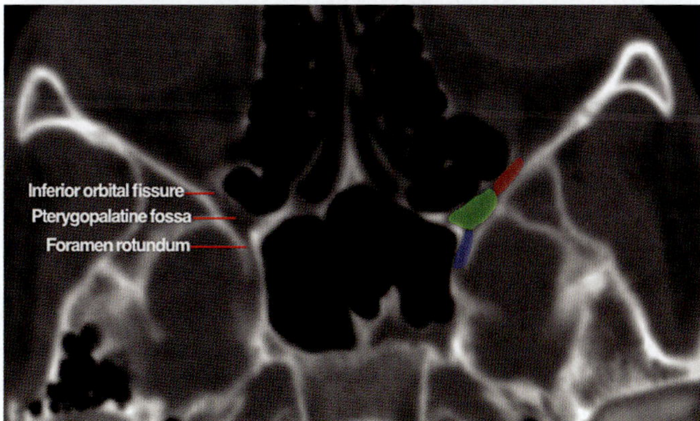

Fig. 3.2.28: Foramen rotundum

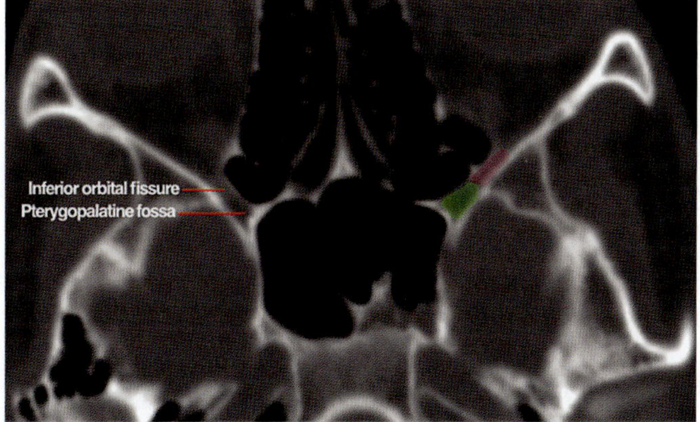

Fig. 3.2.29: Pterygopalatine fossa

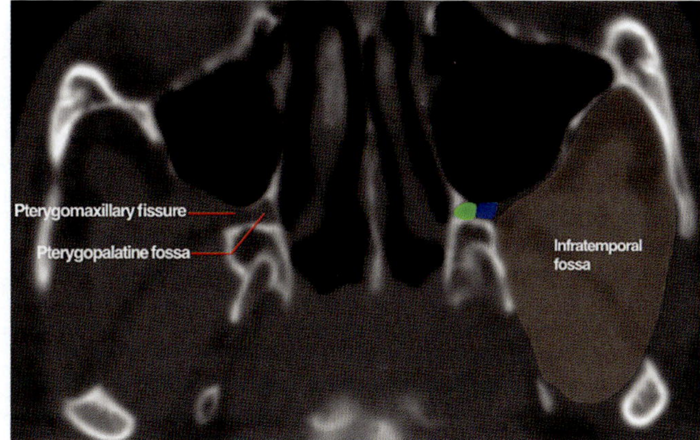

Fig. 3.2.30: Infratemporal fossa

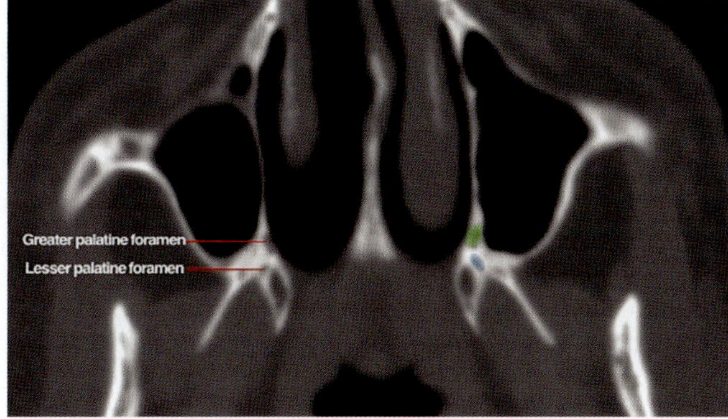

Fig. 3.2.31: Palatine foramen

3.2.B Orbit

Major components of the bony orbital walls are the frontal bone superiorly, zygomatic bone laterally and inferiorly, maxillary bone inferiorly and medially, and ethmoid bone medially. Smaller contributions medially include the lacrimal bone, nasal bone, and a tiny portion of the palatine bone (Figs 3.2.32 to 3.2.37).

The sphenoid bone makes up a large portion of the orbit posteriorly and laterally, forming the complex foramina at the orbital apex. The orbital septum is a thin sheet of fibrous tissue that originates from the orbital rim

Table 3.2.1: Foramen of skull and its contents		
Anterior skull base (ASB)	*Anatomy*	*Contents*
Foramen cecum	ASB to nasal space, in frontoethmoidal suture	Nasal emissary vein
Cribriform foramina	ASB to nasal cavity	Axons of olfactory cells (CN 1)
Anterior and posterior ethmoidal foramina	Openings in ethmoidal bone	Corresponding vessels and nerves
Middle skull base (MSB)		*Contents*
Optic canal	MSB to orbit	Optic nerves and ophthalmic arteries
Superior orbital fissure	Between roof and lateral orbital wall	Opthalmic veins, ophthalmic nerve (CN V1), CN 3,4,6, sympathetic fibres
Foramen rotundum	MSB to sphenopalatine fossa. Located in GWS.	Maxillary nerve (CN V2)
Foramen ovale	MSB to infratemporal fossa. Posterolateral to foramen rotundum in GWS	Mandibular nerve (CN V3) and accessory meningeal artery
Foramen spinosum	MSB to infratemporal fossa. Posterolateral to foramen ovale in GWS	Middle meningeal artery and vein, meningeal branch of CN V3
Foramen lacerum	Located between the sphenoid, apex of petrous temporal and basilar part of occipital. Juncture of the petroclival, sphenopetrosal, and pterygosphenoidal sutures.	Internal carotid artery and its accompanying sympathetic and venous plexus
Groove of greater petrosal nerve		Greater petrosal nerve and petrosal branch of middle meningeal artery
Posterior skull base (PSB)		*Contents*
Foramen magnum	In occipital bone.	Medulla and meninges, vertebral artery, CN 11, dural veins, anterior and posterior spinal arteries
Jugular foramen	PSB to carotid space of SHN. Two parts: Pars nervosa and Pars vascularis	Pars nervosa contains CN9, Jacobson nerve, inferior petrosal sinus Pars vascularis contains CN10, Arnold nerve, CN11, jugular bulb, posterior meningeal artery
Hypoglossal canal	PSB to carotid space of supra-hyoid neck (SHN).	Hypoglossal nerve (CN 12)
Condylar canal	Canal in the condyloid fossa behind the occipital condyle	Emissary veins that pass from the sigmoid sinus to vertebral veins in neck

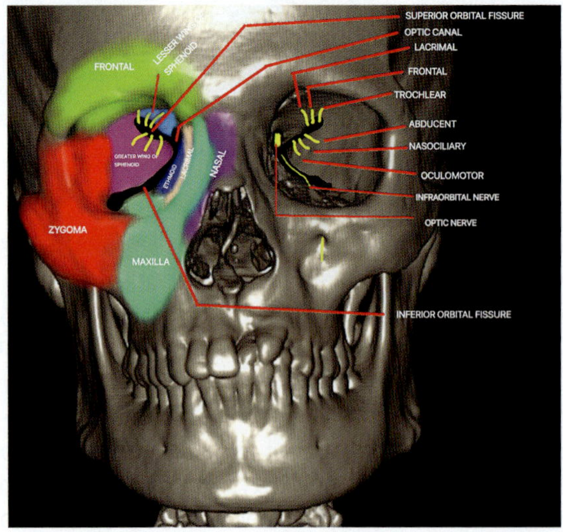

Fig. 3.2.32: Bony orbit

periosteum and blends with the tendon of the levator palpebrae superioris superiorly and inserts into the tarsal plate inferiorly. It serves as barrier to spread of infection from preseptal space to postseptal space.

Globe is an aqueous-filled anterior segment includes anterior and posterior chambers, both anterior to the lens. The vitreous filled posterior segment occupies the bulk of the globe posteriorly. The layers or tunica of the eye include the inner retina, vascular choroid, and outer structural sclera. The anterior refractive constructs include the iris and ciliary body.

Optic nerve is the second cranial nerve and is a continuation of CNS, not surrounded by Schwann cells. It is formed by the central processes from ganglion cells and has 4 parts, namely intraocular, intraorbital, intracanalicular and intracranial. **Orbital spaces** are

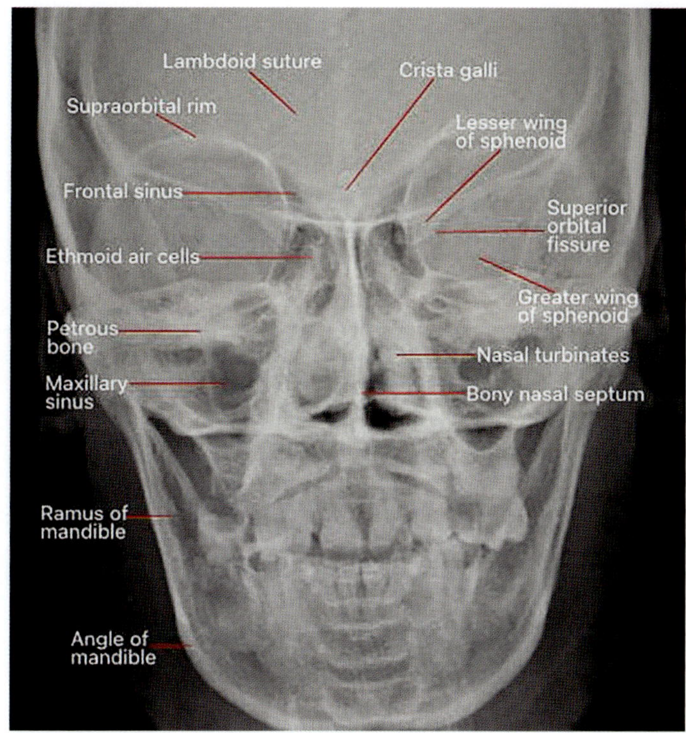

Fig. 3.2.33: X-ray facial bone frontal view

preseptal space which is anterior to orbital septum. Postseptal space with globe is situated posterior to orbital septum. Retro-orbital spaces include intraconal and extraconal spaces. **Intraconal space** is the conical space within the orbit and musculofascial cone, the sides of which are formed by the extraocular muscles and their surrounding fascia which pass posteriorly and converge on the tendinous ring at the orbital apex. It contains ophthalmic artery, cranial nerves 2, 3, 6 and nasociliary branch of trigeminal nerve. **Extraconal space** is external to intraconal space. The orbital bones and their periosteum make up the exterior sides. The extraocular muscles and their associated fascia constitute the internal sides, which pass posteriorly and converge on the tendinous ring near the orbital apex. Contents include cranial nerve 4, branches of ophthalmic and maxillary divisons of trigeminal nerve, branches of ophthalmic artery, infraorbital artery, superior and inferior ophthalmic veins and lacrimal gland. **Myofascial cone** is the physical division between the intraconal and extraconal compartments, but the cone itself is included in the contents of the intraconal space. The organization of myofascial cone allows for the rotational movements of the globe to occur on a fixed axis. The series of MRI images shows the orbit and its contents (Figs 3.2.38 to 3.2.48).

Lacrimal apparatus consists of the lacrimal gland and the nasolacrimal drainage apparatus. The gland secretes into the lateral aspect of the superior fornix which then washes over the eye and is drained at the medial canthus by the lacrimal canaliculi to the lacrimal sac and then to the nasal cavity via the nasolacrimal duct.

3.2.C Nasal Cavity (NC)

It is centrally located and is divided in the midline by the **nasal septum**. The posterior septum is bony and formed by the perpendicular plate of the ethmoid superiorly and vomer bone inferiorly. Anteriorly the septum is cartilaginous (Figs 3.2.51 and 3.2.52). The bony superior, middle and inferior turbinates project into and divide the nasal cavity into inferior, middle, and superior meatuses. The middle turbinate has 3 anatomic parts (Fig. 3.2.64)—the first part is attached superiorly to the cribriform plate via the vertical lamella and the second part courses obliquely to the lamina papyracea and attaches via the basal (ground) lamella, the third part runs horizontally and attaches to perpendicular plate of palatine bone. The second

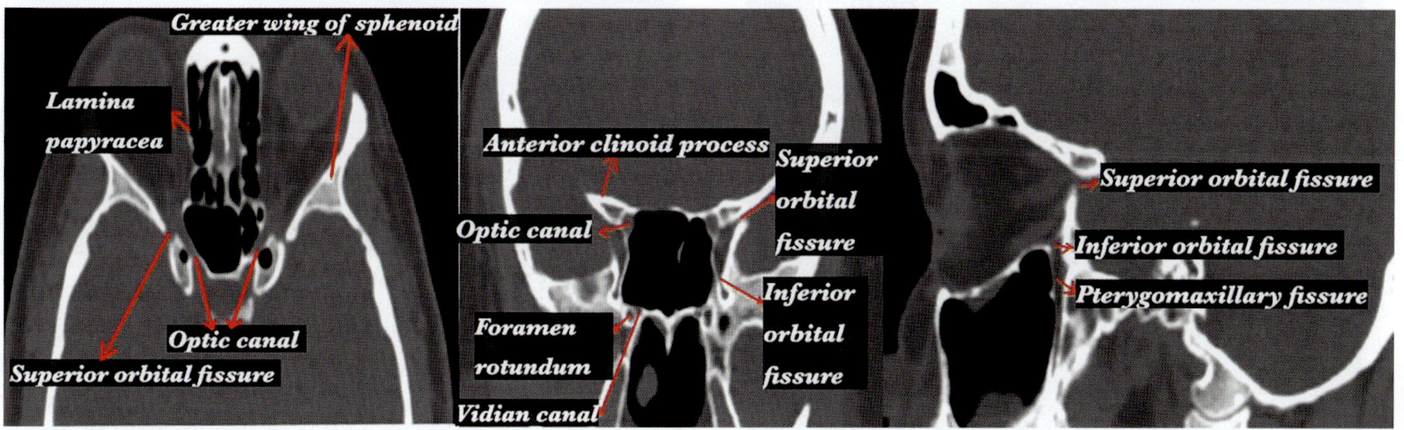

Fig. 3.2.34: CT axial, coronal, sagittal images showing orbital fissures

3

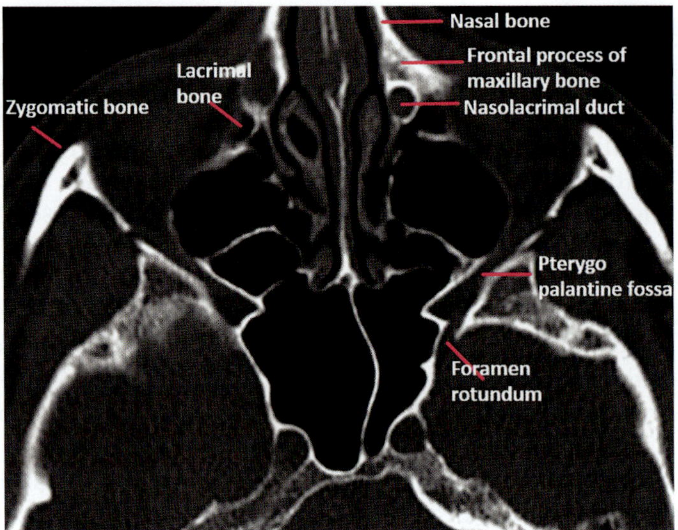

Fig. 3.2.35: Nasolacrimal duct

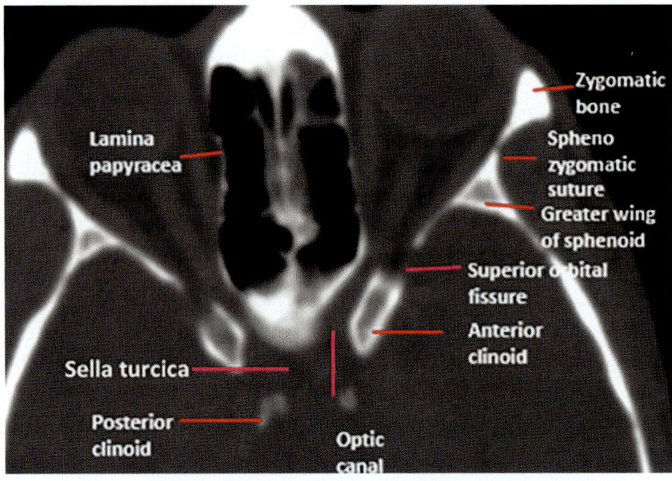

Fig. 3.2.36: CT orbit axial section

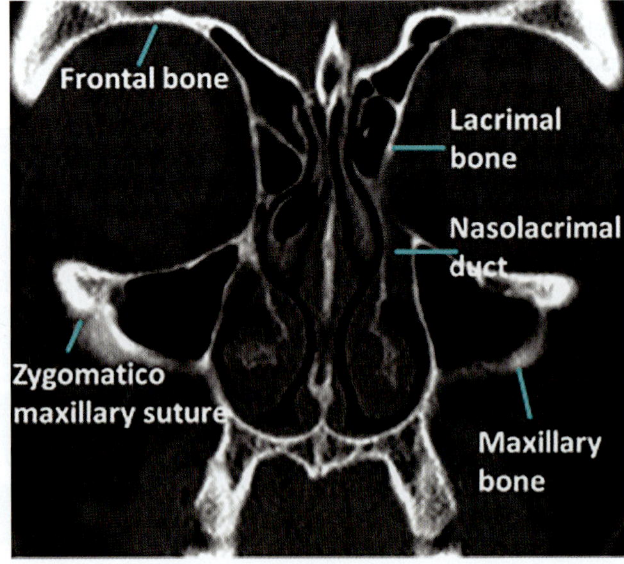

Fig. 3.2.37: CT orbit coronal section

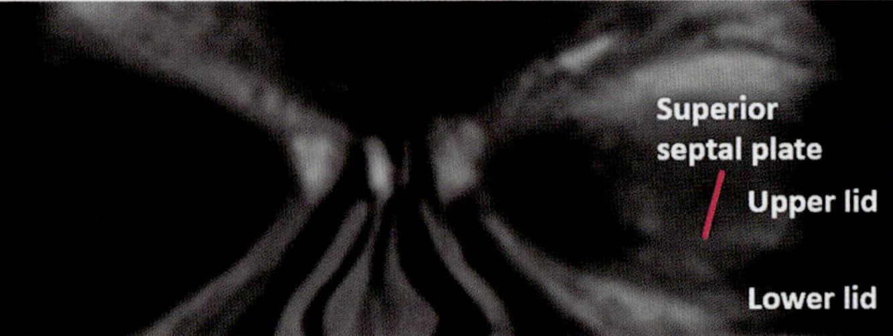

Fig. 3.2.38: MRI orbit coronal section

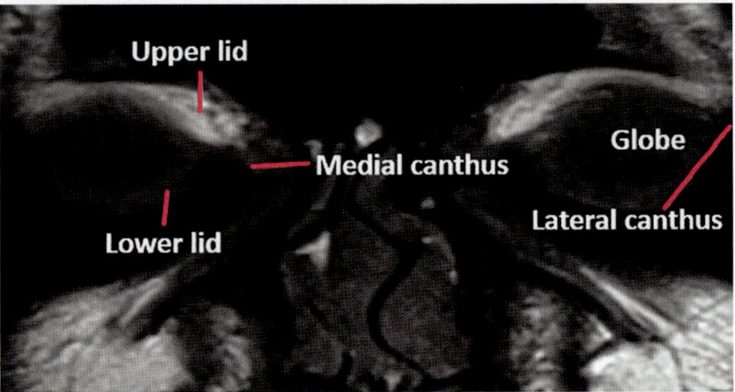

Fig. 3.2.39: MRI orbit T1 image—coronal section

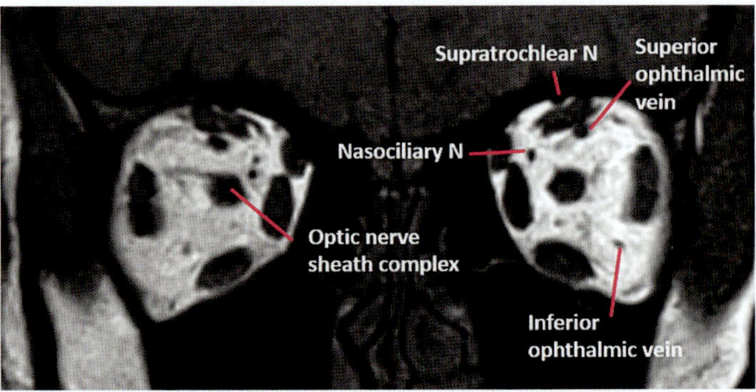

Fig. 3.2.40: MRI orbit T1 image—orbital nerves

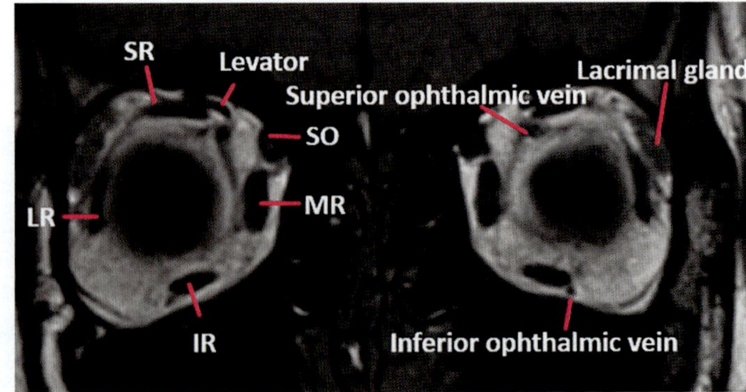

Fig. 3.2.41: MRI orbit T1 image—ocular muscles

part—**basal lamella or the ground lamella** forms the point of division between anterior and posterior ethmoid cells (Fig. 3.2.53). Olfactory fossa is bounded inferiorly by the lamina cribrosa and superiorly by the fovea ethmoidalis with vertical lateral lamella of cribriform

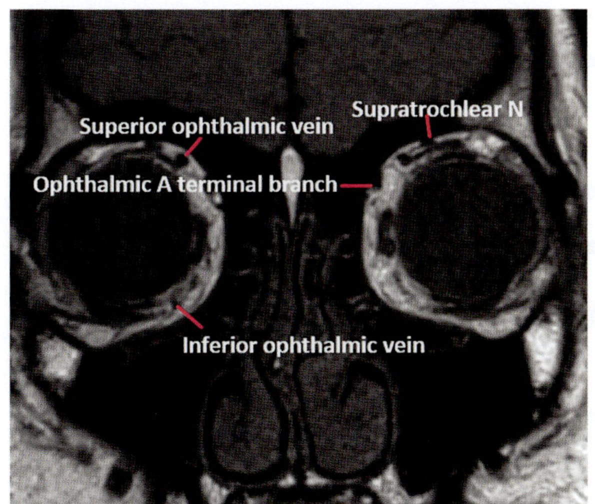

Fig. 3.2.42: Orbit vessels

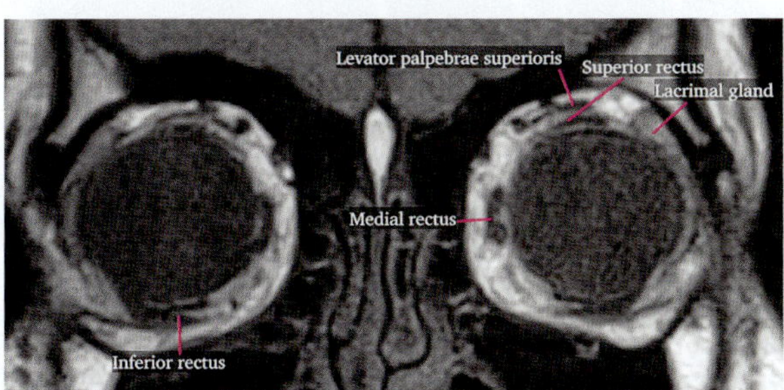

Fig. 3.2.43: Lacrimal gland

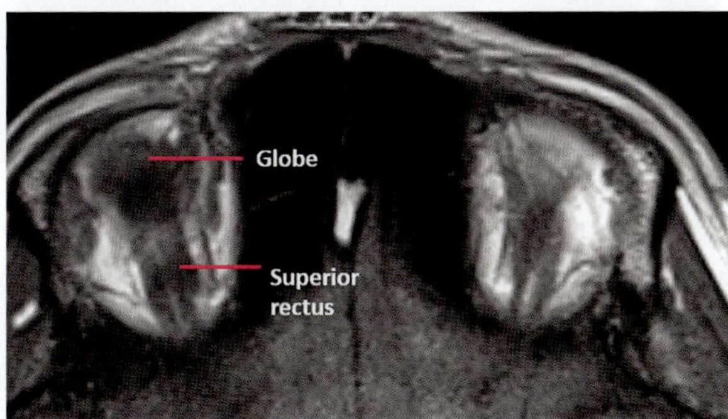

Fig. 3.2.44: MRI orbit T1 image—axial section

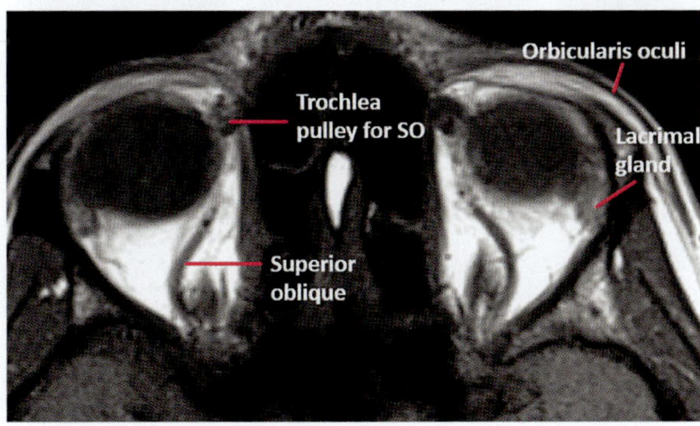

Fig. 3.2.45: MRI orbit T1 image—axial section

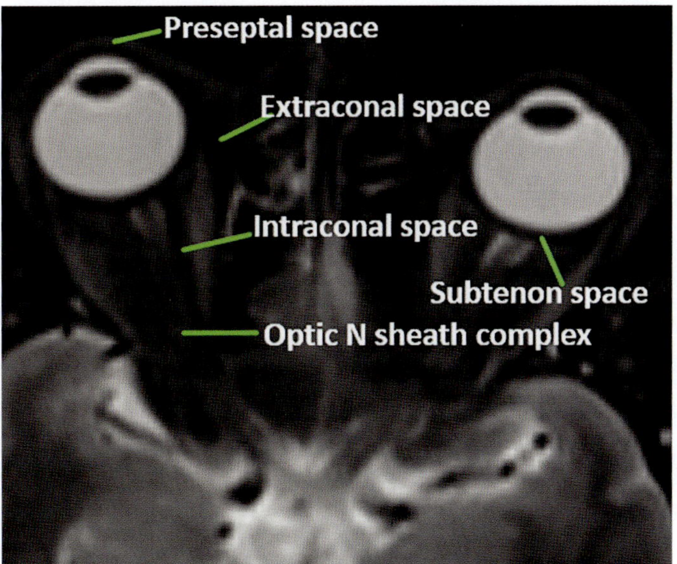

Fig. 3.2.46: Orbit spaces

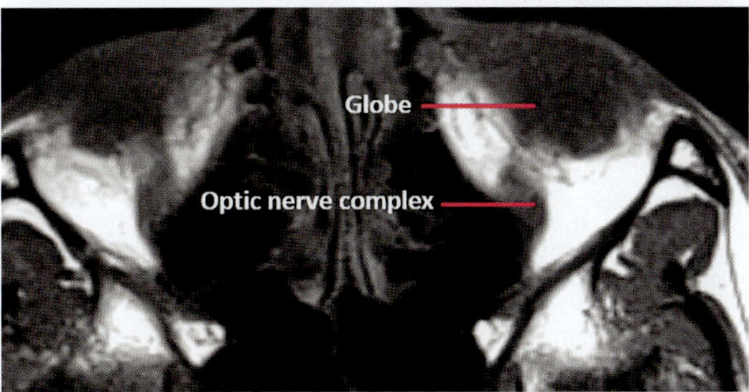

Fig. 3.2.47: MRI orbit T1 image—optic nerve

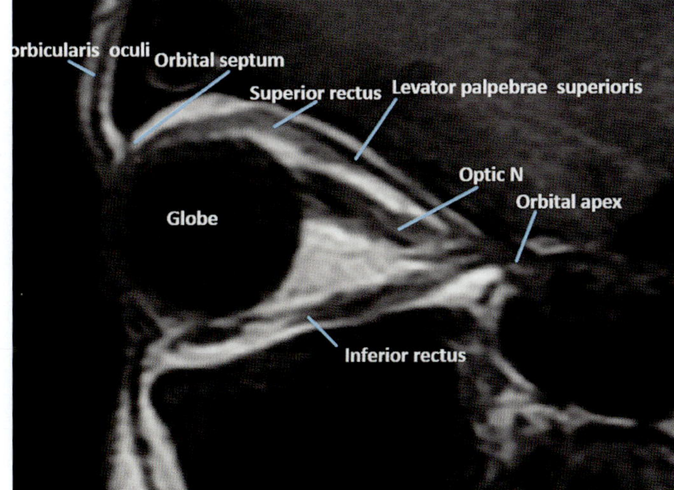

Fig. 3.2.48: MRI orbit T1 image—sagittal image

plate as lateral border. The depth of olfactory fossa is the vertical distance between the lamina cribrosa and fovea ethmoidalis and classified into three types based on **Kero's classification** (Fig. 3.2.60) (Type 1—<3 mm,

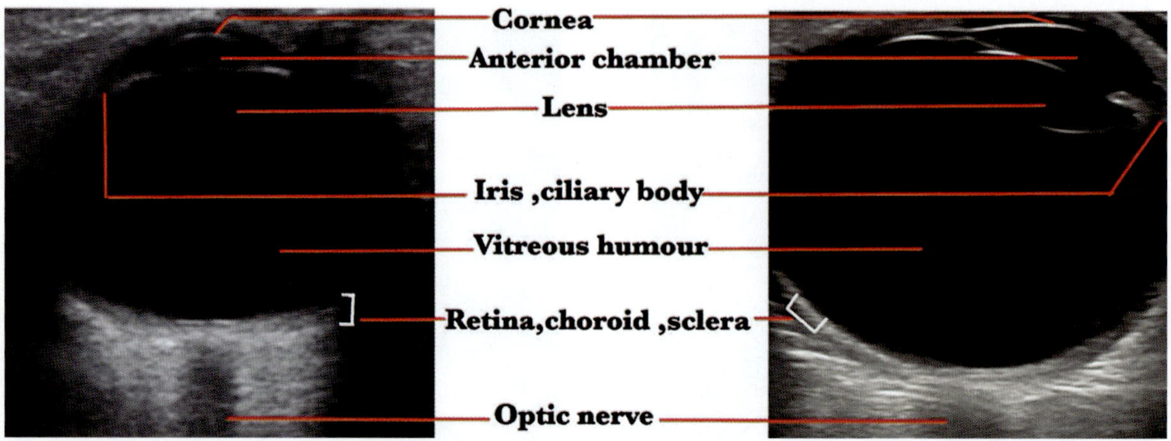

Fig. 3.2.49: Ultrasound of globe

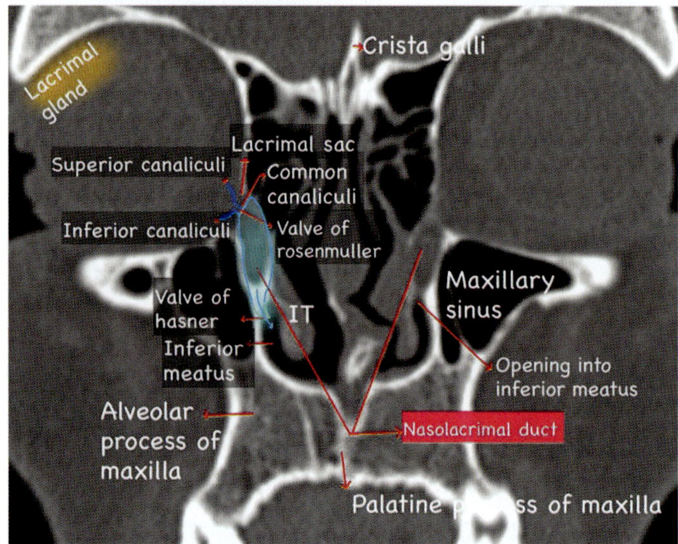

Fig. 3.2.50: Lacrimal apparatus

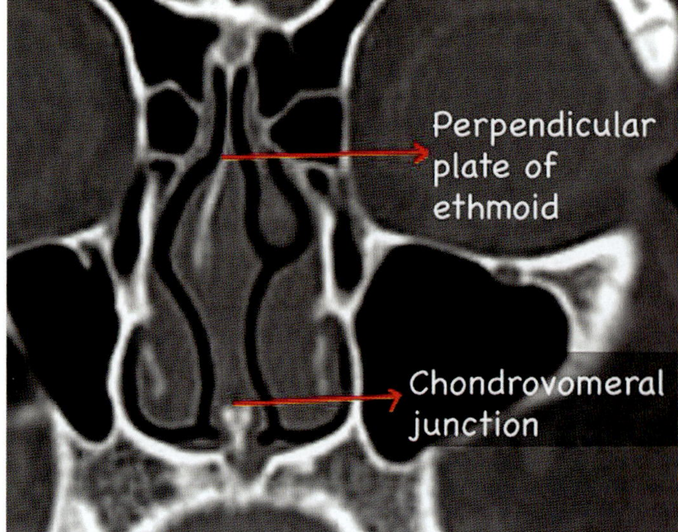

Fig. 3.2.52: CT coronal section—nasal septum

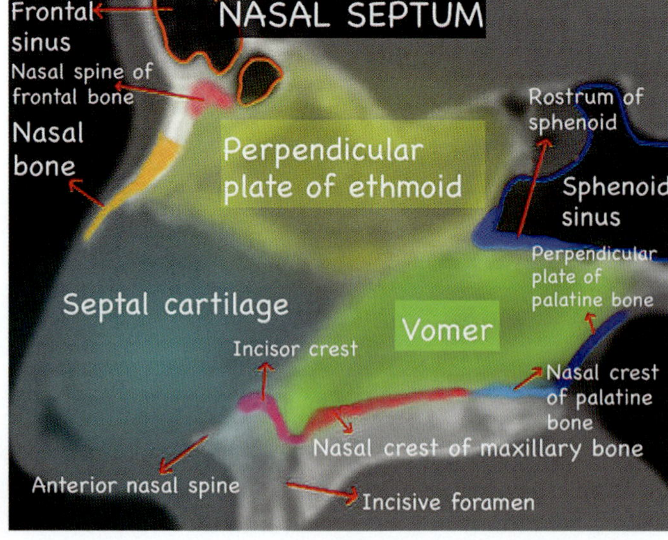

Fig. 3.2.51: CT sagittal section—nasal septum

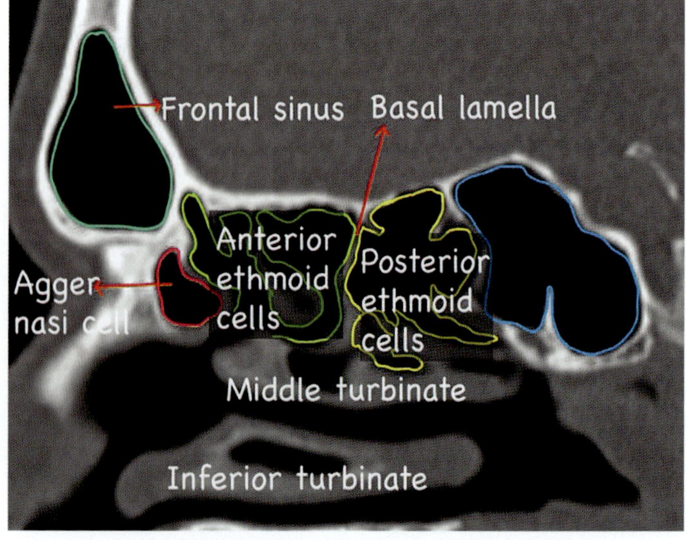

Fig. 3.2.53: Ethmoid sinuses

Type 2–4 to 7 mm, Type 3—>7 mm). As the depth of olfactory fossa increases, the chances of surgical complications also increase. Also, anterior ethmoidal artery, a branch of ophthalmic artery identified by the anterior ethmoidal notch is usually seen abutting the lateral lamella of cribriform plate or fovea ethmoidalis lying at the level of skull base. This location of the artery is safe, less prone to injury at the time of FESS. On the other hand, if the artery is located below the skull base, it is prone for injury. **Chondrovomeral junction:** Anterosuperior margin of the vomer is in the form of a variable groove, which encompasses the adjacent edge of quadrangular cartilage, thereby resulting in deformity mimicking septal spur (Fig. 3.2.52).

3.2.D Paranasal Sinus

The **paranasal sinuses** are group of air-filled spaces surrounding the nasal cavity; which start developing from the primitive choana. The sinuses are named from the facial bones in which they are located. The maxillary and ethmoid sinuses are aerated at birth, while the sphenoid sinuses and frontal sinuses are pneumatized at about the 2nd and 6th year of life respectively. The sinuses reach the adult size at adolescent age. The **maxillary sinuses** lie lateral to the NC and inferior to the orbits. Each drains via its maxillary ostium into the infundibulum, then via the hiatus semilunaris into the middle meatus. The infundibulum represents the superomedial extension of the maxillary ostium. The ethmoidal air cells, also known as the **ethmoidal sinuses,** are located within the ethmoid labyrinth of the ethmoid bone, between the orbit and the nasal cavity. The basal lamella, the lateral connection of the middle turbinate to the lamina papyracea, divides them into anterior and posterior groups. **Agger nasi** cell is a named frontal recess cell that represents the most anterior ethmoid air cell. It is present and pneumatized in the majority of patients and forms a portion of the anterior boundary of the frontal recess. **Haller cells** are infraorbital ethmoid cells and are pneumatized ethmoid air cells. They project along the medial roof of the maxillary sinus and the most inferior portion of the lamina papyracea, below the ethmoid bulla, and lie lateral to the uncinate process. **Frontal cells** are an additional group of frontal recess cells seen along the anterior aspect of frontal recess and been classified based on Kuhn's classification into four types (Fig. 3.2.59). Other variant cells include—supra-orbital ethmoidal cell, frontal bullar cell, suprabullar cell, interfrontal sinus septal cell. The **sphenoid sinuses** are asymmetric air cells in the body of the sphenoid bone. The sphenoid sinuses drain via their ostia into the sphenoethmoidal recess. The sphenoid sinus is classified into conchal, presellar, and sellar (incomplete and complete) types based on the relation to anterior and posterior walls of sella turcica on the sagittal plane. The extension of pneumatization into the clivus is classified into subdorsal, dorsal, occipital, and combined (dorsal + occipital) types based on relation to the posterior wall, the floor of sella, and vidian canal (Fig. 3.2.62). The lateral extension of pneumatization is classified into the greater wing of the sphenoid, pterygoid, and full lateral (greater wing + pterygoid) extension based on the line connecting the medial aspects of foramen rotundum and vidian canal (VR Line). **Onodi cells** are posterior ethmoidal cells extending into the sphenoid bone, either adjacent to or impinging upon the optic nerve. When these Onodi cells abut or surround the optic nerve, the nerve is at risk when surgical excision of these cells is performed. It is also a potential cause of incomplete sphenoidectomy. Important surrounding structures include the maxillary division of CN V in the foramen rotundum laterally, the vidian nerve and artery in the vidian canal inferiorly, the optic nerves and sella superiorly, and the cavernous sinuses laterally.

Table 3.2.2: Types of frontal cells

Type 1	A single anterior ethmoidal cell sitting above the agger nasi cell
Type 2	Two or more anterior ethmoidal cells sitting on the agger nasi cell
Type 3	Single large anterior ethmoidal cell sitting on agger nasi cell and pneumatizing into frontal sinus
Type 4	Cells located entirely within the frontal sinus

Ostiomeatal complex or unit comprises the maxillary sinus ostium, the ethmoidal infundibulum, anterior ethmoid cells and the frontal recess. It is the anterior drainage pathway of the sinuses (Fig. 3.2.58). The **uncinate process** (UP) is an important structure of the ostiomeatal complex. It prevents the direct contact of the inspired air with the maxillary sinus and plays a role in mucociliary activity. The position of the superior attachment of UP can be to one of the following structures: Lamina paperacea, skull base or middle concha (Fig. 3.2.65). Variations in UP can result in impaired mucociliary drainage and complications during surgery. The uncinate process may be medialized, lateralized, or pneumatized/bent. Medialization occurs with giant bulla ethmoidalis. Lateralization of the uncinate process and pneumatization of the uncinate process (uncinate bulla) may obstruct the infundibulum. The series of images from Figs 3.2.53 to 3.2.69 shows anatomy of paranasal sinuses.

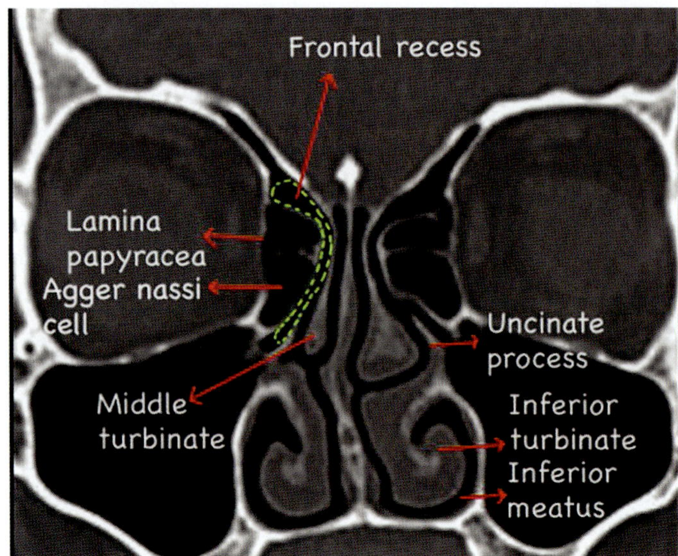

Fig. 3.2.54: CT PNS coronal section: Frontal recess

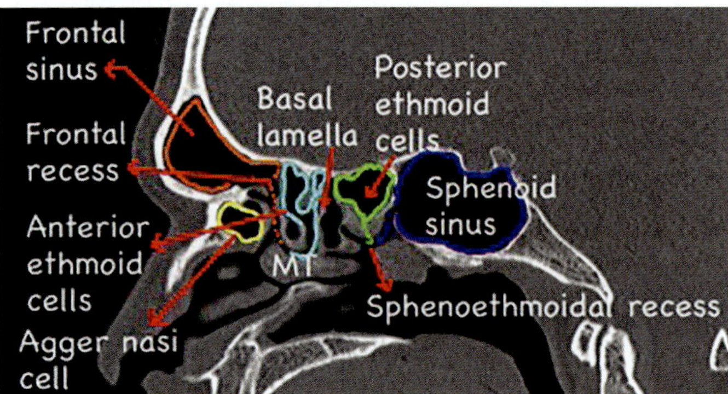

Fig. 3.2.55: CT PNS sagittal image

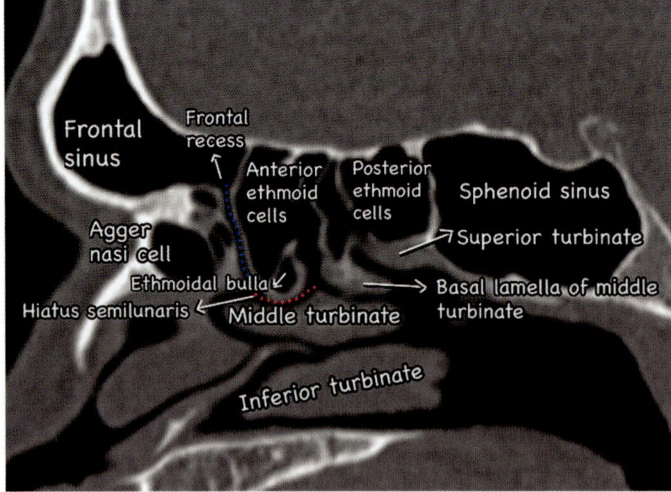

Fig. 3.2.56: CT PNS sagittal image

3.2.E Oral Cavity

The oral cavity is the most proximal portion of the aerodigestive tract, and is continuous posteriorly with the

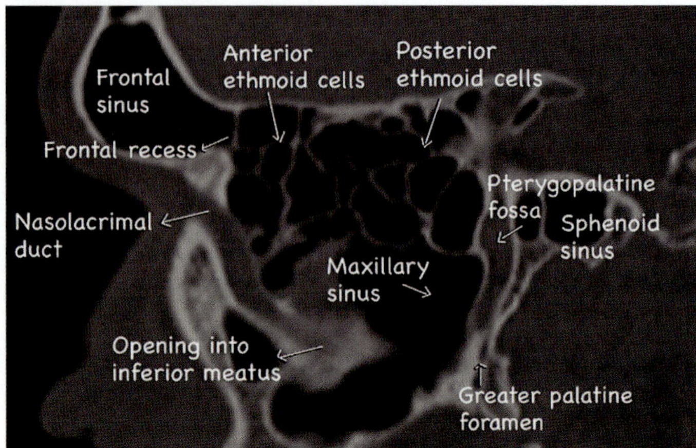

Fig. 3.2.57: CT PNS sagittal image

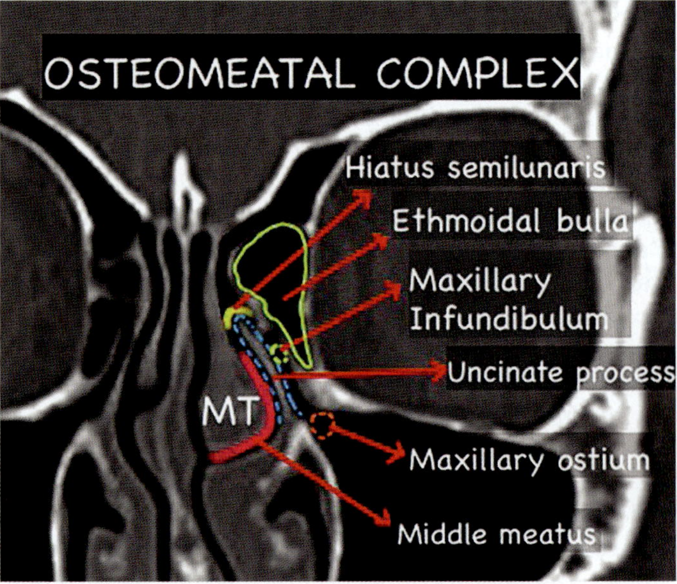

Fig. 3.2.58: CT PNS coronal image—osteomeatal complex

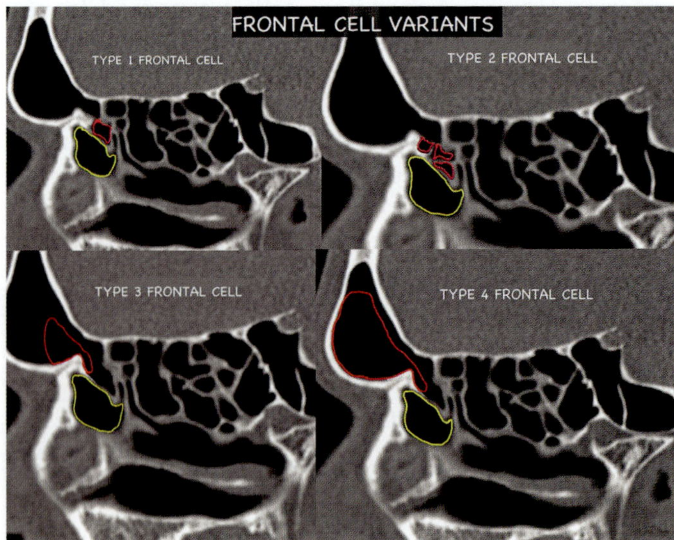

Fig. 3.2.59: Frontal cell variants

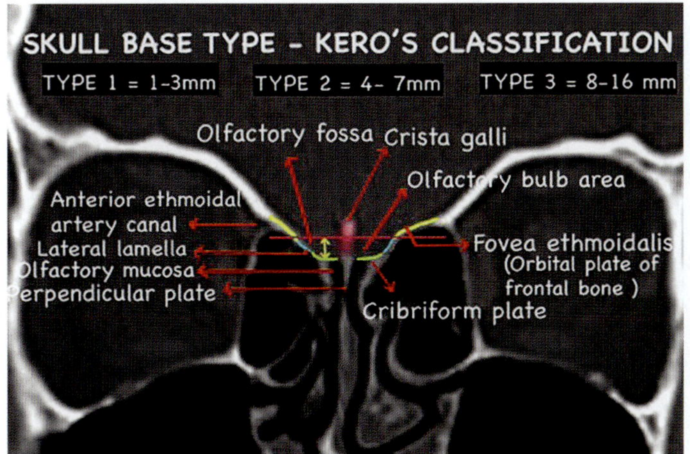

Fig. 3.2.60: Kero's classification—olfactory fossa depth

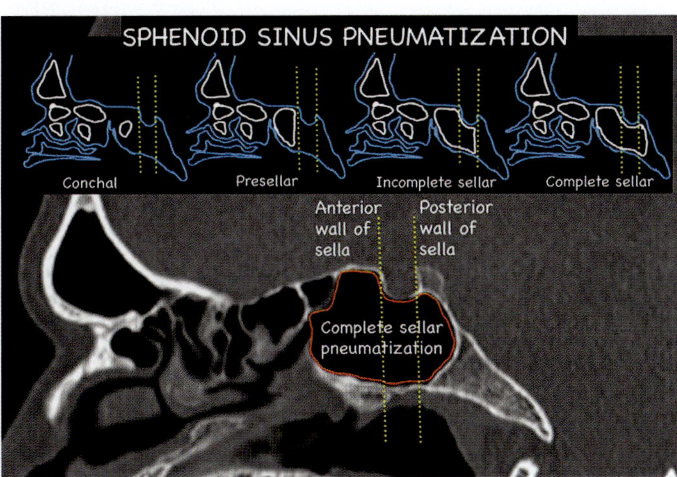

Fig. 3.2.62: Types of sphenoid sinus pneumatisation

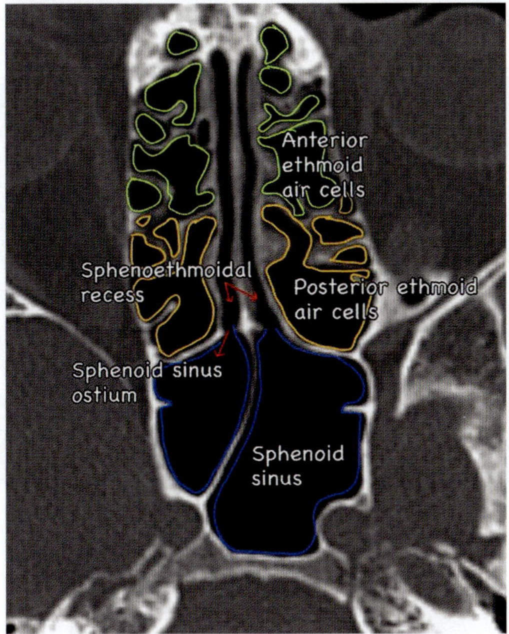

Fig. 3.2.61: Ethmoid air cells

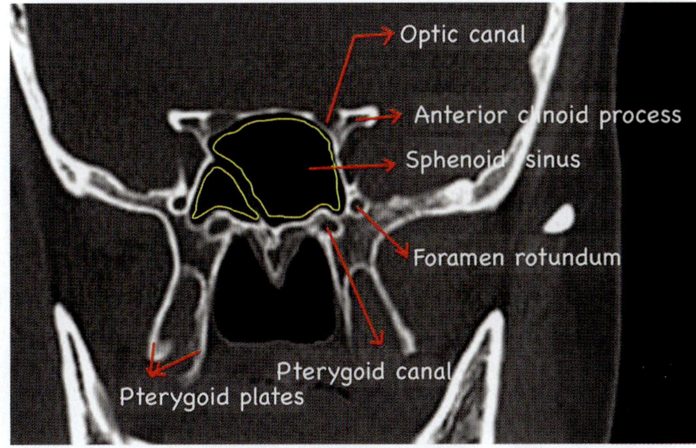

Fig. 3.2.63: Sphenoid sinus

oropharynx. It is anteriorly bound by lips and posteriorly by the circumvallate papillae, anterior tonsillar pillars, and junction of hard and soft palates that divides it from the oropharynx. **The retromolar trigone** is an oral cavity subsite that consists of the mucosa posterior to the last

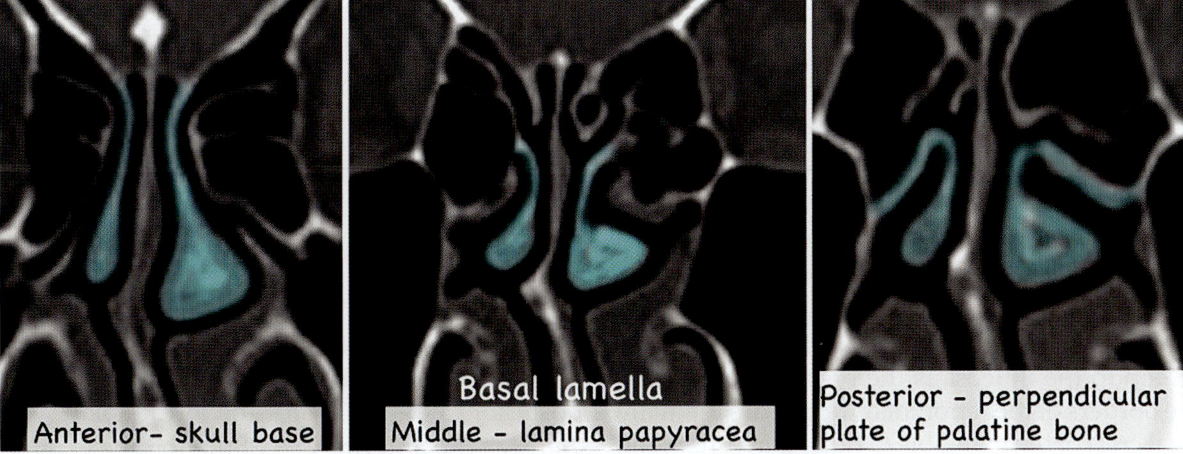

Fig 3.2.64: Middle turbinate at various levels

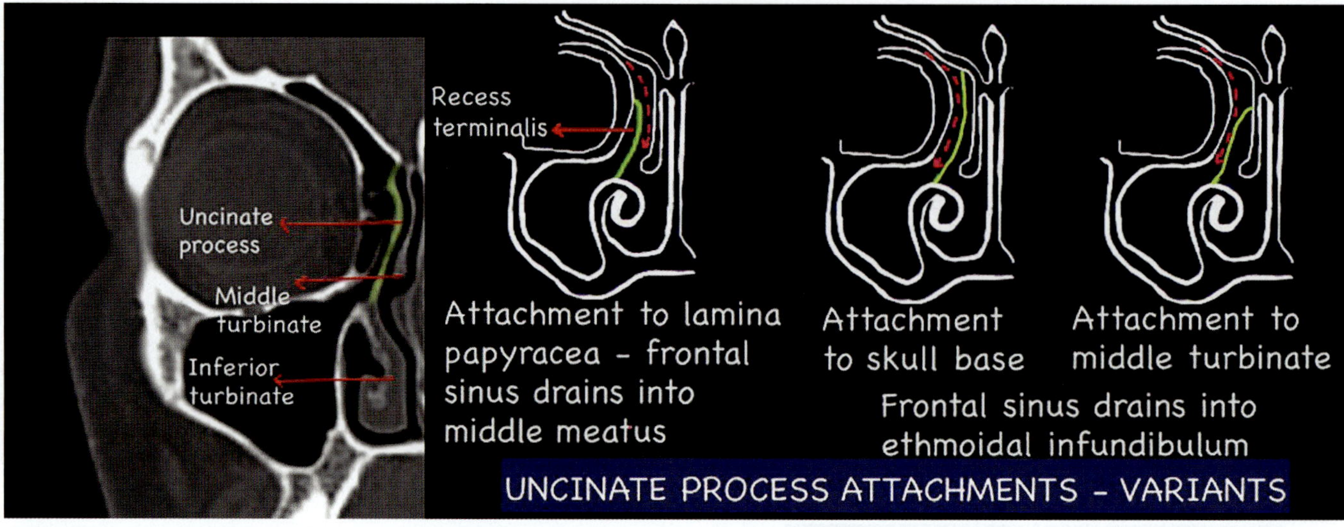

Fig. 3.2.65: Uncinate process variants

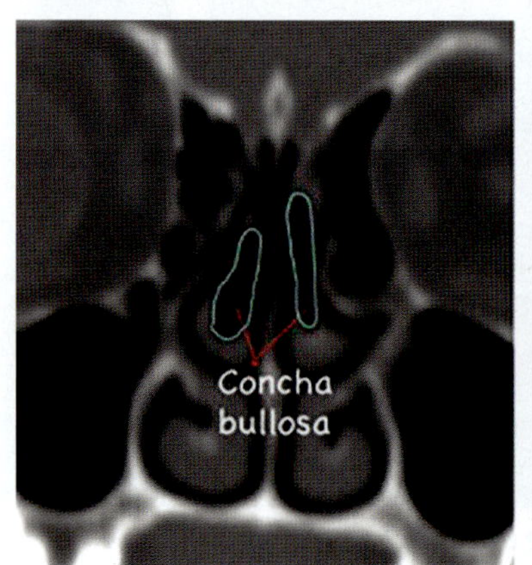

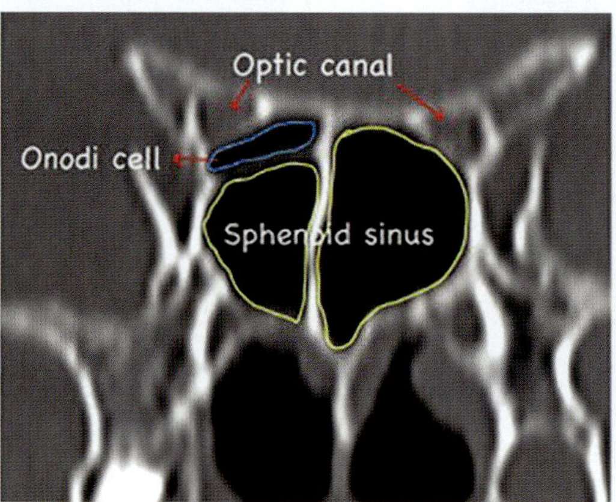

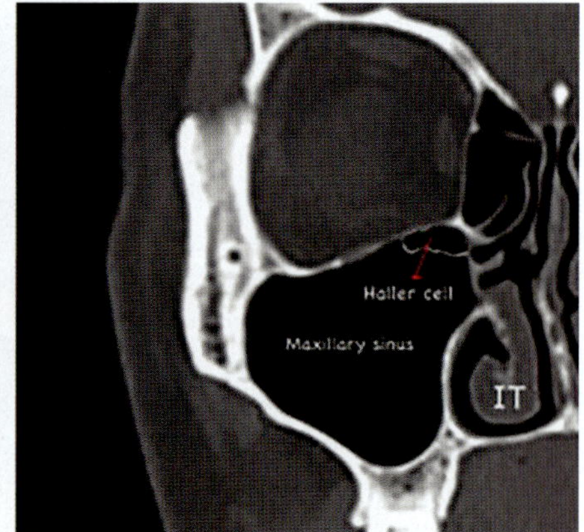

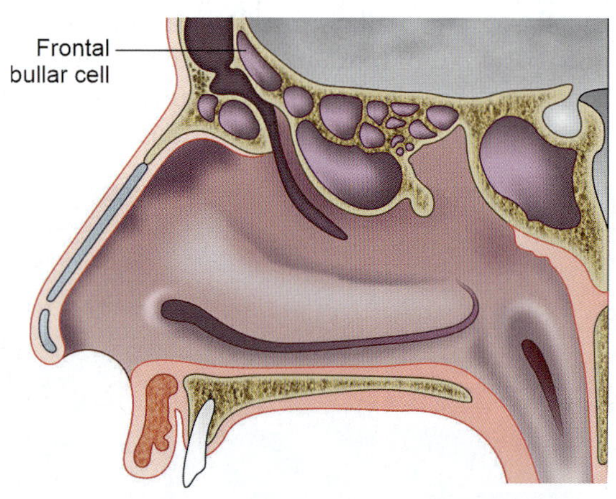

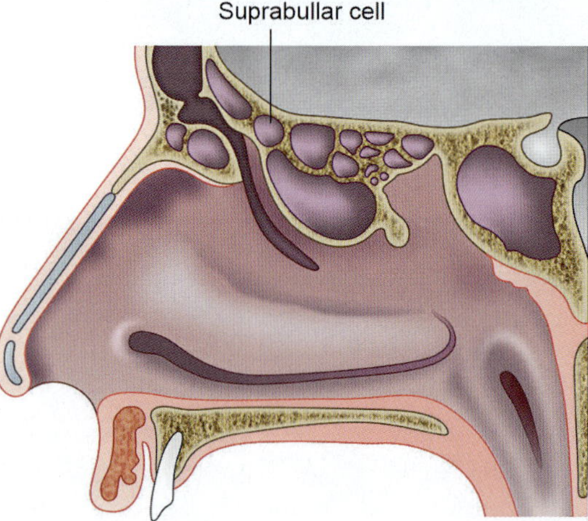

Fig. 3.2.66: Accessory air cells

3

mandibular molar. The upper parts attach the temporalis muscle. Deep to the mucosa is the pterygomandibular raphe. The borders of the retromolar trigone are medially by temporal crest of the mandible (a ridge that runs along the anteromedial face of the coronoid process and ramus to which the temporalis muscle attaches), laterally by anterior border of the ramus of the mandible, basally by posterior to the socket for the third molar.

Tongue: The anterior 2/3 of the tongue is referred to as the oral tongue and lies in the oral cavity. The posterior

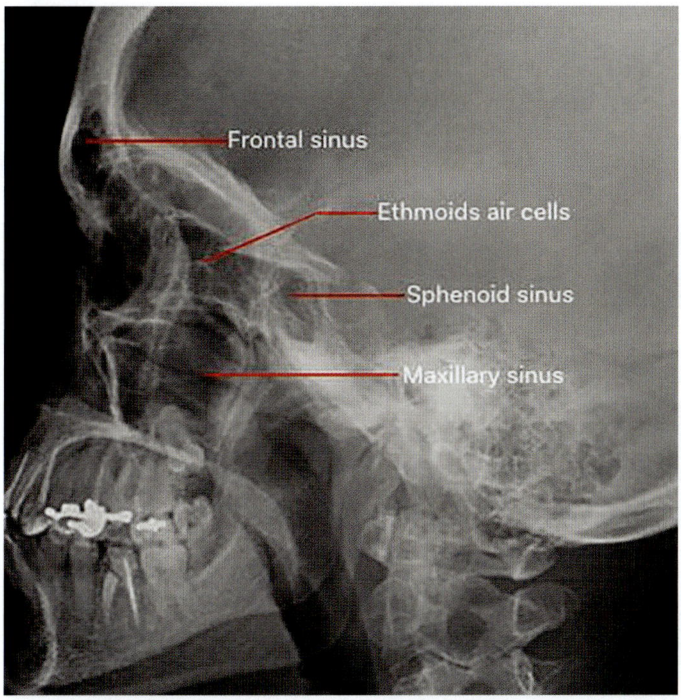

Fig. 3.2.67: X-ray PNS lateral view

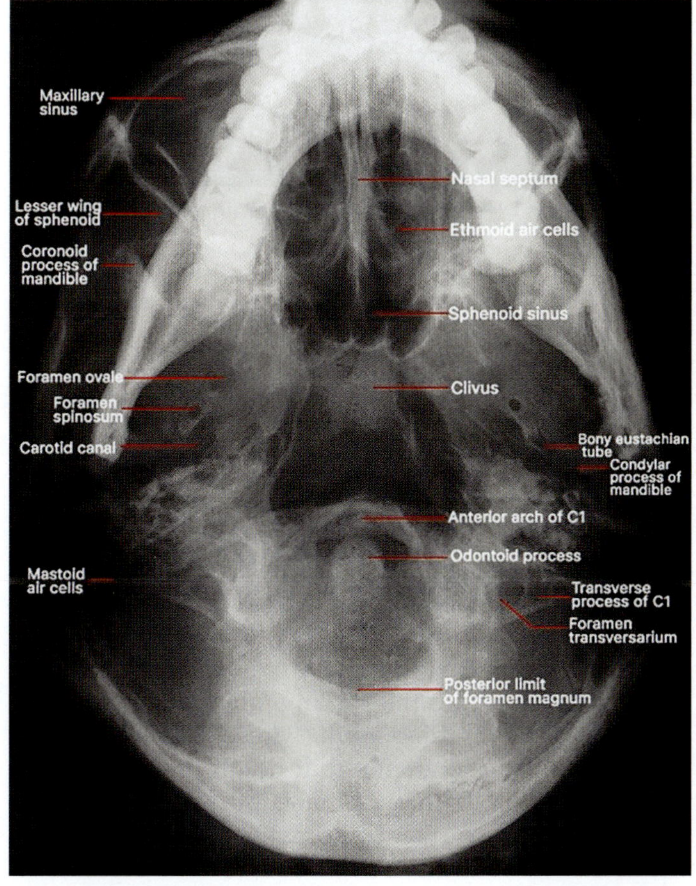

Fig. 3.2.68: X-ray skull—sub-mentor vertex view

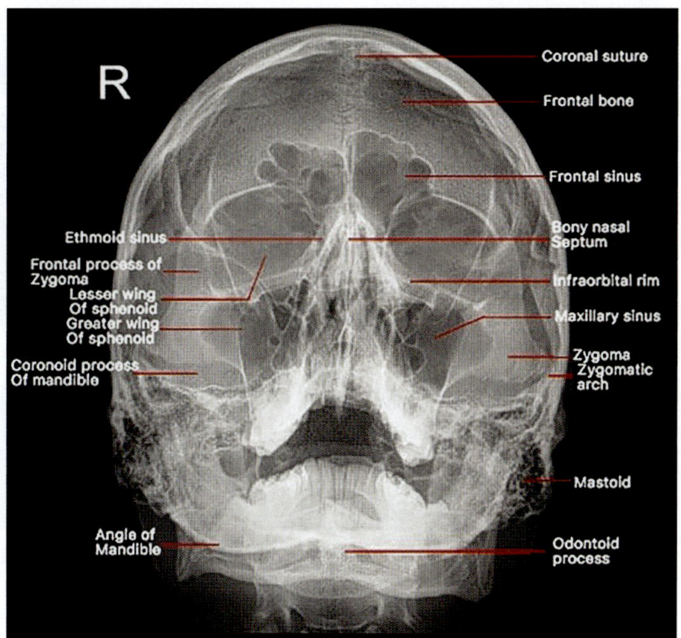

Fig. 3.2.69: X-ray PNS Waters view

1/3 is called the **base of tongue** (lingual tonsil) and is part of the oropharynx. Lingual septum, inferior portion of genioglossus and geniohyoid muscles forms **root of tongue**. The tongue is accompanied by two groups of muscles. The intrinsic muscles are a set of muscles that make up the core of the tongue and are located within it. They are the superior longitudinal, inferior longitudinal, transverse, and vertical muscles, and their major job is to alter the shape of the tongue. The extrinsic tongue muscles of the oral tongue help it perform its function. These include the genioglossus, hyoglossus, styloglossus, and palatoglossus. The genioglossus is the large, fan-shaped muscle and inserts along the entire length of the undersurface of the intrinsic tongue muscles. The tongue has a supporting fibrous framework consisting of the **lingual septum** and the hyoglossus membrane. The midline fibrous lingual septum divides the tongue into two symmetrical muscular halves.

Various enzymes for mastication and digestion are secreted by **salivary glands** in the head and neck. There are two types of salivary glands: Major and minor: The bigger, paired salivary glands in the neck make up the main salivary glands. **Parotid glands** located in parotid space. The parotid gland surrounds the mandibular ramus and extends to a position, anterior and inferior to the ear. It has superficial and deep lobes, separated by the facial nerve, along which pass the external carotid artery and retromandibular vein. It contains several intraparotid lymph nodes. The parotid duct (Stensen's duct) is approximately 5 cm long, passes through the buccal fat and over the anterior border of masseter, then

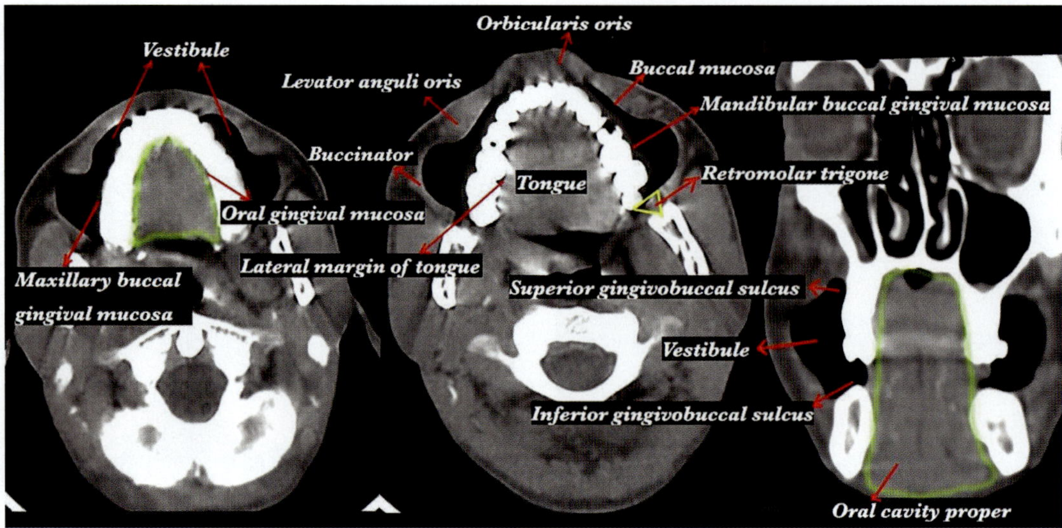

Fig. 3.2.70: Anatomy of oral cavity

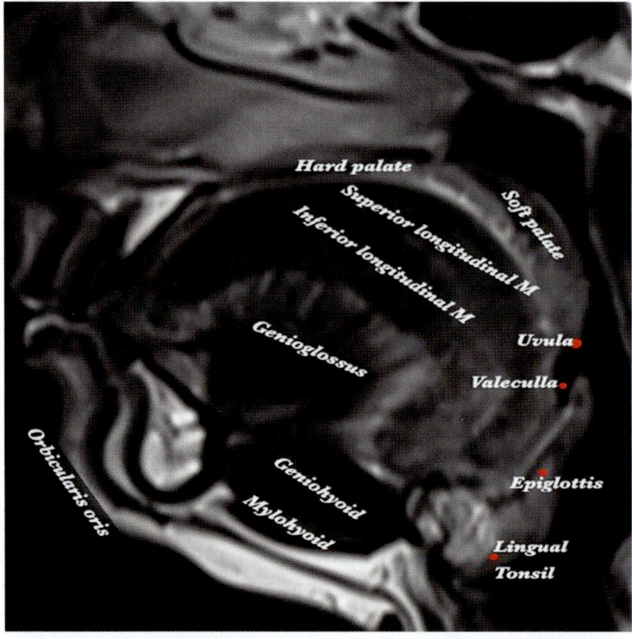

Fig. 3.2.71: Muscles of tongue

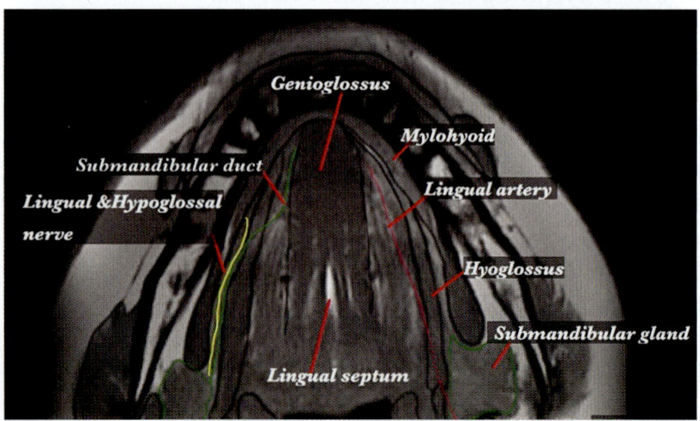

Fig. 3.2.72: Extrinsic muscles of tongue

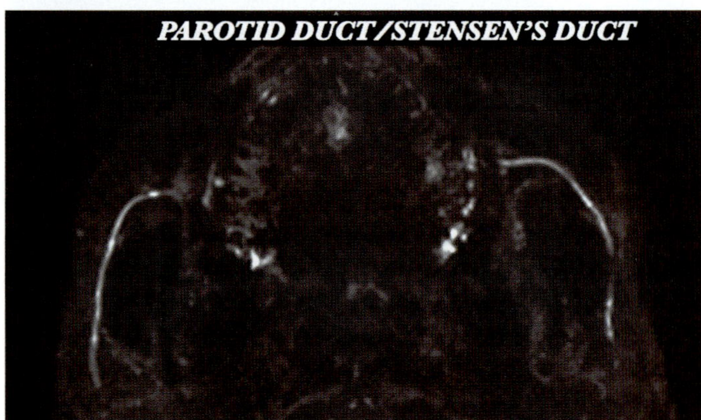

Fig. 3.2.73: MR sialogram

through the buccopharyngeal fascia and the buccinator muscle. It then continues between the buccal mucosa and the buccinator to its opening, located next to the upper second molar tooth (Fig. 3.2.73).

Submandibular glands are paired salivary glands located behind and below the ramus of the mandible in the submandibular triangle. Its lower superficial lobe continues as smaller deep lobe by wrapping around the posterior border of the mylohyoid. The superficial lobe of the submandibular gland is in the submandibular space, and the deep lobe is situated in the sublingual space. The **submandibular duct** (Wharton's duct) runs forward with lingual nerve and vein and hypoglossal nerve and opens into the sublingual papilla at the side of the frenulum of the tongue (Fig. 3.2.74). **Sublingual glands** are salivary glands that lie on the floor of the mouth anterior to the submandibular glands. They secrete predominantly mucous saliva that is drained by a collection of 8–20 excretory ducts collectively termed the duct of Rivinus. The largest of these ducts is Bartholin

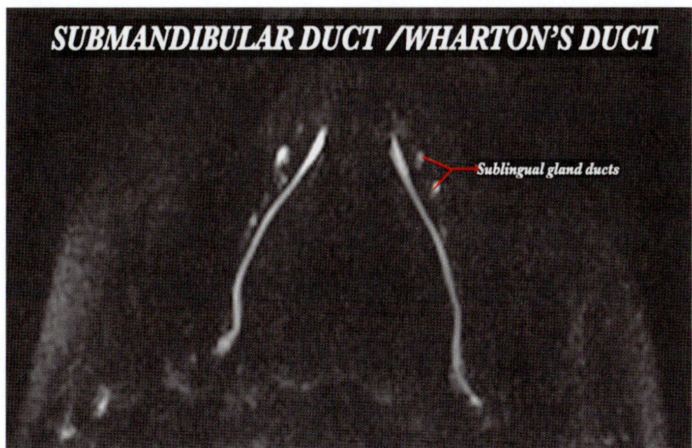

Fig. 3.2.74: MR sialogram

duct. There are up to 600 minor salivary glands located throughout the oral cavity within the lamina propria of the oral mucosa. They are 1–2 mm in diameter and are not encapsulated, unlike the major salivary glands. Instead, they are simply surrounded by connective tissue.

3.2.F Temporal Bone Anatomy

Parts of the middle and posterior fossae are formed by the temporal bones, which make up the lateral skull base. Temporal bone are made up of five osseous elements, namely squamous, mastoid, petrous, tympanic and styloid. The auricle and external auditory canal (EAC), which extends medially to the tympanic membrane, make up the external ear. On CT images, the natural tympanic membrane is frequently seen. The lateral third of the EAC fibrocartilagenous, while the medial two-thirds of the EAC is enclosed by the tympanic portion of the temporal bone. **Middle ear and mastoid:** The ossicular chain is housed in the middle ear, which is bounded laterally by the tympanic membrane, the inner ear structures (which are surrounded by the otic capsule and the cochlear promontory) medially, the tegmen tympani superiorly, and the jugular wall (floor) inferiorly. The tympanic membrane is linked superiorly to the scutum, a pointed bony projection. It is the first bony structure to be eroded as a result of cholesteatoma. Prussak space is the space between scutum and pars flaccida laterally and neck of malleus medially, also called the lateral epitympanic recess. It is the site where pars flaccida cholesteatoma arises. The tegmen is a thin bone plate that connects the middle cranial fossa dura to the middle ear and the mastoid cavity. The series of images from Figs 3.2.75 to 3.2.90 shows anatomy of temporal bone and inner ear and middle ear structures.

Tegmen tympani forms the roof of the middle ear, and the tegmen mastoideum forms the roof of the mastoid.

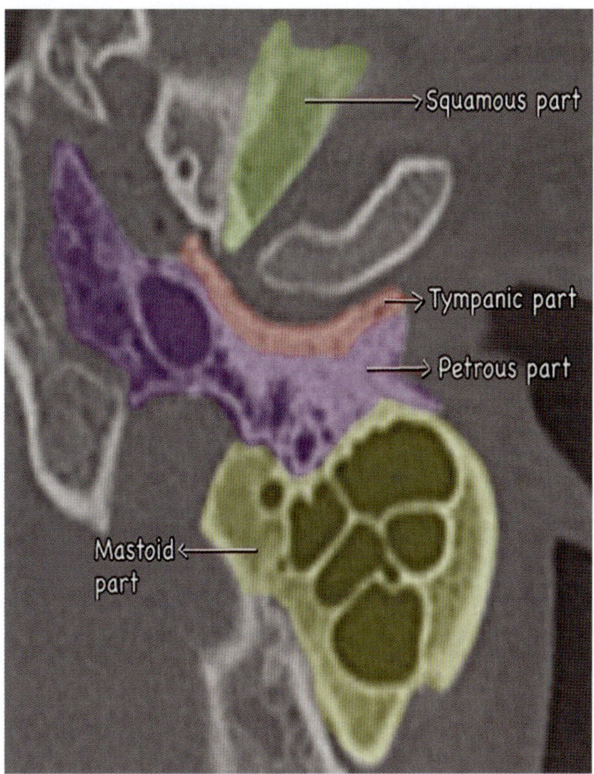

Fig. 3.2.75: HRCT temporal bone

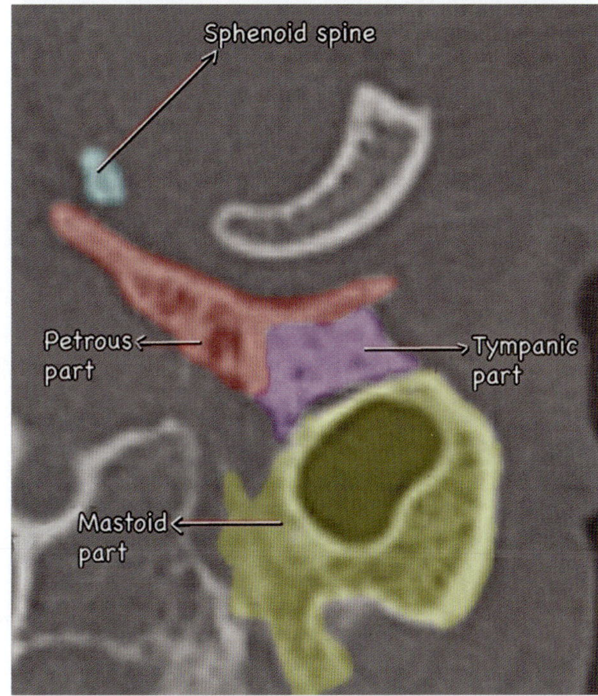

Fig. 3.2.76: HRCT temporal bone

The posterior wall of the middle ear cavity is irregular and includes the facial recess (also referred to as the facial nerve recess), pyramidal eminence where the stapedius muscle exits to its insertion into posterior aspect of

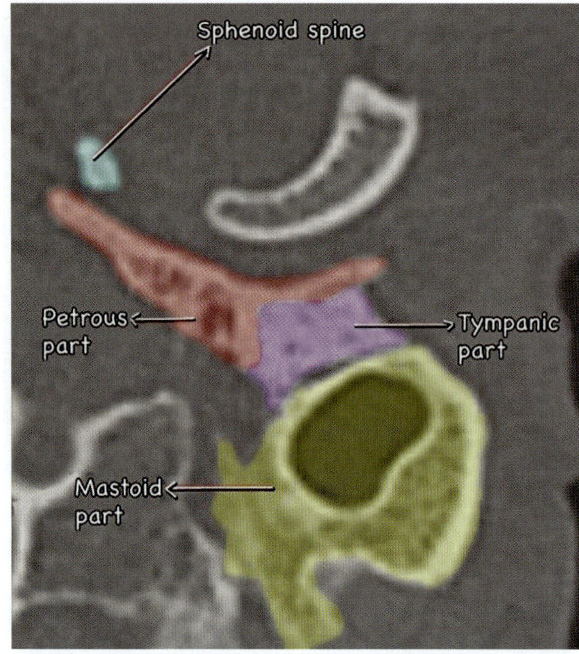

Fig. 3.2.77: HRCT temporal bone

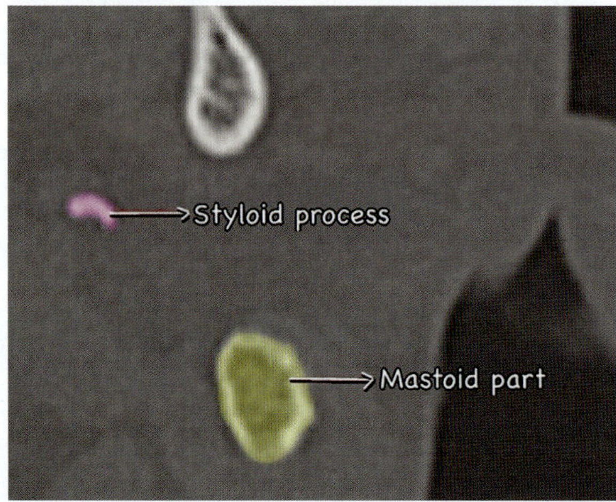

Fig. 3.2.78: HRCT temporal bone

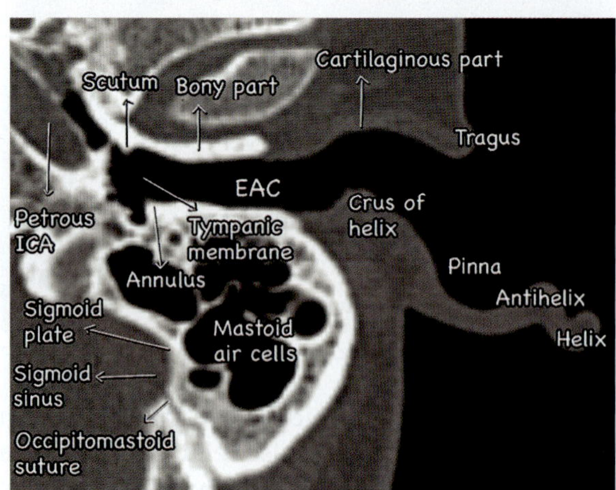

Fig. 3.2.79: External ear

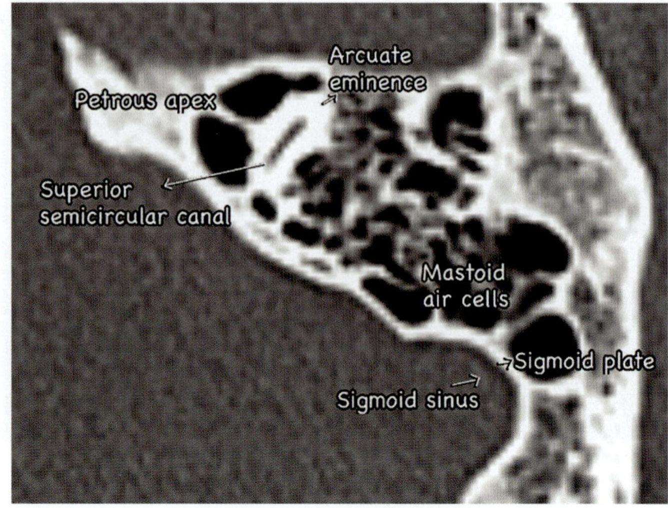

Fig. 3.2.80: Mastoid air cells

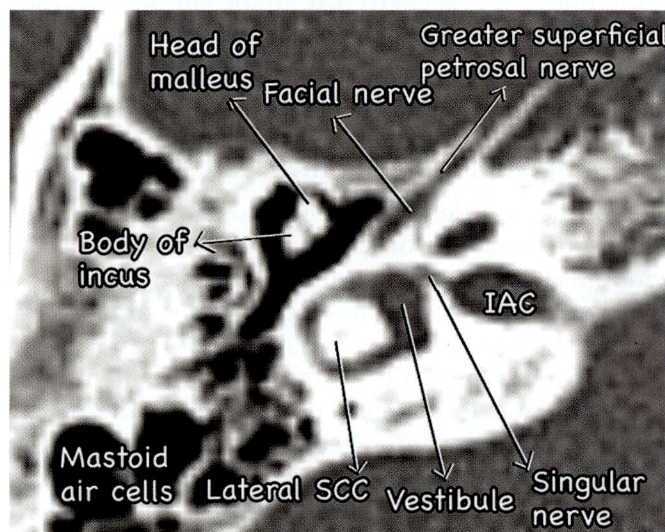

Fig. 3.2.81: HRCT temporal bone

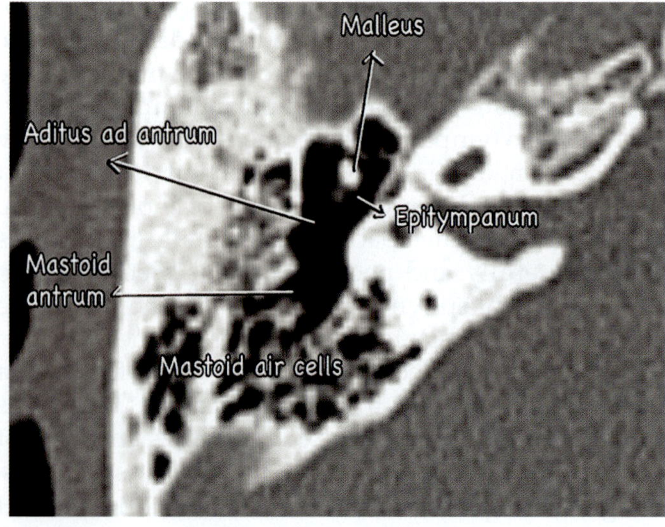

Fig. 3.2.82: Middle ear

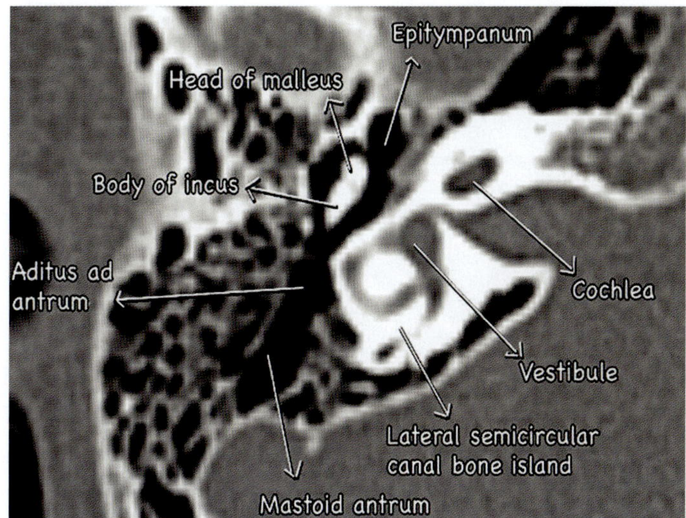

Fig. 3.2.83: Middle and inner ear

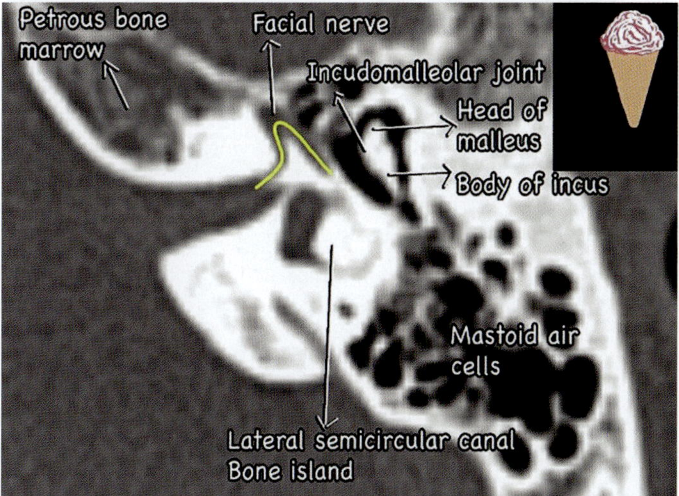

Fig. 3.2.84: Inner and middle ear

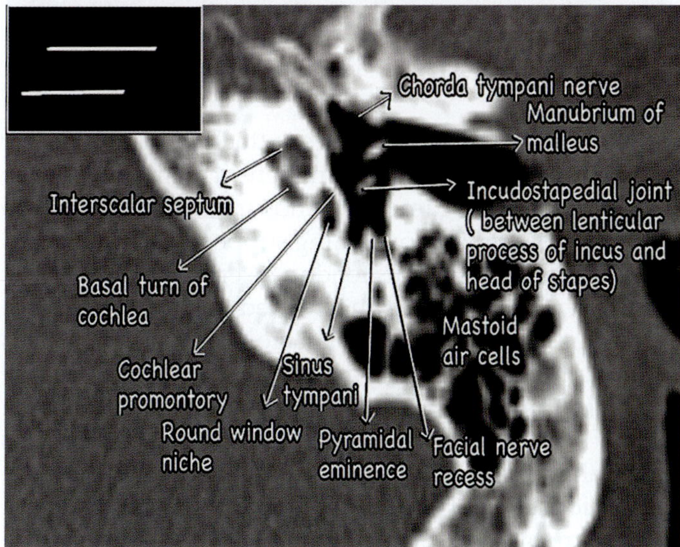

Fig. 3.2.85: Ear ossicles—equal sign

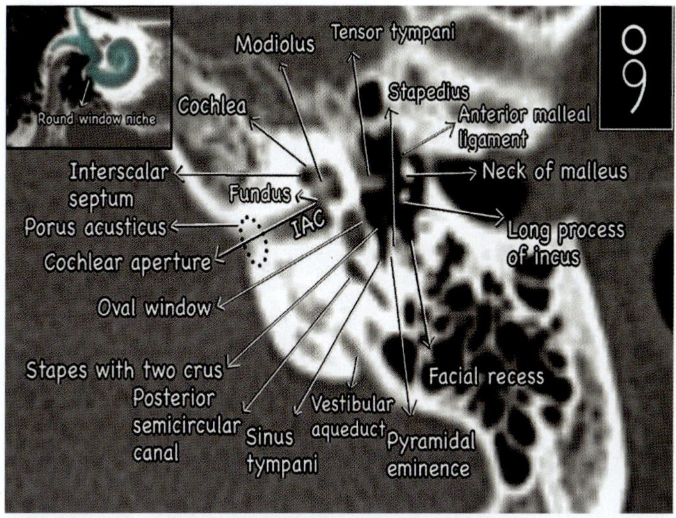

Fig. 3.2.86: Inner and middle ear

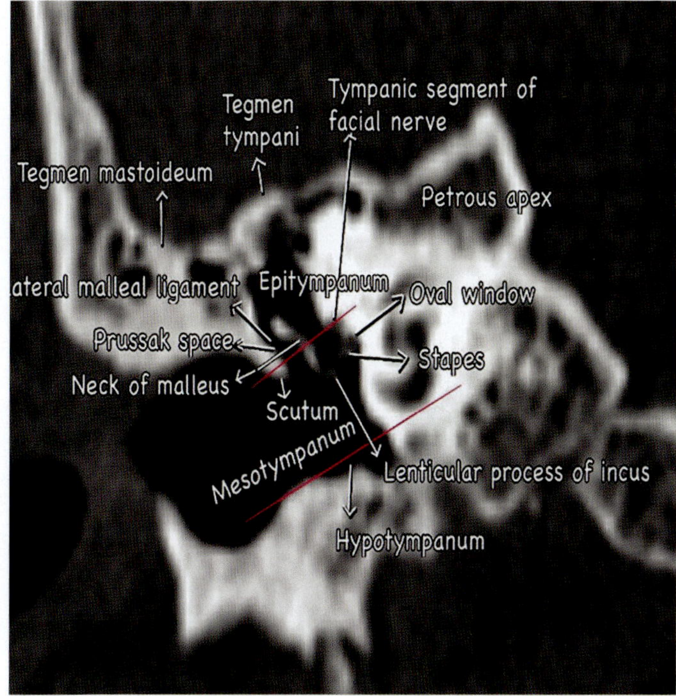

Fig. 3.2.87: Middle ear cavity

neck of stapes, sinus tympani and round window niche from lateral to medial. Sinus tympani could be a blind spot for the surgeon during transmastoid surgery and therefore cholesteatoma at this site may be missed. Basal turn of cochlea opens into round window niche which was the site of cochlear implant in past years but now the implants are inserted just anterior to round window niche. The epitympanum (attic) is superior to the level of the tympanic membrane, the mesotympanum is at the level of the tympanic membrane, and the hypotympanum is inferior to the level of the tympanic membrane. Exact landmarks include two lines, line drawn from

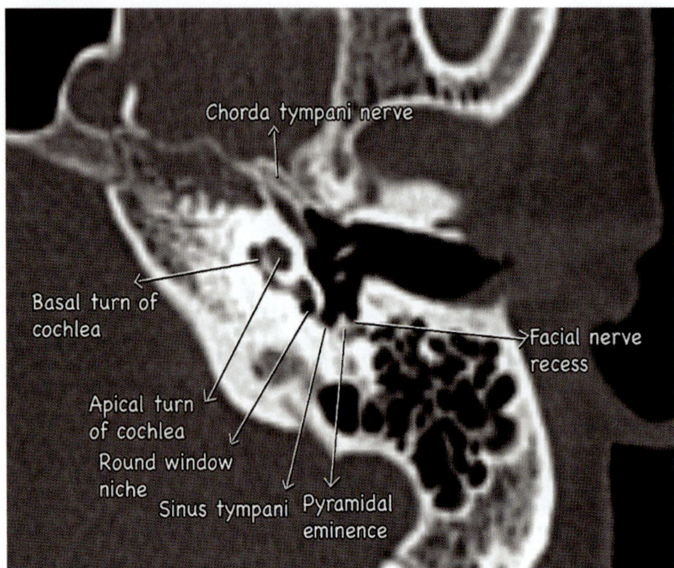

Fig. 3.2.88: CT axial image: Cochlea

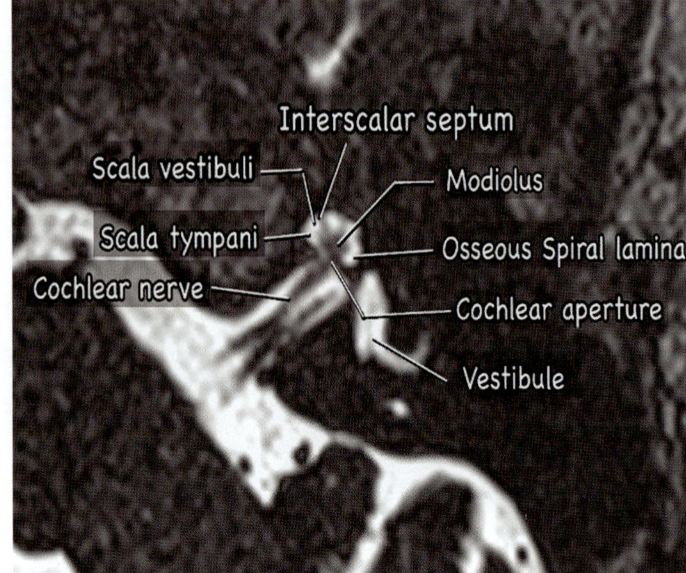

Fig. 3.2.90: Cochlea

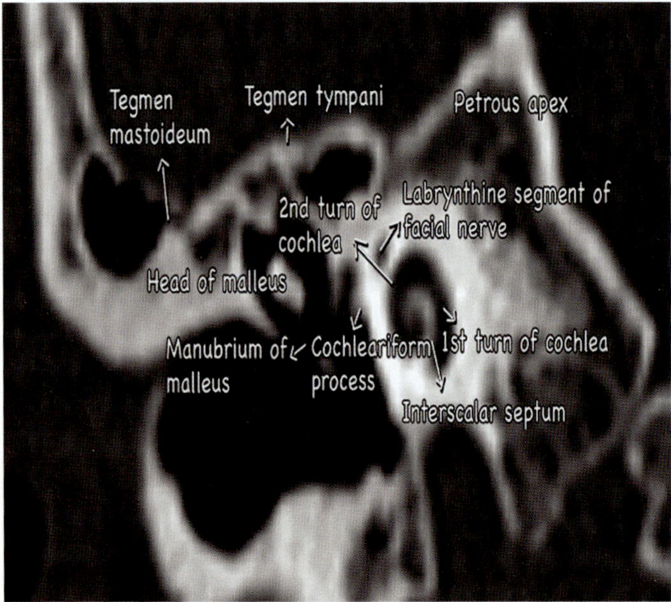

Fig. 3.2.89: CT coronal image: Cochlea

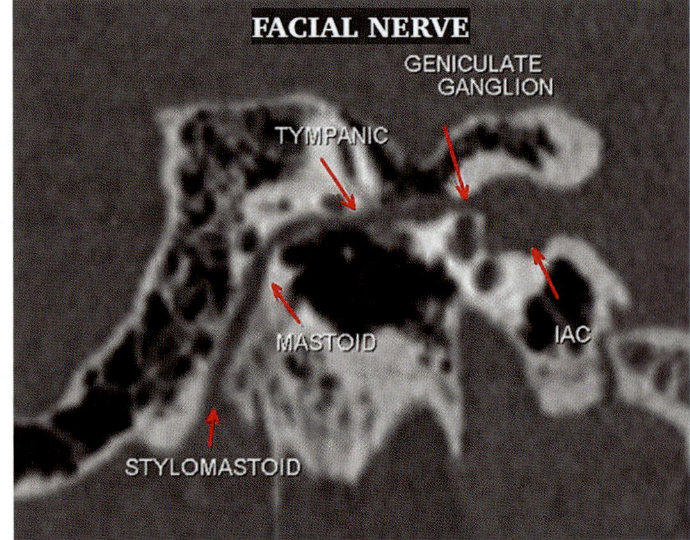

Fig. 3.2.91: Parts of facial nerve

scutum to tympanic portion of facial nerve—dividing epitympanum from mesotympanum, line drawn from tympanic annulus to base of cochlear promontory dividing mesotympanum from hypotympanum. Malleus (head, neck, anterior process, lateral process, and manubrium), incus (body, short process, long process, and lenticular process), and stapes (head/capitellum, anterior crus, posterior crus, and footplate) are the three bones that make up the ossicular chain. These ossicles are supported by anterior, superior and lateral malleal ligament, posterior incudal ligament and tendon of tensor tympani and stapedius muscle. Superior malleal ligament extends from epitympanic roof to head of malleus. Malleus neck provides attachment to anterior and lateral malleal ligament and tensor tympani tendon. Posterior incudal ligament extends from incudal fossa to short process of incus, providing support to incus. Stapes is supported by stapedius tendon inserting on to its neck. Normally, the mastoid is an air-filled cavity divided into numerous compartments by mastoid septations. Aditus ad antrum connects epitympanum to mastoid antrum which is the largest air cell. The Koerner septum, a narrow bony structure generated by the petrosquamous suture that extends posteriorly from the epitympanum and divides the mastoid air cells into medial and lateral compartments, passes through the mastoid air cells. The sigmoid plate separates the medial mastoid air cells from the neighbouring sigmoid sinus. **Inner ear:** The osseous labyrinth, which includes the cochlea, vestibule, and semicircular canals, is located within the petrous part of the ear. The vestibule and semicircular canals are crucial for balance and equilibrium, while the cochlea houses the hearing end organ. The otic capsule is the densest part of the temporal bone that surrounds the osseous labyrinth. The cochlea is a spiral-shaped structure with 2½ to 2¾ turns, with interscalar septae separating the basal, middle, and apical turns. The cochlear promontory is formed when the lateral aspect of the cochlea bulges into the middle ear cavity. Over the cochlear promontory, the Jacobson nerve (a branch of cranial nerve IX) runs. Modiolus is the central bony axis of cochlea which houses the spiral ganglion of cochlear nerve. It is a crown-shaped structure. The bony vestibule is an ovoid region that joins the semicircular canals and is placed above and posterior to the cochlea. Superior, posterior, and lateral (also known as horizontal) canals are all semicircular and positioned orthogonally to one another. At one end of each semicircular canal is a dilatation known as an ampulla. The bony ridge formed by superior semicircular canal at the roof of petrous bone is arcuate eminence, which serves as a landmark for surgeons for entering middle cranial fossa. The endolymphatic duct runs from the posterior aspect of the vestibule to the posterior cerebral fossa, ending in a blind pouch called the endolymphatic sac at the petrous ridge's rear margin. According to the Cincinnati criteria, the bony vestibular aqueduct surrounds the endolymphatic duct and measures up to 1 mm at the midpoint and 2 mm at the operculum. The cochlear aqueduct is a thin bone tube that runs from the basal turn of the cochlea, anterior to the round window, to the subarachnoid region close to the pars nervosa of the jugular foramen, surrounding the perilymphatic duct. The cochlear aqueduct is generally 0.1–0.2 mm wide in the middle and widest at the medial opening. Internal auditory canal transmits the nerves and vessels to inner ear, the medial opening of which is porus acusticus/meatus and lateral opening is the fundus. The fundus of IAC is divided by a horizontal crest, the crista falciformis and a vertical crest, the Bill's bar into superior and inferior, anterior and posterior respectively. Facial nerve resides in anterosuperior, cochlear nerve resides in anteroinferior, superior and inferior vestibular nerve occupying the posterosuperior and posteroinferior compartments, respectively **(Mnemonic: Seven Up Coke Down)**. **The size of IAC depends on the number of nerve bundles. Smaller IAC implies fewer nerve bundles. Usually if IAC is so small that only one nerve is seen, the chance of nerve being the facial nerve is high.** The intratemporal portion of facial nerve consists of four subsegments extending from IAC to the exit of the nerve in stylomastoid foramen. The segments are canalicular segment, labrynthine segment, tympanic segment and mastoid segments and also takes an anterior and a posterior turn called the genu. Anterior genu has the geniculate ganglion. The nerve gives off three branches, namely greater superficial petrosal nerve, stapedius nerve and chorda tympani nerve. The arterial supply to facial nerve is derived from superficial petrosal branch of middle meningeal artery and stylomastoid branch of posterior auricular artery.

3.2.G Mandible

The mandible is the largest and strongest bone in the face, and it is placed inferiorly in the facial skeleton. It serves as a receptacle for the lower teeth and forms the lower jaw. It also forms the temporomandibular joint with the temporal bone on each side. A horizontal body (anteriorly) and two vertical rami (posteriorly) make up the mandible. At the angle of the mandible, the body and the rami meet on each side. The mandible's body is bent and formed like a horseshoe. It has two borders, **alveolar border (superior)** contains 16 sockets to hold the lower teeth. The digastric muscle attaches to the base (inferior). The mandibular symphysis runs through the midline of the body. The fusing of the two halves during development is represented by this little ridge of bone. The symphysis encloses the mental protuberance, a triangular prominence that gives the chin its shape. The mental foramen is located to the side of the mental protuberance (below the second premolar tooth on either side). It serves as a conduit for the transit of neurovascular structures. The mandible has two rami that protrude perpendicularly upwards from the angle of the mandible. Each ramus contains the **head**, it situated posteriorly, and articulates with the temporal bone to form the temporomandibular joint. **Neck** supports the head of the ramus, and site of attachment of the lateral pterygoid muscle. **Coronoid process** is the site of attachment of the temporalis muscle. The **mandibular foramen**, which serves as a route for neurovascular systems, is located on the ramus' internal surface. There are two foramina on the mandible. The **mandibular foramen** is found on the ramus of the mandible's interior surface. The inferior alveolar nerve and the inferior alveolar artery pass through it. They pass through the mandibular foramen, the mandibular canal, and the mental foramen before exiting. The **mental foramen** is located below the second premolar tooth on the mandibular body's exterior surface. The inferior alveolar nerve and artery are able to escape the mandibular canal through this opening. The inferior alveolar nerve becomes the mental nerve when it

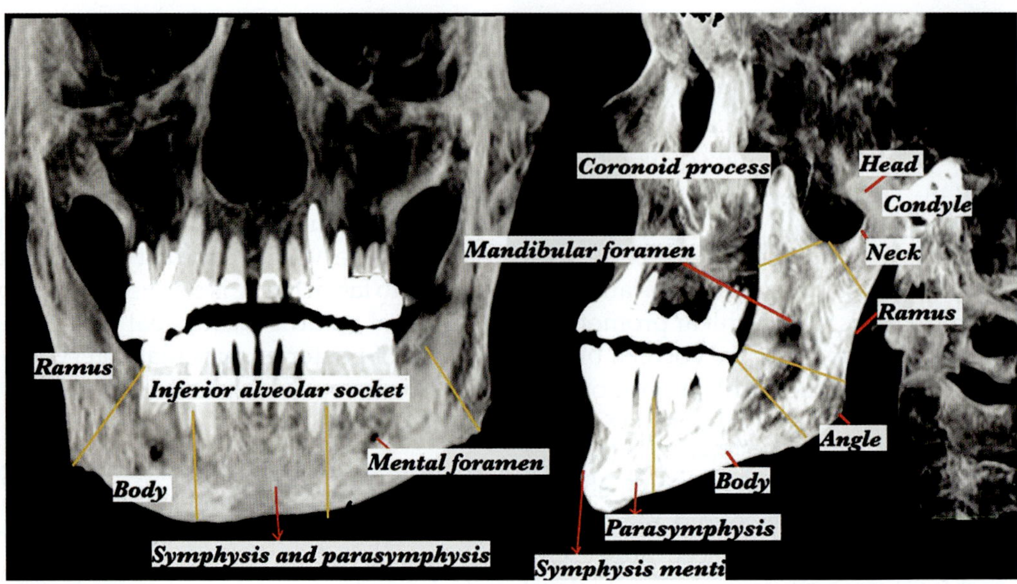

Fig. 3.2.92: Parts of mandible

passes through the mental foramen (innervates the skin of the lower lip and the front of the chin). The mandible serves as a connection point for a variety of muscles, notably the powerful mastication muscles. **Mandibular body** external (lateral) surface gives attachment for mentalis, buccinator, platysma, depressor labii inferioris, depressor anguloris. Internal (medial) surface gives attachment to genioglossus, geniohyoid, mylohyoid and digastric. **Mandibular rami** gives attachment to masseter, temporalis, medial pterygoid and lateral pterygoid. The masseter muscle attaches to the rami, while the temporalis muscle attaches to the coronoid process. The lateral pterygoid attaches to the mandible's neck, while the medial pterygoid attaches to the ramus near the angle of the mandible.

Temporomandibular Joint (TMJ)

TMJ is a complex diarthrodial joint between mandibular condyles and temporal bone with 2 functional movements: Rotation and translation, "ginglymoarthrodial" joint to allow mouth opening (maximum incisal opening). Rotatory movement occurs in inferior compartment between mandibular condyle and articular disc which occurs initially followed by translation movement which occurs in superior compartment between disc and mandibular fossa. Articular surfaces of TMJ are mandibular fossa (articular fossa) located anterior to external auditory meatus and articular eminence (articular tubercle) located anterior to mandibular fossa. Articular disc superior surface is concavoconvex to fit articular eminence and mandibular fossa; disc inferior surface concave to conform to condylar head. Intermediate zone of disc found between anterior and posterior bands. **Anterior band**—anteriorly attaches to joint capsule—portion is integrated into superior aspect of lateral pterygoid muscle. **Posterior band:** Posterior disc margin is bilaminar. Bilaminar zone superior portion composed of loose fibroelastic tissue; attached to posterior mandibular fossa. Inferior portion composed of taut fibrous material; attached to posterior margin of mandibular condyle. Normally the disc is biconcave structure, returns low signal on all sequences, located between the condyle and temporal bone and its posterior band is located at 12 o'clock position with the angle between its posterior limit and vertical orientation of the condyle does not exceed 10°, while some references say 30°. TMJ compartments are superior joint compartment which is between disc and mandibular fossa of T-bone. Inferior joint compartment between disc and condyle—distinct recesses. It has anterior recess which is located anterior to condylar head. Posterior recess is posterior to condylar head, deep to posterior insertion of articular disc onto posterior condylar neck, TMJ capsule and ligaments. Joint capsule is funnel-shaped; extends inferiorly from temporal bone to attach to condylar neck. Temporomandibular ligament: Lateral ligament attached to tubercle on zygoma root above and lateral surface of mandibular neck below. Sphenomandibular ligament, medial ligament that attaches above on spine of sphenoid and below. Pathologic condition is considered to be present if the angle between the posterior band and the vertical orientation of the condyle (twelve o'clock position) exceeds 30 (Rammelsberg, et al). The series of images from Figs 3.2.93 to 3.2.97 shows anatomy of TMJ.

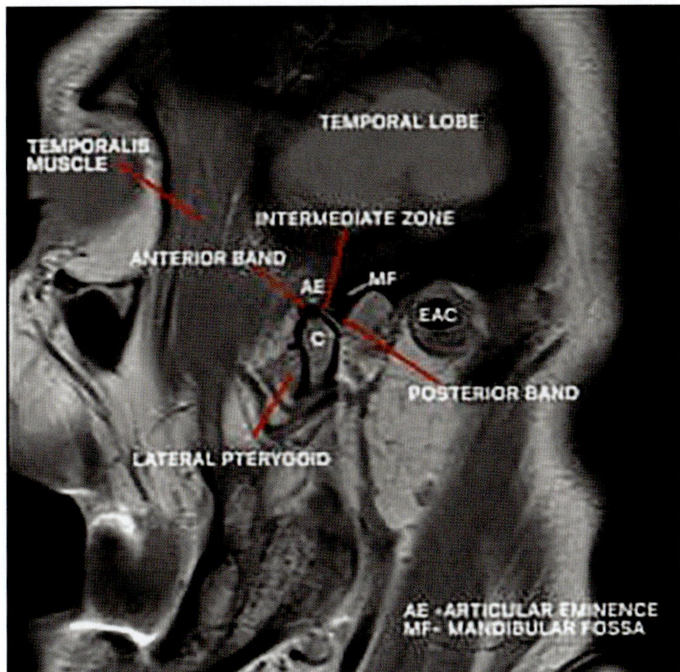

Fig. 3.2.93: MRI T1 sagittal image: TMJ

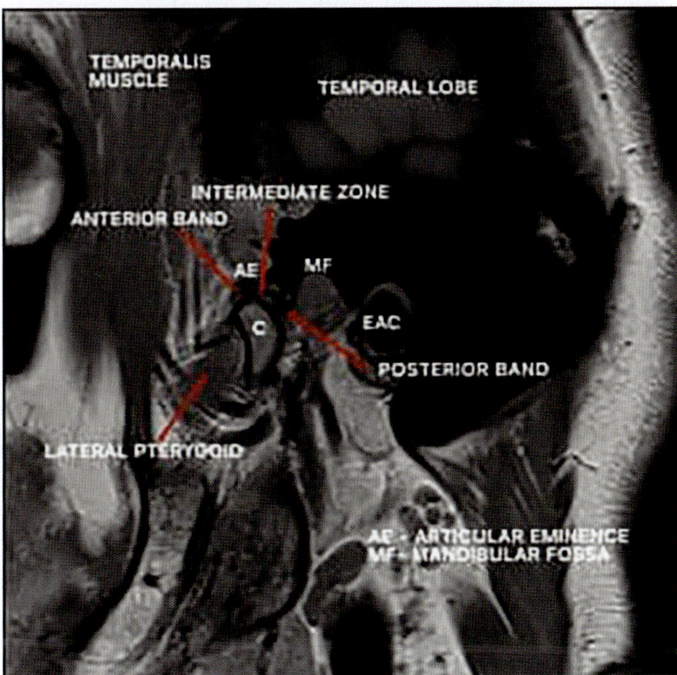

Fig. 3.2.94: MRI T1 sagittal image: TMJ

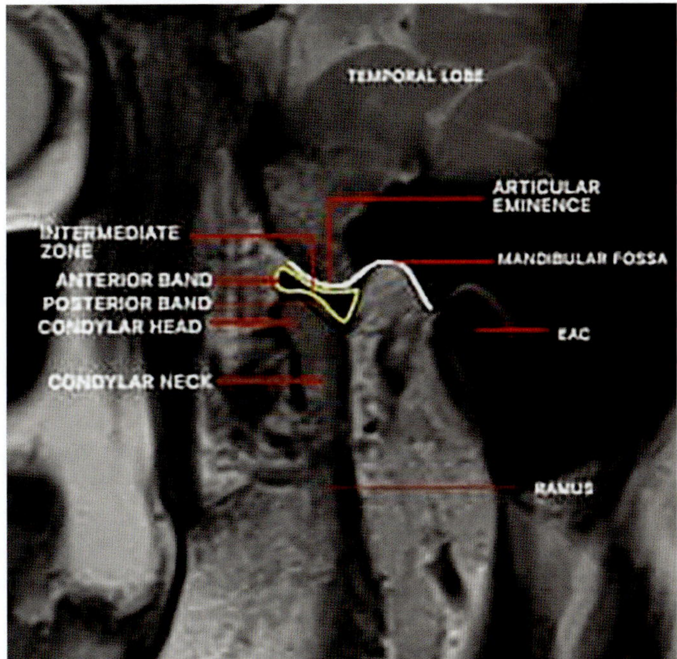

Fig. 3.2.95: MRI T1 sagittal image: TMJ

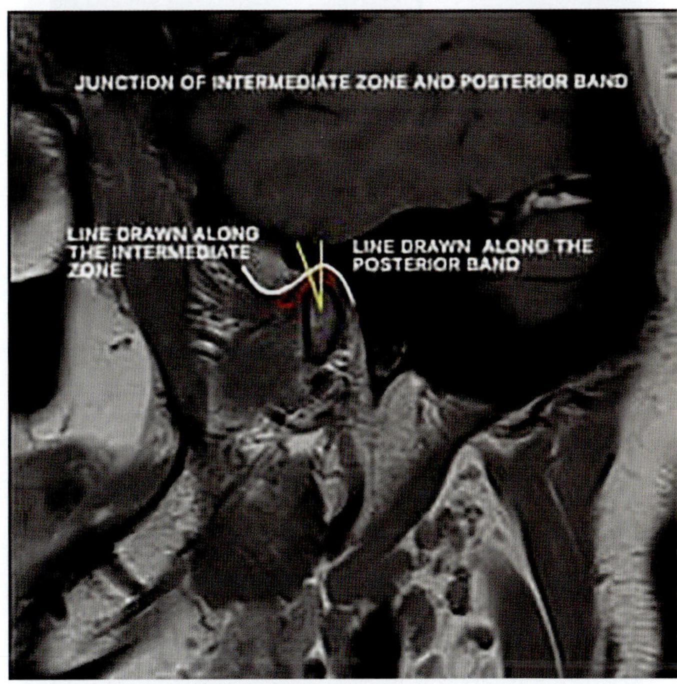

Fig. 3.2.96: MRI T1 sagittal image: TMJ

3.2.H Facial Muscles

Facial muscles are closely intertwined structures and identifying the individual muscles are difficult in cross sectional imaging. They develop from a common embryological origin, arising from the mesoderm of second brachial arch and are innervated by facial nerve. The main function of these muscles is facial expression, differing from other muscles in the body by their direct insertion into dermis through superficial musculoaponeurotic system. Table 3.2.3 provides an overview of facial muscles.

The series of images from Figs 3.2.98 to 3.2.101 shows facial muscles.

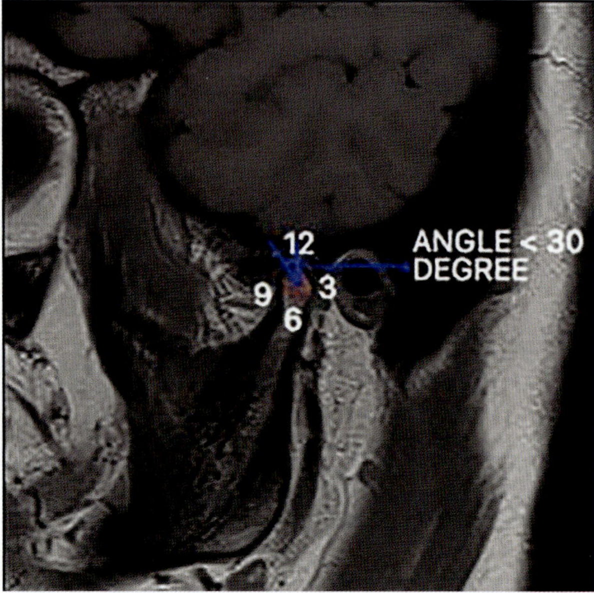

Fig. 3.2.97: MRI T1 sagittal image: TMJ

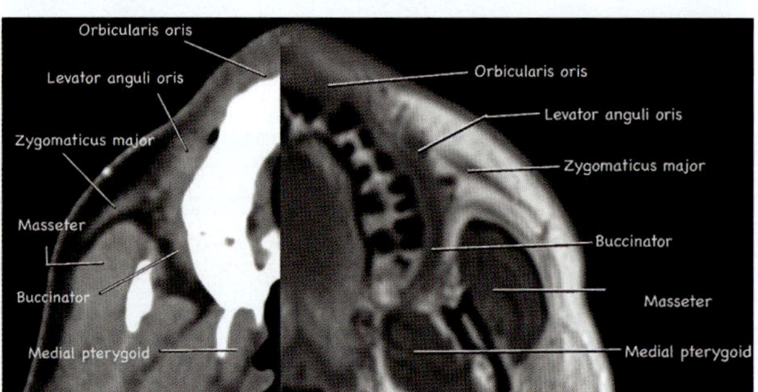

Fig. 3.2.98: CT and MRI: Facial muscles

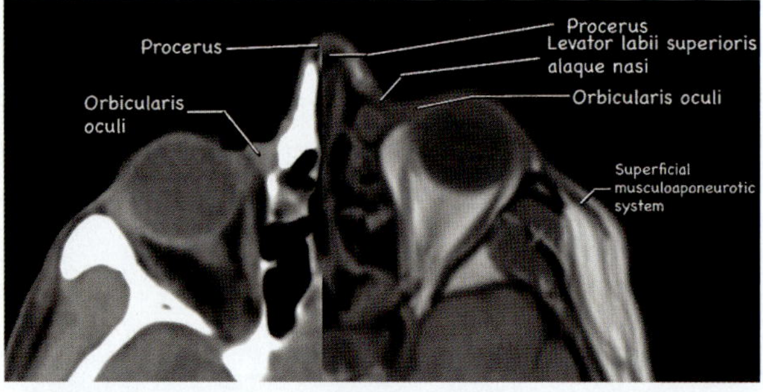

Fig. 3.2.99: CT and MRI: Facial muscles

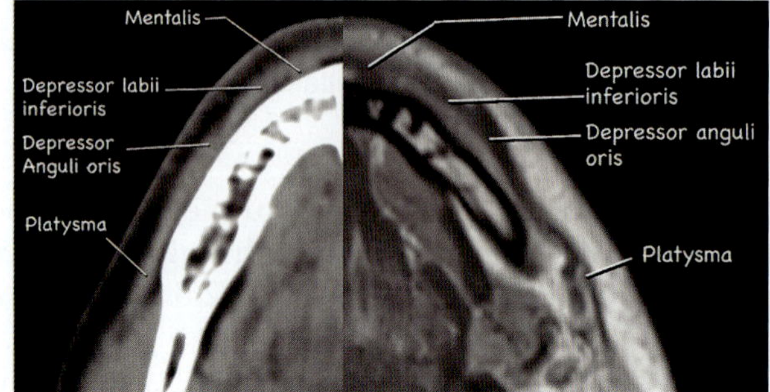

Fig. 3.2.100: CT and MRI: Facial muscles

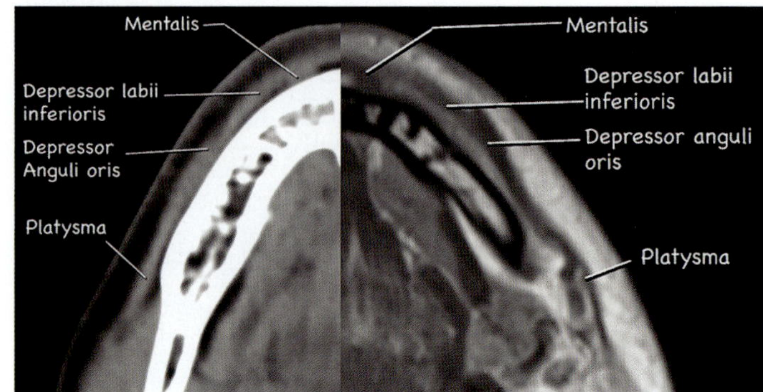

Fig. 3.2.101: CT and MRI: Facial muscles

3.2.I Neck Spaces

The deep spaces of the head and neck refer to compartments delimited by the deep cervical fascia. Because the structure of the deep cervical fascia is slightly different above and below the hyoid bone, the neck spaces are often split into suprahyoid (between the base of the skull and the hyoid bone) and infrahyoid (between the hyoid bone and the clavicles) space. Important SHN space anatomic relationships include their interactions with the skull base, oral cavity and infrahyoid neck. In addition to skull base interactions, the relationships of the SHN spaces to the fat-filled PPSs are key to analyzing SHN masses. Suprahyoid carotid sheath contains ICA, IJV, IX, X, XI, XIIth cranial nerves. Infrahyoid carotid sheath contains CCA, IJV, vagus nerve (Xth cranial nerve). **Parapharyngeal space:** It has bland triangular skull base abutment without critical foramen involved; it empties inferiorly into submandibular space (SMS). **Pharyngeal mucosal space:** It touches posterior basisphenoid and anterior basiocciput, including foramen lacerum; PMS includes nasopharyngeal, oropharyngeal, and hypopharyngeal mucosal surfaces. **Masticator space:** Superior skull base interaction includes zygomatic arch, condylar fossa, skull base including foramen ovale (CNV3), and foramen spinosum (middle meningeal artery); MS ends at inferior surface of body of mandible. **Parotid space:** It abuts floor of external auditory canal, mastoid tip including stylomastoid foramen (CNVII); parotid tail extends inferiorly into posterior SMS. **Carotid space:** It meets jugular foramen (CNIX-XI) floor, hypoglossal canal (CNXII), and petrous internal carotid artery canal; CS can be followed inferiorly to aortic arch. **Retropharyngeal space:** It contacts skull base along lower clivus without involvement of critical structures; it continues inferiorly to empty into DS at T3 level. **Danger space** is immediately posterior to the RPS extends from base of skull to the mediastinum. Anteriorly danger space is separated from the RPS by means of alar fascia, posteriorly it is separated from the prevertebral space

Table 3.2.3: Facial muscles insertion	
Muscles inserting around the orbit	Orbicularis oculi—sphincter of eye, procerus, depressor supercilli, corrugator supercilli
Muscles inserting around the nasal region	Nasalis, depressor septi nasi, dilator naris
Muscles inserting on the upper lip	Levator labii superioris, levator labii superioris alaeque nasi Zygomaticus minor
Muscles inserting on modiolus of mouth	Orbicularis oris, buccinator, risorius, levator angulioris, depressor angulioris, zygomaticus major
Muscles inserting on the lower lip	Mentalis, platysma, depressor labii inferioris

Table 3.2.4: Spaces of neck and its content		
Space	*Contents*	*Lesions*
Pharyngeal mucosal space—PMS (SH)	Mucosa with minor salivary glands, lymphoid tissue, levator and constrictor muscles, cartilaginous eustachian tube	Nasopharyngeal carcinoma, lymphoid hyperplasia, Tornwaldt's cyst, juvenile angiofibroma, tonsil SCC, palatine tonsil inflammation/abscess, lymphoma, minor salivary gland malignancy, Crohn's disease
Parapharyngeal space—PPS (SH)	Fat, minor salivary glands, trigeminal nerve, lymph nodes, internal maxillary/ascending pharyngeal artery	Involved/displaced due to lesions from other spaces, deep lobe parotid neoplasm, masticator space pathology, carotid space mass, PMS mass
Masticator space—MS (SH)	Muscles of mastication, mandibular ramus and body, inferior alveolar nerve	Abscess, bony lesions of mandible, incidental benign conditions—masticator space pseudolesions, pterygoid venous plexus asymmetry, motor denervation fifth cranial nerve (V3), sarcoma, perineural tumour extension
Parotid space—PS (SH)	Parotid gland, intraparotid lymph nodes, facial nerve (CN 7), ECA, retromandibular vein	Focal lesions–pleomorphic adenoma, Warthin tumour, Nodal metastases/lymphoma, salivary gland carcinomas, first branchial cleft cyst Diffuse lesions—parotitis, Sjögren's syndrome, benign lymphoepithelial lesions of HIV, sarcoidosis, lymphoma
Carotid space—CS (both SH and IH)	Cranial nerves (9–12), sympathetic nerves, jugular chain nodes, carotid artery, IJV	Carotid body paraganglioma, Vagal schwannoma, IJV thrombosis, glomus vagale paraganglioma, pseudoaneurysm, neurofibroma
Retropharyngeal space—RPS (both SH and IH)	Lymph nodes, fat, ectopic salivary gland tissue	Reactive/metastatic lymph node, lymphoma, multinodular goitre, ectopic parathyroid adenoma, sympathetic schwannoma
Danger space—DS (both SH and IH)	Loose fatty connective tissue	Potential path for the spread of infection from pharynx into mediastinum
Perivertebral, vertebral (both SH and IH)	Vertebrae, prevertebral muscles, blood vessels paraspinal muscles, phrenic nerve	Vertebral body metastasis, infection, schwannoma, chordoma, plexiform neurofibroma
Visceral space (IH)	Oesophagus, thyroid, parathyroid glands, trachea, nerves and vessels	Benign esophageal lesions and esophageal carcinoma, thyroiditis, thyroid carcinoma, thyroid nodular enlargement, parathyroid adenoma
Posterior cervical space (both SH and IH)	Fat, lymph nodes, CN 11, distal brachial plexus	Lymphadenopathy, third branchial cleft cyst, nerve sheath tumour, nodular fasciitis, thoracic duct cyst, venous diverticulum

SH/SHN: Suprahyoid neck space; IH/IHN: Infrahyoid neck space

by means of prevertebral fascia. **Perivertebral space:** It touches low clivus, encircles occipital condyles and foramen magnum; PVS continues inferiorly to level into thorax and is divided by fascial slip into prevertebral and paraspinal components. The IHN space anatomic relationships are defined by their superior and inferior projections and include the visceral space (VS), posterior cervical space (PCS), CS, RPS, and PVS.

The **visceral space** has no SHN component, instead projecting only inferiorly into the superior mediastinum. The **posterior cervical space** extends superiorly to the mastoid tip and ends inferiorly at the clavicle. It is predominantly an IHN space. **The carotid space** begins at the floor of jugular foramen and carotid canal and extends inferiorly to the aortic arch. Retropharygeal space begins at the ventral clivus superiorly and traverses

SHN, IHN to T3 level. Danger space is immediately posterior to the RPS but continues beyond T3 level into mediastinum. The series of images from Figs 3.2.102 to 3.2.109 shows neck spaces.

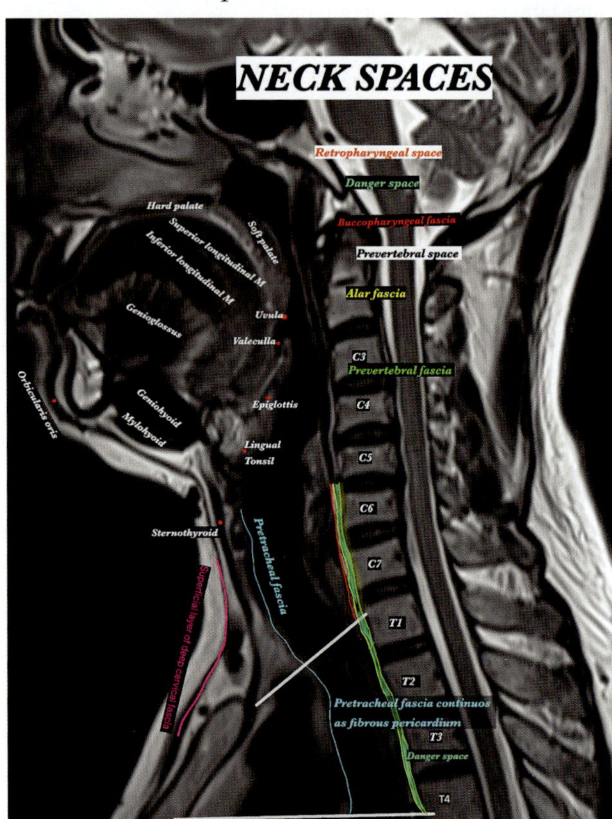

Fig. 3.2.102: MRI T2 sagittal image: Neck spaces

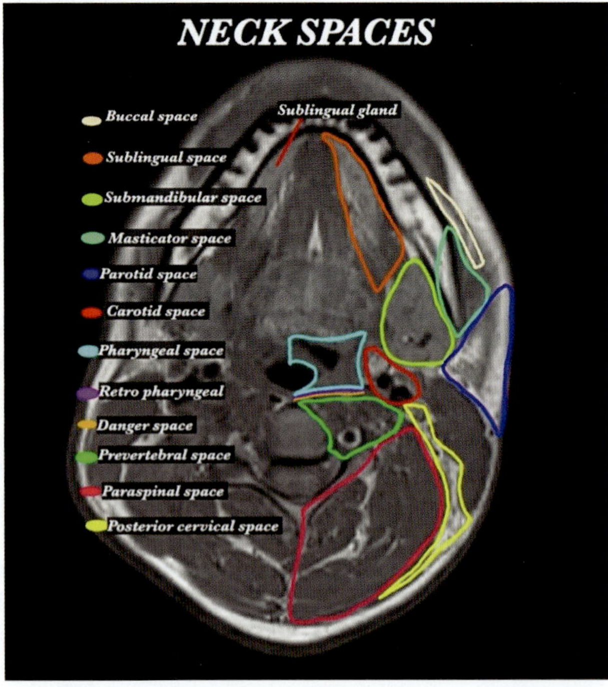

Fig. 3.2.103: MRI T1 axial image: Neck spaces

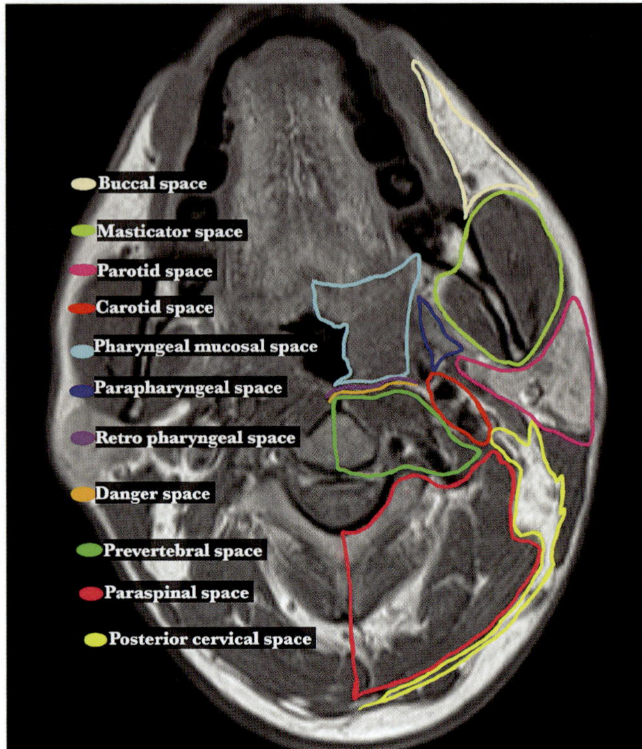

Fig. 3.2.104: MRI T1 axial image: Neck spaces

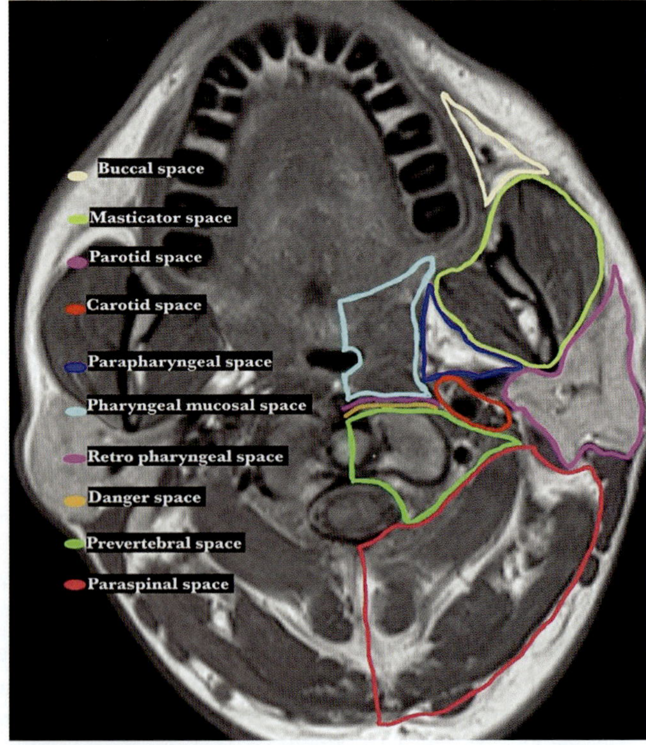

Fig. 3.2.105: MRI T1 axial image: Neck spaces

Neck nodes: Lymph node enlargement/lymphadenopathy may associated with malignancy, acute infection, granulomatous and autoimmune disease. In case of

3

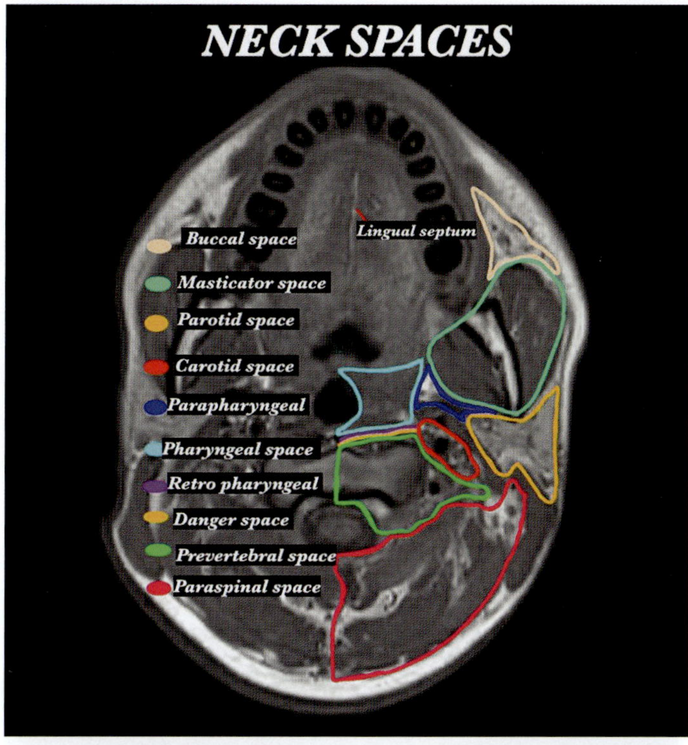

Fig. 3.2.106: MRI T1 axial image: Neck spaces

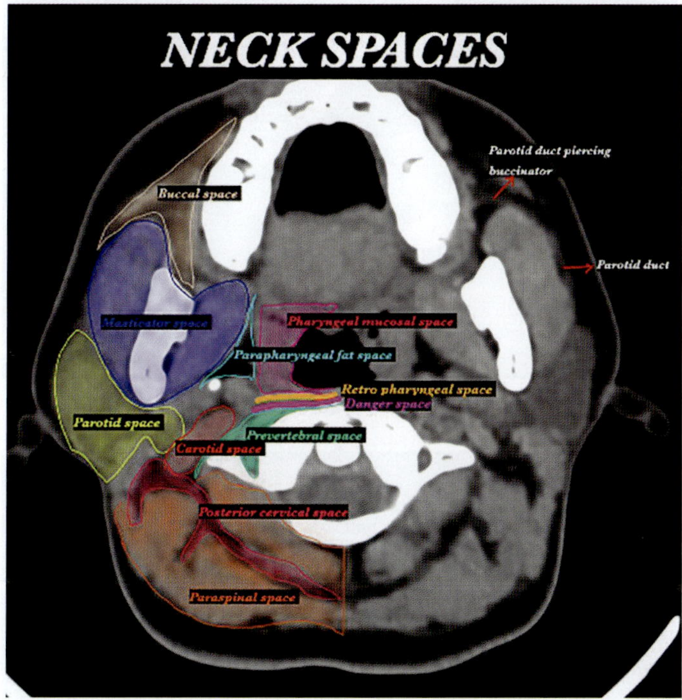

Fig. 3.2.107: CT axial image: Neck spaces

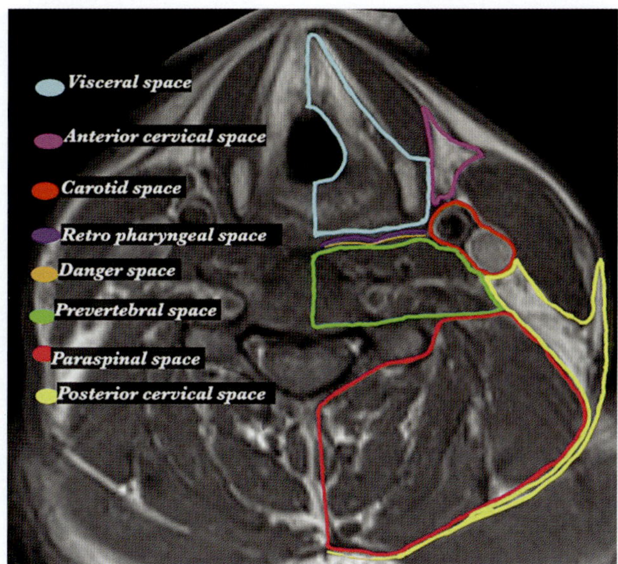

Fig. 3.2.108: MRI T1 axial image: Neck spaces

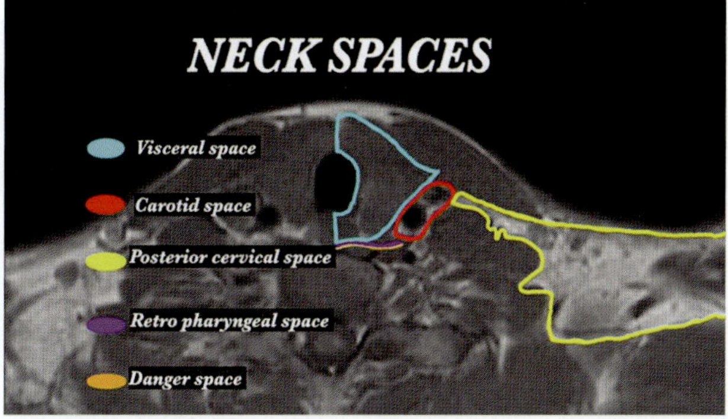

Fig. 3.2.109: Neck spaces

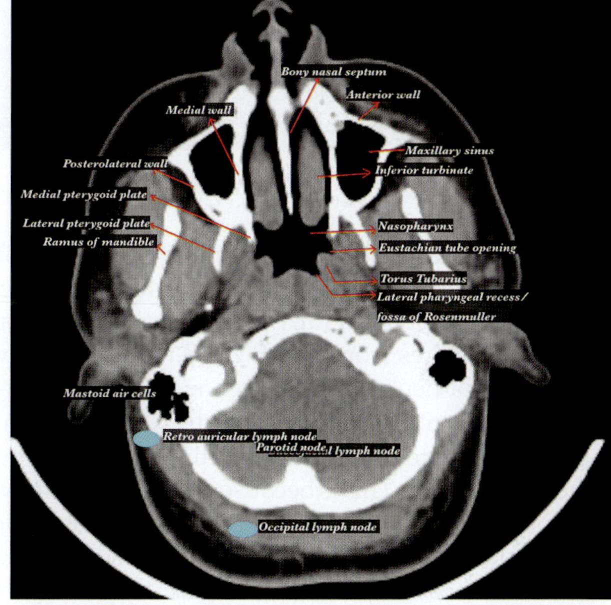

Fig. 3.2.110: CT axial section: Nasopharynx

malignancy, involvement of specific nodal groups is an indicator of pathologically-affected organs and tissues. So, knowledge of the anatomic relationships of the lymphatic nodal levels and the structures they drain is important for appropriate diagnosis and

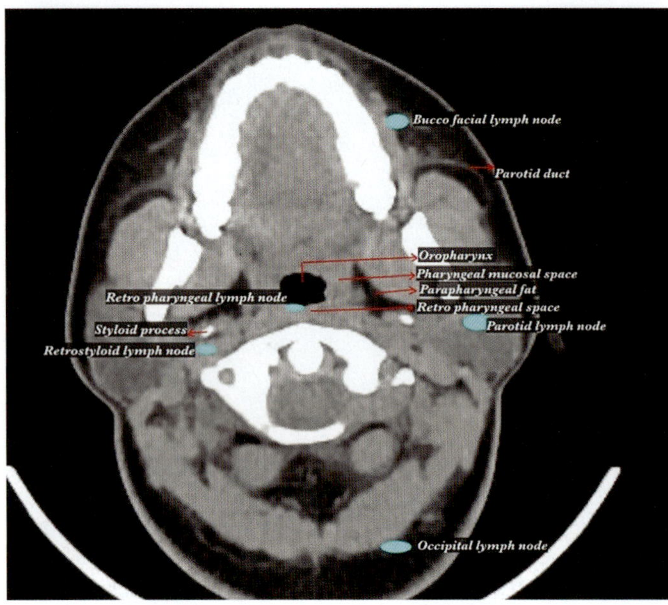

Fig. 3.2.111: CT neck: Lymph nodes

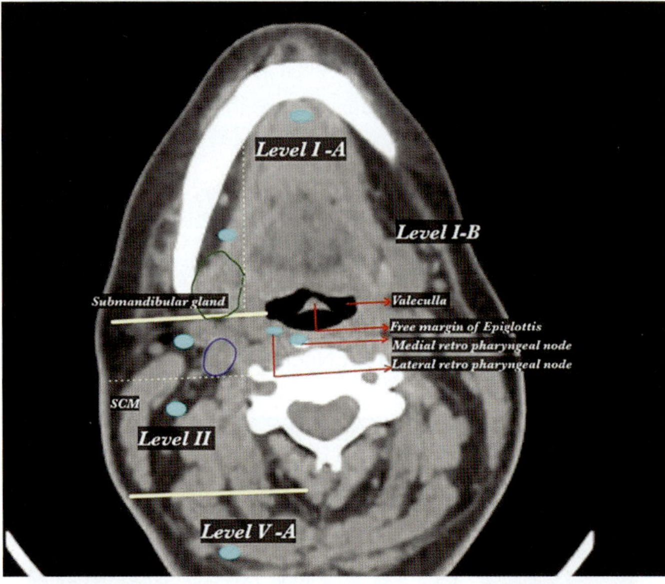

Fig. 3.2.112: CT neck: Lymph nodes

appropriate therapy. Proper knowledge of lymphatic drainage will help in preferring the mode of treatment (whether locoregional therapy or surgery/irradiation). The series of images from Figs 3.2.110 to 3.2.123 shows various levels of neck nodes.

The facial, parotid, mastoid, occipital and retropharyngeal are not included in the simplified level classification system. This is because the level system was first introduced within the framework of neck dissection and these nodes are not normally included in the surgical procedure. If these nodes are enlarged, they are given their anatomical names.

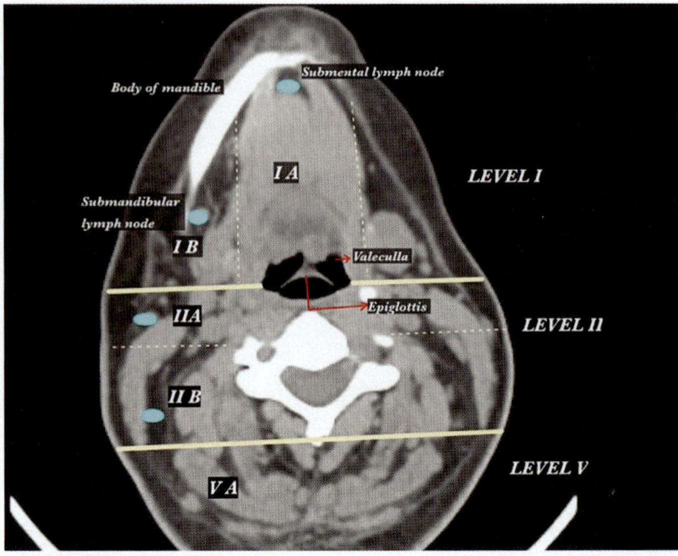

Fig. 3.2.113: CT neck: Lymph nodes

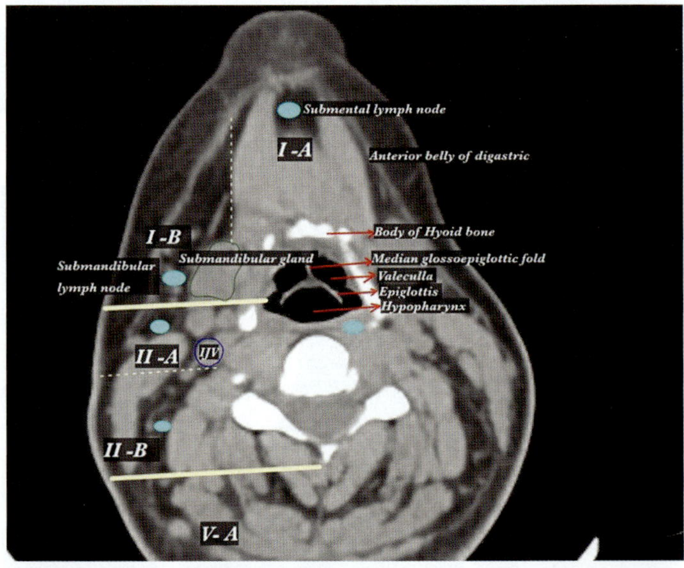

Fig. 3.2.114: CT neck: Lymph nodes

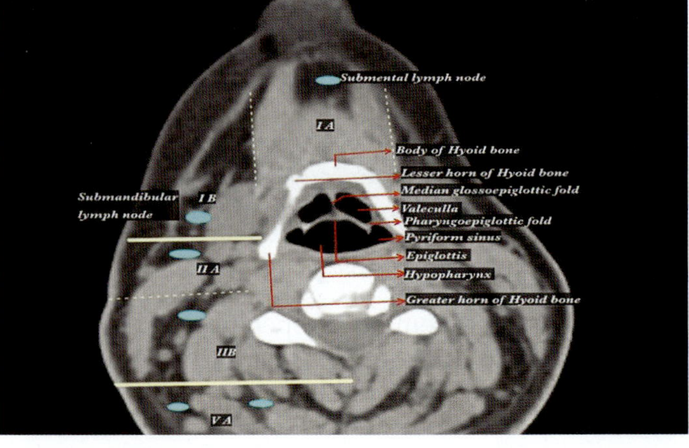

Fig. 3.2.115: CT neck: Lymph nodes

Table 3.2.5: Cervical lymph nodes

Levels of node	*Draining areas*	*Associated malignancies*
Level IA (submental) nodes: Located in the submental space, between the anterior bellies of the digastric muscles	Skin of the mental region, the lower lip, the anterior portion of the oral tongue, and the floor of the mouth	Malignancies of the floor of the mouth, anterior oral tongue, mandibular alveolar ridge, and lower lip
Level IB (submandibular) nodes found in the submandibular space, around the submandibular gland.	Drains the efferent lymphatics from level I-A and also drain the mucosa of the cheek and skin, both upper and lower lips, the mouth floor, and the anterior oral tongue, the lower nasal cavity, both hard and soft palates, and both maxillary and mandibular alveolar ridges.	Malignancies of the anterior nasal cavity, oral cavity, soft-tissues of the mid-face, and submandibular gland
Level II A nodes (upper jugular node): Anterior, lateral, medial or posterior to IJV, if posterior to IJV, it is inseparable from IJV Level-IIB nodes (upper spinal accessory node): Posterior to IJV with fat plane separating nodes and vein	It drains the efferent lymphatics of face, parotid gland, level Ia, level Ib, and retropharyngeal nodes and receives direct drainage from the nasal cavity, pharynx, larynx, external auditory canal, middle ear, and the sublingual and submandibular glands	Malignancies involving the nasal and oral cavities, nasopharynx, oropharynx, hypopharynx, larynx, and major salivary glands
Level III (mid-jugular node): From inferior margin of hyoid bone to inferior margin of cricoid cartilage, anterior to the posterior margin of sternocleidomastoid	Drains the effernt lymphatics from level II and V, and partially from the retropharyngeal, pretracheal, and recurrent laryngeal nodes. It receives direct drainage from the base of the tongue, tonsils, larynx, hypopharynx, and thyroid gland	Malignancies of the oral cavity, pharynx and larynx
Level IV (lower jugular node): From inferior margin of cricoid cartilage to the level of clavicle, anterior to line connecting posterior margin of sternocleidomastoid and posterolateral margin of anterior scalene muscle, lateral to carotid arteries	Drains the effernt lymphatics from level II and V, and partially from the retropharyngeal, pretracheal, and recurrent laryngeal nodes. It receives direct drainage from the hypopharynx, larynx, thyroid gland and esophagus	Malignancies of the hypopharynx, larynx, thyroid, cervical esophagus, and rarely, the anterior oral cavity. Deposits from the anterior oral cavity can manifest without proximal nodal involvement.
Level V-A (upper level V node): From skull base to inferior margin of cricoid cartilage, posterior to posterior margin of sternocleidomastoid. **Level V-B (lower level V node):** From the inferior margin of cricoid cartilage to level of clavicle. Posterior to the line connecting posterior margin of sternocleidomastoid and posterolateral margin of anterior scalene	Drain the efferent lymphatics from the occipital, retro-auricular, and parietal scalp nodes. It receives direct drainage from the skin of the lateral and posterior neck and shoulder, the nasopharynx, oropharynx, and thyroid gland.	Metastatic deposits from malignancies of the nasopharynx, oropharynx, and thyroid
Level VI (visceral node): Between carotid arteries from level of inferior border of hyoid bone to the level of superior margin of manubrium	Drains the integuments of the lower face and the anterior neck (drains the efferent lymphatics from the anterior floor of the mouth, tip of the oral tongue, lower lip, thyroid gland, glottic and supraglottic larynx, hypopharynx, and cervical esophagus)	Malignancies of the lower lip, soft tissues of the chin, such as advanced gingiva-mandibular carcinoma, oral cavity (floor of the mouth and anterior oral tongue), thyroid, glottic and subglottic larynx, the apex of the piriform sinus, and the cervical esophagus.
Level VII (superior mediastinal node): Between carotid arteries below the level of superior margin of manubrium, caudal to the level of innominate vein	Drain the efferent lymphatics from the nasopharynx, eustachian tube, and soft palate	Metastatic deposits from malignancies of the nasopharynx, pharyngeal wall, and oropharynx including tonsillar fossa and soft palate

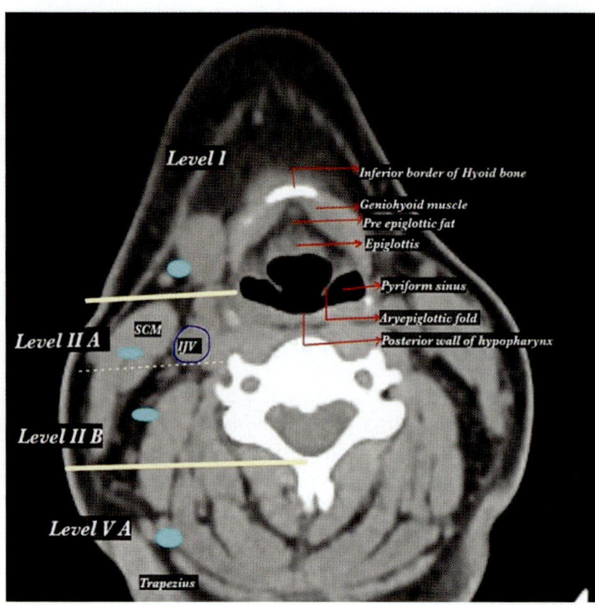

Fig. 3.2.116: CT neck: Lymph nodes

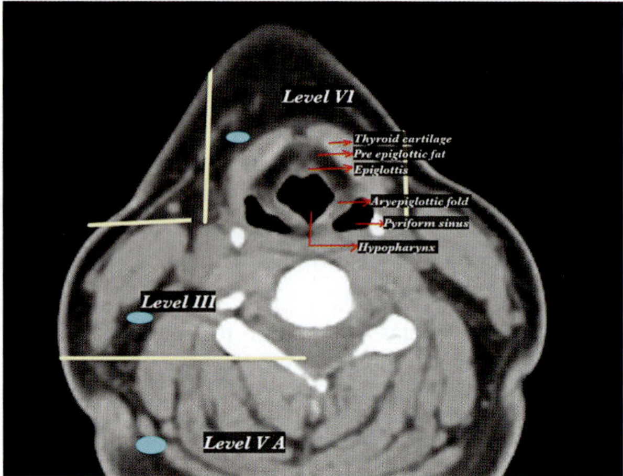

Fig. 3.2.117: CT neck: Lymph nodes

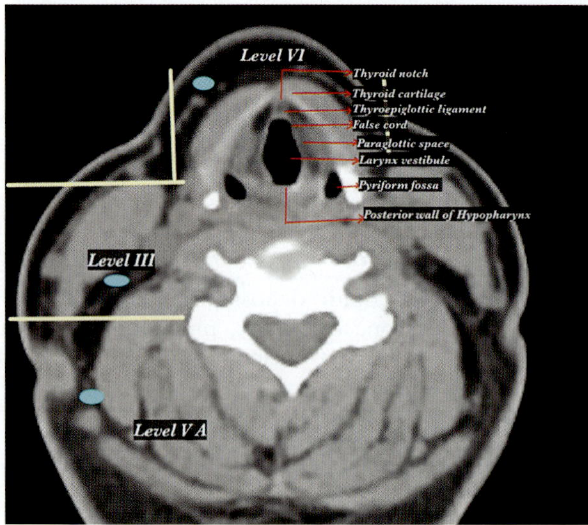

Fig. 3.2.118: CT neck: Lymph nodes

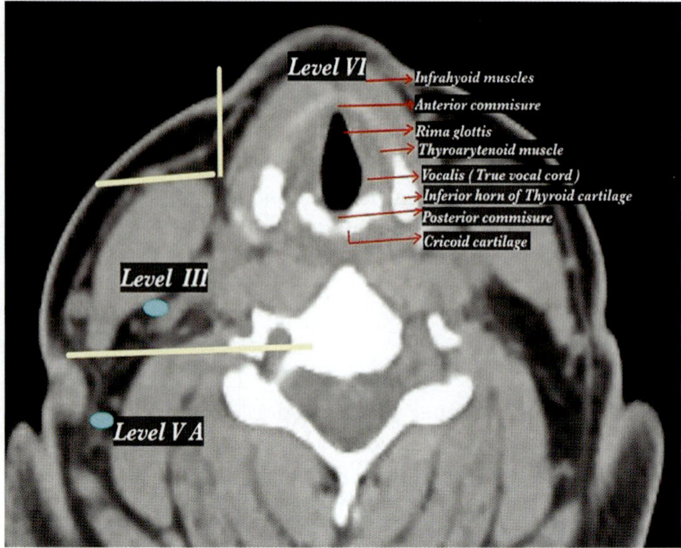

Fig. 3.2.119: CT neck: Lymph nodes

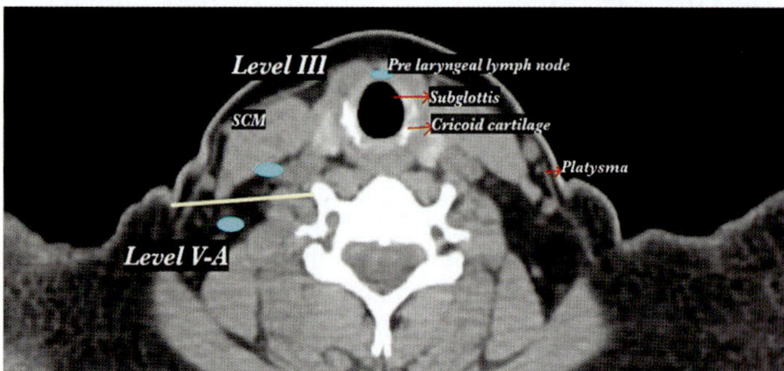

Fig. 3.2.120: CT neck: Lymph nodes

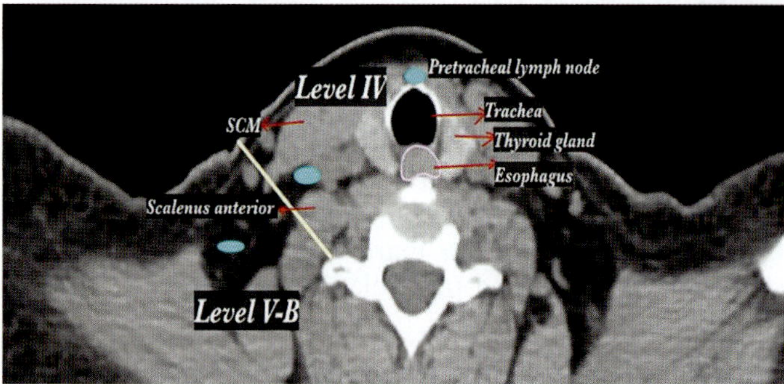

Fig. 3.2.121: CT neck: Lymph nodes

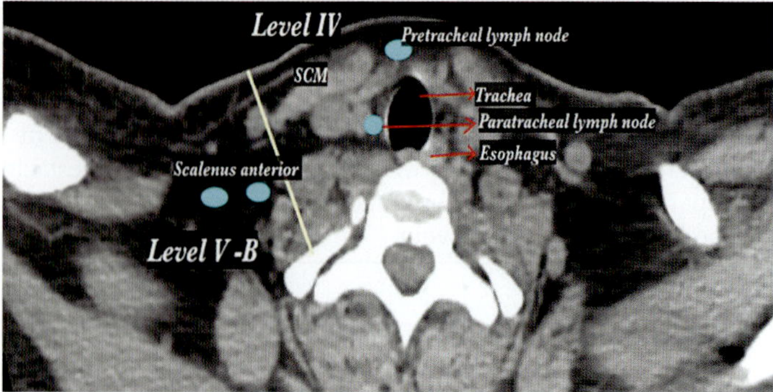

Fig. 3.2.122: CT neck: Lymph nodes

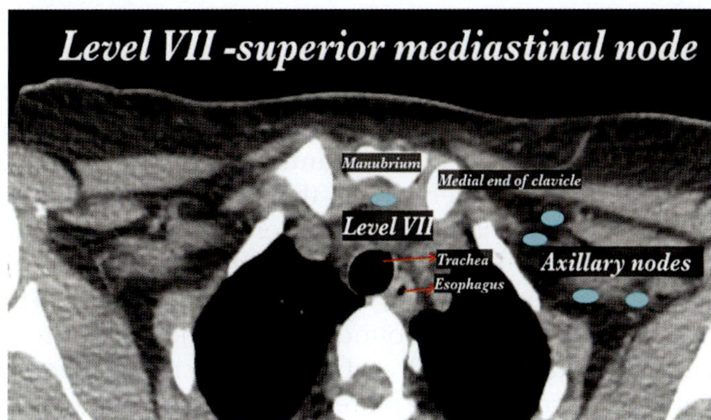

Fig. 3.2.123: CT neck: Lymph nodes

3.2.J Pharynx

The pharynx is a funnel-shaped skeletal muscle tube that runs from the cranial base to the cricoid cartilage's lower edge. The pharynx is located anterior to the cervical spine's vertebral bodies, prevertebral muscles, and retropharyngeal space's loose connective tissue. The neck muscles, lateral sections of the hyoid bone and thyroid cartilage, and the carotid sheath all limit the pharynx laterally. The pharynx and the larynx are anatomically and embryologically connected. The epiglottis and the rest of the supraglottis are pharyngeal in origin, not laryngeal. The pharynx is divided into three parts—the nasopharynx (epipharynx), oropharynx (mesopharynx), and laryngopharynx (hypopharynx). The nasopharynx is essentially a respiratory tract structure that connects the nasal cavity anteriorly. The basisphenoid and basilar part of the occipital bone are abutted by the superior and posterior borders of the nasopharynx. The soft palate separates it from the oropharynx on the lower side. The opening between the nasopharynx and the oropharynx is known as the velopharyngeal portal. The oropharynx and hypopharynx are pharyngeal divisions that help with swallowing. At the level of the anterior tonsillar pillars, the oral cavity extends into the oropharynx at the palatoglossal isthmus (palatoglossal folds). The oropharynx is located behind the oral cavity, stretching craniocaudally from the soft palate to the hyoid bone, where it is arbitrary divided from the hypopharynx. The hypopharynx is located behind and to the side of the larynx, stretching from the pharyngoepiglottic fold to the lower border of the cricopharyngeal muscle at the level of the cricoid cartilage's inferior margin. The epiglottis, aryepiglottic folds, and mucosa atop the muscular process of the paired arytenoid cartilages comprise the laryngeal aditus, which connects with the larynx.

The post-cricoid region is the anterior wall of hypopharynx from the level of superior border of arytenoid cartilage to the inferior border of cricoid cartilage, then it continues as esophageal inlet, lateral to the post-cricoid region we have pyriform sinus, posteriorly lumen of hypopharynx present, anteriorly we have posterior cricoarytenoid muscle. It has mucosa, intramural fat, and a rich venous plexus. A rich venous plexus in this region drains into superior laryngeal veins. It is more prominent in infants and engorges during crying, known as the "postcricoid cushion" on laryngoscopy, it acts as a protection against emesis.

Muscles of pharynx: The superior, middle, and inferior constrictor muscles make up the outer circular layer. The superior constrictor muscle arises from the pterygoid process, the pterygomandibular ligament/raphe, and the posterior end of the mylohyoid line of the jaw. At the pharyngeal tubercle and pharyngeal raphe, the superior constrictor muscle inserts into the base of the skull. The pharyngeal raphe is a tendinous seam in the middle of the throat where the constrictor muscles connect. When the superior constrictor muscle contracts, it constricts the upper portion of the pharynx. The middle constrictor muscle originates from the greater and lesser horn of the hyoid bone and stylohyoid ligament. The middle constrictor inserts into the median pharyngeal raphe as well as blending in with fibers of the superior and inferior constrictors. The middle constrictor muscle contracts to constrict the middle portion of the pharynx. The inferior pharyngeal constrictor muscle further divides into two muscles, the thyropharyngeus, and the cricopharyngeus muscle. The thyropharyngeus muscle originates from the thyroid cartilage and inserts into the median pharyngeal raphe. The cricopharyngeus muscle originates from the cricoid cartilage and blends into the esophageal muscle. When the inferior constrictors contract, they constrict the lower portion of the pharynx. These constrictor muscles work together and contract to push food after swallowing to propel it from the oral cavity into the esophagus.The inner longitudinal layer consists of the palatopharyngeus, salpingopharyngeus, and stylopharyngeus muscle. Figures 3.2.124 and 3.2.125 show anatomy of pharynx.

3.2.K Larynx

The larynx runs from the tip of the epiglottis to the cricoid cartilage's inferior edge. The four main laryngeal cartilages are the epiglottis, thyroid, cricoid, and paired arytenoid cartilages. The epiglottis is the superiormost, leaf-shaped cartilage in the midline. It has a set part and a free margin (stem). The free epiglottic edge is attached to the hyoid bone by the hyoepiglottic ligament, and the epiglottic stem is attached to the inner surface of the thyroid cartilage by the thyroepiglottic ligament. The

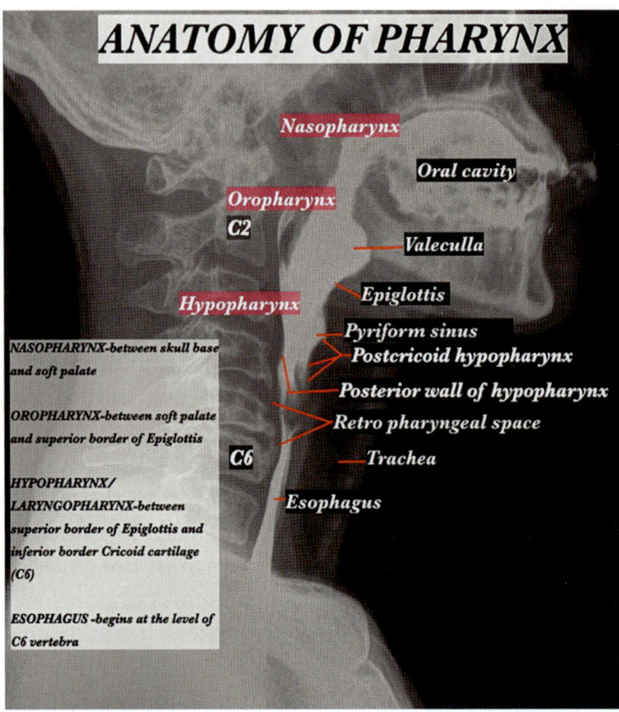

Fig. 3.2.124: X-ray lateral view barium swallow: Pharynx

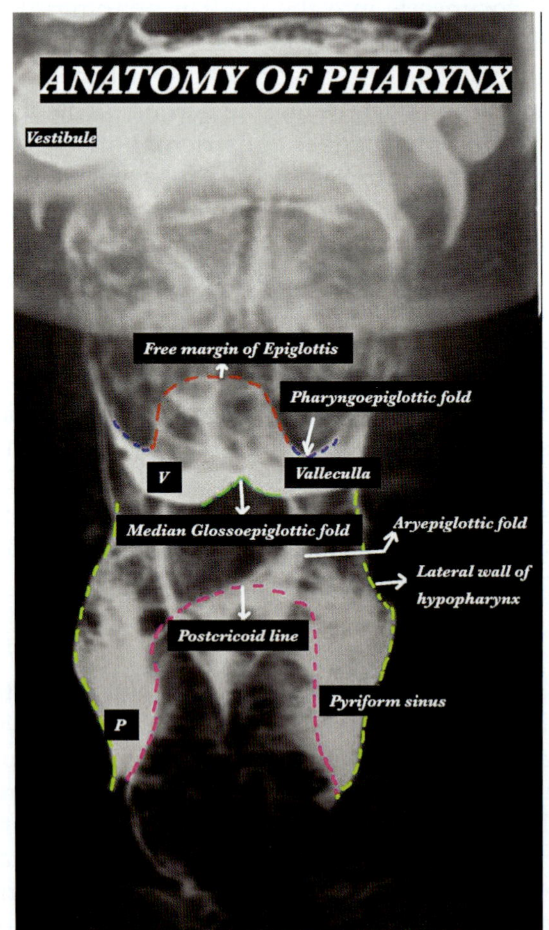

Fig. 3.2.125: X-ray frontal view barium swallow: Pharynx

median glosso-epiglottic fold runs over the hyoepiglottic ligament and projects above the level of the hyoid, and the free margin of the epiglottis is closely connected to the base of the tongue. The superior and inferior cornua are formed by two laminae joined anteriorly and expanded posteriorly in the thyroid cartilage. At the cricothyroid joint, the superior cornua attaches to the thyrohyoid ligament, whereas the inferior cornua articulates medially with the sides of the cricoid. The cricoid is the laryngeal foundation and the inferiormost ring-shaped laryngeal cartilage. The cricoarytenoid joints are formed by the paired arytenoid cartilages that reside along the upper border of the cricoid lamina. The arytenoid's vertical height spans the laryngeal ventricle. The vestibular ligament is attached to the apex of the arytenoid, which corresponds to the level of the false cords. The vocal processes, which attach the vocal ligament running along the inner margin of true vocal cords, protrude anteriorly from the base of the arytenoids. The imaging appearance of these cartilages depends on whether or not they are ossified. The epiglottis and the vocal process of arytenoids are fibrocartilages that do not ossify. Nonossified cartilages have soft tissue attenuation on CT and intermediate signal intensity on T1-weighted (T1W) and T2-weighted (T2W) images. The thyroid, cricoid and arytenoid are hyaline cartilages that show progressive ossification with age. On CT, the ossified cartilages have hyperattenuating inner and outer margins with low attenuation of the medullary cavity. On MRI, the ossified cortical margins are of low signal and the fat-filled medullary cavity is of high signal on T1W and T2W images.

Laryngeal ventricular complex (LVC): It consists of the false cords, genuine cords, and the laryngeal ventricle in between.

Supraglottis is an area between the epiglottis and the laryngeal ventricle.

Glottis extends from the laryngeal ventricle to an imaginary plane 1 cm below this level.

Subglottis extends from the undersurface of true cord to inferior surface of cricoid cartilage.

Anterior and posterior commissure: The anterior commissure is the anterior meeting point of the true vocal cords in midline. It comprises the anterior junction of the two vocal cords, the thyroid cartilage and the Broyle's ligament, a fibrous structure connecting the vocal ligaments to the cartilage.

The posterior commissure is the mucosal surface on the anterior surface of the cricoid cartilage between the arytenoid cartilages. Both the commissures are seen very well on the axial images.

Table 3.2.6: Anatomy at the level of true and false vocal cord	
Findings at the level of false cord (supraglottis)	*Findings at the level of true cord (glottis)*
Presence of paraglottic fat pad, lateral to the false vocal cord	Absence of paraglottic fat pad. Presence of thyroarytenoid muscle, medial border of which forms the vocalis
-	Cricoarytenoid joint seen at this level
-	Anterior and posterior commissures noted
-	RLN noted at this level

The paraglottic space (PGS) and the pre-epiglottic space (PES): The PGS is best seen on axial CT and MR sections through the supraglottis, where it is entirely composed of fat, and is located deep to the mucosal surfaces of the true and false cords, bound laterally by the thyroid and cricoid cartilages. It extends caudally up to the actual vocal cords' undersurface. On coronal pictures, the entire extent is readily seen. The PGS connects the extralaryngeal soft tissues between the thyroid and cricoid cartilages anterolaterally, providing an essential route for extralaryngeal tumor propagation. The pre-epiglottic space (PES) is a fatty, lymphatic-rich region. PES bounded superiorly by hyoepiglottic ligament, anteriorly by the thyrohyoid membrane, inferiorly by the thyroepiglottic ligament, and posteriorly by the epiglottis. The PES and PGS communicate superiorly. Sagittal pictures are preferable for delineating the complete extent of the PES; however, axial imaging can also be used to do so. Findings of vocal cord palsy: Thickening of aryepiglottic fold with widening of pyriform sinus. (If thickening of vocal cord is due to edema/tumour, it results in narrowing of pyriform sinus.)

The series of images from Figs 3.2.126 to 3.2.139 shows laryngeal structures.

Strap muscles of neck: The infrahyoid muscles also known as strap muscles are group of four paired muscles in the anterior neck situated below the hyoid bone,

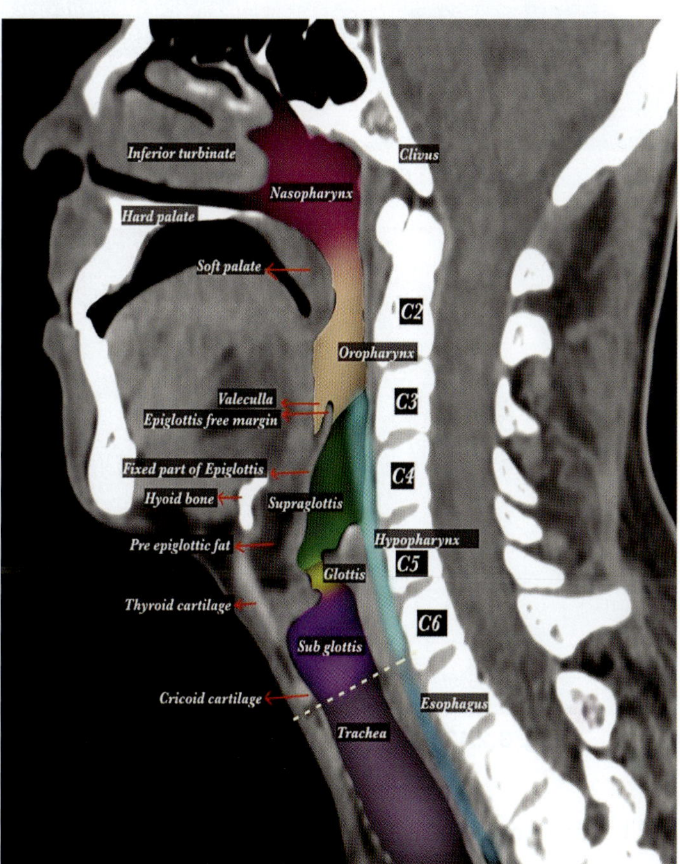

Fig. 3.2.126: CT neck: Sagittal view

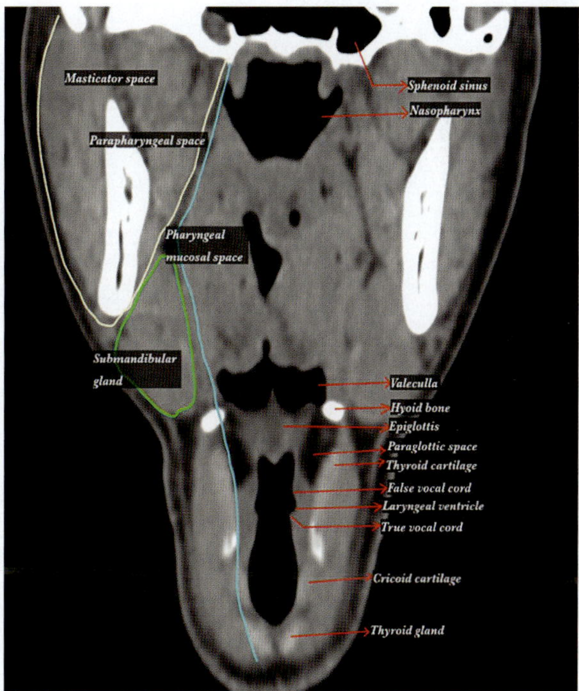

Fig. 3.2.127: CT coronal image: Naso/oropharynx

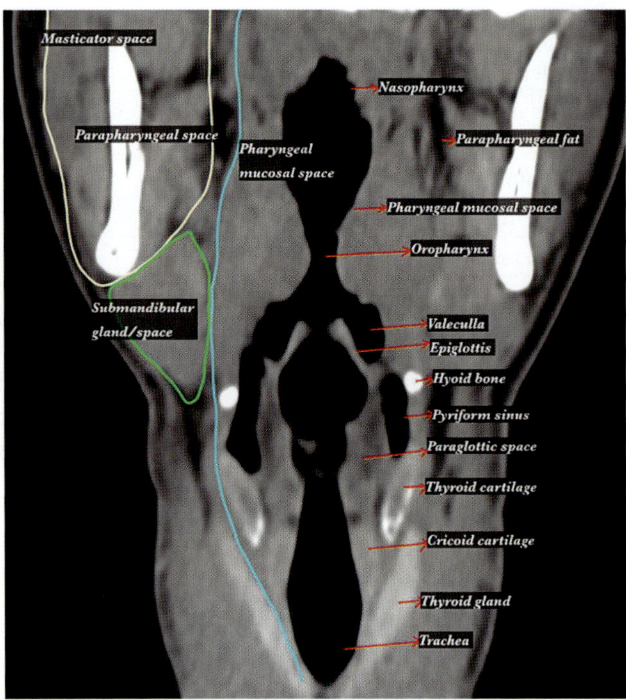

Fig. 3.2.128: CT coronal image: Naso/oropharynx

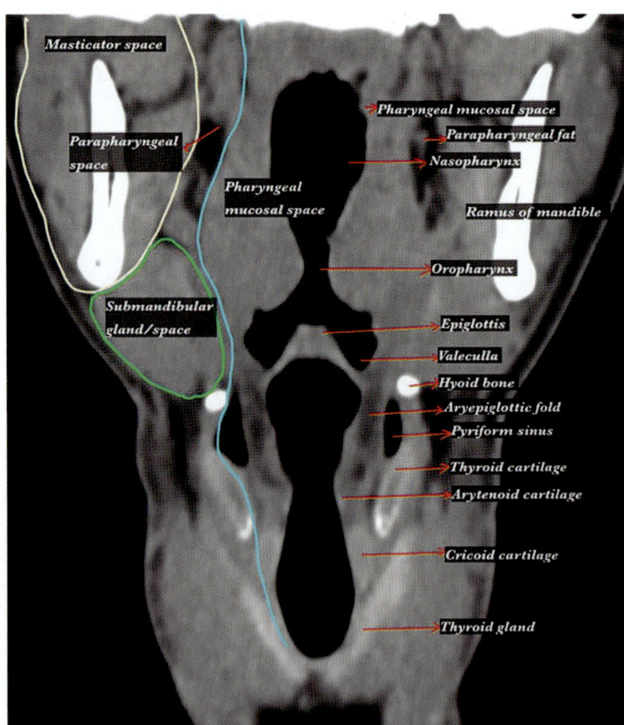

Fig. 3.2.129: CT coronal image: Naso/oropharynx

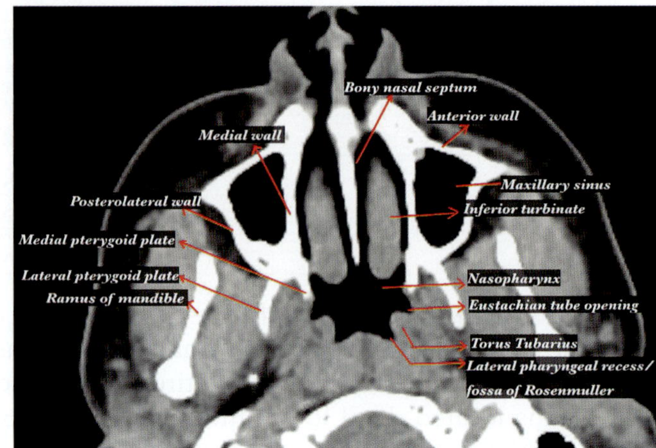

Fig. 3.2.130: CT axial image: Oropharynx

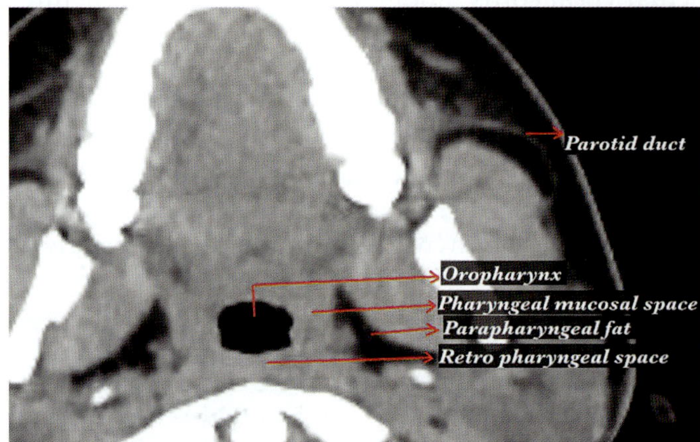

Fig. 3.2.131: CT axial image: Oropharynx

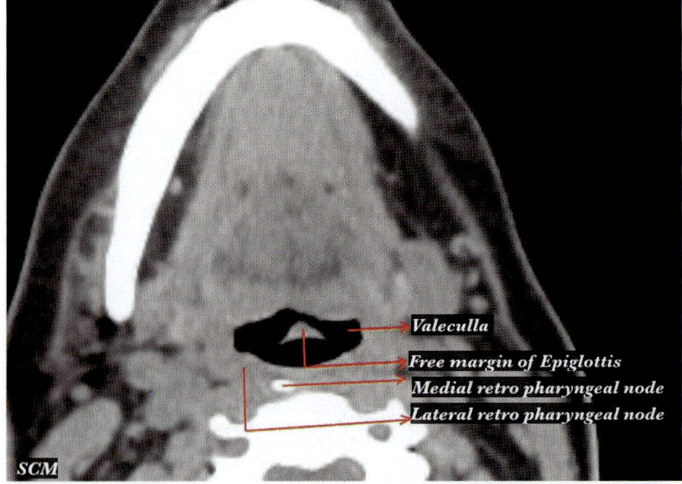

Fig. 3.2.132: CT axial image: Oropharynx

3

within the muscular triangle, which is responsible for depressing the hyoid during swallowing. They are thyrohyoid, omohyoid, sternohyoid and sternothyroid.

3.2.L Cervical Esophagus

Cervical esophagus starts at inferior margin of cricoid cartilage that corresponds to corpus of 6th cervical

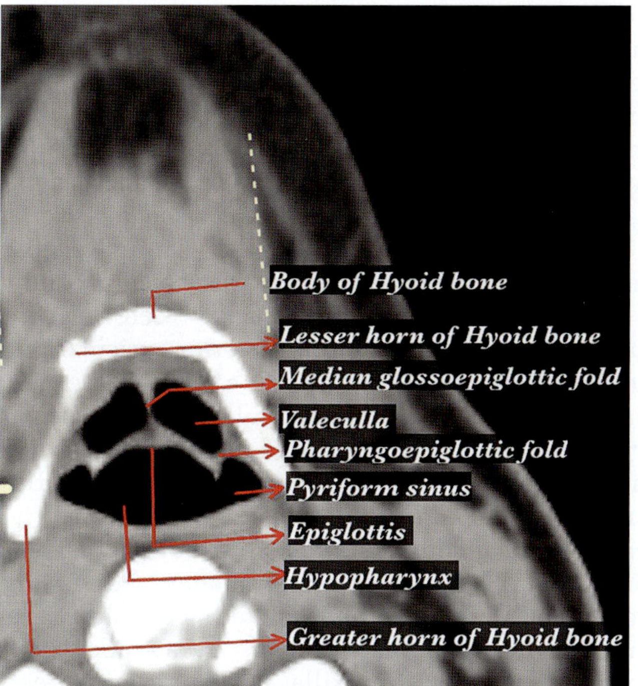

Fig. 3.2.133: CT axial image: Oropharynx

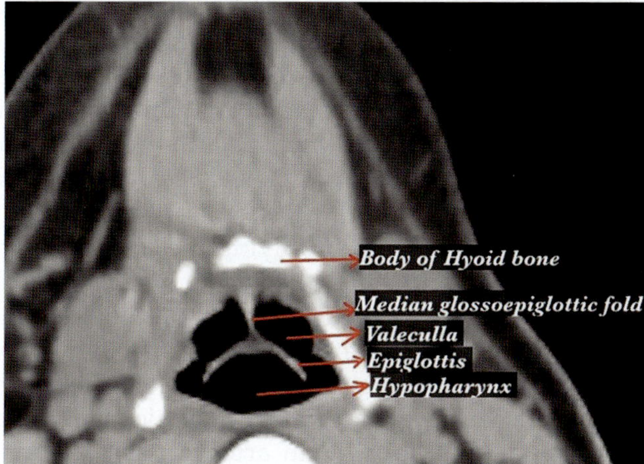

Fig. 3.2.134: CT axial image: Epiglottis

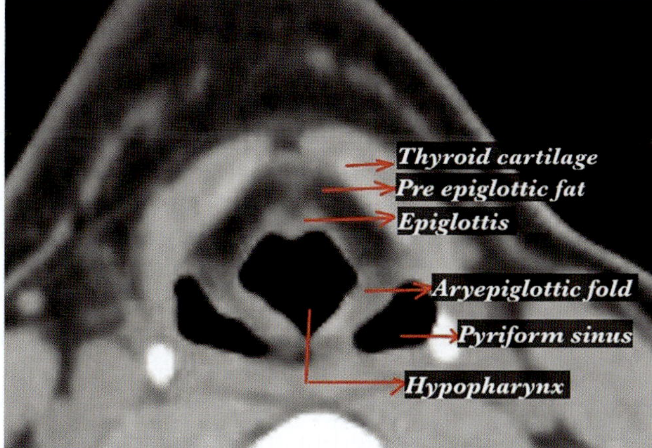

Fig. 3.2.135: CT axial image: Pyriform sinus

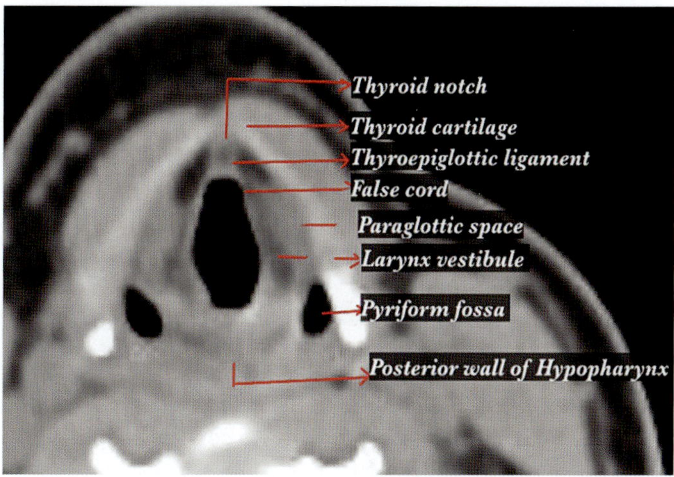

Fig. 3.2.136: CT axial image: Hypopharynx

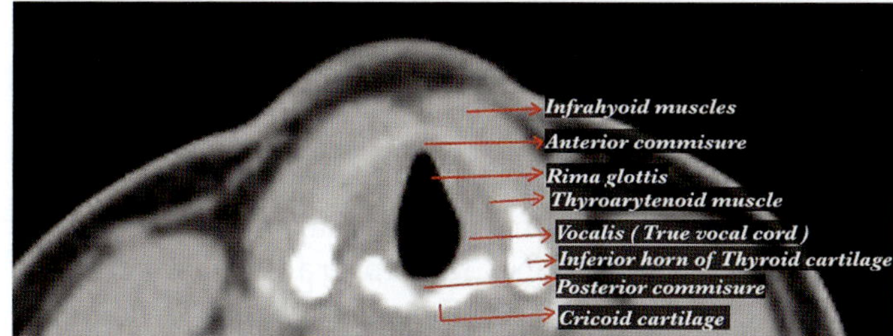

Fig. 3.2.137: CT axial image: Hypopharynx

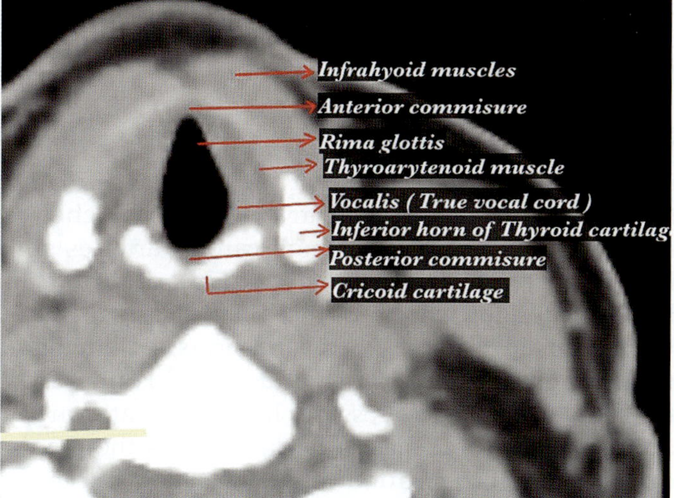

Fig. 3.2.138

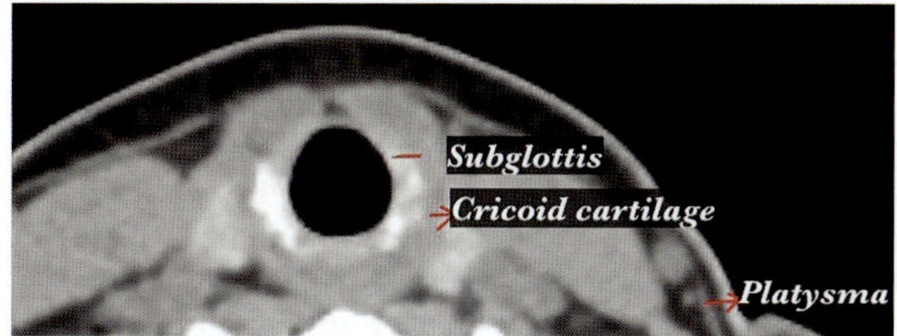

Fig. 3.2.139: Cricoid cartilage

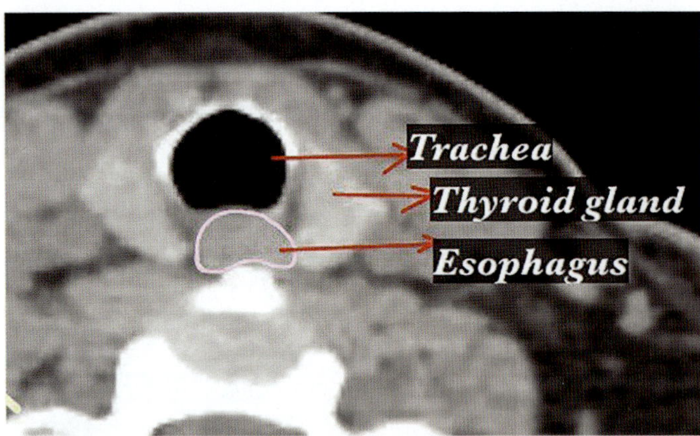

Fig. 3.2.140: Relationship of trachea to cervical esophagus

vertebra. It ends at inferior edge of first dorsal vertebra. It is 5–6 cm long, and its luminal diameter is 1.4–1.5 cm at its narrowest point. It runs in deepest fascial plane of neck, leaning between trachea and pharynx anteriorly and vertebra posteriorly. Esophagus is attached to prevertebral fascia by sagittal septa, which forms retropharyngeal and retro-esophageal spaces. Recurrent laryngeal nerve (RLN) lies in tracheoesophageal groove bilaterally, and esophagus is close to this nerve especially on the left side, which can get injured in cervical esophagectomy. Injury of RLN causes unilateral difficulty in swallowing and hoarseness; bilateral injury causes closure of vocal cords in median position, which needs tracheostomy.

3.2.M Neck Blood Supply

Arterial supply: Arterial supply of the neck is mainly from the external carotid artery and branches of subclavian artery. The common carotid arteries split into the **external** and **internal** carotid arteries at the level of superior margin of the thyroid cartilage (C4), within carotid triangle. The **carotid sinus, a dilated part of common and internal carotid artery,** is important for regulating blood pressure. Internal carotid artery does not have branches in neck, it enters the cranial cavity through the carotid canal and takes part in the formation of circle of Willis. **The ECA** is responsible for supplying the majority of blood to the meninges, scalp, and face. The ECA twists and passes anteriorly and superiorly after its origin, then traverses posteriorly to the mandible's neck. The superior thyroid, ascending pharyngeal, lingual, facial, occipital, and posterior auricular arteries are all branches of the ECA. Within the parotid gland, it divides into the maxillary artery and the superficial temporal artery. Superior thyroid artery supplying to the thyroid gland. It gives a branch called superior laryngeal artery, which pierces the thyrohyoid membrane with the internal laryngeal nerve and supply the larynx. Ascending pharyngeal artery ascends between the internal and external carotid arteries and supplies the pharynx. Lingual artery is a tortuous artery that supplies the tongue by passing deep to the mylohyoid and hyoglossus muscles. Facial artery is also a tortuous artery that courses to the anterior face; it runs deep to the submandibular gland. Sometimes the lingual and facial arteries arise from a common faciolingual (linguofacial) trunk. Occipital artery supplies the occipital region. Posterior auricular artery supplies the region posterior to the ear. Within the parotid gland, sometimes posterior auricular artery and occipital artery can orginate from common trunk. The external carotid artery gives two terminal branches superficial temporal artery and internal maxillary artery. Superficial temporal artery courses superiorly to the temporal region gives multiple branches and terminates by divides into frontal and parietal branches. Internal maxillary artery supplies the structures within the infratemporal fossa, nasal cavity, palate, maxilla, and superior aspect of the pharynx. Internal maxillary artery passes anterior between the mandible ramus and the sphenomandibular ligament, and runs in relation with lateral pterygoid muscle, to the pterygopalatine fossa. It supplies the deep structures of the face. In relation to lateral pterygoid muscle, maxillary artery is divided into three portions: First (mandibular) part: Posterior to lateral pterygoid muscle (gives multiple branches, important one is the middle meningeal artery supplying the dura). Second (pterygoid or muscular) part: Within lateral pterygoid muscle gives multiple branches. Third (pterygopalatine) part: Anterior to lateral pterygoid muscle gives multiple branches, including sphenopalatine artery which is the terminal branch. **Thyrocervical trunk** which is a branch of the first part of subclavian artery arises lateral to the vertebral artery from the anterosuperior wall of the subclavian artery and gives branches like inferior thyroid artery which runs superiorly from the thyrocervical trunk to the inferior portion of the thyroid gland (Fig. 3.2.141). The suprascapular artery and transverse cervical artery both head laterally and cross in front of (anterior to) the scalenus anterior muscle and the phrenic nerve. Suprascapular artery takes part in the scapular anastomosis. Ascending cervical artery ascends medial to the phrenic nerve on the prevertebral fascia. It contributes many small branches into the intervertebral foramina of the neck and lateral muscles of the upper neck. Vertebral artery branch of the first part of subclavian artery traverses through the transverse foramen of C6 to C2 verterbra and takes an arch before entering the transverse foramina of C1 vertebra, from

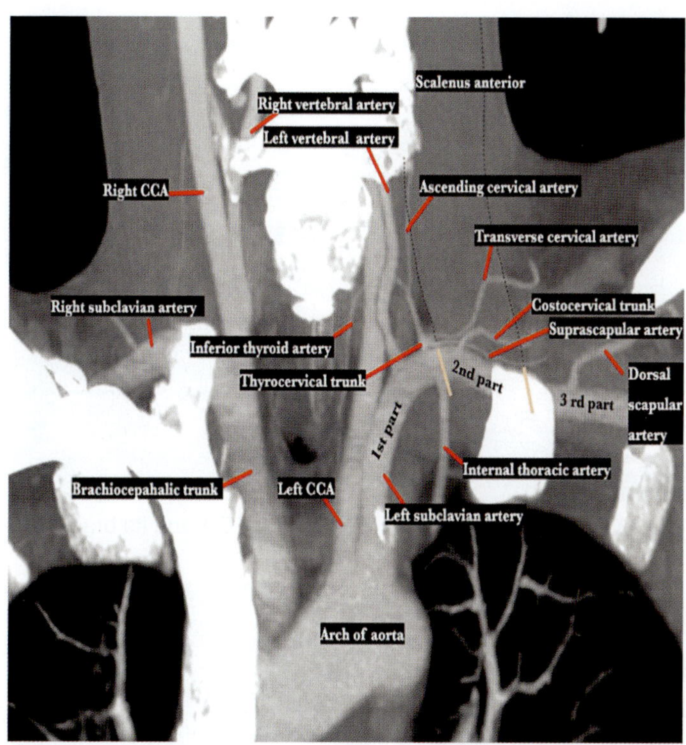

Fig. 3.2.141: CECT coronal MIP image: Aortic arch and its branches

the C1 vertebra again it takes an arch before entering into the posterior fossa. It provides blood supply for the upper part of the spinal cord, brainstem, cerebellum, and posterior part of the brain. Vertebral artery has four segments, first three segments situated in neck without giving branches in neck. Segments of vertebral artery are preforaminal (from subclavian artery to transverse foramen of C6), foraminal (through the transverse foramina of C6 to C2), extradural (from the transverse foramen of axis to the vertebral canal), intradural (from the vertebral canal to the inferior border of pons (Fig. 3.2.142). The series of images from Figs 3.2.143 to 3.2.148 shows branches of ECA.

Venous drainage of face and neck: Venous drainage of face and neck by three major veins—external jugular vein (EJV), internal jugular vein (IJV), anterior jugular vein (AJV). Majority of the external face drained by the external jugular vein and its tributaries. External jugular vein formed by the union of posterior auricular vein (drains the area of scalp superior and posterior to the outer ear) and posterior division of retromandibular vein (retromandibular vein formed by the maxillary and superficial temporal veins, which drain the face). Posterior to the angle of mandible, and inferior to the ear, posterior division of retromandibular vein and posterior auricular vein joins forming the external jugular vein. After formation, the EJV descends down the neck within the superficial fascia and runs anterior

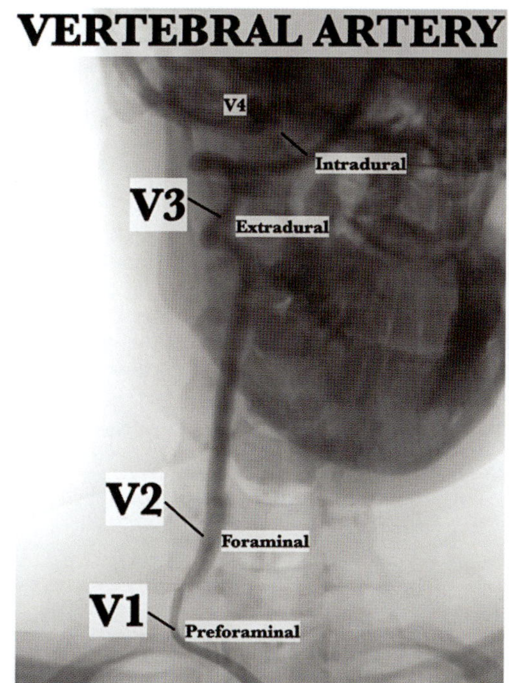

Fig. 3.2.142: DSA: Vertebral artery

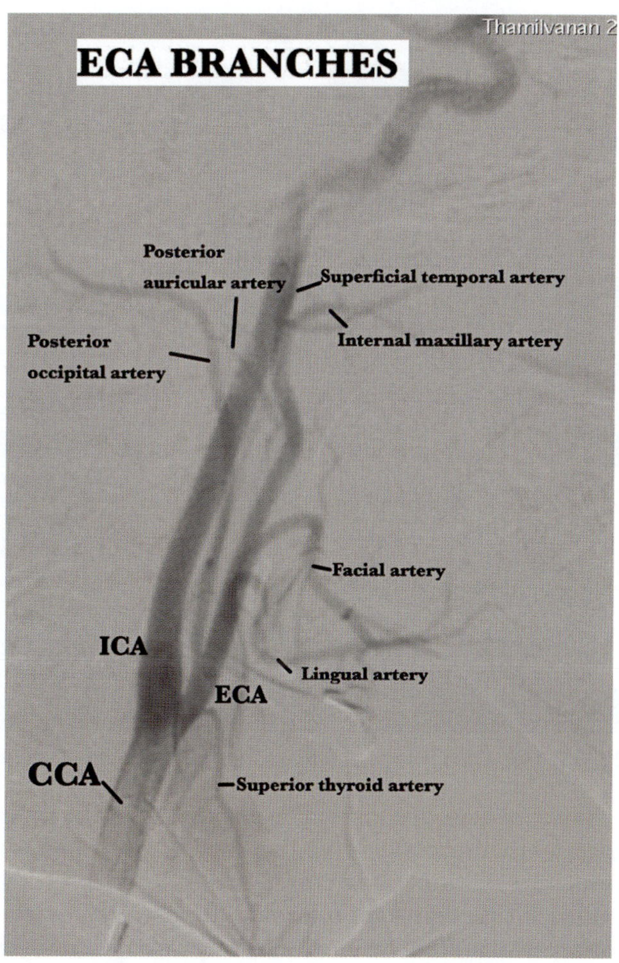

Fig. 3.2.143: DSA-ECA and its branches

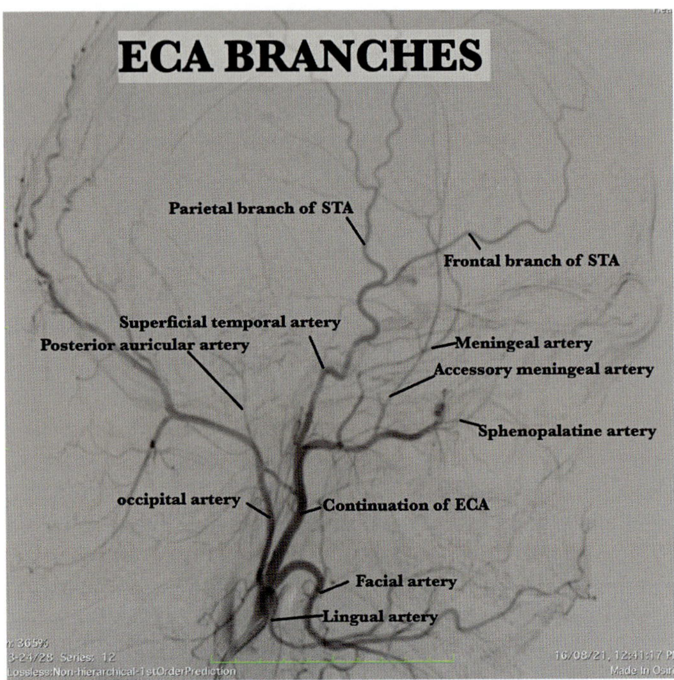

Fig. 3.2.144: DSA-ECA and its branches

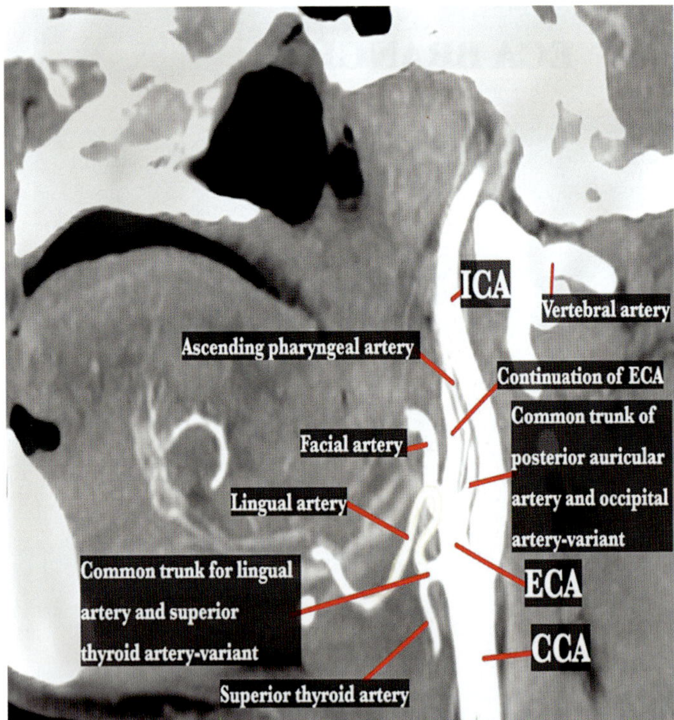

Fig. 3.2.145: CECT sagittal MIP image: ECA and its branches

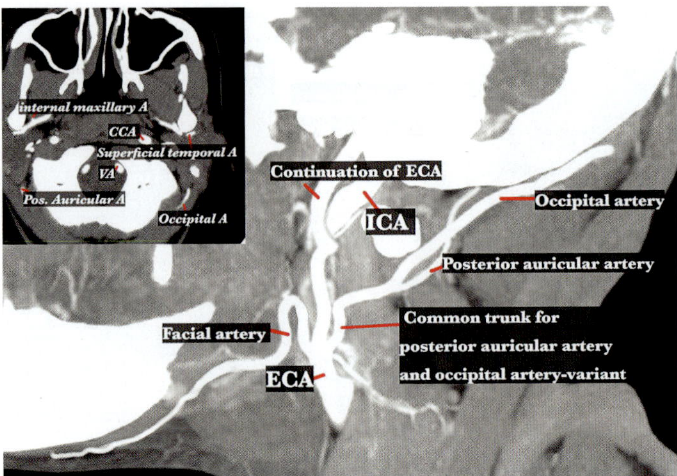

Fig. 3.2.146: CECT sagittal MIP image: ECA and its branches

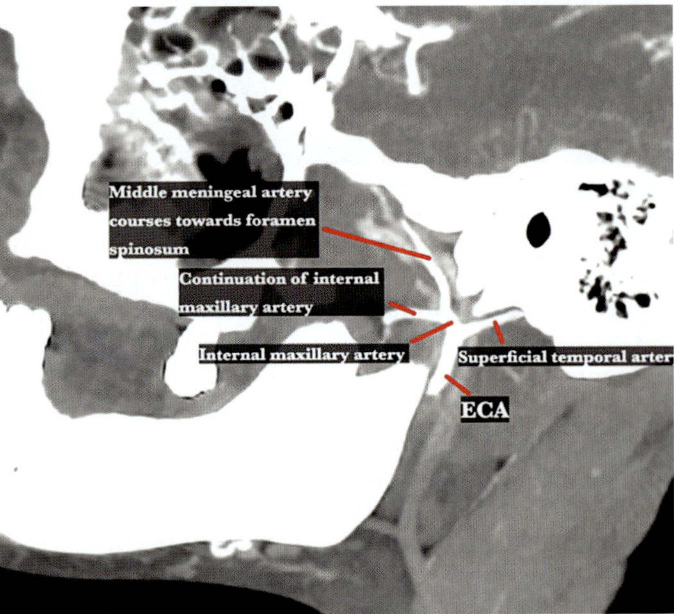

Fig. 3.2.147: CECT sagittal MIP image: ECA and its branches

to the sternocleidomastoid muscle. The vein passes underneath the clavicle in the root of the neck, and drains into the subclavian vein. Along its course down the neck, it receives tributaries like posterior external jugular, transverse cervical and suprascapular veins. Anterior aspect of the neck is drained through multiple superficial veins into anterior jugular vein. **The anterior jugular veins** begin at the hyoid level and may receive communication from the facial veins or the internal jugular vein. The anterior jugular veins descend down the midline of the neck, along the anterior border of the sternocleidomastoid muscles medially or between the midline and the anterior border of these muscles. At the root of the neck, both sides of anterior jugular veins are connected through jugular venous arch, finally AJV emptying into either the subclavian vein / EJV. The internal jugular vein (IJV) is a continuation of the sigmoid sinus, exits the skull via the jugular foramen. The dilated initial part is known as the superior bulb. **The internal jugular vein** descends

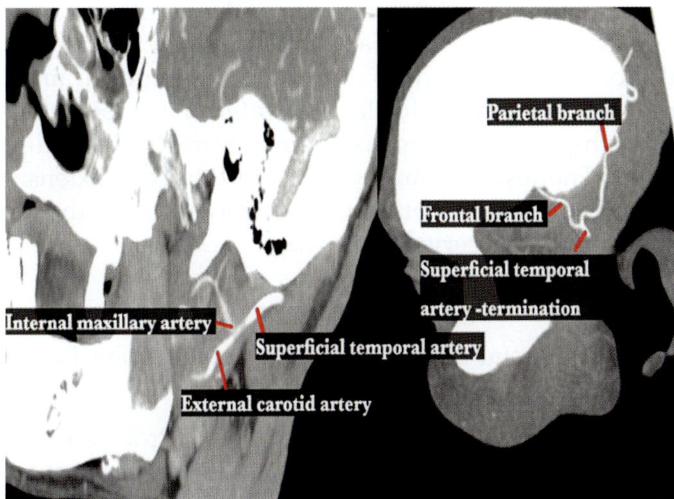

Fig. 3.2.148: Superficial temporal artery

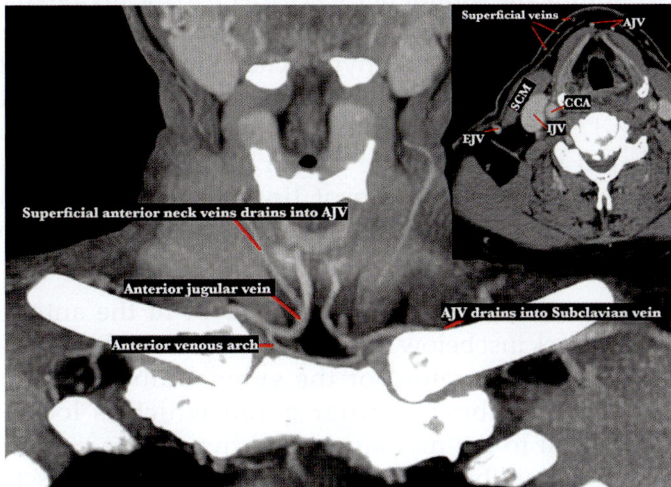

Fig. 3.2.149: Anterior jugular vein

within the carotid sheath in the neck, deep to the sternocleidomastoid muscle and lateral to the common carotid artery. At the base of the neck, posteriorly to the sternal end of the clavicle, the IJV combines with the subclavian vein to form the brachiocephalic vein. Immediately prior to the formation of brachiocepahalic vein, the inferior end of internal jugular vein dilates to form the inferior bulb and it has a valve that stops backflow of blood. During its descent down the neck, the IJV receives blood from the anterior facial vein (facial vein), lingual, occipital, superior and middle thyroid veins. These veins drain blood from the anterior face, trachea, thyroid, oesophagus, larynx, and muscles of the neck. **Anterior facial vein** is the continuation of angular vein which inturn formed by the union of supratrochlear vein and supraorbital vein. The angular vein is linked with the cavernous sinus by the superior and inferior ophthalmic veins which are devoid of valves, so any

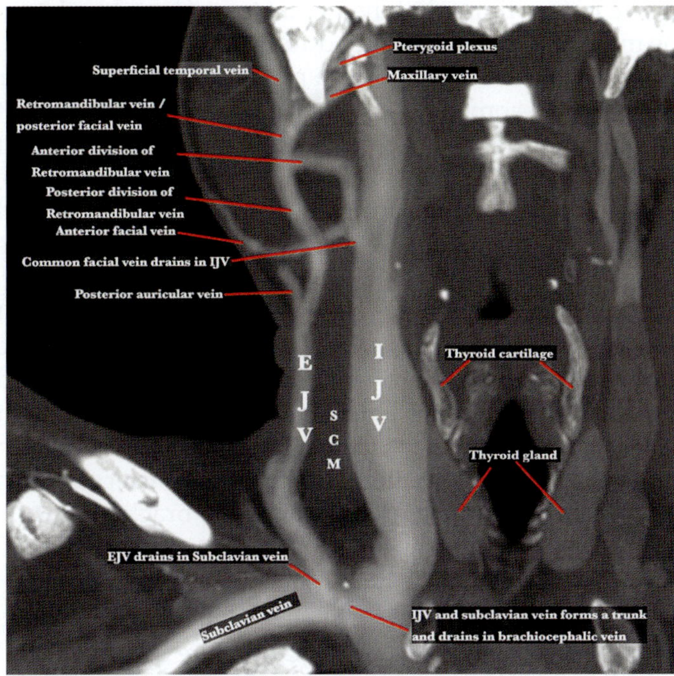

Fig. 3.2.150: EJV and IJV

infection in the face/mouth can spread to the cavernous sinus through angular vein and leads to cavernous sinus thrombosis. The vertebral vein, follows the course of the vertebral artery and exits the spine at the level of the C6 transverse foramen. It receives tributaries from the internal and external vertebral venous plexuses and from the deep and anterior cervical veins and terminates in the brachiocephalic vein near the junction of the internal jugular and subclavian veins.

3.2.N Thyroid Gland

The thyroid gland is located in the anterior neck between the C5-T1 vertebrae. It has right and left lobes, connected by a central isthmus anteriorly. The lobes of the thyroid gland are wrapped around the cricoid cartilage and superior rings of the trachea. The gland is located within the visceral compartment of the neck (along with the trachea, oesophagus and pharynx). Anteriorly it is bounded by infrahyoid muscles, namely the sternothyroid, superior belly of the omohyoid and sternohyoid, laterally by carotid sheath, containing the common carotid artey, internal jugular vein and vagus nerve, medially by larynx, pharynx, trachea and oesophagus. External laryngeal and recurrent laryngeal nerve supplies the thyroid gland. **Zuckerkandl tubercles** is the anatomical variant, it is the projections of normal thyroid tissue from the posterior or posteromedial margin of the thyroid gland that extend posterior to the tracheoesophageal groove. It is an important surgical landmark as the recurrent laryngeal nerve passes immediately medial to it. The tubercle can be mistaken for a thyroid nodule, enlarged parathyroid, or lymph node. When it has a pedunculated or nodular appearance, sometimes due to the lateral impression of the common carotid artery. Another anatomical variant is the pyramidal lobe of thyroid (Lalouette pyramid), superior sliver of thyroid tissue arising from the thyroid isthmus. It is considered as a third thyroid lobe. It arise from the persistent remnant of the thyroglossal duct. Arterial supply includes **superior thyroid artery,** first branch of the ECA. It lies in close proximity to the external branch of the superior laryngeal nerve and **inferior thyroid artery,** branch of thyrocervical trunk. It lies in close proximity to the recurrent laryngeal nerve. In around 10% of people, there is an additional artery known as thyroid ima artery, it arises from the brachiocephalic trunk and supplies the anterior surface and isthmus of the thyroid gland. Venous drainage is by the superior, middle, and inferior thyroid veins, which form a venous plexus around the thyroid gland. The superior and middle veins drain into the internal jugular vein and the inferior drains into the brachiocephalic vein. The thyroid gland is innervated by branches derived from the sympathetic trunk. These nerves do not control the secretory function of the gland, the release of thyroid hormones is regulated by the pituitary gland. The lymphatic drainage of the thyroid is to the paratracheal and deep cervical nodes.

Parathyroid gland: The parathyroid glands are endocrine glands located in the anterior neck. They are responsible for the production of parathyroid hormone (PTH), which acts to increase the level of serum calcium. The parathyroid glands are usually located on the posterior aspect of the thyroid gland, flat and oval shape, situated external to the thyroid gland but within the pretracheal fascia. Most individuals have four parathyroid glands, two superior parathyroid glands and two inferior parathyroid glands, although variation in number from two to six is common. Superior parathyroid glands, derived from the fourth pharyngeal Pouch, located at the middle of the posterior border of each thyroid lobe, approximately 1 cm superior to the entry of the inferior thyroid artery into the thyroid gland. Inferior parathyroid glands, derived from the third pharyngeal pouch. Although inconsistent in location between individuals, the inferior parathyroid glands are usually found near the inferior poles of the thyroid gland. In a small number of people, the inferior parathyroid glands can be found as far inferiorly in the superior mediastinum. Arterial supply is chiefly via the inferior thyroid artery, as this artery supplies the posterior aspect of the thyroid gland, where the parathyroids are located. Collateral arterial supply is from the superior thyroid artery and thyroid ima artery. Venous drainage into the superior, middle, and inferior thyroid veins. The lymphatic drainage is to the paratracheal and deep cervical nodes. The parathyroid glands have an extensive supply of sympathetic nerves derived from thyroid branches of the cervical ganglia.

3.2.O Ultrasonogram of Neck

Use superficial high frequency linear probe for the visualization of neck contents.

Submental region and sublingual region: Probe is kept in the midline in the submental region with neck extended. Transverse grayscale ultrasound of the submental and sublingual region shows mylohyoid muscle which is separating the sublingual space (deep to the mylohyoid) and submandibular space (superficial to the muscle). Bilateral homogeneous, hyperechoic structures lateral to the geniohyoid/genioglossus muscle is the sublingual gland. The submandibular duct course along the lingual vessels. So, the colour Doppler ultrasound helps in differentiation of lingual vessel from the dilated submandibular duct. Figure 3.2.151 shows the ultrasonogram of submental and sublingual region.

Submandibular region: Probe is kept in the anterior lateral neck just below the angle of mandible. Transverse grayscale ultrasound of the submandibular region shows the submandibular gland which is located superficial to the mylohyoid and hyoglossus muscles. The submandibular duct runs between these 2 muscles. The gland is divided into superficial and deep lobes by the free posterior edge of the mylohyoid muscle. Normal lymph nodes can be seen in this region. Figure 3.2.152 shows the ultrasonogram of submandibular region.

Parotid region: Probe is kept along the ramus of mandible in the lateral neck just above the angle of mandible. Transverse grayscale US shows the parotid gland and the mandibular ramus (Figs 3.2.1.53 and 3.2.1.54). Parotid gland can be seen as homogeneous, hyperechoic pattern. On colour Doppler imaging retromandibular vein and external carotid artery can be visualized. The retromandibular vein is usually larger and lateral to the external carotid artery within the parotid gland. Usually the deep lobe of parotid is obscured by shadowing from the mandibular ramus.

Upper cervical region: Probe is kept in the upper anterior neck in paramedian lateral position. We can visualize carotid bifurcation and the internal and external carotid arteries and the internal jugular vein (Fig. 3.2.155).

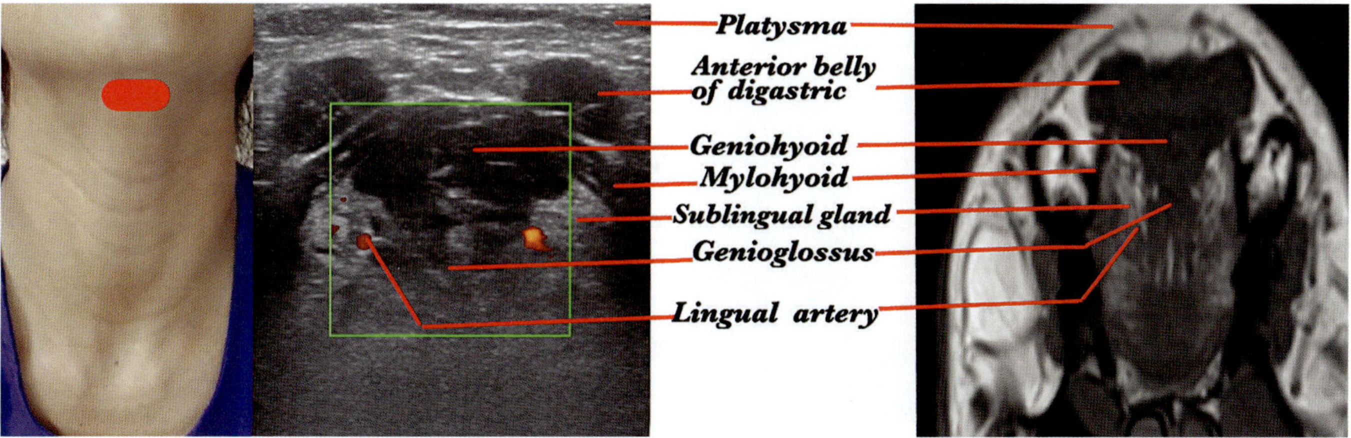

Fig. 3.2.151 Ultrasonogram at submental and sublingual region

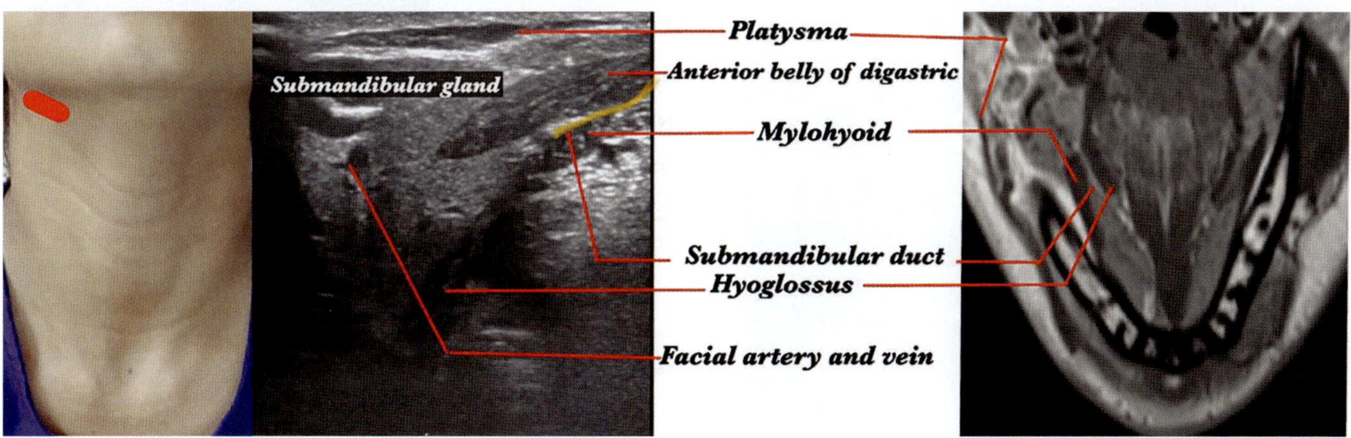

Fig. 3.2.152: Ultrasonogram at submandibular level

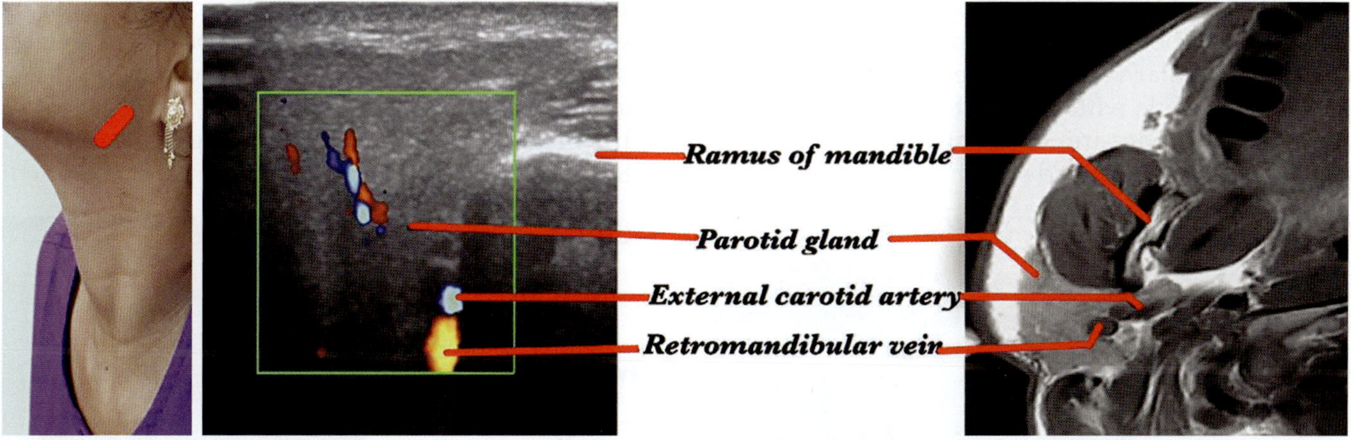

Fig. 3.2.153: Ultrasonogram at parotid level

The external carotid artery is usually more medial and smaller than the internal carotid artery. Below the level of carotid bifurcation we can see the common carotid artery, internal jugular vein, and vagus nerve within the carotid sheath. The uppermost deep cervical lymph node (i.e., the jugulodigastric lymph node) visualized anterior to the carotid arteries. Normal lymph nodes can be elliptical, hypoechoic with echogenic hilum.

Mid-cervical region: Probe is kept in the mid-anterior neck in paramedian lateral position below the level of hyoid bone. We can visualize the common carotid artery, internal jugular vein, and vagus nerve within the carotid

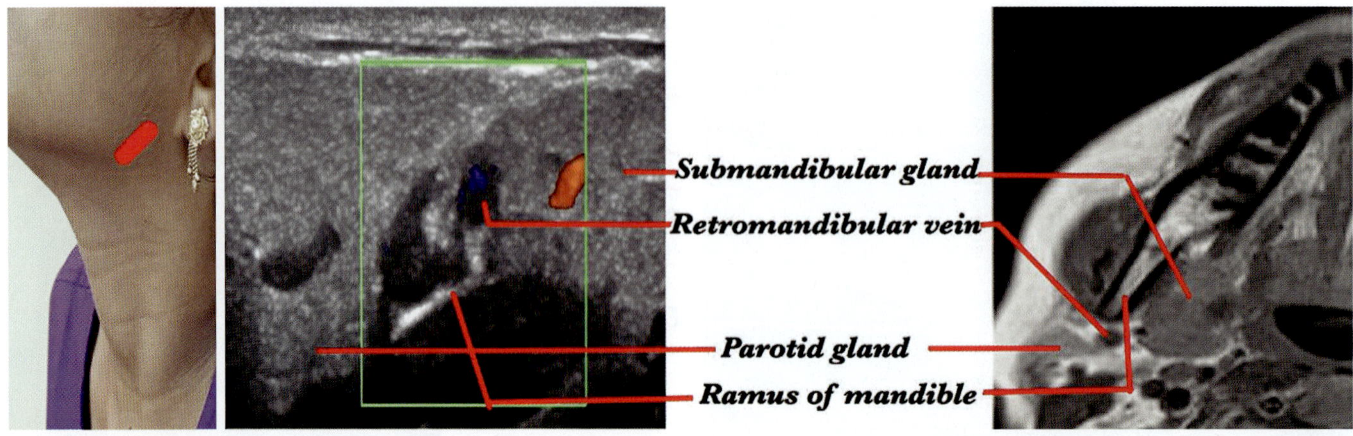

Fig. 3.2.154: Ultrasonogram at parotid level

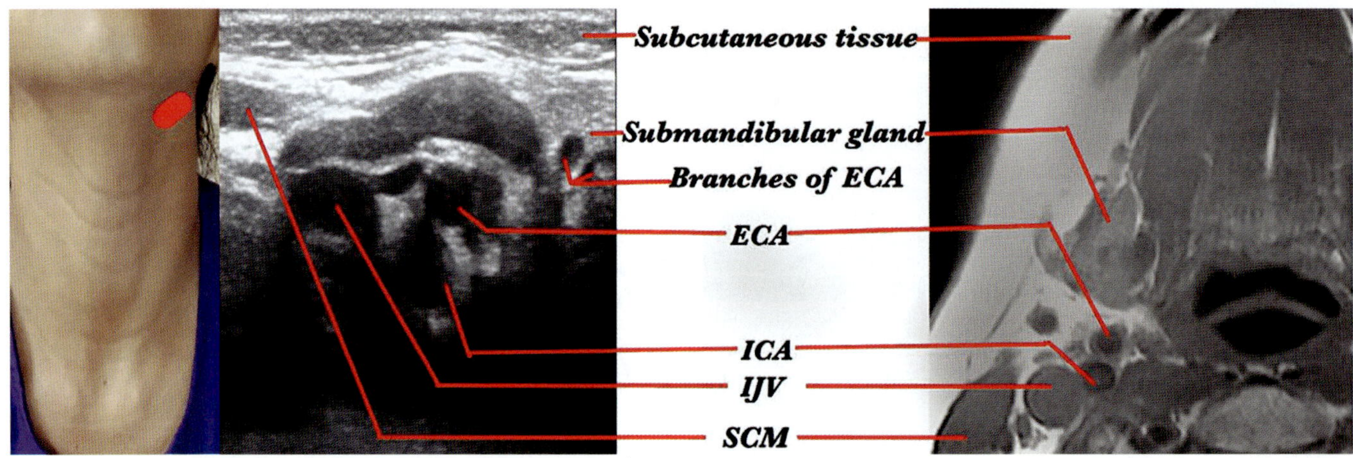

Fig. 3.2.155: Ultrasonogram at upper cervical level

sheath (Figs 3.2.156 and 3.2.157). The vagus nerve is usually located between the common carotid artery and the internal jugular vein and appears as a small, round, hypoechoic nodule with a central echogenic dot. Deep cervical lymph nodes are commonly seen anterior to the major vessels of the carotid sheath.

Lower cervical level and supraclavicular fossa: Probe is kept in the lower anterior neck in paramedian lateral position below the level of cricoid cartilage. We can visualize the common carotid artery, internal jugular vein, thyroid gland, and overlying muscles of the anterior neck (Fig. 3.2.156). At the level of the medial

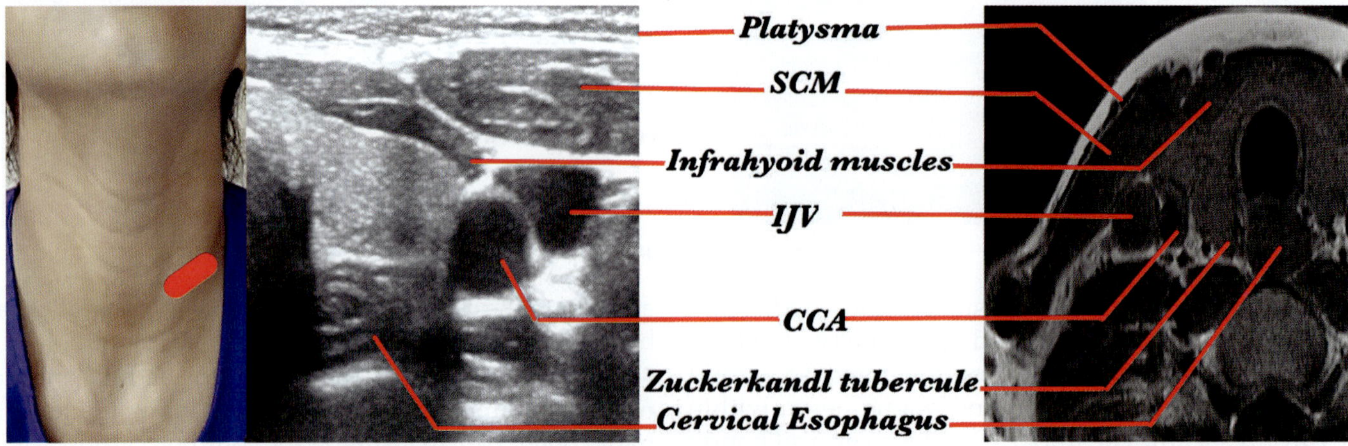

Fig. 3.2.156: Ultrasonogram at mid/lower cervical level

supraclavicular fossa we can visualize the proximity of the proximal internal jugular vein to the subclavian vein at this site, which join to form the brachiocephalic vein. Supraclavicular lymph nodes are commonly seen adjacent to these major vessels. In the lateral supraclavicular fossa, we can visualize the scalenus anterior and medius muscles with the trunks of the brachial plexus between them (Fig. 3.2.158).

Posterior triangle: Probe is kept in the anterior neck in lateral position just lateral to sternocleidomastoid muscle. We can visualize sternocleidomastoid muscle, trapezius and levator scapulae which is the muscle forming the floor of posterior triangle.

Thyroid gland: Probe is kept in the anterior neck in midline below the level of cricoid cartilage. We can visualize both the lobes of thyroid which are connected by the isthmus, the major vessels CCA and IJV which is located lateral to the thyroid gland and the trachea (Fig. 3.2.159). Thyroid gland is usually homogeneous, hyperechoic on ultrasound.

Parathyroid gland: Probe is kept in the anterior neck in midline below the level of cricoid cartilage. Usually normal parathyroid glands not seen. The anatomical location is commonly at the tracheoesophageal groove, posterior to the thyroid gland (Fig. 3.2.159). Transverse grayscale US at a same level shows a small, ovoid, hypoechoic area of soft tissue in the tracheoesophageal groove. Although it is difficult to tell with certainty, this is likely a normal parathyroid gland. Careful analysis should be done to prove they are outside the thyroid capsule and not a thyroid nodule.

Larynx and hypopharynx: Probe is kept in the anterior neck in midline below the level of hyoid bone. Axial grayscale ultrasound of the larynx at the level of the true vocal cords (Fig. 3.2.160) shows that the arytenoid cartilage appears as echogenic foci posteriorly with attachments to the true vocal cords, which have distinct echo-poor appearances and the position of vocal cord during rest and phonation.

Trachea and esophagus: Probe is kept in the anterior neck in midline below the level of cricoid cartilage. We

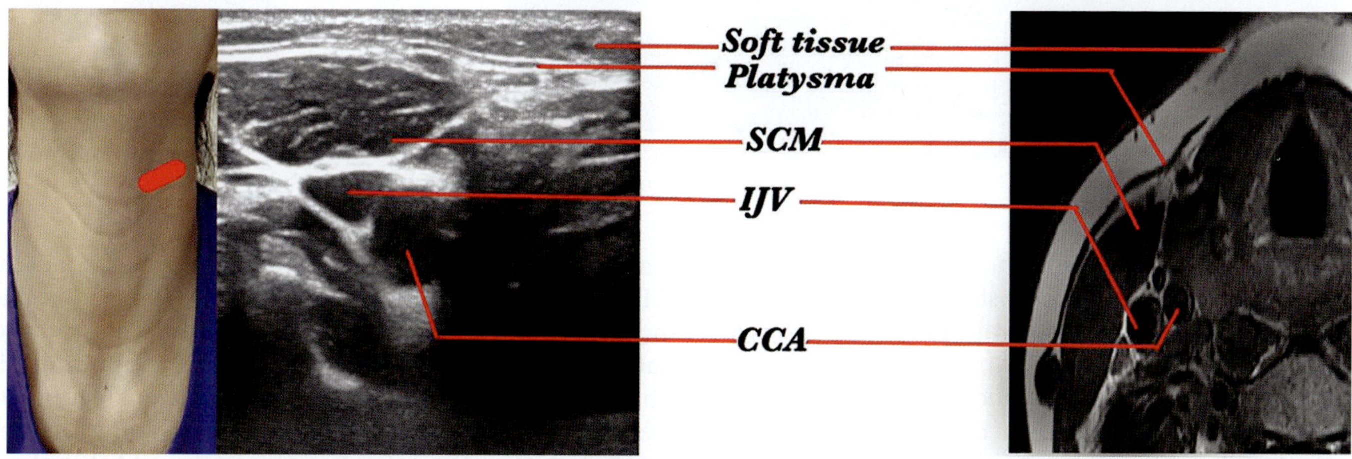

Fig. 3.2.157 Ultrasonogram at midcervical level

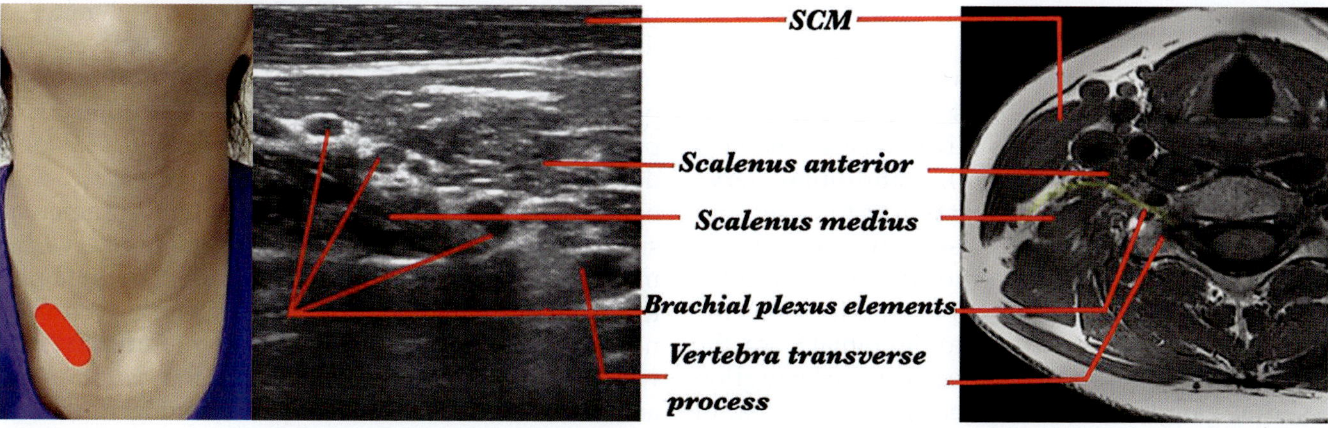

Fig. 3.2.158: Ultrasonogram at lower cervical level and supraclavicular fossa

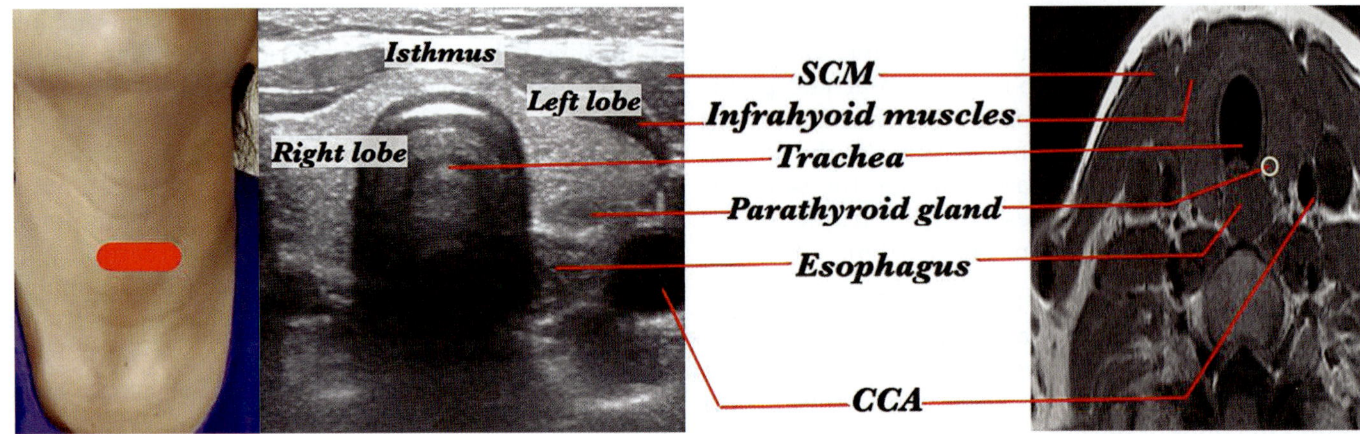

Fig. 3.2.159: Ultrasonogram at thyroid and parathyroid region

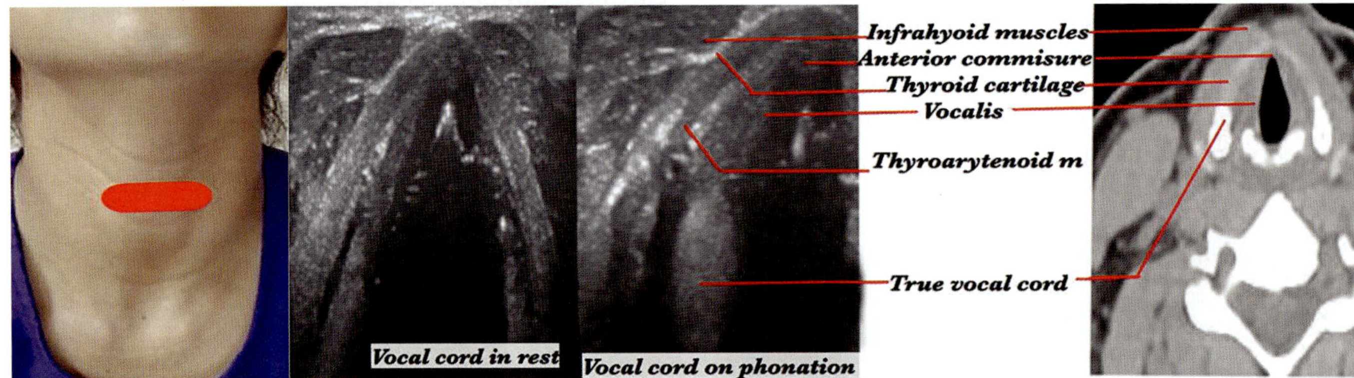

Fig. 3.2.160: Ultrasonogram at true vocal cord level

can visualize the cervical esophagus posterior to the left lobe of the thyroid gland and posterolateral to the trachea (Fig. 3.2.159). The tracheal ring can be seen as hypoechoic band. Cervical esophagus can be identified by the alternating hypo-/hyperechoic rings. The recurrent laryngeal nerve is located in the tracheoesophageal groove but it is difficult to visualize recurrent laryngeal nerve on US.

3.2.P Nerve Supply of Face

CN-V (trigeminal nerve) provides the sensory supply of face and motor supply to the muscles of mastication. It is the largest cranial nerve, has three divisions, namely **ophthalmic (V1), maxillary (V2), mandibular nerve (V3)**. The trigeminal nerve originates from three sensory nuclei (mesencephalic, principal sensory, spinal nuclei of trigeminal nerve) and one motor nucleus (motor nucleus of the trigeminal nerve) extending from the midbrain to the medulla. In the middle cranial fossa, the sensory root expands and form the **trigeminal ganglion (Gasserian ganglion)**. It is located in a depression of the temporal bone called Meckel's cave. The motor root passes inferiorly to the sensory root, along the floor of the Meckel's cave. Its fibres are distributed to the mandibular nerve. The ophthalmic nerve and maxillary nerve travel lateral to the cavernous sinus exiting the cranium via the superior orbital fissure and foramen rotundum respectively. The mandibular nerve exits via the foramen ovale entering the infra-temporal fossa. **Ophthalmic nerve** gives rise to 3 terminal branches, namely **frontal, lacrimal and nasociliary** (Fig. 3.2.161)**,** which innervate the skin and mucous membrane of derivatives of the frontonasal prominence. Frontal and lacrimal nerve passes outside the tendinuous ring, nasociliary nerve passes through the tendinuous ring. Frontal nerve divides into supraorbital nerve and supratrochlear nerve which passes through supraorbital foramen and supratrochlear notch respectively. Nasciliary nerve gives multiple branches, namely small communicating branch to the ciliary ganglion, short ciliary nerve, long ciliary nerve, infratrochlear nerve, posterior ethmoidal nerve which passes through the posterior ethmoidal foramen, anterior ethmoidal nerve which passes through the anterior ethmoidal foramen then through the cribriform plate.

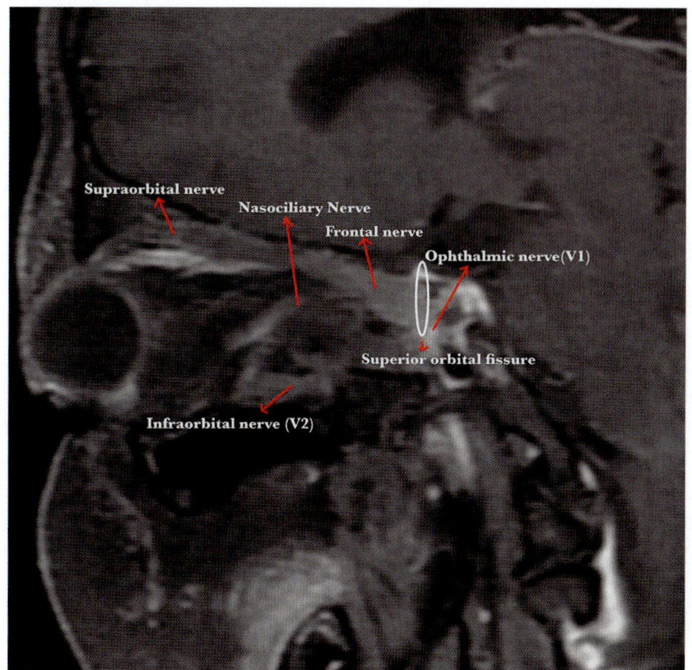

Fig. 3.2.161: Ophthalmic division of trigeminal nerve

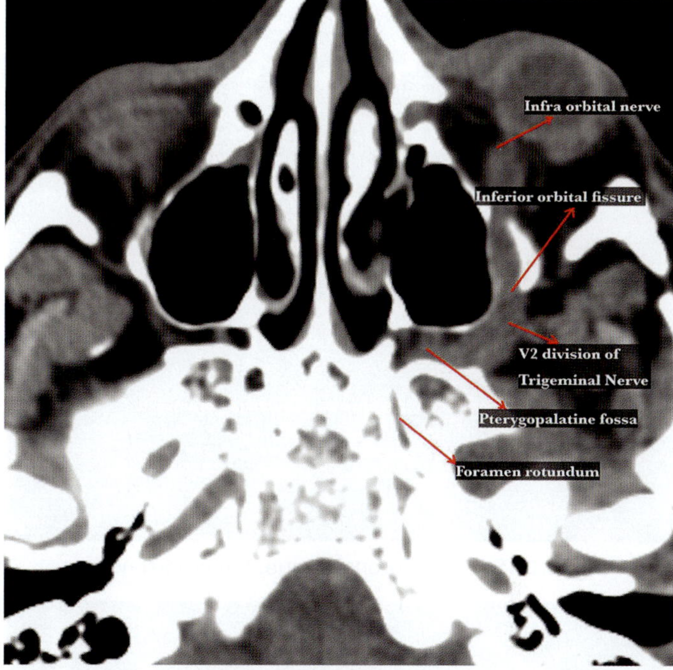

Fig. 3.2.162: Maxillary division of trigeminal nerve

Maxillary nerve courses in the lateral wall of the cavernous sinus inferior to the ophthalmic division. It gives a branch called middle meningeal nerve before passing through the foramen rotundum, then it passes through the pterygopalatine fossa and gives branches to the pterygopalatine ganglion and receives parasympathetic fibre from the ganglion through greater petrosal nerve and then passes through inferior orbital fissure as infraorbital nerve (Fig. 3.2.162). It gives branches like zygomatic nerve, which again divides into zygomaticotemporal and zygomaticofacial nerve, infraorbital nerve which passes through infraorbital foramen, nasopalatine nerve and posterior superior nasal nerve passes through the sphenopalatine foramen, greater palatine nerve, lesser palatine nerve which passes through greater palatine foramen and lesser palatine foramen respectively, and it also gives a pharyngeal branch.

Mandibular nerve courses inferiorly through the foramen ovale and enter the infratemporal fossa. It has sensory root and motor root, motor root bypasses the trigeminal ganglion and passes through the foramen ovale and then unite just below the foramen. It gives off nervus spinosus and nerve to medial pterygoid from the main trunk. It then descends in the infratemporal fossa passing between the tensor veli palatini and lateral pterygoid muscles before dividing into anterior and posterior divisions. Anterior division gives off multiple branches like deep temporal nerves, lateral pterygoid nerves, masseteric nerve, buccal nerve. Posterior division gives off auriculotemporal nerve, lingual nerve, inferior alveolar nerve. Inferior alveolar nerve again gives nerve to mylohyoid, incisive nerve and mental nerve. The series of images from Figs 3.2.163 to 3.2.168 shows divisions of trigeminal nerve and its divisions.

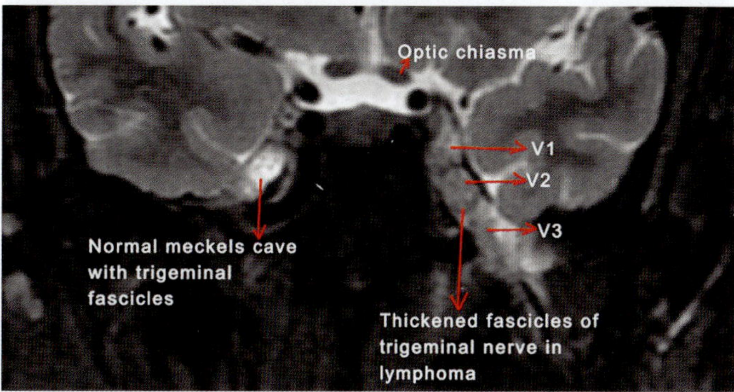

Fig. 3.2.163: MRI coronal image: 5th cranial nerve

3.2.Q Brachial Plexus

The brachial plexus is formed from the **ventral rami of the C5–T1** spinal nerves. These ventral rami are the roots of the brachial plexus. When the C4 nerve supplies the brachial plexus without significant involvement from the T1 nerve, this process is termed a prefixed brachial plexus, while a postfixed brachial plexus refers to a T2 nerve contribution without a significant contribution from the C5 nerve. The first key anatomic landmark, **the neural foramen,** corresponds to the origin of the

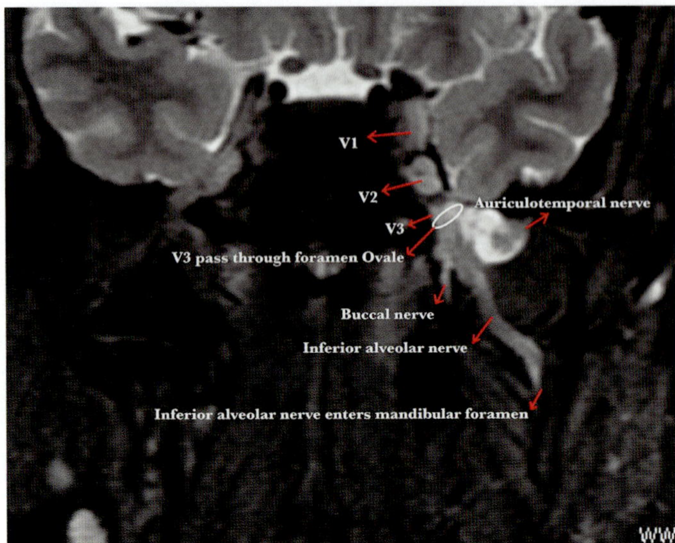

Fig. 3.2.164: MRI coronal image: 5th cranial nerve

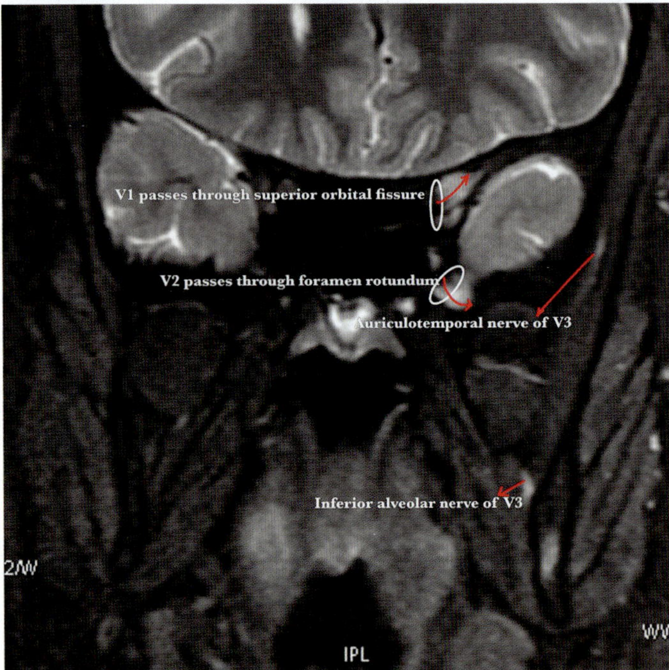

Fig. 3.2.165: MRI coronal image: Enlarged left trigeminal nerve branches in NF1

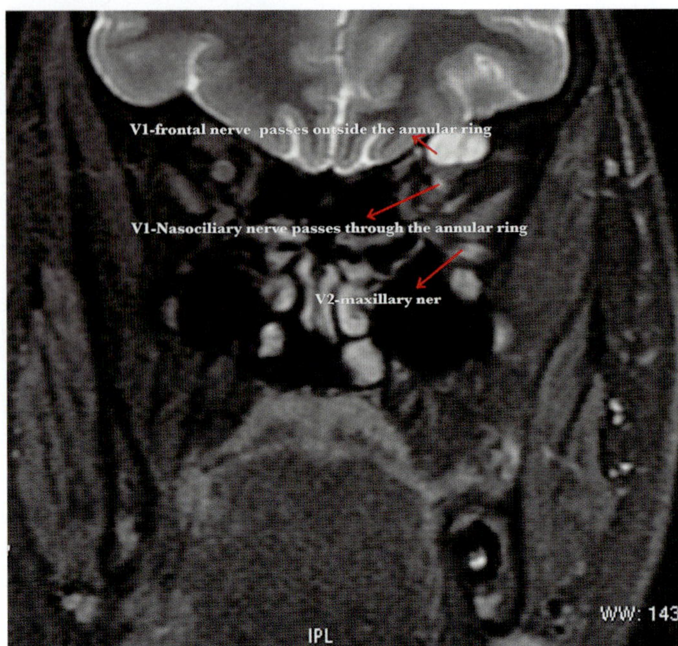

Fig. 3.2.166: MRI coronal image: 5th cranial nerve branches

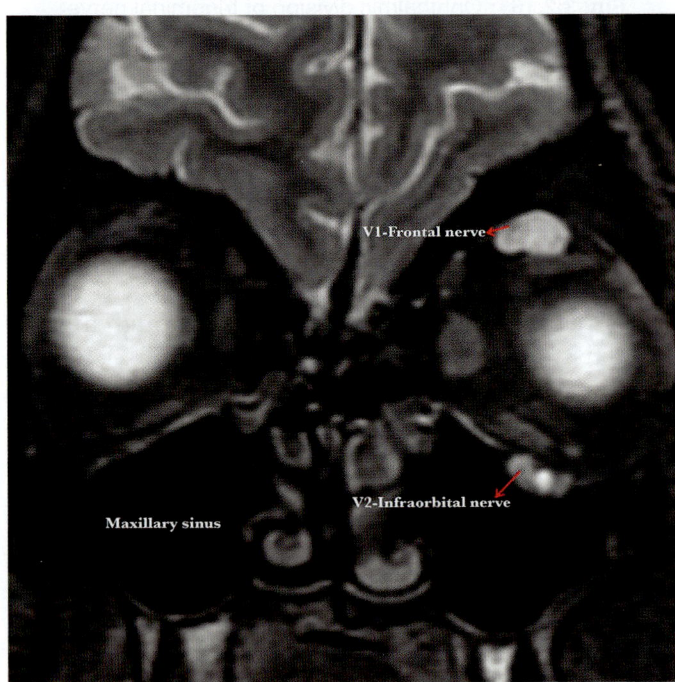

Fig. 3.2.167: MRI coronal image

brachial plexus and is well demonstrated on axial and sagittal views. The ventral and dorsal roots course into the neural foramen, where they merge to form the spinal nerve. The neural foramen also approximates the location of the dorsal root ganglion (DRG), a bulbous structure along the dorsal root located just proximal to the union of the ventral and dorsal roots, which contains the first-order sensory nerve cell bodies. The DRG serves as an important landmark for pre-versus postganglionic injuries. Figures 3.2.171, 3.2.172, 3.2.175 and 3.2.176 show the preganglionic nerve roots. Distal to the neural foramen, the spinal nerve divides into ventral and dorsal rami. The dorsal rami extend posteriorly to innervate the paraspinal muscles. The ventral rami are known as the roots of the brachial plexus and course slightly anteriorly toward the interscalene triangle. The roots appear as five stacked points on sagittal images, and the proximal aspect of the first rib is a useful landmark for locating the roots of the brachial plexus in the sagittal plane, as the T1 root is below the rib, while the C8 root is above the

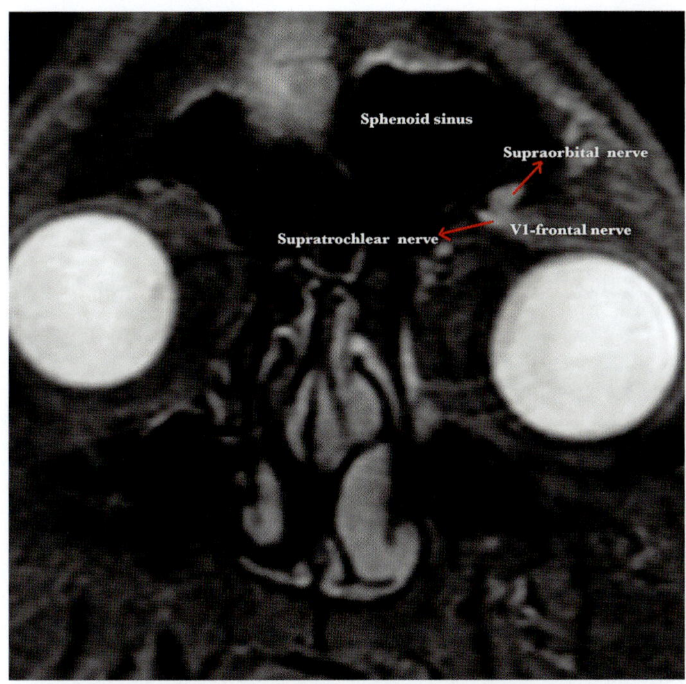

Fig. 3.2.168: Supraorbital and supratrochlear nerve

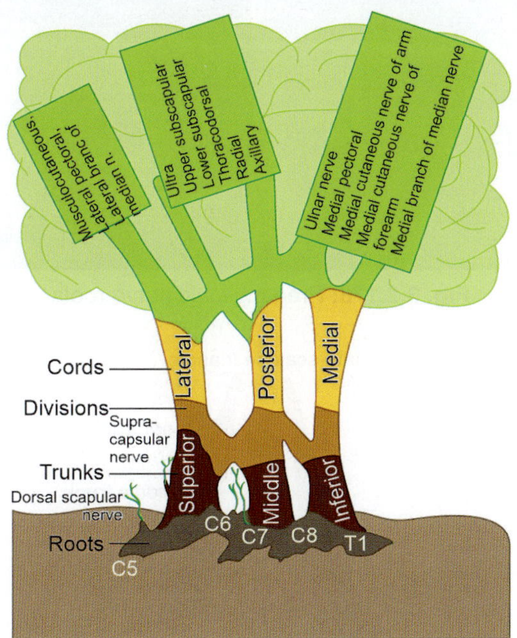

Fig. 3.2.169: Comparing the parts of a tree with brachial plexus, roots, trunks, divisions, cords and branches

rib (Figs 3.2.170 and 3.2.174). The interscalene triangle, the second key anatomic landmark, is formed by the anterior and middle scalene muscles. The upper trunk is formed by the union of the C5 and C6 roots, while the lower trunk represents the union of the C8 and T1 roots. The middle trunk is a continuation of the C7 root. Like the roots, the upper and middle trunks are superior to the artery, while the lower trunk is posterior to the

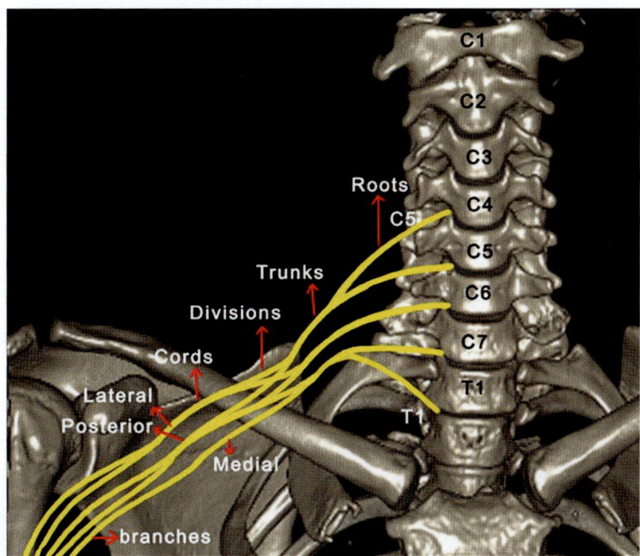

Fig. 3.2.170: The roots, trunks, divisions, cords and branches of brachial plexus in a 3D reformatted CT Image

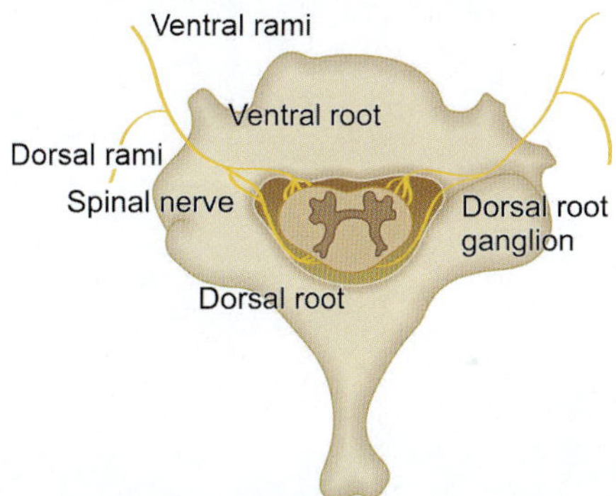

Fig. 3.2.171: Dorsal root ganglion, ventral rami and dorsal rami

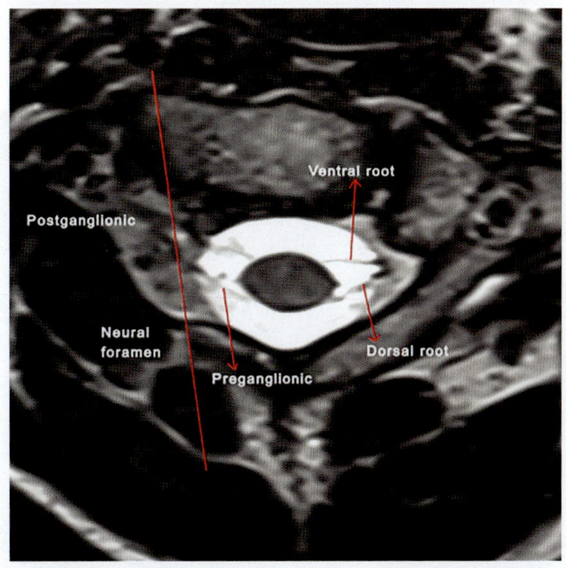

Fig. 3.2.172: MR axial image at cord level highlights the preganglionic and postganglionic nerve root

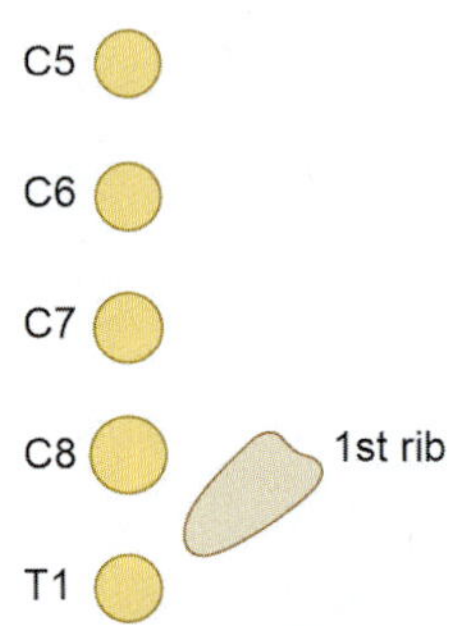

Fig. 3.2.173: The relationship of brachial plexus roots to the 1st rib, T1 root lies inferior to the 1st rib

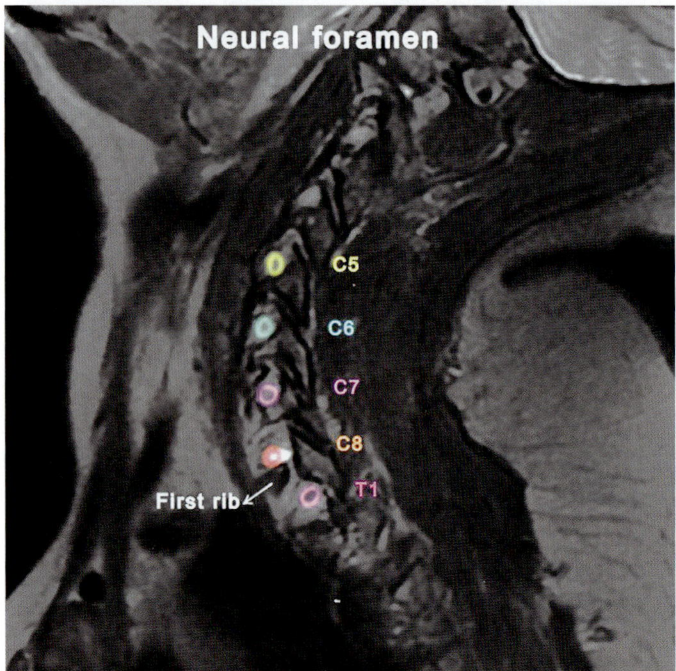

Fig. 3.2.174: MRI sagittal image—nerve roots in neural foramen

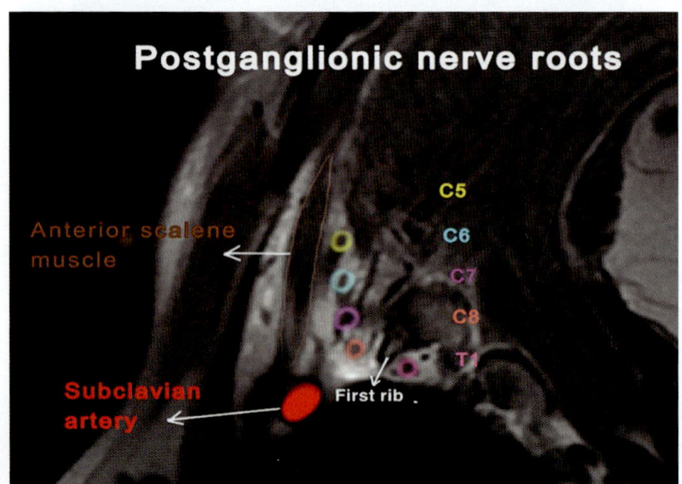

Fig. 3.2.175: Postganglionic nerve roots (entering scalene triangle)

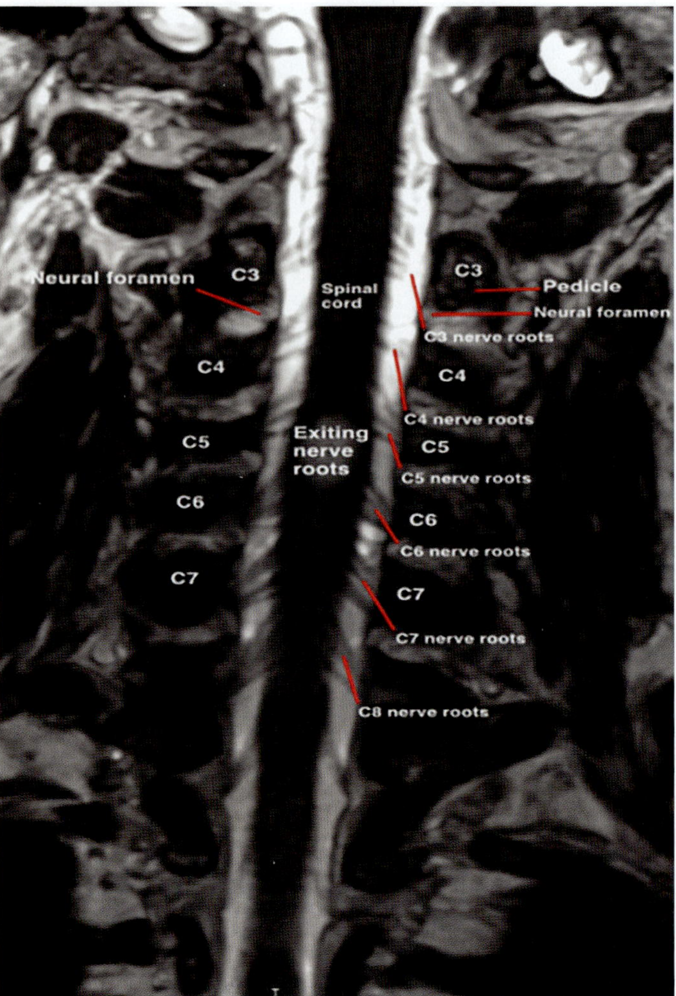

Fig. 3.2.176: Preganglionic nerve roots

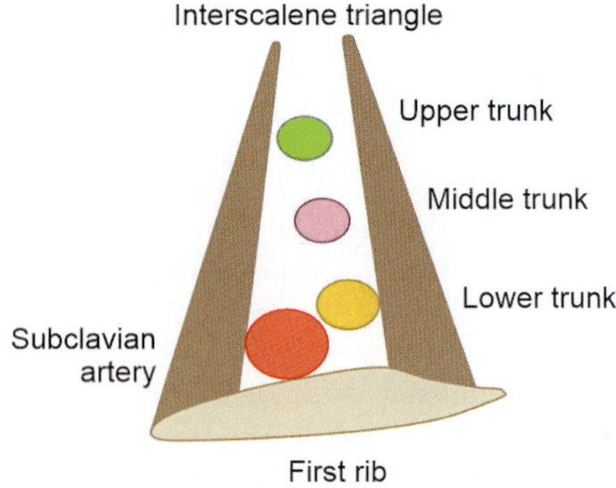

Fig. 3.2.177: The relationship of trunks to the subclavian artery in interscalene triangle

subclavian artery (Figs 3.2.177 and 3.2.178). The trunks appear as three stacked points on sagittal images. The **lateral border of the first rib** is the third key anatomic landmark. As the trunks continue inferolaterally, each trunk separates into an anterior and posterior division at or near the lateral border of the first rib (Figs 3.2.179

and 3.2.180). The divisions of the brachial plexus are functional: The anterior divisions innervate the flexor muscles of the upper limb, and the posterior divisions innervate the extensor muscles of the upper limb. The **medial border of the coracoid process**, the fourth key landmark, serves as the landmark for the cords. As the divisions continue inferolaterally, they form three cords: The lateral, posterior, and medial cords. These cords are named for their relation to the axillary artery, with the posterior cord located between the lateral and medial cords. These three cords, along with the axillary artery, form a three-toed "paw-print" configuration on sagittal images (Figs 3.2.181 and 3.2.182). The fifth and last anatomic landmark is the lateral border of the **pectoralis minor muscle**, where the cords separate into the five terminal branches. In addition to the major components of the brachial plexus, several additional important branches originate or receive contributions

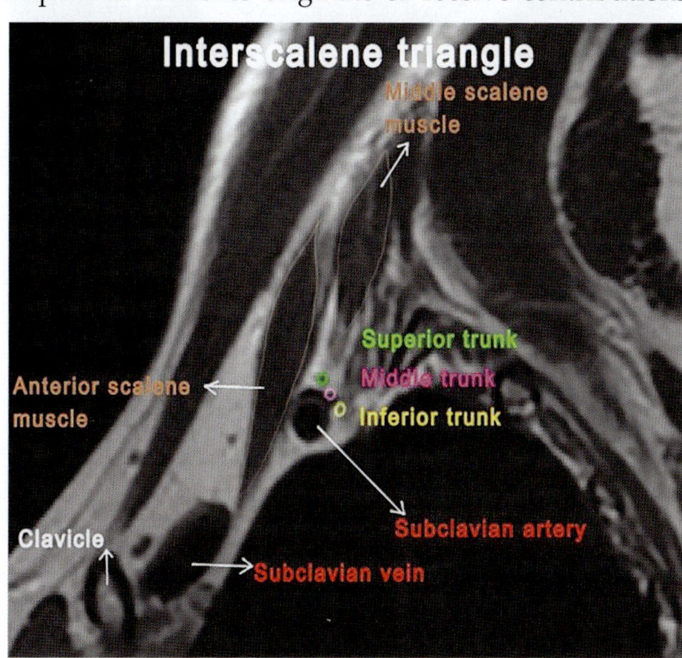

Fig. 3.2.178: The relationship of divisions to axillary artery and midclavicle

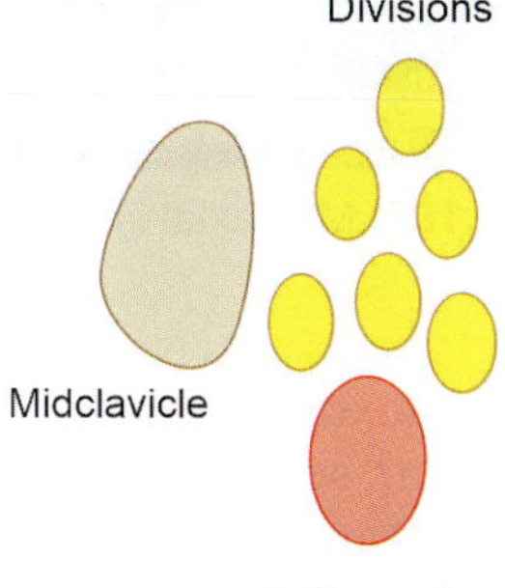

Fig. 3.2.179: Relationship of divisions to axillary artery and midclavicle

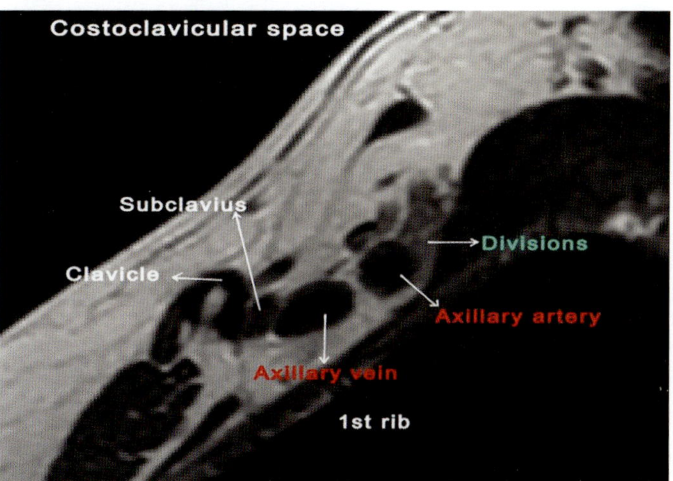

Fig. 3.2.180: Costoclavicular space

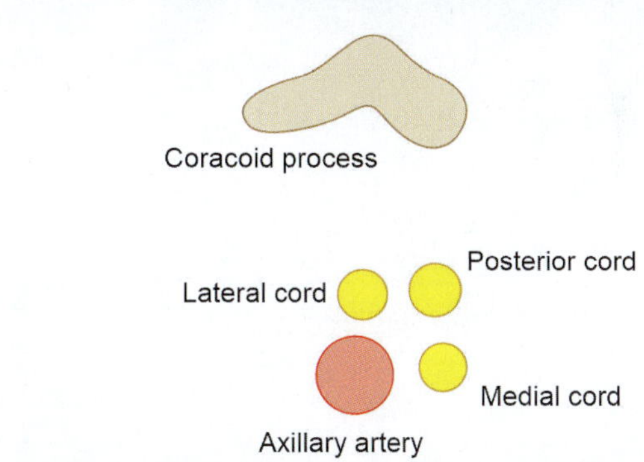

Fig. 3.2.181: The relationship of cord to axillary artery at the level of coracoid process

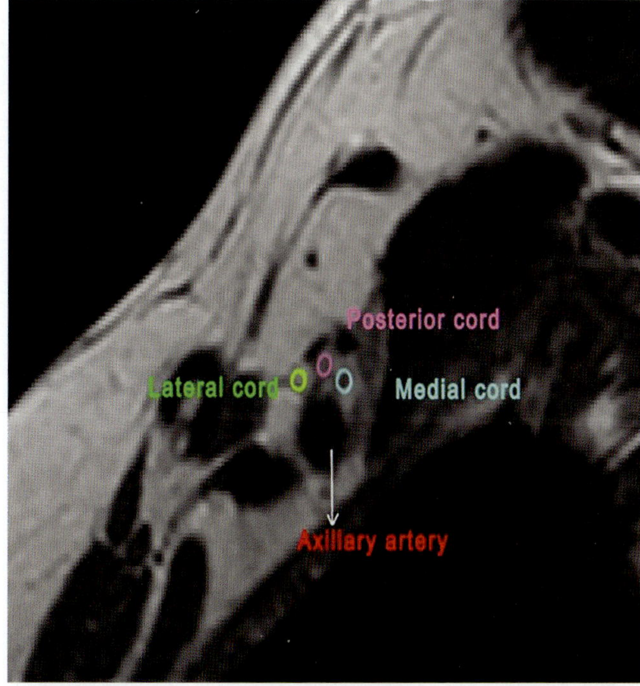

Fig. 3.2.182: Paw print configuration of cords along with axillary artery

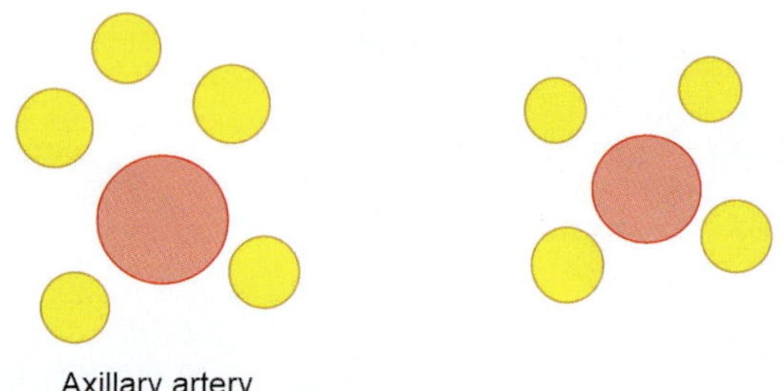

Fig. 3.2.183: Relationship of nerves to axillary artery

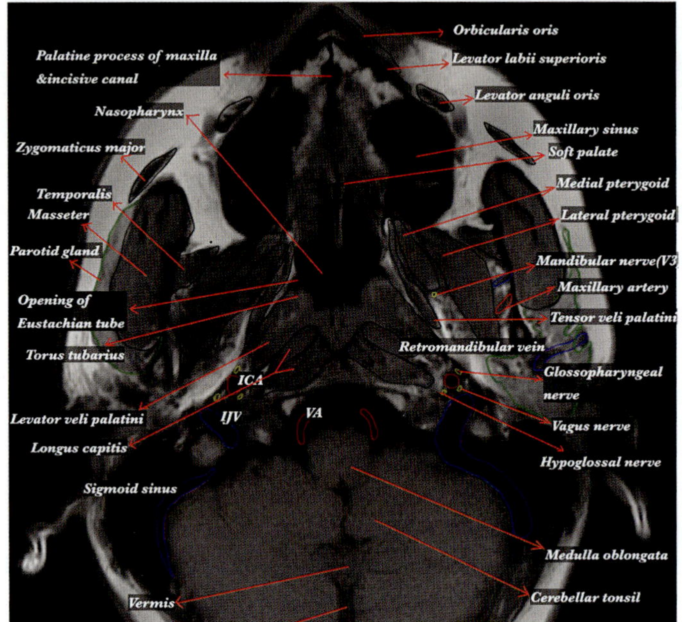

Fig. 3.2.184: MRI axial image: Skull base

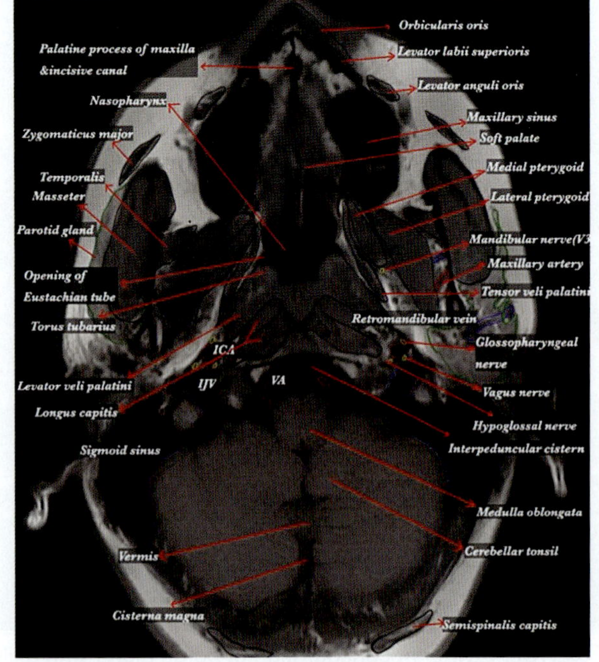

Fig. 3.2.185: MRI axial image: Skull base

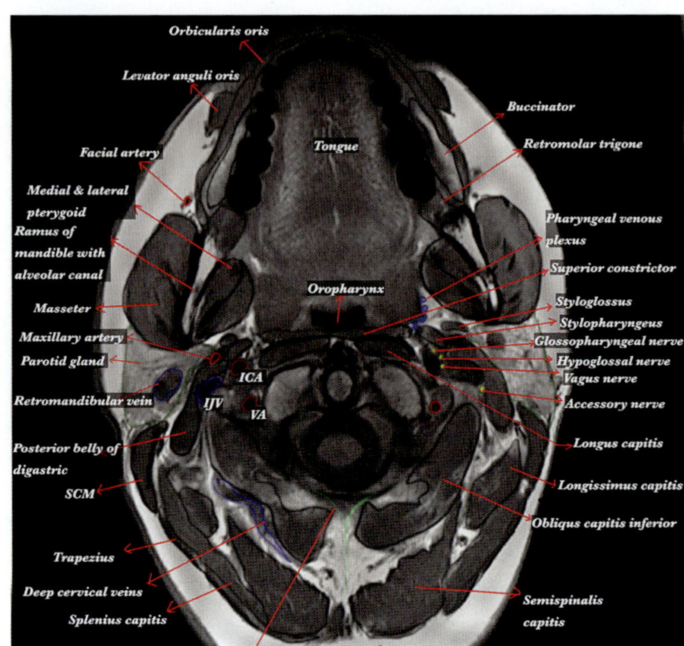

Fig. 3.2.186: MRI axial image: Neck

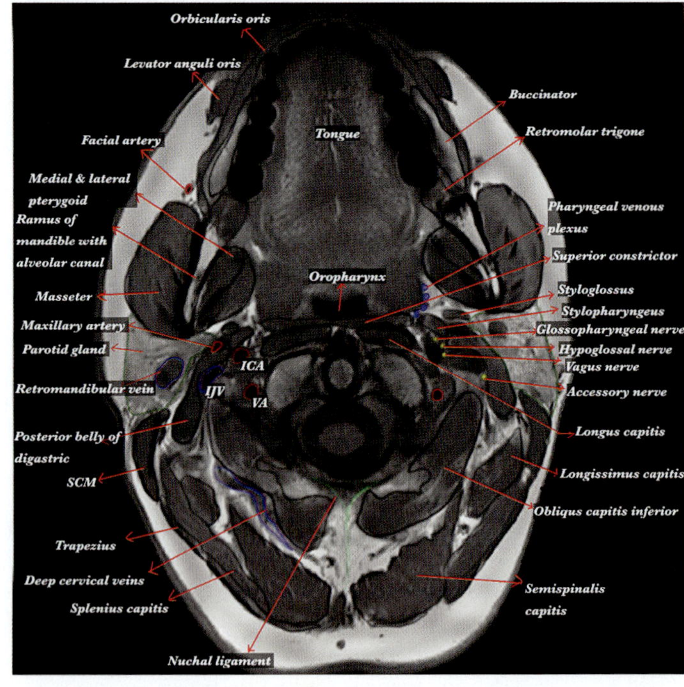

Fig. 3.2.187: MRI axial image: Neck

from the proximal plexus. These include the phrenic, long thoracic, dorsal scapular, and suprascapular nerves. Figures 3.2.169 and 3.2.170 show brachial plexus divisions and branches.

MRI axial sections of neck (Figs 3.2.184 to 3.2.195) showing the neck structures with annotations.

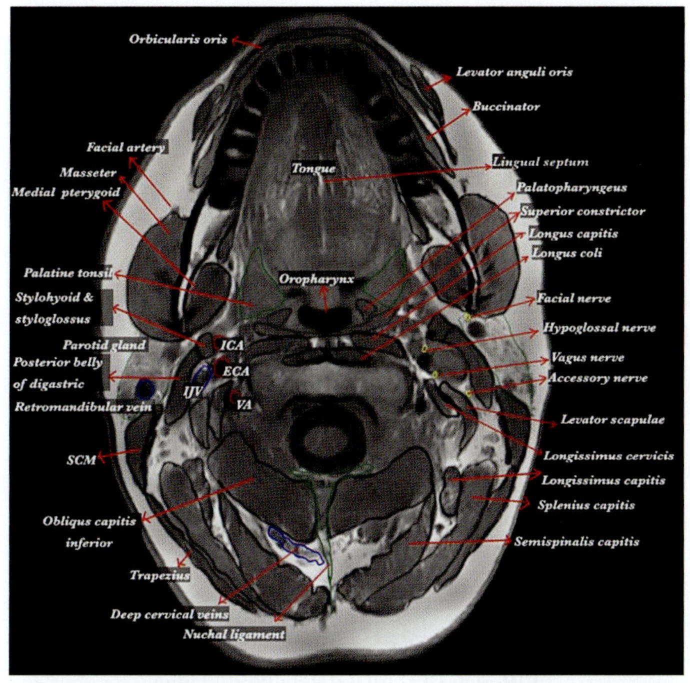

Fig. 3.2.188: MRI axial image: Neck

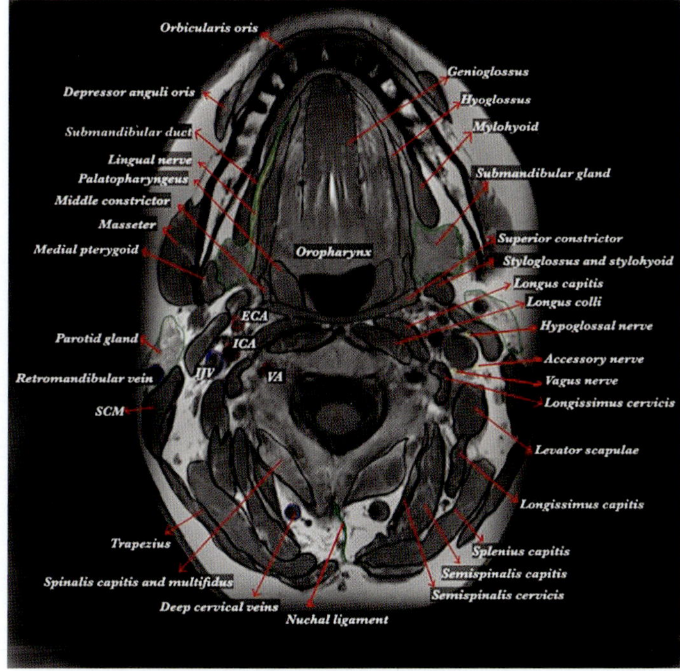

Fig. 3.2.189: MRI axial image: Neck

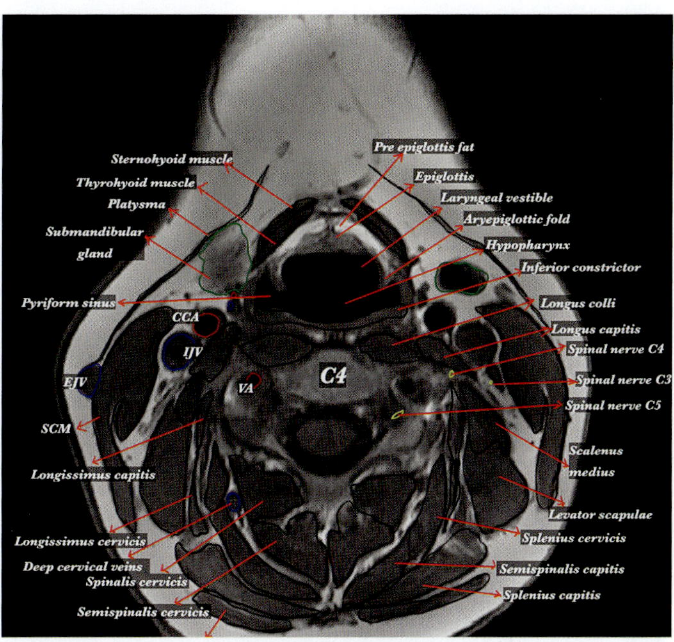

Fig. 3.2.190: MRI axial image: Neck

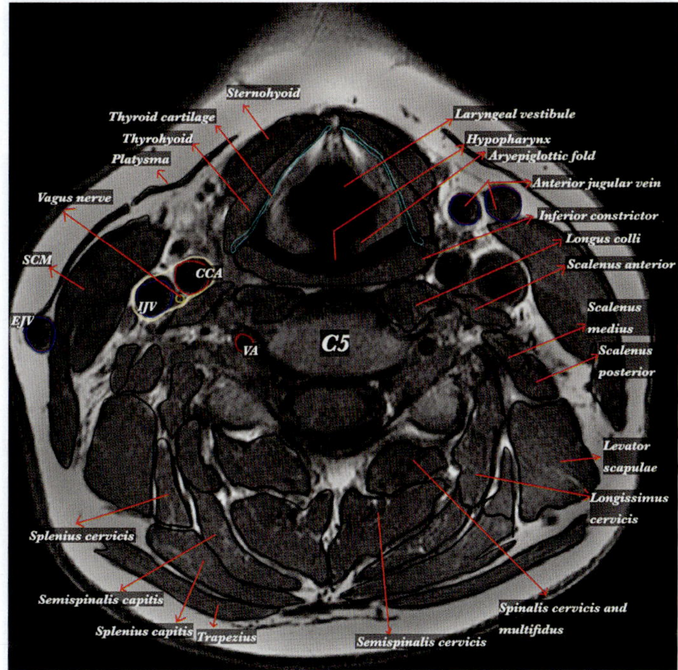

Fig. 3.2.191: MRI axial image: Neck

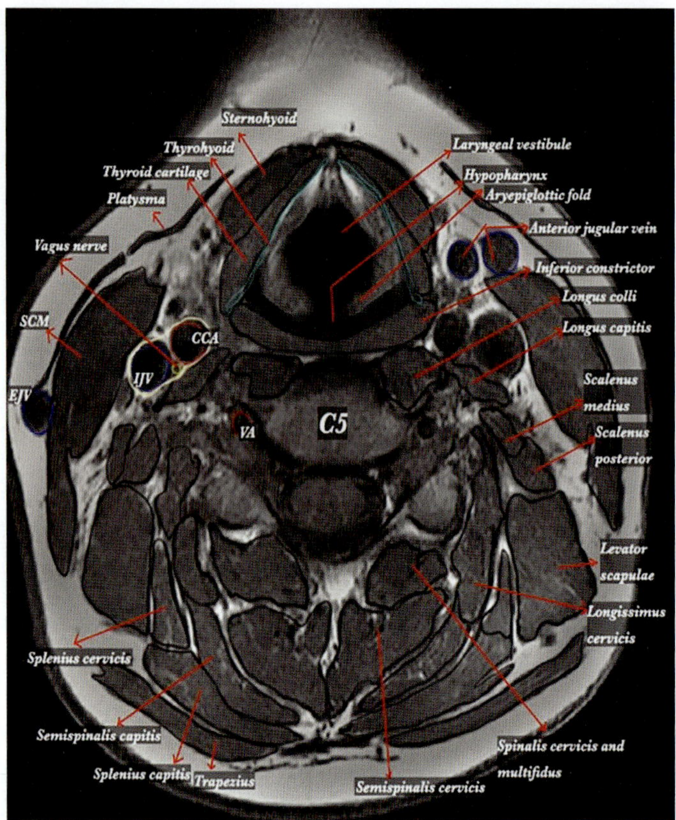

Fig. 3.2.192: MRI axial image: Neck

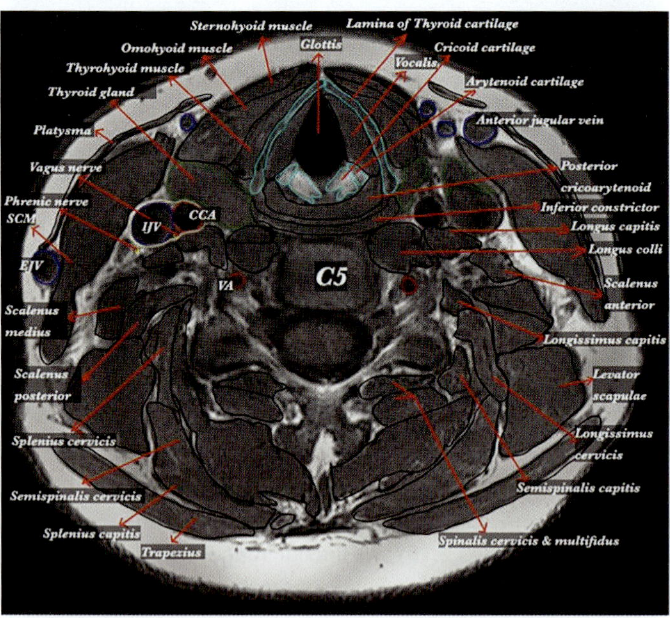

Fig. 3.2.193: MRI axial image: Neck

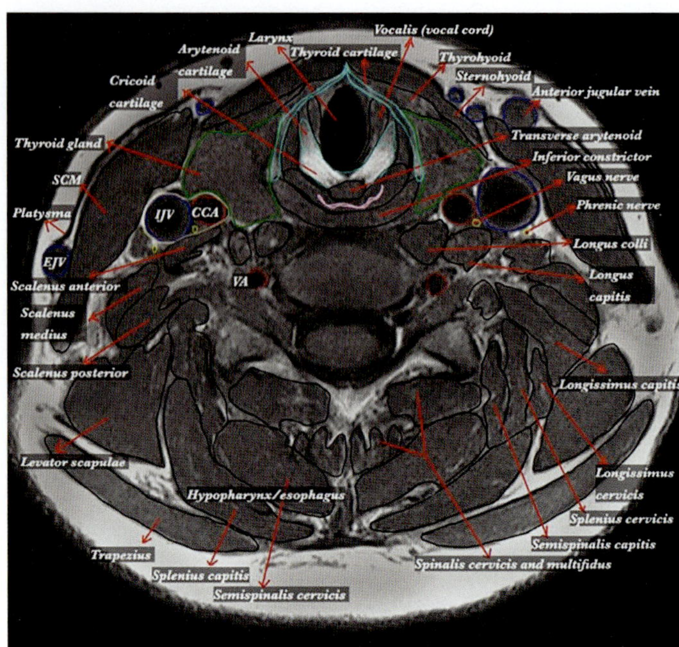

Fig. 3.2.194: MRI axial image: Neck

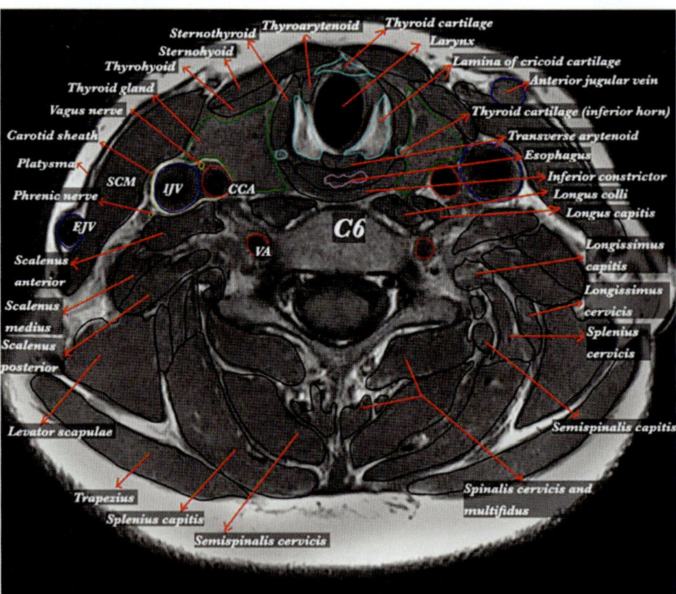

Fig. 3.2.195: MRI axial image: Neck

3.3 CHEST

3.3.A Chest X-ray

The chest X-ray is the most common radiological investigation in the emergency department. The PA and lateral views with the patient standing are the usual radiographic views for evaluating the chest. Anteroposterior (AP) upright or supine projections provide an alternative but less satisfactory image for individuals who are unable to stand. The PA view is commonly used to diagnose a variety of acute and chronic disorders involving all organs of the thoracic cavity, as well as to detect free intraperitoneal gas in patients with acute abdominal discomfort.

PA view: The following are the characteristics of a normal frontal upright chest X-ray: The airway is in the middle. There are no fractures or lytic lesions on the bones. The cardiac silhouette takes up less than half of the thoracic cavity's transverse diameter. The aortic knob is highly defined and the mediastinal breadth is less than 8 cm. The costophrenic angles are extremely acute. The hemidiaphragms are evident bilaterally as smooth curves. The diaphragm on the right is slightly higher than the one on the left. The lung fields appear to be clear. The vascular marks on the lung can be seen from the outside. Because blood flow is diverted to the lung bases by gravity, lung markings are less visible in the apices. The minor fissure appears to be imperceptible or inconspicuous. Where the upper lobes meet anteriorly and posteriorly, the anterior and posterior connection lines are generated. The azygoesophageal recess is the area below the azygos vein arch where the right lung meets the mediastinum between the heart and the vertebral column. The oesophagus surrounds it on the left. All locations where the lung borders the diaphragm, the heart, and other mediastinal structures should be examined on the PA chest-film. At these borders lung-soft tissue interfaces, are seen resulting in a: (1) Line or stripe—for instance, the right para tracheal stripe and (2) Silhouette—for instance, the normal silhouette of the aortic knob or left ventricle. These lines and silhouettes are useful localizers of disease, because they can be displaced or obscured with loss of the normal silhouette. This is called the silhouette sign.

Lateral view: The lateral view reveals the lucent retrosternal space, which overlies the heart and mediastinum on a frontal projection.The retrocardiac space appears lucent on the lateral chest X-ray. The diaphragms normally form smooth curves decreasing from anterior to posterior when viewed from the lateral side. Because it comprises low-density lung tissue, the space above the diaphragm is frequently lucent. Pleural effusions can be seen on lateral views as extensive layering opacities that have replaced the diaphragm's natural curvature in this area. Pleural effusions can sometimes produce a meniscus on the thorax's posterior wall, inverting

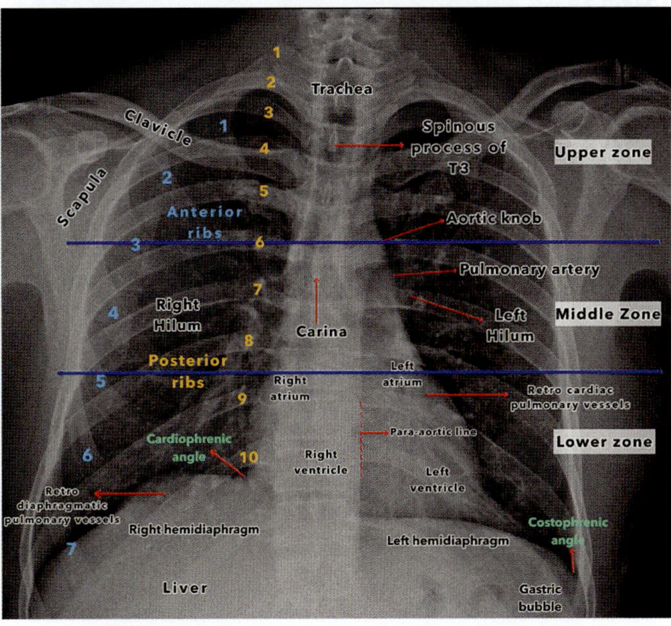

Fig. 3.3.1: Lung zones of PA chest radiograph

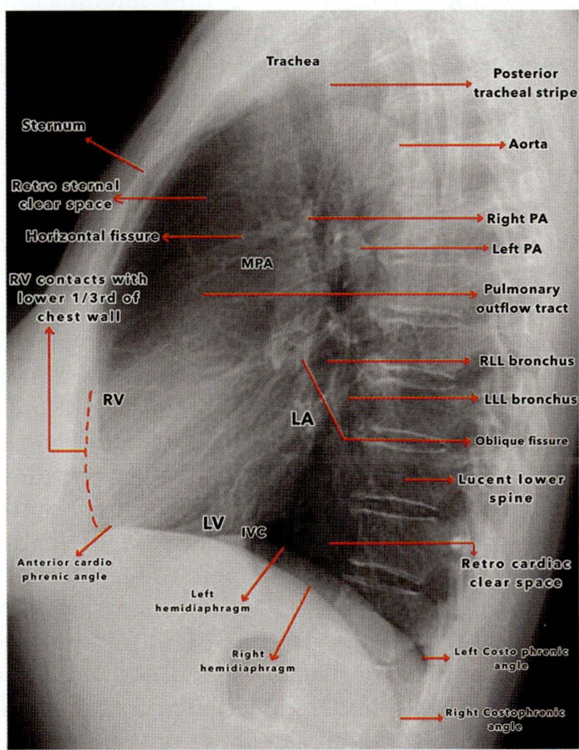

Fig. 3.3.2: Lateral chest radiograph

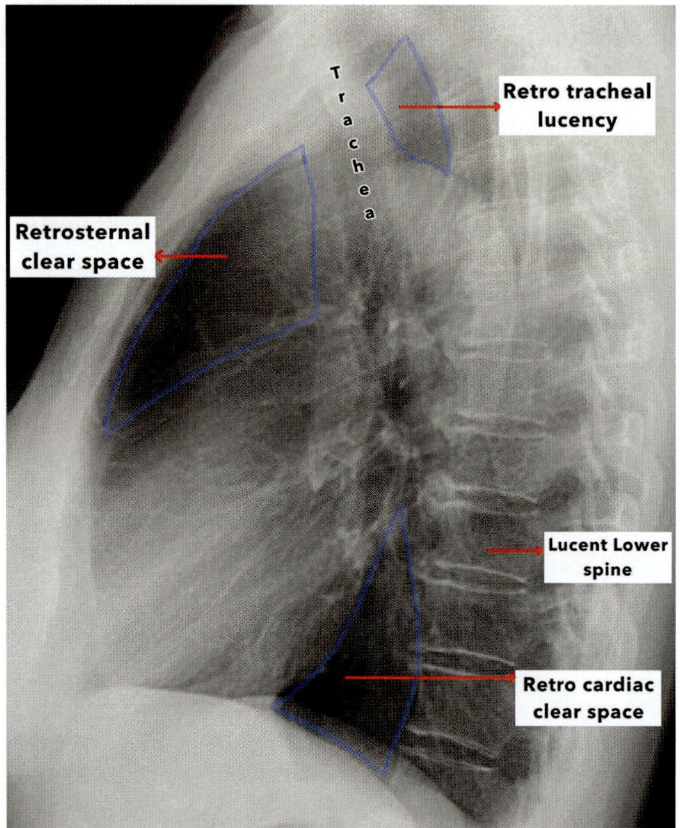

Fig. 3.3.3: Spaces and lucency in normal lateral radiograph

the diaphragm's usual curve. On the lateral view, air beneath the diaphragm (pneumoperitoneum) may also be apparent. The "spine sign" is a common finding, where thoracic spine becomes increasingly lucent as it reaches the diaphragm on a typical lateral chest X-ray.

3.3.B CT Chest—Cross Sectional Anatomy

Bronchopulmonary segments radiology on CT: **Based on Boyden classification**—the segmentation of the lungs into segments based on the tertiary or segmental bronchi is referred to as bronchopulmonary segmental anatomy. Because each segment has its own pulmonary arterial branch, the bronchopulmonary segment is a section of the lung with its own bronchus and artery. Each segment is functionally and physically distinct, allowing for surgical resection of a single segment without impacting adjacent segments. There are **10 segments in the right lung and 8 segments in the left lung (10–8 segments).** Right upper lobe has three segments—apical, anterior and posterior segments. Right middle lobe on the right has two segments—medial and lateral (easy to remember—middle lobe, medial and lateral). Right lower lobe has five segments—superior segment, medial basal, anterior basal, lateral basal and posterior basal segments. Left upper lobe has four segments—anterior, apicoposterior, superior lingular and inferior lingular segments. Left lower lobe has four segments—superior segment, anteromedial basilar, lateral basilar, posterior basilar segments. Left upper lobe apicoposterior segment and left lower lobe anteromedial segment are two regions of the left lung in which two segments are joined as one because they have a common tertiary (segmental) bronchus.

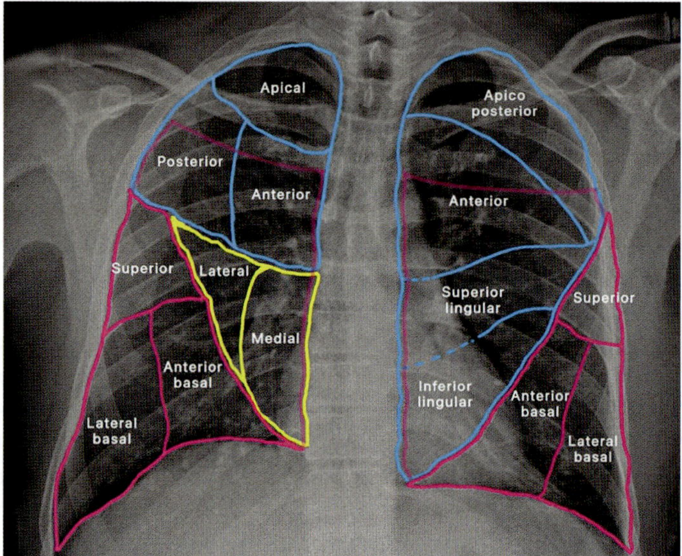

Fig. 3.3.4: Bronchopulmonary segments in normal PA chest radiograph

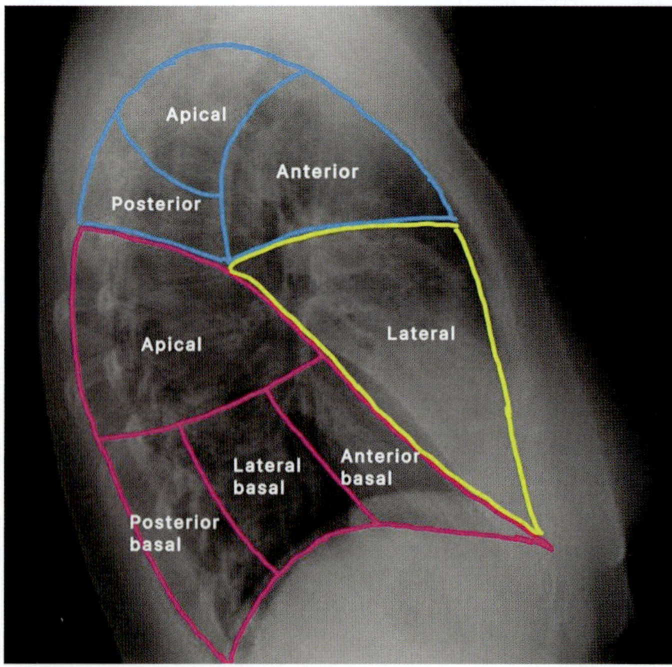

Fig. 3.3.5: Bronchopulmonary segments in normal right lung on lateral chest radiograph

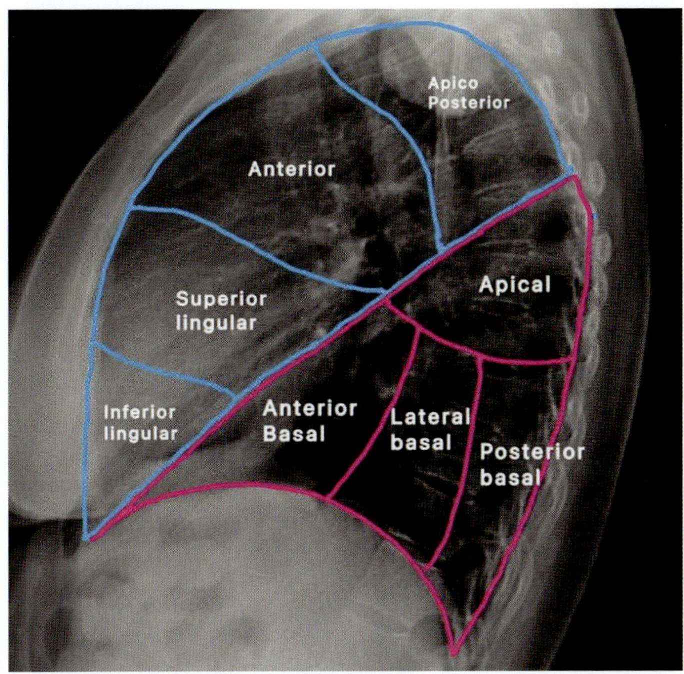

Fig. 3.3.6: Bronchopulmonary segments in normal left lung on lateral chest radiograph

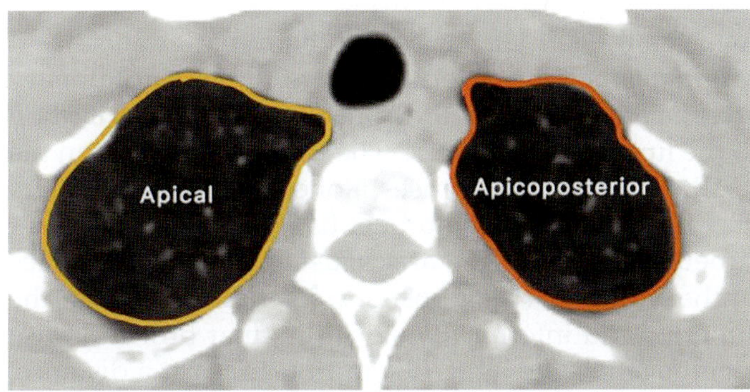

Fig. 3.3.7: Bronchopulmonary segments on axial CT scan (Figs 3.3.7 to 3.3.12)

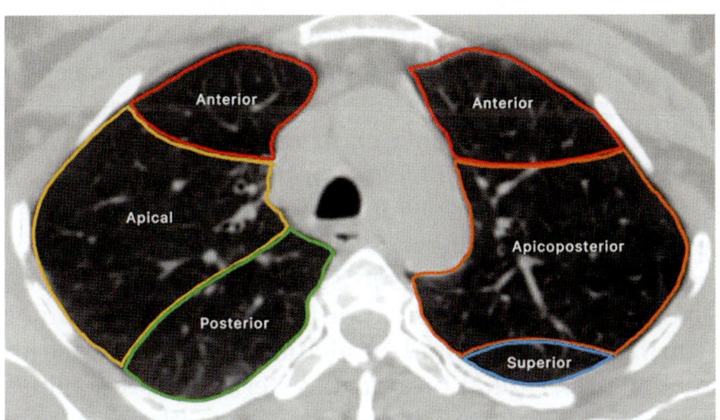

Fig. 3.3.8

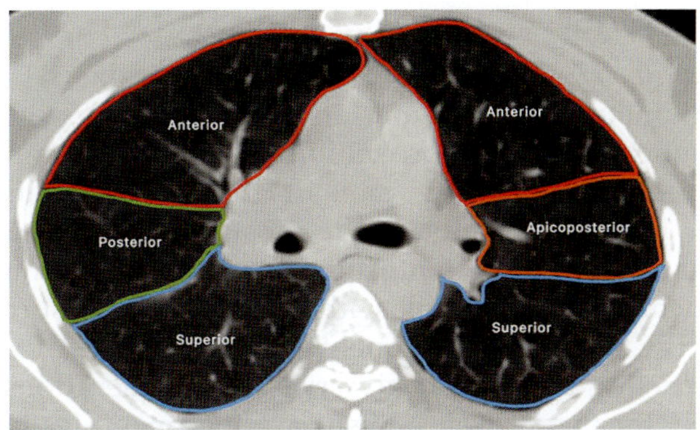

Fig. 3.3.9

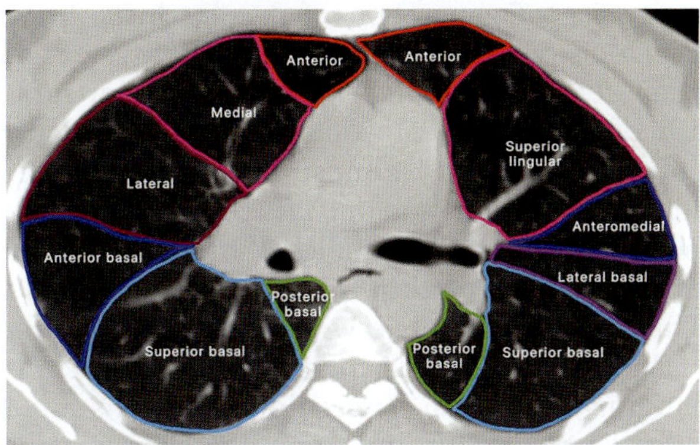

Fig. 3.3.10

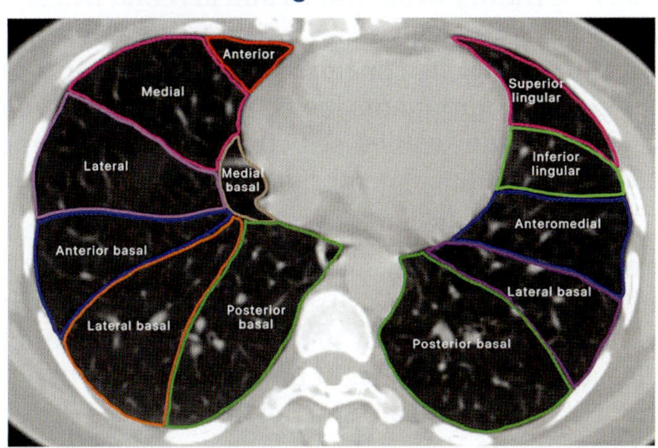

Fig. 3.3.11

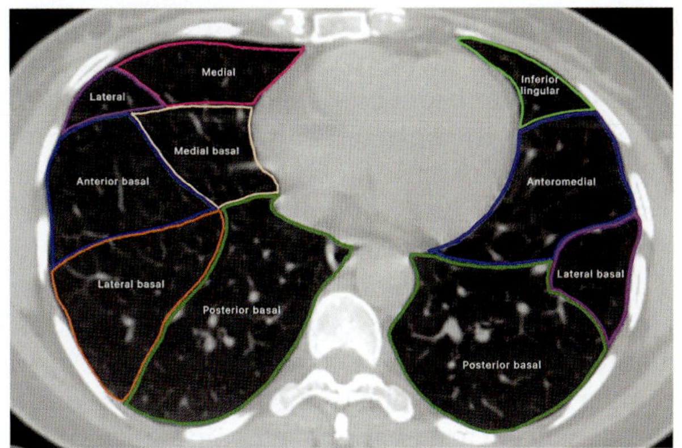

Fig. 3.3.12

3.3.C Airway

Airway structure and types: Bronchi—size >1 cm in diameter, should taper and branch and give rise to noncartilaginous bronchioles. Bronchi <2 mm in diameter not normally visible in HRCT. **Bronchioles**—size 1 mm in diameter. The most distal bronchiole lined by respiratory epithelium is terminal bronchiole. Bronchioles rarely visible within 1 cm of pleural surface on HRCT. **Terminal bronchioles** are the most distal conducting airways. It give rise to ~3 generations of respiratory bronchioles. **Respiratory bronchioles** have increasing numbers of alveoli extend from their walls. They give rise to 3 generations of alveolar ducts. **Alveolar ducts** give rise to series of alveoli adjacent to one another and they terminate in alveolar sacs. **Alveolar sacs** are groups of most distal alveoli and **alveoli. Functional and structural airway zones: Conducting zone:** Its function is air conduction only. Its components include trachea bronchi and bronchioles. It has a **dichotomous** type of **branching pattern** (parent airway divides into 2). **They are asymmetric** with variable diameter in size. There are no alveoli in airway walls and no gas exchanging epithelium. **Transitional zone:** Its function includes air conduction and respiration. Its components include **respiratory bronchioles and alveolar ducts**. The airway walls contain alveoli which enable gas exchange. **Respiratory zone:** Its function is respiration only (gas exchange). Its components include **alveoli and alveolar sacs**. They are thin walled structures and they come in contact with capillary membrane.

Trachea: Except on the left side just above the bifurcation, where the aorta typically forms a smooth depression, the trachea is a midline construction with parallel tracheal walls. The trachea is about 10 to 12 cm long. The trachea divides into the left and right major bronchi at the level of carina that is located around the fifth thoracic vertebra. The subcarinal angle might be anything between 35 and 90 degrees (mean 61 degrees).

Bronchi: The right main bronchus measures approximately 2 cm in length and has a more vertical course than the left main bronchus. It splits into the bronchus intermedius and the right upper lobe bronchus. From the takeoff of the right upper lobe bronchus, the bronchus intermedius continues distally for 3 to 4 cm before bifurcating into bronchi to the middle and lower lobes. The left main bronchus is about 5 cm long and splits into the upper and lower lobe bronchi on the left side. The segmental bronchi branch off from the lobar bronchi. Thus, the right upper lobe bronchus (ULB) is said to be eparterial, since it arises above the point where the right pulmonary artery crosses the right main bronchus (RMB),

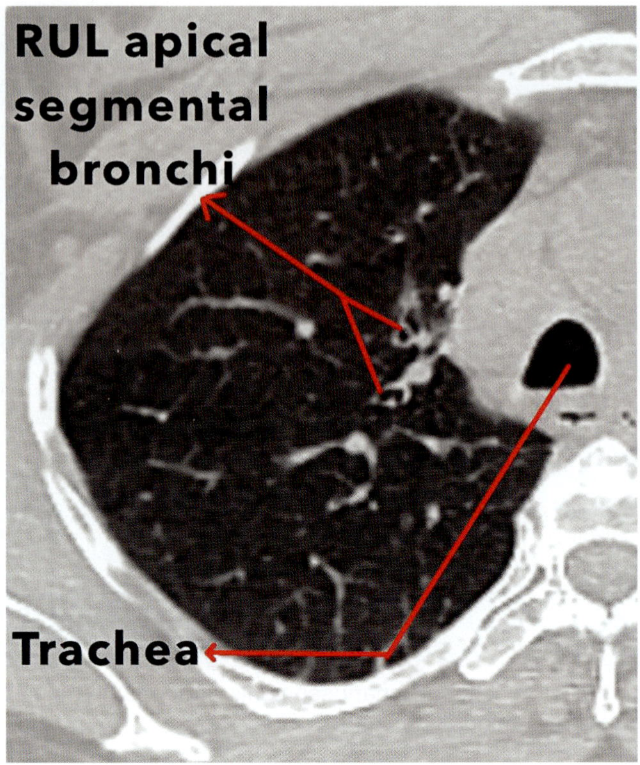

Fig. 3.3.13: Right UL bronchi

whereas the left ULB is said to be hyparterial, since it originates below the point where the left pulmonary artery crosses the LMB. Bronchovascular distribution to the lungs is asymmetric. The RMB is shorter than the LMB. The right ULB arises alone, several centimeters above the middle lobe bronchus (MLB), and the right superior bronchus (B6) arises just inferior to the orifice of the MLB, nearly opposite to it. In the left lung, the superior and inferior divisions (lingular bronchi) arise together from the left ULB, and B6 arises at a distance. Indeed, the common trunk of the left lower lobe is longer than that of the right lower lobe.

3.3.D HRCT Lung

The **secondary pulmonary lobule** is the smallest discrete portion of the lung that is surrounded by connective tissue septa. The normal secondary pulmonary lobule cannot be identified on a chest radiograph or CT. The lung between two lines can only be recognised as a secondary pulmonary lobule when the interlobular septa become apparent as septal lines as a result of thickening by fluid or tissue, such as oedema or cancer. Secondary pulmonary lobule is supplied by lobular bronchiole, preterminal bronchiole that gives rise to smaller preterminal bronchioles, terminal bronchioles and respiratory bronchioles. It has its blood supply from lobular artery and branches. Each lobule is

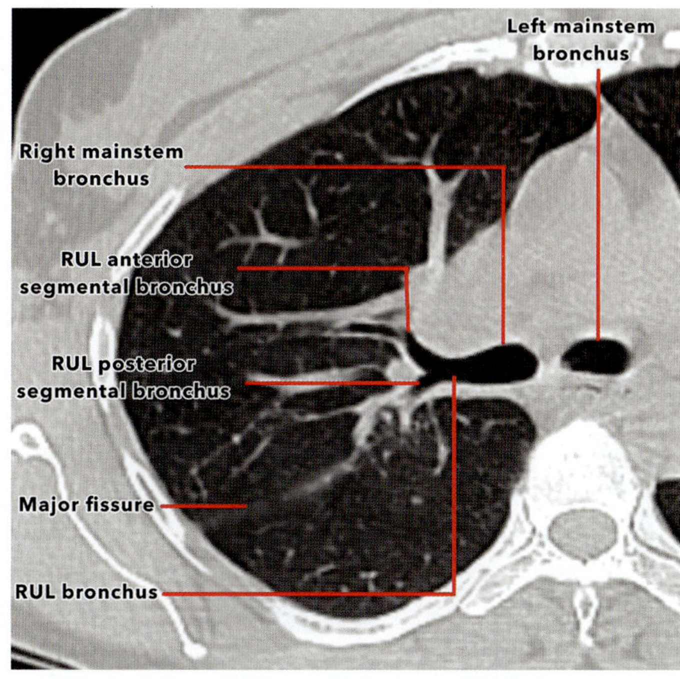

Fig. 3.3.14: CT chest axial image: Bronchial divisions

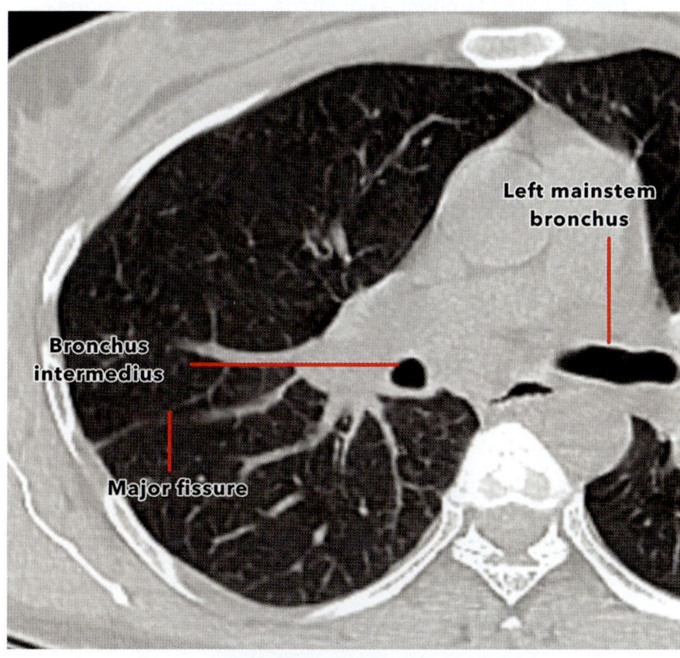

Fig. 3.3.15: CT chest axial image: Bronchial divisions

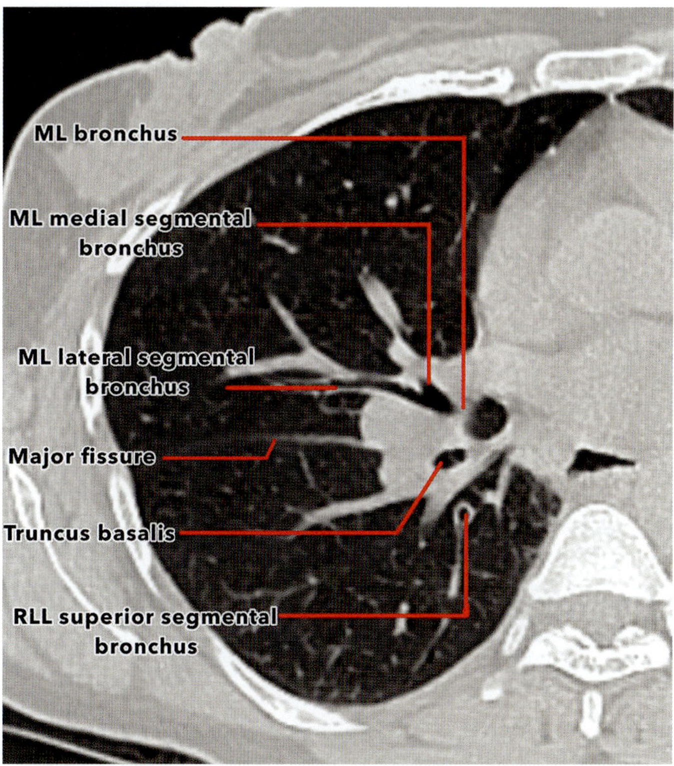

Fig. 3.3.16: CT chest axial image: Bronchial divisions

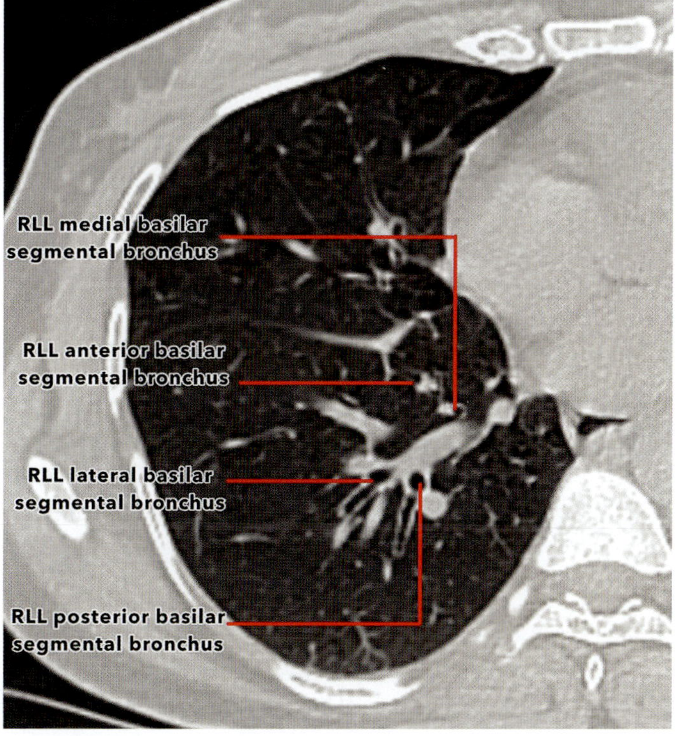

Fig. 3.3.17: CT chest axial image: Bronchial divisions

marginated by interlobular septa containing pulmonary veins and lymphatics. They are irregularly polyhedral in shape measuring 1.0–2.5 cm in diameter. They are most developed and most apparent in lung periphery. They are most often seen in apices, anteriorly, and near mediastinal pleura.

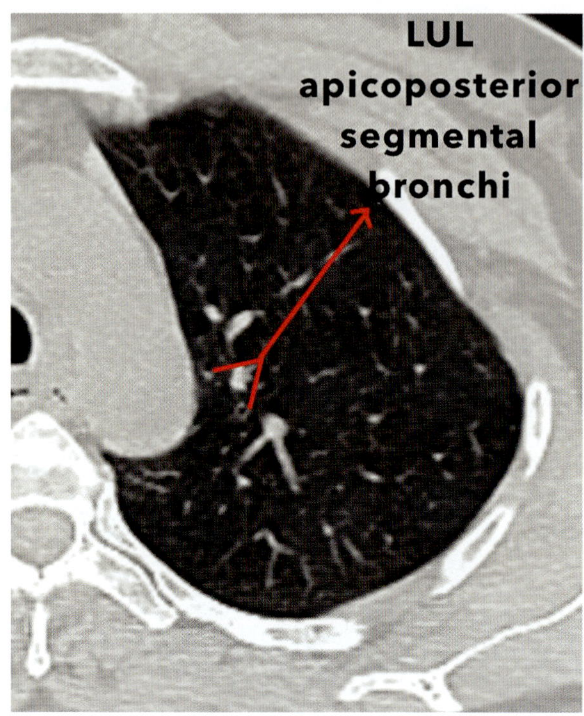

Fig. 3.3.18: CT chest axial image: Bronchial divisions

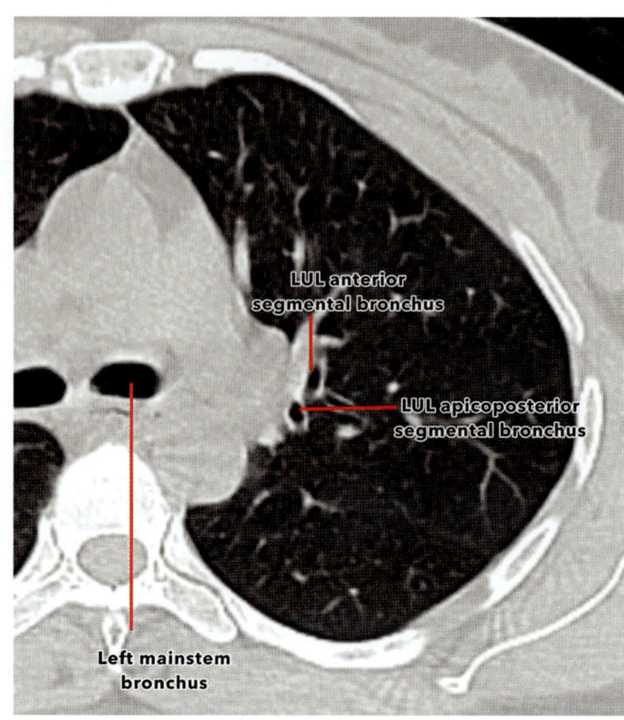

Fig. 3.3.20: CT chest axial image: Bronchial divisions

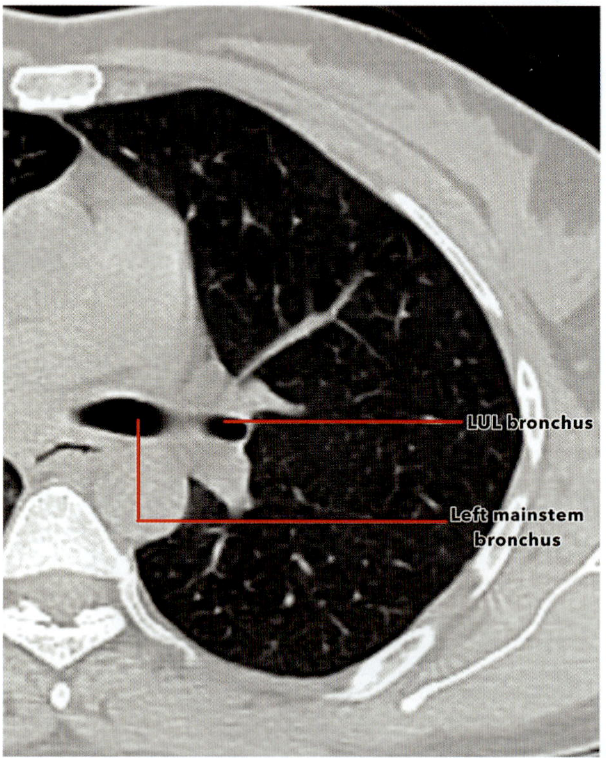

Fig. 3.3.19: CT chest axial image: Bronchial divisions

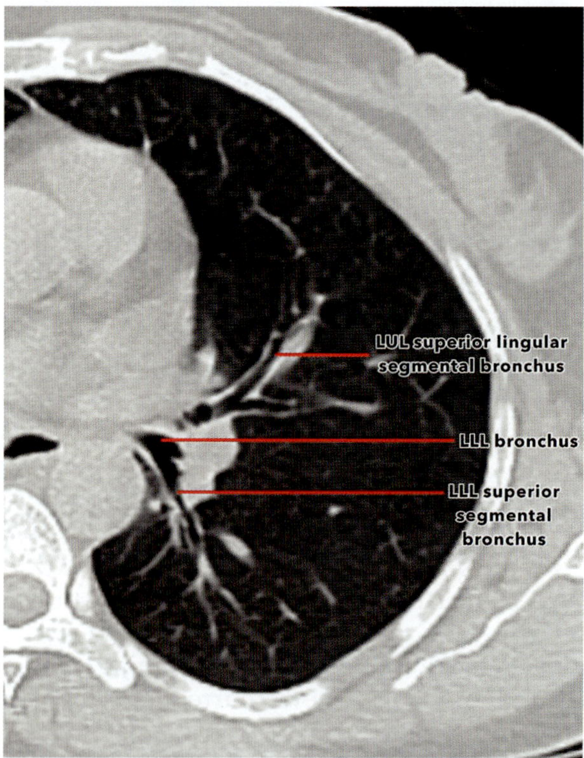

Fig. 3.3.21: CT chest axial image: Bronchial divisions

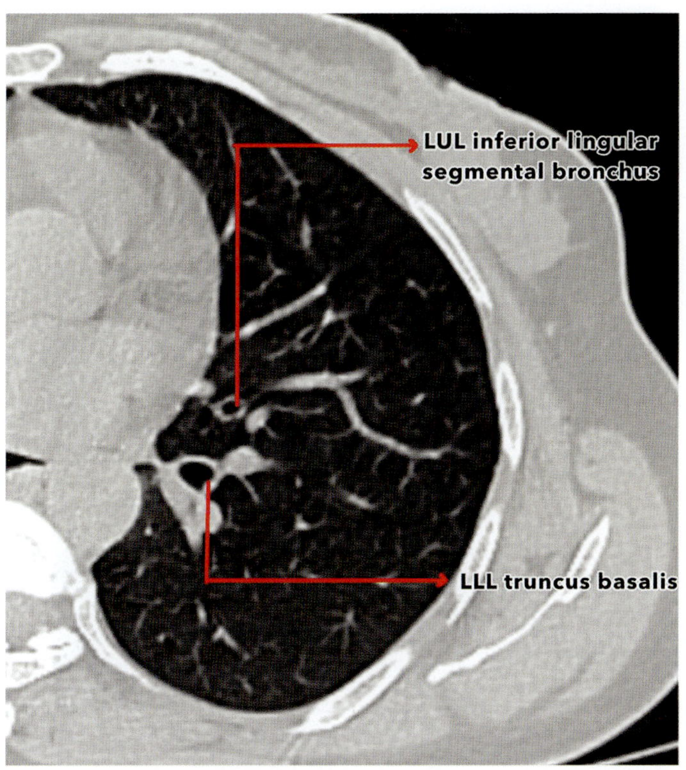

Fig. 3.3.22: CT chest axial image: Bronchial divisions

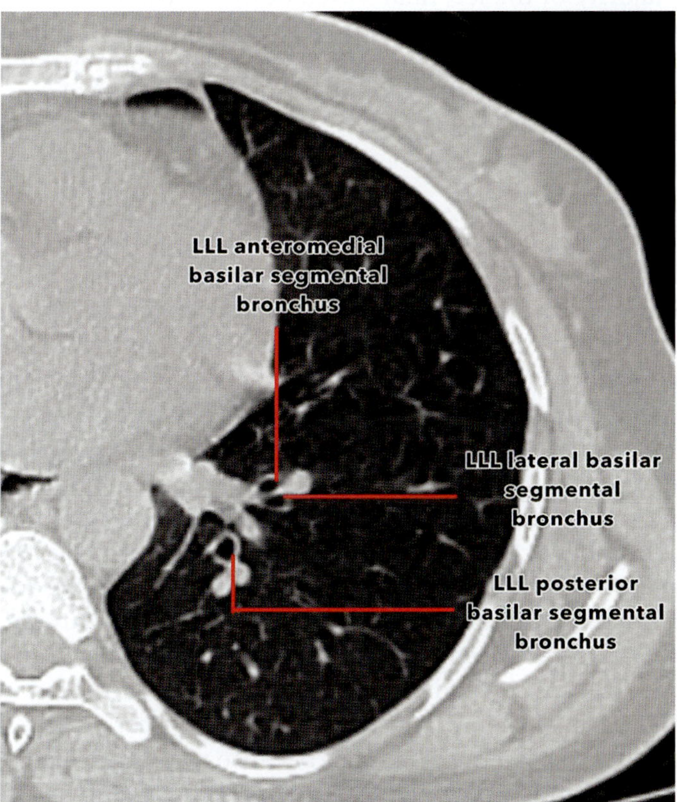

Fig. 3.3.23: CT chest axial image: Bronchial divisions

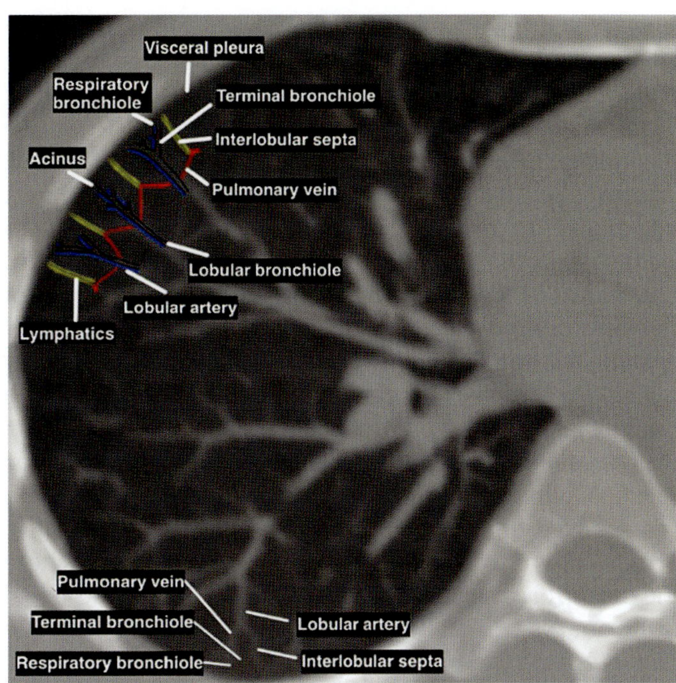

Fig. 3.3.24: Secondary pulmonary lobule

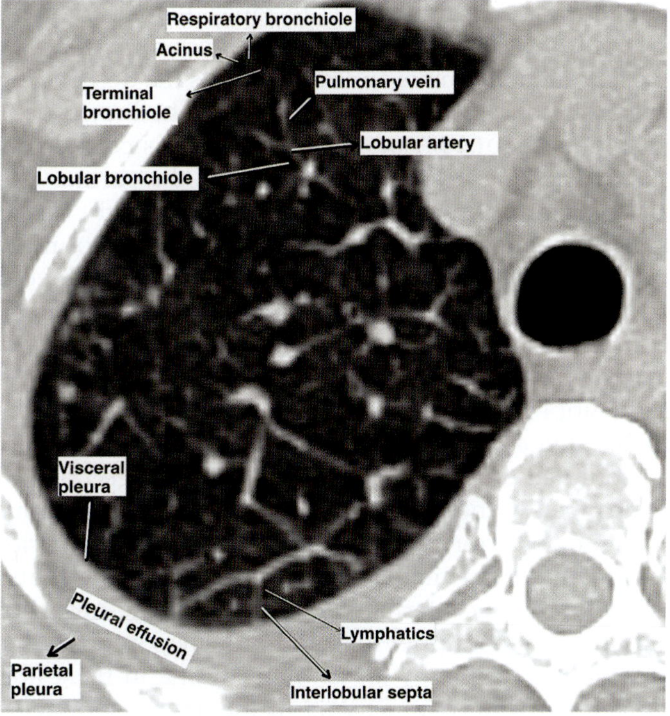

Fig. 3.3.25: CT chest axial section

3.3.E Hilum

The vertically oriented interlobar artery forms the major shadow of the right hilum on a PA radiograph, and structures directly above the interlobar artery include the ascending pulmonary artery (truncus anterior) and superior pulmonary vein. The distal left pulmonary artery, the proximal portion of the left interlobar artery and its segmental arterial branches, and the left superior pulmonary vein and its primary tributaries comprise the upper hilar opacity on the left. **Because the left pulmonary artery arches over the left main and left upper lobe bronchi, the left hilum is typically 1 to 2 cm higher than the highest point of the right hilum.** Enlargement of the hilar lymph nodes leads to increased size and opacity of the hilum, a lobulated contour, and obscuration of the interlobar artery. **Hila are usually concave in shape.** This concavity may disappear and be the first sign of hilar enlargement. In lymphadenopathy, the vessels will be evident through the region of hilar fullness, whereas in pulmonary arterial enlargement, the vessels will converge on the hilar fullness boundaries. This is known as hilar convergence sign. The point where the superior pulmonary vein shadow meets the basal pulmonary artery shadow forms a shallow concave angle termed the **hilar angle**. Because the right and left hilar components are superimposed, the radiographic anatomy of the hila on a lateral projection is complex. The trachea is usually visible all the way down to the carina, where the air column starts to taper. Left pulmonary artery appears as a curved structure as it courses above the left main bronchus and continues as the descending left pulmonary artery. The left upper lobe bronchus is visible in about 75% of cases because it is completely surrounded by vessels at the level of the carina. The air column of the normally more cephalic right upper lobe bronchus can be identified end-on as a rounded radiolucency in 50% of subjects because it is devoid of vascular envelopment on its posterior aspect such that aerated upper or lower lobe parenchyma normally abuts its wall. Consequently, clear identification of the right upper lobe bronchial lumen en face constitutes highly suggestive evidence that the airway is completely surrounded by soft tissue, most likely enlarged lymph nodes. Below the level of the carina, a line continuous with the posterior tracheal wall represents the posterior wall of the right main and intermediate bronchi and is known as the intermediate stem line. The posterior wall of the right upper lobe and bronchus intermedius is rendered visible by air in their lumina in front and by aerated lung parenchyma in the azygoesophageal recess behind. On a lateral radiograph, the intermediate stem line transects the middle or posterior third of the circular, radiolucent left upper lobe bronchus. The superior pulmonary vein anteriorly, the ascending and descending right pulmonary arteries posteriorly, and surrounding connective tissue and lymph nodes make up the right hilar opacity. Because the right pulmonary

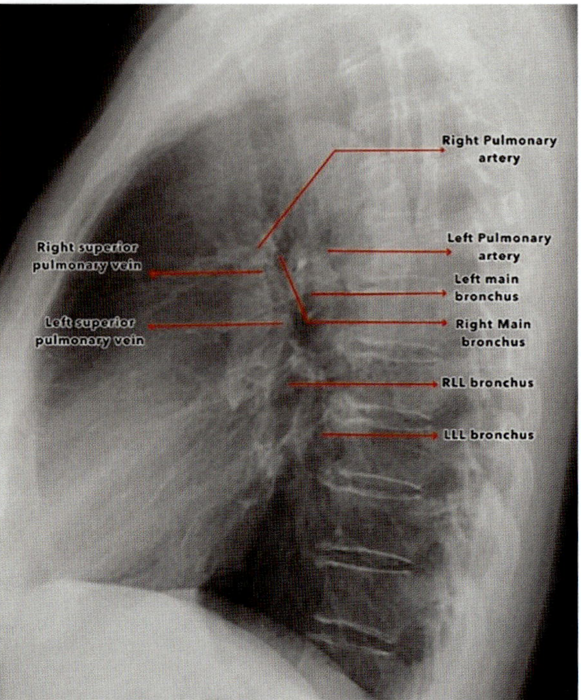

Fig. 3.3.26: Hilum on lateral chest radiograph

artery is a mediastinal vessel that is obscured by other vessels or soft tissue, it is not visible on a lateral radiograph. Behind the intermediate stem line, the majority of the left hilar vasculature is visible. Because of their horizontal orientation, the right and left inferior pulmonary veins are frequently imaged end-on, resulting in a nodular opacity beneath and behind the lower portion of the hila.

3.3.F Pleura

The visceral pleura, which is tightly attached to the lungs, and the parietal pleura, which lines the chest wall, diaphragm, and mediastinum, enclose the pleural space. At the hila, the two come together. The pleura over the convexity of the lungs, as well as the diaphragmatic and mediastinal surfaces, is not normally visible on CR or CT because the combined thickness of the normal parietal and visceral pleural layers is approximately 0.2 mm. Normally, each pleural area stores 8.4 ± 4.3 ml of fluid. A number of factors influence the volume and content of pleural fluids, including starling forces (which provide filtration through the parietal and absorption through the visceral mesothelium), lymphatic drainage, and mesothelial cell activity. Fluid is normally produced in the parietal pleura and drained in the visceral pleura, and it is drawn into the space because recoiling capacity of lung and chest wall acts as an opposing force over the majority of the respiratory volume range.

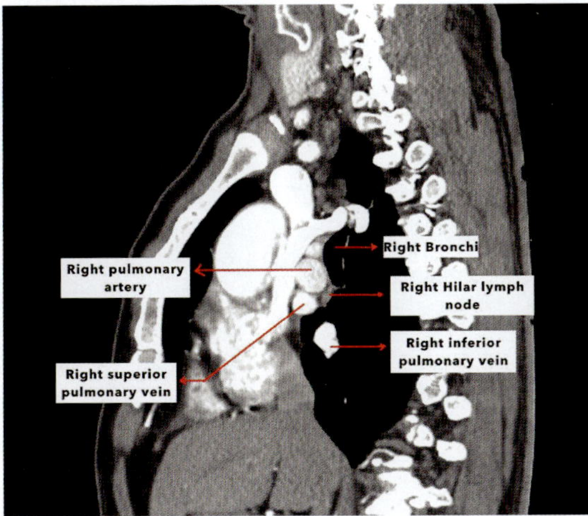

Fig. 3.3.27: Right hilum

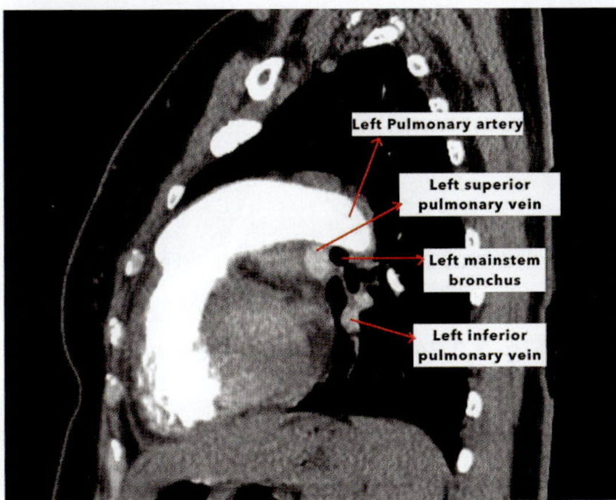

Fig. 3.3.28: Left hilum

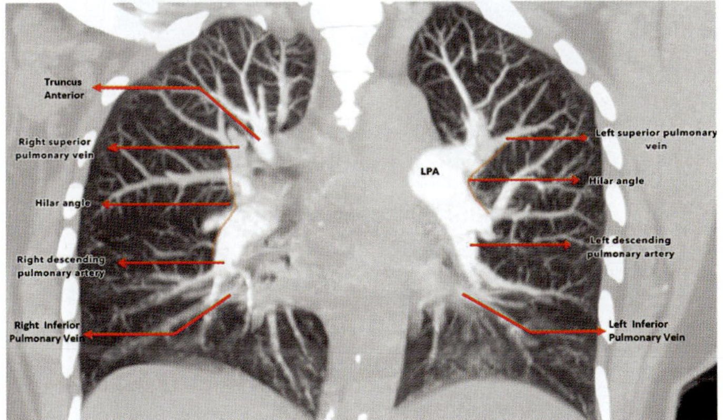

Fig. 3.3.29: Vascular anatomy of CECT chest

3.3.G Fissures

Fissures are pleural invaginations that extend from the lung's outer border into its substance. Fissures that divide the lungs into three right-sided and two left-sided lobes (normal fissures) and those that occur within one of the lobes themselves are traditionally divided into

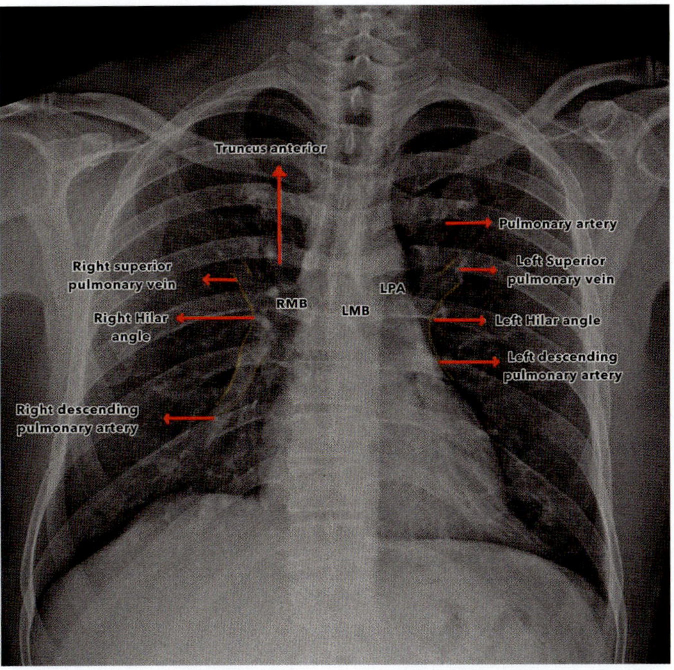

Fig. 3.3.30: Chest X-ray

two categories (accessory fissures). The minor fissure (between the right middle and upper lobes), the right major fissure (between the combined right upper and middle lobes and the right lower lobe), and the left major fissure (between the left upper and lower lobes) are the normal interlobar fissures. The major fissures can be observed on a lateral chest radiograph as lines that extend obliquely downward and forward from the level of the fifth thoracic vertebra and stop a few centimetres behind the anterior pleural gutter at the diaphragm. The interlobar fissures are usually incomplete, and the occurrence of accessory fissures is variable. The azygos fissure, formed by the azygos vein invaginating through the apical region of the right upper lobe, is one of the most well-known accessory fissures. It appears on radiograph as a curvilinear shadow that extends obliquely across the top portion of the right lung and finishes in a teardrop shadow created by the azygos vein itself at a variable distance above the right hilum. Because the vein passes outside the parietal pleura, the fissure is formed by four pleural layers (two parietal and two visceral). The medial basal segment is separated from the rest of the lower lobe by the inferior accessory fissure. It appears as a thin line running from the medial aspect of the hemidiaphragm (most usually right) obliquely cephalad and medially toward the right hilum on 5% to 13% of chest radiographs, most commonly on the right. The superior accessory fissure, more often on the right, divides the superior segment from the lower lobes' basal segments. On around 3% of lateral chest radiographs, the fissure can be seen. The left minor fissure is present in 10–20% of people. The left minor fissure is located slightly more cephalad than the right minor fissure and, like the right minor fissure, is dome shaped (convex superiorly).

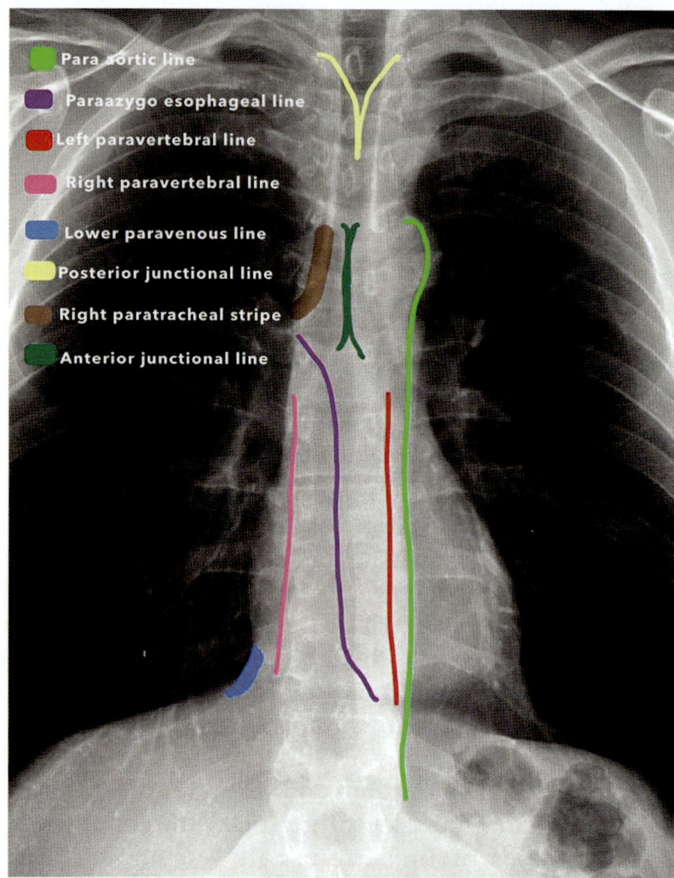

Fig. 3.3.31: Mediastinal lines

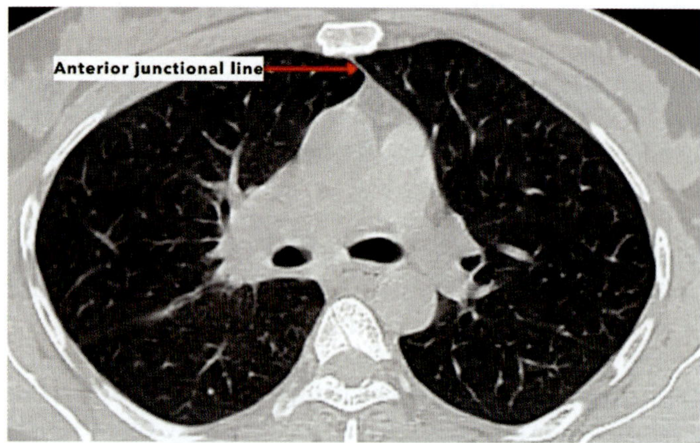

Fig. 3.3.32: CT chest: Mediastinal lines

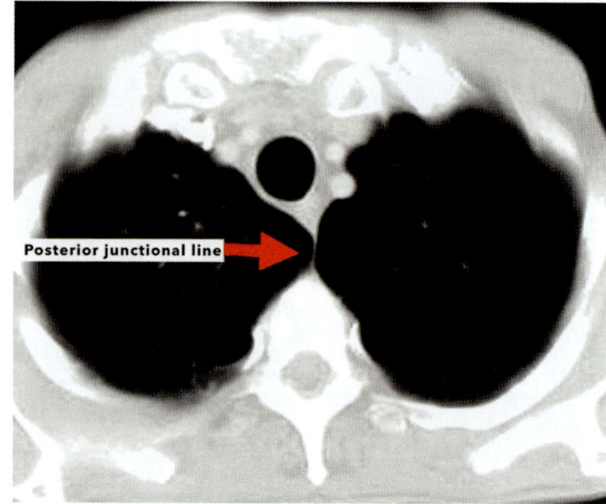

Fig. 3.3.33: CT chest: Mediastinal lines

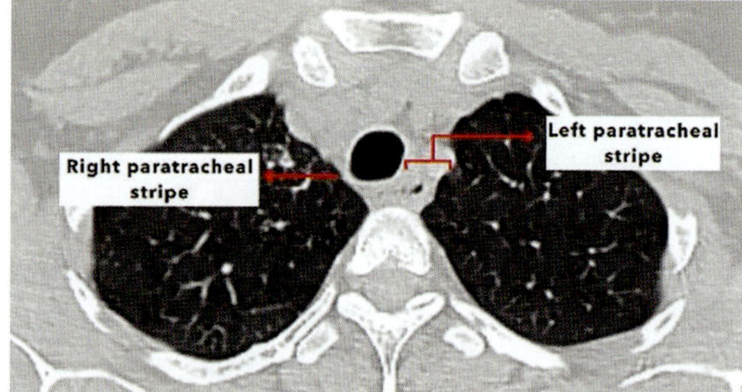

Fig. 3.3.34: CT chest: Mediastinal lines

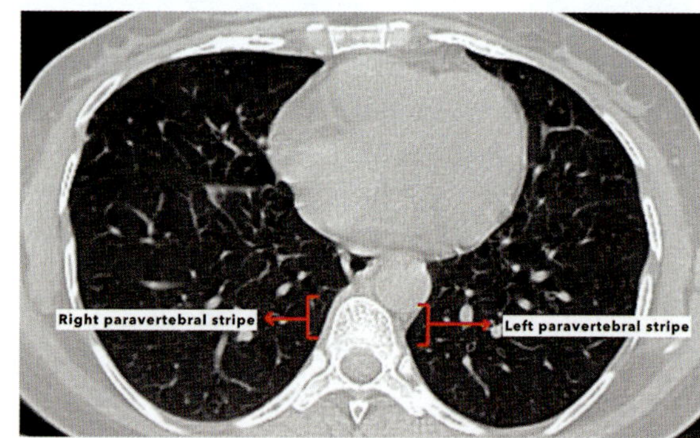

Fig. 3.3.35: CT chest: Mediastinal lines

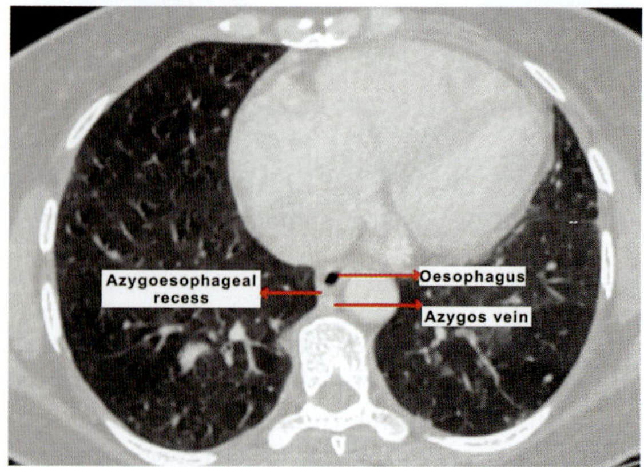

Fig. 3.3.36: CT chest: Mediastinal lines

3.3.H Thoracic Inlet

The thoracic inlet is the point where the structures of the neck and the thorax come together. It runs parallel to the first rib and is higher posteriorly than anteriorly. An opacity that is effaced on its superior aspect and projects at or below the level of the clavicles must be located anteriorly on a frontal chest radiograph, whereas one that projects above the clavicles must be located retrotracheal and posteriorly. The cervicothoracic sign is a combination of these distinct findings. The right and left brachiocephalic veins (which unite behind the right side of the manubrium to form the superior vena cava), the supra-aortic branches, the trachea, the oesophagus, and the recurrent laryngeal nerves on either side of the oesophagus fill the thoracic inlet from front to back. The vascular pedicle is the overall shadow of the great systemic veins and arteries seen on a frontal chest radiograph extending from below the level of the thoracic inlet to the heart. The vascular pedicle's breadth is measured from the SVC's lateral margin as it crosses the right main bronchus to a vertical line drawn inferiorly from where the left subclavian artery emerges from the aortic arch. In a normal upright PA chest radiograph, the vascular pedicle measures less than 6 cm, sometimes it varies. Dilation of the great vessels (supine posture, pregnancy, higher blood volume, left heart failure), mediastinal abnormalities (mediastinal lipomatosis, lymph node enlargement, tumours, fluid collections), or pleural illness can all cause widening of the great arteries (>7 cm).

Thoracic outlet: Thoracic outlet is the space between clavicle and first rib. This narrow passage is crowded with blood vessels, nerves and muscles. The structures passing through the thoracic outlet include—the brachial plexus, the subclavian artery, and the subclavian vein.

3.3.I Mediastinal Anatomy

Except for the lungs, the heart and great vessels, internal mammary vessels, proximal aspect of the azygos venous system, oesophagus, trachea, phrenic nerve, cardiac nerve, supra-aortic and para-aortic bodies, thoracic duct, thymus, and mediastinal lymph nodes are all contained within the mediastinum. Based on the **anatomical classification**, division of the mediastinum is generally conceptualized as comprising 3 or 4 compartments. The **superior mediastinum** is located above the pericardium's upper level and the Ludwig plane (transthoracic plane). This plane spans from the manubriosternal joint (sternal angle or Louis angle) to T4's inferior endplate. Inferior mediastinum: Below the plane of Ludwig. **Anterior mediastinum:** Anterior to the pericardium. **Middle mediastinum:** Within the pericardium. **Posterior mediastinum:** Posterior to the pericardium. The lateral chest radiograph is used to determine the Felson classification. A line drawn along anterior trachea and posterior heart marks the location of the anterior mediastinum. Behind a line that connects points 1 cm behind the front thoracic vertebrae lies the posterior mediastinum. Between the anterior and posterior compartments is the middle mediastinum. The lateral chest radiograph is used for Fraser, Müller, et al classification. The anterior mediastinum of the Felson classification is identical. Between anterior mediastinum and paravertebral region is the middle and posterior mediastinum. The **ITMIG** mediastinal compartments are CT-based mediastinal divisions established based on expert international multidisciplinary consensus. The ITMIG CT-based classifcation includes the prevascular (anterior), visceral (middle), and paravertebral (posterior) compartments. The posterior boundary of the prevascular compartment is the anterior aspect of the pericardium as it wraps around in a curvilinear fashion. Based on these landmarks, the major contents of the prevascular compartment include the thymus, fat, lymph nodes, and left brachiocephalic vein. The anterior boundary of visceral compartment is the anterior aspect of the pericardium, and the posterior boundary is a vertical line connecting a point on the thoracic vertebral bodies 1 cm posterior to anterior margin of spine. The major contents of the visceral compartment include two main components: (1) A vascular component (i.e. the heart, superior vena cava, ascending thoracic aorta, aortic arch, and descending thoracic aorta, intrapericardial pulmonary arteries, and the thoracic duct) and (2) the trachea, carina, esophagus, and lymph nodes.

Thymus: The thymus is visible on the chest radiograph as a mediastinal structure of soft-tissue density. It may be focally or diffusely quite large and mass-like. Typically lung markings can be seen through it; the edges are not sharp, but gradually fade or are wavy because of overlying ribs. Its lower well-defined horizontal border may protrude from the mediastinal contour on the right or the left as a 'sail sign'. It typically has clear lung lateral to it, or clear lung can be seen lateral to it if the patient is oblique enough. A normal thymus does not deviate a normal structure. It should never, for example, cause deviation of the trachea. The thymus appears larger on expiration than on inspiration radiographs. Its anterior location can be seen on a lateral radiograph. The normal thymus can be seen on CT or MRI long after it is no longer visible on a radiograph. On CT it is homogeneous, with a density similar to that of muscle. On T1- and T2-weighted MRI the thymus has a signal greater than that of muscle.

Mediastinal nodes—IASLC Classification (International Association for the Study of Lung Cancer)

Supraclavicular zone: The most cranial station of mediastinal nodes is **Station 1 (supraclavicular)**. The sternal notch, supraclavicular, and lower cervical areas lymph nodes are included. The upper boundary of station 1 is the cricoid cartilage. Station 1 extends inferiorly to the manubrium's upper edge and the clavicles' tops. The midline of trachea is used to distinguish between 1R and 1L lymph nodes.

***Upper zone (superior mediastinal LN):* Station 2 (upper paratracheal):** The left lateral wall of the trachea, rather than the midline, is used to distinguish between 2R and 2L lymph nodes. The apex of ipsilateral lungs and pleural spaces, as well as the upper border of the manubrium, form the upper border of station 2. The inferior edge of the left brachiocephalic vein crosses the trachea at the lower border of station 2 on the right (2R), while the superior border of the aortic arch is at the lower border of station 2 on the left (2L).

Station 3 (prevascular and retrotracheal): Prevascular lymph nodes (3A) are found behind the sternum, in front of the superior vena cava and the left carotid artery. The superior boundary starts at the apex of the chest (like station 2) and extends all the way down to the carina. As the name implies, retrotracheal LNs (3P) are those that are positioned posterior to the trachea and extend from the apex of the chest to the carina.

Station 4 (lower paratracheal nodes) located along the distal trachea, superiorly bordered by station 2, and extending to the carina's level. They are located posterior to the aortic vasculature, and the left lateral wall of the

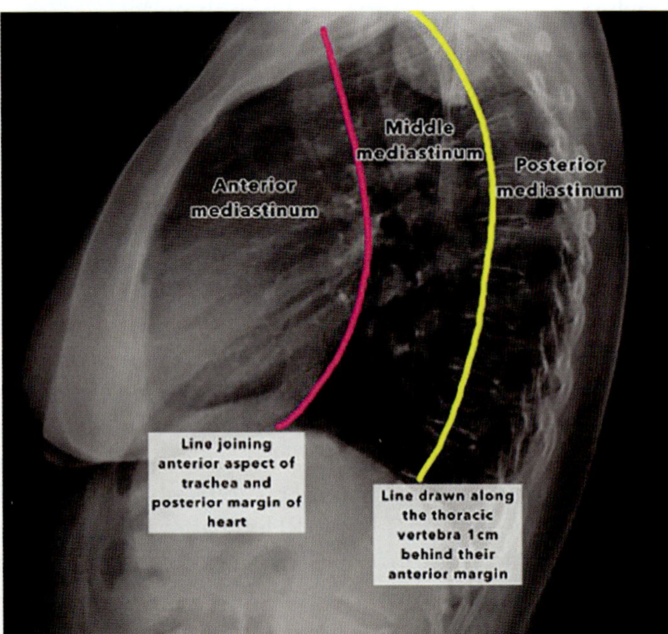

Fig. 3.3.37: Fraser, Muller, et al classification of mediastinum

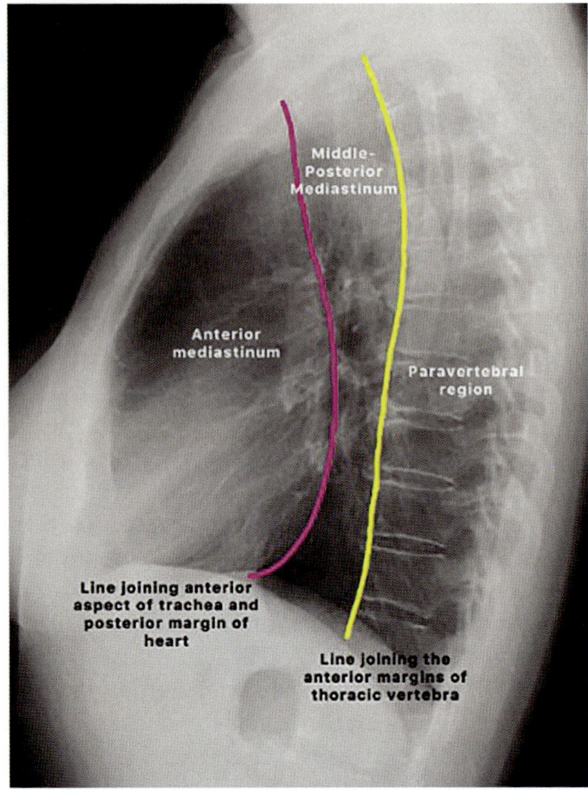

Fig. 3.3.38: Felson classification of mediastinum

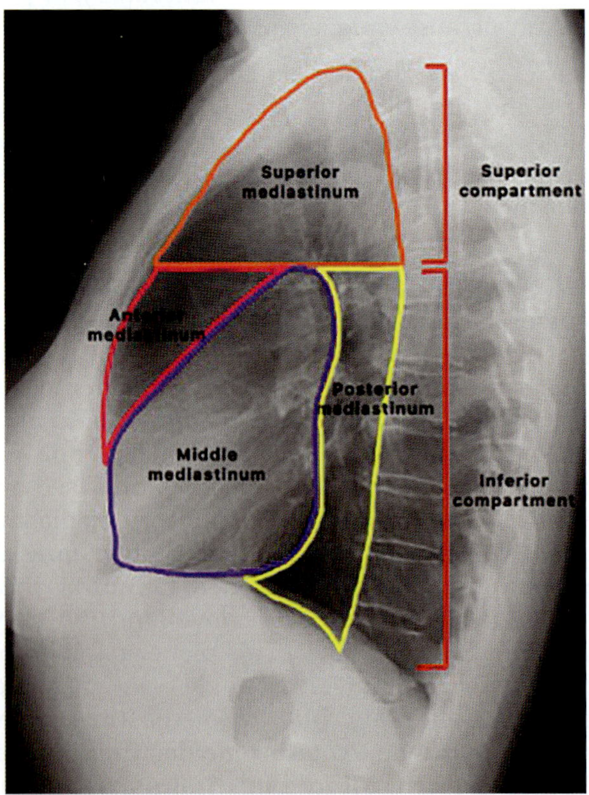

Fig. 3.3.39: Anatomical classification of mediastinum

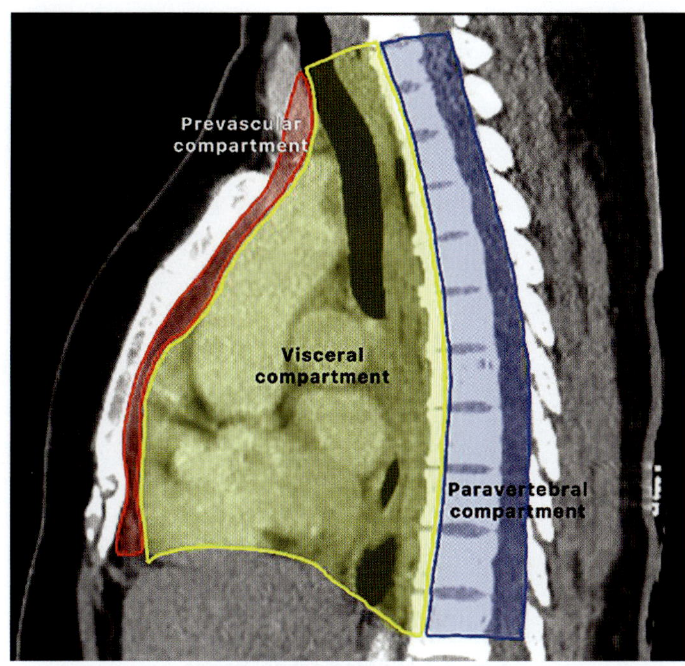

Fig. 3.3.40: ITMIG based classification of mediastinum

trachea, rather than the midline, is used to distinguish between 4R and 4L.

Station 5 (sub-aortic) lymph nodes, also known as aortopulmonary (AP) window LNs, are found lateral to the ligamentum arteriosum, which is the remains of the ductus arteriosus. The top border of station 5 is defined by the lower margin of the aortic arch, while the lower extension is defined by the superior margin of the left pulmonary artery.

Station 6 (para-aortic) LNs are located anterior and/or above the subaortic (AP window) LNs on the anterior and lateral aspects of the ascending aorta and aortic arch. The phrenic nerve can be utilised as a landmark to locate lymph nodes categorized as para-aortic.

Station 7 (subcarinal) is located immediately below the carina and between the mainstem bronchi. The distal aspect of the bronchus intermedius and origin of the left lower lobe bronchus are used to distinguish the right and left inferior extensions of station 7 from the paraesophageal LNs that are found farther caudally. Given that termination of bronchus intermedius is usually lower than the origin of left lower lobe bronchus, this results in an inferior edge that is tilted from the horizontal in most individuals.

Lower zone LNs (inferior mediastinal LNs):

Station 8 (paraesophageal) LNs are those mediastinal lymph nodes found inferior to the subcarinal lymph nodes, along with the anterior or lateral aspects of the esophagus, down to the esophageal hiatus of the diaphragm.

Station 9 lymph nodes are related to the nodes of the pulmonary ligament. These "ligaments" are actually

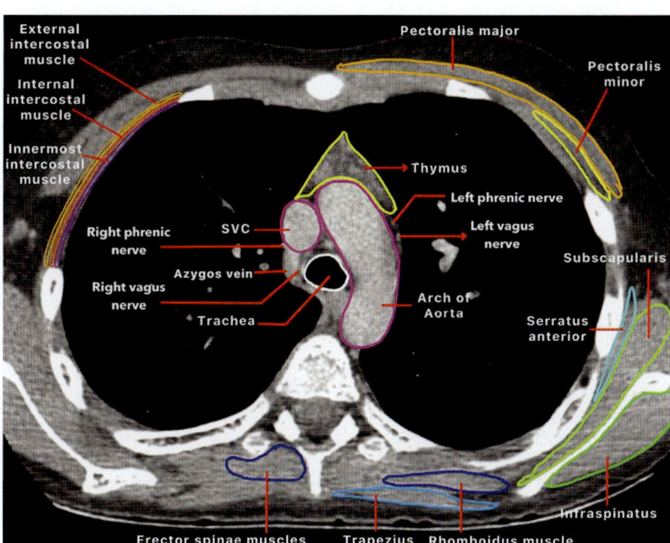

Fig. 3.3.41: CT chest axial image

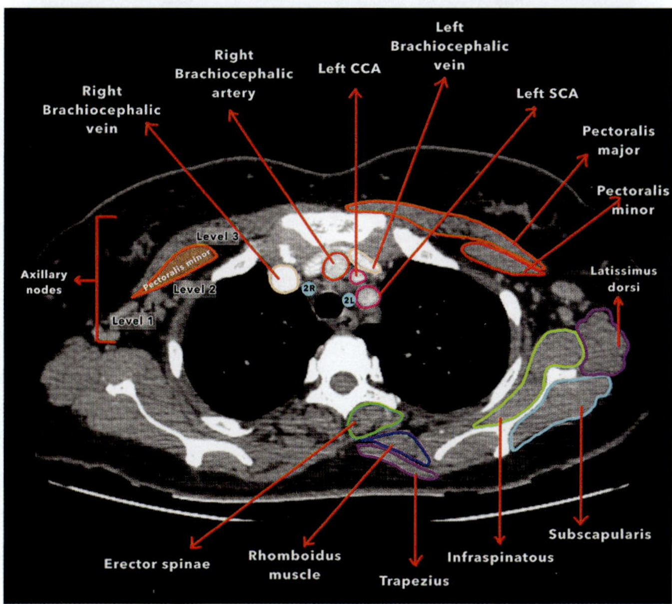

Fig. 3.3.42: CT chest axial image

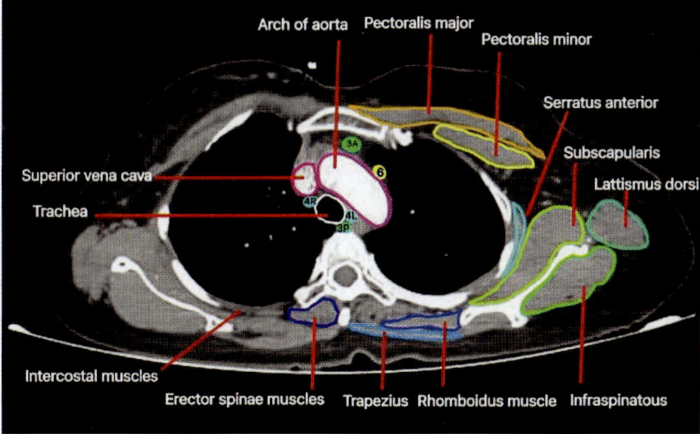

Fig. 3.3.43: CT chest axial image

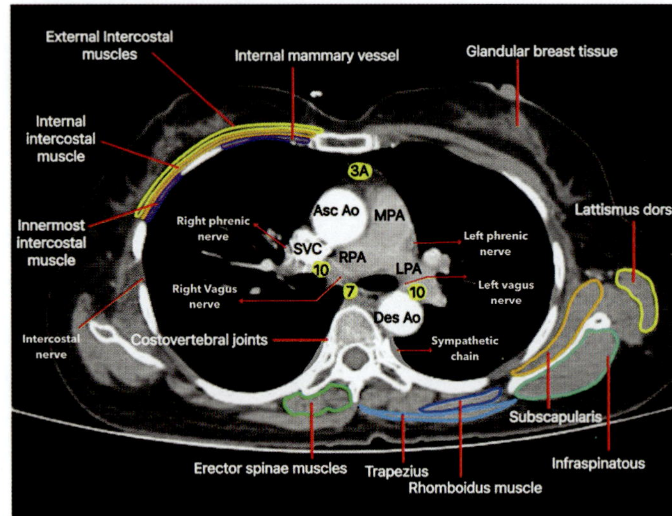

Fig. 3.3.44: Mediastinal lymph node stations

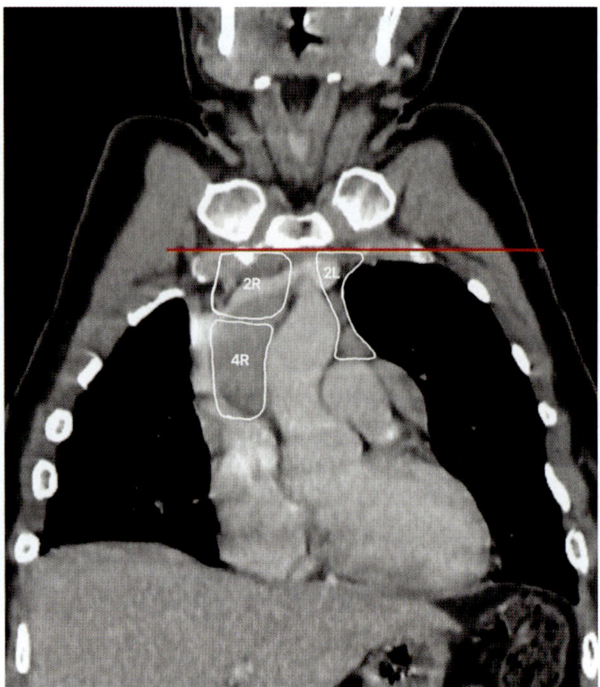

Fig. 3.3.45: Mediastinal nodes

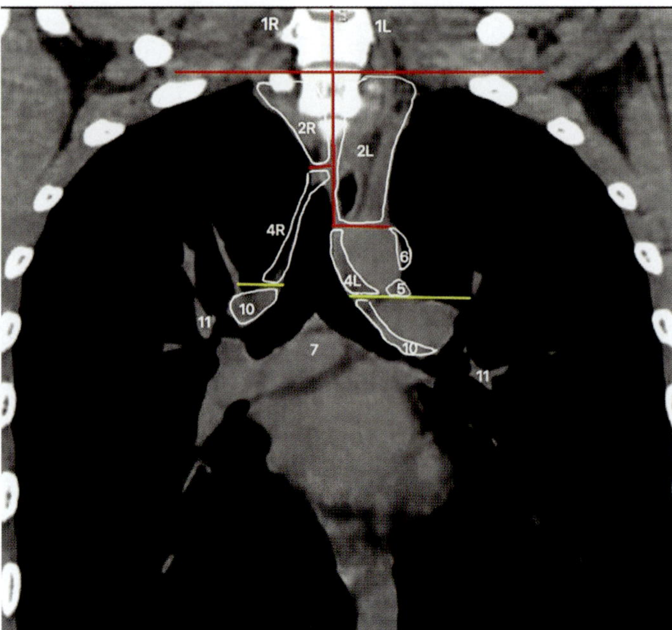

Fig. 3.3.46: Mediastinal nodes

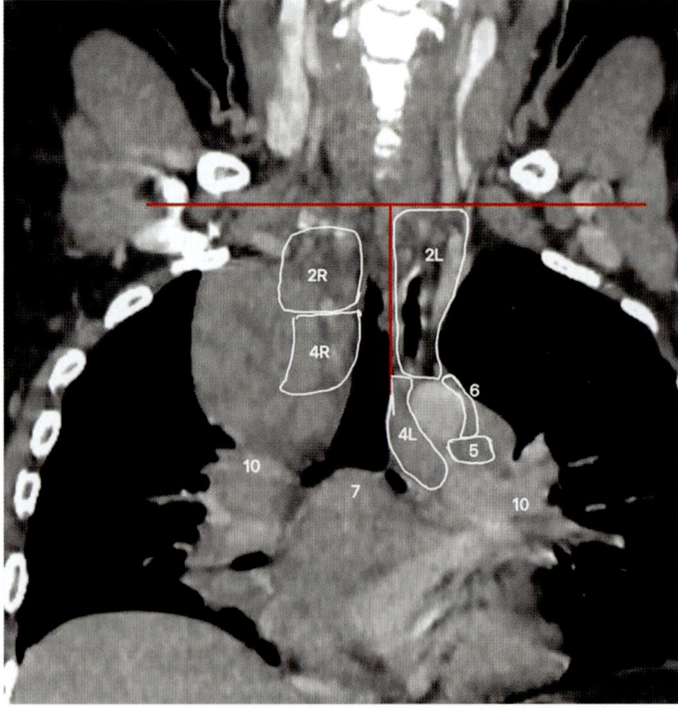

Fig. 3.3.47: Mediastinal nodes

mediastinal parietal pleural reflections that occur below the right and left pulmonary roots (9R and 9L), rather than ligaments.

Hilar Zone + Interlobar and Peripheral Zone (Extra-Mediastinal LNs). These lymph nodes are all outside the pleural reflection of the mediastinum but within the pulmonary visceral pleura.

Station 10 (Hilar) LNs are found along the right and left mainstem bronchi, before they bifurcate, and are designated 10R and 10L, respectively.

Station 11 (interlobar) is made up of LNs located between the lobar bronchi, just beyond the bifurcation of each mainstem bronchi.

Stations 12–14 (peripheral) LNs located along the lobar, segmental, or subsegmental bronchi are referred to as lobar, segmental, or subsegmental lymph nodes. Because these LNs are seldom detected and difficult to

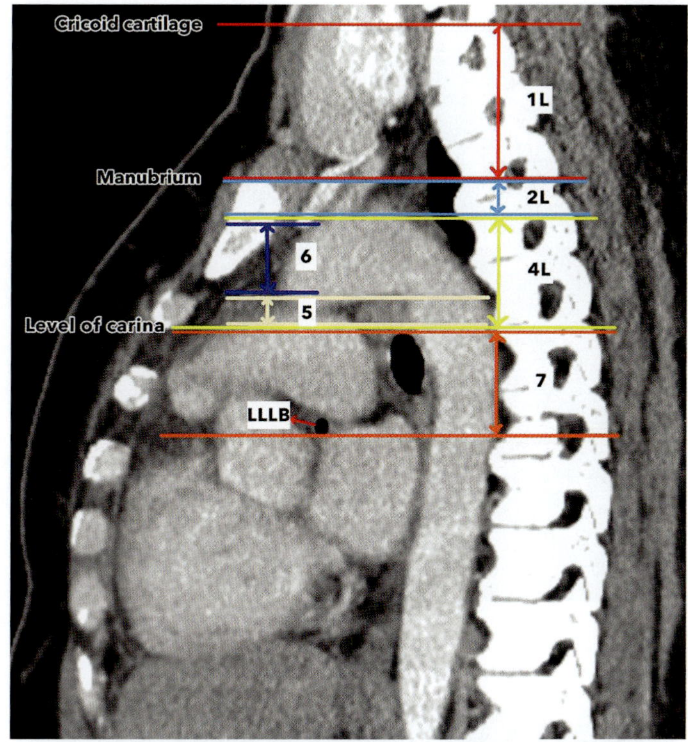

Fig. 3.3.48: Mediastinal nodes

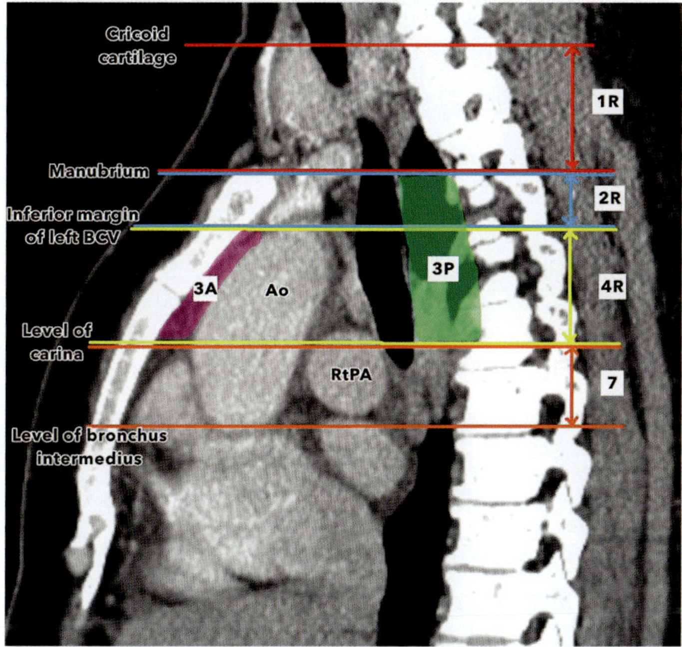

Fig. 3.3.49: Mediastinal nodes

precisely classify on imaging, many people refer to them as peripheral LNs. While the above classification method is the most generally used and is frequently used to describe mediastinal lymph nodes outside of the context of lung cancer, in some cases, such as esophageal cancer staging, different disease-specific maps are acceptable.

3.3.J Thoracic Duct

The thoracic duct arises from a saccular lymphatic reservoir called the 'cisterna chyli', which lies behind the right crus of the diaphragm, anterior to the bodies of L1 and L2. Lymph from the abdomen and lower limbs pass from here into the thoracic duct, which runs superiorly into the posterior mediastinum, passing through the aortic opening in the diaphragm. The thoracic duct ascends anterior to the vertebral column, with the descending aorta to its left and the azygos vein to its right. The right posterior intercostal arteries run across the vertebral column behind the duct, and the terminal parts of the hemiazygos and accessory azygos veins cross behind it to enter the azygos vein. It ascends behind the oesophagus, coming to lie to the left of this at T5 and then running superiorly on its left side into the neck. It then passes laterally behind the carotid vessels, and at the level of C7 the duct arches anteriorly over the left lung, rising 3–4 cm above the clavicle. It then descends to drain into the left subclavian vein at the jugulosubclavian junction.

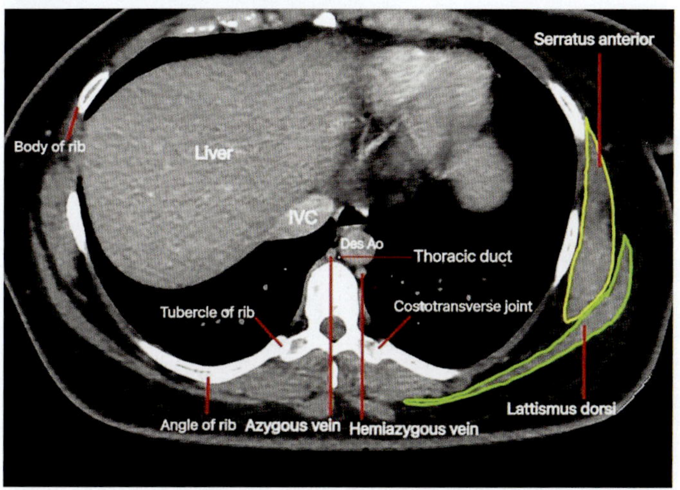

Fig. 3.3.50: Azygous vein

3.3.K Anatomy of Heart

X-ray: The chest X-ray shows the shape and size of the heart and the outline of the large blood vessels in the lungs and chest. X-rays can indicate heart enlargement, which is commonly caused by heart failure or a disorder of heart valves.

Heart borders on X-ray: The cardiac silhouette can be separated into right and left borders from the frontal projection: The right atrium, superior vena cava entering superiorly, and inferior vena cava often seen at its lower boundary comprise the right border. The left ventricle and left atrial appendage create the left boundary, whereas the pulmonary artery, aortopulmonary window, and

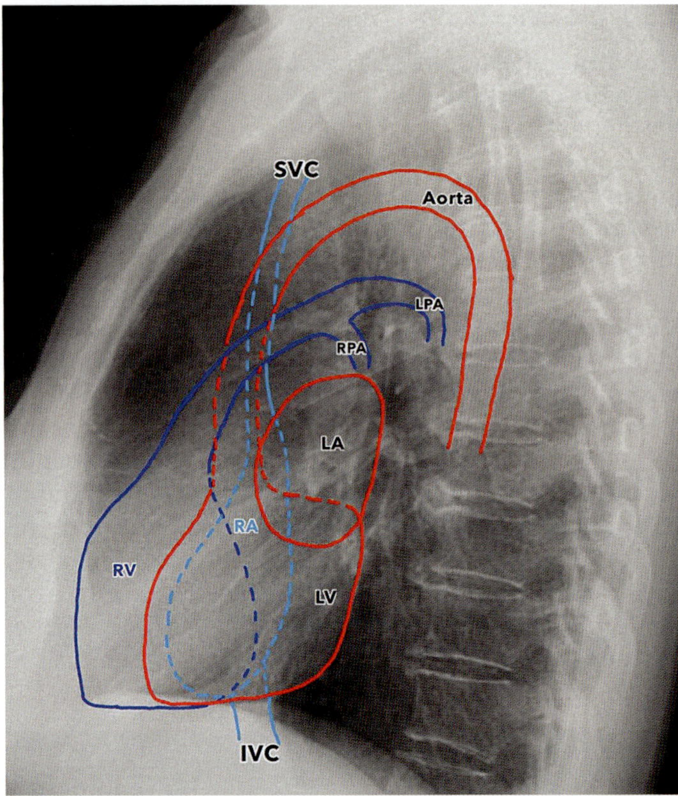

Fig. 3.3.51: Chest X-ray lateral view

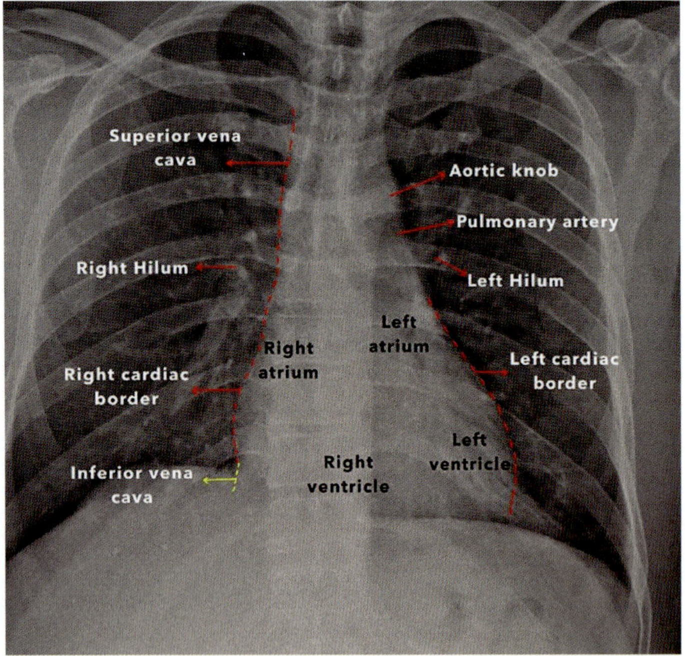

Fig. 3.3.52: Chest X-ray frontal view

aortic notch extend superiorly. On the lateral projection the right ventricle forms the anterior boundary of the cardiac silhouette, whereas the left atrium (superiorly), left ventricle (inferiorly), and the inferior vena cava constitute the posterior border.

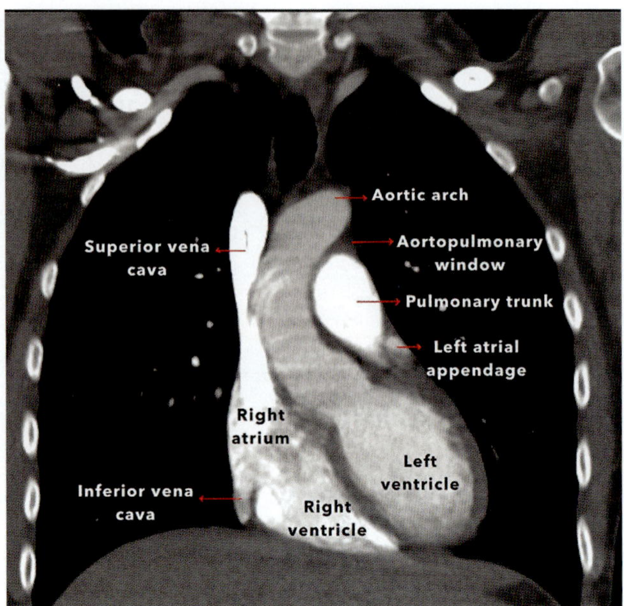

Fig. 3.3.53

Cardiac chambers on cross-sectional imaging

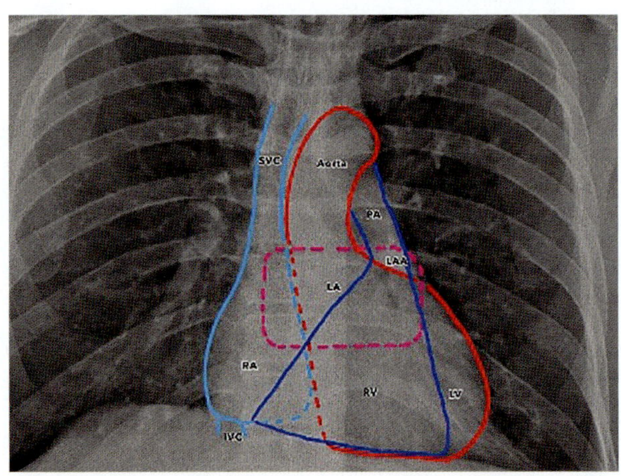

Fig. 3.3.54: Chest X-ray cardiac chambers

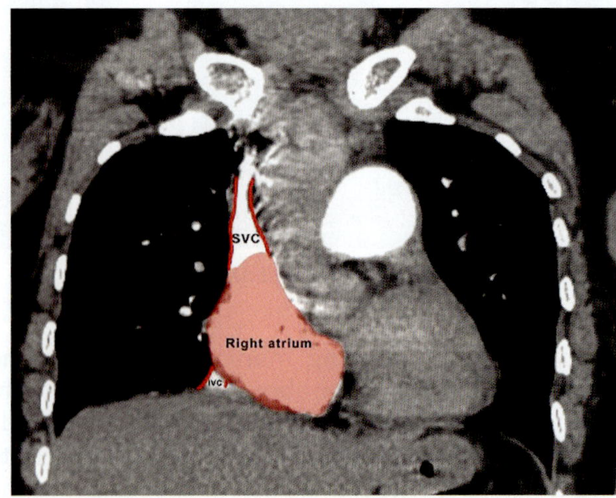

Fig. 3.3.55: Cardiac chambers on cross sectional imaging

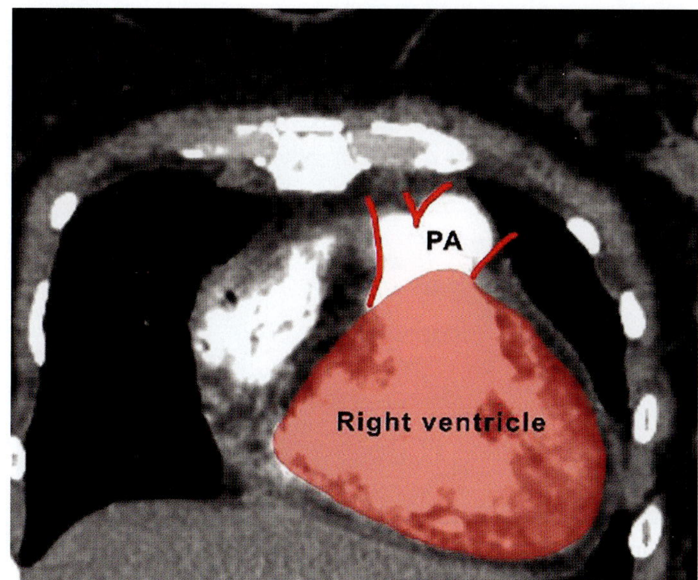

Fig. 3.3.56: Cardiac chambers on cross sectional imaging

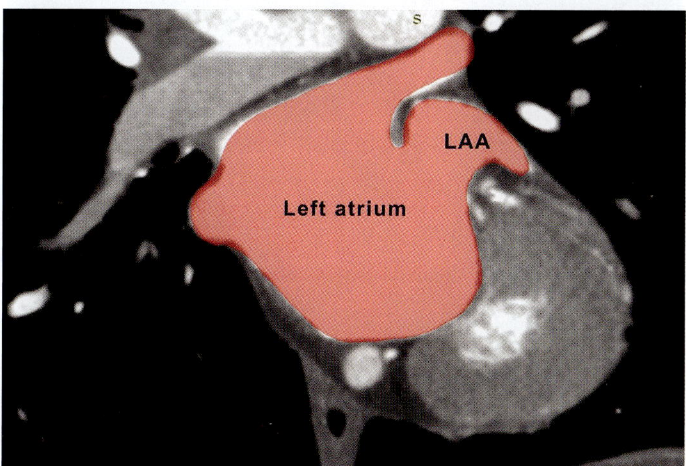

Fig. 3.3.57: Cardiac chambers on cross sectional imaging

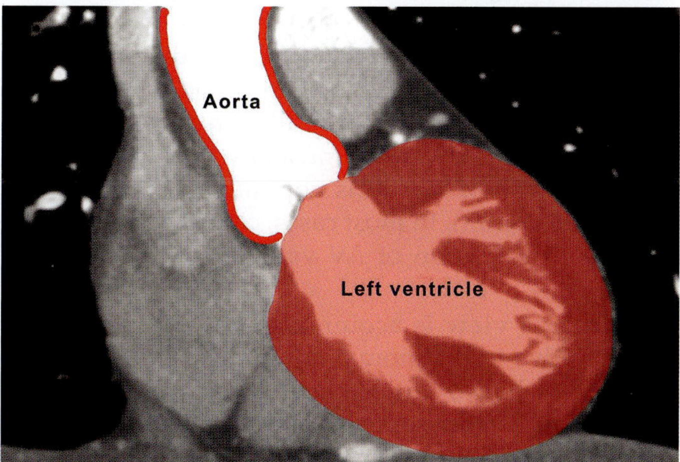

Fig. 3.3.58: Cardiac chambers on cross sectional imaging

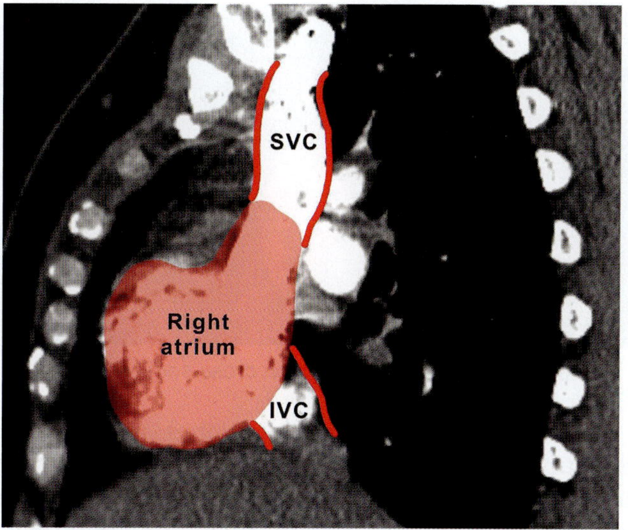

Fig. 3.3.59: Cardiac chambers on cross sectional imaging

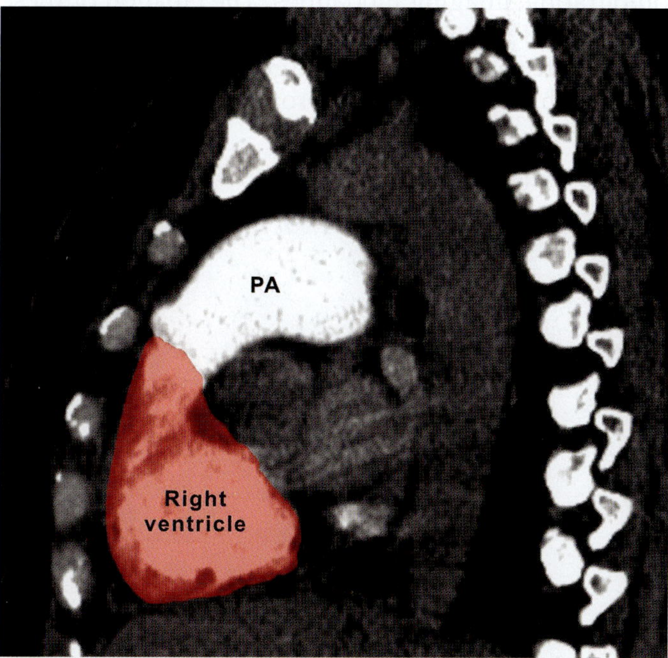

Fig. 3.3.60: Cardiac chambers on cross sectional imaging

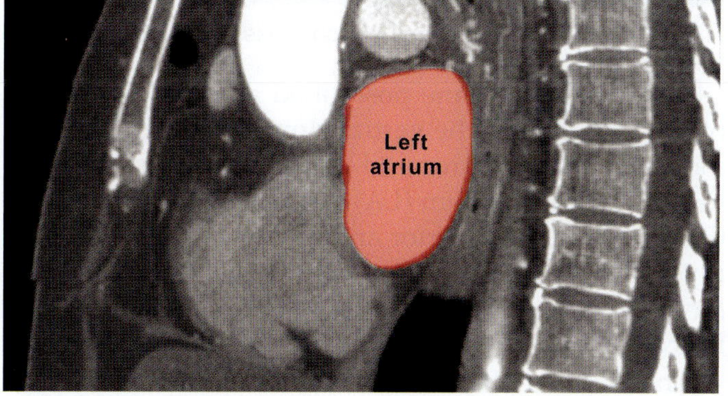

Fig. 3.3.61: Cardiac chambers on cross sectional imaging

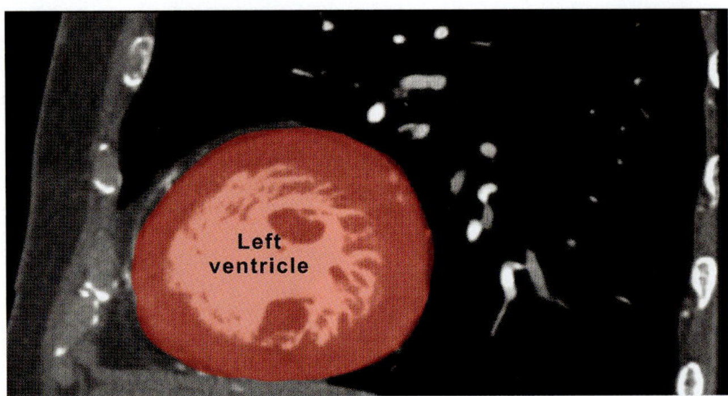

Fig. 3.3.62: Cardiac chambers on cross sectional imaging

Standardized cardiac imaging planes, which include the four-chamber, three-chamber, two-chamber, and short-axis views, are used to assess cardiac morphology, size, and function. These standardized imaging planes, or their approximations, are shared among multiple tomographic imaging modalities. The creation of these planes on CT requires access to multiplanar reformation (MPR) software and knowledge of an accurate and reproducible step-by-step approach based on anatomic landmarks.

Cardiac imaging planes and the left side of the heart

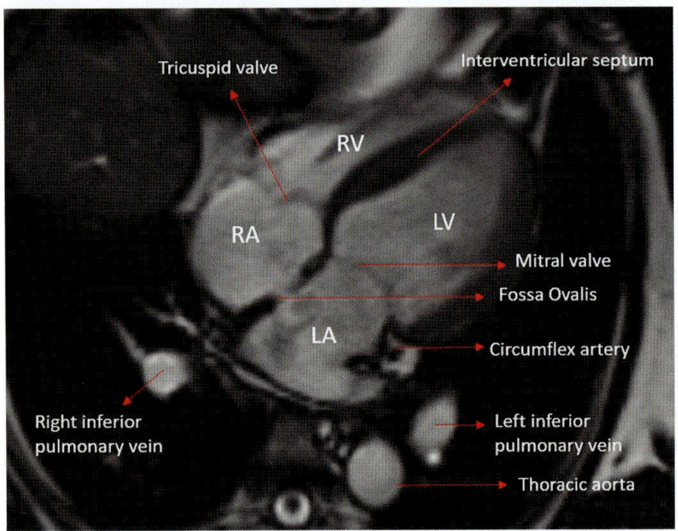

Fig. 3.3.63: Cardiac chambers on cross sectional imaging

A parasagittal plane positioned along the long axis of the LV lumen is the **vertical long-axis view**. Vertical long-axis pictures are used to analyse the connection between the left atrium (LA) and the left ventricle (LV). On this view, the inferior and anterior walls of the LV myocardium are optimised. The bicuspid MV and LV have been widely studied in terms of structure and function.

The four-chamber view, also known as the **horizontal long-axis view**, is a horizontal plane through the heart that basically bisects all four cardiac chambers for assessing chamber size and position of valve. The septal, apical, and lateral LV walls can all be evaluated at the same time. Even in unusually thickened hearts, the lateral wall of the LV is normally thin at the apex (typically 1–2 mm). In most cases, cine mode allows for subjective evaluation of AV valvular and ventricular function.

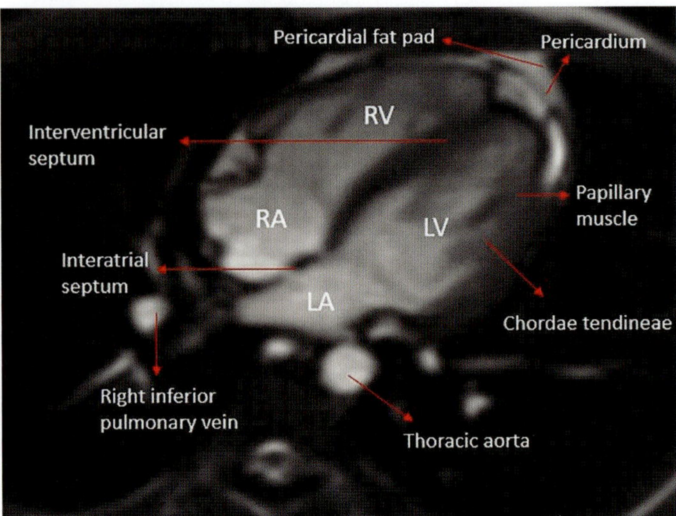

Fig. 3.3.64: Cardiac chambers on cross sectional imaging

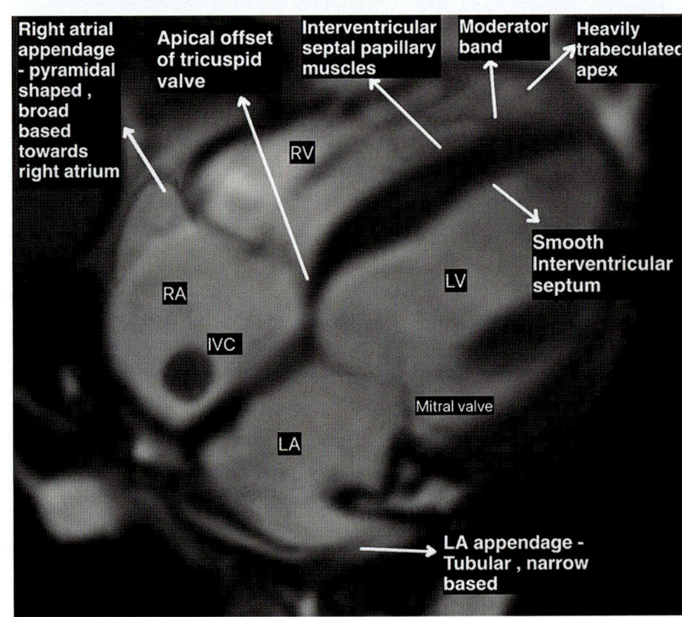

Fig. 3.3.65: MRI cardiac anatomy

Short-axis view is acquired in an oblique coronal plane relative to the thorax, down the barrel of the LV lumen. The basal, middle, and apical regions of LV myocardium can be examined as one moves from the MV to the apex in the short axis. This plane makes measuring LV size and myocardial contractility simple.

3

The RA, RV, and tricuspid valves can be examined in detail if the right side of the heart is increased with contrast material. The coronary sinus, as well as the superior vena cava and inferior vena cava, provide input to the RA. The RV is the most anterior of the heart chambers, with a highly trabeculated apex and papillary muscles that act similarly to those of the LV. The RV's smooth, muscular infundibulum (or conus) is the outflow portion of the RV that lies directly beneath the pulmonary valve.

The moderator band, a muscular band stretching from the interventricular septum to the base of the anterior papillary muscle, is a distinguishing feature of the RV. The right bundle branch conduction system includes the moderator band. Although the moderator band and strongly trabeculated apex distinguish the RV from the LV, other characteristics such as a well-developed infundibulum, septal papillary muscles, and the lack of fibrous continuity of the AV valve and outflow tract are important in distinguishing the RV from the LV. The ability to identify the LV from the RV in complex cases of congenital cardiac disease may be crucial.

Right atrium: On a chest radiograph, the RA forms the majority of the right cardiac border. The RA is morphologically larger than the LA, but it has a 2 mm thinner wall. The presence of an internal ridge called the crista terminalis (externally, sulcus terminalis) that distinguishes the smooth-walled venous RA from the rough-walled appendage is a distinguishing feature of the RA. It begins from the SVC orifice and continues to the anterior aspect of the IVC orifice. The pacemaker of the heart, the sinoatrial (SA) node, is commonly found at the intersection of the crista terminalis and SVC. The extension of the pectinate muscle from the AV junction provides the most precise estimate of heart chamber laterality for determining situs.

Morphological features of RA include: Larger and more triangular appendage, with a broad junction with smooth part of RA; prominent terminal crest between the appendage and smooth venous component; generally located on the same side as trilobed lung; and it follows the rule of venoatrial concordance, i.e. the chamber receiving the IVC inflow is almost always RA.

Right ventricle: The RV is the heart's most anterior chamber. The inlet, which includes the TV, chordae tendineae, and papillary muscles, is separated into three sections: (1) The trabeculated apical myocardium; (2) the smooth-walled infundibulum—conus arteriosus; and (3) the smooth-walled infundibulum—conus arteriosus (also referred to as the RVOT). The RV has a thinner wall (3–4 mm) than the LV, but much more trabeculations. The existence of the moderator band, a muscular extension from the interventricular septum to the RV free wall around the RV apex, is another distinguishing feature of the RV. The right bundle branch is contained by the moderator band, which prevents ventricular overdistention. The RV has three papillary muscles (anterior, posterior, and septal) that attach to the leaflets of the TV (occasionally more) (anterior, posterior, and septal). The largest papillary muscle is the anterior papillary muscle, which comes from the RV's anterior free wall. The septal papillary muscle is the least consistent of the RV's papillary muscles, and it is frequently confused with the ventricular wall. The pulmonary artery is located anterior and to the left of the aorta, emerging from the conus of RV. The muscle infundibulum divides the tricuspid and pulmonary valves, with no fibrous continuity between them, which aids in identifying the morphologic RV.

Morphological features of RV include: The chamber, including the apex, is coarsely trabeculated and contains the moderator band. Papillary muscles (usually three) attach to free wall and interventricular septum. A smooth muscular infundibulum separates the tricuspid and pulmonic valves.

Left atrium: Because of the obliquity of the interatrial septum, the LA is the heart's most posterior chamber and is placed above the RA (IAS). The existence of the IAS, a thin structure that can be difficult to assess adequately on MRI, distinguishes it from the RA. The aortic root and transverse pericardial sinus are directly anterior to the LA, while the tracheal bifurcation, oesophagus, and descending thoracic aorta are directly posterior to the pericardium lining the exterior of the posterior wall of the LA. The LA wall is muscular but smooth internally. From the anterolateral side of the heart, next to the left superior PVs, the LA possesses a finger-like appendage. The pulmonary venous part, septal part, and vestibule are the anatomical divisions of LA.

Morphological features include: Pointed and finger-like appendage with narrow ostial connection with main LA body. Generally located on the same side as bilobed lung.

Left ventricle: The left ventricle (LV) is the heart's outflow chamber, which pumps oxygenated blood into the systemic circulation. It is located posteriorly and to the left of the RV. The LV possesses the thickest myocardium of all the cardiac chambers, and the presence of fine trabeculae carneae on its inner surface distinguishes it from the RV, giving it a comparatively smooth look. The mitral and aortic valves have a fibrous continuity that helps identify the LV from the RV. The existence of anterior (lateral) and posterior (medial) papillary muscles, which are only attached to the LV's free wall, is another distinguishing trait. Chordae tendineae from either MV leaflet are received by each papillary muscle, preventing blood regurgitation into the LA during ventricular systole.

Morphological features include: The trabeculae are thin and delicate, with smooth septal surface. Only free walls are attached to papillary muscles (typically two). Between the mitral and aortic valves, there is fibrous continuity.

Atrial appendages: The LA appendage protrudes anteriorly over the proximal LCx artery from the superolateral side of the LA. It has a smaller base and is more tubular than the generally pyramidal RA appendage. These characteristics make it easy to distinguish between the two appendages, which is useful when the situs is in doubt. The pectinate muscles of the

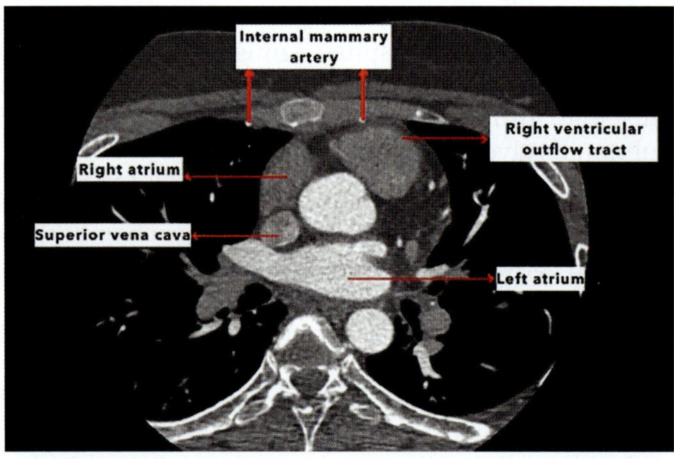

Fig. 3.3.66: Cardiac CT showing cardiac structures

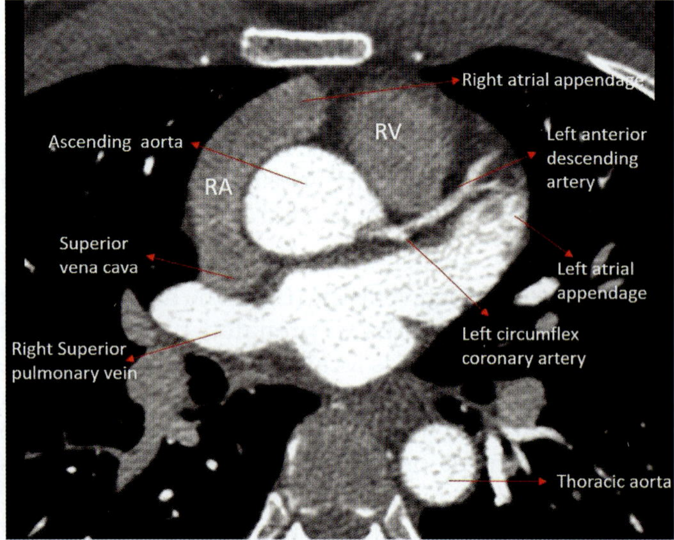

Fig. 3.3.67: Cardiac CT showing cardiac structures

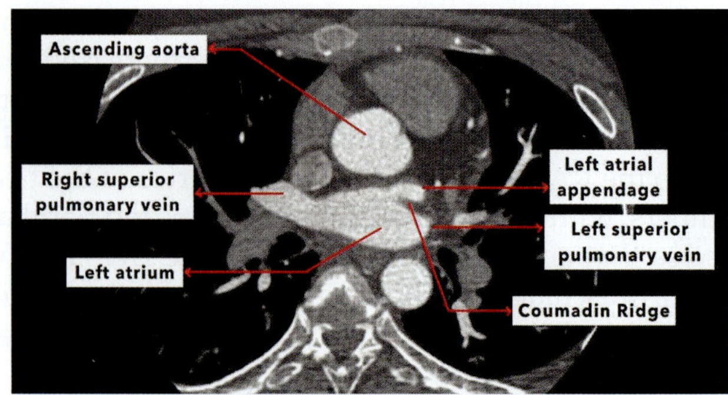

Fig. 3.3.68: Cardiac CT showing cardiac structures

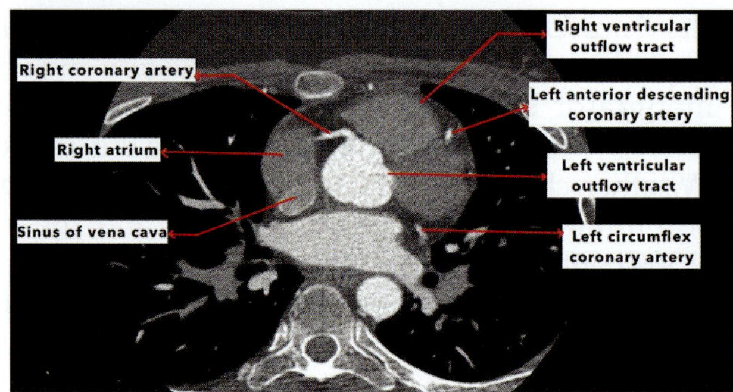

Fig. 3.3.69: Cardiac CT showing cardiac structures

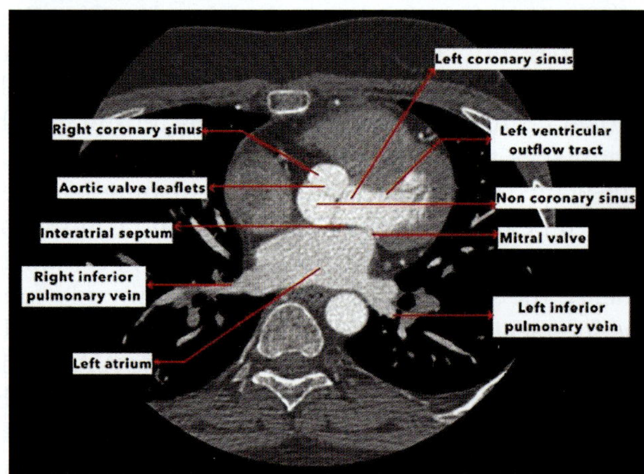

Fig. 3.3.70: Cardiac CT showing cardiac structures

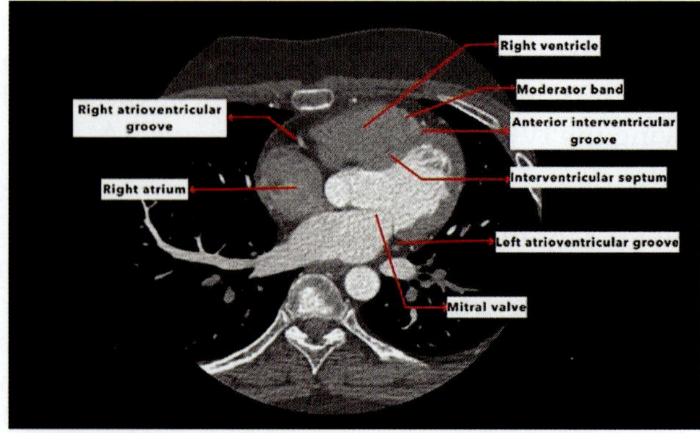

Fig. 3.3.71: Cardiac CT showing cardiac structures

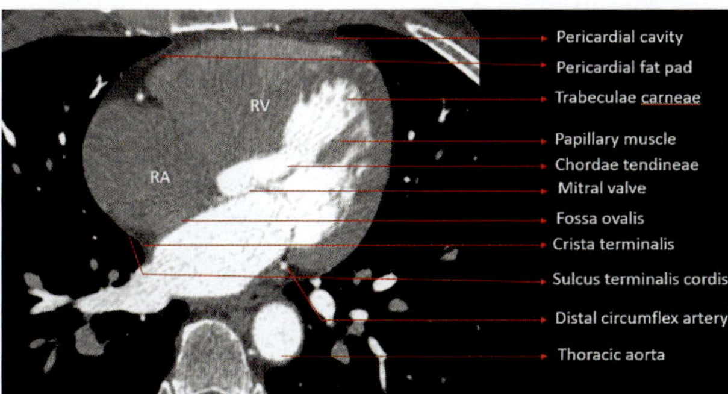

Fig. 3.3.72: Cardiac CT showing cardiac structures

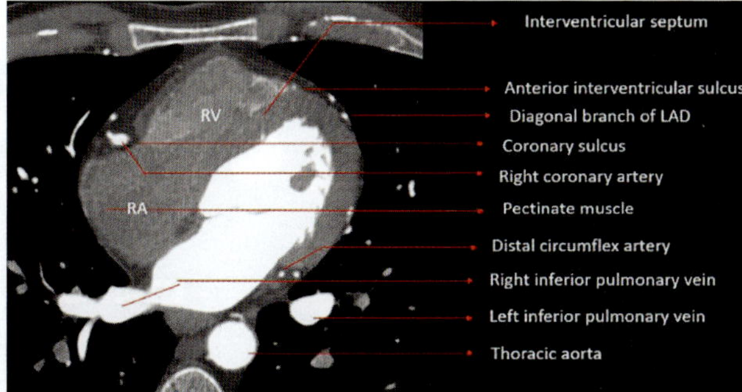

Fig. 3.3.73: Cardiac CT showing cardiac structures

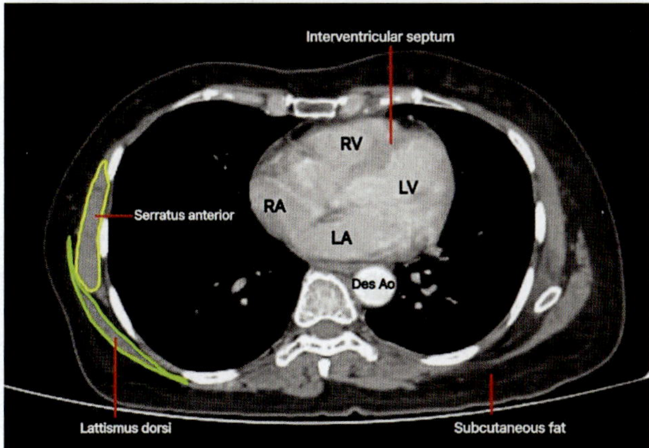

Fig. 3.3.74: Cardiac CT showing cardiac structures

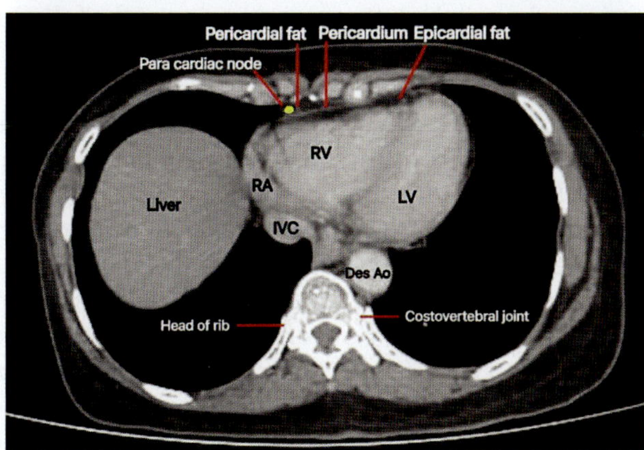

Fig. 3.3.75: Cardiac CT showing cardiac structures

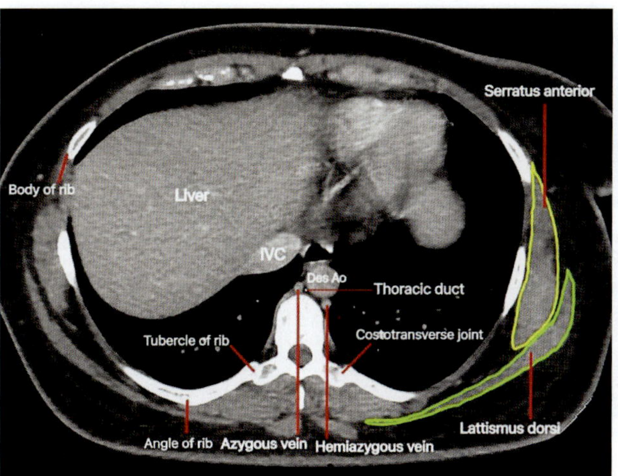

Fig. 3.3.76: Cardiac CT showing cardiac structures

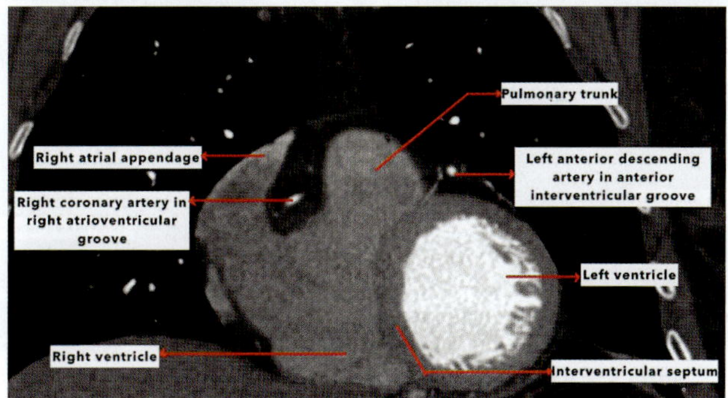

Fig. 3.3.77: Cardiac CT showing cardiac structures

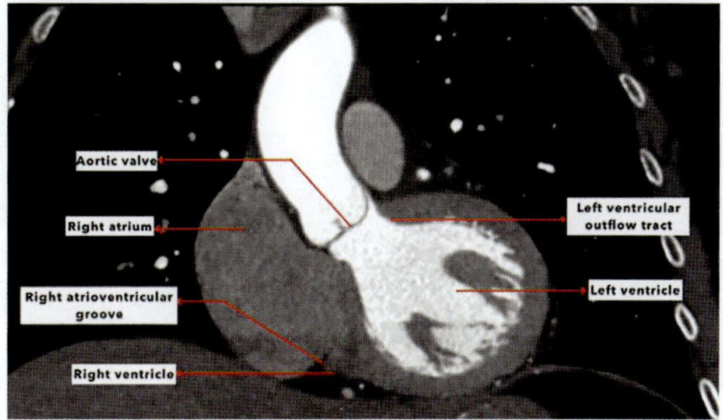

Fig. 3.3.78: Cardiac CT showing cardiac structures

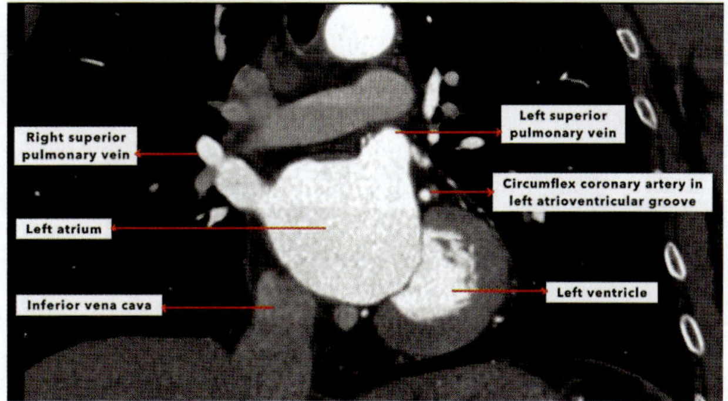

Fig. 3.3.79: Cardiac CT showing cardiac structures

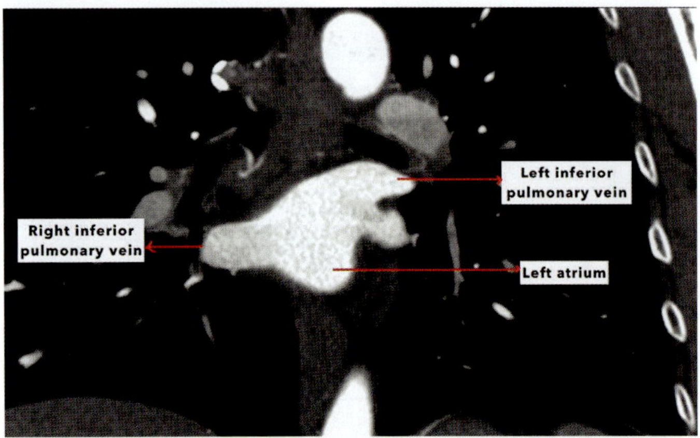

Fig. 3.3.80: Cardiac CT showing cardiac structures

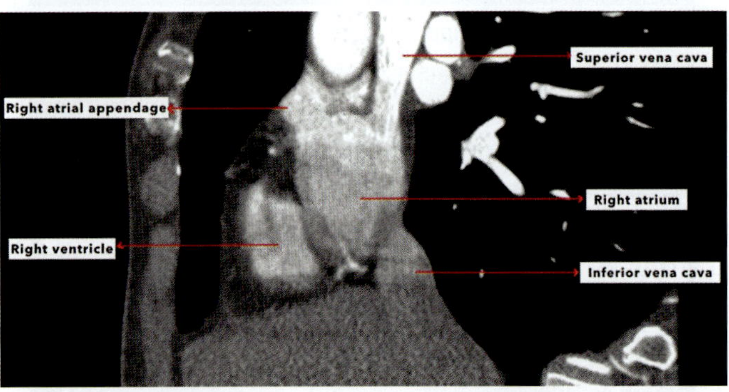

Fig. 3.3.81: Cardiac CT showing cardiac structures

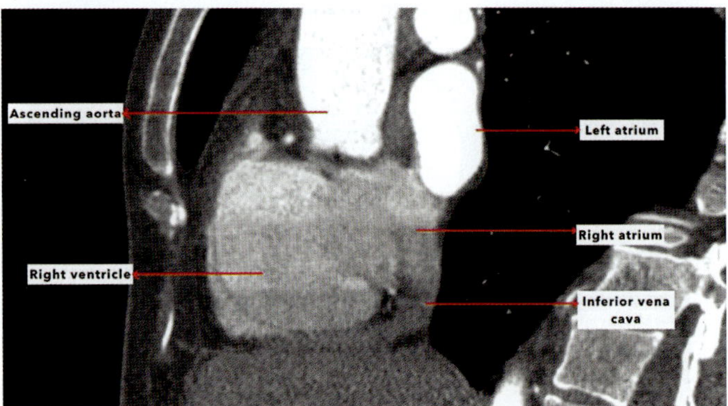

Fig. 3.3.82: Cardiac CT showing cardiac structures

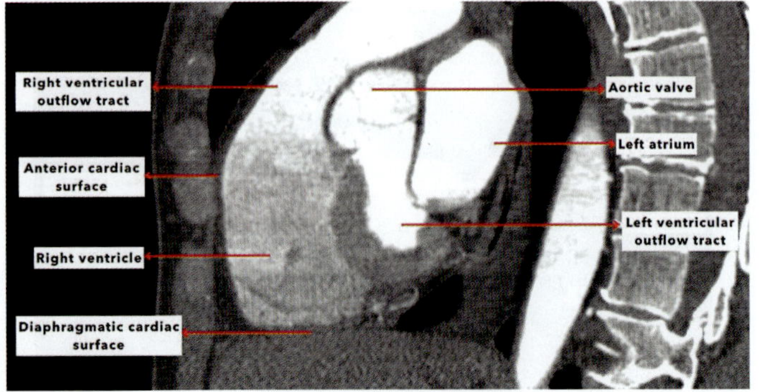

Fig. 3.3.83: Cardiac CT showing cardiac structures

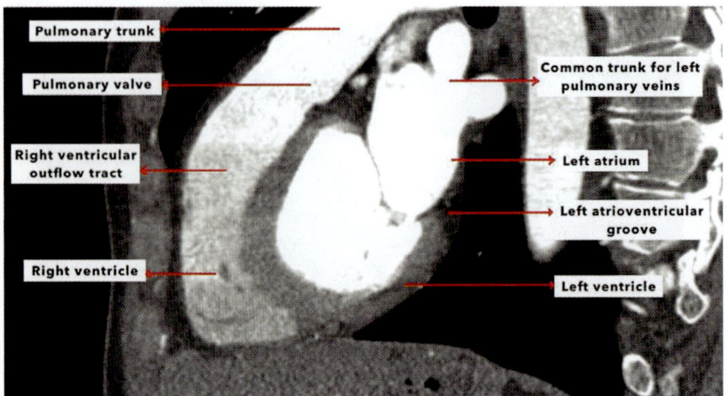

Fig. 3.3.84

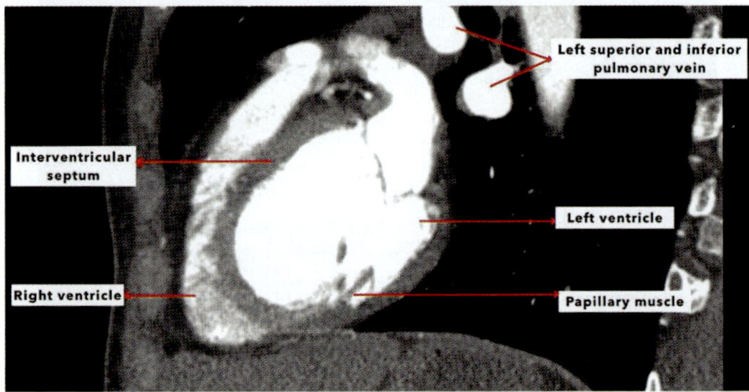

Fig. 3.3.85

LA appendages are larger than 1 mm in most individuals (>97%). The pectinate muscles of the RA appendage are similar to those of the LA appendage, however, they are significantly larger.

Cardiac and pulmonary veins: Cardiac CT angiography is best for imaging the coronary sinus and cardiac veins. The most constant structure is the coronary sinus, which runs along the inferior aspect of the heart in the AV groove before emptying into the RA. The posterior interventricular vein, also known as middle cardiac vein, is the first branch of the CS, and it runs from base to apex in the posterior interventricular groove. The LV's posterior vein and the left marginal vein are the following two branches. The CS then becomes the great cardiac vein, which runs alongside the LCx artery in the left AV groove. It then becomes the anterior interventricular vein, which runs from the base of the heart to the apex close to the Left anterior descending (LAD) artery in the anterior interventricular groove. With multidetector CT, the veins may be mapped in depth, and treatment techniques based on CT findings, such as radiofrequency catheter ablation, can be personalised to individual patients. Two veins (superior and inferior) drain into each side of the LA in most cases. If there are any more PVs present, they must be described before ablation. They are usually single, and they are more common on the right side of the body. Middle PVs emerging on the right side, in particular, show a stronger association to atrial fibrillation.

Cardiac valves: The four cardiac valves are routinely imaged during cardiac CT angiography, and their motion and morphologic characteristics should also be assessed at all cardiac CT angiographic examinations with reconstructed and cine images. The MV separates the LA from the LV. It is normally connected to the morphologic LV. The MV is composed of two leaflets, the anterior and posterior leaflets; the other valves normally have three leaflets. The MV and aortic valve share fibrous continuity. The MV annulus, or valve ring, is embedded in the myocardium and is a component of the cardiac skeleton. The MV apparatus also includes the papillary muscles and associated chordae tendineae. The tricuspid valve connects the RA and RV and is made up of the same components as the MV—leaflets, annulus, commissures (points where two leaflets meet to adhere to the aortic wall), papillary muscles, and chordae tendineae. It is usually associated with the morphologic RV. It is a trileaflet valve (anterior, posterior, and septal leaflets) and is separated from the pulmonary valve by the crista supraventricularis—a muscular ridge—unlike the MV, which is contiguous with the aortic valve. The LV outflow tract is separated from the ascending aorta by the aortic valve. An annulus, cusps, and commissures make up the structure. The aortic valve does not have any papillary muscles or chordae tendineae. The RV outflow tract is separated from the major pulmonary artery by the pulmonary valve, which does not link directly to the tricuspid valve. It has right, left, and posterior leaflets, and functions similarly to the aortic valve. **The location of valves on PA view X-rays are assessed by drawing an imaginary line from the right cardiophrenic angle to the lower border of left hilum. The valve passing through this imaginary line is tricuspid valve. Above this line is aortic and pulmonary valve and below this line lies the mitral valve. The location of valves on lateral radiograph is assessed by drawing an imaginary line from the carina to the cardiac apex. Normally aortic and pulmonary valve are above this line and mitral valve is below this line. Tricuspid valve passes through this line. Cardiac valves anatomy** (Figs 3.3.86–3.3.95).

Layers of heart

Pericardium: The pericardium is a compliant sac that consists of two layers, the parietal and visceral pericardium, separated by a small amount of fluid. It envelops the cardiac chambers and the origins of the great vessels. The pericardium is generally less than 2 mm in thickness. There are two layers of pericardium,

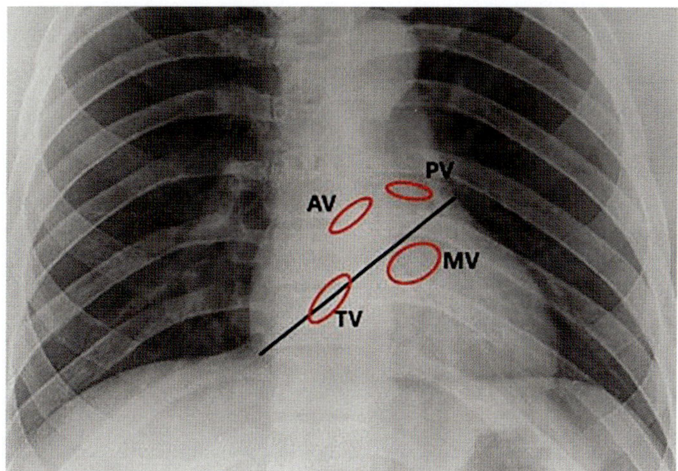

Fig. 3.3.86: Cardiac valves on PA chest Radiograph based on imaginary lined between right cardiophrenic angle and left hilum (*AV–aortic valve, PV–pulmonary valve, TV–tricuspid value and MV–mitral valve)

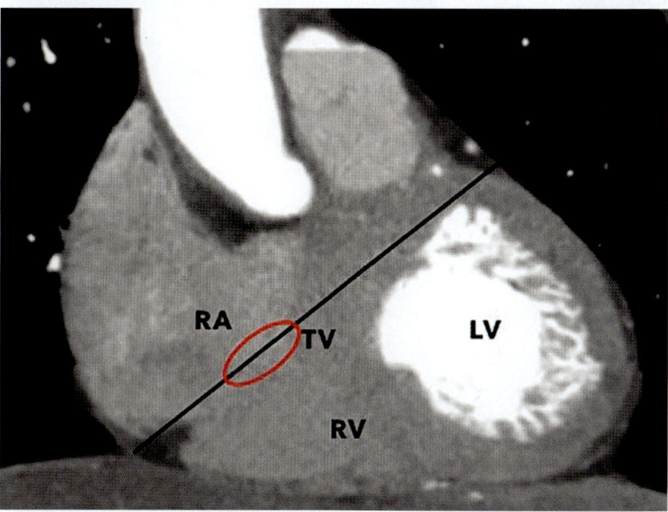

Fig. 3.3.87: Cardiac CT: Cardiac valves

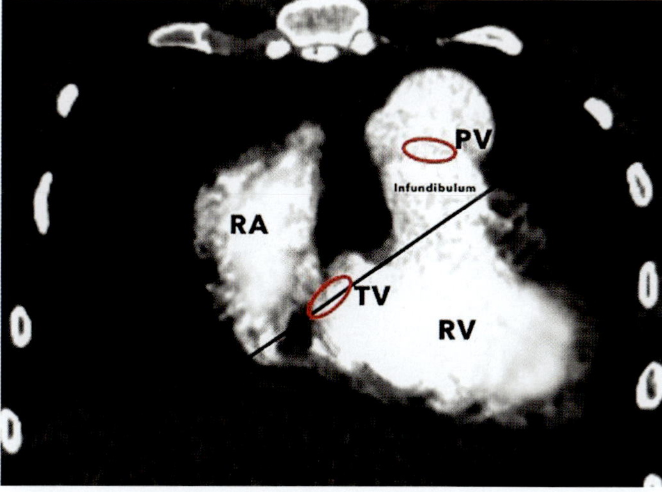

Fig. 3.3.88: Cardiac CT: Cardiac valves

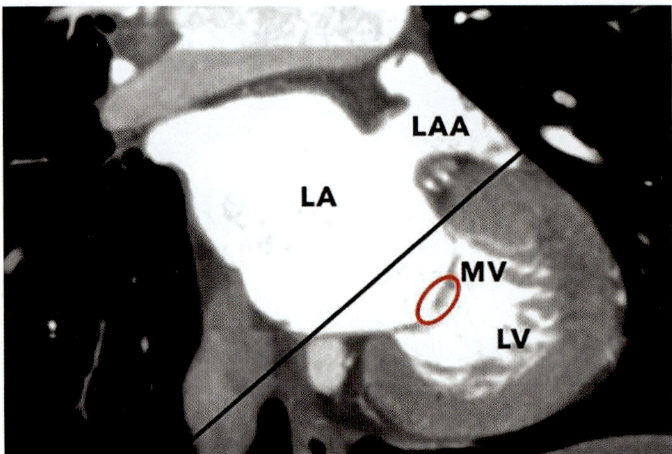

Fig. 3.3.89: Cardiac CT: Cardiac valves

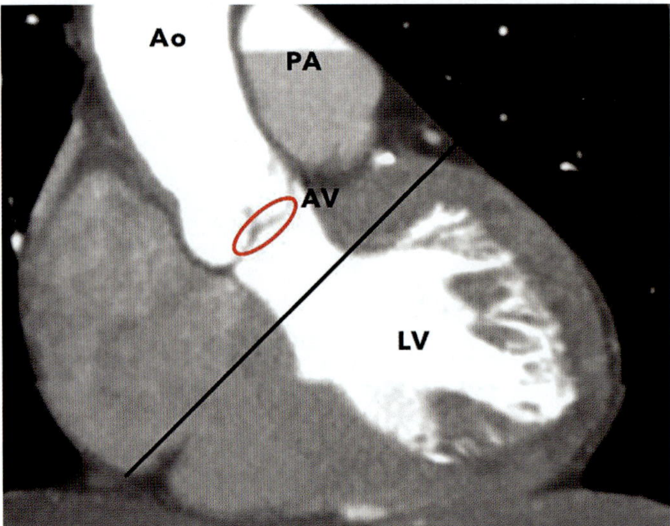

Fig. 3.3.90: Cardiac CT: Cardiac valves

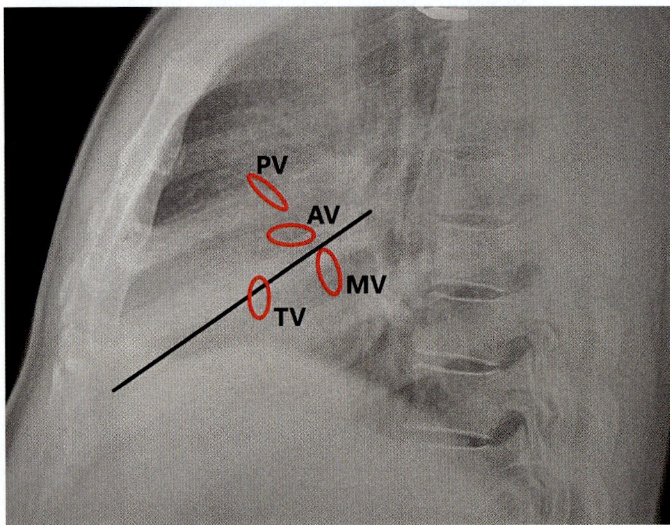

Fig. 3.3.91: Chest X-ray: Cardiac valves

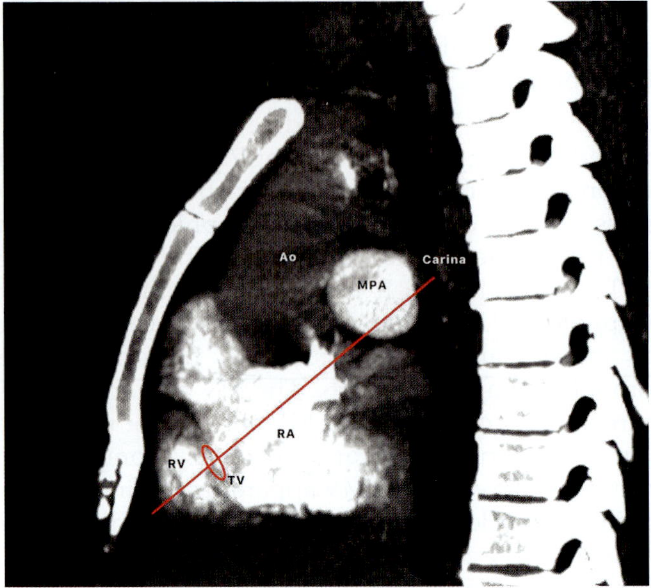

Fig. 3.3.92: Cardiac CT: Cardiac valves

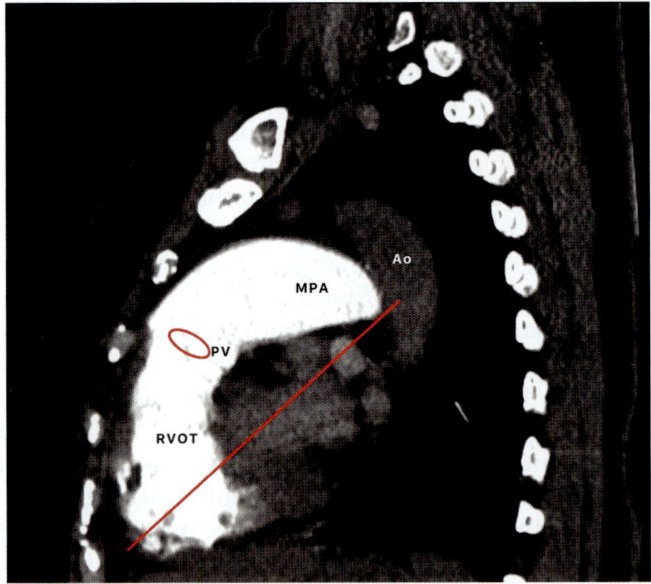

Fig. 3.3.93: Cardiac CT: Cardiac valves

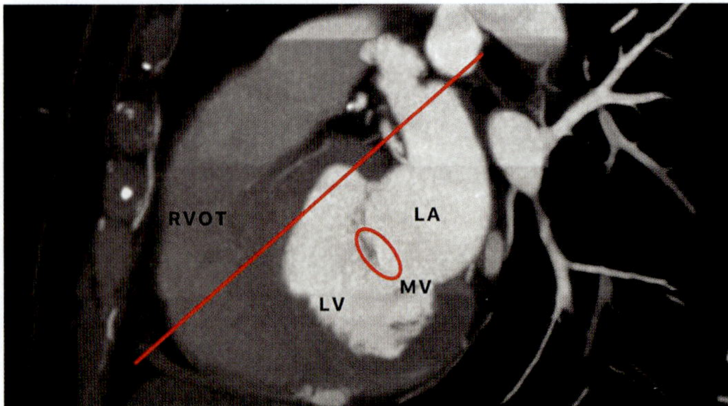

Fig. 3.3.94: Cardiac CT: Cardiac valves

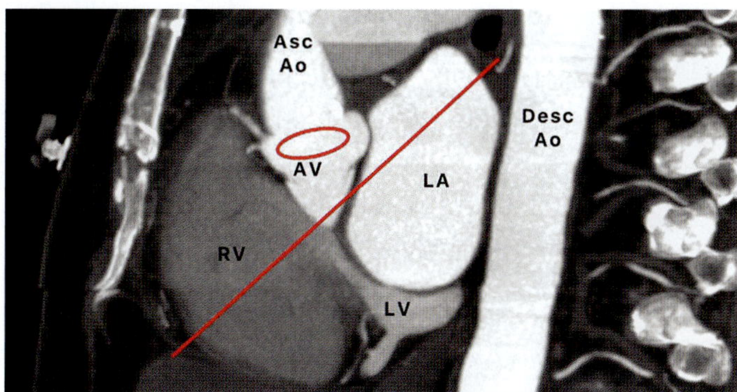

Fig. 3.3.95: Cardiac CT: Cardiac valves

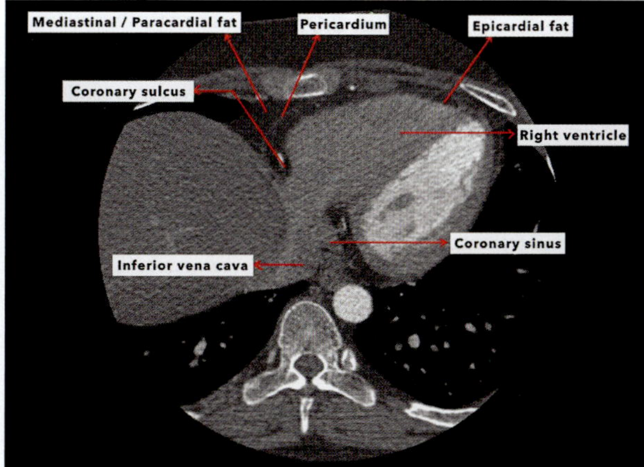

Fig. 3.3.96: Coronary sinus

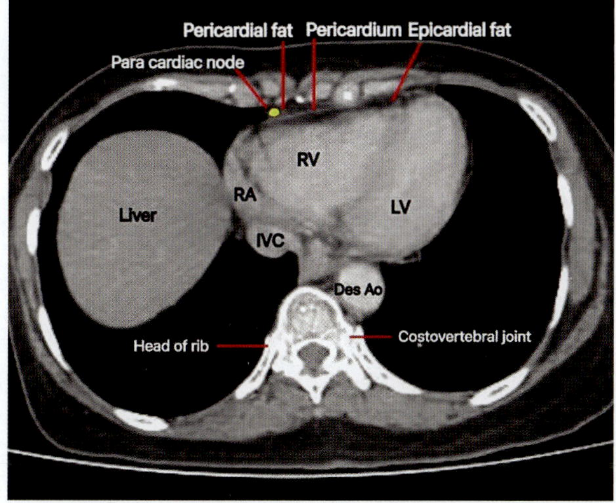

Fig. 3.3.97: Cardiac CT: Pericardium

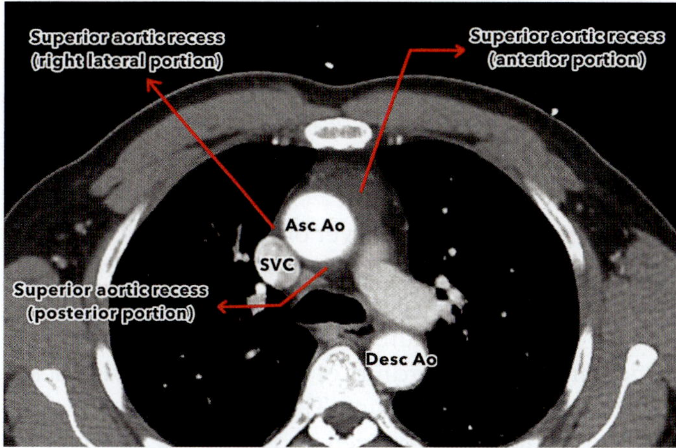

Fig. 3.3.98: Cardiac CT: Cardiac recess

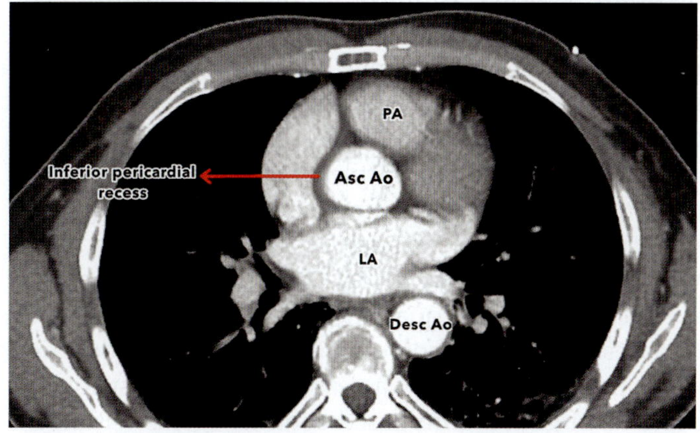

Fig. 3.3.99

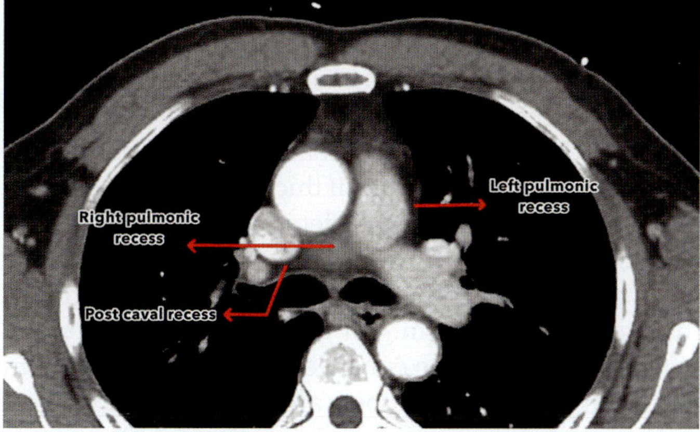

Fig. 3.3.100

fibrous pericardium and serous pericardium. The fibrous pericardium is an outer sac-like structure that defines the boundary of anatomical middle mediastinum and contained phrenic nerve and pericardiacophrenic vessels. The serous pericardium is made up of serous parietal pericardium and serous visceral pericardium. The serous visceral pericardium is adherent to the heart, hence called epicardium. The fluid-filled connections of the visceral and parietal pericardium, which form recesses and sinuses, are regularly seen on multidetector CT. The oblique and transverse sinuses, which are contiguous with the pericardial cavity, are two of the most typically seen sinuses on multidetector CT scans of the heart and thorax. Between the outer wall of the myocardium and the visceral layer of the pericardium is epicardial fat. Pericardial fat is found between the visceral and parietal pericardium, and is anterior to epicardial fat. The epicardial fat has a lot of importance because of its physical proximity to the myocardial and the fact that the two tissues have the same microcirculation.

Myocardium: The middle layer of the heart wall is known as the myocardium. Within the walls of the heart chambers, it is positioned between the endocardium and the epicardial layer of the pericardium. The ventricular myocardium, particularly the myocardium of the left ventricle, is thicker than the atrial myocardium. The coronary arteries feed the myocardium with oxygen and nutrients. The cardiac veins and coronary sinus, as well as the Thebesian veins, facilitate venous drainage of the myocardium. The myocardium appears to be muscle-like in most imaging modalities. Echocardiography has been used as a first-line imaging technique in the evaluation of cardiac morphology and function as well as in the assessment of myocardial contractility and the contractile reserve. Cardiac CT can be used for the assessment of myocardial morphology and myocardial perfusion. In addition, research has conducted with respect to the use as an alternative for myocardial extracellular volume quantification. Cardiac MRI is used to assess wall morphology, inherent tissue properties, myocardial, and also to assess changes in distribution patterns of gadolinium-based contrast agents within the myocardium.

Endocardium: The endocardium is the heart's interior soft tissue lining found within the cardiac chambers, as well as the surface of the cardiac valves. It appears to be a control mechanism for myocardial contractility. The typical endocardium is not seen on imaging because of its small thickness. However, if thickened or altered in the context of sickness, it could be depicted. The endocardium will not be apparent if it is healthy. Cardiac MRI, on the other hand, may aid in the diagnosis of pathologically changed endocardium. An apical filling defect and diffuse late gadolinium enhancement of endocardium in particular if several chambers are involved will suggest endocardial disease, e.g. endomyocardial fibrosis or endocardial fibroelastosis.

Coronary artery anatomy: The right and left coronary arteries emerge from the aortic root's right and left sinuses of Valsalva, respectively. The "noncoronary sinus" refers to the posterior sinus, which rarely gives rise to a coronary artery. Although the coronary arteries' myocardial distribution varies, the right coronary artery (RCA) usually always provides the right ventricle (RV),

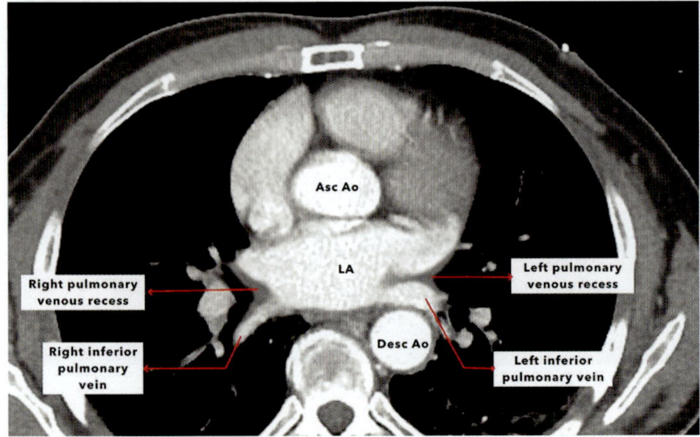

Fig. 3.3.101

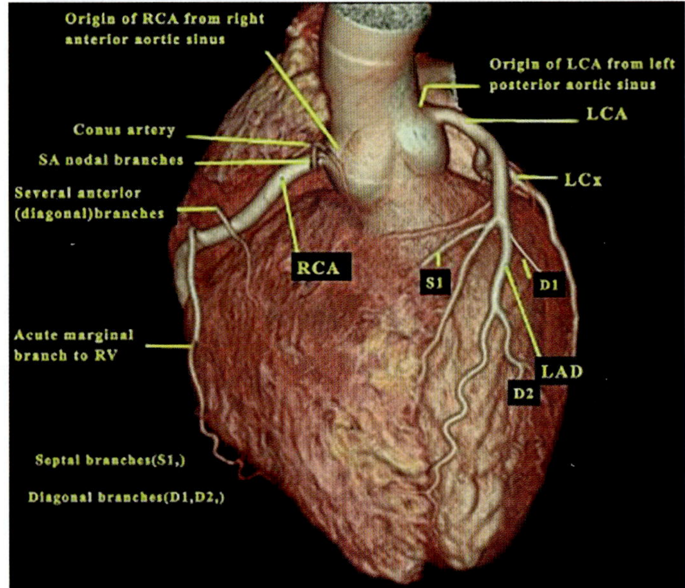

Fig. 3.3.102: 3D virtual image: Coronary arteries

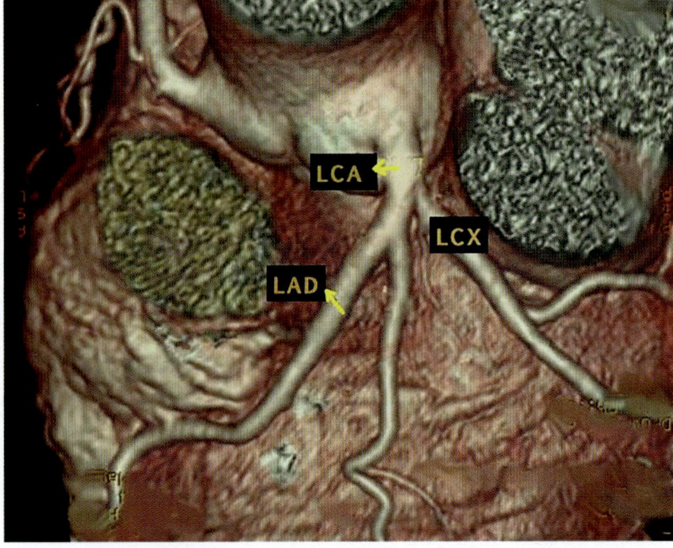

Fig. 3.3.103: 3D virtual image: Coronary arteries

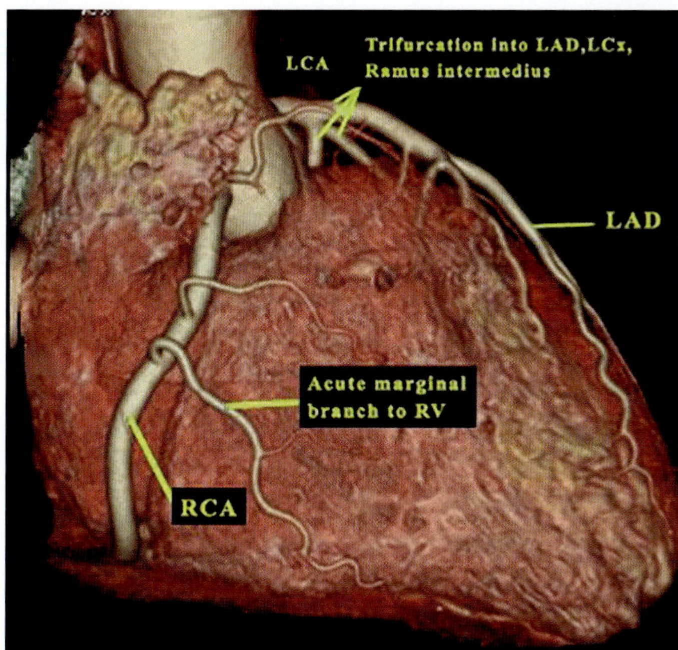

Fig. 3.3.104: 3D virtual image: Coronary arteries

and the left coronary artery (LCA) almost always supplies the anterior portion of the ventricular septum and the anterior wall of the left ventricle (LV). After its origin from the aorta, the RCA passes to the right and posterior to the pulmonary artery and then emerges from under the right atrial appendage to travel in the anterior (right) atrioventricular (AV) groove. Branches include conus branch, sinonodal artery, RV marginal branches, PDA and posterior left ventricular (PLV/PLB) branches. The LCA generally emerges as the left major (LM) coronary artery from the left coronary sinus. The LM coronary artery is a short (5–10 mm) artery that runs to the left and posterior to the pulmonary trunk before bifurcating into the LAD and LCx arteries. The LM coronary artery can sometimes split into three branches: The LAD artery, the LCx artery, and the ramus intermedius artery. Coronary dominance is determined by the artery that supplies the posterior descending artery (PDA) and the posterolateral branch. Heart is said to be right dominant (80–85 percent of the cases) if the PDA and PLB derive from the RCA. If PDA and PLB arise from LCx artery, then the heart is said to be left dominant. If PDA arises from RCA and PLB from LCx, it is termed co-dominance.

Coronary veins: The coronary veins return deoxygenated blood from the myocardium back to the right atrium. Most venous blood returns via the coronary sinus. The coronary sinus is located in the posterior atrioventricular groove and drains into the right atrium's posterior wall to the left of the IVC orifice. Its tributaries are

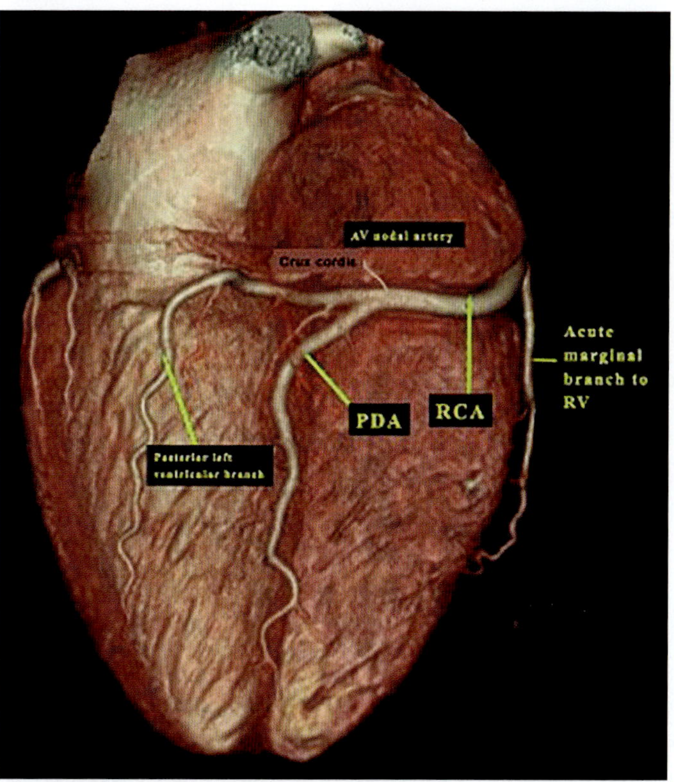

Fig. 3.3.105: 3D virtual image: Coronary arteries

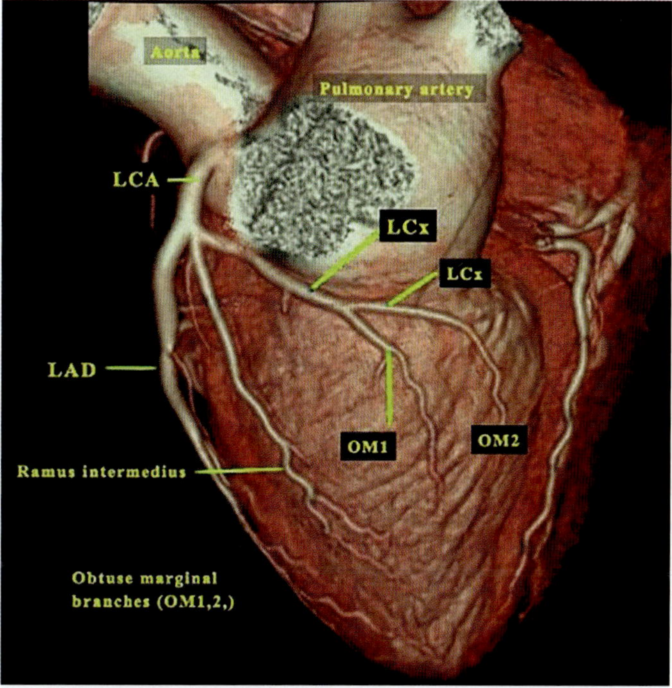

Fig. 3.3.106: 3D virtual image: Coronary arteries

the **great cardiac vein**, which ascends in the anterior interventricular groove and then runs to the left in the atrioventricular groove to become the coronary sinus; the **middle cardiac vein**, which ascends in the posterior

3

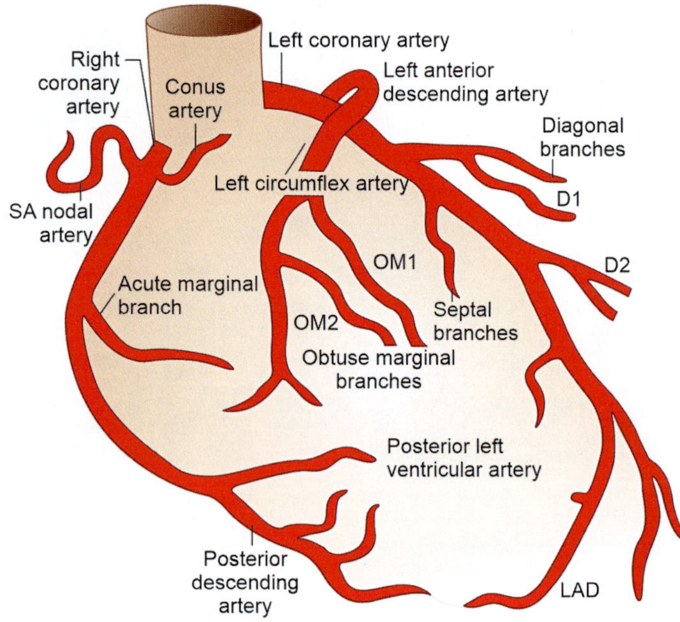

Fig. 3.3.107: Arterial anatomy of heart

interventricular groove, the **small cardiac vein**, which accompanies the marginal branches of the RCA on the inferior surface of the heart and then runs posteriorly in the right atrioventricular groove to enter the right side of the coronary sinus; and the **left posterior ventricular vein**, which accompanies the obtuse marginals of the LCA, running up the posterior aspect of the left ventricle to drain into the coronary sinus. The **anterior cardiac veins** drain much of the anterior surface of the heart and drain into the anterior wall of the right atrium directly. Several small veins, the venae cordis minimae, drain directly into the cardiac chambers.

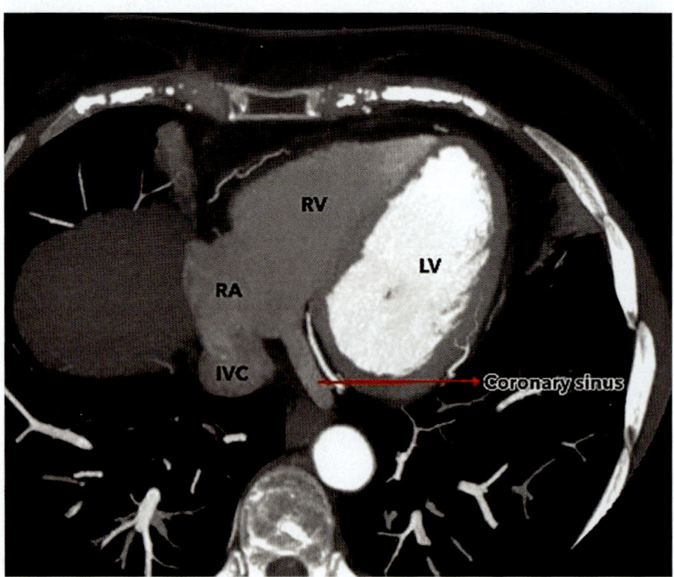

Fig. 3.3.108: Cardiac CT: Coronary vessels

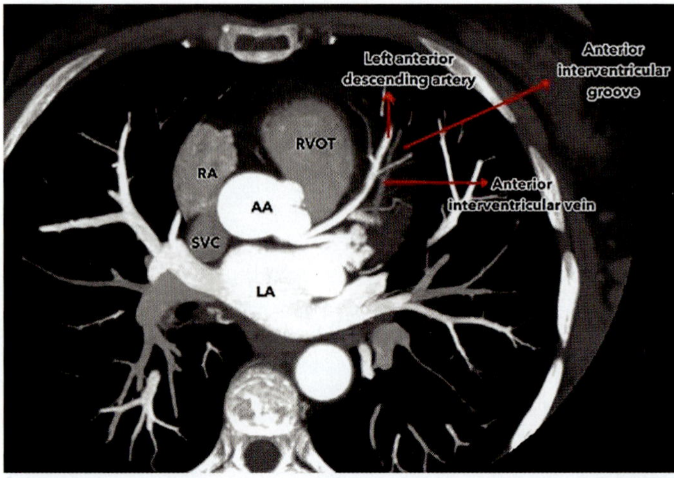

Fig. 3.3.109: Cardiac CT: Coronary vessels

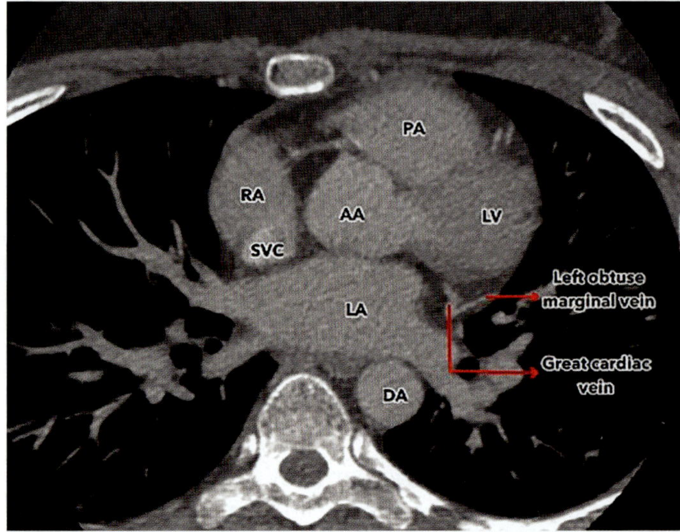

Fig. 3.3.110: Cardiac CT: Coronary vessels

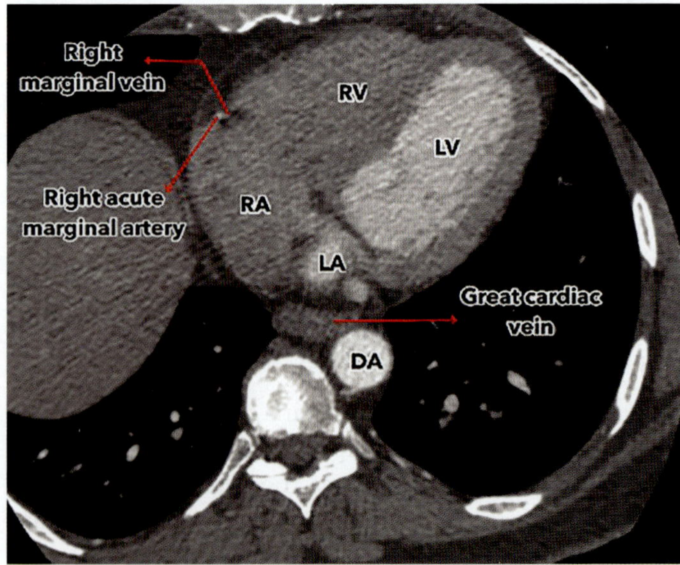

Fig. 3.3.111: Cardiac CT: Coronary vessels

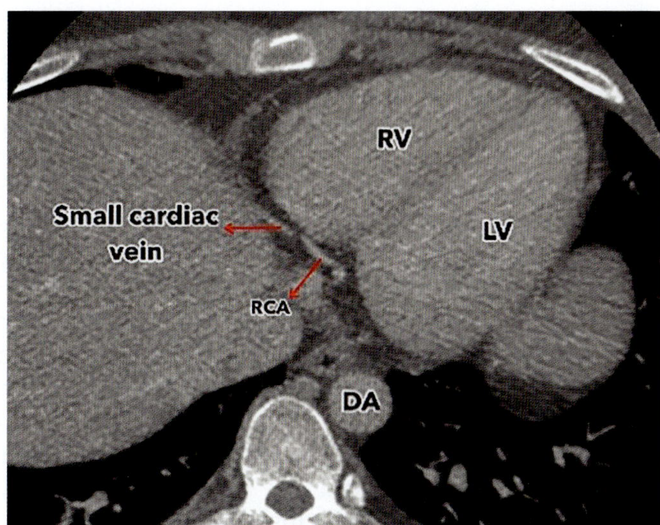

Fig. 3.3.112: Cardiac CT: Coronary vessels

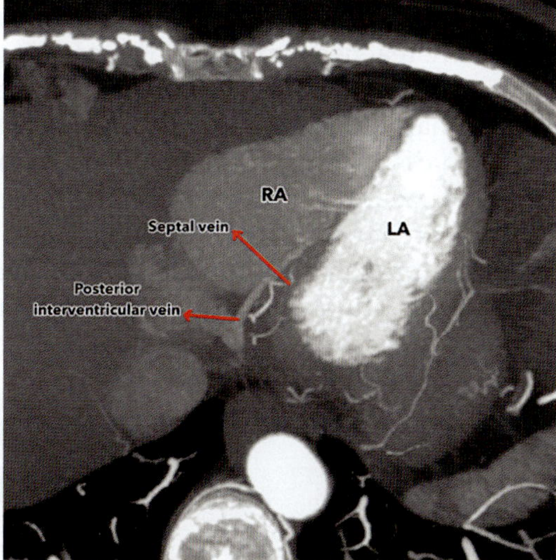

Fig. 3.3.113: Cardiac CT: Coronary vessels

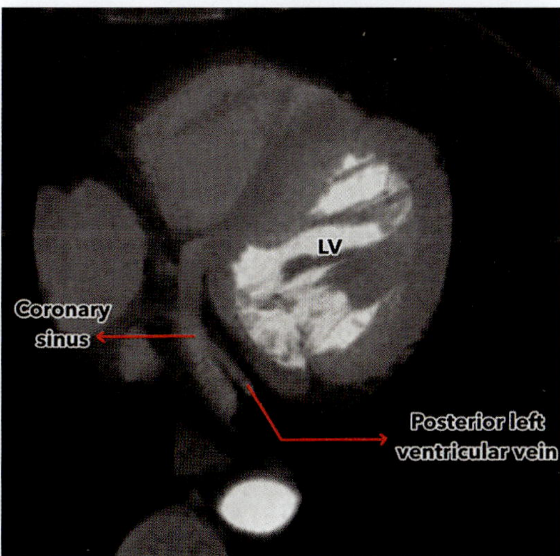

Fig. 3.3.114: Cardiac CT: Coronary vessels

3.3.L Pulmonary Vessels

Pulmonary circulation consists of pulmonary arterial tree, capillary bed, pulmonary veins which is a low pressure, high capacitance system which provides large surface area of gas exchange. Bronchial circulation is low capacitance, high pressure system which provides nutrient to lungs. Main pulmonary artery arises from right ventricle, which bifurcates into right and left main pulmonary arteries at the level of carina, below the aortic arch. The right and left pulmonary arteries divide into two lobar arteries, which subsequently divide into segmental and subsegmental pulmonary arteries. They are parallel to segmental and subsegmental bronchi and named according to bronchopulmonary segments. Right pulmonary artery gives origin to truncus anterior, first branch, which supplies the right upper lobe. Interlobar artery, runs in interlobar fissure, supplies the right middle and right lower lobes. Left main pulmonary artery, after giving off its first branches to left upper lobe (apicoanterior trunk supplies apicoposterior and anterior segments), and superior segmental artery to superior segment of left lower lobe, continues as common basal trunk, which divides into segmental and subsegmental branches supplying the basal segments of left lower lobe. Pulmonary veins are four in number, superior and inferior pulmonary veins on either side, drains into left atrium. Right superior pulmonary vein drains the right upper lobe, right middle lobe. Right inferior pulmonary vein drains the right lower lobe. Left superior pulmonary vein drains the left upper lobe and lingula, left inferior

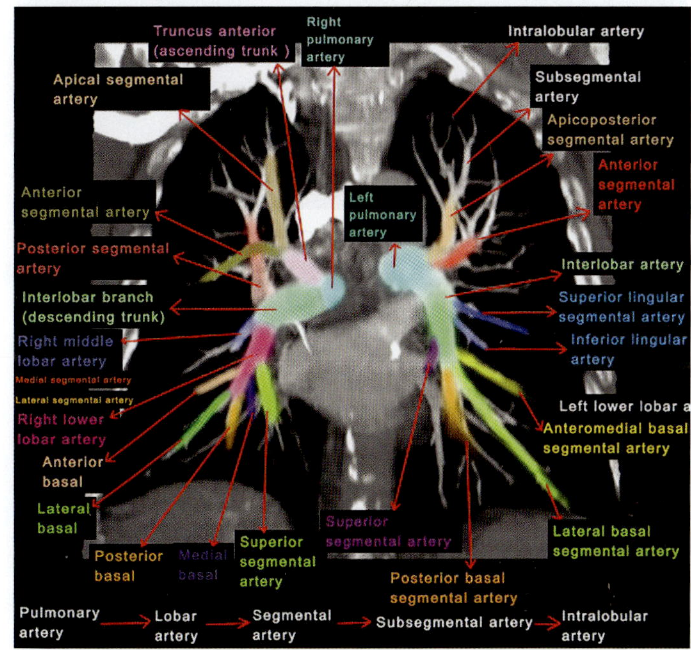

Fig. 3.3.115: Pulmonary arterial anatomy of chest in coronal plane

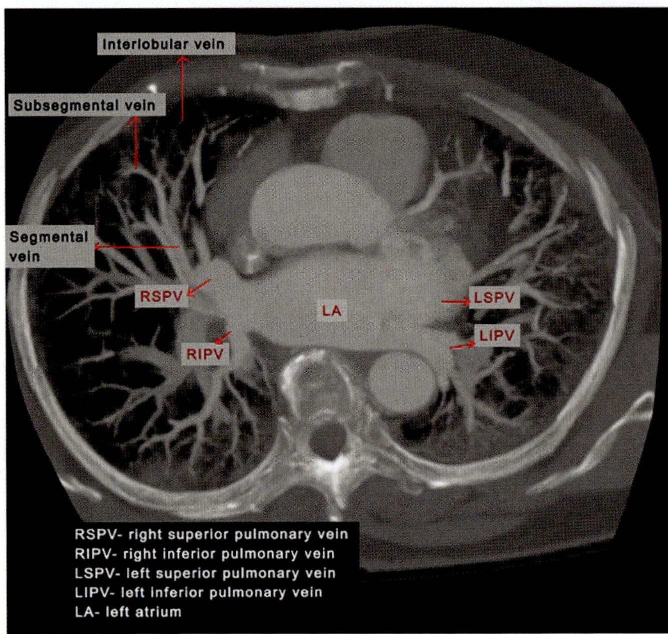

Fig. 3.3.116: Pulmonary vessels

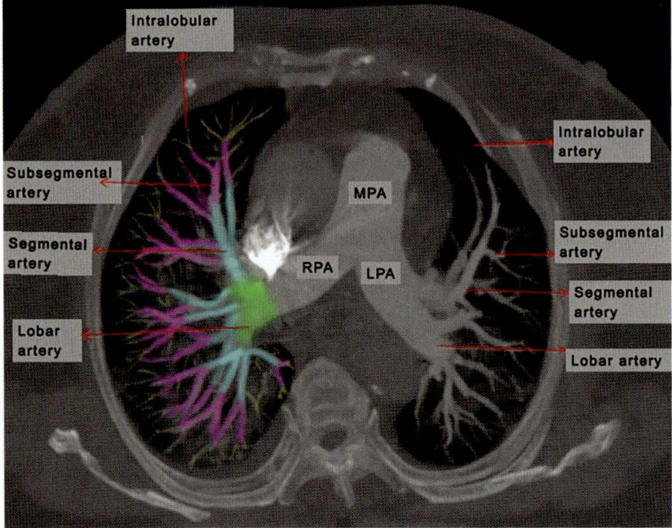

Fig. 3.3.117: Pulmonary vessels

vein drains the left lower lobe. Bronchial arteries (1 on right side and 2 on left side) arise from anterolateral aspect of descending aorta or from intercostal arteries.

Bronchial vessels: In terms of origin and number, the bronchial arteries have a variable range of anatomy. Normal bronchial arteries are tiny vessels that most typically originate from the descending thoracic aorta (orthotopic), usually 1–2 cm above or below the carinal level, mainly at the T5–T6 vertebral plane. They can also originate elsewhere (ectopic), such as from the aortic arch, subclavian artery, thyrocervical trunk, internal mammary artery, and coronary arteries. Ectopic bronchial arteries are distinguished by their proximity to the accompanying bronchi. The right bronchial arteries preferentially emerge from the posteromedial aortic wall in their orthotopic origin, either directly or more usually from a short intercostal-bronchial trunk (ICBT). Both the anterior and lateral aortic walls give rise to the left bronchial arteries, which travel retrotracheally towards each hilum. There are several variations in terms of the number and origin of the bronchial arteries, although four branching types were notably more prevalent. Two left and one right bronchial artery, the latter arising from an ICBT, is the most common (type 1). One artery on each side, the right bronchial artery originating from an ICBT (type 2), two right and two left bronchial arteries (type 3), and two right and one left bronchial artery (type 4) are other common forms. As they ramify in the pulmonary hila, the bronchial arteries have a typical diameter of less than 1.5 mm near the origin and less than 0.5 mm distally. When hypertrophy occurs, the diameter usually reaches 2 mm, and the path is usually more tortuous. Tissues supplied by bronchial arteries drain to pulmonary veins or bronchial veins. Bronchial veins form two distinct systems. The deep veins form a network of veins around the pulmonary interstitium and communicate freely with the pulmonary veins. They also form a bronchial vein trunk that drains to the pulmonary system. The superficial bronchial veins drain to the azygos vein on the right side and to the accessory hemiazygos vein on the left side.

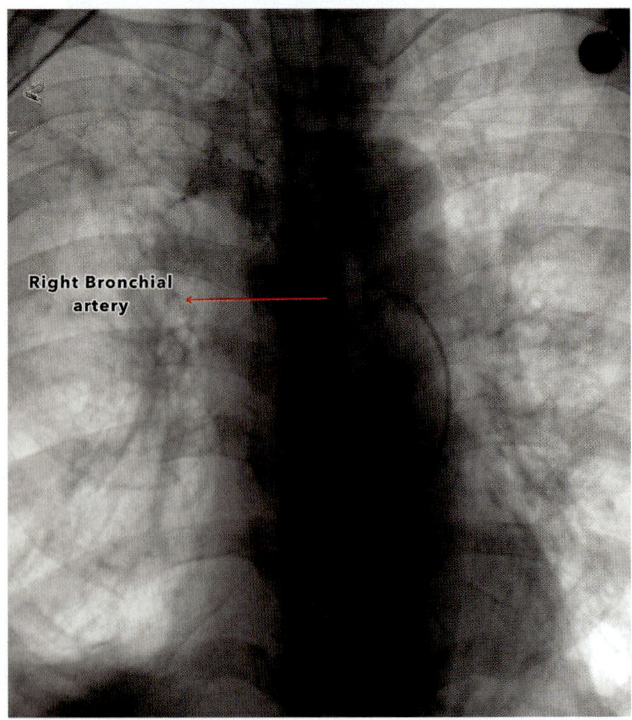

Fig. 3.3.118: DSA: Bronchial artery

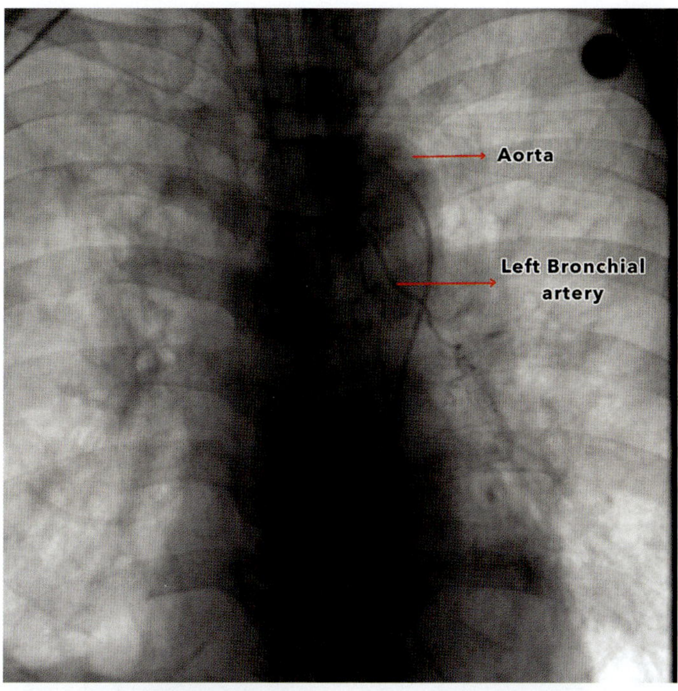

Fig. 3.3.119: DSA: Bronchial artery

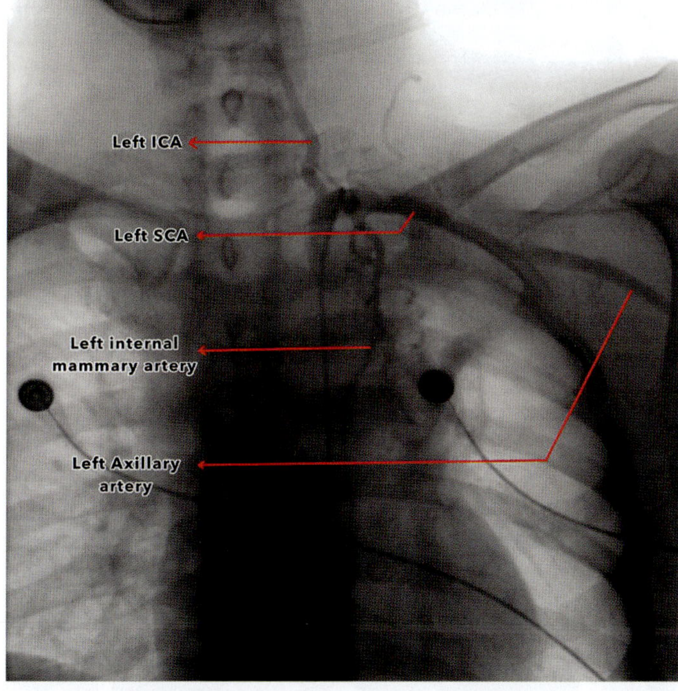

Fig. 3.3.120: DSA: Bronchial artery

3.3.M Nerves in Mediastinum

The vagus nerves are the tenth cranial nerves and pass through the neck in the carotid sheath composed of motor and sensory fibres, the vagus nerve enters the superior mediastinum posterior to the internal jugular vein and brachiocephalic veins. It passes behind the main

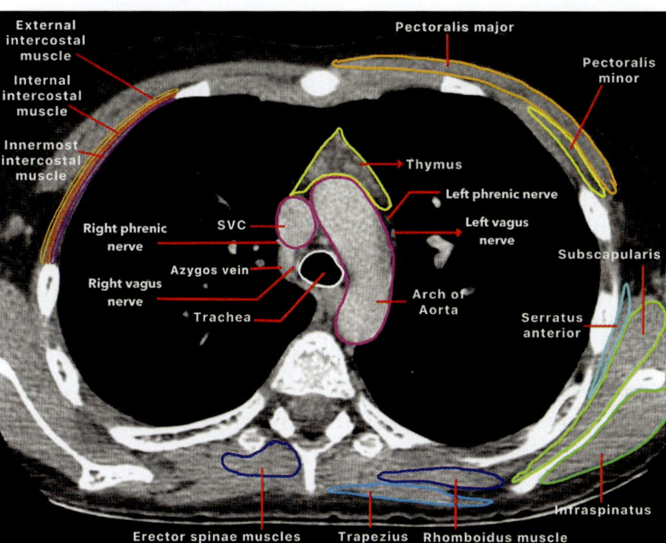

Fig. 3.3.121: CECT chest axial image

bronchi, forming a posterior pulmonary plexus; branches then pass to the oesophagus, forming anterior and posterior oesophageal plexuses, which continue into the abdomen through the oesophageal hiatus as anterior and posterior vagal trunks. The recurrent laryngeal nerves arise from the vagi. On the right, the recurrent laryngeal nerve winds around the subclavian artery, on the left it winds around the aortic arch. The phrenic nerves arise from the third to fifth cervical nerves and are the motor supply to the diaphragm. They enter the chest anterior to the subclavian artery and deep to the vein. The right phrenic nerve runs down in front of the superior vena cava, over the right heart border and inferior vena cava to reach the diaphragm. The left phrenic nerve runs down over the aortic arch and left superior intercostal vein, in front of the left hilum, and runs on the left heart border to reach the diaphragm.

3.3.N Chest Wall

Soft tissues, such as skin, subcutaneous fat, and muscles, are frequently distinguishable on a frontal radiograph of the thorax across the shoulders and along the thoracic wall. The rib cage should be symmetric in the absence of pulmonary or pleural disease or spinal deformity. The inferior interior side of the ribs houses the intercostal arteries, veins, and nerves. To avoid cardiac magnification, a lateral chest radiograph is obtained with the left side against the radiographic detector. As a result, the right ribs are enlarged and appear larger than the left ribs due to their distance (the big rib sign). Unilateral or bilateral cervical ribs can be detected emerging from the seventh cervical vertebra in about 0.5 percent of the population. These are usually coincidental results, but they can lead to thoracic outlet syndrome, which manifests as discomfort and weakness in the C8 nerve root distribution, as well as differences in pulse intensity between the two arms when the affected extremity is in particular positions. Other supernumerary ribs are quite uncommon. The sternum is the thoracic cage's anterior midline component. The manubrium, which articulates with clavicles, the body, and xiphoid process make comprise the xiphoid process. The most frequent congenital anomaly of the sternum is pectus excavatum, or "funnel chest," a depression of the sternum that can cause leftward displacement and axial rotation of the heart if severe. Obscuration of the right heart border on frontal radiographs may be mistaken for right middle lobe airspace illness in certain circumstances. A frontal view of the sternum is difficult to assess, and lateral or oblique views are preferable. A stripe between the posterior cortex of the sternal body and the lung can be identified using retrosternal lung. This fat-based retrosternal stripe is 1 to 3 mm thick and made up largely of fat. Parasternal structures, particularly costal cartilage, may indent the lung, resulting in a lobulated contour posterior to the parasternal stripe. An anomaly, most typically enlarged internal mammary lymph nodes, is indicated by a localised convexity or lobulation that is not at the level of a costal cartilage. The thoracic spine and intervertebral discs should be barely visible on an ideal chest radiograph, with the spinous processes in the midline. Paravertebral interfaces or stripes, which are typically apparent on a frontal radiograph, especially in the lower part of the chest, are caused by contact between the lower lobes and the paravertebral soft tissues. They are usually thin and parallel to the spine. Displacement of the paravertebral stripe may occur with a vertebral abnormality (osteophyte, fracture, infection, neoplasm), paravertebral masses (hematoma, neurogenic tumor, paravertebral abscess), or lymph node enlargement. The intercostal space is bridged by the muscles—the external, internal and innermost intercostal muscles. The neurovascular bundle lies between the internal and innermost muscle layers.

Intercostal arteries: **Posterior**—upper two spaces supplied by superior intercostal arteries from the costocervical branch of the subclavian artery and lower nine from the thoracic aorta.

Anterior—two branches to most intercostal spaces: Upper six spaces supplied by the internal thoracic branch of the subclavian artery; next three by the musculophrenic artery, the continuation of the internal thoracic artery. The lower two spaces have no anterior intercostal artery.

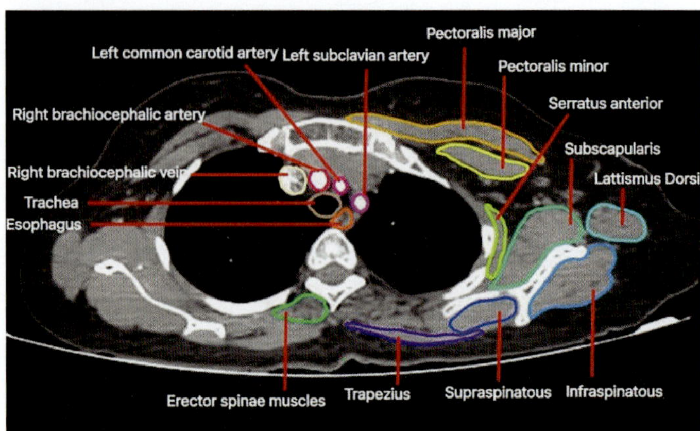

Fig. 3.3.122: CECT chest axial image

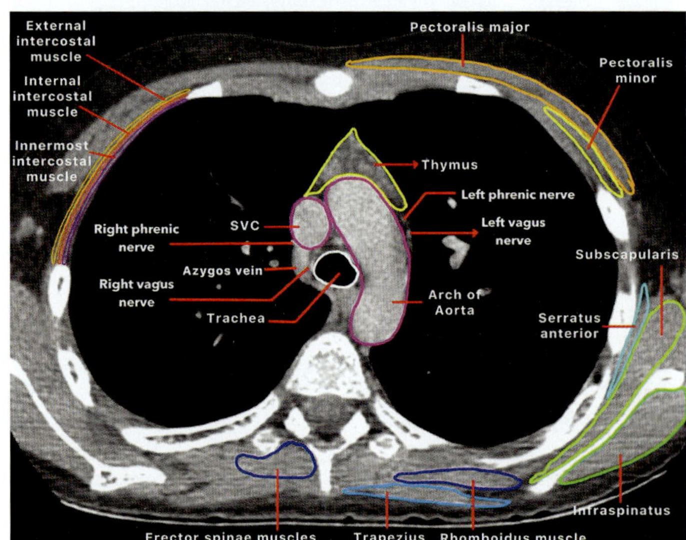

Fig. 3.3.123: CECT chest axial image

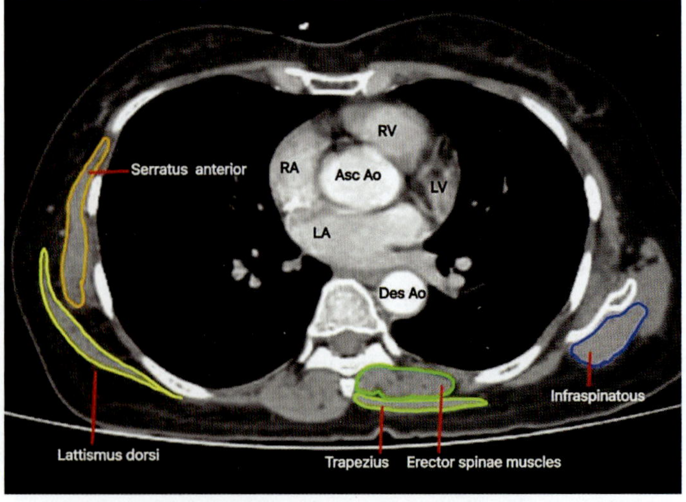

Fig. 3.3.124: CECT chest axial image

3

Intercostal vein: **Posterior**—first intercostal vein arches over the pleura to drain into the brachiocephalic vein. Second to fourth drain to a superior intercostal vein which drains to the azygos vein on the right and to the brachiocephalic vein on the left. Fifth to eleventh on the right drain to the azygos vein. Left fifth to eighth drain to the accessory hemiazygos vein and ninth to eleventh to the hemiazygos vein.

Anterior—veins accompany arteries to internal thoracic and musculophrenic veins.

3.3.O Diaphragm

Diaphragm is the dome-shaped muscle that separates thoracic cavity from abdominal cavity, enclosing the inferior thoracic aperture. The diaphragm has multiple attachments to the body wall. The two diaphragmatic crura attach the diaphragm posteriorly to the upper lumbar vertebral bodies and discs. The crura are joined by a fibrous median arcuate ligament. The diaphragm's muscular fibres start along the inferior thorax's perimeter and converge at a shared insertion point of the central tendon. The crura are tendinous structures that mix together with the vertebral column's anterior longitudinal ligament. The right crus is longer and wider than the left, and it emerges from the front surfaces of the L1-3 bodies. Left crus arises from the corresponding portions of L1-2. Through the diaphragm are a series of 3 major openings that permit the passage of structures between the thoracic and abdominal cavities: Aortic hiatus (T12 level) through which aorta, thoracic duct, azygos vein passes; esophageal hiatus (T10 level) through which esophagus, vagus nerves, small esophageal branches of the left gastric artery passes; vena caval hiatus (T8 level) through which inferior vena cava, right phrenic nerve passes. The upper surface of the dome-shaped diaphragm, which forms an interface with the lung on a chest radiograph, is generally visible; the soft tissues of the belly cover its inferior surface. The level of the cupola of the right hemidiaphragm is projected in a plane ranging from the anterior end of the fifth rib to the sixth anterior interspace in roughly 95% of normal people. The right hemidiaphragm is visible along its whole length in a left lateral view of the chest, whereas the heart obscures the anterior section of the left hemidiaphragm. Right hemidiaphragm is 1.5 to 2.5 cm higher than the left, but the two hemidiaphragms are at the same level in some 9% of the population. In a few normal individuals the left hemidiaphragm is up to 1 cm higher than the right.

3.3.P USG Chest

Scanning technique: Chest ultrasound is made feasible by the interpretation of ultrasound artefacts that arise from the chest wall and pleural surface. The deeper structures can be seen with a 2–5 MHz curvilinear probe. The curvilinear probe can be used to quickly examine the chest wall, pleura, and lungs. A high-resolution 7.5–10 MHz linear probe can be used to provide detailed portrayal of any chest wall, pleural, or peripheral lung abnormalities once an abnormality has been found. With the patient in upright or recumbent positions, raising the arm above the patient's head increases the rib space distance and facilitates scanning. The posterior chest should be imaged when the patient is sitting erect, whereas the anterior and lateral chests can be examined while the patient is lying down. On gray-scale images, the echogenicity of a lesion can be compared with that of the liver and characterized as hypoechoic, isoechoic, or hyperechoic. A complete lung examination consists of 12 imaging regions, 6 on each side. Each hemithorax is divided into anterior, lateral, and posterior zones, demarcated by the anterior and posterior axillary line. Imaging is performed in cephalad and caudad regions of each zone.

Normal anatomy: The layers of muscles and fascia planes show as a sequence of echogenic soft-tissue layers on the normal chest wall. On transverse scans, the ribs appear as curvilinear structures beneath the soft tissue of the chest wall, which is accompanied with posterior acoustic shadowing. The anterior cortex should appear as a continuous smooth echogenic line when the ribs are scanned along the long axis. The visceral and parietal sections of the pleura can be observed as two echogenic lines deep to the ribs using a high-resolution linear probe. The visceral pleura is thicker than the parietal pleura in most cases. The lung is air-filled beyond the pleura–lung interface, preventing further visibility of normal lung parenchyma. However, because of the substantial shift in acoustic impedance at the pleura–lung interface, horizontal artefacts appear below the pleural line as a series of echogenic parallel lines equidistant from one another. In addition, vertically oriented "comet-tail" artefacts, which originate at the pleura-lung contact, are commonly encountered. In a healthy adult, vision of these artefacts is usually limited to the final intercostal area above the diaphragm. The diaphragm can be observed as a 1 mm thick echogenic line above the liver and spleen when investigated through the lower intercostal gaps. On inspiration, a normal downward movement of the diaphragm should be visible.

Observations: When an ultrasound transducer is placed on a normal chest wall with a normally aerated lung, the following is observed: **Pleural line**—the parietal and visceral pleurae appear as a single bright hyperechoic line not wider than 2 mm just deep to the internal intercostal muscles. Respiration causes the pleural border to "slide." During respiration, the visceral pleura rubs against the parietal pleura, creating the sonographic phenomenon of lung sliding (also known as lung gliding or lung sliding sign). It has a larger amplitude near the base than at the peak, where it may be insignificant. With a negative predictive value of 100 percent, the presence of lung sliding rules out pneumothorax at the probe's tip. The image is best viewed in M mode because the superficial parietal layers remain stationary and have a horizontal pattern of lines, whereas the area deep to the pleural line appears "granular" because the pleural line's motion is mirrored throughout this area. This is also called the "seashore sign". The pleura is located below the ribs and appears as white curved lines with a black shadow behind them. This is referred to as the **"Bat sign".** **A-lines:** Horizontal, regularly spaced hyperechogenic lines representing reverberations of the pleural line. These are motionless and are artifacts of repetition. Ultrasound of chest (Figs 3.3.125–3.3.127) **B-lines** occur when sound waves pass through the superficial soft tissues and cross the pleural line encountering a mixture of air and water. They appear as vertical lines extending from the pleural line to the lower edge of the screen without fading. B lines move synchronously with lung during respiration and tend to erase A lines. It is common to see a few B lines at the base of a normal lung, the presence of more than three B lines in a single ultrasound field is considered significant and suggests alveolar interstitial syndrome. **Z lines** are short, broad, ill-defined, vertical comet tail artifacts arising from the pleural line but not reaching the distal edge of the screen and are not B lines. These are found in normal persons as well as in those with pneumothorax. **E lines** are vertical lines seen when there is gas trapped in the subcutaneous space ("E" stands for subcutaneous

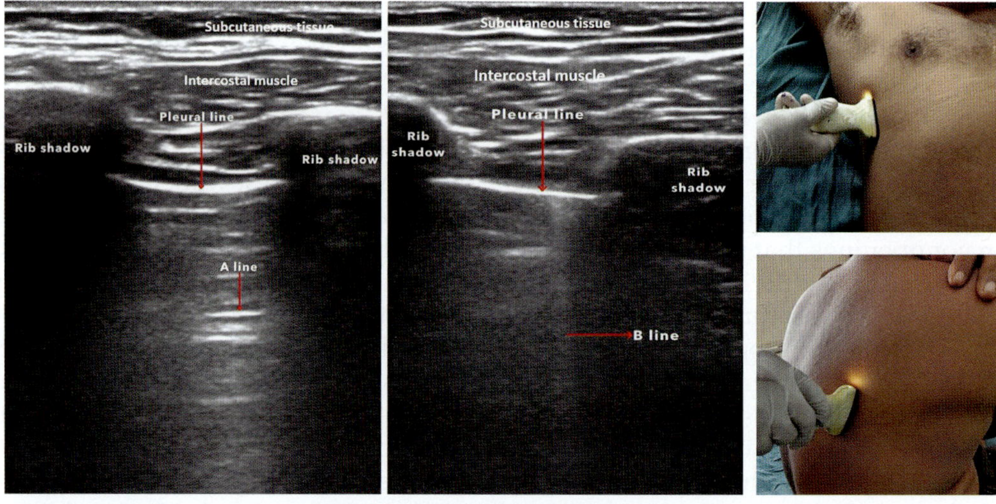

Fig. 3.3.125: Ultrasound of chest

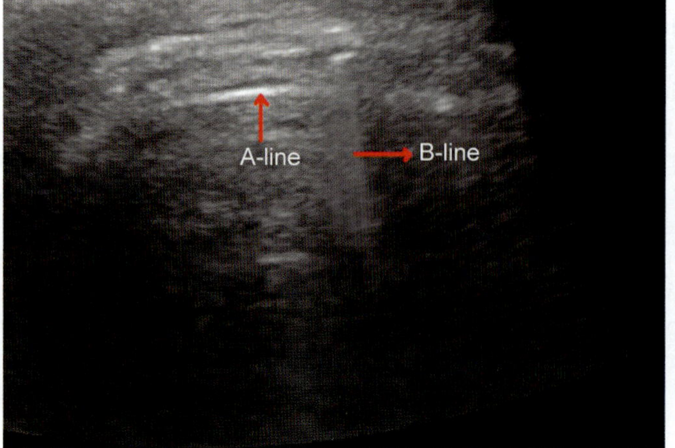

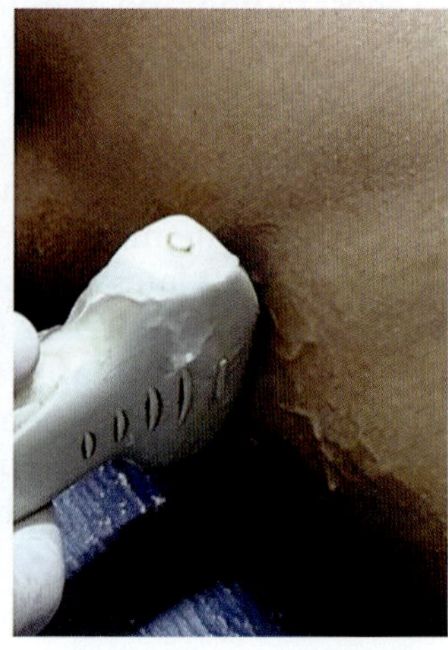

Fig. 3.3.126: Ultrasound of chest

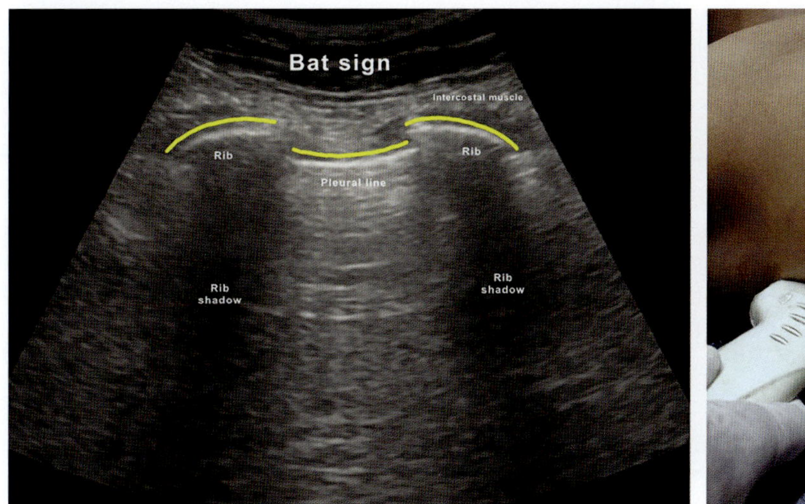

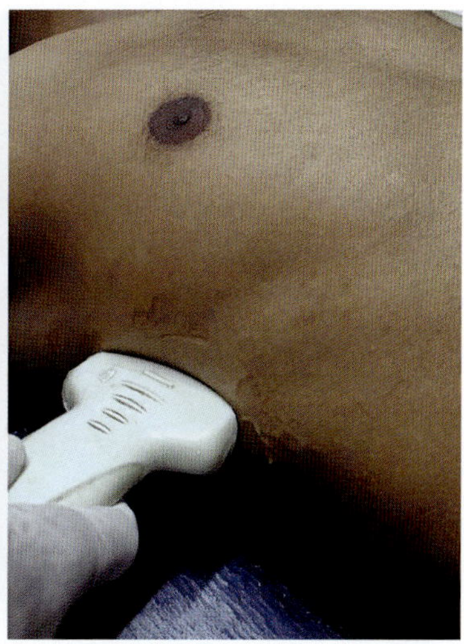

Fig. 3.3.127: Ultrasound of chest

emphysema). These lines do not arise from the pleural line, but from the subcutaneous tissue. E lines are well-defined and also erase A lines, and may, therefore, be mistaken for true B lines. Given the gas does not move, they are not synchronous with respiratory movements.

Diaphragm: The diaphragm appears as a 1 mm thick echoic line; downward movement of the diaphragm should be detected with inspiration, and the splenorenal and hepatorenal recesses must be investigated in each patient. During inspiration, the liver and diaphragm may be covered by the lung, which can be seen while scanning intercostally. This is referred to as the "curtain sign".

3.3.Q Echocardiogram

Echocardiogram is an effective noninvasive investigating modality for imaging heart, with recent advances in imaging techniques have upgraded echocardiogram with added features such as in transesophageal echocardiogram, contrast echocardiogram, bedside echocardiogram still remains as one important imaging modality in emergency setup.

Parasternal long axis view (PLAX): The transducer is placed approximately on the left 3rd intercostal space. The transducer's index mark is directed towards the patient's right shoulder or apex (based on easy orientation). The right (RV) and the left ventricle (LV), as well as the aortic bulb (AB) and the left atrium (LA) can be visualised.

Parasternal short axis (PSAX) (apical level): The transducer is turned 90° clockwise from the previous position and tilted a little upwards and to the left. At times, it will be necessary to place it one intercostal space deeper. The apex of the left (LV) and right (RV) ventricles can be visualised.

Parasternal short axis (papillary muscle level): From the former position the transducer is tilted a little, downwards and to the right. The left ventricle (LV) at the level of the papillary muscles and the right ventricle (RV) can be visualised. **Parasternal short axis (mitral valve level):** Further tilt in the transducer, from the

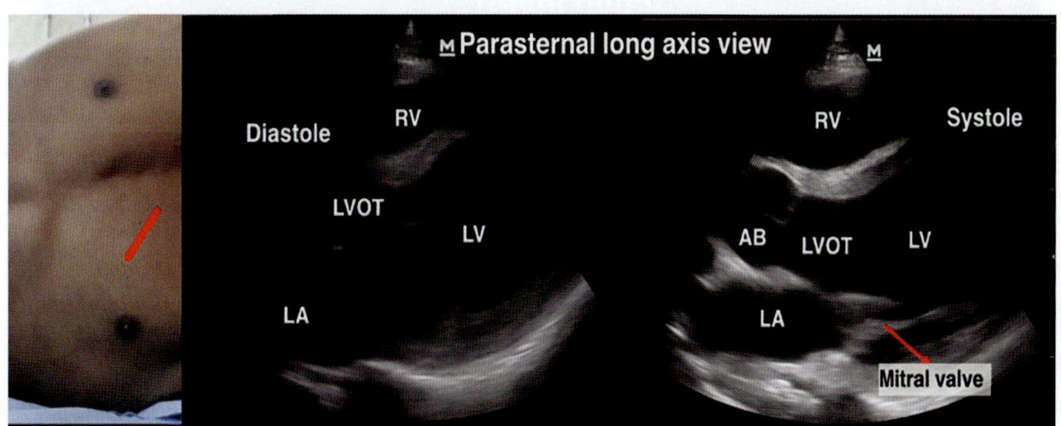

Fig. 3.3.128: ECHO

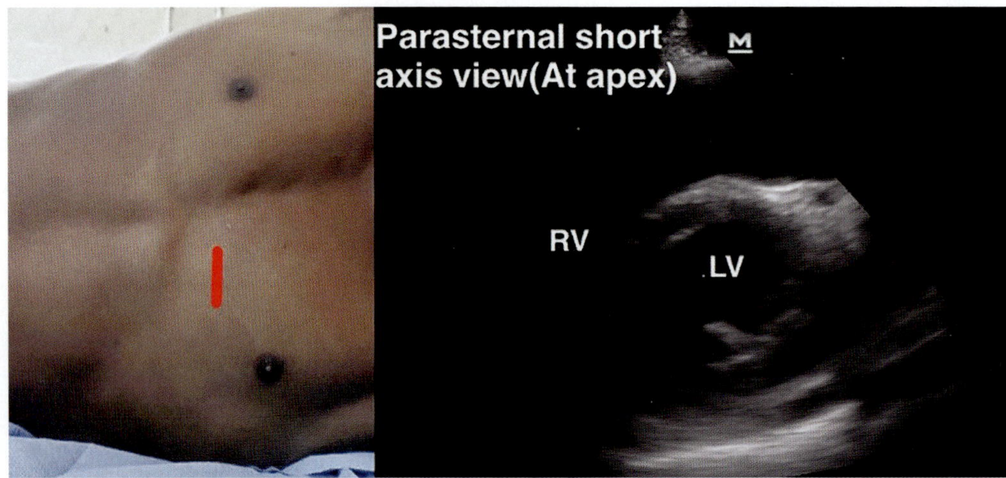

Fig. 3.3.129: ECHO

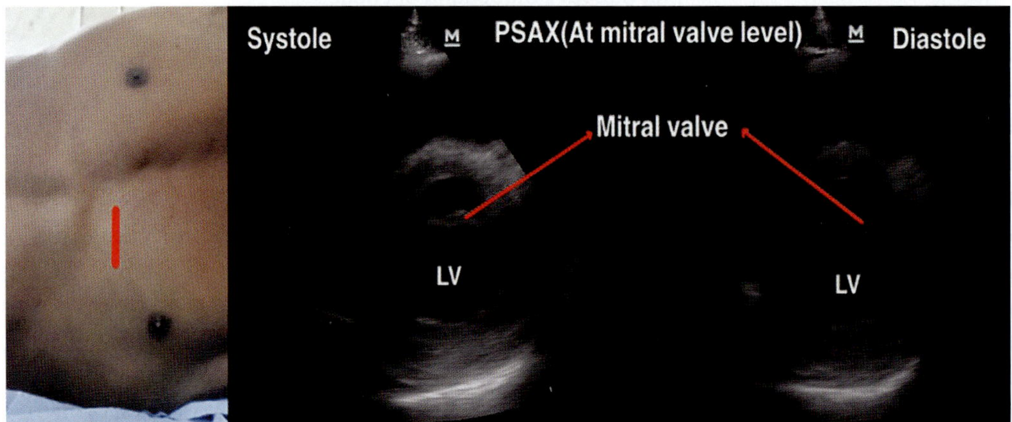

Fig. 3.3.130: ECHO

same position down to the right. A cross section of the left ventricle (LV) at the level of the mitral valve and the right ventricle (RV) can be visualised.

Parasternal short axis (aortic valve level): The transducer is tilted more down to the right. The aortic valve (AV), the pulmonary valve (PV), the left atrium

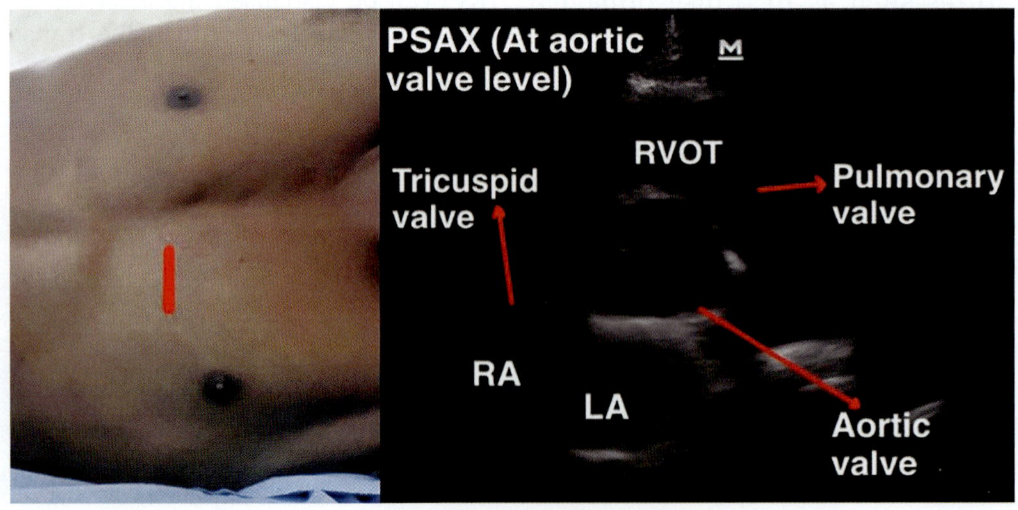

Fig. 3.3.131: ECHO

(LA) and the right atrium (RA), along with the tricuspid valve (TV) and the right ventricular outflow track (RVOT) can be visualised.

Apical four-chamber view (A4C): Place the transducer on the 5th intercostal space (left midclavicular). The left (LV) and the right ventricle (RV), as well as the left (LA) and the right atrium (RA) can be visualised.

Apical two-chamber (A2C) view: Turn the transducer (60° counterclockwise) from the previous position. The left ventricle (LV) and the left atrium (LA) can be visualised

Apical five-chamber view: Show a four-chamber view and then tilt the transducer slightly down. The aortic valve (AV) can be seen in the middle, between chambers.

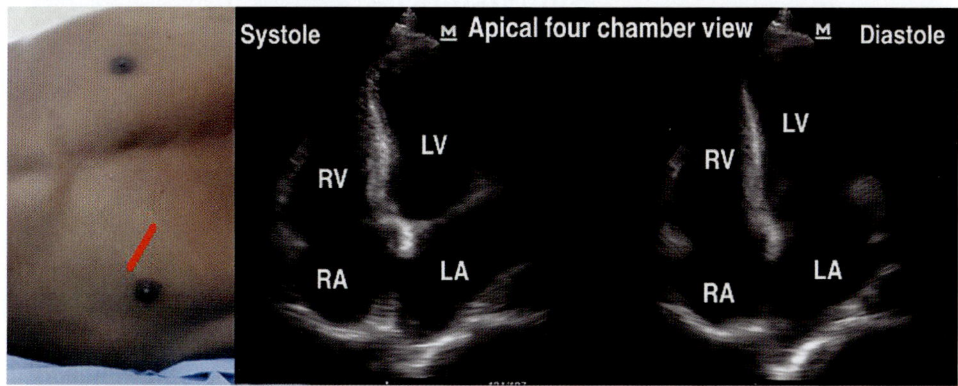

Fig. 3.3.132: ECHO

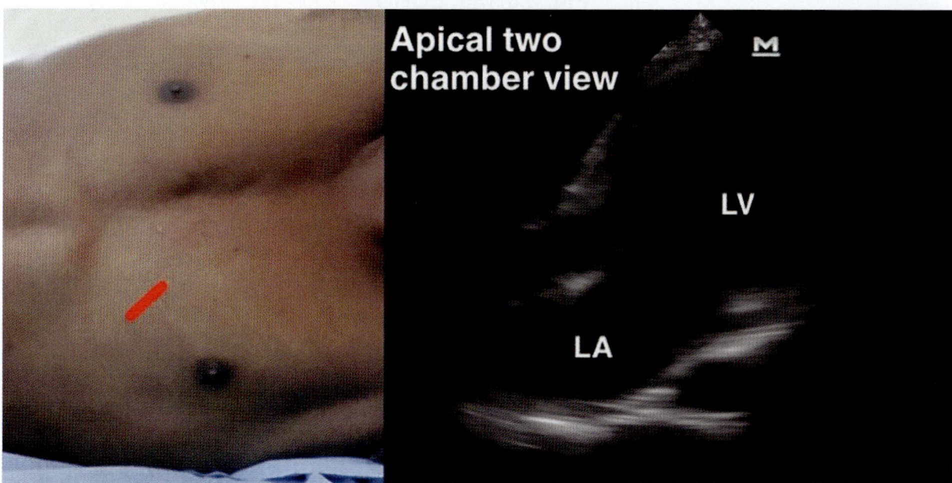

Fig. 3.3.133: ECHO

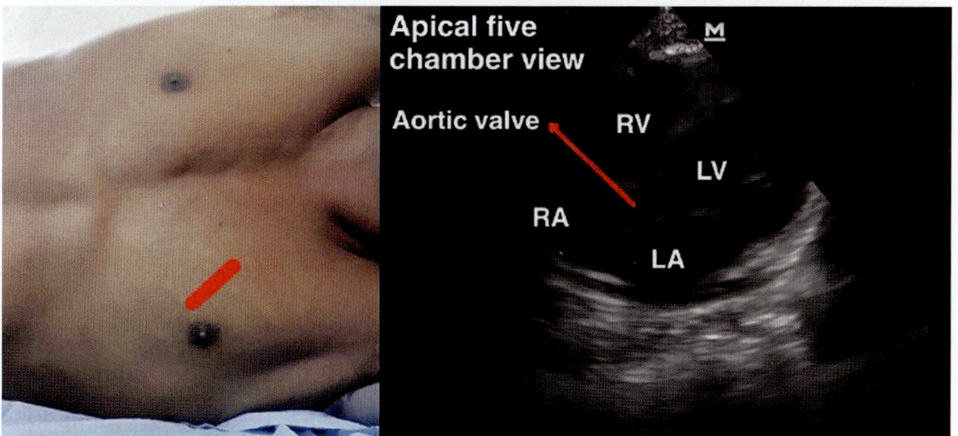

Fig. 3.3.134: ECHO

Tilting the transducer to the opposite direction, the coronary sinus can be displayed.

Subcostal view: The transducer is placed on the subxyphoid region. The transducer's index mark is directed towards the patient's head. The inferior vena cava (VCI) can be visualised. Turn the transducer clockwise slightly to see the right and left ventricle, right (RA) and left atrium (LA).

Subcostal four-chamber view: Turn the transducer (45° clockwise from the previous position). The liver, apex of the left (LV) and right ventricles (RV), as well as the left (LA) and right atrium (RA) can be displayed.

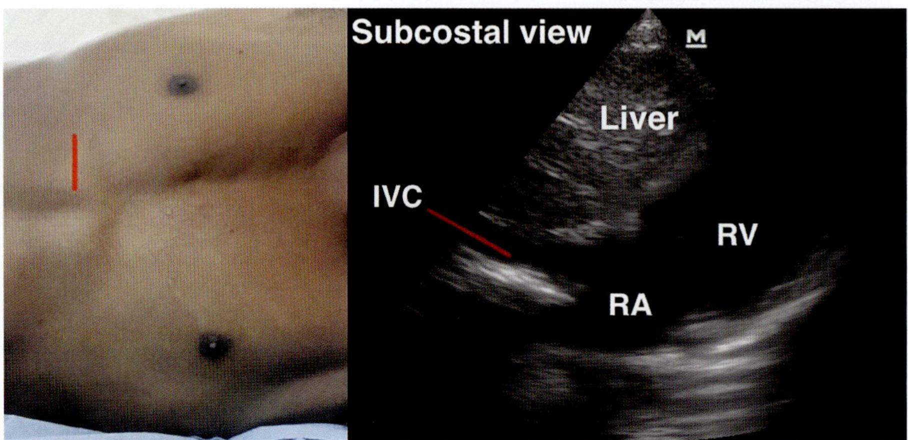

Fig. 3.3.135: ECHO

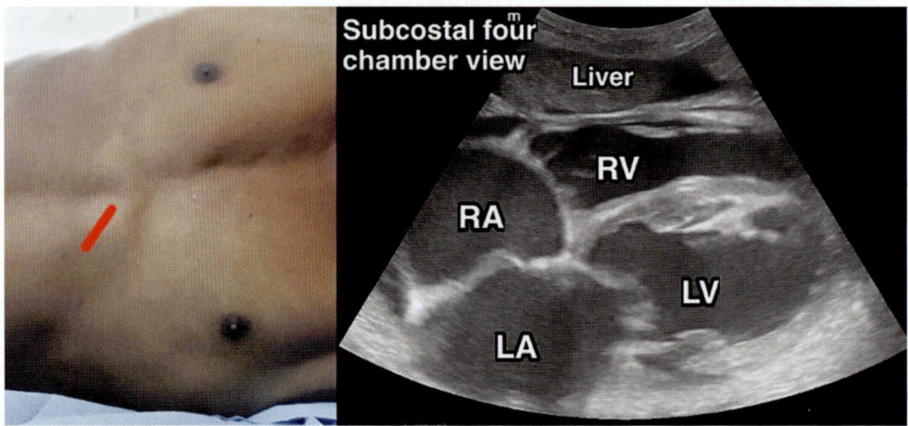

Fig. 3.3.136: ECHO

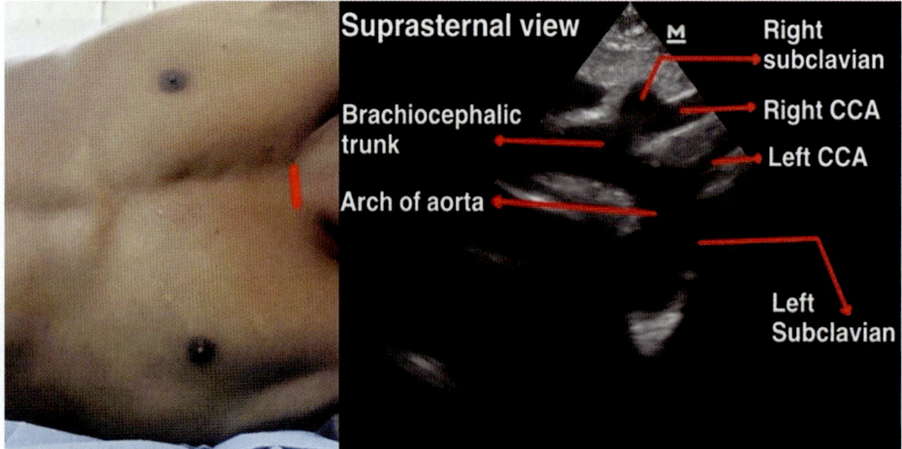

Fig. 3.3.137: ECHO

Suprasternal view: The transducer is placed on the suprasternal region. The transducer's index mark is directed towards the patient's head and turned (45° to the right). The aortic arch (AA), the neck arteries (TB, CL, SL) and the right pulmonary artery (RPA) as well as the left atrium (LA) can be visualised.

Color flow across valve: A—atrio-ventricular valve (Fig. 3.3.142); B—semilunar valve (Fig. 3.3.143).

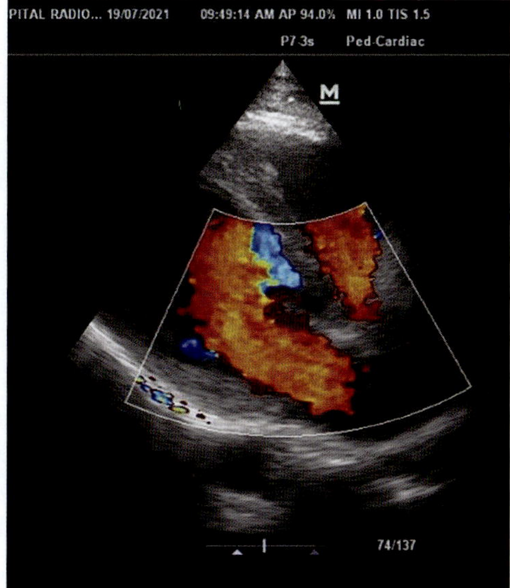

Fig. 3.3.138: ECHO

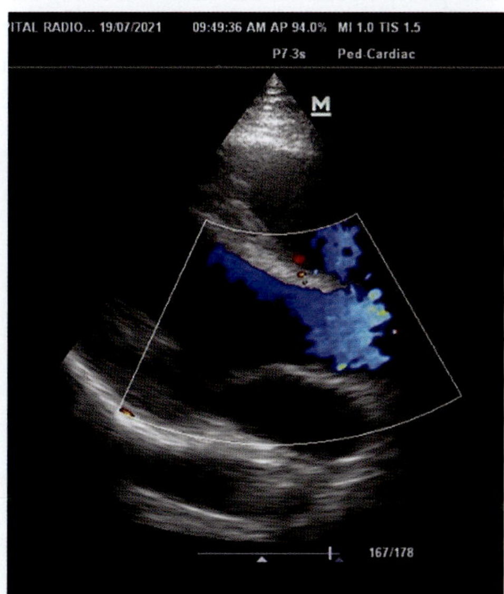

Fig. 3.3.139: ECHO

Measurement of ejection fraction (EF): The EF of the left heart, known as the left ventricular ejection fraction (LVEF), is calculated by dividing the volume of blood pumped from the left ventricle per beat (stroke volume) by the volume of blood collected in the left ventricle at the end of diastolic filling (end-diastolic volume). LVEF

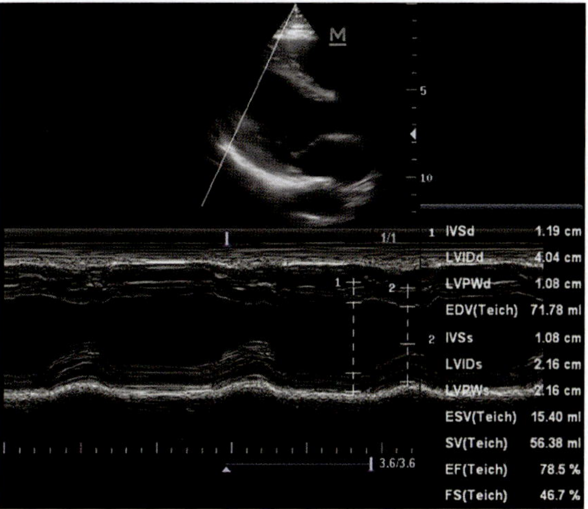

Fig. 3.3.140: Using M–mode on echocardiogram

is an indicator of the effectiveness of pumping into the systemic circulation. Similarly ejection fraction can be measured in right ventricle.

$$EF = (EDV–ESV)/(EDV \times 100)$$

EF: Ejection fraction; EDV: End diastolic volume; ESV: End systolic volume.

Normal EF: 48–78%

Contrast echo: It is similar to conventional echocardiogram, with advantages of clear visualization of cardiac chambers, it can be done using injection of contrast media such as dye or bubbled saline solution through intravenous cannulation. It is very useful tool in evaluating conditions such as pulmonary AV fistula where the contrast appears in left ventricle in 5–7 cycles after opacification of right ventricle and with the persistence of constrast.

3.3.R Breast Anatomy

The breast is a symmetrical organ located on the front of the chest on both sides of the midline. It occupies an area that stretches from the second rib to the sixth rib and from the edge of the sternum to the axilla. The normal breast tissue may also extend into the axilla called the axillary tail of Spence. At the center of the breast there are the nipple and areola. The areola is a flat hyperpigmented area of skin with a round or oval shape and of variable diameter, usually, between 3.5 and 6 cm. The nipple stays at center of the areola and has a variable size and shape (conical, cylindrical). At its apex there are several small depressions that represent the outlets of the ducts. The areolar surface is irregular due to the presence of the 8–12 tubercles of Morgagni, representing sebaceous glands.

The mammary gland is made of three components: Glandular, adipose and fibrous tissues. Functionally, it can be considered a modified apocrine sweat gland, in relation to breast-feeding. The breast parenchyma is contained by a two-layer fold of the subcutaneous superficial fascia, that may be divided in two parts: the superficial layer that covers the gland and contains fibrous septa, called Cooper's ligaments, which penetrate the gland and form the support structure of the parenchyma, and the deep layer, which covers the posterior portion of the gland and separates it from the underlying superficial fascia of the pectoralis major muscle. Cooper's ligaments are the suspensory ligaments of the breast gland and divide the parenchyma into lobes. The glandular tissue consists of a series of ducts and secretory lobules drained by lactiferous ducts. The drainage territory defined by each lactiferous duct is called a segment or lobule. There are generally about 15 to 20 lobes which drain into 8 to 12 ducts. From the distal subsegmental ducts, terminal ductal lobular units (TDLU) arise. TDLU is the functional unit of the glandular tissue.

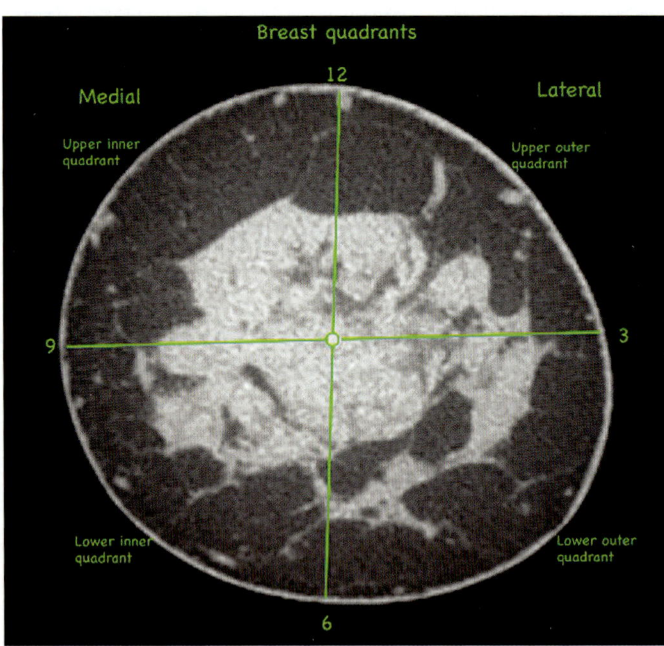

Fig. 3.3.141: Clock positions in left breast

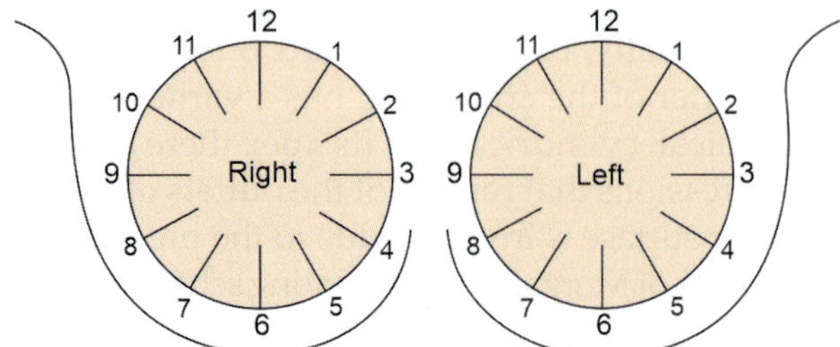

Fig. 3.3.142: Clock positions on breast

Based on the standard procedure recommended for breast imaging in women, the breast is conventionally divided into **4 quadrants:** Upper outer, upper inner, lower outer and lower inner. The lesion location should be provided based on **face of a clock** for future follow-up sessions. The same clock description describes a different location depending on which breast is involved.

In coronal view, three zones have been used that shows the location of any lesion in the transverse plane from the nipple to the axilla.

Zone 1: Adjacent to the nipple (includes first 1/3rd of the breast).

Zone 2: Midway from the nipple (includes 2/3rd of the breast).

Zone 3: Towards the peripheral breast.

In the sagittal plane, regions A, B and C denote the depth/distance of the lesion from nipple (equally divided into 3 parts by 2 vertical lines):

Region A: Near the surface—consists of **premammary (PM)** or subcutaneous fat zone containing subcutaneous fat, blood vessels, Cooper ligaments (CL), and in some cases, a small number of peripheral ducts and lobules.

Region B: Midway between the nipple and chest wall **(mammary zone)** contains all of the central ducts and most of the peripheral ducts and lobules, stromal fat and connective tissue. The anterior mammary fascia (AMF) and the retromammary fascia (RMF) encase the mammary zone.

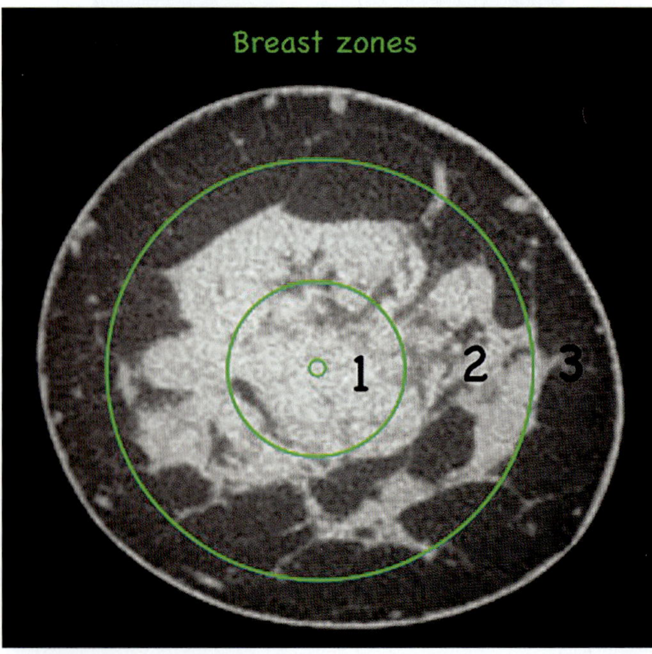

Fig. 3.3.143: Breast zones

3

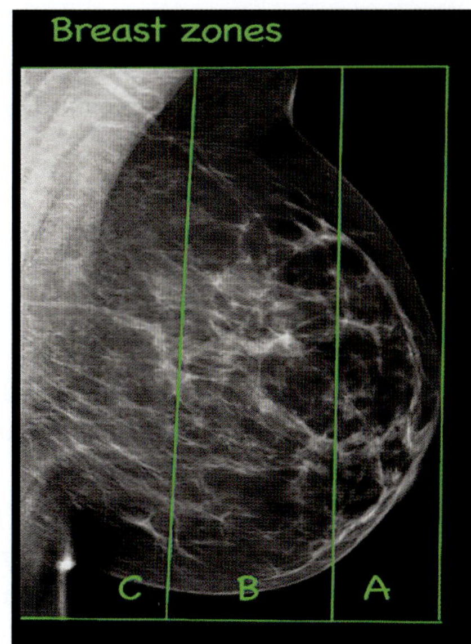

Fig. 3.3.144: Breast zones

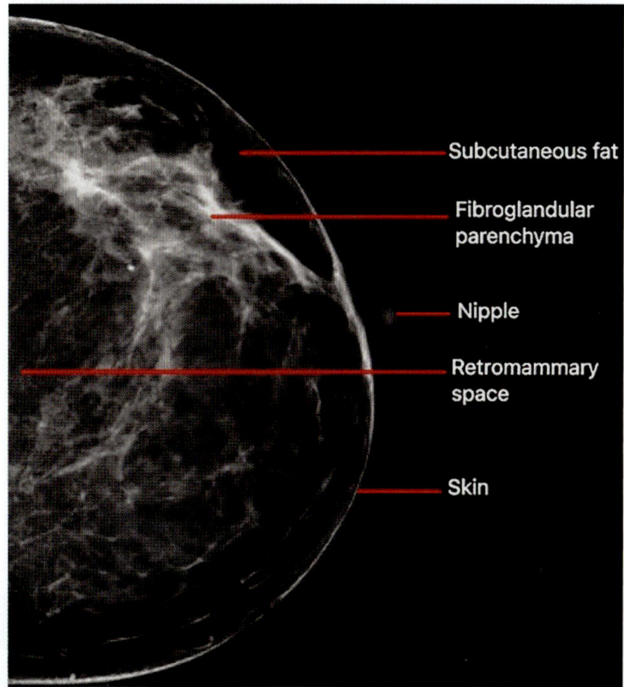

Fig. 3.3.146: Normal breast mammogram on CC view

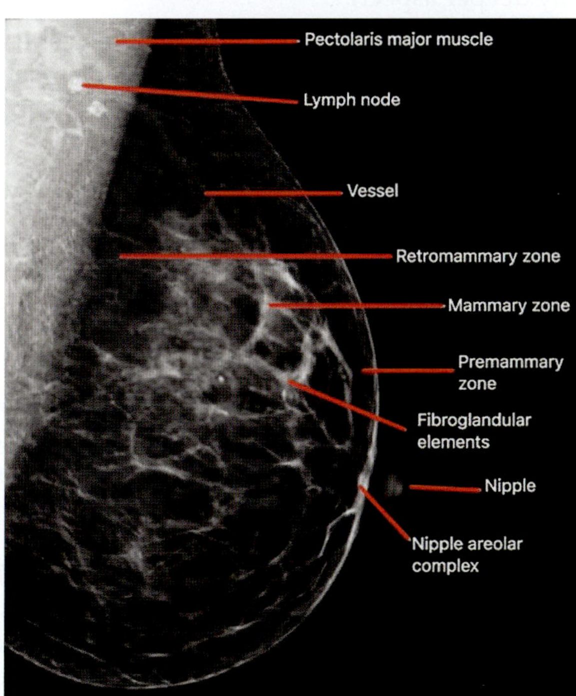

Fig. 3.3.145: Normal breast mammogram in MLO view

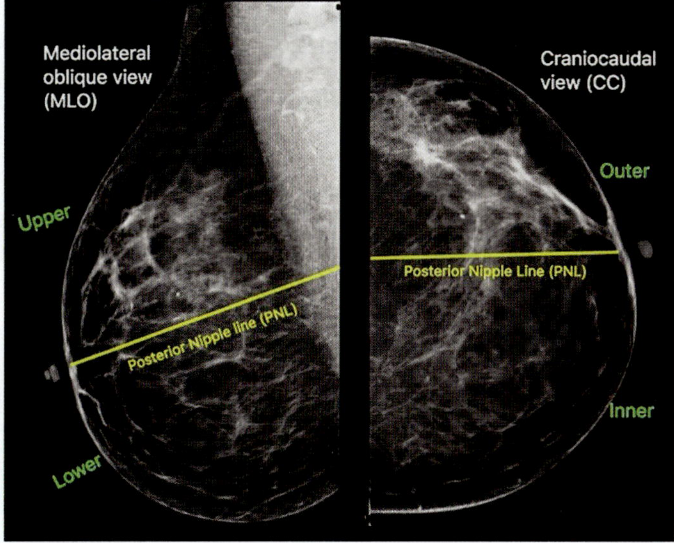

Fig. 3.3.147: Posterior nipple line in MLO and CC view

Region C: Chest wall—the **retromammary zone (RM)** is the deepest of the three zones and contains only fat and ligaments.

Mammography is routinely preformed using mediolateral oblique (MLO) view and craniocaudal (CC) view. **Posterior nipple line (PNL)** refers to a line posteriorly and perpendicularly from the nipple towards pectoral muscle. In an adequately positioned breast, the measurement difference of this line between MLO and CC view should be **ideally within 1 cm**. Each MLO view is divided into upper and lower regions and CC view into outer and inner regions. The nipple should be in profile to avoid mistaking it for a retroareolar lesion.

USG scanning techniques: The most common imaging technique used is grid scanning pattern followed by radial or star-shaped. **In grid scanning,** breast is scanned up and down in rows making sure to overlap each row slightly to ensure no breast tissue is overlooked. Rotate into a sagittal plane and repeat the pattern. **In radial technique**, each quadrant is scanned in a radial fashion

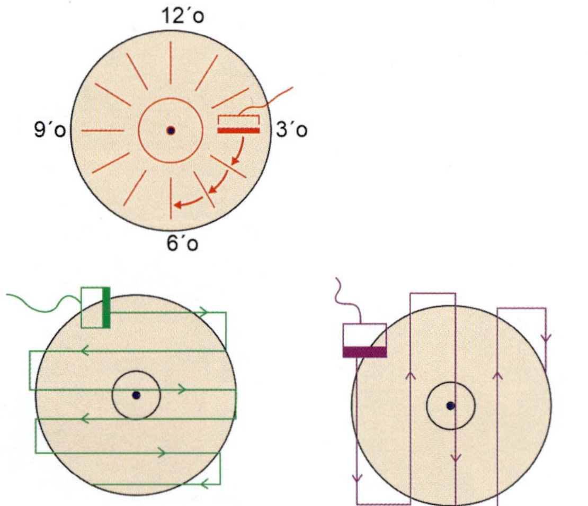

Fig. 3.3.148: Techniques to follow during sonomammogram examination

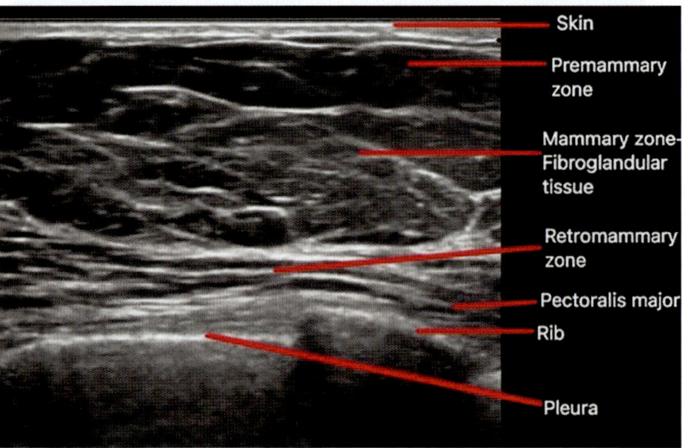

Fig. 3.3.149: Normal breast ultrasound

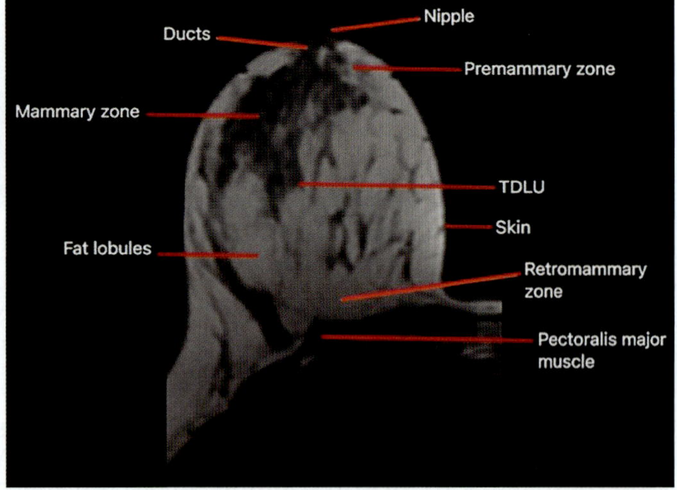

Fig. 3.3.150: MRI breast

3

to accommodate the arrangement of the ducts in the breast. If a pathology is identified, rotate the probe 90 degrees in the anti-radial plane.

From a sonographic point of view, breast is divided into various hyperechoic and hypoechoic layers: Skin—hyperechoic, fat—hypoechoic, breast parenchyma—hyperechoic, retromammary fat—hypoechoic, pectoralis major muscle—hyperechoic.

The skin is usually 1–3 mm in thickness. The ducts are tubular anechoic structures 1–2 mm in thickness. Physiological duct dilatation may occur in pregnancy up to 3 mm.

MRI breast is ideally to be performed 5 to 10 days post-menstrual cycle as the stroma is less dense and there is lower breast water content.

Neurovascular anatomy and lymphatics: The arterial supply is mainly from internal mammary arteries (60%—mainly medial and central aspect), lateral thoracic artery (30%—mainly the upper outer quadrant) and intercostal perforators from 3rd to 5th intercostal arteries (10%—mainly deeper aspect).

Venous drainage is divided into superficial and deep veins. Superficial veins form anastomotic circle near nipple areolar complex and then drain to periphery of breast to join deep venous system. The deep veins generally accompany the large arteries of breast. They mainly include internal mammary vein branches, axillary vein branches and posterior intercostal vein branches. The posterior intercostal veins provide potential direct communication to vertebral venous plexus that may aid metastasis to the spine and brain in breast cancer. The breast is innervated by three nerve groups, medial, lateral and superior mammary branches. The medial and lateral mammary branches arise from the cutaneous branches of the 2–6th intercostal nerves. The superior mammary branches arise from the supraclavicular branches of the cervical plexus.

Lymphatic drainage of breast is about 75% to axillary nodes and about 25% to internal mammary nodes. An abundant lymphatic system called the Sappey plexus is present in the subareolar location that drains into the axillary as well as internal mammary nodes.

3.3.S Axillary Lymph Nodes

They are a group of lymph nodes in the axilla and receive lymph from vessels that drain the arm, the walls of the thorax, the breast and the upper walls of the abdomen. There are five axillary lymph node groups, namely the lateral (humeral), anterior (pectoral), posterior (subscapular), central and apical nodes. The apical nodes are the final common pathway for all of the axillary lymph nodes. **Lateral (humeral) lymph nodes**—posteromedial to axillary vein. **Anterior (pectoral) lymph nodes**—

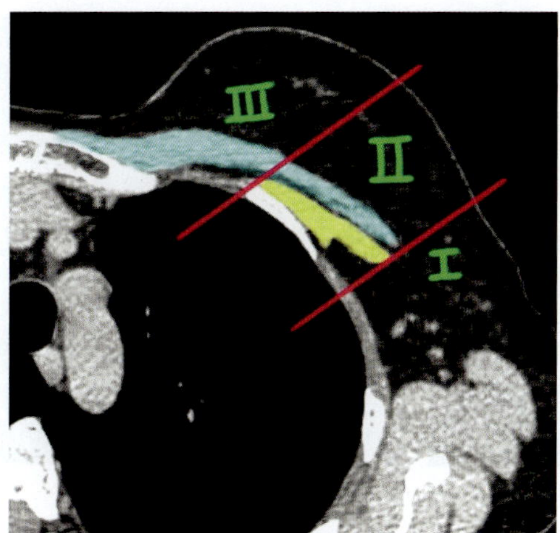

Fig. 3.3.151: Level I, II, III axillary nodes in relation to pectoralis minor

inferior border of pectoralis minor, near lateral thoracic vessels. **Posterior (subscapular) lymph nodes**—along subscapular vessels on inferior margin of the posterior axillary wall. **Central lymph nodes**—fat of the axilla. **Apical (terminal) lymph nodes**—posterior and superior to pectoralis minor, towards the axillary vein.

3.4 SPINE AND SPINAL CORD

3.4.A Vertebra

The spinal cord lies inside the spinal column, which is made up of 33 bones called vertebrae (7 cervical, 12 thoracic, 5 lumbar). Five vertebrae are fused together to form the sacrum (part of the pelvis), and four small vertebrae are fused together to form the coccyx. There are 31 pairs of spinal nerves. Cervical nerves: 8 pairs exit the cervical cord at each vertebral level. The first cervical root exits above the C1 vertebra. The second cervical root exits between the C1–C2 segment and the 3rd to 7th roots exit above the correspondingly numbered vertebra. The eighth cervical nerve root C8 exits between the C7 and T1 vertebra. Thoracic nerves: 12 pairs noted and they exit below the correspondingly numbered vertebra. T1 roots exit between T1 and T2 vertebra. Lumbar nerves: 5 pairs are there and they exit below the correspondingly numbered vertebra (Figs 3.4.1 and 3.4.2). One pair of coccygeal nerves is present. The spinal cord begins at the medulla oblongata and ends in the lumbar region at the level of L1–L2 as it tapers to form a cone called the conus medullaris.

Spinal nerves: Each spinal nerve is connected to the spinal cord by posterior and anterior roots. The posterior root contains the processes of sensory neurons carrying information to the CNS. The cell bodies of the sensory neurons are clustered in a spinal ganglion at the distal end of the posterior root in the intervertebral foramen. The anterior root contains motor nerve fibers, which carry signals away from the CNS. The cell bodies of the primary motor neurons are located in anterior regions of the spinal cord. Medially, the posterior and anterior roots divide into rootlets which are attached to the spinal cord.

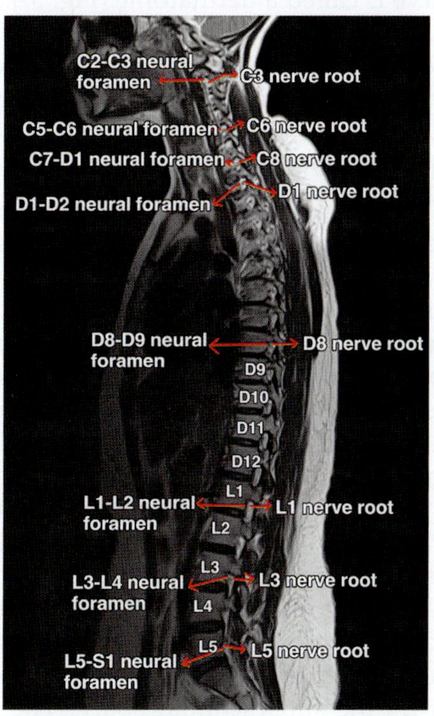

Fig. 3.4.1: MRI vertebra sagittal image

A spinal segment is the area of the spinal cord giving rise to the posterior and anterior rootlets, which will form a single pair of spinal nerves. Laterally, the posterior and anterior roots on each side join to form a spinal nerve. As it emerges from an intervertebral foramen spinal nerve divides into two major branches posterior ramus and anterior ramus. There are two enlargements in spinal cord for brachial and lumbosacral plexus respectively for upper and lower limbs.

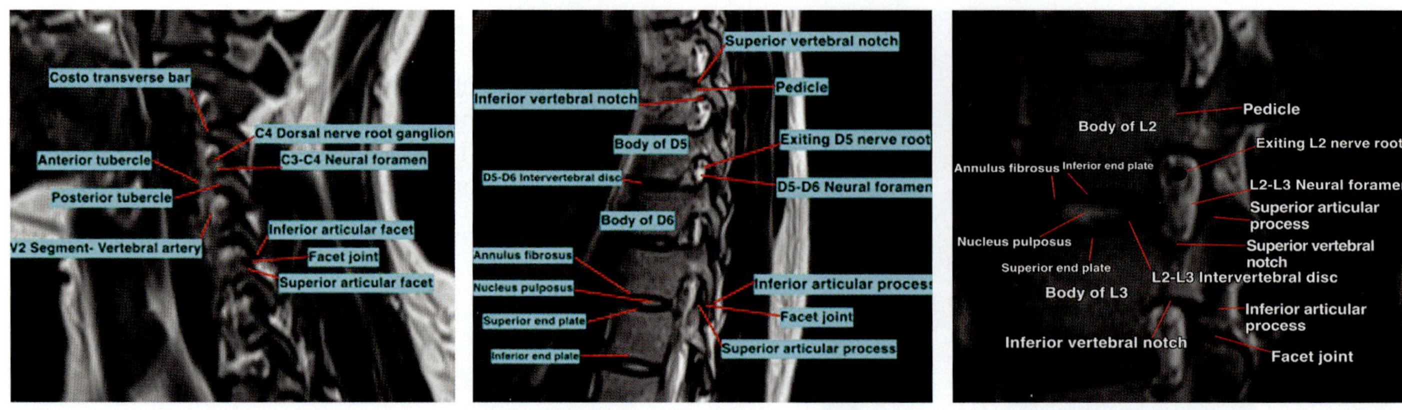

Fig. 3.4.2: MRI cervical, dorsal and lumbar spine

3.4.B Dermatomes

The sensory spinal and cranial nerves have characteristic but often overlapping peripheral distributions. A particular area that is supplied by a particular spinal or cranial nerve is called a dermatome (Fig. 3.4.3). Area of the skin supplied by a branch of a spinal or cranial nerve is called peripheral nerve fields. There is marked overlap between the dermatomes of the adjacent spinal nerves.

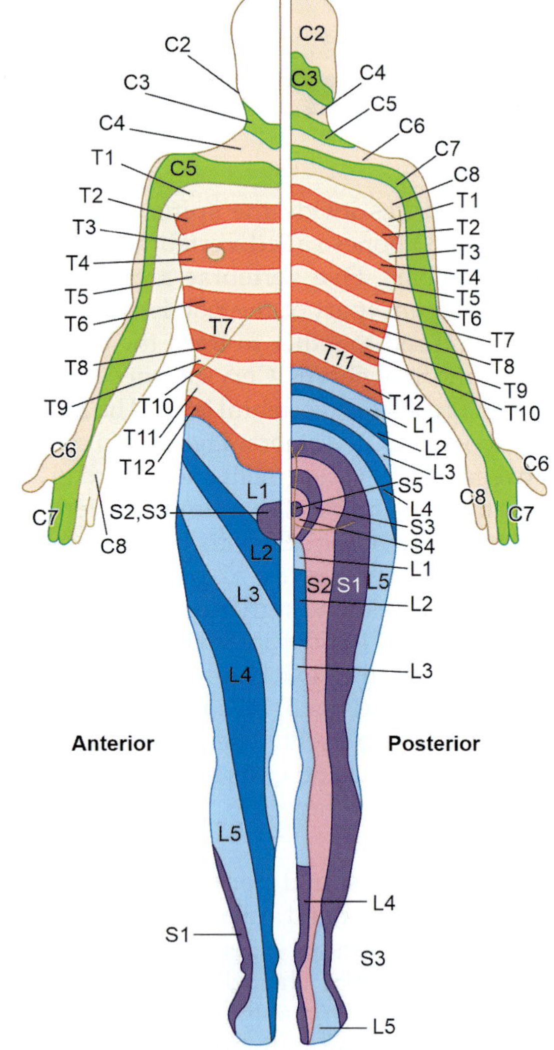

Fig. 3.4.3: Dermatomes

3.4.C Spinal Meninges

The **dura mater** is the outermost meningeal membrane and is separated from the bones forming the vertebral canal by an extradural space. Superiorly, it is continuous with the inner meningeal layer of cranial dura mater at the foramen magnum. Inferiorly, the dural sac narrows at the level of the lower border of vertebra S2 and forms an investing sheath for the pial part of the filum terminale of the spinal cord. This terminal cord-like extension of dura mater attaches to the posterior surface of the vertebral bodies of the coccyx. As spinal nerves and their roots pass laterally, they are surrounded by tubular sleeves of dura mater, which merge with and become part of the outer covering of the nerves. The **arachnoid mater** is a thin delicate membrane against, but not adherent to, the deep surface of the dura. It is separated from the pia mater by the subarachnoid space. The arachnoid mater ends at the level of vertebra S2. The **subarachnoid space** contains CSF. The subarachnoid space around the spinal cord is continuous at the foramen magnum with the subarachnoid space surrounding the brain. The subarachnoid space extends further inferiorly than the spinal cord. The spinal cord ends at approximately the disc between vertebrae L1 and L2, whereas the subarachnoid space extends to approximately the lower border of vertebra S2. Arachnoid trabeculae are continuous with the arachnoid mater on one side and the pia mater on the other side and they span the subarachnoid space and interconnect the two adjacent membranes. **The spinal pia mater** is a vascular membrane that firmly adheres to the surface of the spinal cord. It extends into the anterior median fissure and reflects as sleeve like coatings onto

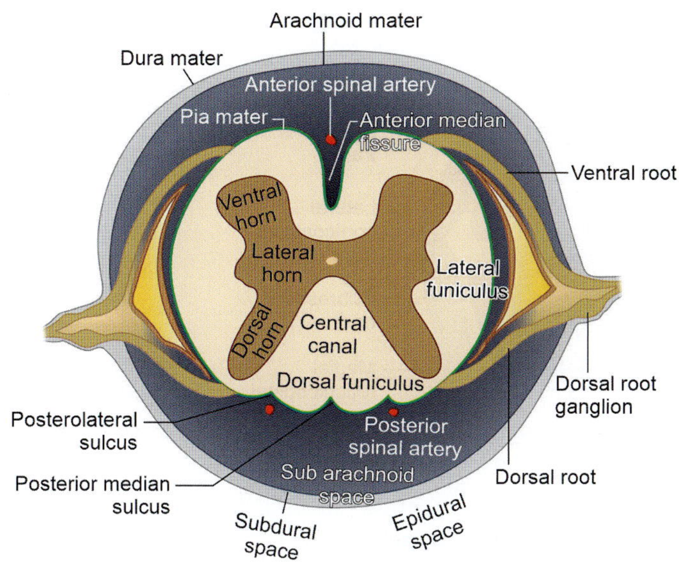

Fig. 3.4.4: Spinal canal

posterior and anterior rootlets and roots as they cross the subarachnoid space. As the roots exit the space, the sleeve-like coatings reflect onto the arachnoid mater. On each side of the spinal cord, a longitudinally oriented sheet of pia mater extends laterally from the cord toward the arachnoid and dura mater known as the denticulate ligament. Medially denticulate ligament is attached to the spinal cord in a plane that lies between the origins of the posterior and anterior rootlets. Laterally each denticulate ligament forms a series of triangular extensions along its free border, with the apex of each extension being anchored through the arachnoid mater to the dura mater.

Arrangement of structures in the vertebral canal: The vertebral canal is bounded anteriorly by the bodies of the vertebrae, intervertebral discs, and posterior longitudinal ligament. Laterally, on each side by the pedicles and intervertebral foramina and posteriorly by the laminae and ligamenta flava, and in the median plane the roots of the interspinous ligaments and vertebral spinous processes. Between the walls of the vertebral canal and the dural sac is an extradural space containing a vertebral plexus of veins embedded in fatty connective tissue.

3.4.D Internal Structure

Spinal cord on a transverse section shows butterfly shaped or H-shaped central gray matter and peripheral white matter. The grey matter houses a CSF containing central canal. The anterior median fissure and posterior median sulcus divides the spinal cord into two equal halves on right and left (Figs 3.4.4 and 3.4.5).

Gray matter: It contains all the cell bodies of neurons and glia and is especially enlarged in the cervical and lumbar regions to provide fibers to large nerve plexuses.

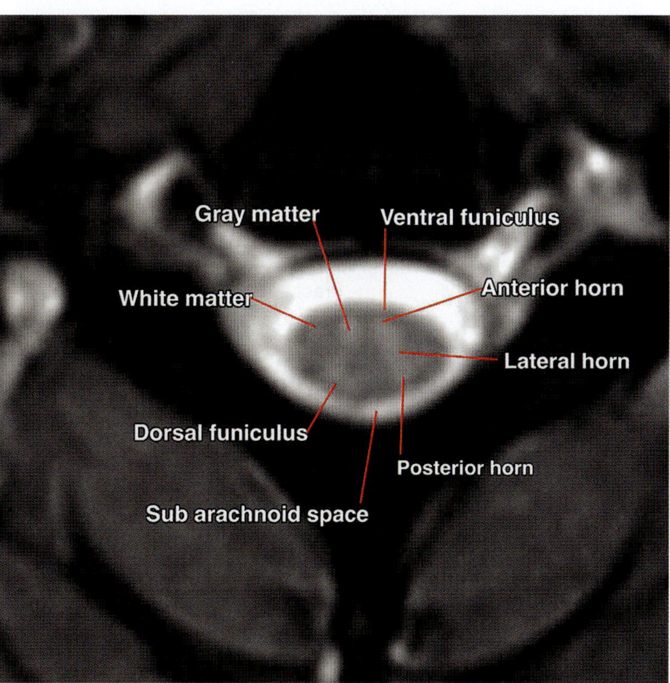

Fig. 3.4.5: MRI T2 axial image-spinal cord

The gray matter of the spinal cord can be classified in different ways as: 1. Four columns concept, 2. six different nuclei concept, and 3. as ten laminae concept by Rexed.

Four columns of the spinal gray matter: Spinal gray matter has four different columns. a. Dorsal horn: Also known as posterior horn. It contains neurons that receive somatosensory afferent fibers carrying information from peripheral sensory organs to brain via ascending pathways. b. Ventral horn: Also known as anterior horn. It contains motor neurons that give efferent to skeletal muscles. c. Intermediate and lateral horns: These contain neurons that send autonomic fibers to viscera and pelvic organs. Lateral horns are seen only in the thoracic region.

Six nuclei group of the spinal gray matter: a. Marginal zone/posterior marginalis (MZ), b. Substantia gelatinosa (SG), c. Nucleus proprius (NP), d. Dorsal nucleus of Clarke (DNC), e. Intermediolateral nucleus (IMN), f. Lateral and medial motor neurons (MN).

White matter: White matter contains tracts and is divided into anterior, dorsal and lateral columns/funiculi as well as anterior spinal commissure. Anterior column: Contains spinothalamic tracts. Posterior/Dorsal column: Vibration, proprioception and fine touch sensation. Lateral column: Contains corticospinal tract (Fig. 3.4.6).

Anterior spinal commissure: Located between the posteriormost extent of the anterior median fissure. Ascending tracts in the spinal cord white matter: These ascending tracts can carry both conscious and unconscious information to the brain.

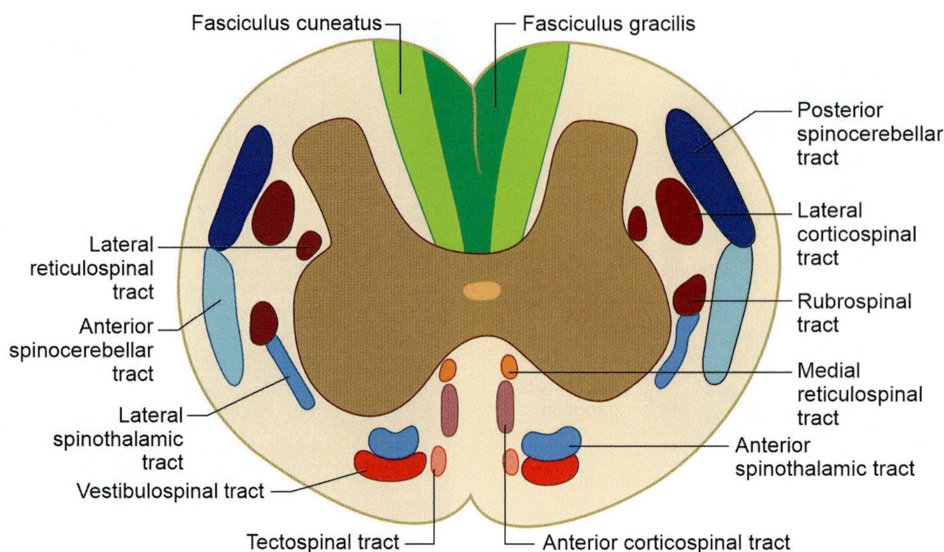

Fig. 3.4.6: Spinal cord internal structures

Conscious information tracts—dorsal column—medial lemniscus pathways and anterolateral pathway. Unconscious information tracts—spinocerebellar tracts, play a very important role in coordination and fine control of movements.

Dorsal column—medial lemniscus pathway: Carries fine touch, vibration and proprioception to brain. The dorsal column exists in the spinal cord and medial lemniscus exists in the brainstem where decussation of tracts occurs. The first order neurons carry information from peripheral nerves to medulla. Second order crosses as it ascends up towards thalamus and third order from thalamus to brain. Signals from upper limbs (above T6) are carried in fasciculus cuneatus which lies laterally and from the lower limbs (below T6) in fasciculus gracilis. Anterolateral pathway: It comprises anterior spinothalamic and lateral spinothalamic tract. The anterior one carries crude touch and pressure and lateral one carries pain and temperature sensations.

Spinocerebellar tracts: Carries unconscious sensation to coordinate and fine tune motor movements. There are four individual pathways within it, namely: a. Posterior spinocerebellar tract: Proprioception from lower limbs to ipsilateral cerebellum. b. Cuneocerebellar tract: Proprioception from upper limbs to ipsilateral cerebellum. c. Anterior spinocerebellar tract: Proprioception from lower limbs and decussate twice to terminate in ipsilateral cerebellum. d. Rostral spinocerebellar tract: Proprioception from upper limbs to ipsilateral cerebellum.

Descending tracts in the spinal cord white matter: The descending tracts also known as efferent or motor tracts are divided into two main groups: a. Pyramidal tracts: Originates in the cerebral cortex and terminates in brainstem and spinal cord. b. *Extrapyramidal tracts:* Originates in brainstem and carry motor impulses to the spinal cord.

Pyramidal tract: Responsible for voluntary control of muscles of face and body. It includes corticobulbar and corticospinal tracts. For the spine we are concerned with corticospinal tract as corticobulbar tracts do not extend till spinal cord and terminates on to various brain stem nuclei. Corticospinal tract divides in the lower part of medulla into two parts: a. Lateral corticospinal tract: It carries decussated/crossed fibers from the contralateral side of cerebral cortex. b. Anterior corticospinal tract: It carries remaining uncrossed ipsilateral fibers from the cerebral cortex which decussate down in the spinal cord.

Extrapyramidal tracts: These tracts originate in brainstem and carry fibers to the spinal cord. They basically control involuntary and automatic control of all muscles. There are four types of extrapyramidal tracts: a. Vestibulospinal tract: Do not decussate and supplies ipsilaterally. b. Reticulospinal tract: Do not decussate and supplies ipsilaterally. c. Rubrospinal tract: Decussates and provide contralateral innervation. d. Tectospinal tract: Decussates and provide contralateral innervation.

3.4.E Craniovertebral Junction

The craniovertebral junction is formed by the occipital condyles, atlas (C1), axis (C2) vertebrae, and their articulations. These structures are approximated at two major joints, the atlanto-occipital and atlanto-axial joints (Figs 3.4.7–3.4.10). The first cervical vertebra (C1), also known as the atlas, is the only vertebra that does not have a body and is not associated with an intervertebral disc. It is a ring-shaped vertebra with bilateral paired lateral masses joined by an anterior and a posterior arch. The dorsal aspect of the anterior arch has an articular surface for the odontoid process of the second cervical vertebra (C2), forming the atlanto-axial joint. Lateral margins of the odontoid process are equidistant from the medial margins of the lateral masses of atlas. The lateral masses have superior and inferior articular facets that articulate superiorly with the occipital condyles and inferiorly with C2, forming the atlanto-occipital and atlanto-axial joints respectively. The superior aspect of the posterior arch just behind the lateral masses of C1 contains a groove that allows passage of the vertebral artery before it enters the foramen magnum. C2 vertebra has a body with odontoid process which articulates with articular facet present in the posterior surface of the anterior arch of the atlas in the midline by a pivot joint. The lateral masses have paired superior articular processes that articulate with the inferior articular facets of the lateral masses of the atlas and inferior articular processes that articulate with the superior articular processes of the third cervical vertebra (C3). The axis has a bifid spinous process.

Bone marrow appearance in MRI depends on the relative proportion of red and yellow marrow in a bone. Red marrow has more cellular element and less fat so it appears hypointense to subcutaneous fat but hyperintense to intervertebral disc and muscle on T1W MRI. Yellow marrow has higher fat content so it has signal intensity comparable to subcutaneous fat and higher than intervertebral disc and muscle on T1. On T2 sequence yellow marrow is slightly hypointense to subcutaneous fat and hyperintense to the disc and muscle. On T2 sequence red marrow is hypointense than yellow marrow appearance on T2 sequence. In children bone marrow is mostly red marrow hence, it is hypointense to subcutaneous fat and hyperintense to disc and muscle on T1 sequence. In adults except the axial and proximal appendicular skeleton all the marrow is converted into yellow marrow hence, it appears isointense to subcutaneous fat and hyperintense to disc and muscle on T1 sequence. On T2 sequence adult marrow is slightly hypointense to subcutaneous fat and hyperintense to the disc and muscle.

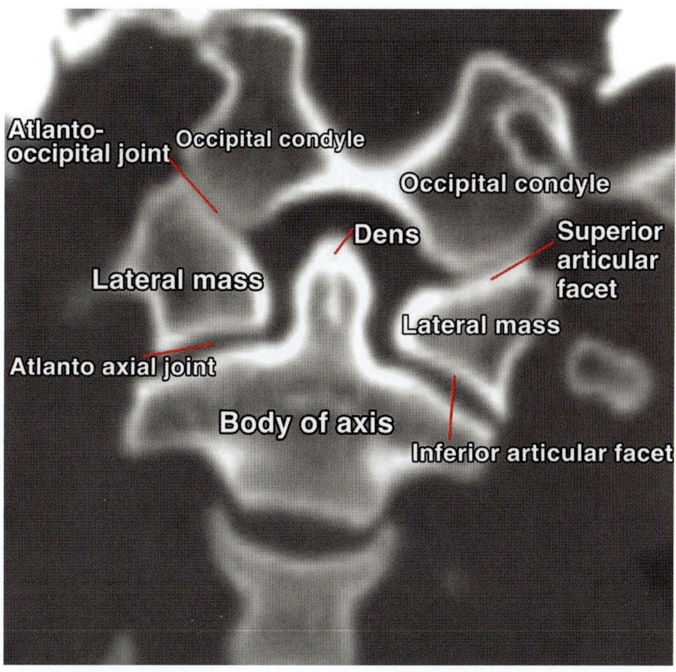

Fig. 3.4.8: Atlanto-occipital and atlanto axial joint

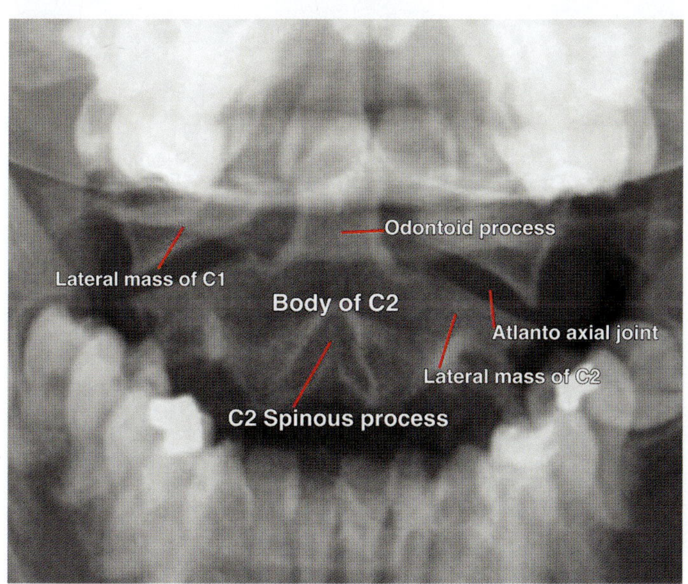

Fig. 3.4.7: X-ray: C2 vertebra

Joints: **Atlanto-occipital joints** are synovial joints formed by convex articular surfaces of the occipital condyles superiorly and concave articular surfaces of superior articular processes of the atlas vertebra inferiorly.

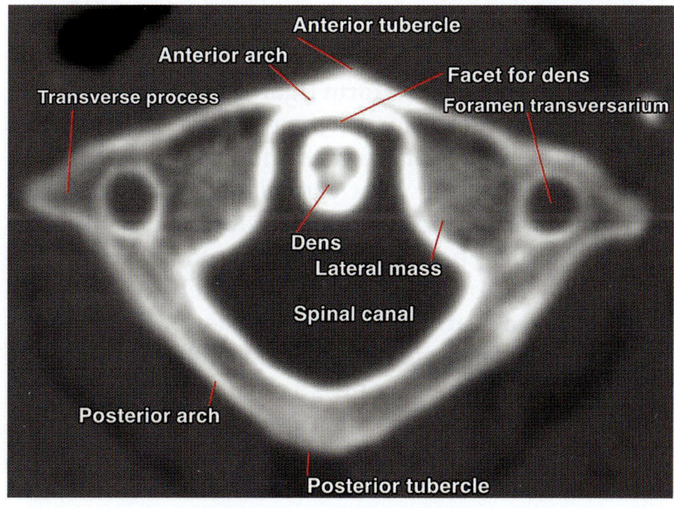

Fig. 3.4.9: Atlas vertebra

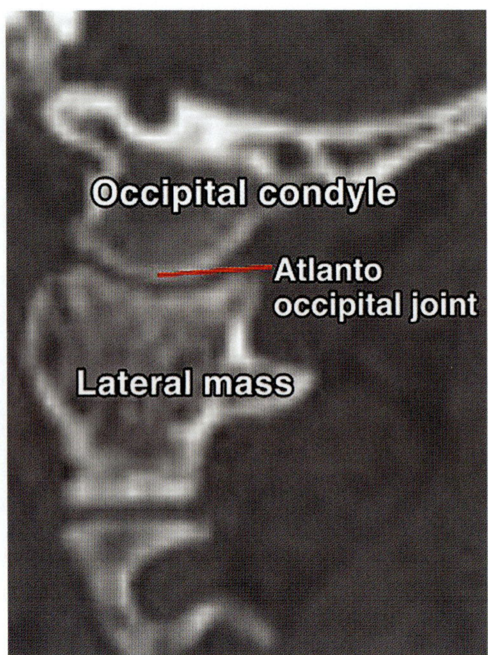

Fig. 3.4.10: Sagittal section of CV junction showing atlanto-occipital joint

On coronal sections joint extends superolaterally and inferomedially. Primary movements of the joint include flexion and extension.

Atlanto-axial joint: It has a four parts including pivot joint between the anterior surface of dens and posterior surface of anterior arch of atlas, posterior surface of dens and transverse band of cruciate ligament, superior articular process of the axis and inferior articular process of the atlas. Primary movement includes axial rotation.

Ligaments: A complex of ligaments stabilizes the atlanto-occipital and atlantoaxial joints (Figs 3.4.11–3.4.13). **Apical ligament** extends from the tip of the odontoid process and is attached with the clivus. **Alar ligament** extends from the superolateral margins of the of odontoid process and is attached with the medial margins of the occipital condyles. **Cruciform ligament** has three bands. Transverse band extends between the medial tubercles of the lateral masses of the atlas and lies posterior to the anterior atlanto-axial joint capsule and stabilizes this joint. Ascending band is attached with the dorsal clivus and descending band has attachment with posterior surface of the body of the axis vertebra. **Tectorial membrane** is a continuation of the posterior longitudinal ligament and has attachment with the clivus. **Posterior occipito-atlantal membrane** is a membranous sheet that is attached on the posterior margin of foramen magnum and superior margin of posterior arch of the atlas vertebra. **Posterior atlanto-axial membrane** is attached with the inferior margin of posterior arch of the atlas vertebra and superior margin of posterior arch of the axis vertebra. **Anterior occipito-atlantal membrane** is a continuation of anterior longitudinal ligament and has attachments with anterior arch of the atlas and clivus.

Meninges and spaces: Triangular and longitudinally oriented ligaments extending from the pia mater along the lateral aspects of the spinal cord and attaching to the thecal sac laterally are known as denticulate ligaments. They run between the ventral and dorsal spinal nerve roots. First denticulate ligaments originate at

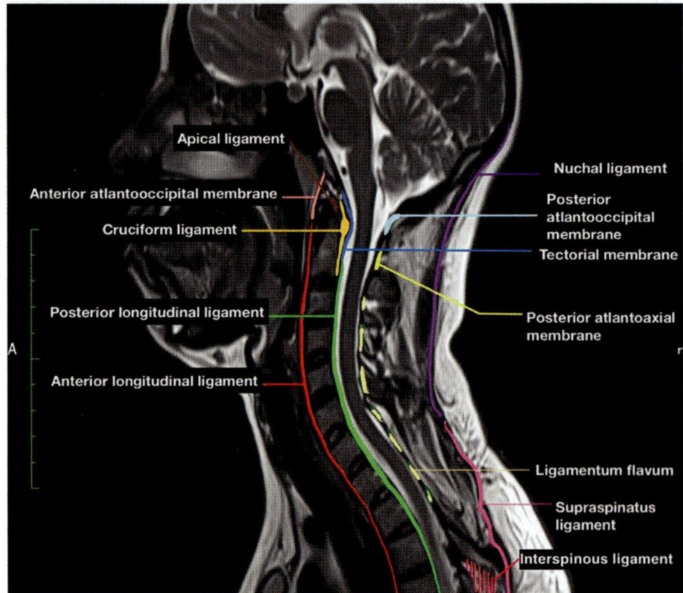

Fig. 3.4.11: MRI cervical spine—ligaments

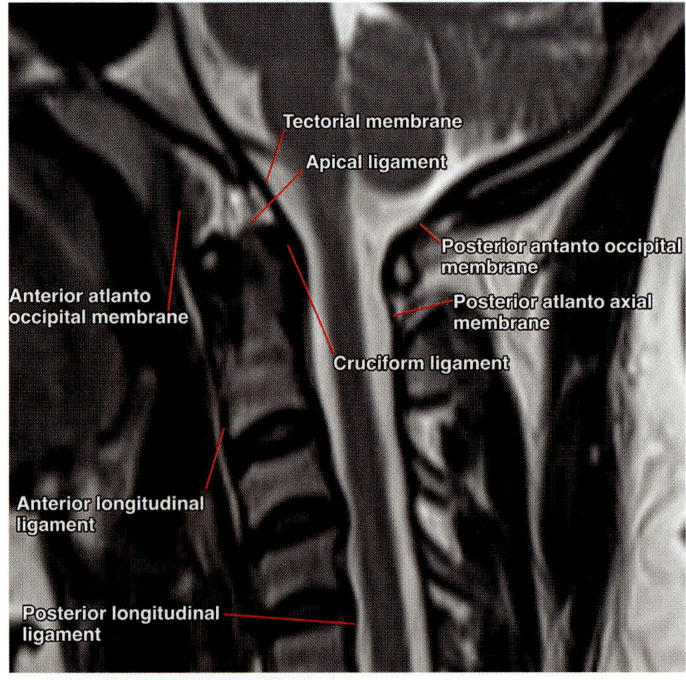

Fig. 3.4.12: MRI cervical spine—ligaments

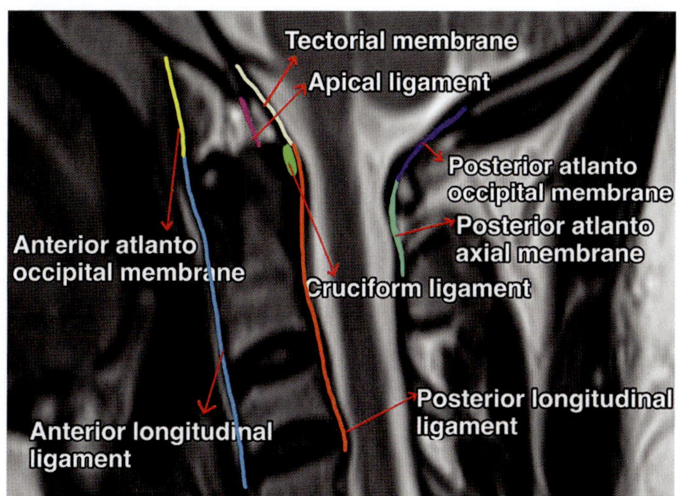

Fig. 3.4.13: MRI cervical spine—ligaments

cervicomedullary junction and attach to the dura mater. Spinal cord occupies approximately half of the spinal canal at cranio-cervical junction and three-quarters of the spinal canal at subaxial level. This arrangement results in subarachnoid space that is wider at cranio-cervical junction than at the subaxial cervical level.

3.4.F Subaxial Cervical Spine

Cervical lordosis is primarily due to the configuration of cervical intervertebral discs because the anterior and posterior heights of the vertebral bodies differ little. From above downwards there is progressive increase in the anteroposterior length and transverse width of the endplates. Posterolateral part of the superior end plate has uncinate process which along with indentation of the inferior end plate of the superior segment forms the uncovertebral joint (Figs 3.4.14–3.4.16 and 3.4.18).

Just inferior to the uncinate process arises the pedicle. Transverse process has anteriorly costal process ending laterally as anterior tubercle and posterior bar ending laterally as posterior tubercle. Both tubercles are connected by costo-transverse bar which completes the foramen transversarium (Fig. 3.4.17). The foramen transversarium of C7 vertebra is more posteriorly placed as well as it is smaller than other subaxial vertebrae. Spinous processes are bifid except the spinous process of C7 vertebra which is monofid. Articular pillar lies at the junction of the pedicle and the lamina. Superior articular facet and inferior articular facets are located in the superior and inferior articular processes respectively. Superior articular facet is located dorsally on the superior articular process and inferior articular process is located ventrally on the inferior articular process. Subaxial cervical spinal canal is bounded anteriorly by posterior margin of vertebral body, laterally by medial margin of pedicles, posterolaterally by anterior margin of laminae, and posteriorly by anterior margin of spinous process. Subaxial cervical spinal canal takes the shape of a triangle or trefoil shape.

Cervical intervertebral disc's ventral height is greater than that of the dorsal height which is responsible for the

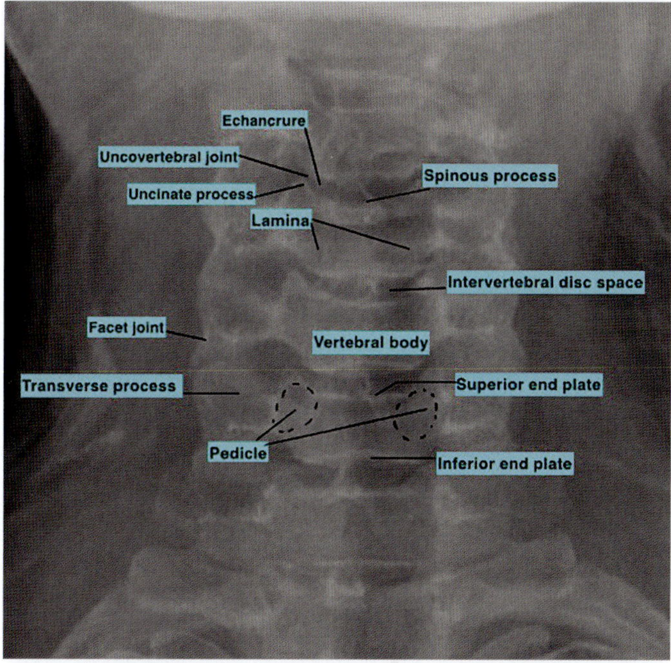

Fig. 3.4.14: X-ray cervical spine frontal view

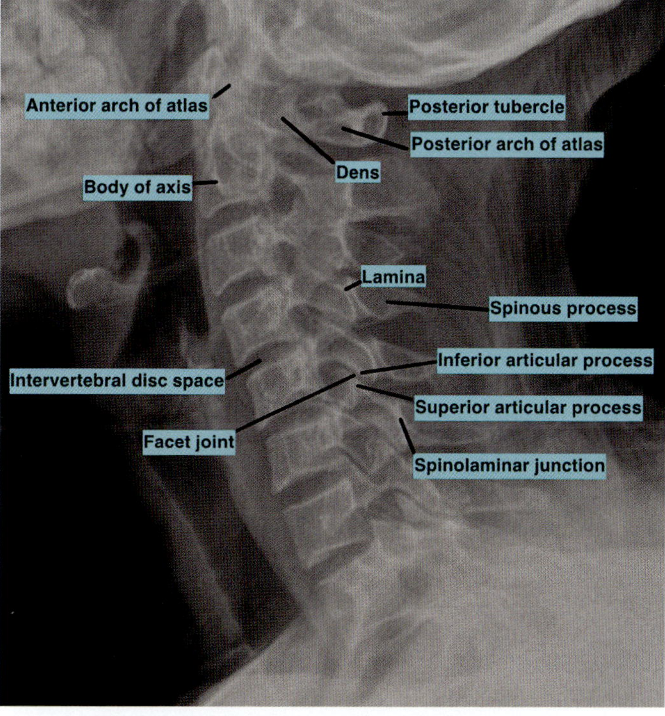

Fig. 3.4.15: X-ray cervical spine lateral view

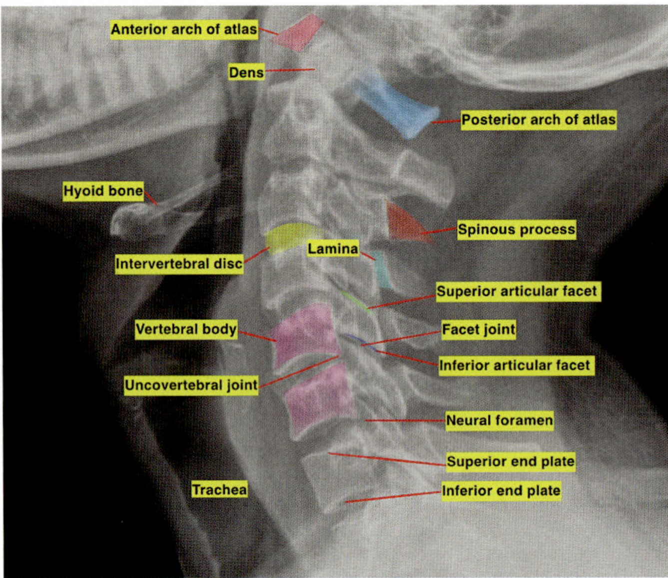

Fig. 3.4.16: X-ray cervical spine lateral view

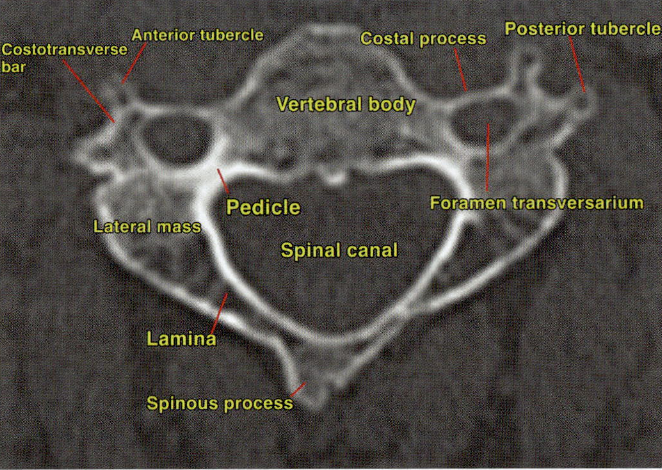

Fig. 3.4.17: CT cervical vertebra

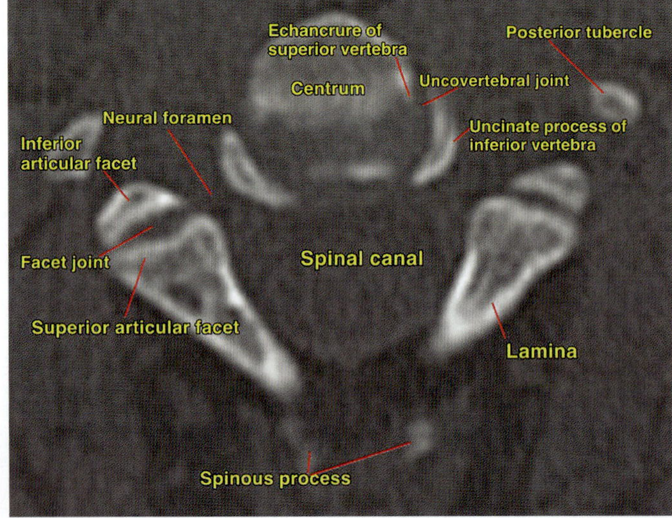

Fig. 3.4.18: CT cervical vertebra

cervical lordosis. Annulus fibrosus is thicker anteriorly than posteriorly. Nucleus pulposus has more collagen than the proteoglycans resulting in more uniform low T2 signal intensity.

Facet joints are formed by superior and inferior articular facet. In the initial subaxial cervical segments, superior articular facet faces posteromedially and inferior articular facet faces inferolaterally (Figs 3.4.20–3.4.22). The orientation of the facet joints is posteromedial in the initial subaxial cervical segments and posterolateral in C6 and C7 segments. Articular facets are lined by articular cartilage and covered by fibrous capsule lubricated by synovial fluid.

Uncovertebral or joints of Luschka are formed by uncinate process located posterolaterally on the superior end plate and echancrure, a shallow depression located posterolaterally on the inferior end plate. Cervical spine is unique in a way that, any uncovertebral osteophyte can cause compression of neural formaen directly. Neural foramina of cervical spine are narrow and nerve roots exit horizontally, hence even minor decrease in foraminal space can cause clinical symptoms at an early stage. **Anterior longitudinal ligament** is attached to anterior tubercle on the anterior arch of the atlas vertebra. It is attached firmly with the anterior margins of the end plates and variably attached with the central portions

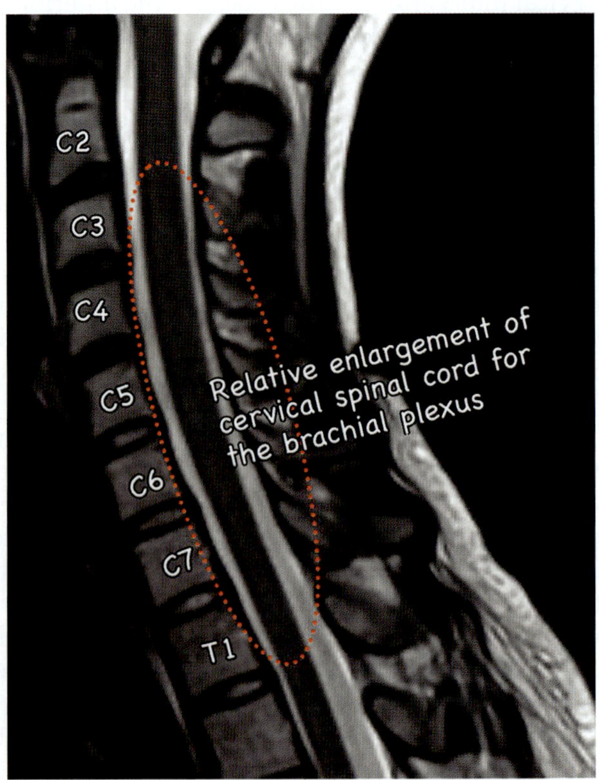

Fig. 3.4.19: MRI cervical spine

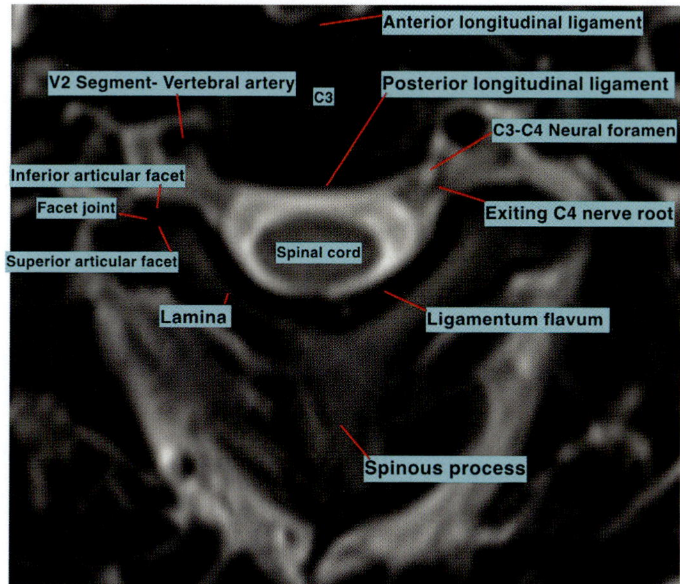

Fig. 3.4.20

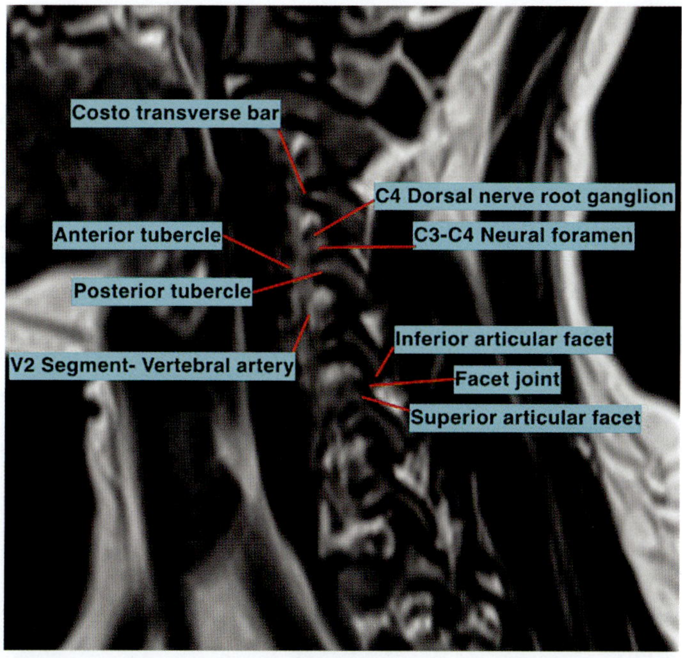

Fig. 3.4.21

of the vertebral body and disc. **Posterior longitudinal ligament** is attached with the body of axis vertebra. It has firm attachments with posterior portion of the annulus fibrosus. Supraspinous and inter transverse ligaments are less prominent in the cervical spine. **Ligamentum flavum** extends on either side of the midline located anterior to laminae and forms medial border of facet joint. **Interspinous ligament** extends from the inferior border of the spinous process to superior border of the spinous process.

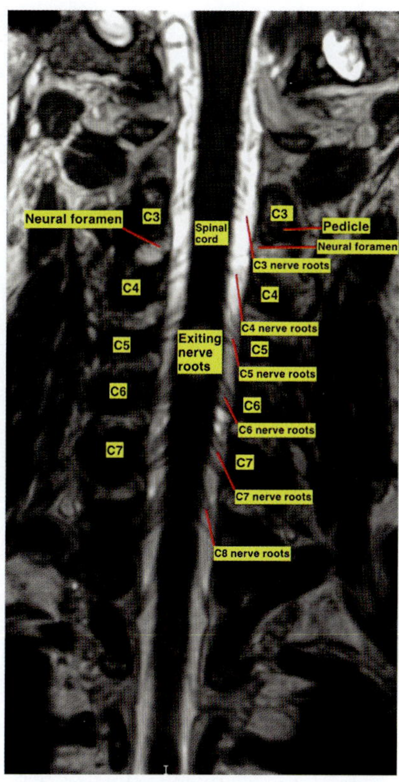

Fig. 3.4.22

3.4.G Dorsal Spine

Dorsal spine has twelve segments. T2–T8 segments have typical thoracic vertebrae. T1 has some cervical features like uncinate process. T9–T12 segments have lumbar transitional features. Thoracic vertebral bodies have wedge shaped configuration with ventral height lesser than dorsal height contributing to thoracic kyphosis (Figs 3.4.23 and 3.4.24). From above downwards transverse width of end plates increases with inferior end plate being wider than superior end plate. In axial plane thoracic bodies demonstrate dorsal concavity resulting in upside down heart configuration. Pedicles arise superiorly from the posterior surface of the vertebral body. Pedicles are broader and elongated than in cervical vertebrae. Typical thoracic vertebrae have deep inferior vertebral notch and shallow superior vertebral notch. Atypical thoracic vertebrae have deep superior vertebral notch. Transverse processes arise at the junction of pedicle and lamina and are oriented posterolaterally. Anterior margin of transverse process has facets for articulating with corresponding ribs known as costal facet. Superior articular processes arise at the junction of pedicle and lamina. Superior articular facet faces dorsally and superolaterally. Inferior articular processes arise from lamina. Inferior articular facets face ventrally and inferomedially. Laminae are thick dorsoventrally and elongated craniocaudally. Spinous processes are

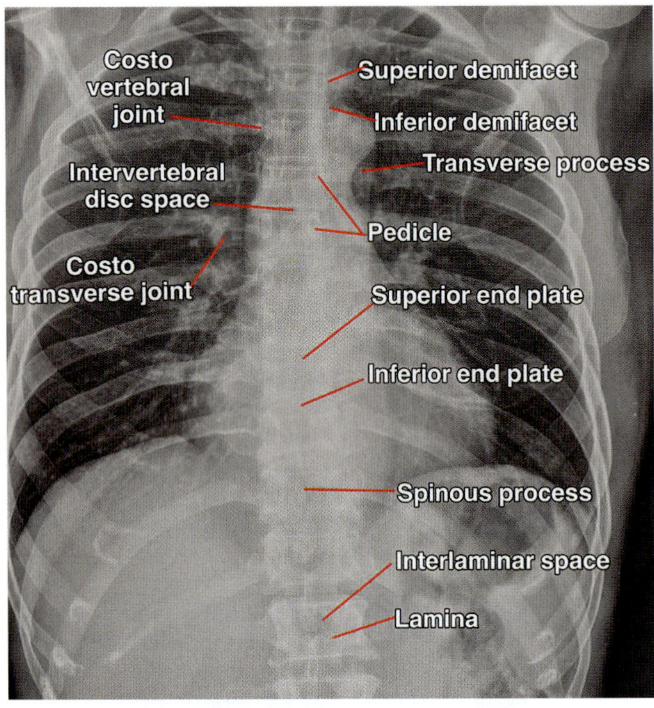

Fig. 3.4.23: Chest X-ray

elongated and rectangular in shape. T1–T4 spinous processes are horizontally oriented, T5–T8 are oriented inferiorly and T8–T12 are oriented horizontally.

Atypical features of atypical thoracic vertebrae include oval costal facet at T10, costal facet located on pedicle in T11, the presence of mamillary and accessory processes in T12.

Thoracic intervertebral discs have similar ventral and dorsal heights. So, thoracic kyphosis is primarily due to the configuration of vertebral bodies. Dorsal spinal canal is bounded anteriorly by posterior margin of vertebral body, laterally by medial margin of pedicles, posterolaterally by anterior margin of laminae, and posteriorly by anterior margin of spinous process. **Facet joints** are formed by the superior and inferior articular facets of the adjacent vertebrae (Figs 3.4.26 and 3.4.28). Articular surfaces are lined by articular cartilages and covered by capsule lined by synovial membrane. Superior articular facet is directed dorsally and superolaterally. Inferior articular facet is directed ventrally and inferomedially. Thoracic facet joints are oriented coronally which transforms into posterolateral orientation at T12. **Costovertebral joints** are synovial joints between the ribs and vertebral bodies (Fig. 3.4.25). Articular facets on the rib heads are convex and they articulate with two costal demifacets located on the superior end plate of the corresponding segment and inferior end plate of the segment lying above. Intra-articular ligament extends between the inter-articular

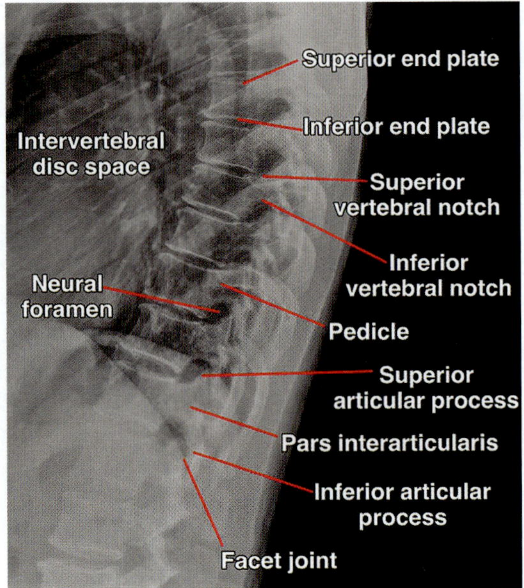

Fig. 3.4.24: Chest X-ray lateral view

crest located between two articular facets on the ribs and adjacent intervertebral disc.

Costotransverse joints are joints between the tubercles facing posteriorly on the ribs and facet facing anteriorly on the anterior margins of the transverse processes. These are planar type of synovial joints (Fig. 3.4.25).

Anterior longitudinal ligament has firm attachments with superior and inferior end plates, sparse attachments with central portion of the vertebral bodies and intervertebral discs. It is thick in the regions of vertebral body and thin in the regions of intervertebral discs. **Posterior longitudinal ligament** has firm attachments

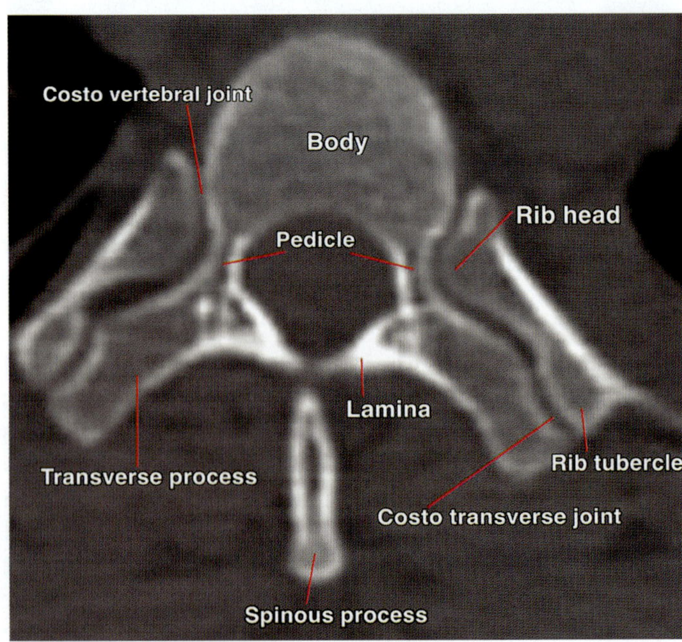

Fig. 3.4.25: CT dorsal spine

3

with intervertebral discs and loose attachments with vertebral bodies. It is wider at intervertebral disc regions and narrower at vertebral body regions resulting in denticulate configuration. It has superficial and deep layers with superficial layer lying posteriorly and wider than the deep layer. Both layers are attached firmly at the midline.

Ligamentum flavum is thicker than seen in the cervical segments and thinner than seen in the lumbar segments (Figs 3.4.29–3.4.31).

Supraspinous ligament has attachments with posterior margins of the spinous processes of adjacent vertebrae. It is formed by combination of tendinous and fascial attachments being formed by the trapezius,

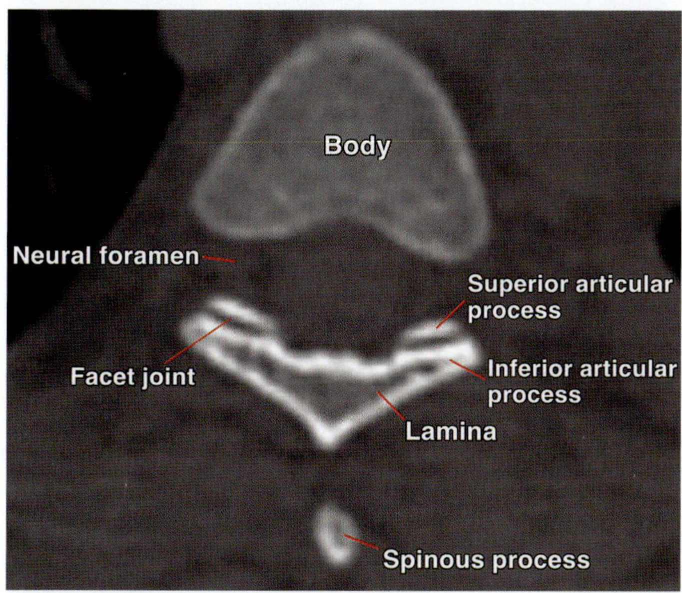

Fig. 3.4.26

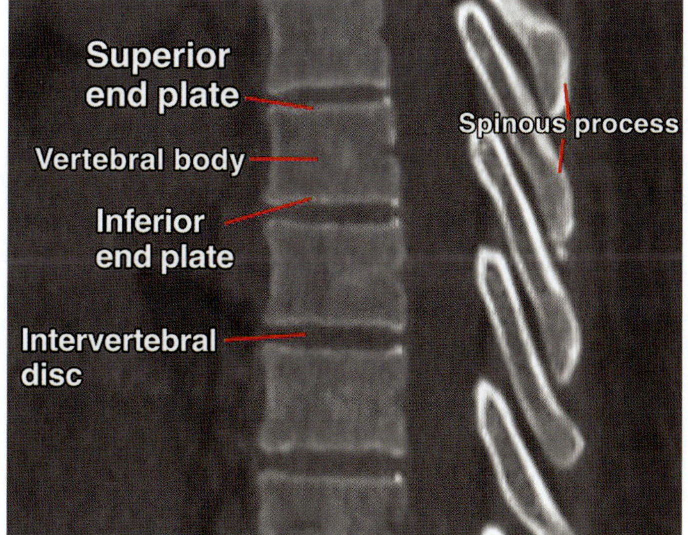

Fig. 3.4.27

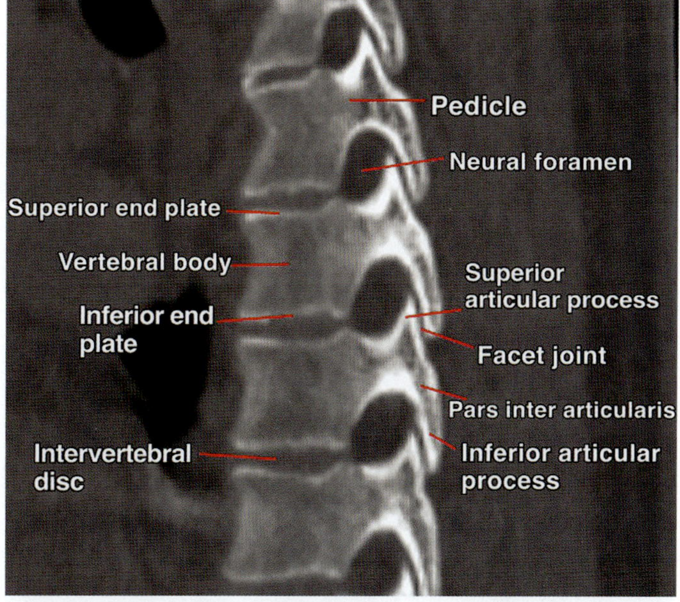

Fig. 3.4.28

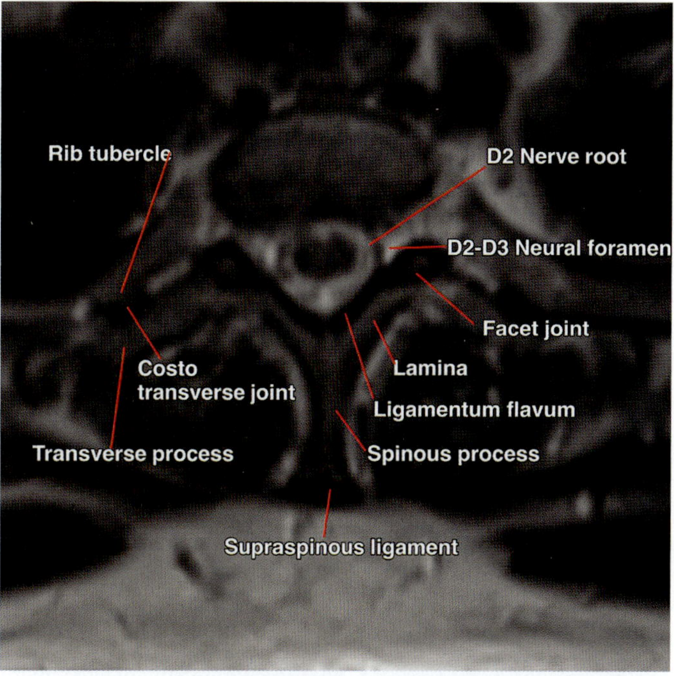

Fig. 3.4.29: MRI dorsal spine

rhomboideus major, splenius cervices and deep fasciae. In the lower thoracic segments it is formed by thoracolumbar fascia and aponeurosis of the trapezius muscle. **Interspinous ligament** is attached with the superior and inferior margins of the adjacent vertebrae. Other ligaments include intra-articular ligament, capsular ligament strengthening costovertebral joints and costotransverse ligament, anterior and lateral costovertebral ligaments strengthening costotransverse joints.

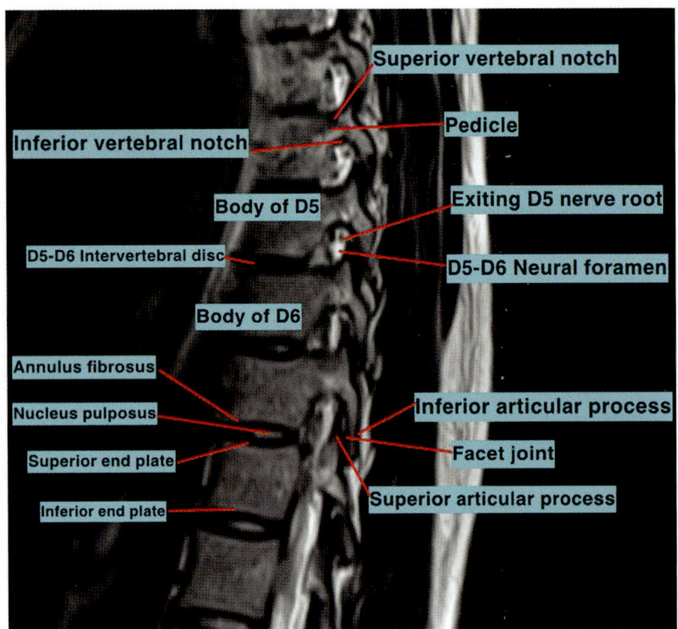

Fig. 3.4.30

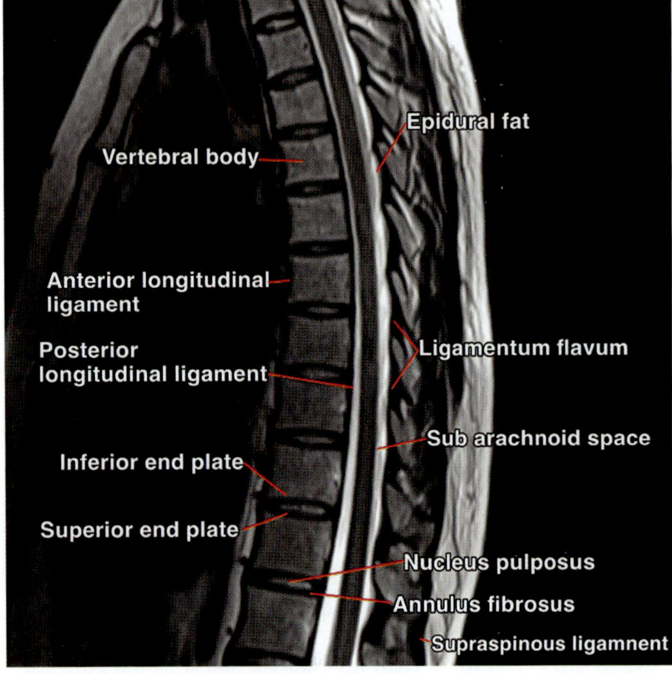

Fig. 3.4.31

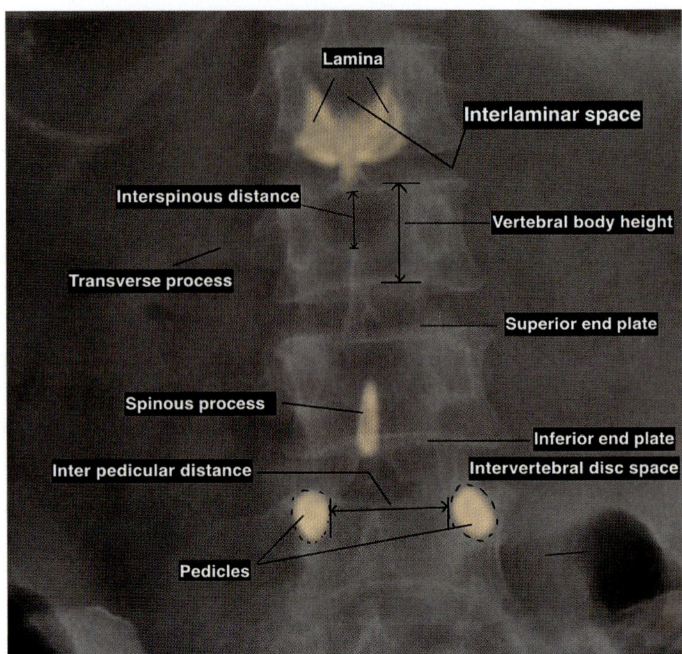

Fig. 3.4.32: X-ray lumbar spine frontal view

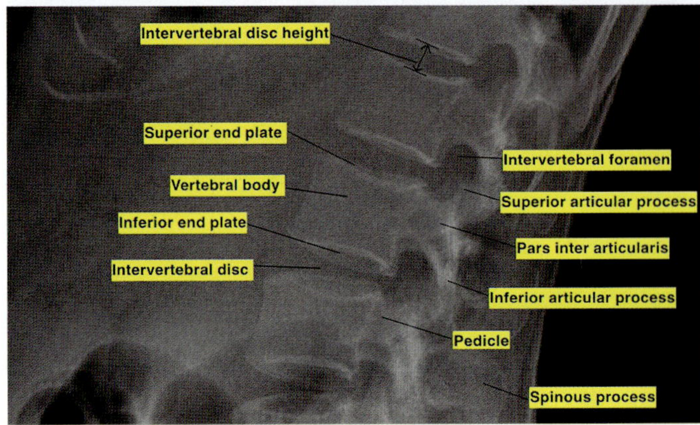

Fig. 3.4.33: X-ray lumbar spine lateral view

3.4.H Lumbar Spine

Lumbar lordosis is due to the configurations of vertebral bodies and intervertebral discs (Figs 3.4.32 and 3.4.33). Ventral height of the lumbar vertebral body is greater than that of the dorsal height. Lumbar intervertebral discs are thicker anteriorly than posteriorly. L1–L4 vertebral bodies have dorsal concavity, whereas L5 vertebral body has dorsal convexity. Lumbar pedicles originate more inferiorly than thoracic pedicles leaving space for shallow superior vertebral notch. Inferior vertebral notch is deep. They are shorter than the thoracic pedicles. Transverse processes are oriented in coronal plane. They arise at the junction of pedicle and lamina anterior to the articular process. There is a process arising from transverse process at its junction with lamina called accessory process which projects posteroinferiorly. Longissimus thoracis and intertransversarii lumborum muscles are attached with the accessory processes.

Laminae of the lumbar spine are thick and broad and are vertically oriented. Superior margins have upward concavity, whereas inferior margins have downward concavity resulting in round to ovoid interlaminar spaces.

Segment of the bone lying between the superior and inferior articular processes is known as pars

3

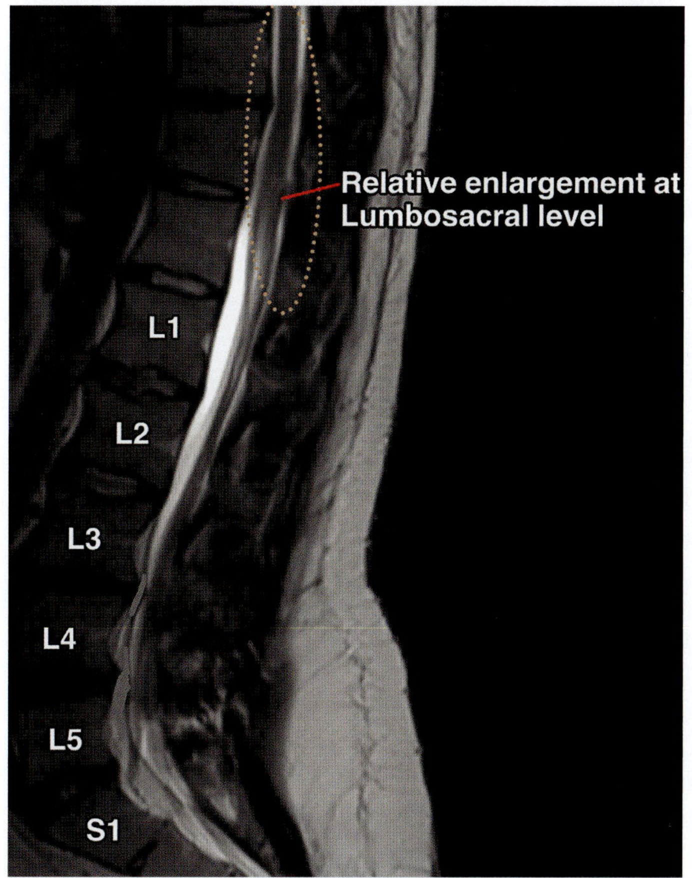

Fig. 3.4.34: Conus-bulbous terminal portion contributing to lumbosacral plexus

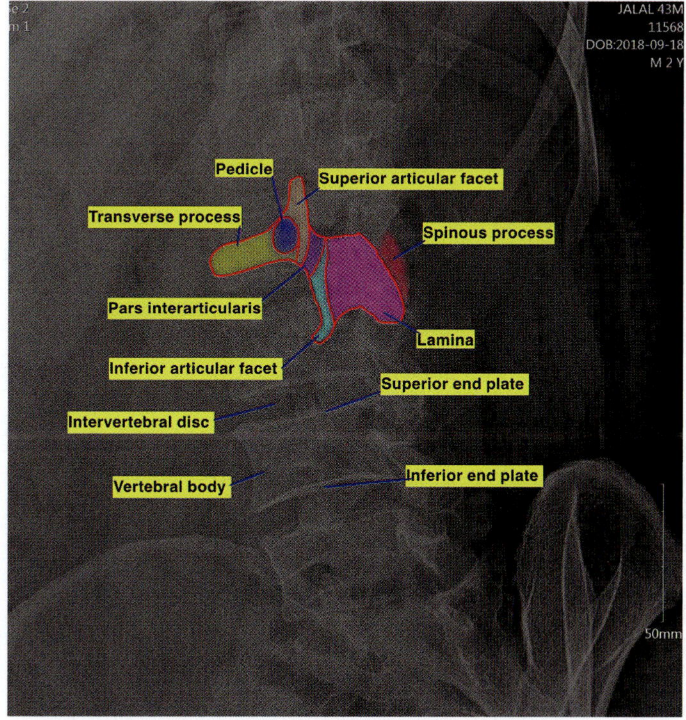

Fig. 3.4.35: X-ray lumbar spine, oblique view

interarticularis which forms the neck of the scottie dog on oblique lateral X-ray of lumbar spine.

Superior articular process is oriented vertically and superior articular facet faces posteromedially. Inferior articular process is oriented vertically and inferior articular facet faces inferolaterally. Bony projection arising from the superior articular process and projecting posteriorly is the mamillary process to which multifidi lumborum muscle is attached. Spinous processes are flat and broad with a rectangular shape and horizontal orientation except L5 spinous process which is oriented inferiorly. Lumbar spinal canal is bounded anteriorly by posterior margin of vertebral body, laterally by medial margin of pedicles, posterorolaterally by anterior margin of laminae, and posteriorly by anterior margin of spinous process (Figs 3.4.36–3.4.40). Upper lumbar spinal canal is round to ovoid in shape, lower lumbar

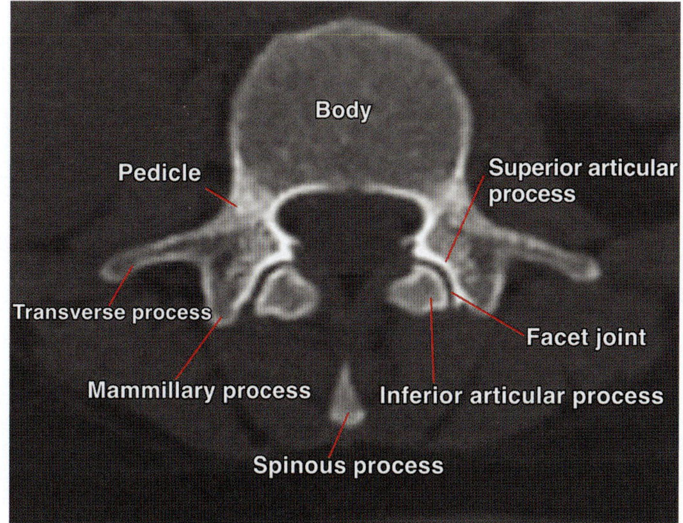

Fig. 3.4.36: CT lumbar spine

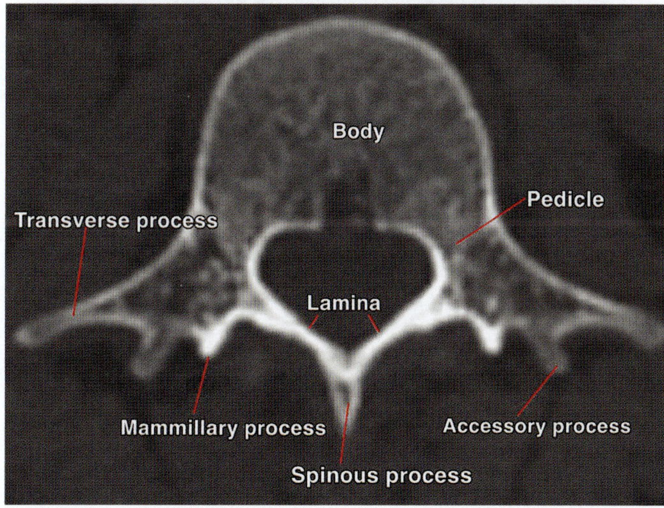

Fig. 3.4.37: CT lumbar spine

3

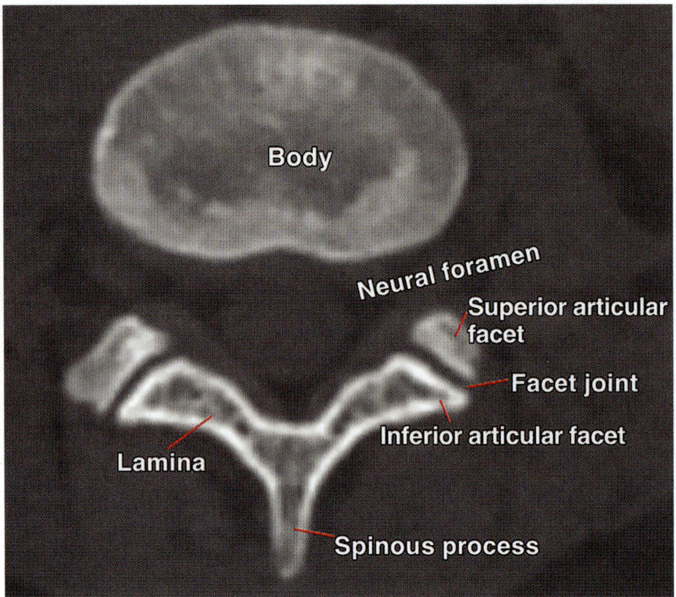

Fig. 3.4.38: CT lumbar spine

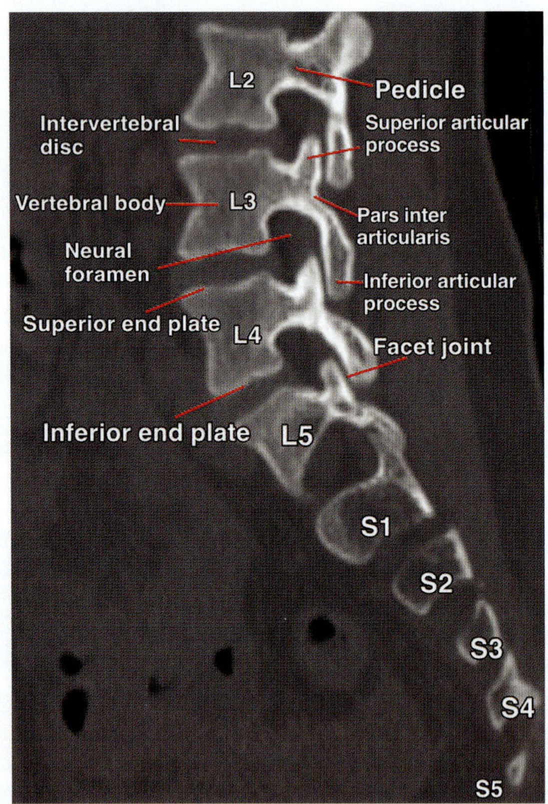

Fig. 3.4.39: CT lumbar spine

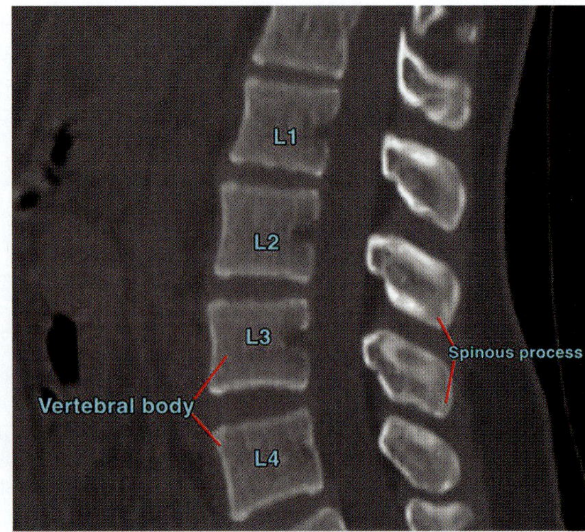

Fig. 3.4.40: CT lumbar spine

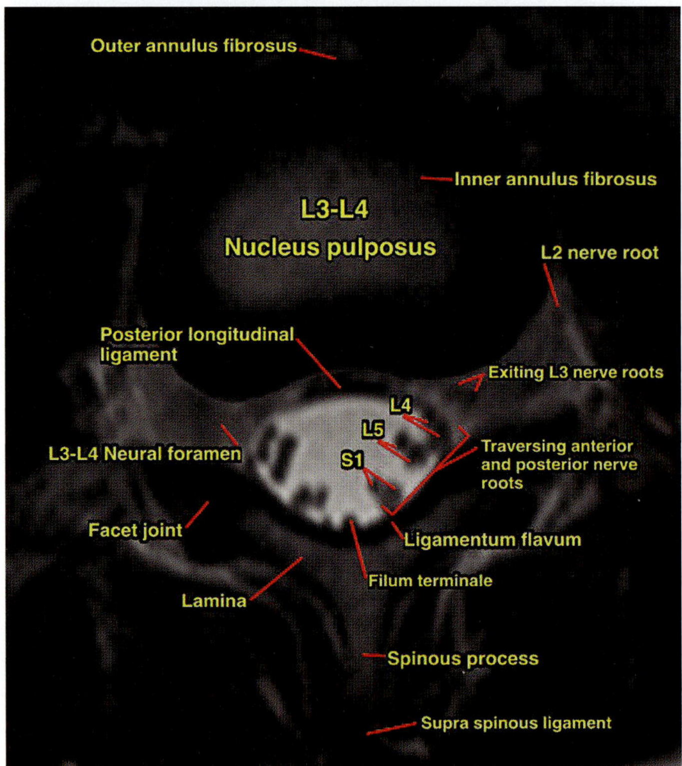

Fig. 3.4.41: MRI lumbar spine

spinal canal is triangle or trefoil in shape. Disc protrusion results in abnormality on sagittal myelograms, whereas ligamentum flavum hypertrophy results in abnormal coronal myelograms (Figs 3.4.46–3.4.47 and 3.4.49).

Intervertebral disc: Lumbar discs and vertebral bodies are responsible for lumbar lordosis. Lumbar intervertebral discs are taller anteriorly than posteriorly. In children the nucleus pulposus and inner annulus fibrosus appear bright on T2 weighted MRI and outer annulus fibrosus appears black on T2 weighted MRI (Fig. 3.4.41). High T2 signal of nucleus pulposus is related to the high proteoglycan and water content. As the age advances, proteoglycans are replaced by collagen fibres and there is decrease in water content resulting in loss of T2 signal intensity ending in black appearing nucleus pulposus indistinguishable from annulus fibrosus.

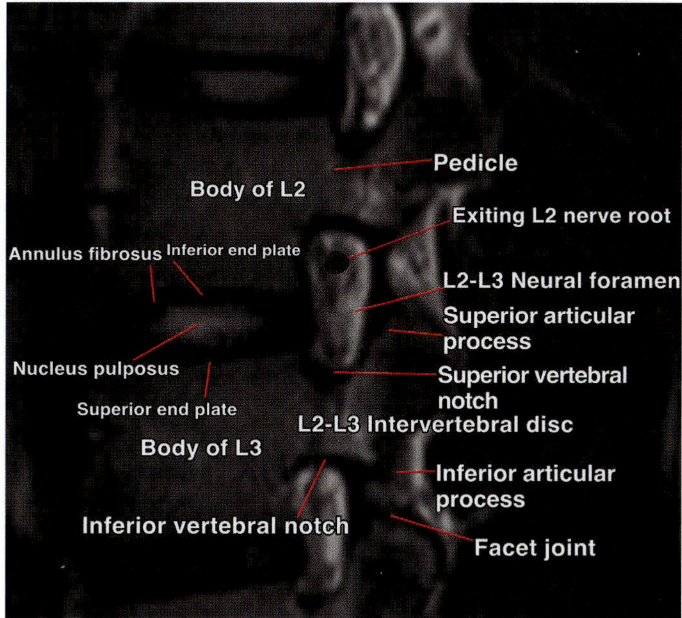

Fig. 3.4.42

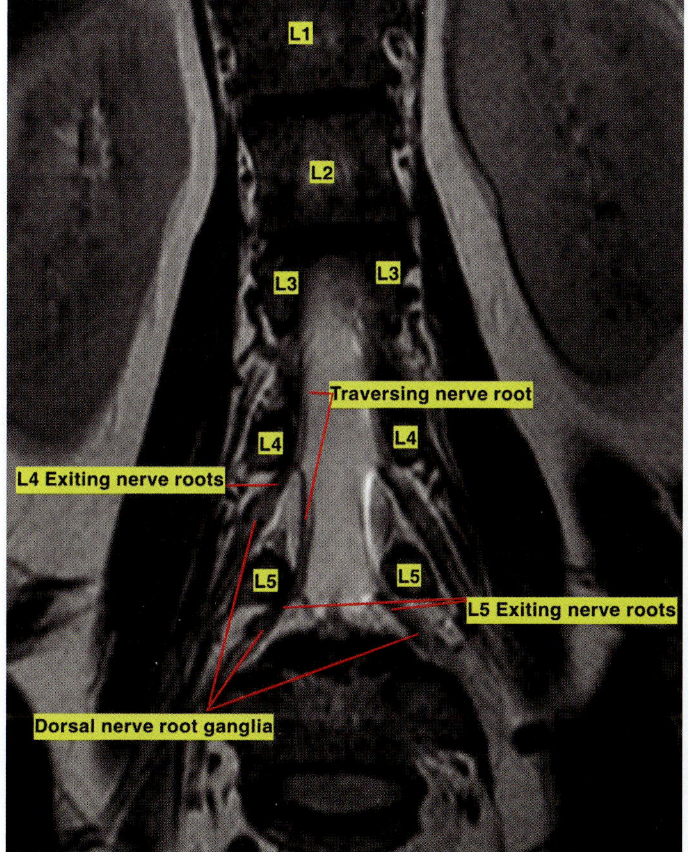

Fig. 3.4.43

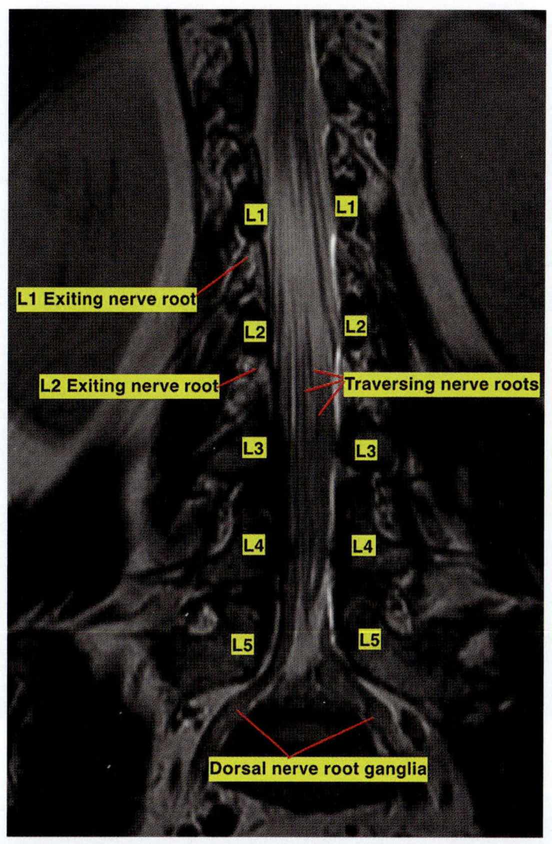

Fig. 3.4.44

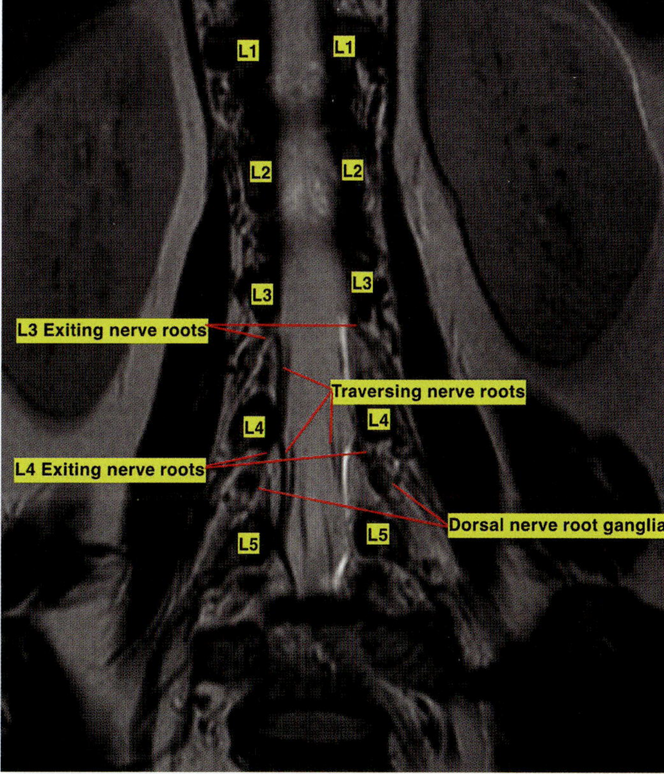

Fig. 3.4.45

Joints: Facet joint is formed between superior and inferior articular facets located on superior and inferior articular processes respectively (Fig. 3.4.35). Superior articular

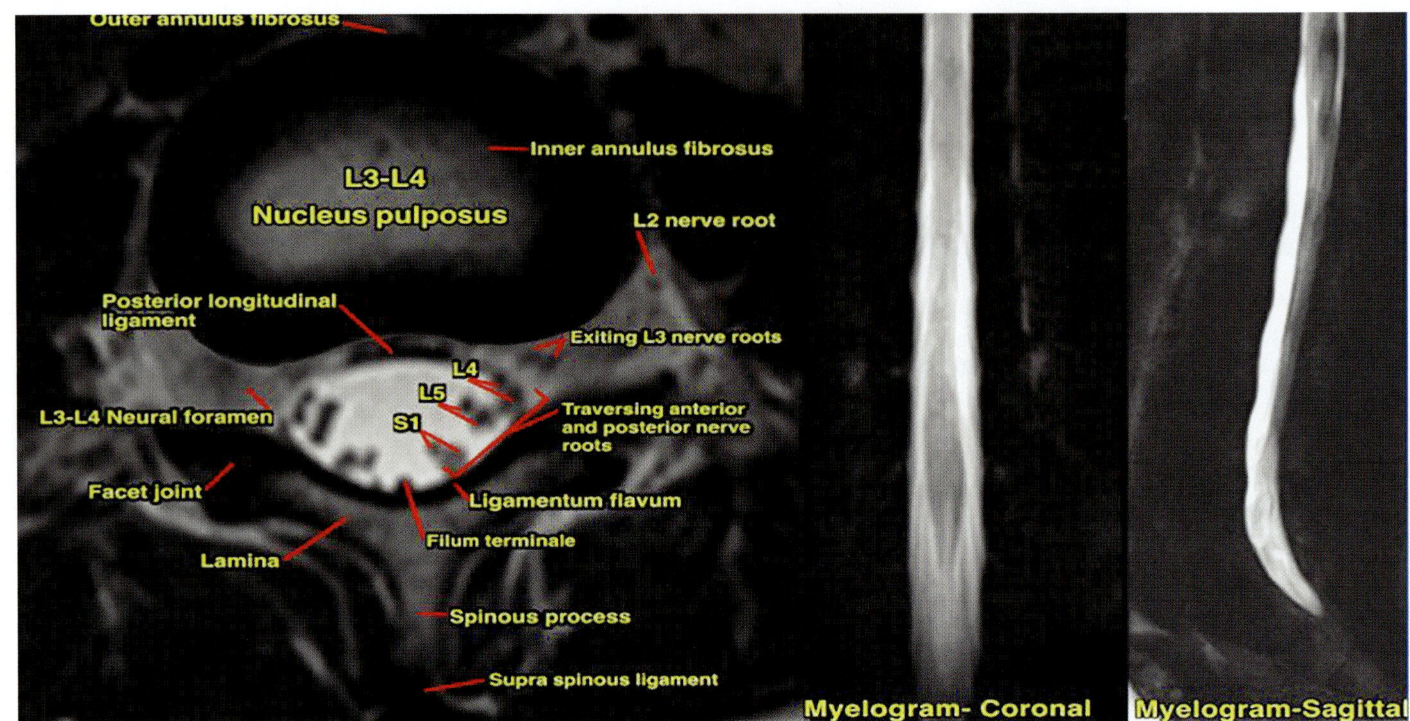

Fig. 3.4.46

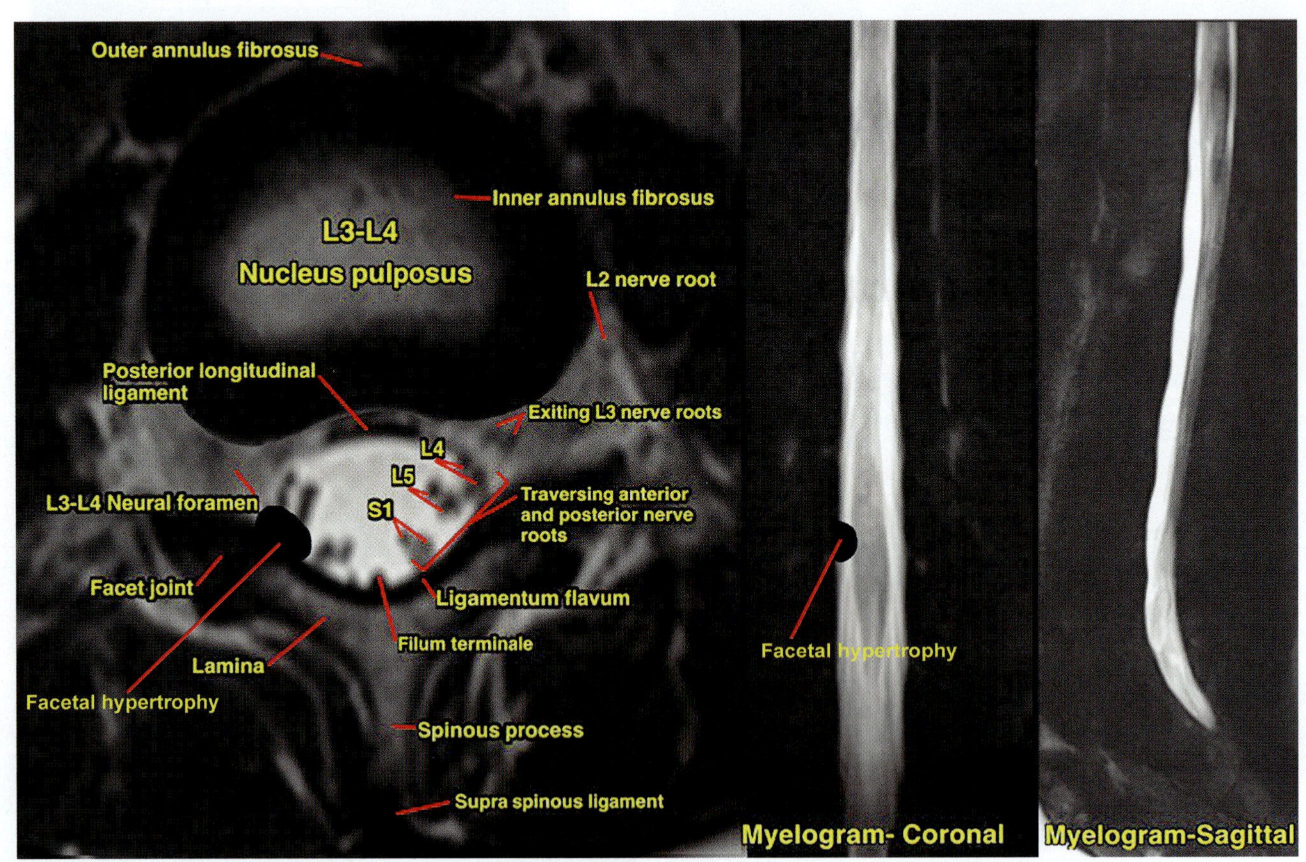

Fig. 3.4.47

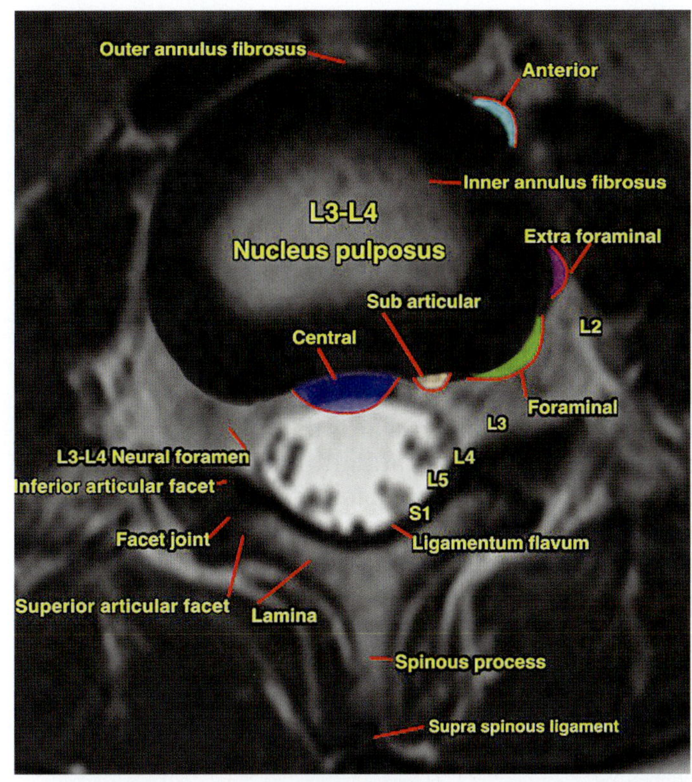

Fig. 3.4.48

facet is oriented dorsally and posteromedially. Inferior articular facet is oriented ventrally and anterolaterally. Articular surfaces are lined by articular cartilages. Facet joints are covered by fibrous capsule lined by synovial membrane. Facet joints are oriented posterolaterally.

Ligaments: In lumbar region **anterior longitudinal ligament** has firm attachments with superior and inferior end plates, sparse attachments with central portion of the vertebral bodies and intervertebral discs. It is thick in the regions of vertebral body and thin in the regions of intervertebral discs. Unique feature of ALL in lumbar region is being wider at intervertebral disc level and narrower at vertebral body level.

Posterior longitudinal ligament has firm attachments with intervertebral discs and loose attachments with vertebral bodies. It is wider at intervertebral disc regions and narrower at vertebral body regions resulting in a denticulate configuration. **Ligamentum flavum** is thickest in the lumbar segments. Medial part of ligamentum flava is thicker than the lateral part. Ligamentum flava are fused at the midline with some discontinuities at the midline to allow passage of veins communicating posterior internal and external vertebral venous plexus. **Interspinous ligament** extends between

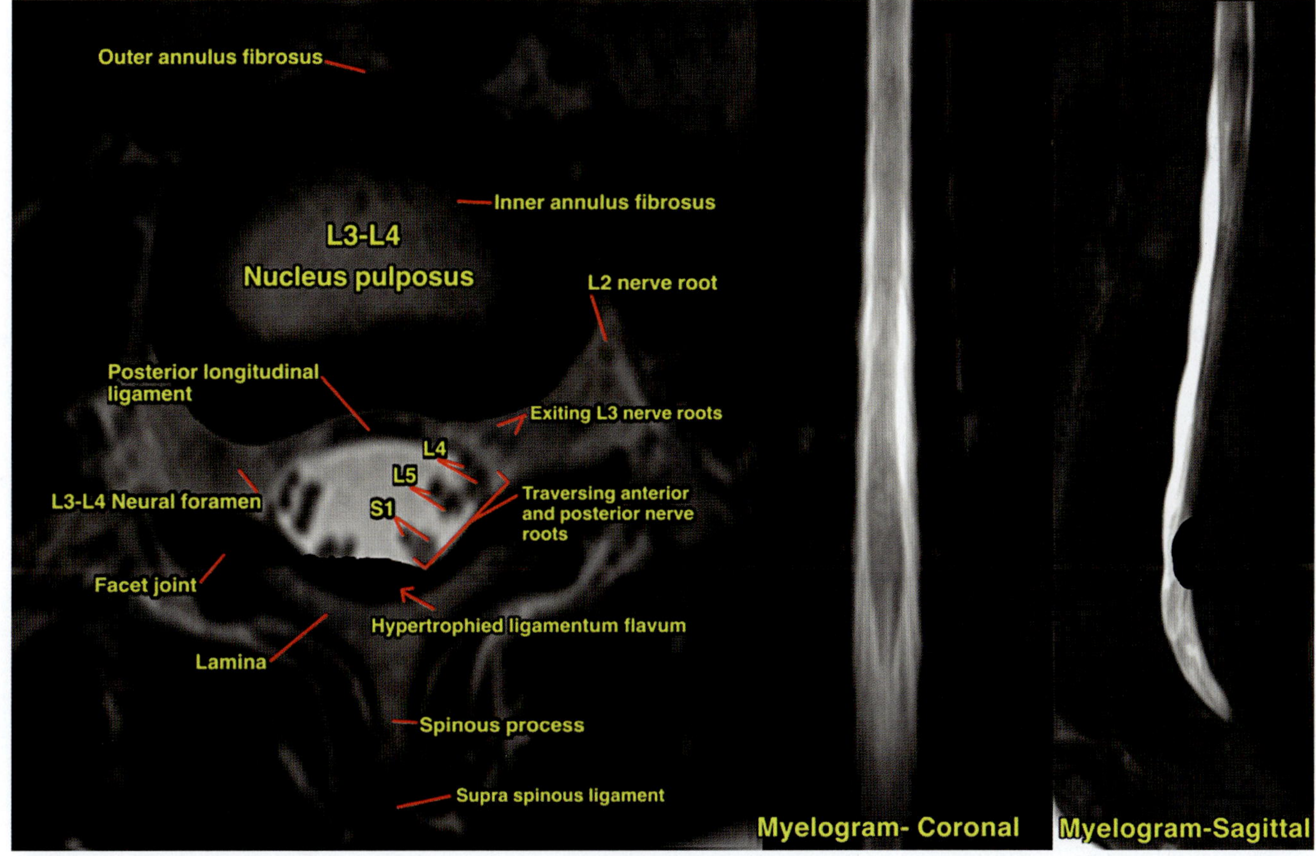

Fig. 3.4.49

the superior and inferior margins of spinous process of the adjacent vertebrae. It has three parts. Anterior part is fused anteriorly with ligamenta flava. Middle part arises from anterior superior margin of spinous process below and attached to posterior inferior margin of the spinous process above. Posterior part arises from posterior superior margin of spinous process below and is attached above to the supraspinous ligament. **Supraspinous ligament** of the lumbar segments extends till L4 vertebra and rarely extends caudal to L4 vertebra. **Iliolumbar ligament** extends from L5 transverse processes to the sacrum and iliac crests. Denticulate ligament is present till above the level of the conus medullaris and is absent at cauda equina. Lumbar intertransverse ligaments are less prominent.

Lumbosacral transitional anatomy: Lumbosacral transitional vertebrae are common in general population. Most common type is sacralization of L5 vertebra. If the first sacral segment shows lumbar features, then it is known as lumbarization. Castellvi lumbosacral transitional vertebra classification divides lumbosacral transitional vertebrae into four types. Type I is dysplastic transverse process with triangular shape and measuring at least 19 mm in width. Type II is elongated transverse process forming diarthrodial joint with sacral ala. Type III is bony fusion of transverse process with sacral ala. Type IV is combination of type II and III. 'a' or 'b' suffixes are added to indicate unilaterality and bilaterality respectively.

Lateral recess and intervertebral foramen: Lateral recess is bounded medially by the thecal sac, laterally by the medial margin of the pedicle, anteriorly by the posterolateral part of the vertebral body, posteriorly by the anterior margin of the superior articular process (Figs 3.4.41–3.4.45). Height of the lateral recess is measured from the anterior margin of the superior articular process to the posterior margin of the vertebral body. From above downwards there is slight progressive decrease in the craniocaudal dimension of the neural foramen. All lumbar neural foramens are keyhole shaped except L5–S1 neural foramen which is shaped like an egg placed upside down. Upper part of the keyhole is rounded and immobile. Superior component of the neural foramen is bounded anteriorly by the posterior margin of vertebral body posteriorly by the anterior margin of the inferior articular process, superiorly by the inferior margin of pedicle. Inferior component is bounded anteriorly by posterior margin of intervertebral disc, posteriorly by the anterior margin of superior articular process. The presence of disc tissue extending

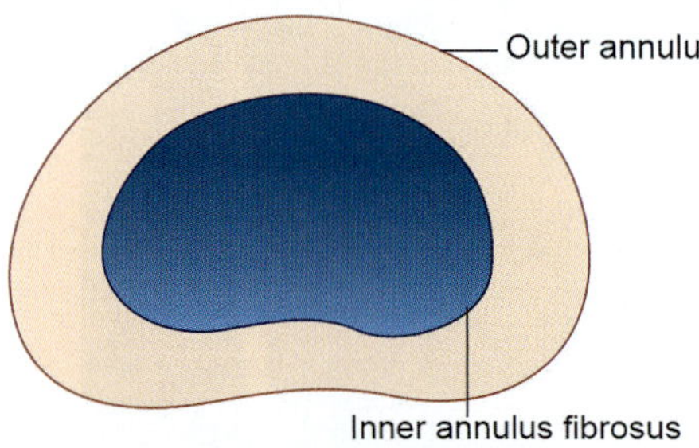

Fig. 3.4.50: Diffuse disc bulge

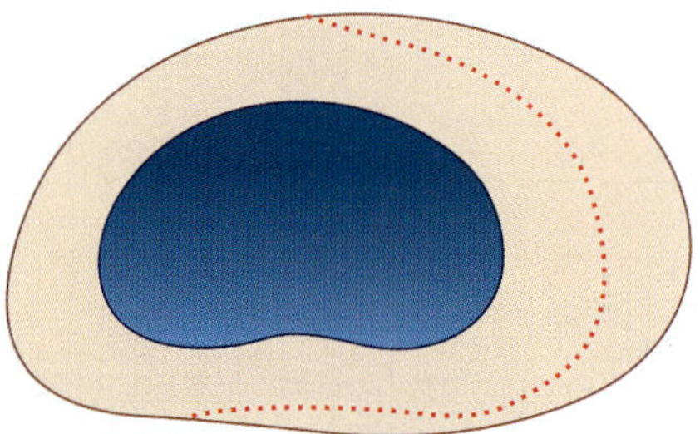
Fig. 3.4.51: Asymmetric disc bulge

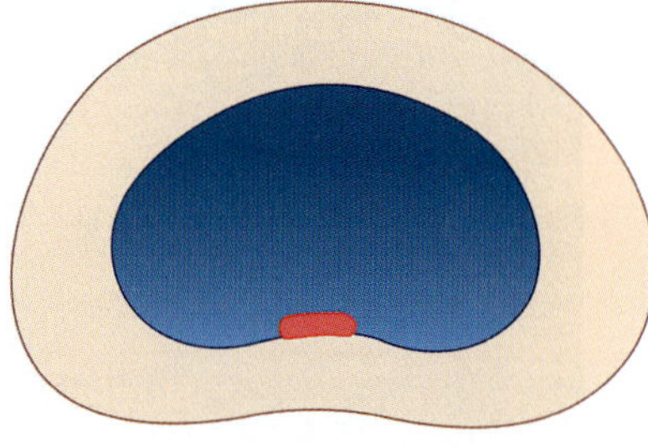
Fig. 3.4.52: Posterior annular tear

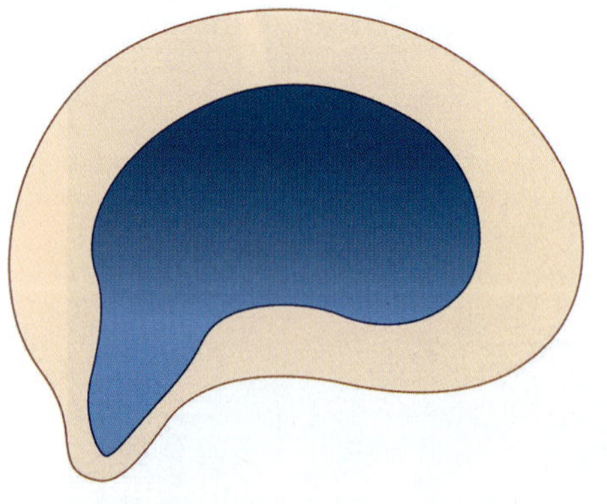
Fig. 3.4.53: Disc protrusion

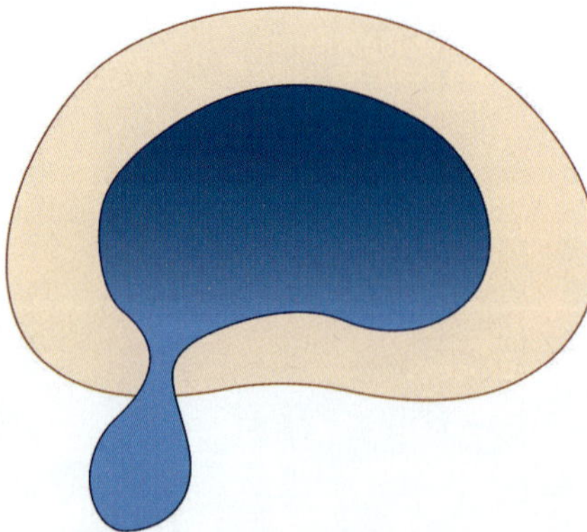
Fig. 3.4.54: Disc extrusion

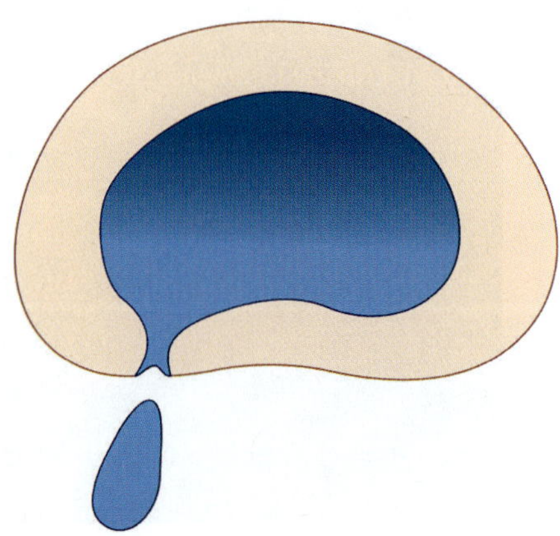
Fig. 3.4.55: Disc sequestration

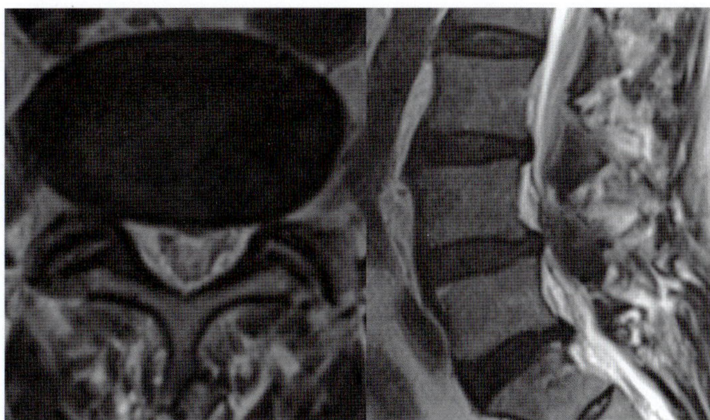

Fig. 3.4.56: MRI lumbar spine—disc herniation

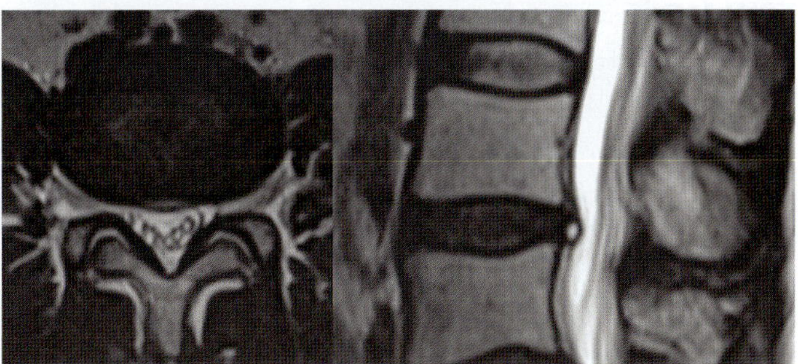

Fig. 3.4.57: MRI lumbar spine—disc herniation

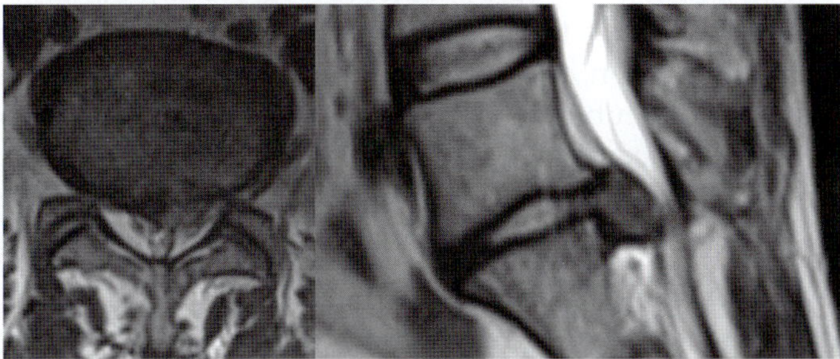

Fig. 3.4.58: MRI lumbar spine—disc herniation

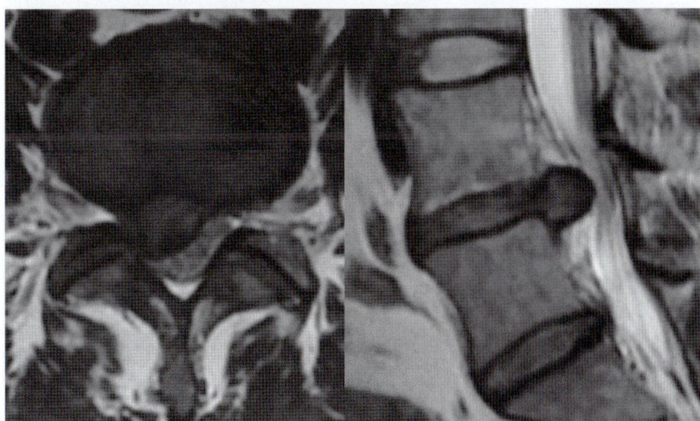

Fig. 3.4.59: MRI lumbar spine—disc herniation

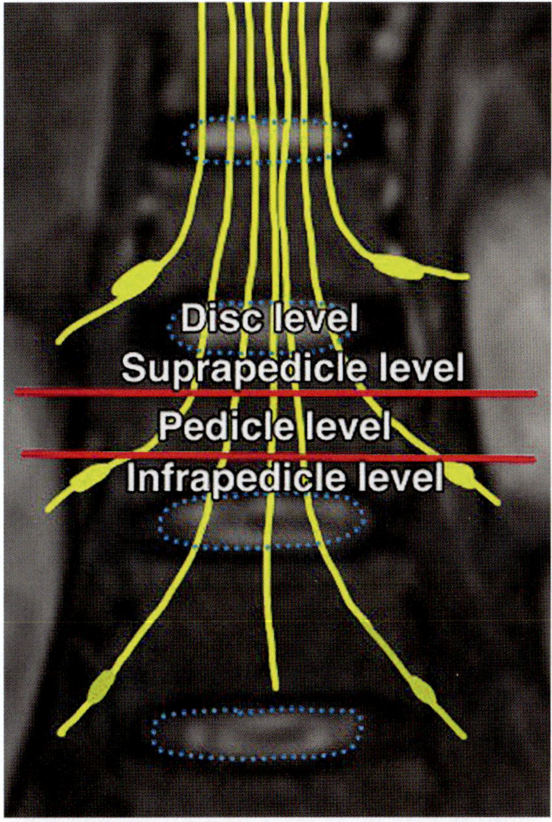

Fig. 3.4.60: MRI lumbar spine—disc herniation

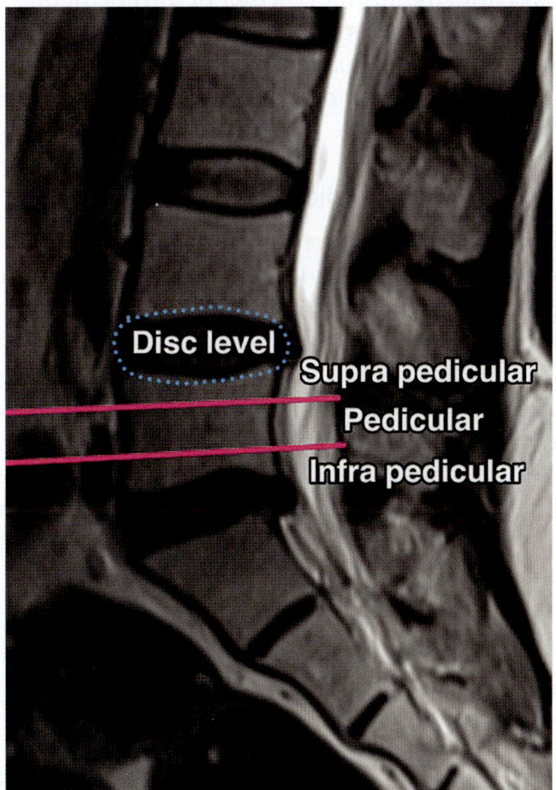

Fig. 3.4.61: MRI lumbar spine—disc herniation

beyond the edges of the ring apophyses, throughout the circumference of the disc, is called "bulging" and is the result of tears in the annulus fibrosus. Asymmetric bulging of disc tissue greater than 25% of the disc circumference is often seen as an adaptation to adjacent deformity (Figs 3.4.50–3.4.52, 3.4.56, 3.4.57). Disc herniation is defined as a focal displacement of disc material (<25% of the disc circumference) beyond the limits of the intervertebral disc space. Neural foramina in lumbar spine are keyhole shaped and and nerve roots descend vertically from the spinal canal via lateral recess exiting along the superior recess of neural foramina. Narrowing of the foramina produce clinical symptoms after a prolonged duration, by which time there is severe narrowing with compression of nerve roots.

Types of disc herniation: Disc protrusion is a type of disc herniation characterized by protrusion of disc content beyond the normal confines of the intervertebral disc, over a segment less than 25% of the circumference of the disc. The width of the base is wider than the largest diameter of the disc material which projects beyond the normal disc margins (Figs 3.4.53 and 3.4.58). **Disc extrusion** (Figs 3.4.54 and 3.4.59) is a type of intervertebral disc herniation is characterized by protrusion of disc in at least one plane, has a broader dome than a neck and/or extends above or below the disc level (into the suprapedicular or infrapedicular zone) (Figs 3.4.60–3.4.61). Sequestration is used to indicate that the displaced disc material has lost continuity with the parent disc and is displaced away from the site of extrusion (Fig. 3.4.55).

3.4.I Modic Classification

Modic classification describes degeneration around the intervertebral disc. It divides the degenerative process into three types (Fig. 3.4.62). Type I is characterized by inflammation and marrow edema. It appears as low signal intensity on T1 and high signal intensity on T2 weighted MR images. Type II describes replacement of red bone marrow by yellow bone marrow due to marrow ischemia. It is T1 hyperintense and T2 iso to hyperintense. Type III describes subchondral sclerosis. It has low signal intensities on both T1 and T2 weighted MR images.

3.4.J Sacrum

Sacrum includes five fused sacral segments with progressive decrease in anteroposterior width and transverse length resulting in triangular shape. Base forms the superior surface. Ovoid articular surface on the base articulates with L5–S1 intervertebral disc.

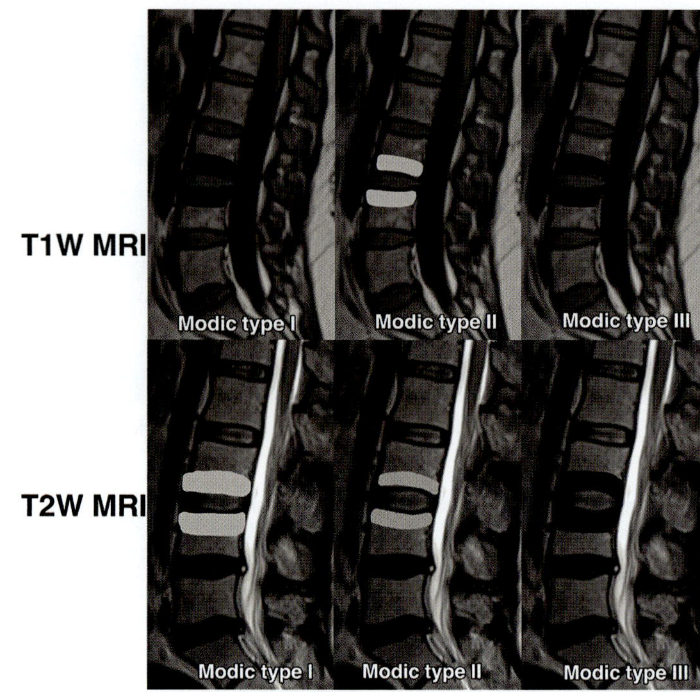

Fig. 3.4.62: Modic stages: Degenerative end plate changes

Anterior margin of the ovoid articular surface forms a ridge which is known as sacral promontory. Wing-like projections extending from the body of S1 are known as alae of the sacrum which are fused portion of costal elements and transverse processes (Fig. 3.4.63). Laminae are fused except that of S4 and S5 laminae resulting in the formation of sacral hiatus. Apex of the sacrum has an ovoid tubercle which articulates with coccyx to form sacrococcygeal joint. Dorsal surface is convex and irregular. Rudimentary spinous processes are known as spinous tubercles. Spinous tubercles are fused in the

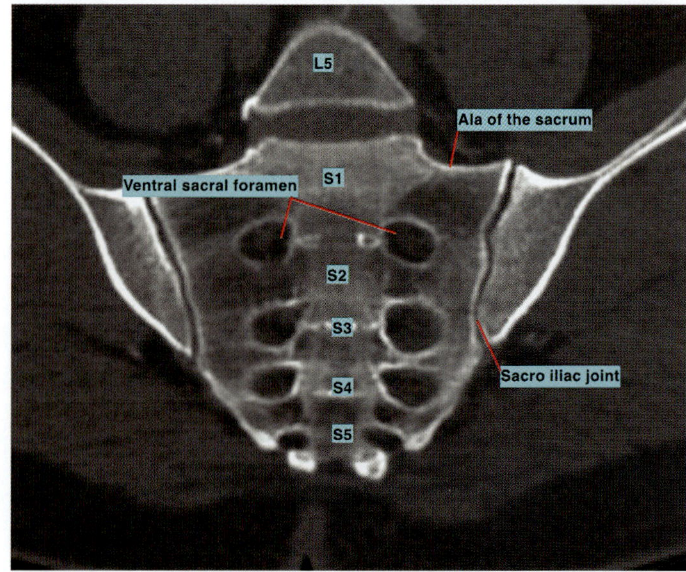

Fig. 3.4.63: CT sacral vertebra

midline to form median sacral crest. Fused articular processes forming a ridge located lateral to the fused laminae is the intermediate sacral crest. Dorsal sacral foramina are located lateral to the intermediate sacral crest. Dorsal sacral foramina are oriented transversely anteromedial to posterolateral and they are irregular. Tubercles arising from the fused transverse processes fuse to form lateral sacral crest.

Ventral or pelvic surface is relatively smooth. Centrally vertebral bodies of sacrum are fused. Fused intervertebral fibrocartilages form transverse ridges four in number. Ventral sacral foramina are located lateral to the vertebral body. Inferior margins of upper two costal elements form arcuate line on plain radiographs.

Lateral surface is "C" shaped in accordance with sacral kyphosis. In the upper part of the lateral surface there is an ear-shaped surface called auricular surface lined by articular cartilage forming cartilaginous portion of the sacroiliac joint. Posterior and superior to the auricular surface is a rough surface which marks the attachment site for the interosseous sacroiliac ligament and posterior sacroiliac ligament, called the sacral tuberosity.

There are typically four ventral and four dorsal sacral foramina. The ventral foramina are funnel or trumpet shaped and transmit the ventral rami of the sacral nerves. The dorsal foramina are smaller in caliber, are more often irregular, and transmit the dorsal rami of the sacral nerves. The ventral foramina are primarily vertically-oriented and course superomedial to inferolateral. This results in an inverted Y-shaped configuration on coronal images. The axes of the S1 and S2 dorsal foramina are oriented anteromedial to posterolateral in the transverse plane. The S3 and S4 dorsal foramina are also oriented primarily in the transverse plane, in a more anterior to posterior fashion. The dorsal foramina of S1 are commonly accessed percutaneously when performing selective nerve root blocks.

Sacroiliac joints (SIJs): The sacroiliac joints (Fig. 3.4.64) are the largest joints of the axial skeleton and are responsible for weight transfer from the upper body to the lower extremities. The SIJs have cartilaginous and ligamentous portions. The cartilaginous portions of the SIJs display features of symphyseal and synovial joints. The superior two-thirds of the cartilaginous portion of the joint are symphyseal and the inferior one-third is synovial. The SIJ capsule is thin and discontinuous posteriorly. The ligamentous portion of the SIJ is best classified as a syndesmosis and is located posterior and superior to the cartilaginous component.

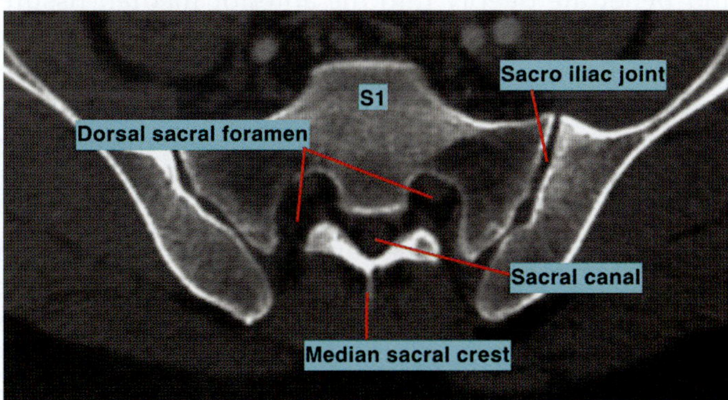

Fig. 3.4.64: CT sacroiliac joint

Ligaments of the sacroiliac joints: Interosseous ligaments are the strongest ligaments supporting the SIJ. They are connected to the sacral and iliac tuberosities at S1, S2 levels. Anterior sacroiliac ligament is made up of two bands and is located at anterior and inferior margin of SIJ. Posterior sacroiliac ligament has two components: Short and long. Short component extends between S1, S2 transverse tubercles and iliac tuberosities and is oriented horizontally. Long component is oriented obliquely and S3, S4 transverse tubercles and posterior superior iliac spines.

Ligaments of the sacral spine: Anterior longitudinal ligament of the lumbar spine continues uninterruptedly below as sacral ALL. It has broad attachment with sacral promontory and as it goes inferiorly the width decreases. It continues as anterior sacrococcygeal ligament. Posterior longitudinal ligament of the lumbar spine continues uninterruptedly below as sacral PLL. It continues as posterior sacrococcygeal ligament. Ligamenta flava attach to the anterior inferior margins of L5 laminae and posterior superior margins of S1 laminae. Interspinous ligament is attached to the inferior margin of L5 spinous process and medial sacral crest. Iliolumbar ligament is attached between the transverse process of L5 and sacrum and iliac crest. Superior bands attach to the transverse processes of L5 and iliac crests. Inferior bands are broad and attach to the L5 transverse processes and sacral alae and are known as lumbosacral ligaments. Sacrospinous ligaments attach to the lateral margins of the sacrum and ischial spines. They form posterior and inferior margins of the greater sciatic foramina. Sacrotuberous ligament extends between the sacrum and ischial tuberosity and forms the superior and posterior margin of lesser sciatic foramen.

3.4.K Spinal Cord Blood Supply

Blood supply to the spinal cord comes from two sources. Arteries arising from vertebral arteries above the level of the cervical segments. They include one anterior and two posterior spinal arteries. Anterior spinal artery arises by the union of two branches arising from the vertebral arteries and run in the anterior median fissure. Posterior inferior cerebellar arteries give off posterior spinal arteries which run in the posterolateral sulcus. Another source of blood supply is from segmental artery which enters the spinal cord via the neural foramen at each level. Segmental arteries arise from vertebral and deep cervical arteries in the neck, from posterior intercostal and subcostal arteries in the thorax, lumbar arteries in the lumbar region, middle and lateral sacral arteries in the sacral region. The blood supply to the cervical subaxial segments is derived from the vertebral arteries. The longitudinal arteries of the cervical spine include the vertebral arteries, deep cervical arteries, ascending cervical arteries, and the costocervical trunks. The vertebral arteries give off the segmental branches within the upper cervical segments. The segmental arteries tend to arise from the deep cervical artery, ascending cervical artery, and costocervical trunk in the lower cervical segments. However, a rich anastomotic network is the rule in the cervical spine, making the cervical spinal cord relatively resistant to infarction. The segmental arteries from vertebral artery origin arise on both sides of the midline and give off anterior and posterior rami. The posterior rami give off spinal and muscular branches. Spinal branches course through the neural foramina and branch into anterior and posterior radicular arteries (Figs 3.4.65–3.4.68). The radicular arteries may supply the nerve roots, dura mater, spinal ganglia, spinal cord. The radicular arteries that supply the spinal cord are referred to as radiculomedullary arteries and tend to travel with the ventral roots. The dominant cervical radiculomedullary artery has been termed the cervical radiculomedullary artery of Lazorthes. A variable number of posterior radiculomedullary arteries make up the posterior spinal arteries. Anterior spinal artery arises from two small branches of the distal vertebral arteries. The anterior spinal artery resides in the anterior median fissure and supplies the anterior two-thirds of the spinal cord. The paired posterior spinal arteries are positioned lateral to the posterior median sulcus and supply the posterior one-third of the spinal cord. The central arteries branch from the anterior spinal arteries and penetrate deeply into the anterior median fissure to supply the central cord. The anterior and posterior spinal arteries contribute to a network of arteries that encircle the spinal cord, the pial arterial plexus or vasa coronae. The longitudinal artery supplying the thoracic spine is the descending thoracic aorta. The segmental arteries of the thoracic spine are nine pairs of posterior intercostal arteries and one pair of subcostal arteries. The intercostal arteries branch into anterior and posterior rami. The anterior rami course laterally to supply the tissues of the intercostal spaces, skin, and mammary glands. The anterior rami anastomose with the superior epigastric and musculophrenic arteries. The posterior

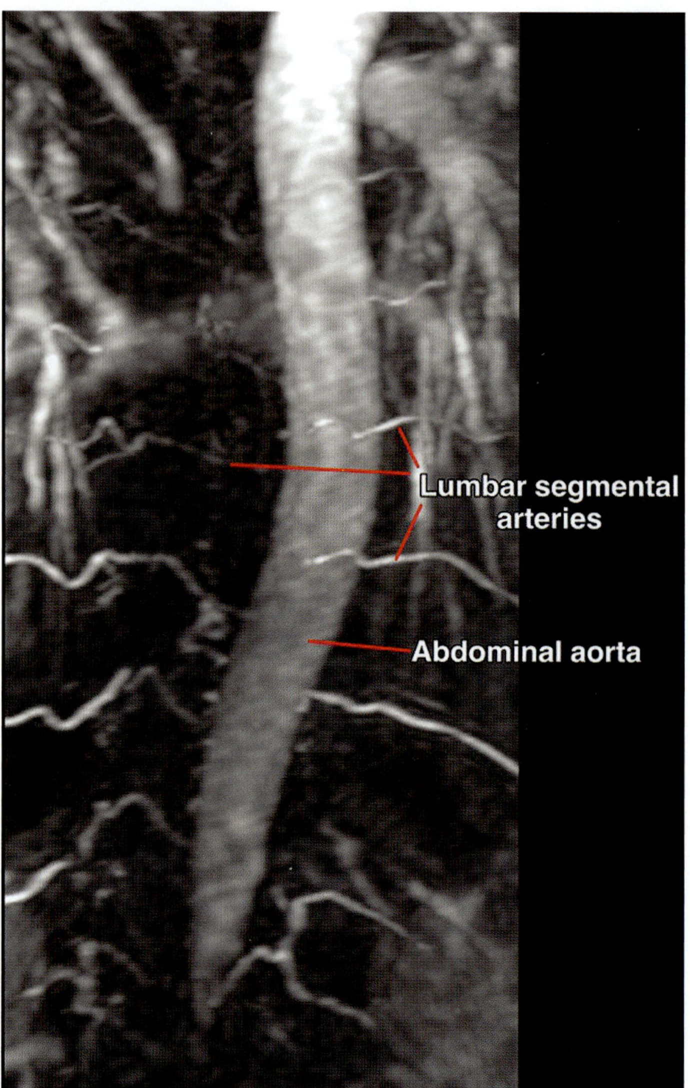

Fig. 3.4.66: MRA: Aortic branches

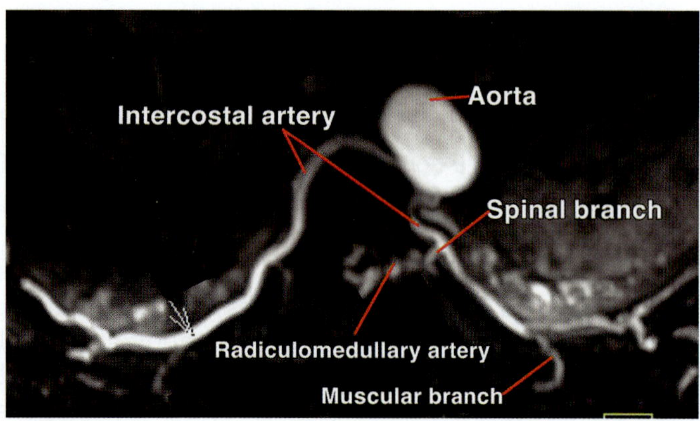

Fig. 3.4.65: MRA: Spinal arteries

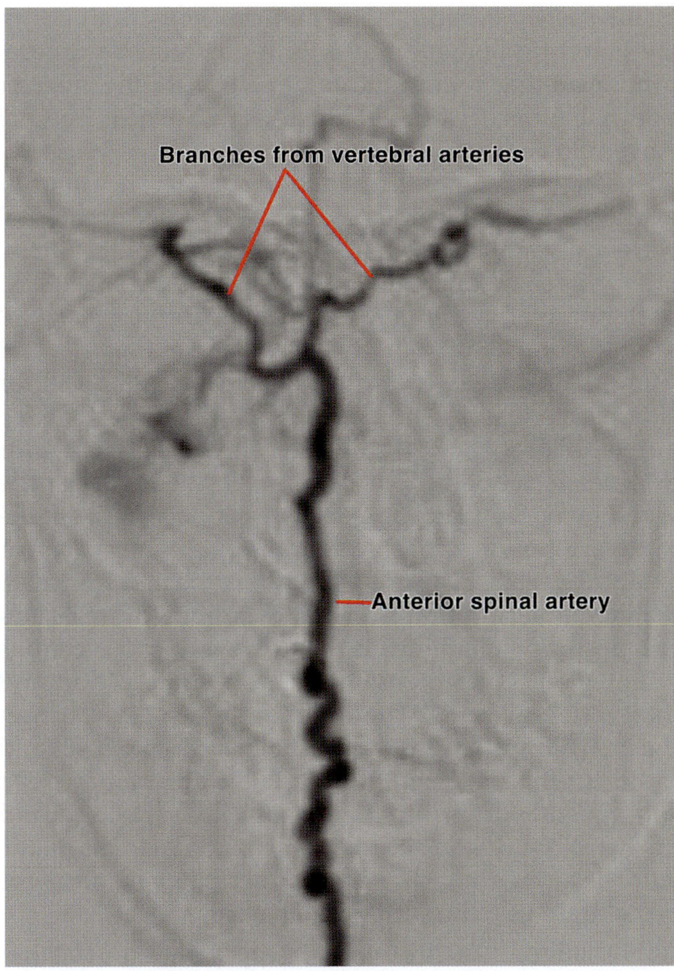

Fig. 3.4.67: DSA: Anterior spinal artery

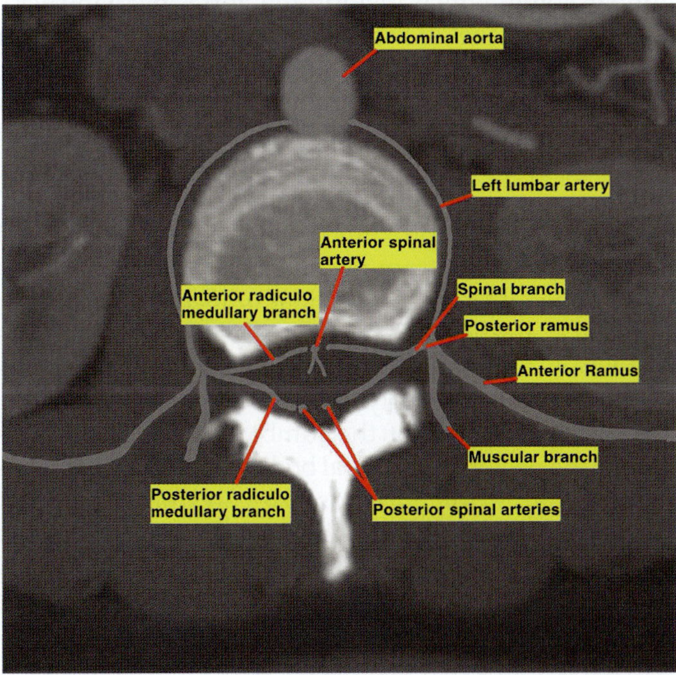

Fig. 3.4.68: CECT axial image: Spinal arteries

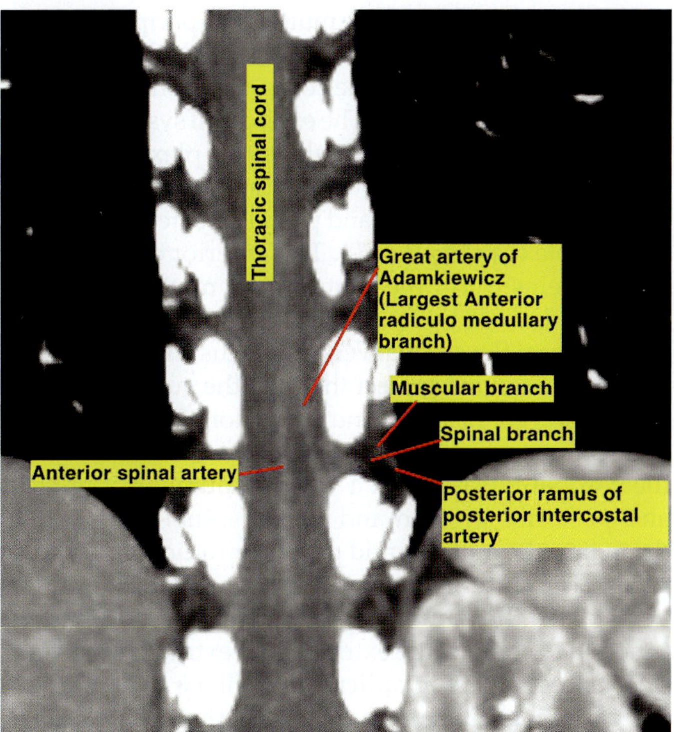

Fig. 3.4.69: CECT coronal image: Spinal arteries

rami give off muscular and spinal branches. The muscular branches course posteriorly, along the lateral margins of the vertebral bodies and supply the soft tissues along the inferior margins of the neural foramina, inferior aspects of the spinal nerves, intercostal muscles, and soft tissues. The spinal branches course through the neural foramina and branch into anterior and posterior radicular arteries. The radicular arteries may supply the nerve roots, dura mater, spinal ganglia, spinal cord. A variable number of radicular arteries send branches along the anterior and/or posterior nerve roots to supply the spinal cord, called the radiculomedullary arteries. Radiculomedullary arteries that supply the anterior spinal artery are called anterior radiculomedullary arteries. Posterior radiculomedullary arteries supply the posterior spinal arteries. The dominant thoracolumbar anterior radiculomedullary artery supplying the lower spinal cord is the great anterior radiculomedullary artery of Adamkiewicz or the artery of Adamkiewicz (Fig 3.4.69). The AKA most commonly arises on the left between T9–T11. The AKA ascends within the spinal canal and takes a characteristic "hairpin turn" as it joins the anterior spinal artery.

Venous drainage of the cervical, thoracic spine and spinal cord is carried out through a heavily interconnected venous network that has three main divisions: Intrinsic, extrinsic, and extradural. The intrinsic system includes the venous network that drains the spinal cord central gray matter and peripheral white matter. The pia mater marks the border of the extrinsic system, which includes the coronal venous plexus and radiculomedullary veins. The extradural system includes the anterior internal vertebral venous plexus, posterior internal vertebral venous plexus, anterior external vertebral venous plexus, and posterior external vertebral venous plexus (Fig. 3.4.70). The anterior and posterior central veins drain the central gray matter. The white matter is drained by small caliber radial veins within the pia that form the coronal venous plexus. Transmedullary anastomotic veins project through the substance of the spinal cord, connecting ventral and dorsal surfaces. Some of the larger caliber longitudinally oriented veins within the coronal plexus form a variable number of anterior and posterior median and lateral spinal veins, which drain into the anterior and posterior radiculomedullary veins. The anterior and posterior radiculomedullary veins drain the spinal cord and spinal nerve roots and function to connect the extrinsic and extradural systems. The largest anterior radiculomedullary vein draining the thoracolumbar spinal cord is the great anterior radiculomedullary vein (GARV). The radiculomedullary veins and anterior and posterior external vertebral venous plexuses drain into the intervertebral veins. The anterior internal vertebral venous plexus resides within two layers of the posterior longitudinal ligament. At pedicle level, it connects through transversely oriented venous anastomoses to the basivertebral veins, the valved system that provides the primary drainage

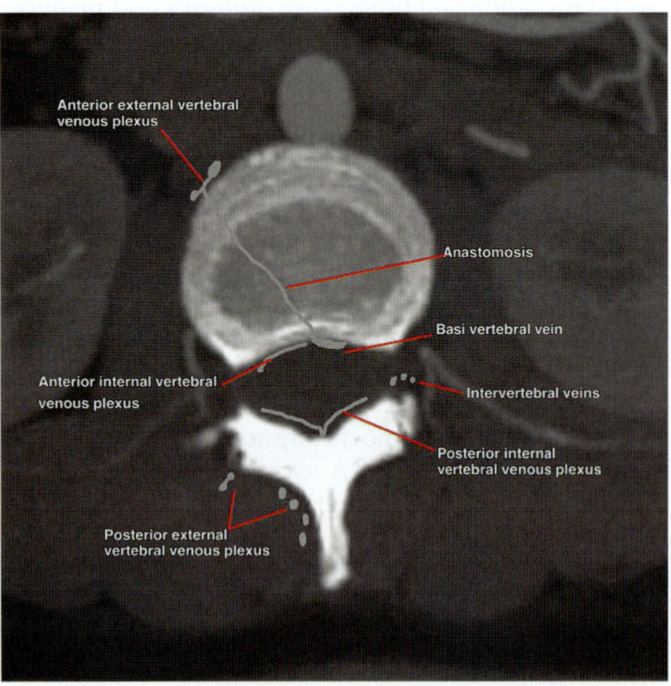

Fig. 3.4.70: CECT axial image-vertebral veins

of the vertebral bodies. The minor venous drainage of the vertebral bodies occurs through small peripheral tributaries that communicate directly with the anterior external vertebral venous plexus. The anterior internal vertebral venous plexus also anastomoses with the posterior internal vertebral venous plexus and anterior external vertebral venous plexus. The posterior internal vertebral venous plexus is composed of longitudinally oriented veins traversing the dorsal epidural space. The posterior internal vertebral venous plexus receives small draining branches from the lateral masses, lamina, and spinous processes. It also connects with the posterior external vertebral venous plexus via small perforating veins through the ligamenta flava. The anterior external vertebral venous plexus is located anterior the vertebral bodies and has extensive connections with the intervertebral and basivertebral veins. The posterior external vertebral venous plexus is located dorsal to the vertebrae and drains the paravertebral muscles and the posterior elements. It has extensive connections with the posterior internal vertebral venous plexus and intervertebral veins. The intervertebral veins connect the internal and external vertebral venous plexuses and drain into the segmental veins. The segmental veins subsequently drain into the azygos vein on the right and the hemiazygos and accessory hemiazygos veins on the left. The azygos, hemiazygos, and accessory hemiazygos veins drain into the superior vena cava.

The segmental branches supplying the lumbar segments arise from the longitudinal arteries of the lumbar spine, which include the aorta, median sacral artery. At the level of the conus medullaris, the anterior and posterior spinal arteries form a dense anastomotic network that has the appearance of a basket. The artery of the filum terminale arises from this anastomotic basket and courses along the ventral aspect of the filum. The cauda equina has a dual arterial supply. The ventral roots are supplied proximally by the vasa corona and radicular branches from the anterior vasa corona. They are supplied distally by radicular branches. The lumbar segmental arteries give off 10 to 20 periosteal arteries that supply the anterolateral walls of the vertebral bodies superiorly and inferiorly. An arcade of arteries arising from posterior rami of the lumbar segmental arteries supply the posterior vertebral bodies. Periosteal branches from the anterior and posterior systems form the metaphyseal anastomosis which supplies the upper and lower portions of the vertebral bodies. The metaphyseal anastomosis gives off small caliber penetrating arteries called metaphyseal arteries, which supply wedge-shaped territories that point centrally. Penetrating branches of the lumbar segmental arteries called equatorial arteries penetrate along the anterolateral margin of the vertebral body and supply the central aspect of the vertebral body. Perforating branches called nutrient arteries enter the posterior wall of the vertebral bodies and supply the central aspect of the vertebral body.

The venous drainage of the lumbar spine, distal cord, and conus is carried out through a densely interconnected venous network that has intrinsic, extrinsic, and extradural divisions. The anterior and posterior radiculomedullary veins drain the spinal cord and spinal nerve roots and function to connect the extrinsic and extradural systems. The great anterior radiculomedullary vein is the largest vein draining the anterior cord in the thoracolumbar region. The radiculomedullary veins and anterior and posterior external vertebral venous plexuses drain into the intervertebral veins. Anterior median spinal vein travels with the anterior spinal artery to the conus and usually continues as the vein of the filum terminale. The venous drainage of the cauda equina, like the arterial supply, has proximal and distal components. The distal radicular veins drain into the lumbar veins at the level the corresponding nerve root exits into the neural foramen. The proximal radicular veins drain into the venous component of the vasa corona and subsequently into the anterior and posterior longitudinal veins of the spinal cord. The venous drainage of the vertebral bodies parallels that of the arterial supply.

3.4.L Paraspinal Muscles

Muscles of the back are divided into superficial, intermediate and deep groups (Figs 3.4.71–3.4.75). Muscles of the superficial group include trapezius, latissimus dorsi, rhomboid major, rhomboid minor,

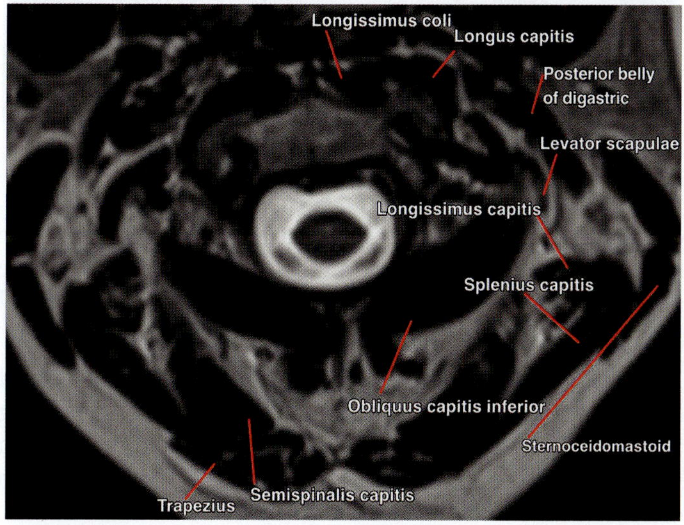

Fig. 3.4.71

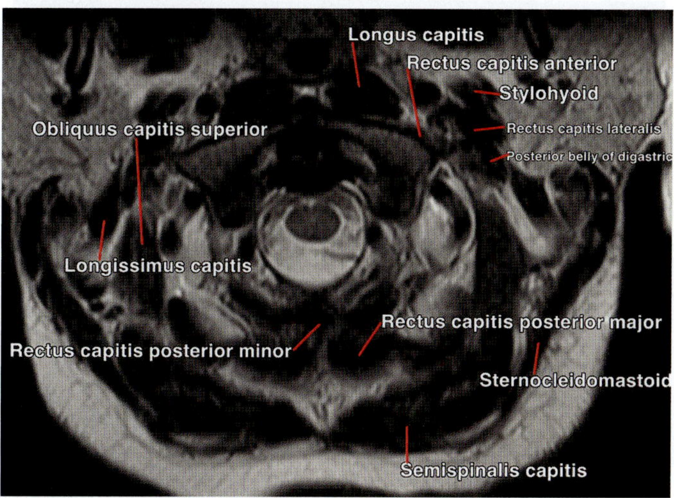

Fig. 3.4.72: MRI axial images: Paraspinal muscles

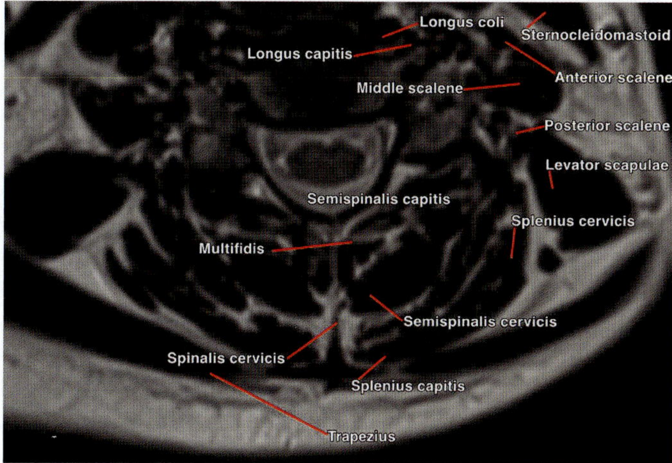

Fig. 3.4.73: MRI axial images: Paraspinal muscles

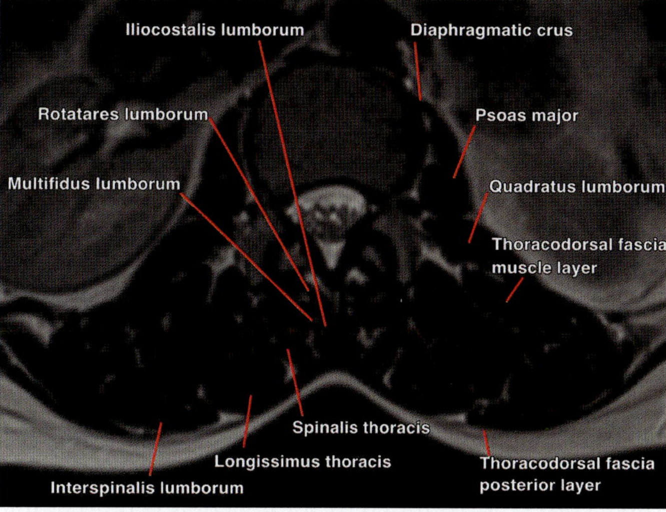

Fig. 3.4.74: MRI axial images: Paraspinal muscles

levator scapulae. Intermediate group of muscles include serratus posterior superior and serratus posterior inferior. The deep or intrinsic muscles of the back extend from

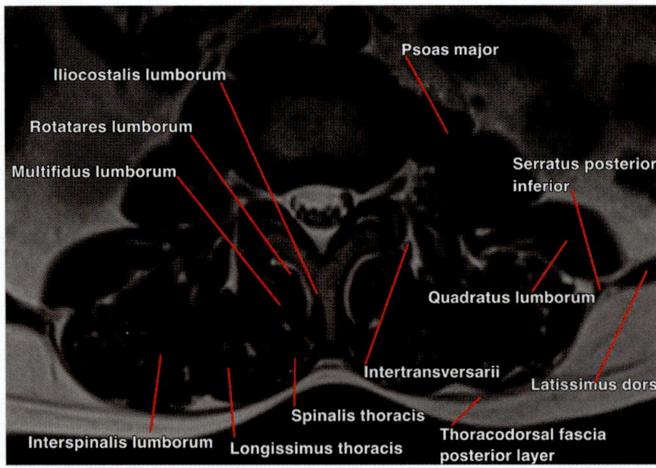

Fig. 3.4.75: MRI axial images: Paraspinal muscles

the pelvis to the skull. They include the extensors and rotators of the head and neck, the splenius capitis and cervicis (spinotransversales muscles), the extensors and rotators of the vertebral column—the erector spinae and transversospinales and the short segmental muscles—the interspinales and intertransversarii. Spinotransversales muscles include splenius capitis and splenius cervicis. Erector spinae muscles include iliocostalis lumborum, iliocostalis thoracis, iliocostalis cervicis, longissimus thoracis, longissimus cervicis, longissimus capitis, spinalis thoracis, spinalis cervicis and spinalis capitis. Transversospinalis muscles include semispinalis thoracis, semispinalis cervicis, semispinalis capitis, multifidus, rotatores lumborum, rotatores thoracis, rotatores cervicis. Short segmental muscles include levatores costarum, interspinales, intertransversarii. Suboccipital group of back muscles include rectus capitis posterior major, rectus capitis posterior minor, obliquus capitis inferior, and obliquus capitis superior.

3.4.M Ultrasonogram of Spine

On a sagittal scan, the spinal cord is a hypoechoic tubular structure with an echogenic center. The central echo complex represents the central canal. At histologic analysis, the central canal corresponds to the border between the myelinated ventral white commissure and the central portion of the anterior median fissure. In healthy newborns, the central canal is overgrown with glial fibrils and is not filled with cerebrospinal fluid. The spinal cord is surrounded by the anechoic cerebrospinal fluid of the subarachnoid space. The arachnoid-dura mater complex of the thecal sac corresponds to the echogenic border of the spinal canal dorsal and ventral to the subarachnoid space (Figs 3.4.76 and 3.4.78).

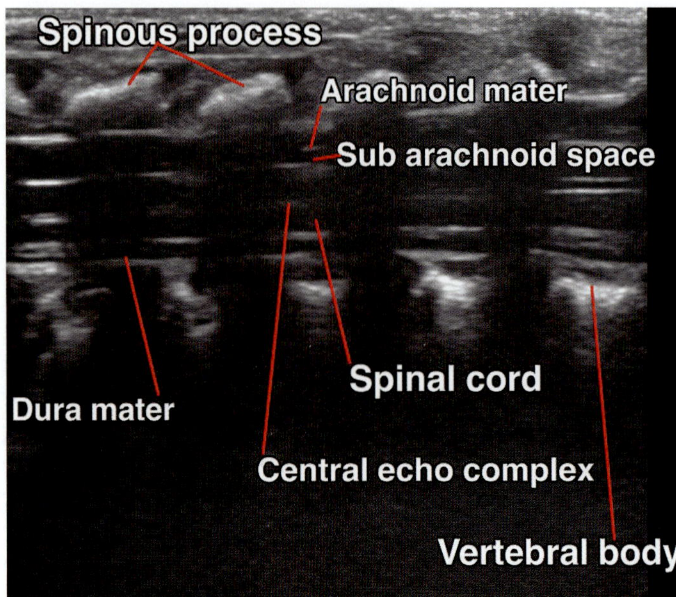

Fig. 3.4.76: USG longitudinal section of spinal cord

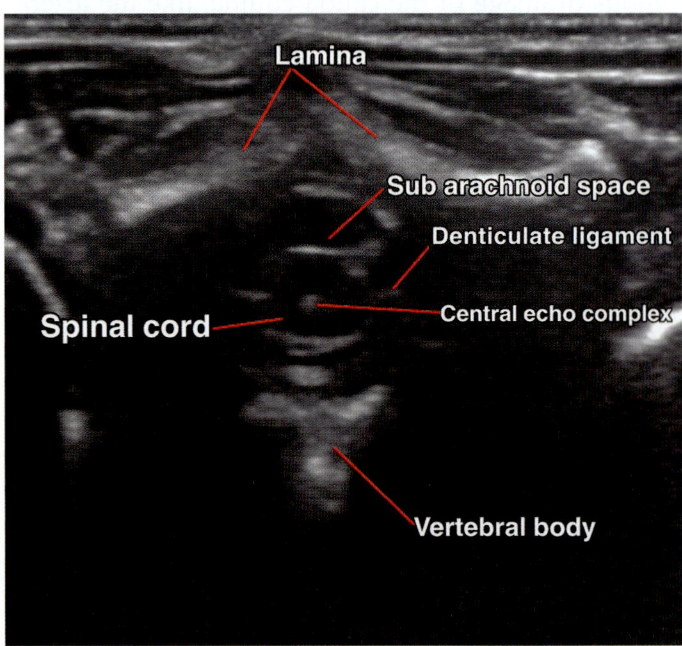

Fig. 3.4.77: USG transverse section of spinal cord

An axial scan of the spinal cord shows the hypoechoic, oval or round spinal cord with the echogenic central echo complex within the anechoic subarachnoid space. The spinal cord gives rise to the paired dorsal and ventral nerve roots (Fig. 3.4.77).

Preparation and positioning: Like all pediatric ultrasound examinations obtaining relevant history and explaining the procedure to the parent or accompanying guardian precedes the study. Examination is carried out in a warm environment with all clothing removed. Warm hands, warmed gel and dim lights assist in making the child

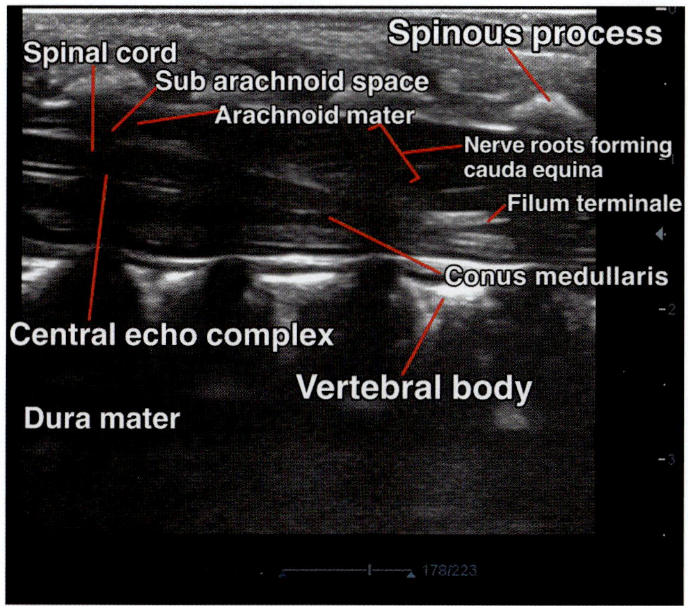

Fig. 3.4.78: USG longitudinal section of spinal cord

more co-operative. Ideally neonate should be fed prior to the ultrasound, however, if pre-procedural feeding is not possible a pacifier dipped in glucose can be helpful to keep the infant still.

Examination is carried out by a posterior approach. The neonate ideally to be placed in prone position over a rolled pillow or bolster, to achieve adequate spinal flexion and increase spacing of spinous processes to provide an ideal acoustic window for examination. Elevation of the neonatal head allows CSF to distend the distal thecal sac improving visualization of distal cord. If prone position compromises neonates' respiration, the neonate can be examined in lateral decubitus position.

In the decubitus position, however, one should remember that the spinal cord and nerve roots may gravitate to the dependent side. The examination can also be carried out with the infant held in an erect position or the parents' shoulder in a burping position, the advantage here being collection of CSF in the lower lumbar region surrounding the lower cord and cauda equina improving resolution also helps outline abnormal CSF filled sacs. This position immensely helps in the LP tap also in case it is needed to rule out infective cause.

Technical details: Probe selection: A high-frequency 17–5 MHz linear transducer is used as it gives a larger image in the near-field and has a higher spatial resolution. In older infants, a lower-frequency may be necessary for better penetration. Panoramic function is used in sagittal imaging of long-segment of the spine and thus aids in identifying the vertebral levels. The cranio-vertebral junction is examined with a small footprint convex high-frequency transducer.

Machine settings: Optimal grey scale settings with keen attention to depth and focus assisted with power Doppler/color Doppler and extended field of view/panoramic functionality.

M-mode can be utilized for documenting the movement of cauda equina/nerve roots under real time scanning, synchronous with neonates breathing movements.

Cine-loops for post-acquisition review study help in increasing diagnostic confidence.

Minimal probe pressure should be with copious use of gel especially if the scanning is between the gluteal masses.

3.5 ABDOMEN

Abdomen is the body space between the thorax and pelvis. At the level of the pelvic bones, the abdomen ends and the pelvis begins.

3.5.A Liver

The **Couinaud** classification of **liver segmental anatomy** divides the liver into eight functionally indepedent segments. Couinaud divided the liver into a functional left and right liver by a main portal fissure containing the middle hepatic vein. This is known as Cantlie's line which runs from the middle of the gallbladder fossa anteriorly to the inferior vena cava posteriorly. The vascular intake, outflow, and biliary drainage are all separate for each segment. Each segment has a portal vein, hepatic artery, and bile duct branch in the middle. The hepatic veins provide circulatory outflow in the periphery of each segment. The right lobe is divided into anterior and posterior parts by the right hepatic vein. The right and left lobes of the liver are separated by the middle hepatic vein and line from inferior vena cava to gall bladder fossa. The Falciform ligament separates the left lobe into a medial (segment 4) and lateral (segments 2 and 3) portion. The portal vein separates the upper and lower halves of the liver. The caudate lobe is a midline, vertically oriented hepatic lobe that is a separate portion of the right and left hepatic lobes on the posterior edge of the liver.

It is located between the inferior vena cava and a ligamentum venosum-created fossa (a remnant of the foetal ductus venosus).

The ligamentum teres, or round ligament, is a fibrous cord formed by the obliterated foetal umbilical vein that goes from the umbilicus into the left lobe of the liver in the free edge of the falciform ligament. The **ligamentum venosum** is a fibrous remnant which travels superiorly from the porta hepatis of the liver to the inferior vena cava (Figs 3.5.1–3.5.12).

Gallbladder is a pear-shaped musculomembranous sac located along the undersurface of the liver. The normal adult gallbladder measures from 7–10 cm in length and 3–4 cm in transverse diameter. Parts of gallbladder—fundus, body, infundibulum (tapered segment between

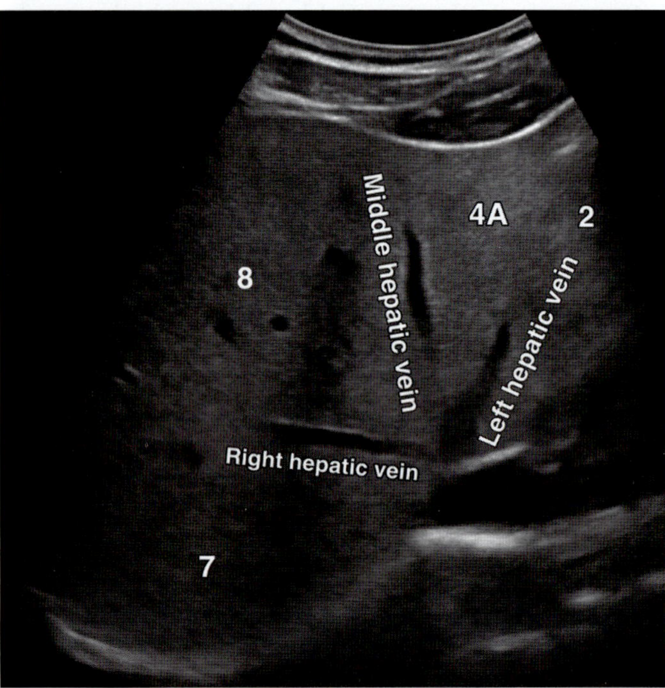

Fig. 3.5.1

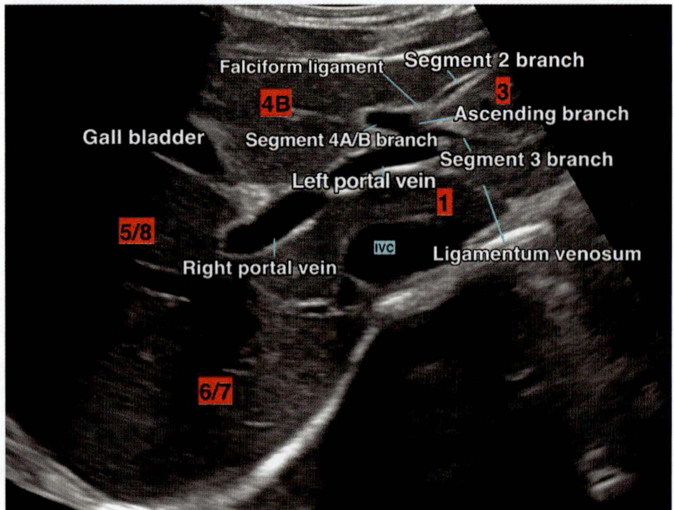

Fig. 3.5.2

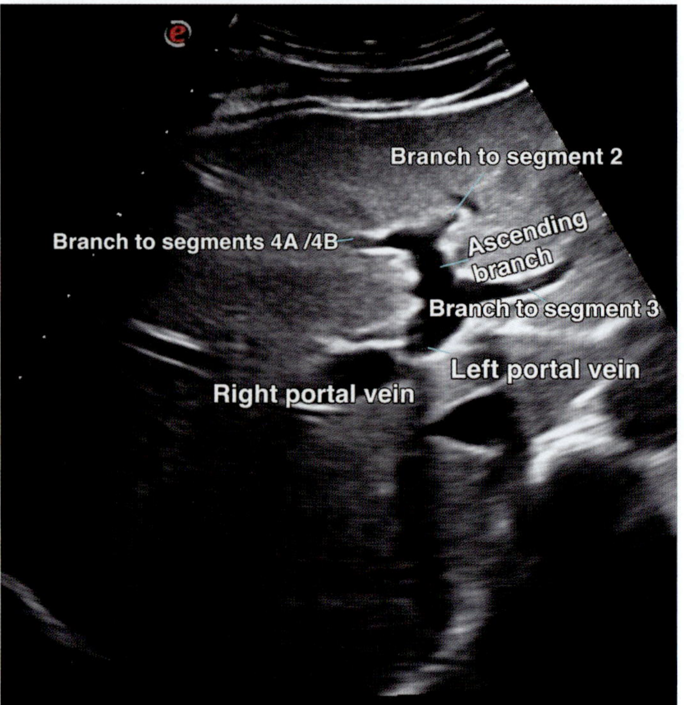

Fig. 3.5.3

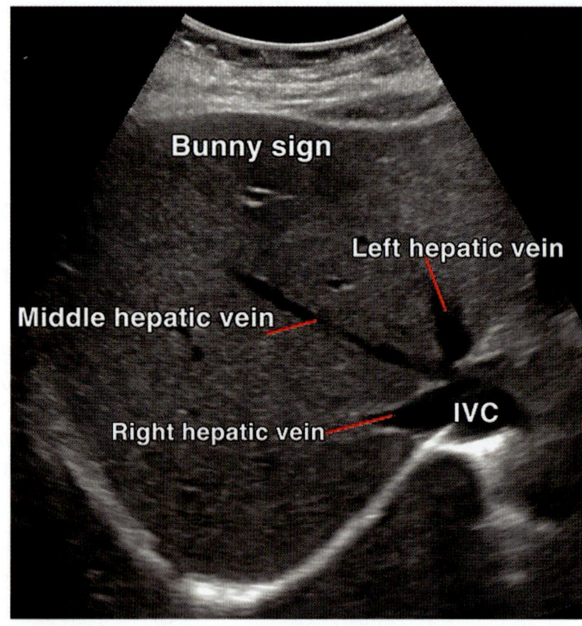

Fig. 3.5.4

body and neck) and neck, which communicates with cystic duct.

Biliary tree anatomy and variants: The anatomy of the biliary system is similar to that of the portal vein. The right hepatic duct drains the right liver lobe's segments (5–8). The right posterior duct (RPSD), which drains the posterior segments VI and VII, and the right anterior

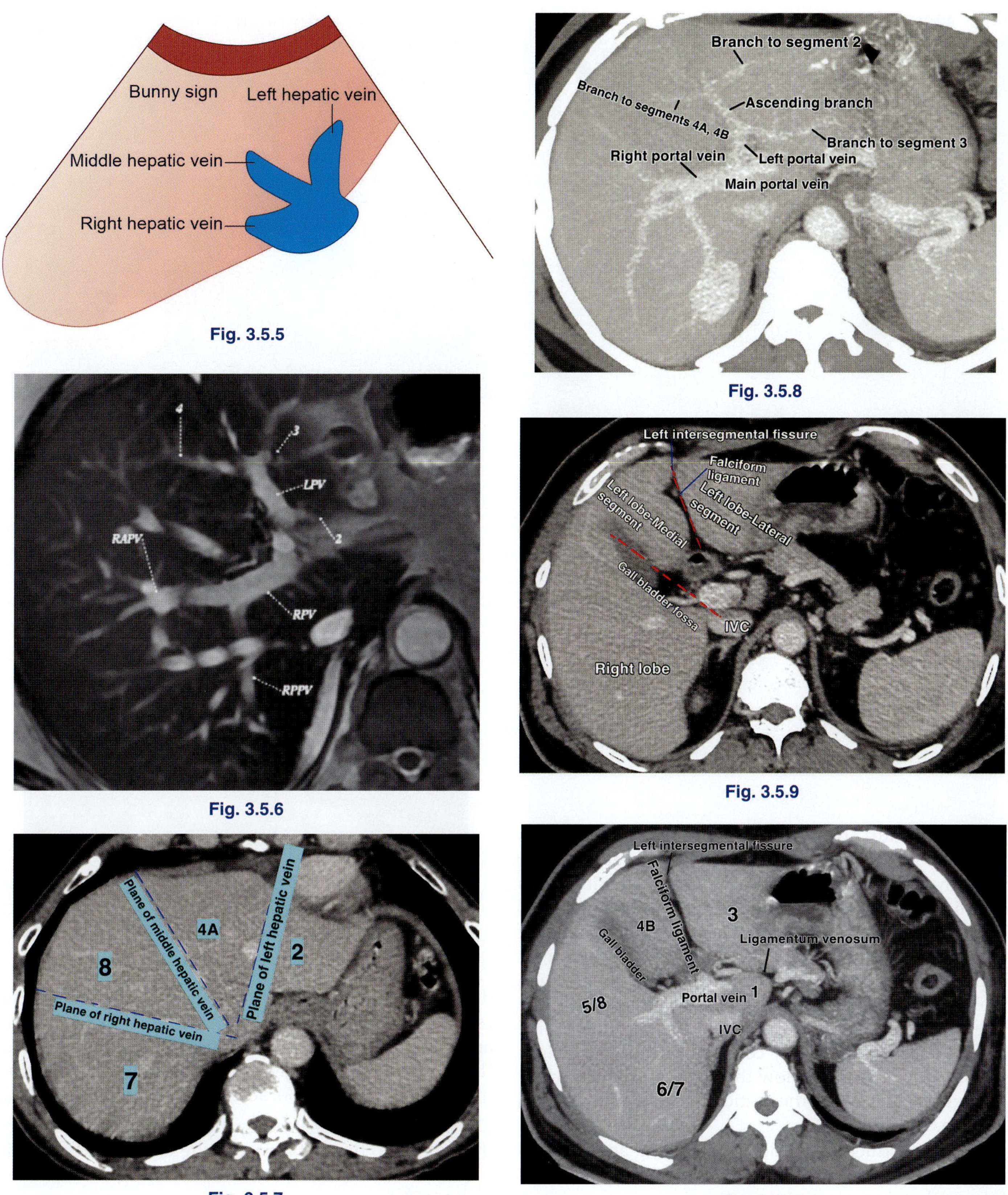

Fig. 3.5.5

Fig. 3.5.6

Fig. 3.5.7

Fig. 3.5.8

Fig. 3.5.9

Fig. 3.5.10

duct (RASD), which drains the anterior segments 5 and 8, are the two major branches of the right hepatic duct.

The right anterior duct follows a more vertical path than the right posterior duct, which follows a nearly

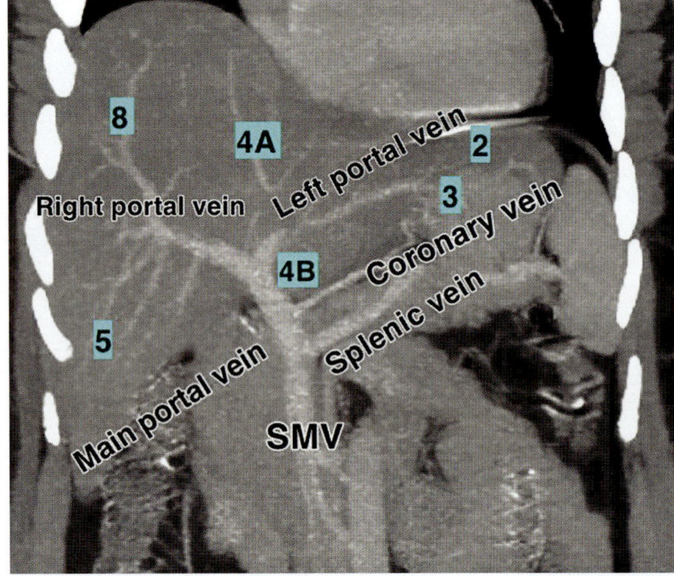

Fig. 3.5.11

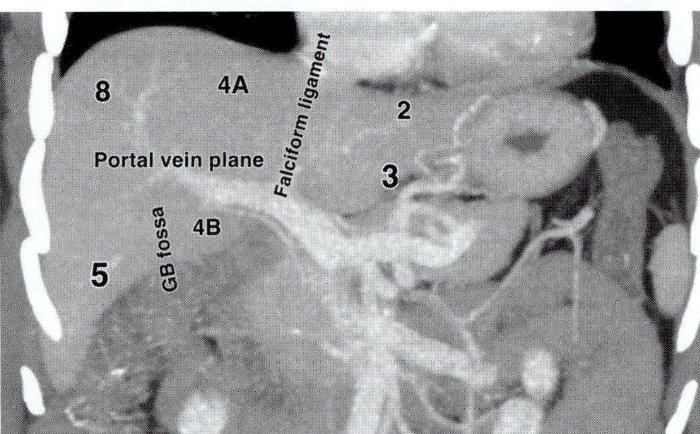

Fig. 3.5.12

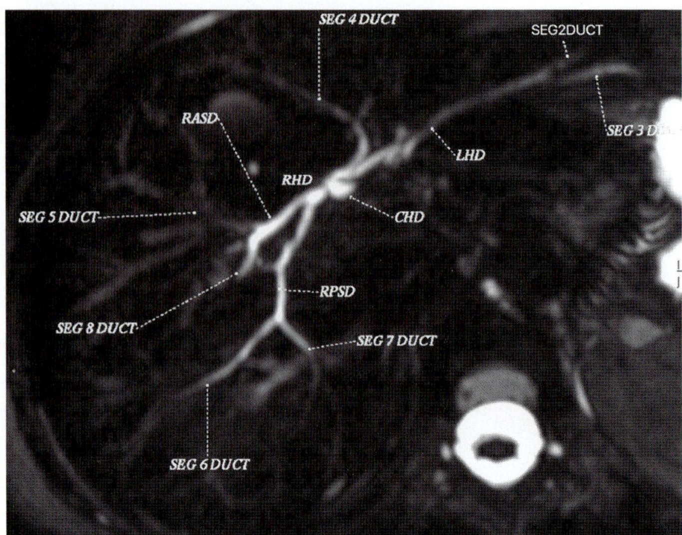

Fig. 3.5.13: MRI of biliary duct branches

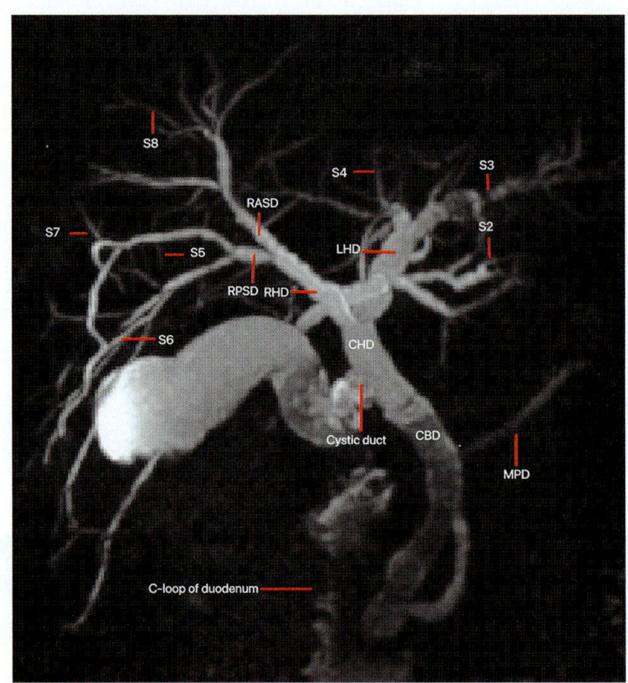

Fig. 3.5.14: Coronal MR: Biliary anatomy

horizontal path. The right posterior duct normally runs posterior to the right anterior duct and unites with it to form the right hepatic duct. Segmental tributaries draining segments 2–4 produce the left hepatic duct. The common hepatic duct is formed by the confluence of the right and left hepatic ducts. In most cases, the right hepatic duct is shorter than the left hepatic duct. When the angle between the right and left hepatic ducts is less than 90°, it is said to be narrow. The bile duct that drains the caudate lobe normally connects to the left or right hepatic duct's origin. Below the confluence of the right and left hepatic ducts, the cystic duct joins the common hepatic duct.

The cystic duct is typically 2–4 cm long and 1–5 mm in diameter. It contains spiral valves of Heister's and frequently takes a tortuous course.

Variant anatomy is quite common: RPSD draining into LHD (~15%), RASD draining into LHD (~6%), RPSD draining into anterior (not posterior) aspect of RASD (~12%), "triple confluence": Union of RPSD, RASD and LHD to form CHD (~11%), aberrant hepatic duct (typically RPSD draining into CHD) ~6%, low insertion of RHD into CHD (~2%), accessory hepatic ducts (~2%).

Cystic duct variants: Low cystic duct insertion—10% of the time, into the distal part of the CHD. Medial cystic insertion—into the left, rather than the right, side of the CHD (15%).

Parallel cystic duct course: Courses parallel to the CHD for at least 2 cm (~10%).

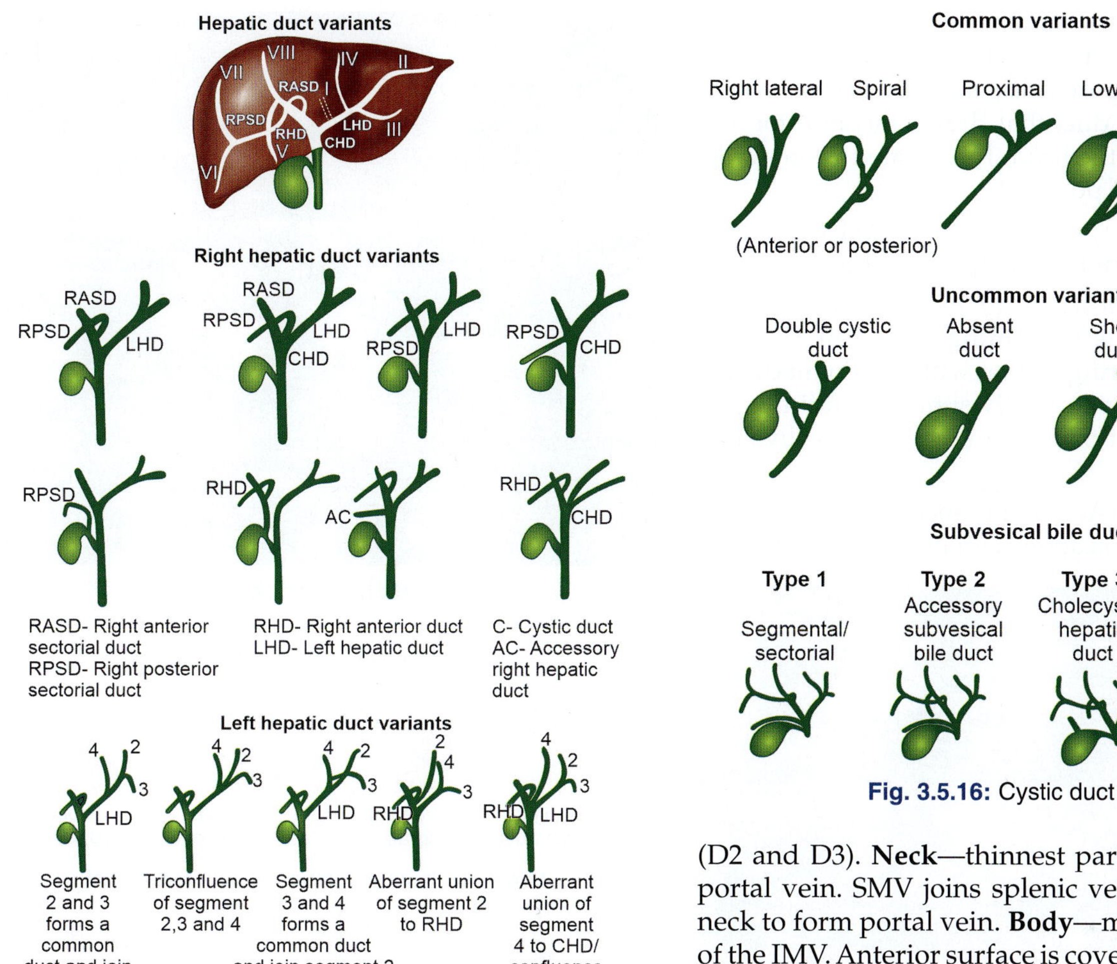

Fig. 3.5.15: Hepatic duct variants

Fig. 3.5.16: Cystic duct variants

Subvesical ducts: (A) Segmental/sectorial—bile duct with unusual superficial course in proximity to gallbladder fossa, but otherwise typical anatomy, (B) Accessory subvesical bile duct—bile duct supernumerary from the formal biliary tree, (C) Cholecystohepatic duct—bile duct drains directly to gallbladder, (D) Aberrant subvesical bile ducts—network of small bile ducts within the connective tissue/capsule of the gallbladder fossa.

3.5.B Pancreas

The pancreas may have the shape of a dumbbell, tadpole, or sausage. Situated in the retroperitoneum in the anterior pararenal space. Lies in an oblique position posterior to the stomach. The pancreas is bordered by the lesser sac above, the transverse colon anteriorly, and the peritoneal cavity below. It can be divided into four main parts: **Head**—thickest part; lies anterior to the plane of the SMA and to the right of the superior mesenteric vein. **Uncinate process**—extension of the head, posterior to the plane of the SMA attached to "C" loop of duodenum (D2 and D3). **Neck**—thinnest part; lies anterior to the portal vein. SMV joins splenic vein behind pancreatic neck to form portal vein. **Body**—main part; lies to right of the IMV. Anterior surface is covered with peritoneum forming the posterior surface of the omental bursa (lesser sac). Splenic vein lies in the groove on posterior surface of body. **Tail**—lies to the left of the IMV and between layers of the splenorenal ligament in the splenic hilum.

Two major pathways of **pancreatic innervation:** The plexus pancreaticus capitalis 1 and 2. Plexus pancreaticus capitalis 1 arises from the right celiac ganglion and travels posteriorly past the portal vein to enter the pancreatic uncinate process at upper medial margin. It has been part of the posterior hepatic plexus, involved in perineural invasion of adenocarcinoma of the head of the pancreas. Plexus pancreaticus capitalis 2 arises from the superior mesenteric artery plexus and runs largely via the posteroinferior pancreaticoduodenal artery and the jejunal trunk to reach the uncinate process. For adenocarcinomas of the uncinate process, this is the main route of extrapancreatic perineural invasion. **Pancreatic duct:** The pancreatic duct runs from the tail to the head and enters the common bile duct at the hepatopancreatic ampulla at a 60° angle. **Main pancreatic duct** is a portion of the dorsal duct proximal to the dorsal–ventral fusion point, drains at the ampulla of Vater. **Pancreatic duct of Wirsung**—it is a segment of the ventral duct between the dorsal–ventral fusion point and the major papilla that is located at the distal end of the main pancreatic duct. **The accessory pancreatic duct (of Santorini)** is a branch of the dorsal duct that drains the anterior and superior portions of the head. It is located distal to the dorsal–ventral fusion point.

Variation in course of pancreatic duct: (A) Descending, (B) vertical, (C) sigmoid, (D) loop-shaped course.

Variation in configuration of pancreatic duct: (A) Bifid configuration with dominant duct of Wirsung drainage, (B) bifid configuration with dominant duct of Santorini drainage without divisum, (C) rudimentary non-draining duct of Santorini (D) pancreas divisum, (E) ansa pancreatica.

Pancreatic divisum: (A) Small branches of ventral duct may retain communnication with dorsal duct, (B) duct of Wirsung is completely absent, (C) no communication between dominant dorsal duct and small ventral duct.

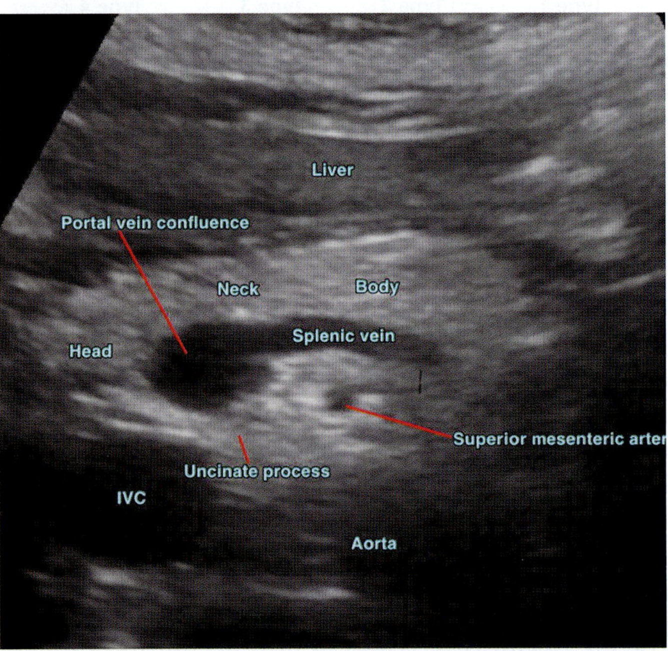

Fig. 3.5.17: USG parts of pancreas

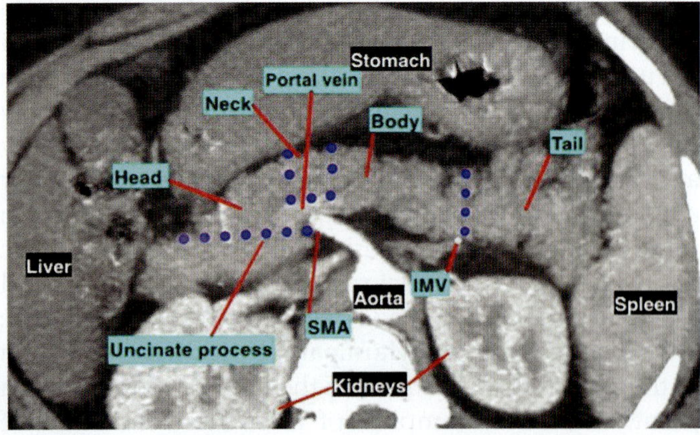

Fig. 3.5.18: CT parts of pancreas

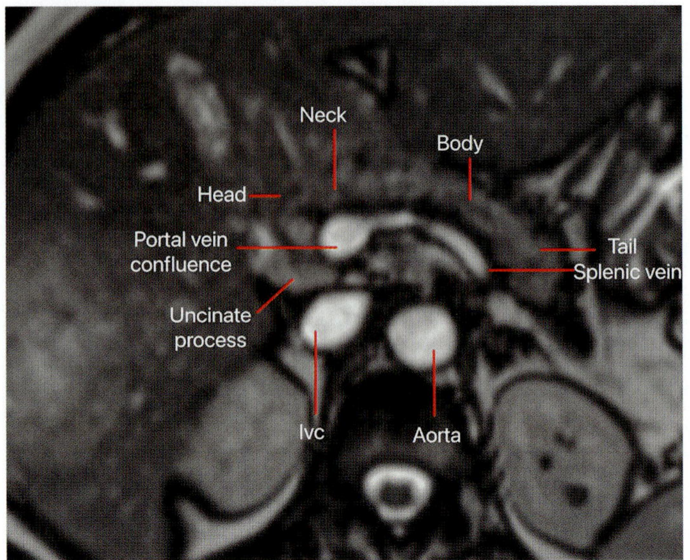

Fig. 3.5.19: MRI parts of pancreas

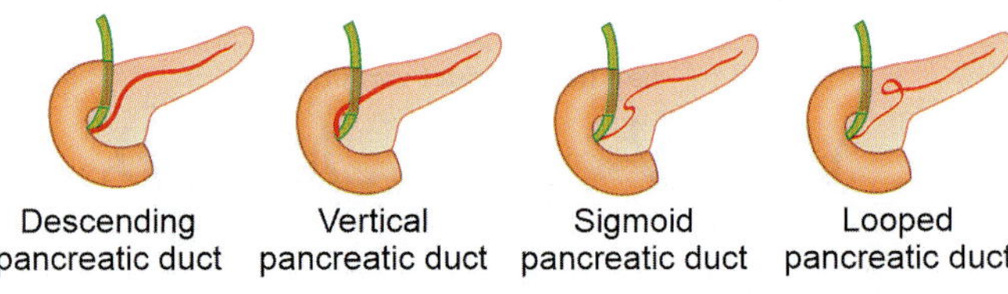

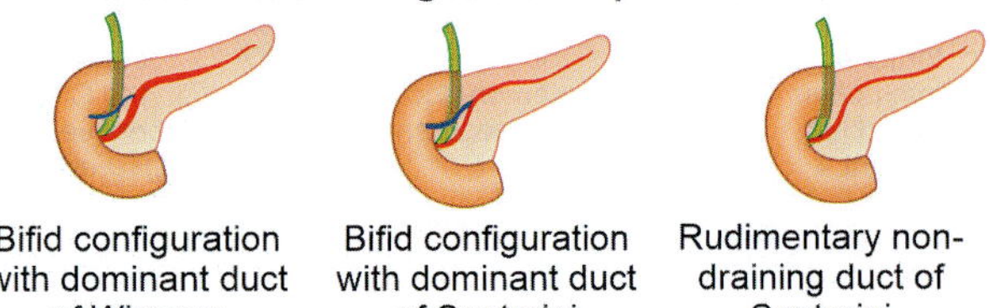

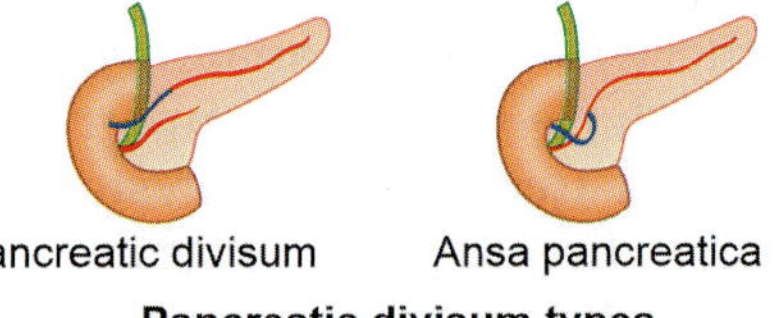

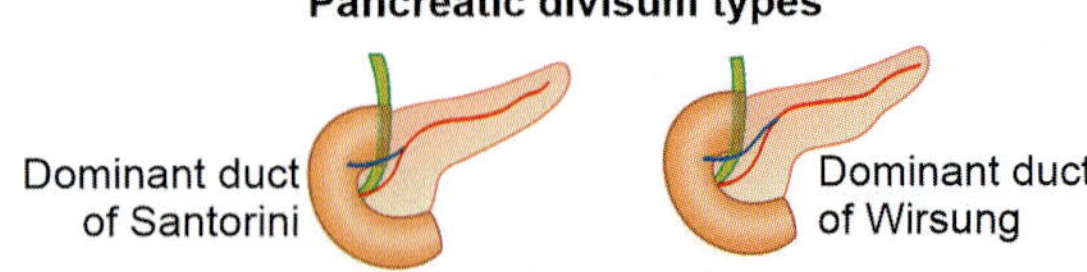

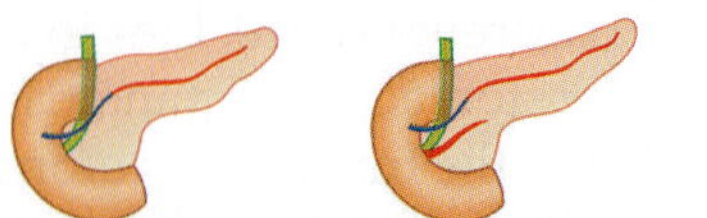

Fig. 3.5.20: Pancreatic duct variants

3.5.C Spleen Anatomy

The spleen is a wedge-shaped organ lying mainly in the left upper quadrant (left hypochondrium and partly in the epigastrium) and is protected by the left 9th to 11th ribs. The spleen is completely covered by peritoneum, except at the hilum, which forms a number of ligaments: Gastrosplenic ligament, splenorenal ligament. The splenic parenchyma consists of lymphatic follicles and reticuloendothelial cells, surrounding the arteries (white pulp) and an interspersed network of vascular sinusoids (red pulp). The ratio of white to red pulp increases with age due to accumulated antigenic exposure and stimulation. **On CECT**, the differing circulatory routes through the splenic pulp result in an unique inhomogeneous enhancement pattern in arterial/early portal venous phase termed **tigroid splenic enhancement** (red pulp enhances early, white pulp enhances later). In later phases, uniform enhancement is noted. Splenic lobules are remains of foetal splenic lobulation that persist as variances in normal form throughout adulthood. They are most typically found near the spleen's medial border, and they are sometimes fed by a branch of the splenic artery. The splenic margins often have notches or clefts, which are vestiges of the grooves that separated the foetal lobules. They usually have sharp edges and can reach a depth of 2–3 cm. Although splenic lobules have no clinical significance, they should not be mistaken for splenic laceration in individuals who have experienced abdominal trauma.

The absence of free abdominal or perisplenic fluid, as well as normal splenic enhancement are important imaging findings that distinguish these variants from laceration.

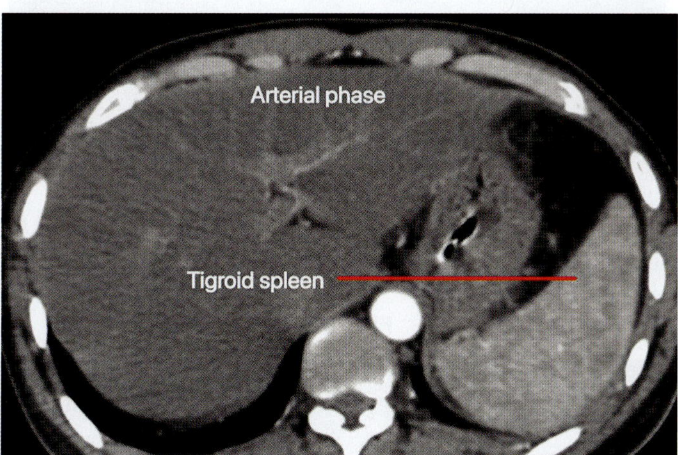

Fig. 3.5.21: Spleen arterial phase

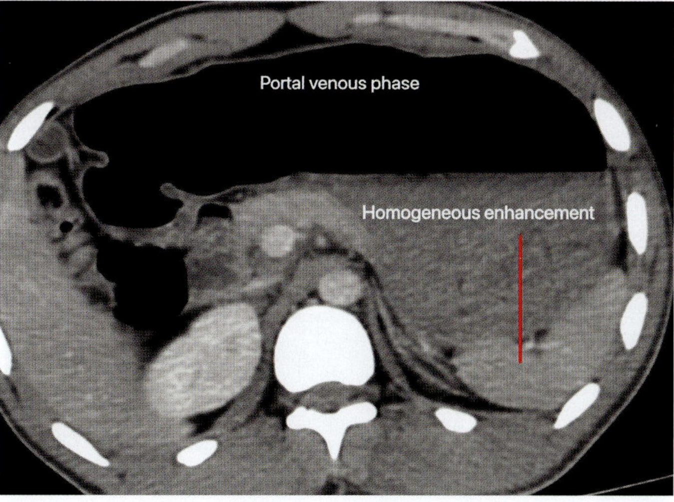

Fig. 3.5.22: Spleen venous phase

3.5.D Peritoneum Anatomy

The peritoneum is the body's largest and most complexly structured serous membrane. It is a thin, translucent serous membrane. The peritoneal cavity is the area between the parietal peritoneum, which lines the abdominal wall, and the visceral peritoneum, which surrounds the abdominal organs. The peritoneal cavity is closed in men, while it communicates with the extraperitoneal pelvis via the fallopian tubes, uterus, and vaginal canal in women. The **greater sac** is further subdivided into supramesocolic and the inframesocolic spaces by the transverse colon and its mesentery, which are then subdivided into multiple compartments and recesses due to peritoneal reflections. **Supramesocolic space** is further subdivided into right and left compartments.

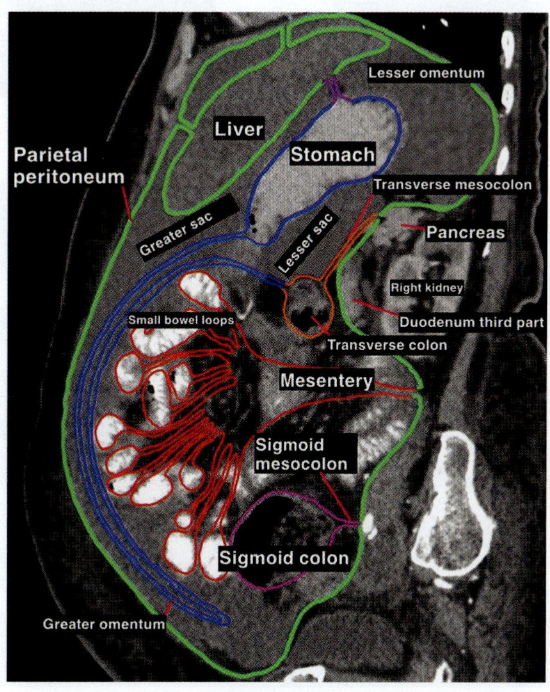

Fig. 3.5.23

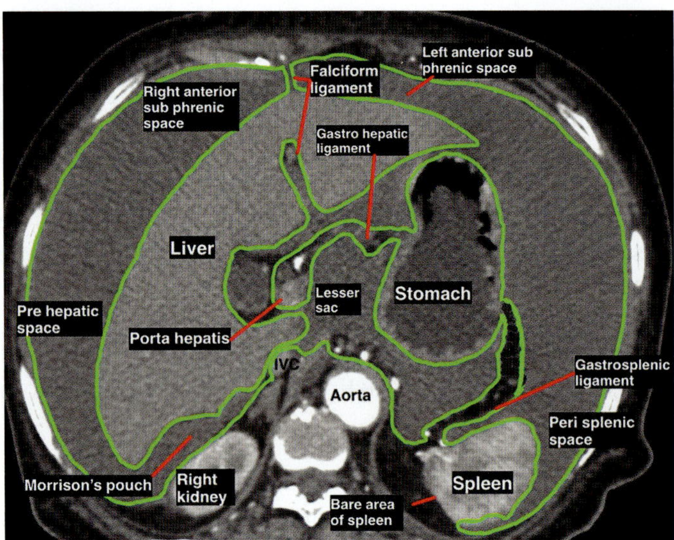

Fig. 3.5.24

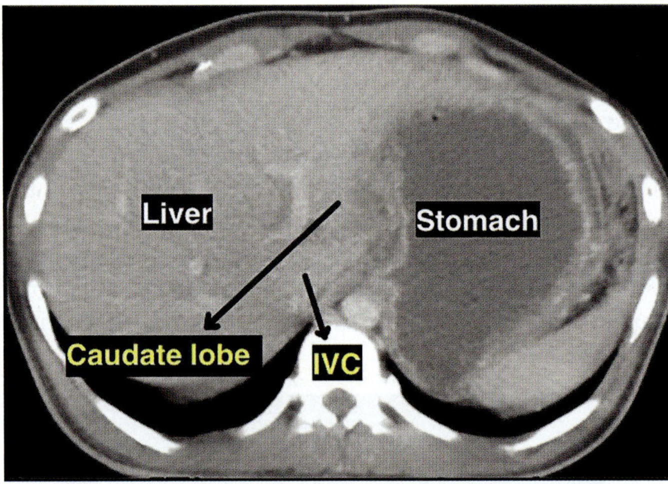

Fig. 3.5.25

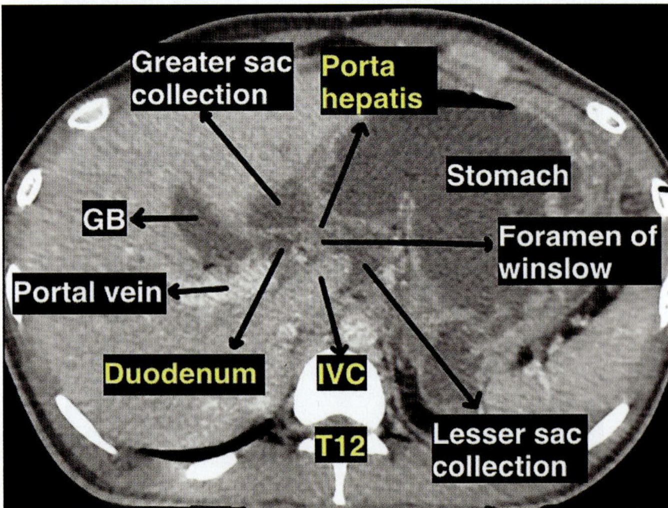

Fig. 3.5.26

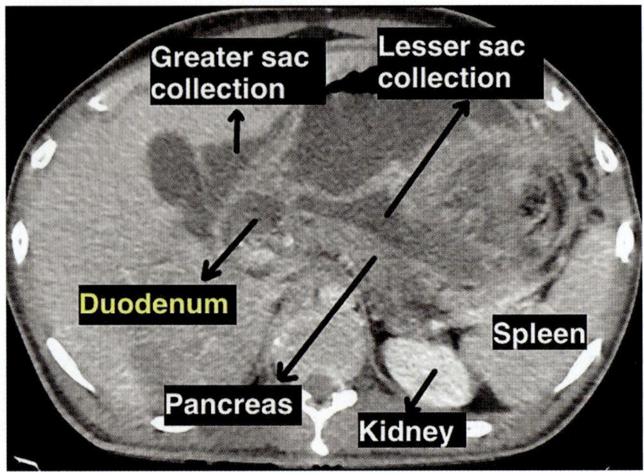

Fig. 3.5.27

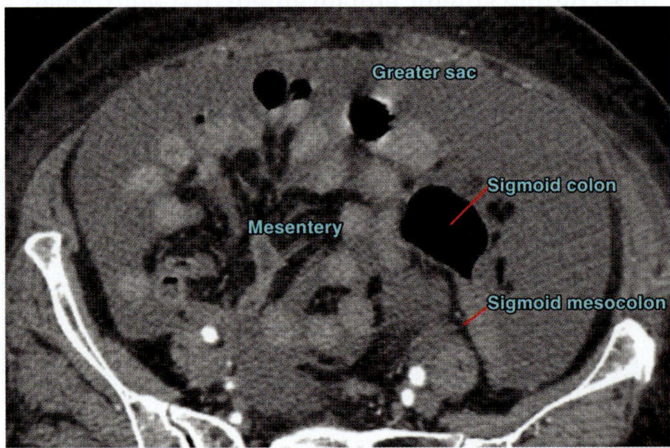

Fig. 3.5.28

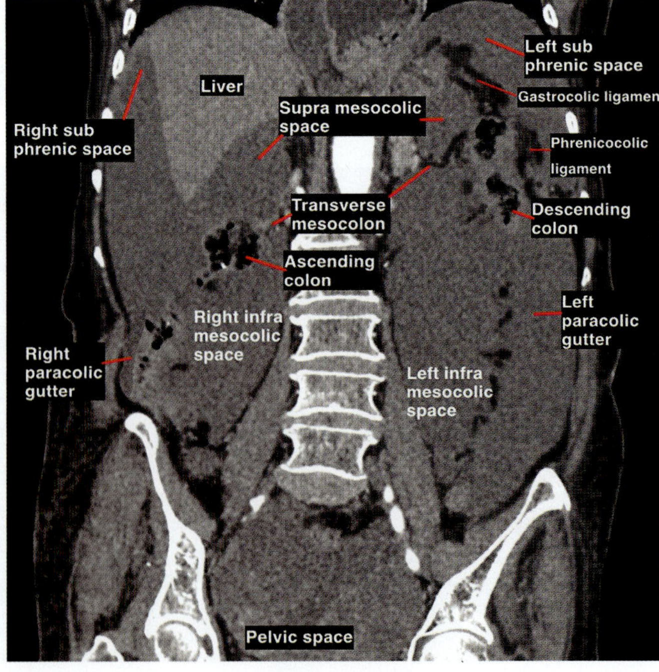

Fig. 3.5.29

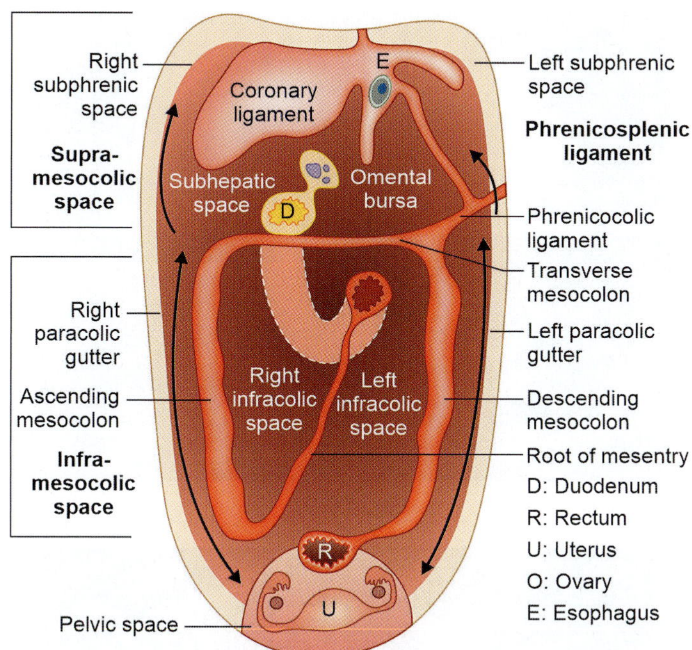

Fig. 3.5.30

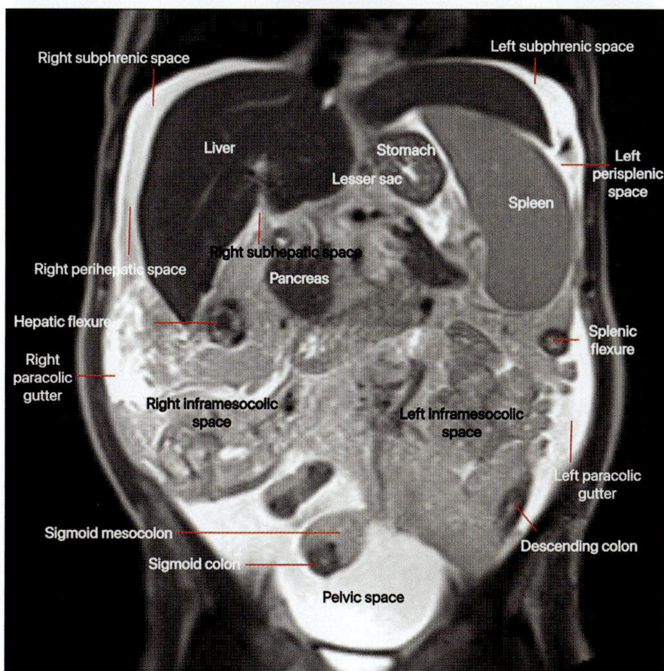

Fig. 3.5.31

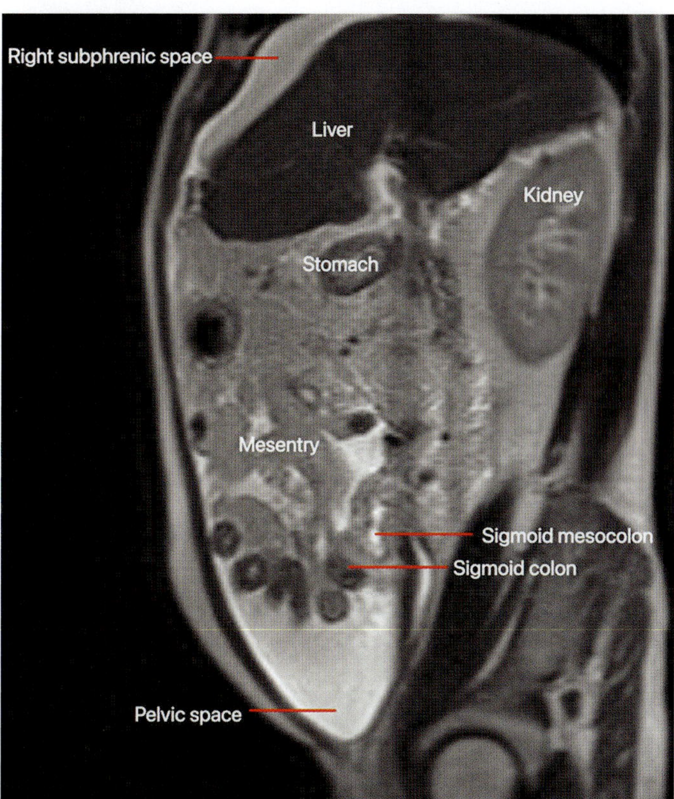

Fig. 3.5.32

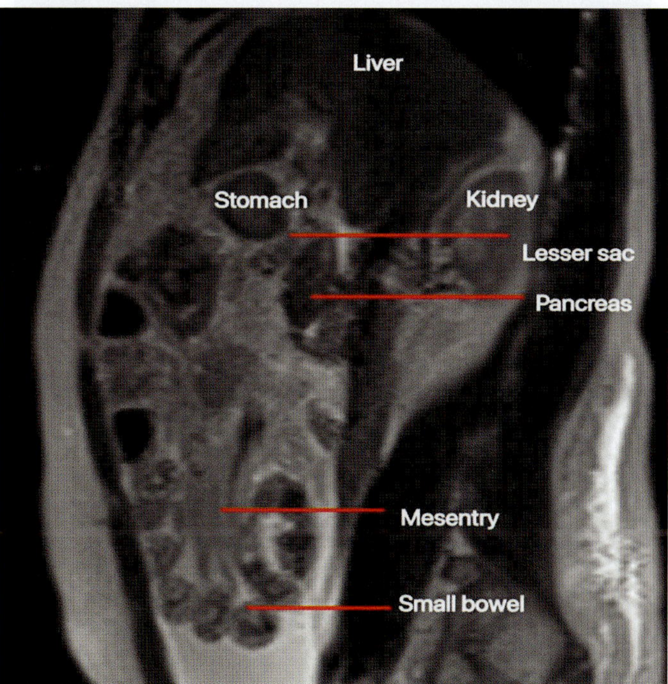

Fig. 3.5.33

Right supramesocolic space: Right perihepatic space including the right subphrenic space and right subhepatic space/Morrison's pouch. **Lesser sac** bounded by caudate lobe of liver superiorly, IVC posteriorly, free border of lesser omentum, CBD, portal vein and hepatic artery anteriorly. It communicates with the greater sac through the epiploic foramen. **Left supramesocolic space:** Left anterior perihepatic space, left posterior perihepatic space, left anterior subphrenic space, left posterior subphrenic space. **Inframesocolic space:** Infracolic space—right and left, paracolic gutters—right and left, pelvis containing lateral paravesical

3

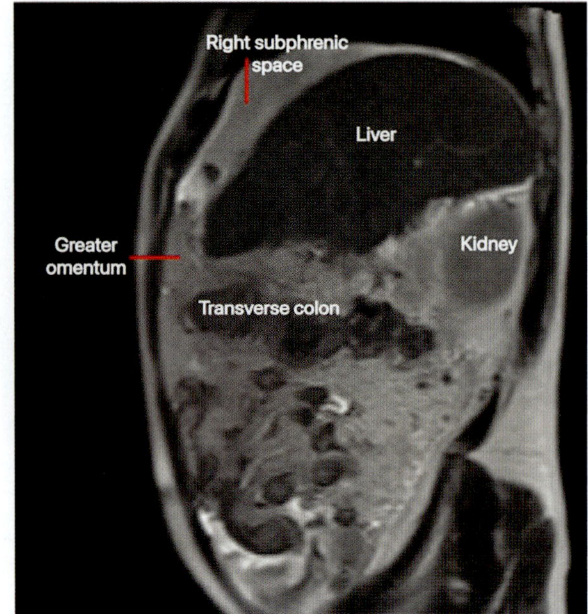

Fig. 3.5.34

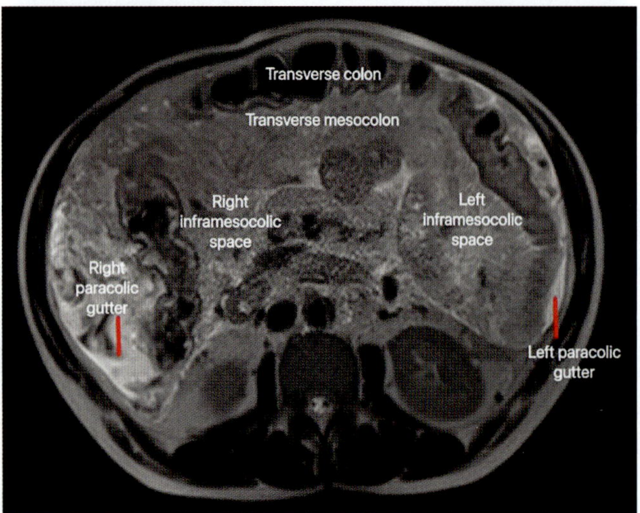

Fig. 3.5.35

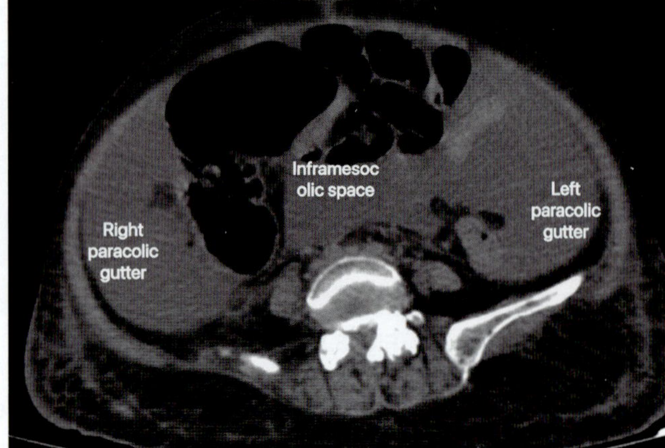

Fig. 3.5.36

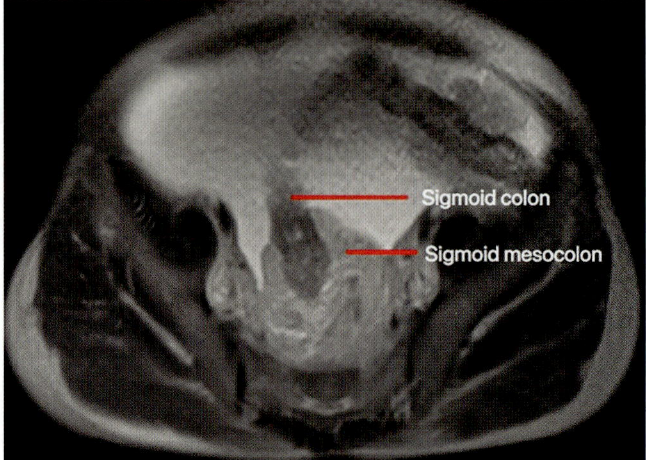

Fig. 3.5.37

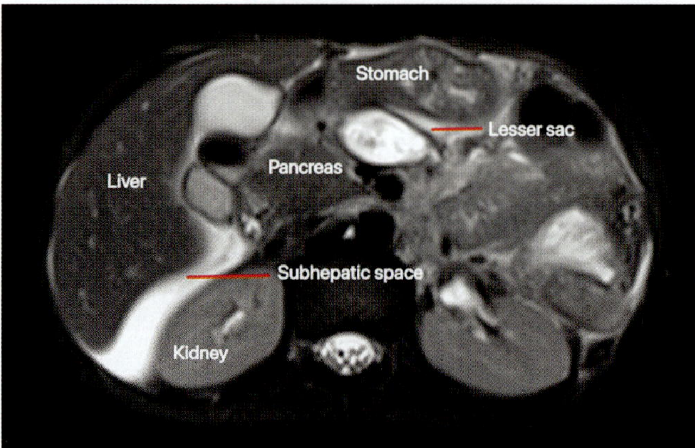

Fig. 3.5.38

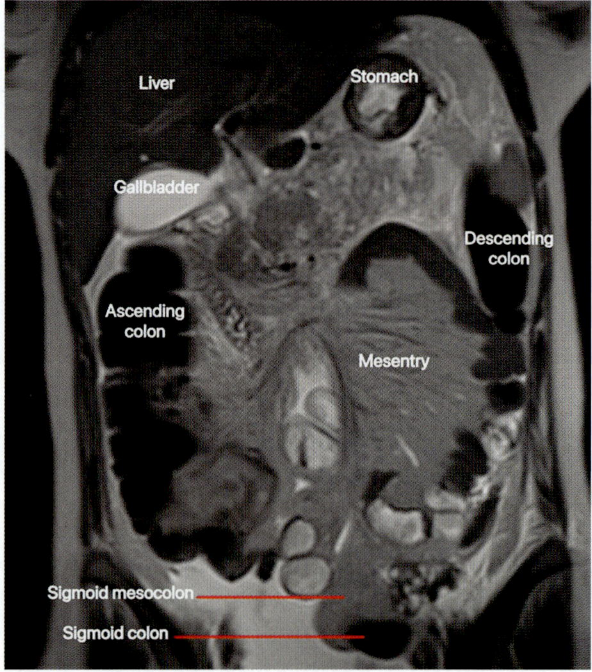

Fig. 3.5.39

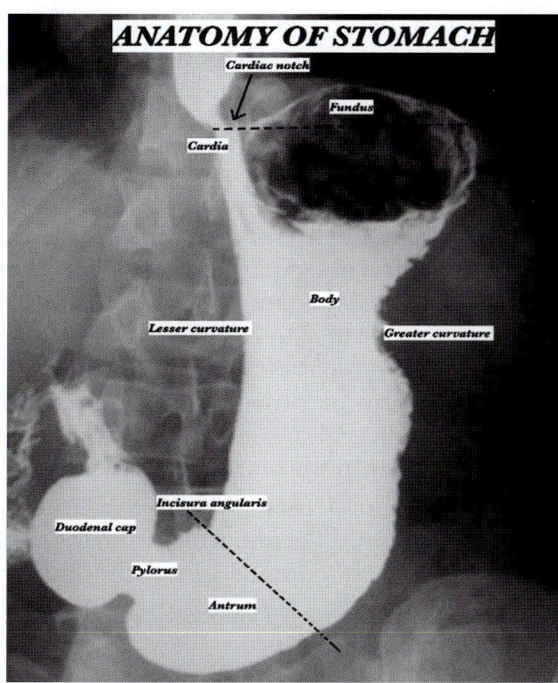

Fig. 3.5.40a: Stomach parts on barium swallow

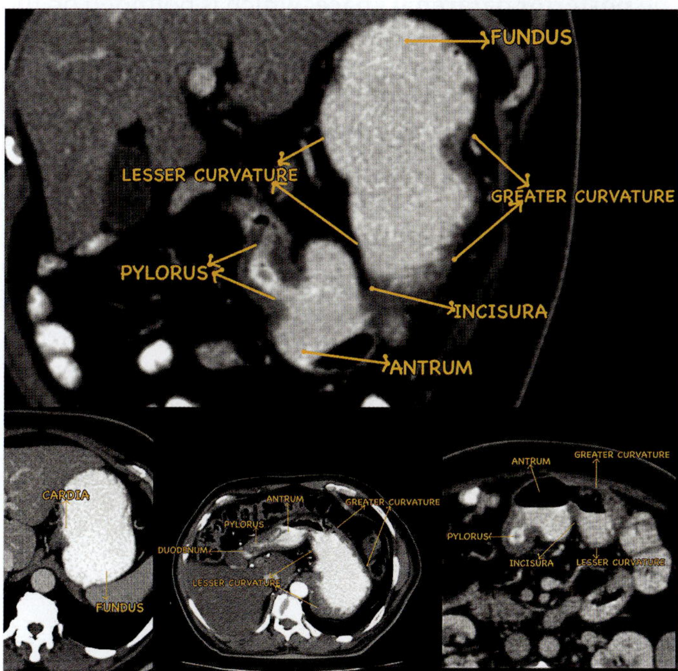

Fig. 3.5.40b: Parts of stomach in CT oral contrast study

space, rectovesical space in men, rectouterine sapce in women. Figures 3.5.23 to 3.5.39 show peritoneal spaces.

The **omentum** is a mesentery, or double layer of peritoneum, that runs from the stomach to the duodenal bulb and connects to other organs. The **lesser omentum** connects the stomach and duodenal bulb to the liver and is made up of two continuous ligaments called the gastrohepatic and hepatoduodenal ligaments. The stomach is connected to the **greater omentum,** which hangs like an apron from the transverse colon. **Mesentery** is a double peritoneum layer that surrounds and links an organ to the abdominal wall. Blood vessels, lymph nodes, nerves, and fat are all included in the mesenteric contents. The mesentery covers the most mobile elements of the intestine (e.g. the small bowel linked to the retroperitoneum), and the retroperitoneal regions of the colon may contain remnant mesocolon as a result of the colon's failure to absorb embryonic mesentery. The **transverse mesocolon** is a broad, meso-fold of peritoneum, which connects the transverse colon to the posterior wall of the abdomen.

3.5.E Stomach

The stomach is a muscular organ located in the upper abdomen between the oesophagus and the duodenum. **The cardia, fundus, body, antrum, and pylorus** are the five segments of the stomach.The gastric cardia surrounds the lower oesophagus and is the most proximal portion. When the patient is upright, the fundus is the most superior region of the stomach, and when the patient is supine, the fundus is the most dependent portion. The stomach bubble observed on upright radiographs is due to the fundus, which is also the most prevalent site for intraluminal contents accumulation on CT, particularly blood products. The lesser curvature can be found on axial imaging to the right and posteriorly, whereas the greater curvature can be found to the left and anteriorly. The gastric antrum is the stomach's most muscular section, has the most peristalsis, and is hence the thickest gastric segment. Rugal folds on the inner mucosal surface increase the surface area of the stomach lining, which improves its efficiency. **The incisura angularis** marks the transition to antral-type mucosa between the stomach body and the antrum. The superior arch-shaped edge of the stomach's fundus is known as the **fornix gastricus**.

Arterial supply: Right gastric artery (inferiorly) and left gastric artery (superiorly) to lessser curvature. Cardia—left gastric artery, greater curvature—right gastroepiploic artery (inferiorly) and left gastroepiploic artery and short gastric arteries (superiorly), fundus of the stomach—short gastric arteries.

Venous drainage: Left and right gastric veins drain to portal vein, short gastric and left gastroepiploic veins drain into splenic vein, right gastroepiploic vein drains into superior mesenteric vein.

3.5.F Small Bowel

It has distinctive mucosal folds, valvulae conniventes, and is made up of three functional units: Duodenum, jejunum, ileum. The duodenum runs from the pylorus to the duodenojejunal flexure, where a mesentery marks the transition to the small bowel proper. Around the head of the pancreas, the duodenum curls in a C shape. It is divided into four sections—first, second, third, and fourth. These are 2 cm, 8 cm, 8 cm, and 4 cm in length, respectively.

The first part starts at the level of the L1 lumbar vertebra, the second at L2, the third at L3, and the fourth at L2.

Jejunoileal fold pattern reversal: Indicates celiac disease.

Table 3.5.1: Jejunum vs ileum

Jejunum	*Ileum*
Upper left part of greater sac	Lower right part of greater sac
Greater calibre, thicker walls, more vascular (normal diameter <3 cm)	Lesser calibre, thinner walls, less vascular (normal diameter <2 cm)
Mucosal folds (valvulae conniventes), thicker, more numerous, deeper, greater caliber, number—4–6/inch	Mucosal folds,less thick, lesser in number, superficial lesser caliber, number—2–4/inch
Mesenteric fat—less	Mesenteric fat— more
—	Prominent Peyer patches in ileum

3.5.G Large Intestine

From the cecum to the rectum, it is a long tube. It contains three outer longitudinal muscular layers known as taenia coli that are approximately 30 cm shorter than the length of the large bowel, resulting in characteristic sacculations interrupted by incomplete rings known as haustra. Cecum, appendix, ascending colon, right colic flexure, transverse colon, left colic flexure, descending colon, sigmoid colon, rectum are the parts of the large bowel.

3.5.H Appendix

The appendix or vermiform appendix (plural: Appendices) is a blind muscular tube that arises from the posteromedial surface of cecum. It is a blind diverticulum that varies in length from 2 to 20 cm and is located on its own mesentery, the mesoappendix.Retrocecal (65–70%), pelvic (25–30%), pre- or post-ileal (5%), promontory, paracaecal, and subcecal are all possible positions for the appendix tip within the abdominal cavity.

The appendicular artery provides blood to the appendix (branch of the ileocolic artery from the superior mesenteric artery). The venous blood drains into the superior mesenteric vein via the corresponding veins.

3.5.I Retroperitoneum

The retroperitoneum is divided into three compartments: The **posterior pararenal space**, which is bounded on the back by the transversalis fascia; the **anterior pararenal space**, which is bounded on the front by the parietal peritoneum; and the **perirenal space**, which is bounded on the front by the perirenal fascia. The pancreas, as well as the ascending and descending colon, form the majority of the structures in the anterior pararenal region, which arise from the dorsal mesentery. The kidneys and adrenal glands are located in the perinephric space, which is bounded on the front by **Gerota fascia** and the back by **Zuckerkandl fascia**. The transversalis fascia runs posteriorly while the lateroconal fascia runs laterally, enclosing the tiny posterior pararenal space. The aorta

Fig. 3.5.41: Large bowel parts

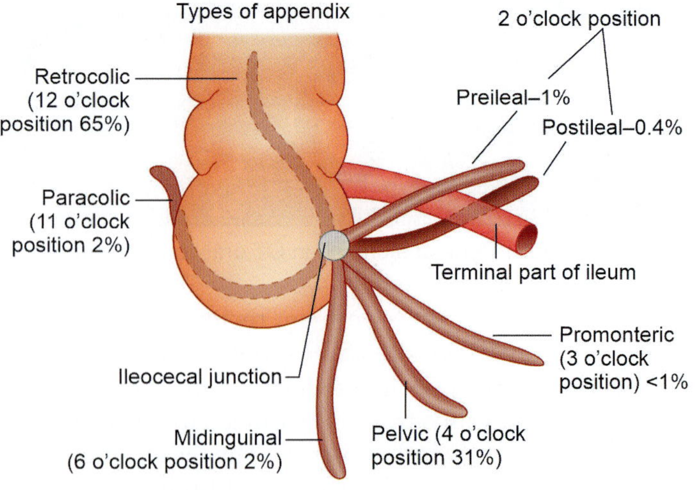

Fig. 3.5.42: Appendix positions

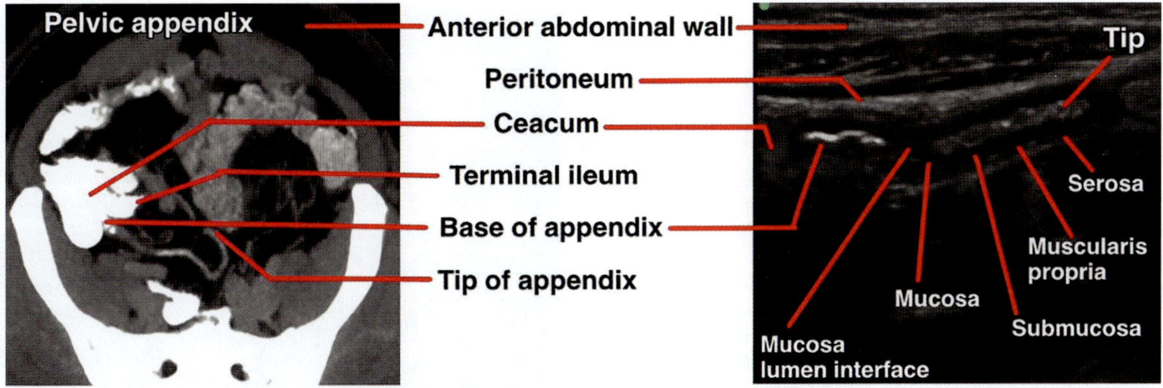

Fig. 3.5.43: Parts of appendix on CT and ultrasound

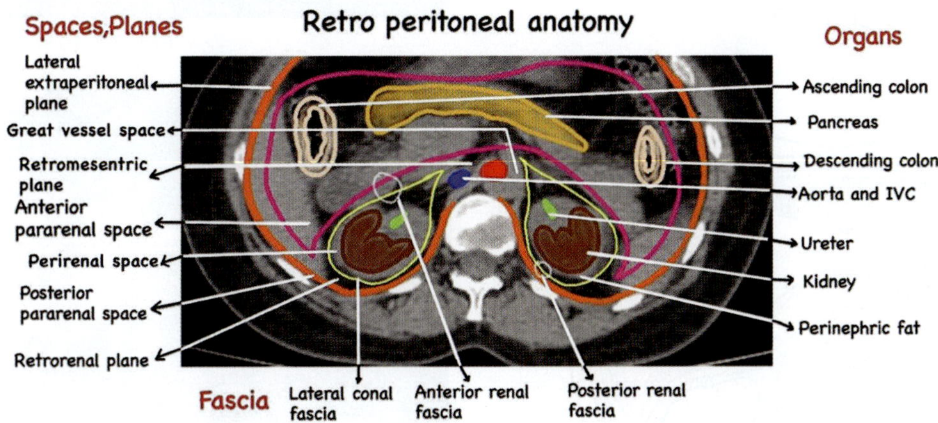

Fig. 3.5.44

and inferior vena cava are surrounded by a fourth space known as the **great vessel space**. The perirenal spaces and ureters limit this region laterally, but it continues superiorly into the posterior mediastinum. Between the anterior pararenal space and the perirenal space is the retromesenteric plane, which has the potential to expand. Because the great vessel space interrupts it, it does not cross the midline. The **psoas major muscle** is one of the muscles of the posterior abdominal wall and lies not in the retroperitoneum but posterior to it, in the iliopsoas compartment (Figs 3.5.44–3.5.52).

3.5.J Kidneys

The kidneys lie retroperitoneally in the paravertebral gutters of the posterior abdominal wall. They lie obliquely with their upper poles more medial and more posterior than their lower. The kidneys measure 10–15 cm in length, 3–5 cm wide, 3 cm in antero-posterior thickness, the left being commonly 1.5 cm longer than the right.

The kidney is bean-shaped with a superior and an inferior pole, anterior and posterior surfaces, and lateral and medial borders. The renal parenchyma, which includes the renal cortex and medulla, and the renal sinus, which includes the renal pelvis, calyces, renal arteries, nerves, lymphatics, and perirenal fat. The cortex and medulla are the two layers of the renal parenchyma. The renal cortex is located on the periphery of the capsule, while the renal medulla is composed of 10–14 renal pyramids separated by renal columns, which are an inward extension of the renal cortex. The renal lobes, which are made up of the renal pyramid, the overlaying renal cortex, and the surrounding renal columns, produce urine. Each renal lobe empties into a minor calyx at a papilla, and four or five of these join to form a major calyx. The renal pelvis is formed by the joining of two or three major calyces in each kidney.

Arterial supply: Renal arteries (from the abdominal aorta), venous drinage—renal veins (to inferior vena cava), the sympathetic and parasympathetic renal nerve plexus is generated from the abdominopelvic splanchnic nerves.

Ultrasound: Although the cortex is normally less echogenic than the liver or spleen, it is iso or hyperechoic in comparison to these organs in the young infant.

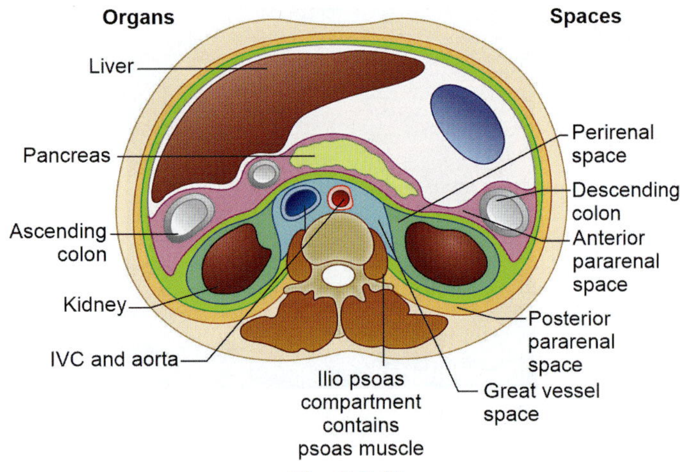

Fig. 3.5.45

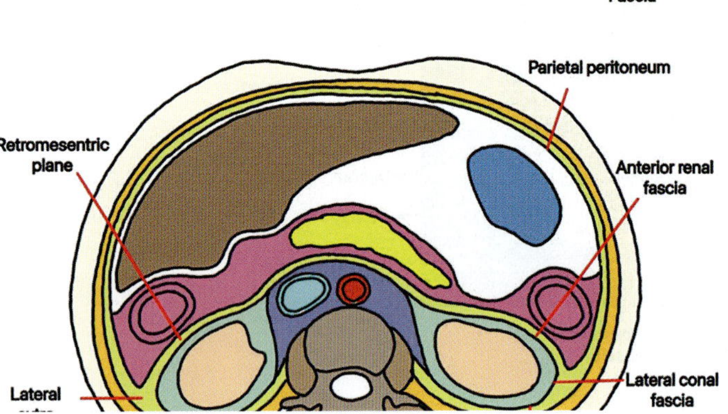

Fig. 3.5.46

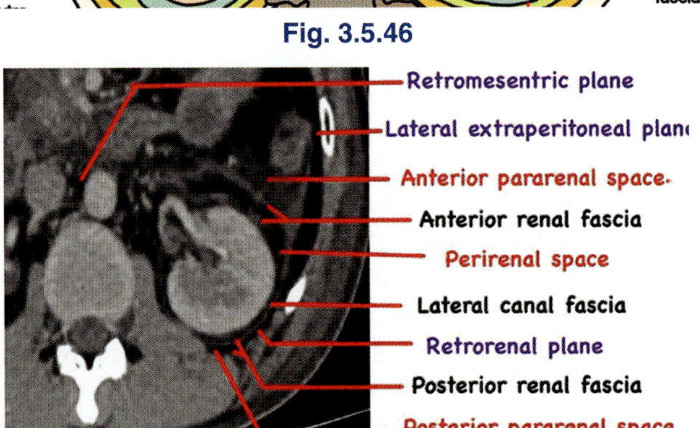

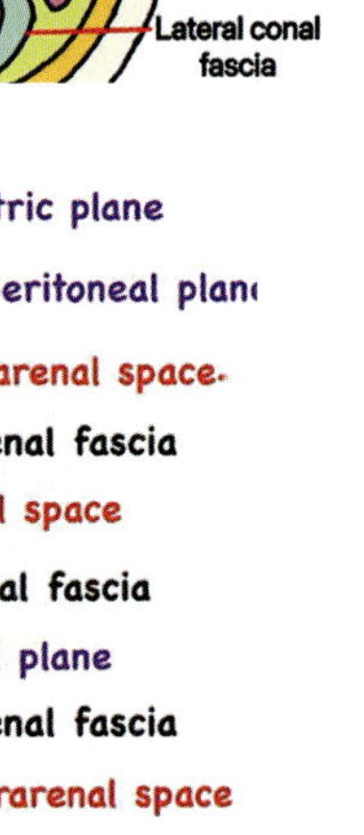

Fig. 3.5.47

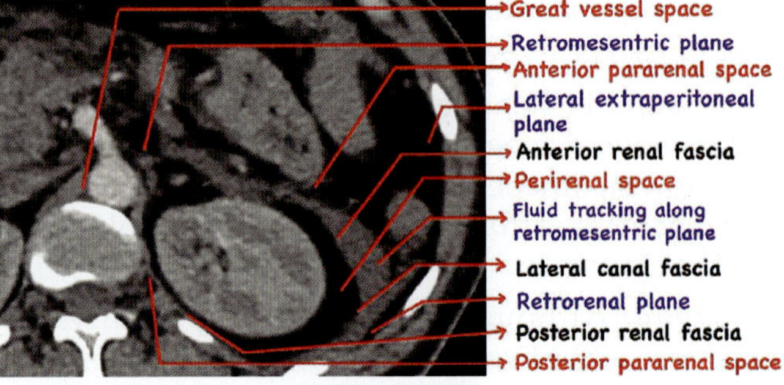

Fig. 3.5.48

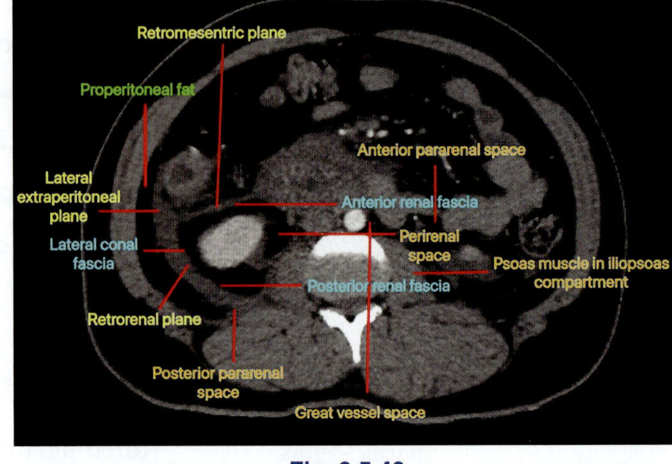

Fig. 3.5.49

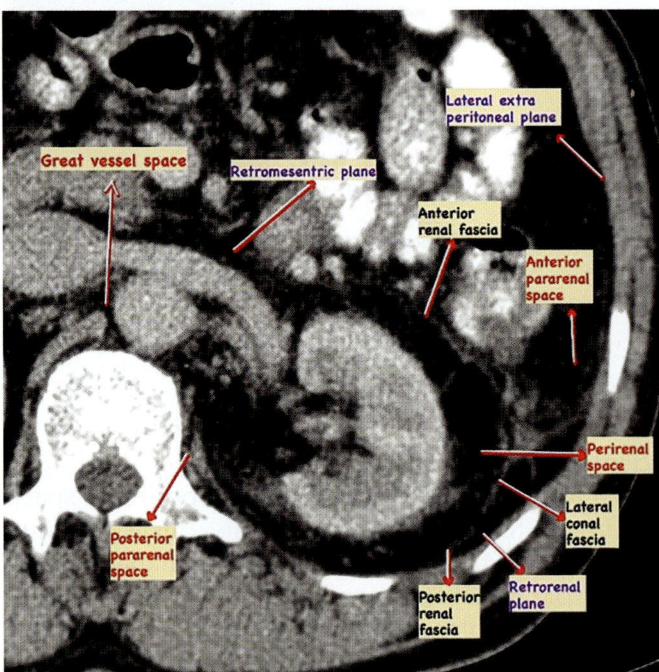

Fig. 3.5.50

Fig. 3.5.51

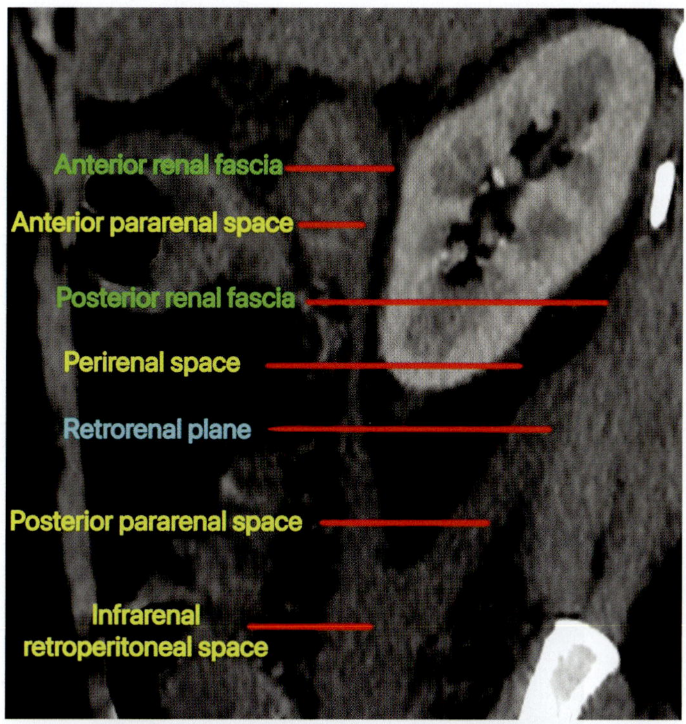

Fig. 3.5.52: Interfacial plane of the retroperitoneum

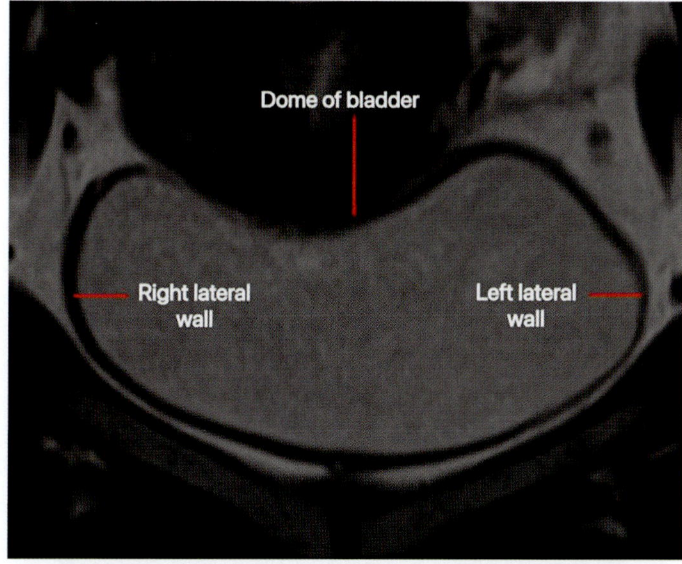

Fig. 3.5.53: MRI pelvis coronal section showing urinary bladder

The cortex has a thickness of more than 6 mm, and the medullary pyramids are slightly less echogenic. After 15 weeks of pregnancy, corticomedullary differentiation is evident, but at 20 weeks, clear distinction between cortex and medulla is evident. Because of the many tissue interfaces, the renal sinus contains fat, calyces, infundibulae, and veins, and is highly echogenic. It is possible that the renal pelvis is intrarenal or extrarenal. It may seem dilated when extrarenal. The collecting system's visualisation is variable. When the person is highly hydrated and/or in a condition of diuresis, it is most visible. Allowing you to distinguish between them.

Three phases of enhancement can be seen on both CT and MRI: The arterial corticomedullary phase is characterised by a substantial enhancement of the cortex and the greatest contrast between the cortex and the medulla. The contrast is homogenous throughout the kidney in the venous nephrographic phase. Delayed excretory phase: where contrast is seen in the collecting system. MRI: On T1-weighted images the renal cortex has a slightly higher signal than the medulla. On T2-weighted images the renal cortex is slightly lower in signal than the medulla (Figs 3.5.58–3.5.63).

The ureter: Course along posterior abdominal wall in retroperitoneum, just behind parietal peritoneum. Proximal ureters lie in perirenal space. In lower abdomen, lie on psoas muscles. In pelvis, lie along lateral walls near internal iliac vessels.

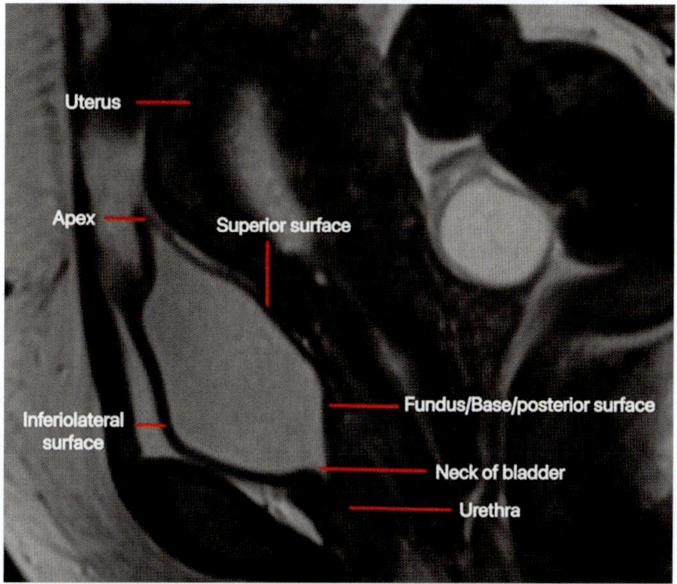

Fig. 3.5.54: MRI pelvis sagittal section showing parts of bladder

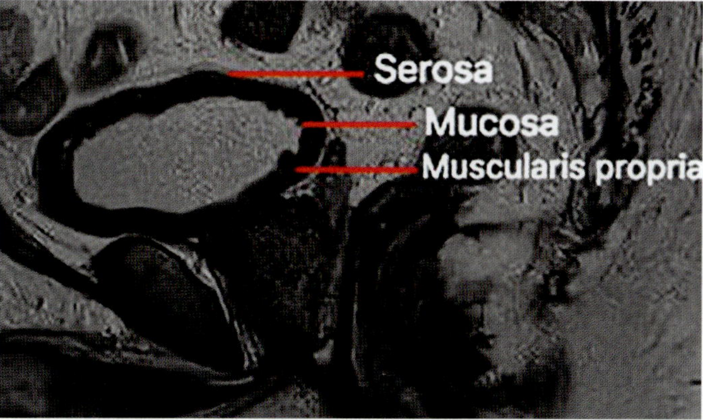

Fig. 3.5.55: MRI pelvis showing layers of bladder wall

At the level of ischial spines, ureters curve anteromedially to enter bladder at level of seminal vesicles (men) or cervix (women). Ureters travel obliquely through the muscular wall of the bladder, creating a valve effect that prevents urine reflux. Each one is 25–30 cm long and consists of abdominal, pelvic, and intravesical components.

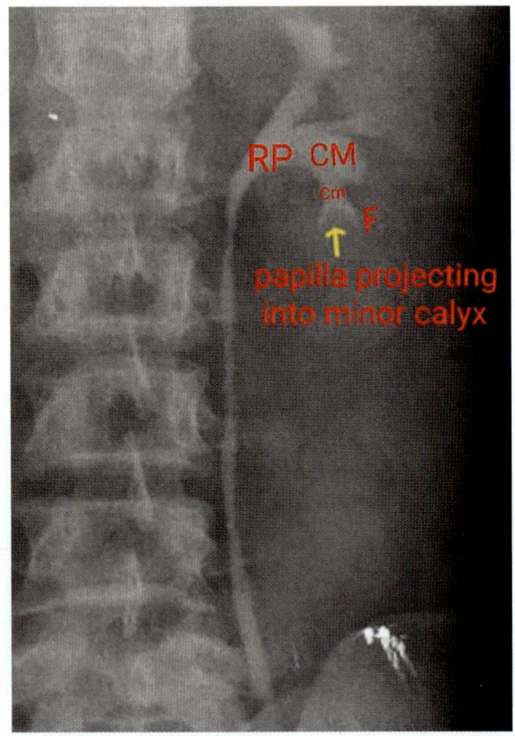

Fig. 3.5.56: IVU anatomy (*RP: Renal pelvis; CM: Major calyx; Cm: Minor calyx; F: Fornix)

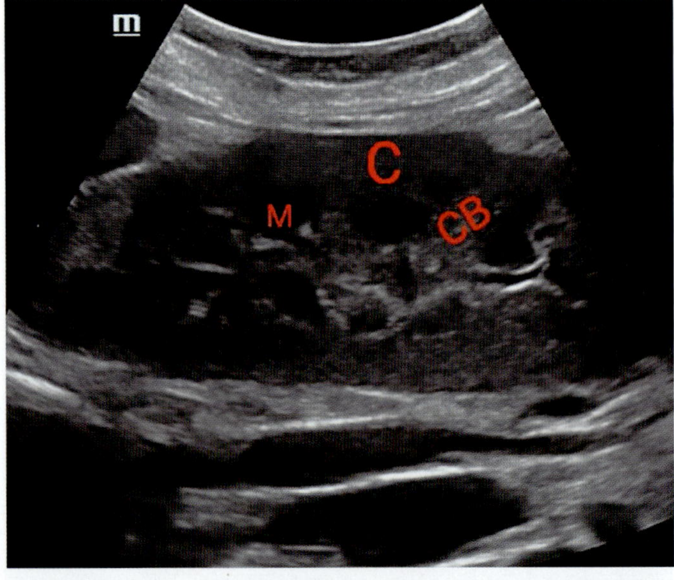

Fig. 3.5.57: Renal ultrasound (M–medulla, C–cortex, CB–column of Bertin)

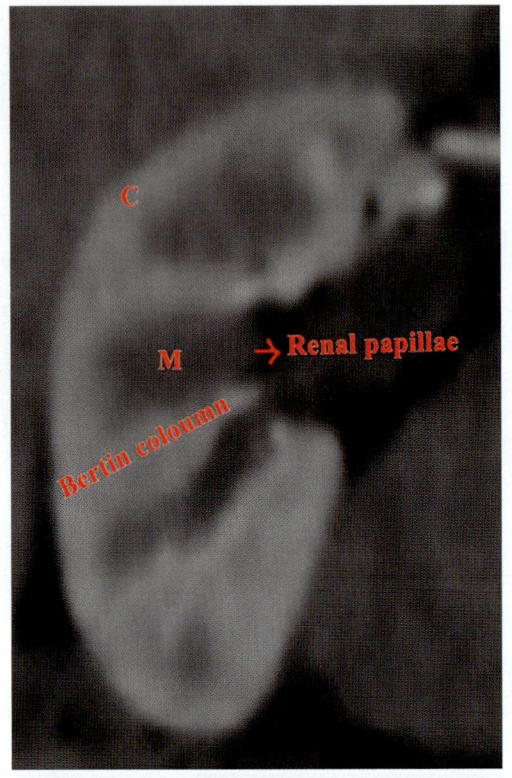

Fig. 3.5.58

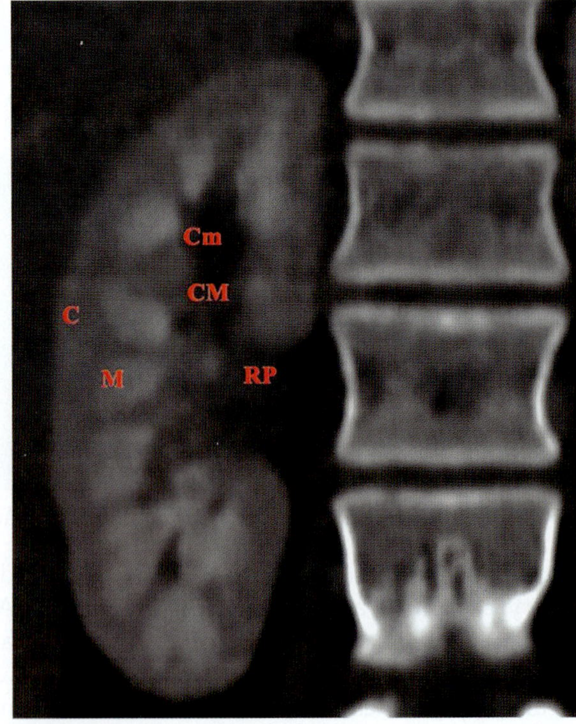

Fig. 3.5.59: RP: Renal pelvis; CM: Major calyx; Cm: Minor calyx M: medulla, C: cortex

The ureter has a diameter of around 3 mm, but it narrows at three points: The pelvis–ureter junction,

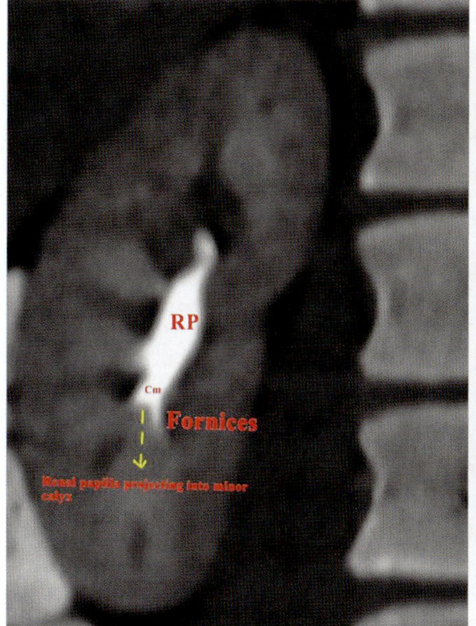

Fig. 3.5.60

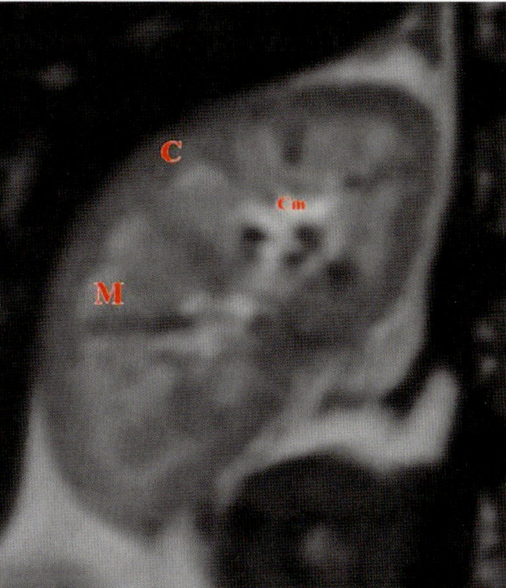

Fig. 3.5.61

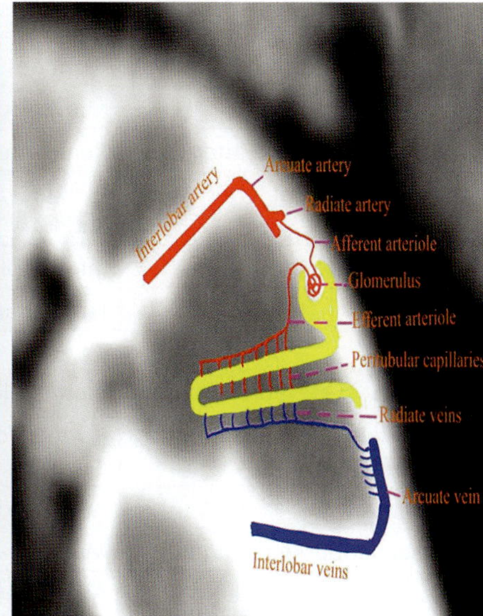

Fig. 3.5.62

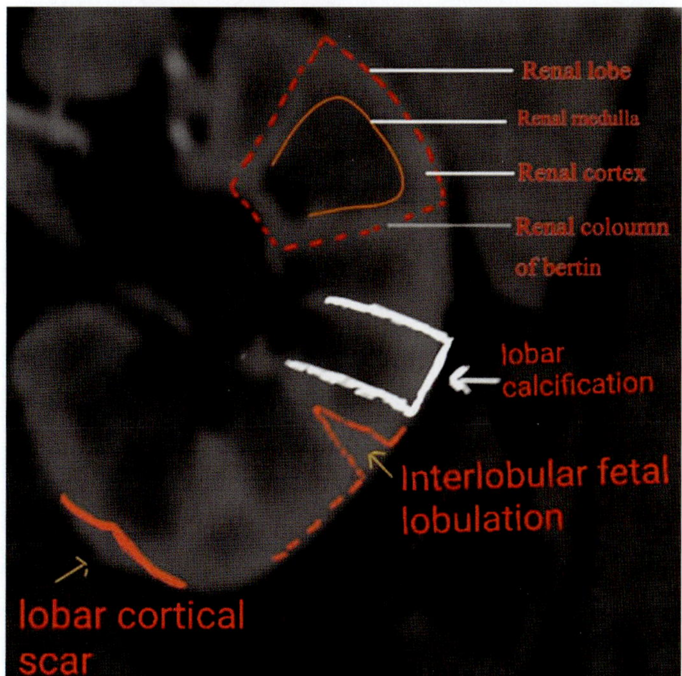

Fig. 3.5.63

the pelvic brim, and the intravesical ureter, which goes through the muscular bladder wall.

Bladder: The urinary bladder is a distal part of the urinary tract and is an extraperitoneal structure located in the true pelvis. The distended bladder has a round or oval form with a peritoneum-covered dome. The apex of the bladder, connected to the umbilicus by the urachus during embryologic development, is directed antero-superiorly; the bladder neck is positioned inferiorly.

On the interior surface of the base, the trigone is a triangular region of smooth mucosa. The ureteric orifices form the superolateral angles, while the internal urethral orifice forms the inferior angle. The internal urethral sphincter surrounds the urethra, which arises from the bladder's neck.

The adrenal glands: The adrenal glands lie retroperitoneally above each kidney.

Each gland is composed of a body and medial and lateral limbs.

Normal measurements: 5 × 3 × 1 cm (length × breadth × thickness)

On cross-section it is linear or V-shaped, with a larger medial limb and a smaller lateral limb.

On MRI: They are iso- or slightly hypointense compared to liver on both T1- and T2-weighted images. They lose signal on fat suppression or fat subtraction techniques.

Arterial supply: Three arteries supply these glands on each side: The superior adrenal artery originates from the inferior phrenic artery, while the middle adrenal artery originates from the aorta and the inferior adrenal artery originates from the renal artery.

Venous drainage: The right adrenal vein drains to the IVC and the left adrenal vein drains to the left renal vein.

3.5.K Abdomen Vascular Anatomy

The abdominal aorta is the major blood vessel in the abdominal cavity, carrying oxygenated blood from the thoracic cavity to the abdominal organs and lower limbs.

Table 3.5.2: Branches of abdominal aorta

Branches (unpaired)	*Branches (paired)*
Celiac artery (T12)	Middle adrenal arteries
Superior mesenteric artery (L1)	Renal arteries (L1–L2)
Inferior mesenteric artery (L3)	Gonadal arteries (between L2 and L3)
Median sacral artery	Inferior phrenic arteries
	Lumbar arteries

Table 3.5.3: Mesenteric vascular connections

Connections between celiac axis and SMA	*Connections between SMA and IMA*
Arc of Buhler	Arc of Riolan
Pancreaticoduodenal arcade	Marginal artery of Drummond
Dorsal pancreatic artery	Arc of Barkow
The right hepatic artery and the SMA have a communication channel.	

At L4, it divides into the right and left common iliac arteries. Coeliac trunk (CT) is wide ventral branch of aorta and normally divides into left gastric artery (LGA), common hepatic artery (CHA) and splenic artery. Coeliac trunk may also give off one or both inferior phrenic arteries. Gastroduodenal artery (GDA) arises from hepatic artery and divides into right gastro-epiploic and superior pancreaticoduodenal arteries. Superior pancreaticoduodenal arteries are usually double—anterior

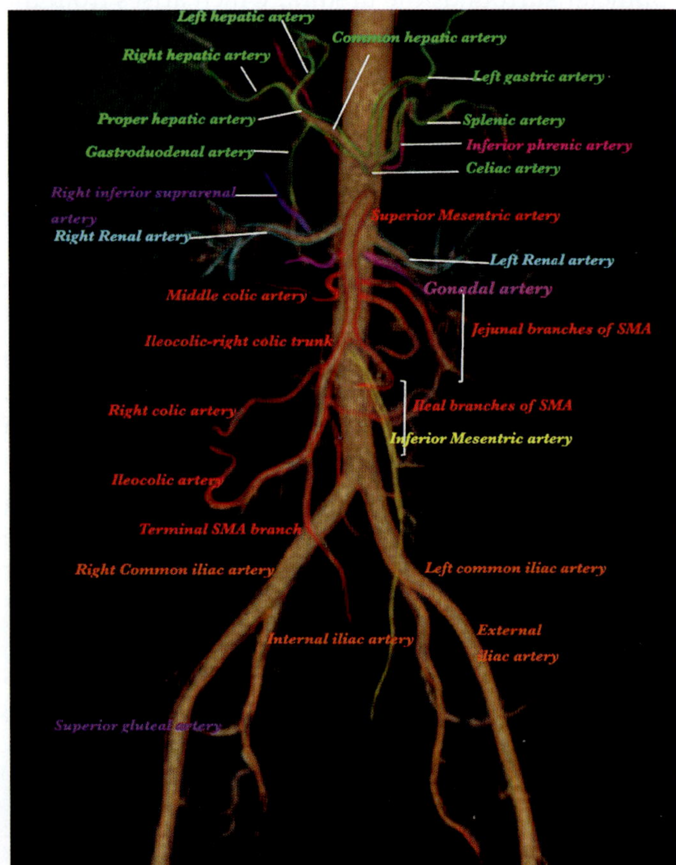

Fig. 3.5.64: Branches of abdominal aorta

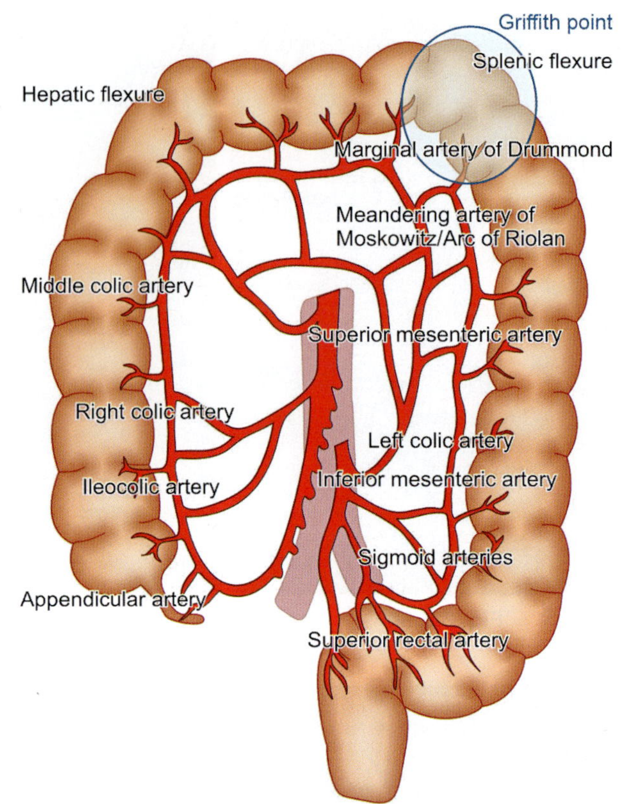

Fig. 3.5.65: Arterial supply of large intestine

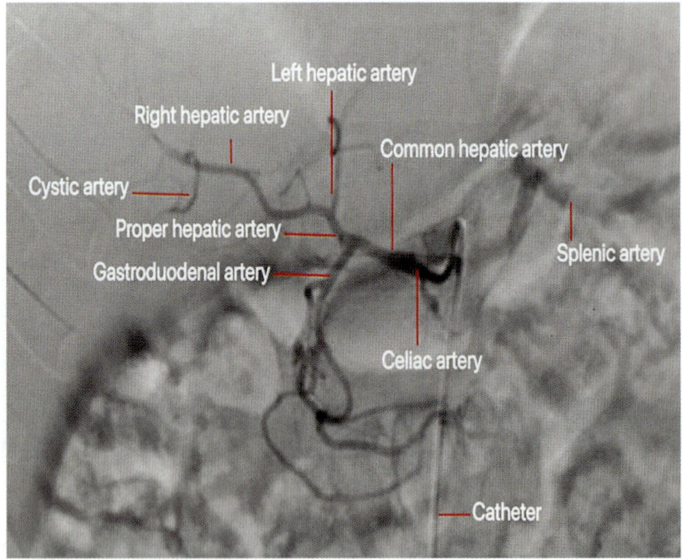

Fig. 3.5.66: Celiac artery and branches

3

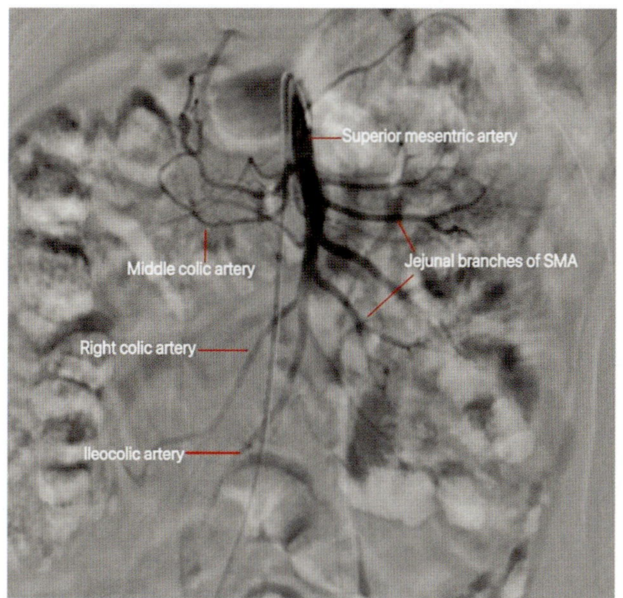

Fig. 3.5.67: SMA and branches

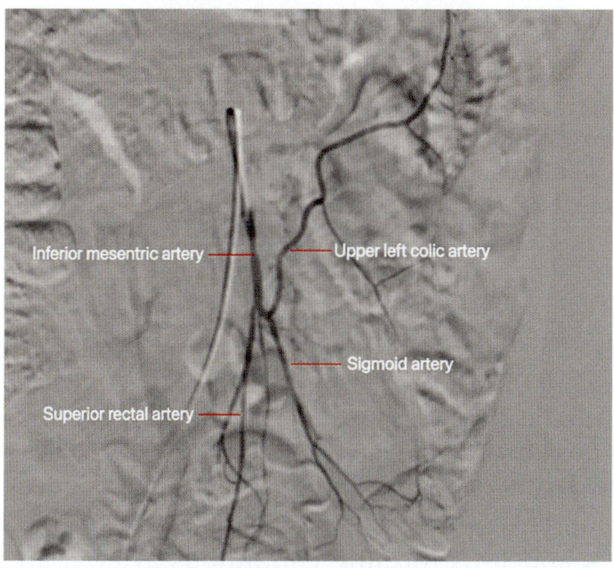

Fig. 3.5.68: IMA and branches

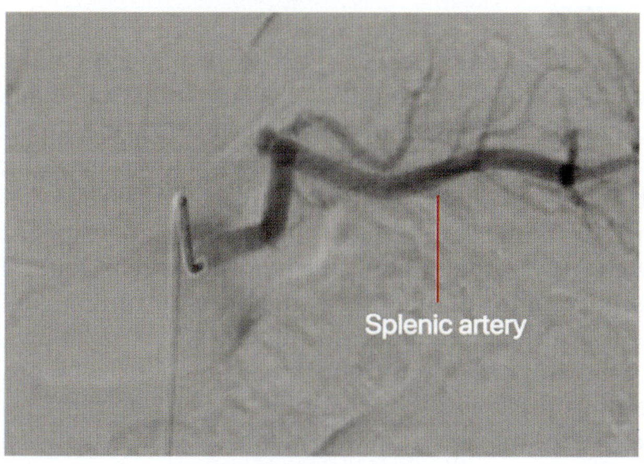

Fig. 3.5.69: Splenic artery

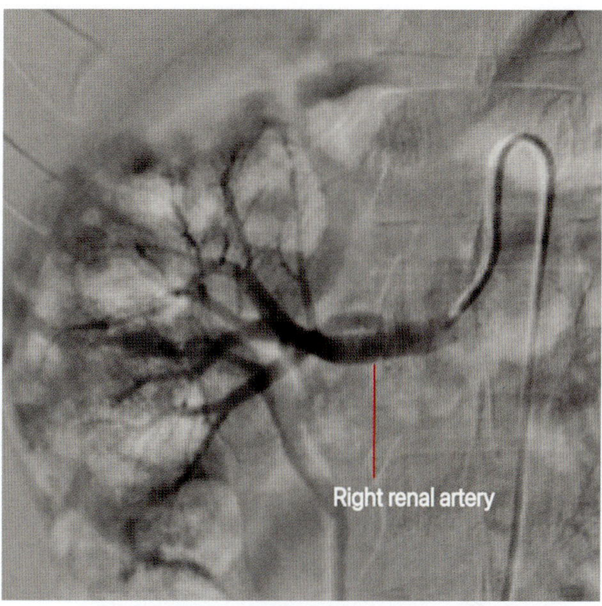

Fig. 3.5.70: Renal artery and branches

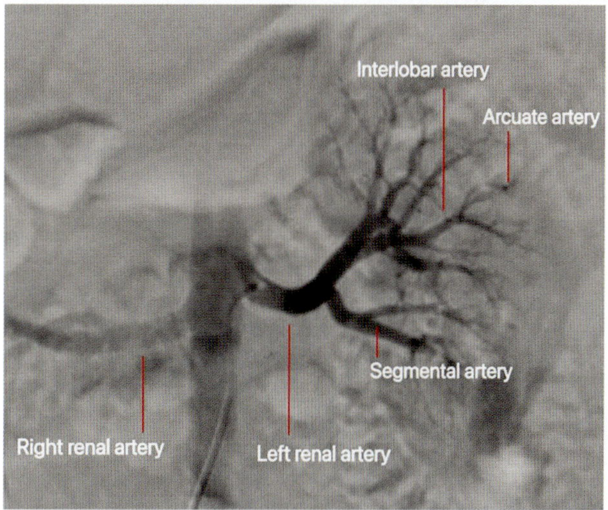

Fig. 3.5.71: Renal artery and branches

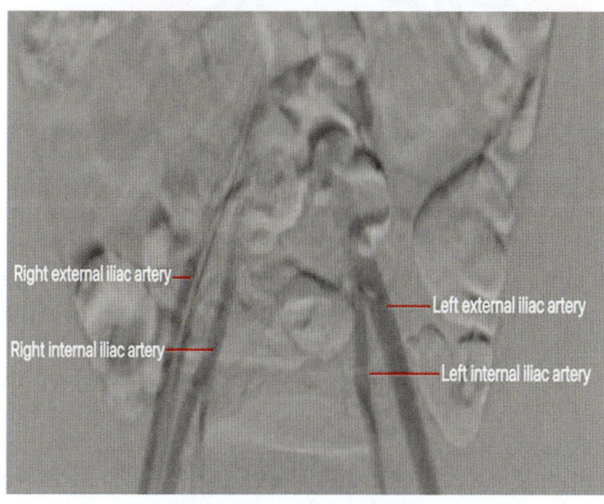

Fig. 3.5.72: Iliac vessels

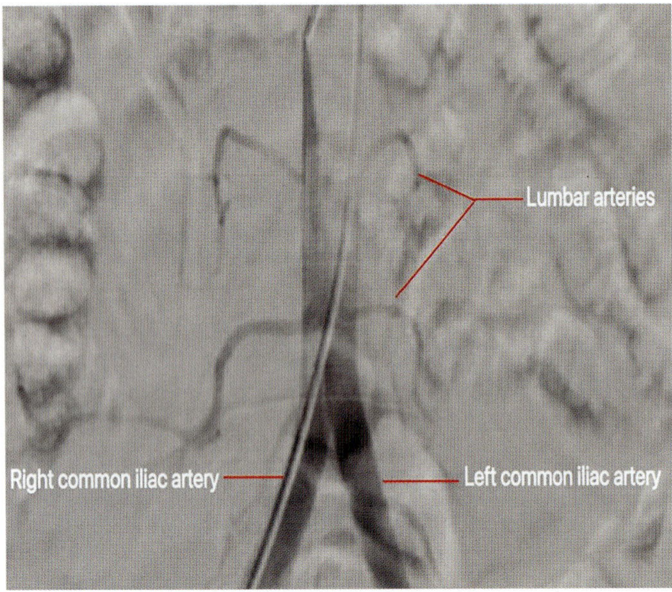

Fig. 3.5.73: Lumbar arteries

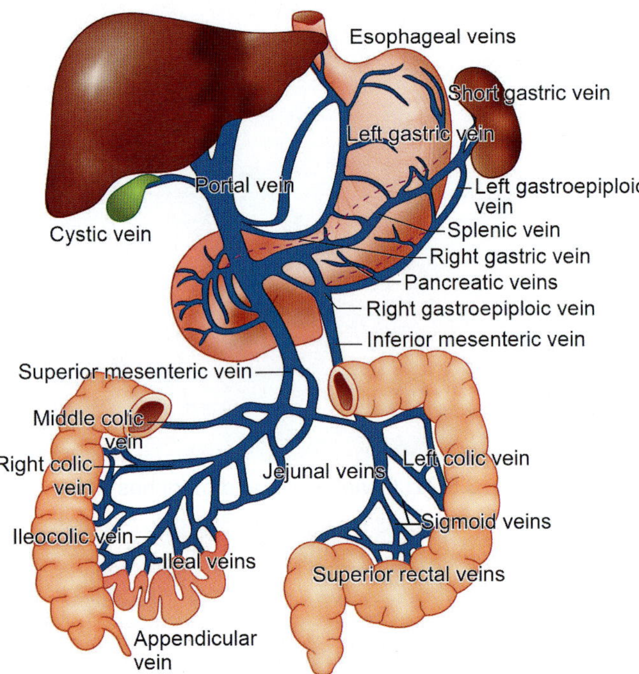

Fig. 3.5.74: Portal venous system

and posterior. The classic hepatic arterial anatomy, with the proper hepatic artery branching into right and left hepatic arteries, is seen in 55% patients.Superior mesenteric artery (SMA) arises from the front of aorta about 1 cm below the coeliac trunk at the level of L1 vertebrae. Inferior phrenic arteries arise from the aorta just above the celiac trunk. Renal arteries arise laterally from the aorta, just below the superior mesentric artery.

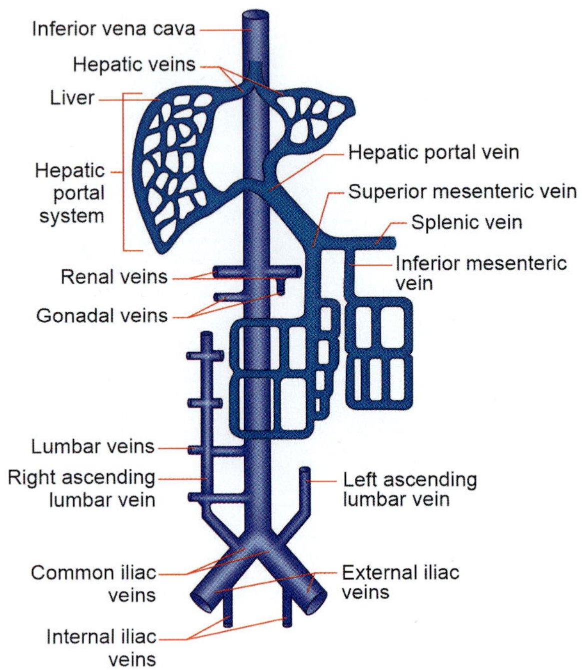

Fig. 3.5.75: Systemic venous system

The right is longer and often higher. The left renal artery is little lower. One or two accesory renal arteries frequently occur, especially on the left, usually from the aorta above or below the main artery. There are two venous systems that drain abdominal structures, the portal venous system and the systemic venous system.

Inferior mesentric artery (IMA) originates at the level of L3 vertebrae.

Arch of Riolan/meandering artery of Moskowitz: Anastomosis between middle colic branch of SMA and left colic branch of IMA, it runs proximally to the root of mesentry.

Marginal artery of Drummond: Anastomoses between SMA and IMA forming continuous arterial arcade along inner border of colon, it runs distal to the root of mesentry.

Systemic venous system: The inferior vena cava is a venous drainage system that connects all regions below the diaphragm. At the L5 vertebral level, the vessel is formed by the union of the common iliac veins. It gets tributaries from the external and internal iliac veins, which form the common iliac veins. They are responsible for draining the lower limbs and gluteal area. The posterior abdominal wall is drained by lumbar veins. The kidneys, left adrenal gland, and left testis/ovary are all drained through the renal veins. In men and women, the right testicular/ovarian vein drains the right testes and ovary (the left testicular/ovarian vein empties into the left renal vein) respectively.

The right suprarenal vein is responsible for draining the right adrenal gland (the left adrenal vein drains into the left renal vein). The diaphragm is drained by the inferior phrenic veins.

The liver is drained via hepatic veins. It is found on the posterior abdominal wall and exits the abdomen by entering the diaphragm at T8 (the caval hiatus). The inferior vena cava drains into the right atrium of the heart from within the thorax.

Portal venous system: The portal vein is formed by the confluence of the splenic vein with the superior mesenteric vein at the level of L2, which is posterior to the pancreas' neck. The portal vein passes posteriorly to the superior part of the duodenum and the bile duct as it ascends to the liver. It also receives tributaries from the right and left gastric veins, cystic veins and para-umbilical veins. Splenic vein receives tributaries from short gastric veins, left gastro-omental vein, pancreatic veins and inferior mesenteric vein. Superior mesenteric vein receives tributaries from right gastro-omental vein, anterior and posterior inferior pancreaticoduodenal veins, jejunal vein, ileal vein, ileocolic vein, right and middle colic veins.

The main sites of portosystemic collateral pathways are:

Left gastric: Left gastric (coronary) vein and short gastric veins to distal esophageal veins, located between the medial wall of the gastric body and the posterior margin of the left hepatic lobe in the lesser omentum, generally accompanied by esophageal/paraesophageal varices.

Esophageal: Distal esophageal submucosal venous plexus dilated.

Paraesophageal: Coronary vein to azygos and hemiazygos veins and vertebral venous plexus.

Perisplenic: Splenic vein to the left renal vein, passing via the splenocolic ligament; may result in a spontaneous splenorenal shunt.

Retrogastric: Left gastric (coronary) vein or gastroepiploic vein to esophageal or paraesophageal veins, located in posterior/posteromedial aspect of gastric fundus.

Retroperitoneal-paravertebral: Colic or mesenteric branches of the superior mesenteric vein to retro-peritoneal/lumbar veins to the inferior vena cava.

Paraumbilical: Left portal vein drains to paraumbilical veins in the anterior ridge of falciform ligament.

At anterior abdominal wall: Paraumbilical and omental veins drains to subcutaneous periumbilical veins and superior and inferior epigastric veins; collaterals appear to radiate from the umbilicus (caput medusae).

Mesenteric: Dilated branches of superior mesenteric vein.

Anal canal: Superior rectal vein (from the inferior mesenteric vein) to upper anal canal veins (hemorrhoids).

In abdominal aortoiliac stenosis/occlusion: The commonest collateral pathways to the lower extremities Superior mesenteric artery → inferior mesenteric artery → superior rectal artery → middle and inferior rectal arteries → internal iliac arteries or obturator/internal pudendal arteries → common femoral arteries

Intercostal, subcostal, and lumbar arteries → superior gluteal and iliolumbar arteries → internal iliac arteries external iliac arteries

Intercostal, subcostal, and lumbar arteries circumflex arteries → external iliac arteries

Subclavian arteries → internal thoracic arteries → superior epigastric arteries → inferior epigastric arteries → external iliac arteries

3.5.L Abdomen Lymph Nodes

Knowledge of the location and nomenclature of the common nodal stations in the abdomen are essential for complete report of radiological findings. The major lymphatics and lymph nodes of the abdomen, such as the external iliac nodes, celiac, and superior mesenteric

Table 3.5.4: Regional lymph nodes for specific types of cancer

<table>
<tr><td>Gastric cancer greater curvature of stomach: Greater curvature</td><td>Pancreatic cancer: Peripancreatic, hepatic artery, celiac axis, pyloric, splenic region</td><td>Colorectal cancer: Pericolic/perirectal, Iileocolic, right colic, middle colic, left colic, inferior mesenteric artery, superior rectal</td></tr>
<tr><td colspan="3">Gastric cancer lesser curvature of stomach: Lesser curvature, lesser omental, left gastric, cardio-esophageal, common hepatic, hepatoduodenal ligament</td></tr>
<tr><td>Pancreatic and splenic area: Pancreaticolienal, peripancreatic, splenic</td><td>Hepatocellular carcinoma: Hepato-duodenal ligament, caval lymph nodes, hepatic artery</td><td>Renal cell carcinoma: Renal hilar, paracaval, paraaortic, periaortic, retroperitoneal</td></tr>
<tr><td colspan="3">Additional lymph nodes for lymphoproliferative disorders. Retrocrural, inferior diaphragmatic, anterior diaphragmatic, middle diaphragmatic, gastro-esophageal</td></tr>
</table>

nodes, are positioned along and have the same name as the major blood vessels. The lumbar nodes, also known as the para-aortic and para-caval nodes, receive afferents from the lower abdominal viscera, abdominal wall, and lower extremities, and are commonly involved in inflammatory and neoplastic disorders. The cisterna chyli, which might be a distinct sac or a plexiform convergence, is formed when the lumbar trunks unite with an intestinal trunk (around the L1 level). The thoracic duct is formed when the cisterna chyli and other major lymphatic trunks combine at level L1–L2 behind the crura to produce the thoracic duct, which goes through the aortic hiatus to enter the mediastinum.

The thoracic duct empties into the left subclavian or innominate vein after collecting up additional lymphatic trunks within the thorax.

Abdominal lymph nodes (Figs 3.5.76 to 3.5.81).

3.5.M Lumbosacral Plexus

The **lumbar plexus** is formed when the ventral rami of the L1–L4 spinal nerve roots combine in or posterior to the psoas major muscle in the psoas compartment

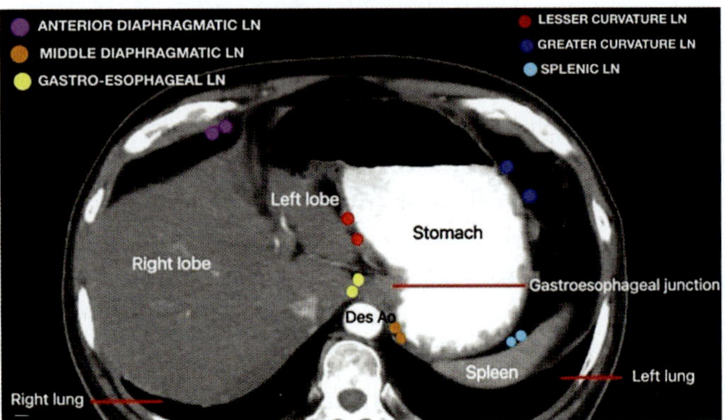

Fig. 3.5.76

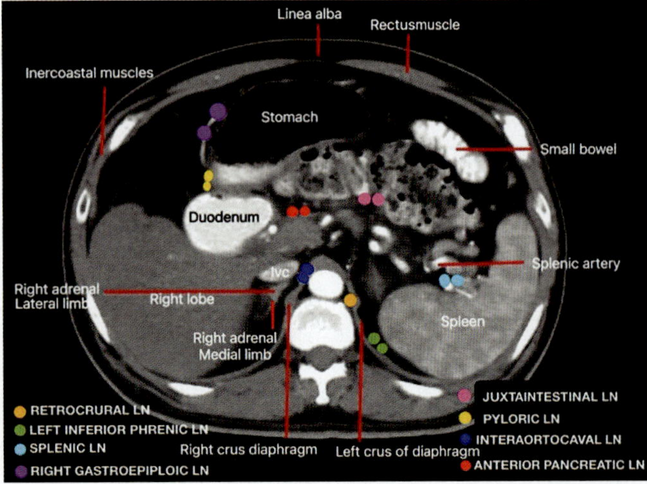

Fig. 3.5.77

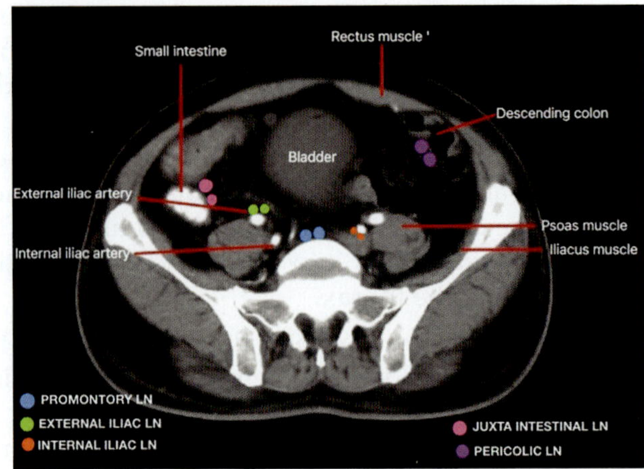

Fig. 3.5.78

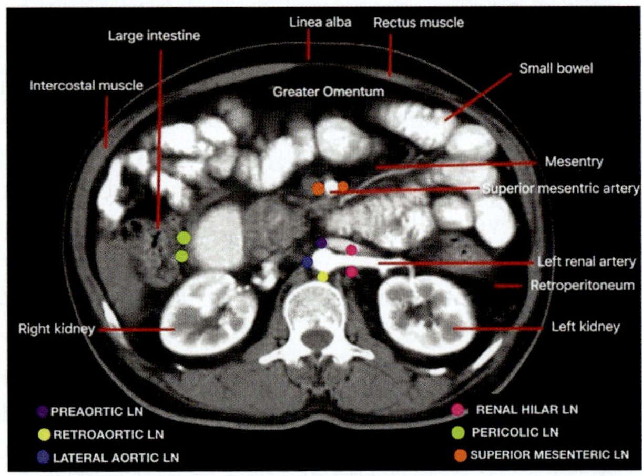

Fig. 3.5.79

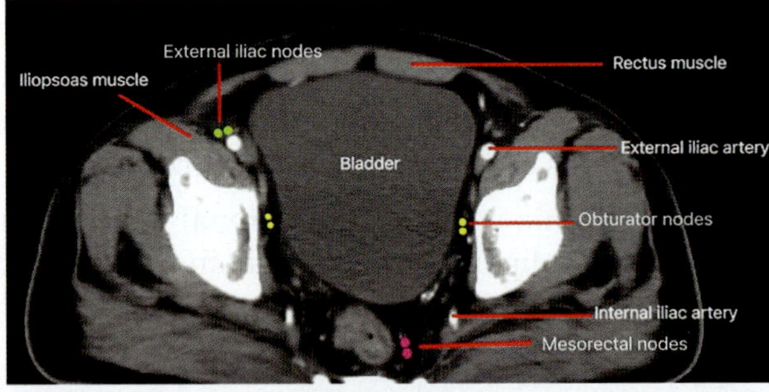

Fig. 3.5.80

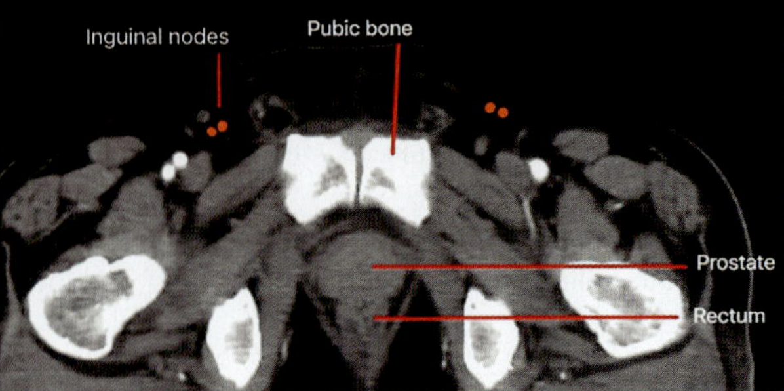

Fig. 3.5.81

Table 3.5.5: Lumbosacral plexus			
Nerve	*Roots*	*Muscular innervation*	*Sensory innervation*
Lumbar plexus			
Iliohypogastric	L1	Lower fibres of transverse abdominal and internal oblique muscles	Lateral gluteal region and area above pubis
Ilioinguinal	L1	Lower fibres of transverse abdominal and internal oblique muscle	To pubic symphysis, root of penis and anterior scrotum in men, superior and medial aspect of femoral triangle, mons pubis and labia majora in women
Genito-femoral	L1, L2	Cremaster muscle	Thigh adjacent to inguinal ligament and around femoral triangle, spermatic cord and scrotum in men, labia majora in women
Obturator	L2–L4	Adductor magnus, adductor brevis, adductor longus, obturator externus, pectineus and gracilis muscles	Medial and distal thigh
Femoral	L2–L4	Quadriceps, pectineus, sartorius	Upper anterior thigh, hip and knee joints
Sacral plexus			
Lateral femoral cutaneous	L2, L3	None	Anterior and lateral thigh
Sciatic nerve	L4–S3	Biceps femoris, semitendinosus, semimembranosus, adductor magnus muscles	Gluteal region, posterior thigh, perineum, hip joint, popliteal fossa, lower leg
Pudendal	S2–S4	Sphincters of urinary bladder and rectum	External genitalia
Superior gluteal	L4–S1	Gluteus medius, gluteus minimus, tensor fasciae lata muscles	None
Inferior gluteal	L4–S1	Gluteus maximus	None

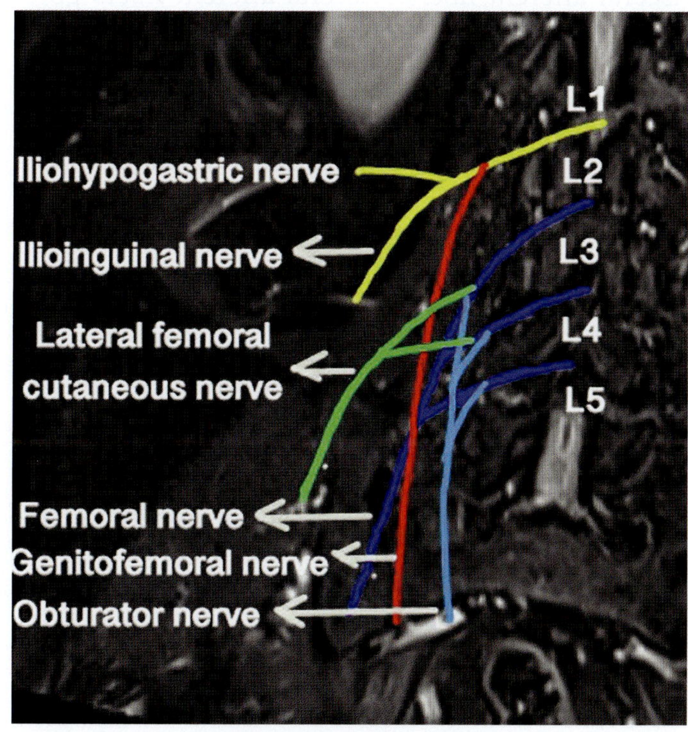

Fig. 3.5.82: Lumbar plexus

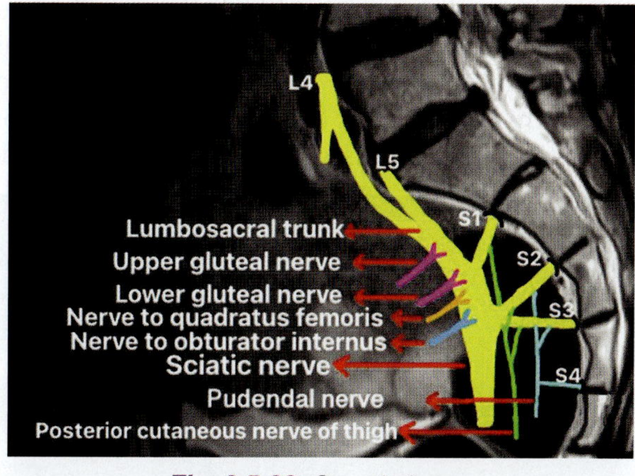

Fig. 3.5.83: Sacral plexus

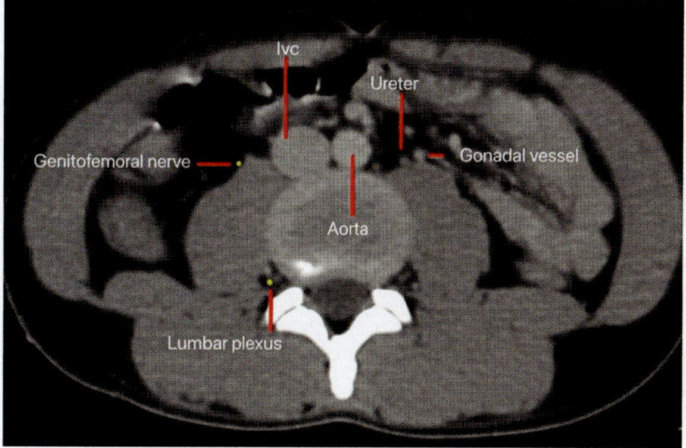

Fig. 3.5.84: Axial CT: Lumbar plexus

at the level of the L2–L5 transverse processes. The iliohypogastric, ilioinguinal, genitofemoral, femoral, and lateral femoral cutaneous nerves arise from the lumbar plexus and exit lateral to the psoas major muscle, as well as the obturator nerve and lumbrosacral trunk (which course medial to the psoas major muscle). The **sacral plexus** is formed when the ventral rami of the L4–S3 spinal nerve roots combine anterior to the piriformis muscle, giving rise to the sciatic, pudendal, superior gluteal, and inferior gluteal nerves. The lumbrosacral plexus is formed when the lumbar and sacral plexuses unite in the lumbrosacral trunk.

The neural network connection created within or posterior to the psoas muscle is the muscular landmark for the lumbar plexus. As a result, nerves can be categorised as follows based on where they leave in relation to the psoas muscle margins: (i) Medial to psoas—obturator nerve and lumbosacral trunk; (ii) Lateral to psoas—iliohypogastric, ilioinguinal, genitofemoral, femoral, and lateral femoral cutaneous nerves.

Celiac ganglia: Celiac ganglia are found anterior to the diaphragm's crura, bilaterally over the anterolateral wall of the aorta, and just caudal to the celiac artery's origin. Depending on the operator's preferences and the safest route of access, both anterior and posterior approaches may be used for celiac ganglion block. Because the needle point is anterior to the spinal arteries and spinal canal, the anterior approach has a lower chance of neurologic problems. This enables for a single puncture, a shorter operation time, and the use of less neurolytic chemical.

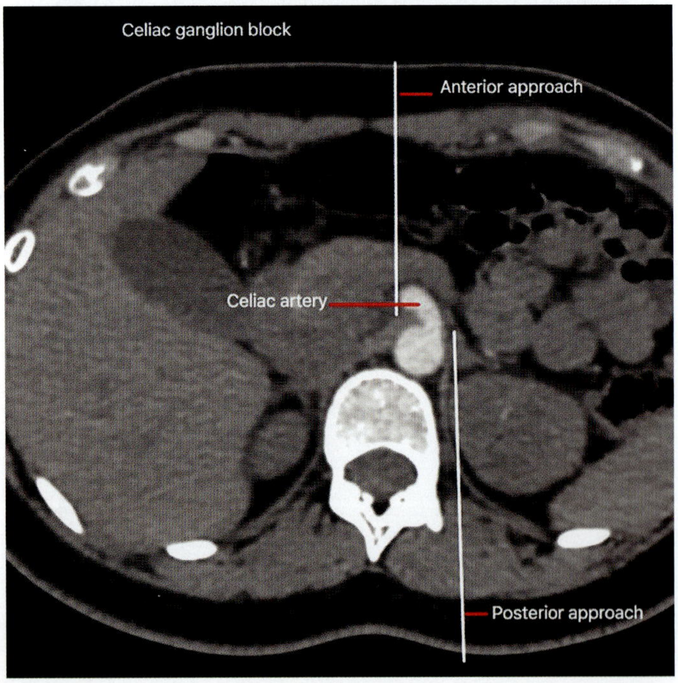

Fig. 3.5.85: Celiac ganglion block—anterior and posterior approach

The lumbar splanchnic nerves are splanchnic nerves that arise from the lumbar part of the sympathetic trunk and travel to an adjacent plexus near the aorta. They originate from L1 and L2. These nerves contain preganglionic sympathetic and general visceral afferent fibers. The site of synapse is found in the inferior mesenteric ganglion and the postsynaptic fibers innervate the smooth muscle and glands of the pelvic viscera and hindgut.

The sacral sympathetic nerves emerge anteriorly from the ganglia from the sacral section of the sympathetic trunk. They travel to the inferior hypogastric plexus on their corresponding side, where preganglionic nerve fibres synapse with postganglionic sympathetic neurons, whose fibres ascend to the superior hypogastric plexus, aortic plexus, and inferior mesenteric plexus, where they are distributed to the anal canal. They also innervate pelvic organs and vessels from the inferior hypogastric plexus. The preganglionic and postganglionic sympathetic fibres in the sacral sympathetic nerves are mainly preganglionic. There are also general visceral afferent fibres in them.

The pelvic splanchnic nerves arise from the anterior rami of the sacral spinal nerves S2, S3, and S4, and enter the sacral plexus. They travel to their side's corresponding inferior hypogastric plexus, located bilaterally on the walls of the rectum. They contain both preganglionic parasympathetic fibers as well as visceral afferent fibers. Visceral afferent fibers go to spinal cord following pathway of pelvic splanchnic nerve fibers. A ganglion in the upper portion of the **superior mesenteric plexus** is known as the superior mesenteric ganglion. It is located near the superior mesenteric artery's origin. The inferior mesenteric ganglion is a ganglion located near where the inferior mesenteric artery branches from the abdominal aorta.

3.5.N Anterior Abdominal Wall

Scarpa's fascia is a fibrous layer that runs deep beneath the skin and subcutaneous fat of the lower anterior abdominal wall. This fascia unites with the deep fascia of the perineum (Colles' fascia) and extends to the penis and scrotum (or labia majora). The linea alba, pubic crest, inguinal ligament, and iliac crest are all inserted into the external oblique muscle, which arises on the anterior aspect of the lower ribs. The lumbar fascia, iliac crest, and lateral two-thirds of the inguinal ligament form the internal oblique muscle, which inserts into the linea alba and the costal border. The transversus abdominis muscle arises from the lower ribs and inserts into the linea alba, interdigitating with the diaphragm, lumbar fascia, iliac crest, and lateral part of the inguinal ligament. The rectus abdominis muscle is a thick ribbon of muscle that runs from the costal cartilages to the pubic crest on either side of the midline. At intervals along its length, it has three to four tendinous junctions that adhere to the anterior rectus sheath. The aponeuroses of the other abdominal wall muscles surround the rectus muscle and join to the linea alba to form the rectus sheath. **Preperitoneal fat** only a layer of fat separates the muscles of the anterior abdominal wall from the peritoneum and the abdominal contents. This is referred to as extraperitoneal fatty tissue or preperitoneal fat. **Divarication of the recti** is a stretching of the linea alba with abnormal widening of the gap between the two medial sides of the rectus abdominis muscle (increased inter-recti distance). **Pannus**—dense layer of fatty tissue, consisting of excess subcutaneous fat within the lower abdominal region (Figs 3.5.86–3.5.87).

CT of the abdomen: Three muscles can be seen anterolaterally—the external oblique is outermost, with the internal oblique and transversus abdominis deep to it. The rectus muscle and its rectus sheath can be seen in the anterior paramedian position (Figs 3.5.88, 3.5.89 and 3.5.91).

Inguinal canal: Passage through anterior abdominal wall, transmits spermatic cord in males and round ligament in females formed embryologically by evagination of processus vaginalis.

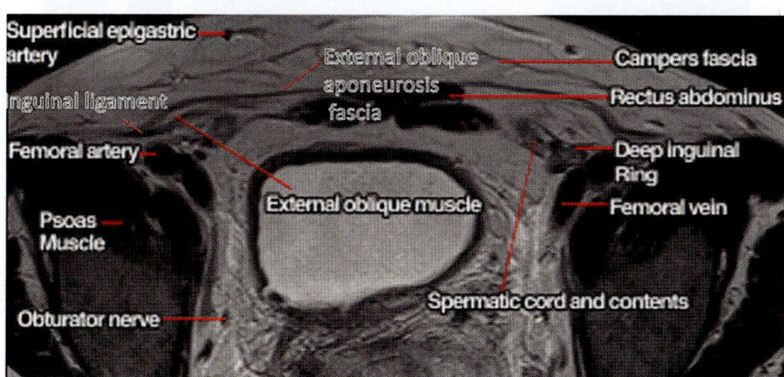

Fig. 3.5.86

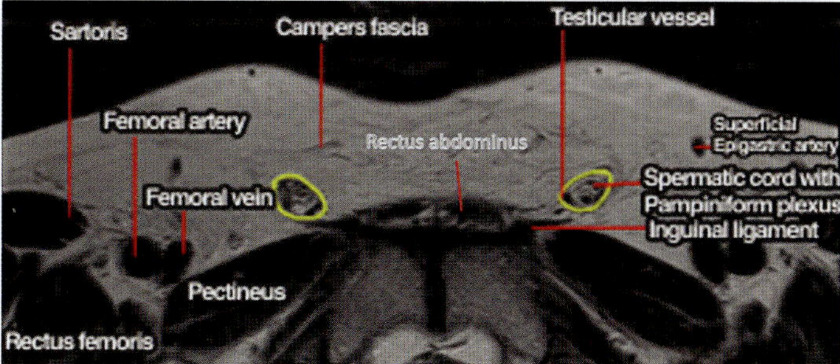

Fig. 3.5.87

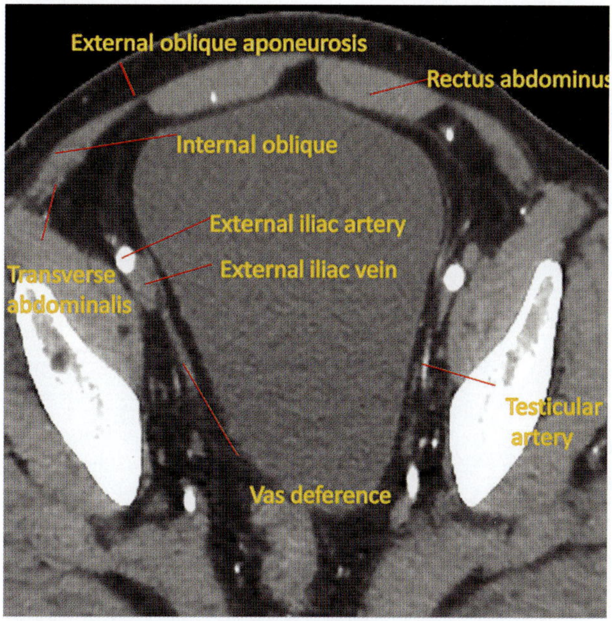

Fig. 3.5.88

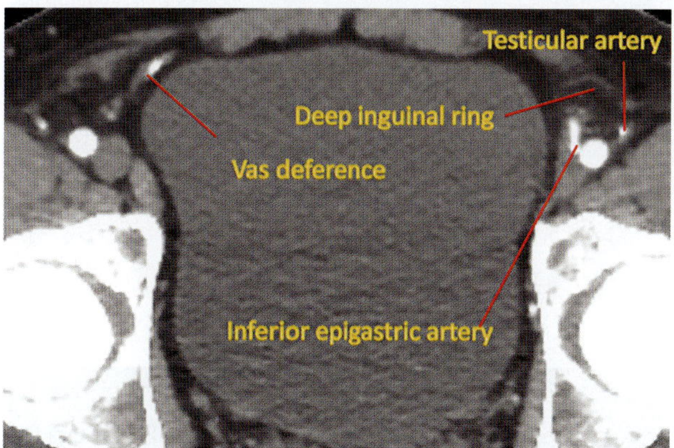

Fig. 3.5.89

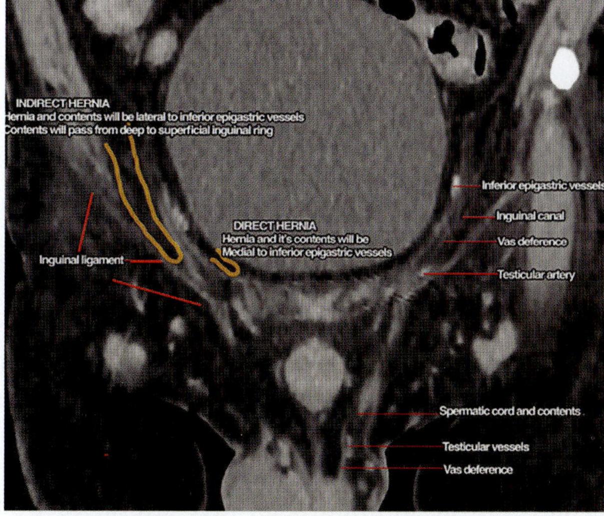

Fig. 3.5.90: Direct and indirect inguinal hernia

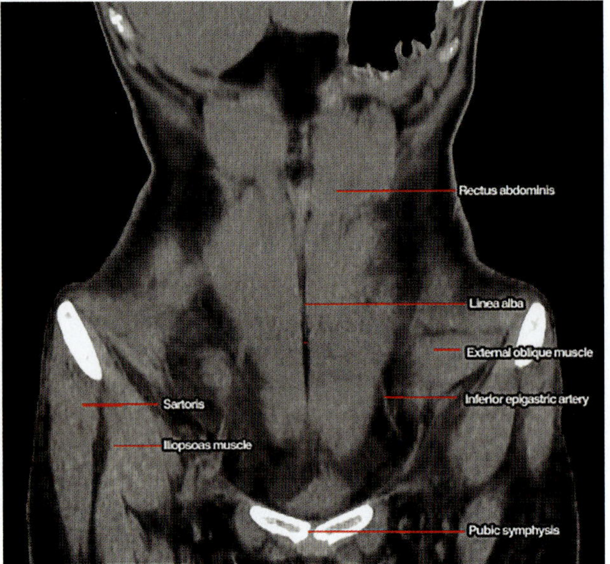

Fig. 3.5.91: Anterior abdominal wall muscles

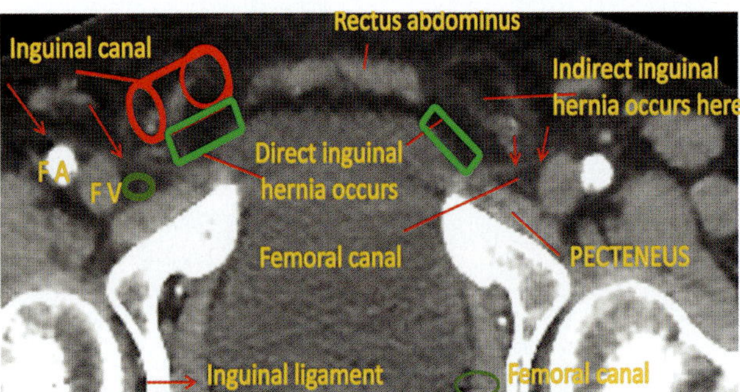

Fig. 3.5.92: Inguinal canal

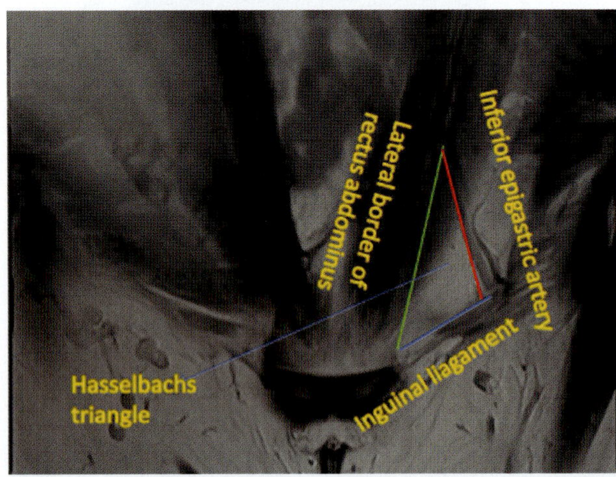

Fig. 3.5.93: Hesselbach triangle

Internal or deep ring: Opening through transversalis fascia located above mid-portion of inguinal ligament lateral to inferior epigastric artery.

External or superficial ring: Triangular opening in external oblique aponeurosis, just lateral to pubic tubercle.

3

Hesselbach triangle: Area of weakness in pelvic wall. Site of direct inguinal hernias. **Medial border:** Lateral edge of rectus sheath.

Lateral border: Inferior epigastric artery, **inferior border:** Inguinal ligament.

Normal variants mimicking focal bowel thickening in CT scan (Figs 3.5.94 to 3.5.98)

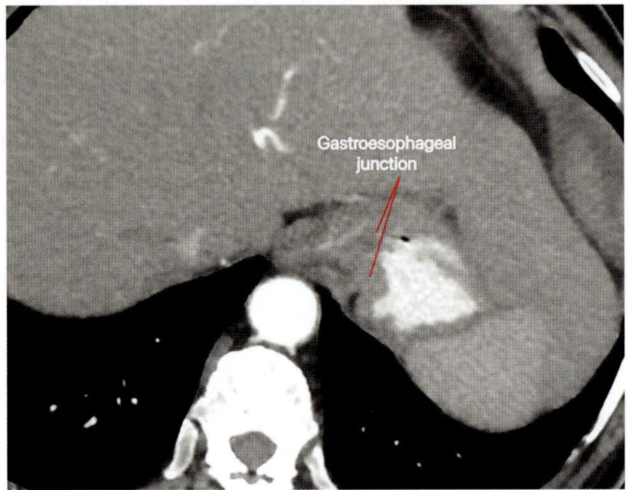

Fig. 3.5.94: Gastroesophageal junction

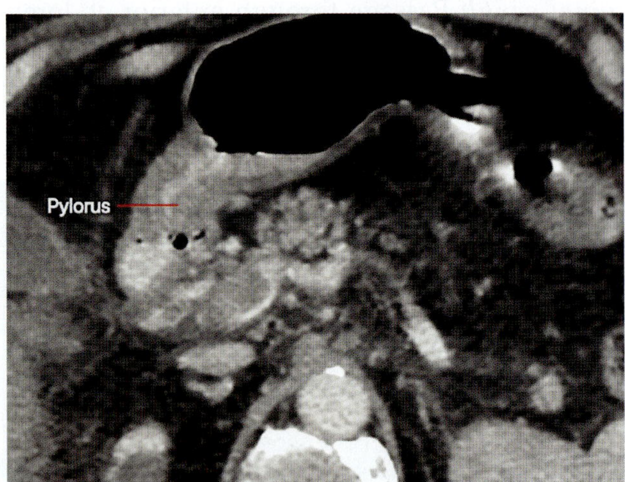

Fig. 3.5.95: Pylorus

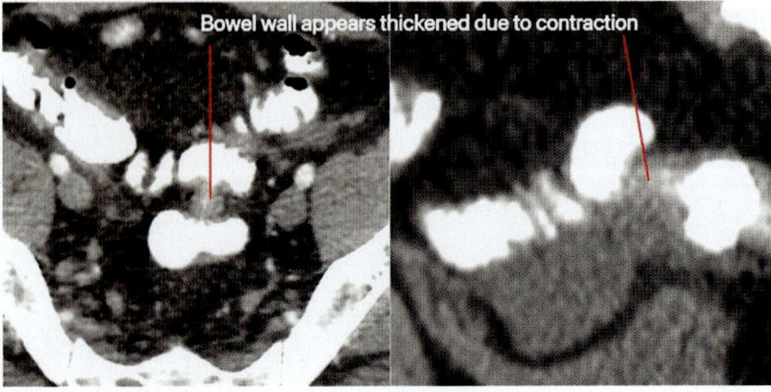

Fig. 3.5.96

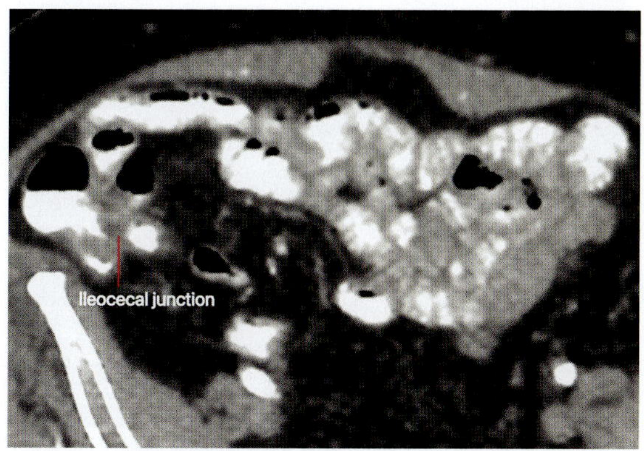

Fig. 3.5.97: Ileocecal junction

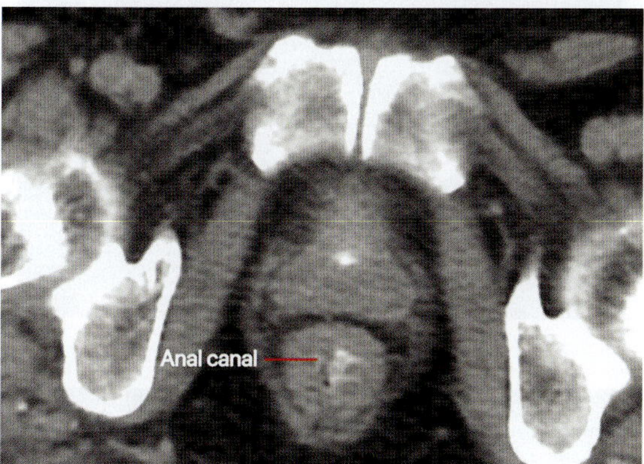

Fig. 3.5.98: Anal canal

CT axial sections abdomen (Figs 3.5.99 to 3.5.112)

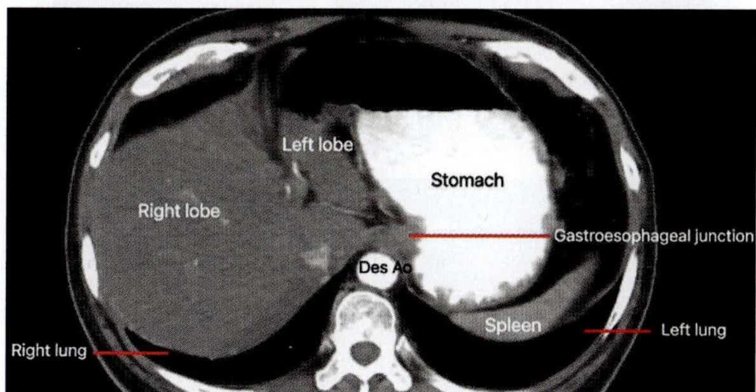

Fig. 3.5.99

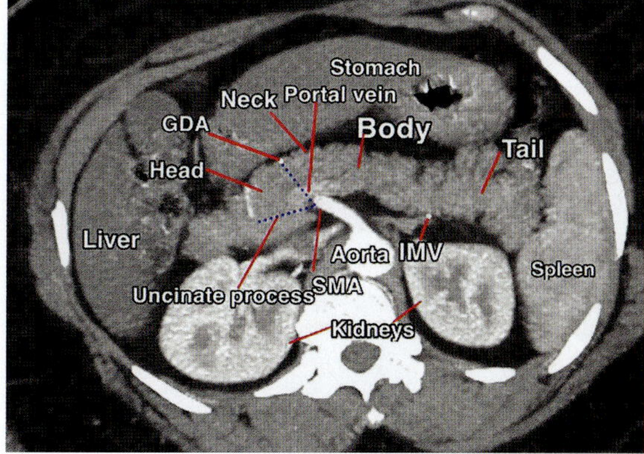

Fig. 3.5.100

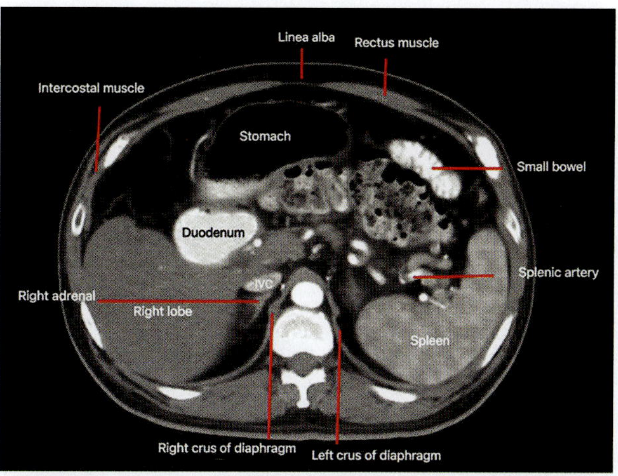

Fig. 3.5.101

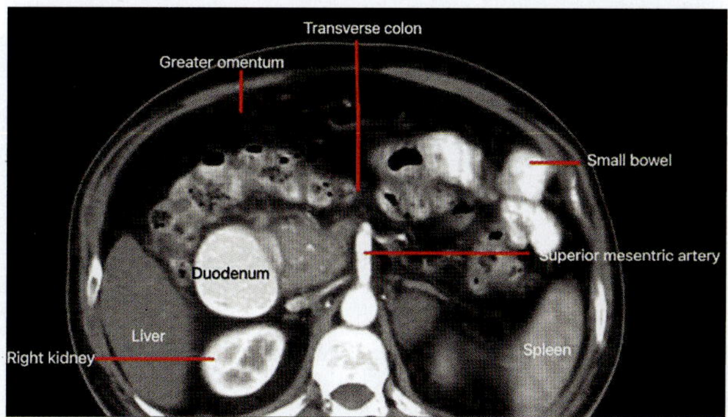

Fig. 3.5.102

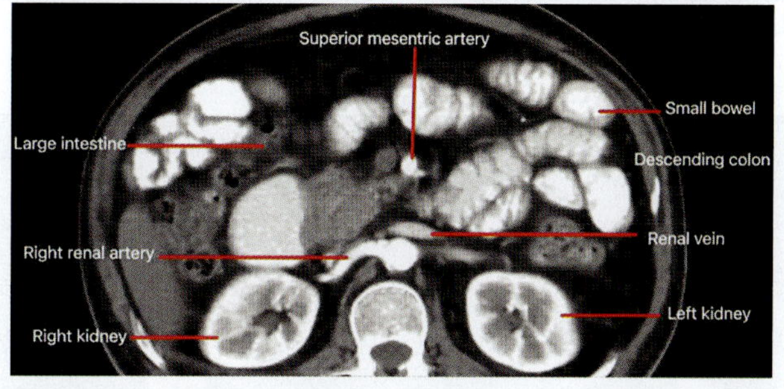

Fig. 3.5.103

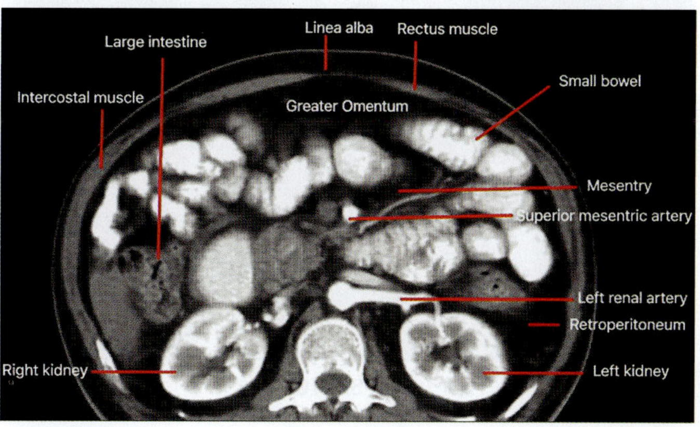

Fig. 3.5.104

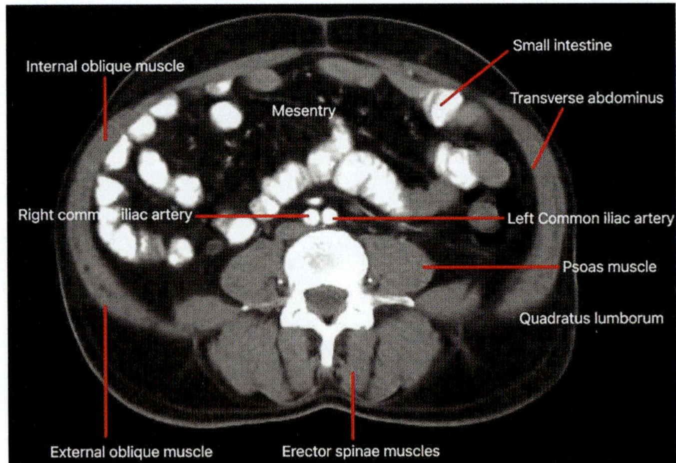

Fig. 3.5.105

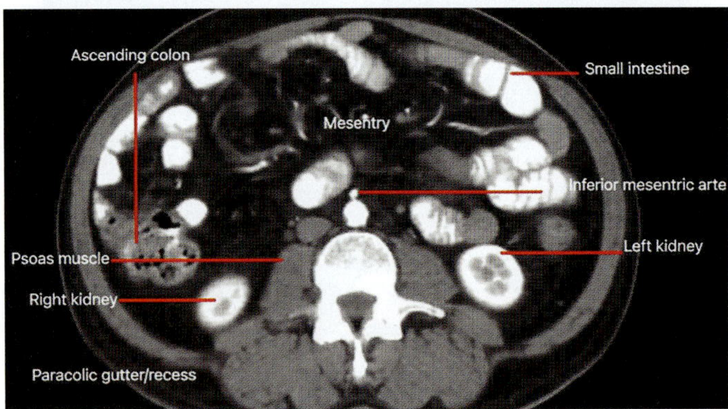

Fig. 3.5.106

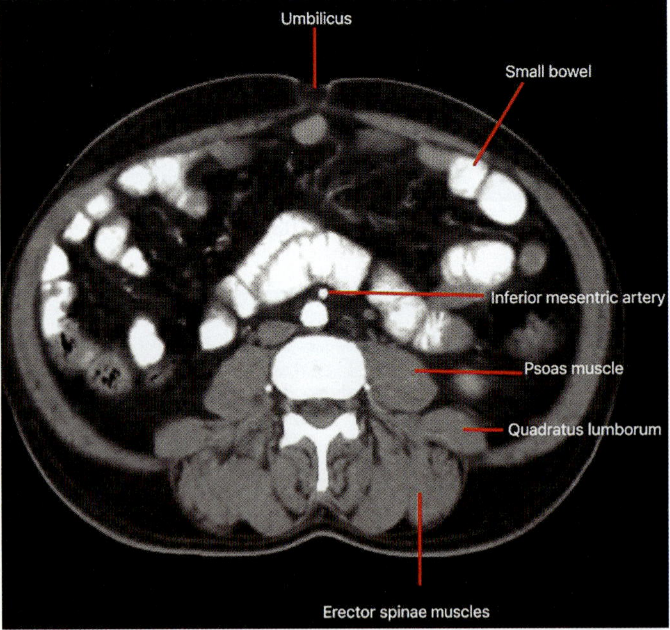

Fig. 3.5.107

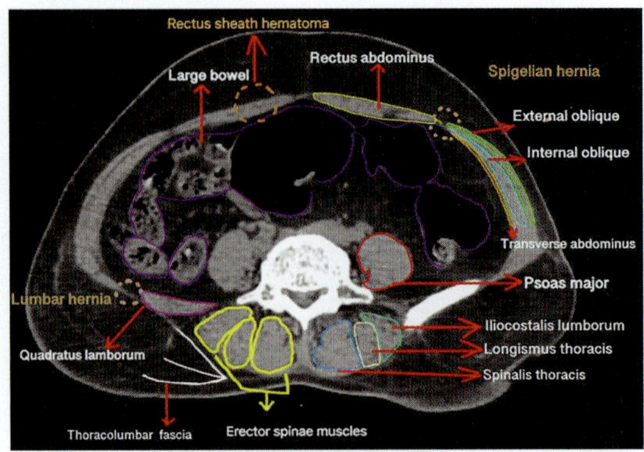

Fig. 3.5.108

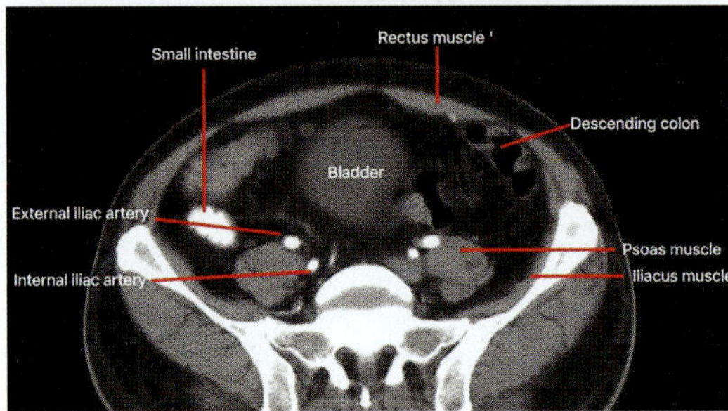

Fig. 3.5.109

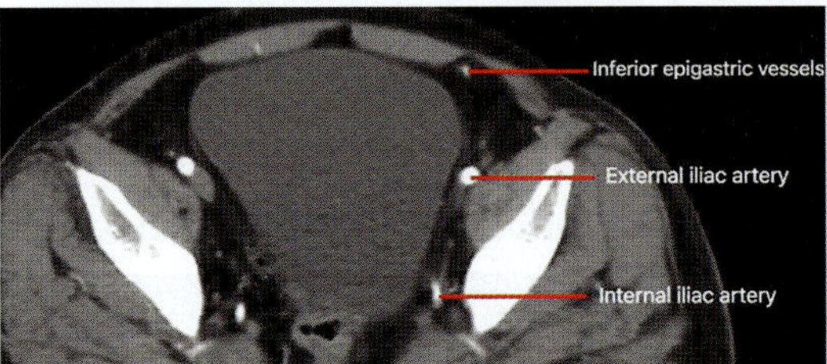

Fig. 3.5.110

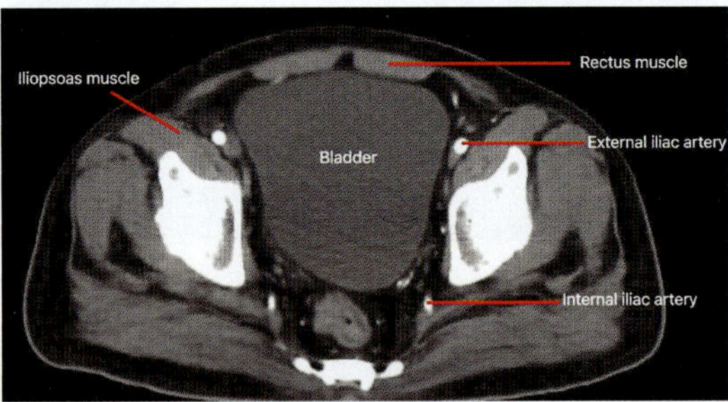

Fig. 3.5.111

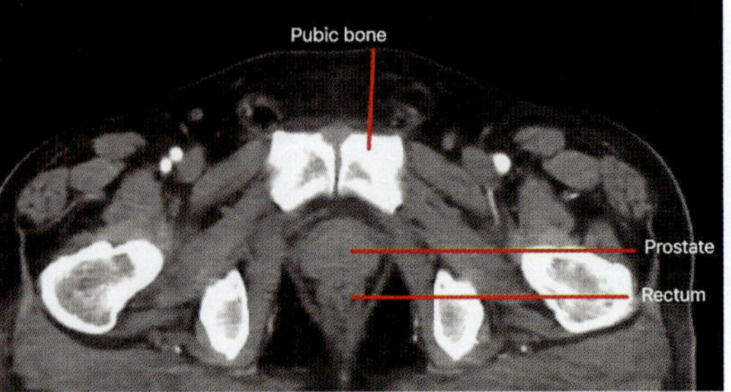

Fig. 3.5.112

3.6 PELVIS

Pelvic inlet: The pelvic inlet, is the anatomical limit between the true pelvis below and the false pelvis above. The pelvic inlet involves three of the four units of which the bone pelvis is composed. The pelvic brim involves the first sacral segment, the iliac and pubis portion, but not the ischium.

Pelvic outlet: The pelvic outlet, also called the inferior pelvic aperture, defines the lower margin of the lesser (true) pelvis. The pelvic outlet is the inferior opening of the pelvis that is bounded by coccyx, the ischial tuberosities, and the pubis symphysis.

Pelvic cavity: The pelvic cavity (the true pelvis) predominantly contains the urinary bladder, the colon, and the internal reproductive organs. This space is enclosed between the pelvic inlet and the pelvic outlet.

3.6.A Male and Female Bony Pelvis

Pelvic peritoneum/retroperitoneum: In the female, the peritoneum is reflected from the superior surface of the bladder to the anterior surface of the uterus is known as **anterior cul-de-sac** (Fig. 3.6.3). The peritoneum is further reflected from the posterior part of the uterus to the rectum, and this fold is known as the **pouch of Douglas** or posterior **cul-de-sac.** In the male, the peritoneum is reflected off the bladder to the rectum, forming the **rectovesical pouch** or cul-de-sac. These peritoneal pouches usually contain loops of bowel (Figs 3.6.5 and 3.6.6).

The retropubic space (otherwise known as the perivesical space, cave of Retzius) is an extraperitoneal space located posterior to the pubic symphysis and anterior to the urinary bladder. It is separated from the anterior abdominal wall by the transversalis fascia and extends to the level of the umbilicus.

Pelvic spaces: The pelvic spaces (Fig. 3.6.6) contain loose connective tissue but are important surgical dissection planes. Vesicovaginal/vesicocervical space—between lower urinary tract and vagina/cervix. Rectovaginal space contains fascia which provides support for the

Table 3.6.1: Difference between male and female pelvis

Male pelvis	*Female pelvis*
Pubic arch (angle formed by inferior pubic rami at symphysis pubis) <90°	Flattened pubic arch (>90°)
Hemi-shaped pelvic inlet with narrow outlet	Oval pelvic inlet with larger pelvic outlet
Round obturator foramen	Oval obturator foramen
Narrow sciatic notch	Wide sciatic notch
Larger, thicker cortex lines	Thinner cortex, more delicate bones

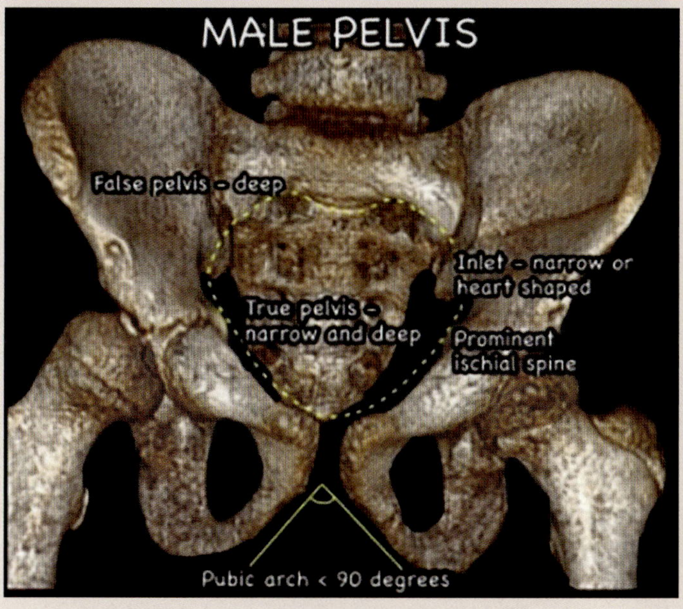

Fig. 3.6.1

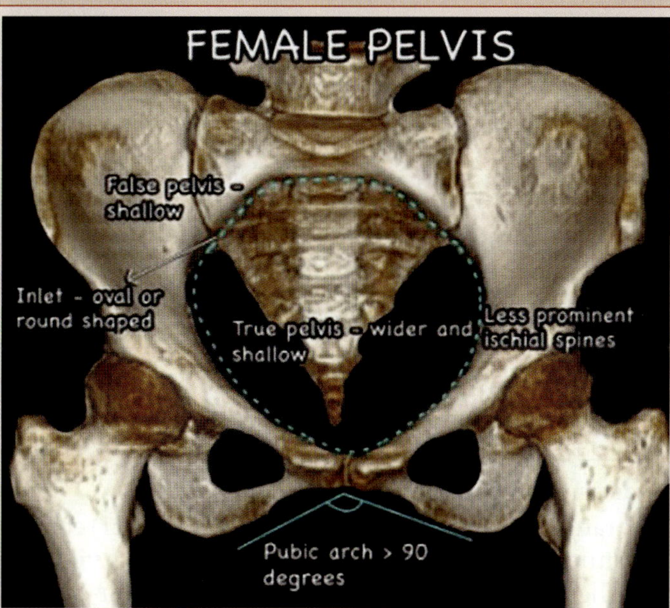

Fig. 3.6.2

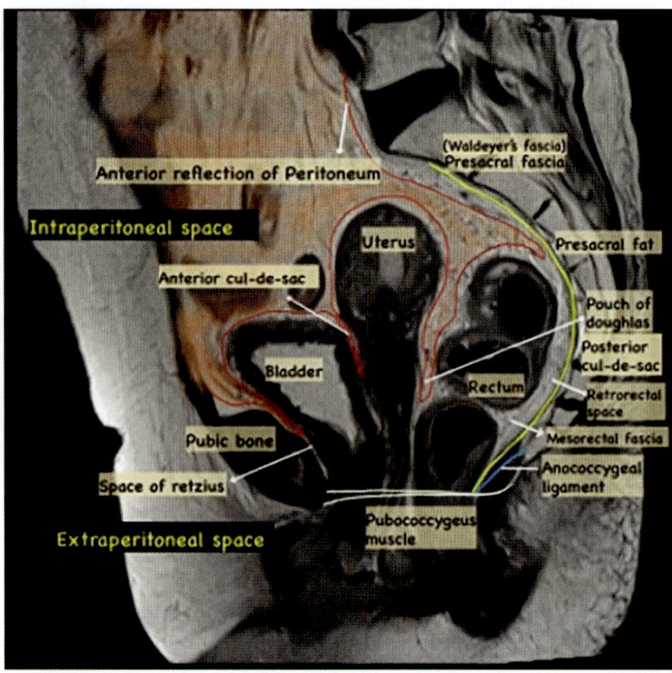

Fig. 3.6.3: Female peritoneum

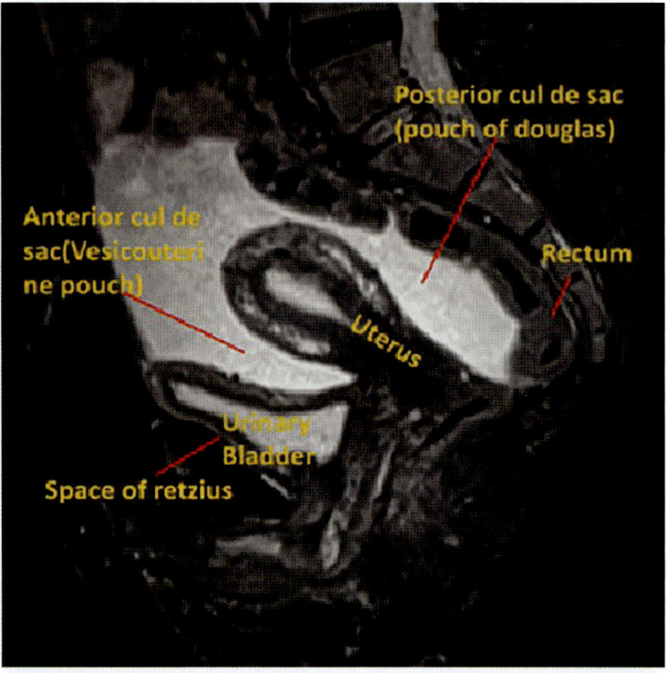

Fig. 3.6.4

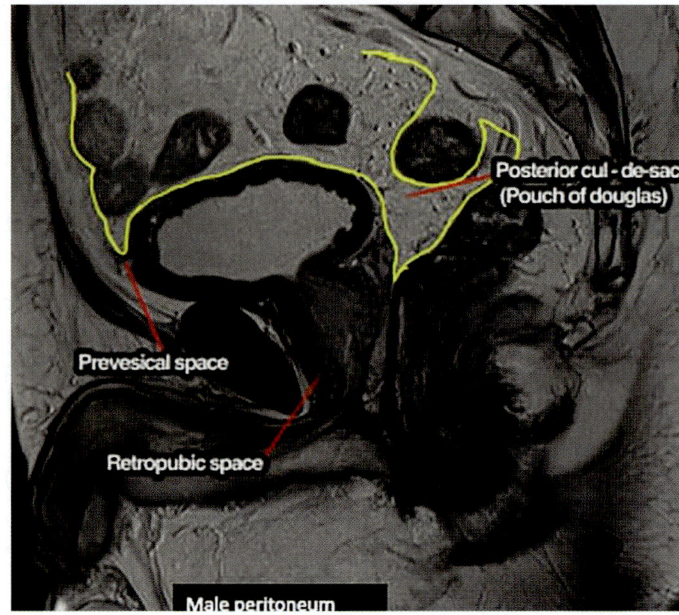

Fig. 3.6.5: Male peritoneum

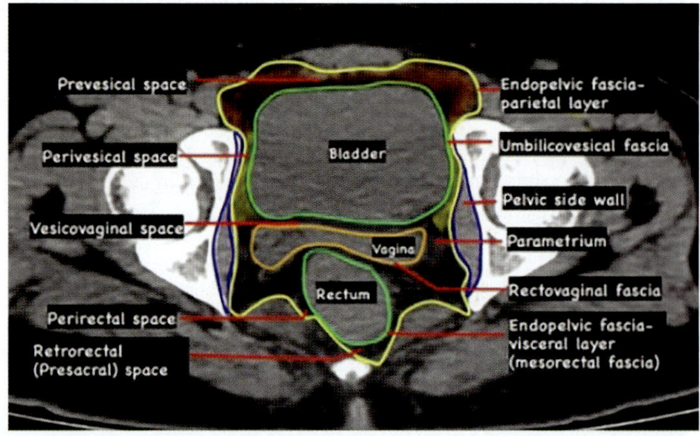

Fig. 3.6.6: Pelvic spaces

rectum. Paravesical and pararectal spaces. Presacral space—between rectum and sacrum/coccyx. Extends as far as aortic bifurcation.

Parametrium and paracervix (Figs 3.6.7–3.6.11) consist of connective areolar tissue enveloping the visceral branches of hypogastric vessels during their course toward the uterus and vagina. Parametrium refers to the tissue located cranially to the ureter, between the uterine corpus and the pelvic sidewall, surrounding the uterine artery. The parametrium includes the superficial uterine pedicle (uterine artery and superficial uterine vein) and related connective tissue and lymphatic channels. The connective tissue crossing below the ureter is considered paracervix, which can be identified with the cardinal ligament. The parametrium is divided into lateral, anterior and posterior parametrium. The **lateral parametrium** consisting of connective tissue and a lateral part that reaches the pelvic wall, and is made of fatty tissue and lymph nodes surrounding the vessels and nerves. The **anterior parametrium** is the constant bilateral anterior expansion of parametrium around the cervical-vescical branches of the uterine artery, or the superficial portion of the vesicouterine ligament, which is composed of vascular and fatty tissue connecting the bladder to the cervix and contributing

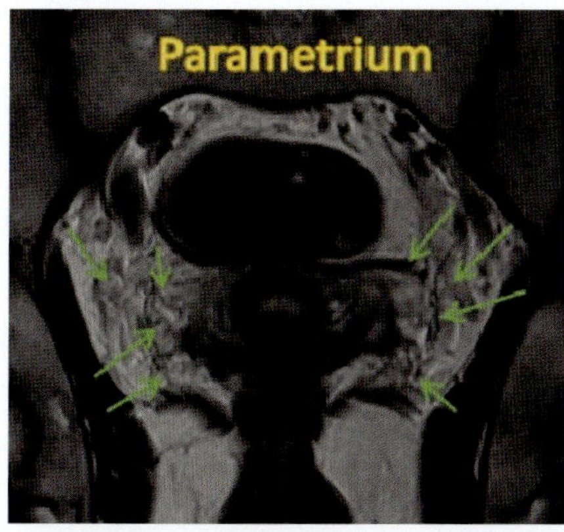

Fig. 3.6.7

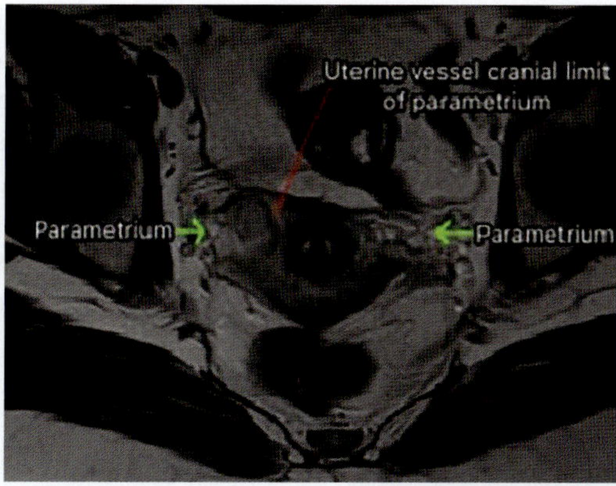

Fig. 3.6.8: Parametric with cranial limit

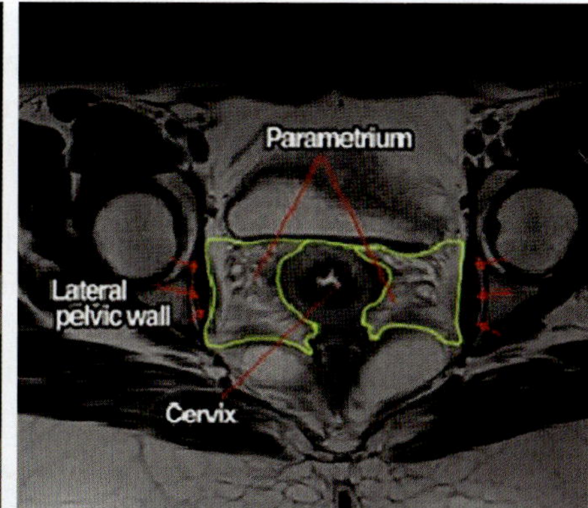

Fig. 3.6.9

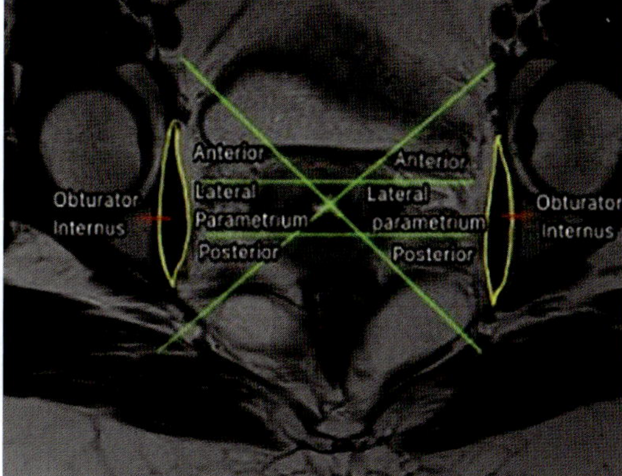

Fig. 3.6.10: Anterior, lateral and posterior parametrium

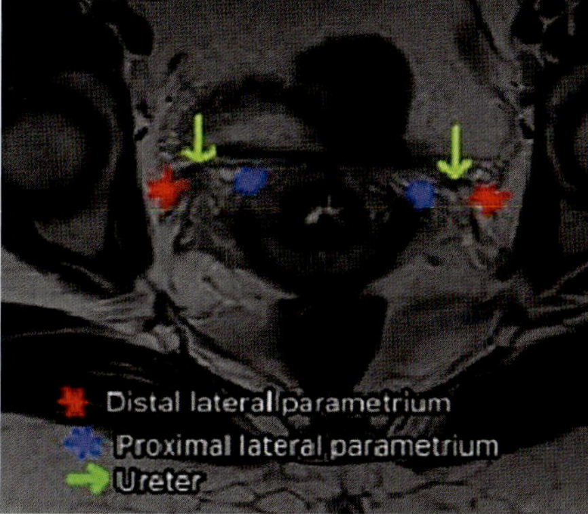

Fig. 3.6.11: Lateral parametrium

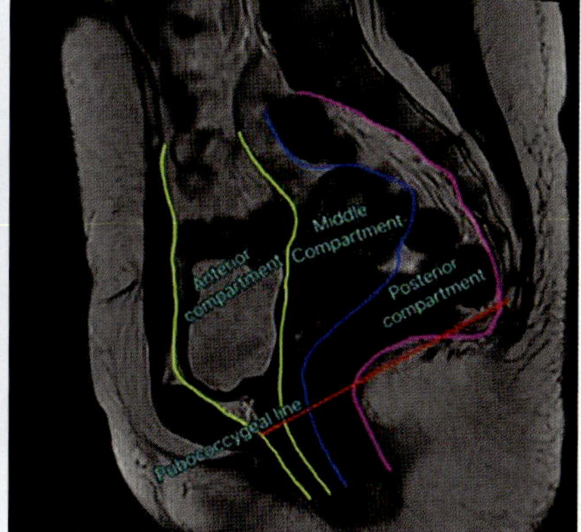

Fig. 3.6.12: Compartments in pelvis

to the roof of the ureteral tunnel near the bladder. The posterior parametrium is the posterior expansion of the parametrium at the uterosacral and rectovaginal ligament level. The **posterior parametrium** is composed of dense connective fibers originating from the posterior-lateral pelvic sidewalls and converging towards the upper dorsolateral portions of the uterine cervix and the dorsolateral portions of the superior and middle vagina, respectively. Therefore, the upper part of the posterior parametrium corresponds to the uterosacral ligament joining the uterine torus, while its lower part extends until the superior vaginal walls. The lateral wall of parametrium is formed by obturator internus and its fascia. The posterior wall of the parametrium is formed by pyriformis muscle. Paracolpium—the connective tissue and other tissue surrounding the vagina. Space of Retzius/prevesical/retropubic space—separated from the anterior abdominal wall by transversalis fascia.

3.6.B Female Reproductive System

The uterus: The uterus is extraperitoneal (Fig. 3.6.14). It has a fundus, a body and a cervix. The uterine cavity is triangular in coronal section, but its anterior and posterior walls are opposed, giving it a slit-like appearance in the sagittal plane. Just above the cervical canal, the uterine cavity narrows to an isthmus.The uterus continuous with the vagina via the cervical canal.

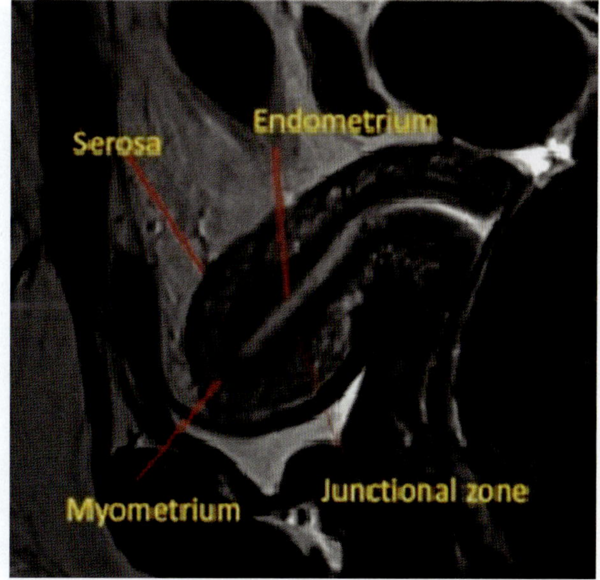

Fig. 3.6.13: Layers of uterus

Cervix: The internal OS is at the upper end of the cervical canal and the external OS at its lower end. The inner lining of the uterus is the endometrium, which undergoes cyclical changes of proliferation and desquamation in the premenopausal female (Fig. 3.6.16).

Peritoneum covers the fundus, body, cervix and upper part of the vagina posteriorly. From here it is reflected on to the anterior surface of the rectum, forming the pouch of Douglas. Anteriorly, the peritoneum is reflected from the upper part of the uterus to the superior surface of the bladder. On either side of the uterus, the peritoneum is reflected to the lateral pelvic walls covering the fallopian tubes. The fold of peritoneum so formed is called the broad ligament. Transabdominal ultrasound enables evaluation of the entire pelvis. Size and position of the uterus can be determined as well as gross pathology. Transvaginal US allows detailed evaluation of the internal structure of the uterus. The muscular myometrium forms most of the uterine wall. It is composed of three layers that can be identified by—**Ultrasound:** 1. inner layer or junctional zone—thin, compact hypoechoic layer surrounds echogenic endometrium forming a subendometrial halo. 2. Intermediate layer—thickest, uniform low to moderate echogenicity. 3. outer layer—less echogenic than intermediate layer, separated from it by arcuate vessels. **CT scan:** Seen as a homogeneous soft tissue mass dorsal to the bladder. Maybe a central

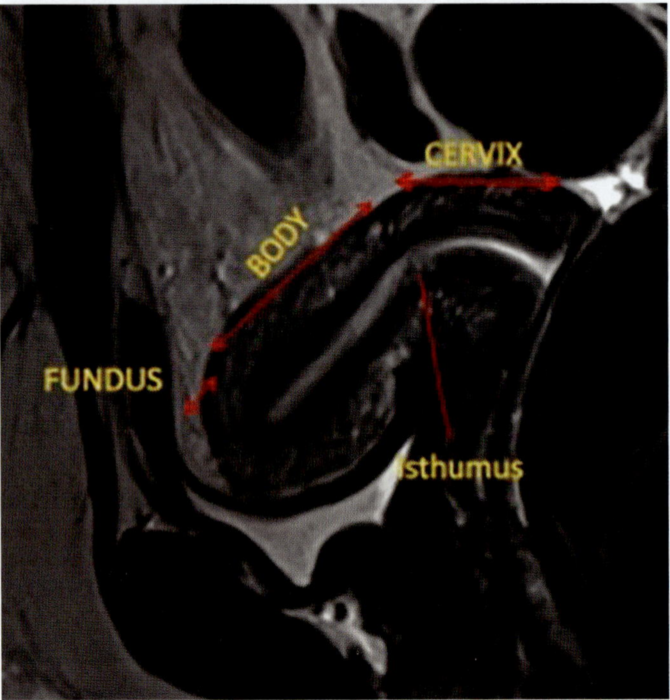

Fig. 3.6.14: Parts of uterus

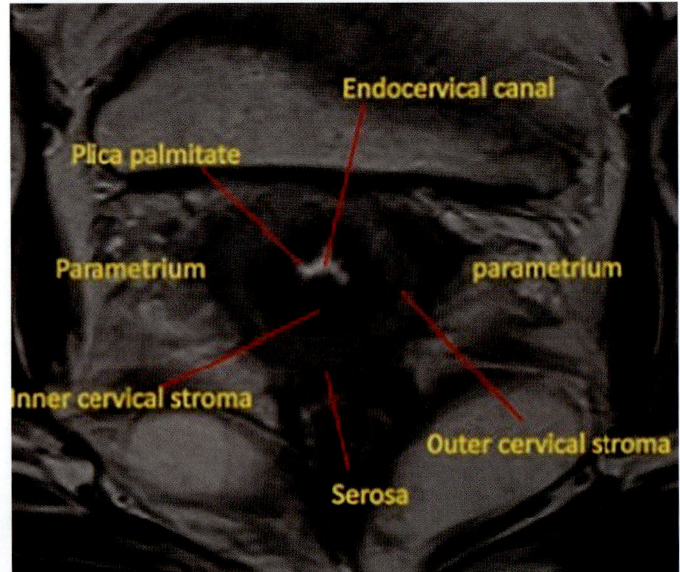

Fig. 3.6.15: Axial section of uterus

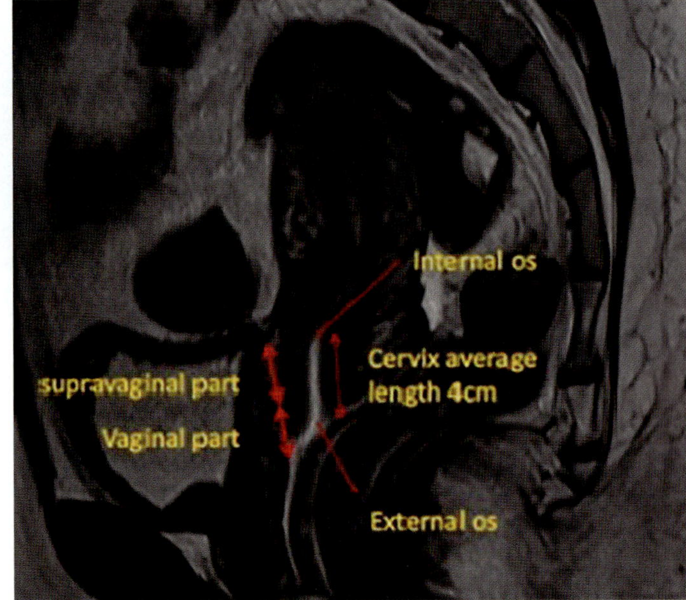

Fig. 3.6.16: Cervix

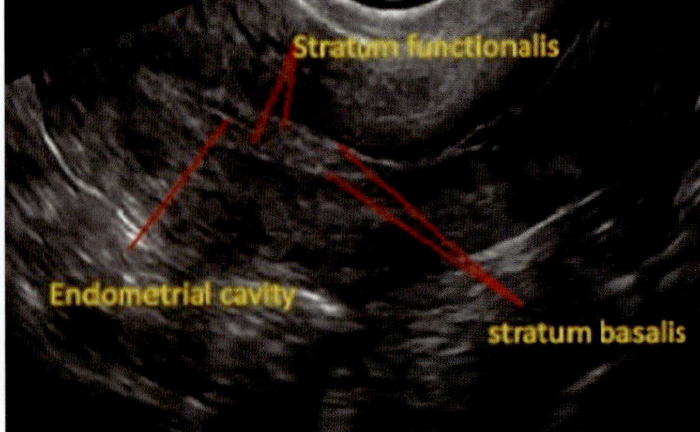

Fig. 3.6.17: Layers of endometrium

area of low attenuation. If a vaginal tampon is used seen as a tubular air-filled structure. Postintravenous contrast the uterus enhances and the ureters can be identified laterally to the cervix. The broad ligament appears as a thin soft tissue density extending anterolaterally from the uterus to the pelvis sidewalls. **MRI scan:** Uterus appears, T1 uniform signal of both the uterus and cervix, T2–three distinct zones: Endometrium—high signal. Junctional zone–low signal 2–8 mm, thick inner myometrium, low water content. Outer myometrium—intermediate signal (Figs 3.6.13–3.6.15).

Ligamentous support of the uterus: Pubocervical ligaments which run anteriorly from the cervix, around the base of the bladder to the pubic bone. Transverse cervical (cardinal) ligaments which run laterally from cervix and lateral aspect of vaginal fornix to pelvic sidewall (Figs 3.6.18–3.6.24).

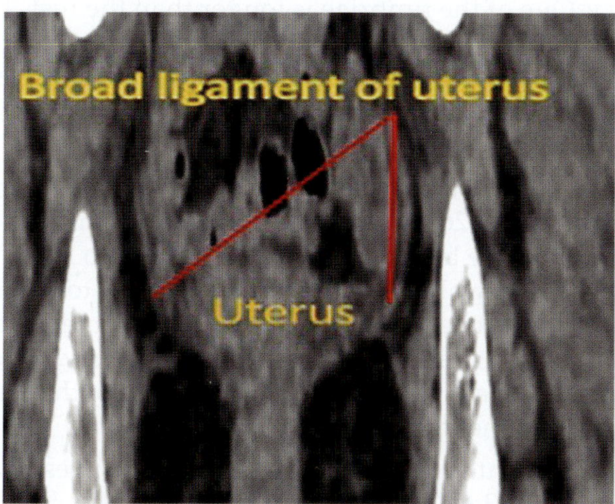

Fig. 3.6.18: Broad ligament of uterus

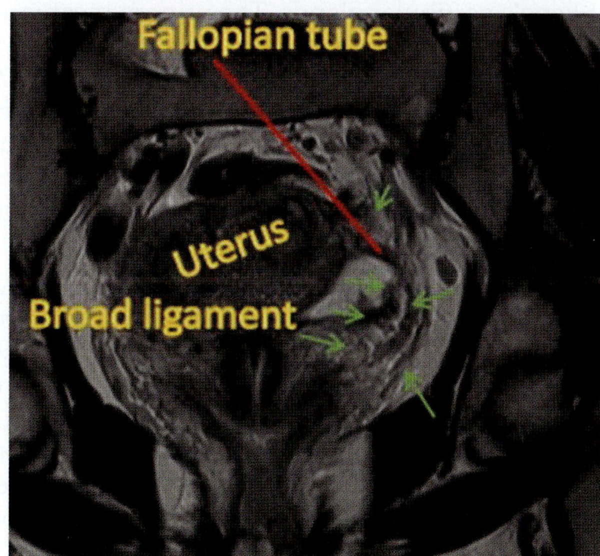

Fig. 3.6.19: Broad ligament of uterus

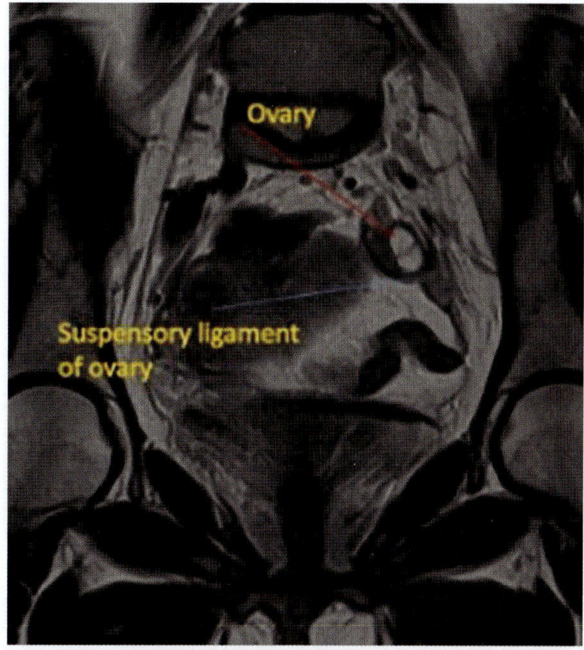

Fig. 3.6.20: Suspensary ligament of ovary

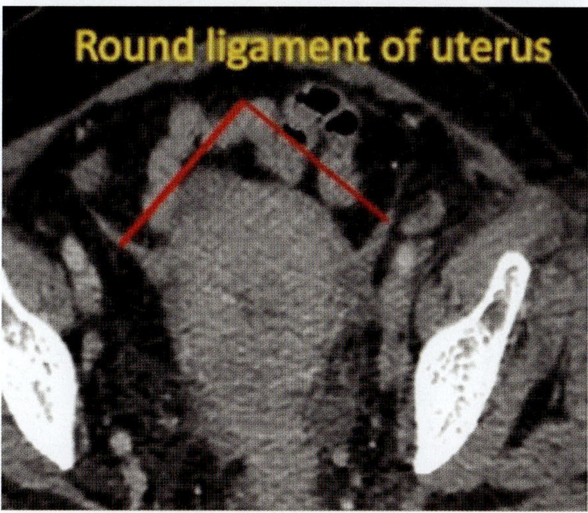

Fig. 3.6.21: Round ligament of uterus

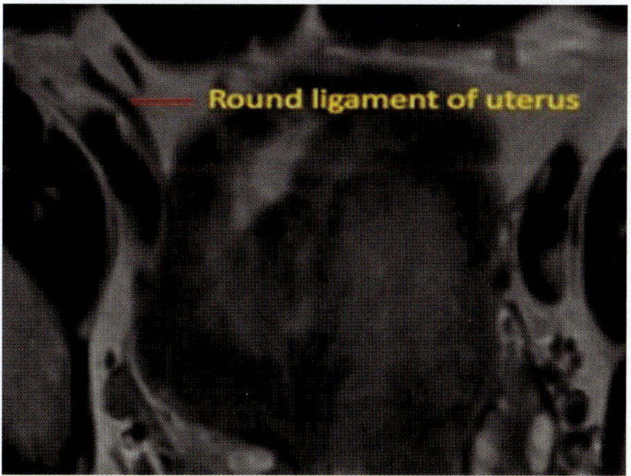

Fig. 3.6.22: Round ligament of uterus

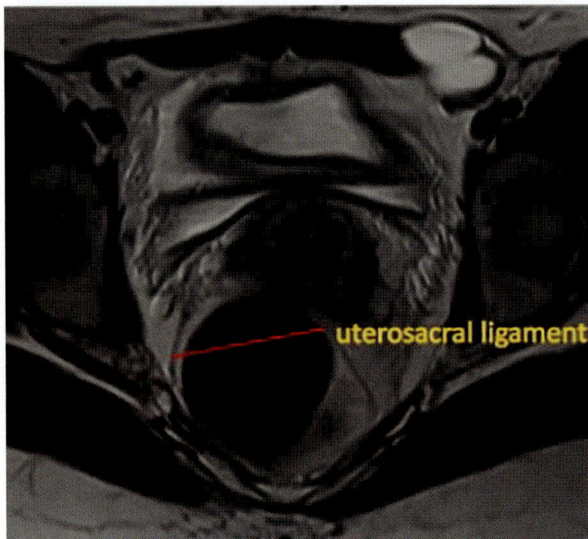

Fig. 3.6.23: Uterosacral ligament

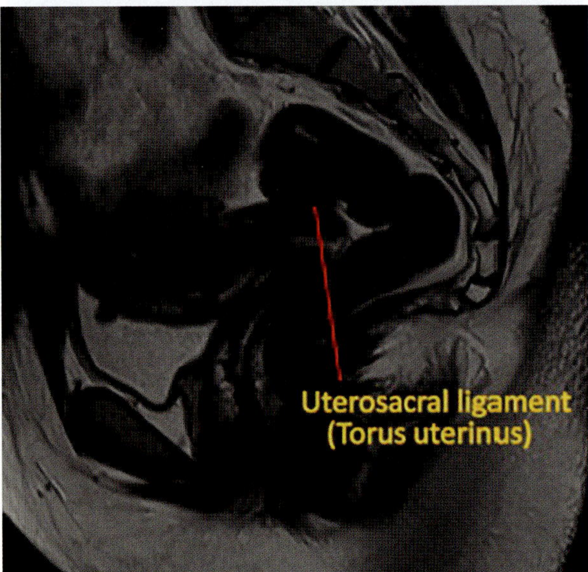

Fig. 3.6.24

Uterosacral ligaments which run posterosuperior to the midsacrum on the upper surface of the levator ani muscle. The round ligament is a fibromuscular band that passes from the upper lateral part of the uterus to the inguinal canal, ending in the labium majoris.

Uterine tubes: They are having four parts as follows (Fig. 3.6.25): The uterine parts are intramural/interstitial—this is the part within the wall of the uterus and opens into it. The isthmus—this is long and narrow and leads to the ampulla—this is a wide, dilated tortuous part at the outer end where fertilization of the ovum usually occurs; and the infundibulum—this is the outer extremity of the tube. It is funnel-shaped and its rim is fimbriated. It extends out beyond the broad ligament through the abdominal ostium and opens into the peritoneal cavity.

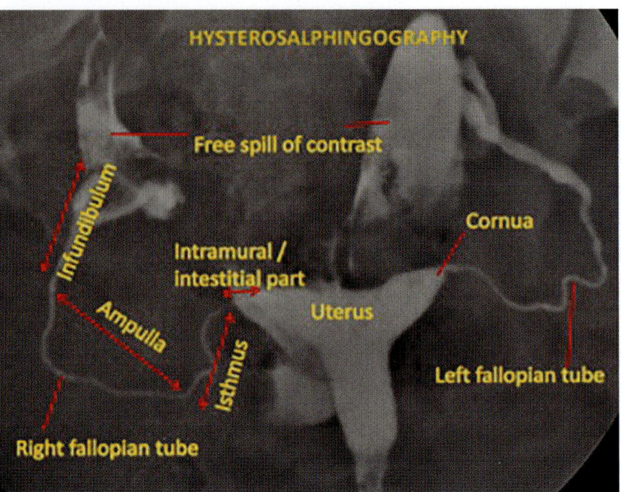

Fig. 3.6.25

The fimbriae spread over the upper surface of the ovary. One of the fimbriae is longer than the rest. This is called the ovarian fimbria as it is attached to the ovary. Cornua of uterus—the superolateral angle of the body project outwards at the junction of the body and the fundus.

Blood supply of the uterus and uterine tubes: The uterine artery (Fig 3.6.26), a branch of the internal iliac, runs medially in the base of the broad ligament to reach the lower lateral wall of the uterus. It ascends tortuously within the broad ligament to supply the uterus and tubes and anastomoses with the ovarian artery. Venous drainage is via a venous plexus in the base of the broad ligament to the internal iliac vein.

Vulva: The vulva consist of the mons pubis, vestibular bulbs (Figs 3.6.31–3.6.38), vulval vestibule, urinary meatus, the vaginal opening, hymen, and Bartholin's and Skene's vestibular glands. The urinary meatus also opens into the vulval vestibule. Other features of the vulva include the pudendal cleft, sebaceous glands, the urogenital triangle, and pubic hair. The vulva provides a double layer of protection for this by the folds of the outer and inner labia. Some of the pelvic floor muscles along with muscles of urogenital triangle provides support the structures of the vulva.

Vagina: The vagina is an extraperitoneal structure (Figs 3.6.27–3.6.30). This muscular canal extends from the uterus to the vestibule, opening between the labia minora behind the urethra and clitoris. Superiorly the cervix of the uterus projects into its anterior wall at an acute angle. The cervix invaginates the upper vagina and arbitrarily divides it into a shallow anterior and deep posterior and lateral recesses or fornices. The ureters pass medially above the lateral fornices.The vagina traverses levator ani and the urogenital diaphragm, which have

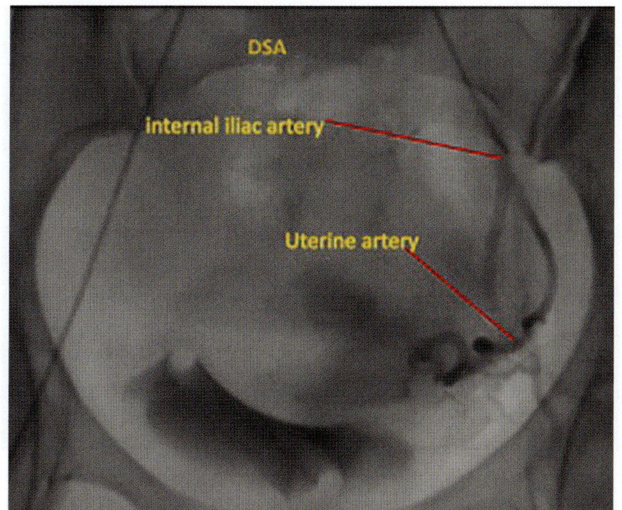

Fig. 3.6.26

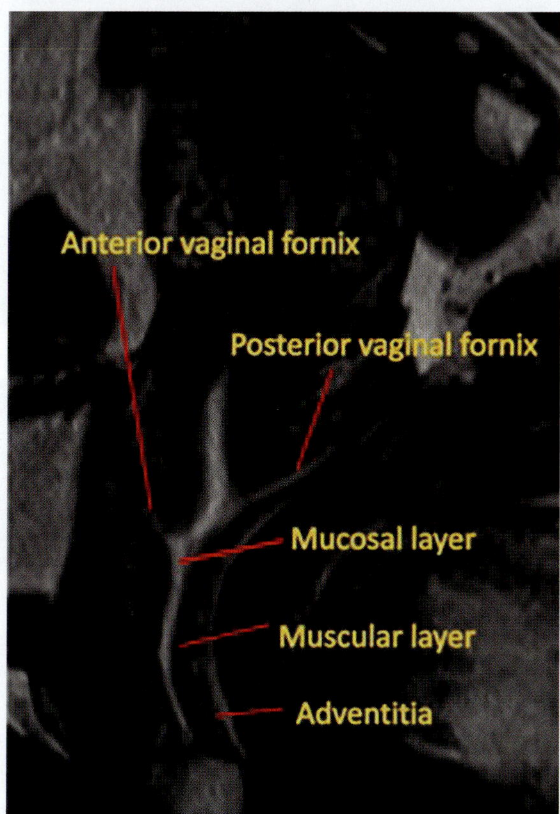

Fig. 3.6.27

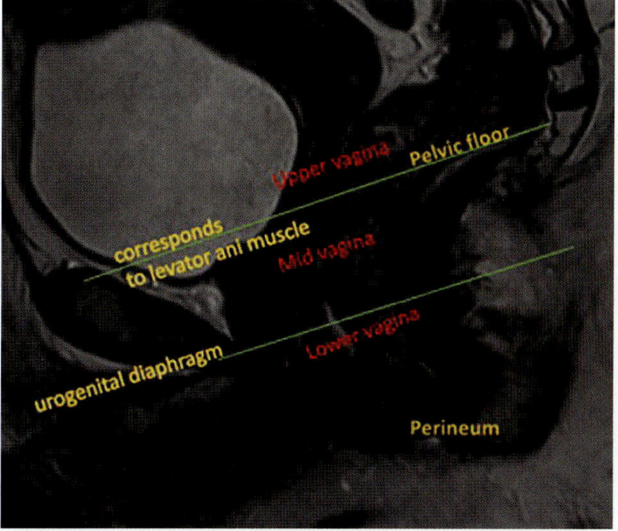

Fig. 3.6.28

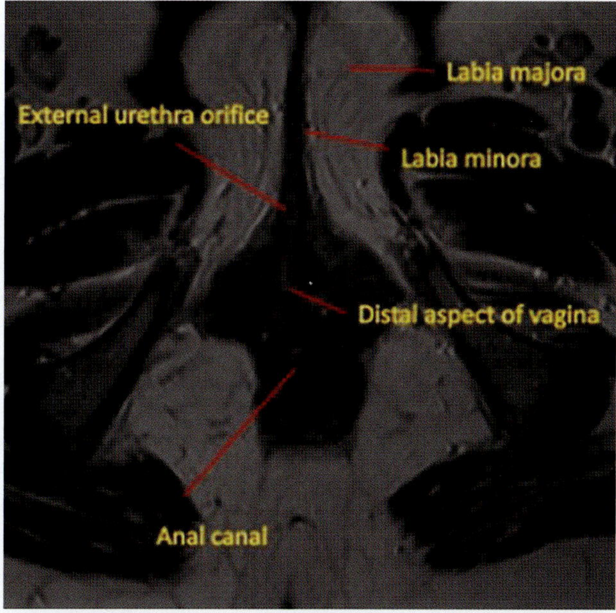

Fig. 3.6.29

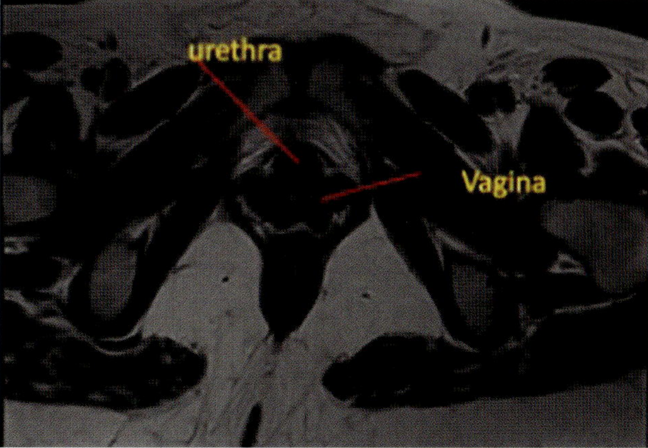

Fig. 3.6.30

a sphincter-like action. The levator muscles insert into a fibromuscular node called the perineal body, which lies between the lower vagina and the anal canal.The layers of vagina on MRI—mucosa has high signal intensity, low signal—muscular layer, high signal—adventitia. The vagina demonstrates an H-shaped configuration on transaxial imaging and consists of a fibromuscular tube extending upward and backward from the vulva to the

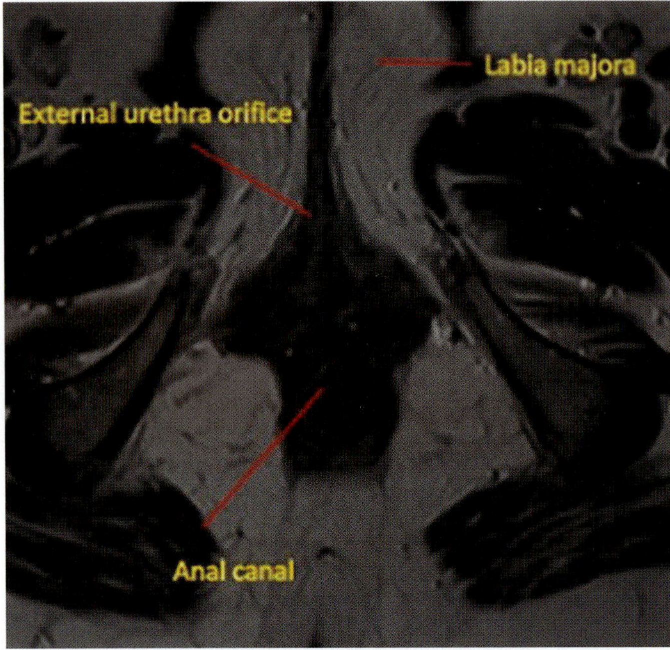

Fig. 3.6.31

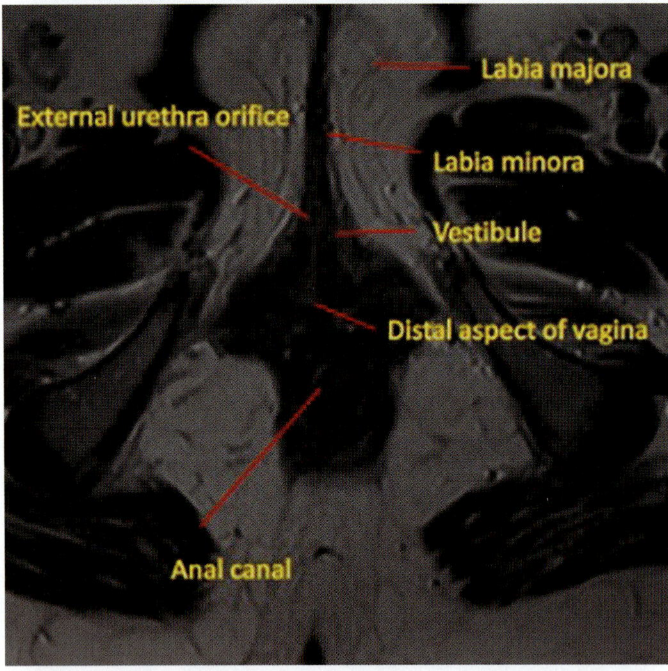

Fig. 3.6.32

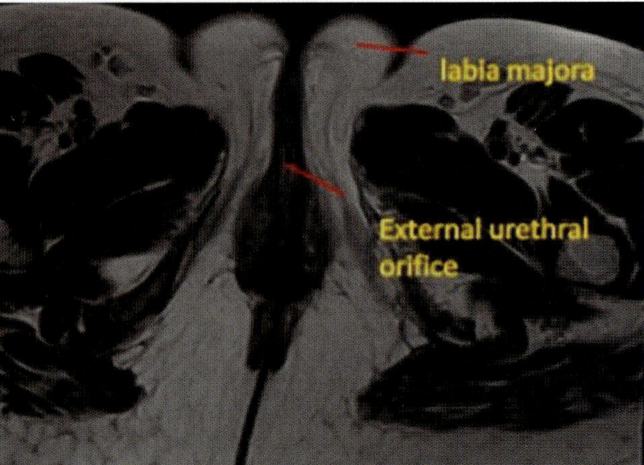

Fig. 3.6.33

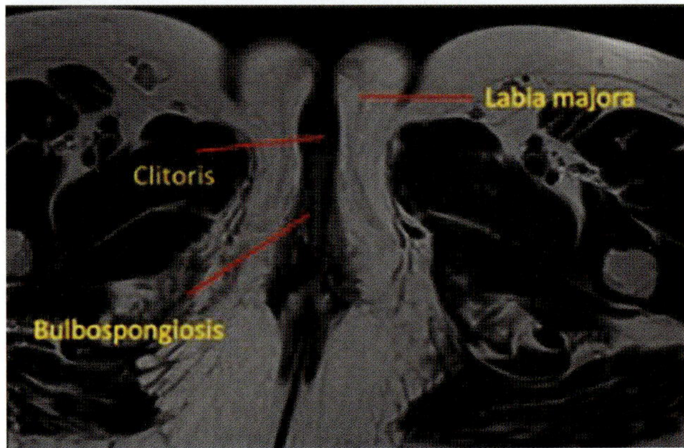

Fig. 3.6.34

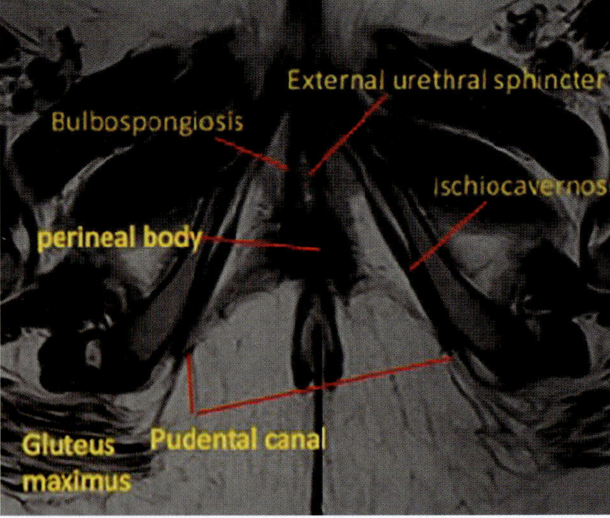

Fig. 3.6.35

uterus. It measures 7 to 9 cm in length and is divided into thirds. The upper third of the vagina corresponds to the lateral vaginal fornices and is supported by the levator ani, transverse cervical, pubocervical, and sacrocervical ligaments. The middle third corresponds to the vagina at the level of the bladder base (which is supported by the urogenital diaphragm), and the lower third is defined as vagina below the level of the bladder base at the level of the urethra (which is supported by the perineal body).

Blood supply: Vaginal branches of the internal iliac and the uterine arteries supply the vagina. Venous drainage is via a plexus on its lateral walls to the internal iliac vein.

Lymph drainage: The upper two-thirds drain to internal and external iliac nodes. The lower third drains to superficial inguinal nodes.

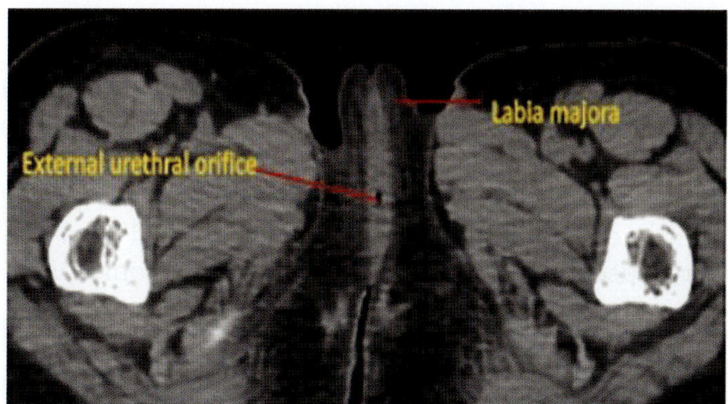

Fig. 3.6.36

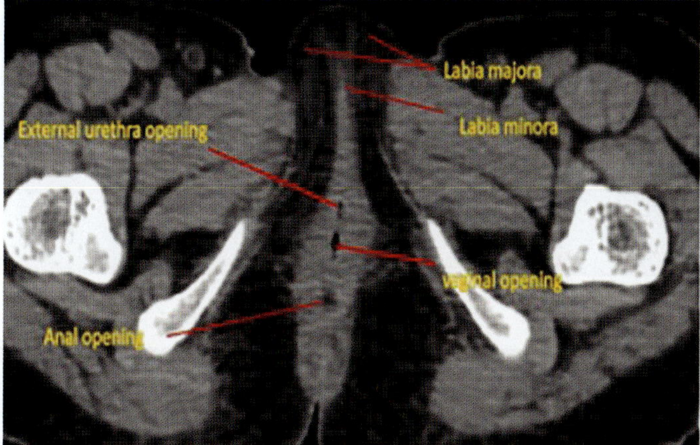

Fig. 3.6.37

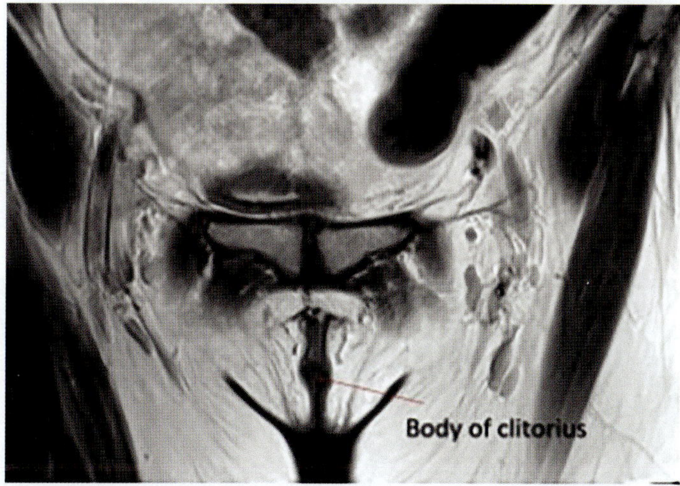

Fig. 3.6.38

Ovaries: These are paired oval organs measuring approximately 3 cm × 2 cm × 2 cm. They are usually orientated somewhat vertically and thus can be described as having upper and lower poles. Ovaries located on the posterior surface of the broad ligament in close contact with the infundibulum of the fallopian tube and attached to its ovarian fimbria.

The anterior surface of the ovary is attached to the posterior surface of the broad ligament by a short meso-ovarium that fuses with the surface of the ovary. The lower pole of the ovary is attached to the uterus by the ovarian ligament. A superolateral extension of the broad ligament, the suspensory ligament of the ovary, runs from the upper pole of the ovary to the pelvic sidewall. **Blood supply:** Arterial supply is via the ovarian artery, which arises directly from the aorta (Figs 3.6.41–3.6.43). **Venous drainage** is via the right ovarian vein into the inferior vena cava, and via the left ovarian vein into the left renal vein. **Lymph drainage** Along the ovarian vessels to para-aortic nodes. **Ultrasound:** On ultrasound the ovary has a homogeneous echotexture with central echogenic medulla. Several small anechoic follicles are seen peripherally in the cortex. Echogenic foci are common. These are non-shadowing and can diffuse. They are caused by a specular reflection from the walls of tiny unresolved cysts. Focal calcification may be seen. Doppler shows a low-velocity, low-resistance arterial waveform (Fig. 3.6.39).

MRI scan: T1: Uniform intermediate signal with low signal follicles. T2: Multiple high signal follicles with low signal capsule and medulla slightly higher signal than cortex. Postmenopausal ovaries are of homogeneous signal on both T1 and T2. Postgadolinium the stroma of the ovary enhances, making the low-signal follicles more prominent (Fig. 3.6.40).

3.6.C Male Reproductive System

Prostate: The prostate gland is an inverted pyramid shaped structure and it surrounds the proximal urethra (Fig. 3.6.44), urethra traverses the prostate close to its anterior surface at base and then more centrally. It has a base superiorly, apex inferiorly and has three surfaces: Anterior, inferolateral and posterior. The base of the prostate continues as the bladder. It ends inferiorly at the apex at the urogenital diaphragm. The anterior surface forms the posterior limit of the retropubic space. The puboprostatic ligaments connect the prostate to pubic bone. It is separated from the rectum by the rectovesical fascia (Denonvilliers fascia). The seminal vesicles lie posterior and superior to the prostate gland. Their ejaculatory ducts pierce the posterior surface of the prostate below the bladder and drain into the prostatic urethra. The prostate gland lacks a true capsule and the so-called prostate capsule is a pseudocapsule formed from fibromuscular tissue surrounding 3 distinct layers of fascia: The anterior, lateral, and posterior fasciae. Anteriorly and apically this pseudocapsule is deficient. Laterally the fascia fuses with the levator fascia. The

3

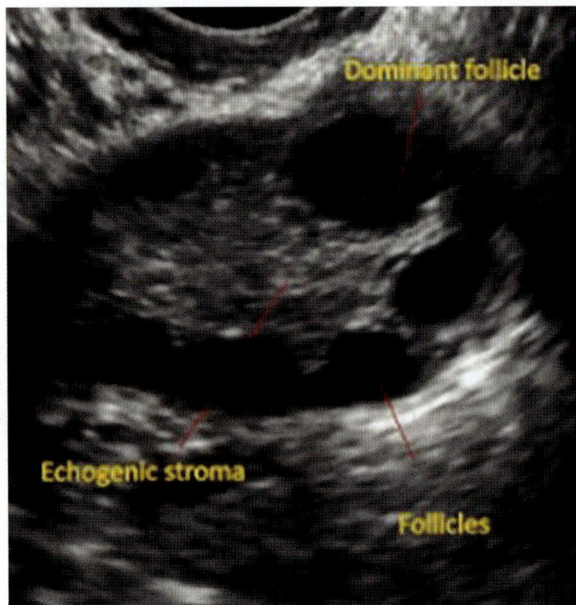

Fig. 3.6.39

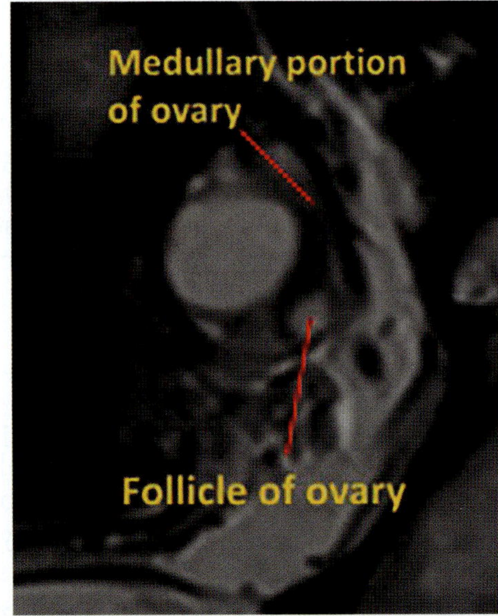

Fig. 3.6.40: MRI ovary

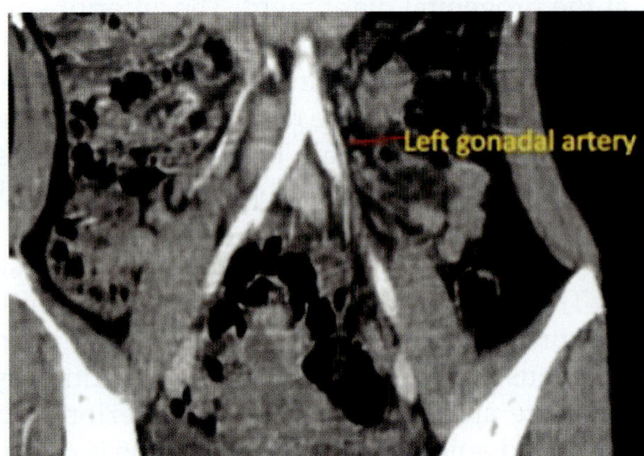

Fig. 3.6.41

prostatic venous plexus (Santorini's plexus) lies between and passes through, the pseudocapsule and fascia. Neurovascular bundles travel posterolaterally at 5 and 7 o'clock and give off branches into the prostate at the apex and base.

Zonal anatomy of prostate has four zones: Peripheral zone, central zone, transition zone, and anterior fibromuscular zone (or stroma). Zonal anatomy of the

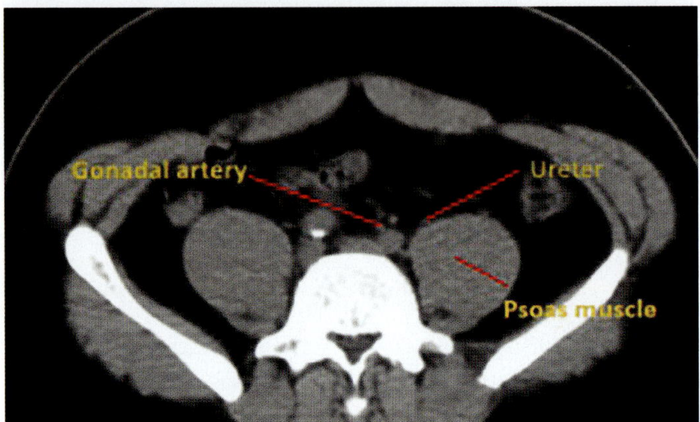

Fig. 3.6.42

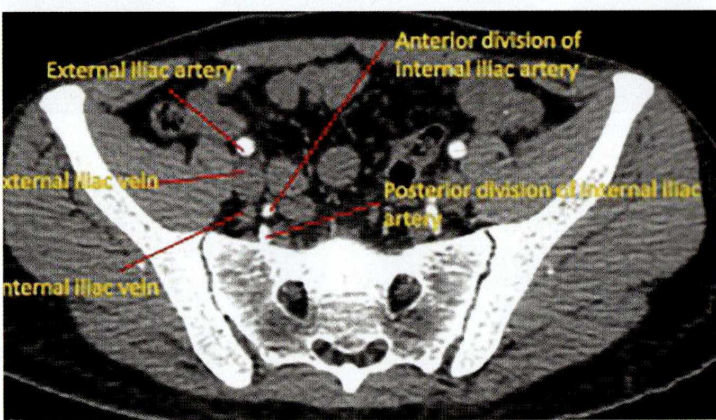

Fig. 3.6.43

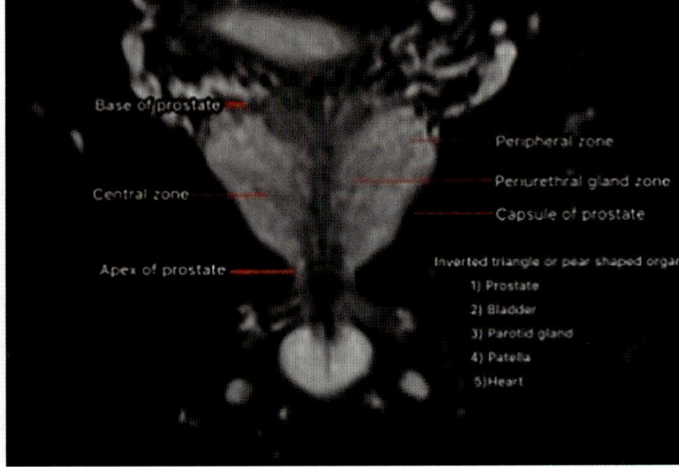

Fig. 3.6.44: MRI of prostate in coronal section

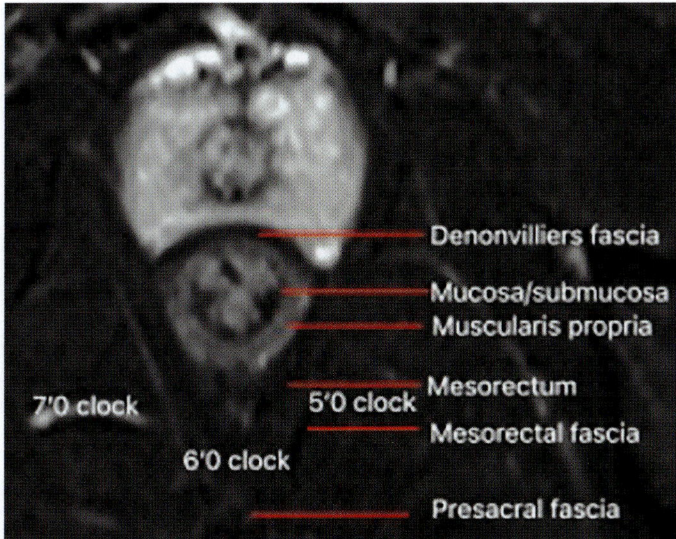

Fig. 3.6.45: Prostate with fascia

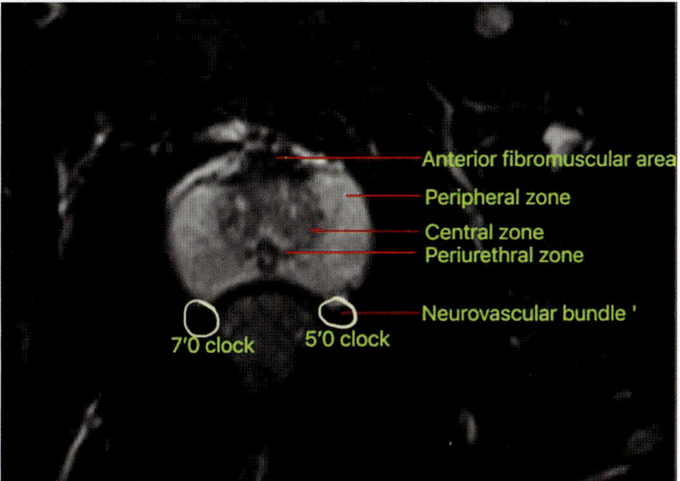

Fig. 3.6.46: Prostate axial sections

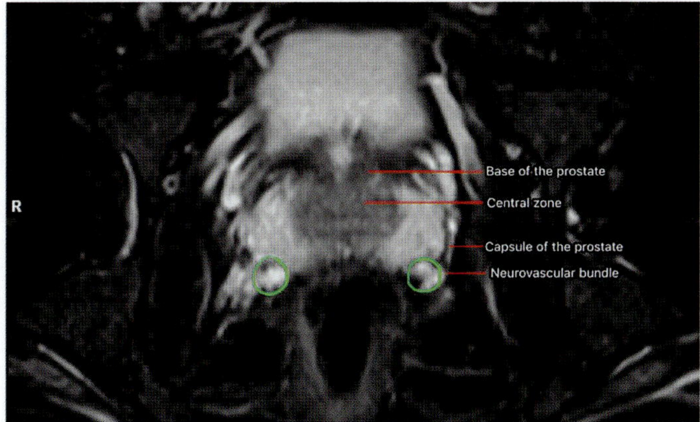

Fig. 3.6.47

prostate gland is best seen on MRI T2-weighted images. **Central gland:** The transition and central zones cannot be differentiated on MRI due to similar signal intensity of the prostate. They are collectively referred to as the central gland. **Transition zone:** The transition zone forms 5% of the gland in young adults and is the innermost section of the prostate and prostate consists of two small lobules and surrounds urethra superiorly to verumontanum the posterior part of urethra at base and anterolateral part at midland. **Central zone:** The central zone is comprises up to 25% of the glandular tissue and is located at the base of the prostate between the peripheral and transition zones surrounding the ejaculatory ducts and narrowing to an apex at the verumontanum. **Anterior fibromuscular stroma:** AFS is a thick sheath of tissue and it continues with detrusor vesicae which forms anterolateral border of glandular prostate. It does not contain glandular tissue and contacts the urethra anteriorly at the base. AFMS is connected to the inferior edge of pubic symphysis by puboprostatic ligament. On MRI imaging T2 sequence, the anterior fibromuscular stroma is hypointense due to a lack of glandular tissue. **Arterial supply** by prostatic branch of the inferior vesical artery and a branch of the anterior division of the internal iliac artery. Sometimes supplied by the middle rectal arteries. **Venous drainage** by prostatic venous plexus in communication with the pudendal plexus to the deep dorsal vein (to the internal iliac vein) with some communication to the Batson vertebral venous plexus. **Ultrasound:** The prostate is most frequently imaged by transrectal ultrasound. The peripheral zone is the most reflective, although it may be indistinguishable from the rest of the gland (Figs 3.6.48–3.6.49). The urethra is seen as a central anechoic structure, surrounded by a hypoechoic area comprising smooth muscle, periurethral glands and the transition zone. **CT scan:** The prostate is seen as a soft tissue mass, separated from the obturator internus muscles by a well-defined fat plane. CT cannot delineate the zonal anatomy of the gland. **MRI:** The gland is of homogeneous low signal on T1W sequences. Zonal anatomy is best demonstrated on T2W sequences central and transition zones (sometimes loosely termed the 'central gland') have relatively low T2 signal. Peripheral zone and seminal vesicles return high T2 signal. MRI is used to stage prostate cancer, with T2W imaging being most useful (Figs 3.6.45, 3.6.47, 3.6.50, 3.6.51).

Seminal vesicle: The seminal vesicles (SVs) are paired accessory sex glands of the male reproductive system. The seminal vesicle is very high in fructose produces over two-thirds of the ejaculate. The seminal vesicle is 10–15 cm long tubular structure but it measures 4–5 cm in length due to coiled nature. It is located superiorly and posteriorly to the prostate (Fig. 3.6.52).

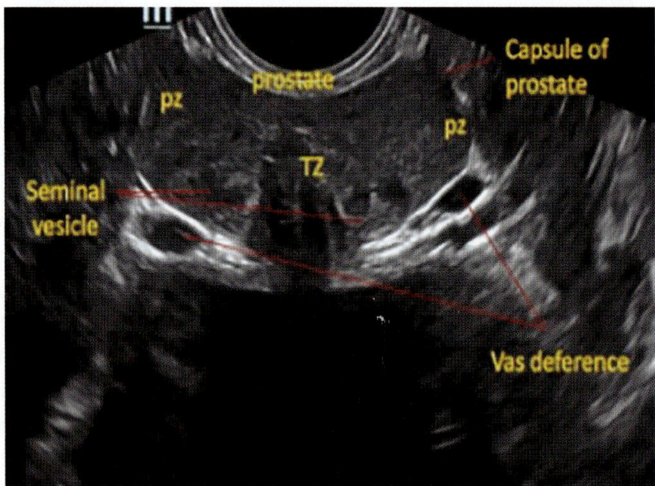

Fig. 3.6.48

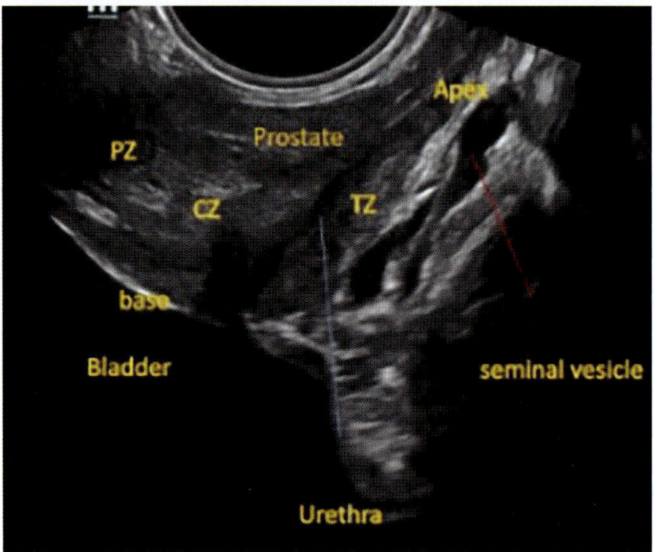

Fig. 3.6.49

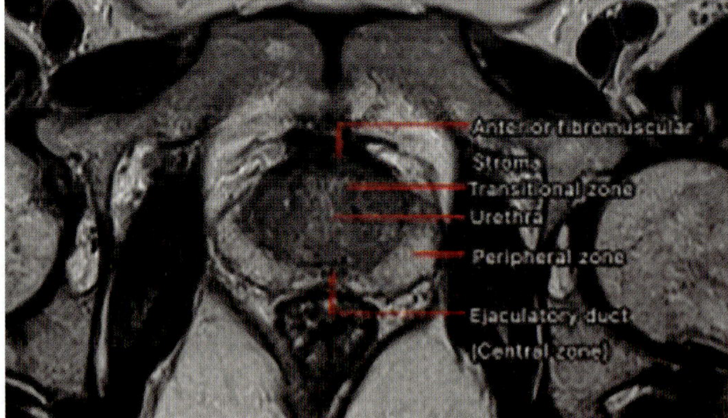

Fig. 3.6.50

The excretory duct of the seminal vesicle unites with the ductus deferens to form the ejaculatory duct.

The SVs are seen as elongated septate cystic structures above the prostate. The distal portion of the VD is seen as a slightly dilated tubular structure (the ampulla of the VD) medial to the SV. At contrast-enhanced computed tomography (CT), the SVs are seen as fluid-containing

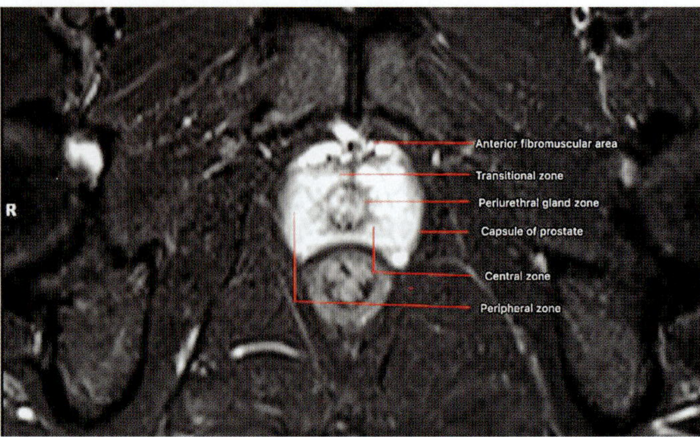

Fig. 3.6.51

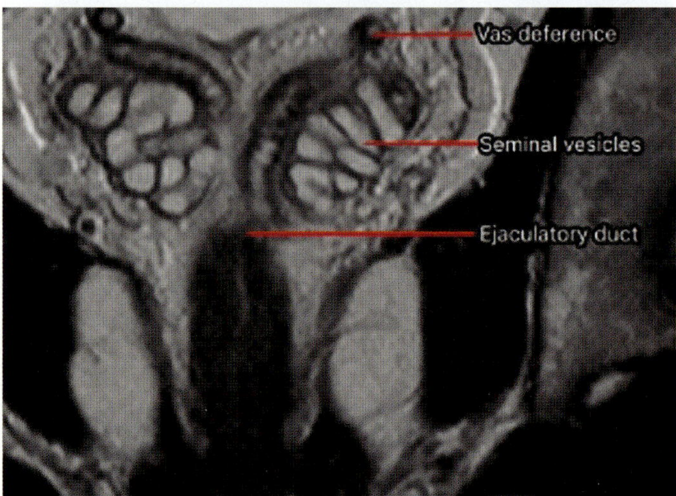

Fig. 3.6.52

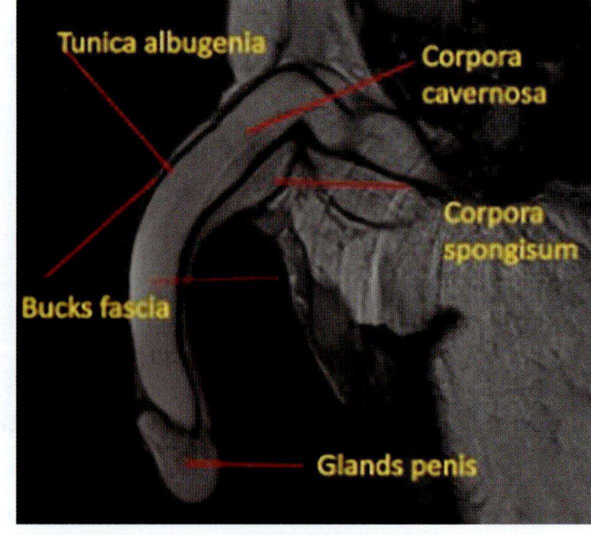

Fig. 3.6.53

structures of bow tie configuration. The SVs are seen as elongated fluid-containing structures with thin septa. Ultrasound: Seminal vesicles are tubular structures containing fluid, located above and lateral to the base of the prostate gland. Ejaculatory ducts are sometimes identified as a triangular hypoechoic 'beak' as they project into the central zone of the prostate gland.

MRI: The seminal fluid demonstrates low signal intensity on T1-weighted images and high signal intensity on T2-weighted images (bunch of grapes appearance).

Vas deferens (VD): A muscular tube, about 30–45 cm long, connecting the epididymis to the ejaculatory duct. Origins from the tail of the epididymis and pass through the inguinal canal and pelvis to fuse with the duct of the seminal vesicles, to form the ejaculatory duct in the prostate gland.

Penis: The penis is the external midline urinary and reproductive structure of the male urogenital system. The penis is composed of three cylindrical endothelium-lined cavernous spaces: The paired corpora cavernosa, and the single, ventral, and midline corpus spongiosum. The penis has three parts: Root—the most proximal, fixed part of the penis. It is located in the superficial perineal pouch of the pelvic floor, and is not visible externally. The root contains three erectile tissues (two crura and bulb of the penis), and two muscles (ischiocavernosus and bulbospongiosus). The bulb of the penis has no bony attachment, it is attached to the perineum. Body—the free part of the penis, located between the root and glans. It is suspended from the pubic symphysis. It is composed of three cylinders of erectile tissue, two corpora cavernosa, and the corpus spongiosum. Glans is conical in shape, and is formed by the distal expansion of the corpus spongiosum. This contains the opening of the urethra, termed the external urethral orifice, blood supply is derived mainly from branches of the internal pudendal artery, perineal artery and branches of common penile artery (bulbourethral artery, cavernosal artery and dorsal artery of penis). Venous drainage—deep dorsal vein (unpaired) drains the corpus cavernosum and corpus spongiosum and superficial dorsal vein (unpaired) drains the prepuce and penile skin. The variable MR signal intensity of these structures is due to rate of blood flow within the cavernous spaces that constitute the corporal bodies. The three corpora of the penis are of intermediate T1-weighted and high T2-weighted signal intensity. The corpora cavernosa are isointense relative to one another. The corpus spongiosum is a separate space and may normally have flow and signal intensity characteristics different from those of the cavernosa. On axial T2-weighted images, the deep arteries which are located in corpora cavernosa are seen as small, round areas of hypointensity (due to faster flow) within the medial, dorsal portions of the cavernosa (Figs 3.6.53, 3.6.54 and 3.6.58).

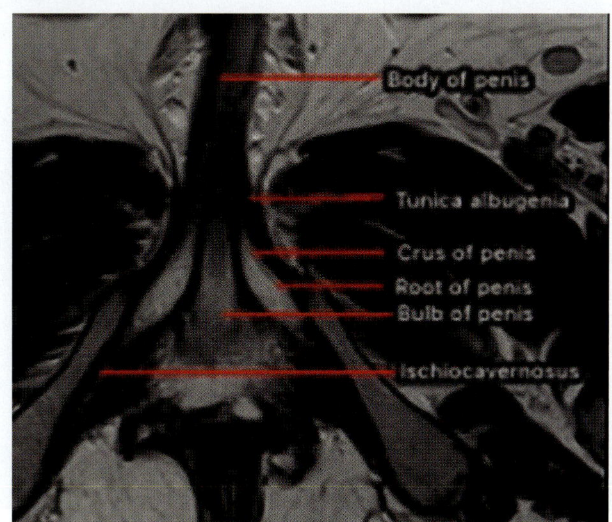

Fig. 3.6.54

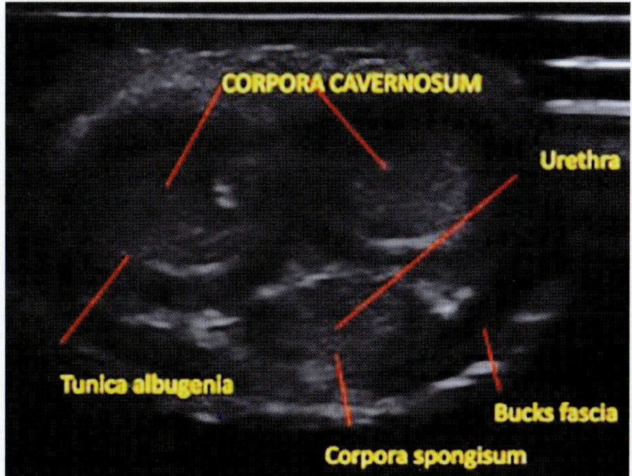

Fig. 3.6.55

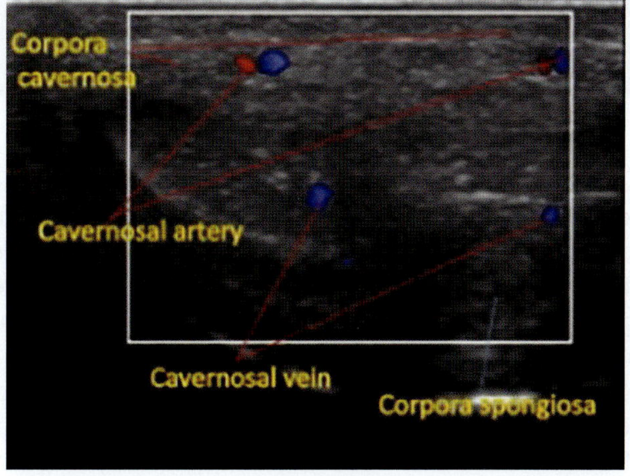

Fig. 3.6.56

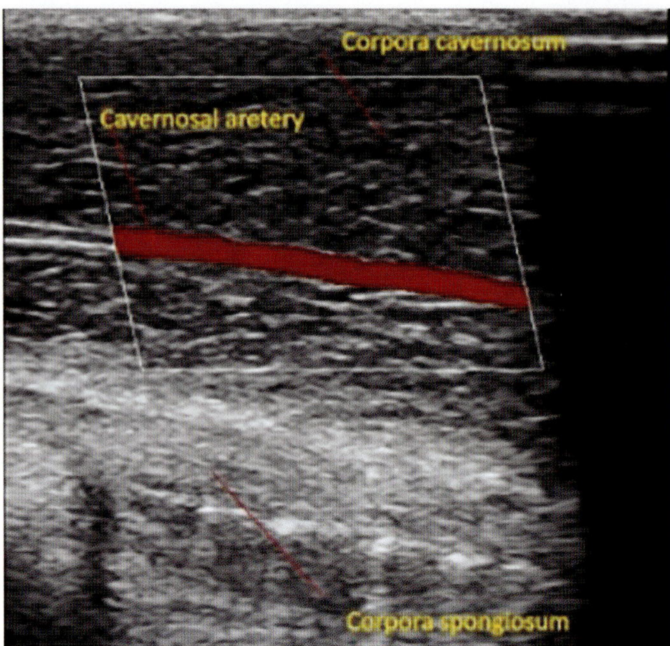

Fig. 3.6.57

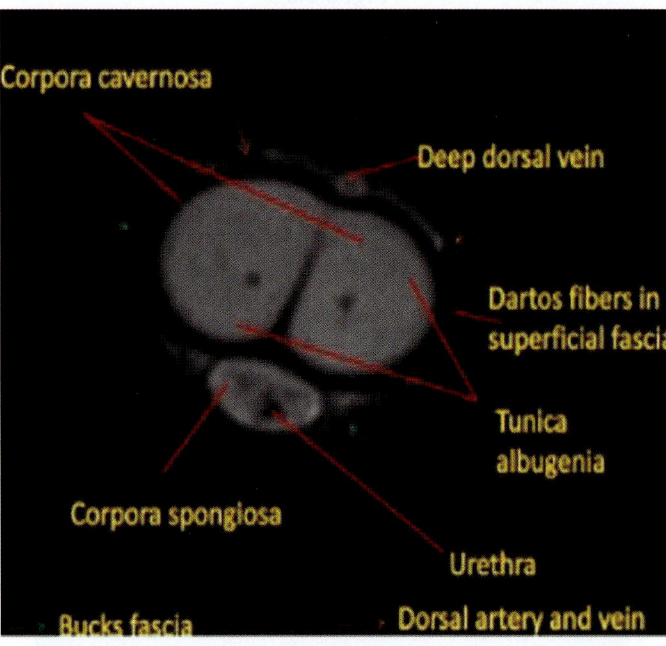

Fig. 3.6.58

Arterial supply is derived from the branches of the internal pudendal artery and include the perineal artery and common penile artery which further gives off artery of the bulb of the penis, cavernosal artery (deep artery of penis) and dorsal artery of penis.Venous drainage is via superficial and deep dorsal veins.

Ultrasound: The corpora demonstrate low-level echoes. The urethra appears as a circular echogenic structure, with a central anechoic area, and is best seen when distended. Colour flow Doppler ultrasound allows visualization of the penile arteries, which is important in the assessment of erectile dysfunction (Figs 3.6.55–3.6.57).

MRI scan: Variable appearances depending on the imaging sequence and the state of erection. On T1W sequences, the corpora are indistinguishable and return signal that is lower than fat (Fig. 3.6.58).

Scrotum: The scrotal wall is composed of multiple layers, including the skin, multiple muscle and fascial layers, and the tunica vaginalis. The tunica vaginalis is a two-layered serous membrane and is derived from the processus vaginalis of the peritoneum: The visceral layer envelops the testicles and epididymis, the parietal layer forms the inner lining of the scrotal sac. Hydroceles has the fluid collection, form in the potential space between the layers of the tunica vaginalis. MR imaging: The scrotal sac is hypointense on both T1- and T2-weighted images.

Testes: The testes (singular: testis), also known as the testicles, are the male gonads and are contained within the scrotum. The paired testes are responsible for the production of sperm and testosterone (Fig. 3.6.59).

Normal adult testes are ovoid and measure approximately 3 cm (AP) × 2–4 cm (TR) × 3–5 cm (length), with a volume of 12.5–19 mL. From the mediastinum testis, several radiating septa extend into the testis forming 250–400 lobules. Each of these lobules contains 2–3 seminiferous tubules. Seminiferous tubules carry the sperm via tubuli recti into a dilated space within the mediastinum testis which is known as the rete testis, which drains into the epididymis through 10–15 efferent ductules. Efferent ducts is located in the head of the epididymis (globus major) unite to form a single duct (globus minor) in the body and tail region, which

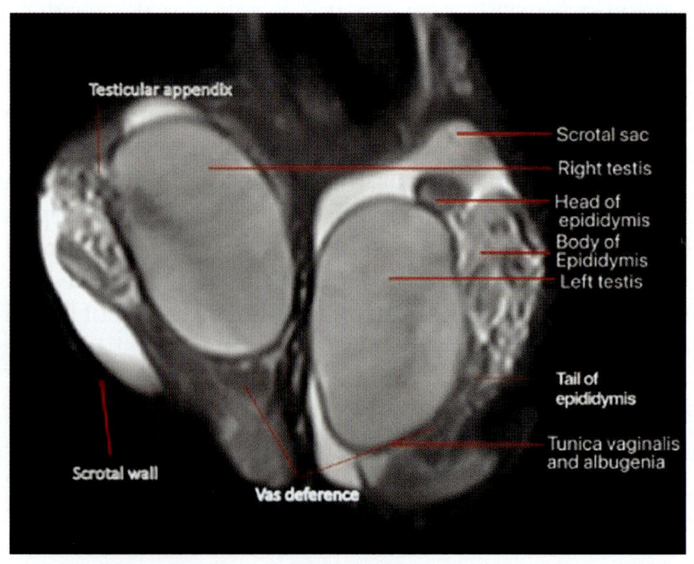

Fig. 3.6.59

continues as the ductus deferens (vas deferens). The testes are supplied by testicular arteries, arising from the aorta, just below the origin of renal arteries. The testes are drained by a plexus of veins (pampiniform plexus), which continue as the testicular veins. The right testicular vein directly drains into the inferior vena cava (IVC), while the left testicular vein drains into the left renal vein.

Ultrasound: Oval structure having a homogeneously granular echotexture with uniform medium-level echoes. Vessels coursing through the testis are often identified as hypoechoic linear structures. The mediastinum testis can be identified as an echogenic line posteriorly, parallel to the epididymis. Occasionally the rete testis is prominent as multiple anechoic tubular structures adjacent to the epididymis. The appendix testis may be seen, especially in the presence of a hydrocoele (Figs 3.6.60–3.6.63).

MRI: On T1W sequences, the testis is of homogeneous low signal intensity. On T2W sequences, normal testicular tissue returns high signal intensity. The tunica albuginea, mediastinum testis and fibrous septa are of low signal intensity on T2W sequences. The epididymis is of variable intensity.

Urethra

The male urethra drains urine from the bladder.The male urethra measures 18–20 cm in length. It origins at the internal urethral orifice in the trigone of the bladder and opens in the fossa navicularis of the glans penis at the external urethral meatus, and is the narrowest part of the urethra.

The male urethra can be divided into anterior and posterior portions.

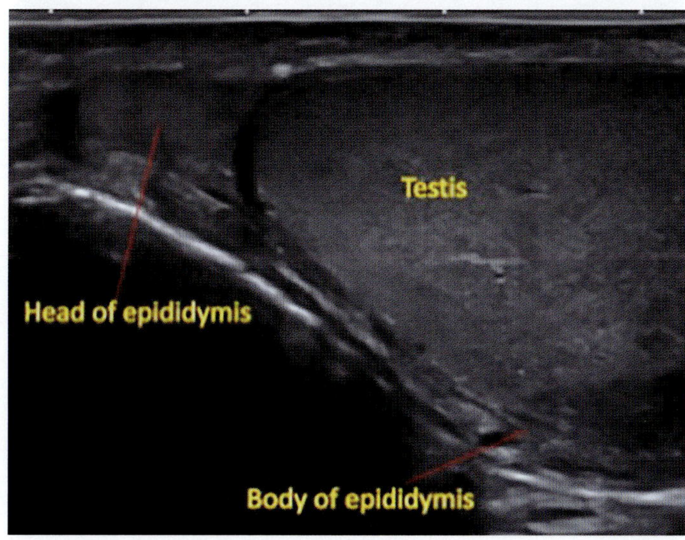

Fig. 3.6.60

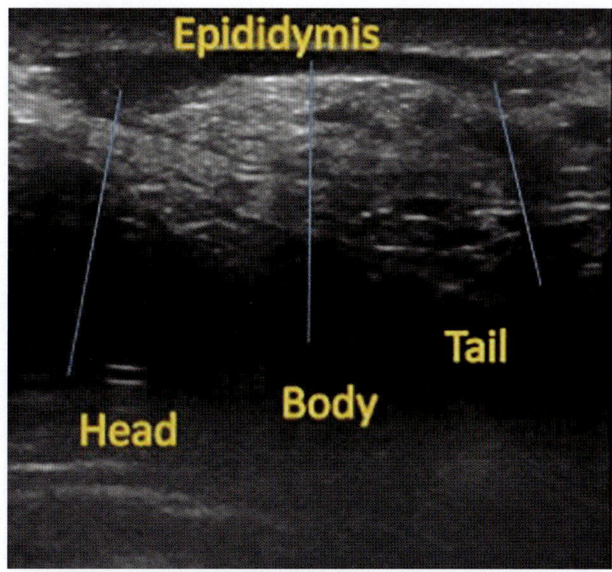

Fig. 3.6.61

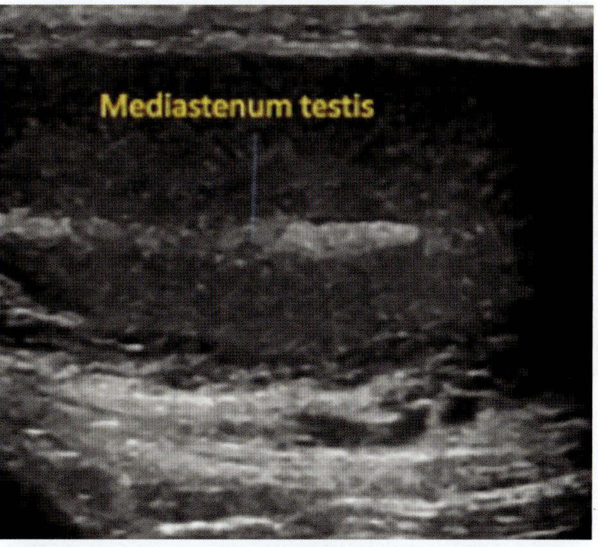

Fig. 3.6.62

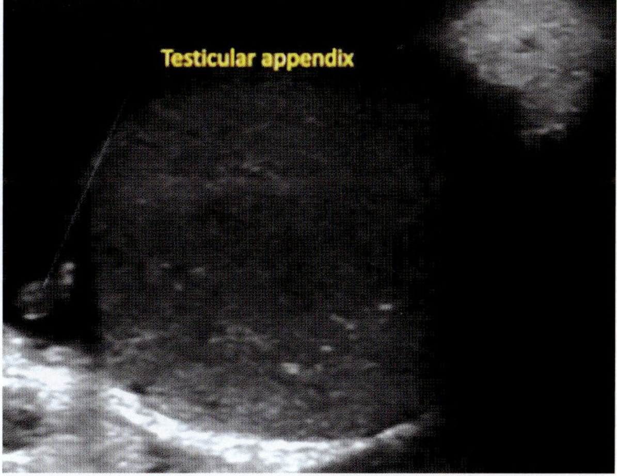

Fig. 3.6.63

Table 3.6.2: Urethra	
Male urethra (Fig. 3.6.64)	*Female urethra*
It is about 20 cm long	It is about 4 cm in length
It is divided into 3 regions	It is not divided into regions
It opens out at the tip of the penis by urogenital aperture	It opens in urinary aperture in front of vaginal aperture
It carries urine as well as semen to exterior	It carries only urine to exterior

Table 3.6.3: Male urethra	
Posterior urethra	*Anterior urethra*
Prostatic urethra: Approximately 3.5 cm long; passes through prostate gland; includes urethral crest and verumontanum	**Bulbar urethra:** Extends from inferior aspect of urogenital diaphragm to penoscrotal junction
Membranous urethra: Approximately 1 cm long Traverses urogenital diaphragm (external urethral sphincter and Cowper's glands)	**Penile urethra:** Extends from penoscrotal junction, passes through corpus spongiosum, and ends at external meatus. Glands of Littré parallel to anterior urethra
Landmarks: Proximal-distal end of verumontanum, distal-conical tip of bulbar urethra	**Fossa navicularis:** Distal 1.5 cm of penile urethra, mild widening in distal urethra

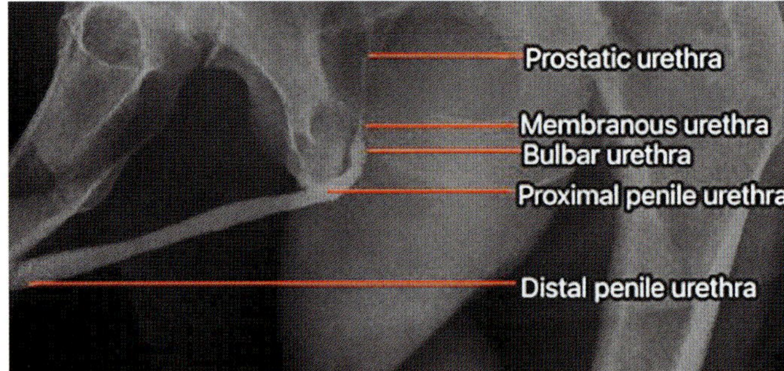

Fig. 3.6.64

3.6.D Rectum

The rectum connects the sigmoid colon to the anal canal. The rectum begins at the S2–S3 and ends at the perineum. It is about 12 to 16 cm long and may be subdivided into three parts: The upper third lies intraperitoneally, middle third retroperitoneally, lower third under the pelvic diaphragm and therefore extraperitoneal. The rectum ends at the anorectal transition. The anorectal transition may be defined by 2 anatomic landmarks: The first there is an abrupt increase in thickness of the inner muscular layer, which corresponds to the upper limit of the internal sphincter of the anus. The other is the superior border of the puborectalis the sling or U-shaped portion of the levator ani muscle complex or pelvic diaphragm. The definition of the upper limit of the rectum is an intraoperative definition, corresponding to the lower limit of the large bowel that can be mobilised away from the spinal column (Figs 3.6.65–3.6.73).

The mesorectal fascia, a layer of connective tissue, enclosing the perirectal fat that surrounds the rectum.

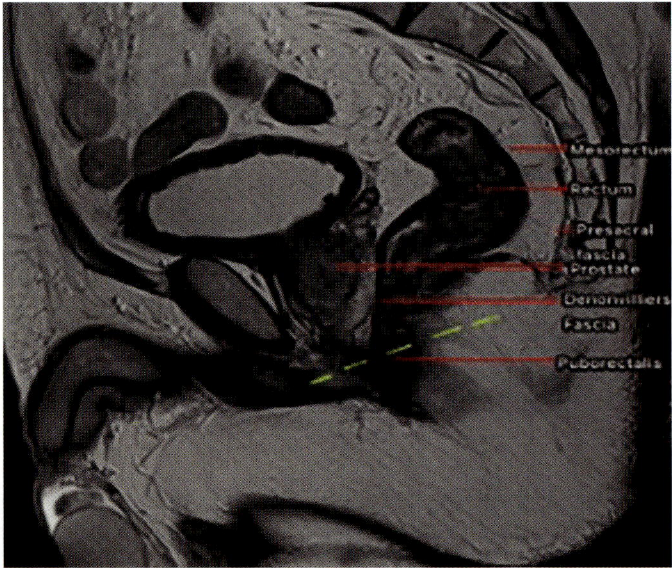

Fig. 3.6.65

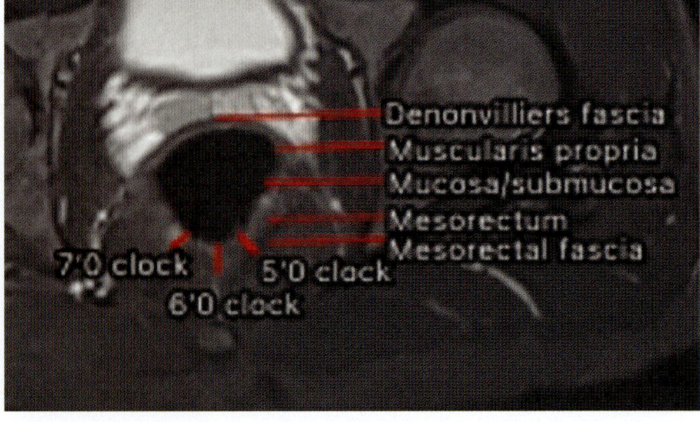

Fig. 3.6.66

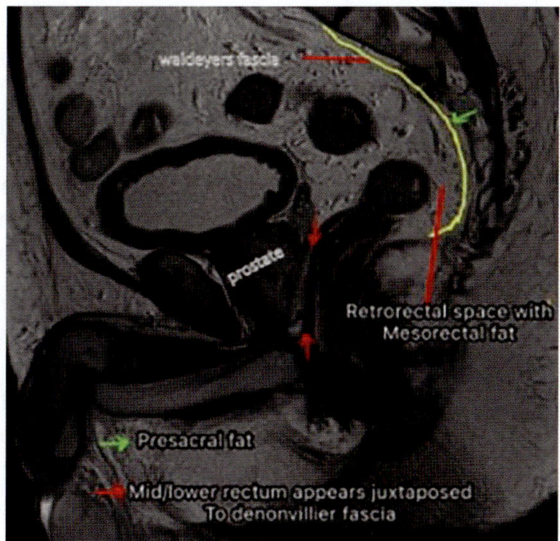

Fig. 3.6.67

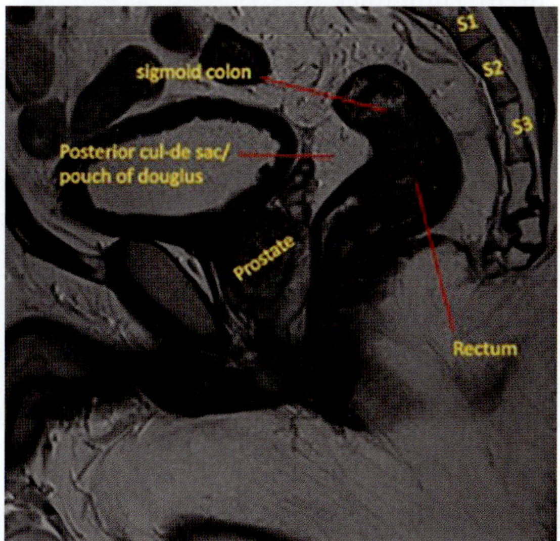

Fig. 3.6.68

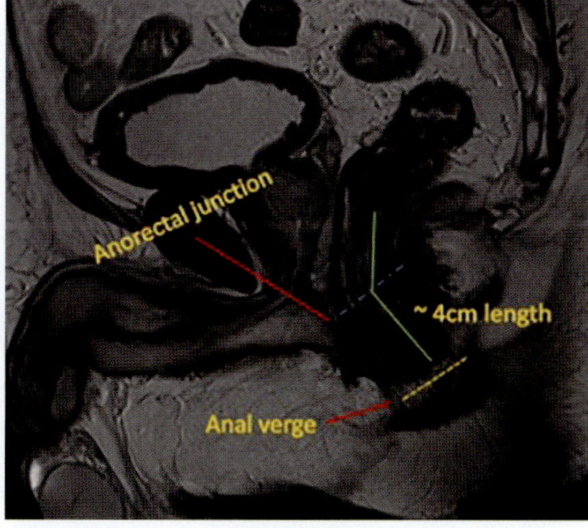

Fig. 3.6.69

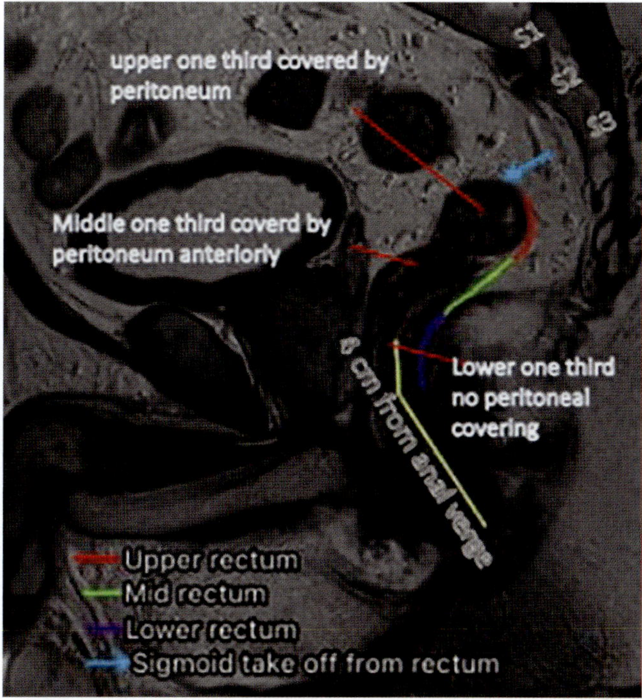

Fig. 3.6.70

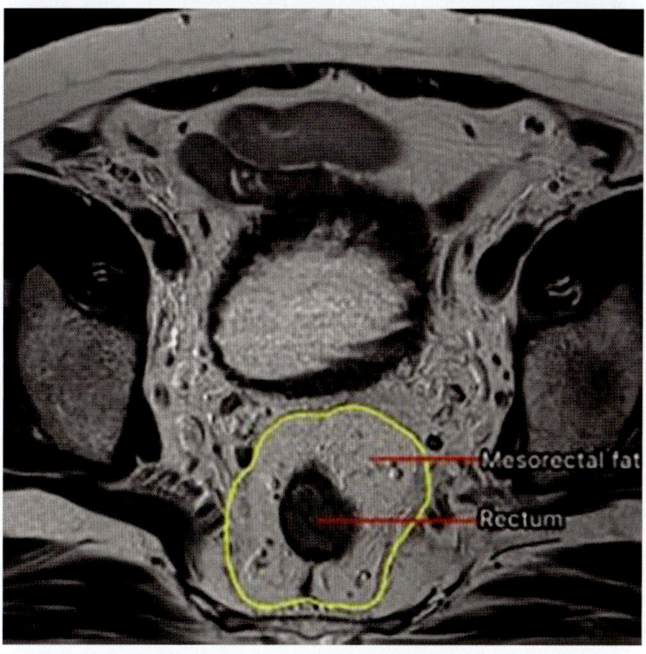

Fig. 3.6.71: Mesorectal fascia

It is an important anatomical structure in rectal cancer staging, as it forms the circumferential resection margin for the non-peritonealised portion of the rectum.

3.6.E Anal Canal

The anal canal is the last part of the gastrointestinal tract. It is about 3 to 5 cm long and lies completely

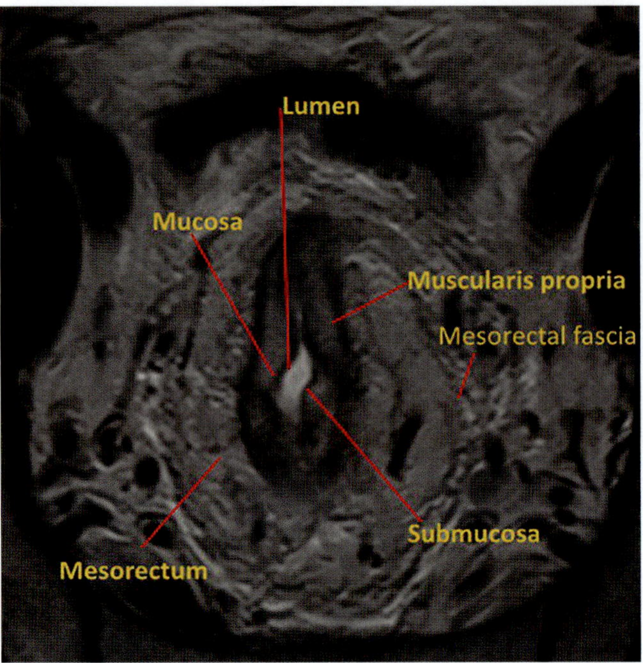

Fig. 3.6.72

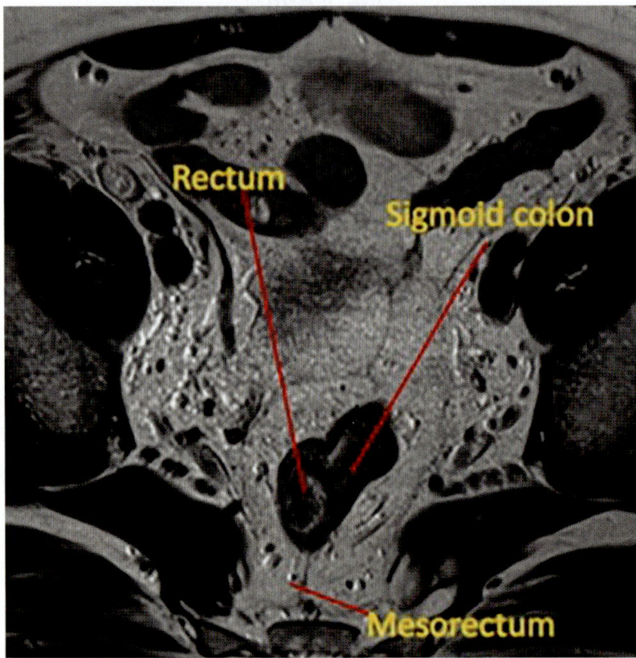

Fig. 3.6.73: In axial sections, rectum is seen as transverse, while sigmoid colon is longitudinally oriented as shown in this figure

extraperitoneal. It begins at the anorectal junction distally from the perineal flexure and ends at the anus. The transitional point from the rectum to anus is identified by the anorectal ring, which is the area where the muscles of the intrinsic and extrinsic sphincters binds superiorly with the puborectalis muscle. The division between the internal and external anal sphincters is identified by the pectinate line. It is divided into three anatomical zones; columnar, intermediate and cutaneous. The dentate (pectinate) line divides the anal into upper (two-thirds) and lower (one-third) parts, each one being supplied by completely different neurovascular structures (Figs 3.6.74–3.6.76). **Arterial supply:** Above dentate line (superior 2/3)—superior rectal artery, below dentate line (inferior 1/3)—middle and inferior rectal arteries.

Venous drainage: Above dentate line (superior 2/3)—superior rectal vein, finally draining into portal circulation.

Below dentate line (inferior 1/3)—middle and inferior rectal veins, finally draining into systemic circulation via vena cava.

The anal sphincter is divided into internal and external anal sphincters. Internal anal sphincter: Continuation of inner rectal muscle and has thickened, circular muscle fibers, up to 5 mm thick.

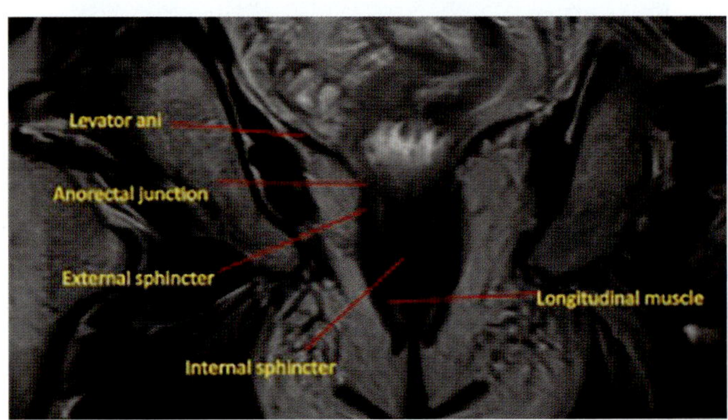

Fig. 3.6.74

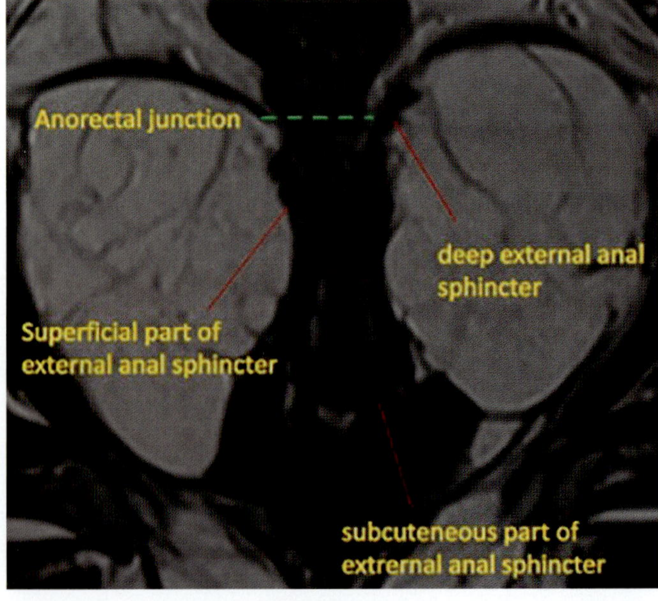

Fig. 3.6.75

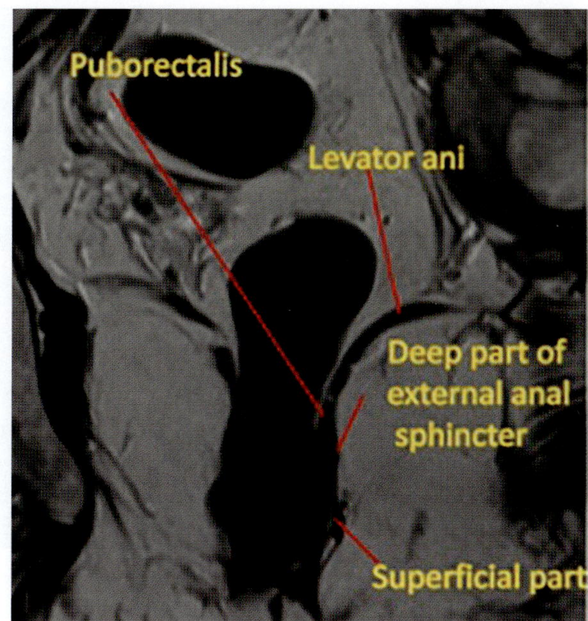

Fig. 3.6.76

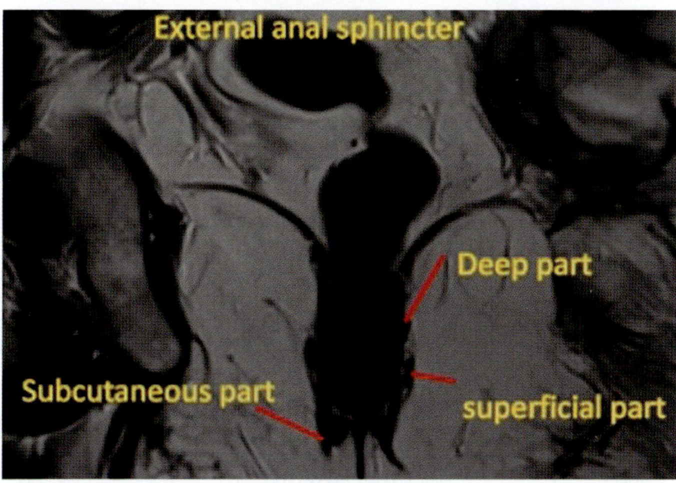

Fig. 3.6.77

External anal sphincter has 3 parts, **deep part** is composed of circular muscle fibers and blends with the puborectalis part of levator ani (posteriorly and laterally). The aforestated region is called the anorectal ring and is palpable on rectal examination. Superficial part has elliptical muscle fibers and attaches from the tip of the coccyx posteriorly to the perineal body anteriorly. It is the only part of the sphincter with bony attachment. Subcutaneous part is composed of circular muscle fibers. Lower ends of this part curve inwards, lying below the end of the internal sphincter (Figs 3.6.77–3.6.80).

3.6.F Pelvic Wall

Anterior pelvic wall: Continuation of upper abdominal muscles **External oblique muscle:** Largest and most

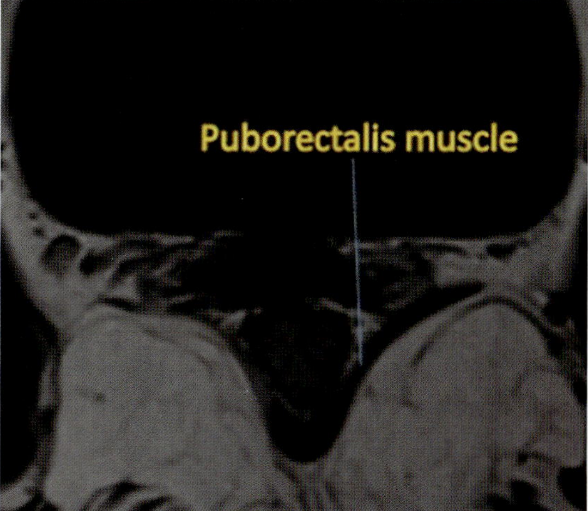

Fig. 3.6.78

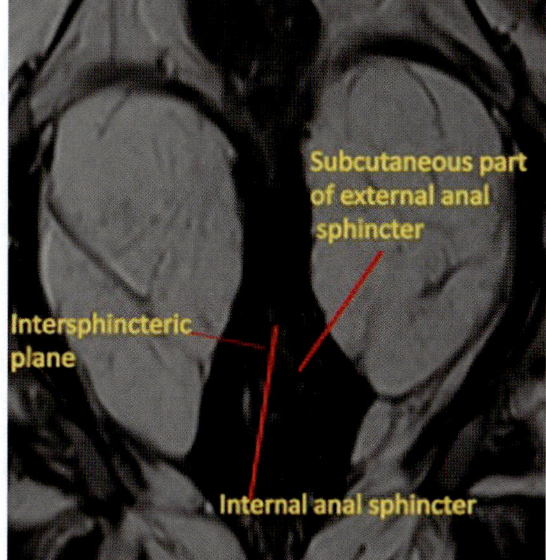

Fig. 3.6.79

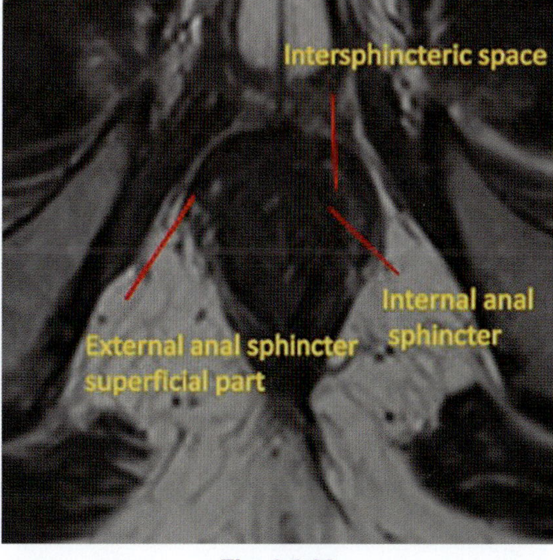

Fig. 3.6.80

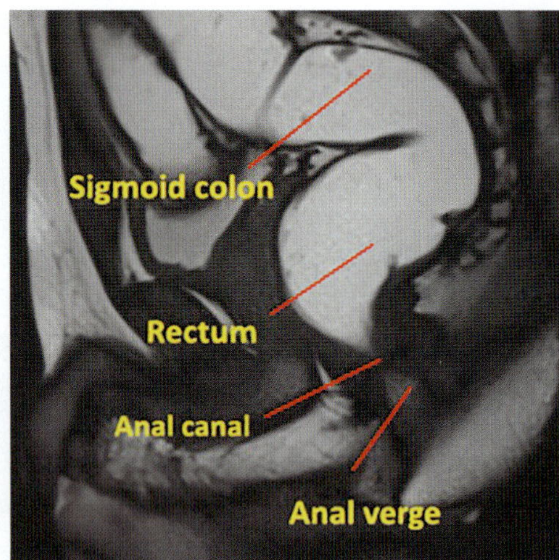

Fig. 3.6.81

superficial of the flat muscles and the fibers course inferomedially. **Internal oblique muscle:** Middle flat muscle runs superomedially at right angles to external oblique muscle in abdomen. Muscle fibers become more horizontal in pelvis and become inferiorly directed more caudal. **Transversus abdominis muscle:** Innermost flat muscle with horizontal course. **Rectus abdominis muscle:** Vertically directed strap muscle. **Linea alba:** Midline fibrous raphe formed by aponeurosis of flat muscles.

Posterior pelvic wall (false pelvis): Psoas and iliacus muscles fuse caudally to form iliopsoas muscle which inserts on lesser trochanter and is powerful hip flexor.

Lateral wall of pelvis: The lateral wall is composed of the pelvic outermost layer of the hip bone below the pelvic inlet, the obturator membrane, the sacrotuberous and sacrospinous ligaments, and the obturator internus muscle with its covering fascia (Figs 3.6.82–3.6.83).

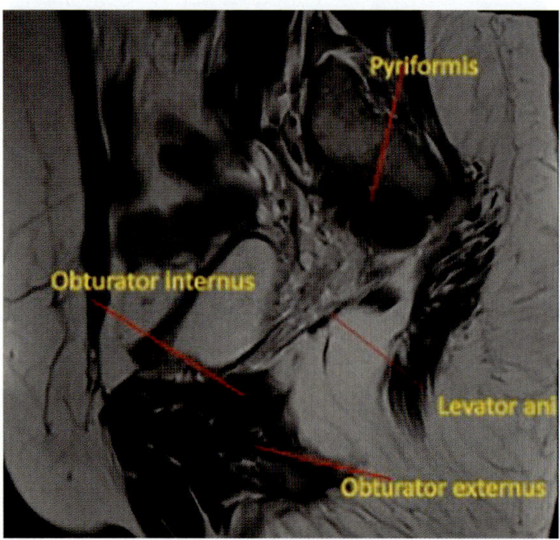

Fig. 3.6.82

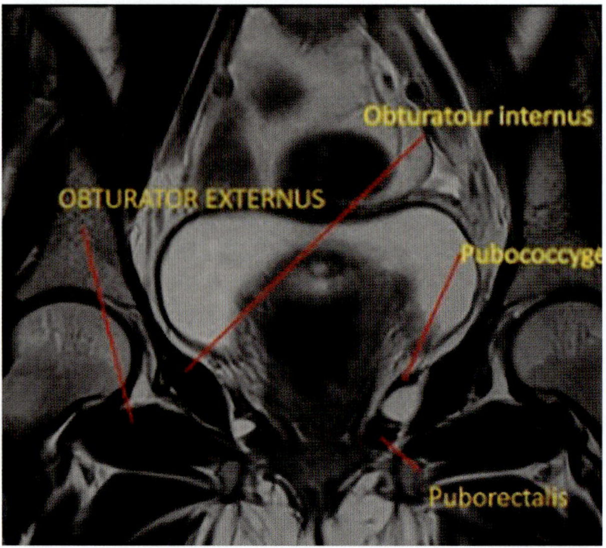

Fig. 3.6.83

3.6.G Pelvic Floor

The pelvic floor is broadly divided into three compartments. The bladder and urethra form the anterior compartment. The vagina and uterus form the middle compartment and the posterior compartment comprises the rectum and anal canal.

The **H** and **M** lines are reference lines for the pelvic floor on imaging studies and help detect and grade pelvic floor prolapse on defecography studies (Fig. 3.6.85).

The H line is drawn from the inferior margin of the pubic symphysis to the posterior aspect of the anorectal junction, and represents the diameter of the levator hiatus, and a normal value is <6 cm. The M line is drawn perpendicularly from the posterior end of the H line to the pubococcygeal line, and represents the descent of the hiatus, and a normal value is <2 cm.

The pubococcygeal line (PC line) corresponds to the pelvic floor. The **pelvic floor** levator ani is a funnel-shaped structure. It attaches to the walls of the lesser pelvis, separating the **pelvic cavity** from the **perineum** inferiorly (region which includes the genitalia and anus). There are two holes in the pelvic floor. They are **urogenital hiatus**—an anteriorly situated gap, which allows passage of the urethra (and the vagina in females) (Figs 3.6.84–3.6.88).

Rectal hiatus: A centrally positioned gap, which allows passage of the anal canal. Between the urogenital hiatus and the anal canal lies a fibrous node known as the **perineal body**, which joins the pelvic floor to the perineum. There are **three** main components of the pelvic floor: Levator ani muscle, coccygeus muscle and fascia coverings of the muscles. **Levator ani muscles (largest component)**: The levator ani is a broadsheet

3

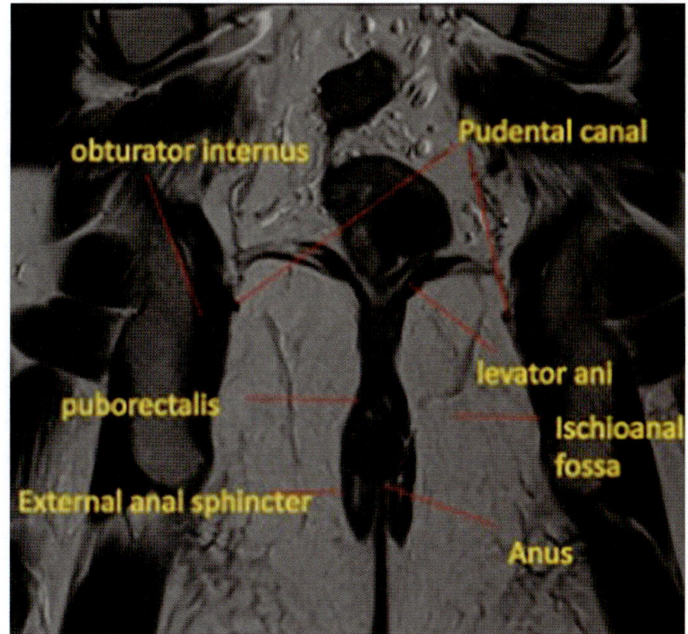

Fig. 3.6.84

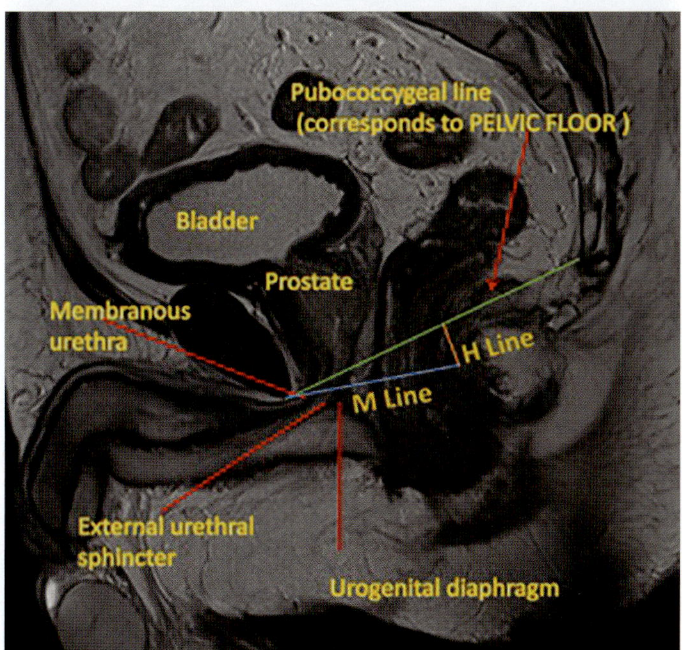

Fig. 3.6.85

of muscle. It is composed of three separate paired muscles; pubococcygeus, puborectalis and iliococcygeus. **Puborectalis:** The puborectalis muscle is a U-shaped sling, extends from the bodies of the pubic bones, past the **urogenital hiatus**, around the anal canal, and some fibers form another U-shaped sling that flank the urethra in the male and the urethra and vagina in the female. **Pubococcygeus:** The muscle fibres of the pubococcygeus form the main constituent of the levator ani. It arises from

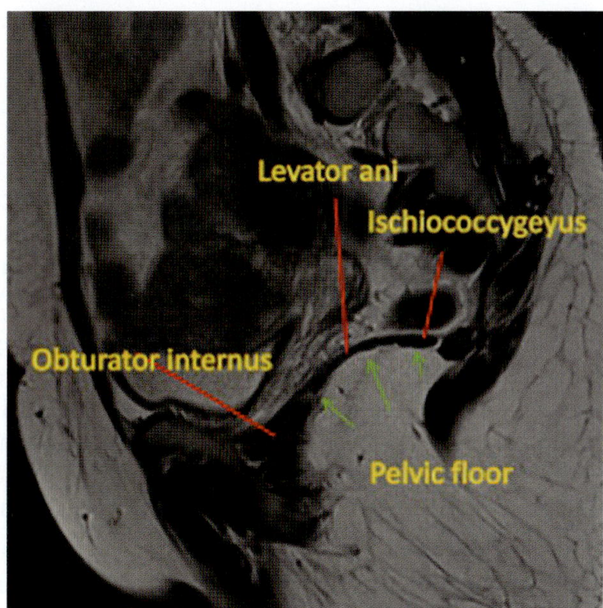

Fig. 3.6.86

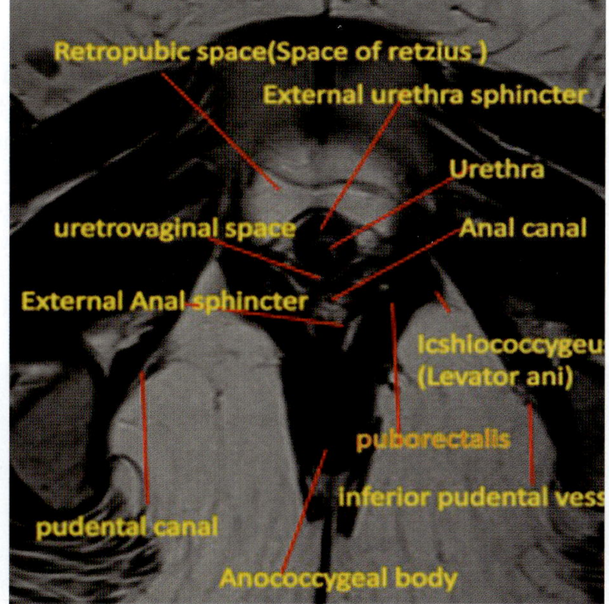

Fig. 3.6.87

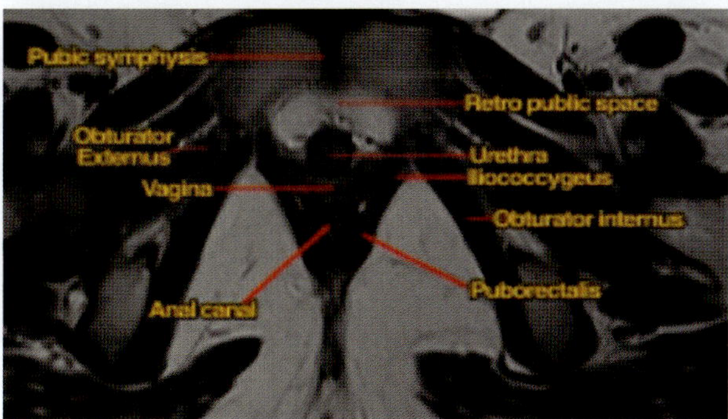

Fig. 3.6.88

the body of the **pubic bone** and the anterior aspect of the **tendinous arch**.

3.6.H The Perineum

The **perineum** is the diamond-shaped space between the pubis, the ischial tuberosities and the coccyx. It is divided into two compartments by the transverse perineal muscles, which arise from the ischial tuberosity and run medially to insert into the perineal body (Fig. 3.6.89).

Urogenital triangle: The anterior urogenital triangle contains a tough sheet of fascia—the perineal membrane—which is pierced by the urethra and in females by the vagina as well. The external urethral sphincter is reinforced by this layer. Its inferior surface gives attachment to the bulb and crura of the penis or clitoris (bulbocavernosus and ischiocavernosus).

Anal triangle: The posterior compartment is the **anal triangle**. It contains the anus and its sphincters, with the **ischiorectal fossa** on either side. The ischiorectal fossa is the space below and lateral to the posterior part of the levator ani and medial to the inner wall of the pelvis (it is bounded posteriorly by sacrotuberous ligaments and the gluteus maximus muscle, laterally by the fascia of the obturator internus muscle and anteriorly by the perineal body). It contains mainly fat. It is of importance in pathological conditions of the rectum. The anococcygeal body extends from the anus to the coccyx posteriorly. It receives fibres from the anal sphincter and levator ani muscles. The **perineal body**, also known as the central tendon of the perineum, is a key midline fibromuscular structure, with important muscular attachments, which acts to stabilize the structures of the pelvis and perineum. It is located between the anal canal and the bulb of the penis, or, in females, the vagina. The perineal body has a trilaminar structure: Superficial layer—muscle fibers of the external anal sphincter which pass anteriorly into the bulbospongiosus muscle. Intermediate layer—superficial transverse perineal muscle. Deep layer—deep transverse perineal muscle (Figs 3.6.90–3.6.96).

Pudendal canal: The pudendal canal is also known as Alcock's canal, fascia derived from the obturator internus muscle and found in the lower lateral wall of the ischiorectal fossa. The contents are pudendal nerve with internal pudendal artery and vein (Figs 3.6.97–3.6.99).

Fig. 3.6.89

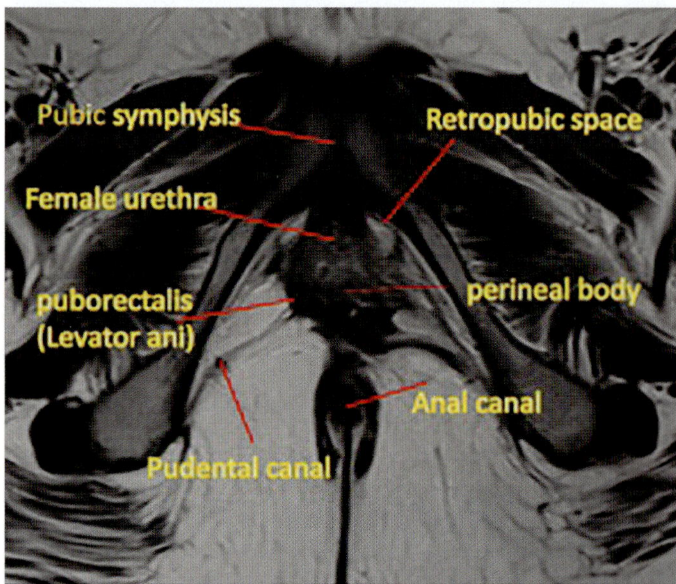

Fig. 3.6.90

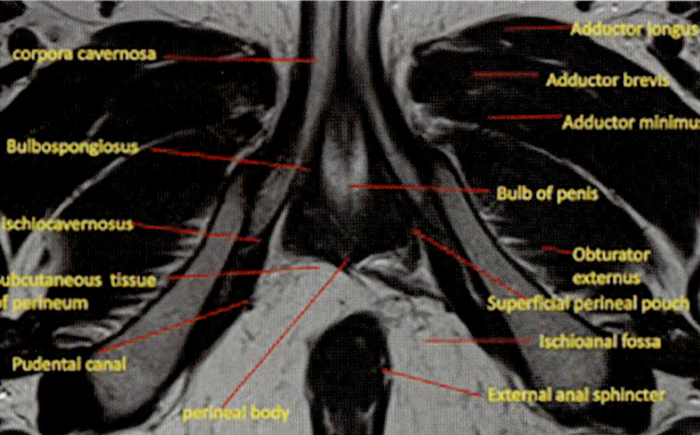

Fig. 3.6.91

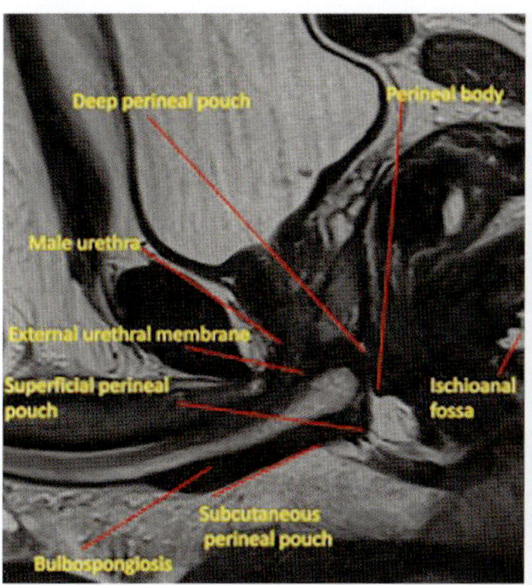

Fig. 3.6.92

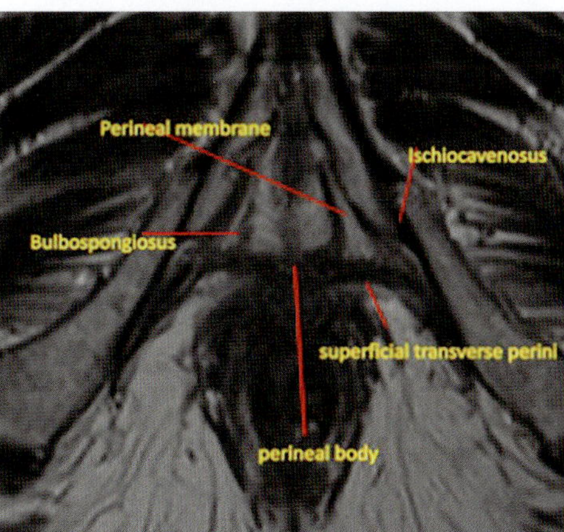

Fig. 3.6.93

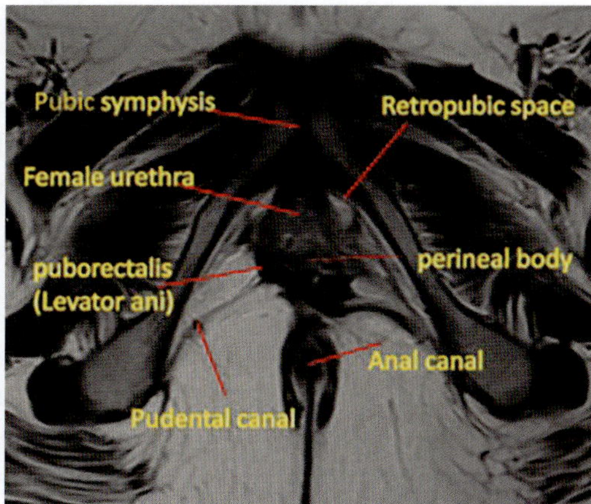

Fig. 3.6.94

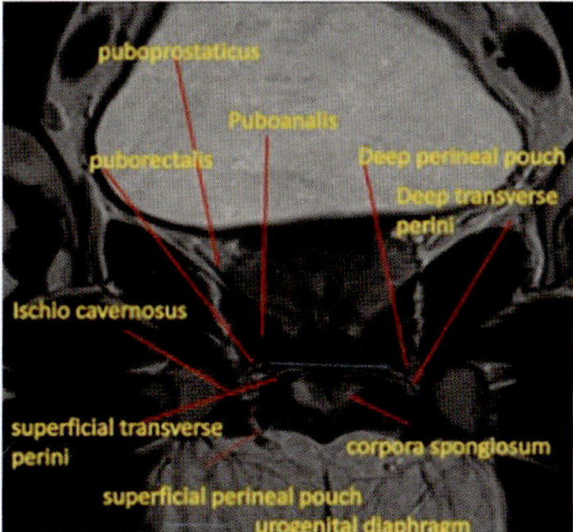

Fig. 3.6.95

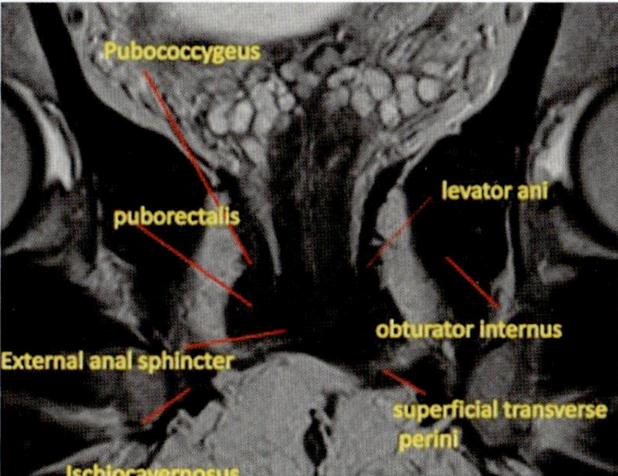

Fig. 3.6.96

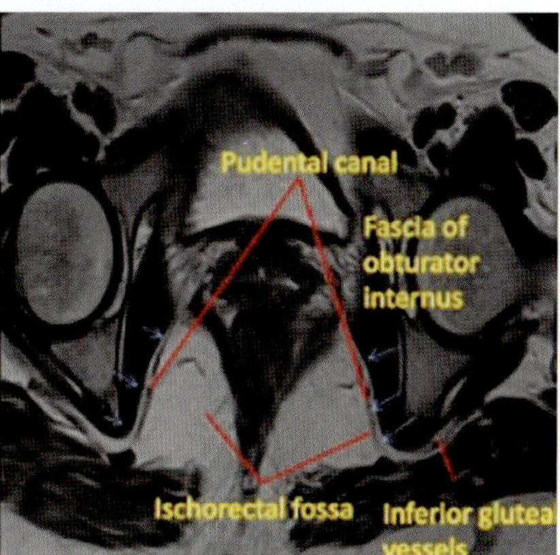

Fig. 3.6.97

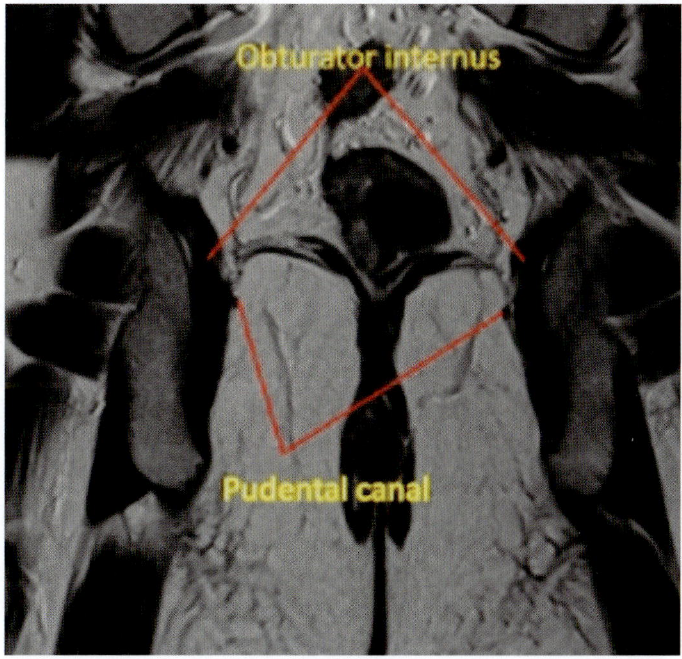

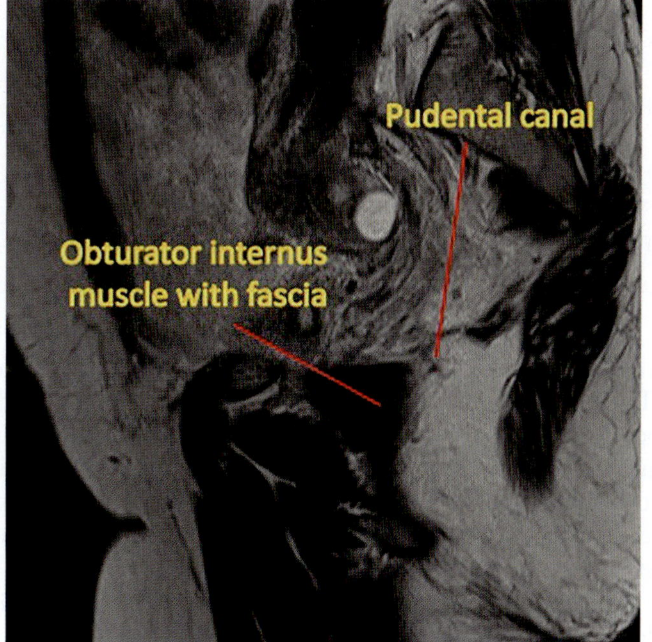

Fig. 3.6.98

Fig. 3.6.99

3.7 OBSTETRICS IMAGING

In obstetrics, prenatal ultrasound is quintessential for monitoring fetus and mother. A complete obstetric ultrasound includes an evaluation of the uterus, the adnexa, and the intrauterine contents.

3.7.A First Trimester Scan

There is no evidence to offer routine ultrasound simply to confirm an ongoing early pregnancy in the absence of any clinical issues, pathological symptoms or specific indications. Therefore, it is recommended to offer the first ultrasound examination between 11 and 13 weeks six days, as this gives viability, establish gestational age, number of fetuses and to evaluate gross fetal anatomy.

Table 3.7.1: Intrauterine pregnancy (the nomenclatures used in first trimester ultrasound)

Recommended terminology	*Definition*
Viable pregnancy	One that may potentially result in liveborn baby
Nonviable pregnancy	One that cannot possibly result in liveborn baby; examples include ectopic and failed intrauterine pregnancies (IUPs)
Pregnancy of unknown location	Positive pregnancy test (urine or serum) with no signs of intrauterine or extrauterine gestation on transvaginal ultrasound
IUP of uncertain viability	IUP with embryo <7 mm without cardiac activity or mean sac diameter <25 mm without embryo
Definite IUP	Intrauterine gestational sac with yolk sac ± embryo ± cardiac activity
Probable IUP	Intrauterine echogenic sac-like structure without yolk sac or embryo
Definite ectopic	Extrauterine gestational sac with yolk sac ± embryo ± cardiac activity
Probable ectopic	Inhomogeneous adnexal mass or extrauterine sac-like structure

The gestational sac can first be visualized at approximately 5.0 weeks of gestation on transvaginal ultrasound (TVS). Gestational sac is a fluid collection in the mid-portion of uterus within the echogenic decidua. A thin line of collapsing endometrial cavity may be visible. This combined gestational sac and collapsed endometrial cavity is called intradecidual sign (which indicates the sac is in echogenic decidua of uterus) (Fig. 3.7.1).

A reliable sign to differentiate from pseudosac is double decidual sign/double sac sign. The two layers of decidua, i.e. decidua capsularis and decidua parietalis, are seen surrounding the gestational sac. The decidua basalis invaded by the trophoblasts to become the future placenta. At 5 weeks on TVS, yolk sac seen as echogenic ring within the gestational sac (Fig. 3.7.2).

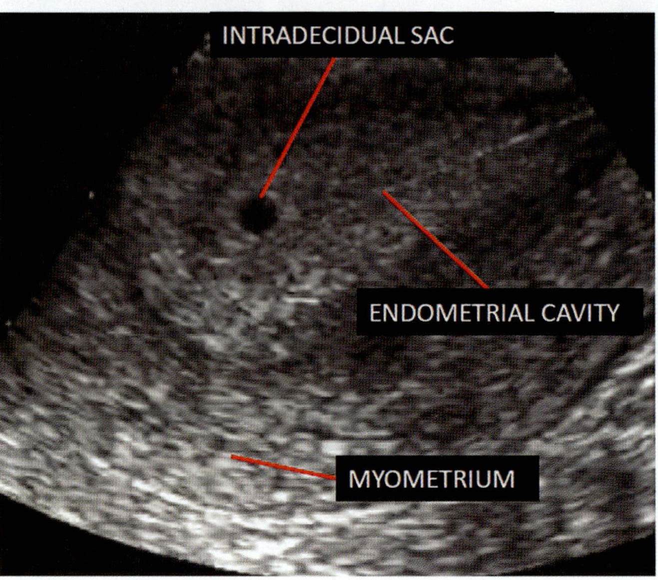

Fig. 3.7.1: Intradecidual sac sign

Between 5th and 6th weeks early embryo may be identified approximately measuring 2–4 mm in length. The yolk sac and embryonic pole gives the appearance called double bleb sign. By the end of 6th week or mid 7th week , when the embryonic pole measures 5 mm, on TVS cardiac activity is visible.

Gestational Age Measurement

Before the embryonic pole appears, mean sac diameter (MSD) of gestational sac is used to assess the age. To obtain

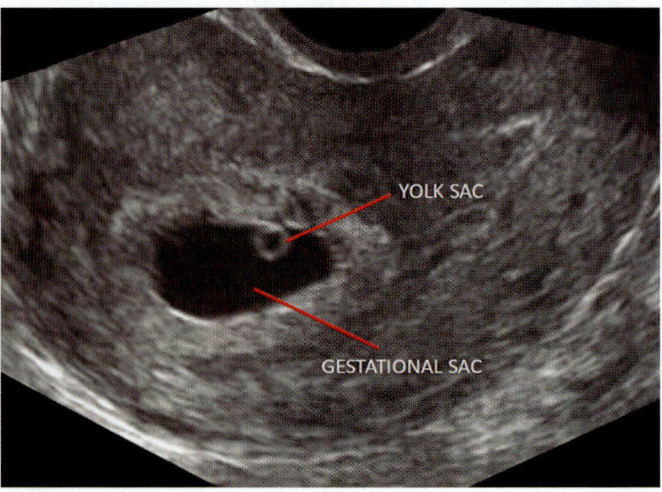

Fig. 3.7.2: Yolk sac

3

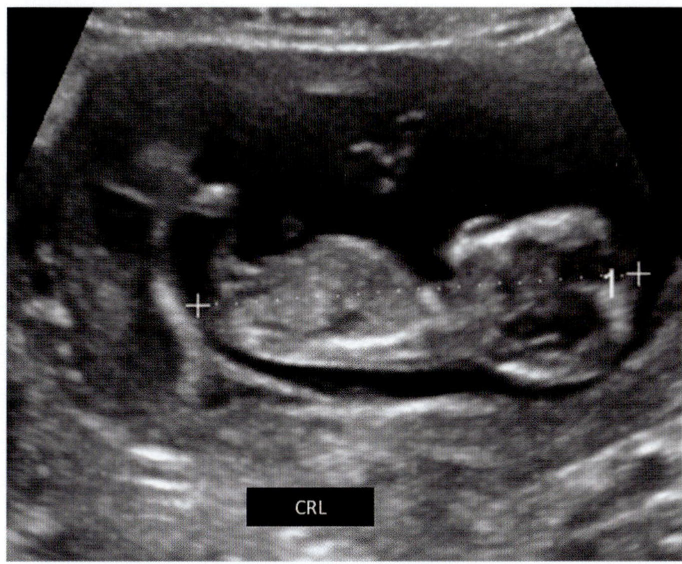

Fig. 3.7.3: Crown rump length

the MSD an average of the height, width and depth of the fluid part of the sac is used. The MSD increases 1 mm per week. If the embryonic pole (as mentioned earlier, embryonic pole appears by the end of 6th week) is visualized, crown rump length (CRL) is used to assess the age. It can be obtained by measuring embryo along its longest axis, preferably in a sagittal view with the fetus in neutral position, care must be taken not to include yolk sac (Fig. 3.7.3). The accuracy of CRL decreases with gestational age, by 7th–11th weeks gestational measurements should be within 4 dates by LMP (last menstrual period). By 12–13 weeks it is within 7 dates of LMP.

Twin Pregnancy

Two separate fertilization always gives rise to dichorionic diamniotic (DCDA) twins. When single embryo splits, it may result in difference of chorionicity and amniocity based on which day the separation happens, when it occurs on 1–3 days—dichorionic diamniotic (DCDA) twins, at 4–8 days—monochorionic diamniotic (MCDA) twins, at 8–13 days—monochorionic monoamnitic (MCMA) twins, after 13 days results in conjoined twins. A thick membrane consisting of two chorions and two amnions is depicted between DC twins, whereas only two layers of amnion separate MC twins. In DC twins, the chorionic tissue extending from the placenta into the base of the thick membrane creates (Fig. 3.7.5) the **twin-peak sign (lambda sign)**, which helps to detect the true chorionicity even when there is a single placental mass. In MC-DA twins, the amnions abut the placenta without intervening chorion, creating a **T sign** (Fig. 3.7.4). In MC-MA twins, both embryos or fetuses

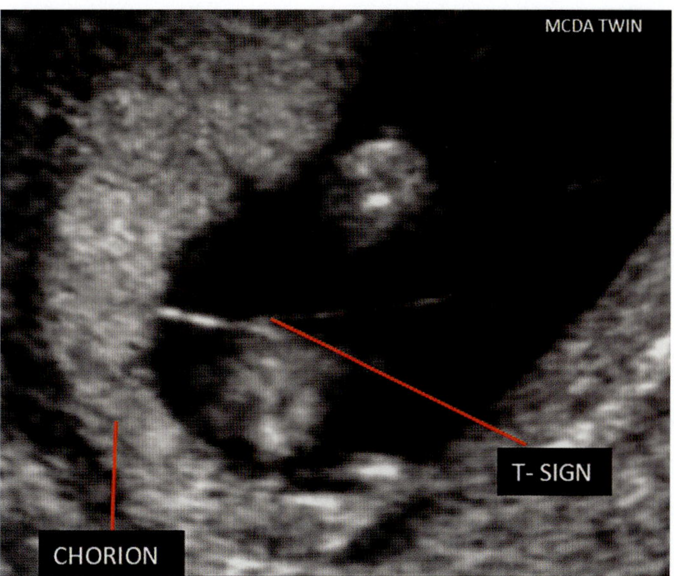

Fig. 3.7.4: T sign of monochorionic monoamniotic pregnancy

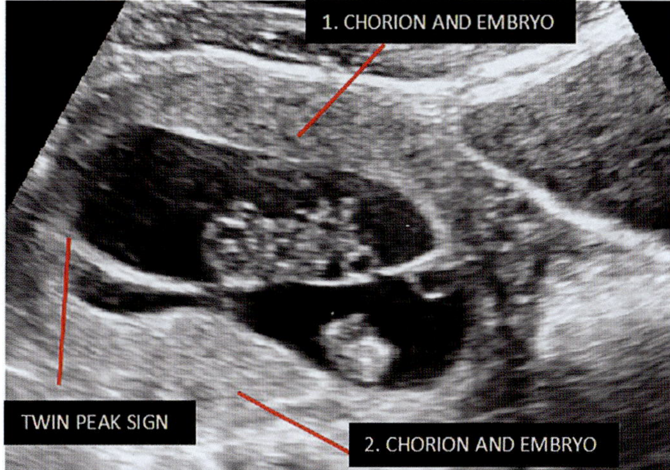

Fig. 3.7.5: Lambda sign or twin-peak sign of monochorionic diamniotic pregnancy

are in a common space surrounded by a single chorion and a single amnion. Usually, the number of yolk sacs should correspond to the number of amnions.

Nuchal Translucency

The nuchal translucency (NT) is defined as a sonolucent area enclosed by a membrane that extends from the posterior aspect of the embryo's head to a variable point along the spine (Figs 3.7.6 and 3.7.7).

Table 3.7.2: Guidelines for NT measurement

1	The edges of NT must be clear for proper placement of the calipers.
2	The fetus in midsagittal plane.

3	The image must be magnified such that it is filled by the fetal head, neck, and upper thorax.
4	The fetal neck shall be in neutral position, there should be no flexion and not extention.
5	The amnion is seen as a separate from the NT line.
6	The calipers on the ultrasound equipment must be used to perform the NT measurement.
7	The calipers should be placed on inner margins of nuchal space such that the horizontal crossbars is not protrusion into the space.
8	Placement of caliper must be perpendicular to long axis of fetus.
9	The value should be measured at the widest space of the NT.

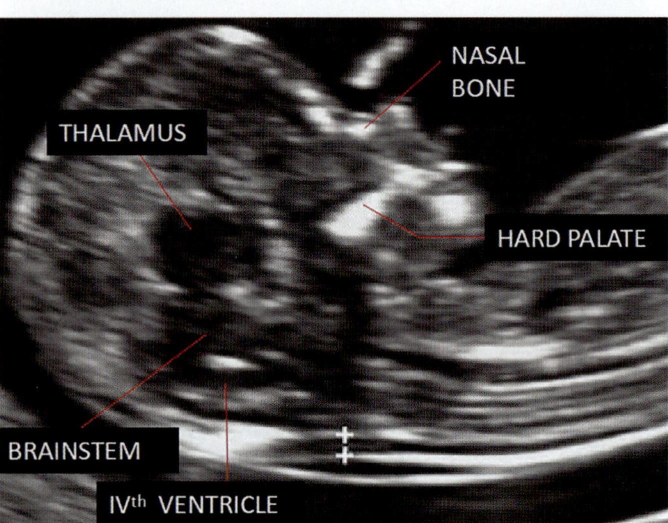

Fig. 3.7.6: NT measurement

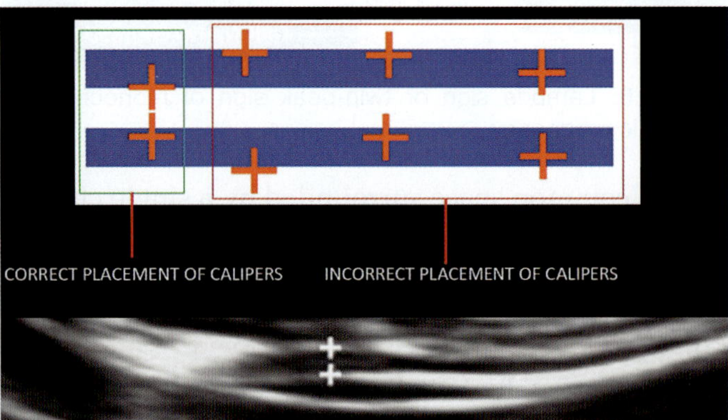

Fig. 3.7.7: Caliper placement for NT measurement

It is a good marker for aneuploidy. This combined with biochemical markers increases the chances of detection of aneuploidy. The NT is performed between about 11 and 14 weeks' gestational age or when the CRL is between 45–84 mm. It is the one of the soft markers for trisomy 21. Values of NT is plotted against the nomograms. Generally values less than 2.2–2.8 mm correlates with decreased risk of aneuploides.

3.7.B Targeted Imaging for Fetal Anomalies (TIFFA) Scan

The main objective of a routine second trimester (between 18–22 weeks) is to provide diagnostic information for the delivery of better antenatal care with the good outcomes for mother and fetus.

1. To determine gestational age
2. To perform fetal measurements
3. To detect congenital malformations and multiple pregnancy

Fetal biometry: The following sonographic parameters can be used to estimate gestational age and for fetal size assessment—biparietal diameter (BPD), head circumference (HC), abdominal circumference (AC) or diameter, femur diaphysis length (FDL).

Biparietal Diameter (BPD)

Many techniques has been described (e.g. outer edge to inner edge, the leading edge technique and outer edge to outer edge), at the broadest part of the skull (Fig. 3.7.8).

Prerequisites: Axial view of the fetal head at the level of the thalami; ideal angle of insonation should be ninety degrees to the midline echoes; both hemispheres must be symmetrical; continuous midline echo of falx cerebri which is broken in middle by the cavum septi pellucidi and thalamus; No cerebellum sholud be visualized.

Head Circumference (HC)

Using the ellipse calipers head circumference can be measured directly by keeping the ellipse around the outside of the skull bone echoes (Fig. 3.7.8).

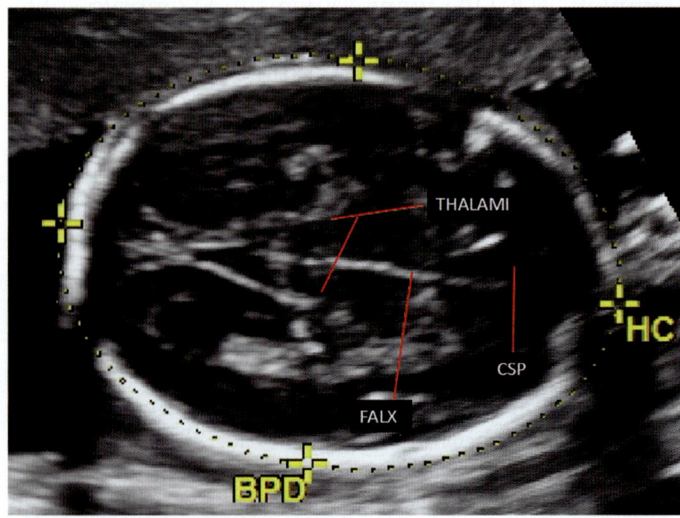

Fig. 3.7.8: BPD and HC measurement

Alternatively, the HC can be measured from the BPD and OFD (occipitofrontal diameter) as follows: The BPD is measured as described above and the OFD is measured by placing the calipers in the middle of the bone echo at both the occipital and frontal skull bones.

The caliper placement is same as that of described in calculation of biparietal diameter.

Abdominal Circumference (AC)

The AC is measured at the outer surface of the skin line, either directly with ellipse calipers or from linear measurements made perpendicular to each other, usually the anteroposterior abdominal diameter (APAD) or the transverse abdominal diameter (TAD) (Fig. 3.7.9). In TAD method, the calipers are placed on the outer borders of body outline, across the abdomen at its widest point. In APAD, the calipers are placed on the outer borders of the body outline, from the anterior abdominal wall to posterior aspect (skin covering the spine).

Prerequisites: Transverse section of the fetal abdomen (as circular as possible); umbilical vein at the level of the portal sinus; stomach bubble visualized.

Femur Diaphysis Length (FL)

Calipers are placed at the ends of the ossified diaphysis (should not include distal femoral epiphysis). Beware of triangular spur artificats at the end of bone, if it occurs exclude it, angle of insonation should be between 45 and 90 betweeen ultrasound beam and femur (Fig. 3.7.10).

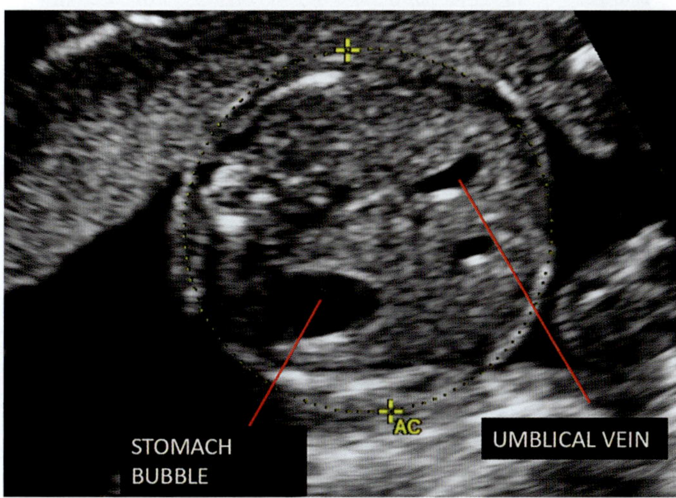

Fig. 3.7.9: AC measurement

Table 3.7.3: Basic mid-trimester fetal anatomical survey (ISUOG)

Head	Intact cranium, CSP, falx in midline, thalami, ventricles, cerebellum, cisterna magna
Face	Both orbits, median facial profile, mouth and upper lip intact
Neck	No mass is present (e.g. cystic hygroma)
Chest/Heart	Normal appearing size/shape of chest and lungs, heart activity present, four-chamber view of heart in normal position, aortic and pulmonary outflow tracts, no features of diaphragmatic hernia
Abdomen	Position of stomach, bowels, both kidneys present
Skeletal	Spine in sagittal and transverse views. Arms, hands, feet and legs are present and normal relationship
Placenta and cord insertion site	Position, no masses present, accessory lobe, if any present
Umbilical cord	Three-vessel cord
Genitalia	Male or female, look for presence, document only if any anomaly is present, do not disclose it to the patient or mention in report if normal (PCPNDT Act)

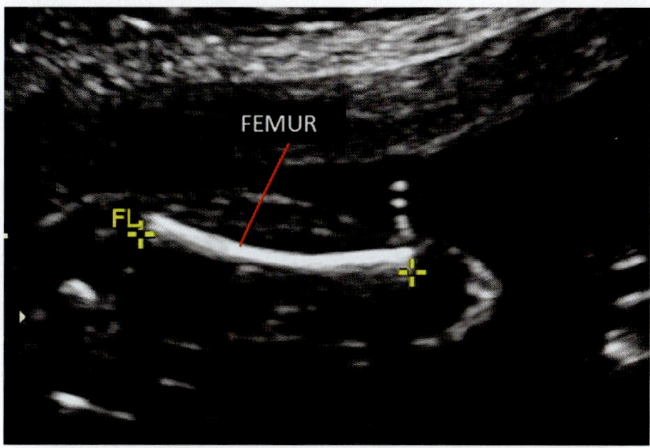

Fig. 3.7.10: FL measurement

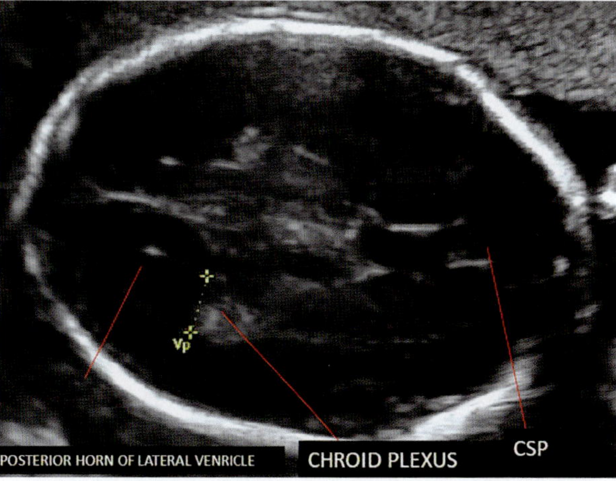

Fig. 3.7.11: Brain—transventricular plane

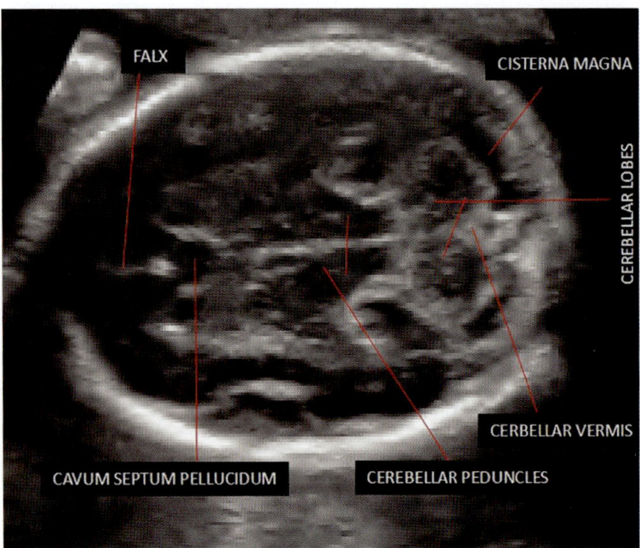

Fig. 3.7.12: Brain—posterior fossa view

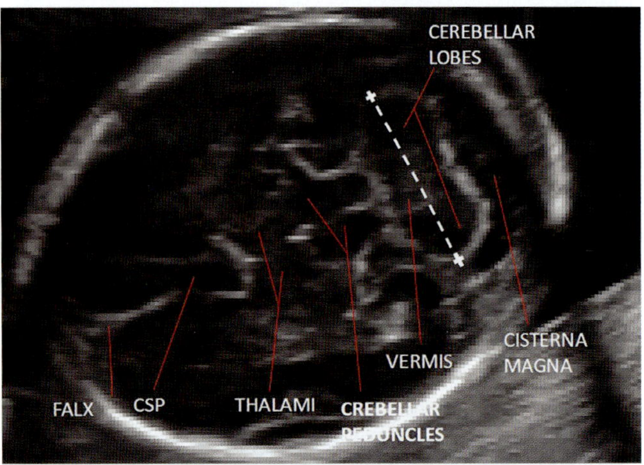

Fig. 3.7.13: Brain—cerebellar view

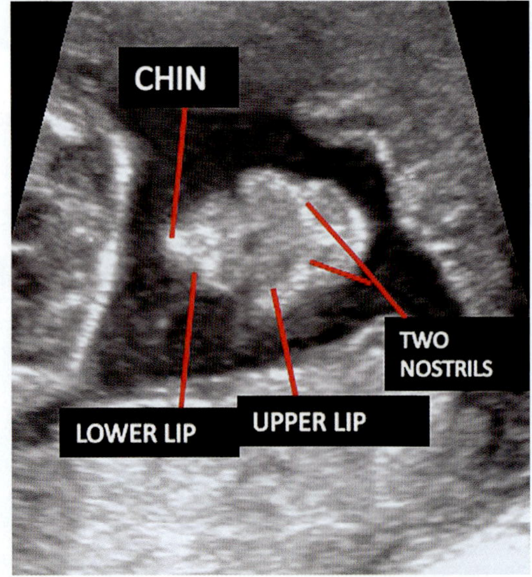

Fig. 3.7.14: Face—in profile view

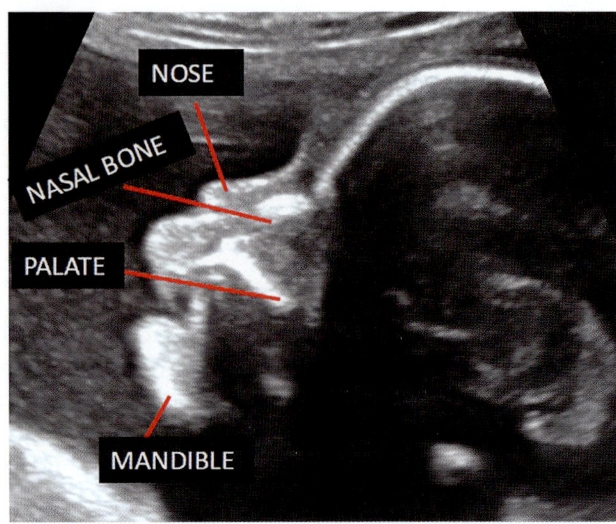

Fig. 3.7.15: Face—sagittal view showing nasal bones

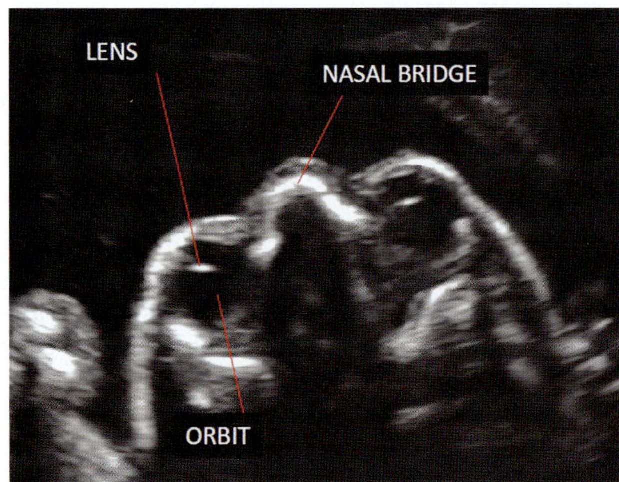

Fig. 3.7.16: Axial section showing both orbits

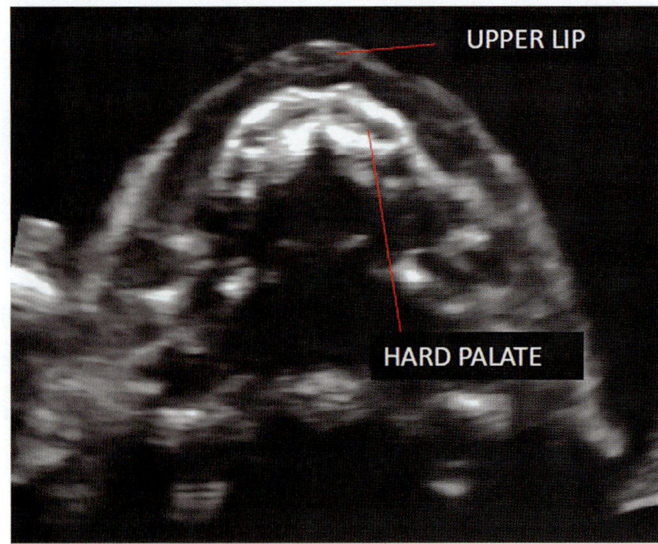

Fig. 3.7.17: Axial section showing upper lip and hard palate

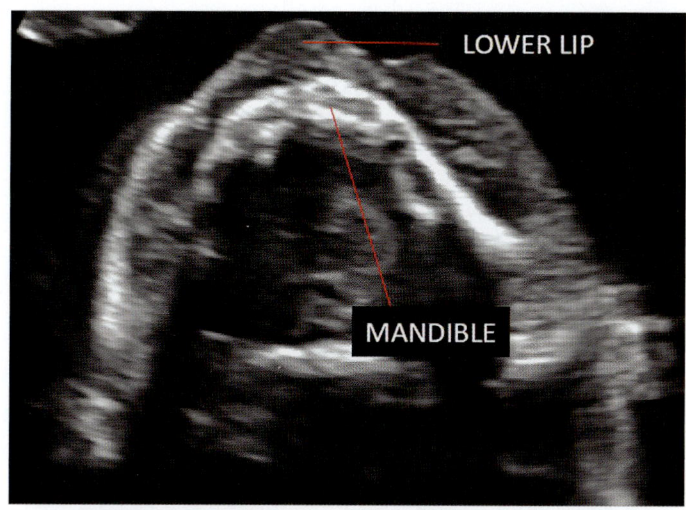

Fig. 3.7.18: Axial section showing lower lip and mandible

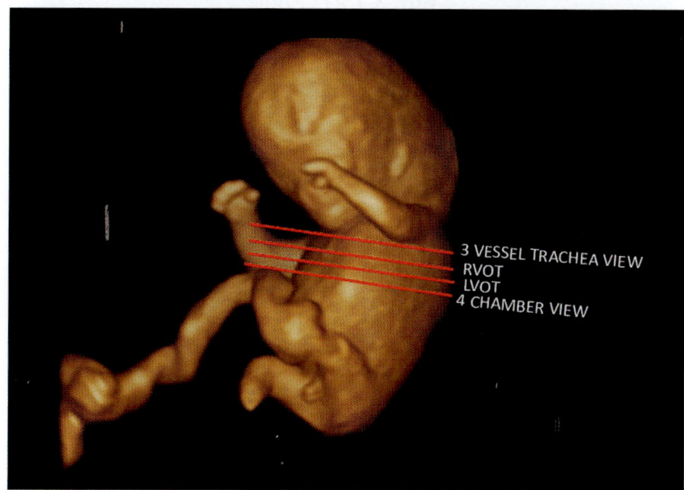

Fig. 3.7.19: Graphic image for serial axial sweeping

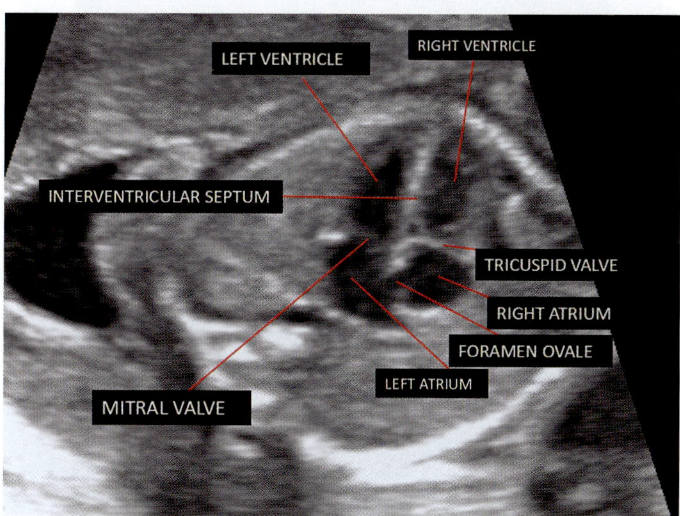

Fig. 3.7.20: Four-chamber view

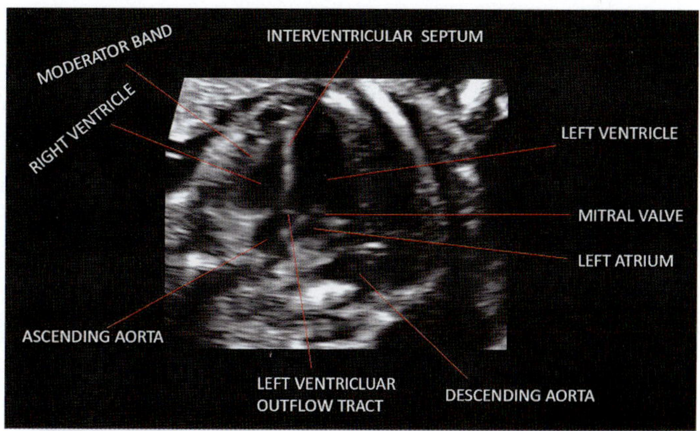

Fig. 3.7.21: LVOT view

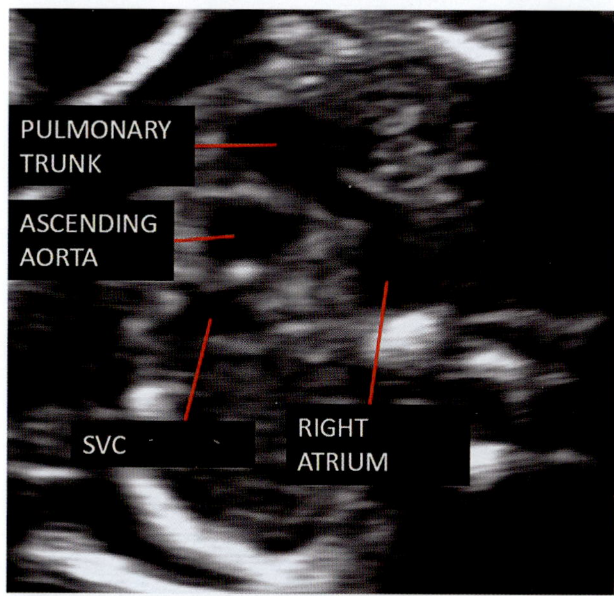

Fig. 3.7.22: RVOT view

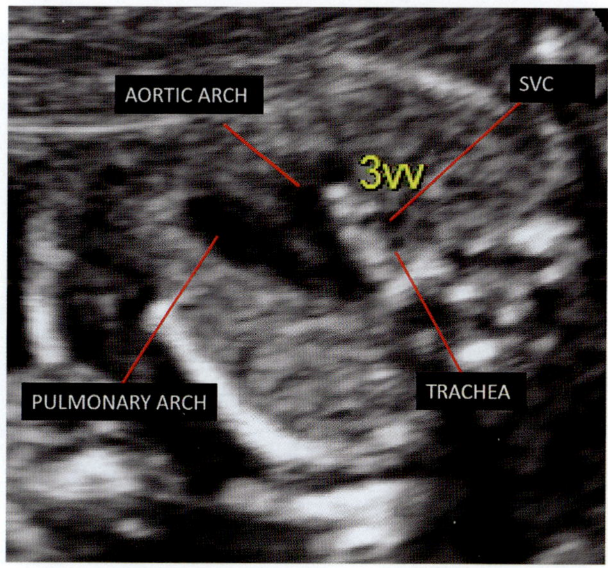

Fig. 3.7.23: 3-vessel trachea view

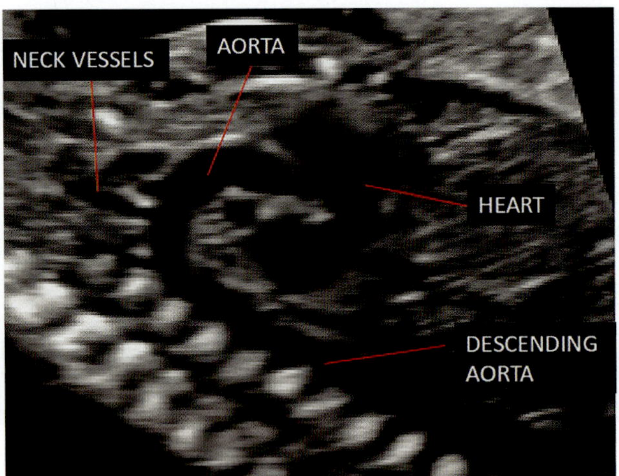

Fig. 3.7.24: Aortic arch

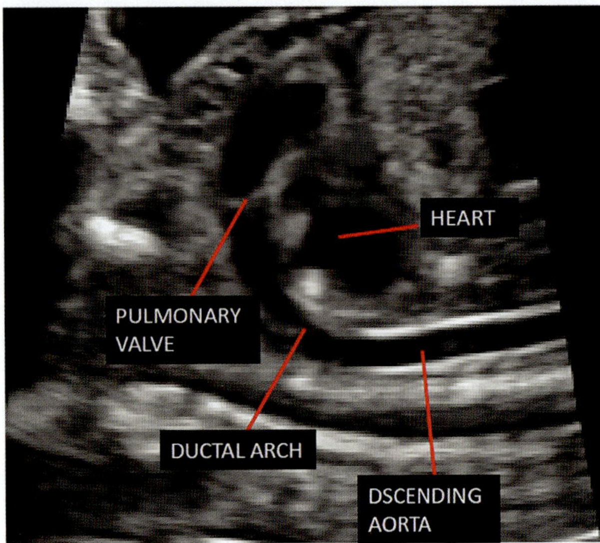

Fig. 3.7.25: Ductal arch

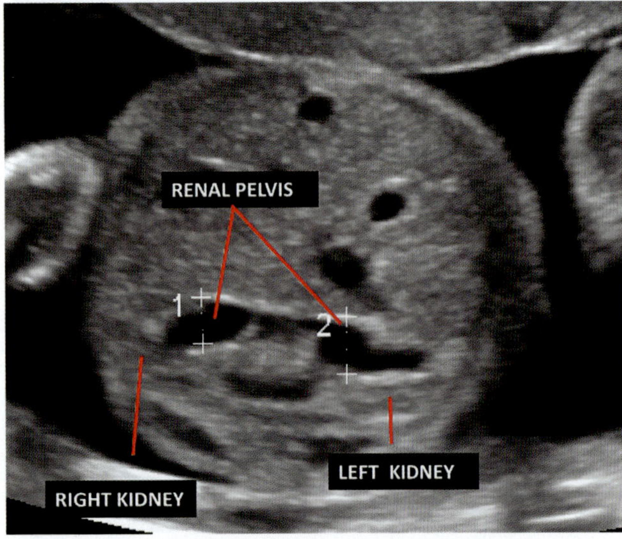

Fig. 3.7.26: Both kidneys and renal pelvis

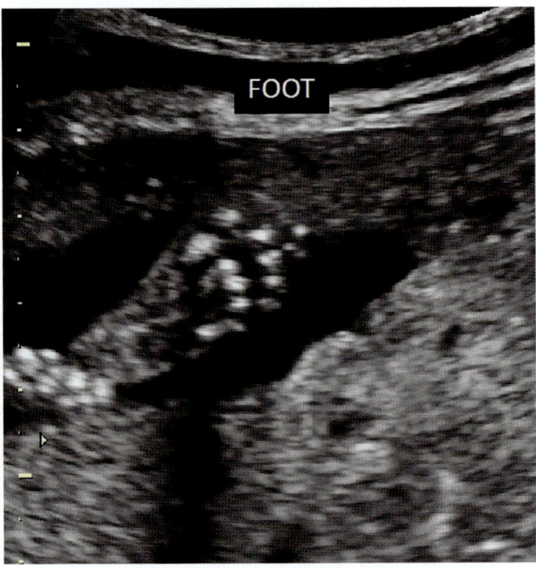

Fig. 3.7.27: Foot

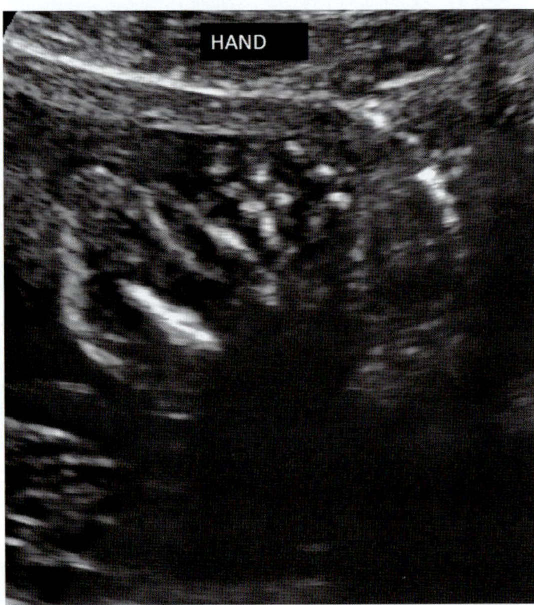

Fig. 3.7.28: Hand

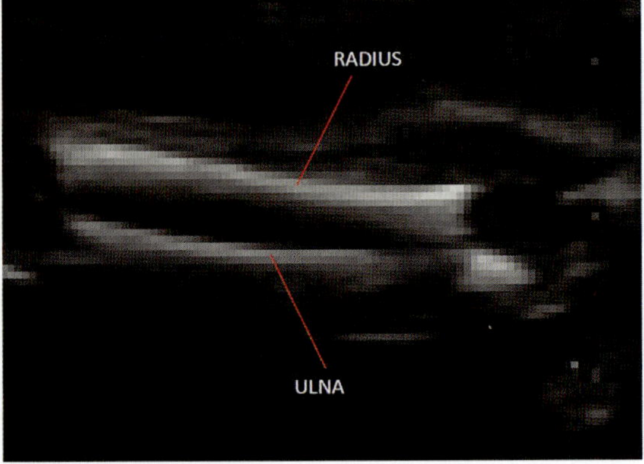

Fig. 3.7.29: Radius and ulna

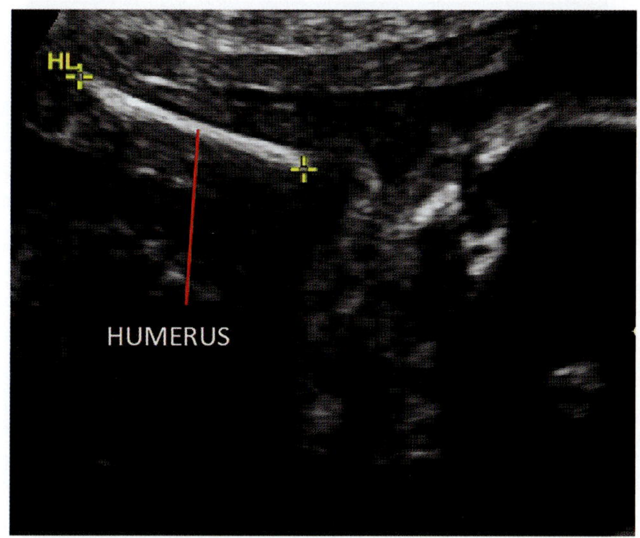

Fig. 3.7.30: Humerus

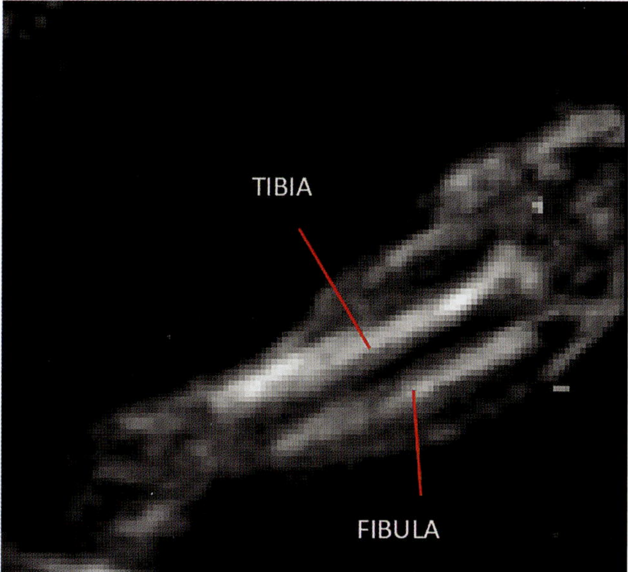

Fig. 3.7.31: Tibia and fibula

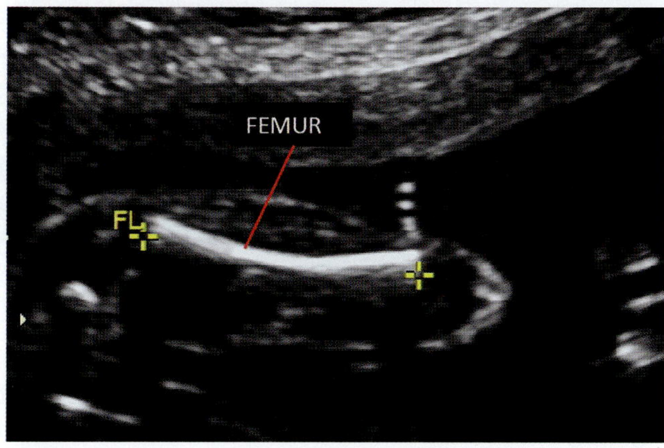

Fig. 3.7.32: Femur

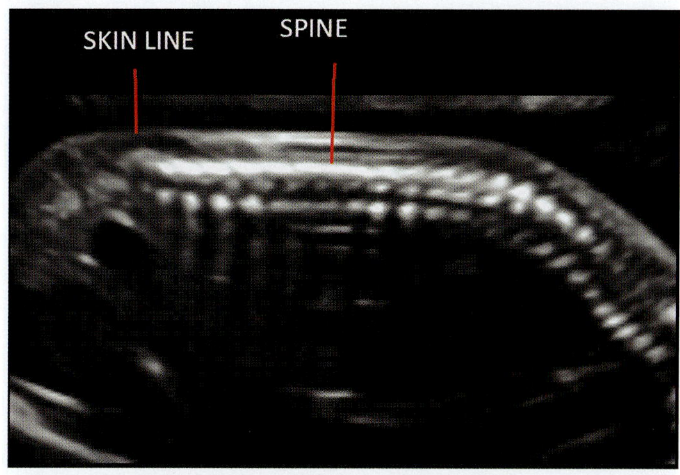

Fig. 3.7.33: Spine: Longitudinal view

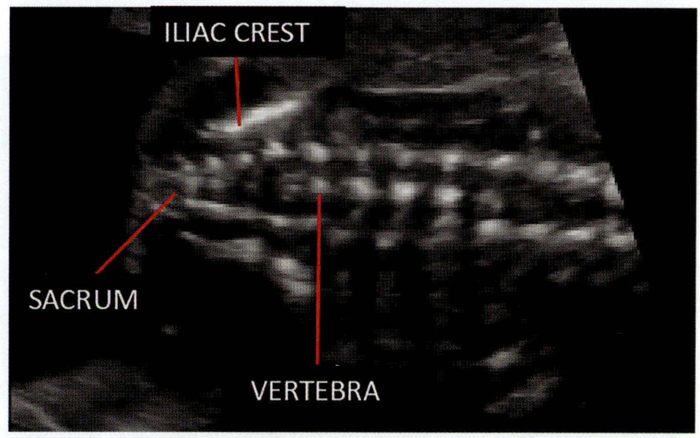

Fig. 3.7.34: Spine: Coronal view

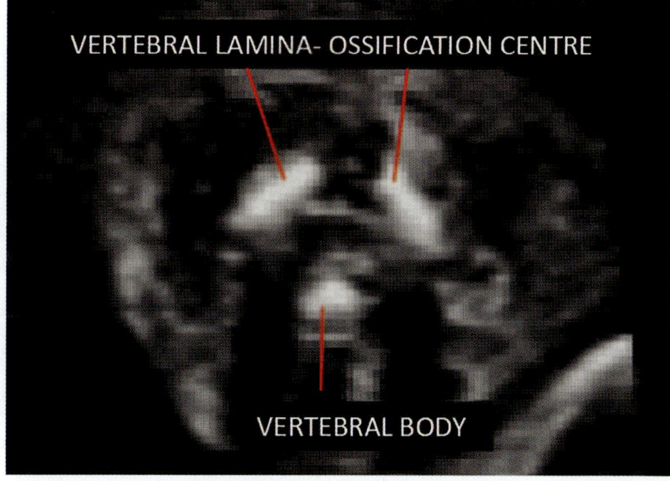

Fig. 3.7.35: Spine: Axial view

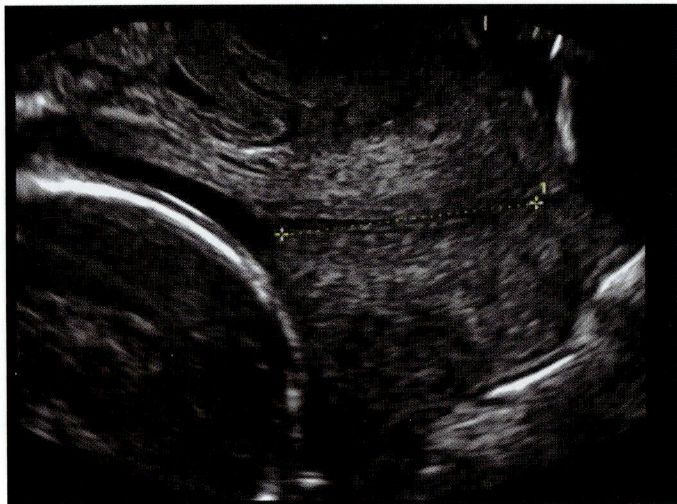

Fig. 3.7.36: Cervix length

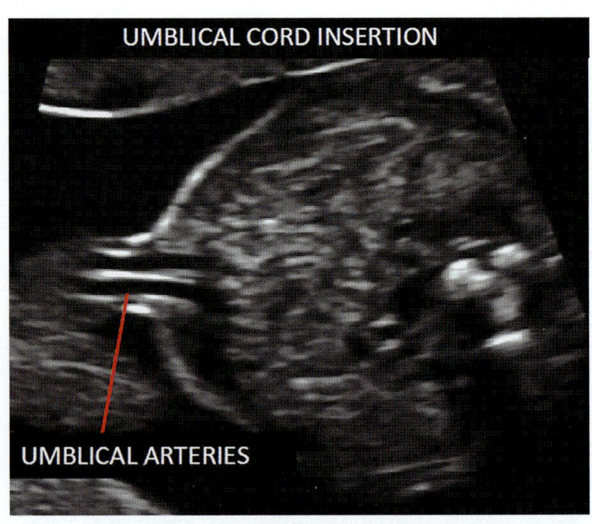

Fig. 3.7.37: Umbilical cord insertion

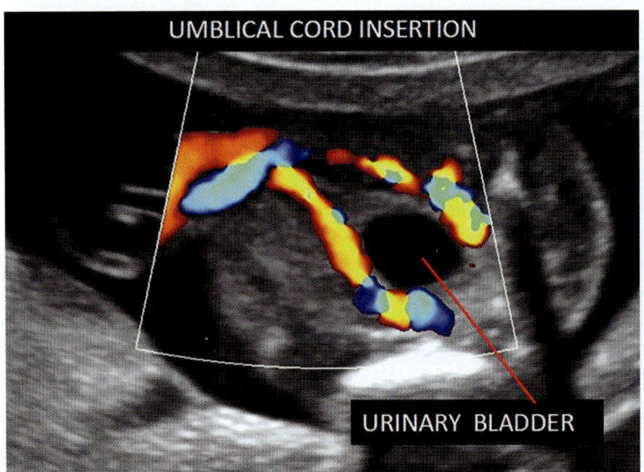

Fig. 3.7.38: Umbilical artery on either side of bladder converging towards umbilicus

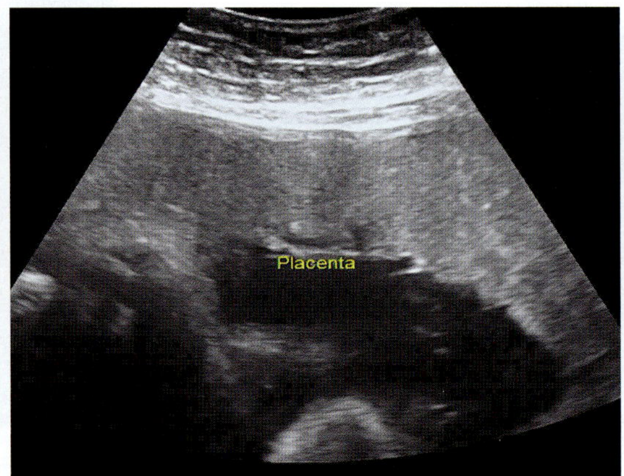

Fig. 3.7.39: Placenta

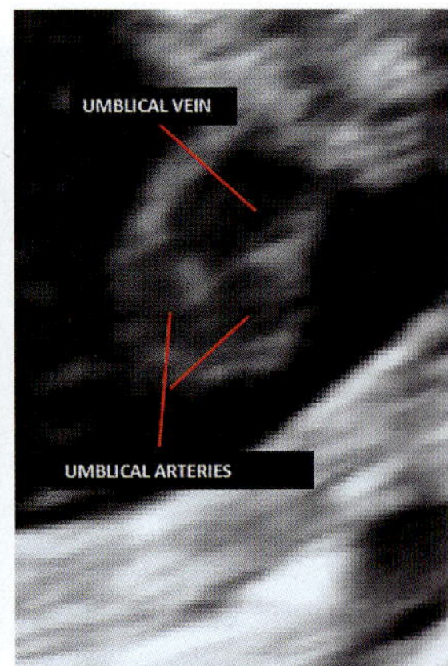

Fig. 3.7.40: Umbilical arteries and veins

Amniotic Fluid Index Calculation: Four Quadrant Method

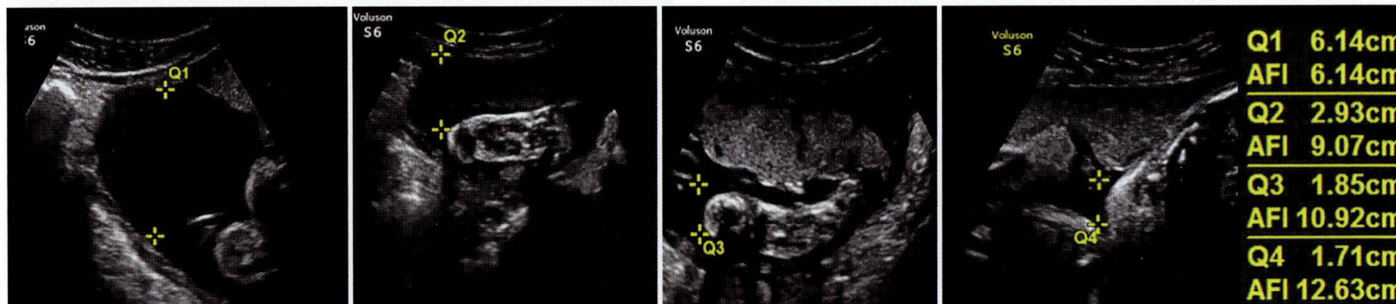

Fig. 3.7.41: Amniotic fluid index calculation—four-quadrant method

Situs Determinaton Methods

1. Based on fetal position

3

Cardiac axis: The axis is angle between the line that connects sternum to spine and a line drawn along the ventricular septum. The axis ranges between 30 to 45 in the second and third trimesters. In the first trimester, the range is greater, lies from 34.6 to 56.7 (mean ± standard deviation = 47.6 ± 5.6) (Fig. 3.7.42).

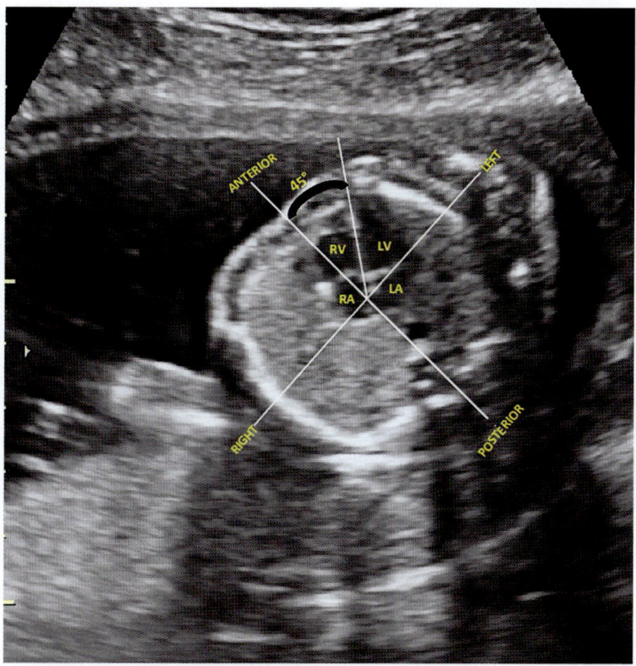

Fig. 3.7.42: Normal cardiac axis

Scan the uterus, look at where the fetal head is in the uterus and confirm the present part.

Then determine the lie of the fetus inside the uterus by getting a sagittal view of the fetal spine. (Longitudinal lie—when the fetal spine aligns with the mother's spine; transverse lie—when the fetal spine is perpendicular on the mother's spine; oblique lie when the fetal spine is oblique to the mother's spine.) After finding the exact location of the fetus, determine the position of the left side of the fetus relative to the mother's abdomen (the left side of the fetus is front [near the transducer], posterior [near the posterior wall of the uterus], the right side [near the uterine wall to the mother's right], the left side [near the mother's uterine wall]). Get the opposite view of the fetal abdomen by rotating the transducer 90 degrees from the sagittal view of the lower thoracic spine. The fetal stomach is located on the left side of the abdomen, the descending aorta is posterior to left, and the inferior vena cava anterior to right. By sliding the transducer into the fetal chest, a four-chambered heart image is taken. Note that the apex of the heart is facing the left side of the baby's chest. Determining whether the abdomen, descending aorta, and apex of the heart are located on the left side of the fetus and the inferior vena cava is located on the right side establishes the normal visceral situs (Fig. 3.7.43).

2. Cordes Method

The key steps to this technique are orientation of the fetal sagittal plane with the head to the right of the video screen and then a 90° clockwise transducer rotation to obtain the transverse image. This results in a transverse image presented in the standard caudal to cranial perspective. If the left hand of the operator is placed in front of the ultrasound screen positioned as an 'L' shape with the tips of fingers pointing towards the fetal sternum and the palm placed on the fetal spine, the thumb will now be pointing towards the left side of the fetus (Fig. 3.7.44).

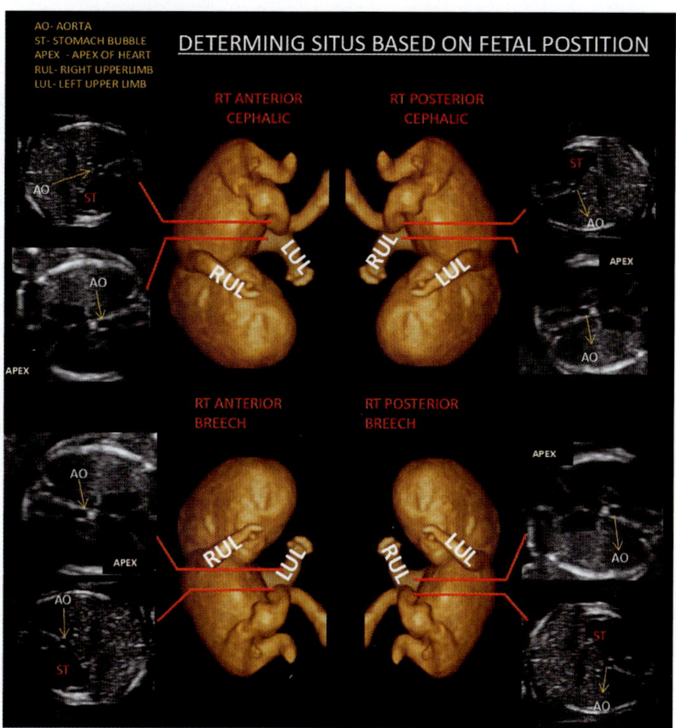

Fig. 3.7.43: Situs determination based on fetal position

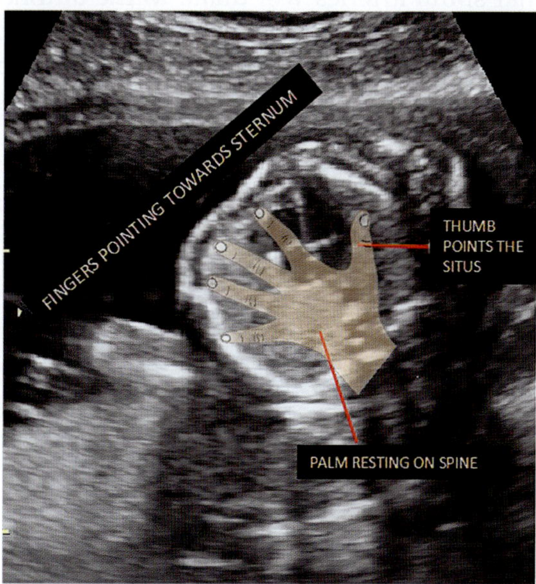

Fig. 3.7.44: Cordes method

3. Clock Method

In this way, the radiologist should sit to the right of the patient, hold the probe in the right hand and perform a transabdominal examination. The left side of the probe should be on the left side of the ultrasound screen.The thoracic cavity is thought of as a dial clock and the fetal spine refers to a 12-hour position. If the fetus is in a breech position, the cardiac axis should be approximately 7 hours long and similarly, if the embryo is in the cephalic position, the cardiac axis should be approximately 5 hours long. If the fetus is lying on the lie, the probe indicator should point to the patient's head to obtain a sagittal image and a fetal structure close to the doctor (in other words, the closest part of the baby to the mother's right side) accepted as the presenting part (Fig. 3.7.45).

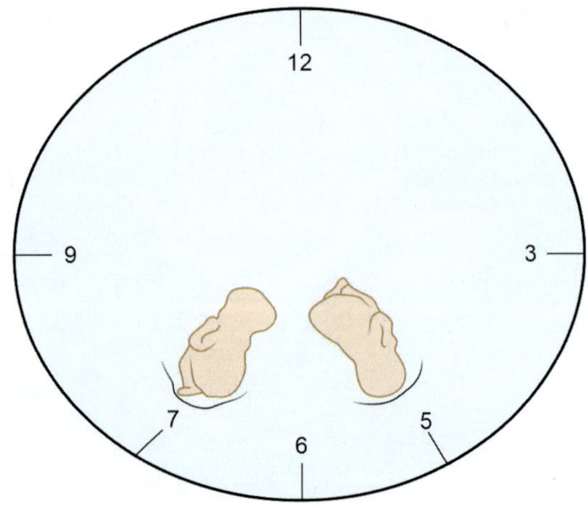

Fig. 3.7.45: Clock method

3.7.C Obstetrics Doppler

Umbilical Artery Doppler (Fig. 3.7.47)

It is a low resistance circulation and reflects the status of placental circulation. There is increase in amount of blood flow in end diastolic flow in advancing gestation. It can be obtained from any portion of umbilical cord, but ISUOG suggests taking measurements from free loop of cord. The absent or reversed diastolic flow is commonly associated with fetal growth restriction and oligohydaminos.

Uterine Artery Doppler (Fig. 3.7.46)

The maternal changes to pregnancy is the result of trophoblastic invasion of the maternal spiral arteries in the first half of pregnancy. As a result of invasion, the maternal spiral arteries will dilate to the autonomous nervous system response. It can be imaged in colour Doppler as it crosses the internal iliac artery and vein just before it enters at the uterine–cervical junction.

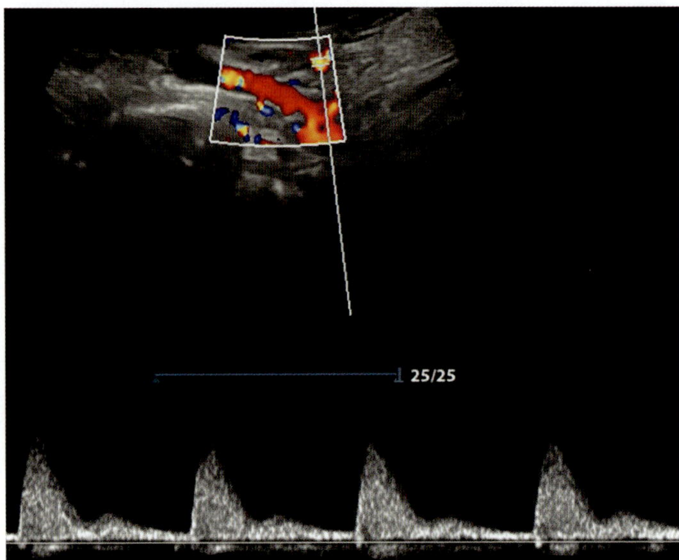

Fig. 3.7.46: Uterine artery Doppler

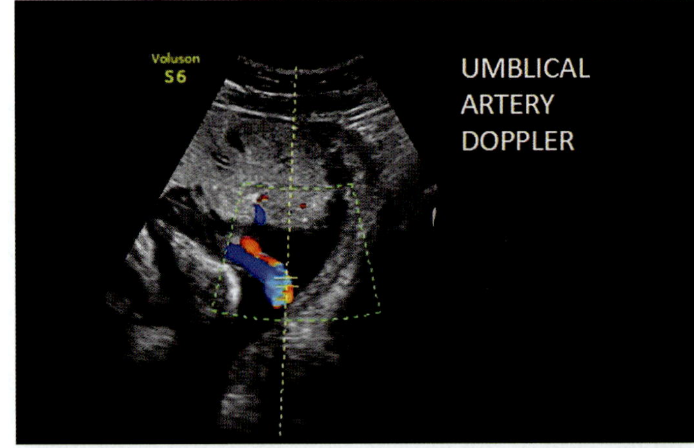

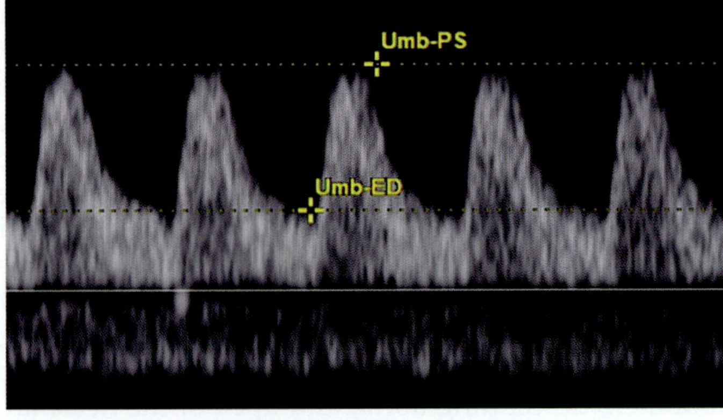

Fig. 3.7.47: Umbilical artery Doppler

Middle Cerebral Artery (MCA) Doppler (Fig. 3.7.48)

It is the most accessible cerebral vessel, carries more than 80% of cerebral blood flow. The cerebral circulation is a high resistance circulation with continuous forward flow throughout the cardiac cycle. At the plane of thalami

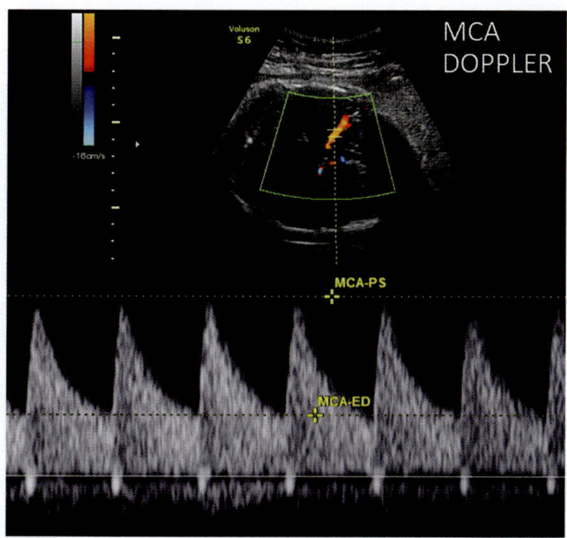

Fig. 3.7.48: MCA Doppler

Table 3.7.4: Some major anomalies and their earliest detection in weeks*

Anomalies	*Earliest detection*
Anencephaly	9–11 weeks with 100% accuracy
Cephaloceles	11–12 weeks
Holoprosencephaly	11–14 weeks
Ventriculomegaly	11–14 weeks
Open spina bifida (OSB)	11–12 weeks
Dandy-Walker malformation (DWM)	13–14 weeks, rescan @ 20–22 weeks to exclude
Cleft lip and palate—retronasal triangle	11–14 weeks
Ocular anomalies	12–16 weeks
Micrognathia	Only severe anomalies in first trimester, others at 18–21 weeks
Malformations of the heart	50% in 11–13 weeks
Congenital diaphragmatic hernia (CDH)	12–14 weeks
Gastroschisis	12–14 weeks
The body stalk anomaly	11–13 weeks
Megacystis	11–13 weeks
Bilateral renal agenesis (BRA)	12–14 weeks
ARPKD	13–16 weeks
Achondroplasia	>24 weeks
Thanatophoric dysplasia and achondrogenesis	11–13 weeks
Other skeletal dysplasias	18–22 weeks
CPAM	8–16 weeks

*All detected anomalies should be confirmed in 2nd trimester scan. Most of the major anomalies can be detected and confirmed in 2nd trimester scan only

and wings of sphenoid, the proximal and distal middle cerebral arteries are seen in their long axis with course parallel to ultrasound beam. Waveforms are obtained from proximal third portion of the vessel, immediately after the origin of circle of Willis.

In the presence of fetal hypoxemia, central redistribution of blood flow occurs resulting in increased blood flow to brain which leads to low resistance flow in MCA (brain sparing effect).

Ductus Venosus Doppler (Fig. 3.7.49)

At the same plane as for measuring abdominal circumference, ductus venosus waveforms can be obtained. As it branches from the portal vein, a high velocity turbulent flow creates an aliasing artefact, where the measurement is taken.

The waveform is biphasic with the first phase is ventricular systole and the second phase is early diastole and the nadir corresponds to late diastole or atria kick.

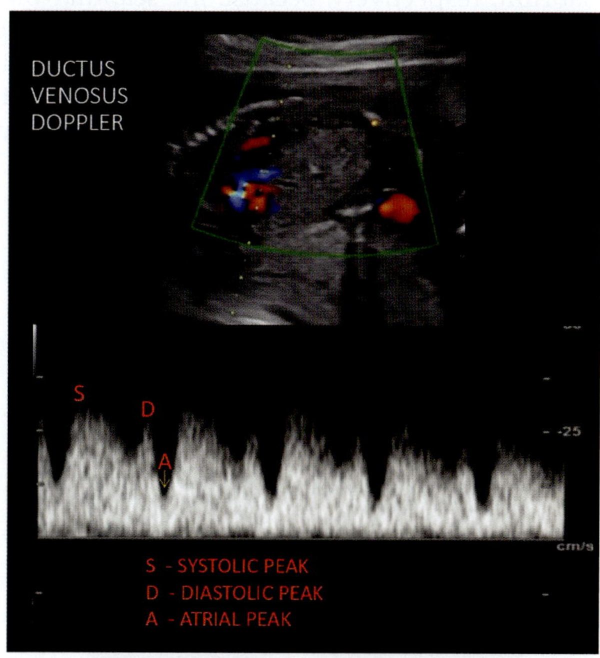

Fig. 3.7.49: Ductus venosus Doppler

3.8 UPPER LIMB

3.8.A SHOULDER

The shoulder joint is a complex and freely movable joint due to the articulation at the glenohumeral joint. It has shoulder girdle that connects upper limb to the axial skeleton via the sternoclavicular joint. The shoulder girdle is composed of the clavicle and the scapula, which articulates with the proximal humerus of the upper limb. Joints are present in the shoulder region: The acromioclavicular (AC), scapulothoracic joints, and glenohumeral joint. Acromioclavicular joint is atypical synovial joint (lined by fibrocartilage, whereas synovial joint is usually lined by hyaline cartilage). A weak, synovium-lined joint capsule is attached to the articular margins superior acromioclavicular ligament, inferior acromioclavicular ligament reinforces joint capsule. The scapulothoracic joint is the articulation of the scapula gliding across the posterior thoracic cage, rather than a genuine joint. The usual coronal and sagittal imaging planes are orientated along the supraspinatus tendon and labrum, respectively, because the scapular blade is tilted 30° anteriorly relative to the body. The single joint that joins the upper limb to the axial skeleton is the sternoclavicular joint, which is a synovial saddle joint. It connects the clavicle to the sternum's manubrium and is supported by the costoclavicular ligament. Primary ossification centre in the clavicle appears in membrane by 5–6 weeks of gestation and fuses by 7th week of gestation. Secondary ossification centre occurs in the sternal end by 15–17 years and fuses by 25 years. The oblique coronal plane is usually perpendicular to the glenoid fossa or parallel to the supraspinatus tendon's long axis. The glenoid face is parallel to the oblique sagittal plane (or orthogonal to the oblique coronal plane). Anatomic angulation is rarely used for acquiring axial pictures.

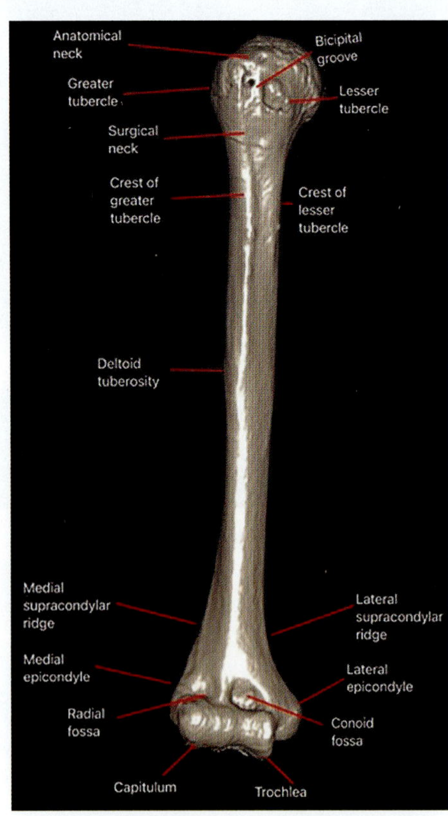

Fig. 3.8.1: Anatomy of humerus

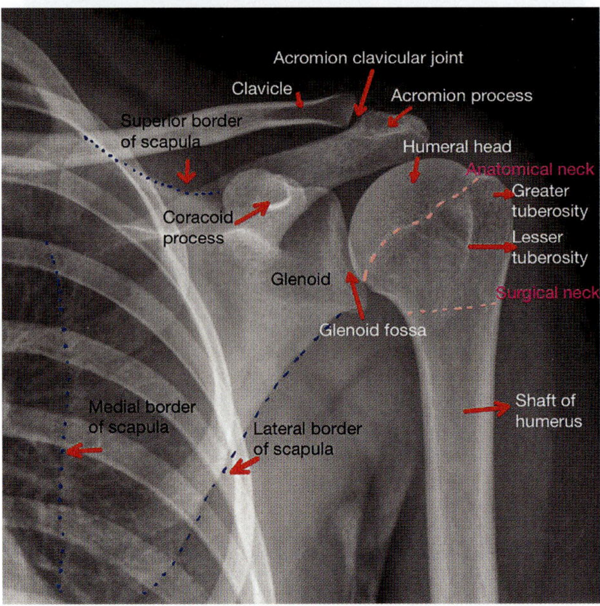

Fig. 3.8.2: Shoulder X-ray: AP view

MRI shoulder axial sections (superior to inferior—Figs 3.8.3–3.8.10).

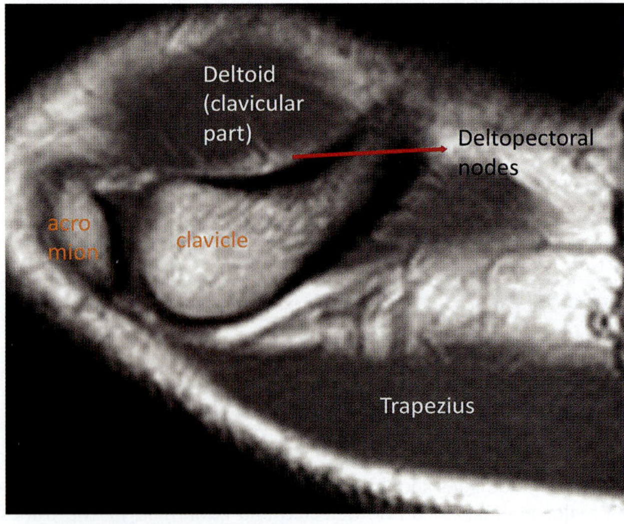

Fig. 3.8.3

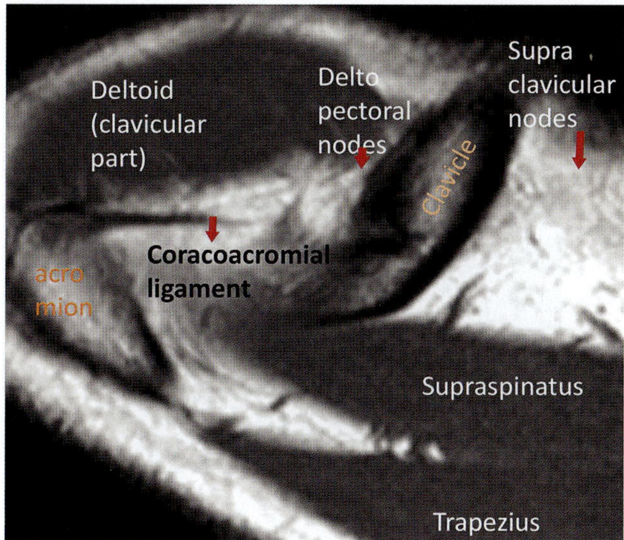

Fig. 3.8.4

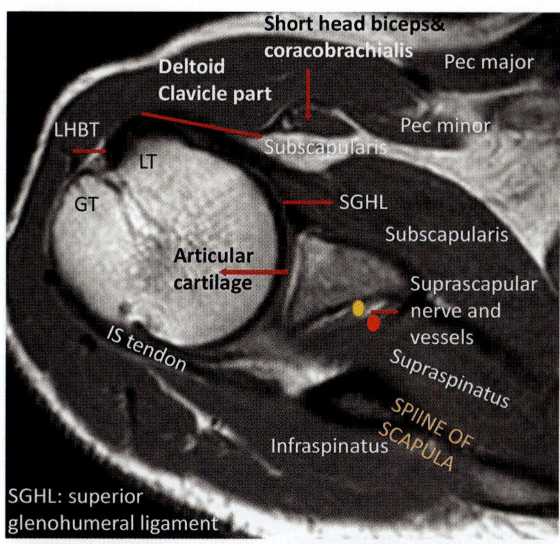

Fig. 3.8.7

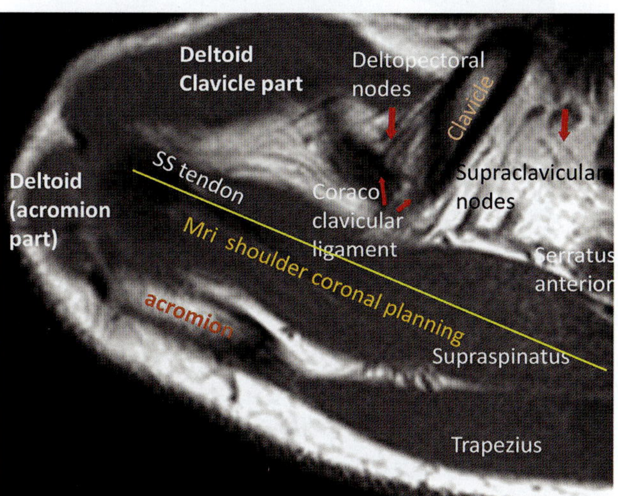

Fig. 3.8.5

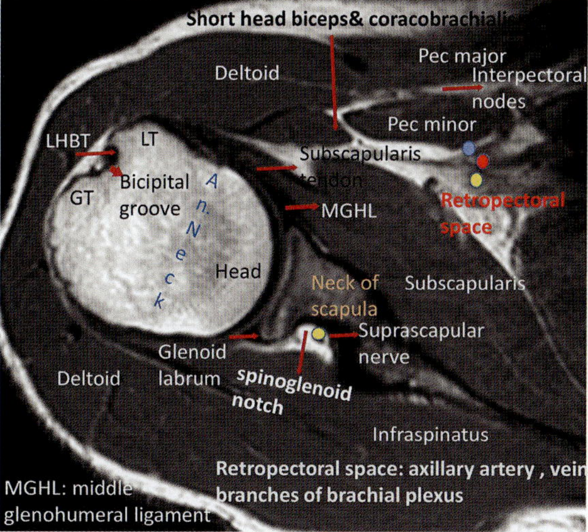

Fig. 3.8.8

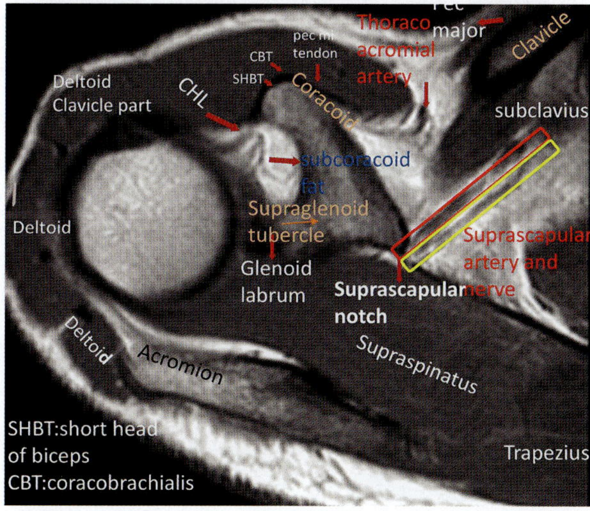

Fig. 3.8.6

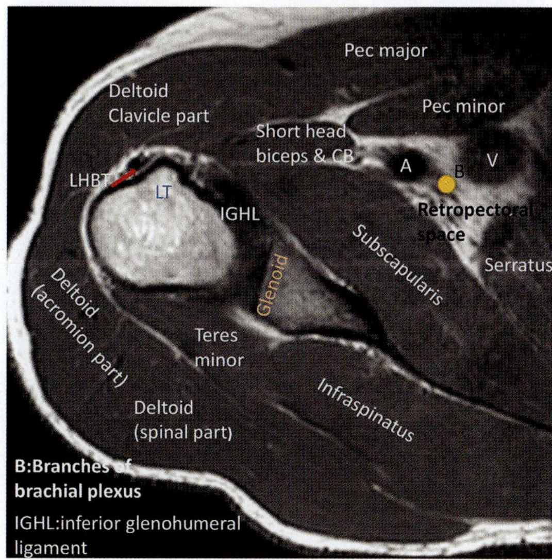

Fig. 3.8.9

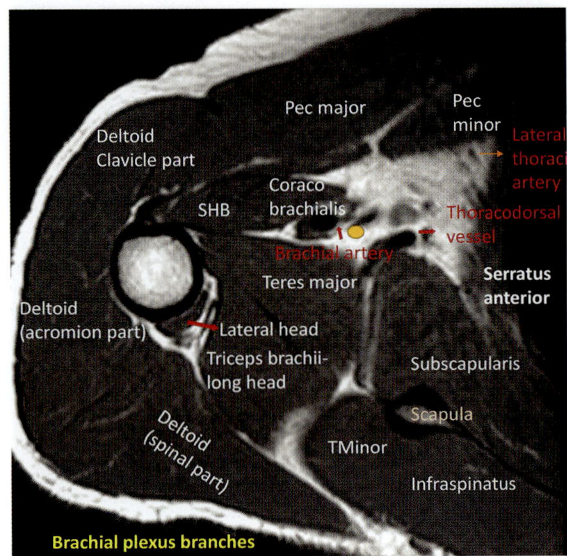

Fig. 3.8.10

Coronal (anterior to posterior—Figs 3.8.11–3.8.18).

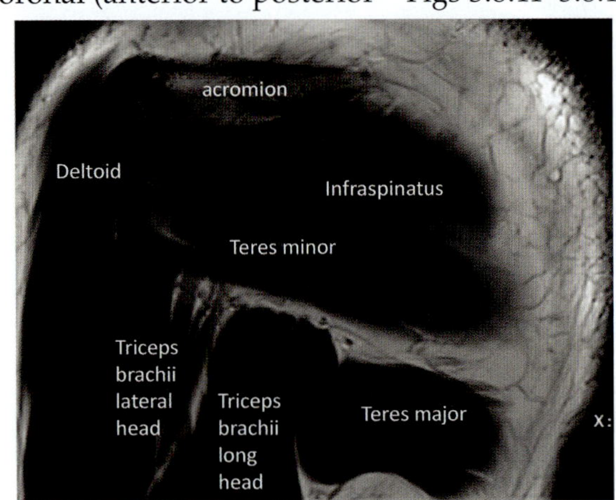

Fig. 3.8.11

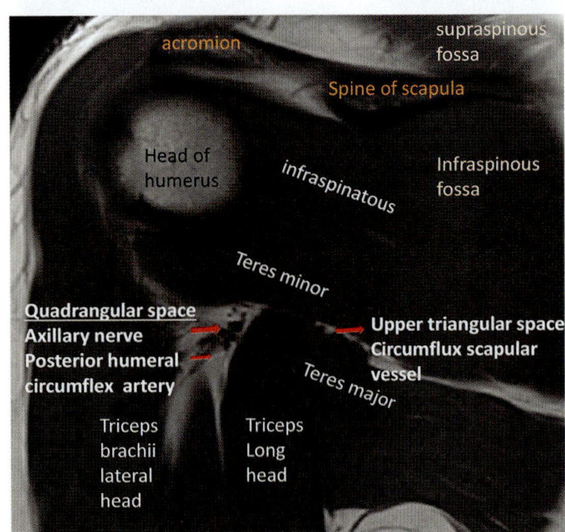

Fig. 3.8.12

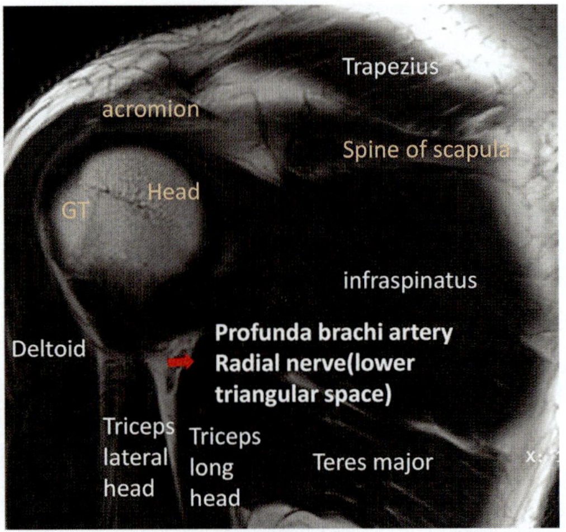

Fig. 3.8.13

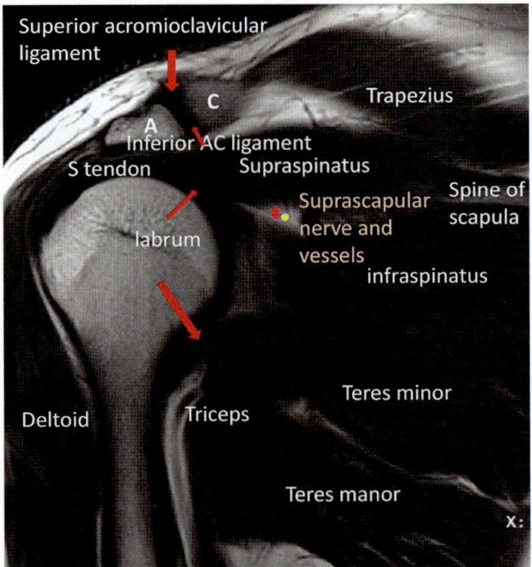

Fig. 3.8.14

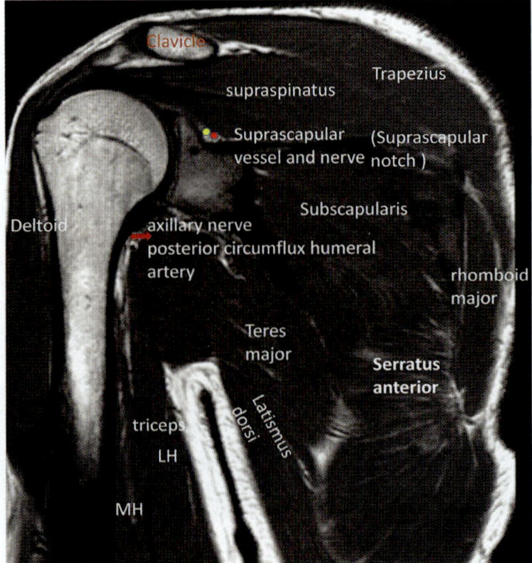

Fig. 3.8.15

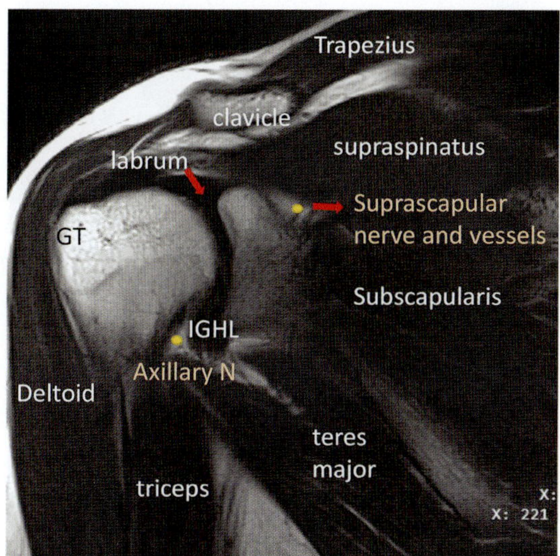

Fig. 3.8.16

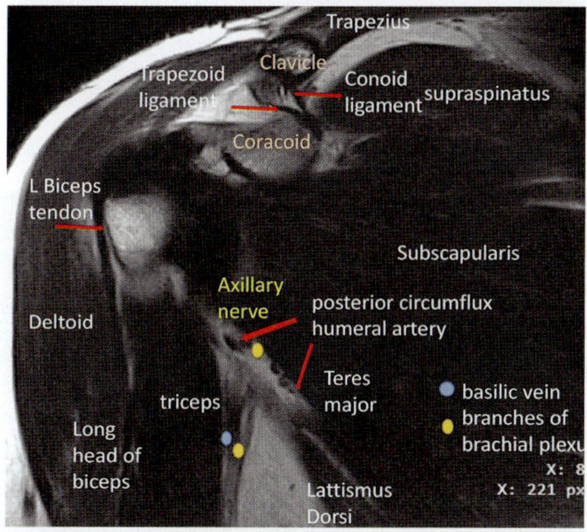

Fig. 3.8.17

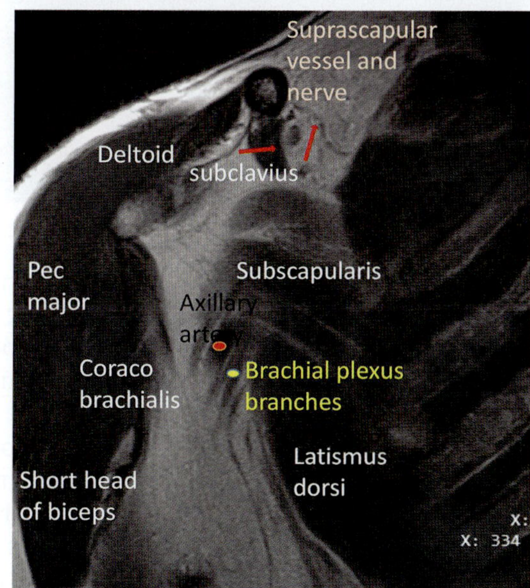

Fig. 3.8.18

Sagittal oblique (lateral to medial—Figs 3.8.19–3.8.25).

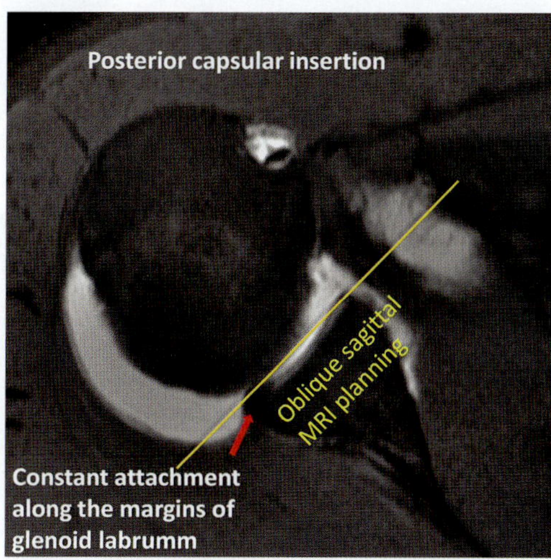

Fig. 3.8.19

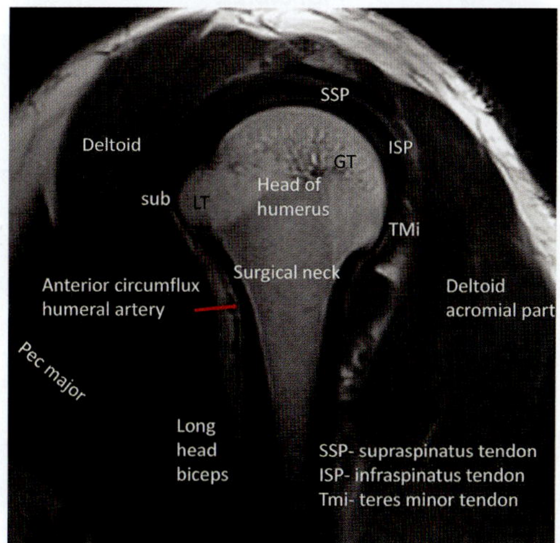

Fig. 3.8.20

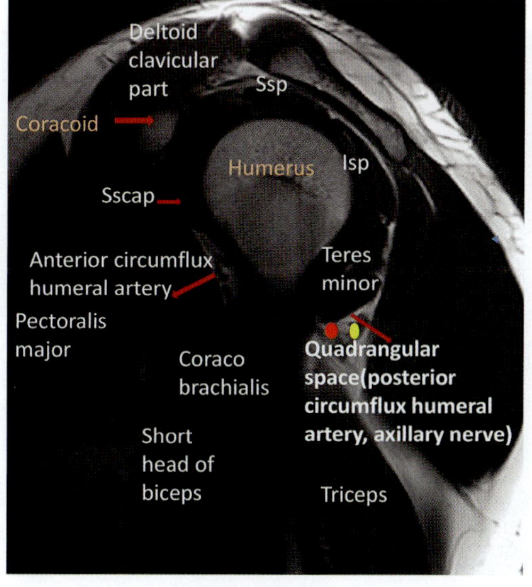

Fig. 3.8.21

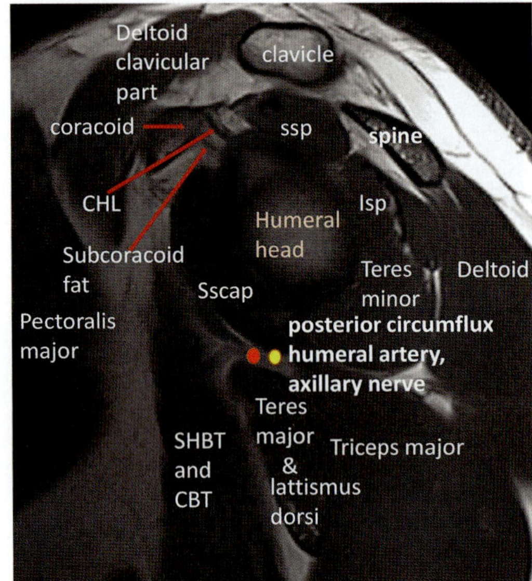

Fig. 3.8.22

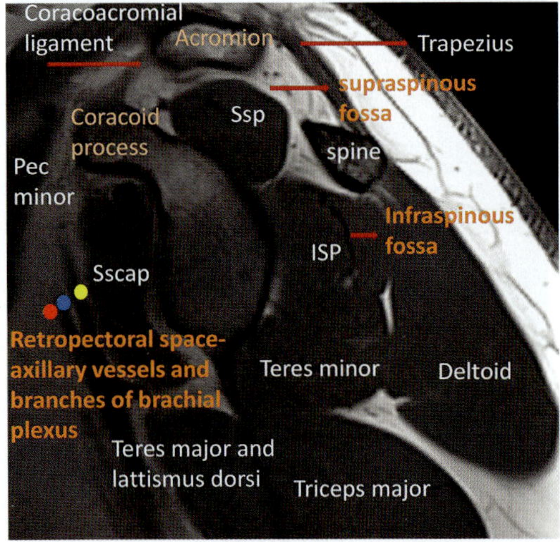

Fig. 3.8.23

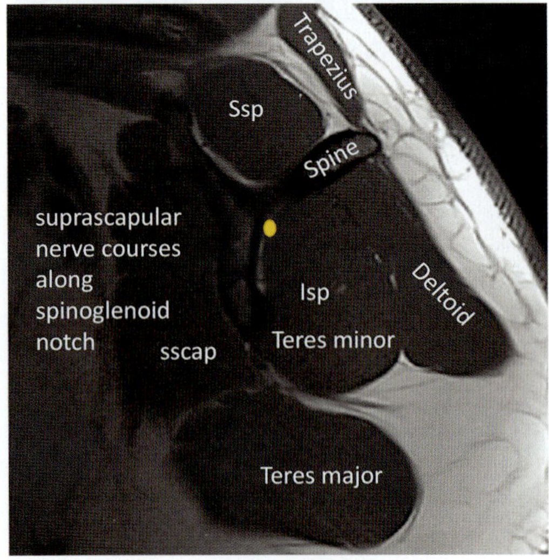

Fig. 3.8.24

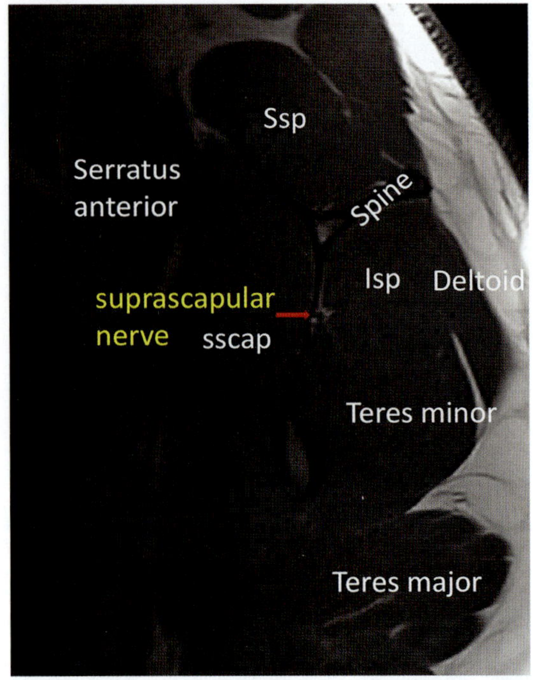

Fig. 3.8.25

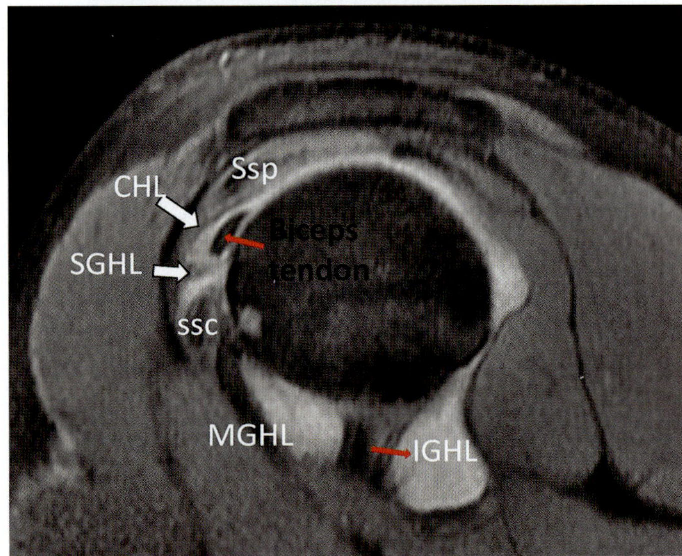

Fig. 3.8.26

The rotator cuff: The rotator cuff is an extrinsic glenohumeral joint stabiliser. The rotator cuff is made up of four muscles that link as tendons to the proximal humerus and are easily recognisable in the coronal oblique, sagittal oblique, and axial planes: Supraspinatus, infraspinatus, teres minor and subscapularis (mnemonic—SITS). The supraspinatus, infraspinatus, and teres minor muscles all insert into the greater tuberosity. The subscapularis attaches to the lesser tuberosity of the proximal humerus and is found anterior to the scapula (Fig. 3.8.27).

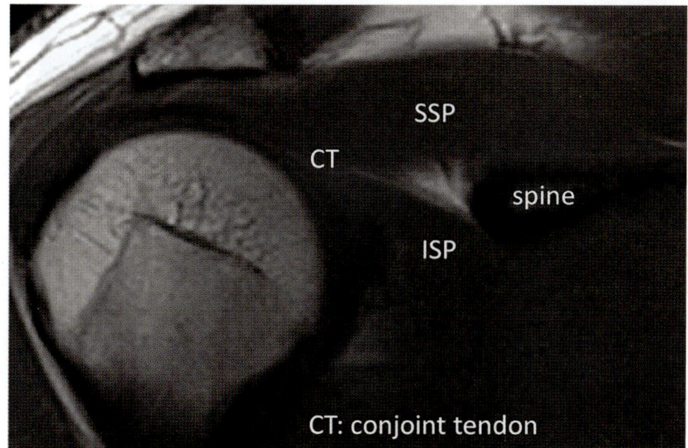

Fig. 3.8.27: Conjoint tendon

Significance: Rotator cuff tears, tendinitis, tendinopathy are common. Rotator cuff tear: Most commonly injured rotator cuff muscle is supraspinatus followed by infraspinatus and teres minor. Footprint is the site of insertion of the tendons on greater tuberosity. Critical zone is a potentially undervascularised portion of the distal supraspinatus tendon, located at 8–15 mm from the attachment at greater tuberosity, relatively decreased vascular supply at this site may predispose to tear/age related degeneration. Rotator cuff interval: The rotator interval is the distance between the supraspinatus tendon's anterior leading edge and superior edge of the subscapularis tendon. As it approaches the supraglenoid tubercle of the scapula, the long head of the biceps brachii tendon becomes intra-articular in this

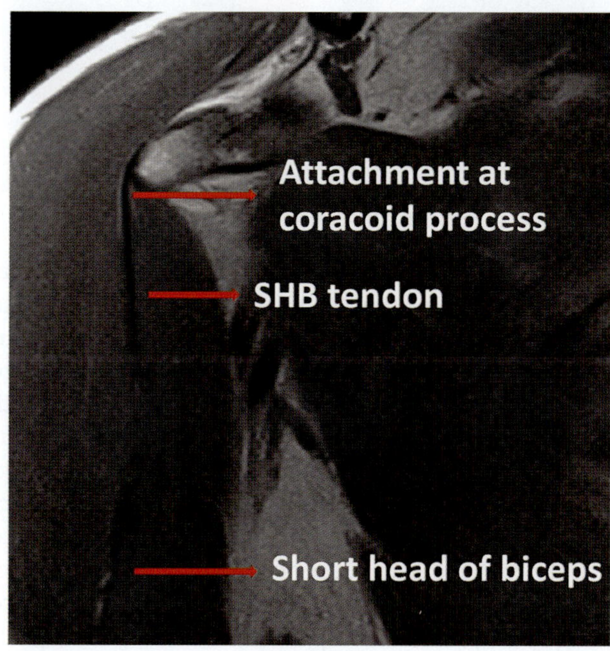

Fig. 3.8.28

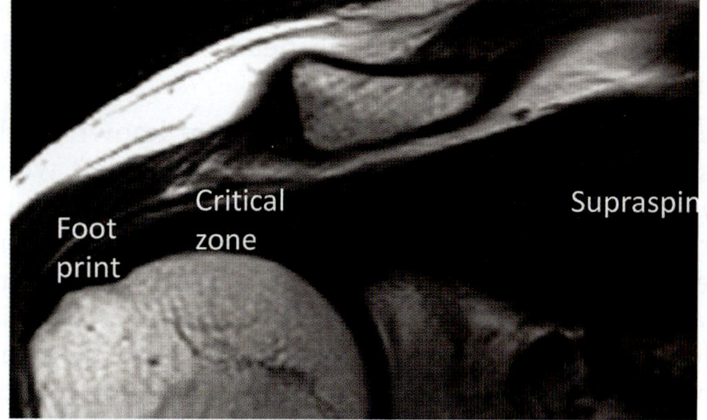

Fig. 3.8.29

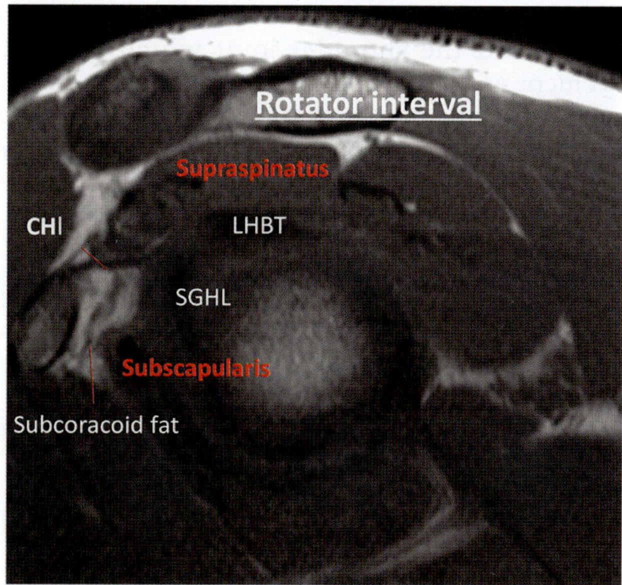

Fig. 3.8.30: Rotator intervel

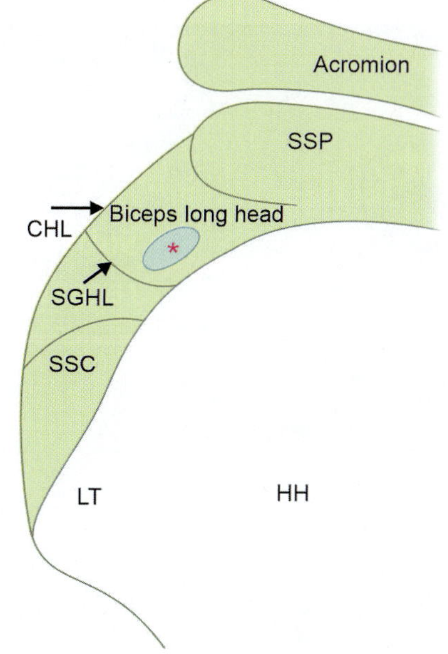

Fig. 3.8.31: Pictorial representation of rotator interval

area. Contents are coracohumeral ligament, superior glenohumeral ligament, long head of biceps brachii tendon, subcoracoid fat.

Biceps pulley: The biceps pulley, often known as the "sling," is a capsuloligamentous complex that works to anchor the biceps tendon's long head in the bicipital groove. It prevents the medial subluxation of the long head of biceps tendon from the bicipital groove and stabilises the tendon during biceps flexion. The superior glenohumeral ligament, the coracohumeral ligament, and the distal attachment of the subscapularis tendon, the transvere humeral ligament, make comprise the pulley complex.

Shoulder bursae refers to sac filled with the synovial fluid around the shoulder joint which facilitates movement and reduce friction at tendon–tendon and bone, bone–bone interfaces (Figs 3.8.32–3.8.35). There

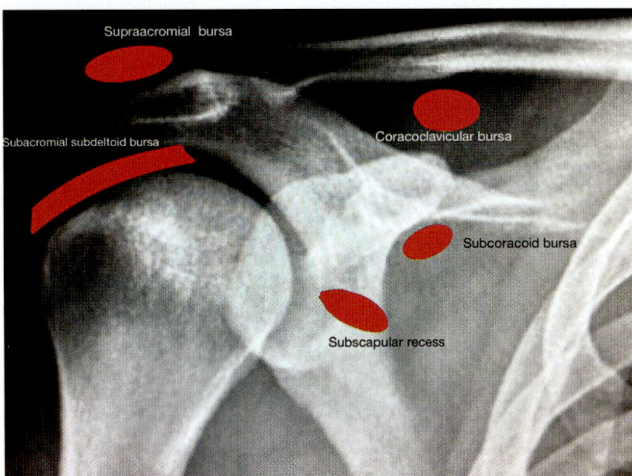

Fig. 3.8.32

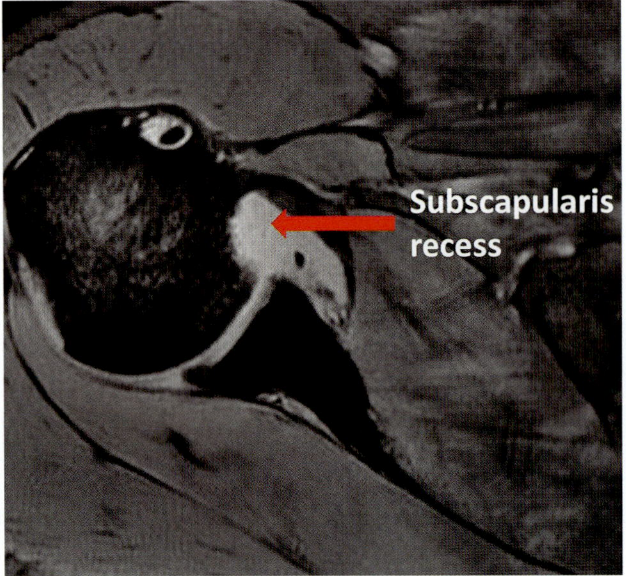

Fig. 3.8.33

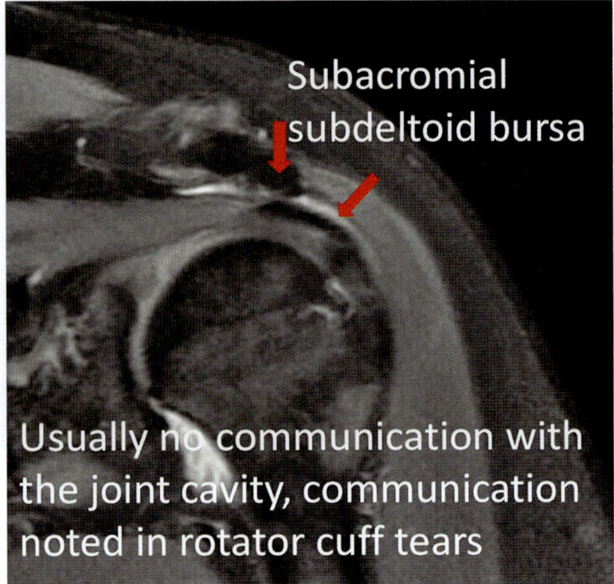

Fig. 3.8.34: Subacromial subdeltoid bursa

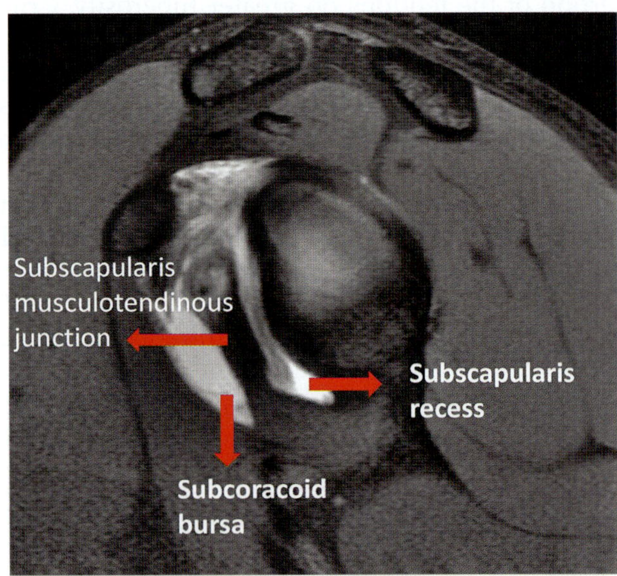

Fig. 3.8.35: Subscapularis recess

are 5 main bursae around shoulder joint. They are: 1) Subacromial and subdeltoid bursae, 2) Subcapsular recess, 3) Subcoracoid bursa, 4) Coracoclavicular bursa, 5) Supra-acromial bursa. Subacromial and subdeltoid bursae normally communicate with each other. Neither subcoracoid bursa nor subacromial, subdeltoid bursa communicate with the glenohumeral joint cavity. Communication noted in full thickness rotator cuff tears esp. supraspinatus. Fluid distended subcoracoid bursa can suggest the presence of shoulder pathologies like rotator cuff tear, biceps pulley lesion, subcoracoid impingement, adhesive capsulitis. Fluid in subscapularis recess may be normal due to its communication with

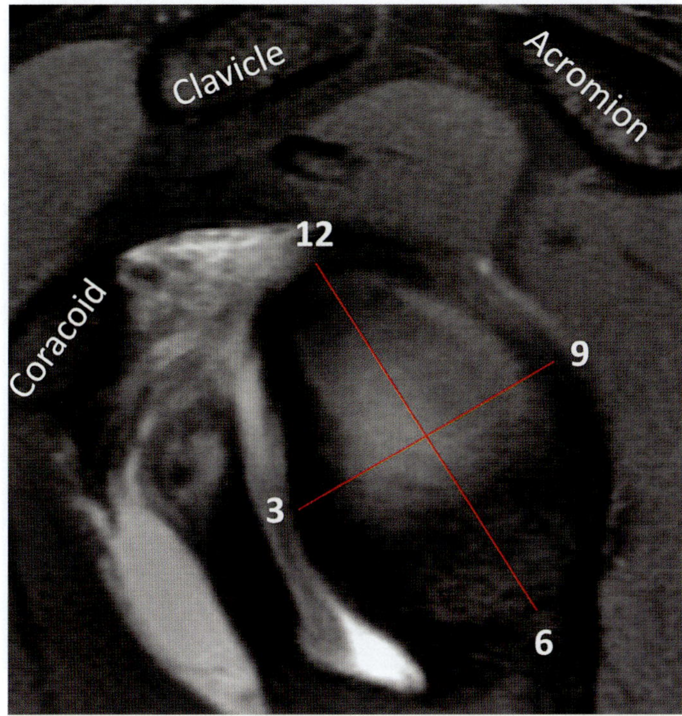

Fig. 3.8.36: Glenoid fossa

glenohumeral joint but can be distended in rotator cuff tears like subscapularis. Supra-acromial and coracoclavicular bursa are locations of calcific tenditis and not identified as sources of shoulder pathology.

Acromial shape: There are four types of acromion process (Fig. 3.8.37). It is said that undersurface of acromion has impact on rotator cuff injury and hence it is useful to know the types: Type 1—flat undersurface, type 2 —curved undersurface, type 3–hooked undersurface, type 4–convex undersurface. Acromion with hooked undersurface (type 3) or convex undersurface (type 4) may contribute to impingement and subsequent rotator cuff tears.

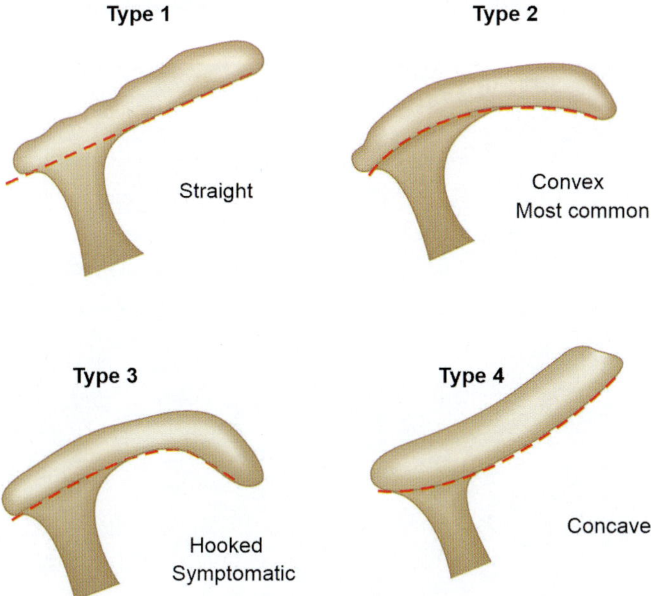

Fig. 3.8.37 Types of acromion

Anatomical spaces around the shoulder region: There are 3 potential spaces around the shoulder region—quadrangular space, lateral (lower) triangular space and medial (upper) triangular space. These spaces transmit nerves and vessels from anterior to posterior portion of shoulder region.

The coracoid process, coracoacromial ligament, and acromion combine to produce the coracoacromial arch. Structures located within the coracoacromial arch include: 1) Subacromial–subdeltoid bursa, 2) supraspinatus tendon, 3) superior part of infraspinatus tendon, 4) long head of biceps tendon, 5) coracohumeral ligament, 6) superior glenohumeral ligament.

Shoulder joint ligaments: The glenohumeral joint is a synovial joint that connects the glenoid to the humeral head. The fibrocartilaginous labrum, which forms a rim around the glenoid's perimeter, deepens the shallow glenoid articulation by 50%. A layer of hyaline articular cartilage covers both the glenoid and the humeral head. The joint capsule inserts along the anatomic neck of the humerus and along the neck of the glenoid. In front, it is reinforced by three glenohumeral ligaments (GHLs) (the superior, middle, and inferior), which converge from the humerus to be attached by the long head of the biceps tendon to the supraglenoid tubercle. Ligaments are stabilizer of glenohumeral joint, glenohumeral ligaments strengthen the anterior joint capsule (Figs 3.8.38–3.8.44).

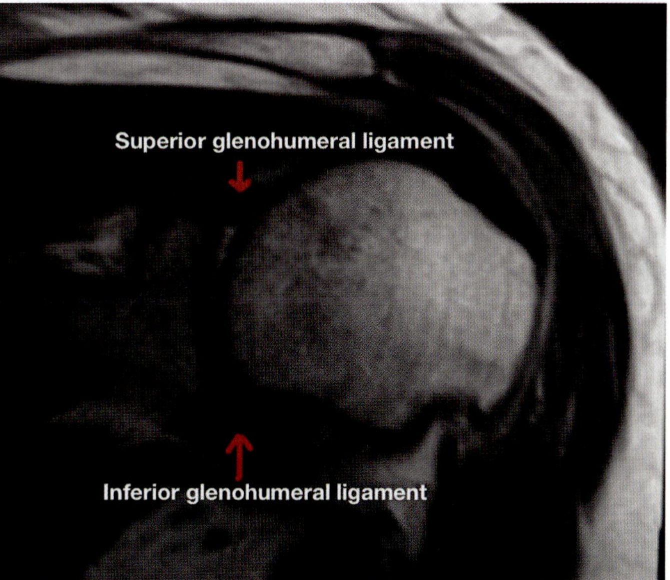

Fig. 3.8.38

Superior glenohumeral ligament (SGHL): Originates from the anterosuperior glenoid (anterior to biceps) and coracoid process and ends in lesser tuberosity, stabilizes biceps tendon.

Middle glenohumeral ligament (MGHL): Arises from the anterosuperior glenoid behind SGL extends along deep surface of subcapsularis tendon.

Inferior glenohumeral ligament (IGHL): Arise from the lower two-thirds of the glenoid labrum to the lower aspect of the anatomical humeral neck, three parts—anterior band, posterior band and axillary pouch, most important ligamentous structure that stabilizes shoulder joint and prevents dislocation at extreme range of motions.

The other important ligaments are the acromioclavicular, coracoacromial, and the coracoclavicular.

Coracoacromial ligament extends from distal two-thirds of coracoid to acromion tip forms a part of coracoacromial arch also reinforces inferior aspect of acromioclavicular joint.

Acromioclavicular ligament (ACL) reinforces acromioclavicular joint capsule. Have superior and inferior component.

Coracoclavicular ligament is the major static stabilizing ligament of the acromioclavicular joint. Ligament divides into two parts—conoid ligament: Arises from coracoid process of scapula and attaches to conoid tubercle on undersurface of clavicle. Trapezoid ligament: Arises from upper surface of coracoid and attaches to trapezoid ridge on undersurface of clavicle. Forces are transferred from upper limb to glenoid by this ligament.

Coracohumeral ligament (CHL): Supportive ligament of shoulder joint, arises from coracoid process runs across glenohumeral joint capsule blends with rotator cuff tendons—supraspinatus and subscapularis and covers the long head of biceps tendon superiorly, inserts on lesser and greater tuberosities.

Transverse humeral ligament joins both greater and lesser tuberosities and stabilizes biceps tendon in bicipital groove. This ligament is strengthened by coracohumeral ligament.

Glenoid labrum: Fibrocartilaginous rim around the periphery of the glenoid that deepens the articulating surface of the glenoid by about one-third and provides increased stability to the joint. The labrum also provides sustenance to the glenoid cavity and aids in the lubrication of the shoulder joint. With all pulse sequences, the signal intensity is low. The labrum is commonly split into four or six regions for the purpose of locating anomalies, or in terms of time zones on a clock face.

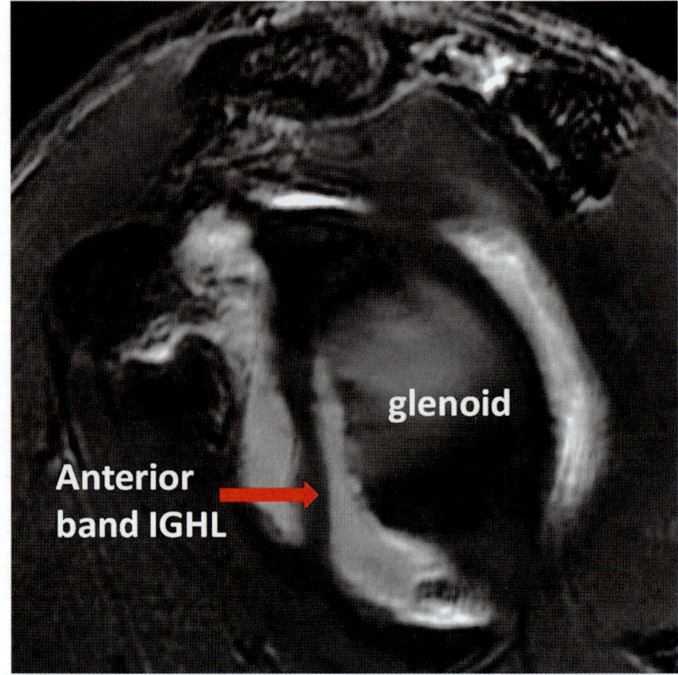

Fig. 3.8.39

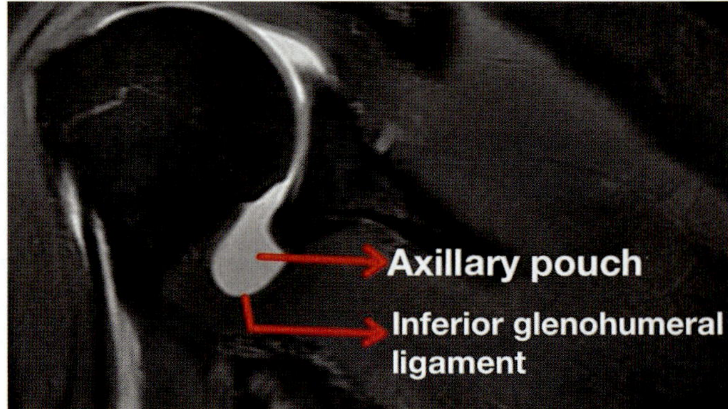

Fig. 3.8.40

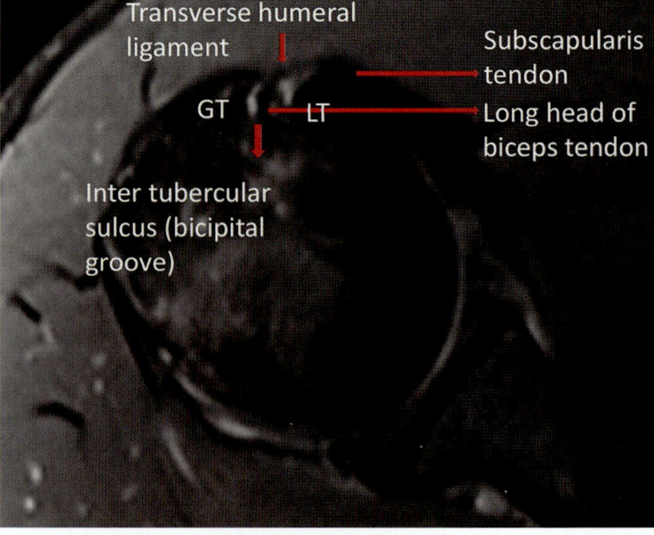

Fig. 3.8.41

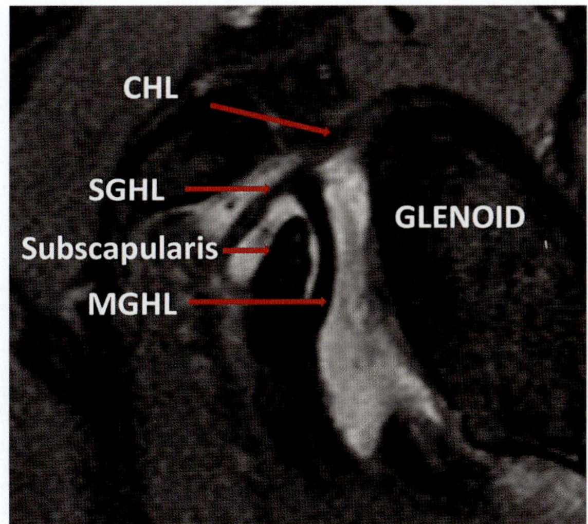

Fig. 3.8.42

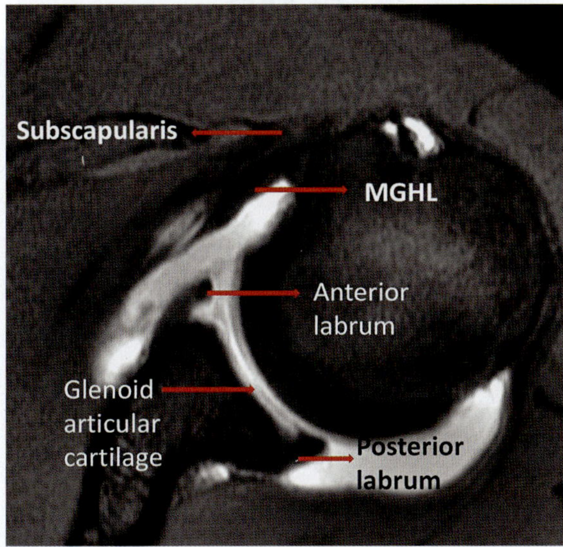

Fig. 3.8.43

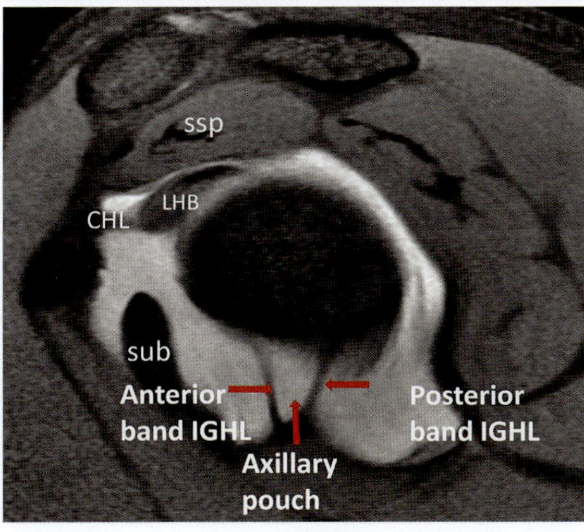

Fig. 3.8.44

The labrum is compared to the face of a clock for the divide into clock zones, with the superior portion at 12 o'clock and the inferior portion at 6 o'clock. Both shoulders are traditionally positioned with the anterior section at 3 o'clock and the posterior portion at 9 o'clock. **Capsular insertion:** Type 2, type 3 anterior capsular insertion are more prone for joint instability (Figs 3.8.45–3.8.49). The anterior joint capsule varies in the way it inserts onto the glenoid: Zlatkin categorized this into three types, types 1–3, depending on the proximity of capsular insertion to the glenoid margin. In type 1 capsular attachment is at or near the glenoid labrum. In type 2 capsular attachment anterior capsule less than 1 cm medial to glenoid labrum. In type 3 anterior capsule is attached above 1 cm medial to glenoid labrum.

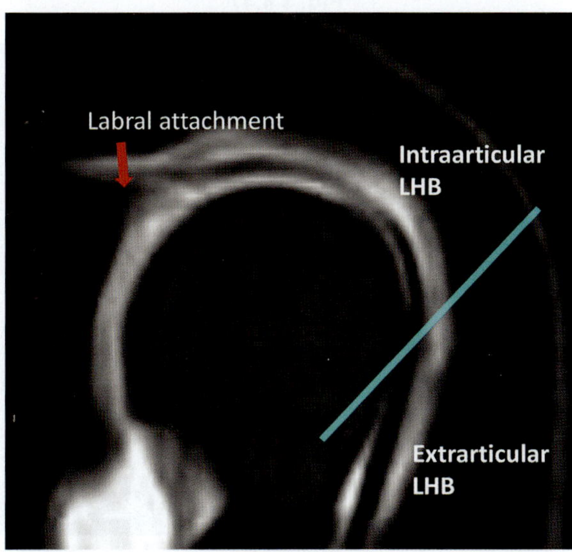

Fig. 3.8.45

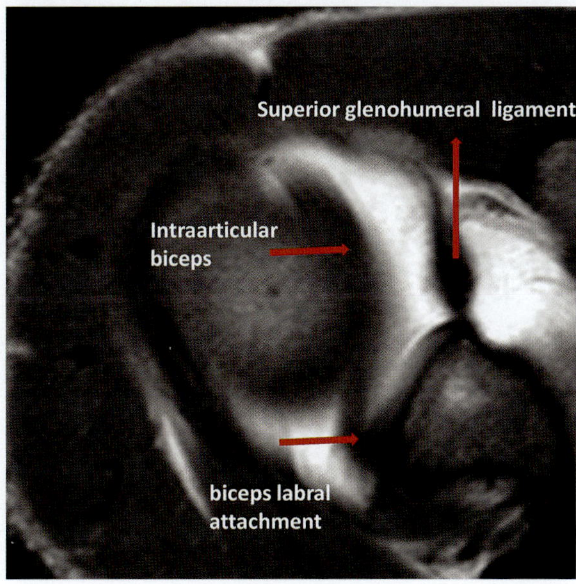

Fig. 3.8.46

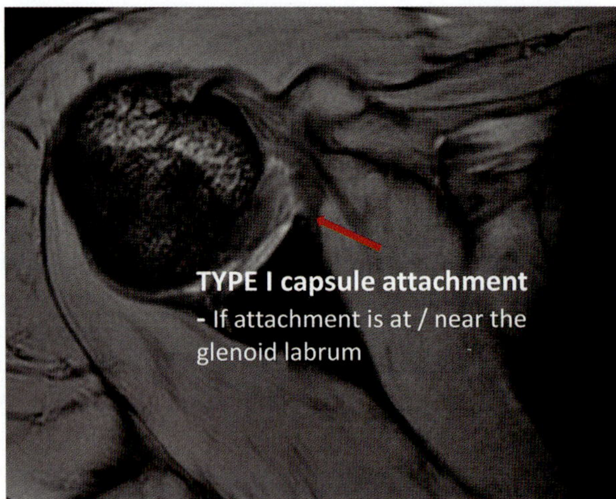

Fig. 3.8.47

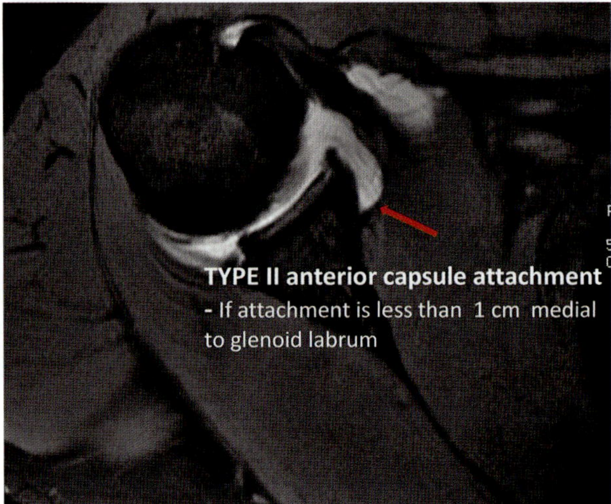

Fig. 3.8.48

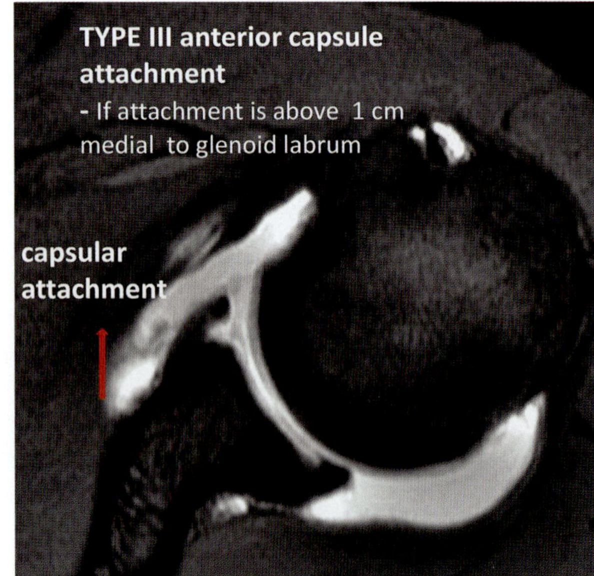

Fig. 3.8.49

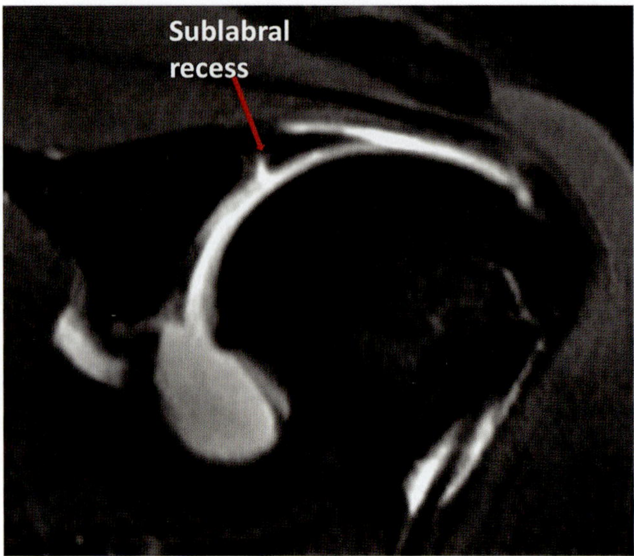

Fig. 3.8.50

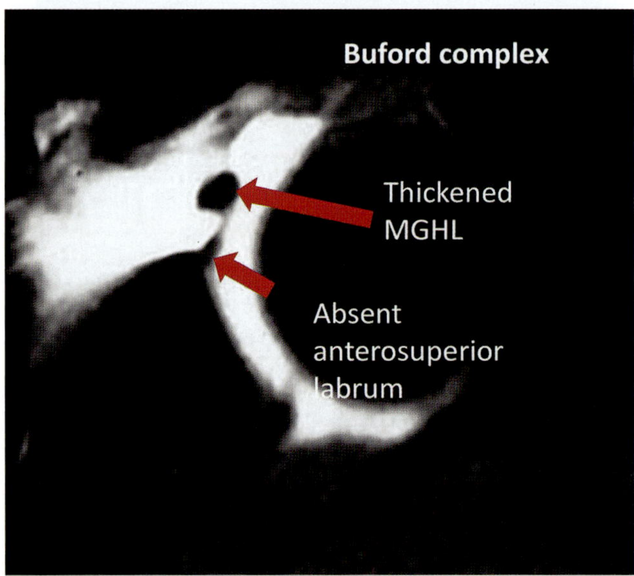

Fig. 3.8.51

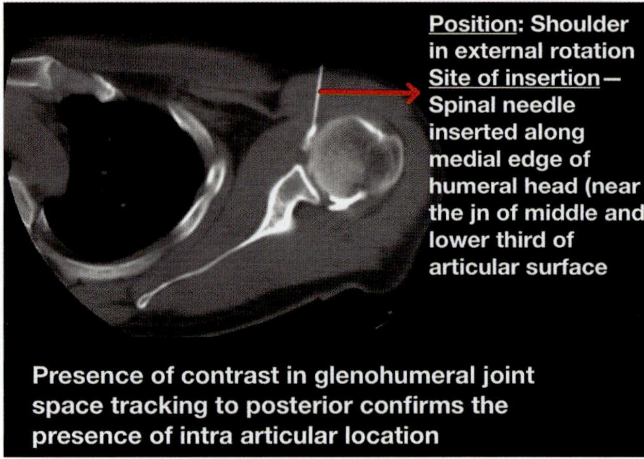

Fig. 3.8.52: CT guided shoulder arthrography

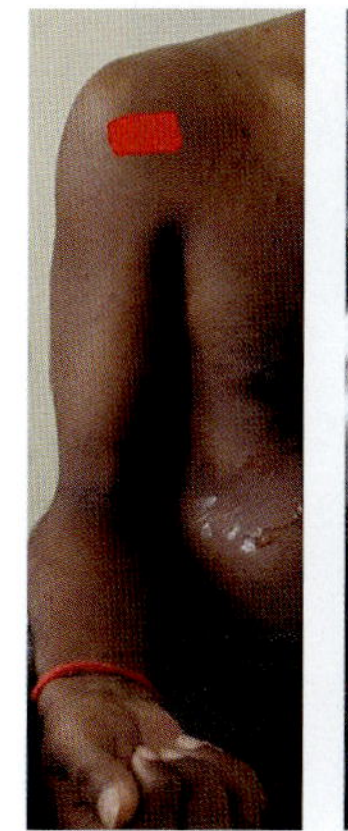
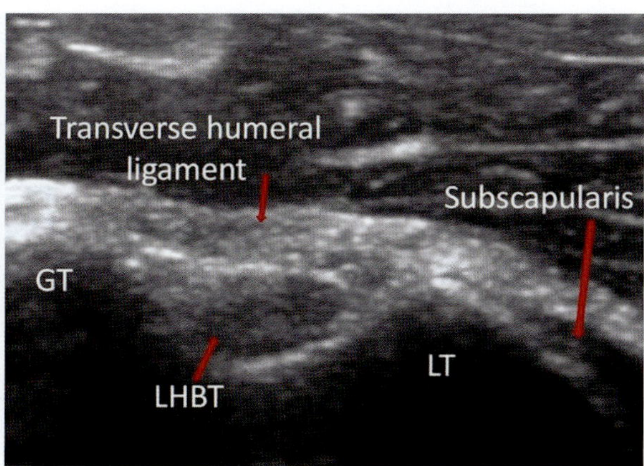

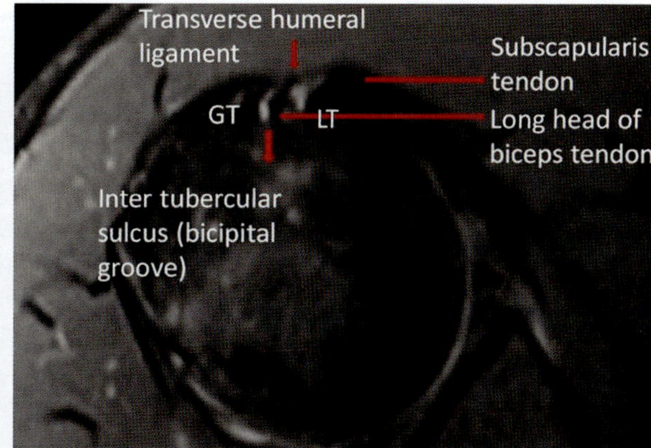

Fig. 3.8.53: Subscapularis muscle

Labral variants: Sublabral recess: Defect of the anterosuperior labrum which does not extend posterior to the biceps tendon attachment (not to be confused with SLAP tear). Buford complex: Congenital absence of anterosuperior labrum with thickened middle glenohumeral ligament (Figs 3.8.50–3.8.51).

Ultrasound

Subscapularis: Patient position: Place the forearm in external rotation after fixing elbow close to body, probe position: Move the probe medially (from previous position). Primary structure: Axial subscapularis (attachment to lesser tuberosity). Sagittal—multipennate nature of subscapularis (Figs 3.8.53 and 3.8.55). **Long head of biceps tendon (LHBT/LHB):** Patient position: Place the arm in slight internal rotation, elbow flexed at 90°, palm facing up. Probe position: Locate greater and lesser tuberosities of proximal humerus and find the tendon between two tuberosities, use short and long axis planes. Primary structure: Transverse LHBT (axial plane), longitudinal LHBT (sagittal plane), oblique plane to look for rotator interval (Fig. 3.8.54). **Acromioclavicular joint:** Patient position: Arm neutral, elbow flexed at 90°, palm facing up. Probe position: In coronal plane over the shoulder. Primary structure: Acromioclavicular joint, superior acromioclavicular ligament (Fig. 3.8.58). **Coracoacromial ligament:** Patient position: Arm neutral, elbow flexed at 90°, palm facing up. Probe position: Fix the probe in acromion process and move the probe medial on transverse plane till you visualize coracoid process. Primary structure: Coracoacromial ligament (Fig. 3.8.59). **Supraspinatus:** Patient position: Arm posteriorly placing the palmar side of hand on gluteal muscle with the elbow flexed and directed posteriorly. Probe position: Over greater tuberosity.

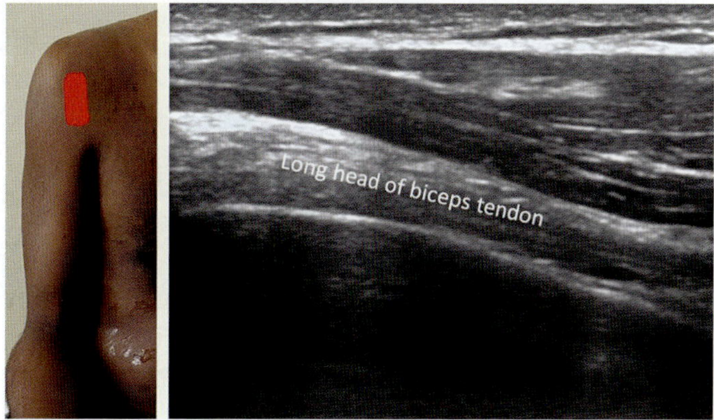

Fig. 3.8.54: Long head of biceps tendon

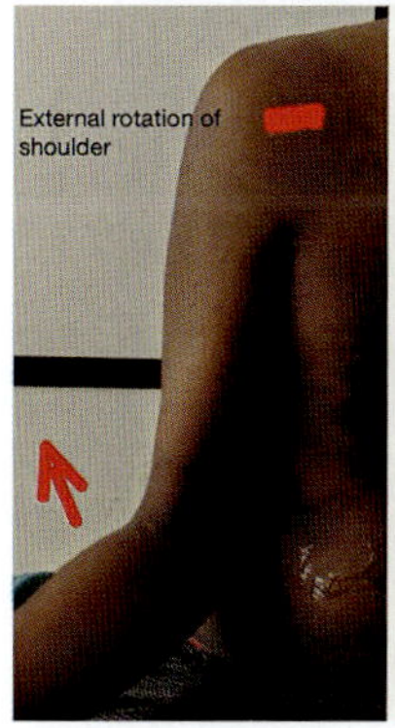

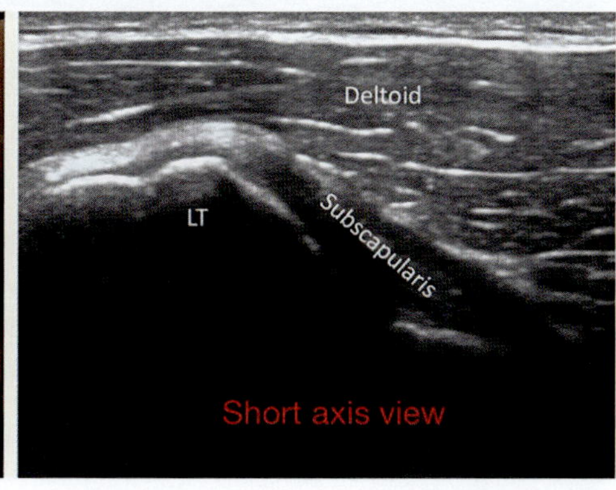

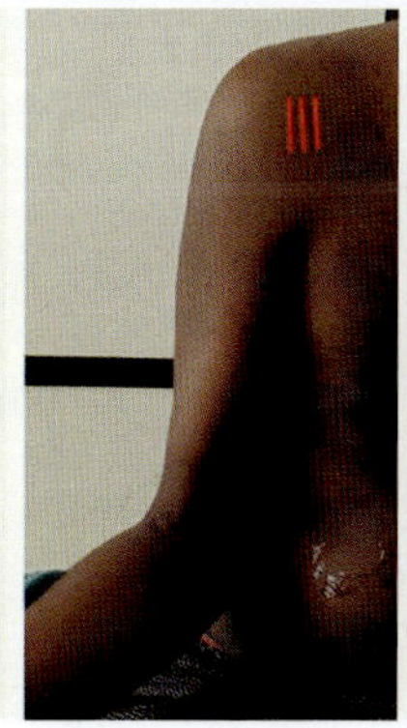
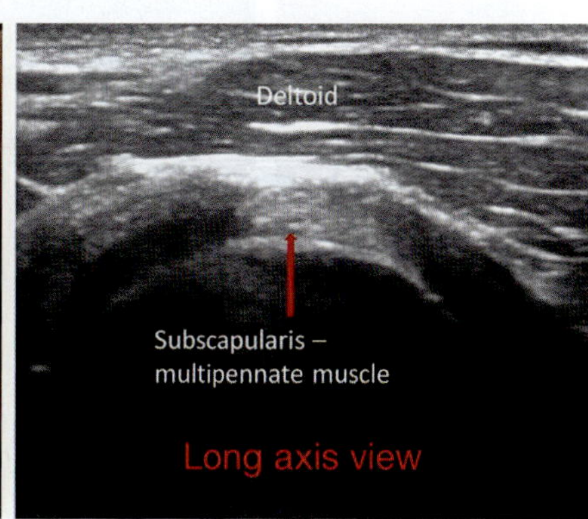

Fig. 3.8.55: Subscapularis muscle

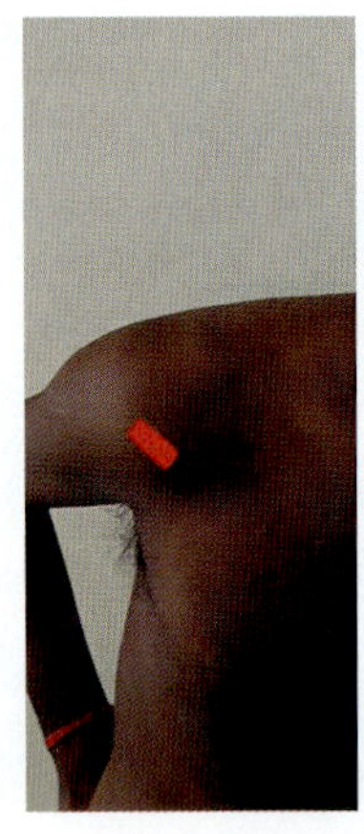
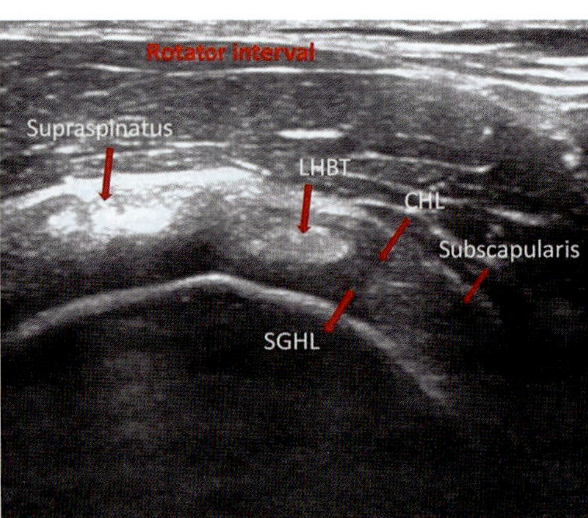

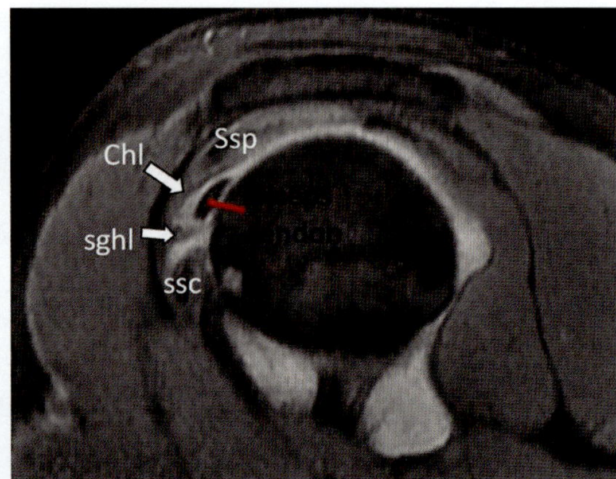

Fig. 3.8.56: Ultrasound for rotator interval (*ssc: subscapularis ; Ssp: Supraspinatous)

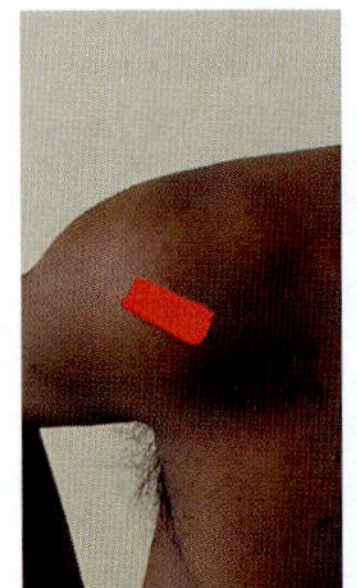
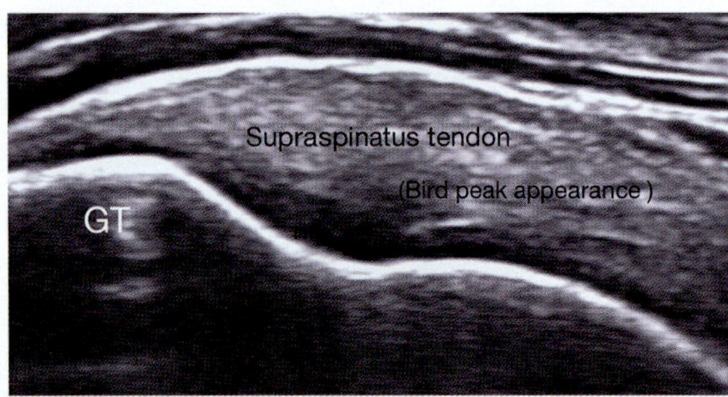

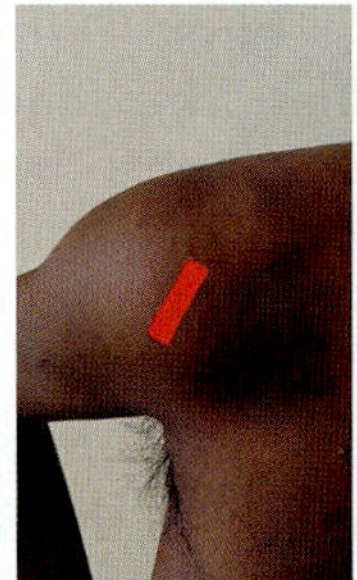
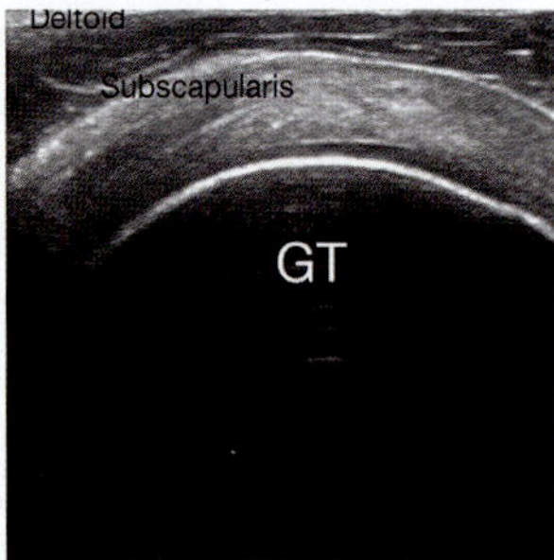

Fig. 3.8.57: Supraspinatus muscle

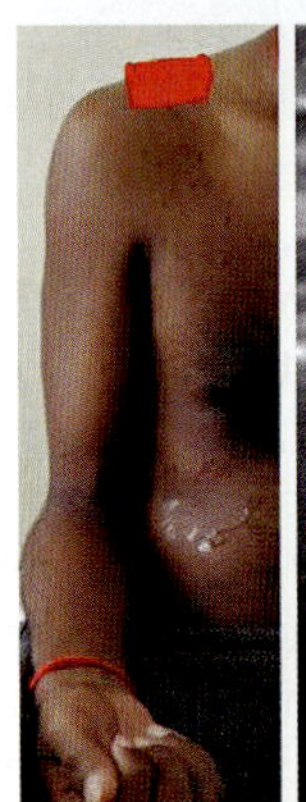
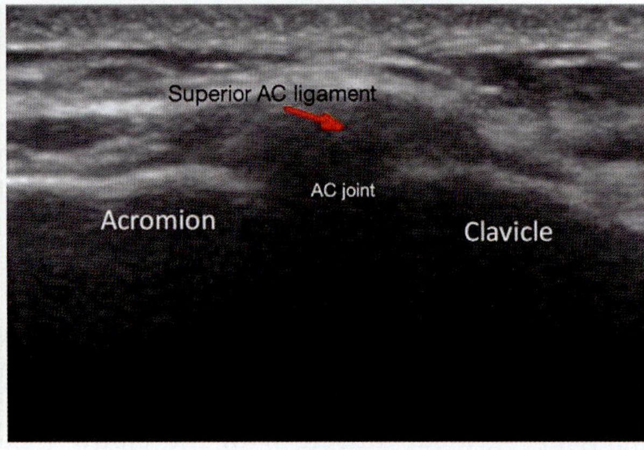

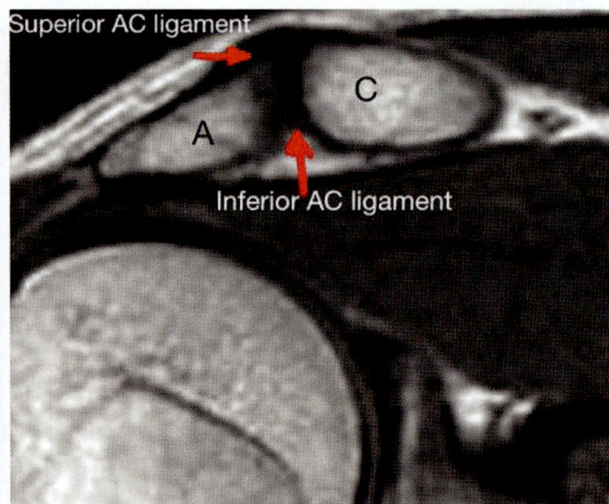

Fig. 3.8.58: Acromioclavicular joint

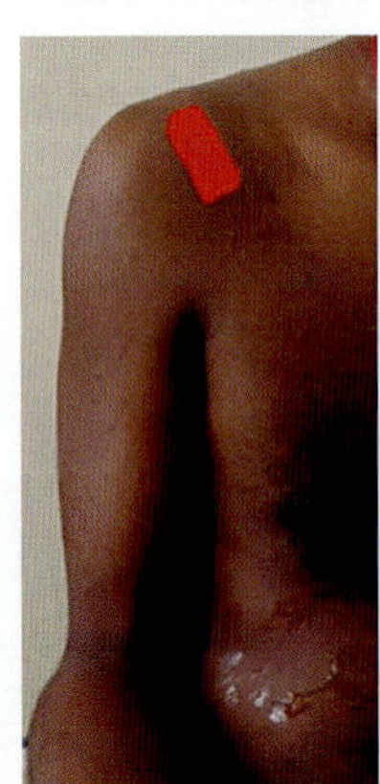
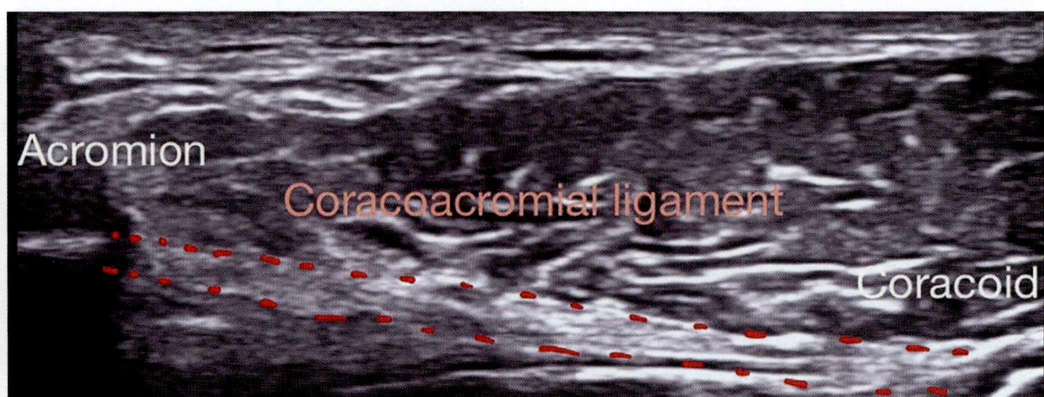

Fig. 3.8.59: Coracoacromial ligament

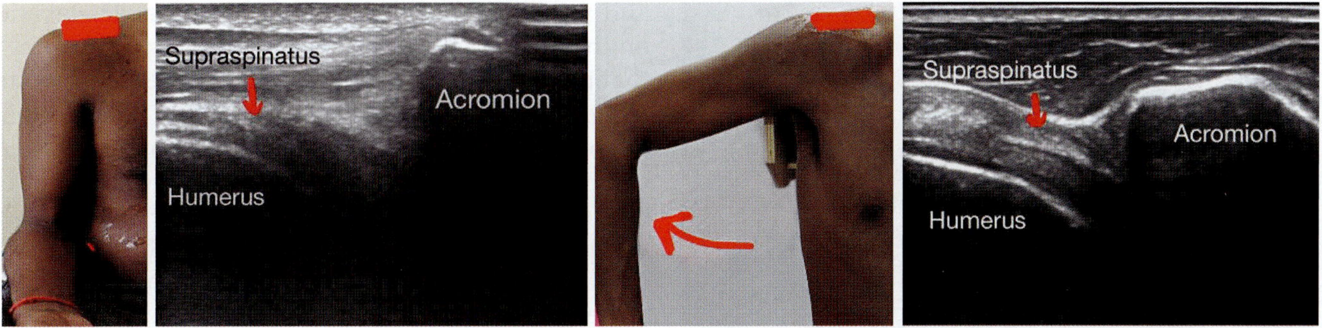

Fig. 3.8.60: Supraspinatus muscle

Primary structure: Supraspinatus in long and short axis (Figs 3.8.57 and 3.8.60) **Infraspinatus and teres minor:** Patient position: Place the palm over opposite shoulder. Probe position: Over the posterior aspect of glenohumeral joint and sweep towards greater tuberosity. Primary structure: Infraspinatus superiorly and teres minor inferiorly (Figs 3.8.61 and 3.8.62). **Posterior glenohumeral joint recess:** Patient position: Arm neutral, elbow flexed at 90°, palm facing up. Probe position: Over the posterior aspect of glenohumeral joint. Primary structure: Posterior labrum capsular complex and posterior joint

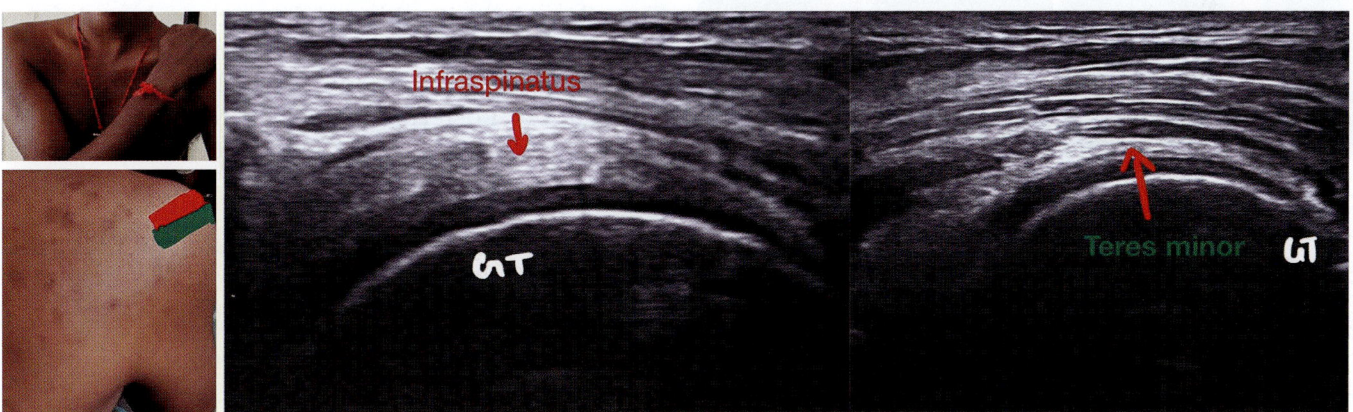

Fig. 3.8.61: Infraspinatus muscle

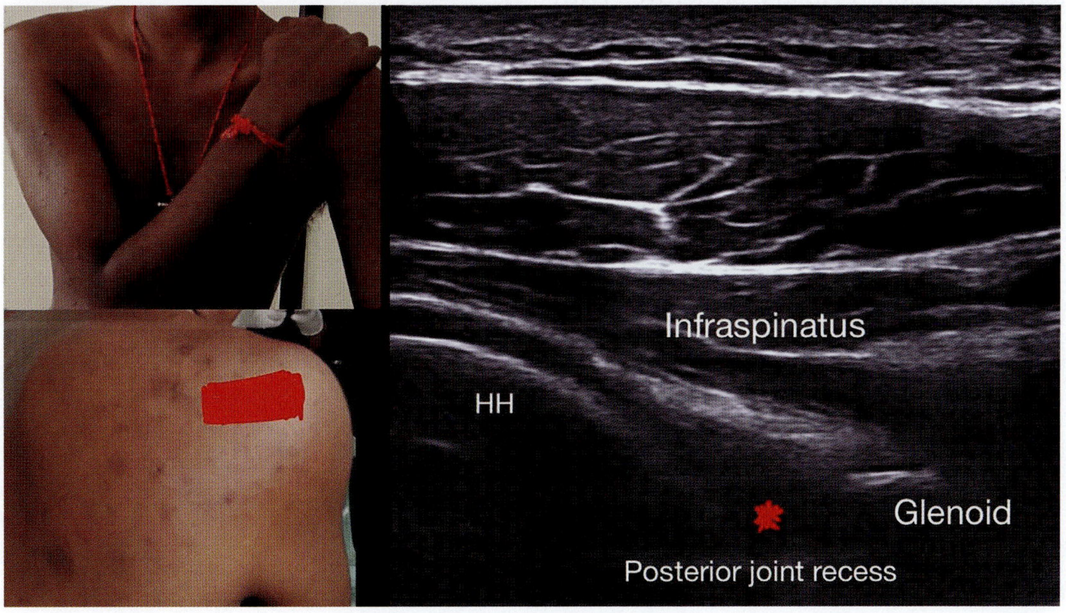

Fig. 3.8.62: Infraspinatus muscle

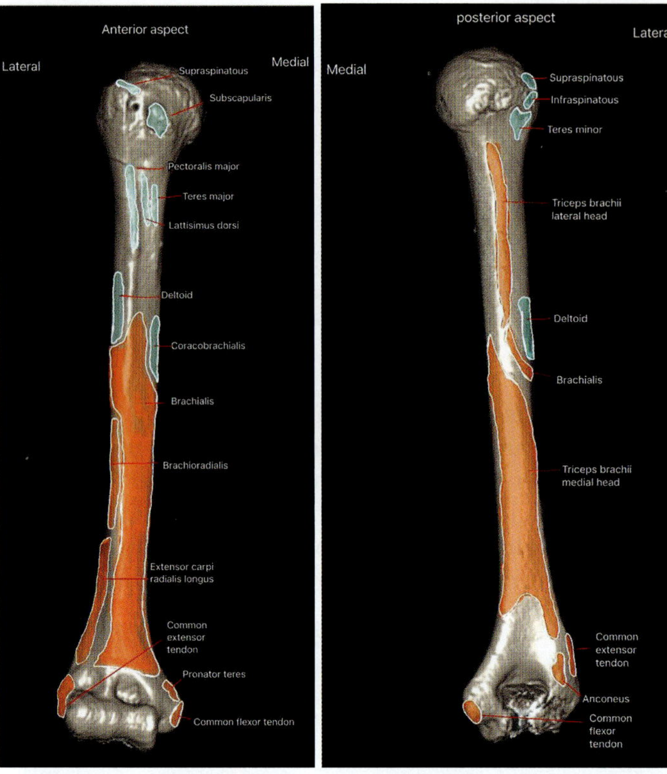

Fig. 3.8.63 **Fig. 3.8.64**

recess assess for joint effusion. It is the site for ultrasound guided contrast injection for arthrography. Subacromial impingement test: Dynamic assessment of subacromial impingement can be done. Patient position: Initially place arm neutral, elbow flexed at 90°, palm facing up. Probe position: Place the probe in coronal plane over the lateral margin of acromion. Ask the patient to abduct the arm in internal rotation. Primary structure: With this maneuver the supraspinatus and bursa can be seen passing deep to acromion.

3.8.B Arm

Deltoid tuberosity is roughened protuberance on the humeral diaphysis for attachment of the deltoid muscle. Spiral groove accommodates the radial nerve. Lateral and medial supracondylar ridges are linear elevations on the lateral and medial aspects of the distal humerus that provide attachment for the fascial septa of the arm.

Compartments: The arm is encircled by a sheath of deep fascia. Lateral and medial intermuscular septae extend from it to the respective supracondylar ridges of the humerus, dividing the arm into separate anterior and posterior fascial compartments. Each compartment contains its own muscles and neurovascular supply. Anterior (flexor) fascial compartment contents are biceps brachii, coracobrachialis and brachialis muscles, and supplied by brachial artery and musculocutaneous nerve. Posterior (extensor) fascial compartment contains triceps brachii muscle and supplied by profunda brachii and ulnar collateral arteries and radial nerve.

Axial sections: Superior to inferior—Figs 3.8.65–3.8.68.

3.8.C Elbow

The elbow joint is a hinge joint and made up of three articulations: Radiohumeral, ulnohumeral and proximal radioulnar articulation. Joint capsule encloses all three articulation. Posteriorly attached to capitulleum and olecranon. Anteriorly attached to coronoid process and annular ligament.

Table 3.8.2: Muscles around the elbow joint

Forearm flexors at elbow	Forearm extensors at elbow
Primary: Biceps brachii, brachialis, brachioradialis *Secondary:* Pronator teres, palmaris longus, flexor digitorum superficialis, extensor carpi radialis longus and brevis	*Primary:* Triceps brachii *Secondary:* None
Forearm pronators at elbow	Forearm supinators at elbow
Primary: Pronator teres, pronator quadratus *Secondary:* Brachioradialis	*Primary:* Supinator, biceps brachii *Secondary:* None

Cubital fossa: Triangular-shaped potential space in anterior elbow that permits passage of structures from

Table 3.8.1: Ossification centers in shoulder region

Primary ossification centre				*Secondary ossification centre*		
Bones	*Site*	*Appear*	*Fusion*	*Site*	*Appear*	*Fusion*
Scapula	Middle of the coracoid process	1st year of life	15 years	The inferior angle, the medial border, and the root of the coracoid process	14–20 years	22–25 years
Humerus		8th week		Head Greater tubercle	1 year 3 years 5 years	Fused together by 6 years. Fusion with shaft at 20 years
Clavicle	Membrane	5th, 6th weeks	7th week	Sternal end	15–17 years	25 years

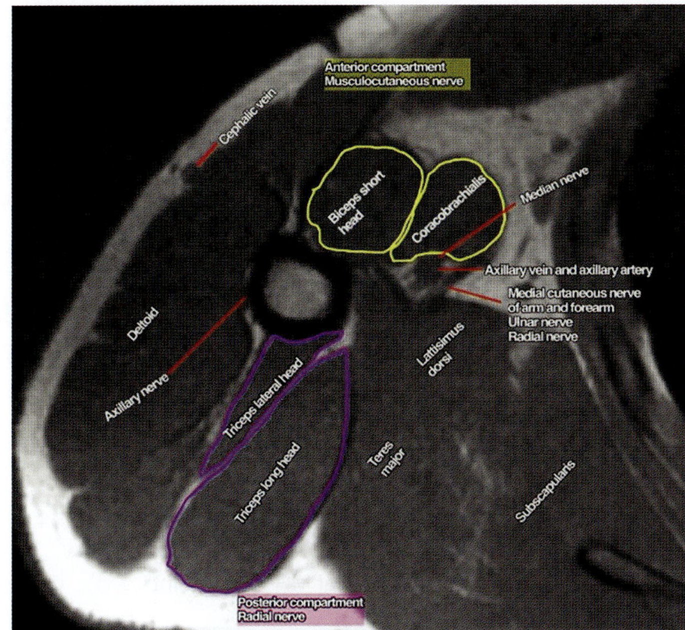

Fig. 3.8.65

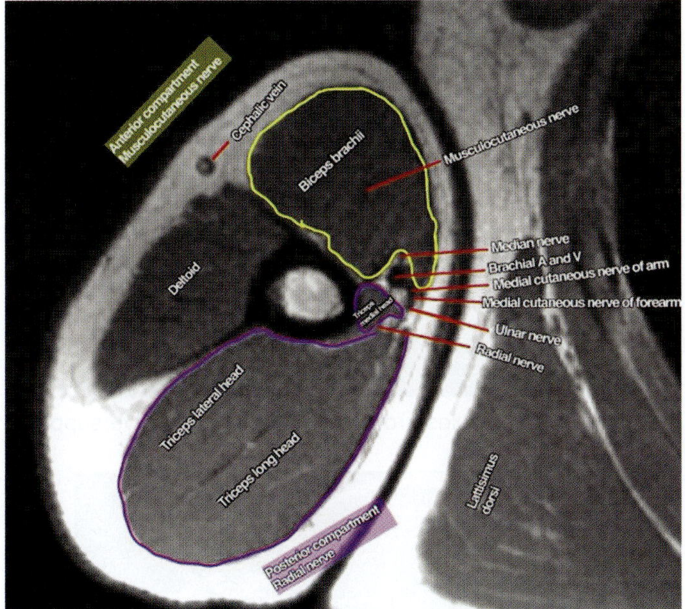

Fig. 3.8.66

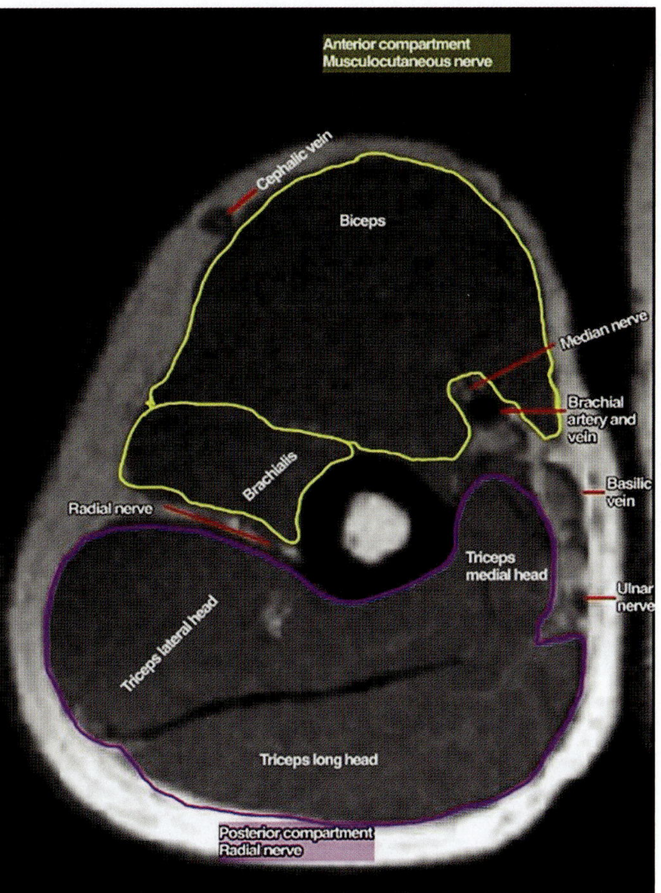

Fig. 3.8.67

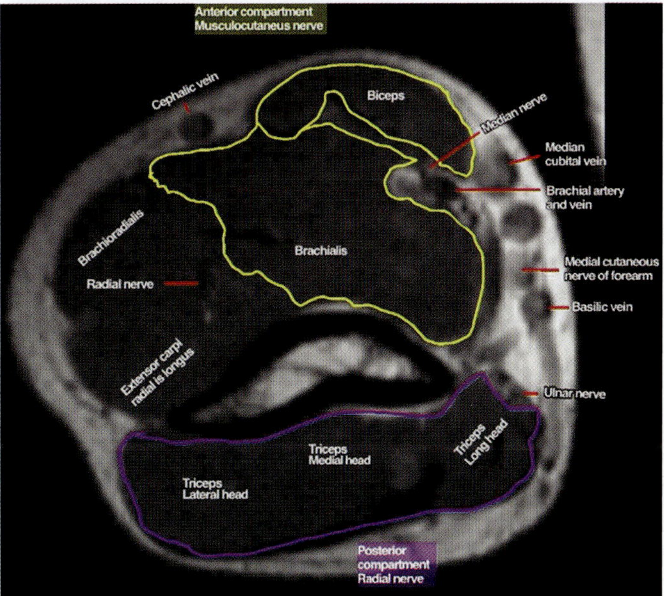

Fig. 3.8.68

the arm to the forearm. Base formed by imaginary horizontal line connecting the epicondyles of the humerus. Apex formed by point at which the borders of the brachioradialis and pronator teres muscles cross. Contents (from lateral to medial) are biceps brachii tendon, brachial artery, which divides into the radial, ulnar artery and median nerve.

Cubital tunnel: Roof formed by flexor carpi ulnaris (FCU) fascia and arcuate ligament of Osborne (cubital retinaculum) that travels from the medial epicondyle to the olecranon. Floor formed by posterior and transverse bands of MCL and elbow joint capsule. Walls formed by medial epicondyle and olecranon. Content: Ulnar nerve (Fig. 3.8.73).

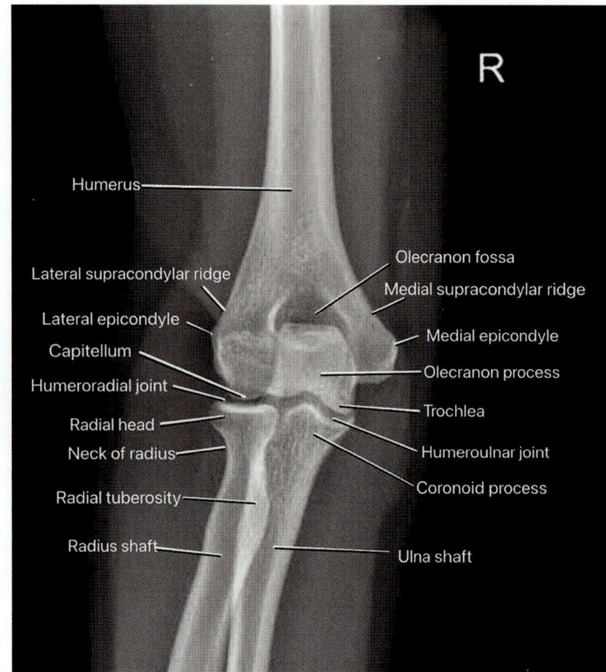

Fig. 3.8.69: Elbow X-ray AP view

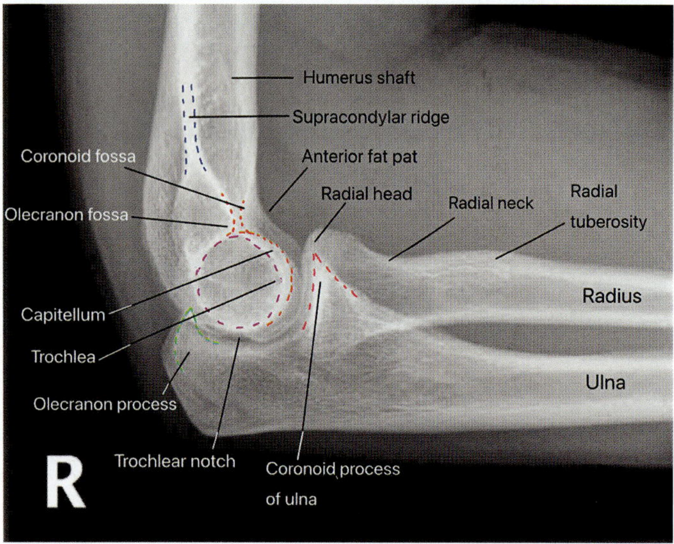

Fig. 3.8.70: Elbow X-ray lateral view

Ligaments: The ulnar (medial) collateral ligament is responsible for medial elbow joint stability and resistance to valgus strain. It is composed of three discrete bundles: Anterior bundle, posterior bundle, and transverse bundle. It extends from medial epicondyle to ulna. The lateral collateral ligament has two components: (1) Radial collateral ligament which extends from lateral epicondyle to annular ligaments and restrains against varus strain. (2) Lateral ulnar collateral ligament which extends from lateral epicondyle to radial collateral ligament and restrains against posterolateral instability.

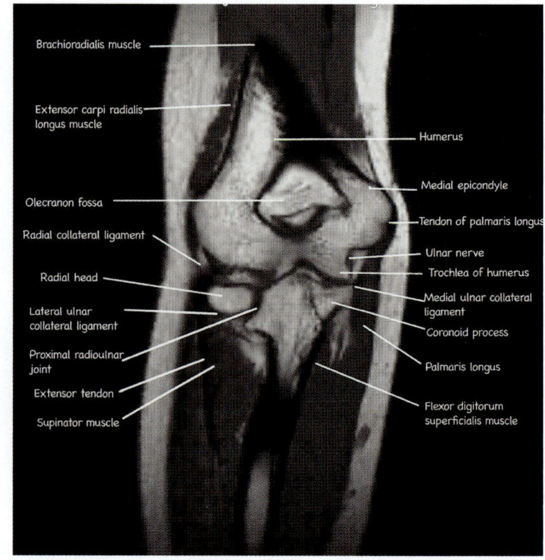

Fig. 3.8.71: Coronal MR-elbow joint

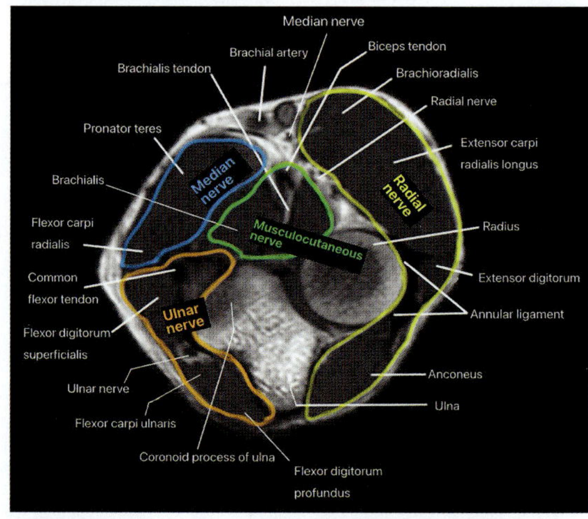

Fig. 3.8.72: Muscles around elbow joint and nerve supply

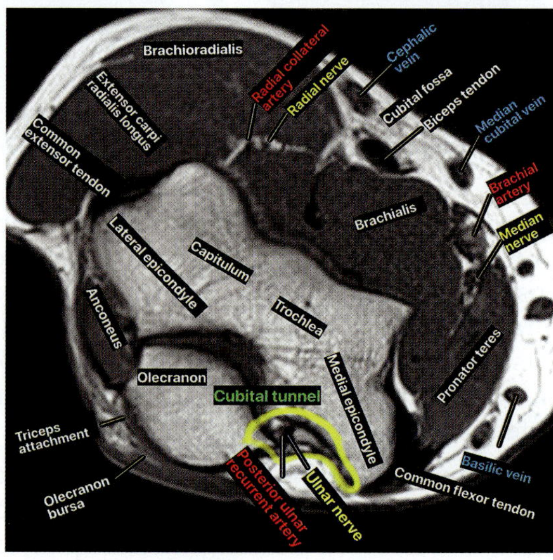

Fig. 3.8.73 Cubital tunnel

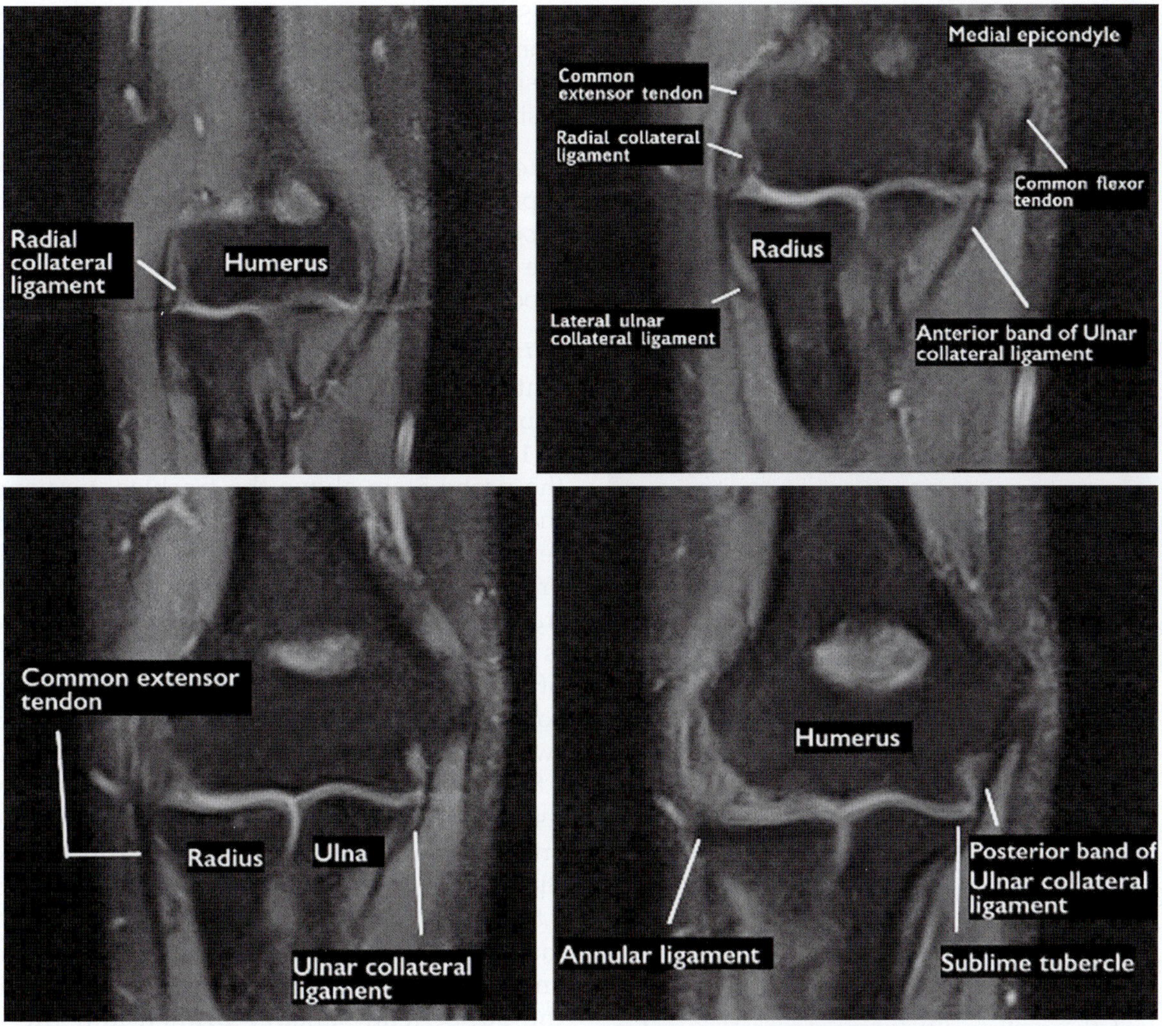

Fig. 3.8.74 Elbow joint ligaments in coronal section (anterior to posterior)

Ligaments of proximal radioulnar joint: (1) Annular ligament which attaches to anterior and posterior aspects of radial notch of ulna, (2) Quadrate ligament extending from radial neck to ulna (Figs 3.8.74–3.8.76).

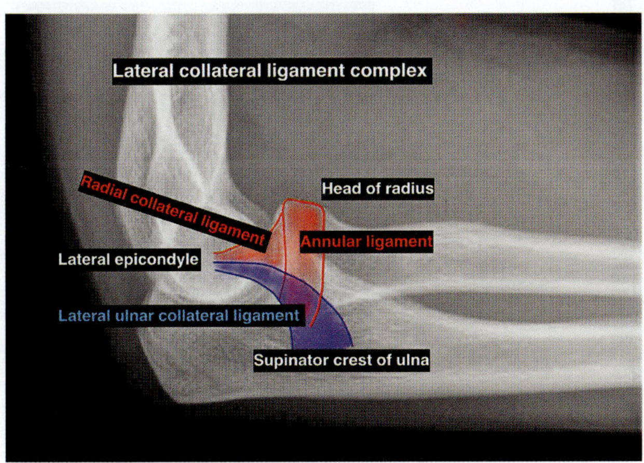

Fig. 3.8.75

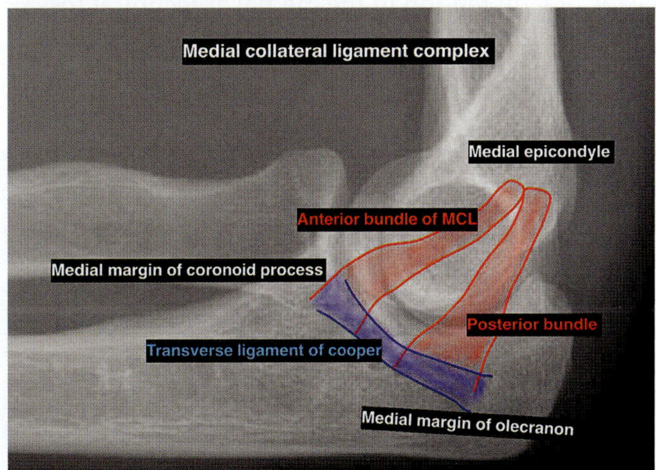

Fig. 3.8.76

Bursae: The elbow bursae are a group of synovial-lined bursae that surround the elbow joint. Bursae surrounding the olecranon and in the cubital fossa are two types of

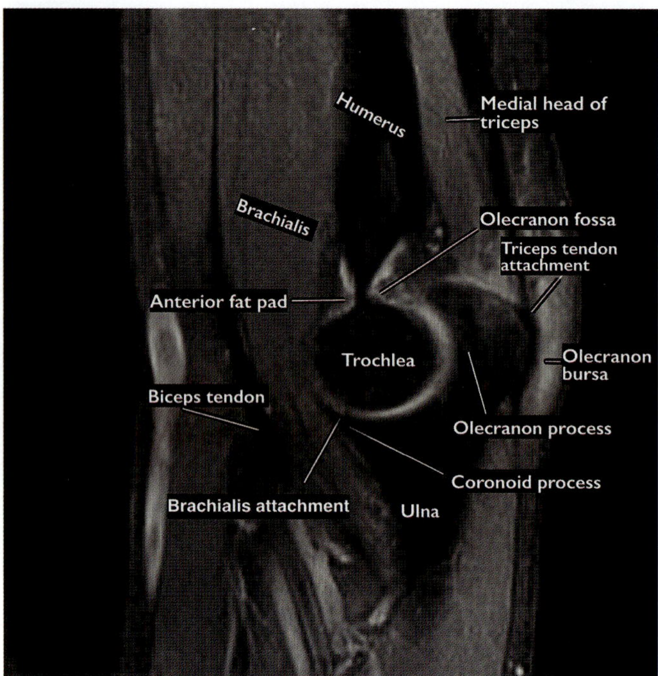

Fig. 3.8.77: Olecranon bursa

bursae. Olecranon bursae: (1) Superficial olecranon bursa: Lies between the olecranon and the subcutaneous tissue. (2) Subtendinous olecranon bursa: Lies between the tip of the olecranon and deep to the triceps brachii tendon. (3) Intratendinous olecranon bursa: lies within the triceps brachii tendon near its insertion onto the olecranon. Cubital bursae: (1) Bicipitoradial bursa: Lies between the distal biceps brachii tendon and the tuberosity of the radius. (2) Interosseous bursa: Lies along side the brachialis muscle and adjacent to the biceps brachii tendon in the medial antecubital fossa.

Normal variants: Supracondylar (avain) spur: Bony spur 5 cm proximal to medial epicondyle. Ligament of Struthers: Accessory origin of pronator teres arising from supracondylar spur. Os supratrochleare: Accessory ossicles in olecranon fossa. Patella cubiti: Sesamoid in distal triceps tendon.

Imaging pitfalls: On MR imaging: Pseudodefect of capitellum: Normal groove between the posterolateral aspect capitellum and lateral condyle. Pseudodefect of the trochlear groove: Localised defect in the trochlea groove between olecranon and coronoid process junction.

Ultrasound of elbow joint:

Anterior elbow (A): Patient is made seated with elbow support and forearm in full extension and supination. **(A1)** Transverse plane images are obtained by placing the probe 5 cm above the trochlea, perpendicular to the humeral shaft. Images of the supracondylar region reveal the biceps and brachialis muscles medially brachial artery and median nerve (Fig. 3.8.79). **(A2)** On transverse plane the anterior distal humeral epiphysis is a wavy hyperechoic line covered by a thin layer of hypoechoic articular cartilage; the lateral third corresponds to the humeral capitellum (round), medial two-thirds is the humeral trochlea (V-shaped) (Fig. 3.8.80). **(A3)** The distal biceps tendon is examined on its long-axis to avoid confusion between the tendon and the adjacent artery, tendon appears echogenic. Biceps tendon gets inserted in radial tuberosity (Fig. 3.8.81). **(A4)** Radial nerve: Follow the radial nerve's main trunk in its short-axis between the brachioradialis and brachialis muscle down to its bifurcation into the superficial sensory branch and the posterior interosseous nerve on the anterolateral elbow. The posterior interosseous nerve demonstrated using short axis planes as it pierces the supinator muscle and passes two heads of supinator muscle (Fig. 3.8.82).

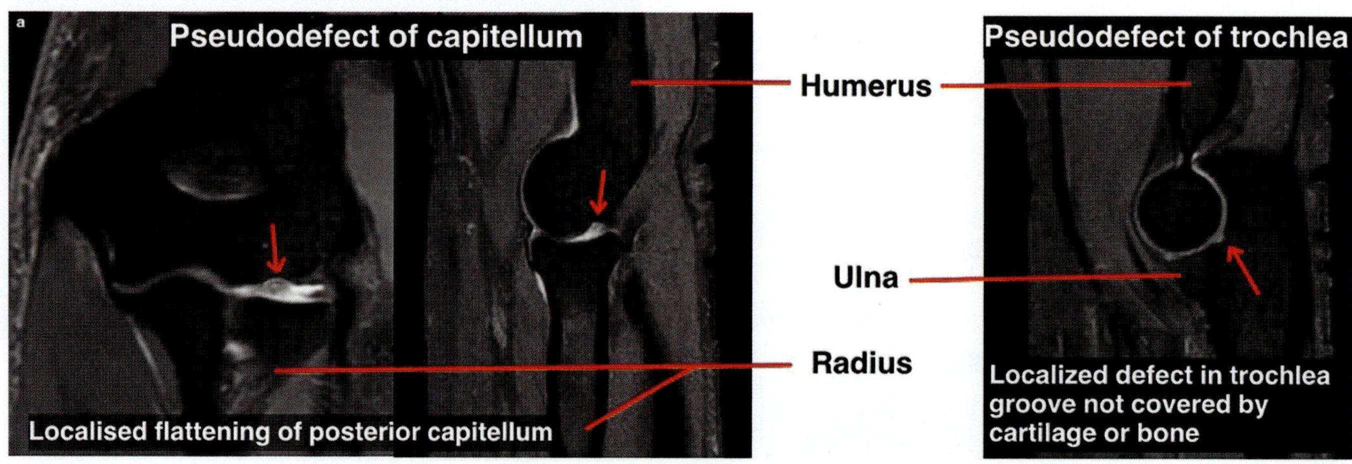

Fig. 3.8.78

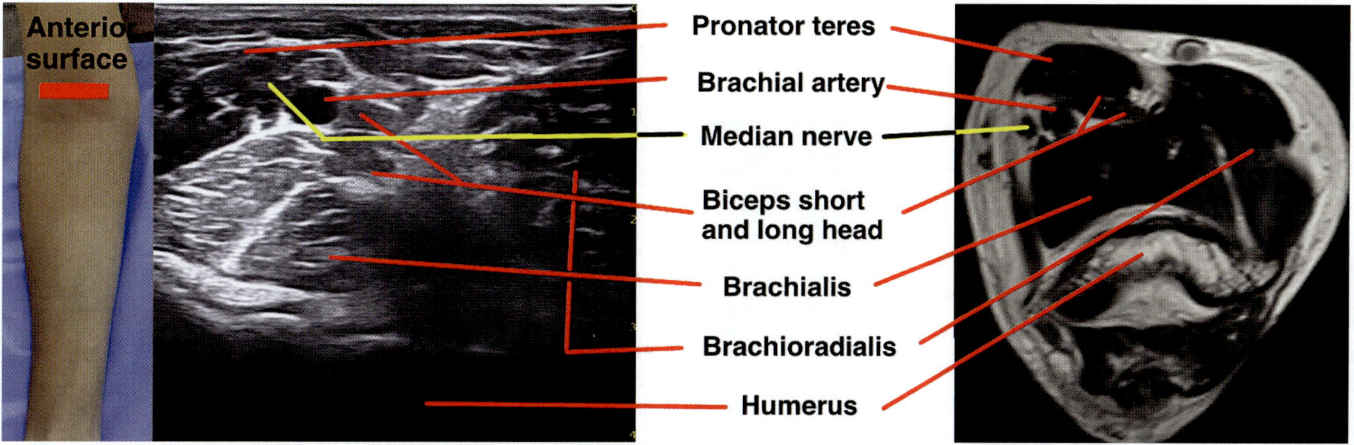

Fig. 3.8.79

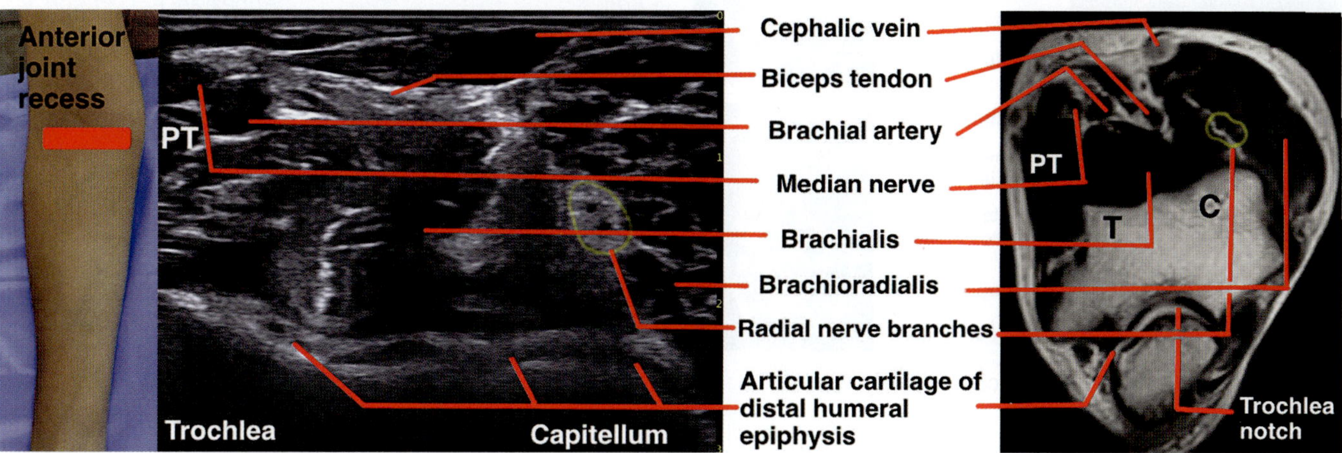

Fig. 3.8.80

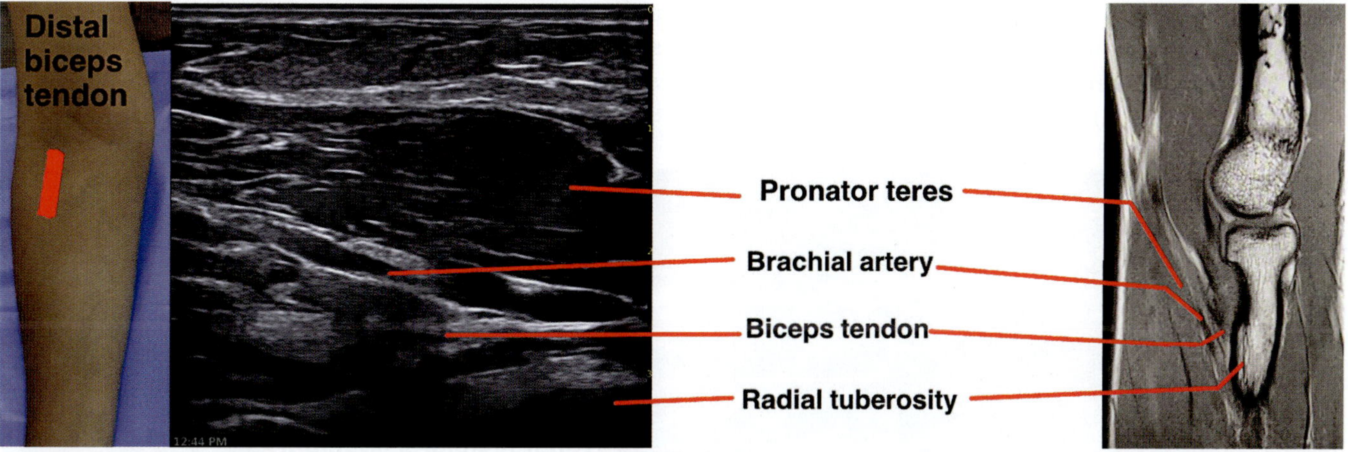

Fig. 3.8.81

Medial elbow: The patient's forearm kept in forceful external rotation with elbow extended or slightly flexed, resting on a table. The probe's cranial edge is placed over the medial epicondyle in coronal plane and common flexor tendon is examined which is shorter and larger than common extensor tendon. Anterior bundle of the medial collateral ligament present deep to this tendon (Fig. 3.8.83).

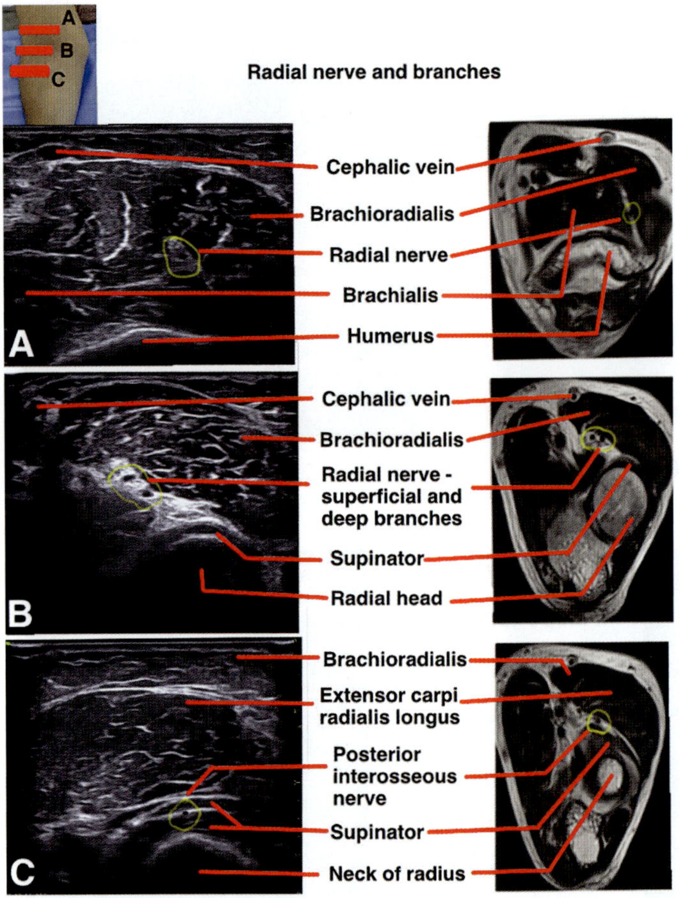

Fig. 3.8.82: Radial nerve course in elbow joint

Lateral elbow: Elbow kept in extension or flexion and cranial edge of the probe placed on the lateral epicondyle, common extensor tendon is visualized on its long-axis in coronal plane. Due to a similar fibrillar echotexture, the lateral ulnar collateral ligament and the overlying extensor tendon cannot be distinguished in normal conditions (Fig. 3.8.84).

Posterior elbow (P): (P1) The posterior elbow may be examined by keeping the joint flexed 90°. The triceps muscle and tendon are assessed superior to the olecranon Probe is gently moved forward and backward to shift elbow joint fluid into the olecranon recess. Because minor bursal effusions may be pushed away, gentle pressure is given with the probe to evaluate the superficial olecranon bursa (Fig. 3.8.85). (P2) Ulnar nerve and cubital tunnel: Patient's elbow placed in forceful internal rotation with extended elbow (olecranon facing the examiner). The ulnar nerve is examined in its short-axis from the distal arm through the distal forearm. Changes occur in the shape of the nerve across the epicondylar groove (a) and the cubital tunnel (b) (Fig. 3.8.86).

Table 3.8.3: Ossification centres in elbow CRITOE

Bones	*Appearance*	*Fusion*
Capitellum	1 year	14–17 years
Radial head	4–5 years	14–17 years
Internal (medial) epicondyle	5–7 years	15–18 years
Trochlea	8–9 years	14–17 years
Olecranon	8–10 years	14–17 years
External (lateral) epicondyle	11–12 years	14–17 years

3.8.D Forearm

Forearm is encircled by a sheath of deep fascia, attached to the posterior subcutaneous border of the ulna. A lateral intermuscular septum passes from the deep fascia to the radius. The interosseous membrane passes between the interosseous borders of the radius and ulna. Together, the deep fascia, lateral intermuscular septum and interosseous membrane divide the forearm into separate anterior and posterior fascial compartment. Anterior (flexor) fascial compartment is divided into superficial, intermediate and deep layers. All four

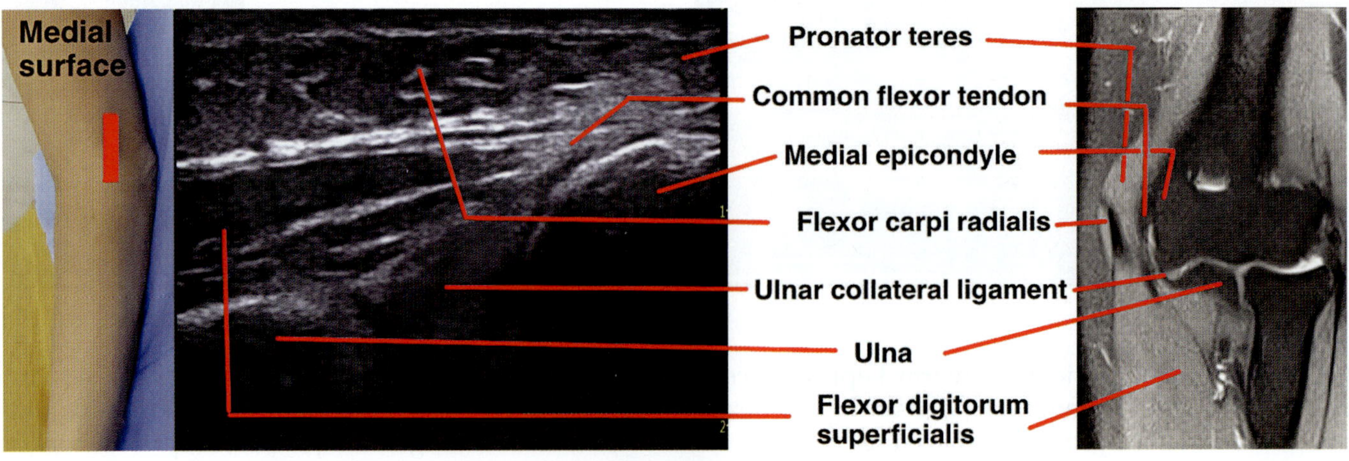

Fig. 3.8.83

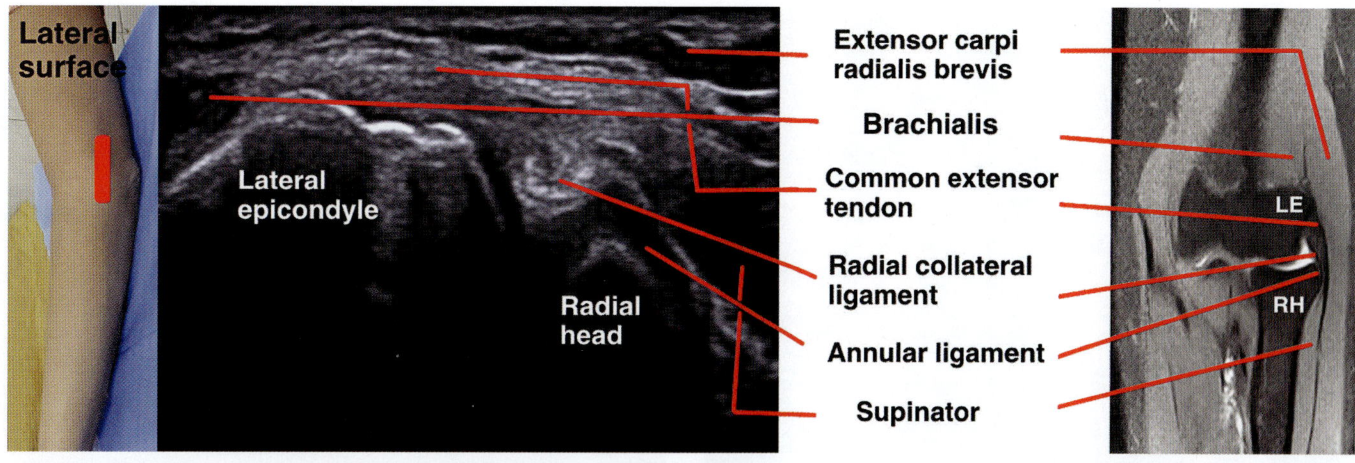

Fig. 3.8.84

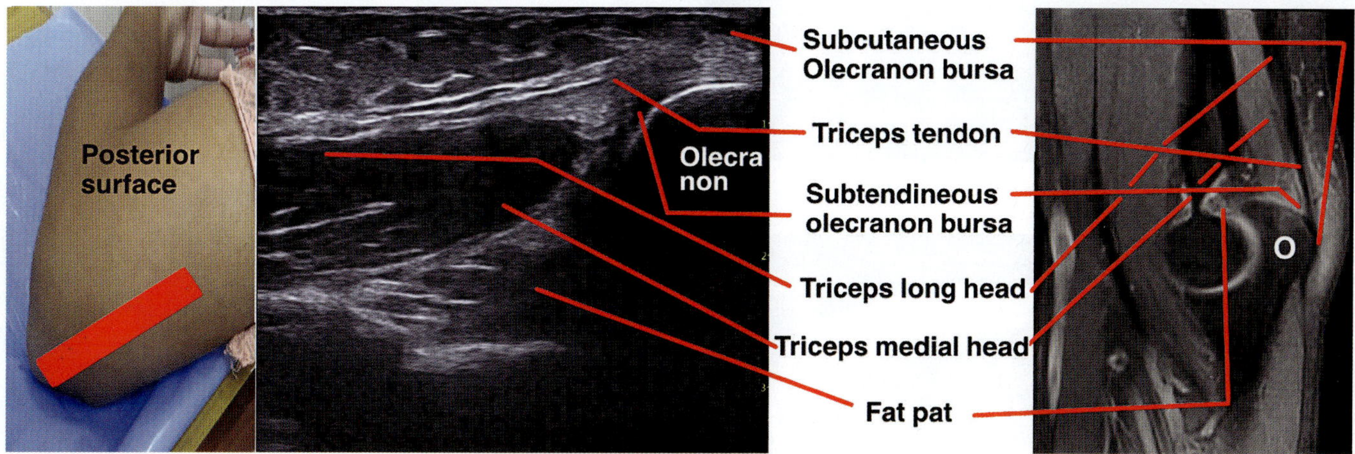

Fig. 3.8.85

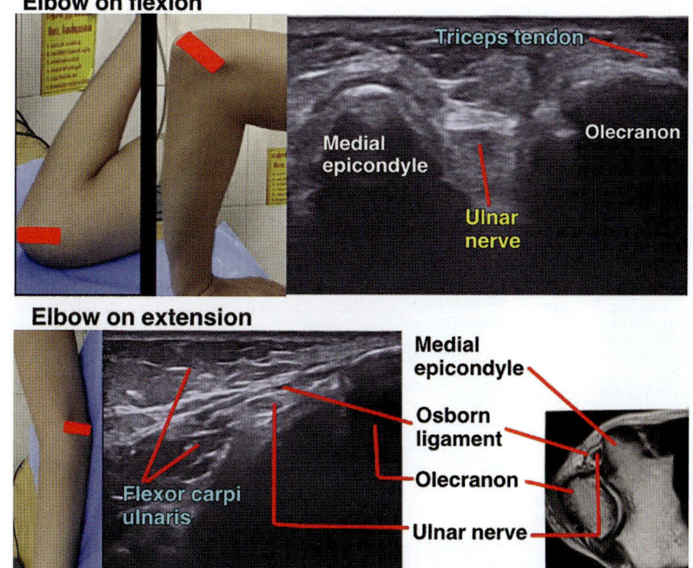

Fig. 3.8.86: Dynamic imaging of ulnar nerve in cubital tunnel

muscles in the superficial layer have a common origin from the medial epicondyle of the humerus, the common flexor origin. Supplied by radial and ulnar arteries and median nerve, whereas ulnar nerve supplies flexor carpi ulnaris and the medial part of the flexor digitorum profundus. Posterior (extensor) fascial compartment is divided into superficial and deep layers. All muscles in the superficial layer have a common origin from the lateral epicondyle, the common extensor origin and lateral supracondylar ridge of the humerus. Supplied by anterior and posterior interosseous arteries, branches of the common interosseous branch of the ulnar artery and radial nerve.

The radial tunnel is a space that extends 5 cm from radial head and the supinator's distal edge. This tunnel is related to the brachioradialis, extensor carpi radialis longus, and extensor carpi radialis brevis on the lateral side, and the biceps tendon and brachialis on the medial side. The deep head of the supinator and the capsule of the radiocapitellar joint forms the floor, while the

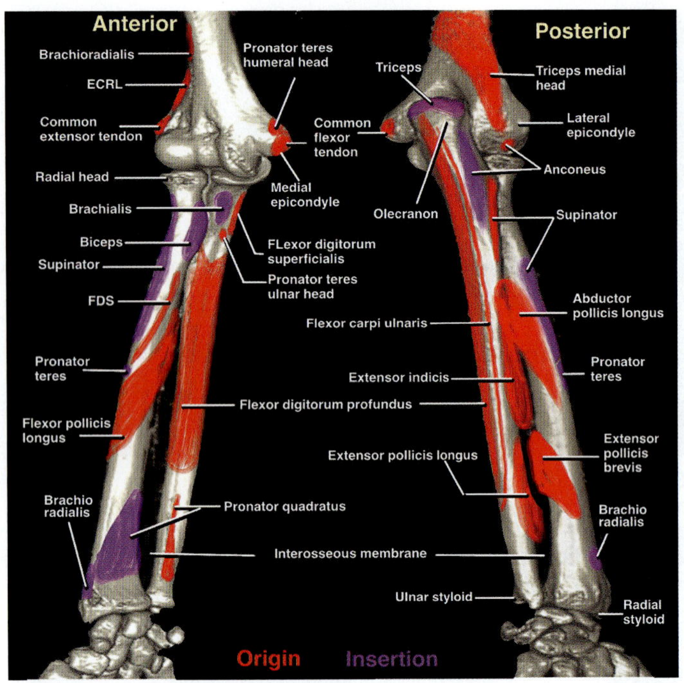

Fig. 3.8.87: Muscles of forearm

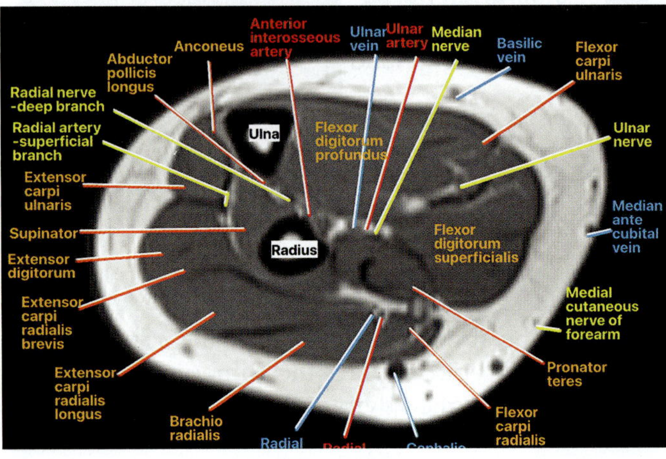

Fig. 3.8.88

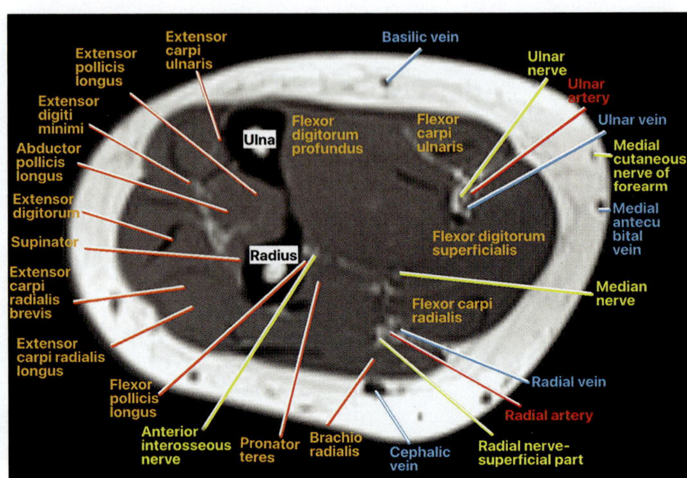

Fig. 3.8.89

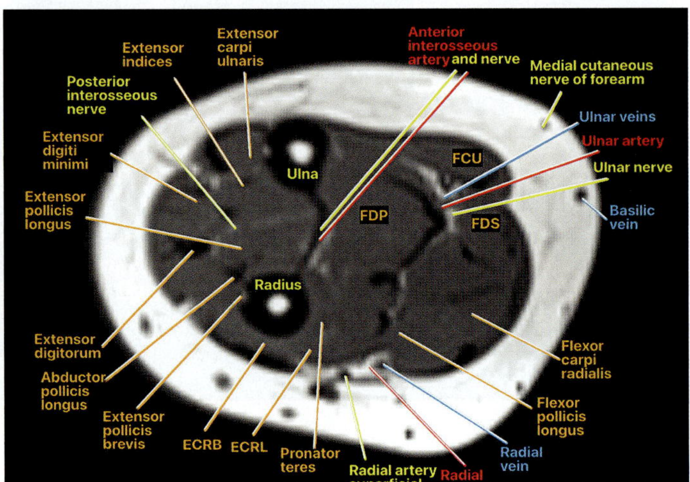

Fig. 3.8.90

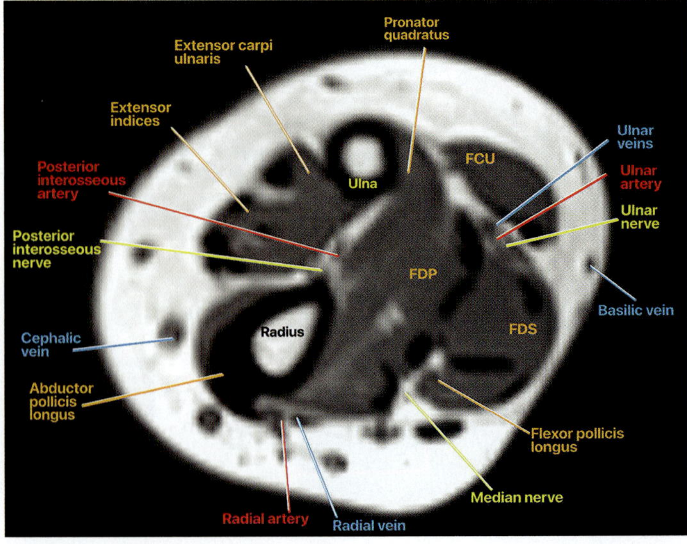

Fig. 3.8.91

superficial head of the supinator and the radial recurrent vessels forms the roof. Ossification centre:Appears in diaphysis on 8th week of gestation for both ulna and radius.

Axial sections (superior to inferior—Figs 3.8.88–3.8.92).

Coronal sections (anterior to posterior—Figs 3.8.93–3.8.100).

3.8.E Wrist Joint (Radiocarpal Joint)

This is a synovial ellipsoid joint with articulation between the distal radius and the scaphoid, lunate and triquetral carpal bones. The flexor tendons and extensor tendons are the two primary types of tendons in the wrist. There are six compartments formed by the extensor tendons.

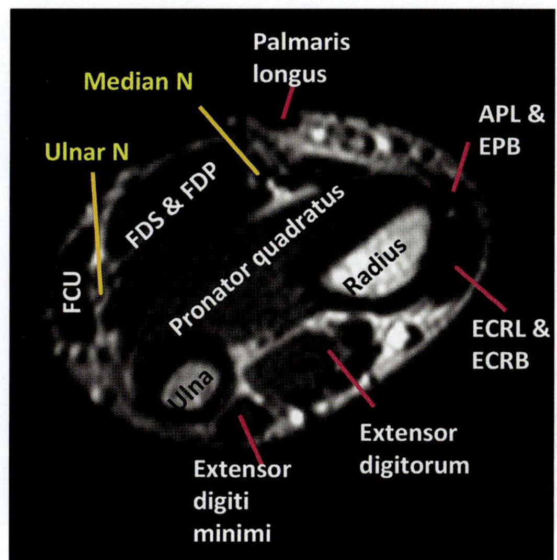

Fig. 3.8.92

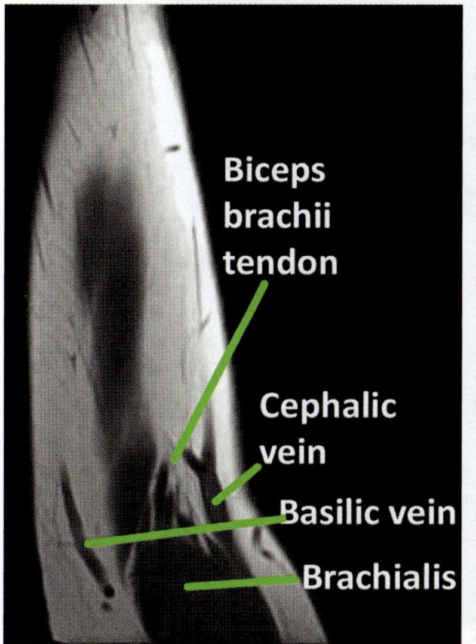

Fig. 3.8.93

Fig. 3.8.94

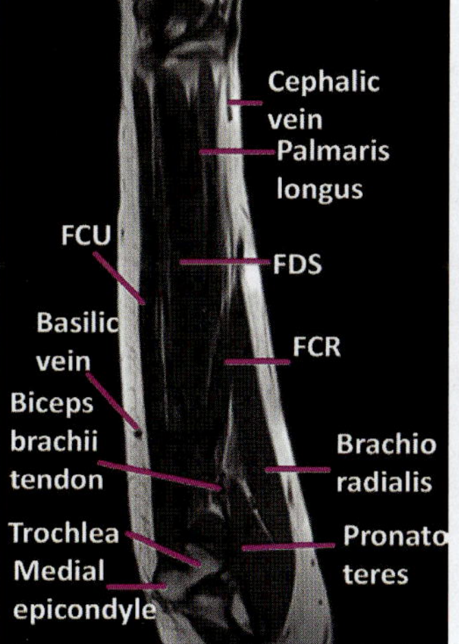

Fig. 3.8.95

Fig. 3.8.96

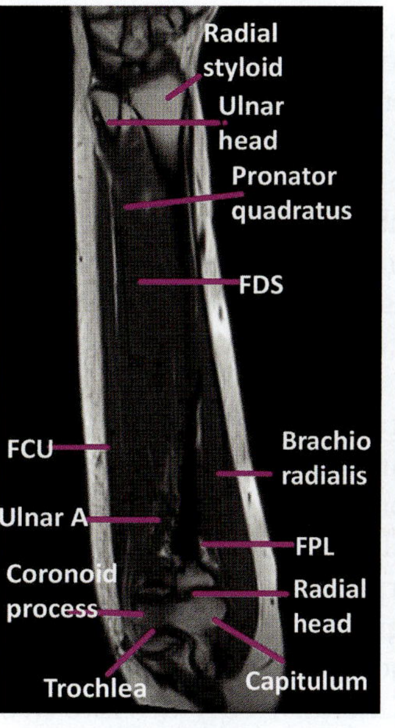

Fig. 3.8.97

Fig. 3.8.98

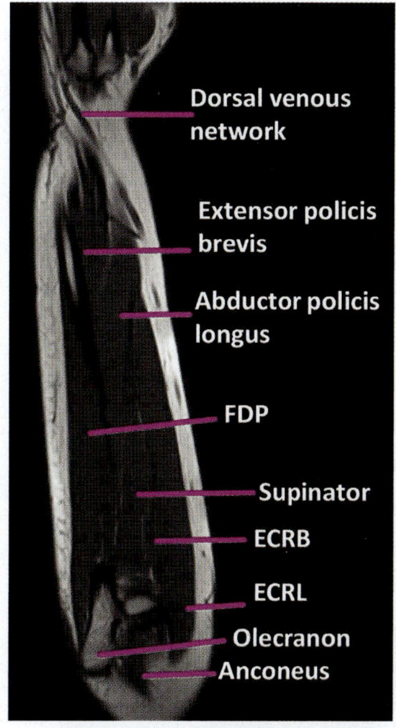

Fig. 3.8.99

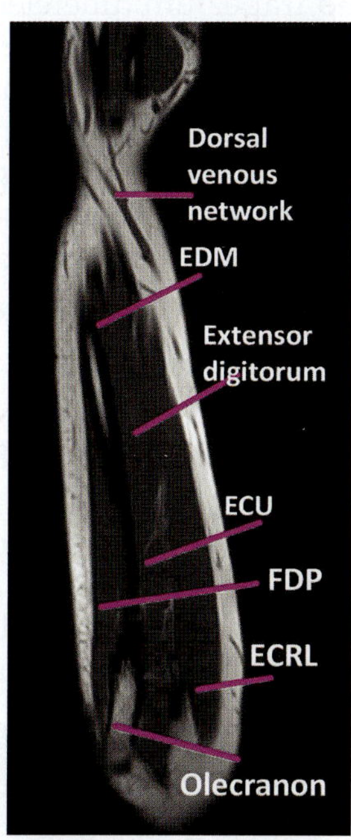

Fig. 3.8.100

Table 3.8.4: Extensor compartment muscles in wrist

Compartment	*Tendons*
1	Abductor pollicis longus, extensor pollicis brevis
2	Extensor carpi radialis longus, extensor carpi radialis brevis
3	Extensor pollicis longus
4	Extensor indicis, extensor digitorum
5	Extensor digiti minimi
6	Extensor carpi ulnaris

Abductor pollicis longus (1st compartment tendon) crosses from medial to lateral aspect and attaches base of 1st metacarpal. Extensor pollicis longus—3rd compartment muscle crosses over to 1st compartment and attaches to distal phalanx of thumb. The extensor retinaculum and the dorsal tubercle of the radius (Lister tubercle) are the two key structures define the extensor anatomy of wrist joint and separates the second and third compartments. The extensor retinaculum is a thick fibrous band that runs across the dorsum of the wrist obliquely. The carpal tunnel allows passage for majority of flexor tendon which is bounded volarly by the flexor retinaculum tendon. The flexor retinaculum crosses the front of the carpal bones and converting its anterior concavity into the carpal tunnel, through which the flexor tendons of the digits and the median nerve pass. The pisiform and the hook of hamate are related medially to the retinaculum. Laterally, it divides into two laminae: One superficial, which adheres to the scaphoid and trapezium tubercles, and one deep, which attaches to the trapezium groove's medial lip. The flexor tendons do not have their own compartments, unlike the extensor tendons. Three flexor tendons are still visible outside the carpal tunnel. The flexor carpi ulnaris tendon, attached to the pisiform bone, as well as the flexor carpi radialis and palmaris longus tendon, are among them.

Axial sections (superior to inferior—Figs 3.8.101–3.8.106)

Coronal sections (palmar to dorsal—Figs 3.8.107–3.8.118).

Sagittal sections (medial to lateral—Figs 3.8.119–3.8.122)

Guyon's canal: This is a fibro-osseous tunnel that permits the passage of the ulnar nerve as well as the ulnar artery and vein. The flexor retinaculum forms the floor, and the palmar carpal ligament forms the roof. It has a proximal radial wall formed by the pisiform and a slightly distal ulnar wall formed by the hook of hamate.

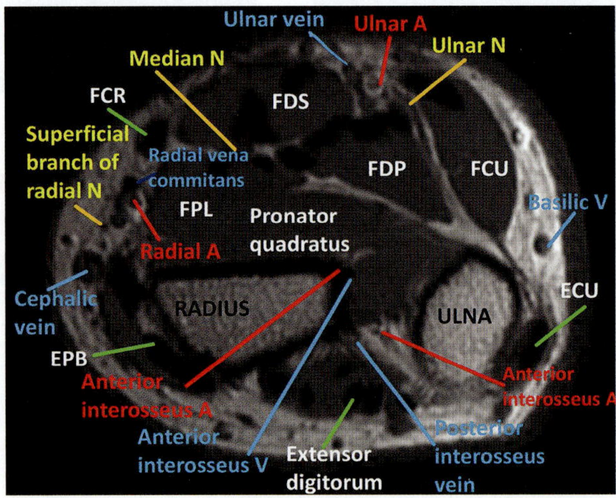

Fig. 3.8.101

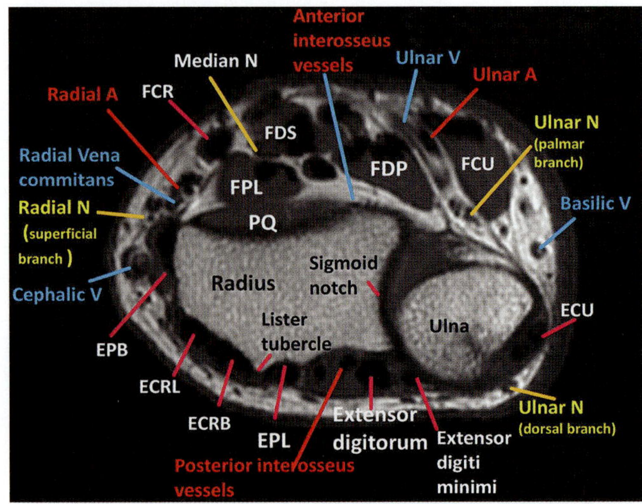

Fig. 3.8.102

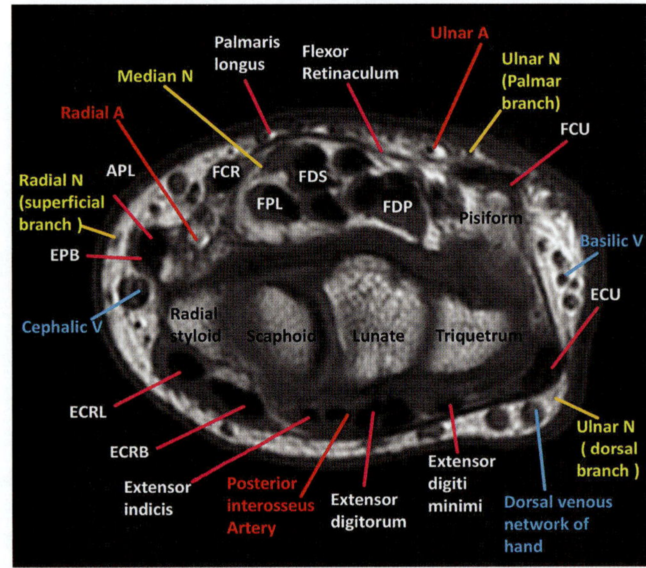

Fig. 3.8.103

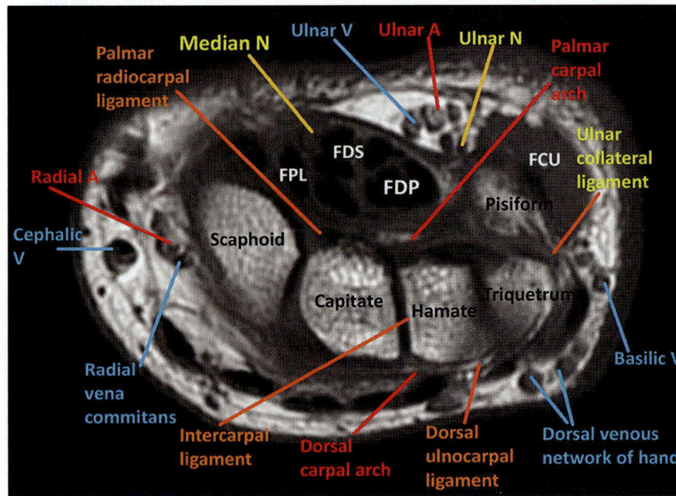

Fig. 3.8.104

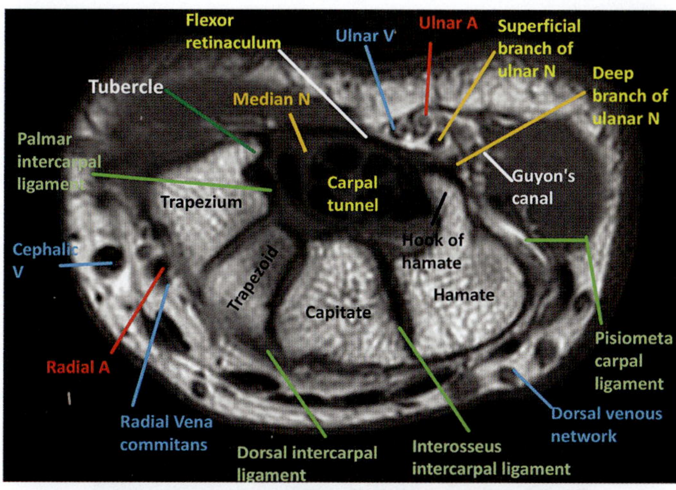

Fig. 3.8.105

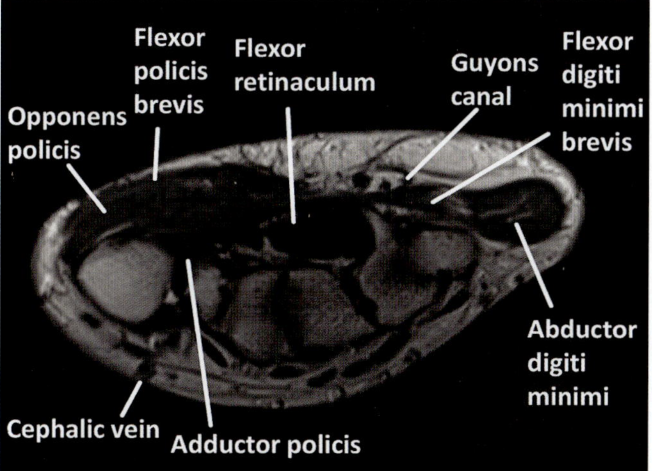

Fig. 3.8.106

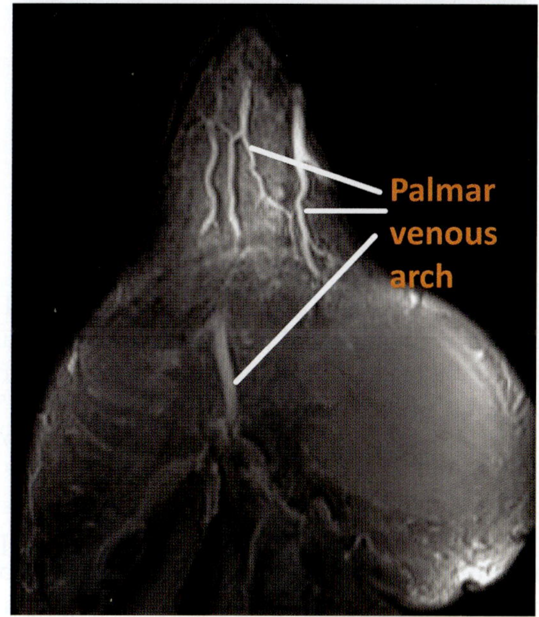

Fig. 3.8.107

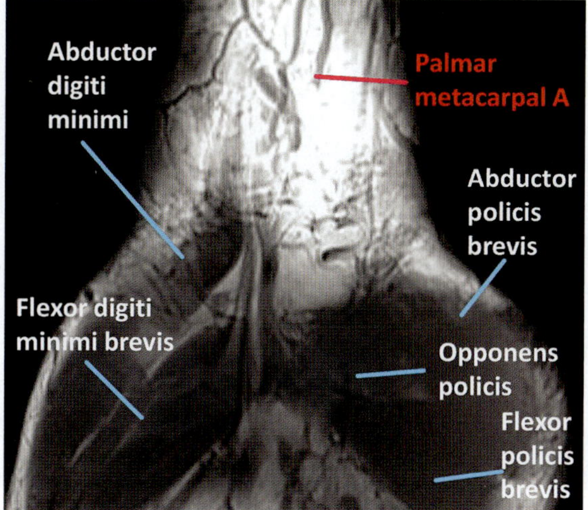

Fig. 3.8.108

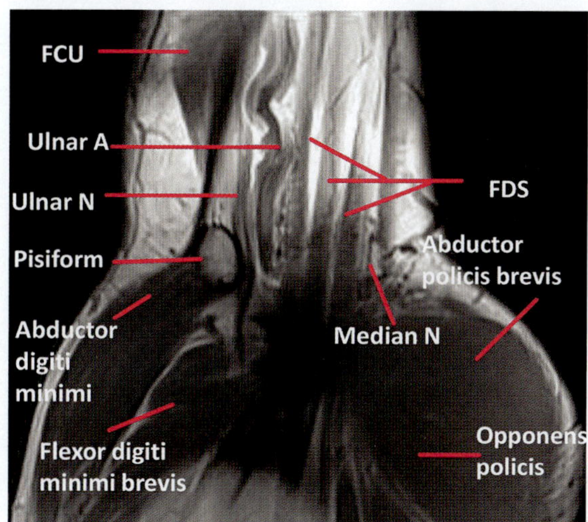

Fig. 3.8.109

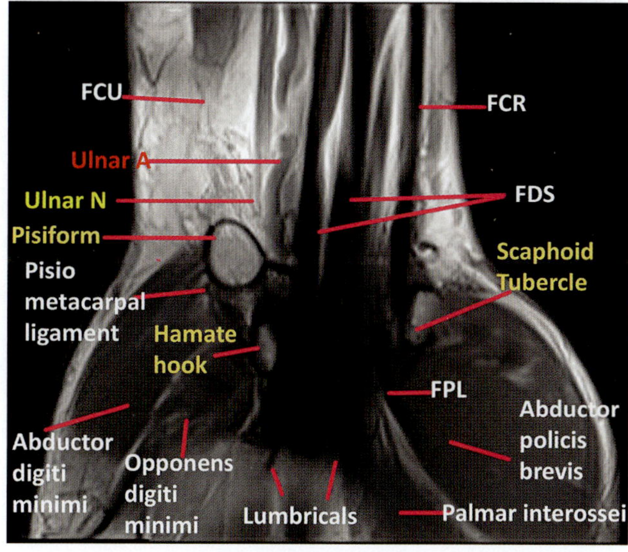

Fig. 3.8.110

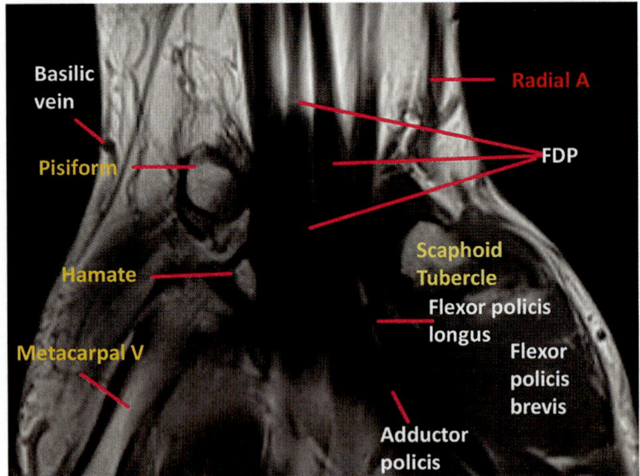

Fig. 3.8.111

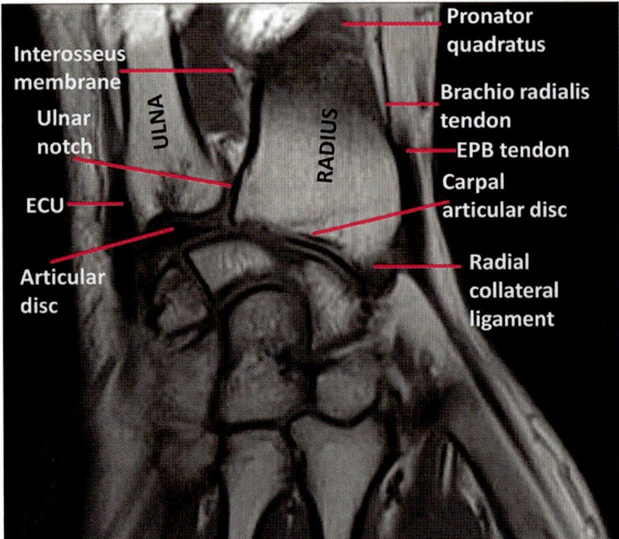

Fig. 3.8.112

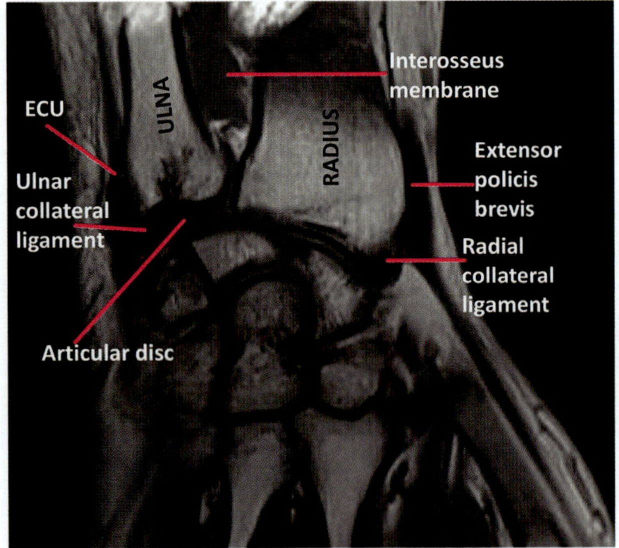

Fig. 3.8.113

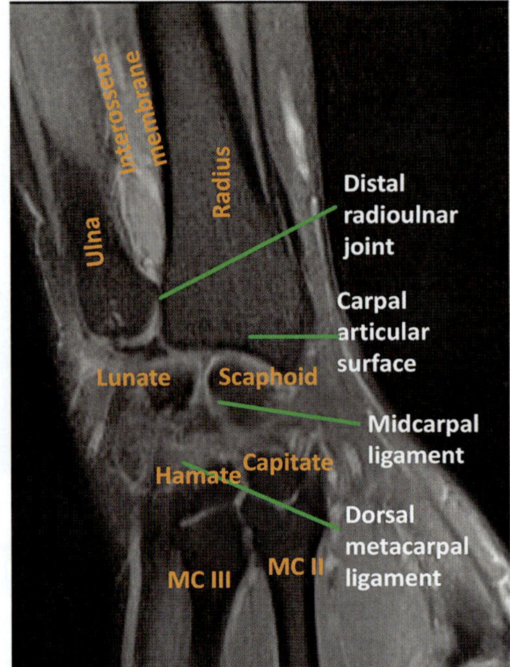

Fig. 3.8.114

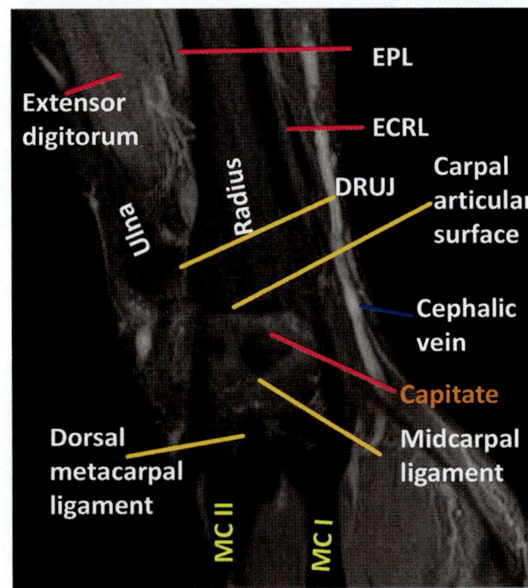

Fig. 3.8.115

TFCC: The triangular fibrocartilage complex (TFCC) originates from the medial border of distal radius and inserts into the base of ulnar styloid. The central disc is avascular and peripheral blood vessels penetrate TFCC margins. It serves to stabilize the distal radioulnar joint (DRUJ) by acting as cushion for the ulnar head and lunate during the axial loading of the wrist and ulnar deviation of the wrist. The TFCC is composed of ligament, cartilage and tendon. These include the triangular fibrocartilaginous articular disc, volar and dorsal radioulnar ligaments, volar ulnotriquetral

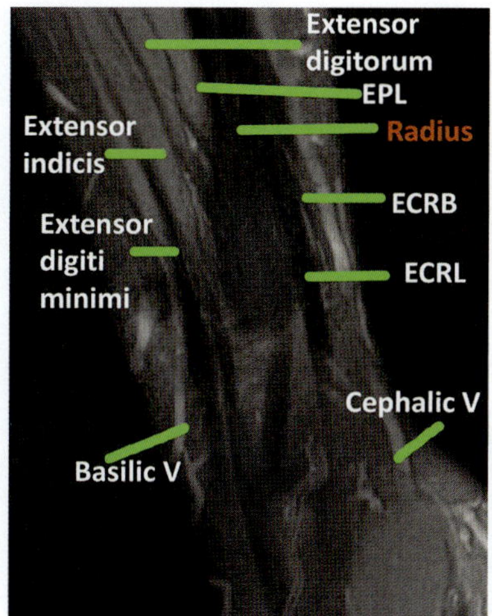

Fig. 3.8.116

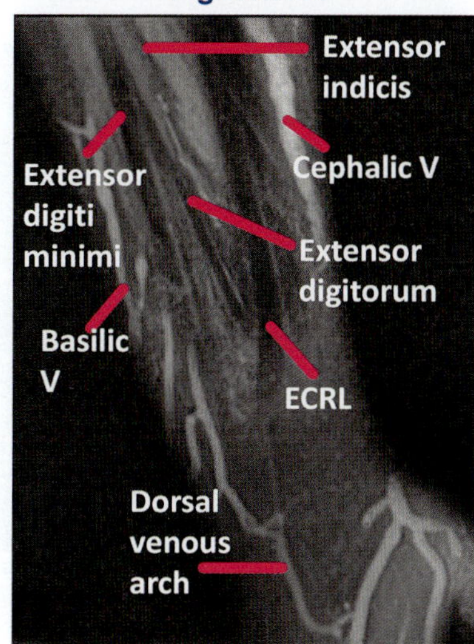

Fig. 3.8.117

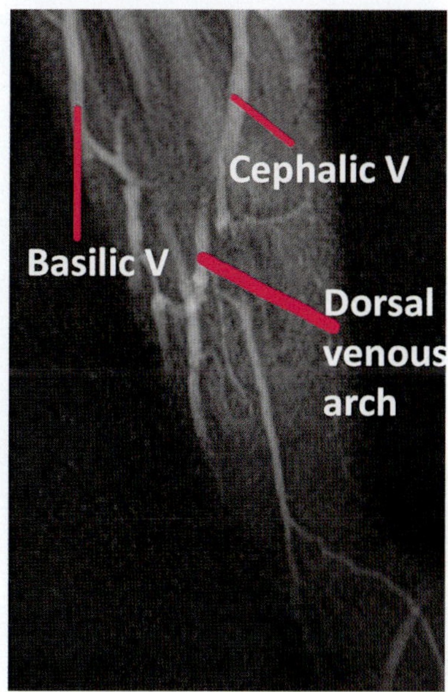

Fig. 3.8.118

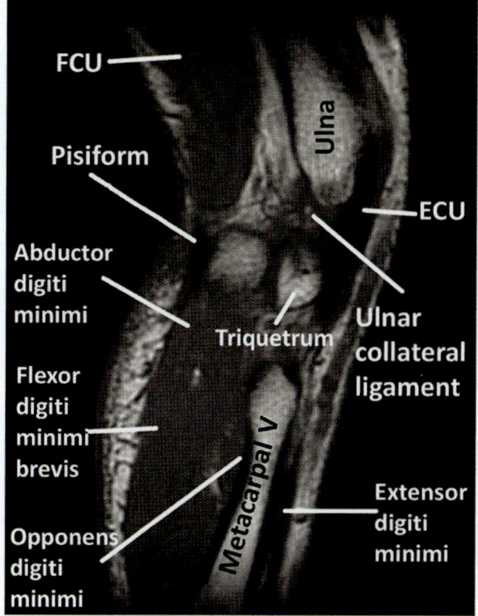

Fig. 3.8.119

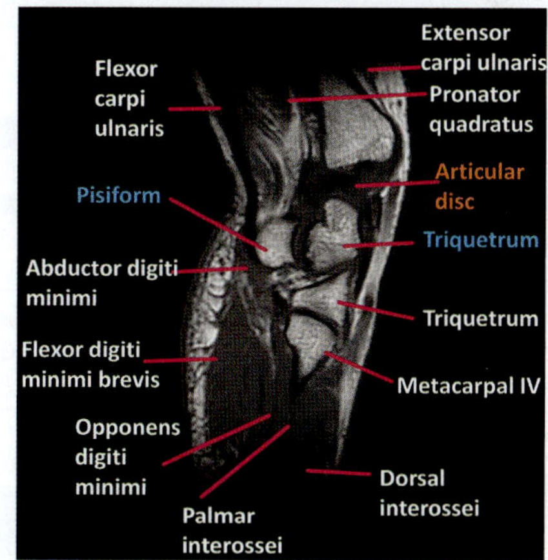

Fig. 3.8.120

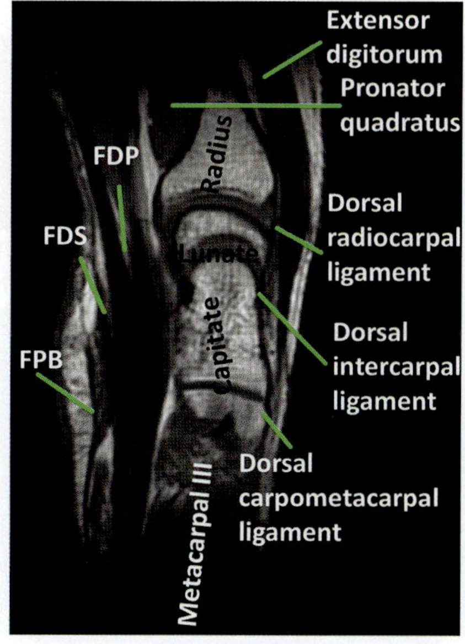

Fig. 3.8.121

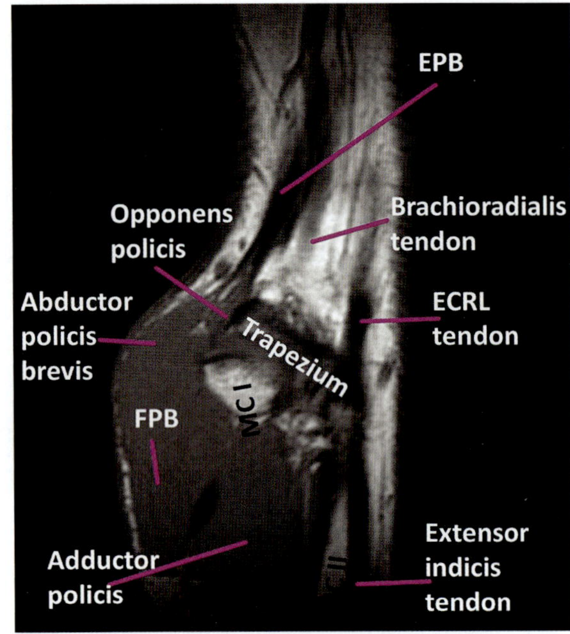

Fig. 3.8.122

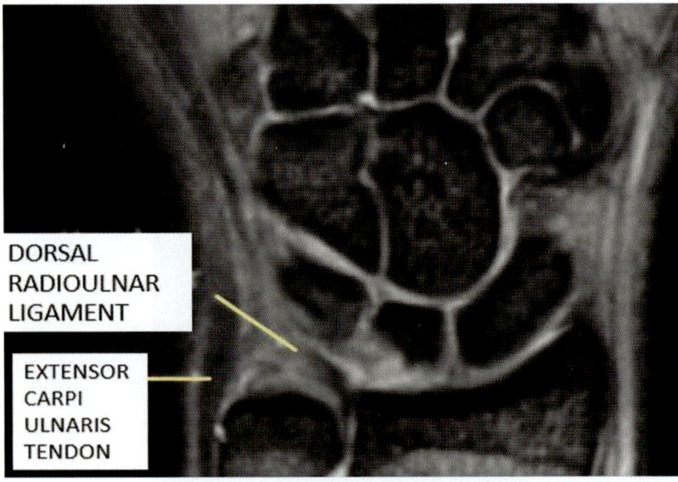

Fig. 3.8.125

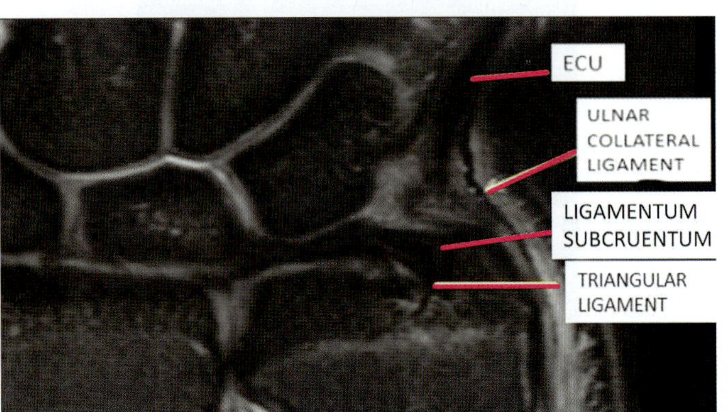

Fig. 3.8.123

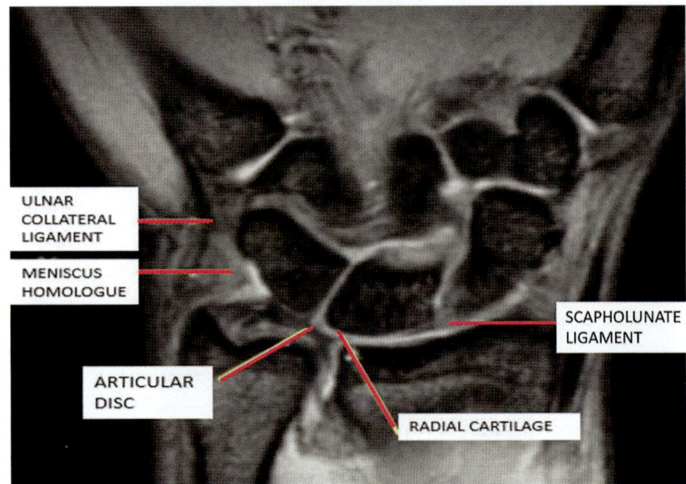

Fig. 3.8.126

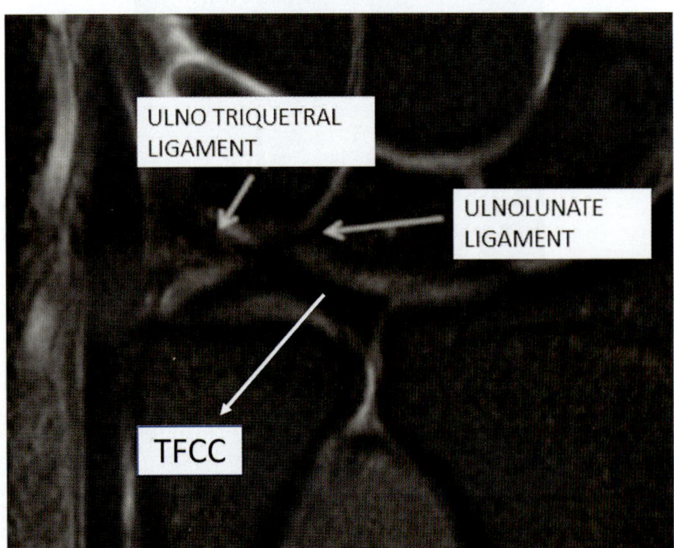

Fig. 3.8.124

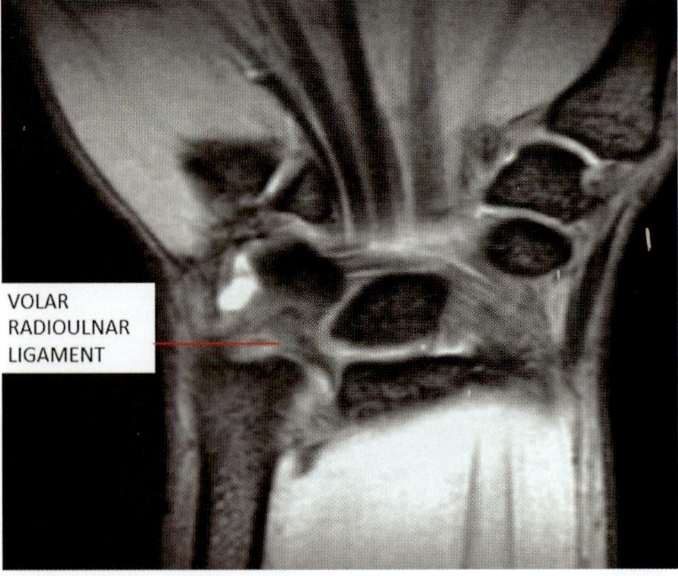

Fig. 3.8.127

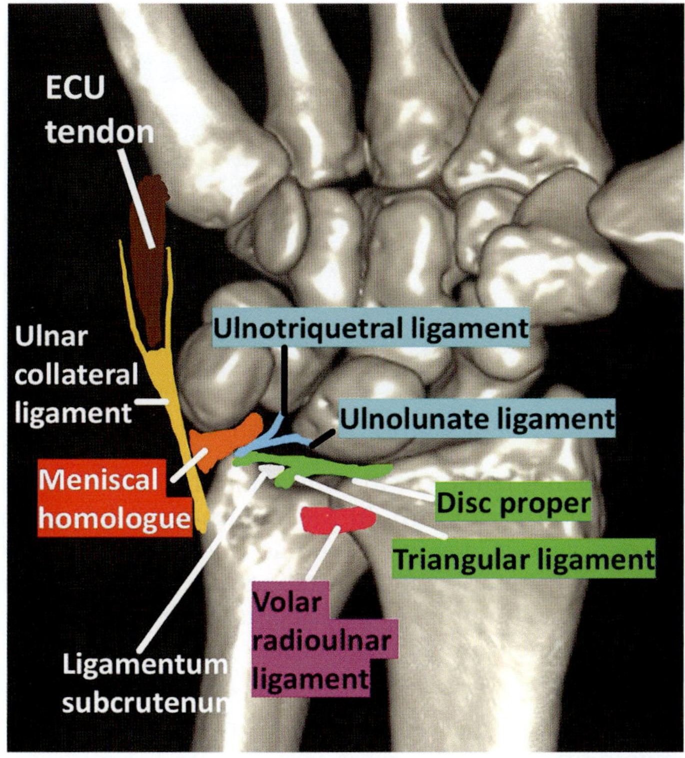

Fig. 3.8.128: Ligaments of wrist

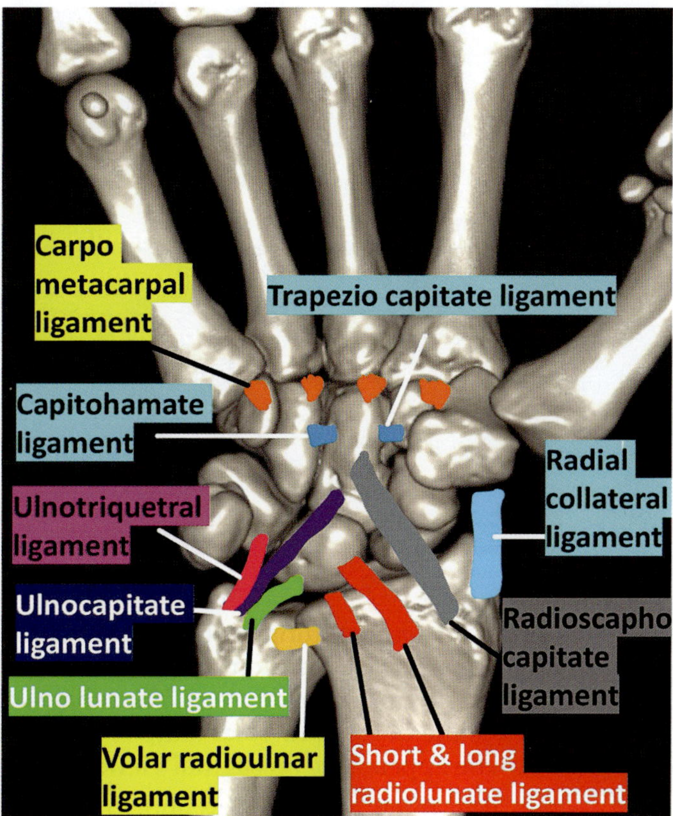

Fig. 3.8.130: Ligaments of wrist

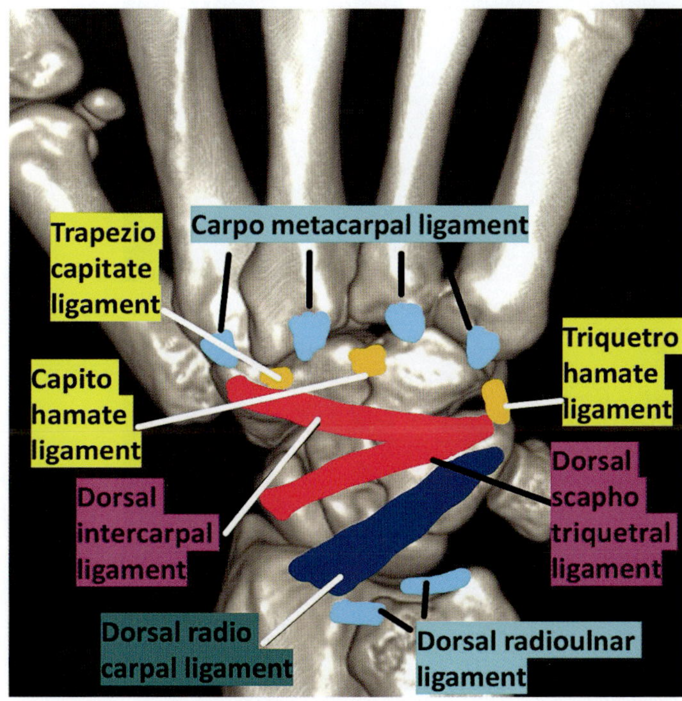

Fig. 3.8.129: Ligaments of wrist

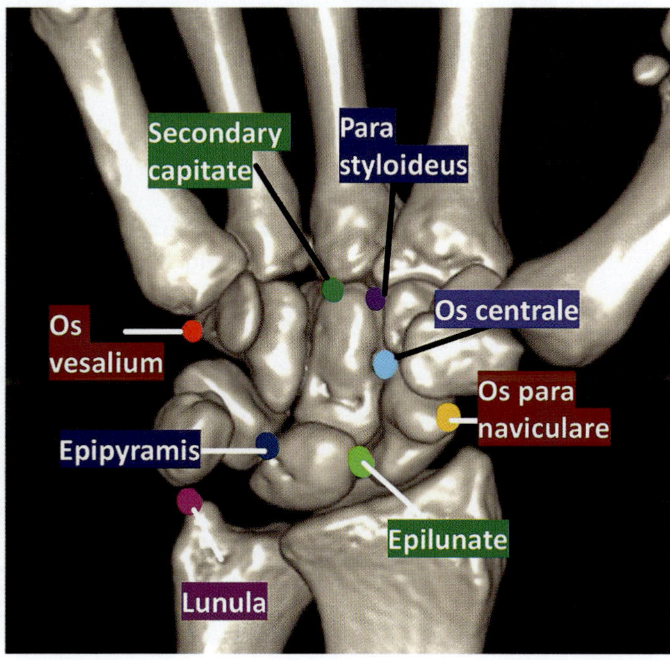

Fig. 3.8.131

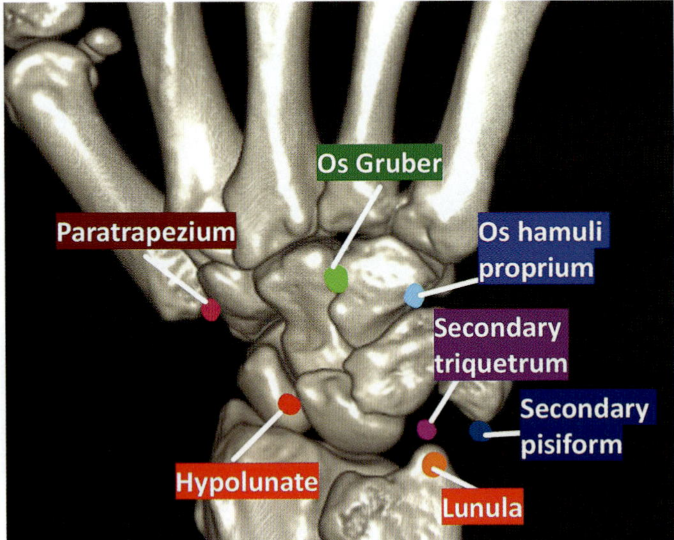

Fig. 3.8.132

and ulnolunate ligaments, ulnar collateral ligament, extensor carpi ulnaris (ECU) tendon sheath. The central component is a triangular fibrocartilage. The ulnar side is broader while the dorsal and volar sides are thicker, giving it a bowtie appearance on sagittal view.

Disc proper: It is thick at periphery and thin at the centre. It has the radial attachment in the sigmoid notch. The peripheral attachment to ulna is at 2 sites, with the proximal lamina at the fovea and the distal lamina at the ulnar styloid tip. In MRI, normally it has got a striated appearance which should not be mistaken for tear or degeneration. Between the two laminae of ulnar attachment, there is an intermediate signal intensity called **ligamentum subcrutenum**.

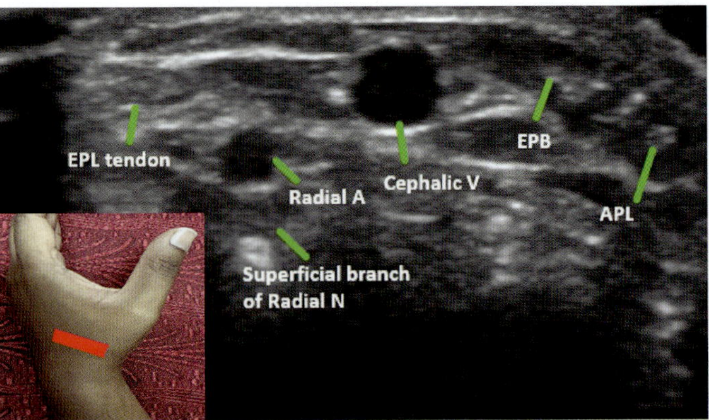

Fig. 3.8.133: 1st compartment

Volar and distal radioulnar joints: They have their attachment in the radial sigmoid notch to the ulnar styloid tip.

Meniscus homologue: It is a fibrous tissue on the ulnar aspect of TFCC which spans from the ulnar styloid tip to the triquetrum and pisiform. The peripheral zone

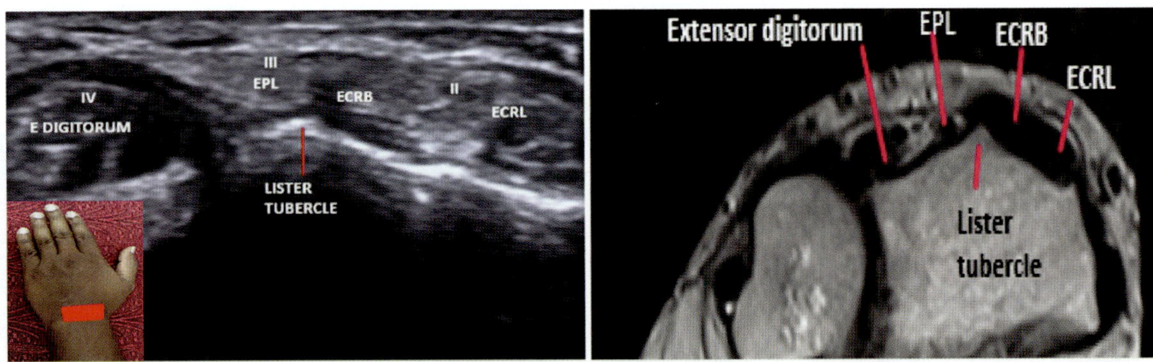

Fig. 3.8.134: 2nd, 3rd and 4th compartments

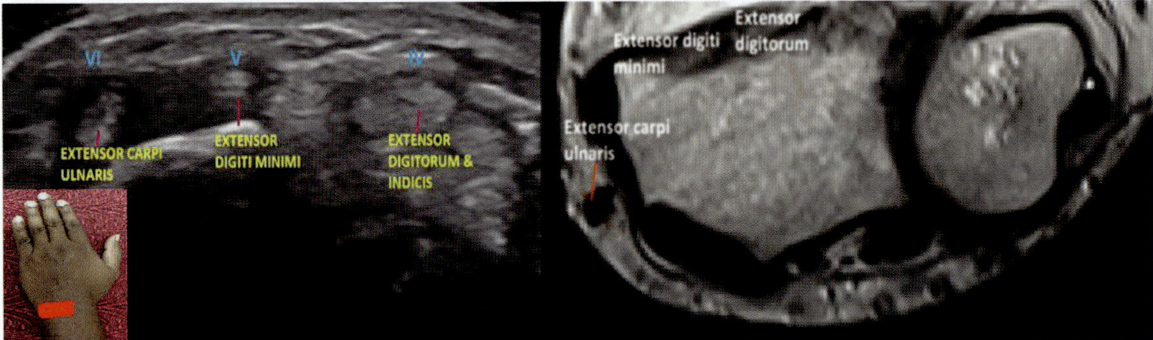

Fig. 3.8.135: 4, 5, and 6th compartments

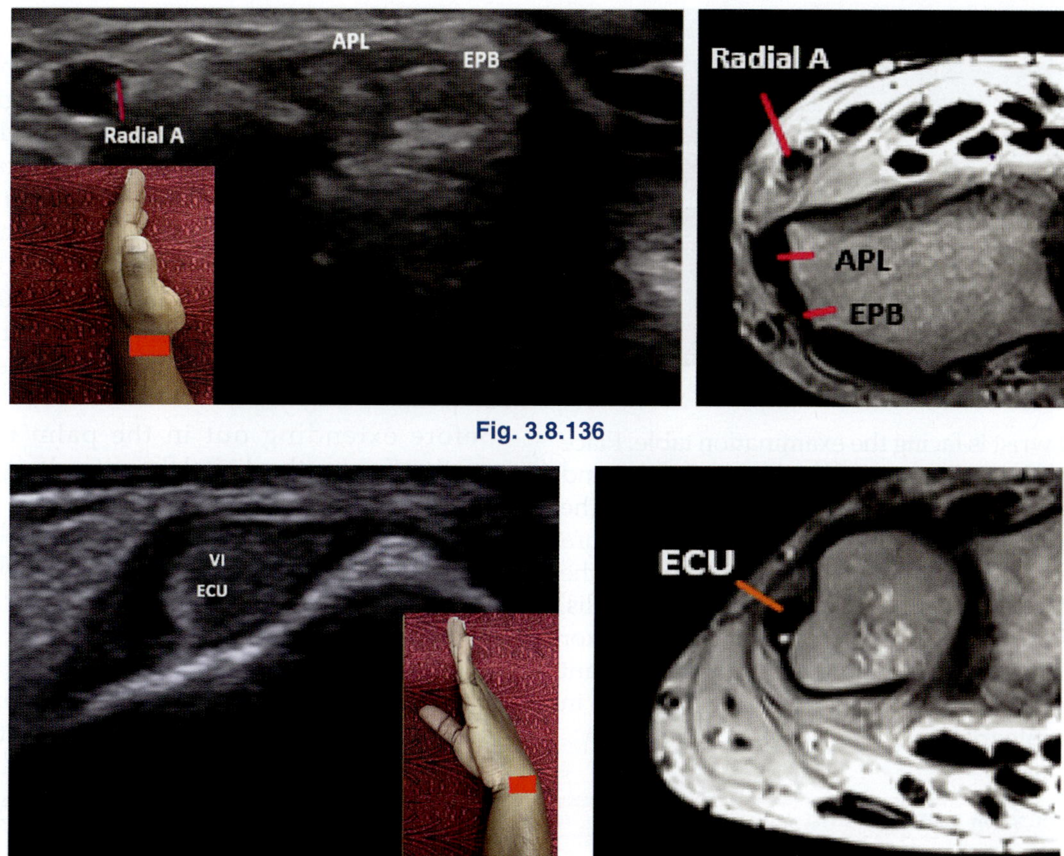

Fig. 3.8.136

Fig. 3.8.137: 6th compartment

is vascular (repair zone) and the center is relatively avascular (debridement zone). The central component is a triangular fibrocartilage. The ulnar side is broader while the dorsal and volar sides are thicker, giving it a bowtie appearance on sagittal view.

Ultrasound wrist

Dorsal wrist: To properly identify the extensor tendons, place the transducer in a transverse plane over the dorsal part of the wrist. **First compartment:** Place the probe on the lateral aspect of the radial styloid to evaluate the tendons—abductor pollicis longus ventrally and extensor pollicis brevis dorsally—while keeping the patient's wrist halfway between pronation and supination (Fig. 3.8.133). **Second compartment:** Shift the probe medially on transverse planes with the palm towards the examination table to represent the second compartment—the extensor carpi radialis longus and extensor carpi radialis brevis tendons (Fig. 3.8.134). **Third compartment:** To distinguish the second compartment from the third compartment, locate the Lister tubercle over the dorsal radius as a bone landmark. Extensor pollicis longus tendon detected at the medial side of the Lister tubercle. It crosses the extensor carpi radialis brevis and extensor carpi radialis longus tendons (Fig. 3.8.134). **Fourth and Fifth compartments:** Examine the fourth compartment muscles, namely extensor digitorum communis and extensor indicis proprius and fifth compartment muscle extensor digiti minimi by placing the transducer in the transverse plane across the mid-dorsal wrist. Individual tendons of the fourth compartment can be distinguished through dynamic testing during finger flexion and extension. The extensor digiti minimi can also be identified using dynamic scanning (Figs 3.8.134 and 3.8.135). **Sixth compartment:** Wrist is placed in slight radial deviation to examine extensor carpi ulnaris (Figs 3.8.135 and 3.8.137).

Scapholunate ligament: Examine the ulna's styloid process and the triangular fibrocartilage complex that fills the space between the styloid and the radius: this structure can be assessed in part using transverse and oblique coronal images. Image the dorsal section of the scapholunate ligament by sweeping the probe distally from the level of the Lister tubercle on transverse planes. The ulnar deviation of the wrist may be beneficial in determining the ligament's integrity (Fig. 3.8.138). **Palmar aspect (proximal carpal tunnel):** Ensure that the

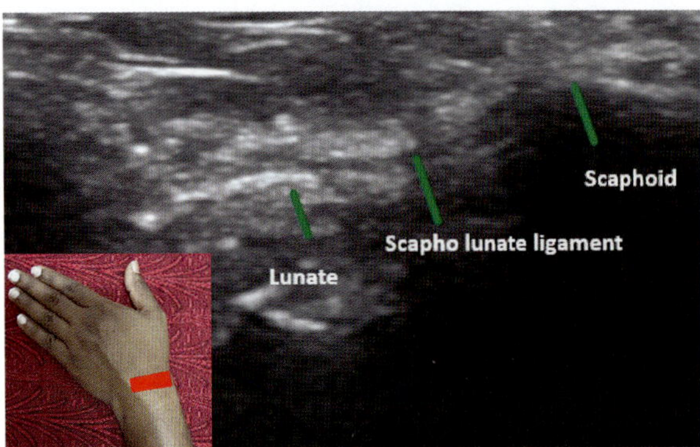

Fig. 3.8.138: Scapholunate ligament

patient's dorsal wrist is facing the examination table. Place the probe above the palmar crease in the axial plane and locate the scaphoid tubercle on the radial side and the pisiform on the ulnar side. Examine the flexor retinaculum and each of the nine long flexor tendons enclosed within the carpal tunnel (four from the flexor digitorum superficialis, four from the flexor digitorum profundus, and the flexor pollicis longus radially). Dynamic scanning of the relevant finger during passive flexion and extension may aid in determining its integrity.

Ossification centre

Table 3.8.5: Ossification centres in wrist			
Bones	*Appearance*	*Bones*	*Appearance*
Capitate	1–4 months	Scaphoid	4–6 years
Hamate	2–4 months	Trapezium	4–6 years
Triquetrum	2–3 years	Trapezoid	4–6 years
Lunate	3–5 years	Pisiform	8–11 years
Bones	Site	Appearance	Fusion
Radius	Distal epiphysis	1st year	19–20 years
Ulna	Distal epiphysis	5–6 years	18–20 years

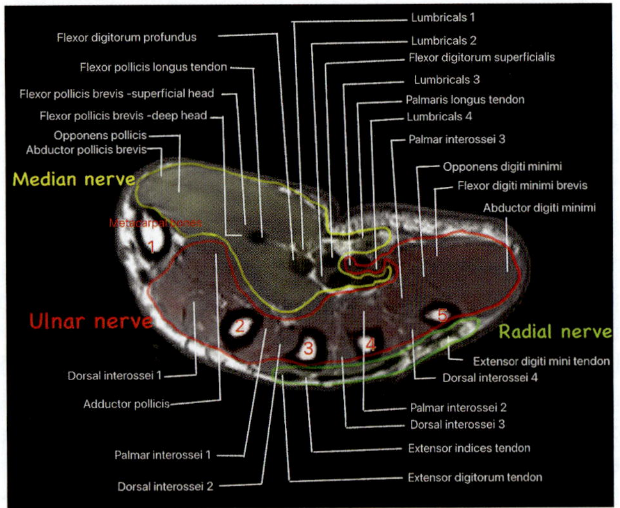

Fig. 3.8.139: Muscles around the hand and nerve supply

3.8.F Hand and Fingers

Fingers tendon: Both extrinsic and intrinsic extensor muscles work together to extend the digits. Extrinsic muscles begin in the forearm and elbow and terminate in the hand. Extensor digitorum communis, extensor indicis proprius (EIP), and extensor digiti quinti minimi (EDQM) are involved in extension of metacarpophalangeal (MCP) joint, however, they can also extend the PIP and DIP joints. The interosseous and lumbrical muscles, which originate and insert in the hand, are intrinsic muscles. Their job is to extend the PIP and DIP joints and flex the MCP joint.

Before extending out in the palm toward their respective fingers, the digital flexor tendons pass through the carpal tunnel. The flexor digitorum superficialis (FDS) inserts in the midportion of the middle phalanx, and the flexor digitorum profundus (FDP), lies volar to the FDS and inserts on the volar base of the distal phalanx, are the two flexor tendons on each finger. The flexor tendons runs along osteofibrous canals surrounded by a synovial sheath that supply nutrition and lubrication to the tendons from the metacarpal neck to the DIP joint.

Pulleys: Five annular pulleys (A1–A5), which are transverse, well-defined areas of thickening of the tendon sheath, and three cruciform pulleys (C1–C3), which are produced by crisscrossing fibres of the annular pulley components, make up the fibrous portion of the canal. The first annular pulley (A1) starts in the MCP joint's palmar plate and extends to the proximal phalanx's base. The second annular pulley (A2) rises from the volar aspect of the proximal phalanx's proximal section and extends to the proximal phalanx's distal third. The third annular pulley (A3) is a tiny pulley that stretches over the PIP joint region. The fourth annular pulley (A4) is found in the centre of the middle phalanx, while the fifth annular pulley (A5) is found in the DIP joint region. The A2 and A4 pulleys are the largest, thickest, and most consistent in form and distribution. The shape and predominance of cruciform pulleys are the most varied. At the distal end of the A2 and A4 pulleys, the first (C1) and third (C3) cruciform pulleys frequently blends. The principal purpose of the annular pulleys is to secure the tendon sheaths to the bony skeleton, preventing palmar "bowstringing" and supporting the tendon during finger bending. The cruciform pulleys are designed to allow distortion of the tendon sheath without impinging on the tendon itself during flexion.

Joints of fingers: Magnetic resonance (MR) imaging can provide important information for diagnosis and evaluation of finger pathologies. Familiarity with the fine anatomy of the normal finger is crucial for identifying pathologic entities. PIP joint: The PIP joint is a hinged joint with a bicondylar anatomy that allows a wide range of flexion and extension movements. The surrounding soft tissues, particularly the collateral ligaments and the volar plate, act as primary joint stabilisers. Dynamic stability

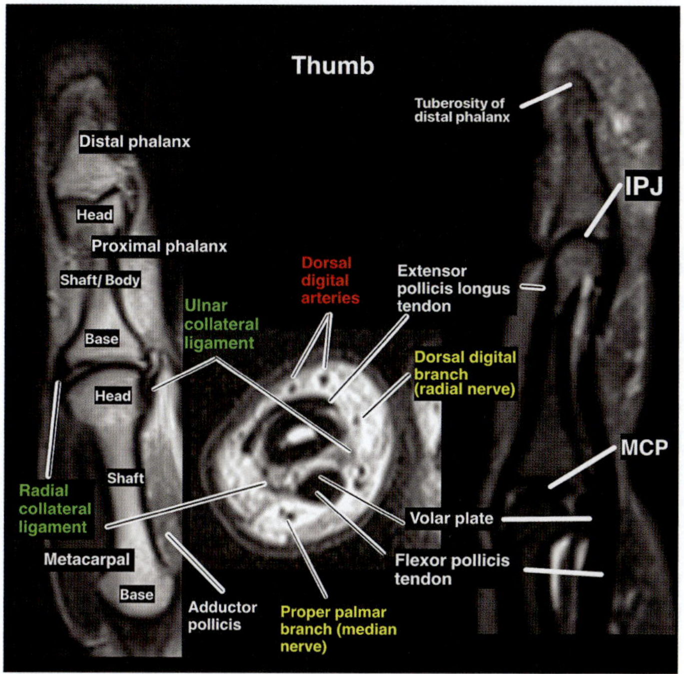

Fig. 3.8.140: MRI anatomy of thumb

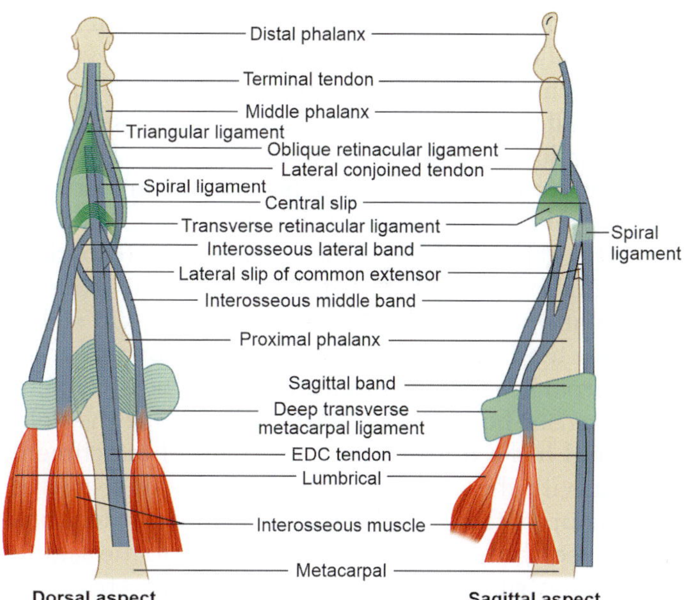

Fig. 3.8.142: Extensor hood mechanism of fingers

is aided by the extensor mechanism, flexor tendons, and retinacular ligaments. **Volar plate:** The palmar aspect of the MCP and the interphalangeal joint capsule are made up of a thick fibrocartilaginous tissue called the volar plate. Originates from metacarpal head and inserted to periarticular surface of proximal phalanx , via U-shaped due to two lateral bands, which are called the "checkrein"

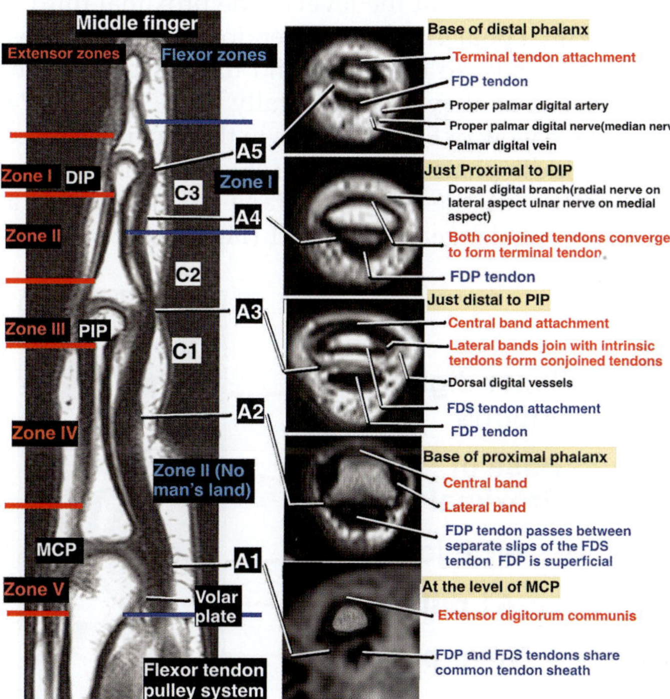

Fig. 3.8.141: MRI anatomy of middle finger and flexor, extensor zones

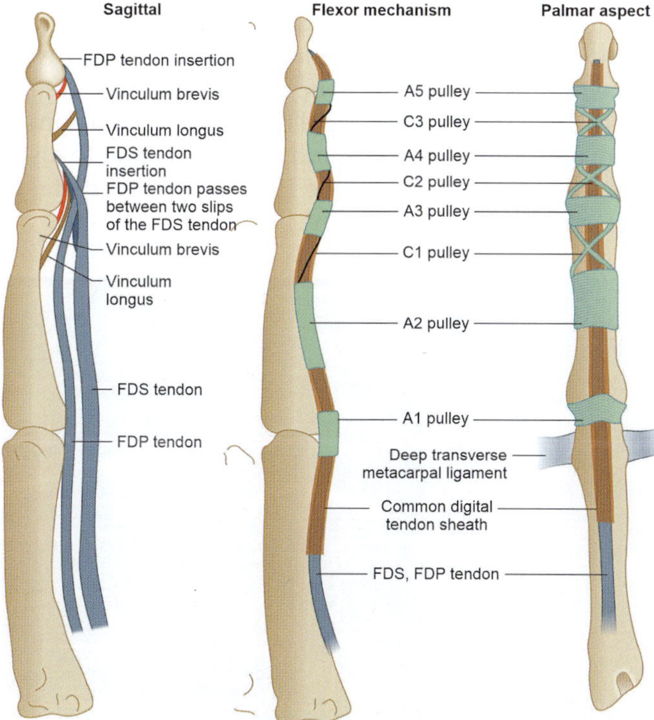

Fig. 3.8.143: Flexor mechanism of fingers

ligaments. **MCP Joint:** The unicondylar MCP joint's bony structure allows for extensive radial and ulnar deviation, as well as moderate rotation. In flexion, the MCP joint's collateral ligaments are stiff, whereas in extension, they are lax, allowing abduction and adduction. The deep transverse metacarpal (interglenoid) ligament connects the volar plate to the neighbouring MCP joints, making it a significant joint stabiliser. The extensor hood (especially its sagittal bands), which helps to anchor the extensor tendon at this level, also helps to keep the joint stable. Extensor tendons are stabilised over the dorsum of the metacarpal head by the extensor hood at the MCP joint. The extensor hood, which starts primarily at the volar plate and has a dorsal tendinous point of attachment, gliding with the extensor system as the finger moves, is made up of the sagittal bands. The intrinsic tendons' transverse fibres, which are located distal to the sagittal bands, contribute to the extensor hood's structure. Extrinsic and intrinsic tendons integrate into the dorsal apparatus and are spread circumferentially around the dorsum of the fingers distal to the MCP joint. In the central and lateral slips or bands, the extrinsic extensor tendon is continued. The middle phalanx's base is where the central slip gets inserted. The lateral slips are formed mostly by intrinsic tendons.

Zoning system in fingers and hands: Verdan original tendon injury zones is useful in hand surgery. For thumb no established zone classification exists. **Zones in flexor tendon:** Moving from proximal to distal–Zone I extends distal to FDS insertion, Zone II extends from beginning of common digital sheath to FDS insertion, Zone III extends from end of carpal tunnel to beginning common digital sheath, Zone IV includes carpal tunnel. Preferred zoning system for thumb: Zone I extends from proximal to distal aspect of oblique pulley, Zone II extends from distal to distal aspect of oblique pulley.

Zones of extensor tendon: Zone I lies at the level of DIP joints, Zone II lies between PIP and DIP, Zone III lies at the level of PIP, Zone IV lies between MCP and PIP, Zone V lies at the level of MCP joint, Zones VI lies between CMC joint and MCP joint.

Ligaments

Extensor ligaments: Lumbrical tendon passes volar to transverse metacarpal ligament and interossei tendon passes dorsal to transverse metacarpal ligament.

Retinacular ligaments: It retain and position the common extensor mechanism during PIP and DIP flexion. Contains oblique band (oblique retinacular ligament of Landsmeer) and transverse band.

Collateral ligaments: Stabilize MCP joint during motion. Components are radial collateral ligaments and ulnar collateral ligaments. RCL is more horizontal compared to UCL. Each have 2 parts: Proper and accessory ligaments. Accessory ligament attaches from metacarpal head to palmar plate. Proper ligament attaches from posterior tubercle of metacarpal head (dorsal to mid-axis) to base of the proximal phalanx.

USG fingers: Palmar aspects: **(P1)** Longitudinal ultrasound of the digital flexor sheath at A1 pulley level. (Fig. 3.8.144) **(P2)** Extended field of view longitudinal ultrasound showing the flexor digitorum tendon from A2 to A5 pulley and FDP attachment in the distal phalanx (Fig. 3.8.147). **(P3)** Transverse ultrasound of the flexor digitorum tendons at the level of the proximal third of the proximal phalanx, the FDS tendon divides into two slips which pass to the radial and ulnar aspects of the FDP tendon as they course distally (Fig. 3.8.145). **(P4)** Transverse view of FDS insertion in the proximal aspect of the middle phalanx (Fig. 3.8.146). **(P5)** Longitudinal ultrasound of the ulnar surface of the thumb at metacarpophalangeal joint level (Fig. 3.8.148). **Dorsal**

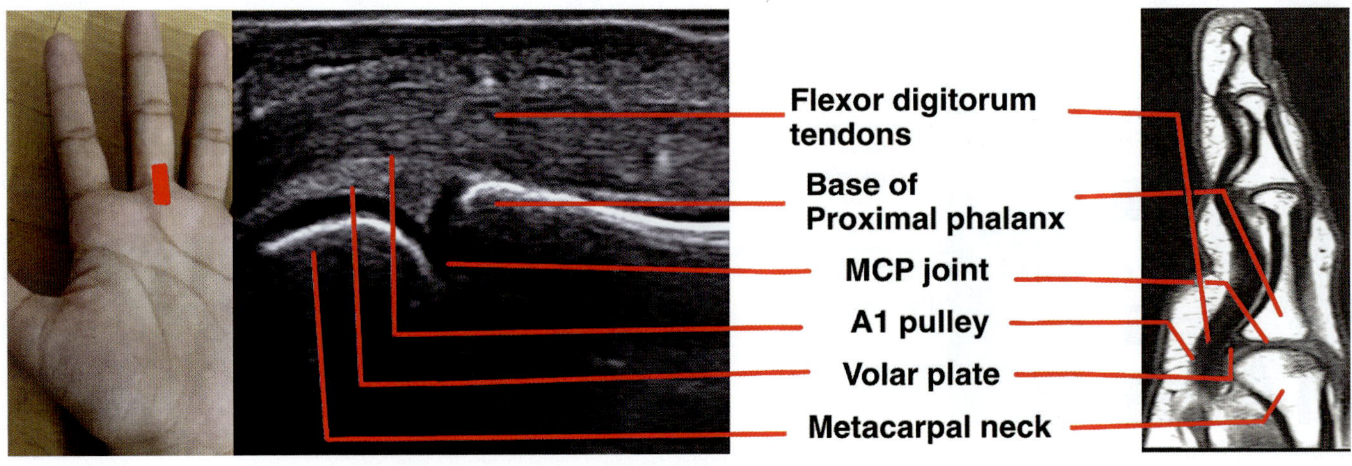

Fig. 3.8.144

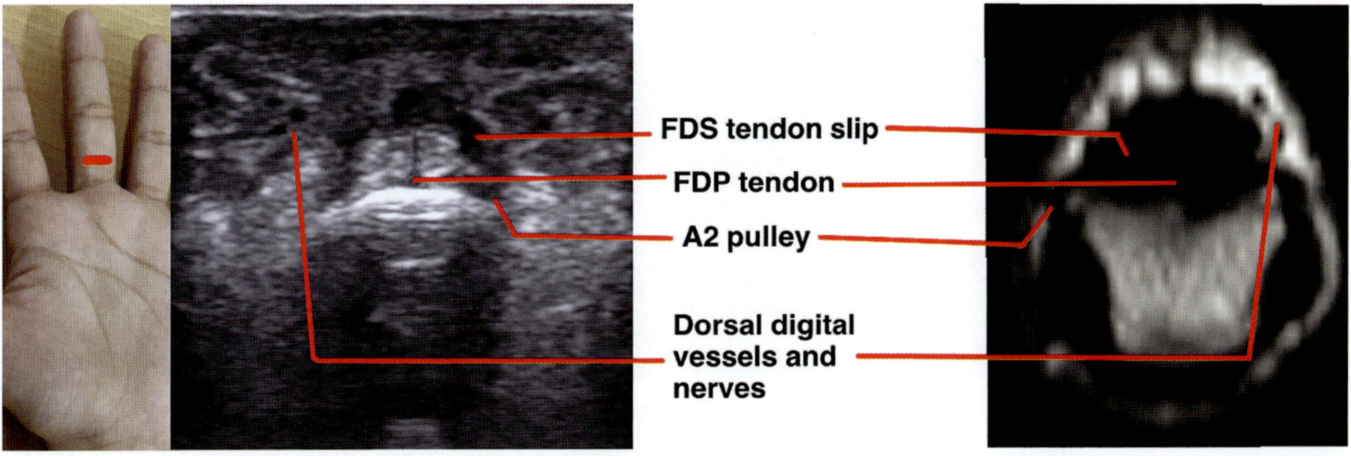

Fig. 3.8.145

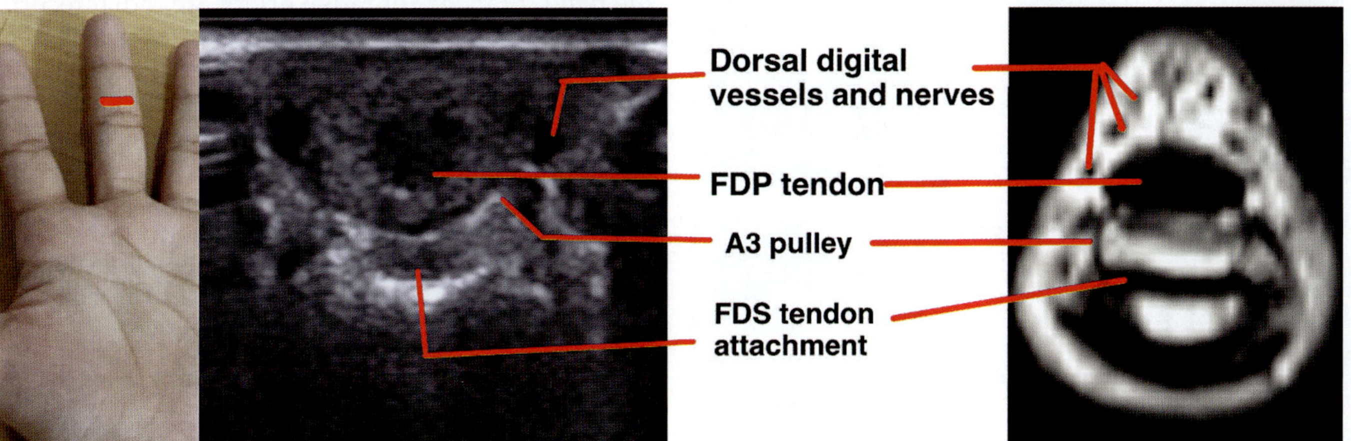

Fig. 3.8.146

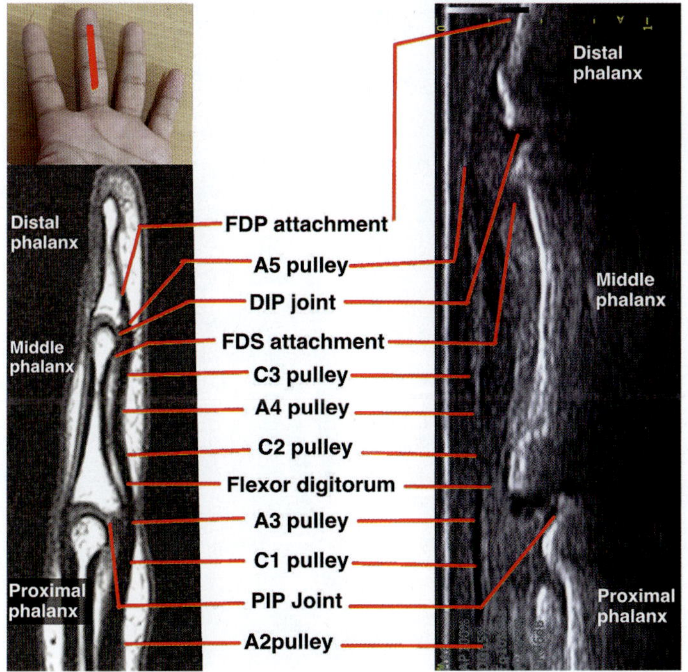

Fig. 3.8.147

aspects: Longitudinal view of the digital extensor hood (Fig. 3.8.149).

Table 3.8.6: Ossification centres in hand

Bones	*Site*	*Appearance*	*Fusion*
Metacarpals	Distal end (head)	1–2 years	15–20 years
	Diaphysis	9th week of gestation	
Phalanges	Proximal end (base)	2–3 years	14–18 years
	Diaphysis	8–12 weeks of gestation	

3.8.G Neurovascular Structures

Arteries of upper limb: Aortic arch has three branches—right brachiocephalic trunk, left common carotid artery and left subclavian artery. Right subclavian artery arises from the right brachiocephalic trunk, behind the right sternoclavicular joint passing upward behind the scalenus anterior muscle. Subclavian artery has 5 branches—vertebral artery, thyrocervical trunk, costocervical trunk, dorsal scapular artery, internal

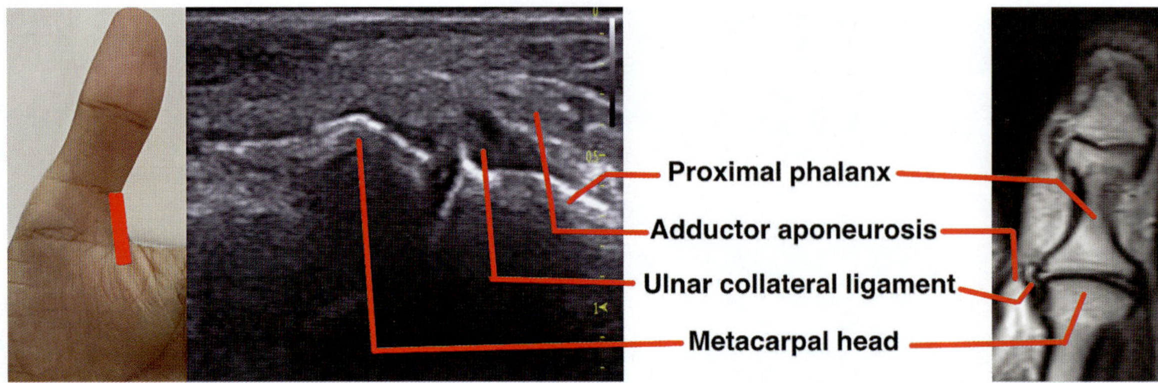

Fig. 3.8.148

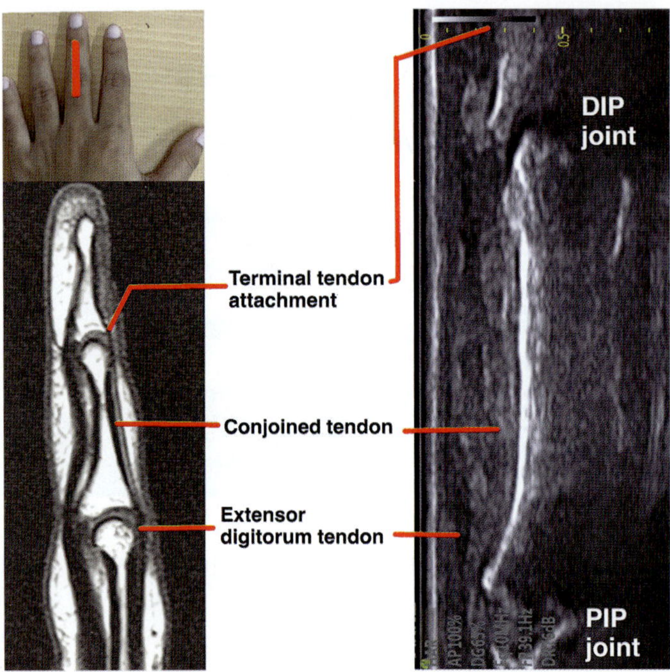

Fig. 3.8.149

mammary artery. Thyrocervical trunk gives rise to three branches—inferior thyroid artery, transverse cervical artery, suprascapular artery. Subclavian artery continues as axillary artery beyond the outer border of first rib. Axillary artery has 6 branches; superior thoracic artery, thoracoacromial artery, lateral thoracic artery, anterior circumflex and posterior circumflex humeral artery, suprascapular artery. Axillary artery continues as brachial artery at the lower border of teres major muscle. It courses down the arm, medially to the humerus and gradually moving to the front of bone. It terminates 1 cm below the elbow by dividing into radial and ulnar artery. Brachial artery has 7 branches, profunda brachii artery, muscular branches, nutrient artery, superior ulnar collateral artery, inferior ulnar collateral artery, radial artery and ulnar artery. Radial artery is the direct continuation of brachial artery, about 1 cm below the bend of elbow, coursing along the radius bone, reaching the hand. Branches of radial artery are radial recurrent artery, muscular branches palmar carpal branch. Ulnar artery is the larger of two branches, it begins at the level of neck of radius, passing downward and medially, reaching the ulnar side of forearm. It then continues as superficial palmar arch. Branches are anterior ulnar recurrent artery, posterior ulnar recurrent artery, common interosseous artery, anterior and posterior interosseous artery, muscular branches, palmar carpal branch (Figs 3.8.150–3.8.155).

Veins of upper limb: There are two groups of veins, superficial and deep venous system, with free

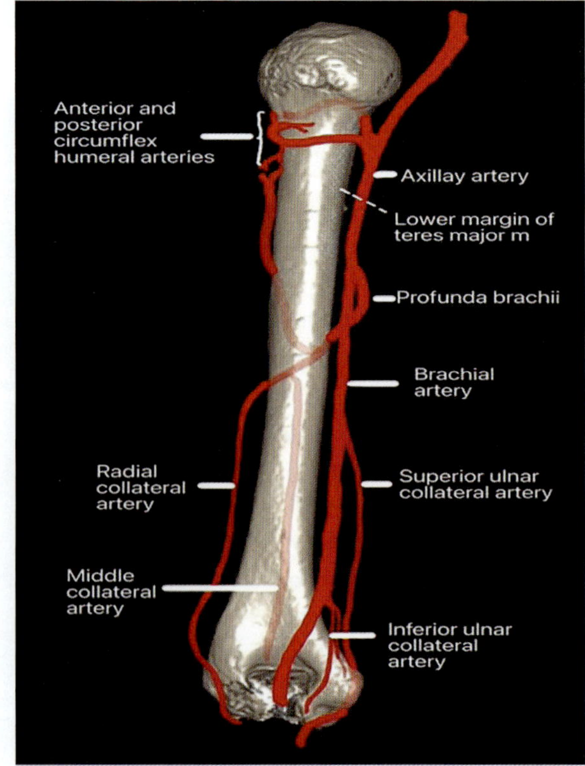

Fig. 3.8.150: Arterial supply around shoulder joint, arm

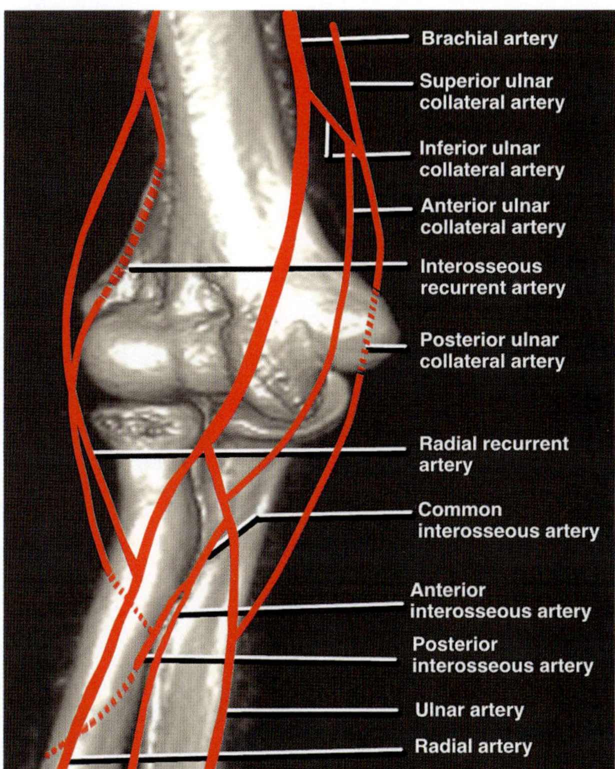

Fig. 3.8.151: Arterial supply around elbow

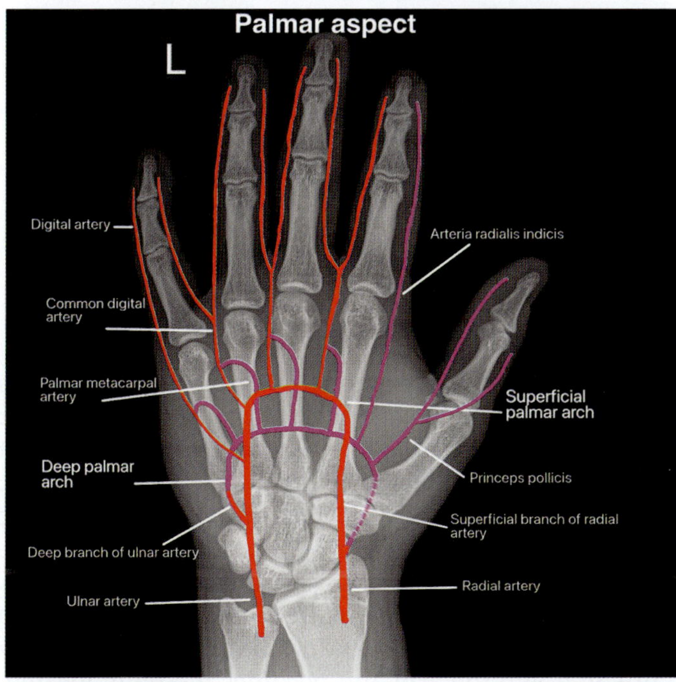

Fig. 3.8.152: Arterial supply of palmar aspect of hand

anastomosis between them. Deep veins accompany the arteries. Superficial veins are cephalic, basilic and median antebrachial veins. Dorsal venous network of hand, continues laterally as cephalic vein and medially it continues as basilic vein. Cephalic vein runs along

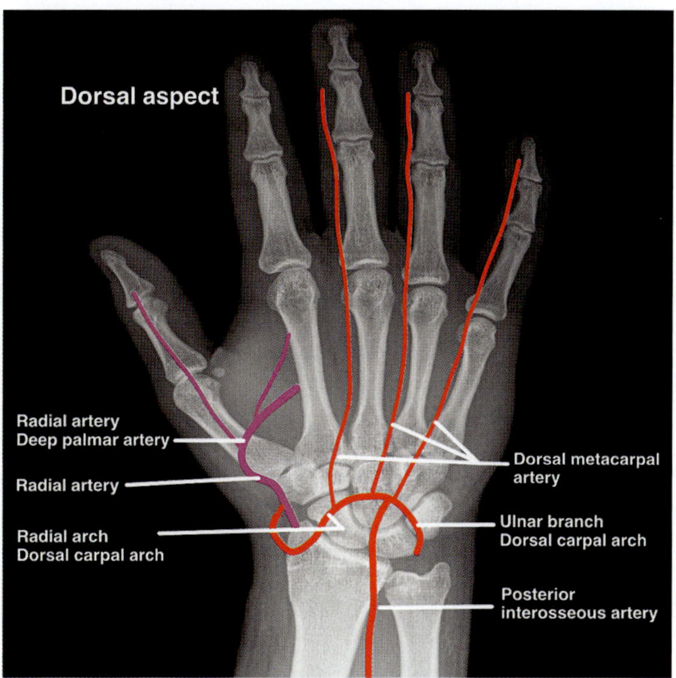

Fig. 3.8.153: Arterial supply of dorsal aspect of hand

the radial border of forearm. Median cubital vein from cephalic vein is given, in front of elbow, has communications with the deep veins of forearm, and it passes medially to communicate with basilic vein. The cephalic vein ascends subcutaneously lateral to biceps. It ends in the axillary vein in the infraclavicular fossa. Basilic vein originates in ulnar aspect of dorsal venous network, follows a subcutaneous path in the dorsal side of forearm, then moves forward to the ventral surface. It is joined by medial cubital vein in front of elbow and ascends between the biceps and pronator teres muscle. At the shoulder level, it perforates the deep fascia and continues as axillary vein. Median vein of forearm, formed by superficial palmar venous plexus and ends in basilic or median cubital vein. Deep veins accompany the arteries, radial and ulnar veins join to form brachial veins, and join the axillary vein, or axillary vein is continuation of basilic vein, and it lies medially to the axillary artery, which then continues as subclavian vein which is joined by internal jugular vein to form brachiocephalic vein. It lies anterior and inferior to subclavian artery (Fig. 3.8.154).

Nerves of upper limb: The axillary nerve (C5 and C6) is a direct continuation of the posterior cord from the brachial plexus. The axillary nerve is found in the axilla, posterior to the axillary artery and anterior to the subscapularis muscle. It leaves the axilla via the quadrangular space at the inferior edge of the subscapularis, frequently accompanied by the posterior circumflex humeral

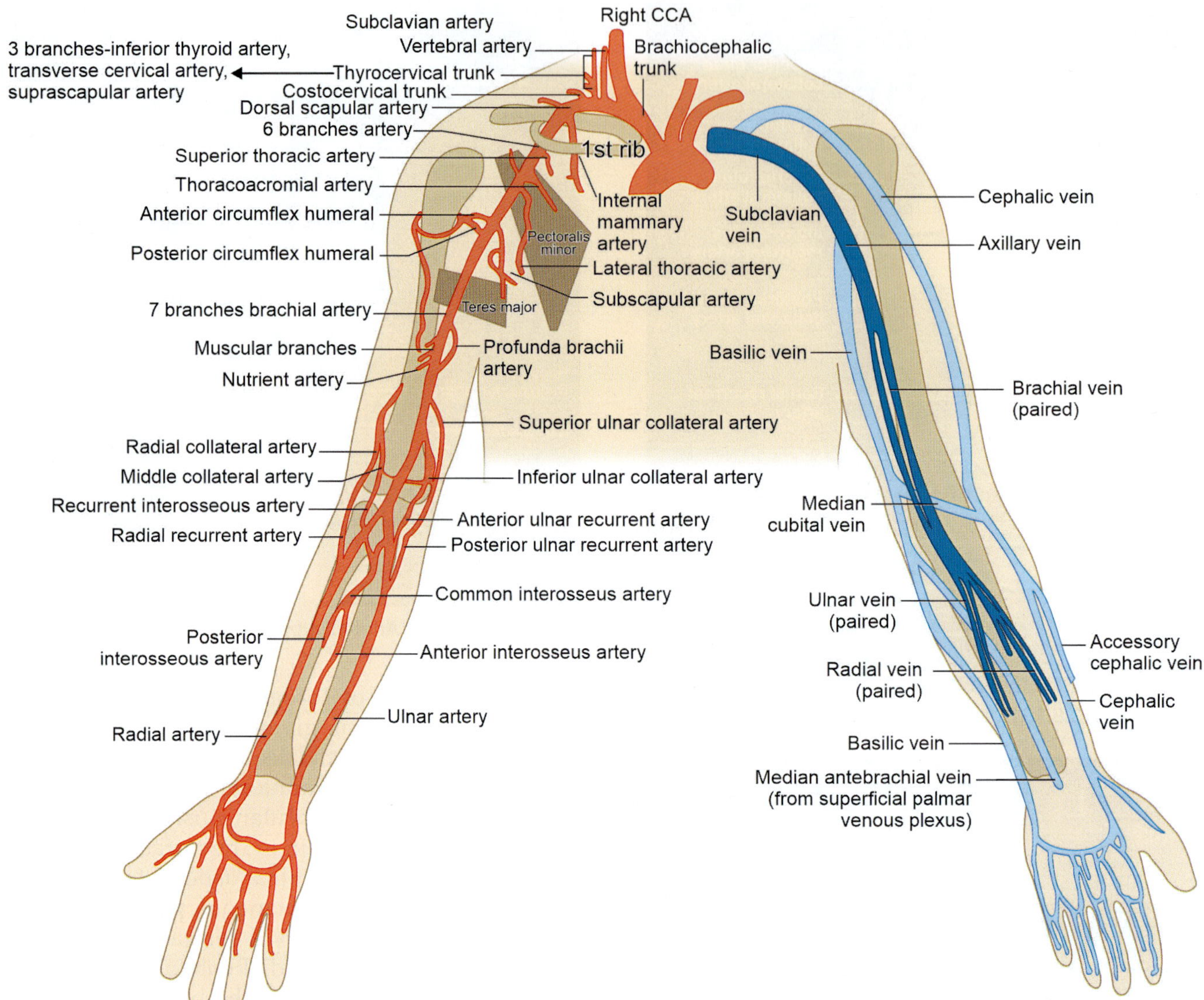

Fig. 3.8.154: Arterial and venous drainage of upper limb

artery and vein. After passing medially to the surgical neck of the humerus, the axillary nerve separates into three branches: Posterior terminal branch, anterior terminal branch, and articular branch. **Suprascapular nerve**, a branch from C5 nerve root traverses across. Suprascapular notch, supraspinatus fossa, spinoglenoid notch and infraspinatus fossa. As the nerve traverses across suprascapular notch, it gives branches to supraspinatus muscle, it supplies infraspinatus after it traverses through spinoglenoid notch. The musculocutaneous nerve arises at the inferior border of the pectoralis minor muscle as the terminal branch of the lateral cord of the brachial plexus (C5, C6, C7). It emerges from the axilla, pierces the coracobrachialis muscle near its insertion on the humerus, and travels down the upper arm's flexor compartment, superficial to the brachialis and deep to the biceps brachii. The nerve then emerges lateral to the biceps tendon and brachioradialis after piercing the deep fascia lateral to the biceps brachii. It continues into the forearm as the lateral cutaneous nerve. **Medial cutaneous nerve of forearm** accompanies basilic vein in the arm. The medial and lateral cords of the brachial plexus in the axilla give rise to the median nerve. The median nerve in the arm descends initially lateral to the brachial artery. The nerve crosses the brachial artery halfway down the arm and becomes medially located. The median nerve is found in the anterior cubital fossa, deep to the bicipital aponeurosis and anterior to the brachialis muscle. As it exits the cubital fossa, it passes between the heads of the pronator teres muscle. The nerve runs between the flexor digitorum profundus and flexor digitorum superficialis muscles in the forearm.

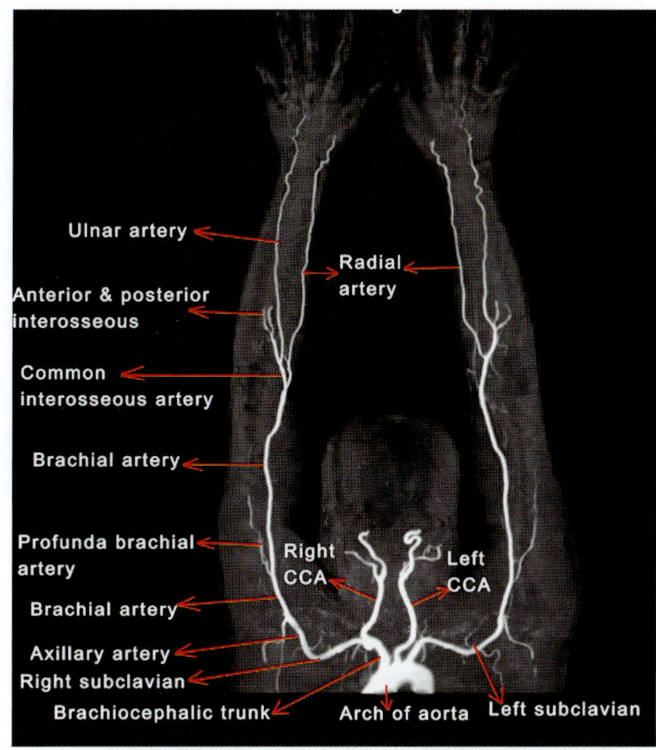

Fig. 3.8.155: CT angiogram upper limb

The median nerve gives off two major branches in the forearm—anterior interosseous nerve branch at the level of pronator teres and palmar cutaneous nerve. Median nerve enters the hand via the carpal tunnel and terminate into two branches—recurrent branch supply thenar muscle 1st and 2nd lumbricals. Palmar digital branch (sensory) supply to lateral half of palm, 1–3 digits and lateral half of 4th digit on palmar aspect and distal to PIP joint to fingertips for 1–3 digits and lateral half of 4th digit on dorsal aspect. The **radial nerve** (C5–T1) is the terminal continuation of the posterior cord of the brachial plexus. Situated posteriorly to the axillary artery in axilla. It exits axilla inferiorly (via the triangular interval), descends down the arm, travel in the radial groove of humerus. Gives sensory branches, namely lower lateral cutaneous nerve of arm and posterior cutaneous nerve of arm. Radial nerve travels anterior to the lateral epicondyle of the humerus, through the cubital fossa and gives off the posterior interosseous (deep motor) branch and a superficial (sensory) branch. The posterior interosseous nerve enters the radial tunnel underneath a musculotendinous arch, the arcade of Frohse which is a connection between the deep and superficial heads of the supinator and moves from the anterior to the posterior surface of the forearm. Radial nerve gives sensory supply from radiocarpal joint to just distal to PIP joint for 1–3 digits and lateral half of 4th digit on dorsal aspect. The ulnar nerve (C8,T1) is a continuation of the medial cord. Ulnar nerve descends lateral to axillary artery and medial to axillary vein. In arm nerve lies medial to the brachial artery where it penetrates the medial fascial septum to enter the posterior compartment of the arm. It passes posterior to the elbow through the cubital tunnel and gives articular branch. In the forearm, the ulnar nerve pierces the two heads of the flexor carpi ulnaris, and travels deep to the muscle, alongside the ulna. In forearm gives muscular branch—innervates anterior compartment muscles. At the wrist, the ulnar nerve travels superficially to the flexor retinaculum, and is medial to the ulnar artery. It enters the hand via the ulnar canal (Guyon's canal). In the hand, the nerve terminates into deep branches which supply hypothenar muscles, all interossei, 3rd and 4th lumbricals and adductor pollicis and superficial branch gives sensory supply from radiocarpal joint to fingertips of 5th and medial half of 4th finger both palmar and dorsal aspects (Figs 3.8.156–3.8.160).

Lymphatics: Superficial channels that accompany the basilic and cephalic veins to a series of nodes around the elbow, namely: (1) superficial and deep cubital lymph nodes, (2) Epi/supratrochlear lymph nodes medial to the brachial vein, just superior to the medial epicondyle. Deep channels that accompany the arteries and drain via deep lymph node in the forearm to the axillary nodes. Lymph then drains up the arm, passing through a few deep brachial lymph nodes and deltopectoral lymph nodes with the cephalic vein at the deltopectoral groove, before draining into infraclavicular lymph nodes that predominantly drain lateral upper limb and lateral two digits and axillary lymph nodes that predominantly drain medial upper limb and medial three digits (Fig. 3.8.161).

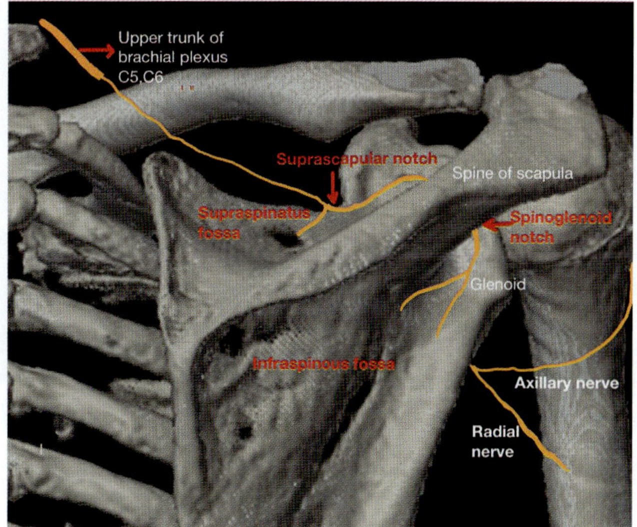

Fig. 3.8.156: Nerve supply around shoulder region

3

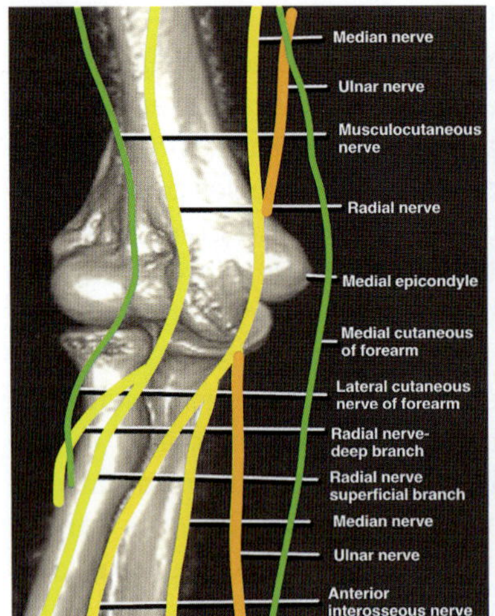

Fig. 3.8.157: Nerve supply around elbow

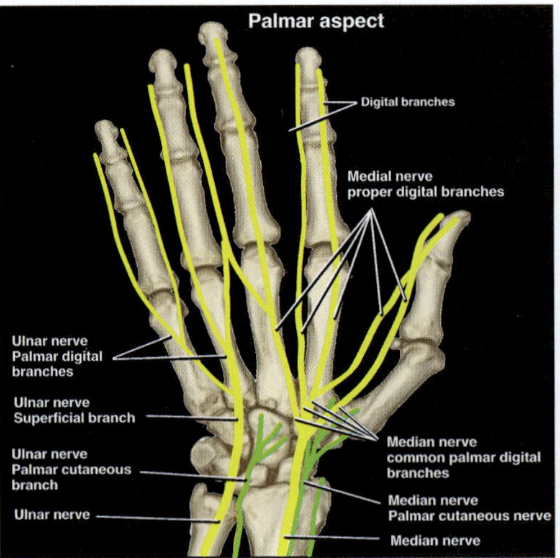

Fig. 3.8.158: Nerve supply of dorsal aspect of hand

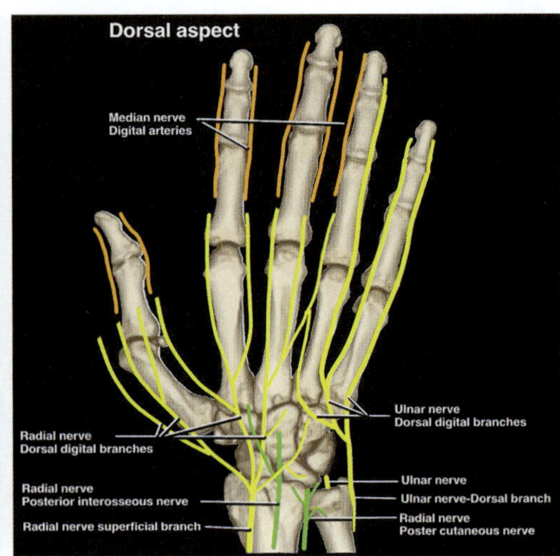

Fig. 3.8.159: Nerve supply of dorsal aspect of hand

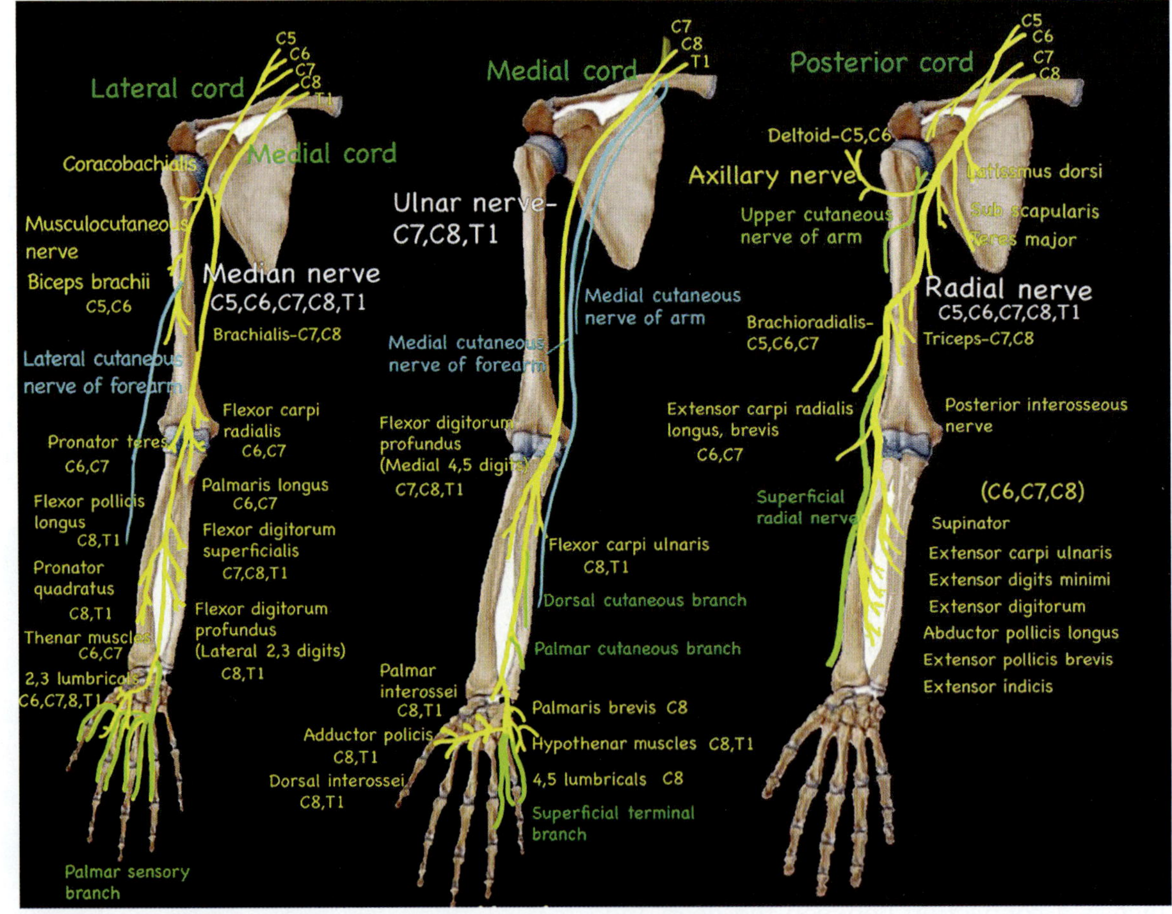

Fig. 3.8.160: Upper limb nerves

Table 3.8.7: Nerve entrapment syndromes

Entrapment syndrome	Nerve compressed	Site of compression
Quadrangular space syndrome	Axillary nerve	Quadrangular space
Suprascapular entrapment neuropathy	Proximal suprascapular nerve	Suprascapular notch
Cubital tunnel syndrome	Ulnar nerve	Cubital tunnel
Pronator teres syndrome	Median nerve	Between the two heads of the pronator teres muscle
Kiloh-Nevin syndrome	Anterior interosseous nerve	Ulnar head of pronator teres
Supinator syndrome	Posterior interosseous nerve	Arcade of Frohse in radial tunnel
Carpal tunnel syndrome	Median nerve	Carpal tunnel
Wartenberg's syndrome	Superficial sensory radial nerve	At wrist by scissoring action of brachioradialis and ECRL tendons during forearm pronation
Ulnar tunnel syndrome/Guyon's canal syndrome/handlebar palsy	Ulnar nerve	Guyon's canal
Radial tunnel syndrome	Posterior interosseous nerve	Lateral intermuscular septum

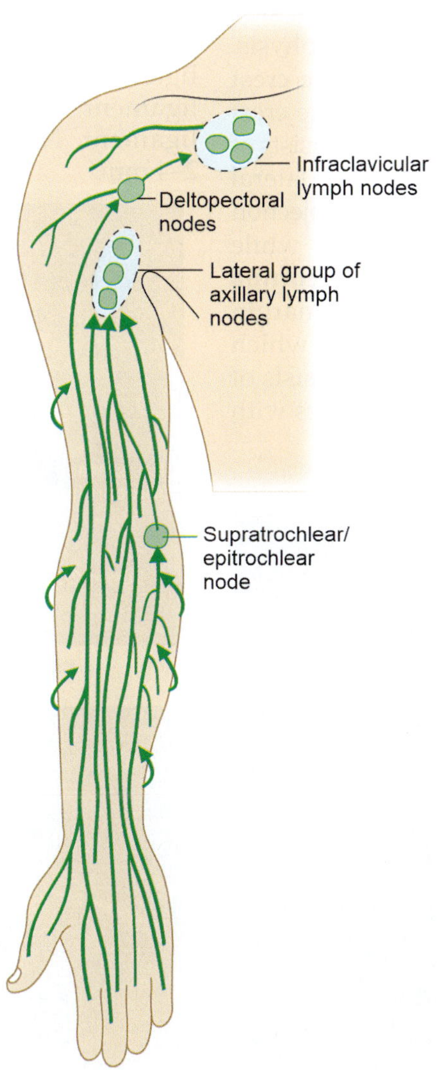

Fig. 3.8.161: Lymphatics of upper limb

3.9 BONY PELVIS, SACROILIAC JOINT, HIP JOINT AND THIGH

3.9.A Bony Pelvis

It is composed of three bones—hip bone, sacrum and coccyx (Fig. 3.9.1). Hip bone has three parts—ilium, ischium and pubis. **Ilium** has an **ala** and **external gluteal fossa, internal iliac fossa**. The superior prominence is **iliac crest** which corresponds to L4–L5 level and anterior protuberance includes—anterior superior iliac spine and anterior inferior iliac spine. The posterior protuberances are the posterior superior and inferior iliac spines. **Ischium** has a **body and ramus**, posteriorly forming the **ischial tuberosity** which is the site of origin of hamstring muscles. **Ischial spine** is a prominence oriented posteromedially which is the site of attachment of sacrospinous ligament forming the boundary between greater and lesser sciatic foramen. **Pubis** consists of a **body and two rami**—the superior and inferior pubic rami. The two pubic bodies of either side articulate in the midline forming the pubic symphysis. The superior aspect of pubic body is the **pubic crest and pubic tubercle** is the lateral aspect of pubic crest where the inguinal ligament attaches. Sacrum consists of 5–6 rudimentary vertebra which are fused. The lateral wings of sacrum are called the ala. The superior projection of S1 vertebra is called the **sacral promontory** while the inferior articular facet of S5 is called the **cornua** which articulates with coccyx. The superior margin of neural foramina are called the **sacral arcs** which should be symmetric. The triangular coccyx consists of 3–5 fused rudimentary vertebra which articulates with sacrum.

Fig. 3.9.1: X-ray pelvis

Sacroiliac joint: The sacroiliac joint (SIJ) is a synovial joint between ilium and the sacrum. The main function of the sacroiliac joint is transferring the weight between the axial and lower appendicular skeletons. The SI joint is symmetrical joint (i.e. is paired) with an oblique coronal orientation and is located at the S1–3 level. Movement at the sacroiliac joint is minimal and limited to gliding and rotation. The sacroiliac joint is formed by the irregular articular surfaces of the sacrum and the ilium, which provide some strength to the joint. The upper one-third is a syndesmosis. The lower two-thirds are lined by articular cartilage—although only the lower third is lined by synovium, and the middle third resembles a symphysis (Figs 3.9.2 and 3.9.3). Being a synovial joint it is surrounded by a capsule. Stability is conferred by the irregular articular surfaces and mainly through extra-capsular ligaments. Ligaments and joints complete the greater and lesser sciatic foramina. The ligaments are interosseous sacroiliac ligament, anterior sacroiliac ligament, posterior sacroiliac ligament, iliolumbar ligament, sacrospinous ligament and sacrotuberous ligament. Normal sacroiliac joint space is between 2–4 mm.

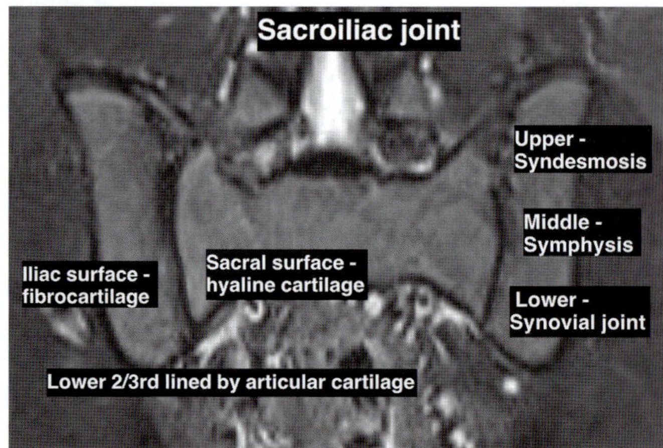

Fig. 3.9.2: Coronal MRI of sacroiliac joint

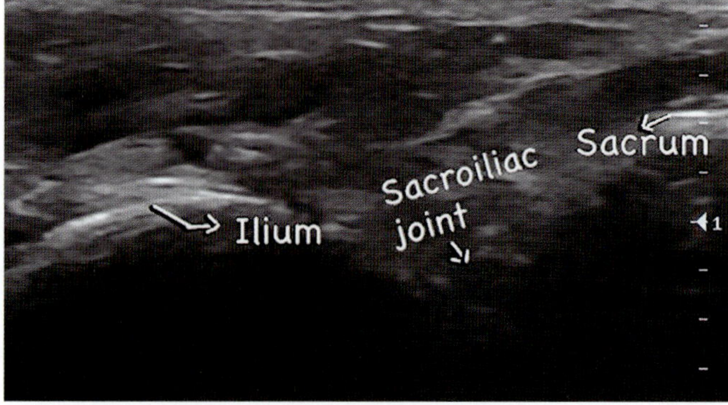

Fig. 3.9.3: Ultrasound of sacroiliac joint

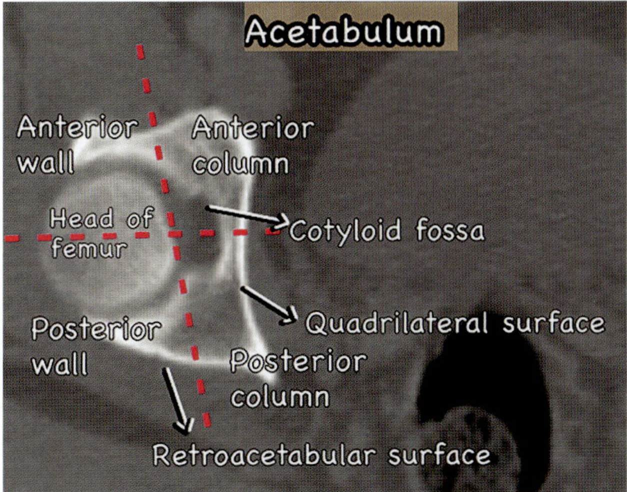

Fig. 3.9.4

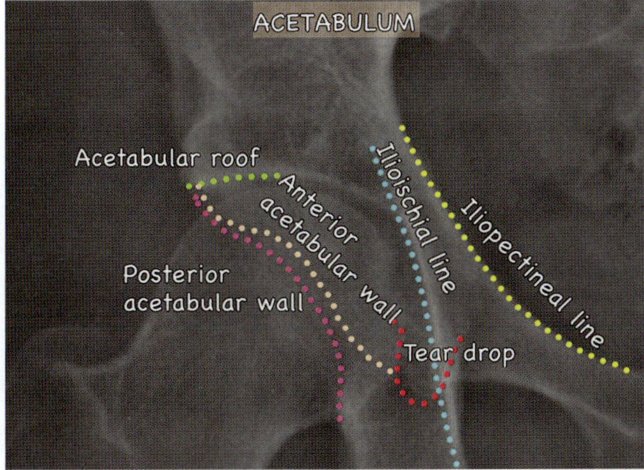

Fig. 3.9.5

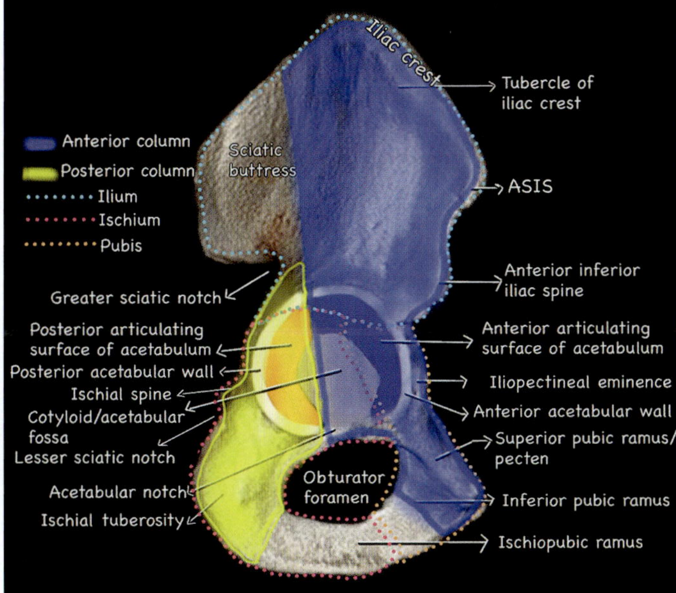

Fig. 3.9.6: 3D image of hip bone with columns of acetabulum

3.9.B Hip Joint

The hip joint, the most stable joint, is a ball and socket type of synovial joint between the **acetebulum of hip bone and head of femur**. The acetabulum is formed by three bones—**ilium (2/5), ischium (2/5) and pubis (1/5)** which together form the innominate bone, at the junction of which lies the epiphyseal plate—**triradiate cartilage**. Acetabulum is considered as **inverted Y shaped** structure with **two limbs formed by the anterior iliopubic and posterior ilioischial column and the stem formed by ilium.** The rim of acetabulum is covered by labrum (fibrocartilage) which increases the depth of the joint, thereby increasing the stability of the joint but causes a reduction in the movement of the joint. The actual hyaline articular cartilage-covered area (lunate surface) of acetabulum is C-shaped and forms an incomplete ring due to the acetabular notch. This notch is traversed by the **transverse ligament**. From the transverse ligament arises the **ligamentum teres** which passes to the femoral head. **Labrocartilaginous cleft is between the articular cartilage and labrum.** The cartilage devoid nonarticular area in the centre of acetabulum is acetabular fossa filled with fibrofatty tissue—**pulvinar**. The flat, medial wall of acetabulum which faces the pelvic organs is **quadrilateral plate or surface**. Anterior column of acetabulum includes anterior border of iliac wing, pelvic brim, anterior superior iliac spine, anterior inferior iliac spine, anterior wall of acetabulum and superior pubic ramus. Posterior column of acetabulum includes ischial portion of innominate bone (inclusive of greater and lesser sciatic notch), posterior wall of acetabulum and ischial tuberosity (Figs 3.9.4 to 3.9.6). **Femoral head** articulates with acetabulum and is covered by articular cartilage except at the **fovea capitis**

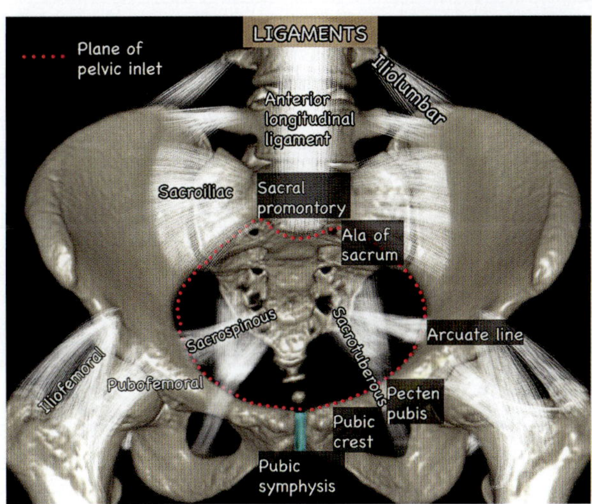

Fig. 3.9.7: Pelvic ligaments

3

where the ligamentum teres attaches. Joint capsule has 2 layers—synovial and fibrous layer. The fibrous layer forms capsular ligaments. The **joint capsule** is attached to acetabular labrum superiorly and inferiorly to intertrochanteric line and intertrochanteric crest on anterior and posterior aspect of femur respectively (Figs 3.9.9–3.9.12). **Perilabral recess** lies between labrum and capsule. The joint volume is about 8–20 cc and flexion and internal rotation of hip joint maximizes joint volume.

Table 3.9.1: Ligaments of hip (Fig. 3.9.7)

Iliofemoral (Bigelow) ligament	Strongest ligament in body.Extends from anterior inferior iliac spine to intertrochanteric crest of femur. It prevents anterior translation.
Ischiofemoral ligament	Weakest. Triangular band of fibres directed posteriorly extending from ischium to blend with the posterior joint capsule attaching on the intertrochanteric line of femur. It prevents posterior translation.
Pubofemoral ligament	Anteroinferior in direction. Attached to obturator crest and superior pubic ramus, iliopubic eminence and distally blends with the joint capsule and deep surface of iliofemoral ligament.
Zona orbicularis	Deep and circular fibres around the femoral neck.

Table 3.9.2: Bursa around hip joint (Fig. 3.9.8)

Iliopsoas bursa	Largest bursa of hip joint. Lies beneath the musculotendinous portion of iliopsoas muscle. May communicate with hip joint in 10% individuals.
Obturator externus bursa	Lies between zona orbicularis and ischiofemoral ligament.
Trochanteric bursa	Also known as subgluteus maximus bursa as it lies deep to gluteus maximus muscle. Largest among bursa covering the hip joint.
Subgluteus medius bursa	Seen on the lateral aspect of hip joint, covers the lateral facet of greater trochanter. Deep to gluteus medius tendon.
Subgluteus minimus bursa	On the lateral aspect of hip joint, covering the anterior facet of greater trochanter. Deep to gluteus minimus tendon.
Gluteofemoral bursa	On the lateral aspect of hip joint, lying beneath the iliotibial band.

Blood supply of hip joint: Supplied by branches of medial and lateral circumflex femoral, superior and inferior gluteal arteries, acetabular branch of obturator artery (supplies ligamentum teres).

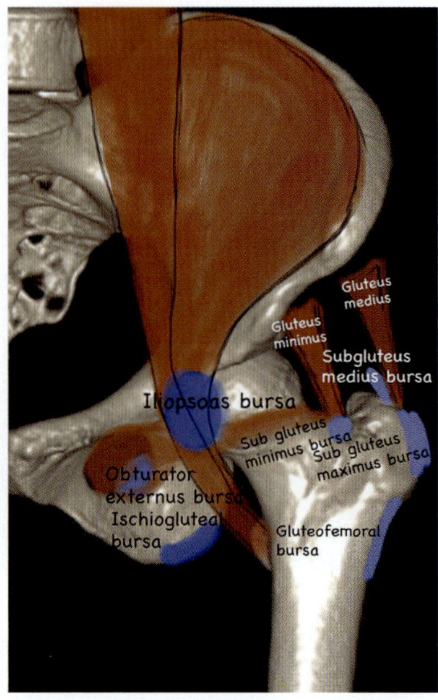

Fig. 3.9.8: Bursa around hip joint

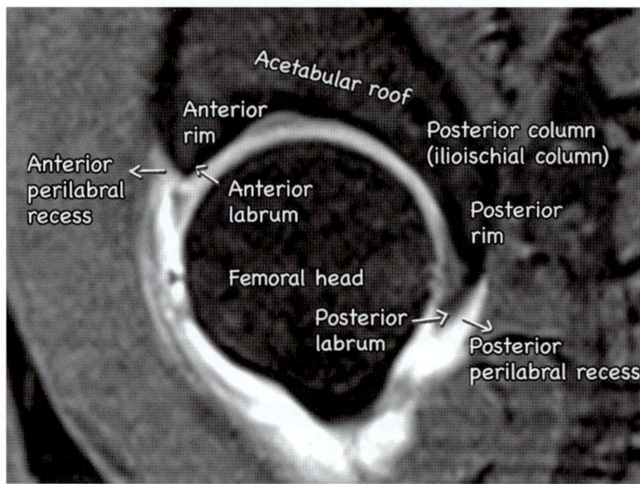

Fig. 3.9.9: MR arthrogram with labrum and perilabral recess

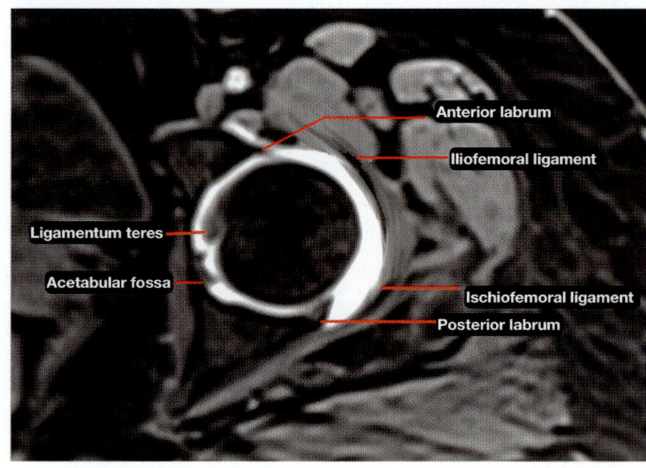

Fig. 3.9.10: MR arthrogram-labrum and ligaments

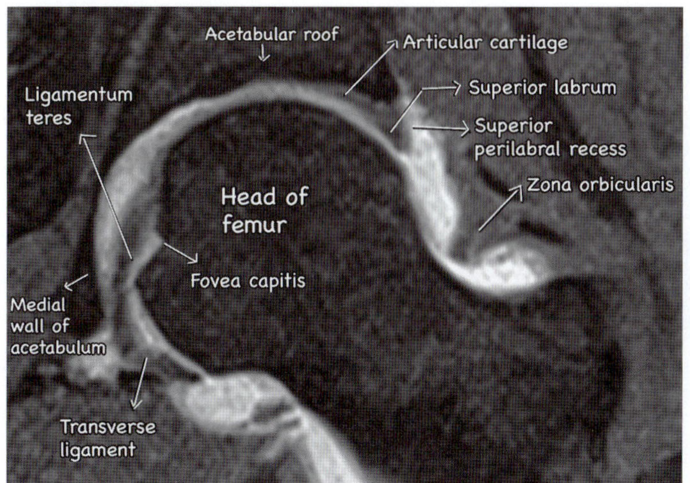

Fig. 3.9.11: MR arthrogram of hip joint—superior labrum, ligamentum teres, zona orbicularis

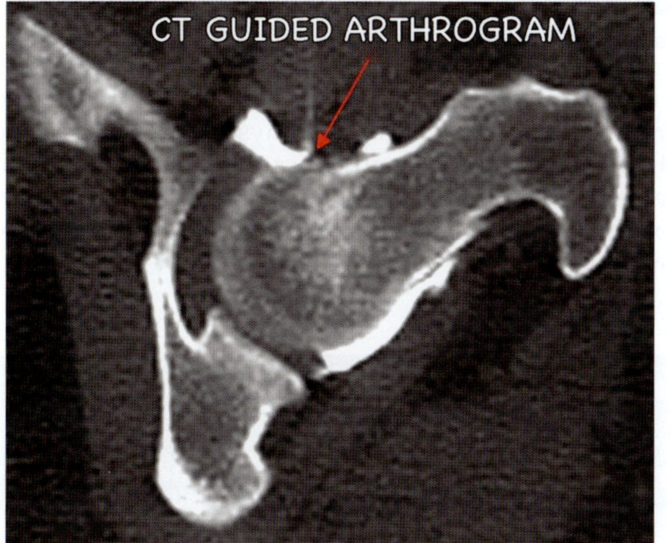

Fig. 3.9.12

Table 3.9.3: Important bony landmarks and their muscular attachments	
Pubis (Figs 3.9.13 and 3.9.14)	Rectus abdominis, adductor longus—together forms a common aponeurosis, adductor brevis, adductor magnus, gracilis, pectineus and obturator externus.
Ischial tuberosity	Divided into upper and lower parts. Origin of Hamstrings Upper superolateral part—semimembranosus. Upper inferomedial part for the long head of biceps femoris and semitendinosus. Lateral lower area—adductor magnus hamstring part.
Anterior inferior iliac spine	Straight head of rectus femoris, Iliacus and Iliofemoral ligament.
Greater trochanter has four bony facets—superoposterior, lateral, posterior and anterior (Fig. 3.9.15)	Gluteus minimus, gluteus medius, gluteus maximus, vastus lateralis, piriformis Gemellus superior, obturator internus, gemellus inferior, obturator externus, quadratus femoris.
Lesser trochanter	Iliopsoas.

Table 3.9.4: Major conduits to lower limb	
Abdomen	**Beneath the inguinal ligament** **Muscles:** Iliacus, psoas major, pectineus. **Nerves:** Femoral, femoral branch of genitofemoral nerve, lateral cutaneous nerve of thigh **Vessels:** Femoral artery and vein. **Lymphatics**
Pelvis	**Obturator canal:** Obturator nerve and vessels. **Greater sciatic foramen:** **Muscle:** Piriformis. **Nerves:** Sciatic nerve, superior and inferior gluteal nerve, pudendal nerve. **Vessels:** Superior and inferior gluteal vessels, internal pudendal artery.
Perineum	**Lesser sciatic foramen:** Tendon of obturator internus.

Subgluteal space: It is a space located between the middle and deep gluteal aponeurosis, containing important neurovascular structures like superior gluteal artery/nerve (supra piriform space), sciatic nerve, inferior gluteal nerve, inferior gluteal artery, ascending circumflex femoral artery, posterior cutaneous nerve of thigh in the infrapiriform space and muscles like piriformis, superior gemellus, obturator internus, inferior gemellus, quadratus femoris. This space is important because in cases of deep gluteal syndrome, the cause of pain lies in this space. One important cause of pain in this space is from the presence of fibrous bands which has to be differentiated from the normal neurovascular bundle located in this space.

Ischiofemoral space: It is the shortest distance between medial cortex of lesser trochanter and lateral cortex of ischial tuberosity.

Quadratus femoris space: It is the shortest distance between the posteromedial iliopsoas tendon/lesser trochanter and superolateral hamstring tendons for the passage of quadratus femoris muscle. These spaces are important for the reason that ischiofemoral impingement occur at these sites. Ischiofemoral impingement is one of the rare causes for chronic pelvic pain. The muscle involved primarily is quadratus femoris muscle. If the ischiofemoral space is <2 cm in supine pelvic X-rays, <1.9 cm in standing pelvic X-rays, then ischiofemoral impingement is likely. On MR imaging, due to different

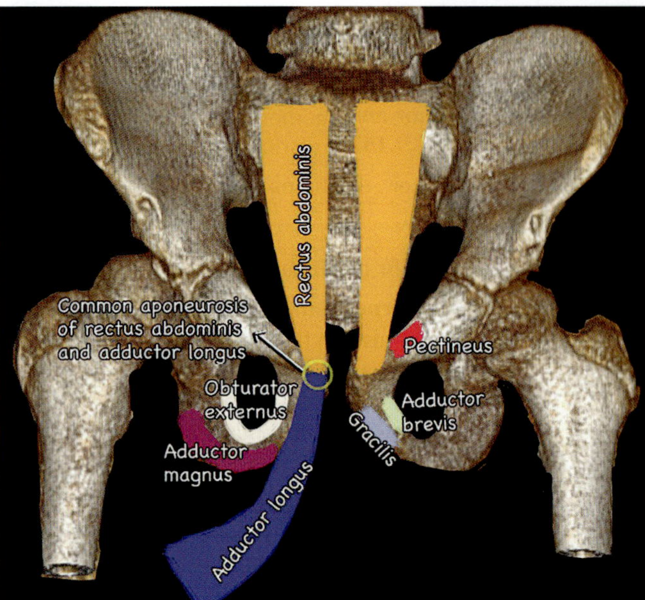

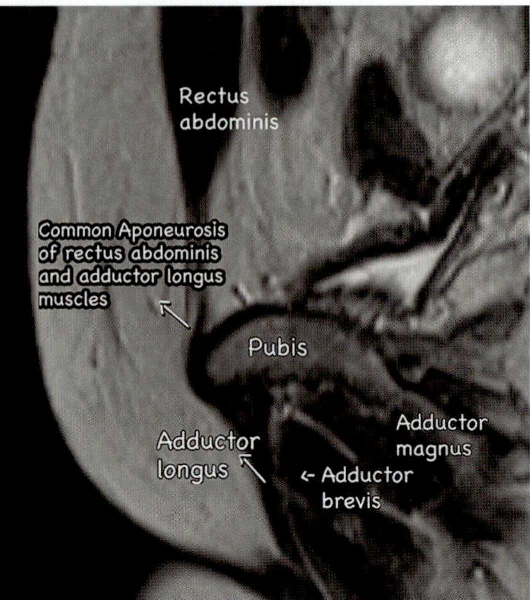

Fig. 3.9.13: Pubic muscle attachments

leg positioning, there are no standard values for assessing these spaces.

Bone marrow: The signal intensity changes in bone marrow depend on the age of the patient. Depending on the presence of hematopoietic or fatty marrow, the signal intensity varies. The conversion of hematopoietic to fatty marrow occurs in an organized fashion. At the time of birth, almost it is completely hematopoietic, showing organized conversion to yellow marrow proceeding from, proximal and distal epiphyses, followed by the diaphysis, distal metaphysis, and then the proximal metaphysis. In adults, the bone marrow is almost fatty, except for hematopoietic marrow in proximal femoral metaphysis.

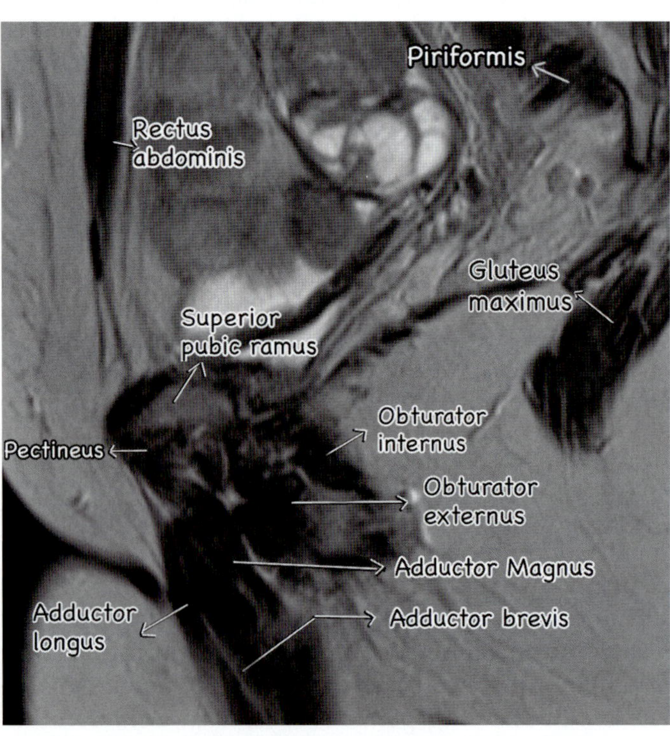

Fig. 3.9.14: Sagittal view of pubic muscle attachments

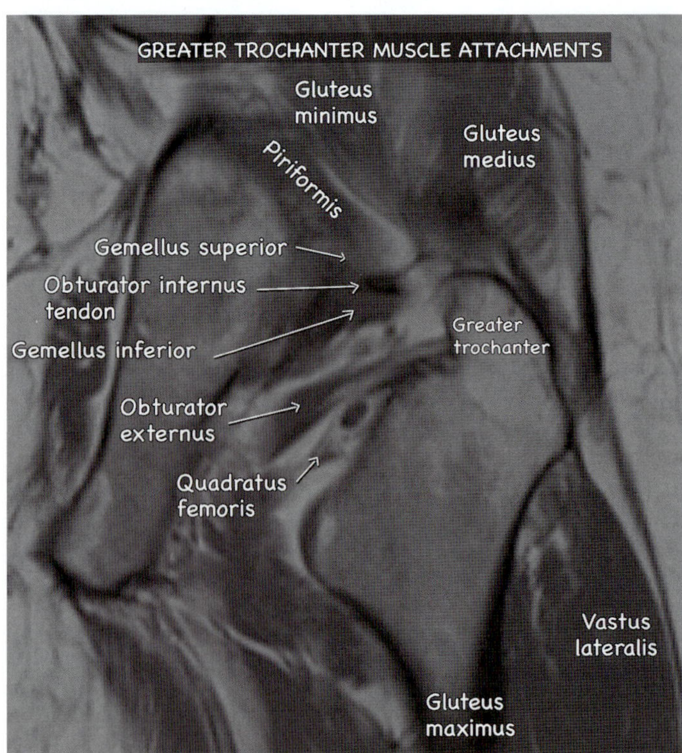

Fig. 3.9.15

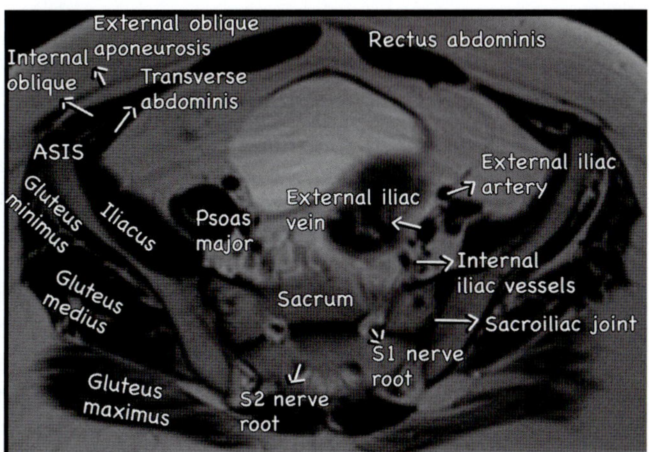

Fig. 3.9.16: MR—axial sections of pelvis

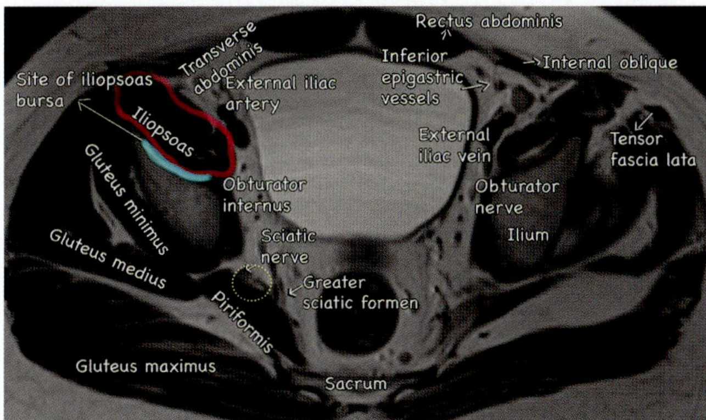

Fig. 3.9.17

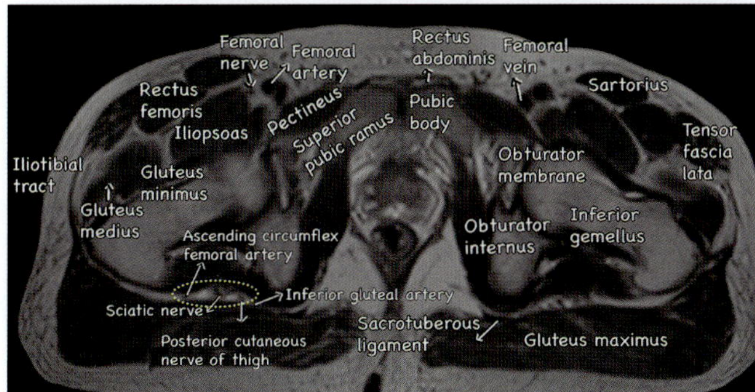

Fig. 3.9.18

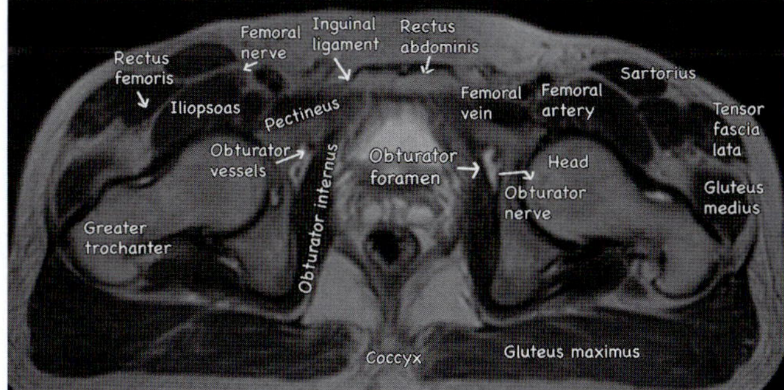

Fig. 3.9.19

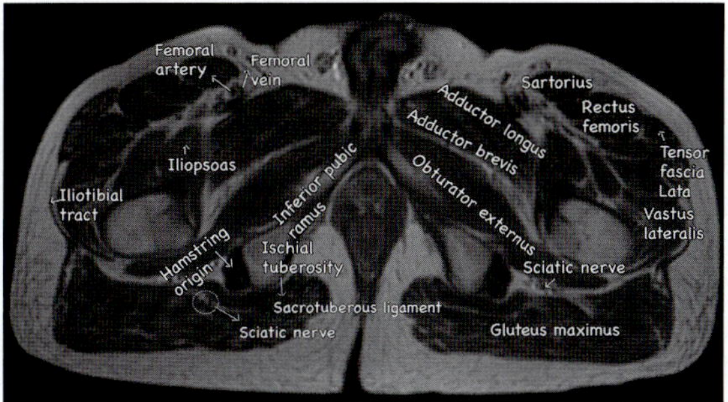

Fig. 3.9.20

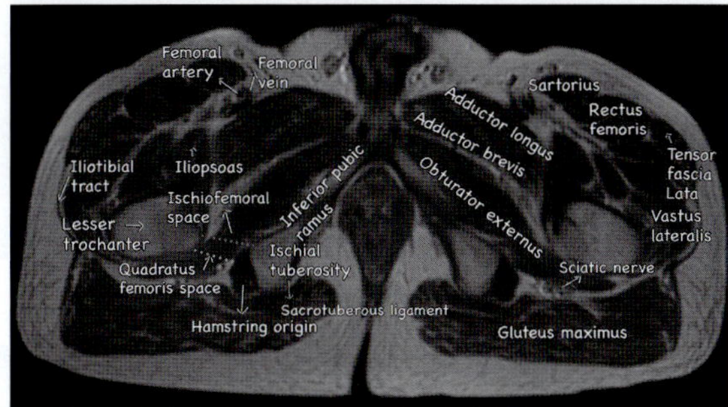

Fig. 3.9.21

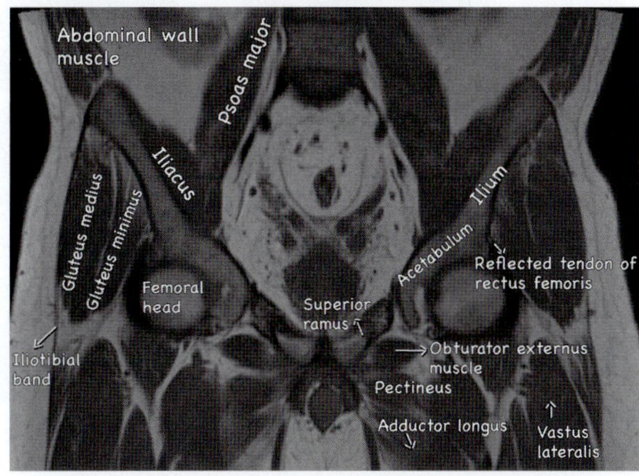

Fig. 3.9.22: MR coronal sections of pelvis

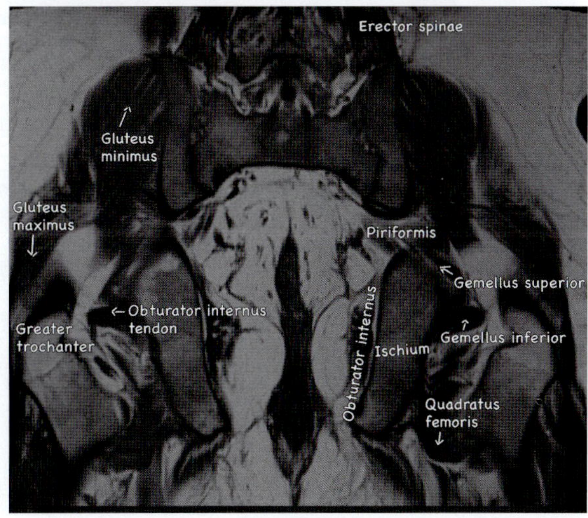

Fig. 3.9.23

3

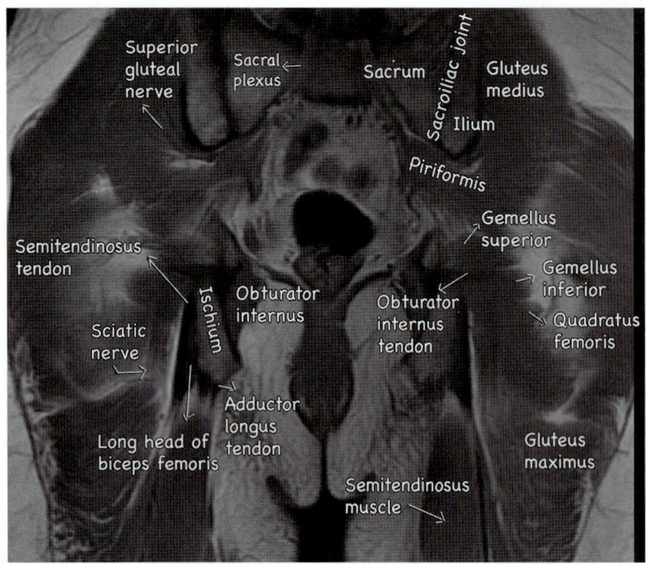

Fig. 3.9.24

Ultrasound Examination of Hip Joint

Anterior side of hip (Figs 3.9.25–3.9.33): Keep the patient in supine and transducer in oblique longitudinal plane over the femoral neck to examine the anterior synovial recess. The fibro cartilaginous anterior glenoid labrum can be visualized as homogenous hyperechoic triangular structure just cranial to the joint recess. By keeping the transducer over the anterior superior iliac spine in axial plane the tendons of Sartorius and tensor fasciae latae can be identified medial and lateral to ASIS respectively. The lateral femoral cutaneous nerve of thigh can be identified just medial to the attachment of inguinal ligament into the ASIS. From medial to lateral femoral vein, femoral artery and nerve are identified just medial to the iliopsoas muscle, further medial pectineus muscle seen over the pubis. At the anterior inferior iliac spine place the transducer to visualize the direct tendon of the rectus

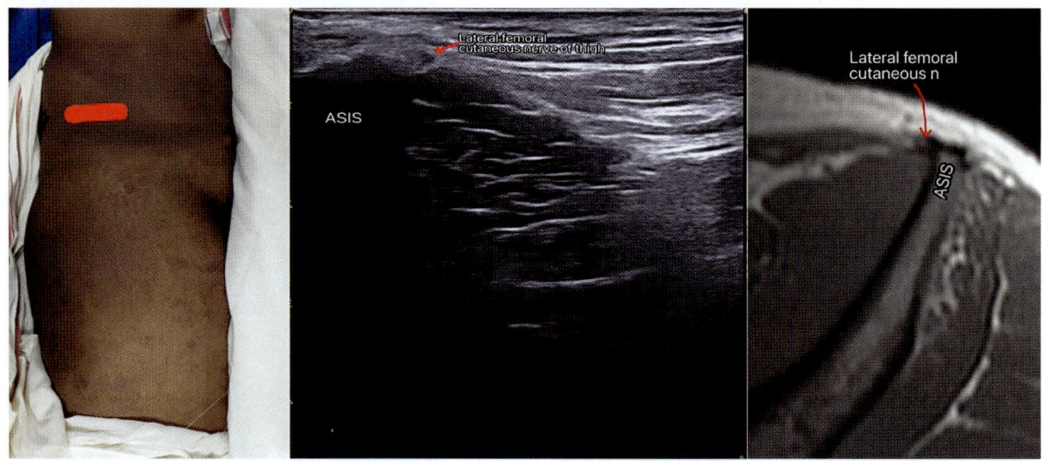

Fig. 3.9.25: Ultrasound images of anterior side of hip

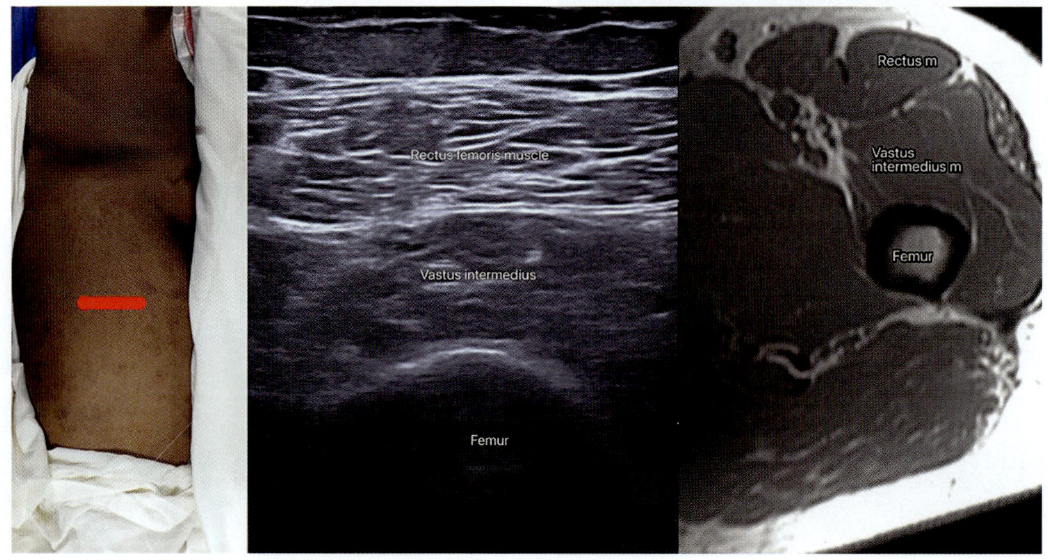

Fig. 3.9.26

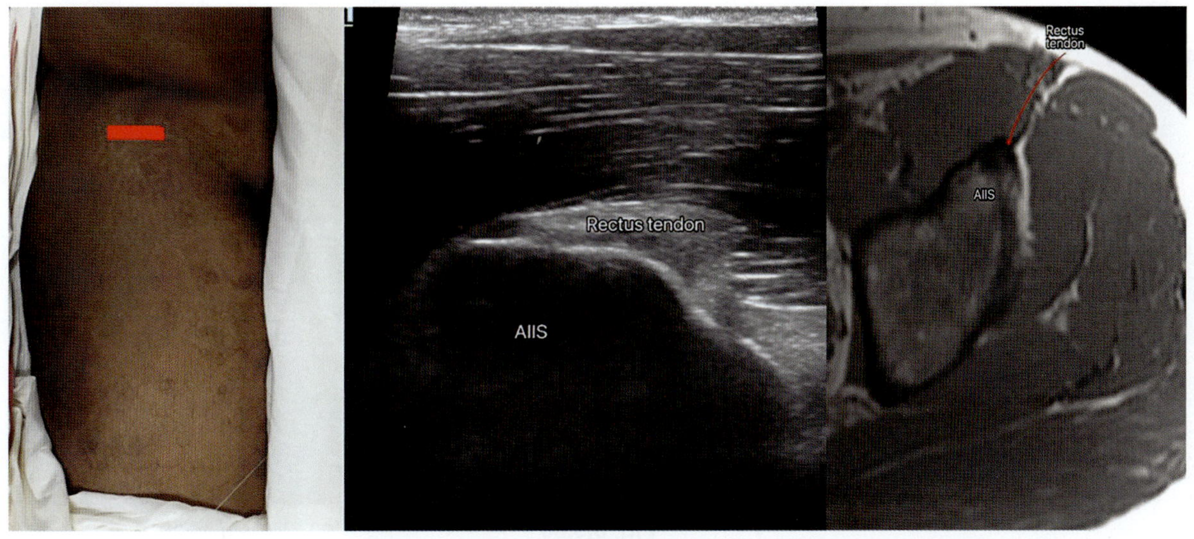

Fig. 3.9.27

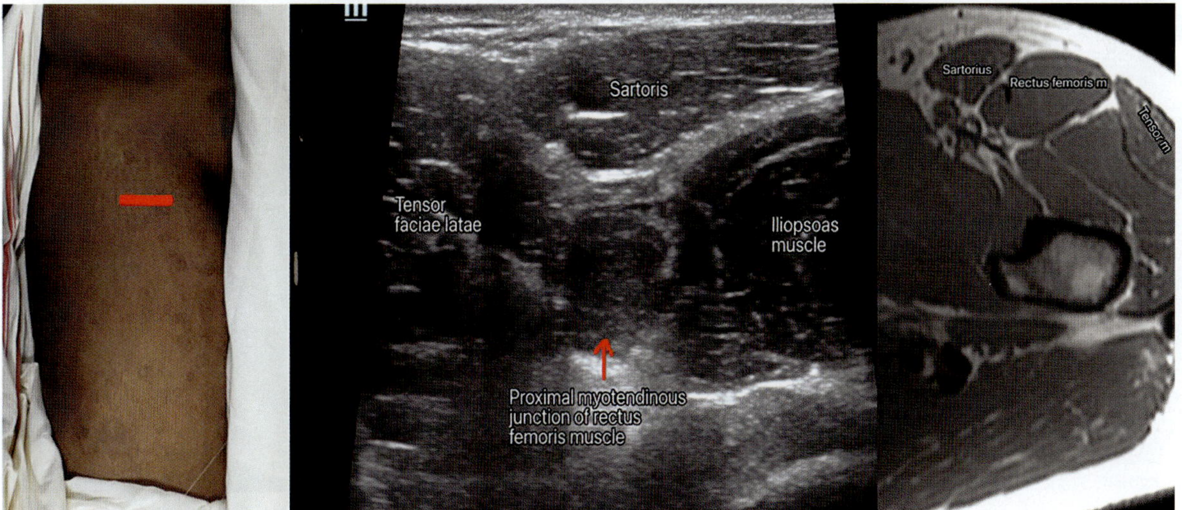

Fig. 3.9.28

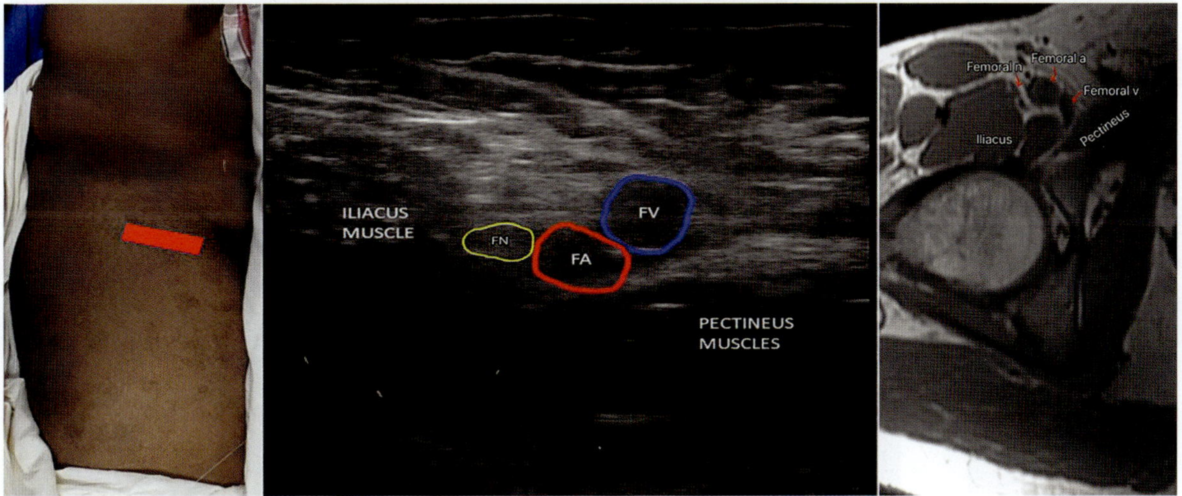

Fig. 3.9.29

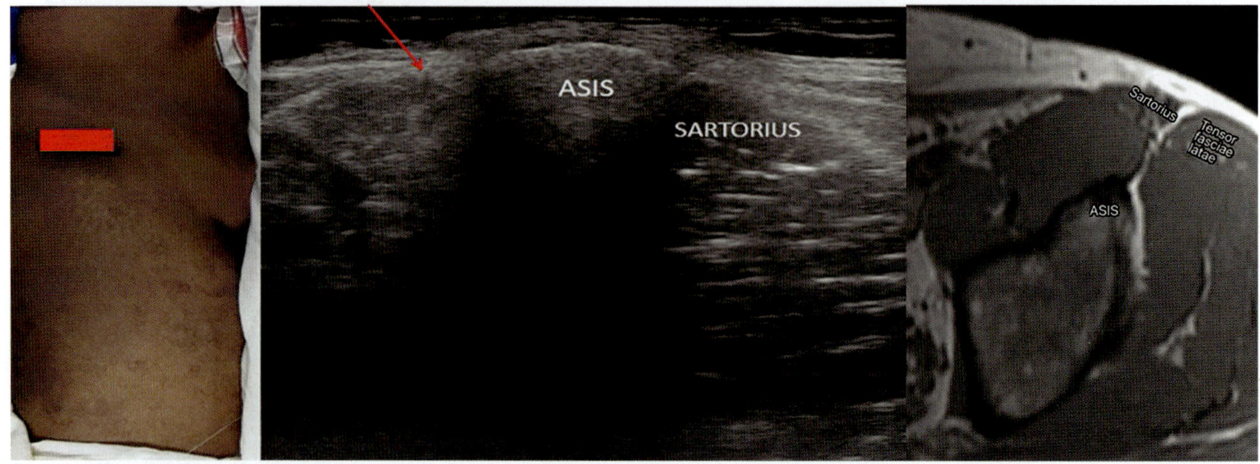

Fig. 3.9.30

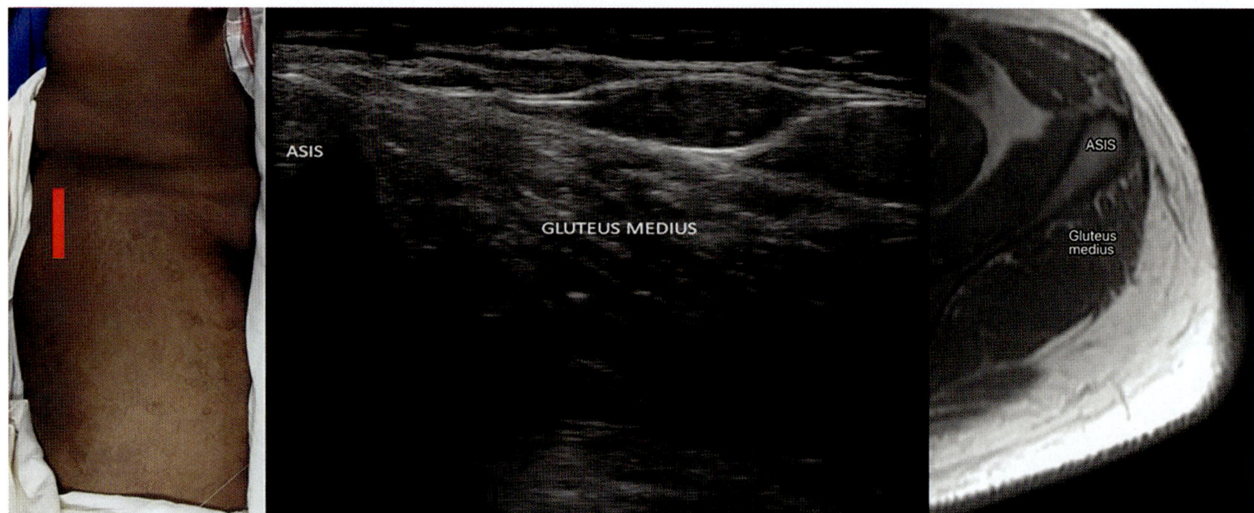

Fig. 3.9.31

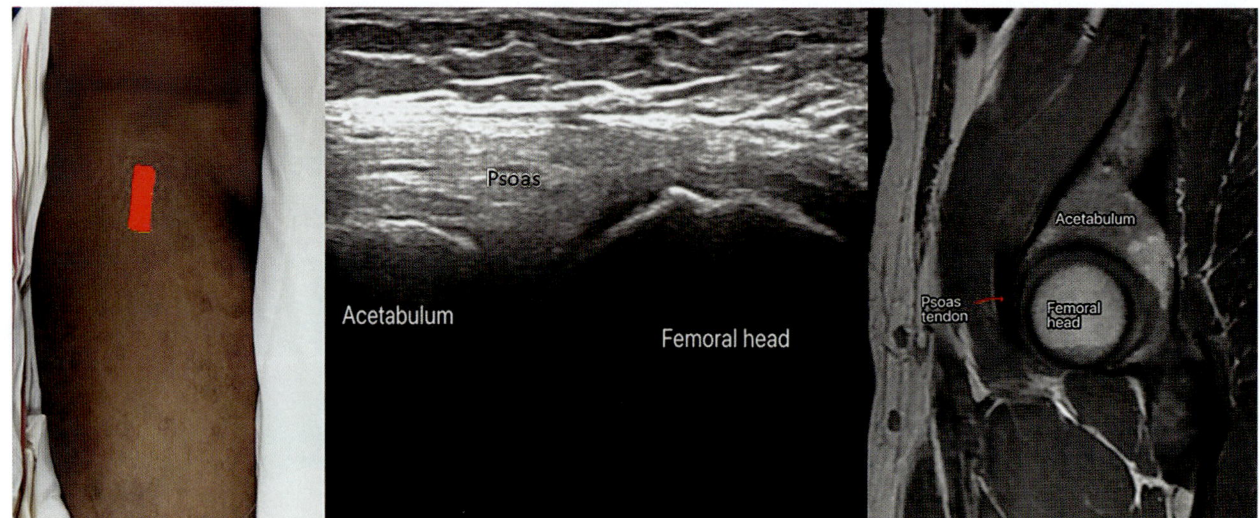

Fig. 3.9.32

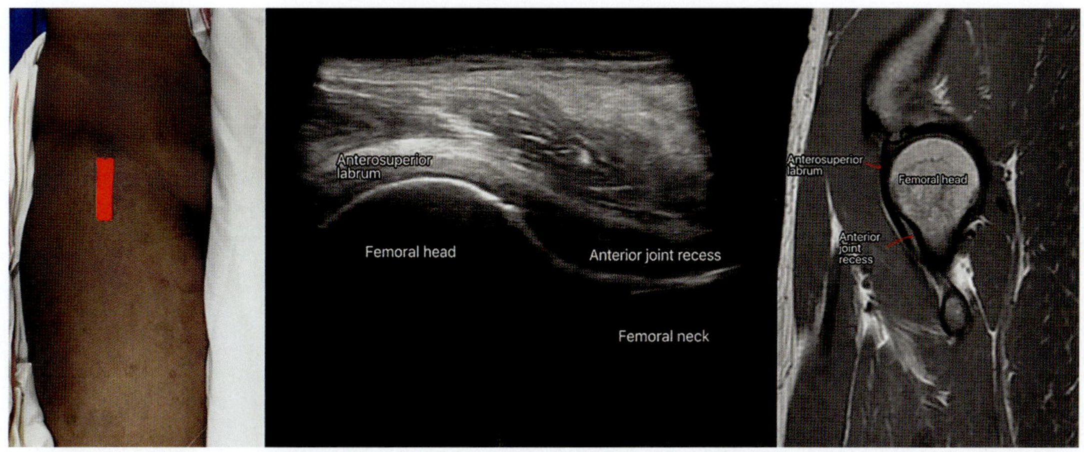

Fig. 3.9.33

femoris. As we progress distally, the muscle belly can be identified between the Sartorius and tensor fasciae latae.

Medial side of hip (Fig. 3.9.34): By keeping the patients leg in externally external rotation and abducted hip and flexed knee we can visualize the adductors and their insertion into the pubis.

Lateral side of hip (Figs 3.9.35 and 3.9.36): Ask the patient to lie on the opposite hip to examine the lateral aspect. By scanning just cranial to the greater trochanter we can

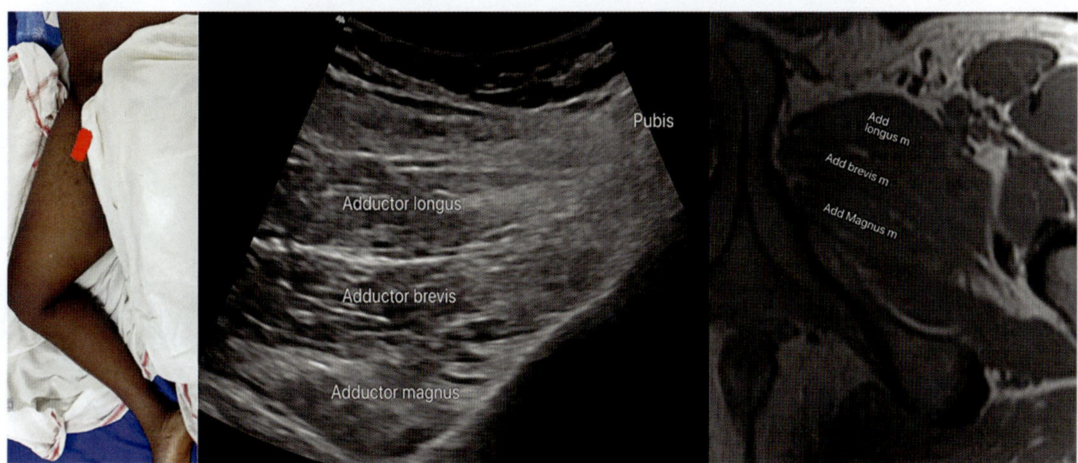

Fig. 3.9.34: Ultrasound of medial side of hip

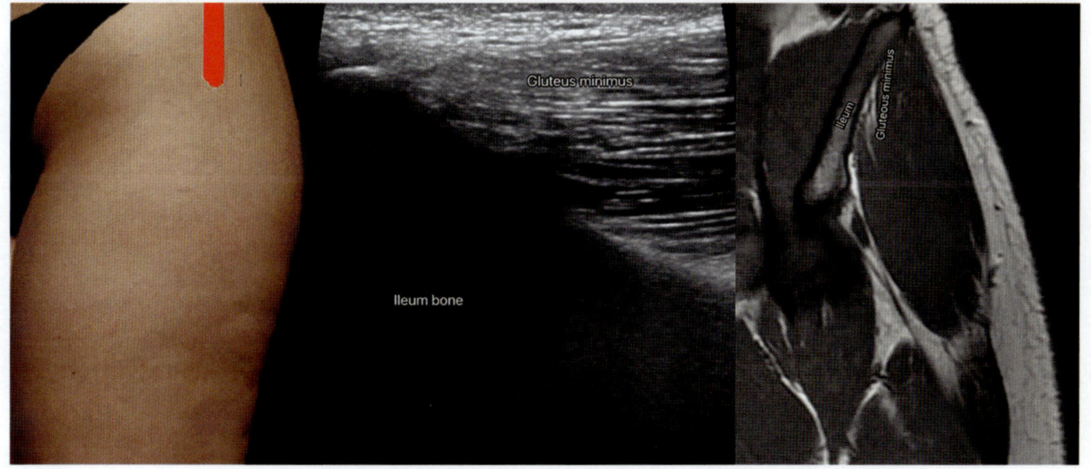

Fig. 3.9.35: Ultrasound of lateral side of hip

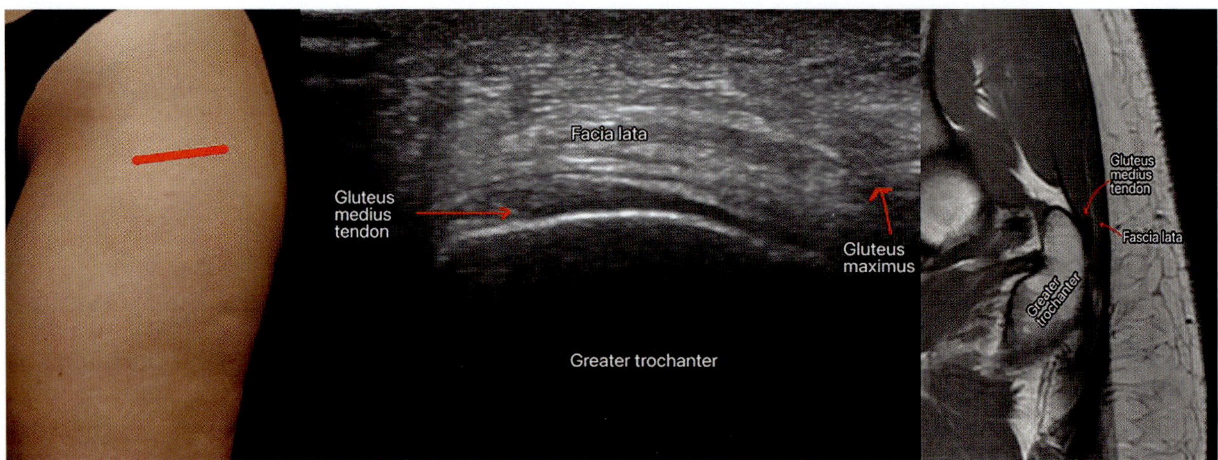

Fig. 3.9.36: Ultrasound of lateral side of hip

see the gluteus medius and minimus. As we move the probe down we can see the gluteus minimus tendon as an anterior structure and inserts into the anterior facet of the greater trochanter. By keeping over the lateral facet we can see the gluteus medius tendon as a curvilinear fibrillary band.

Posterior side of hip (Figs 3.9.37 to 3.9.40): Ask the patient to lie prone and by using low frequency

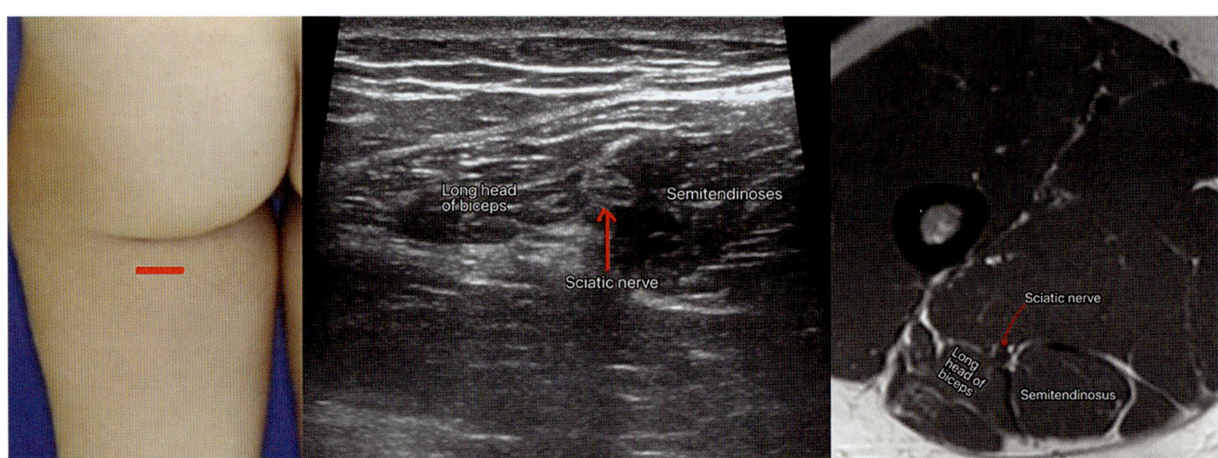

Fig. 3.9.37: Ultrasound images of posterior side of hip

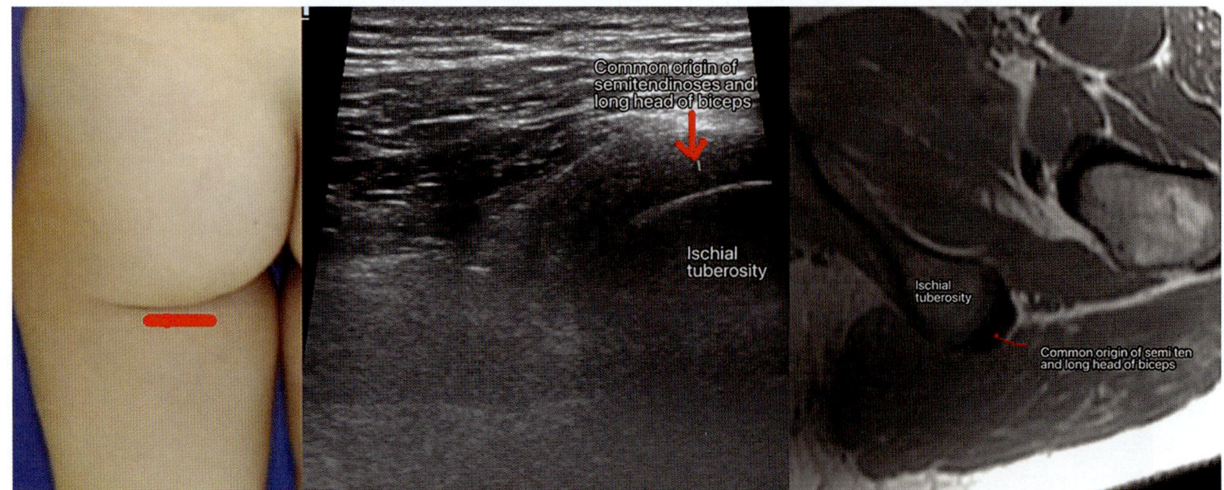

Fig. 3.9.38

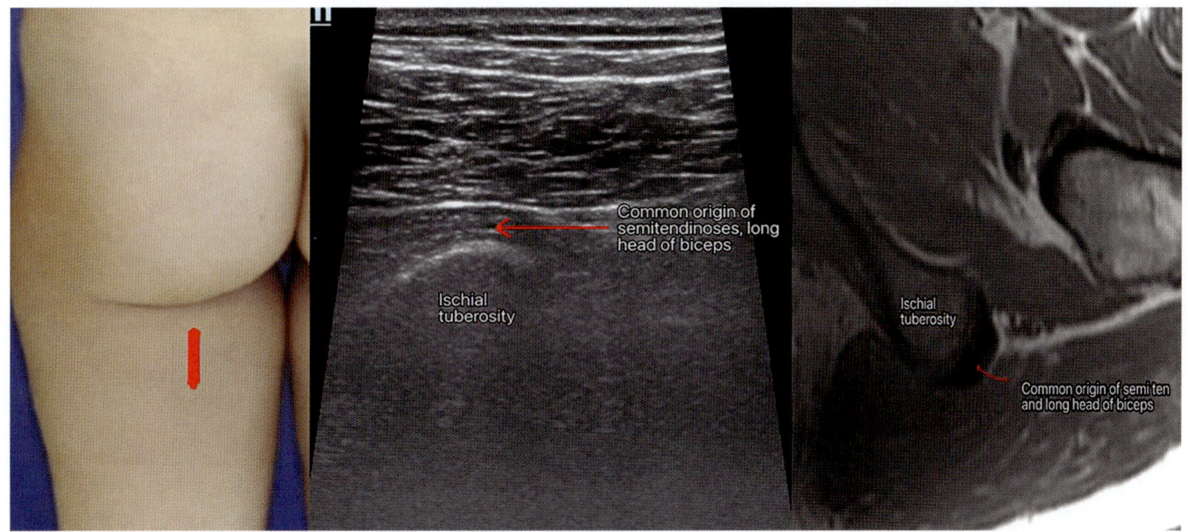

Fig. 3.9.39

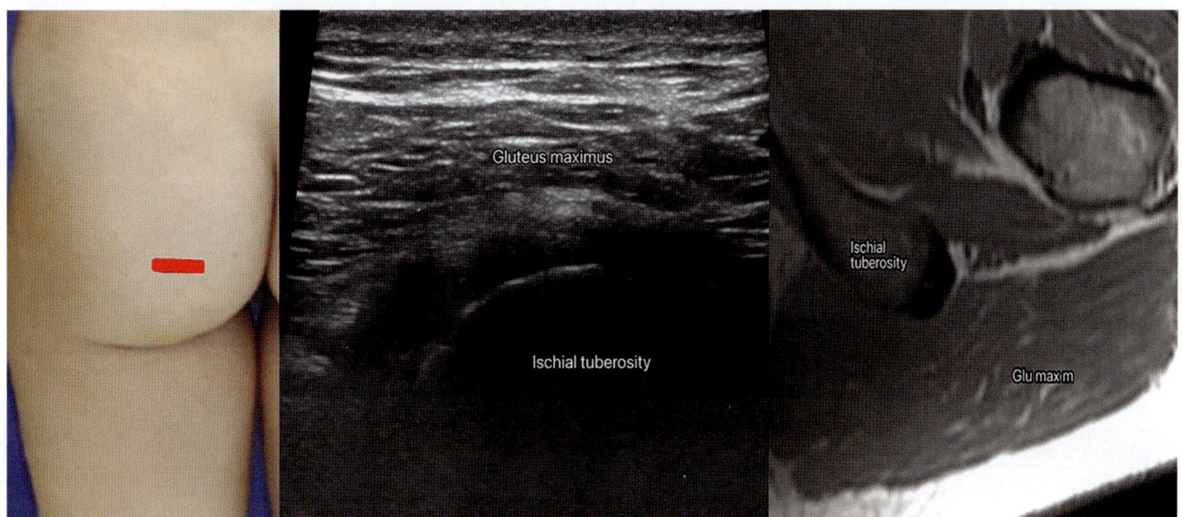

Fig. 3.9.40

probes gluteus maximus can be evaluated both long and short axis. By moving the probe just below we can identify the ischial tuberosity and insertion of the semimembranosus, semitendinosus and long head of biceps can be identified. Lateral to them sciatic nerve is seen as a flattened structure seen emerging from the piriformis muscle.

Pediatric hip: The baby is placed in supine or lateral position depending on the convenience and the images acquired in the coronal flexion view or the coronal neutral view. A high frequency linear probe is used and image is acquired at the triradiate cartilage.

Measurements are:

1. Bony rim of acetabulum (If the bony rim is angular, this point is easily recognized. If it is rounded, the point is taken when the concavity of bony acetabular roof changes into convexity of the ilium).
2. Centre of the labrum.
3. Lower limb of iliac bone (point where iliac bone meets the triradiate cartilage).

Alpha angle (Fig. 3.9.41): It is the angle between bony rim of acetabulum and lower limb of iliac bone.

Beta angle (Fig. 3.9.42): It is the angle between the bony rim of acetabulum and centre of labrum.

3.9.C Thigh

Thigh is the region between hip and knee joint. It has been divided into three compartments—anterior, medial and posterior compartments by extensions from fascia lata.

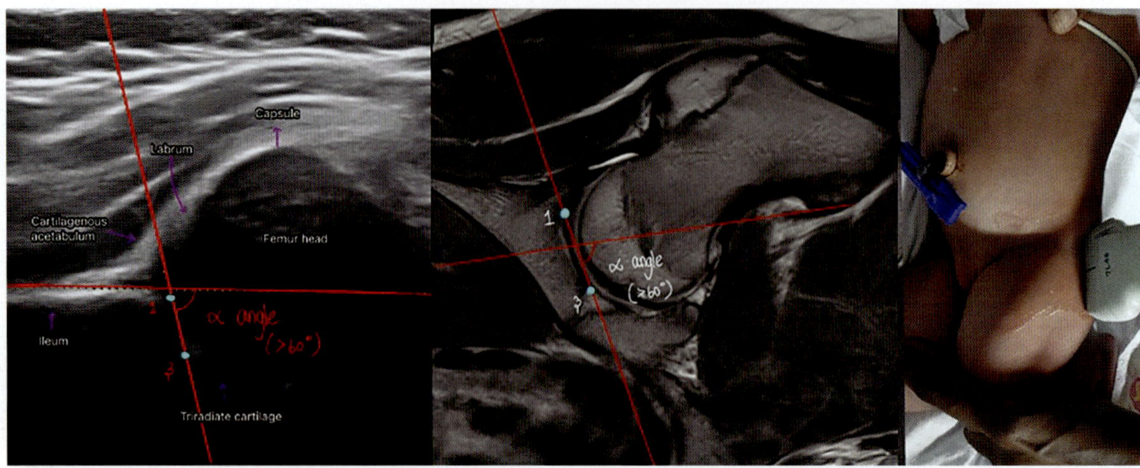

Fig. 3.9.41: Ultrasound and corresponding MRI—alpha angle

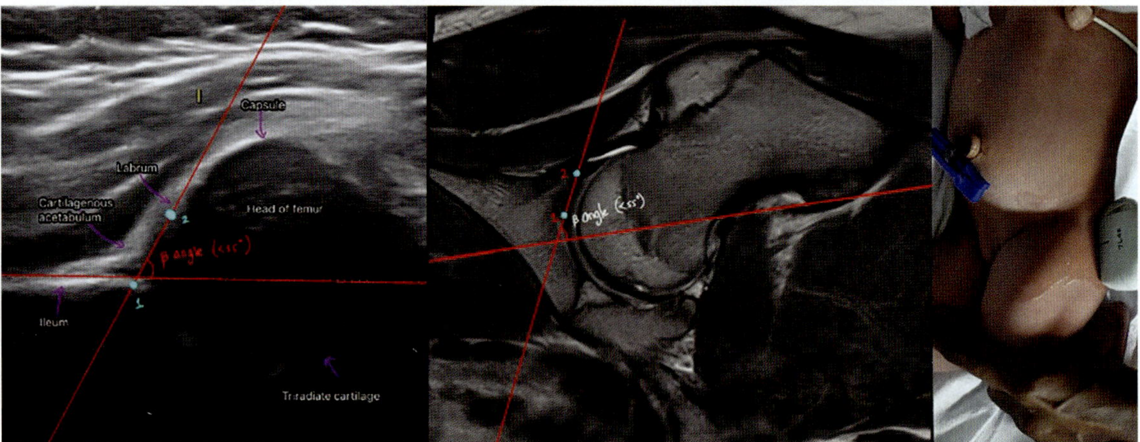

Fig. 3.9.42: Ultrasound and corresponding MRI—beta angle

Table 3.9.5: Muscles and nerves of thigh (Figs 3.9.43 to 3.9.47)

Compartment	*Muscles*	*Nerve of the compartment*	*Functions*
Medial compartment	Gracilis, pectineus, adductor longus, adductor brevis, adductor magnus, obturator externus.	Obturator nerve except pectineus which is also supplied by femoral nerve	Hip adduction, also helps in flexion and internal rotation, obturator externus—lateral rotator of hip joint
Anterior compartment	Iliacus, psoas major, sartorius, rectus femoris, vastus lateralis, vastus medius, vastus intermedius	Femoral nerve	Iliopsoas—flexion at hip joint Vastus muscles—extension of knee joint, rectus femoris—flexion of hip and extension of knee, sartorius—flexes both hip and knee joint
Posterior compartment	Biceps femoris—long and short head, semimembranosus, semi-tendinosus	Sciatic nerve (tibial nerve) except short head of biceps femoris supplied by common fibular nerve	Extension at hip joint and flexion at knee joint

Watershed muscles—have dual nerve supply: Biceps femoris (long and short head)—long head supplied by tibial nerve and short head by common fibular nerve, pectineus supplied by femoral and obturator nerve and adductor magnus (adductor and hamstring part) supplied by obturator and tibial nerve respectively.

Adductor canal: Also known by the **subsartorial** or **hunterian** canal bounded anteromedially by sartorius, anterolaterally by vastus medialis muscle, posteriorly bounded by the adductor longus and magnus muscle. It is a triangular passage seen in midthigh. The exit of this triangle is adductor hiatus which is a gap between adductor portion and ischiocondylar portion of adductor magnus. It is through this hiatus the vessels and nerves pass from thigh to popliteal fossa. Femoral artery, vein and saphenous nerve pass through this hiatus to popliteal fossa.

Table 3.9.6: Ossification centers of pelvis

Site	*Appearance*	*Fusion*
Ilium	8 weeks of gestation	
Ischium	18–22 weeks of gestation	7–9 years
Pubis	18–22 weeks of gestation	
Acetabulum	Puberty	20–25 years
Capital femoral epiphysis	3–6 months	
Shaft	7 weeks of gestation	
Greater trochanter	2–4 years	14–18 years
Lesser trochanter	Puberty	

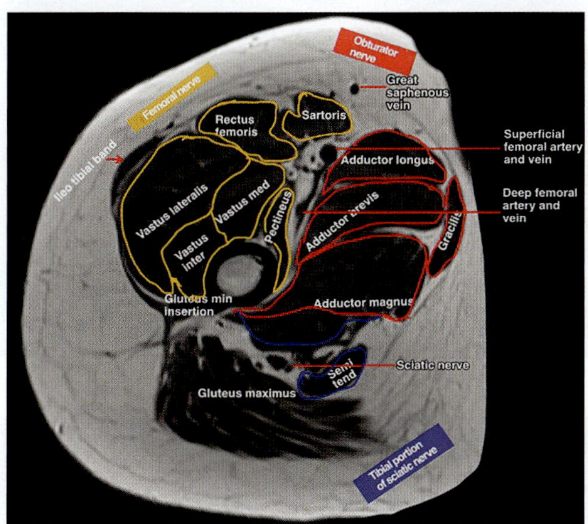

Fig. 3.9.43: MRI axial sections of thigh

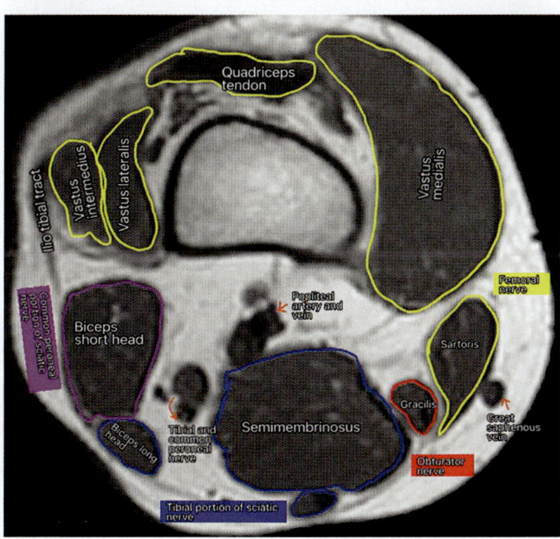

Fig. 3.9.44

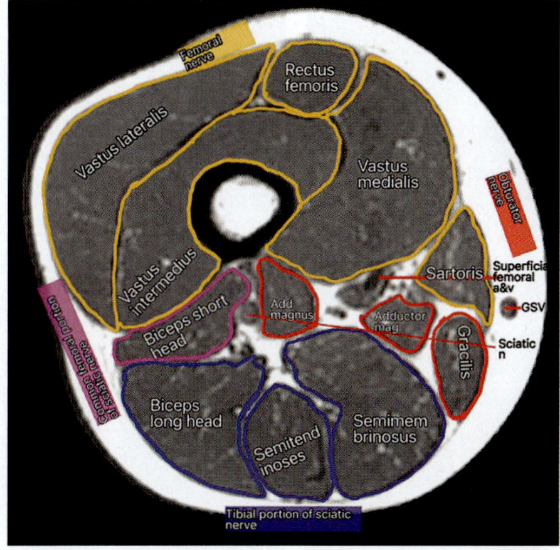

Fig. 3.9.45

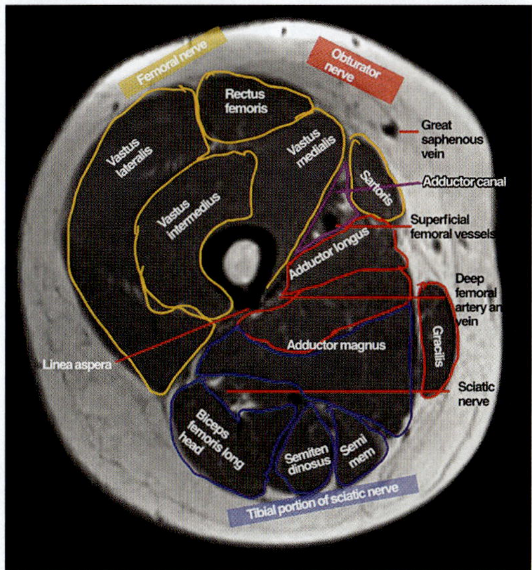

Fig. 3.9.46

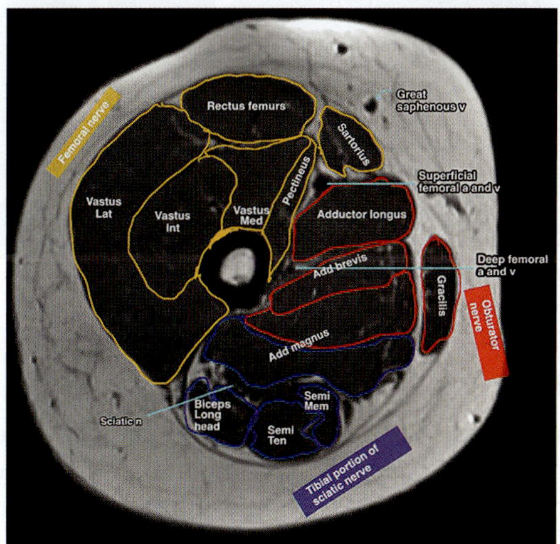

Fig. 3.9.47

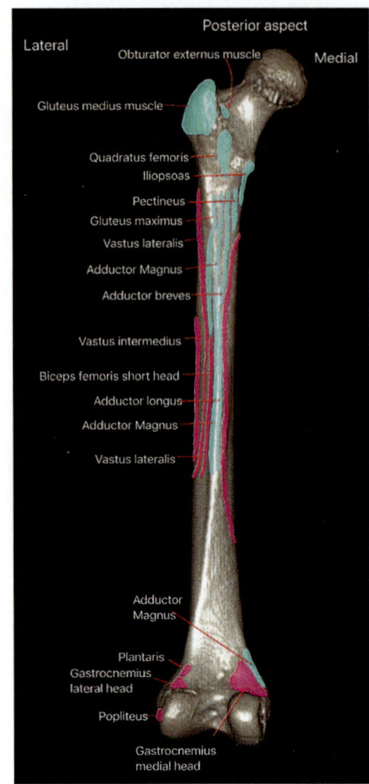

Fig. 3.9.48: Muscle attachments posterior aspect

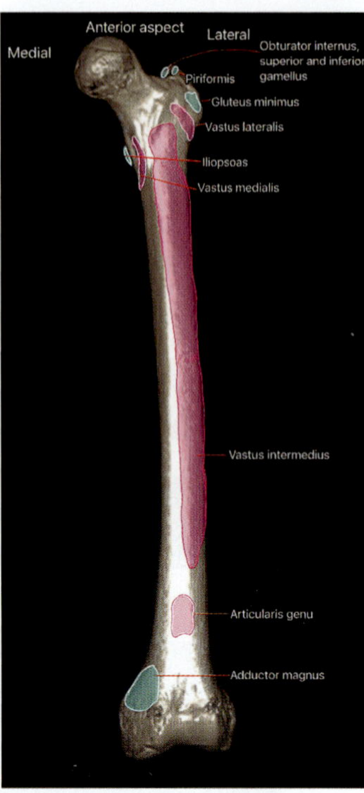

Fig. 3.9.49: Muscle attachments anterior aspect

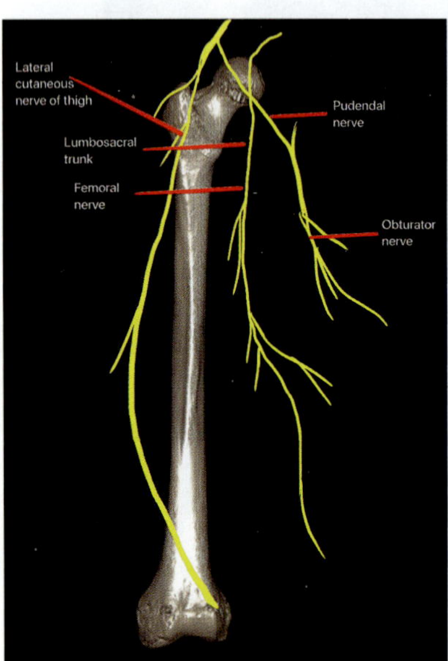

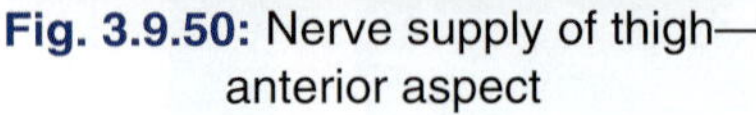

Fig. 3.9.50: Nerve supply of thigh—anterior aspect

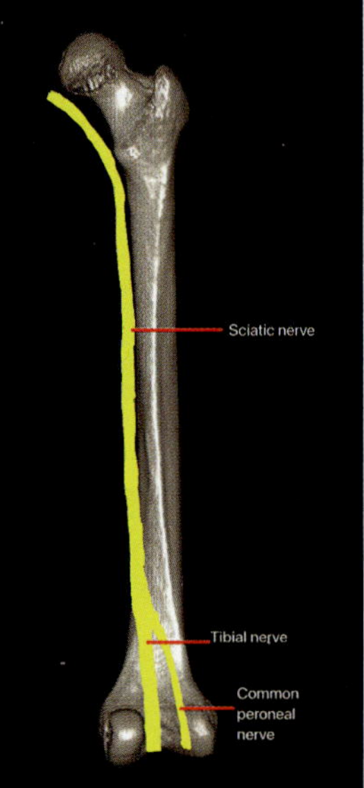

Fig. 3.9.51: Nerve supply of thigh—posterior aspect

3.9.D Knee Joint

The knee joint is a modified hinge joint between the femur, tibia, and patella. It is the largest synovial joint in the body and allows flexion and extension of the leg as well as some rotation in the flexed position. Saddle joint between the patella and femoral condyles.

Synovial membrane: Synovial surfaces surround all articular areas, capsule surrounds the entirety of joint. An intracapsular extrasynovial space exists between menisci. It is actively supported by: (1) Quadriceps attachment, (2) laterally by iliotibial band (ITB), (3) medially by tibial collateral ligament, (4) posteriorly reinforced by oblique popliteal ligament, (5) posterolaterally pierced by popliteus.

Axial Sections of Knee Joint

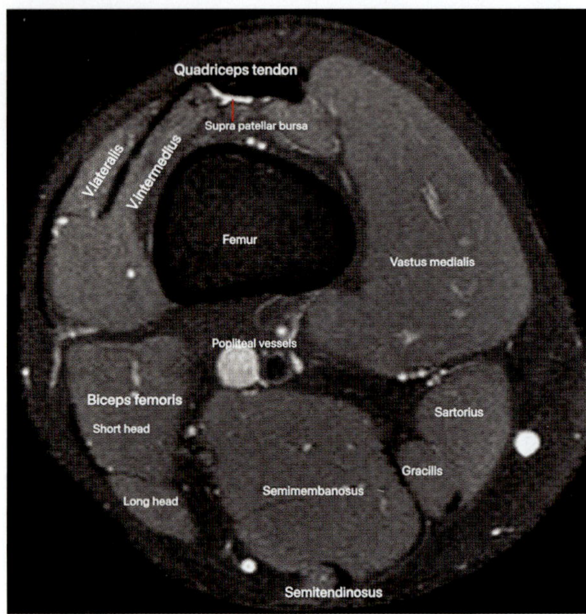

Fig. 3.9.52

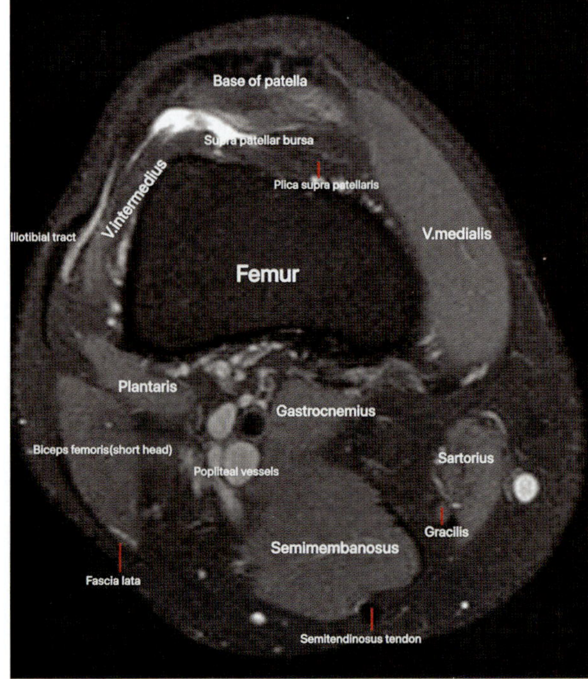

Fig. 3.9.53

3

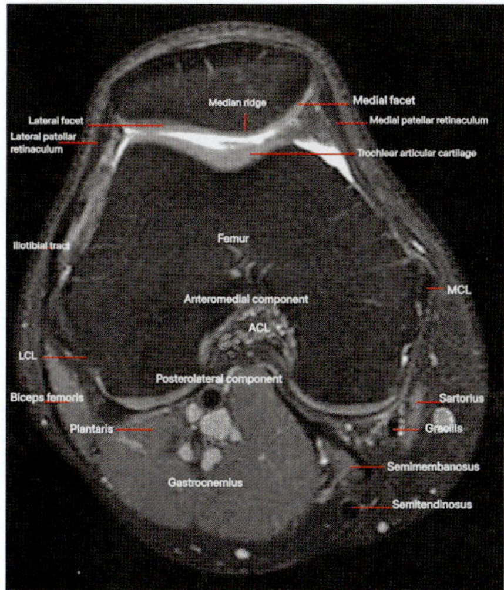

Fig. 3.9.54

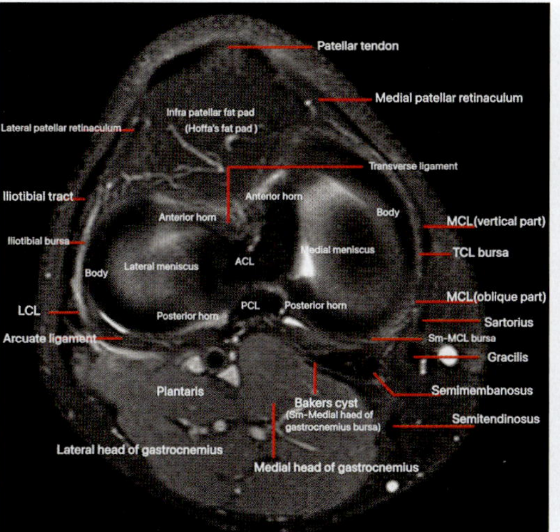

Fig. 3.9.55

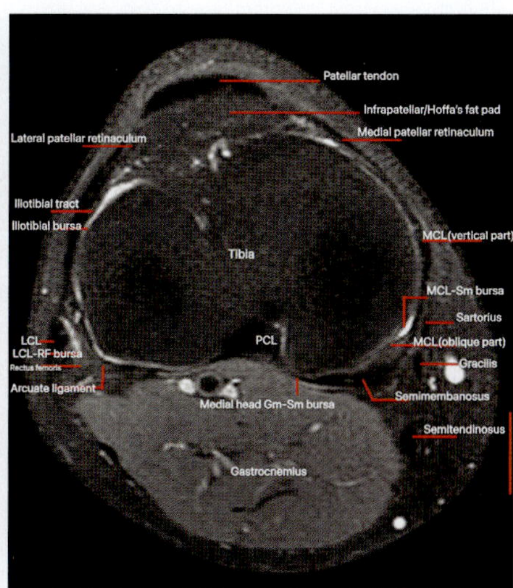

Fig. 3.9.56

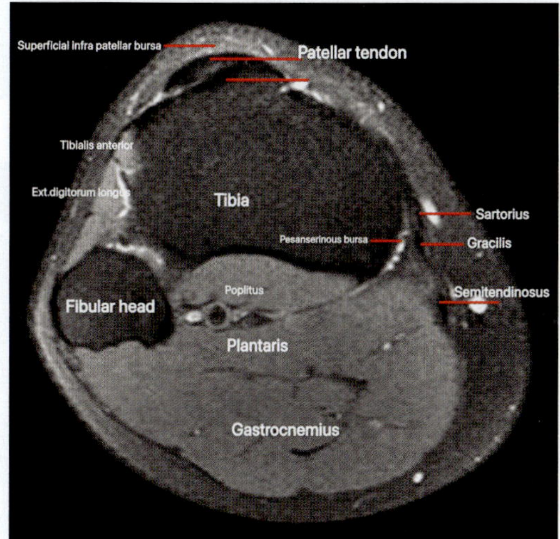

Fig. 3.9.57

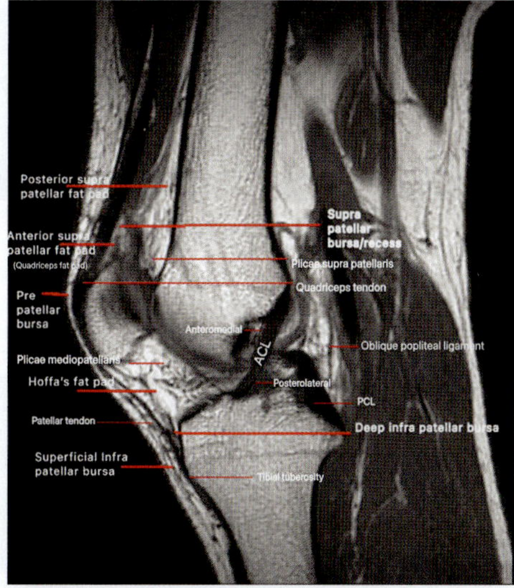

Fig. 3.9.59

Sagittal Sections of Knee Joint

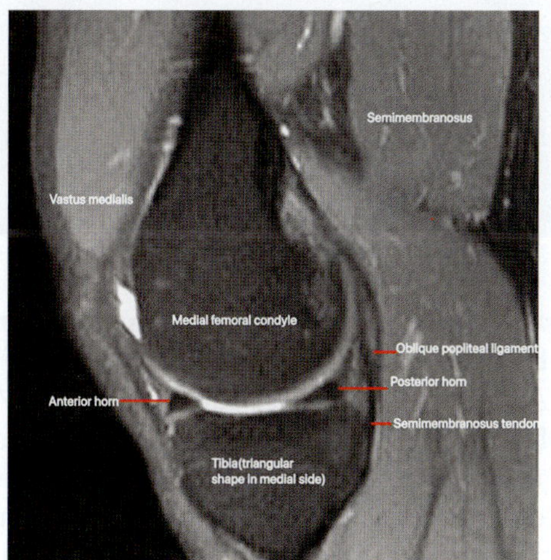

Fig. 3.9.58

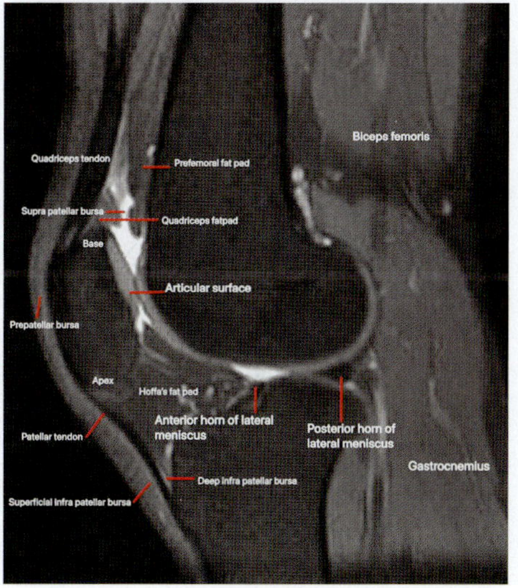

Fig. 3.9.60

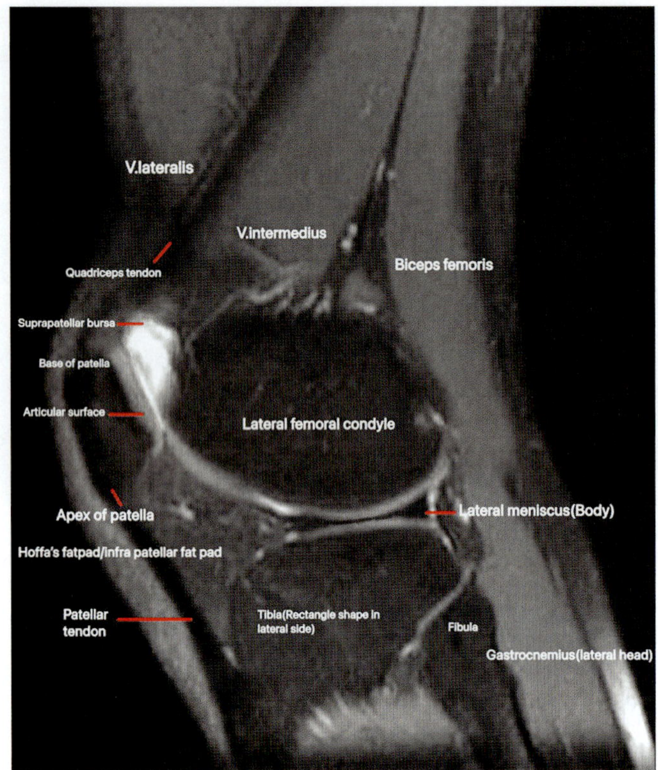

Fig. 3.9.61

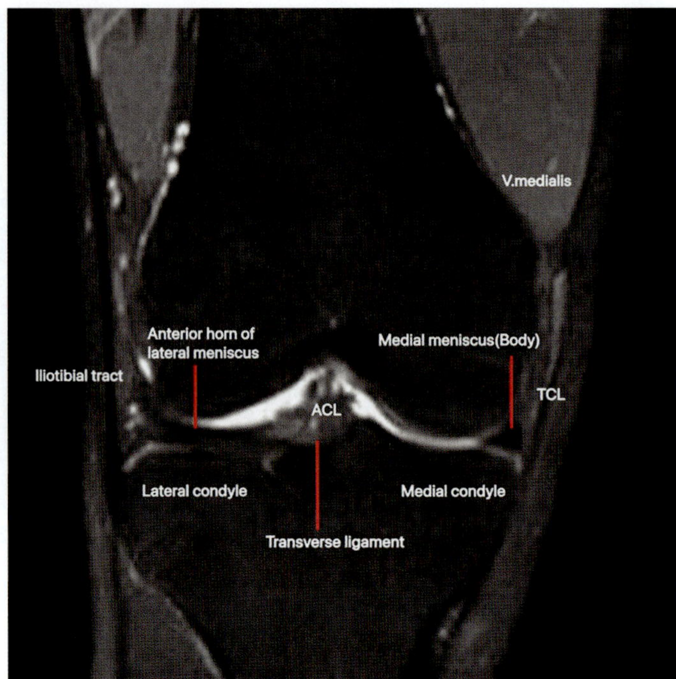

Fig. 3.9.63

Coronal Sections of Knee Joint

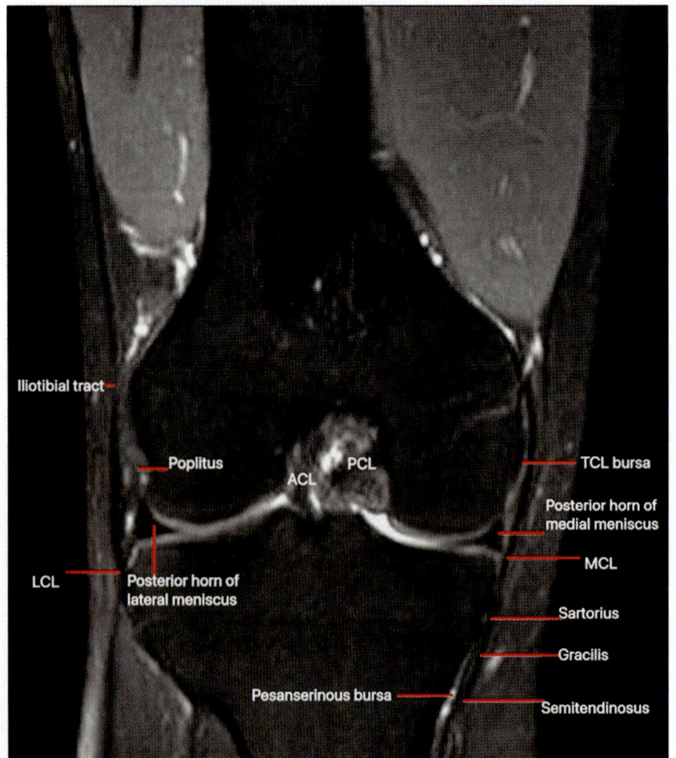

Fig. 3.9.62

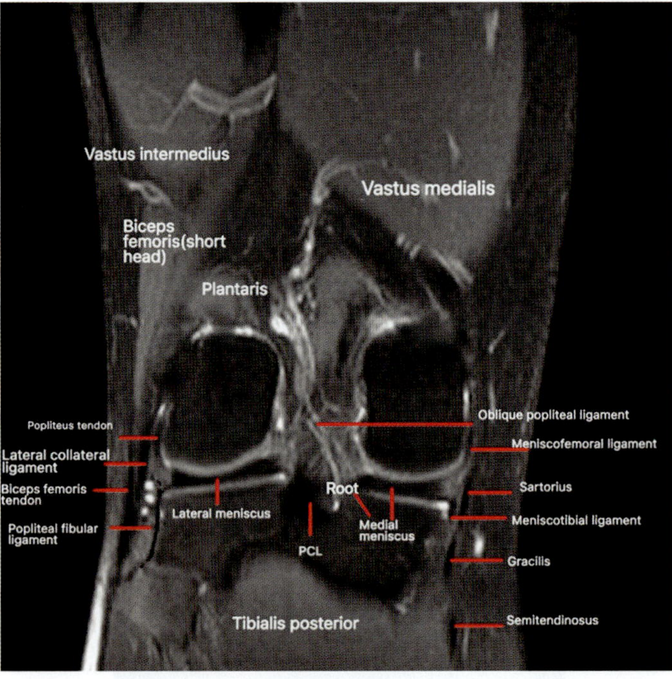

Fig. 3.9.64

Intracapsular ligaments: **Anterior intermeniscal ligament**—it connects the anterior limbs of the two menisci. Anterior (Humphrey) and posterior (Wrisberg) meniscofemoral ligaments—the lateral meniscus is attached to the medial femoral condyle via the anterior and posterior meniscofemoral ligament of Humphrey and Wrisberg. Cruciate ligaments: Cross each other to form an "x" shape. Anterior cruciate ligament: From the anterior tibial plateau to the lateral femoral condyle. Posterior cruciate ligament: From the posterior tibial intercondylar area to the medial femoral condyle.

Extracapsular ligaments: Patellar retinacular ligaments, medial collateral ligament, lateral collateral ligament, oblique popliteal ligament, arcuate popliteal ligament, popliteofibular ligament, patella ligament.

Cruciate ligaments

Anterior cruciate ligament: It is intra-articular and extra-synovial ligament. ACL prevents anterior translation of tibia. ACL is composed of 3–5 layers of fibers. It originates from postero-medial aspect of the lateral femoral condyle and it inserts into the anterior aspect of intercondylar eminence. It fan out femoral attachment to tibial attachment. It is divided into femoral attachment site, mid-part and tibial attachment. ACL has two components: (1) Antero-medial bundle; (2) Postero-lateral bundle. Between the fibers there can be fat, synovium or fluid will be there. Due to that ACL hyperintense on PD/T2 sequences.

Posterior cruciate ligament: It is also intra-articular and extra-synovial ligament. PCL prevents posterior translation of tibia. It originates from inner surface of the anterior aspect of the medial femoral condyle and it inserts at far posterior aspect of the tibial plateau. PCL has two components: (1) Antero-lateral bundle, (2) Postero-medial bundle.

Menisci: Anterior and posterior roots, anterior and posterior horns and body. Each menisci is divided into three zones—peripheral vascular zone which heals well, a middle zone with vascularity in the periphery and a central avascular zone with poor healing capability. Medial meniscus-shape—"C"-shaped and wider than lateral meniscus. Horns are equilateral triangles in cross section; anterior horn is smaller than posterior horn. Body of menisci—seen as continuous bow-tie sign for at least 2 contiguous sagittal sections of 4 mm thickness. Absent bow tie sign can be seen in bucket-handle meniscal tear. Anterior root of medial meniscus—attaches to tibial plateau, anterior to ACL (from anterior to posterior, the attachments are—anterior root of medial meniscus, ACL, anterior root of lateral meniscus). Posterior root of medial meniscus—attaches anteromedial to PCL in the slope of the intercondylar fossa. The posterior root of lateral meniscus is anterior to the root of medial meniscus. Lateral meniscus-shape—"C-shaped and smaller than medial meniscus". Horns are equilateral triangles in cross section; anterior horn is smaller than posterior horn. Anterior root of lateral meniscus—attaches in tibial plateau, posterior to anterior horn of medial meniscus. The root has a striated appearance due to divergent fibers and can mimic a tear. Posterior root of lateral meniscus—attaches to the lateral tibial spine anterior to attachment of posterior root of medial meniscus.

Medial meniscus has anterior, body and posterior horn. Both medial and lateral menisci are divided into red-red, red-white and white-white zone depending on their blood supply. Outer 1/3rd has rich blood supply and has good chances of healing. Posterior medial meniscus root ligament (PMMRL) attaches immediately anterior to the posterior cruciate ligament. PMMRL is responsible for maintain the hoop stress and it also prevents the meniscal extrusion.

Lateral meniscus is more circular than medial meniscus and it forms tight C-shape. It is symmetric in width from anterior to posterior. Posterior horn is higher than anterior horn. It is relatively more mobile and more loosely attached to the joint capsule.

Medial supporting ligamentous structure: The medial supporting ligamentous structures of the knee are divided into 3 layers. Layers of 1 and 2 fused anteriorly, with layers of 2 and 3 fused posteriorly. The deep crural fascia makes up the superficial layer (layer 1) on the medial side of the knee. This fascia is connected with the fascia overlying the vastus medialis muscle in the anterior, and with the sartorius muscle in the posterior. The superficial section of the medial collateral ligament, also known as the tibial collateral ligament, makes up layer 2. Layer 3 consists of the joint capsule, the deep portion of the MCL, which is also called the mid-third medial capsular ligament, the menisco-femoral ligament, the menisco-tibial ligament and the patella-meniscal ligament. These ligaments represent the thickening of medial joint capsule, firmly adheres to the superficial MCL fibers posteriorly.

Medial collateral ligament: Extra-capsular in location. It has superficial and deep component. Superficial portion is thick, it extends from femoral condyle to proximal tibia. Deep component has meniscal attachment. It originates from the medial femoral epicondyle antero-inferior to the adductor tubercle. Insertion: It has two insertion sites at the upper medial surface of the tibia: (a) Soft tissue along the antero-inferior band of the semimembranous tendon then continues inferiorly to attach to the tibial periosteum deep to the pes-anserine attachment, (b) posterior aspect of the medial collateral ligament blending into the posterior oblique ligament and knee capsule. It stabilizes the valgus stress. The MCL's surface layer is made up of vertically aligned fibres. It is also referred to as the MCL's vertical component. The posterior oblique section of the MCL is found posterior to the vertical component of the MCL. This section of the MCL's posterior oblique is fused to layer 3 and linked to the posteromedial meniscus. The posterior oblique ligament is another name for this conjoined structure. This structure accepts fibres from the semimembranosus tendon and synovial sheath around the back of the knee. The oblique popliteal ligament envelops the posterior side of the femoral condyle.

Lateral supporting ligamentous structures: The lateral supporting ligamentous structures are divided into 3 layers. Layer 1 consists of ilio-tibial band, lateral fascia, short and long head of biceps tendon. Layer 2 consists of lateral patellar retinaculum and patella-femoral ligament. Layer 3 consists of postero-lateral corner complex. It consists of popliteus tendon, fibular collateral ligament (FCL), popliteal fibular ligament (PFL) and the posterolateral joint capsule. The posterolateral capsule is reinforced by fabellofibular ligament and arcuate ligament.

Lateral collateral ligament: Extra-capsular in location. It does not have meniscal attachment. It originates from a small bone depression just posterior to the lateral femoral epicondyle and inserted in lateral aspect of the fibular head as conjoined tendon with biceps femoris.

Patellar retinaculum: **Lateral patellar retinaculum** has superficial and deep part. Superficial part originates from vastus lateralis fascia, lowest fibers of ilio-tibial band and deep part originates from lateral patellar ligament, transverse ligament. It inserts onto the lateral aspect of patellar ligament, patella and quadriceps tendon and finally blends with lateral tibial condyle through knee joint capsule.

Medial patellar retinaculum: It has superficial and deep part. Superficial part originates from vastus medialis, Sartorius, and medial collateral ligament and deep part originates from medial patellar femoral retinaculum and adjacent fascia. It inserts onto the medial aspect of patellar ligament patella and quadriceps tendon and finally blends with medial tibial condyle through kene joint capsule, resisting lateral patellar dislocation.

Corner complex:

Posteromedial corner complex: Components are semimenbranous tendon, oblique popliteal ligament, posterior oblique ligament, posterior-medial capsule and posterior horn of medial meniscus.

Posterolateral corner complex (Fig. 3.9.65): The three major static stabilizers of the PLC are the fibular (lateral) collateral ligament (FCL), the popliteus tendon (PLT) and the popliteofibular ligament (PFL). The PLC's lateral supporting structures were separated into three layers: The iliotibial band, its anterior expansion, and the biceps femoris were defined as the superficial layer.

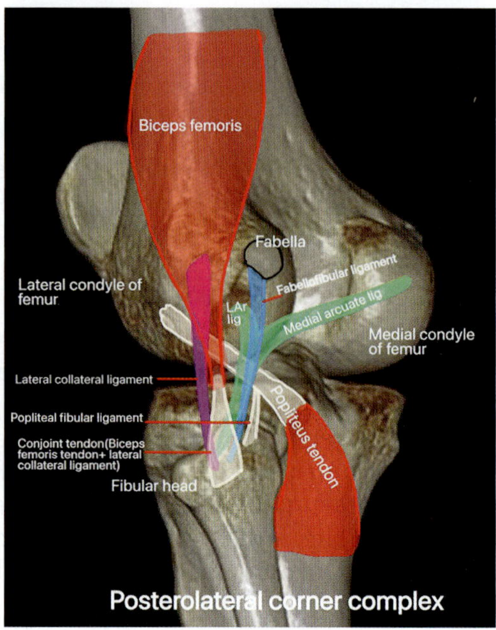

Fig. 3.9.65

The lateral patellar retinaculum, the two patellofemoral ligaments, and the patellomeniscal ligament make up the intermediate layer. The deep layer was described as being composed of the lateral capsule, lateral collateral ligament (LCL), coronary ligament (lateral meniscotibial ligament), arcuate ligament, popliteus muscle-tendon unit, popliteofibular ligament (PFL), and fabellofibular ligament. Three main stabilizers include the lateral collateral ligament, popliteus tendon, and popliteofibular ligament. Function: The structures of the PLC are primarily responsible for resisting varus angulation—sometimes referred to as varus rotation—and external tibial rotation. They act as secondary stabilizers, in conjunction with the cruciate ligaments, to prevent anterior and posterior translation during the early phase of flexion.

Bursa Around Knee Joint

Anterior bursa: Suprapatellar bursa, prepatellar bursa, superficial infrapatellar bursa, deep infrapatellar bursa. Medial and posteromedial bursa—pes anserine bursa, tibial collateral bursa, semi-membranous—tibial collateral bursa, semi-membranous—gastrocnemius bursa. Lateral and posterolateral bursa—iliotibial bursa, popliteal recess, fibular collateral—biceps femoris bursa.

Suprapatellar recess: It is the largest recess in the knee joint and it communicates freely with remainder of the joint.

Plicae: Synovial plicae are remnants of synovial folds which separate anatomical compartments of the knee during fetal development and fail to regress. The plicae

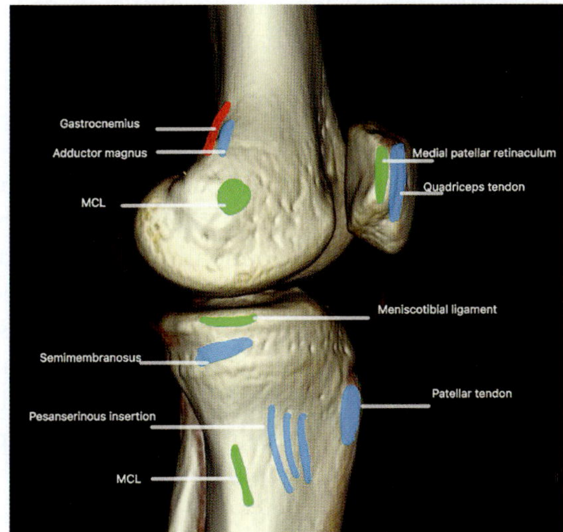

Fig. 3.9.66: Muscle attachments—medial aspect

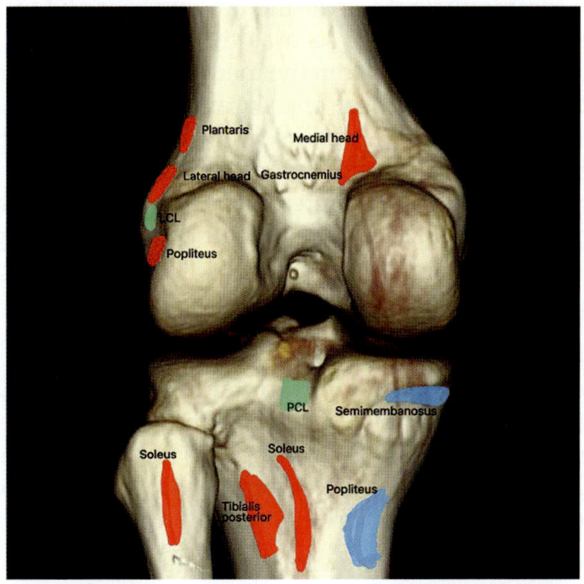

Fig. 3.9.68: Muscle attachments—posterior aspect

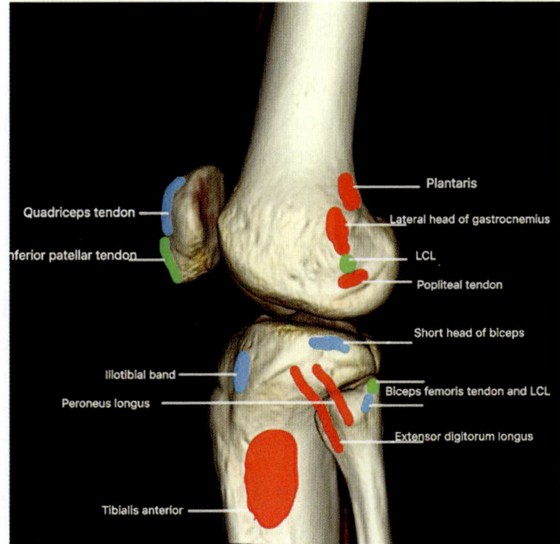

Fig. 3.9.67: Muscle attachments—lateral aspect

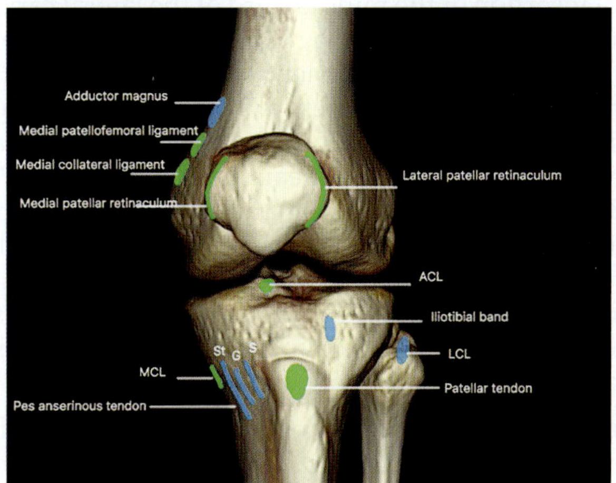

Fig. 3.9.69: Muscle attachments—anterior aspect

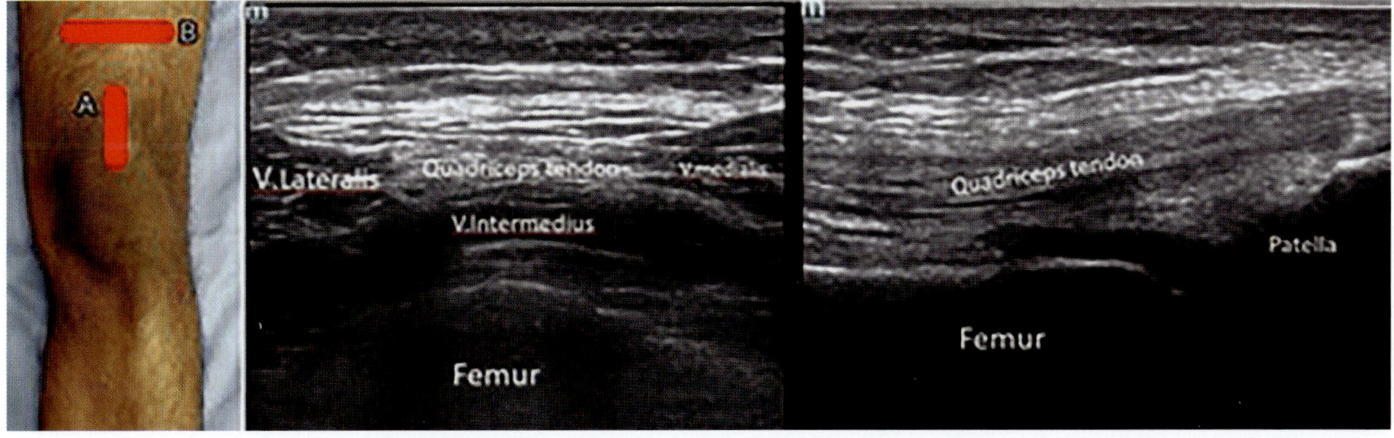

Fig. 3.9.70: Ultrasound of anterior knee—quadriceps tendon

seen commonly include the medial, superior and inferior patellar plicae and are seen as thin fibrous bands. The medial plica extends from the medial joint capsule to the medial patellar facet seen on axial and sagittal images. The superior plica is seen to course through the suprapatellar recess. The inferior plica extends from the inferior pole of patella to the roof of intercondylar notch through the Hoffa's fat pad. Plica may get thickened and produce pain.

Fat pad around knee joint: Infrapatellar (Hoffa's) fat pad, suprapatellar fat pad, quadriceps fat pad.

Avulsion sites

Possible site of avulsion from femur: (a) Posterolateral intercondylar notch (ACL origin), (b) Mid-medial intercondylar notch (PCL origin), (c) Medial epicondyle (MCL origin), (d) Avulsion fragment from the superior aspect of patella (quadriceps tendon avulsion).

Possible site of avulsion from tibia: (a) Tibial tuberosity avulsion/Osgood–Schlatter disease (patellar tendon insertion), (b) Segond fracture (cortical avulsion of the tibial insertion of the middle third of the lateral capsular ligament), (c) Reverse Segond fracture (avulsion of the deep capsular component of the medial collateral ligament), (d) Bony fragment in the intercondylar notch (tibial insertion of the ACL), (e) Avulsed fragment arise from the posterior tibial plateau (tibial insertion of PCL), (f) Bone fragment arising from the styloid process fibular head/arcuate sign (arcuate complex injury), (g) Avulsion of posterolateral aspect of fibular head (biceps femoris tendon insertion site), (h) Sinding-Larsen-Johansson syndrome/jumpers knee (avulsed bony fragment arising from the inferior aspect of patella).

Gerdy's tubercle: Site on the lateral condyle of the proximal tibia (where it is located anterolaterally) where the iliotibial band and anterior tibialis muscle inserts. Termed lighthouse to the knee, because it serves as an important surgical landmark. Avulsion of Gerdy's tubercle indicates iliotibial band injury.

Ultrasound Examination of the Knee Joint

Anterior knee

Quadriceps tendon (Fig. 3.9.70): With the patient reclined, the anterior aspect of the knee is inspected. By inserting a tiny pillow beneath the popliteal gap, a knee flexion of around 20°–30° can be achieved. The quadriceps tendon is visible in sagittal US pictures taken in the midline while retaining the probe's distal edge over the patella. Due to the tight apposition and distal union of the quadriceps tendon, this tendon appears multilayered in long-axis and short-axis planes.

Suprapatellar recess (Fig. 3.9.71): The suprapatellar fat pad is located close cranially to the patella, deep in the distal portion of the quadriceps tendon. The prefemoral fat pad presents as a big hyperechoic area immediately superficial to the femur. The suprapatellar synovial recess is a thin hypoechoic S-shaped region that is deep to the quadriceps tendon and suprapatellar fat pad and superficial to the prefemoral fat in normal situations.

Femoral trochlea (Fig. 3.9.72): On axial planes, the femoral V-shaped trochlea and the overlying articular cartilage are evaluated with full knee flexion. The quadriceps tendon is forced anteriorly by the femoral trochlea and takes a curved path over it in this posture.

Medial Side of Knee

Medial patellar retinaculum (Fig. 3.9.73): Axial planes are used to image the medial and lateral retinacula on each side of the patella—they show as bilayered structures that cannot be distinguished from the underlying joint

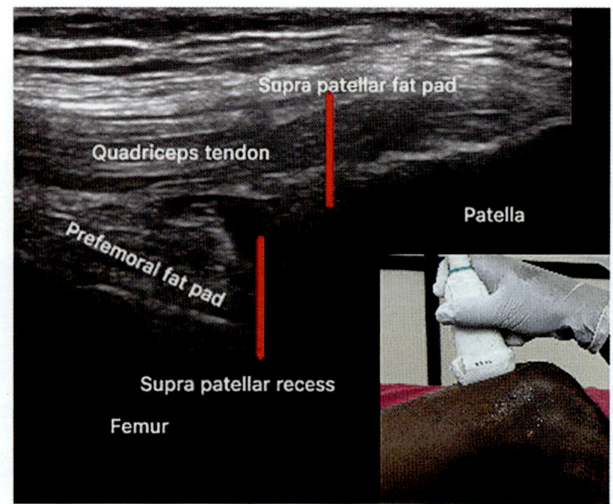

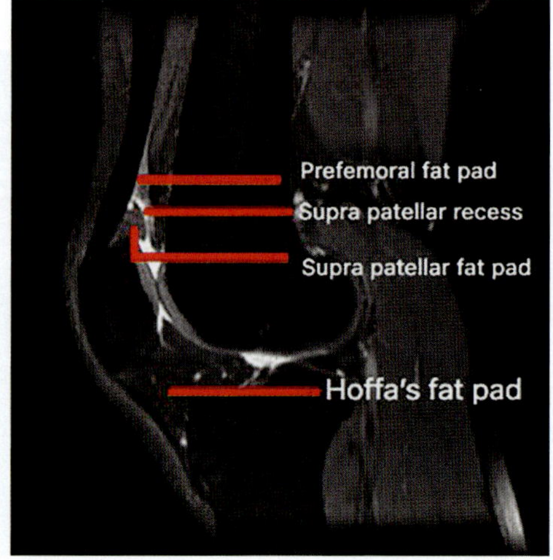

Fig. 3.9.71: Suprapatellar recess

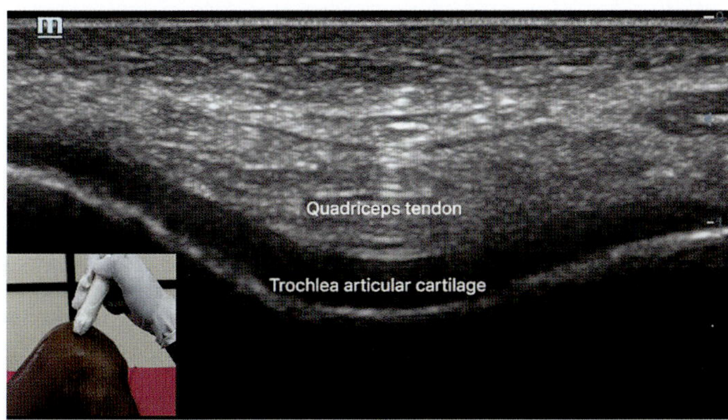

Fig. 3.9.72: Femoral trochlea

capsule. By tilting and pushing the transducer internally while maintaining the knee extended, an attempt can be made to examine the medial articular facet of the patella with ultrasound.

Medial collateral ligament (Fig. 3.9.74): The patient is advised to rotate the leg externally while maintaining 20°–30° of knee flexion for medial knee assessment. Position the transducer obliquely above the medial collateral ligament's long axis. This ligament should be thoroughly examined along its full length. During valgus stress, dynamic scanning can help determine its integrity.

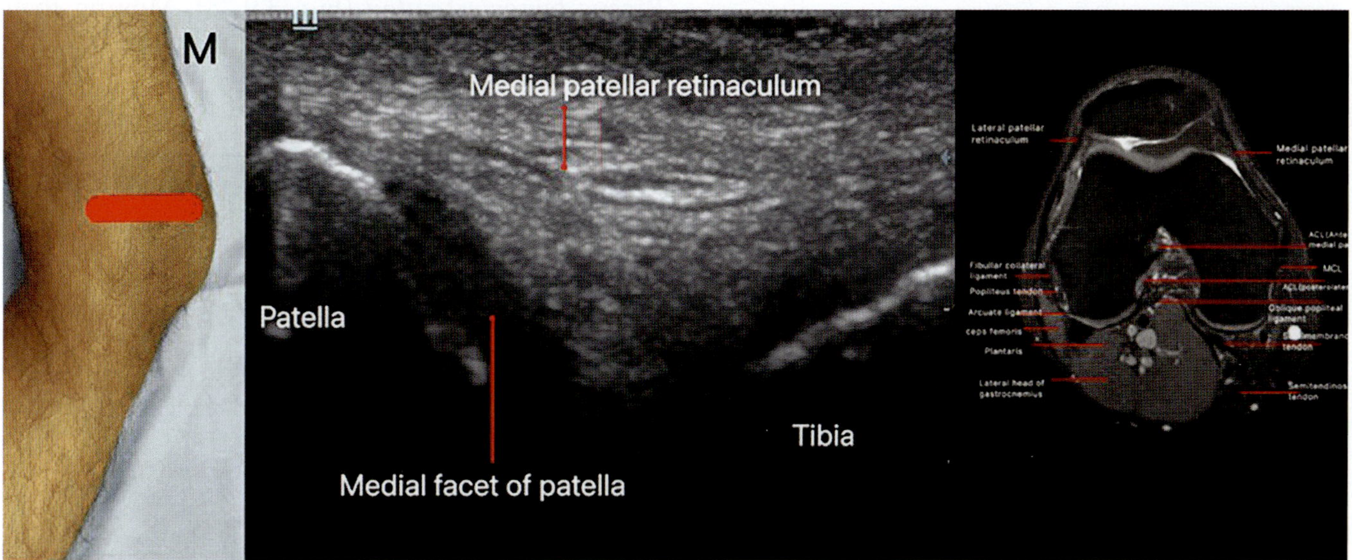

Fig. 3.9.73: Medial patellar retinaculum

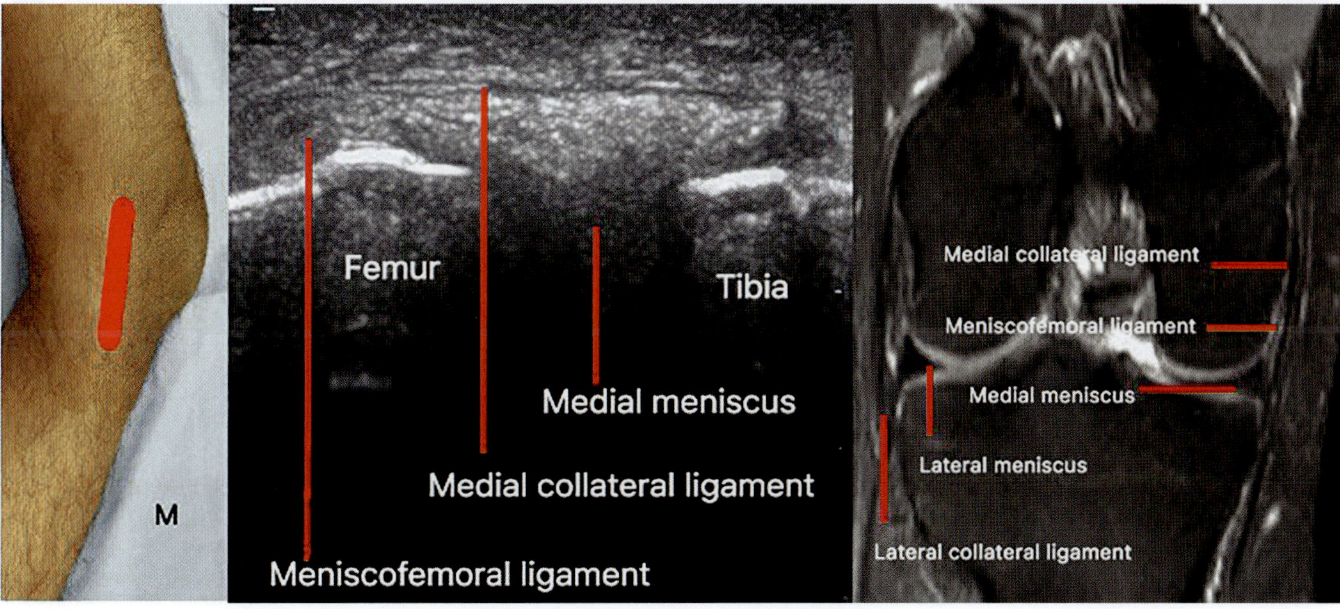

Fig. 3.9.74: Medial collateral ligament

Inferior Side of Knee Joint

Patellar tendon (Fig. 3.9.75): Using long- and short-axis planes, examine the patellar tendon from its cranial origin to its distal insertion. Because the lower pole of the patella has a V-shaped appearance, it is important to remember that the tendon inserts not only on the apex of the bone, but also on the inferolateral and inferomedial borders. Because tendinopathy can occur outside of the midline, short-axis US pictures of the proximal patellar tendon should also be taken. Examine the intracapsular Hoffa fat pad deep to the patellar tendon, as well as the deep infrapatellar bursa between the distal patellar tendon and the anterior side of the tibial epiphysis.

Lateral Side of Knee

Iliotibial band (Fig. 3.9.76): Internally rotate the patient's leg while maintaining 20°–30° of knee flexion for lateral knee assessment. To approach the Gerdy's tubercle, follow the iliotibial band down its long axis. If you are not sure whether the probe is in the right place, remember that the iliotibial band is placed between the anterior and middle third of the lateral portion of the knee and is orientated along the major axis of the thigh.

Lateral collateral ligament (Fig. 3.9.77): Place the lower edge of the probe on the peroneal head with the knee extended, then rotate the top edge of the probe anteriorly until the lateral collateral ligament appears as long as feasible in the US image. The popliteal tendon can be seen in its bony groove just deep to the proximal section of the lateral collateral ligament.

Biceps femoris tendon (Fig. 3.9.78): Moving to the posterolateral aspect of the knee, examine the biceps femoris muscle and tendon by means of long- and short-axis planes. Careful evaluation of the myotendinous

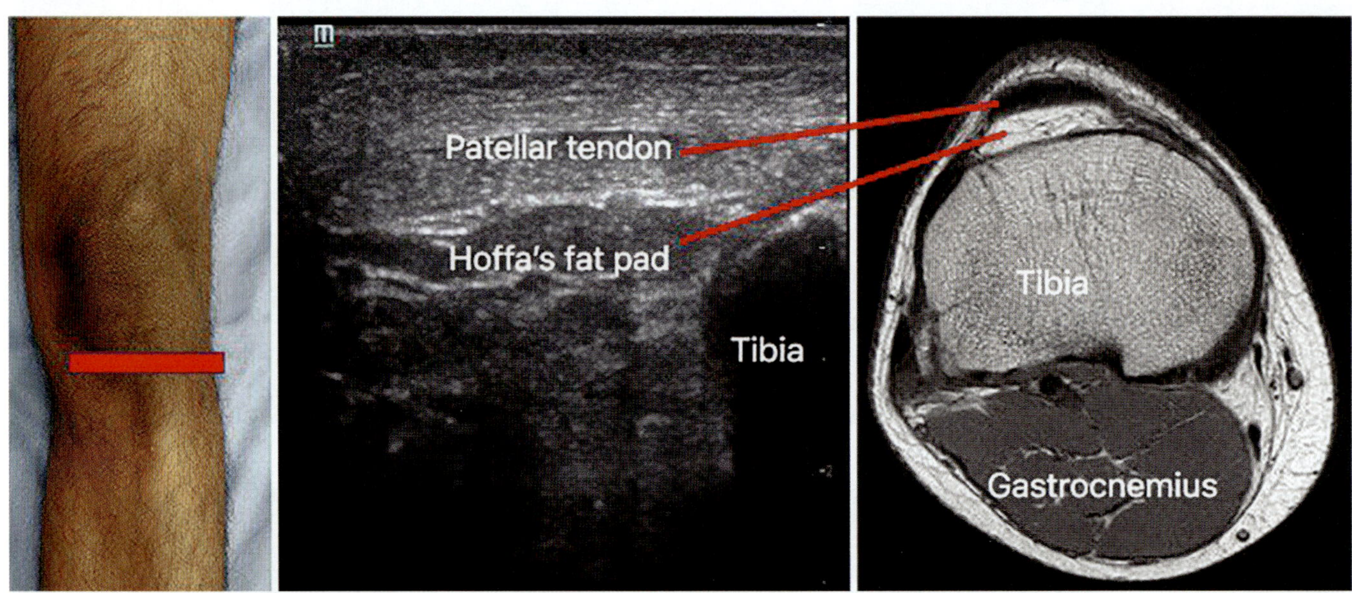

Fig. 3.9.75: Patellar tendon

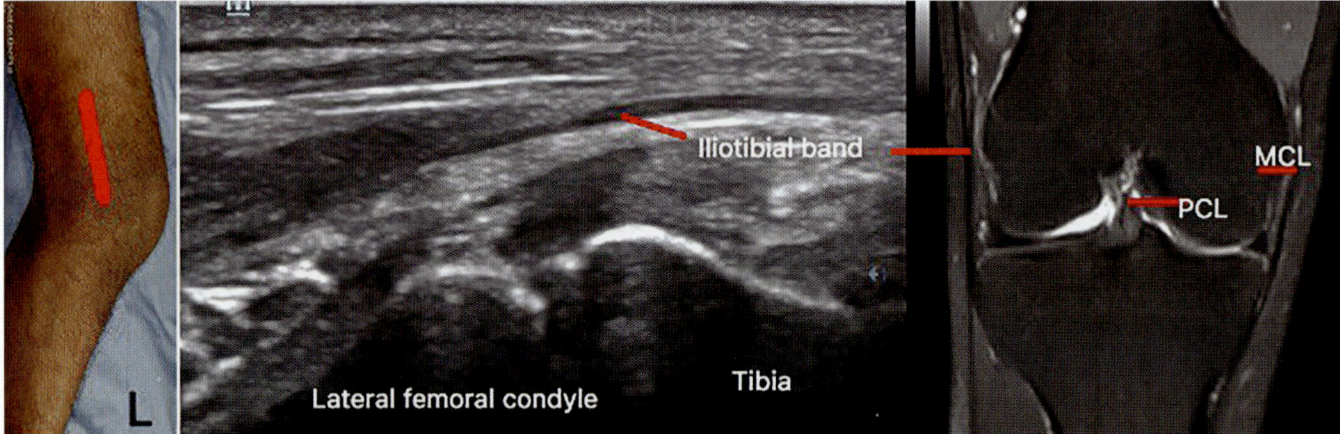

Fig. 3.9.76: Iliotibial band

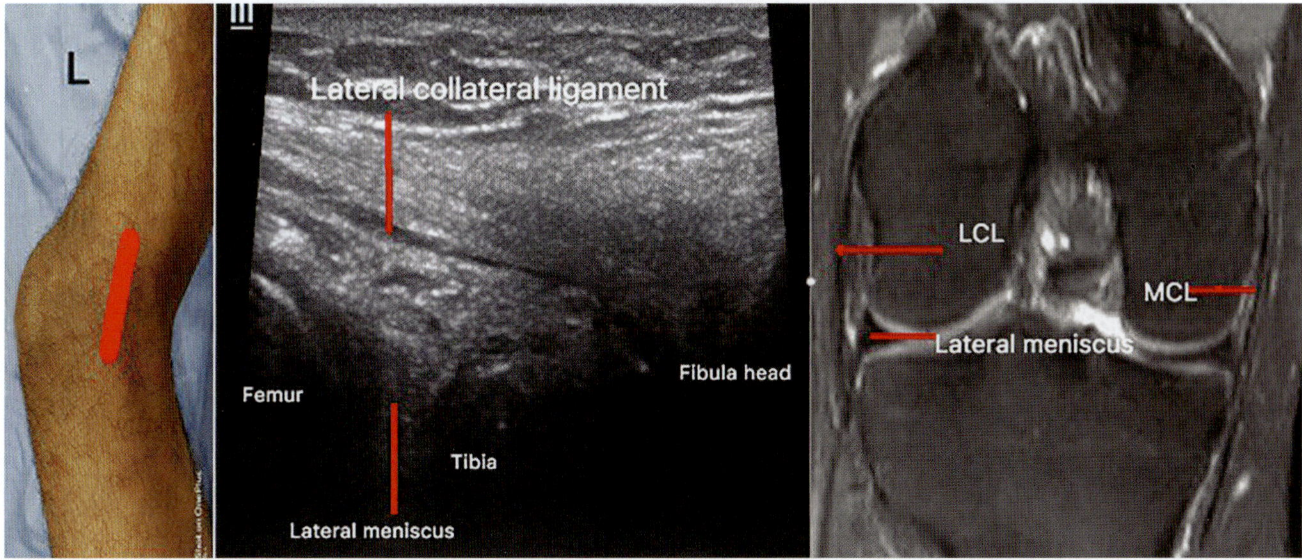

Fig. 3.9.77: Lateral collateral ligament

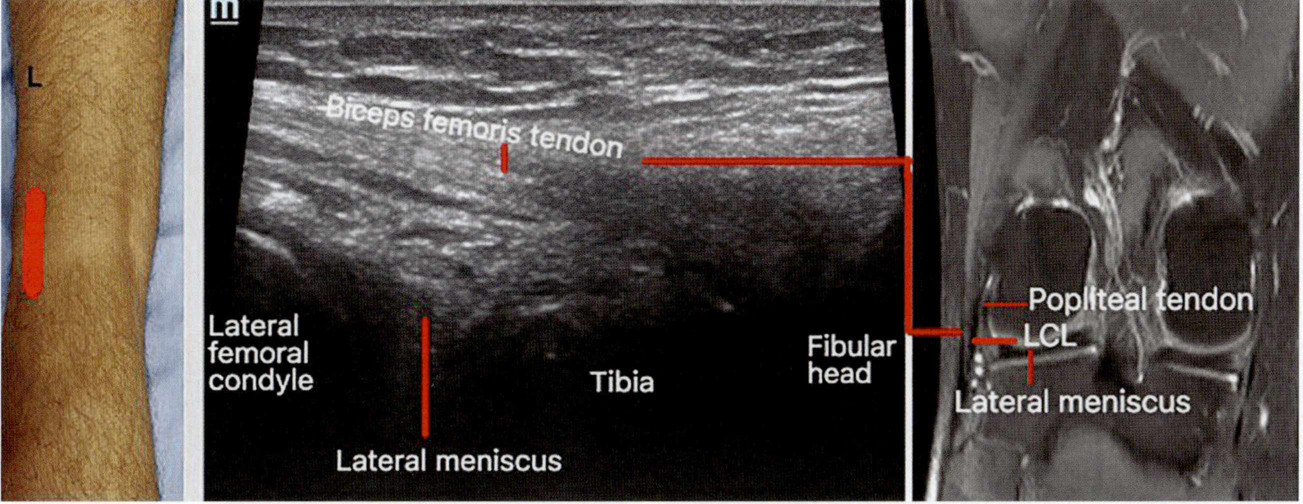

Fig. 3.9.78: Biceps femoris tendon

junction of the two heads of the biceps femoris muscle because this is a common site of sport-related tears. The biceps femoris tendon can be followed straight downward from its origin to the fibular head.

Peroneal nerve (Fig. 3.9.79): Determine where the common peroneal nerve arises from the sciatic nerve. Follow the common peroneal nerve along the lateral part of the popliteal space to the fibular head and neck on its short axis. The peroneal nerve can be discovered behind the biceps femoris.

Knee Joint Normograms

Tibial offset distance

Landmarks: This can be measured by drawing a line vertically from the lateral edge of the lateral femoral condyle on knee radiograph in AP projection (Fig. 3.9.80). This line will pass through the tibial condyle. Normal range: The distance between the line parallel to the lateral edge of the tibia and femur should be less than 5 mm. Remarks— tibial depression fractures are to be suspected if the width is more than 5 mm.

Patellar height measurement: Numerous methods are described to assess the patellar height.

1. **Insall-Salvati ratio:**

   Landmarks: Ratio of patellar tendon length to the maximum vertical length of patella. It is measured in lateral radiographs taken in 30° flexion or sagittal MRI images. The ratio of B to A is the Insall–Salvati ratio (Fig. 3.9.81).

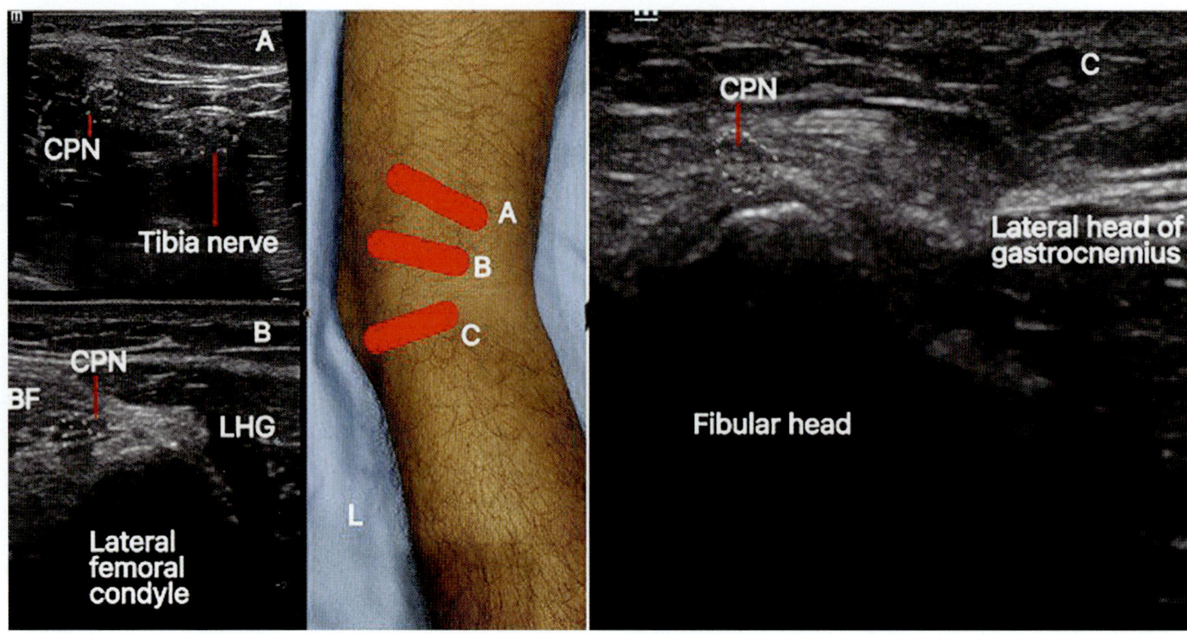

Fig. 3.9.79: Peroneal nerve

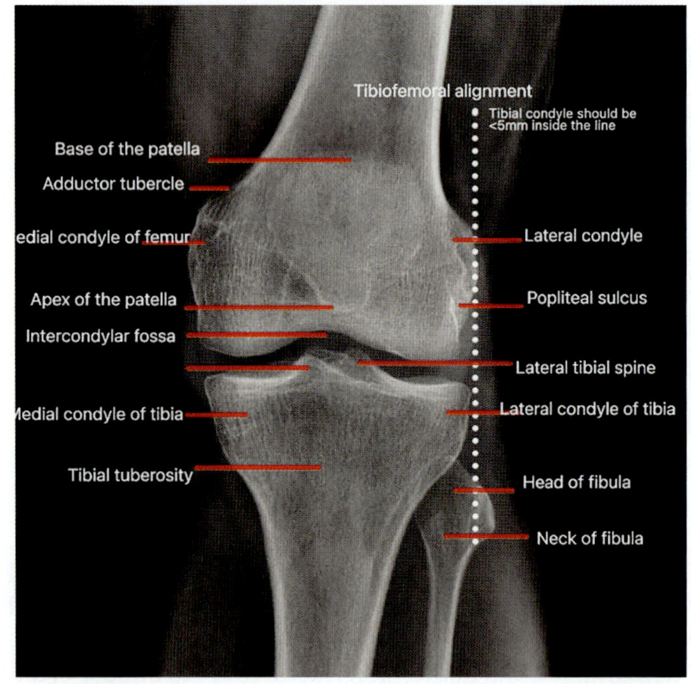

Fig. 3.9.80: X-ray AP view—tibial offset distance

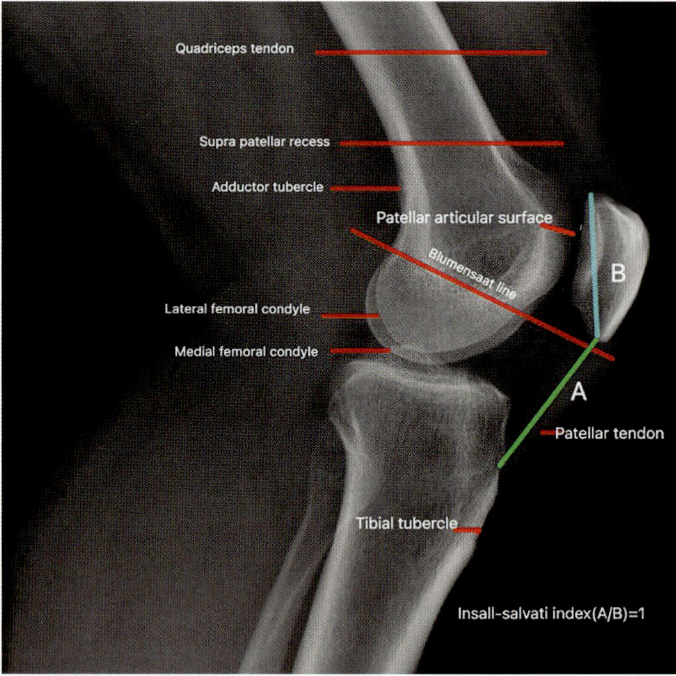

Fig. 3.9.81: X-ray lateral view–Insall-Salvati ratio and Blumensaat line

Normal range: Normal range is between 0.8 and 1.2. The ratio of more than 1.2 is indicative of patella alta and less than 0.8 is patella baja.

Significance: Patella when elevated relative to the femoral trochlea is termed as patella alta. This structural abnormality results in a reduction of the contact surface leading to maltracking.

2. Modified Insall–Salvati ratio:

Landmarks: It is the ratio between the length of the patellar tendon to the articular surface of the patella. It is measured in lateral radiographs taken in 30° flexion or sagittal MRI images.

Normal range: Normal measurement is 1.2 and the ratio above 2 is considered as patella alta.

Table 3.9.7: Muscles and nerves of leg (Figs 3.9.82–3.9.86)

Compartment	*Muscles and vessels*	*Nerve of the compartment*	*Functions*
Anterior	Tibialis anterior, extensor **h**allucis longus (EHL), Anterior tibial vessels (**A**rtery, **N**erve) Extensor **D**igitorum longus (EDL), **P**eroneus tertius Mnemonic: THE HOSPITALS ARE NOT DIRTY PLACES	Deep peroneal nerve	Dorsiflexors Additional actions: Tibialis anterior—inverts foot EHL—extends great toe EDL—extends interphalangeal and metatarsophalangeal joints of lateral 4 toes Peroneus tertius—everts foot
Posterior	Superficial muscles—gastrocnemius, soleus, plantaris, popliteus Deep muscles—**T**ibialis posterior, flexor **D**igitorum longus, posterior tibial vessels (**A**rtery and **V**ein), Flexor **H**allucis longus Mnemonic: TOM DICK AND VERY NAUGHTY HARRY	Tibial nerve	Plantar flexion except popliteus—which acts at knee joint helping in Unlocking Additional actions: Tibialis posterior—everts foot Flexor digitorum longus—flexes interphalangeal and metatarsophalangeal joints of lateral 4 toes Flexor hallucis longus—flexes great toe
Lateral	Peroneal **L**ongus (**P**ostero**L**ateral) Peroneal brevis	Superficial peroneal nerve	Everts foot and also assists in plantar flexion

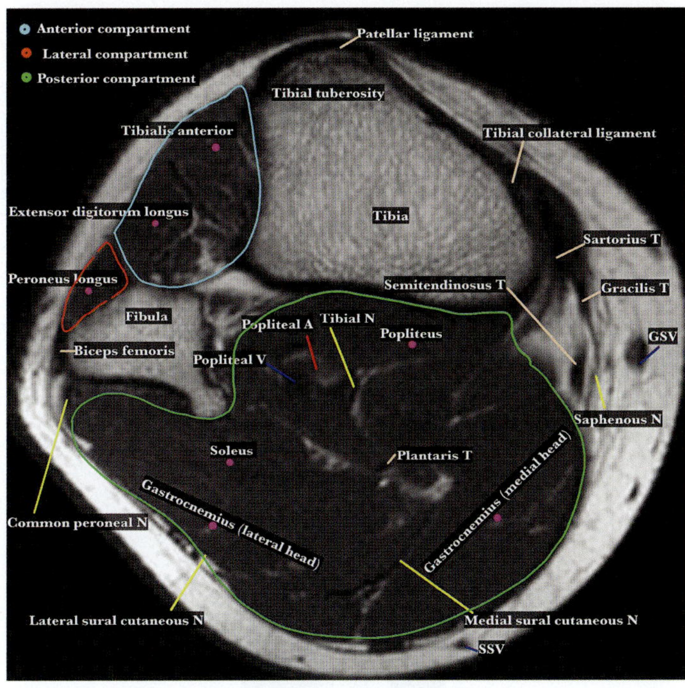

Fig. 3.9.82: Axial sections of MRI of leg

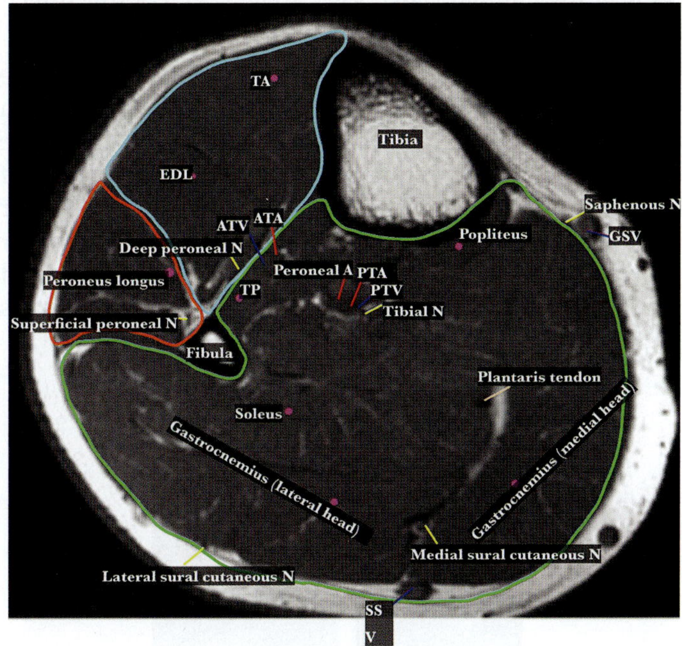

Fig. 3.9.83

Significance: The morphology of the lower pole of patella is highly variable. To eliminate this factor modified Insall-Salvati ratio is advocated which takes into account only the articular surface of the patella.

Blumensaat line: *Landmark:* It is drawn on lateral radiograph of knee in 30° flexion. A line drawn through the roof of the intercondylar notch should intersect the lower pole of the patella. The line corresponds to the roof of the intercondylar fossa of the femur seen on the lateral radiograph. It is the sclerotic line but not always straight.

Significance: Iriuchishima classified the morphology of the Blumensaat line. It is a straight line in approximately 30% of the population, appears as a small hill in 19% of the population and appears as a large hill in 44% of the population. Protrusion extending to half-length of

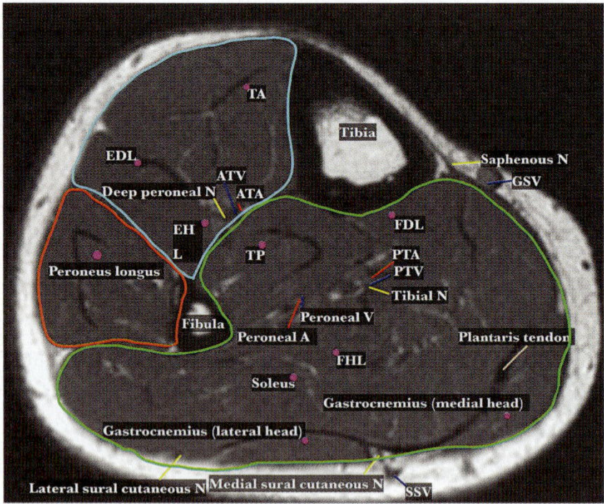

Fig. 3.9.84

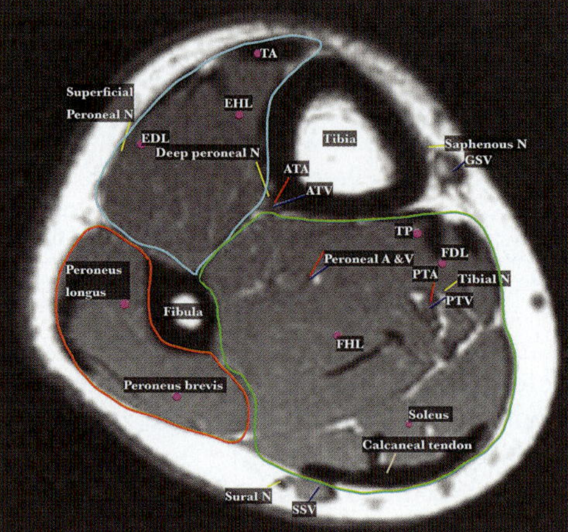

Fig. 3.9.85

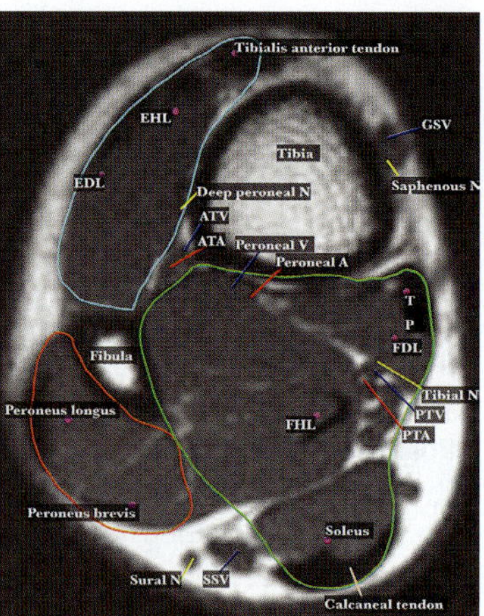

Fig. 3.9.86

the line is termed small hill type while longer than half is called large hill type. On a lateral radiograph taken in 30 degree of knee flexion, a line drawn through the roof of the intercondylar notch should intersect the lower pole of the patella. When the patella is above this line, it is representative of patella alta.

Leg: It is the region between knee and ankle joint. The osseous anatomy of leg is formed by tibia and fibula forming proximal and distal tibiofibular joint. The proximal tibiofibular joint is formed between head of fibula and lateral condyle of tibia. The distal tibiofibular joint is by the articulation of **fibula with tibia at fibular notch, this joint is strengthened by anterior and posterior tibiofibular ligaments and interosseous ligament.** The medial border of tibia is predominantly subcutaneous, with proximal portion covered by pes anserinus. **Saphenous nerve and great saphenous vein run along the medial border of tibia** (Figs 3.9.87–3.9.88).

Table 3.9.8: Ossification centres of knee and leg

Site	*Appearance*	*Fusion*
Distal femoral epiphysis	9th month of intrauterine life	20 years
Tibia—proximal end	During intrauterine life	20 years
Tibia—distal end	2nd year	18 years
Fibula—proximal end	4 years	25 years
Fibula—distal end	2 years	20 years

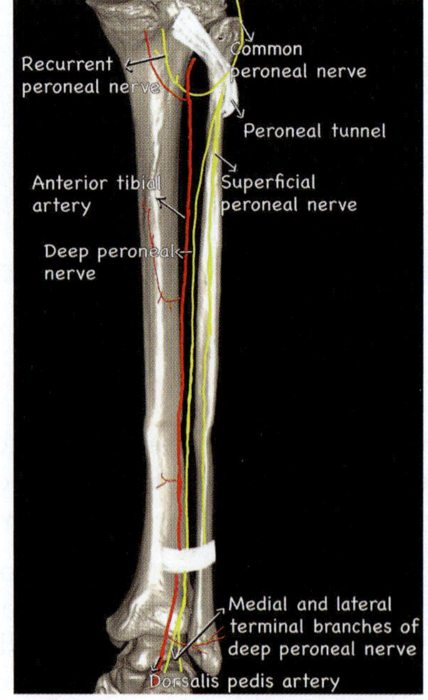

Fig. 3.9.87: Nerve supply of leg (anterior aspect)

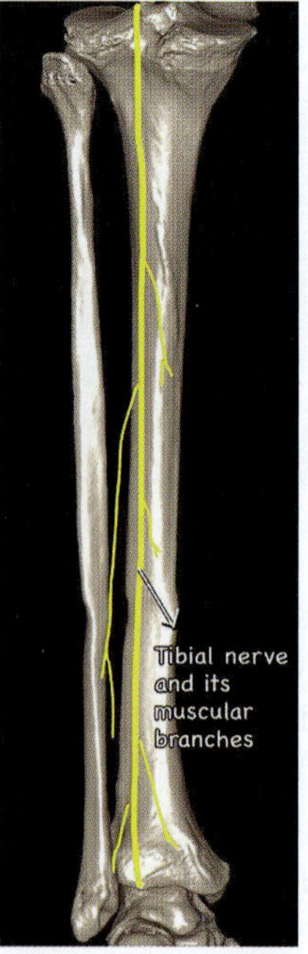

Fig. 3.9.88: Nerve supply of leg (posterior aspect)

3.9.E Ankle Joint and Foot

Ankle Joint (Talocrural Joint)

The ankle joint is articulation between the foot and the leg involving the distal tibia, fibula and body of talus (Fig. 3.9.89). The lower end of the tibia with its medial malleolus and the lateral malleolus of the fibula with inferior transverse tibiofibular ligament, form a deep recess ('mortise') for articulation of body of the talus (Fig. 3.9.90). It is a hinge type of synovial joint allowing dorsiflexion and plantar flexion.

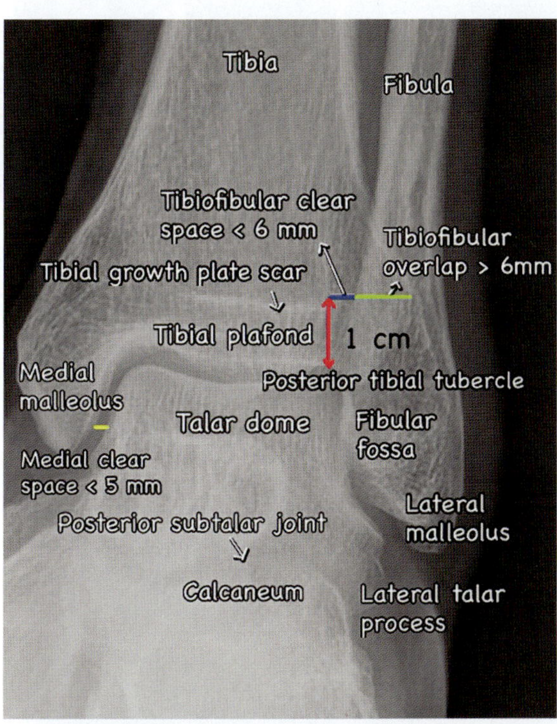

Fig. 3.9.89: X-ray AP view of ankle joint

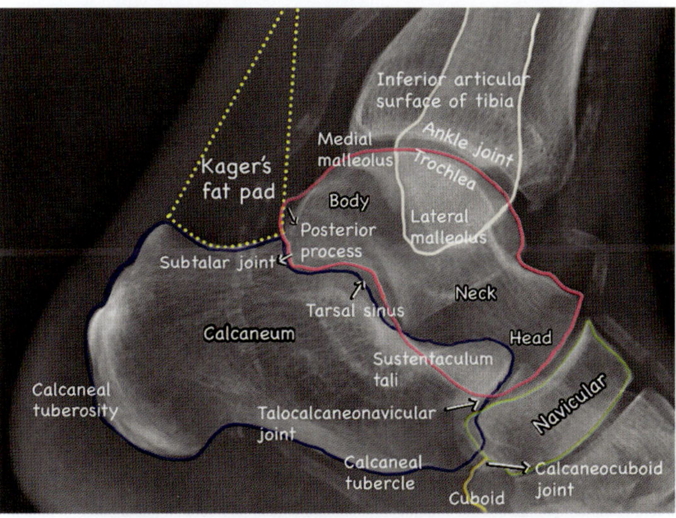

Fig. 3.9.90: X-ray lateral view of ankle joint

Ligaments of ankle joint (Figs 3.9.91 and 3.9.92): **Syndesmotic ligaments** (Fig. 3.9.93): There are 4 tibiofibular syndesmotic ligaments—anterior and posterior tibiofibular ligament, interosseous ligament, inferior transverse ligament. Basett ligament is the distal anterior tibiofibular ligament. **Lateral collateral ligaments** (Fig. 3.9.96): There are 3 lateral ligaments—anterior talofibular, calcaneofibular and posterior talofibular

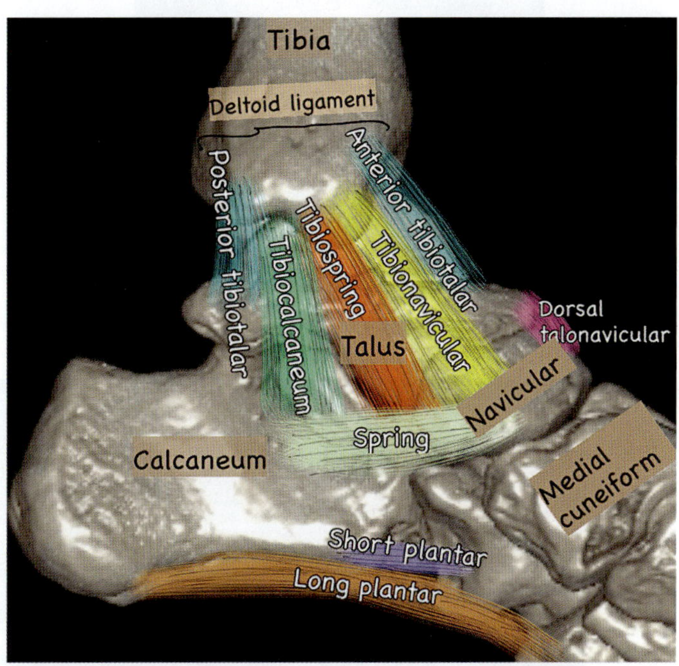

Fig. 3.9.91: Medial ligaments of ankle joint

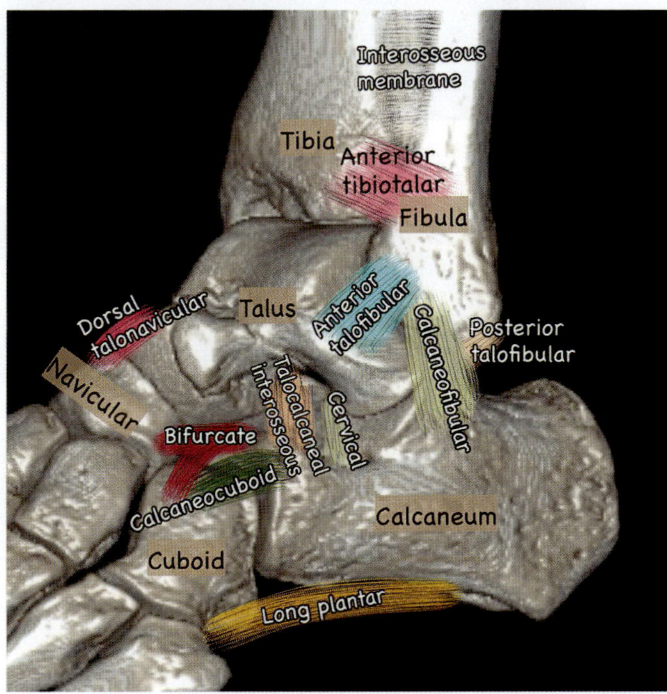

Fig. 3.9.92: Lateral ligaments of ankle joint

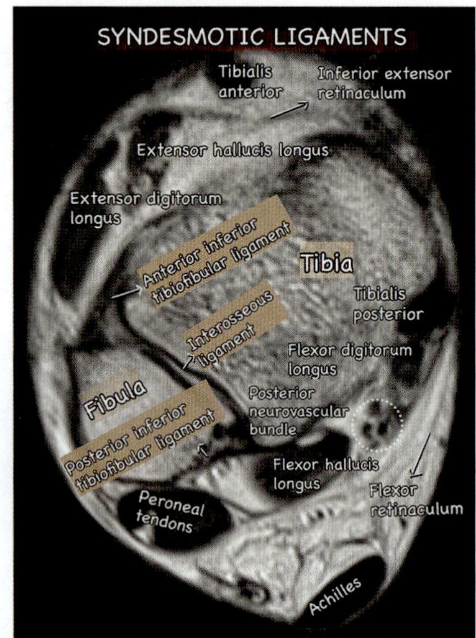

Fig. 3.9.93

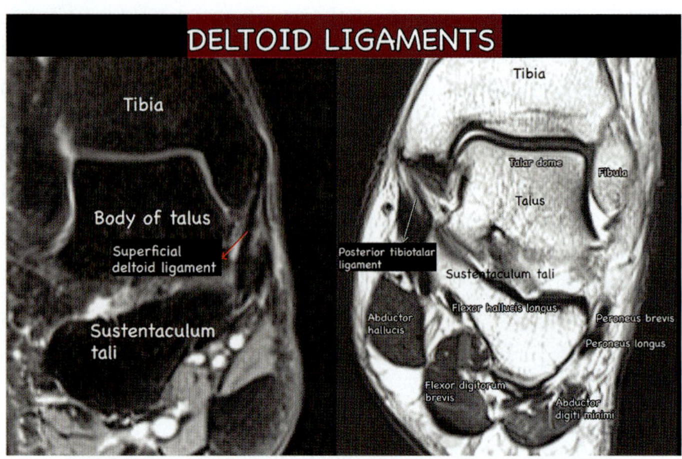

Fig. 3.9.94

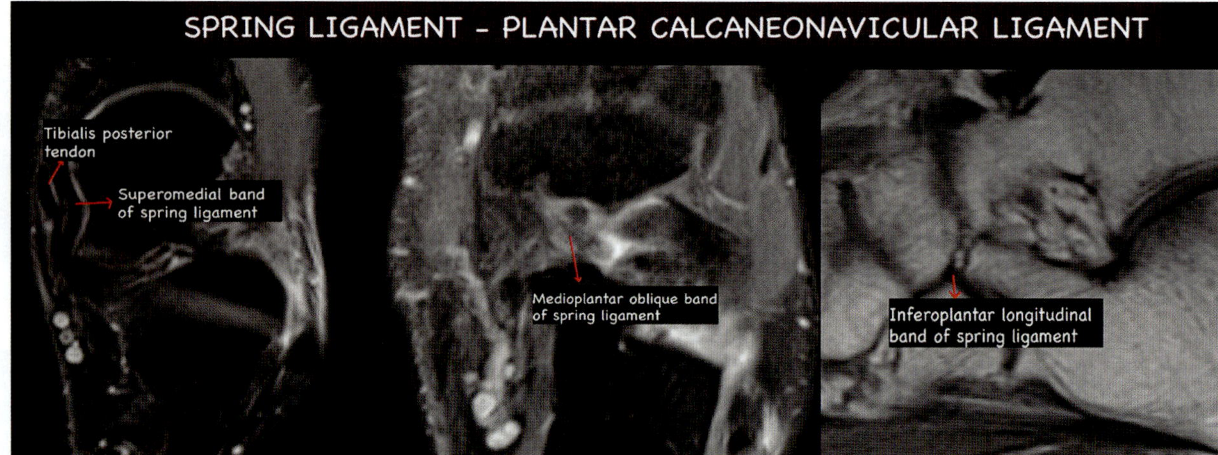

Fig. 3.9.95

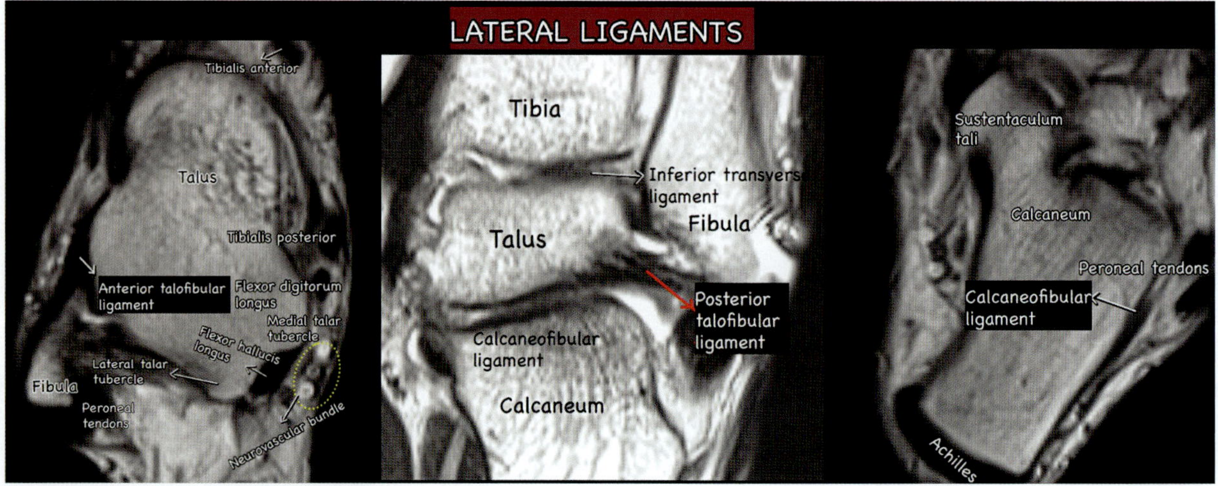

Fig. 3.9.96

ligaments. The weakest ligament of ankle joint is the anterior talofibular ligament. **Medial collateral ligament (deltoid ligament)** (Fig. 3.9.94): Consists of superficial and deep components. Superficial components include tibiocalcaneal, tibionavicular, tibiospring ligaments. Deep components are anterior and posterior tibiotalar bands. Spring ligament (Fig. 3.9.95) is plantar calcaneonavicular ligament. Ligaments are seen as thin, linear, low signal intensity structures and usually delineated by the surrounding high signal intensity fat. Some ligaments like anterior tibiofibular, tibiotalar components of deltoid ligament, posterior talofibular ligament may appear heterogenous due to interposition of fat between the ligamentous fibres.

Muscles and tendons around ankle joint (Fig. 3.9.97): There is an anterolateral, posteromedial and lateral compartment of the ankle typically superficial to the joint. The posteromedial compartment, in order of anterior to posterior has the tendons of tibialis posterior and flexor digitorum longus, the posterior tibial vessels, the tibial nerve and flexor hallucis longus tendon.

The anterior compartment under the extensor retinaculum consists of the tibialis anterior tendon, extensor hallucis longus tendon, anterior tibial vessels, deep peroneal nerve, extensor digitorum longus tendon.

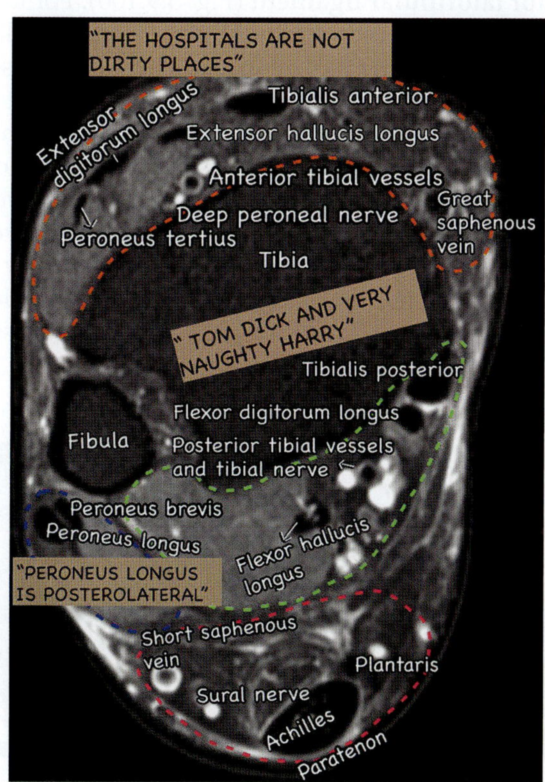

Fig. 3.9.97: MRI axial section—muscles and tendons around ankle joint

The peroneal compartment consists of peroneus longus, peroneus brevis, and the terminal branch of peroneal artery. **Superficial to the peroneal compartment is the sural nerve and small saphenous vein.** The peroneal tendons, peroneus brevis anterior to the peroneus longus, course around the lateral malleolus within its slightly concave aspect called the fibular groove. The peroneus brevis tendon passes along the lateral margin of the foot to insert at the base of the fifth metatarsal; the peroneus longus tendon courses beneath the cuboid to insert at the base of the first metatarsal and medial cuneiform.

Posteriorly, the Achilles tendon is formed by merging of the gastrocnemius and soleus tendons, which extends inferiorly to insert on the dorsal margin of the calcaneus. Injury occurs either at the insertion of the Achilles in association or at the musculotendinous junction 6 cm proximal to the insertion on the calcaneus, where tendon fibres intertwine and create a zone of relative ischaemia. The tibialis posterior tendon is the second most commonly injured tendon in the foot. The tendinous continuation of the muscle belly within the deep posterior compartment of the calf rounds the medial malleolus and passes forward to a dominant insertion at the base of the navicular, and six further lesser insertions in the forefoot, at the bases of the cuneiforms and the bases of metatarsals two to four. The flexor hallucis is a dominant flexor and inverter of the foot, with an extensive course to insert at the base of the distal phalanx of the great toe.

Retinaculum: These are localized band-shaped thickening of deep fascia, providing mechanical strength to prevent the bowstringing of tendons during contraction. Usually seen as bands of low signal intensity in both T1 and T2 sequences.

Flexor retinaculum: Extends from medial malleolus posteroinferiorly for attachment on the medial process of calcaneum. Proximally continuous with the deep fascia of leg and distally continuous with the plantar aponeurosis. It converts the grooves on tibia and calcaneum into canal for passage of flexor tendons. It forms the lateral border of tarsal tunnel.

Tarsal tunnel: It is fibro-osseous tunnel with its roof formed by flexor retinaculum, and floor formed by medial surfaces of tibia, talus and calcaneum seen on the medial aspect of ankle. The contents of tarsal tunnel are tibialis posterior, flexor digitorum longus, neurovascular bundle composed of posterior tibial artery, vein and tibial nerve, flexor hallucis longus tendon.

Peroneal retinaculum: Superior peroneal retinaculum: It is a short band originating from lateral malleolus inserting on the lateral surface of calcaneum and deep fascia of leg, binding peroneal tendons to retrofibular groove.

Inferior peroneal retinaculum: It is continuous anteriorly with the inferior extensor retinaculum, posteriorly inserts on the lateral surface of calcaneum, with some fibres fusing with fibular trochlea on calcaneum. This retinaculum binds the peroneal tendons to calcaneum.

Extensor retinaculum

Superior extensor retinaculum: Lies immediately proximal to the anterior aspect of ankle joint, attaching medially to tibia and laterally to anterior fibula and distally continuous with inferior extensor retinaculum. It binds the tendons of anterior compartment.

Inferior extensor retinaculum: It is Y-shaped, lying anterior to ankle joint with stem of Y lying medially and two limbs lying laterally. The stem of Y is attached to upper calcaneum. The proximal medial limb has two layers—deep and superficial layer. Distal medial band is continuous with plantar aponeurosis. Deep peroneal nerve and dorsalis pedis vessels lie deep to all layers of inferior extensor retinaculum.

Bursa

Retrocalcaneal bursa/subachilleal bursa: Situated between the posterosuperior calcaneum and antero-inferior Achilles tendon. Retrocalcaneal bursitis is a part of triad of Haglund syndrome which includes insertional Achilles tendinopathy, retrocalcaneal bursitis and posterosuperior calcaneal exostosis.

Subcutaneous calcaneal bursa/retroachilleal bursa/ superficial retrocalcaneal bursa: This bursa is located between the calcaneal tendon and skin.

Kager fat pad: Also known as precalcaneal fat pad, pre-Achilles fat pad is seen within the well-defined Kager's triangle which is bordered anteriorly by flexor hallucis longus muscle, posteriorly by Achilles tendon and inferiorly by calcaneum. This fat pad can be distorted by infection, inflammation, edema, hemorrhage, adjacent soft tissue abnormalities.

Ultrasound Examination of Ankle Joint

Anterior ankle

Extensor tendons (Fig. 3.9.98): The patient lies supine or can be seated with knee flexed to 45 degrees such that the plantar surface of foot lies flat on the bed. The probe is held in transverse plane and swept upwards and downwards to examine the tendons of anterior compartment with the neurovascular bundle. The tendons from medial to lateral are tibialis anterior, extensor hallucis longus and extensor digitorum longus with anterior tibial vessels, deep peroneal nerve lying between extensor hallucis longus and digitorum longus. The tendons must be examined throughout the whole length from the myotendinous junction to their insertion.

Anterior recess of ankle joint (Fig. 3.9.99): With the patient in same position, the transducer is placed in longitudinal place over the dorsum of ankle for looking the anterior recess of tibiotalar joint. Also the talar dome can be examined by moving the probe medially and laterally.

Anterior talofibular ligament (Fig. 3.9.100): For looking the anterior talofibular ligament, the forefoot is slightly inverted for stretching the lateral ligaments. The transducer is placed parallel to the examination bed with posterior edge over the distal lateral malleolus to view the anterior talofibular ligament. The intactness of the ligament can be checked by performing sonographic anterior drawer test by placing the patient prone with foot hanging over the examination table and pulling the forefoot anteriorly while maintaining the foot in plantar flexion and inversion. In case of ligament tear, anterior shift of talus against tibia will reveal the gap in the substance of ligament.

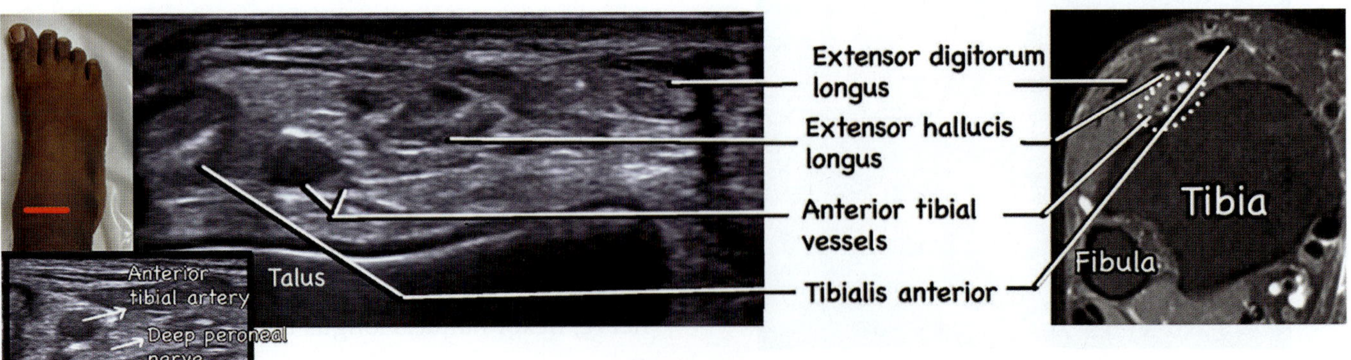

Fig. 3.9.98: Extensor tendons

Anterior tibiofibular ligament (Fig. 3.9.101): In the same position, with posterior edge of transducer on lateral malleolus, the anterior edge rotated upwards to see the anterior tibiofibular ligament.

Calcaneofibular ligament (Fig. 3.9.102): In the same position, the transducer is placed in oblique coronal plane with superior edge on the tip of lateral malleolus, and inferior edge lying slightly posteriorly, the foot is dorsiflexed to view the calcaneofibular ligament.

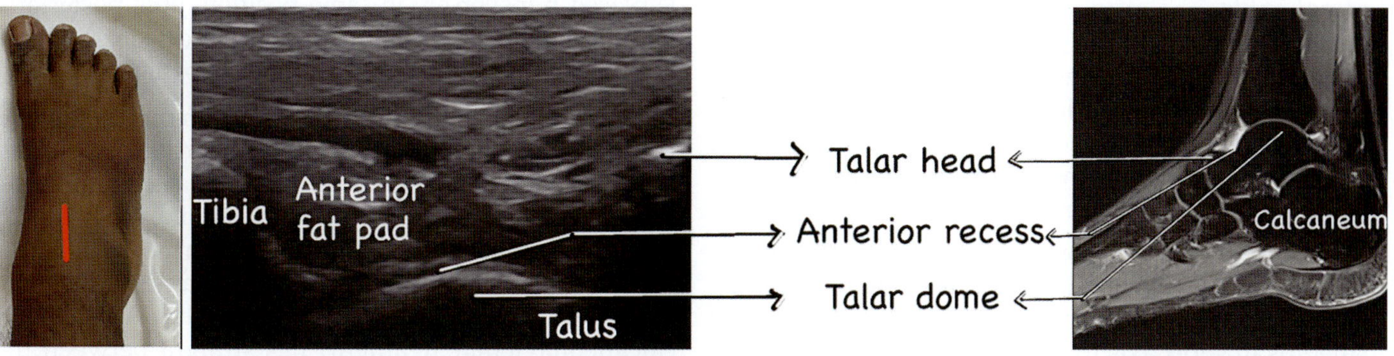

Fig. 3.9.99: Anterior recess of ankle joint

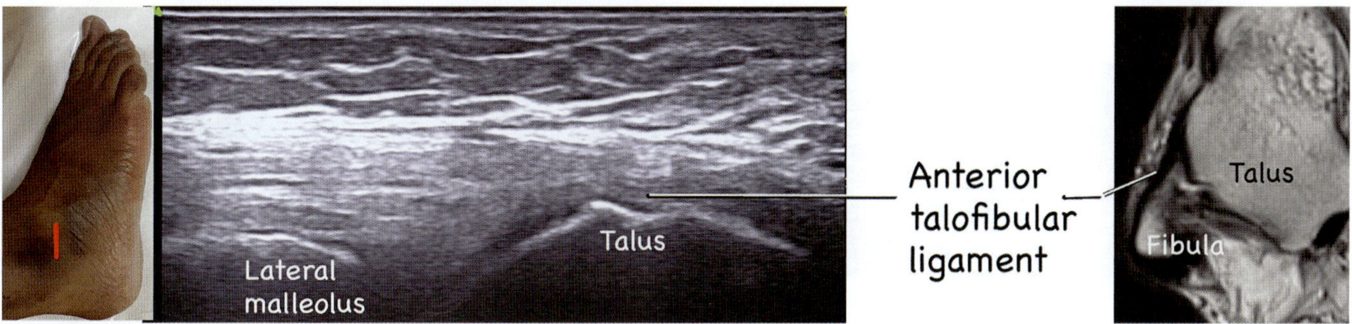

Fig. 3.9.100: Anterior talofibular ligament

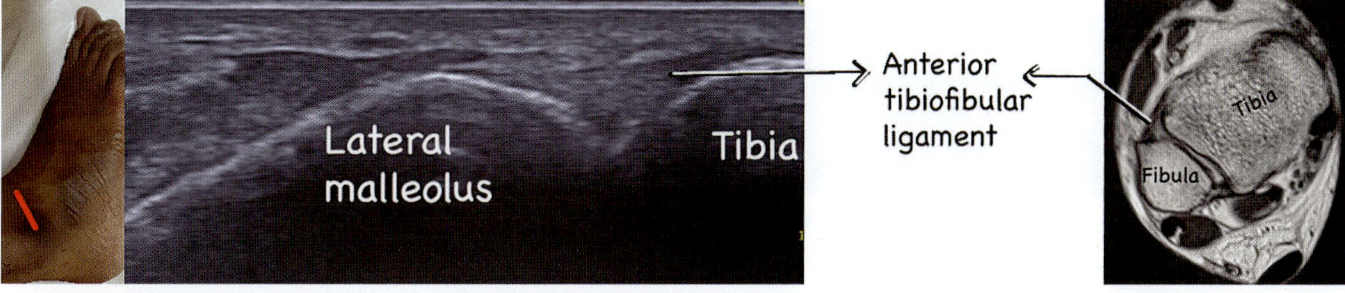

Fig. 3.9.101: Anterior tibiofibular ligament

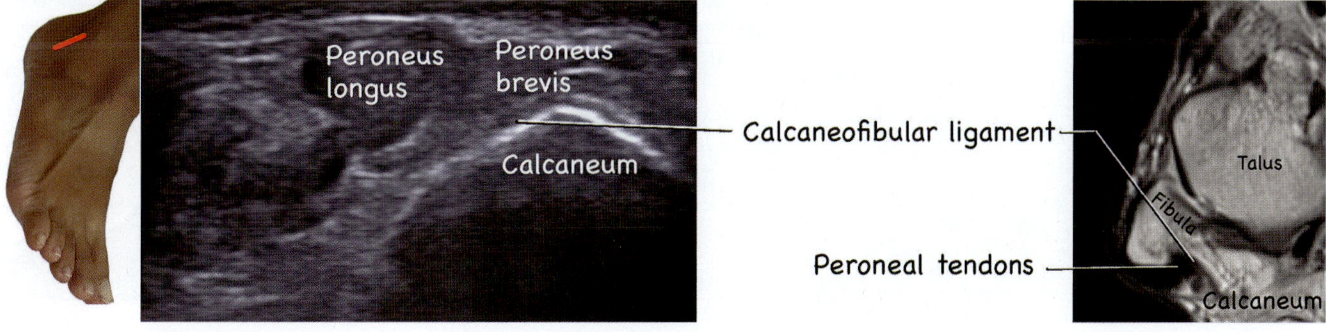

Fig. 3.9.102: Calcaneofibular ligament

Dorsal midtarsal ligaments: The dorsal talonavicular, dorsal calcaneocuboid, calcaneocuboidonavicular ligaments can be examined by placing transducer longitudinally over the dorsum of foot between the corresponding bones.

Lateral ankle

Peroneal tendons (Fig. 3.9.103): The peroneal tendons can be examined by placing the transducer transversely behind the lateral malleolus to examine them in short axis. The ultrasound beam must be maintained perpendicularly to avoid the anisotropy. The entire extent of tendon to be examined.

Medial ankle: Tibialis posterior and flexor digitorum longus tendon: The medial ankle is examined in frog leg position, the transducer is placed behind the medial malleolus in short axis to examine the tibialis posterior and flexor hallucis longus tendon.

Tarsal tunnel and tibial nerve (Fig. 3.9.104): The transducer is placed further inferiorly to examine the tarsal tunnel with the tibial nerve and posterior tibial artery and vein.

Flexor hallucis longus tendon (Fig. 3.9.105): The transducer is placed transversely in same position, little posteriorly to examine the flexor hallucis longus tendon in short axis between the medial and lateral tubercle of talus.

Deltoid ligament (Fig. 3.9.106): To examine the deltoid ligament, the transducer is placed in coronal plane with superior edge over the tip of medial malleolus and the inferior edge is tilted posteriorly to examine the tibiotalar and tilted anteriorly to examine the tibiocalcaneal ligament while the foot is in dorsiflexion. The tibionavicular ligament is best seen in neutral position. The spring ligament (plantar calcaneonavicular ligament) lies straight between the sustentaculum tali and navicular bone.

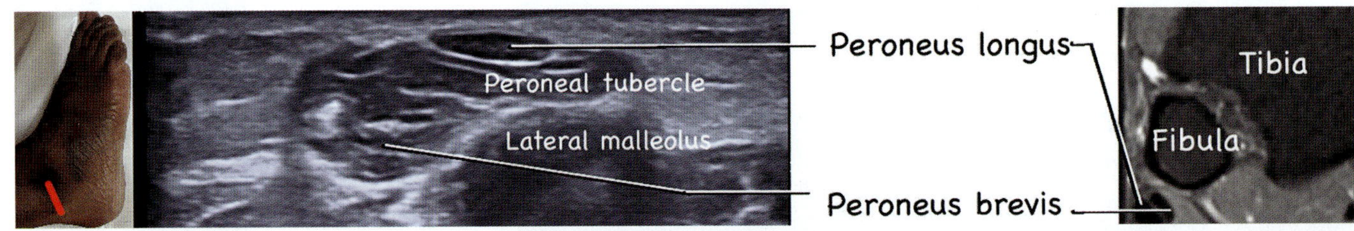

Fig. 3.9.103: Peroneal tendons

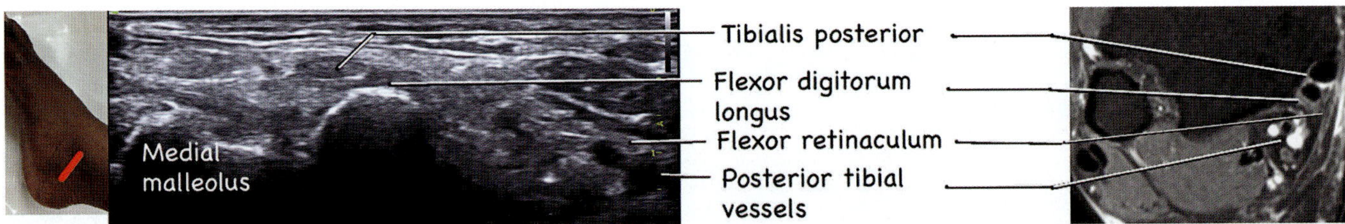

Fig. 3.9.104: Tarsal tunnel and tibial nerve

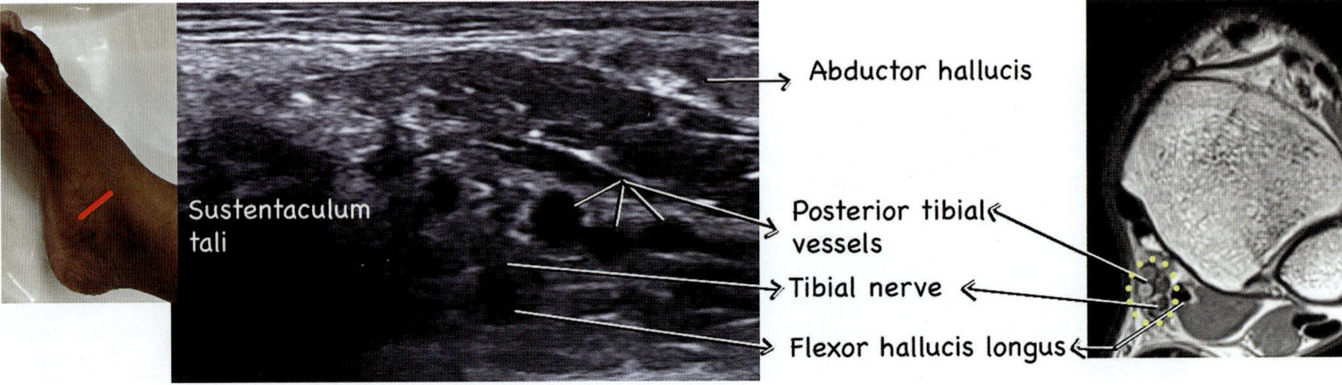

Fig. 3.9.105: Flexor hallucis longus tendon

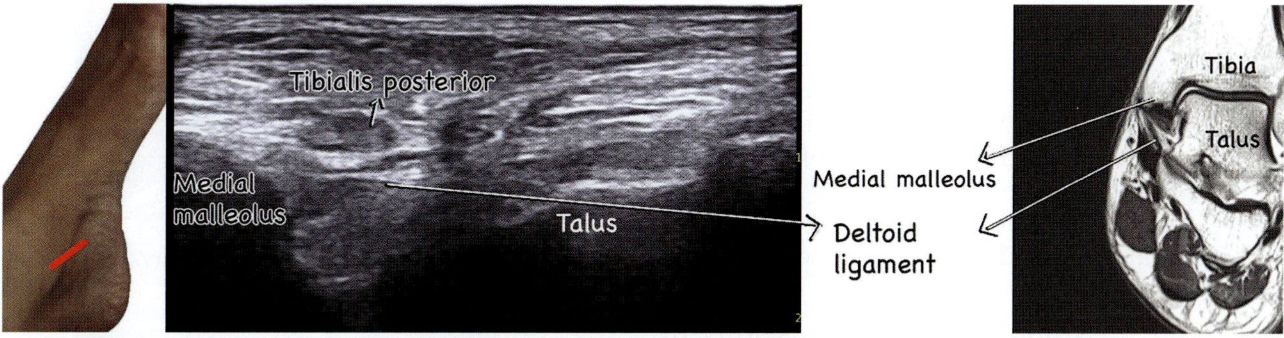

Fig. 3.9.106: Deltoid ligament

Posterior ankle

Posterior joint recess and flexor hallucis longus tendon (Fig. 3.9.107): This is examined by placing the patient in prone position with foot resting on toes and probe is placed medial to Achilles tendon in oblique sagittal plane to examine the posterior joint recess. Also the tendon of flexor hallucis longus tendon in long axis can be examined.

Achilles tendon (Fig. 3.9.108): The Achilles tendon can be examined in prone position, with the foot hanging out the examination table. The Achilles tendon has to be examined in both transverse and longitudinal planes from the myotendinous junction to the calcaneal insertion. Also the retrocalcaneal and retroachilles bursa has to be examined.

Plantar fascia (Fig. 3.9.109): To examine the plantar fascia, the transducer is placed over the plantar aspect of hindfoot. Longitudinal placement of transducer just medial to midline is used for examining the plantar fascia.

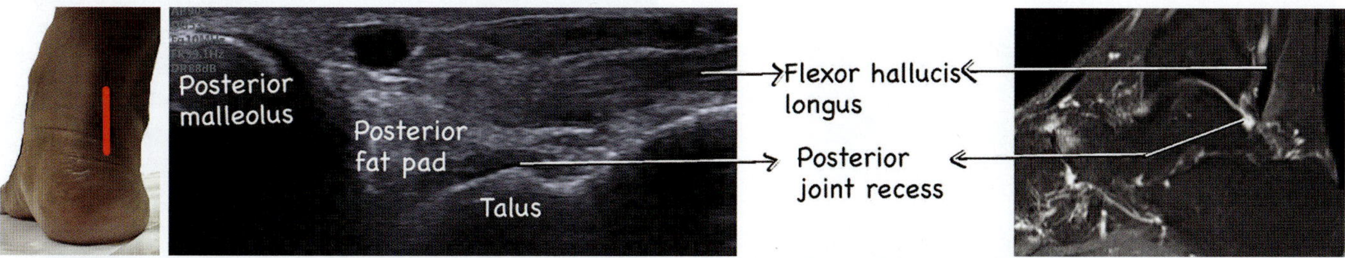

Fig. 3.9.107: Posterior joint recess and flexor hallucis longus tendon

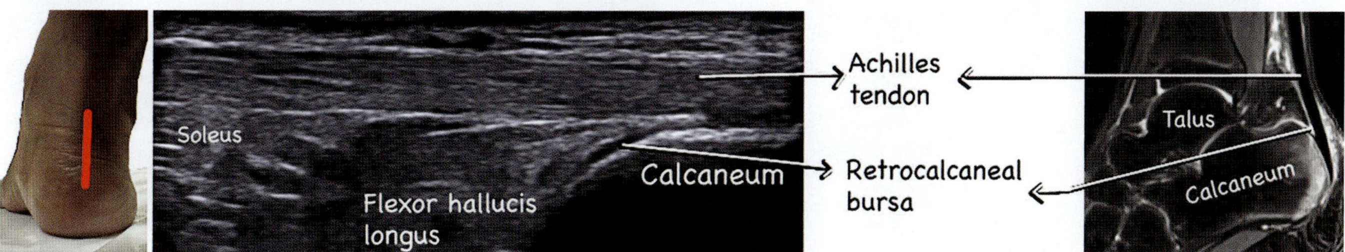

Fig. 3.9.108: Achilles tendon

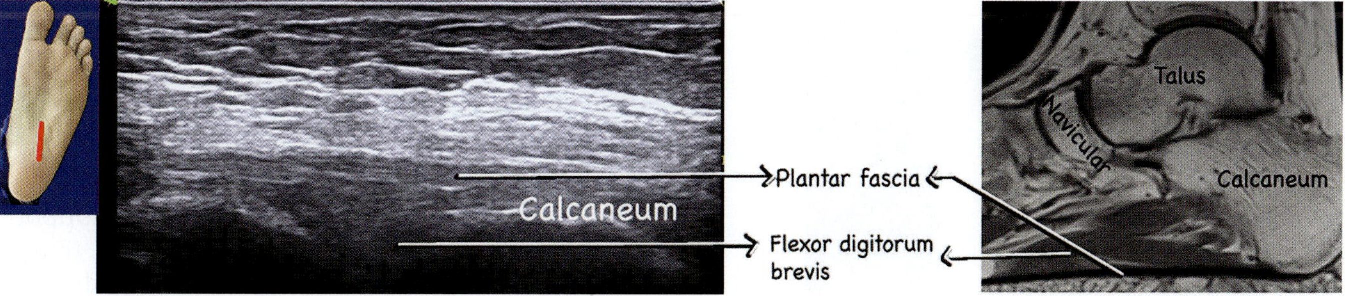

Fig. 3.9.109: Plantar fascia

Foot

Foot has been divided into three major divisions: Hindfoot, midfoot and forefoot and two columns—medial and lateral column (Fig. 3.9.110). Hindfoot consists of talus and calcaneum. Midfoot consists of navicular, calcaneum and cuboid. Forefoot consists of metatarsals and phalanges. Calcaneum, cuboid, 4th and 5th digit forms the lateral column. Rest of the bones form the medial column.

Chopart joint: It is midtarsal joint, consisting of talonavicular and calcaneocuboid joints.

Lisfranc joint: It is the tarsometatarsal joint, the articulation between the tarsal bones and bases of metatarsals. The first three metatarsals articulate with the cuneiforms and last two metatarsals articulate with cuboid. The 2nd metatarsal is usually recessed relative to 1st and 3rd metatarsal providing added bone stability. Dorsal tarsometatarsal ligaments, interosseous tarsometatarsal ligaments and plantar tarsometatarsal ligaments all support the tarsometatarsal joint. Of these, the Lisfranc ligament is most important. **Lisfranc ligament is a thick, broad ligament extending obliquely from medial cuneiform to medial surface of 2nd metatarsal base.** It has three bands—dorsal, interosseous and plantar. Interosseous Lisfranc ligament is the strongest of three bands and most important stabilizer.

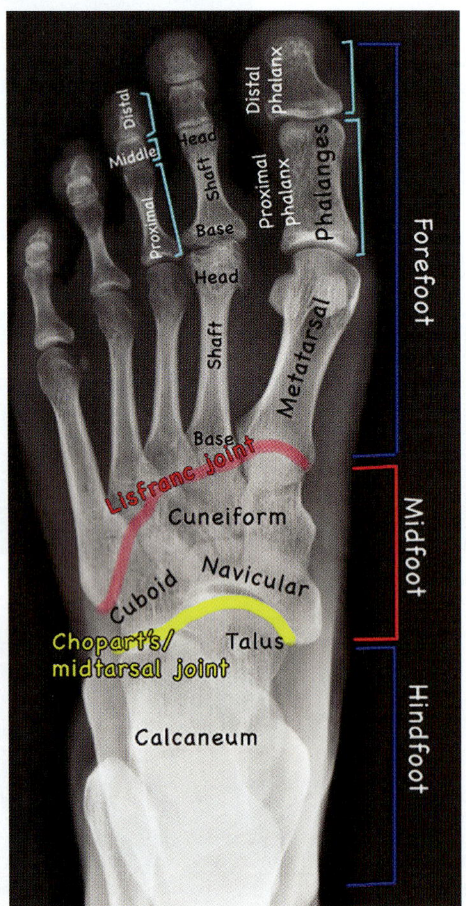

Fig. 3.9.110: X-ray AP view of foot

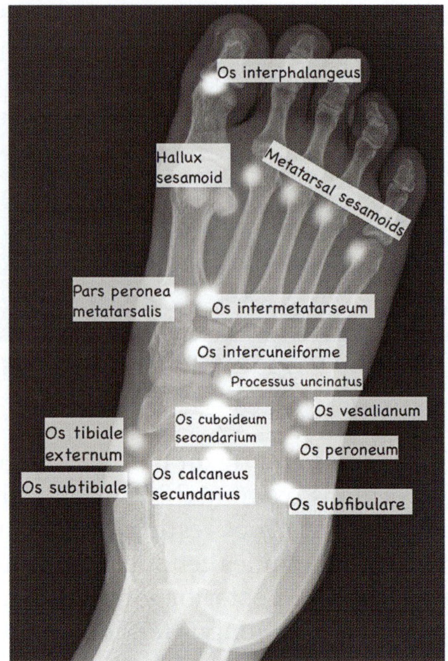

Fig. 3.9.111: Accessory ossicles of foot—AP view

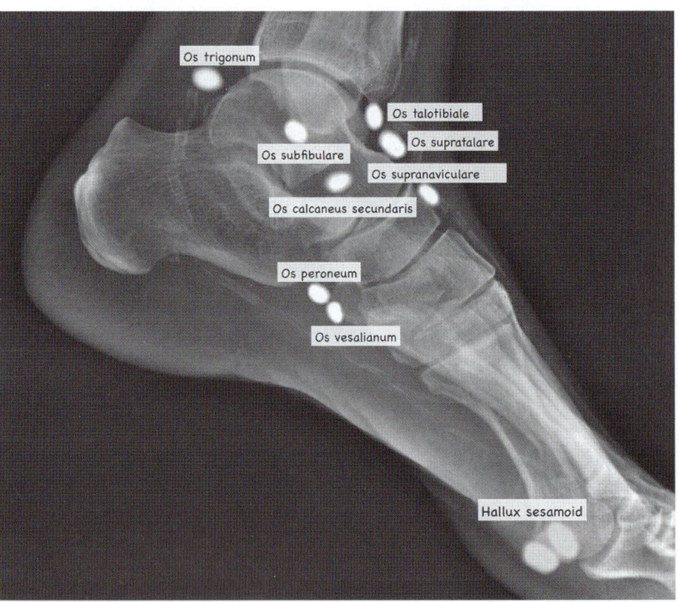

Fig. 3.9.112: Accessory ossicles of foot—lateral view

Osseous anatomy of talus and calcaneum

Talus: It is most superior of bones of foot supported by calcaneum and articulates with tibia and fibula to form ankle joint. It has a **head, neck and body** almost forming a snail shape. Head of talus articulates with

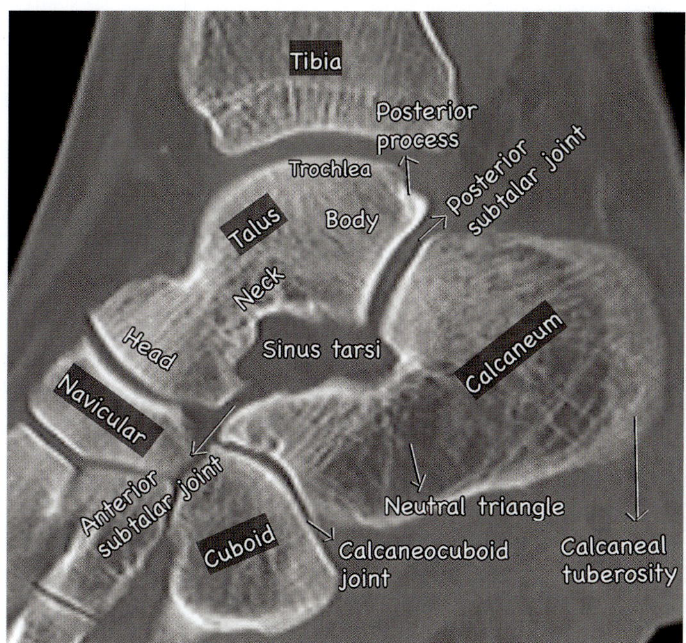

Fig. 3.9.113: CT bone window—sagittal view with parts of talus

navicular bone anteriorly (Fig. 3.9.113). Inferiorly there are three facets on the head for articulation with calcaneum with medial most of the three facets articulating with spring ligament. Neck of talus has a deep groove called the **sulcus tali**. The body of talus is elevated on the superior surface (trochlear/talar dome) for articulation with tibia and fibula. The lateral aspect of body of talus which articulates with the lateral malleolus of fibula forms a bony projection called lateral process. Also, there is another projection facing backwards and medially called the posterior process. The posterior process has two tubercles—medial and lateral—between which pass the tendon of flexor hallucis longus. The inferior surface of body of talus has facet for articulation with calcaneum. There are no muscular attachments on talus resulting in **tenuous vascularity**. Blood supply is by anterior tibial artery (head and neck), posterior tibial artery (medial side of body and sinus), peroneal artery (lateral side of body and sinus).

Calcaneum: It is a box-shaped, largest tarsal bone forming the skeletal framework of heel. The posterior surface of calcaneum has three facets, the upper, middle and lower. The middle facet is the site of attachment of Achilles tendon. The upper facet is separated from Achilles tendon by retrocalcaneal bursa. Lower facet is the weight-bearing region, curves forward onto the plantar surface forming the **calcaneal tuberosity**. The anteriormost projection of calcaneal tuberosity on plantar surface is the **calcaneal tubercle** where the short plantar ligament attaches. Laterally, calcaneum has two raised areas—**fibular trochlea**—anterior to the middle of lateral surface where the peroneal tendons get bound as they pass over the lateral side of calcaneum. Another raised area, posterosuperior to the fibular trochlea is the **trochlea for attachment of calcaneofibular ligament**. The medial surface of calcaneum has projection on the upper margin—sustentaculum tali—which is a shelf of bone supporting the posterior part of head of talus. Superior surface of calcaneum has anterior and posterior talar articulating facets. Between the two facets, there is deep groove called the calcaneal sulcus.

Sinus tarsi: The calcaneal sulcus together with the sulcus tali forms sinus tarsi on the lateral side of foot (Fig. 3.9.114). It contains the cervical, interosseous talocalcaneal ligaments, medial, lateral and intermediate roots of inferior extensor retinaculum, neurovascular structures and fat. Inflammation or hemorrhage in synovial recess can result in sinus tarsi syndrome.

Subtalar joint: Also called the talocalcaneal joint, comprising of articulations between talus and calcaneum. Anterior subtalar joint is the articulation between head of talus and anterior facet of calcaneum (Fig. 3.9.115). Middle subtalar joint is the articulation between sustentacular facet of talus and middle facet on sustentaculum tali of calcaneum (Figs 3.9.116 and 3.9.117). Posterior subtalar joint is between posterior facet of talus and posterior facet of calcaneum.

Plantar fascia/aponeurosis: It is a strong, fibrous investing layer on sole of foot extending from calcaneal tuberosity to divide into central, medial and lateral components distally, supporting the longitudinal arch of the foot. The central component is thickest and

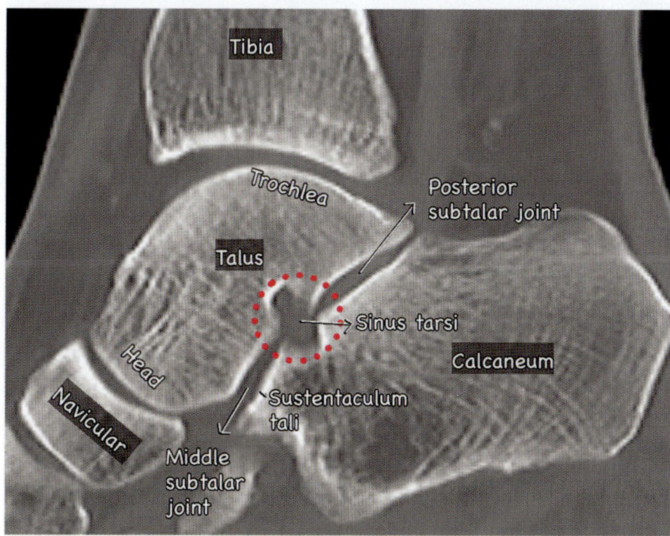

Fig. 3.9.114: CT bone window—sagittal view with sinus tarsi

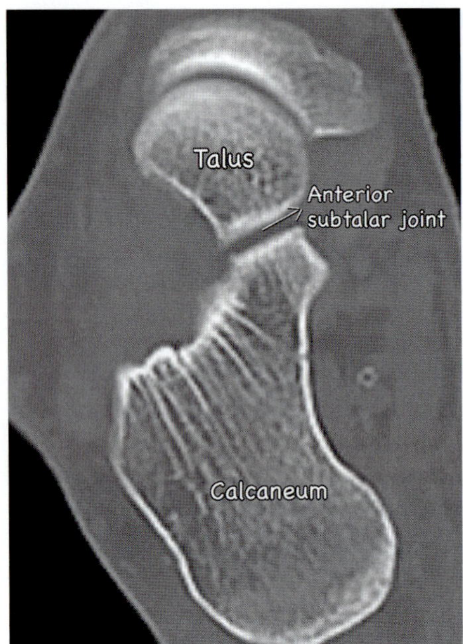

Fig. 3.9.115: CT bone window—anterior subtalar joint

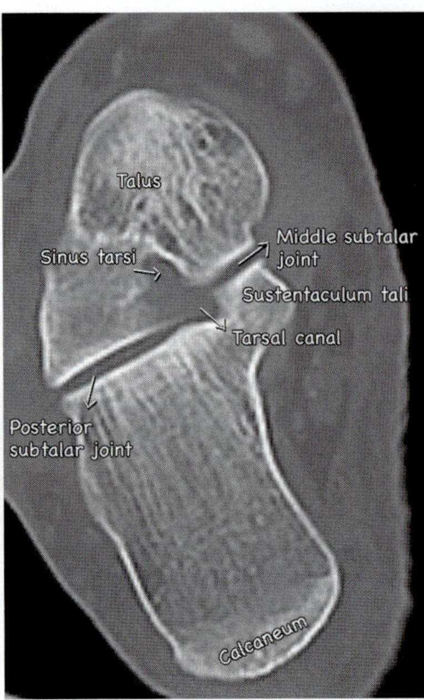

Fig. 3.9.116: CT bone window—middle and posterior subtalar joint

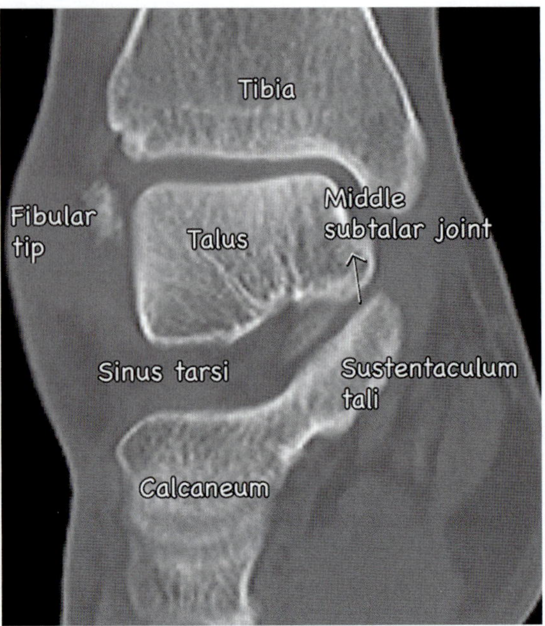

Fig. 3.9.117: CT bone window coronal section—sinus tarsi and middle subtalar joint

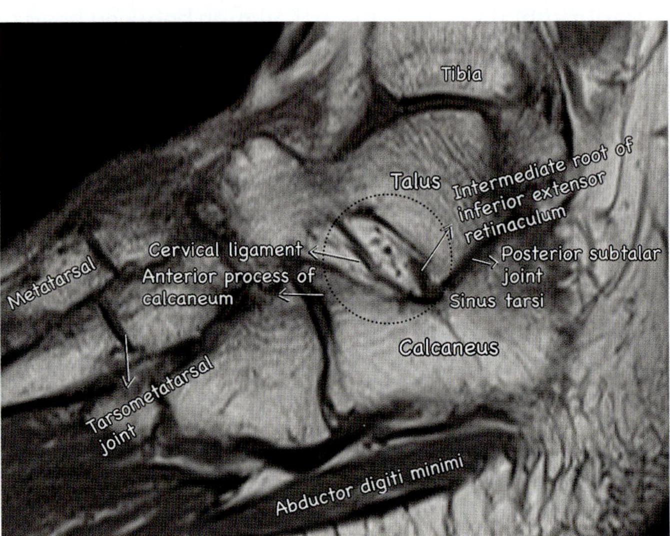

Fig. 3.9.118: MRI sagittal section of hindfoot

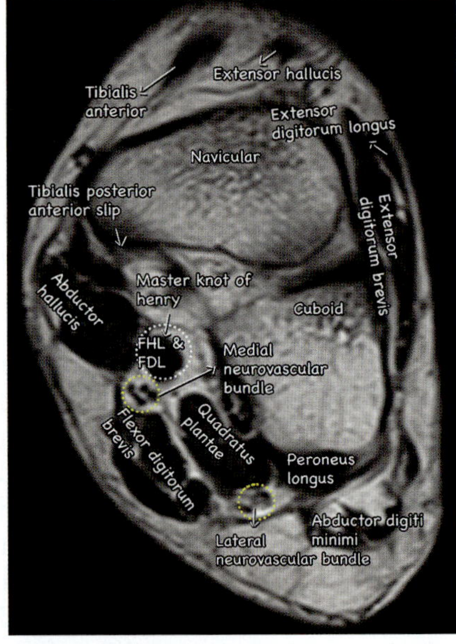

Fig. 3.9.119: MRI axial section—knot of Henry

divides distally into five digitations which insert on the metatarsophalangeal joint. The medial portion is the thinnest and arises from the midportion of central bundle proximally and distally inserts on the metatarsal joint capsule. Lateral component is comparatively thicker, arising from the lateral margin of calcaneal tubercle and inserts into the fifth metatarsal joint capsule. The average thickness of plantar fascia in the central component is about 4 mm.

Knot of Henry (Fig. 3.9.119): The superficial crossing of flexor digitorum longus tendon obliquely over the tendon of flexor hallucis longus tendon occurs at the level of midfoot. This cross over site is the knot of Henry. It is one of the sites of flexor hallucis longus tenosynovitis. Coronal plane is better for viewing this tendons. In total, flexor hallucis longus passes through three fibro-osseous tunnel—medial and lateral talar tubercles, under sustentaculum tali and medial and lateral sesamoids of 1st metatarsal.

Intrinsic muscles of foot

There are 4 plantar muscle layers and 2 dorsal muscle layers.

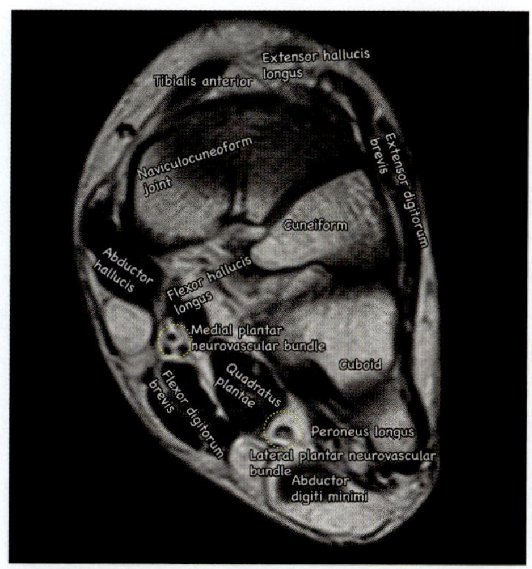

Fig. 3.9.120: MRI axial section of midfoot

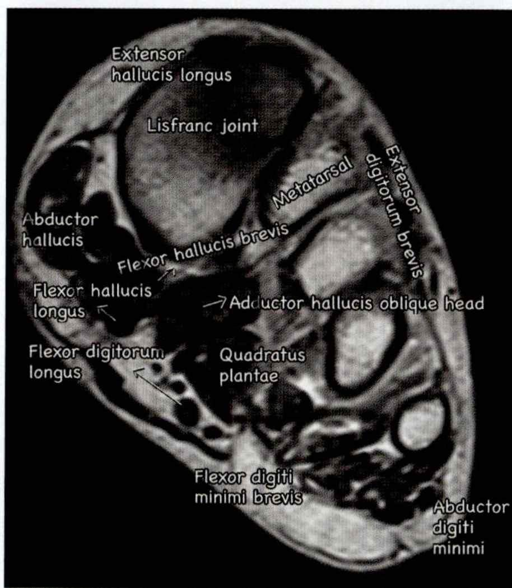

Fig. 3.9.121: MRI axial section at the level of Lisfranc joint

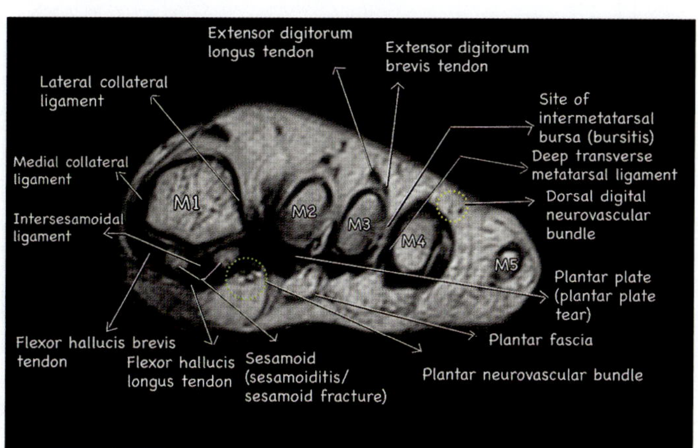

Fig. 3.9.122: MRI axial section at the level of metatarsal head

Table 3.9.9: Plantar foot muscles (arranged in 4 layers)	
Layer	*Muscles*
1	Abductor hallucis, flexor digitorum brevis, abductor digiti minimi, peroneus brevis
2	Quadratus plantae, flexor digitorum longus, flexor hallucis longus, lumbricals
3	Flexor hallucis brevis, adductor hallucis, flexor digiti minimi brevis, tibialis posterior
4	Plantar interossei (3), dorsal interossei (4)

Table 3.9.10: Dorsal foot muscles (arranged in 2 layers)	
Superficial layer	Tibialis anterior, extensor hallucis longus, extensor digitorum longus, peroneus tertius
Deep layer	Extensor hallucis brevis, extensor digitorum brevis

Plantar plate (Fig. 3.9.126): It is a fibrocartilaginous thickening of plantar capsule extending from first

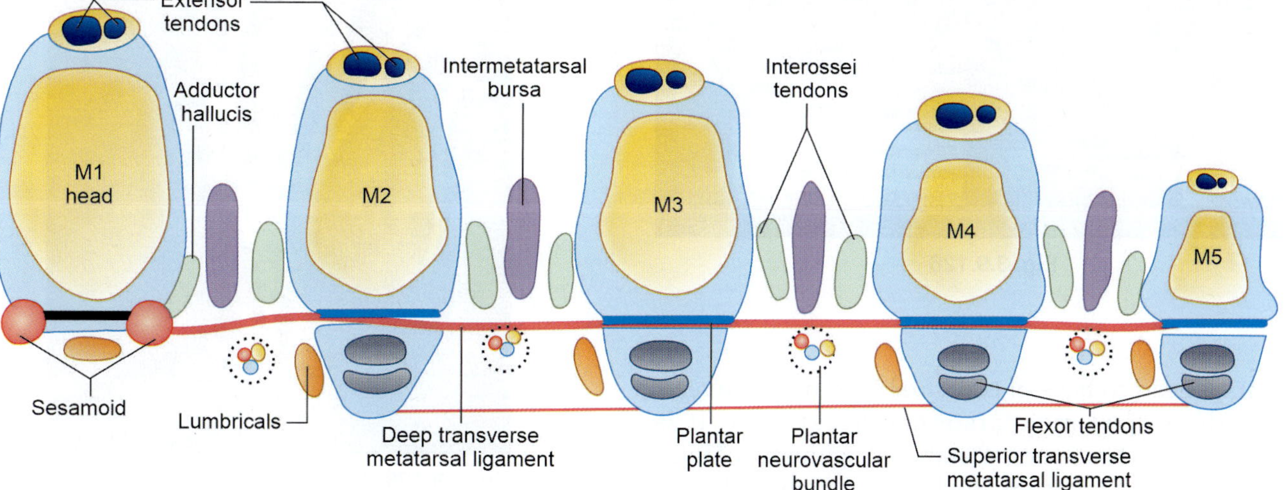

Fig. 3.9.123: Schematic representation of structures at first metatarsal head

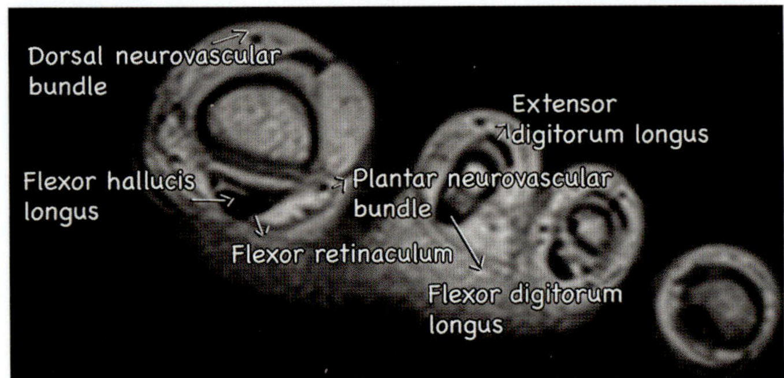

Fig. 3.9.124: MRI axial section of distal foot

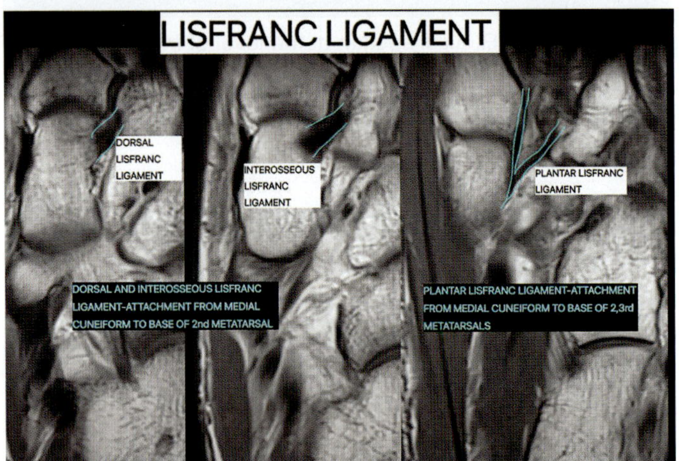

Fig. 3.9.125

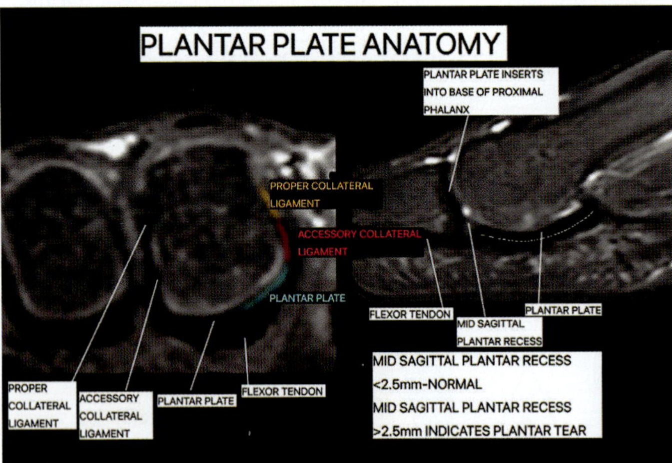

Fig. 3.9.126

metatarsal head to base of proximal phalanx. It invests sesamoids in first metatarsophalangeal joint. It is attached to deep transverse metatarsal ligament, plantar fascia, flexor tendon sheath, medial and lateral collateral ligaments.

3

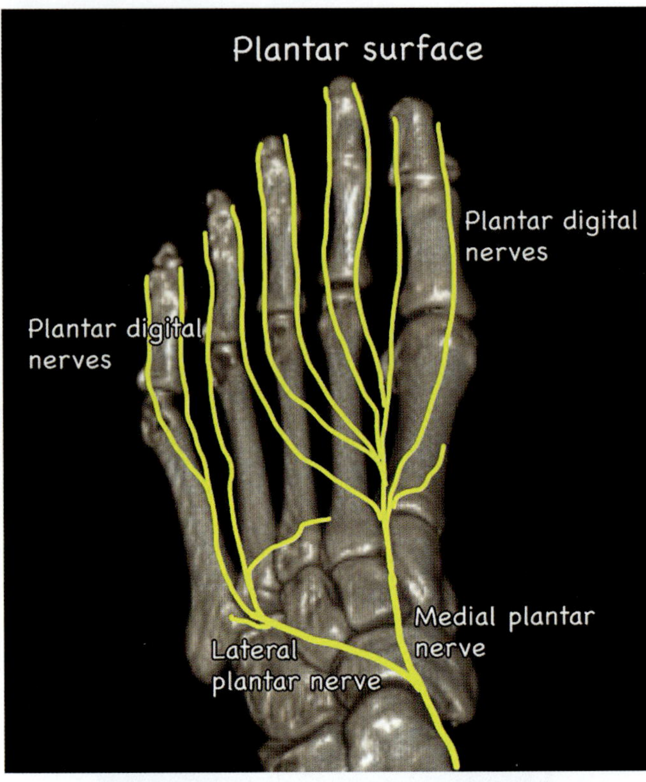

Fig. 3.9.127: Nerve supply of plantar surface of foot

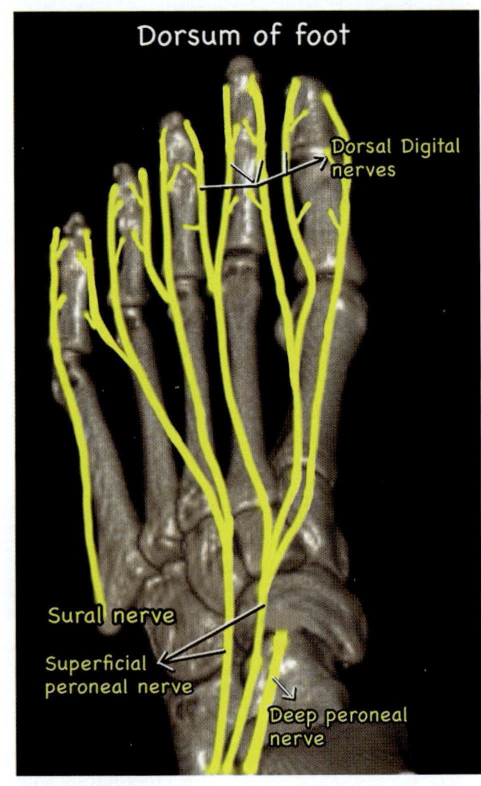

Fig. 3.9.128: Nerve supply of dorsum of foot

Bursa in the foot: Bursa between 1st and 2nd metatarsal bases, bursa at 5th metatarsal base, 1st and 5th metatarsophalangeal bursa, intermetatarsophalangeal bursa. Intermetatarsophalangeal bursa is adjacent to plantar digital neurovascular bundle. So, inflammation of intermetatarsophalangeal bursa can irritate the plantar digit nerve, thereby mimicking Morton neuroma.

3.9.F Arteries, Veins and Nerves of Lower Limb

Arterial system of the lower limb (Figs 3.9.129 and 3.9.130)*:* The external iliac artery continues as femoral artery under the inguinal ligament. It enters the femoral triangle where the profunda femoris artery arises from the posterolateral aspect and gives off three main branches: Perforating branches, lateral circumflex femoral artery, medial circumflex femoral artery. Superficial femoral artery continues down through adductor canal and enters the posterior compartment of the thigh as the popliteal artery. The popliteal artery travels via the popliteal fossa between the gastrocnemius and popliteus muscles, gives genicular branches as it lowers the posterior thigh. It joins the anterior tibial artery and the tibioperoneal trunk at the lower border of the popliteus. Through a fissure in the interosseous membrane, the anterior tibial artery passes anteriorly between the tibia and fibula. In foot, ATA lies deep to the extensor retinaculum midway between the malleoli and becomes the dorsalis pedis artery. Dorsalis pedis artery (DPA) lies deep and medial to extensor digitorum longus and passes over the dorsal aspect, then reaches the sole of the foot. In sole DPA anastomoses with the lateral plantar artery to form the deep plantar arch. The posterior tibial

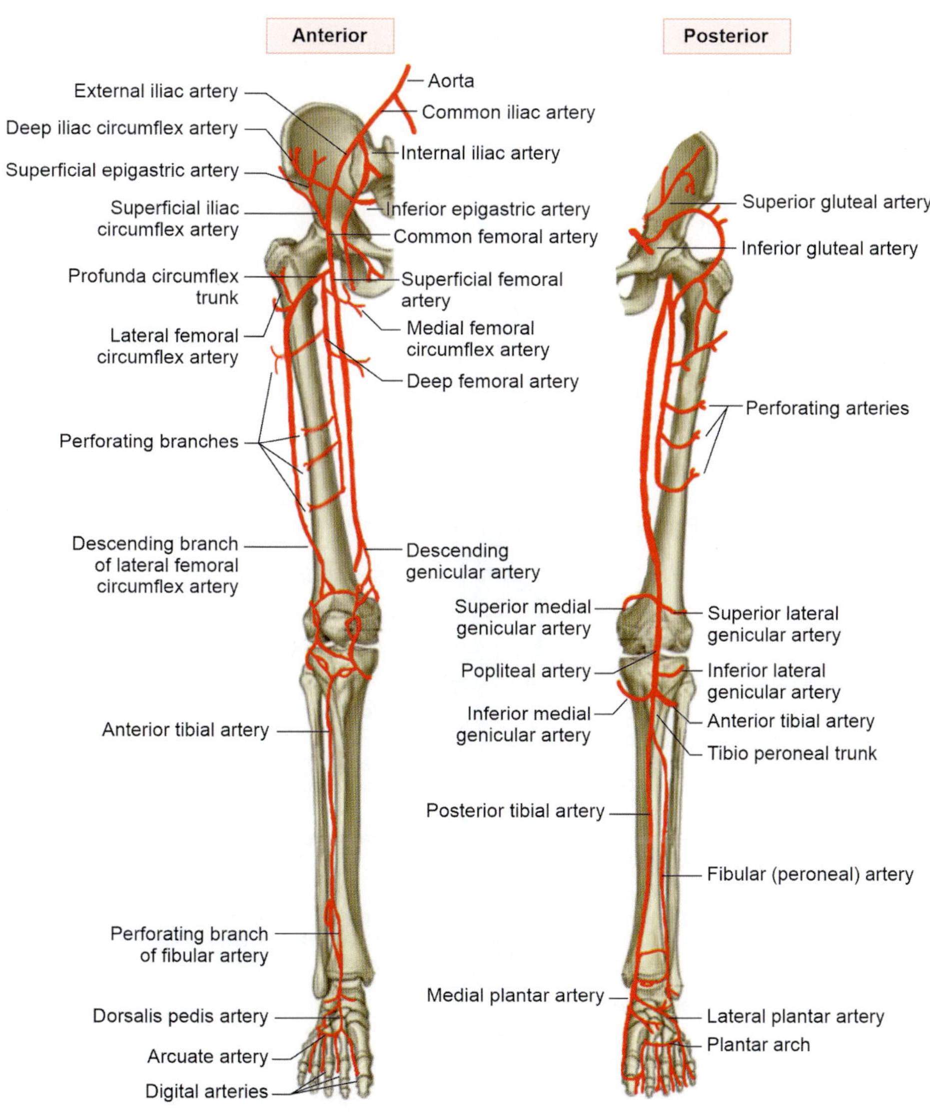

Fig. 3.9.129: Arterial system of lower limb

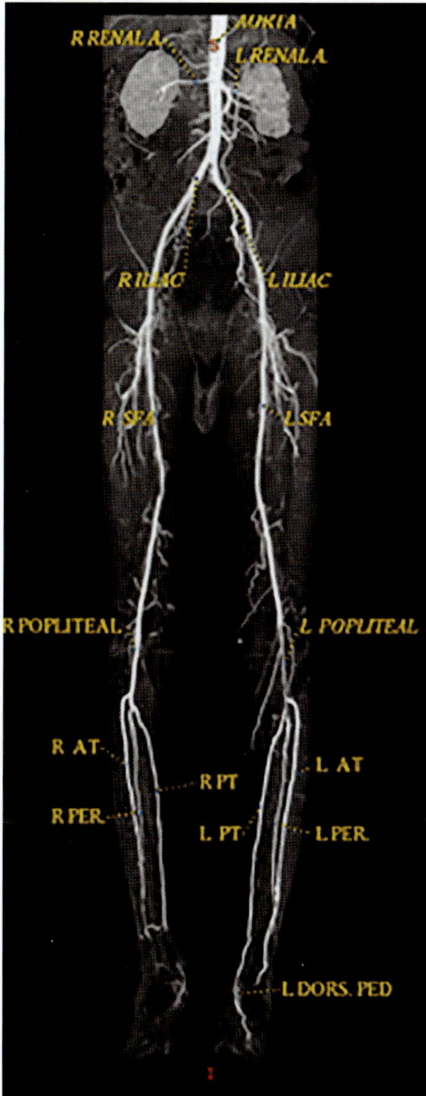

Fig. 3.9.130: CT angiogram of lower limb

3

and fibular arteries split the tibioperoneal trunk. The inferior course of the posterior tibial artery runs over the surface of the deep posterior leg muscles. It enters the sole of the foot through the tarsal tunnel and splits into the lateral and medial plantar arteries, along with the tibial nerve. Fibular (peroneal) artery descends posteriorly to the fibula, within the posterior compartment of the leg. It gives rise to perforating branches, which penetrate the intermuscular septum. Additional blood supply to lower limb is by the following arteries: The obturator artery arises from the internal iliac artery in the pelvic region. It descends via the obturator canal to enter the medial thigh, bifurcating into two branches: Anterior branch and posterior branch. The superior and inferior gluteal arteries also arise from the internal iliac artery, entering the gluteal region via the greater sciatic foramen. The superior and inferior gluteal artery leaves the foramen above and below the piriformis muscle respectively.

Venous system of lower limb (Fig. 3.9.131): There are two types of veins in the lower limb—deep and superficial.

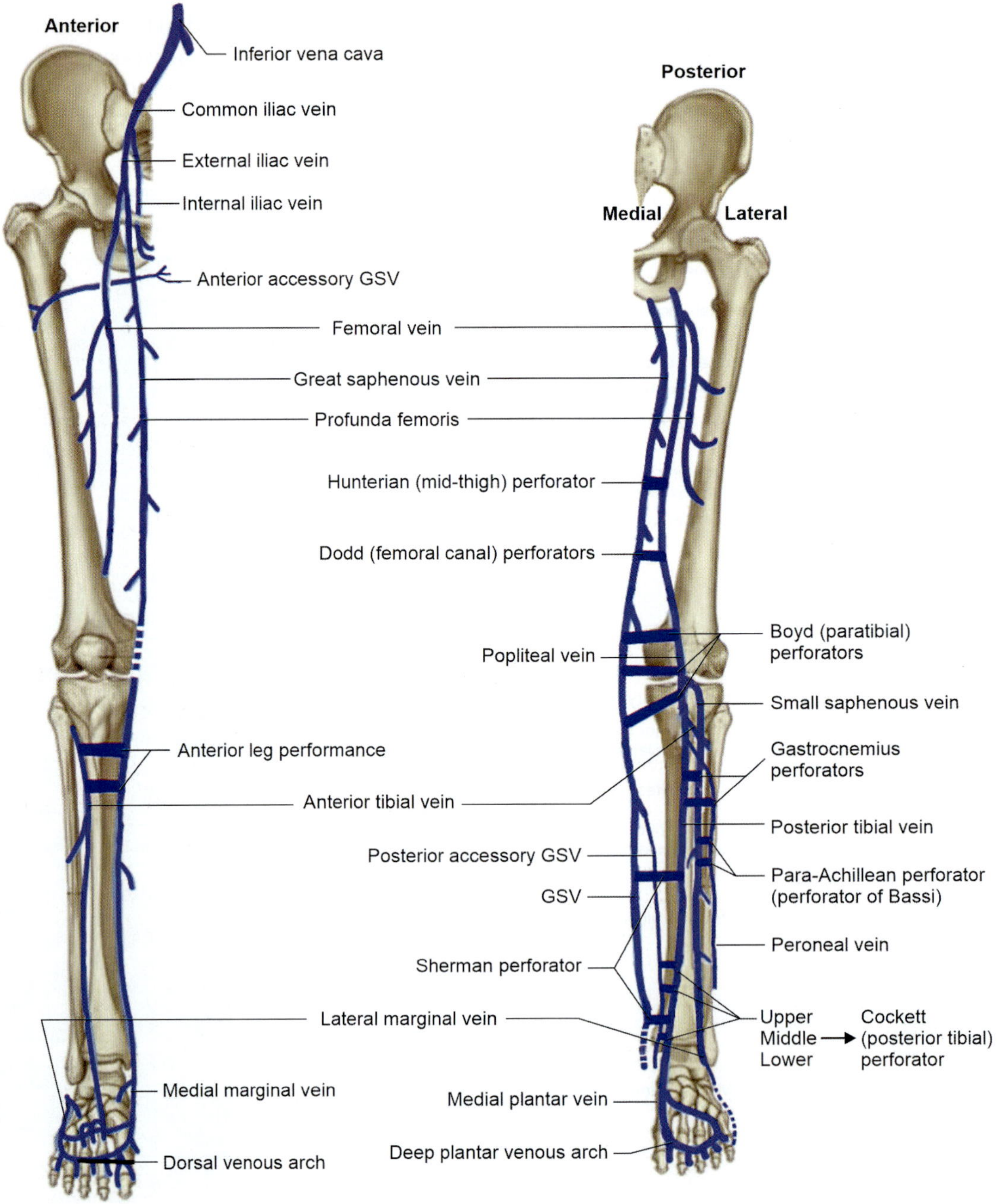

Fig. 3.9.131: Venous system of lower limb

Deep veins run alongside the major arteries beneath the deep fascia of the lower limb. The dorsal venous arch is the major venous structure of the foot, and it drains mostly into the superficial veins. The anterior tibial vein is formed by veins from the arch that penetrate deep into the leg. Medial and lateral plantar veins arise in the plantar aspect of the foot and combine to form the posterior tibial and fibular veins. The posterior tibial vein joins the posterior tibial artery at the medial malleolus and enters the leg posteriorly. The anterior tibial, posterior tibial, and fibular veins join to produce the popliteal vein on the back of the knee. As the femoral vein, the popliteal vein enters the thigh through the adductor canal. It runs beside the femoral artery and is located anteriorly. The other major venous component in the thigh is the deep vein (profunda femoris vein). It drains blood from the thigh muscles by perforating veins. It subsequently discharges into the femoral vein's distal part. The femoral vein exits the thigh and runs beneath the inguinal ligament, where it becomes the external iliac vein. The inferior and superior gluteal veins drain the gluteal area. The internal iliac vein receives the blood from these veins. The subcutaneous tissue contains superficial veins. They finally reach the deep veins and drain. The great saphenous vein and the small saphenous vein are the two major superficial veins. The dorsal venous arch of the foot and the dorsal vein of the great toe combine to generate the great saphenous vein. It ascends up the medial side of the leg, passing anteriorly to the medial malleolus at the ankle, and posteriorly to the medial condyle at the knee. As the vein moves up the leg, it receives tributaries from other small superficial veins. The great saphenous vein terminates by draining into the femoral vein immediately inferior to the inguinal ligament. The dorsal venous arch of the foot and the dorsal vein of the little toe combine to generate the small saphenous vein. It travels along the back of the leg, passing behind the lateral malleolus and along the calcaneal tendon's lateral border. It travels between the two heads of the gastrocnemius muscle and empties into the popliteal vein, which is located in the popliteal fossa.

Perforators of lower limb (Figs 3.9.132 and 3.9.133): The perforating veins of the lower limb perforate the deep fascia to connect the superficial venous systems with the deep, draining into it. There are numerous perforators with variable location.

Perforators of the foot (venae perforantes pedis) include dorsal foot perforators, intercapitular veins, plantar foot perforators, lateral and medial foot perforators.

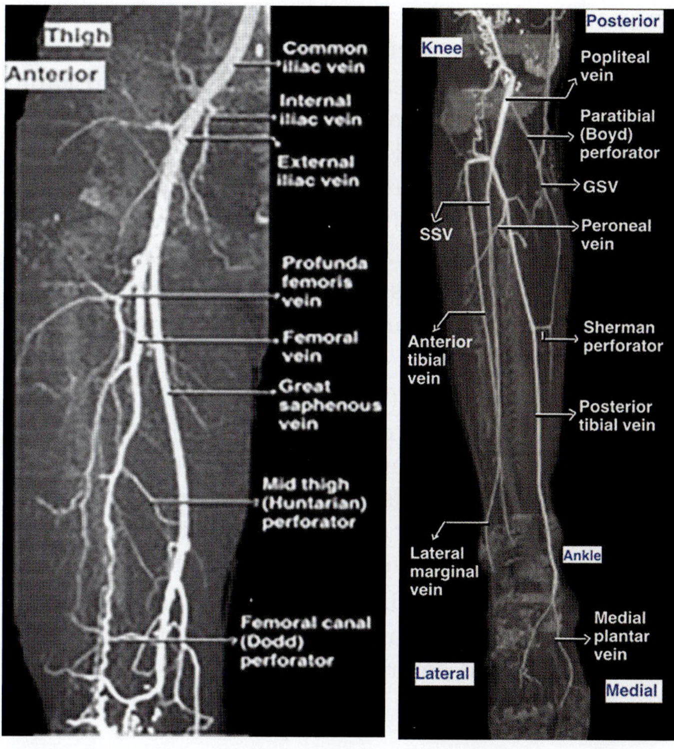

Fig. 3.9.132: CT venogram of thigh with perforators

Fig. 3.9.133: CT venogram of leg and foot with perforators

Perforators of the ankle (venae perforantis tarsalis) include medial, lateral and anterior ankle perforators. **Perforators of the leg (venae perforantes cruris):** Medial leg perforators: (i) Paratibial PV join the main trunk or tributaries of the great saphenous vein (GSV) with the posterior tibial veins and course close to the medial surface of the tibia. These correspond to the so-called **Sherman PV** (at the lower and mid leg) and **Boyd PV** (at the upper leg). (ii) Posterior tibial PV posterior tibial perforators **(Cockett perforators—upper, middle, and lower)** connect the posterior accessory great saphenous vein with the posterior tibial veins. Anterior leg perforators pierce the anterior tibial compartment and connect the anterior tributaries of the GSV to the anterior tibial veins. Lateral leg perforators connect veins of the lateral venous plexus with the fibular veins. Posterior leg perforators are medial gastrocnemius perforators (in the medial calf), lateral gastrocnemius perforators (in the lateral calf), intergemellar perforators (connecting the SSV with the calf veins, also called "mid-calf perforator of May"), para-Achillean perforators (connecting the SSV with the fibular veins; also called "perforator of Bassi"). **Perforators of the knee (venae perforantes genus)** include medial and lateral knee perforators, suprapatellar perforators, infrapatellar perforators and popliteal fossa perforators. **Perforators of the thigh (venae perforantes femoris):** Medial thigh perforators include perforators of the femoral canal (Dodd), inguinal perforators. Posterior thigh perforators include posteromedial thigh perforators (Hunterian canal perforator), sciatic perforators, posterolateral thigh perforators, "perforator of Hach" and pudendal perforators. There are also anterior and lateral thigh perforators. **Perforators of the gluteal muscles (venae perforantes glutealis)** are grouped as superior, mid and lower perforators.

Nerves of lower limb (Fig. 3.9.134): The major nerve supply of lower limb is derived from lumbar and sacral plexus. The three major nerves of lower limb are the **femoral (posterior divisions of ventral rami of L2, L3, L4), obturator (anterior divisions of ventral rami of L2, L3, L4) and sciatic nerve (L4, L5, S1, S2, S3).**

Femoral nerve: It is the **largest branch** of lumbar plexus coursing inferiorly from its origin, medial to psoas major muscle and emerges between psoas and iliacus, then passes behind the inguinal ligament, to enter the lower limb where it divides into **anterior and posterior divisions**. The femoral nerve lies lateral to femoral artery outside the femoral sheath. The femoral nerve supplies **the muscles of anterior compartment of thigh via numerous motor branches, skin on the anterior and medial aspects of thigh and skin on the medial side of leg and foot.** In the abdomen just before passing behind the inguinal ligament, femoral nerve gives a branch to iliacus and pectineus. Then passing behind the inguinal ligament, it gives off anterior and posterior divisions. From the posterior division arise the **saphenous nerve which is the largest and longest cutaneous branch of the femoral nerve and the longest nerve in the body.** The saphenous nerve descends initially lateral to femoral artery in the adductor canal, and then courses anterior to the artery to lie medial to it, and emerges through the aponeurotic covering at the distal end of the canal with contributions to subsartorial plexus, peripatellar plexus and distally descends with the great saphenous vein along the medial border of tibia, and then passes anterior to the ankle to supply the skin on the medial side of

Table 3.9.11: Nerve entrapment in lower limb

Nerve	*Site of entrapment*
Common peroneal nerve	Fibular neck (superficial location), origin of peroneus longus muscle
Deep peroneal nerve	Anterior tarsal tunnel, dorsum of foot (between the first and second tarsometatarsal joints)
Superficial peroneal nerve	10–15 cm above the ankle joint where the nerve pierces the deep fascia
Tibial nerve	Tarsal tunnel
Medial plantar nerve	Tarsal tunnel or distal to tarsal tunnel, knot of Henry
Lateral plantar nerve	Tarsal tunnel or distal to tarsal tunnel
Inferior calcaneal nerve (Baxter nerve—first branch of lateral plantar nerve)	Medial calcaneal tuberosity, compression by hypertrophied abductor hallucis muscle, at the medial edge of quadratus plantae muscle
Interdigital nerve (Morton neuroma)	Intermetatarsal space mostly second and third intermetatarsal space
Joplin neuroma (medial plantar proper digital neuropathy)	First metatarsophalangeal joint and plantar aspect of hallux
Sural nerve	Lateral aspect of foot as it passes behind the lateral malleolus (most commonly resulting from trauma involving the distal fibula, talus and calcaneum)
Lateral femoral cutaneous nerve (meralgia paresthetica)	Under the inguinal ligament
Sciatic nerve	Between greater sciatic notch and ischial tuberosity Piriformis syndrome (compression at greater sciatic notch by piriformis muscle)
Obturator nerve	Point of entry to obturator foramen under the superior pubic ramus
Femoral nerve	Under the inguinal ligament
Pudendal nerve	Compression of pudendal nerve either at Alcock's canal (Alcock's canal syndrome) or at ischial spine under sacrospinous and sacrotuberous ligament

3

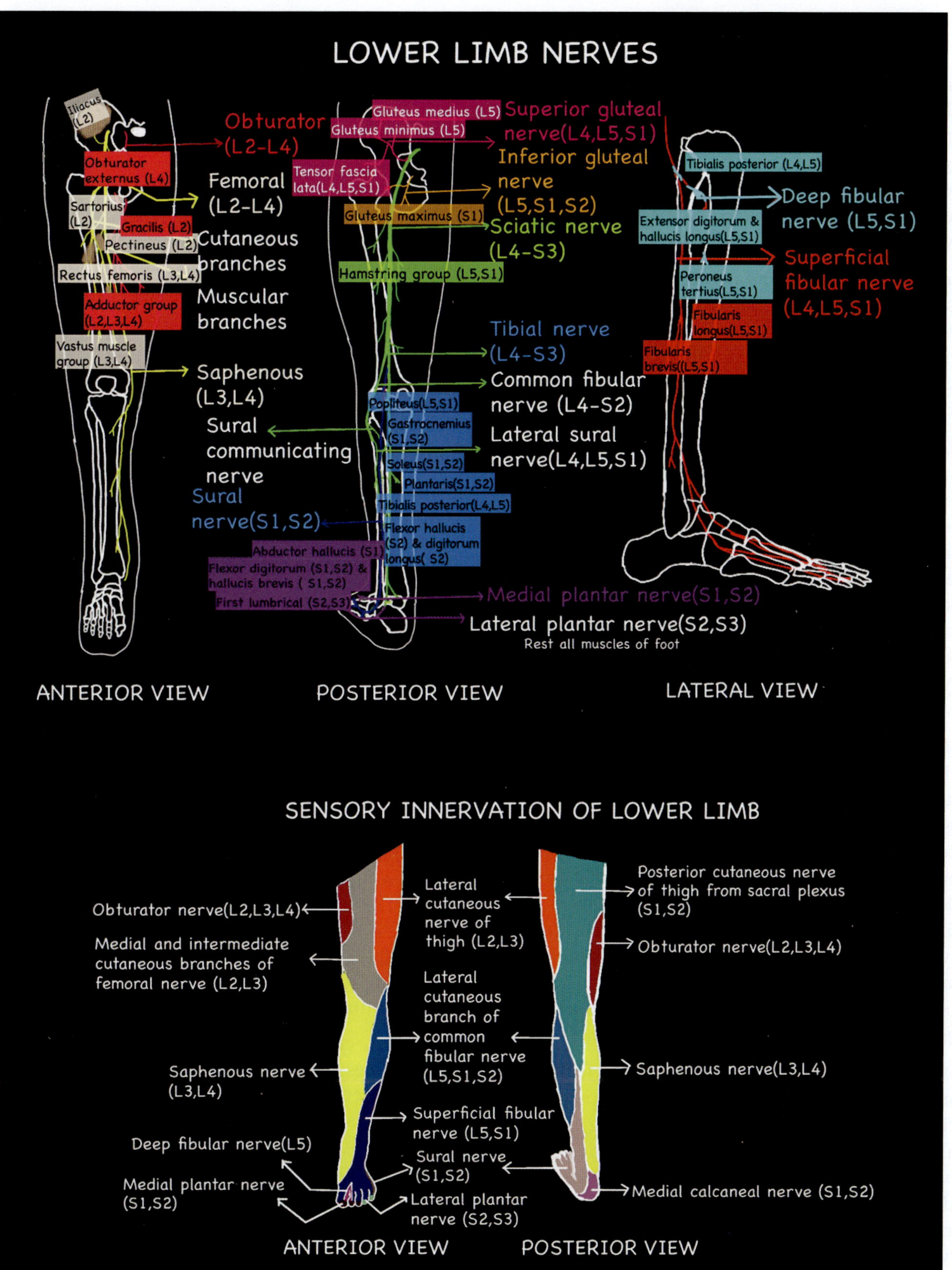

Figs 3.9.134: (Upper part): Lower limb nerves **and 3.9.135:** (Lower part): Sensory innervation of lower limb

the foot, often as far as the first metatarsophalangeal joint.

Obturator nerve: Obturator nerve is another major branch from lumbar plexus, continuing along the lateral pelvic wall, and enters the medial compartment of thigh through the obturator canal and divides into anterior and posterior branches. It is the nerve supply to all the adductor muscles of thigh and also provides cutaneous innervation to skin on the medial side of thigh.

Lateral femoral cutaneous nerve of thigh: This nerve arises from the lumbar plexus (L2, L3) and leaves abdomen passing between inguinal ligament and pelvic bone, medial to anterior superior iliac spine or sometimes pass directly through the inguinal ligament supplying the skin on lateral side of thigh.

Sciatic nerve: The sciatic nerve is the thickest nerve of the body, arising from the sacral plexus, leaves the pelvis via greater sciatic foramen below the piriformis, descends on the posterior aspect of thigh finally dividing into tibial and common peroneal nerve. The point of division of the sciatic nerve into its tibial and common fibular components is variable, the common site is at the junction of the middle and lower thirds of the thigh, near the apex of the popliteal fossa, but the division may occur at any level above this point and, rarely, may occur below it.

Tibial branch of sciatic nerve: The tibial nerve after its origin from the sciatic nerve, courses through the popliteal fossa and is the motor supply to all the muscles of posterior compartment of thigh (except short head of biceps femoris supplied by common fibular nerve), posterior compartment of leg and intrinsic muscles of sole of foot. It provides sensory innervation to the articular branches to knee, ankle joints and cutaneous innervation to posterolateral side of lower half of leg and lateral side of ankle, foot and little toe and skin on sole of foot and toes via the medial and lateral plantar nerves.

Common fibular branch of sciatic nerve: It provides motor innervation to short head of biceps femoris, anterior and lateral compartments of leg, first two dorsal interossei muscles of foot. It provides sensory innervation to skin over the lateral aspect of leg, ankle and dorsum of foot and toes. It actually divides into superficial and deep branch with superficial branch innervating the muscles of lateral compartment of leg and deep branch innervating the anterior compartment of leg.

Sural nerve: It is one of the important sensory nerves of lower limb, a cutaneous branch of tibial nerve originating high in the leg. It has close relationship with short saphenous vein, passing posterior to lateral malleolus and innervating the skin on the lateral side of foot and dorsolateral surface of little toe.

Superior gluteal nerve: It is a branch from sacral plexus formed by the dorsal branches of L4, L5 and S1 ventral rami. It leaves the pelvis via the greater sciatic foramen above piriformis, and divides into superior and inferior branches and provides innervation to gluteus medius and gluteus minimus.

Inferior gluteal nerve: It also arises from sacral plexus, formed from the dorsal branches of L4, L5, S1 and S2 ventral rami. It passes via greater sciatic foramen below the piriformis and provides innervation to gluteus maximus muscle.

3.9.G Lymphatic System

The lymphatic system is the collective term given to the lymphatic vessels and lymphoid tissues in the body.

Lymphatic vessels: A percentage of the blood that enters a tissue capillary bed does not return via the veins, but instead creates interstitial fluid in the extracellular space, which is returned to the circulation via the lymphatic vessels (also known as lymphatics), which make up the lymph vascular system. The fluid in the lymphatic system is referred to as lymph. When referring to the lymph emptying the gut and liver, which contains chylomicrons from digested food, it is referred to as chyle. Lymphatic capillaries constitute the foundation of the lymphatic system, which eventually combine to produce bigger precollectors and collector lymphatic veins. These collecting vessels join to form lymphatic trunks, which then drain into the body's two major trunks, the thoracic duct and right lymphatic duct, on the left and right sides, respectively. Lymph flow is estimated to be 2–4 litres per day on average.

Lymphatic capillaries: The lymphatic capillaries are the smallest vessels in the system, arising as blind-ending single layer endothelial tubes in the tissue capillary beds. In comparison to capillaries, lymphatic capillaries are dilated and have a wider range of caliber. Anchoring filaments link the capillary walls to the surrounding structural tissues, preventing dynamic collapse.

Precollecting and collecting lymphatics: The lymphatic capillaries converge to produce the collecting lymphatics (or collectors), which have both valves and smooth muscle, and walls that resemble veins, but the tunica layers are more difficult to discern than the venous wall. The number of valves more than in the veins. In some lymphatic networks, capillaries merge first to create precollector lymphatics, which are similar to capillaries in that they have a single-layer endothelial wall but differ in that they have valves but no smooth muscle layer. Peristaltic waves are created by smooth muscle in the collector walls, guaranteeing unidirectional lymph flow. A lymphangion is a contractile unit that ensures lymph travels to the next lymphangion through a shared interposing valve between two valves. Skeletal muscle action, the inspiratory fall in intrathoracic pressure, and a pressure gradient towards the veins into which the biggest lymphatics drain all contribute to this one-way flow. As afferent lymphatics, the collecting lymphatics enter into the cortex of local lymph nodes (prenodal collecting lymphatics). The efferent lymphatics (postnodal collecting lymphatics) leave the nodes, either passing to further nodes in the chain or merging with other efferent lymphatic vessels to form the lymphatic trunks.

Lymphatic trunks (Fig. 3.9.136): The lymphatic trunks, comprise four paired sets (one trunk for each side of the body), the multilevel intercostal trunks and an unpaired left-sided intestinal trunk: jugular trunks drain the neck, subclavian trunks: drain the upper limbs, bronchomediastinal trunks: drain the chest, intercostal trunks: drain the chest wall, lumbar trunks, intestinal trunks: drains the gut. Most of the lymphs from beneath the diaphragm drain into the cisterna chyli, before it finally returns to the main systemic circulation via the thoracic duct on the left, and on the other side of the body, the right lymphatic duct. For the most part, subcutaneous lymphatic vessels accompany veins, whilst deeper lymphatics accompany arteries. The initial lymphatics in the microvilli of the gut wall are specially named—due to their unique function in absorbing and transporting fats—and are called lacteals.

Fig. 3.9.136: Lymphatic system

Alymphatic organs: With the exception of cartilage, bone marrow, bone, placenta, cornea, brain, and teeth, lymphatic vessels can be found throughout the body. The presence of lymphatic vessels in the bone is debatable, and if they exist, they are far more scarce than in other bodily tissues. Although new research has shown that the brain possesses a lymphatic system. There is a lymphatic system in the meninges. The presence of a lymphatic drainage system in the eye has been a source of debate for many years. The presence of lymphatics in the eye appears to have gained acceptance in recent years, however, many specifics remain uncertain.

Functions: The lymphatic system's main job is to return exuded capillary fluid and protein to the circulatory system. Every day, around 25–50 percent of plasma proteins re-enter the central veins from the lymphatic system. The draining lymphatics in the GI tract play an important role in delivering cholesterol and long-chain fatty acids (as chylomicrons) to the liver.

Imaging modalities: Visualization of the lymphatic system by medical imaging has lagged behind radiology

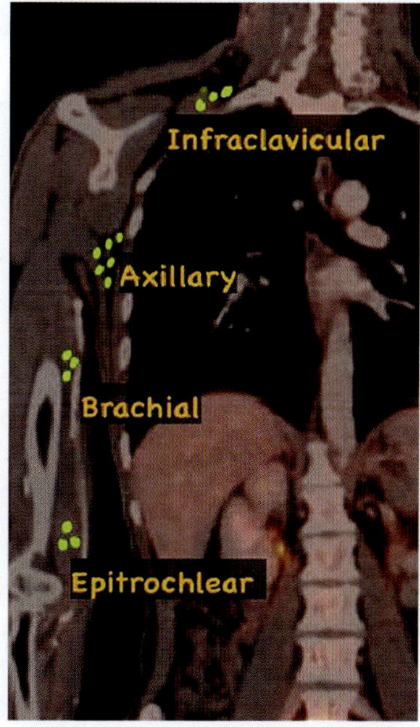

Fig. 3.9.137: Lymphatic chain of upper limb

of many other body systems due to the small caliber of many of the lymphatics. Methods employed: Extremity lymphangiography, lymphoscintigraphy, indocyanine green lymphangiography and MR lymphangiography.

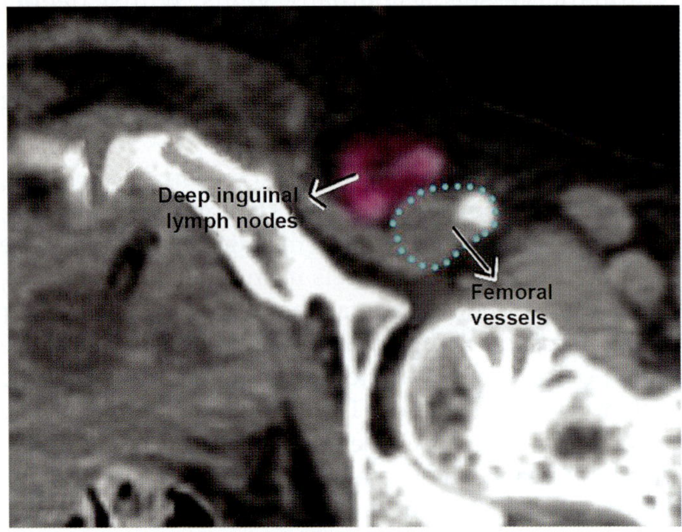

Fig. 3.9.138

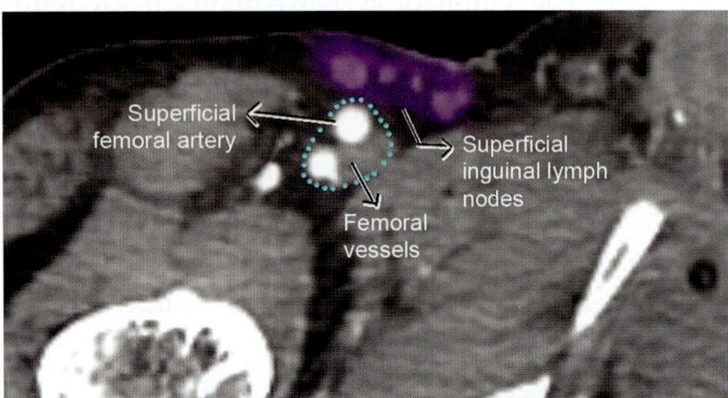

Fig. 3.9.139

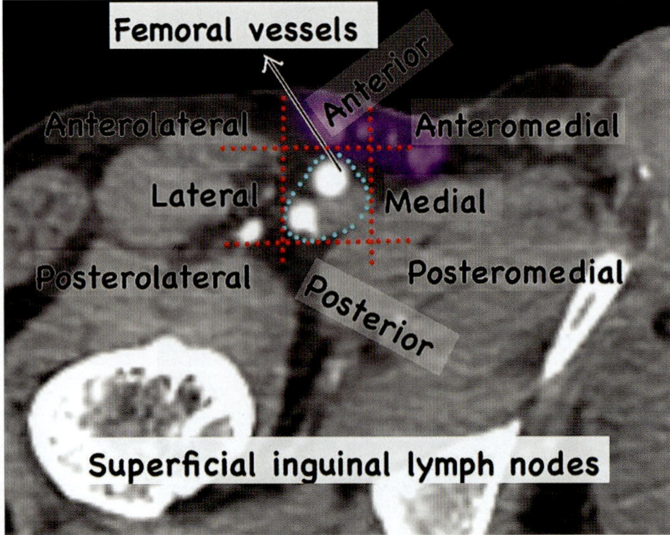

Fig. 3.9.140

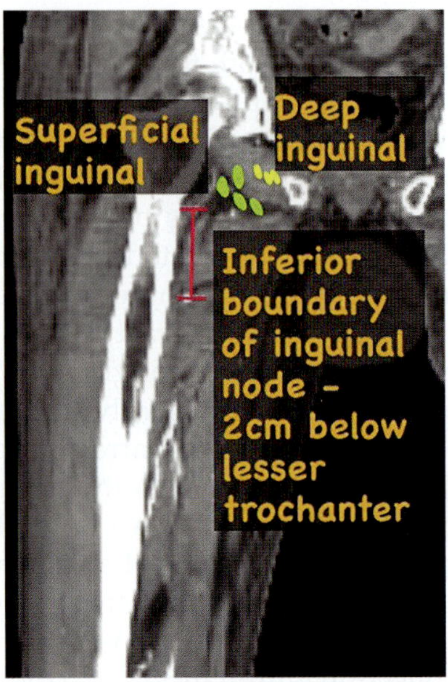

Fig. 3.9.141

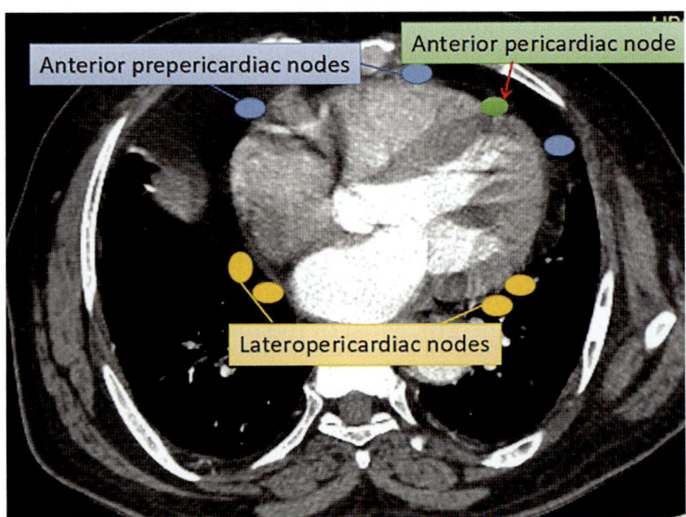

Fig. 3.9.142

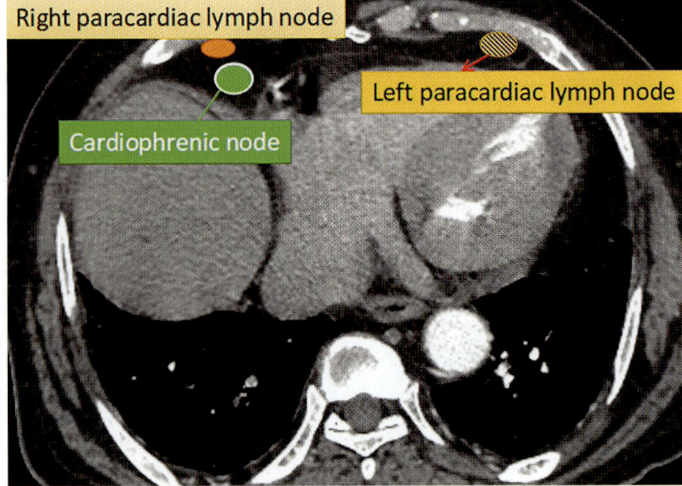

Fig. 3.9.143

Major lymphatic groups in imaging shown in Figs 3.9.138 to 3.9.148.

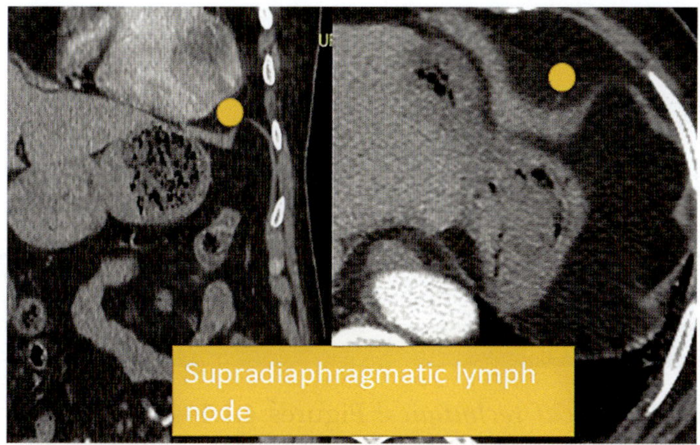

Fig. 3.9.144

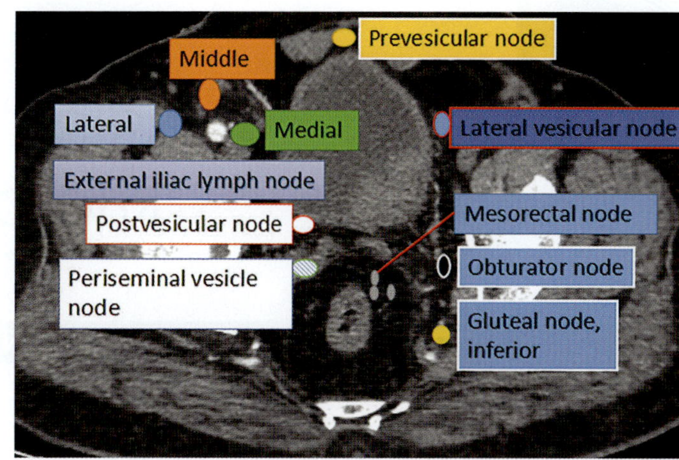

Fig. 3.9.147

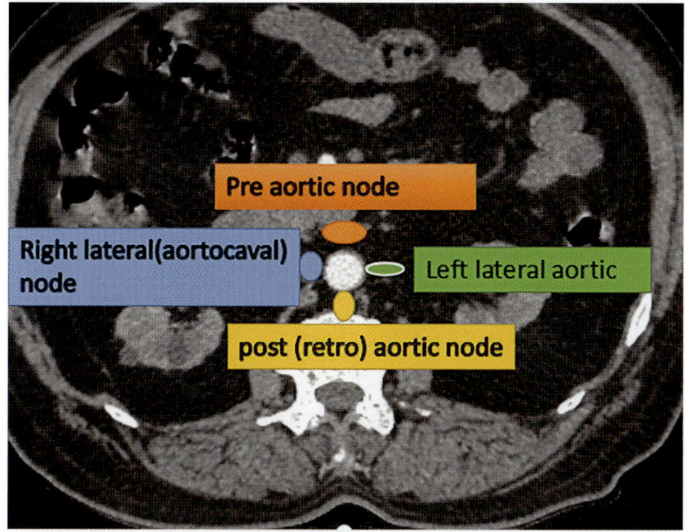

Fig. 3.9.145

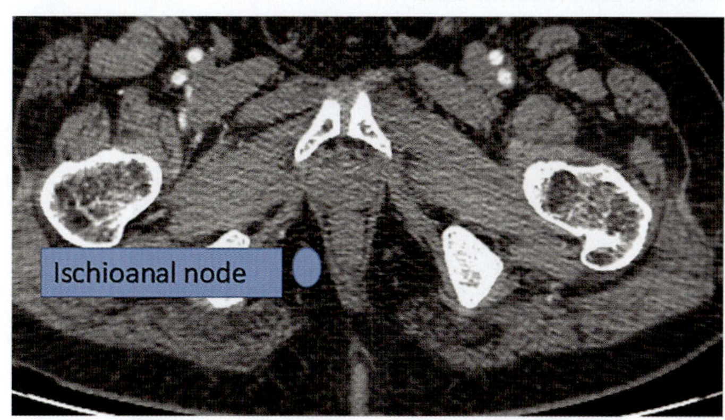

Fig. 3.9.148

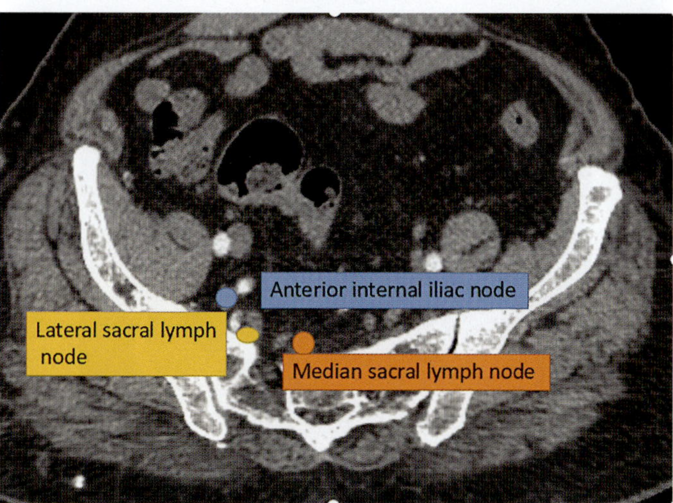

Fig. 3.9.146

Imaging Approach for Radiology Cases

4.1 CENTRAL NERVOUS SYSTEM

Case No. 1

Clinical history: A one-year-old child with macrocephaly and developmental delay.

Radiological techniques: Figures 4.1.1–4.1.4 are MRI brain images in T2 axial, T1 sagittal sequences and antenatal ultrasound images respectively.

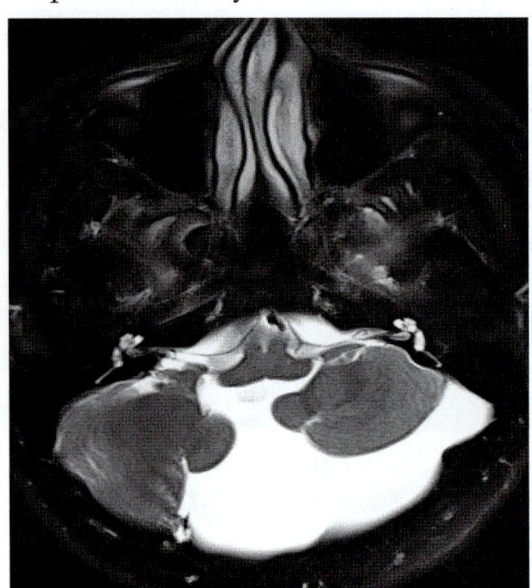

Fig. 4.1.1

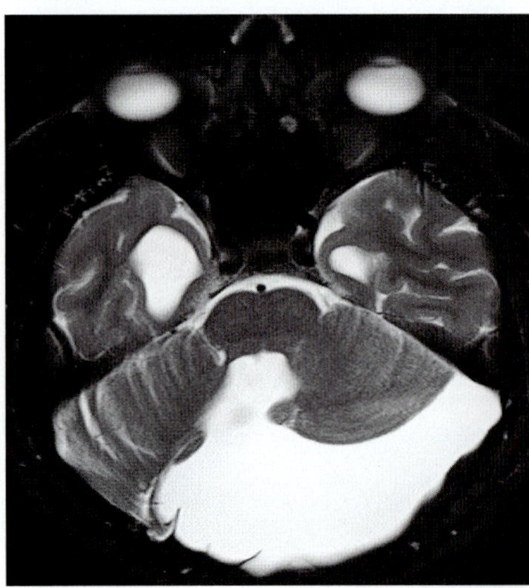

Fig. 4.1.2

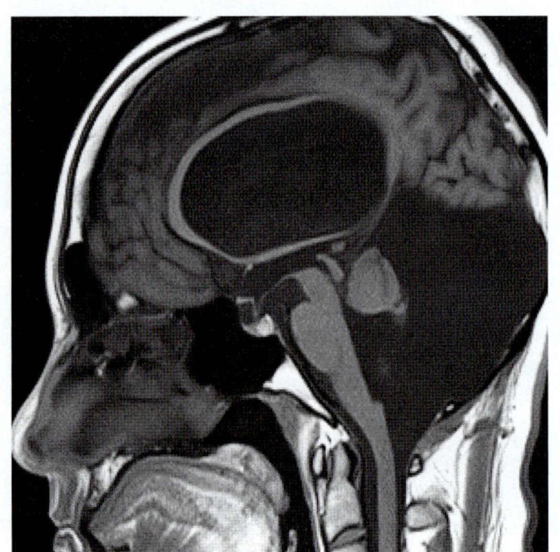

Fig. 4.1.3

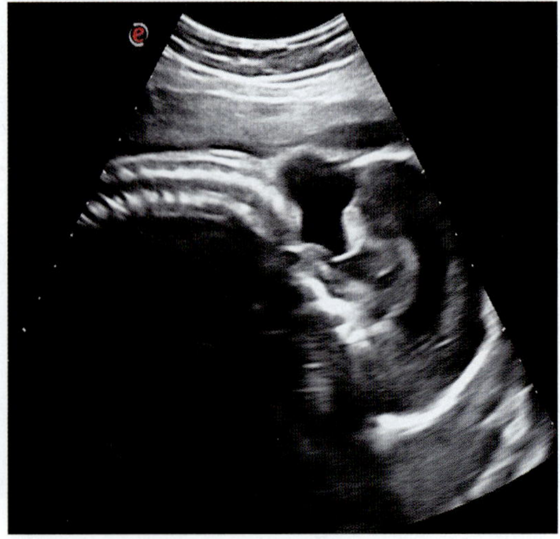

Fig. 4.1.4

Observation: There is **hypoplasia of the vermis and counter-clockwise cephalad rotation of vermian remnant. Cystic dilatation of 4th ventricle extending posteriorly into the retro cerebellar space** and cerebellar hemispheres displaced anterolaterally. **It consists of enlarged posterior fossa and torcular-lambdoid inversion** (the torcular that lies above level of the lambdoid due to abnormally high tentorium—torcular Herophili). Tentorium cerebelli displaced superiorly. Tegmento-vermian angle is more than 45 degrees. There is also gross hydrocephalus.

Interpretation: A—1-year-old child with lesion in 4th ventricle, C—Cystic lesion in the 4th ventricle communicating with enlarged posterior fossa, B—Vermian hypoplasia, cephalad rotation of vermian remnant and torcular-lambdoid inversion. Tegmento-vermian angle >45°, D—Dandy-Walker malformation.

Table 4.1.1: Differential diagnosis for Dandy-Walker malformation

Isolated vermian hypoplasia with rotation (HVR): Old term = Dandy-Walker variant. Characterised by partial vermian hypoplasia specifically on its inferior portion. Remainder of the vermis, cerebellar hemispheres, 4th ventricle—normal. Normal cognitive, language, social, and behavioural outcomes.

Variable vermian hypoplasia, small posterior fossa cyst, keyhole vallecula

Reduced vermian tissue below fastigium-declive line. Superior rotation of vermis. **Increased** tegmento-vermian angle (18–45°). **Posterior fossa normal size.** Diagnosis cannot be made definitely until the 18th week of gestation as inferior vermis does not form until then.

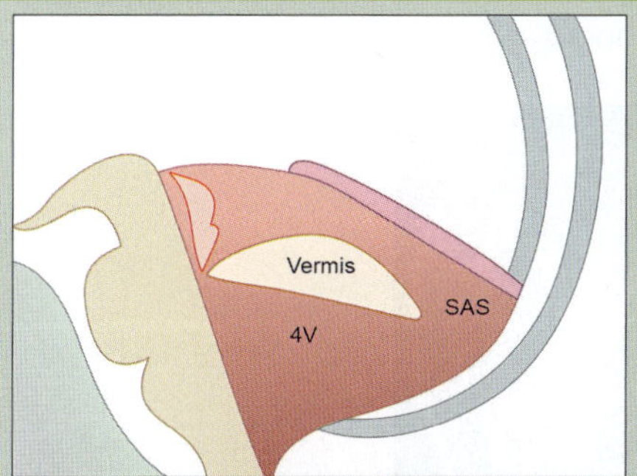

Fig. 4.1.5: Dandy-Walker variant

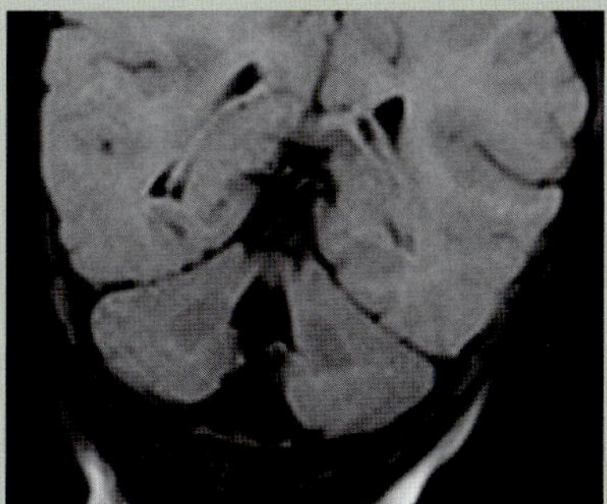

Fig. 4.1.6: Dandy-Walker variant

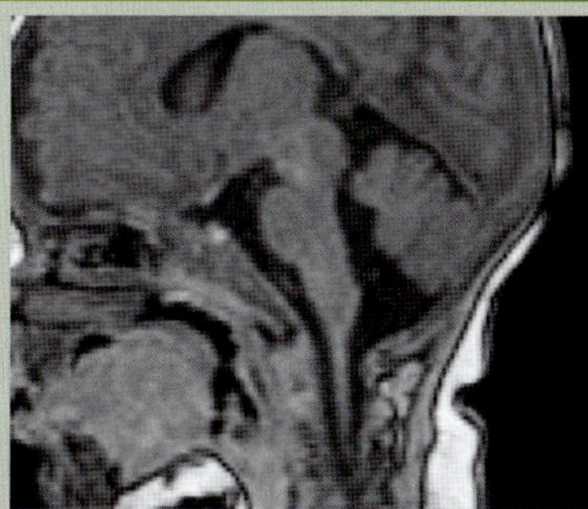

Fig. 4.1.7: Dandy-Walker variant

Persistent Blake pouch cyst

Also known as rudimental fourth ventricle tela choroidea. Posterior ballooning of inferior medullary velum into the cisterna magna. Can present in childhood or adulthood as hydrocephalus.

Infra vermian cyst that communicates with 4th ventricle. Normal size and morphology of vermis. Elevated vermis. Increased tegmentovermian angle (18–45°). Normally positioned torcula.

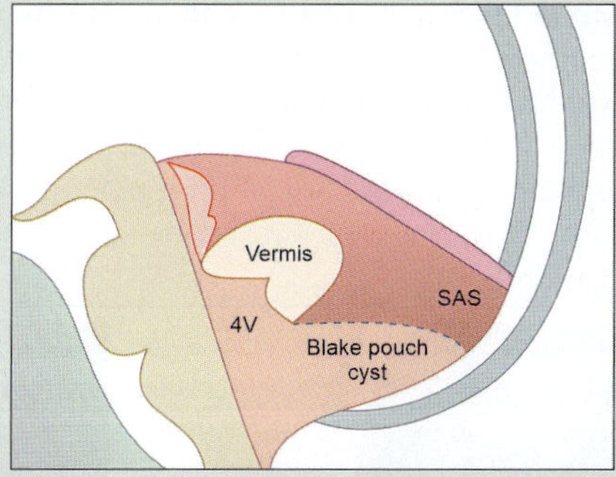

Fig. 4.1.8: Persistent Blake pouch cyst

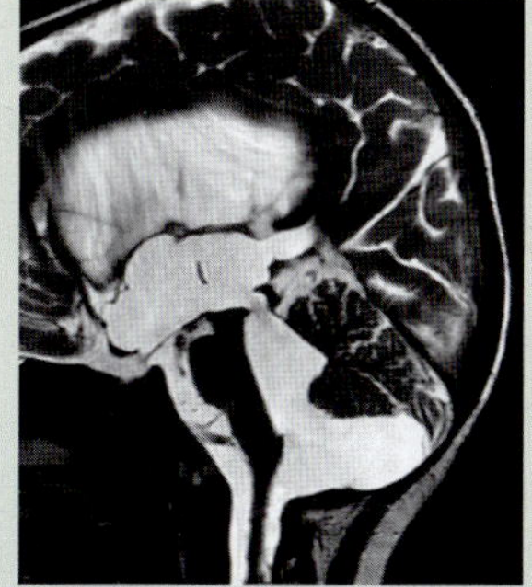

Fig. 4.1.9: Persistent Blake pouch cyst

Mega cisterna magna: Normal variant; occurs in 1% postnatally. Truly focal enlargement of CSF filled subarachnoid space in inferior and posterior portions of posterior cranial fossa. If an isolated finding with normal ventricles, prognosis is good.

Enlarged retrocerebellar CSF (>10 mm). No mass effect on vermis or cerebellum. Normal vermis. Communication seen with the 4th ventricle/basal subarachnoid spaces.

Normal tegmento-vermian angle (<18°). Fluid crossed by veins, falx cerebelli. May scallop/remodel occiput (more common than posterior fossa arachnoid cyst).

Contd...

Table 4.1.1: Differential diagnosis for Dandy-Walker malformation *(Contd...)*

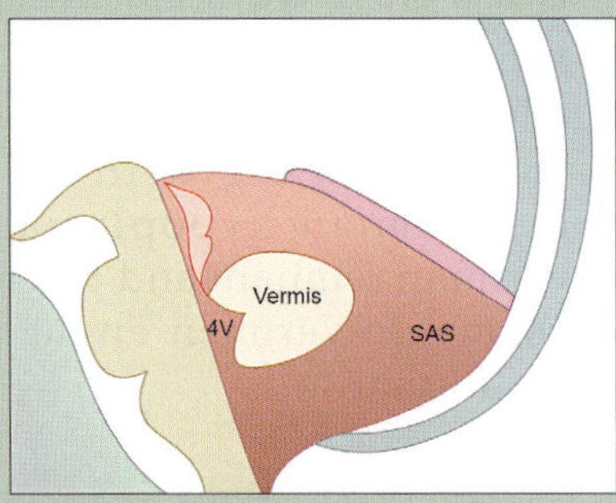

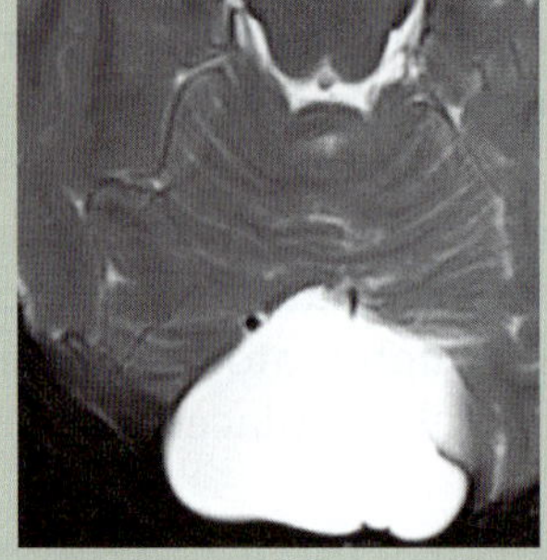

Fig. 4.1.10: Mega cisterna magna **Fig. 4.1.11:** Mega cisterna magna

Posterior fossa arachnoid cyst: Common benign condition; mostly asymptomatic.

Sporadic, also seen with increased frequency in MPS. Not truly in the Dandy-Walker continuum. Most common location—middle cranial fossa. Retrocerebellar location: 30–40%. Surgery or shunting in symptomatic patients. Rare complication—spontaneous rupture in subdural space.

Well-circumscribed cyst with imperceptible wall.

Location: Cerebellopontine angle > retrovermian. **No communication with 4th ventricle. No crossing veins or falx cerebelli. Causes mass effect,** may **remodel bone**. Cisternography shows communication of cyst with subarachnoid spaces.

Tegmento–vermian angle: 0°

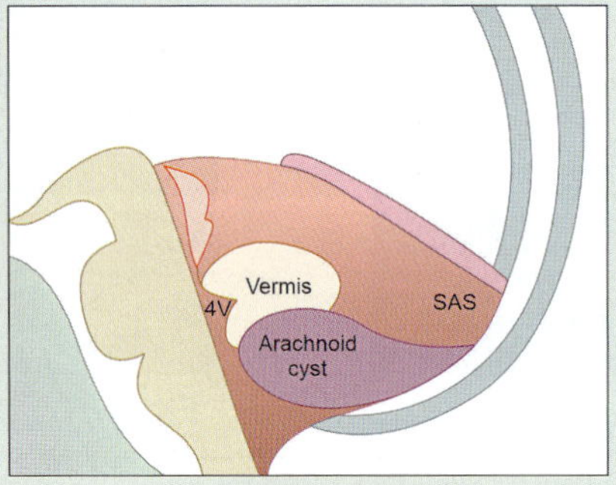

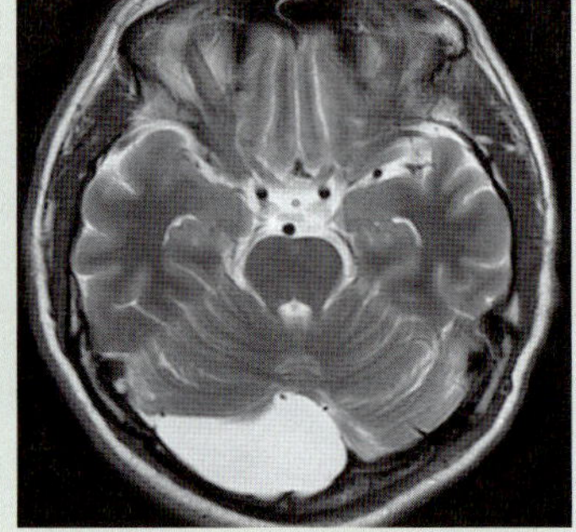

Fig. 4.1.12 Posterior fossa arachnoid cyst **Fig. 4.1.13:** Posterior fossa arachnoid cyst

Molar Tooth Malformation (Joubert Syndrome and Related Disorder)

Predominantly autosomal recessive disorder with variable degree of cerebellar vermal agenesis. Considered as ciliopathy. Typically presents in infancy and childhood.

Midline vermian clefting seen (vermian agenesis) on all sections. **Molar tooth appearance with foreshortened midbrain** on axial images. **Open umbrella-shaped/triangular/bat-wing** configuration 4th ventricle. Thickened superior cerebellar peduncle seen. Tentorium is in the normal location. Sagittal images show **deep ponto mesencephalic junction and high riding 4th ventricle** (normally seen at the level of lower pons and upper medulla).

DTI—superior cerebellar peduncles fail to decussate in mesencephalon. Classic clinical presentation—developmental delay, ataxia, oculomotor and respiratory abnormalities.

Genetic counselling, physical and occupational therapy will be needed.

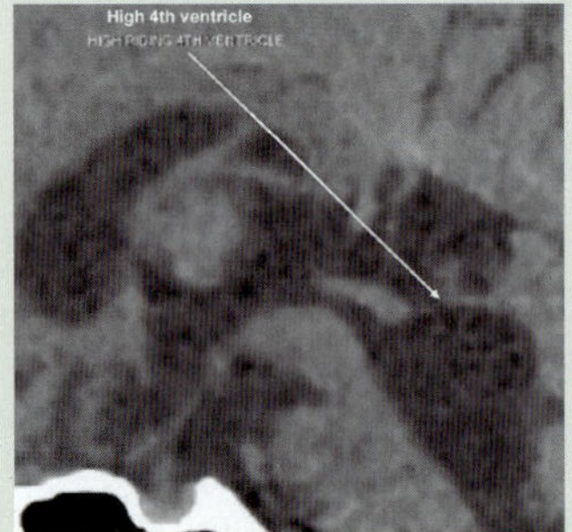

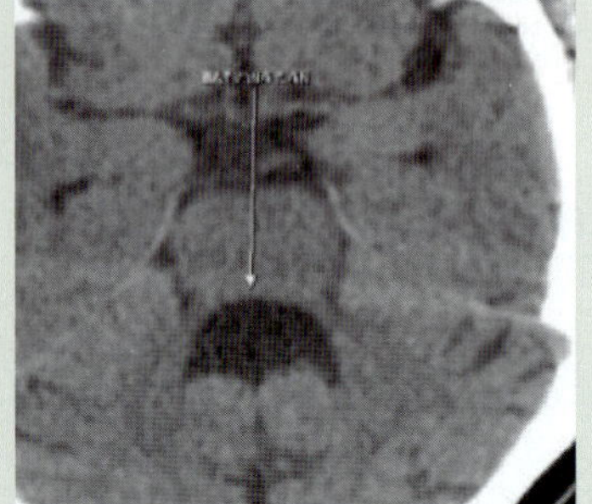

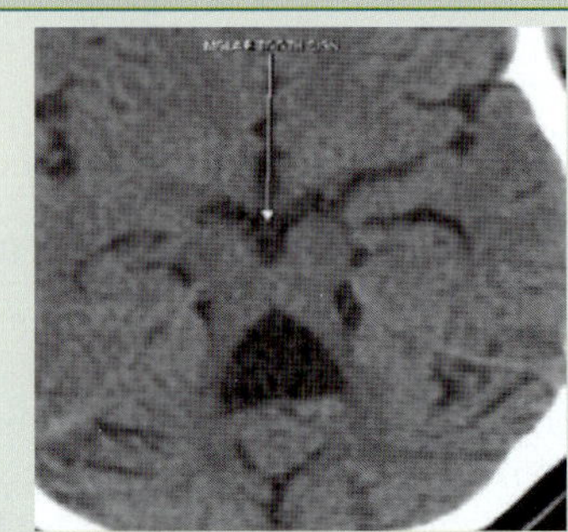

Fig. 4.1.14: Molar tooth malformation **Fig. 4.1.15:** Molar tooth malformation **Fig. 4.1.16:** Molar tooth malformation

Contd...

Table 4.1.1: Differential diagnosis for Dandy-Walker malformation *(Contd...)*
Posterior fossa epidermoid cyst Congenital inclusion cyst arising from ectodermal inclusions during neural tube closure. Most common location—**intradural (90%) with CP angle in 40–50% cases.** Most common symptom—headache. Rare malignant degeneration into squamous cell carcinoma reported. Microsurgical resection can be done. CSF like mass that insinuates cisterns and encases neurovascular structures. NECT—round and lobulated hypodense mass with 10–25% having clacification. Dense epidermoid—secondary to hemorrhage, high protein, saponification of cyst debris. May have bone erosion. T1—slightly hyperintense to brain; **white** epidermoid—hyperintense to brain due to high triglycerides and unsaturated fatty acids; **black** epidermoid—hypointense to CSF due to presence of solid crystal cholesterol and keratin. Characteristic hyperintensity seen in DWI and this distinguishes from arachnoid cyst. MRS-resonances from lactate; no NAA/choline/lipid.
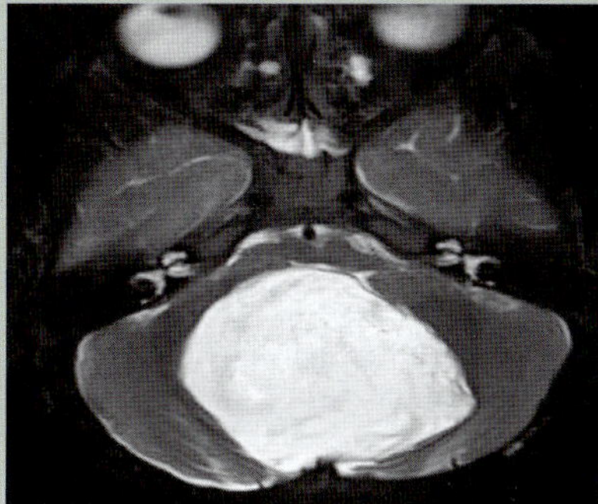 **Fig. 4.1.17:** Posterior fossa epidermoid cyst 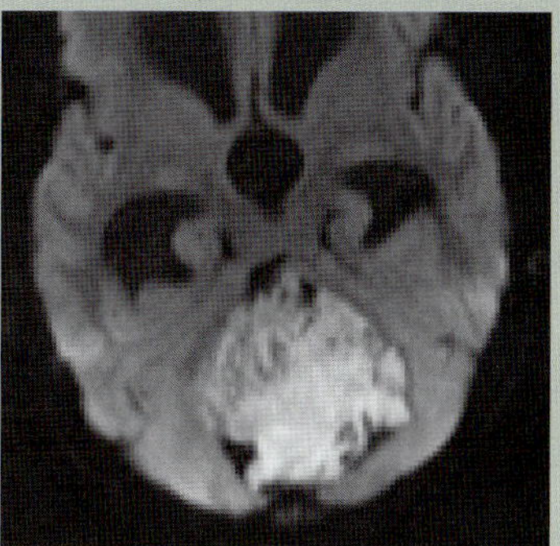 **Fig. 4.1.18:** Posterior fossa epidermoid cyst
Trapped 4th ventricle Obstruction occurs to the entry and exit path of CSF through the ventricle. Symptoms include diplopia, ataxia, nystagmus. Treatment of the cause and shunting of the ventricle can be done. Focally dilated cystic structure of 4th ventricle that follows CSF signals. The remaining ventricluar system appears normal. Transependymal CSF seepage occurs around trapped ventricle. Keyhole sign is seen in herniation of trapped 4th ventricle. 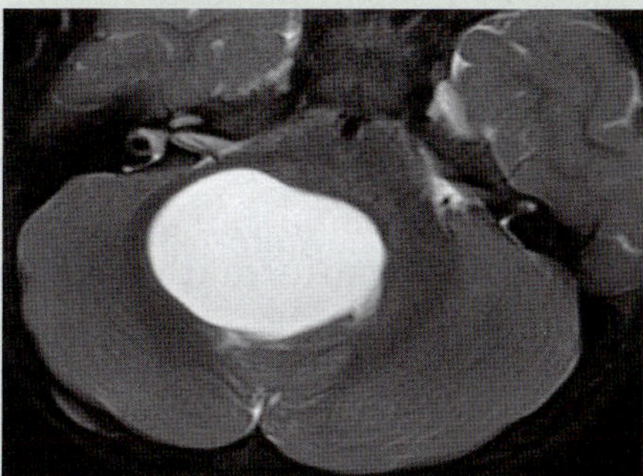 **Fig. 4.1.19:** Trapped 4th ventricle 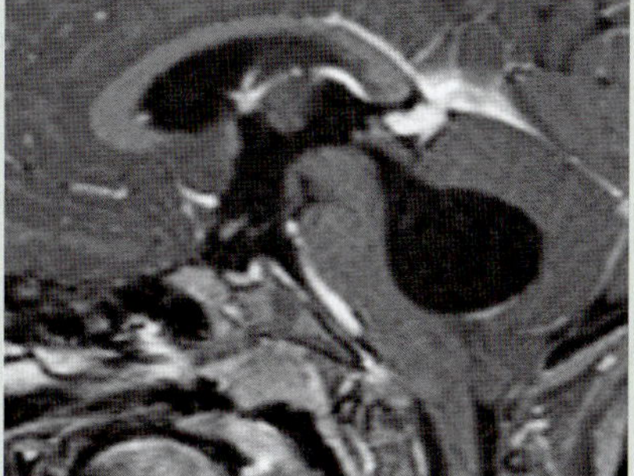 **Fig. 4.1.20:** Trapped 4th ventricle
Other cystic lesions in posterior fossa include: 4th ventricular neurocysticercosis.
Brain stem hypoplasia
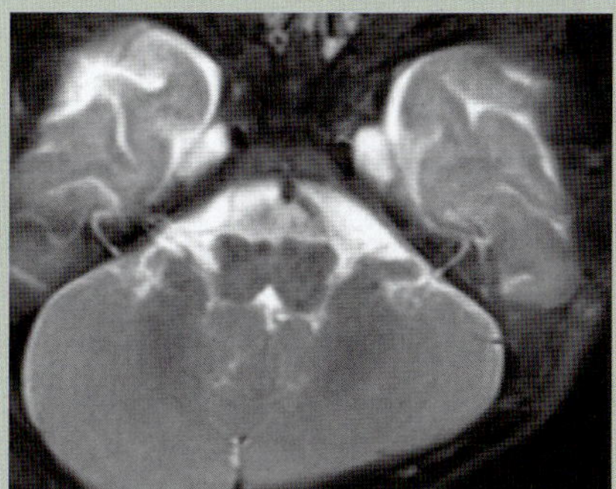 **Fig. 4.1.21:** Brain stem hypoplasia

Contd...

Table 4.1.1: Differential diagnosis for Dandy-Walker malformation *(Contd...)*		
Cerebellar hypoplasia with heterotropia		
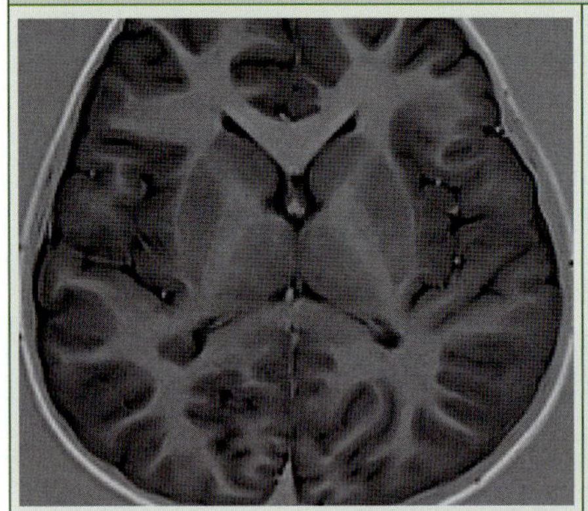 **Fig. 4.1.22:** Cerebellar hypoplasia with heterotropia	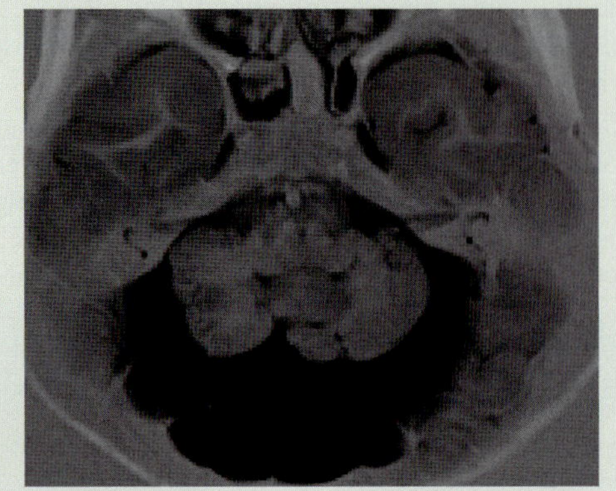 **Fig. 4.1.23:** Cerebellar hypoplasia with heterotropia	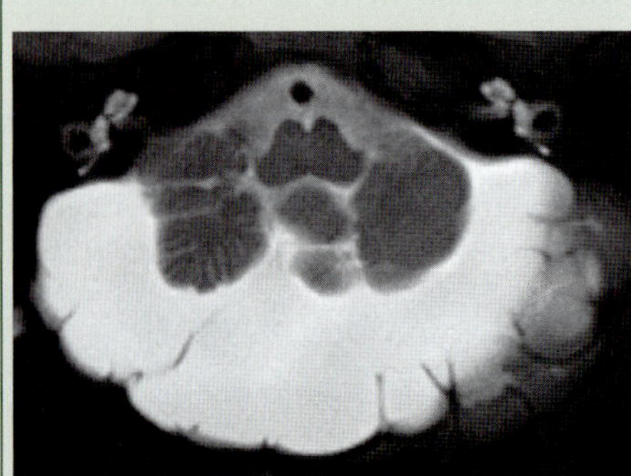 **Fig. 4.1.24:** Cerebellar hypoplasia with heterotropia
Other common posterior fossa malformations: Rhombencephalosynapsis, Lhermitte duclos, butterfly pons, dural AVF, tegmental cap dysplasia, PHACES syndrome, split pons, horizontal gaze palsy, progressive scoliosis.		

Principal Diagnosis: Dandy-Walker Malformation

Discussion: Dandy-Walker continuum is a spectrum of anomalies that includes Dandy-Walker malformation, vermian hypoplasia, Blake pouch cyst and mega cisterna magna. Two measurements are important in distinguishing these entities: **Tegmento-vermian angle and fastigium-declive line. Most common posterior fossa malformation** is Dandy-Walker spectrum of disorder. Slight female predominance. Majority sporadic; Autosomal dominant and X linked cases reported; 80% diagnosed by 1 year. Accompanied by >18 types of chromosomal abnormality; can occur as a result of maternal diabetes, warfarin use, fetal infection by CMV, rubella, or Zika virus. Most common presentation—increased intracranial pressure; cerebellar signs—uncommon. Accounts for 1–4% of all hydrocephalus cases. Intelligence normal in 35–50% of patients with classic DWM. Thin sagittal views of MRI crucial.

Imaging: Radiography—enlarged calvaria, particularly posterior fossa. CT: Variable sized 4th ventricle cyst communicating with enlarged posterior fossa, torcular-lambdoid inversion, occipital bone may appear scalloped. T1WI—floor of 4th ventricle present which opens to variable-sized CSF cyst; anterior medullary velum, fastigium, choroid plexus—absent. Vermian agenesis or hypogenesis. Increased tegmento-vermian angle >45°. **MRV**—elevated torcular Herophili. **USG**—identical to MR; can diagnose in fetus. **Cisternography**—delineates cyst wall. Associated anomalies—callosal agenesis or dysgenesis, cortical dysplasia, heterotopias, myelination delays, PHACES, neurocutaneous melanosis, midline anomalies, etc.

Management: A Dandy-Walker malformation has high **mortality rate**, about 70% in live-born fetuses, due to associated abnormalities. It carries poorer prognosis if diagnosed prior to 21 weeks of gestation and better prognosis if diagnosed postnatally. In the absence of associated syndromes, there is a recurrence risk is in range of 1–5% in subsequent pregnancies.

Treatment: To inform neurosurgeon for CSF diversion where hydrocephalus is a significant problem; VP shunt ± cyst shunt/marsupialization.

Pontine tegmental cap dysplasia (PTCD): It is a rare congenital malformation of the hindbrain where

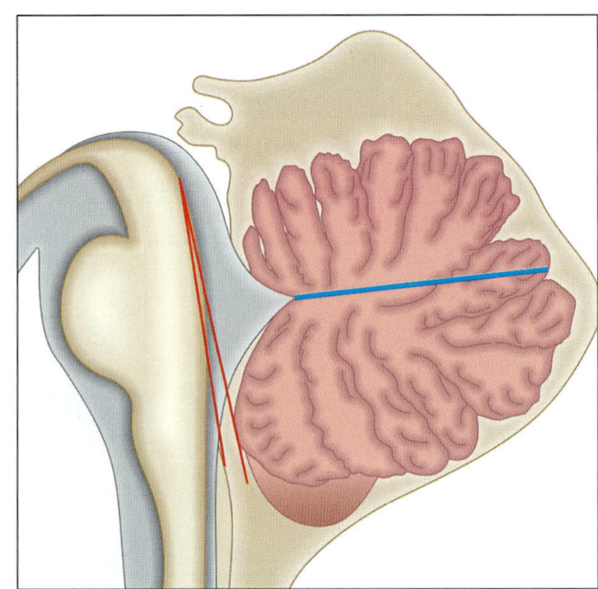

Fig. 4.1.25: Tegmento-vermian angle (red lines) and fastigium-declive line (blue lines)

Table 4.1.2: Summary of posterior cranial fossa malformations

	Vermis position	*Vermis size*	*Torcular position*	*Cerebellar hemispheres*	*Fourth ventricle*	*Hydro-cephalus*
Dandy-Walker malformation	Rotated	Hypoplastic	Elevated	Often small	Dilated, enlarged; lacks normal fastigial point	Yes
Vermian dysgenesis	May be rotated	Hypoplastic (inferior portion)	Normal	Normal	Abnormal in shape; lacks normal fastigial point	No
Blake pouch cyst	Rotated	Normal	Normal	Normal	Enlarged; communicates with posterior fossa via vallecula	Yes
Mega cisterna magna	Normal	Normal	Normal	Normal	Normal	No
Arachnoid cyst	May be displaced	Normal or compressed	Normal	Normal or compressed	Normal or compressed	Possible
Joubert syndrome	Normal	Hypoplastic	Normal	Small	Large	No

ectopic dorsal transverse pontine fibres project from the tegmentum into the 4th ventricle. On MRI, the lateralised course of the superior cerebellar peduncle results in a **"molar tooth" appearance** of the midbrain.

A butterfly-shaped pons due to pontine hypoplasia and midline pontine cleft are features of horizontal gaze palsy with progressive scoliosis (HGPPS) disorder.

The differential diagnosis for cerebellar hypoplasia is diffuse cerebellar atrophy—progressive loss of volume, pontocerebellar hypoplasia, unilateral cerebellar hypoplasia, isolated inferior vermian hypoplasia, vermian aplasia (Joubert syndrome), Dandy-Walker malformation.

4.2 CENTRAL NERVOUS SYSTEM

Case No. 2

Clinical history: A one-day-old neonate with seizures, respiratory failure, flaccidity or decerebrate posturing with a vegetative state.

Radiological techniques and observation: **Observation:** Figures 4.2.1 to 4.2.6 are T1 coronal, T1 sagittal, T2 axial, and MR angiography images demonstrating macrocephaly with largely **absent cerebral mantle affecting bilateral ICA territory.** CSF fills all supratentorial spaces. Brainstem and cerebellum are displaced inferiorly. Thalamus and basal ganglia not fused. **Falx is at midline.** Frontal and parietal lobes **are not able to be identified. Large head with fluid-filled cranial vault ("water-bag" brain) and small nubbins of remnant brain noted in occipital region, thalamus and brainstem with a normal falx cerebri and posterior fossa are typical findings of hydranencephaly.** No obvious peripheral thin cerebral mantle seen. MR angiography show **absence of distal intracranial part of ICA and its branches.**

Interpretation: A—Neonate with lesion involving bilateral ICA territory, C—CSF dense fluid filling the cranial vault, B—Normal falx and posterior fossa structures, no obvious peripheral thin cerebral mantle seen, attenuated ICA, D—Hydranencephaly.

Principal diagnosis: Hydranencephaly

Discussion: Hydranencephaly—perhaps also rather unkindly termed a **'water-bag brain'** is a condition of the newborn, in which the **cerebral hemispheres are essentially absent, due to compromise of the anterior circulation of the brain *in utero*.** Range of

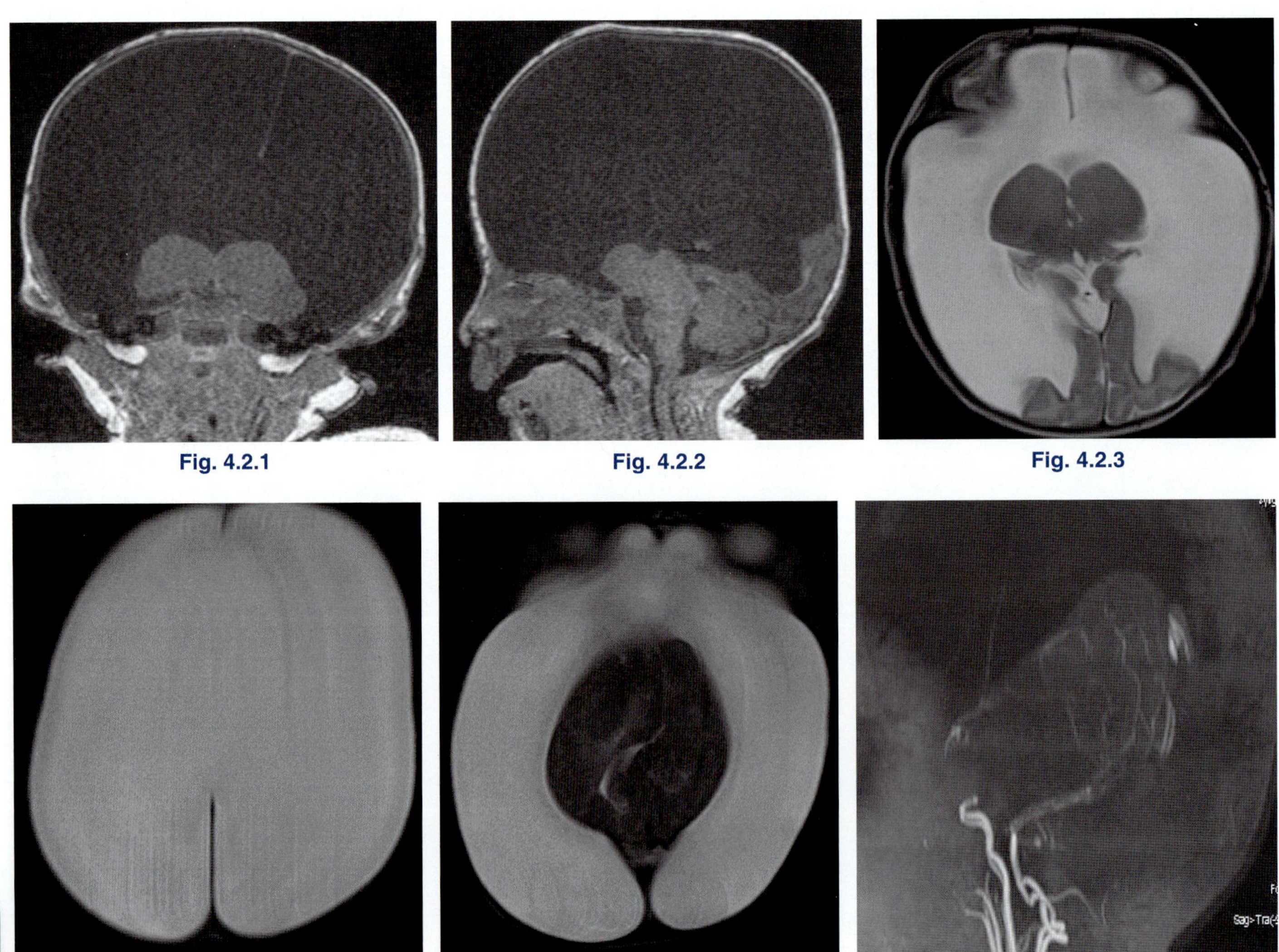

Fig. 4.2.1 Fig. 4.2.2 Fig. 4.2.3

Fig. 4.2.4 Fig. 4.2.5 Fig. 4.2.6

Differential Diagnosis		
Bilateral open lip schizencephaly Rare, almost always sporadic. No known gender predilection. Divided into two morphological types: Open and closed lip. Open lip schizencephaly is the most common form in bilateral cases, and seen usually in MCA territory. Presents with seizures, developmental delay, etc. One-third of children has non-CNS abnormalities.	Fetal USG and foetal MR can be used to diagnose this condition. CSF density extending from the right lateral ventricle body to the frontal cortex with open dysplastic grey matter lined cleft. Septo-optic dysplasia, grey matter heterotopia, absent septum pellucidum, and corpus callosum dysgenesis are all frequently accompanied with other brain anomalies. Normal appearing falx and tentorium will be seen.	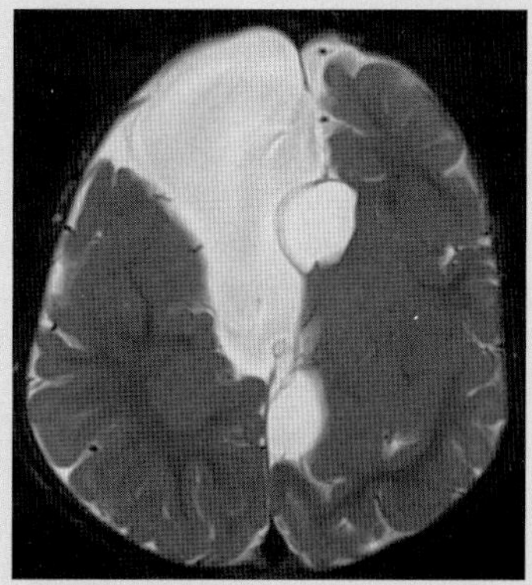 **Fig. 4.2.7:** Right open lip schizencephaly

Alobar holoprosencephaly: The most severe of the three holoprosencephaly categories, with loss of basic cerebral hemisphere structure and varied quantities of remnant cortex. Failure of complete separation of the two hemispheres, as well as failure of transverse cleavage of the diencephalon and telencephalon, is a rare congenital malformation. Proboscis, mono-orbit/cyclopia, mono-nostril, hypotelorism, cebocephaly, and ethmocephaly are severe facial deformities (the face predicts the brain). In the neonatal period, it is generally lethal. **Pancake brain with poor gyration and sulcation and single midline horseshoe mono ventricle** (or holo sphere). Cerebral mantle fused anteriorly. Fused thalami fused basal ganglia. Dorsal cyst of holoprosencephaly. Lateral and third ventricles are absent. **Absent midline structures and septum pellucidum.** Agenesis or hypoplasia of the corpus callosum. **Absent interhemispheric fissure and falx cerebri.** Absent olfactory tract. Absent, fused or normal optic nerves. Middle and anterior cerebral arteries can be replaced by tangled branches of internal carotid and basilar vessels.

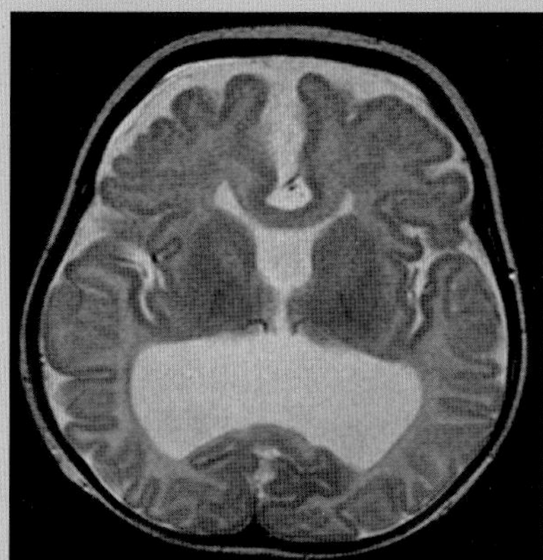

Fig. 4.2.8: Interhemispheric variant of prosencephaly

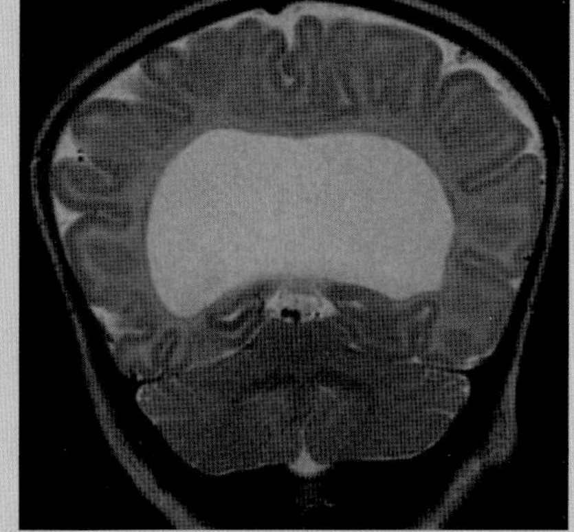

Fig. 4.2.9: Interhemispheric variant of prosencephaly

Differential Diagnosis	
Severe obstructive hydrocephalus obstructive intraventricular type (refers to CSF cannot exit the ventricular system/obstruction to CSF absorption). The ventricles upstream are dilated, causing a mass effect on the adjacent brain. Aqueduct stenosis, tectal glioma, posterior fossa tumour, cerebellar infarct, or cerebellar haemorrhage are some of the causes. Treatment temporary or permanent CSF diversion-shunting; 3rd ventriculostomy; In mechanical causes—resect the mass Bifrontal horn to intracranial diameter ratio >0.33. Temporal horn width >3 mm. Transependymal edema or periventricular oozing. Thin rim of cortical mantle seen. Thinned and elevated corpus callosum depression of the Fornices. Ballooning of the suprapineal recess may be seen. US features: Dangling choroid sign; separation of >3 mm between the choroid plexus and margin of the ventricle.	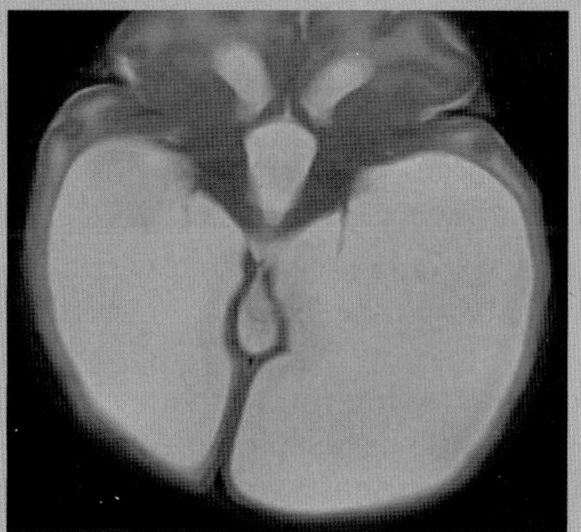 **Fig. 4.2.10:** Severe obstructive hydrocephalus

4

Contd...

Large arachnoid cyst: Refer to case 21 Well-circumscribed cyst extending from left middle cranial fossa almost to vertex with imperceptible wall and mass effect on left cerebral hemisphere and left lateral ventricle and scalloping of overlying calvarium. No diffusion restriction. Cisternography will show communication of cyst with subarachnoid spaces.	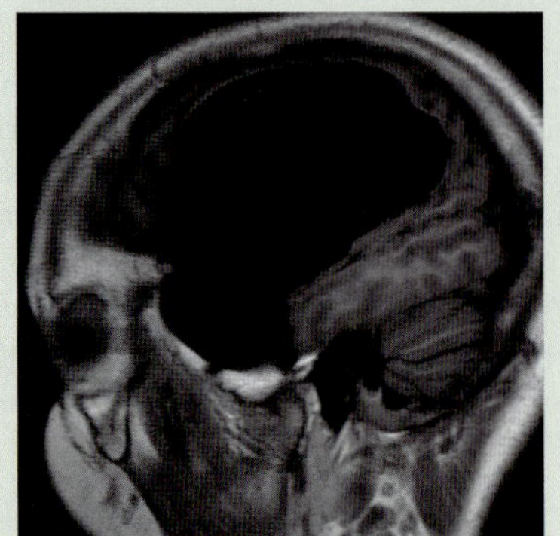 **Fig. 4.2.11:** Arachnoid cyst	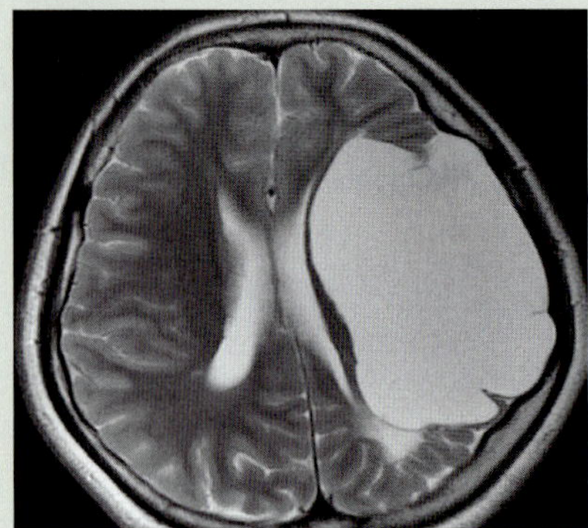 **Fig. 4.2.12:** Arachnoid cyst

Differential Diagnosis

Multicystic encephalomalacia

Corresponds to a variant of encephalo-malacia which has numerous loculated lacy pseudocysts within the white matter and cortex are present due to result of an extensive brain insult. Common feature observed in neonatal HIE.

Multiple cysts of various sizes and shapes are found in the white matter and inner layers of the cortex on both sides of the brain. Except for Wallerian degeneration of the corticospinal pathways, relative sparing is evident infratentorial areas, which includes the cerebellum and spinal cord. The basal ganglia, inferior temporal lobes, and orbital surfaces of the frontal lobes are among the supratentorial structures that are relatively spared. Ex vacuo dilation of the lateral ventricles with intact ventricular walls.

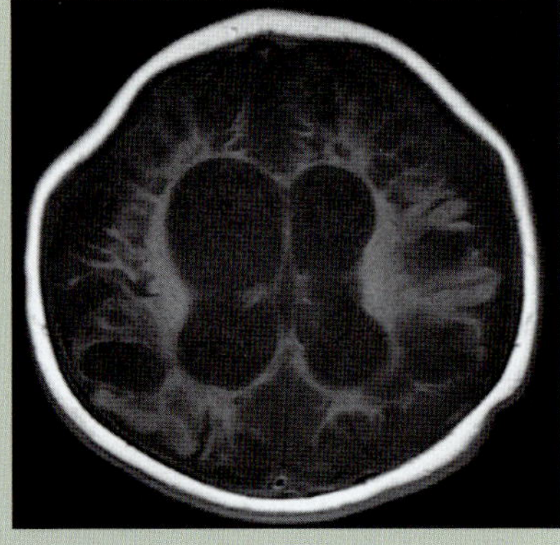

Fig. 4.2.13: Multicystic encephalomalacia

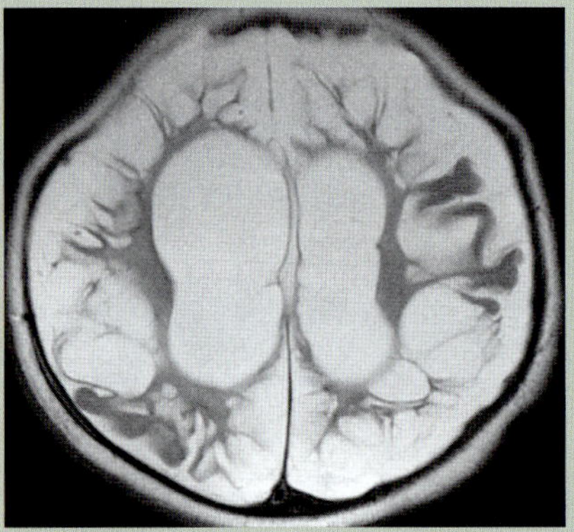

Fig. 4.2.14: Multicystic encephalomalacia

causes—anoxia, hypoxia, leukomalacia, infection and maternal exposure to toxins, etc. Only fluid is seen in supratentorial brain instead of normal brain parenchyma, so the term 'water-bag brain', **although the falx cerebri remains, either completely or partially.** Some occipital lobe tissue may be present. Bilateral and symmetrical; a rare condition—only one hemisphere is destroyed—termed **"hemihydranencephaly"**. CSF continues to be elaborated but not normally resorbed. Usually sporadic; Associated with arthrogryposis, renal aplastic dysplasia, poly valvular developmental heart defects, trisomy 13, etc. **Fowler syndrome**—rare AR disorder in which hydranencephaly is accompanied by glomeruloid vasculopathy of the CNS vessels and neurogenic muscular atrophy.

Imaging: Essentially no remaining cortical tissue—often islands of residual tissue **preserved at occipital poles and orbitofrontal regions; medial temporal tissue may be identified,** as the medial temporal lobes are supplied by the basilar circulation. Preserved thalami and posterior

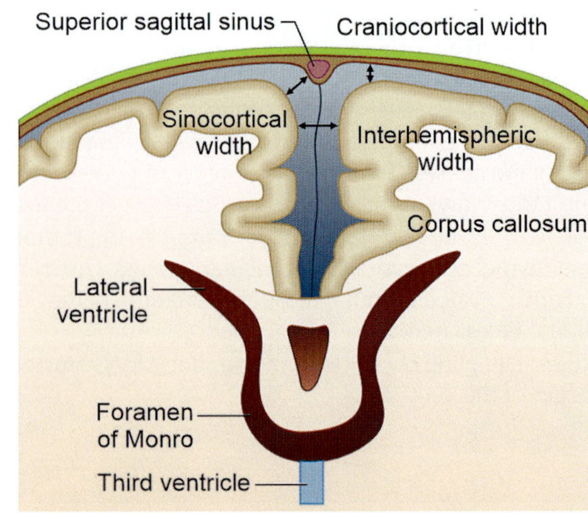

Fig. 4.2.15: Measurements in CSF spaces

Table 4.2.1: Ventricular indices

Evan's index (A/B): Ratio of maximum width of frontal horns of lateral ventricle and maximum internal diameter of skull at the same level. **Normal <0.3** 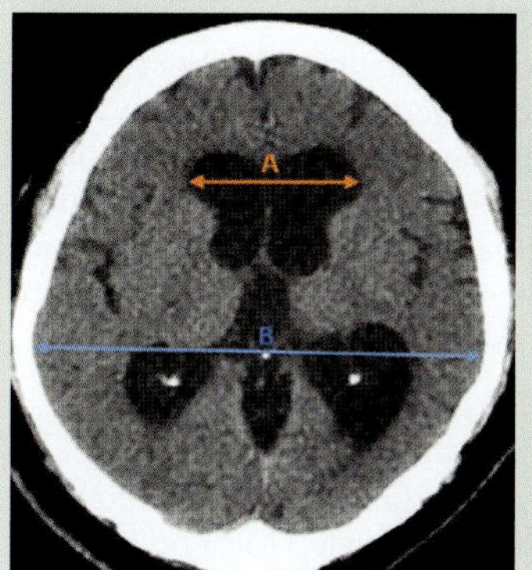 **Fig. 4.2.16:** Evan's index	Bifrontal index (A/B): Ratio of maximum width of lateral ventricle in relation to inner skull width at the same level. **Normal 0.2–0.3** 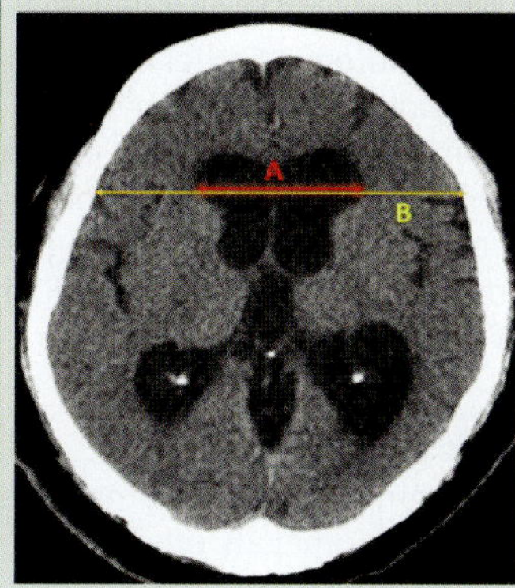 **Fig. 4.2.17:** Bifrontal index	Bicaudate index (A/B): Ratio of width of two lateral ventricles at the level of caudate nucleus to distance between outer tables of skull at the same level. **Normal 0.05–0.1** 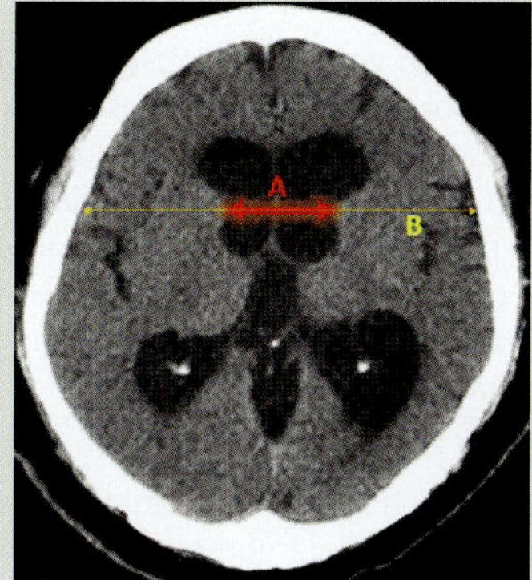 **Fig. 4.2.18:** Bicaudate index	Fronto-occipital horn ratio [(A+B)/2C]: (Bifrontal horn dimension + Bioccipital horn dimension)/2 × Biparietal calvarial dimension . 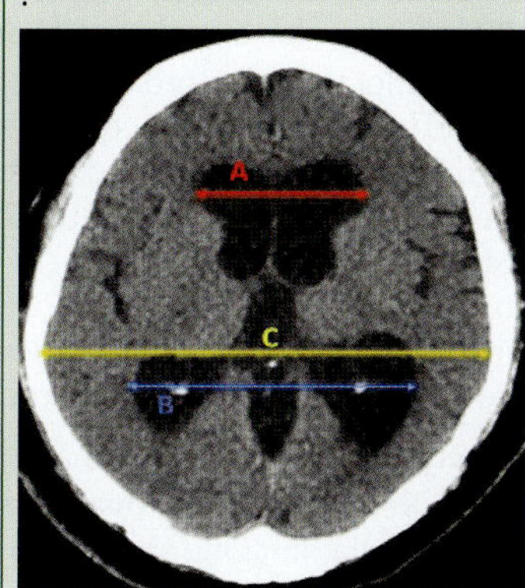 **Fig. 4.2.19:** Fronto-occipital horn ratio
Huckman's index (A/B): Minimum width of lateral ventricles + maximum bifrontal diameter. **Normal 3.3 to 5** 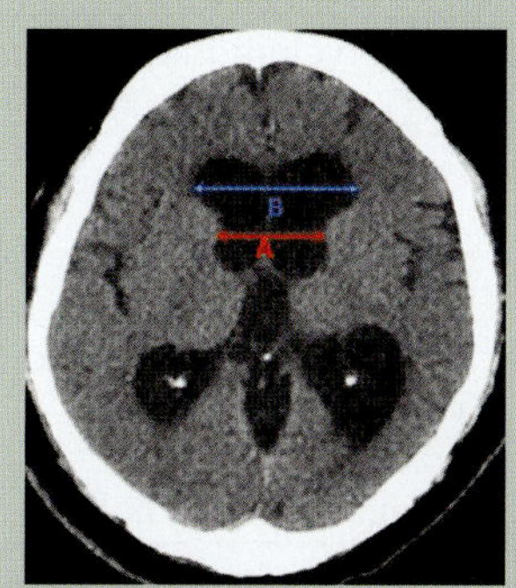 **Fig. 4.2.20:** Huckman's index	**Cella media index (A/B):** At the cella media, the ratio of the biparietal diameter of the skull to the maximal external diameter of the lateral ventricles (i.e., central part of lateral ventricles) **Normal >4** 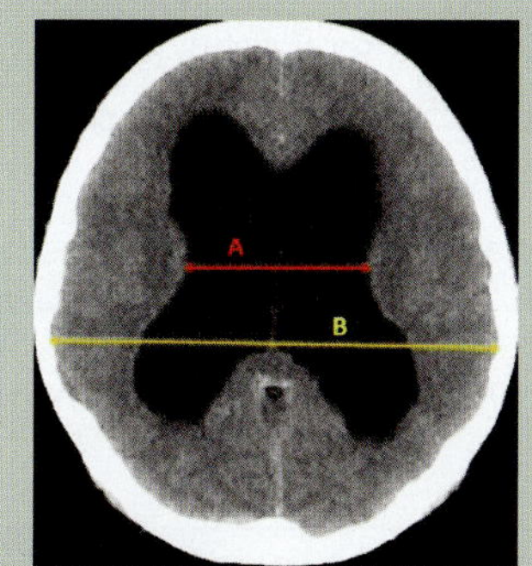 **Fig. 4.2.21:** Cella media index	**Third ventricle index (A/B):** Ratio of maximum width of each lateral margin of 3rd ventricle to transverse diameter of brain at the same level. 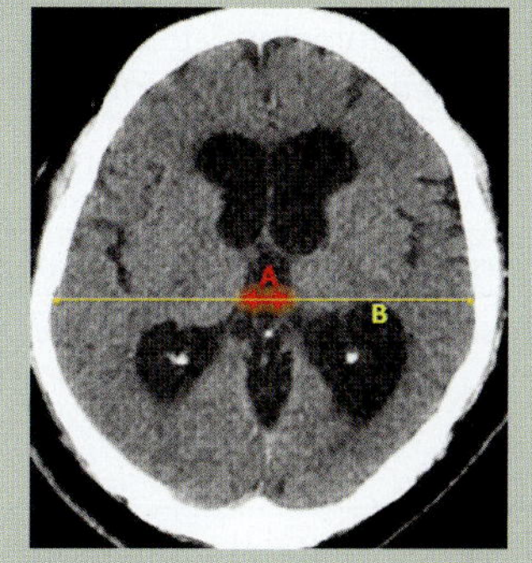 **Fig. 4.2.22:** Third ventricle index	Callosal angle: Measured on coronal image perpendicular to the anterior and posterior commissure plane at the level of posterior commissure. **Normal 100–120 degree.** 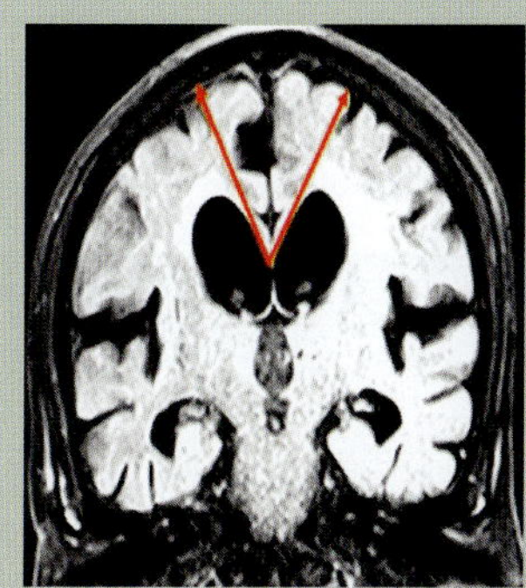 **Fig. 4.2.23:** Callosal angle

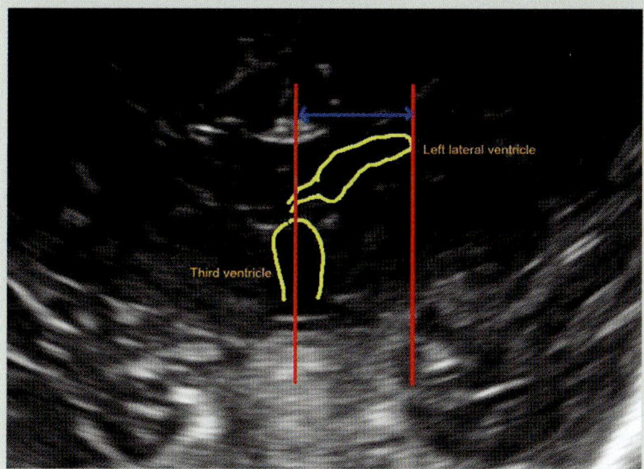

Fig. 4.2.24: Ventricular measurements: The ventricular index, as developed by Levene and used for preterm infants, is widely accepted. The distance between the falx and the lateral border of the lateral ventricle is measured coronally in the plane of the 3rd ventricle, posterior to the foramen of Monro. In full-term infants, the Virkola measurement is employed.

fossa. Falx is **usually present.** Hemi cranium is filled with fluid, in which choroid can often be identified. Antenatal ultrasound or vascular imaging demonstrate absence of middle cerebral arteries.

Normal values of CSF spaces in newborn: Sinocortical width <3 mm, craniocortical width <4 mm, interhemispheric width <6 mm, width of third ventricle <10 mm, width of lateral ventricle—frontal horn

Table 4.2.2: Types of hydrocephalus	
Intraventricular obstructive hydrocephalus The outlet foramina proximal to the fourth ventricle is obstructed. It could be congenital or acquired, acute or chronic. Acute obstructive hydrocephalus—ballooned ventricles, "blurred" ventricle borders, periventricular fluid accumulation (CSF, ISF, or both), halo/fingers of fluid around ventricles—T2 hyperintense, does not suppress on FLAIR. Large ventricles, no periventricular halo, callosal impingement, and atrial diverticula are all characteristics of chronic compensated obstructive hydrocephalus	**Extraventricular obstructive hydrocephalus** **Terminology:** Earlier called "communicating" hydrocephalus; Outside the ventricular system, obstruction can occur anywhere from the foramina of the 4th ventricle to arachnoid granulations. Subarachnoid bleeding (aneurysm > trauma) is the most prevalent cause, followed by meningitis (bacterial, granulomatous), and metastatic disease. Use CISS to check for blocking membranes if your imaging shows no clear cause
Overproduction hydrocephalus Rare, Results from CSF overproduction: Choroid plexus tumor > > hyperplasia; Imaging shows pan ventricular enlargement	Arrested hydrocephalus No/minimal overt symptoms, no stigmata of elevated ICP, Ventriculomegaly often incidental, unexpected MR finding. May be stable for years, may cause subtle neurologic deterioration, Rarely there may be sudden fatal decompensation
Normal pressure hydrocephalus Ventriculomegaly with normal CSF pressure, altered fluid dynamics; Accounts for ≈ 5% of dementias; Presentation: Dementia, gait apraxia, incontinence (minority). Imaging diagnosis difficult- Disproportionately enlarged ventricles vs sulci, MR may show exaggerated aqueductal "flow void", elevated stroke volume, indium-111 DTPA cisternography - Persistant intraventricular tracer at 24 hours.	**Syndrome of inappropriately low-pressure acute hydrocephalus** Progressive neurologic deterioration, acute progressive obstructive hydrocephalus, CSF opening pressure very low or negative. **Imaging:** Like acute obstructive hydrocephalus with elevated ICP, quadri-ventricular enlargement, small/inapparent sulci common. Differential diagnosis–acute obstructive hydrocephalus with elevated ICP, idiopathic intracranial hypotension, critical post-craniotomy CSF hypovolemia
Normal variants: Age related changes, asymmetric lateral ventricles, cavum septi pellucidi and vergae, cavum velum interpositum, enlarged subarachnoid spaces (BESS—benign enlargement of subarachnoid spaces).	

Table 4.2.3: Holoprosencephalies (based on DeMyer's three degrees of severity)				
	Alobar holoprosencephaly	*Semilobar holoprosencephaly*	*Lobar holoprosencephaly*	*Middle interhemispheric variant of holoprosencephaly (syntelencephaly)*
Facial anomalies	Severe (cleft lip, cleft palate, hypotelorism, cyclopia, proboscis, ethmocephaly, cebocephaly, single nostril, microcephaly, trigonocephaly, micrognathia)	Mild (cleft lip, cleft palate, hypotelorism)	Very mild (hypotelorism)	Very mild (hypotelorism)
Thalami	Completely fused	Partially fused	Fusion +/–	Fused in 1/3 to 1/2
Ventricular system	Single mono ventricle. No occipital or temporal horns. No third ventricle.	Single ventricle but rudimentary occipital horn, temporal horn. Partially formed third ventricle.	Separate lateral ventricle with occipital and temporal horns and third ventricle. Colpocephaly.	Normal or hypoplastic anterior horn. Third ventricle formed.
Septum pellucidum	Absent	Absent	Absent	Absent
Corpus callosum	Absent	Absent	Absent	Body absent Genu variably present Splenium present

Contd...

Table 4.2.3: Holoprosencephalies (based on DeMyer's three degrees of severity) *(Contd...)*

Interhemispheric fissure	Absent	Rudimentary	Dysplastic with dysplastic frontal lobe, frontal horn fused	Absent in the posterior frontal and parietal region
Olfactory bulb and optic tract	Absent	Absent	Absent	Present
	Alobar holoprosencephaly	*Semilobar holoprosencephaly*	*Lobar holoprosencephaly*	*Middle interhemispheric variant of holoprosencephaly (syntelencephaly)*
Pachygyria, lissencephaly	+	+	+	+/–
Aprosencephaly and atelencephaly (AP/AT); these two rare lethal malformations are intermediate in the continuum between anencephaly and holoprosencephaly. AP/AT is now considered the most severe end of the holoprosencephaly spectrum. These three extreme malformations are usually diagnosed at fetal MR, sonography, or postmortem examination.				

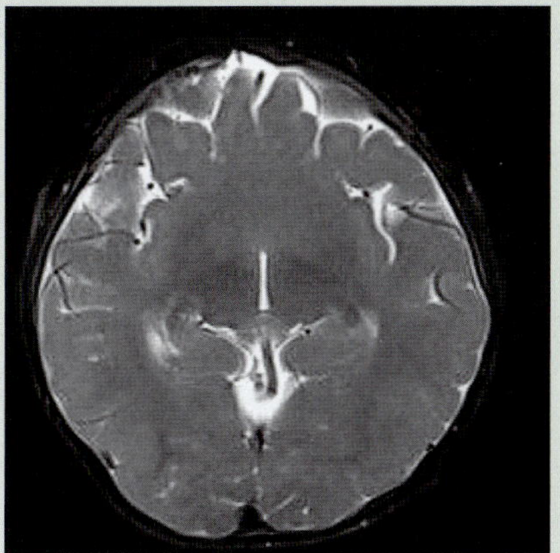

Fig. 4.2.25: Holoprosencephaly

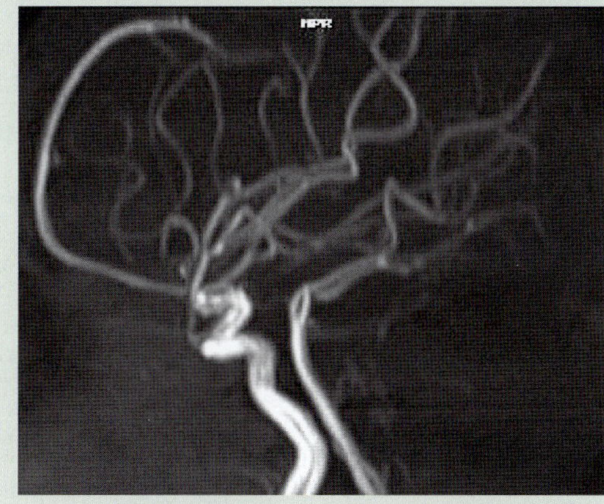

Fig. 4.2.26: Holoprosencephaly

<13 mm. Increased in benign enlargement of subarachnoid spaces in infancy (BESSI) or external hydrocephalus is the most common cause of macrocephaly in infants. Obs-USG measurement findings—normal width of lateral ventricular atrium <10 mm. In hydrocephalus, BPD >95th percentile; commensurate dilatation of temporal horn with lateral ventricles (most reliable sign).

Table 4.2.4: Types of holoprosencephaly

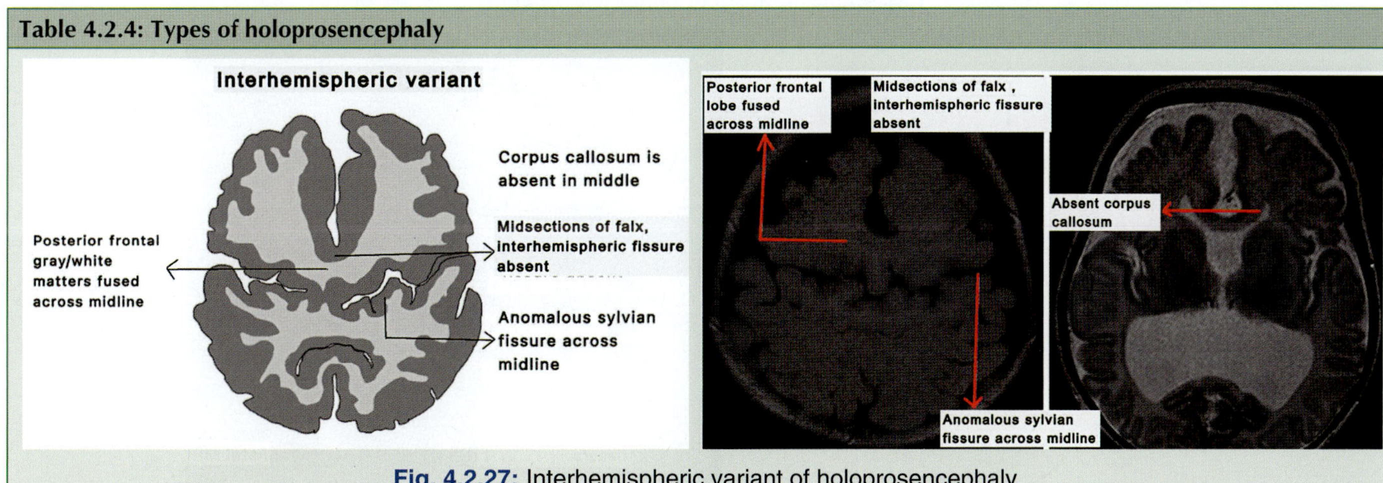

Fig. 4.2.27: Interhemispheric variant of holoprosencephaly

Contd...

4

Table 4.2.4: Types of holoprosencephaly *(Contd...)*

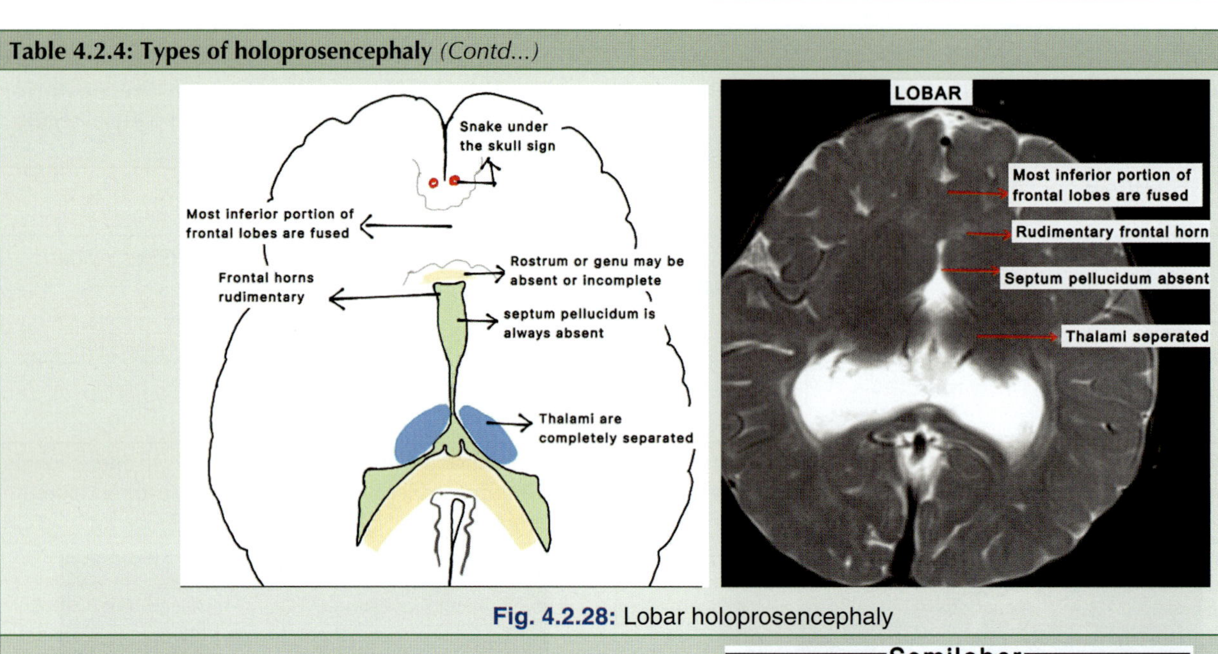

Fig. 4.2.28: Lobar holoprosencephaly

Azygos ACA seen directly beneath the frontal bone
Snake under the skull sign
Fused frontal lobes
Single lateral ventricle with rudimentary occipital,temporal horn
Partially formed third ventricle
Thalamus partially fused
Absent corpus callosum
Rudimentary interhemispheric fissure
Semilobar
Fused frontal lobes
Thalamus partially fused
Partially formed third ventricle
Single Lateral ventricle with rudimentary occipital, temporal horn
Rudimentary interhemispheric fissure

Fig. 4.2.29: Semilobar holoprosencephaly

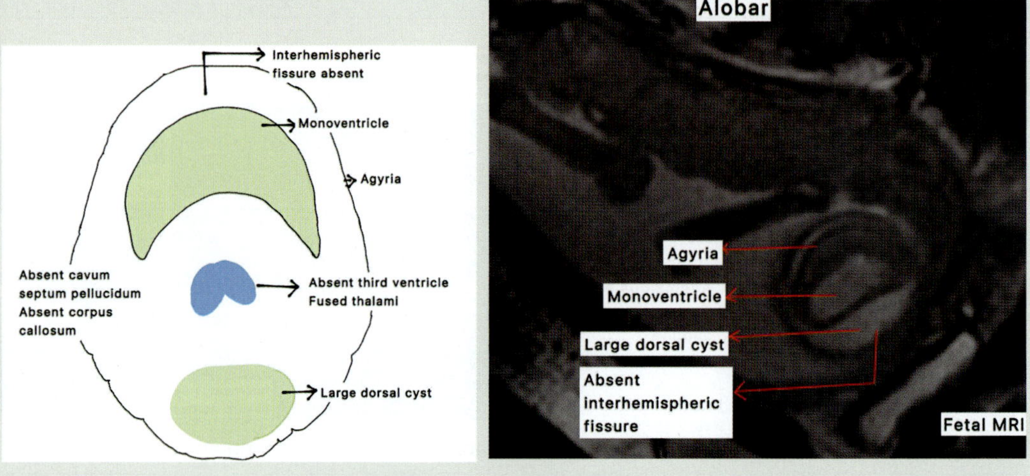

Fig. 4.2.30: Alobar holoprosencephaly

4.3.1 CENTRAL NERVOUS SYSTEM

Case No. 3.1

Clinical history: A 7-year-old female with short stature and visual disturbances.

Radiological technique: Figures 4.3.1.1 to 4.3.1.6 are MRI brain—T1 coronal, T2 FS coronal, T2 axial, T1 sagittal images respectively showing absent septum pellucidum. Coronal imaging shows flat roofed frontal ventricles and downward pointing anterior horns of bilateral lateral ventricles. T1 coronal and T2 FS coronal clearly show severe thinning of the entire left optic nerve up to the optic chiasma. Right optic nerve appears normal. Anterior lobe of pituitary, posterior pituitary bright spot and pituitary stalk appear normal. Corpus callosum appears normal.

Interpretation: A: Young child (<10 years). C: Absent septum pellucidum, flat-roofed frontal ventricles and downward pointing anterior horns. B: Severe thinning of entire left optic nerve up to optic chiasma. D: Septo-optic dysplasia.

Principal diagnosis: Septo-optic dysplasia.

Further investigations: Use CISS/FIESTA/SPACE sequence to better see cisternal segment of optic nerves.

Management: Hormone replacement therapy.

Brief discussion: Septo-optic dysplasia/de Morsier syndrome.

Age and sex: Generally detected in infants, M = F. **Clinical presentation:** Abnormal endocrine function (60%): Pituitary deficiencies. Thin pituitary stalk, small anterior lobe of pituitary and posterior pituitary ectopia. Normal endocrine function (40%): Often have schizencephaly, seizures, bilateral optic nerve hypoplasia (70%).

Associated abnormalities: 75–90% have brain abnormalities. **Most common** = **schizencephaly**, seen in 50% of patients with SOD. Perisylvian polymicrogyria, midline malformations (callosal dysgenesis, etc.), ocular anomalies (coloboma, anophthalmia, microphthalmia), olfactory tract/bulb hypoplasia and incomplete hippocampal rotation.

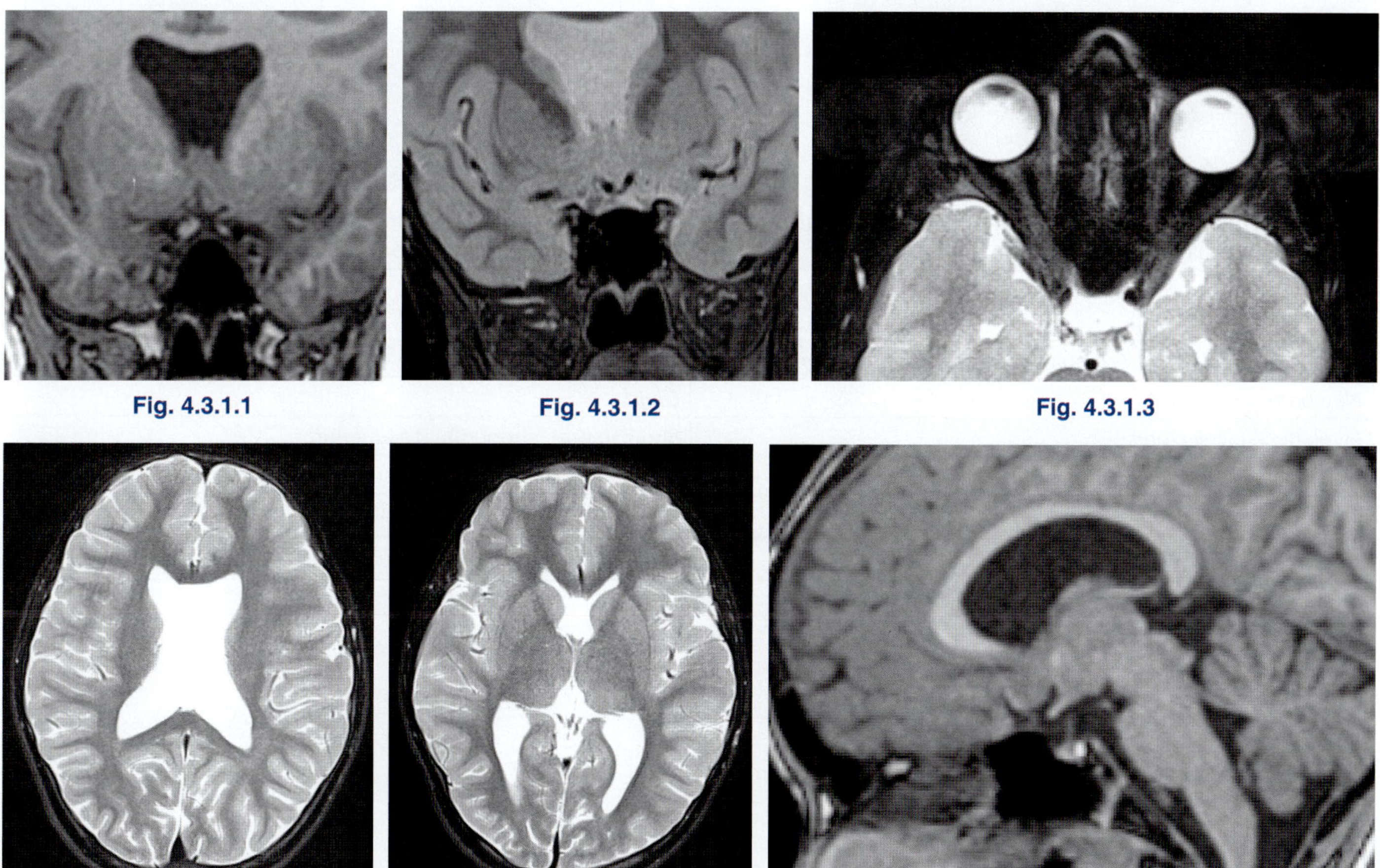

Fig. 4.3.1.1 Fig. 4.3.1.2 Fig. 4.3.1.3

Fig. 4.3.1.4 Fig. 4.3.1.5 Fig. 4.3.1.6

Complications: Hypothalamic and pituitary crisis, sudden death (hypercortisolism)

Grading

i. *Isolated optic nerve hypoplasia:* Visual defect only; intelligence and growth normal
ii. *Optic nerve hypoplasia and septal deficiency:* Same as isolated
iii. *Optic nerve hypoplasia and septal and pituitary deficiency:* May have developmental delay
iv. *Complete septal agenesis:* Worse developmental prognosis
v. Optic nerve, chiasmatic, and hypothalamic deficiency—intrauterine or perinatal insult (especially meningitis).

Table 4.3.1.1: Differential diagnosis for septo-optic dysplasia

1. Optic—infundibular dysplasia—normal septum pellucidum, with small pituitary gland.
2. Lobar holoprosencephaly (optic hypoplasia is rare)
3. Kallmann syndrome: Absent olfactory nerves ± visual, septal, pituitary abnormalities

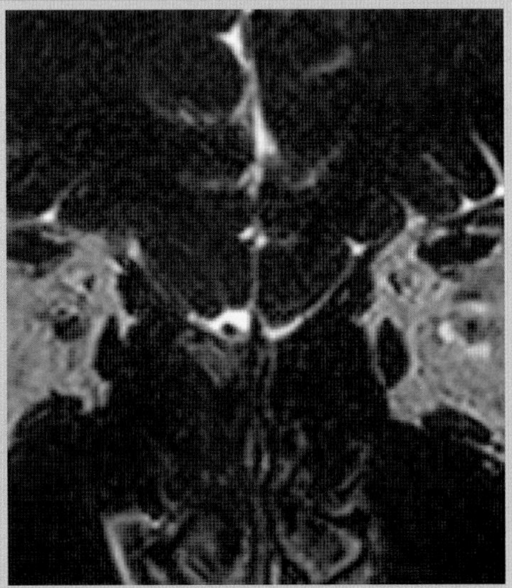

Fig. 4.3.1.7: Kallmann syndrome—absent left olfactory nerve and olfactory sulcus

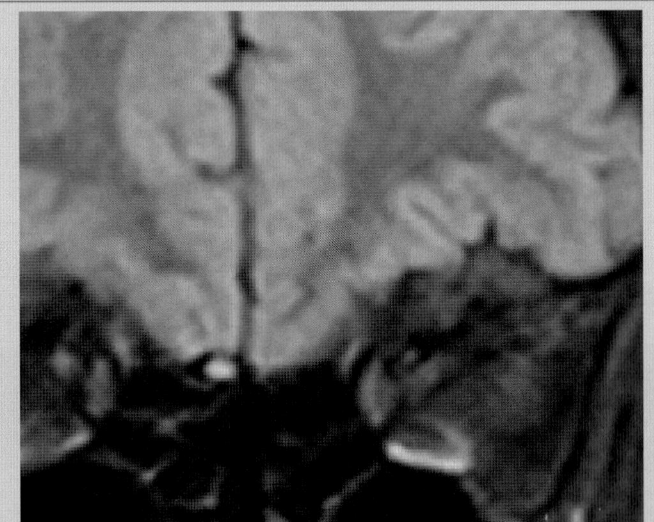

Fig. 4.3.1.8: Kallmann syndrome

Table 4.3.1.2: Clinical presentation in septo-optic dysplasia: Newborn vs child

Newborn	*Child*
Hypoglycemic seizures	Short stature, endocrine dysfunction
Apnea, cyanosis and hypotonia	Normal or color blindness, visual loss, nystagmus, strabismus
Prolonged conjugated jaundice	± Mental retardation, spasticity
Microphallus (in boys)	Microcephaly, anosmia

4.3.2 CENTRAL NERVOUS SYSTEM

Case No. 3.2

Clinical history: A 2 years old female child was brought with developmental delay.

T2 axial, FLAIR axial, coronal, sagittal images (Figs 4.3.2.1 to 4.3.2.7) show a few gyri in the parietotemporal region. Multiple small gyri associated with cortical thickening in the frontoparietal regions. Diffuse decrease of white matter is noted in bilateral cerebral hemispheres. Mild enlargement of bilateral lateral ventricles with altered shape noted. Temporal and trigone of lateral ventricle show scalloping.

Interpretation: A: 2-year-old female child, pathology in bilateral cerebral hemispheres. C: A few gyri in the parietotemporal region. Multiple small gyri associated with cortical thickening in the frontoparietal regions B: Diffuse loss of white matter is in bilateral cerebral hemispheres. Mild enlargement of bilateral lateral ventricles, D: Pachygyria microgyria complex.

Principal diagnosis: Pachygyria microgyria complex.

Discussion—polymicrogyria: It is due to late neuronal migration and cortical organisation abnormality. Neurons enter the cortex, but their distribution is abnormal,

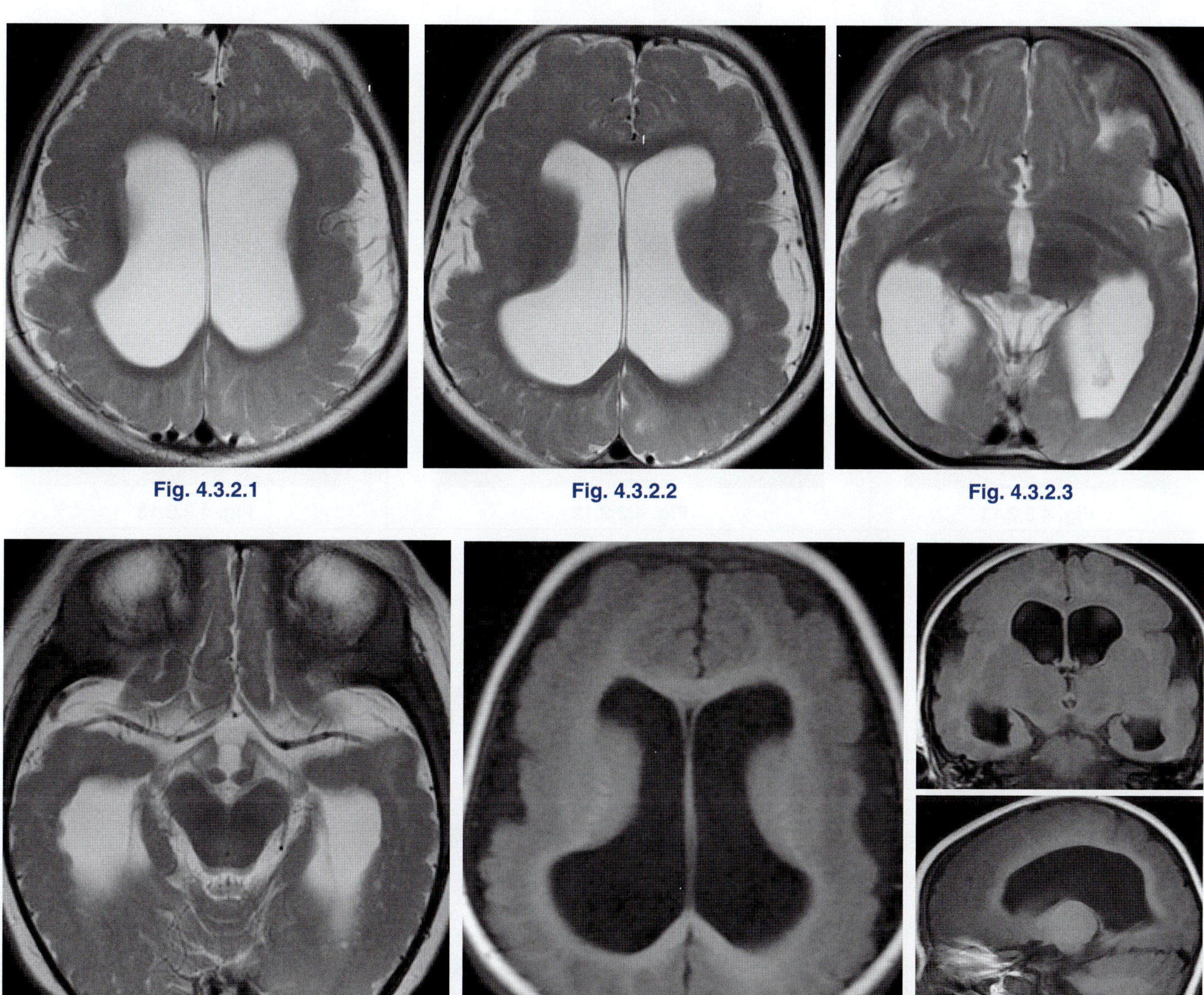

Fig. 4.3.2.1

Fig. 4.3.2.2

Fig. 4.3.2.3

Fig. 4.3.2.4

Fig. 4.3.2.5

Figs 4.3.2.6 and 4.3.2.7

Table 4.3.2.1: Differential diagnosis for cortical developmental disorders

Heterotopia is characterized by interruption of normal neuronal migration from near the ventricle to the cortex, thus resulting in normal neurons in abnormal locations. Classified under type 2 cortical developmental malformation classification. On MRI—heterotopic tissue has same signal intensity as gray matter on all sequences. fMRI—activation in heterotopic nodules which is equivalent to epileptogenic EEG discharge. MRS—decrease in NAA/Cr ratio in the heterotopic gray matter.

Heterotopia with trans mantle sign (Figs 4.3.2.8 to 4.3.2.10)

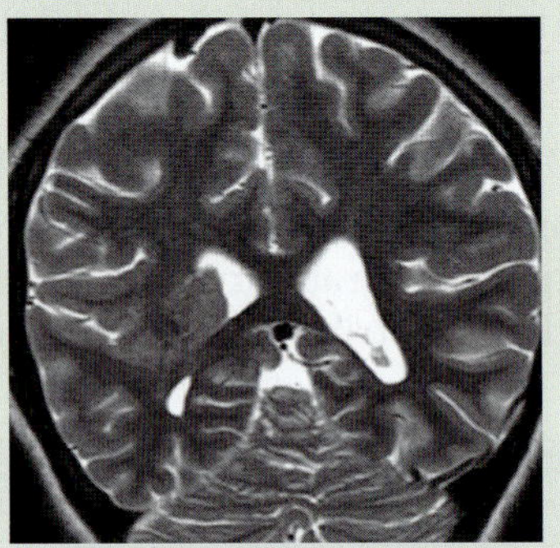
Fig. 4.3.2.8

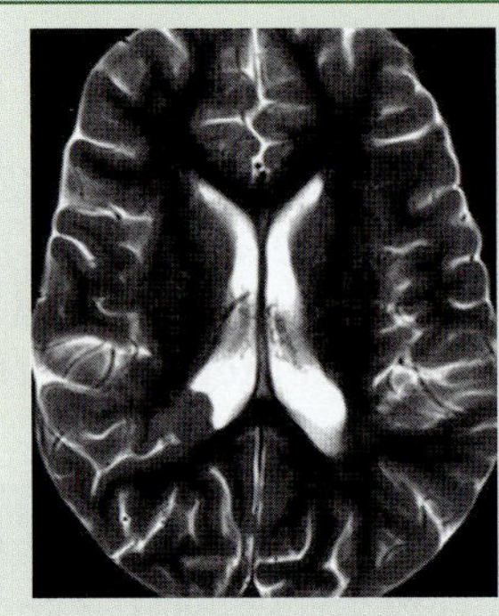
Fig. 4.3.2.9

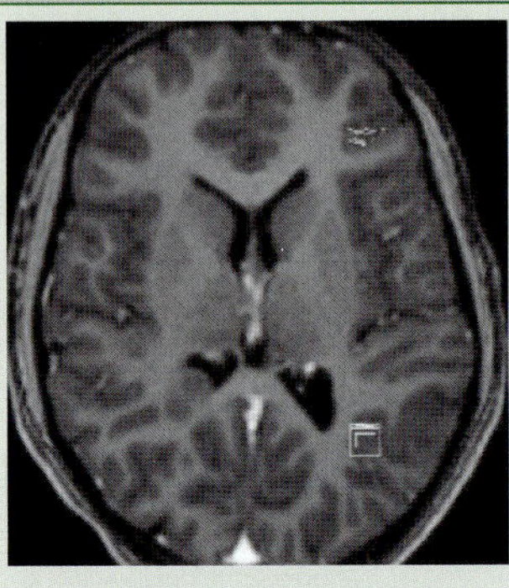
Fig. 4.3.2.10

Temporal and trigone of lateral ventricles show scalloping, suggestive of subependymal nodular heterotopia (Figs 4.3.2.11 to 4.3.2.13)

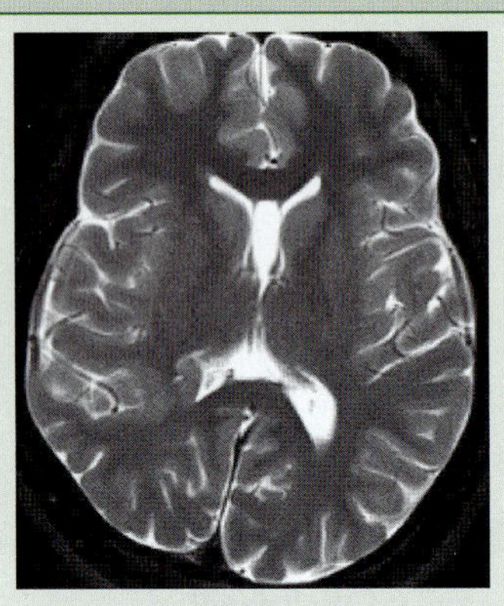
Fig. 4.3.2.11

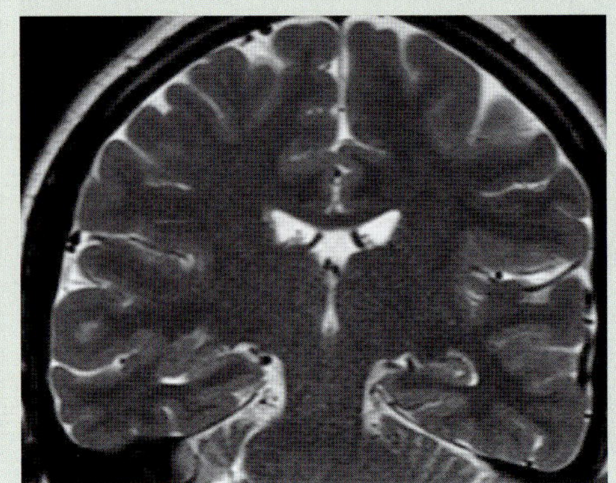
Fig. 4.3.2.12

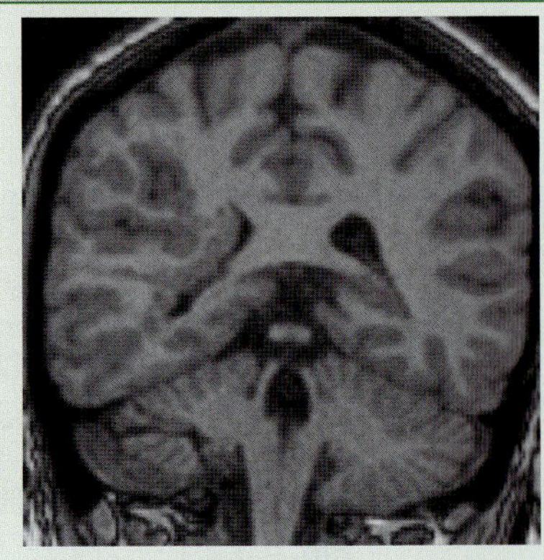
Fig. 4.3.2.13

Band heterotopia: It is a subtype of diffuse gray matter heterotopia. It affects only women. It is also called double cortex syndrome. Anterior predominance points to DCX mutations. LIS1 mutations are considered to be the cause of the posterior predilection. MRS–NAA levels in heterotopic grey matter are lower.

Figures 4.3.2.14 to 4.3.2.17 show a band of grey matter runs parallel to and deep to the cortex, with either normal or pachygyria over the cortex. On all sequences, the signal strength is the same as normal cortex.

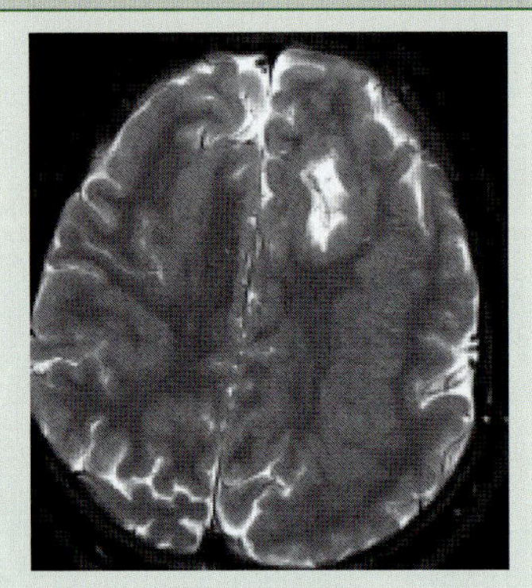
Fig. 4.3.2.14

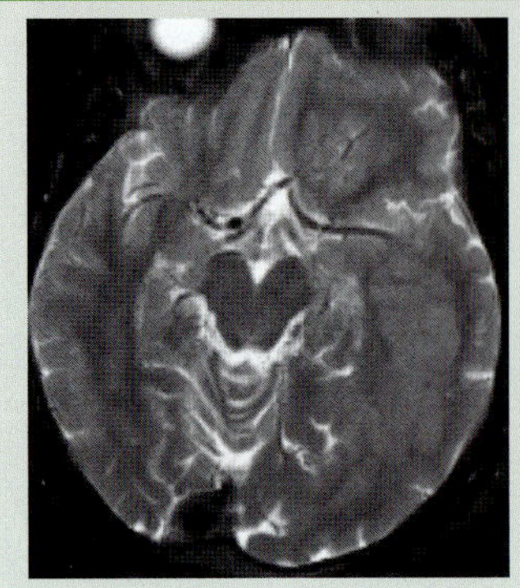
Fig. 4.3.2.15

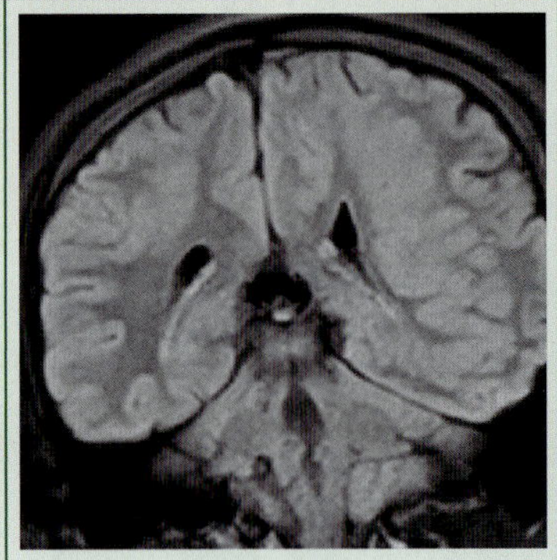
Fig. 4.3.2.16

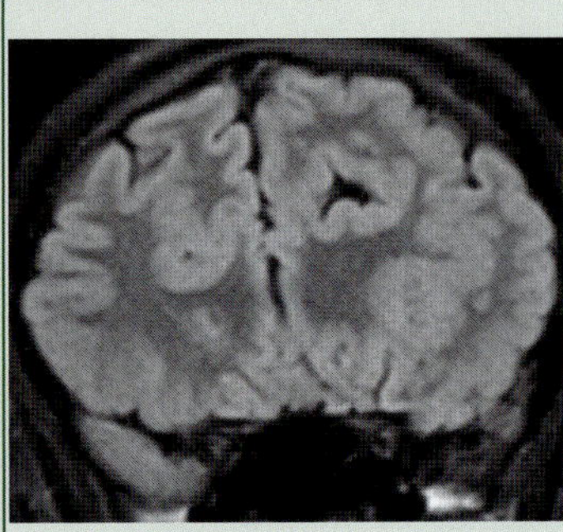
Fig. 4.3.2.17

Contd...

Table 4.3.2.1: Differential diagnosis for cortical developmental disorders *(Contd...)*		
Holoprosencephaly, hydranencephaly—Refer to Case 4.2		
Lowe syndrome (Figs 4.3.2.18 to 4.3.2.23): Oculocerebrorenal syndrome of Lowe affects brain, eyes, and kidneys. X-linked recessive multisystem disorder.	CT brain will be normal initially and shows dense calcified lenses secondary to cataract development. In the newborns, MRI brain scans reveal delayed myelination and the subsequent development of distinctive dilated perivascular spaces in the white matter of the subcortical and periventricular regions with surrounding gliosis. MRS: Unusually increased myo-inositol peak (3.56 pm) may arise as a result of gliosis from brain tissue injury or phosphatidyl inositol 4,5-biphosphate accumulation due to OCRL1 protein loss of function in Lowe syndrome.	
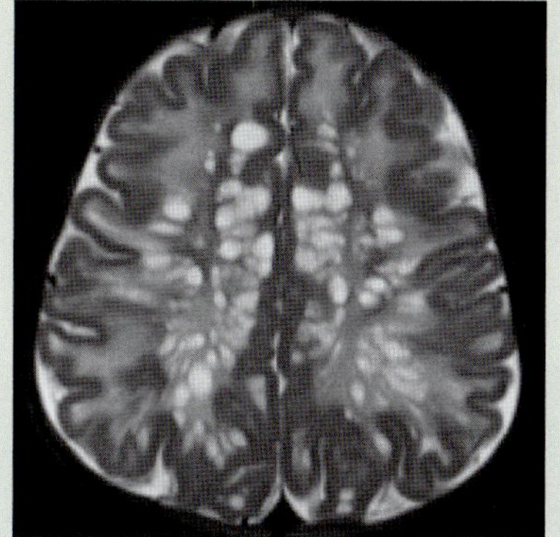 Fig. 4.3.2.18: Lowe syndrome	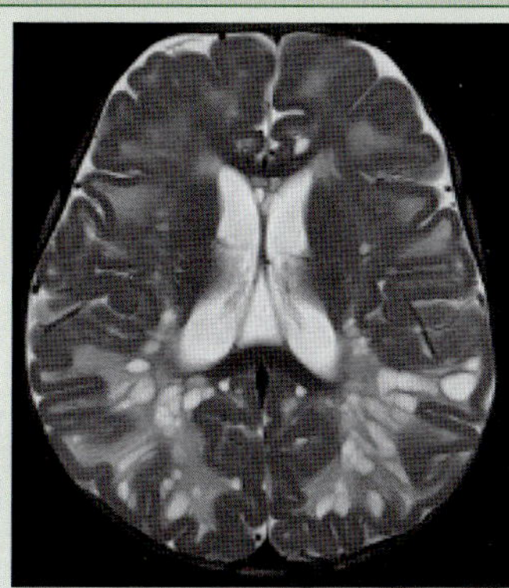 Fig. 4.3.2.19: Lowe syndrome	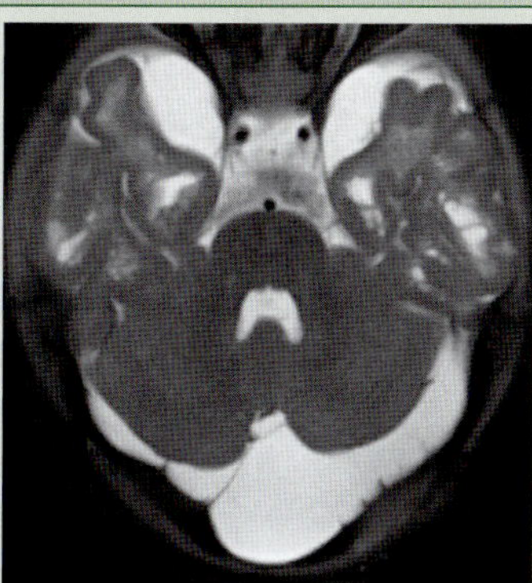 Fig. 4.3.2.20: Lowe syndrome
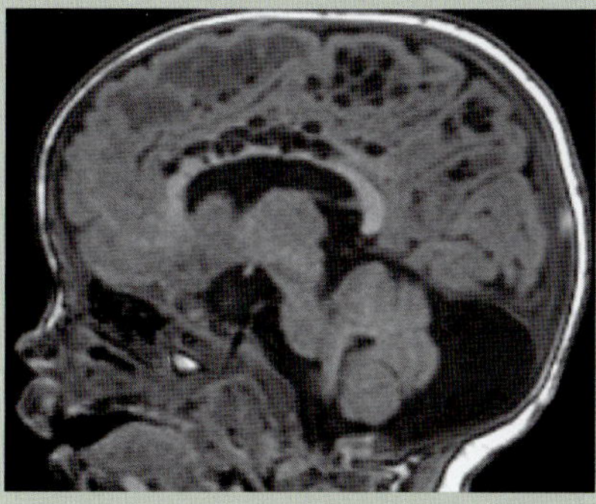 Fig. 4.3.2.21: Lowe syndrome	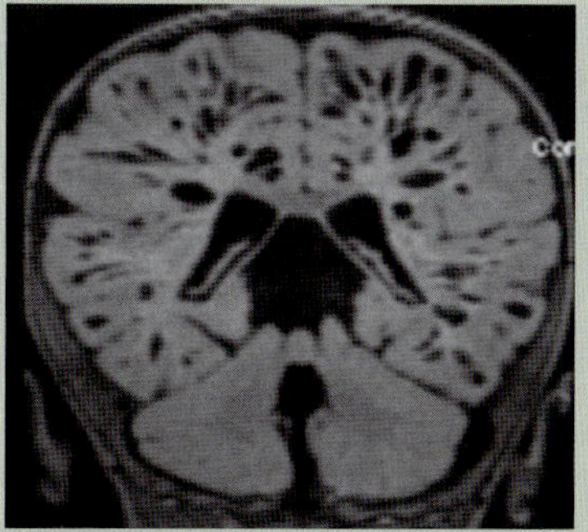 Fig. 4.3.2.22: Lowe syndrome	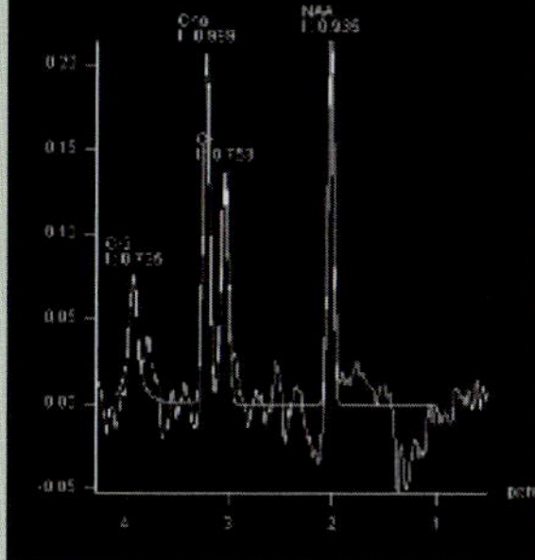 Fig. 4.3.2.23: Lowe syndrome
The lissencephaly-pachygyria spectrum—they are spectrum of disorders that result in smooth brain surface. They include agyria (no gyri) pachygyria (broad gyri) and lissencephaly (smooth brain surface). Type I (classic) lissencephaly is characterised by hypotonia and a lack of mobility. It appears as an hourglass or figure-8 shape, or as a smooth outer surface with a few poorly formed gyri (pachygyria). It is strongly associated with band heterotopia. Muscle-eye-brain (MEB) illness, Walker-Warburg syndrome and Fukuyama syndrome are all examples of type II lissencephaly, which causes muscular dystrophy-like diseases. It possesses a cobblestone complex, which is a microlobulated surface. The cortex is thinner than in type I and there is no band heterotopia.		
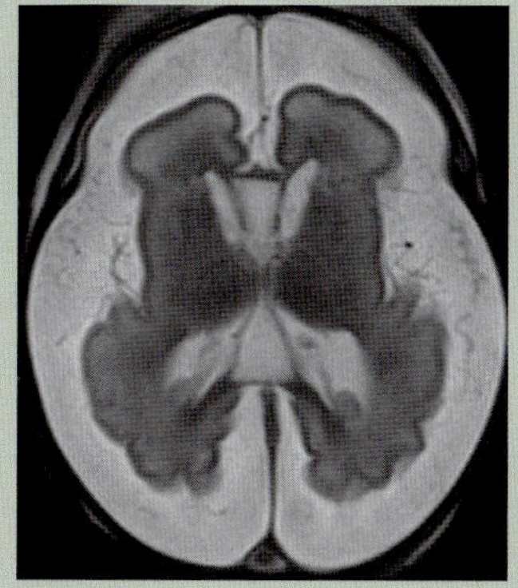 Fig. 4.3.2.24: Type I lissencephaly	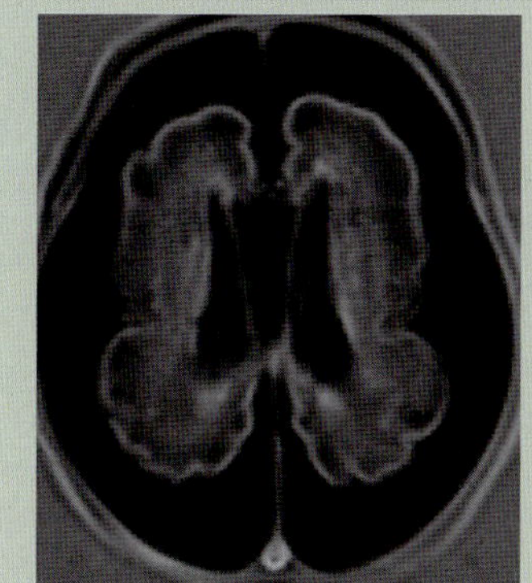 Fig. 4.3.2.25: Type I lissencephaly	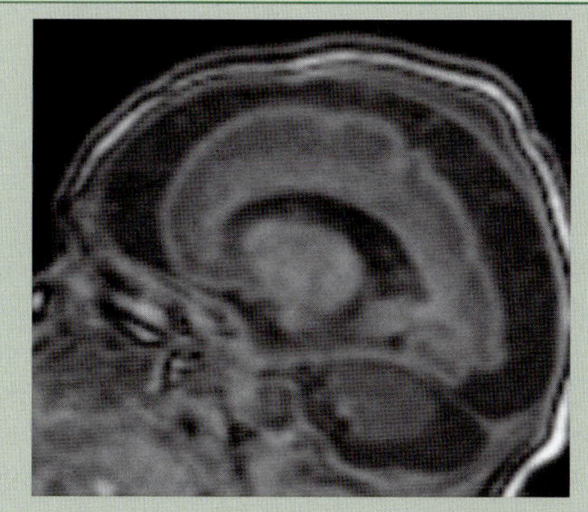 Fig. 4.3.2.26: Type I lissencephaly

Contd...

Table 4.3.2.1: Differential diagnosis for cortical developmental disorders *(Contd...)*

Megalencephaly (Fig. 4.3.2.27)—disorder of neuronal proliferation, migration and differentiation resulting in abnormal large bilateral cerebral hemispheres. Syndromes associated with megalencephaly are achondroplasia, epidermal nevus syndrome, Beckwith-Wiedemann syndrome, Klippel-Trénaunay-Weber syndrome, NF1 and TS. Differential diagnosis for megalencephaly: **Sotos syndrome** (AD type of cerebral gigantism presenting as prominent trigone, colpocephaly, ventriculomegaly, corpus callosal dysgenesis, persistent cavum velum interpositum) and **Zellweger syndrome** (cerebrohepatorenal syndrome)		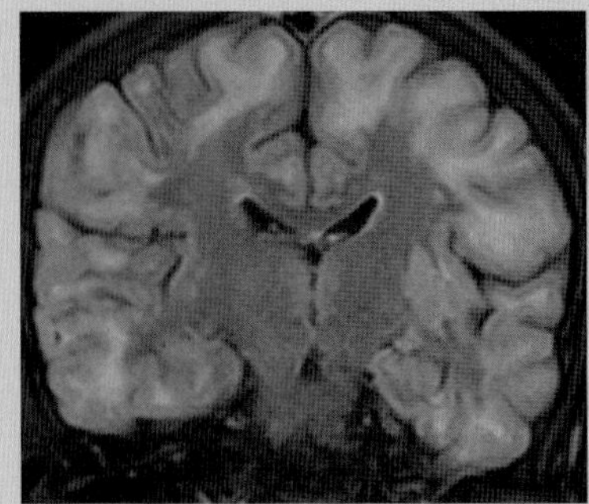 **Fig. 4.3.2.27:** Megalencephaly
Hemimegaloencephaly: Affected hemisphere is large (in polymicrogyria, affected hemisphere is small). MRI—a **thickened cortex with ipsilateral ventricular dilatation on the side of the megalencephaly.** Syndromes associated with hemi-megalencephaly include epidermal nevus syndrome, Klippel-Trénaunay syndrome, McCune-Albright syndrome, Proteus syndrome, unilateral hypomelanosis of Ito, CLOVES syndrome. Rarely with NF1, tuberous sclerosis. Right hemimegalencephaly is noted in Figs 4.3.2.28 to 4.3.2.30		
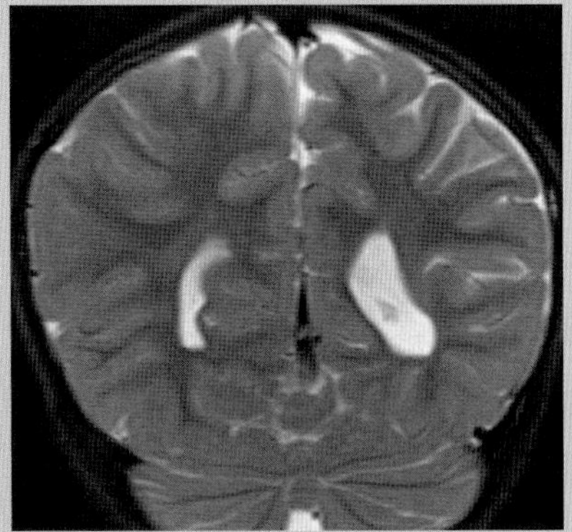 **Fig. 4.3.2.28:** Hemimegaloencephaly	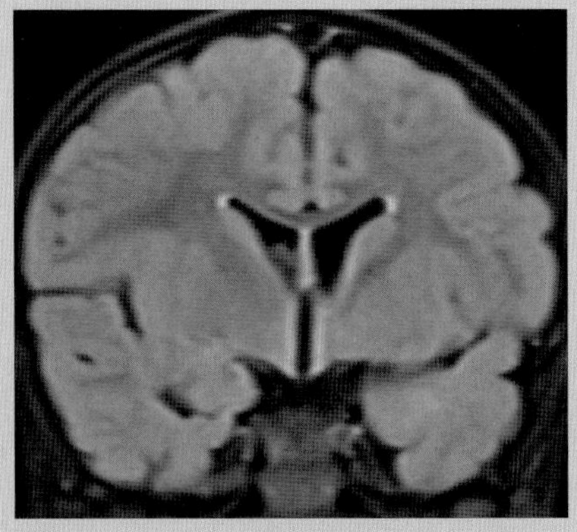 **Fig. 4.3.2.29:** Hemimegaloencephaly	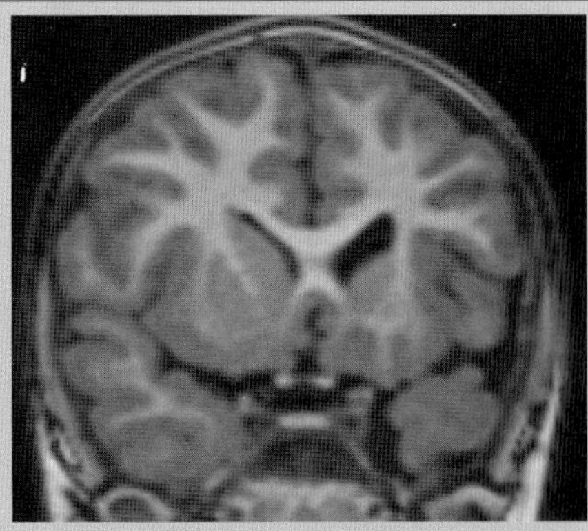 **Fig. 4.3.2.30:** Hemimegaloencephaly
Microcephalus with simplified gyral pattern—disorder of stem cell proliferation, head circumference <3 SD below mean. Normal cortical thickness, smooth linear cortical margin, normal primary and secondary sulci		
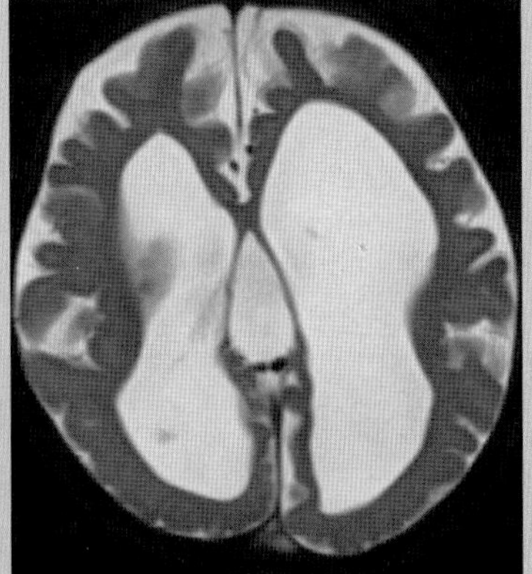 **Fig. 4.3.2.31:** Microcephalus with simplified gyral pattern	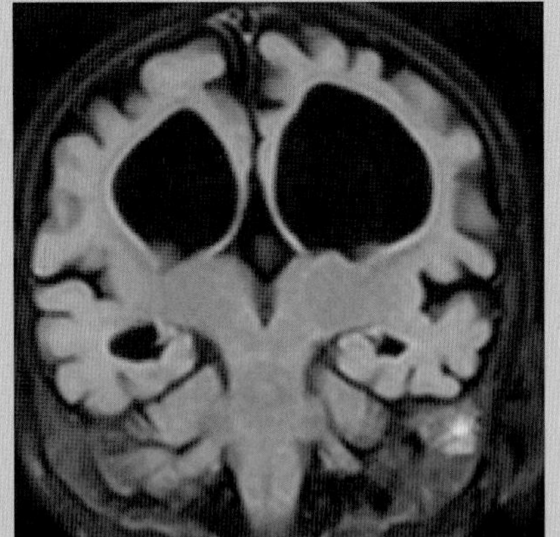 **Fig. 4.3.2.32:** Microcephalus with simplified gyral pattern	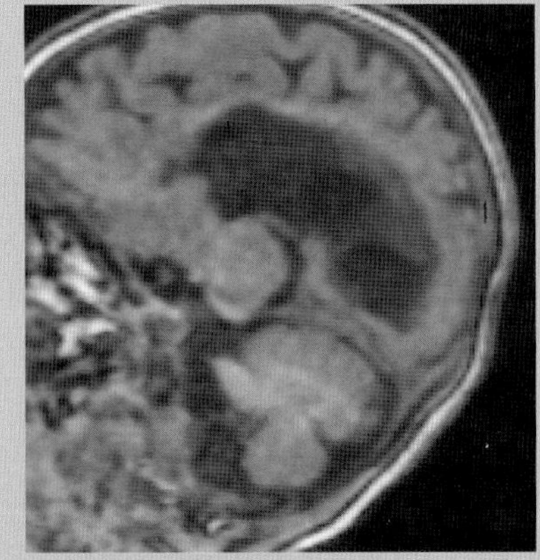 **Fig. 4.3.2.33:** Microcephalus with simplified gyral pattern
Schizencephaly: The gray matter lined cleft that extends from ventricular ependyma to pial surface of cortex. Most common associated anomaly is absent septum pellucidi (75%), dysgenetic corpus callosum. It is of two types—open and closed lipped. Trans mantle gray matter lining clefts seen as a dimple in the wall of ventricle if cleft is narrow. 50% are bilateral, of which 6% are open lipped both sides. Gray matter lining clefts may appear hyperdense. Calcification if associated with CMV or COL4A1 mutations. Prior to myelination, T2W more clearly defines the lesion.		

Contd...

Table 4.3.2.1: Differential diagnosis for cortical developmental disorders *(Contd...)*

Open lip: The lips of the cleft is widely separated. GM lining cleft may be harder to discern than in closed lip	**Closed lip**: The lips of the cleft is closely apposed. Lining gray matter can appear dysplastic on margin of cleft/at GM-WM junction areas.
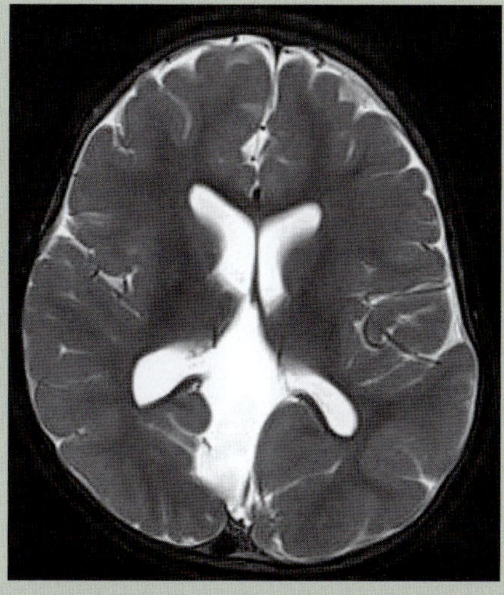 **Fig. 4.3.2.34:** Unilateral right occipital closed lip schizencephaly	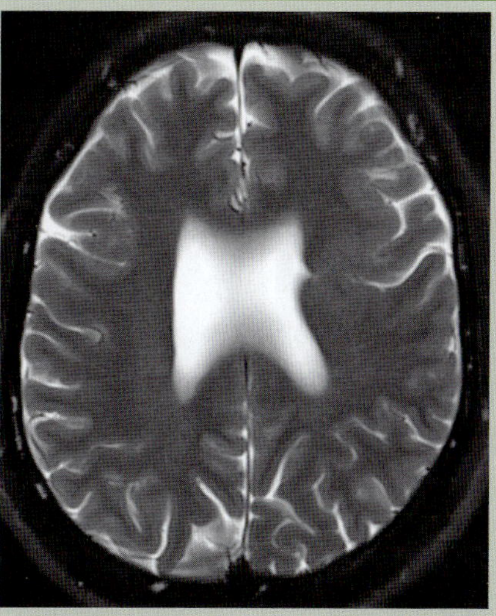 **Fig. 4.3.2.35:** Unilateral left frontal closed lip schizencephaly

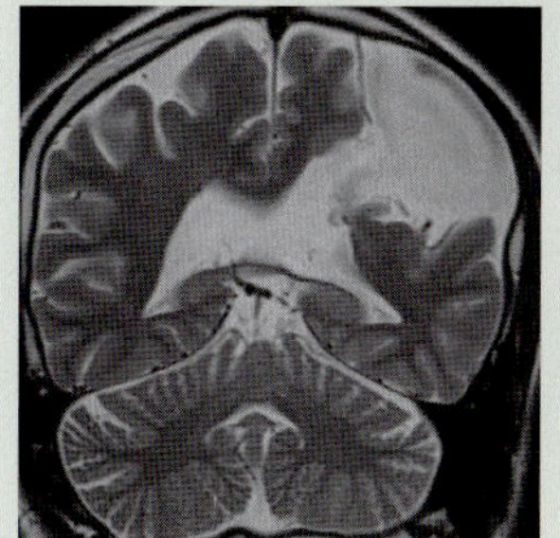 **Fig. 4.3.2.36:** Unilateral left frontoparietal open lip schizencephaly	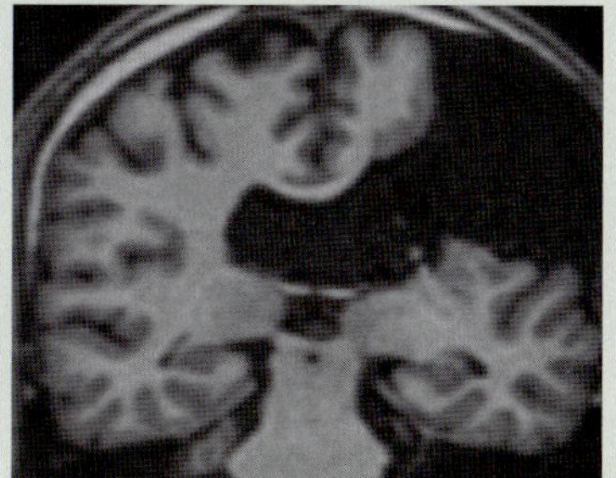 **Fig. 4.3.2.37:** Unilateral left frontoparietal open lip schizencephaly	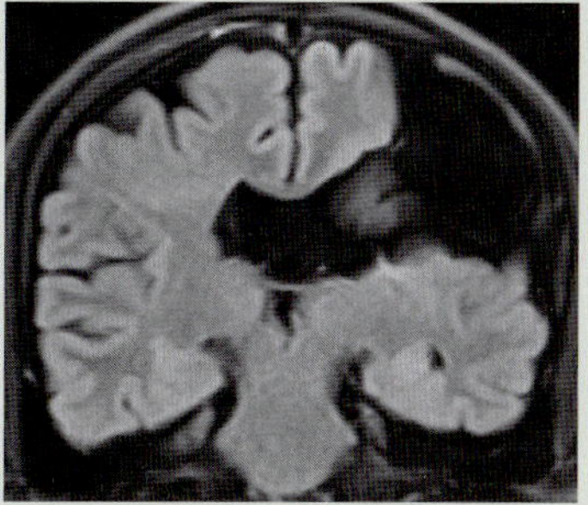 **Fig. 4.3.2.38:** Unilateral left frontoparietal open lip schizencephaly	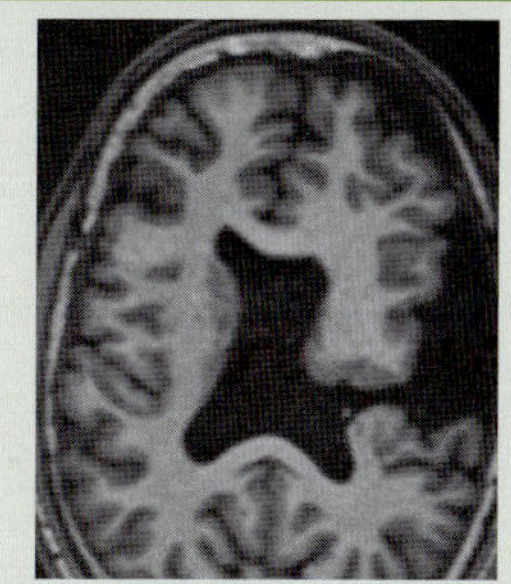 **Fig. 4.3.2.39:** Unilateral left frontoparietal open lip schizencephaly
Unilateral left frontoparietal open lip schizencephaly seen from Figs 4.3.2.36 to 4.3.2.39			
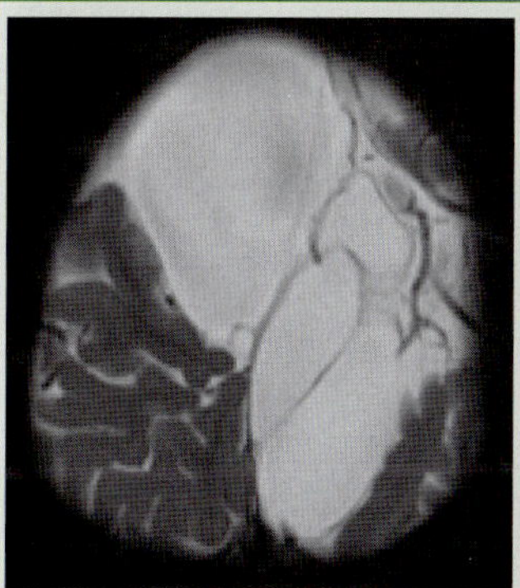 **Fig. 4.3.2.40:** Polymicrogyria	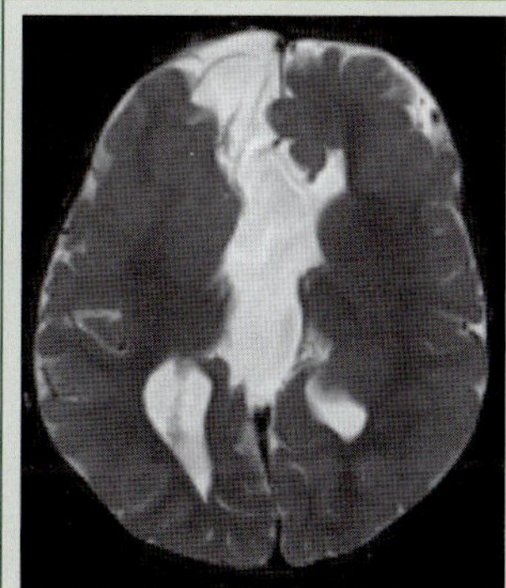 **Fig. 4.3.2.41:** Polymicrogyria	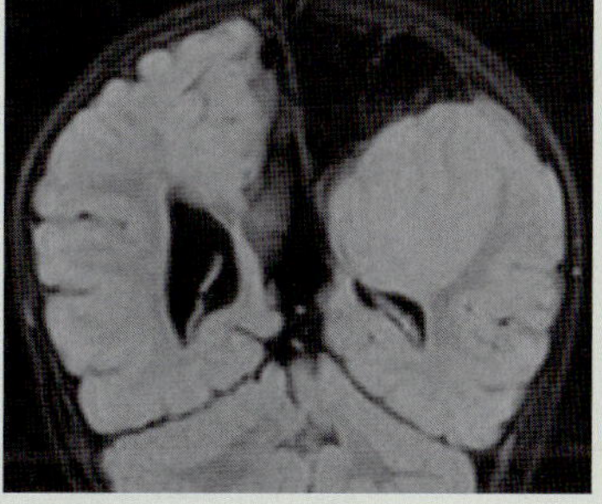 **Fig. 4.3.2.42:** Polymicrogyria	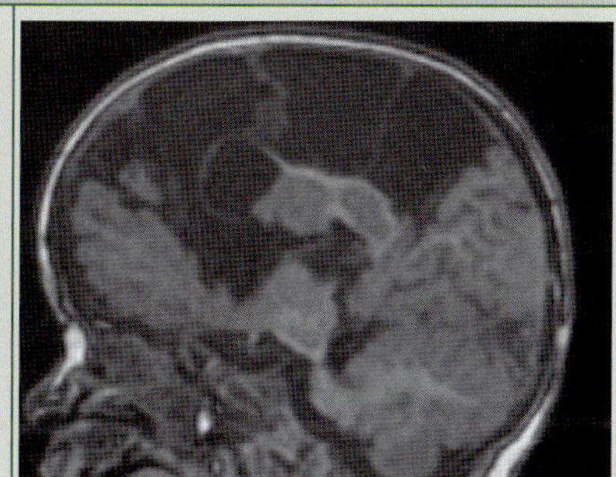 **Fig. 4.3.2.43** Polymicrogyria
Polymicrogyria with schizencephaly is seen from Figs 4.3.2.40 to 4.3.2.43			

Contd...

Table 4.3.2.1: Differential diagnosis for cortical developmental disorders *(Contd...)*

Tubulinopathies (Figs 4.3.2.44 to 4.3.2.47) are a group of cortical abnormalities caused by mutations in the tubulin protein, which controls neuronal migration throughout brain development. Micro lissencephaly, agyria-pachygyria, central pachygyria, polymicrogyria-like cortical dysplasia, and simplified gyral pattern are five major cortical malformation types identified in tubulinopathies.

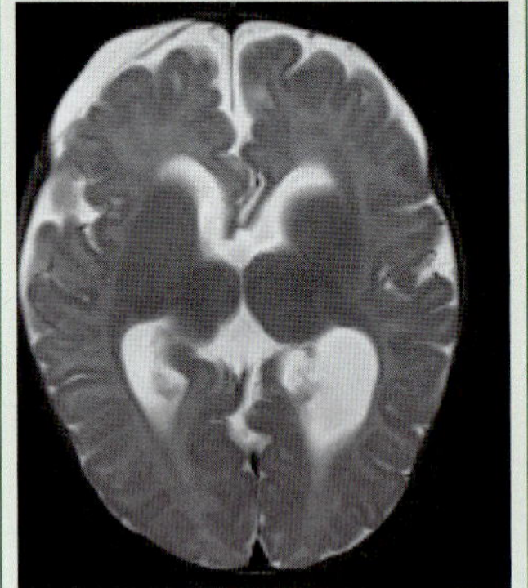

Fig. 4.3.2.44: Tubulinopathy

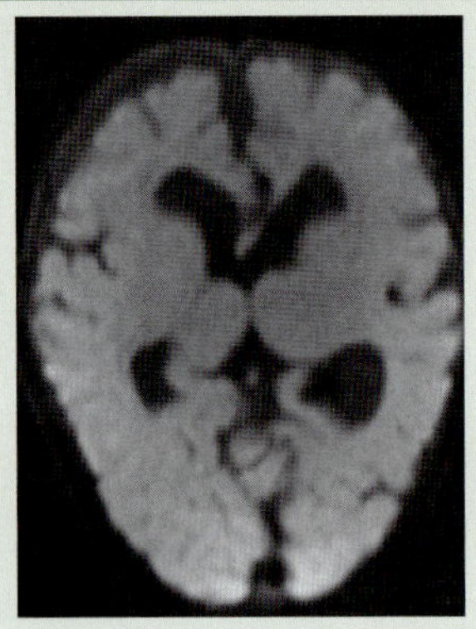

Fig. 4.3.2.45: Tubulinopathy

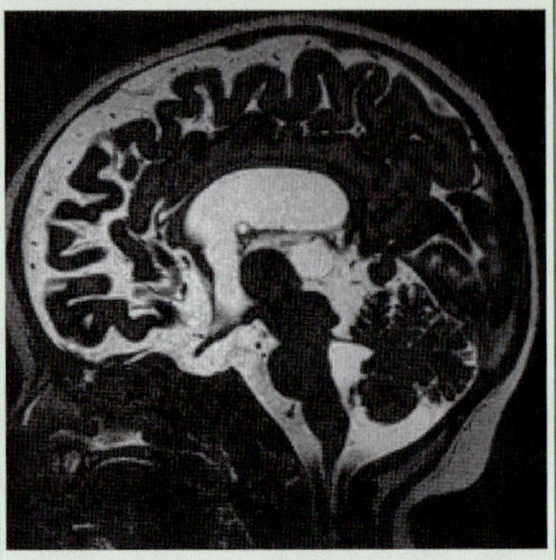

Fig. 4.3.2.46: Tubulinopathy

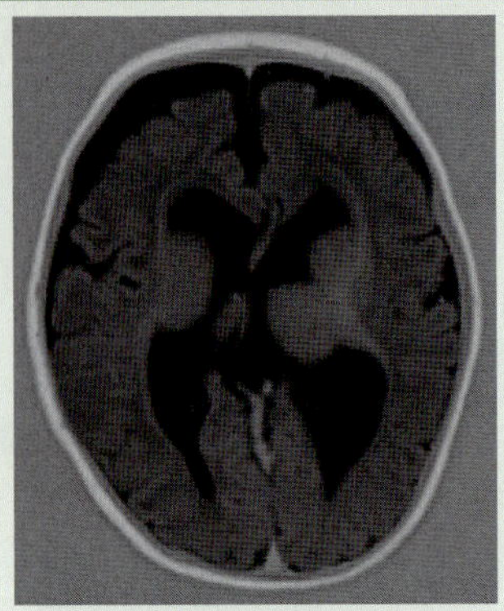

Fig. 4.3.2.47: Tubulinopathy

Kallmann syndrome—Refer to case 4.3.1

Arnold-Chiari malformation with corpus callosal dysgenesis (Figs 4.3.2.48 to 4.3.2.52): Refer to case 4.45

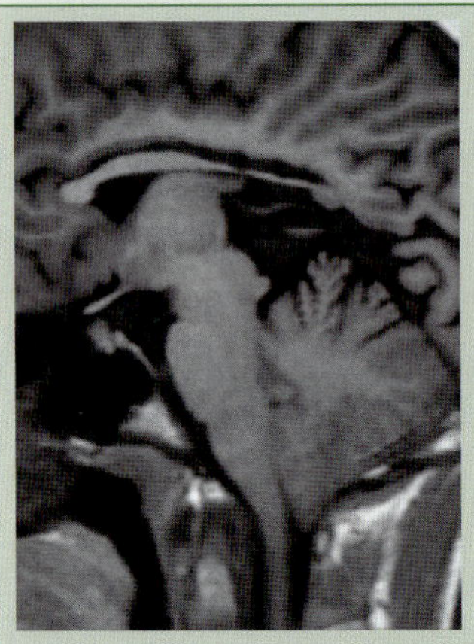

Fig. 4.3.2.48: Arnold-Chiari malformation with corpus callosal dysgenesis

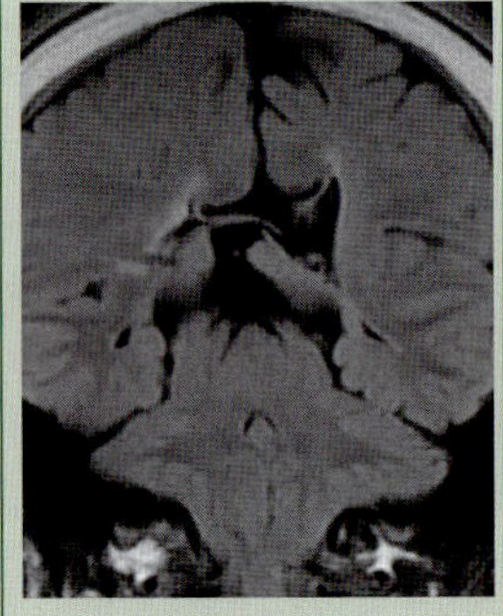

Fig. 4.3.2.49: Arnold-Chiari malformation with corpus callosal dysgenesis

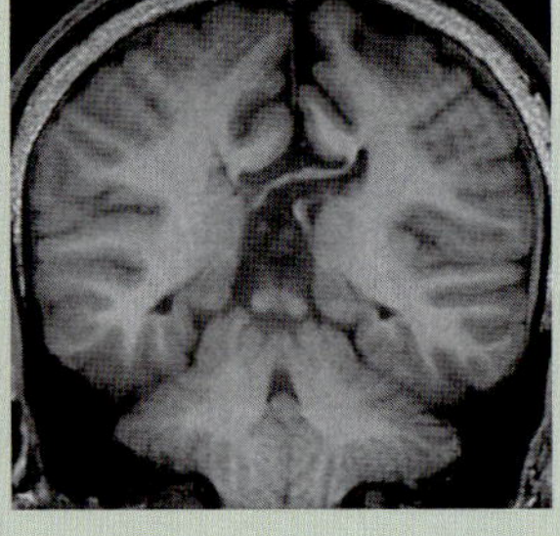

Fig. 4.3.2.50: Arnold-Chiari malformation with corpus callosal dysgenesis

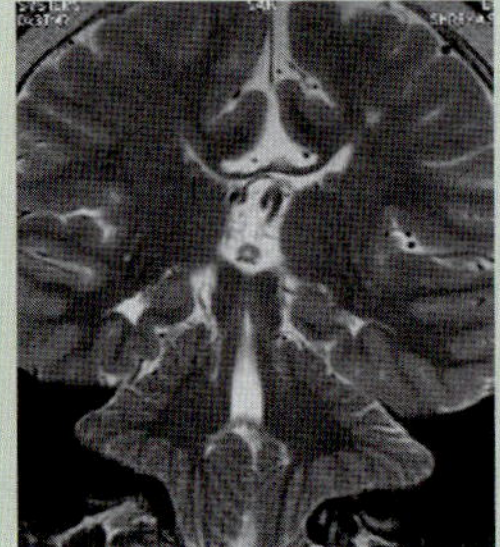

Fig. 4.3.2.51: Arnold-Chiari malformation with corpus callosal dysgenesis

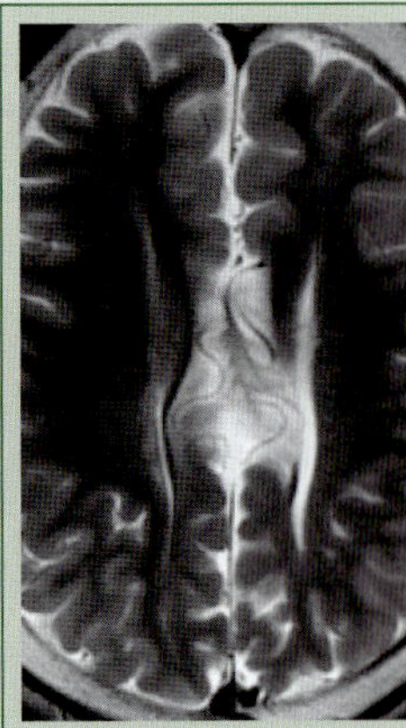

Fig. 4.3.2.52: Arnold-Chiari malformation with corpus callosal dysgenesis

Atretic cephalocele (Figs 4.3.2.53 to 4.3.2.55): Refer to case 4.5 for detailed explanation

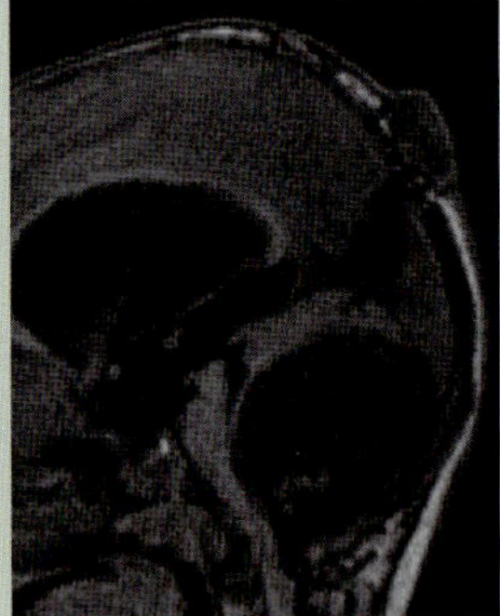

Fig. 4.3.2.53: Atretic cephalocele

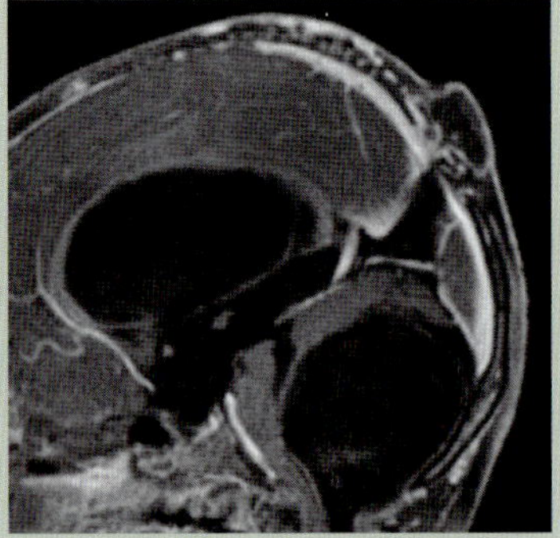

Fig. 4.3.2.54: Atretic cephalocele

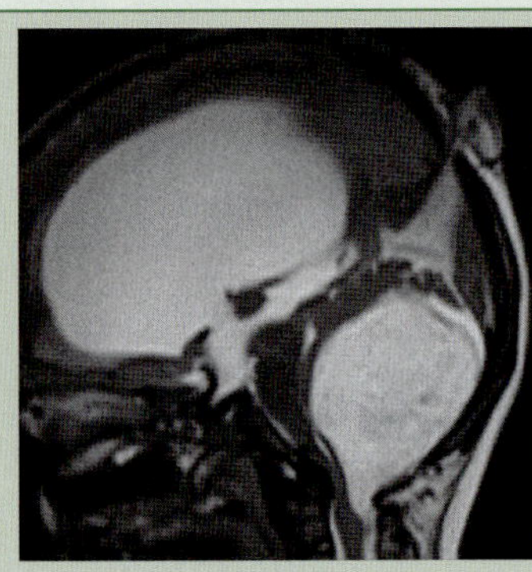

Fig. 4.3.2.55: Atretic cephalocele

Contd...

Table 4.3.2.1: Differential diagnosis for cortical developmental disorders *(Contd...)*

Cobblestone malformations are associated with hypomyelination, cerebellar dysgenesis and pontine hypoplasia. Often associated with congenital muscular dystrophy: Refer to case 4.37

Crossed cerebellar diaschisis: It is a condition in which a cerebellar hemisphere's perfusion, metabolism, and function are affected due to contralateral focal supratentorial lesion/infarct (mostly). Contralateral perfusion abnormalities was observed in 20% of instances when CT perfusion was conducted after an acute stroke. CBF and CBV maps, in particular, show only a mild-to-moderate decrease in these parameters, which are not low enough to be classified as infarctions. A comparable role can be played by MR perfusion. Crossed cerebellar atrophy, or volume loss in the contralateral cerebellar hemisphere, can occur in chronic stages.Wallerian degeneration. FDG-PET imaging in the afflicted cerebellar hemisphere reveals hypometabolism, which is characteristic of this condition.

Right cortical dysplasia with posthemispherectomy status (Figs 4.3.2.56 to 4.3.2.60)

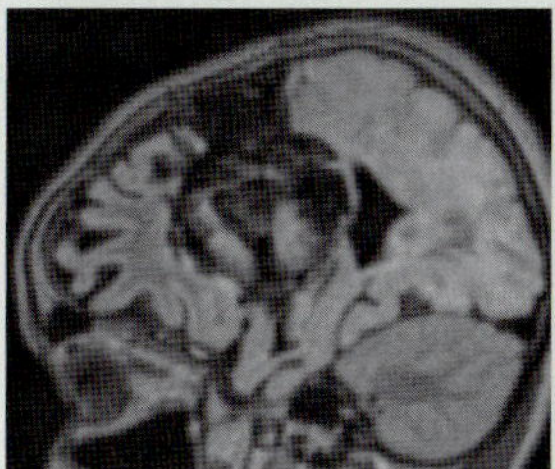
Fig. 4.3.2.56

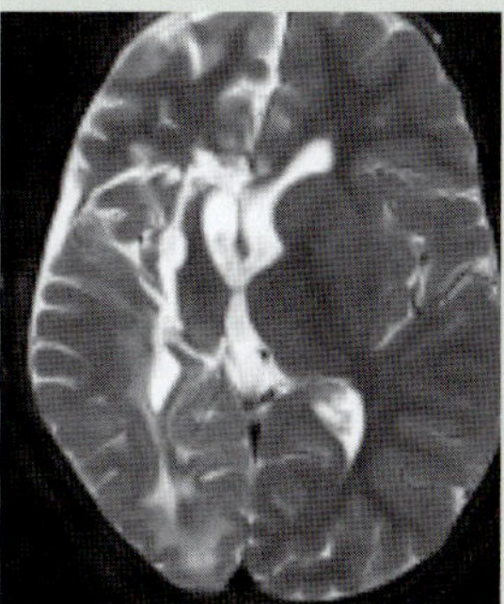
Fig. 4.3.2.57

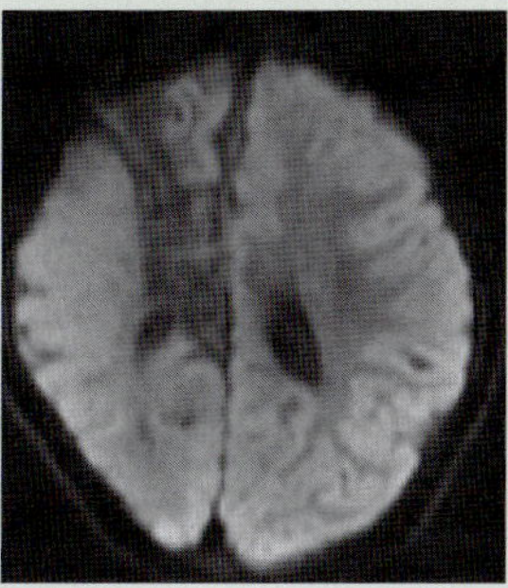
Fig. 4.3.2.58

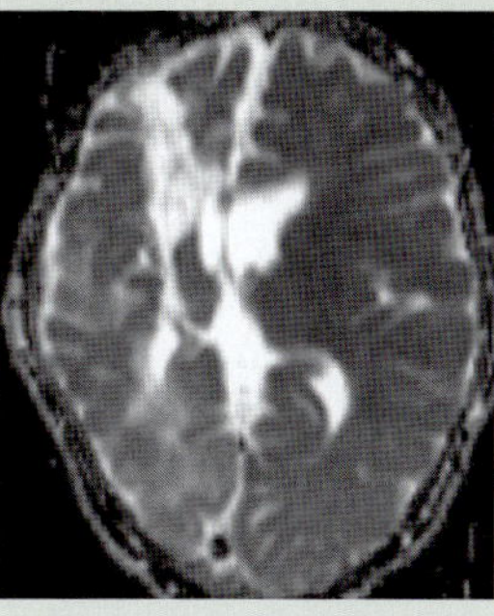
Fig. 4.3.2.59

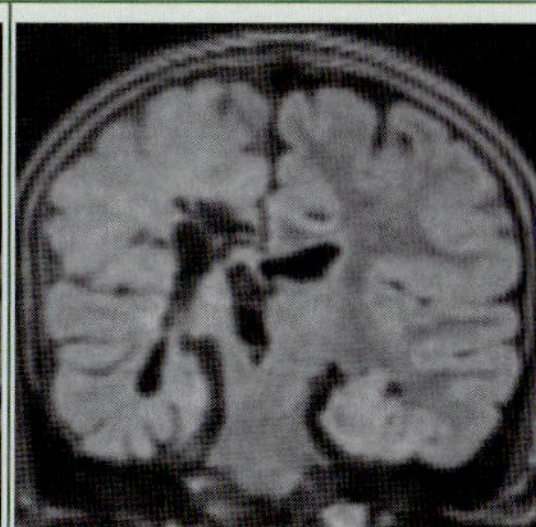
Fig. 4.3.2.60

Corpus callosal malformations: Congenital, acquired (infarction of ACA)
Agenesis: Complete absence of corpus callosum (hippocampal commissure absent, anterior commissure often present)
Hypogenesis, dysgenesis: Rostrum, splenium often absent, corpus callosum agenesis

Corpus callosum agenesis occurs when an insult occurs between 8 and 12 weeks of pregnancy. In a racing car sign, the WM tracts that normally cross the midline are orientated vertically (called Probst bundles), dividing the lateral ventricles widely. DSA will show ACA with an abnormal vertical course

Figures 4.3.2.61 to 4.3.2.65 show the ventricles run parallel rather than in the traditional "bow-tie" shape, giving the image of a racing car; "Texas longhorn"/moose head/viking helmet appearance on coronal imaging due to colpocephaly; dilated high-riding 3rd ventricle communicating with the interhemispheric cistern or project superiorly as a dorsal cyst. Cortex shows Probst bundles, absent cingulate gyrus leading to radial gyri, everted cingulate gyrus,limbic system, hypoplastic fornices and hypoplastic hippocampi. All these findings denote corpus callosal agenesis.

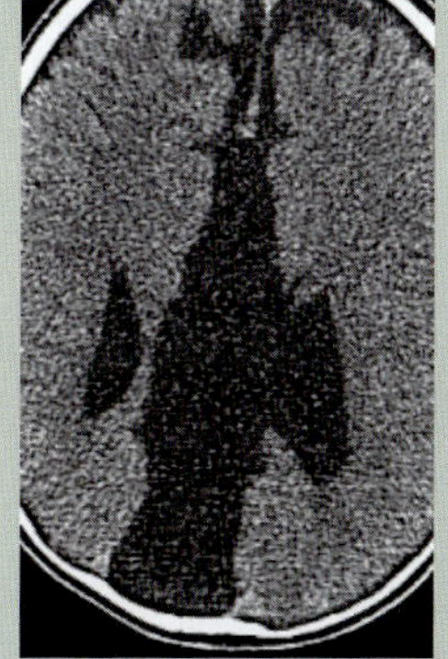
Fig. 4.3.2.61: Corpus callosum agenesis

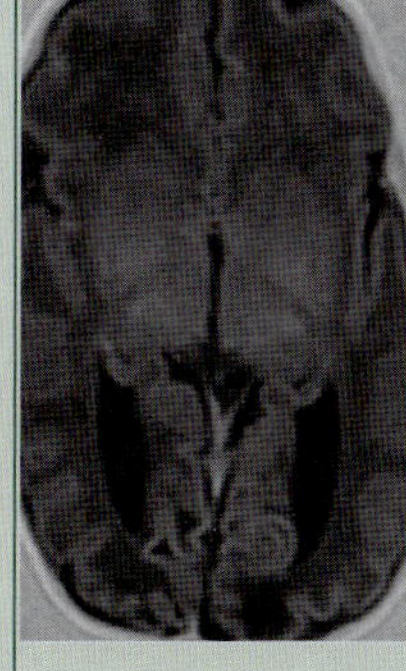
Fig. 4.3.2.62: Corpus callosum agenesis

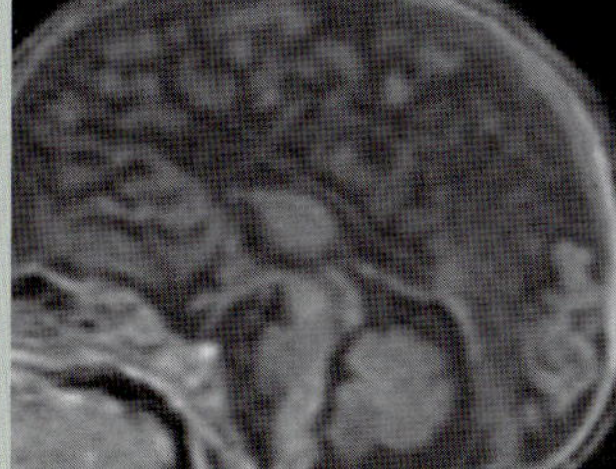
Fig. 4.3.2.63: Corpus callosum agenesis

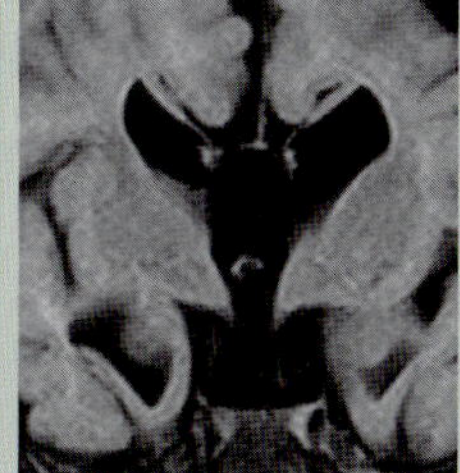
Fig. 4.3.2.64: Corpus callosum agenesis

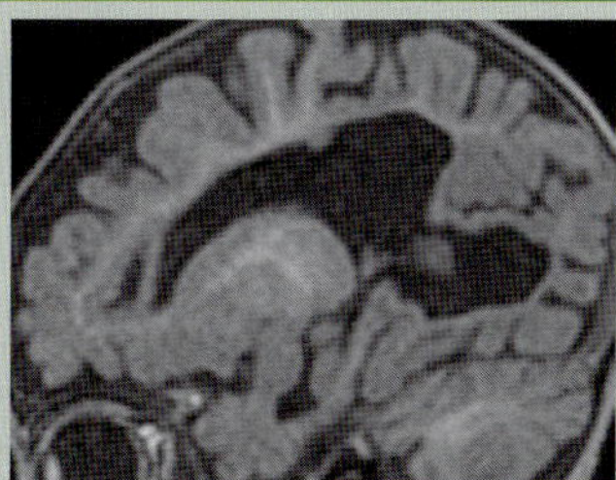
Fig. 4.3.2.65: Corpus callosum agenesis

Corpus callosum agenesis with choroid plexus papilloma (Figs 4.3.2.66 to 4.3.2.70)

Contd...

Table 4.3.2.1: Differential diagnosis for cortical developmental disorders *(Contd...)*

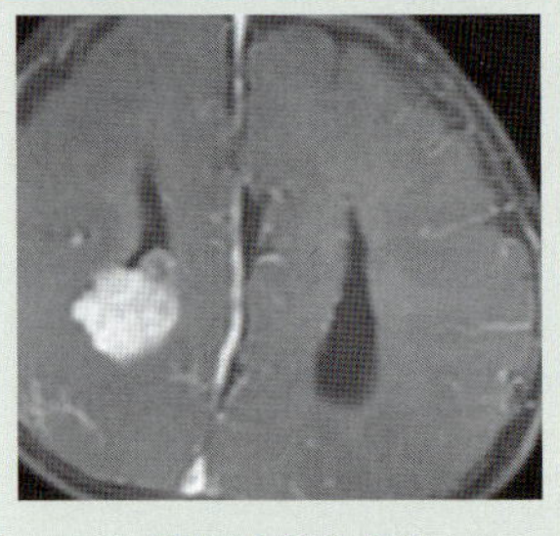
Fig. 4.3.2.66

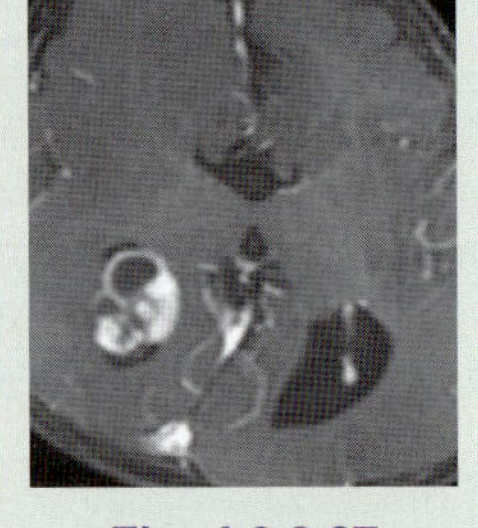
Fig. 4.3.2.67

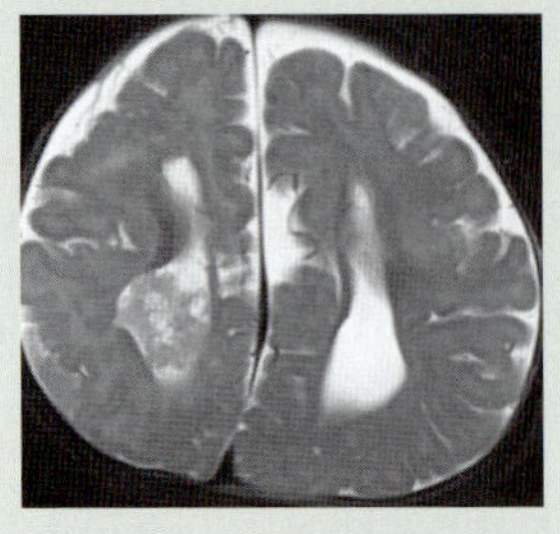
Fig. 4.3.2.68

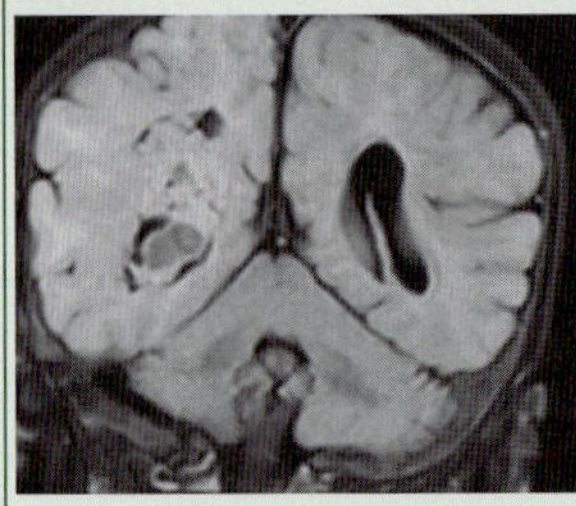
Fig. 4.3.2.69

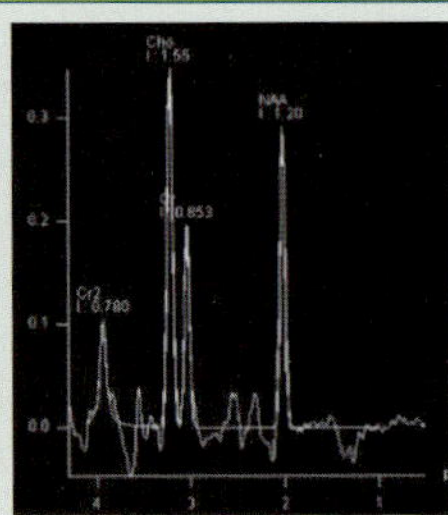
Fig. 4.3.2.70

Corpus callosum hypoplasia without dysplasia: (Figure 4.3.2.71) Here all major anatomic features intact including a distinctive rostrum, genu, corpus, and splenium. In severe cases, more caudal characteristics of corpus callosum will gradually wane resulting in hypoplastic and foreshortened posterior part of corpus callosum (i.e., corpus or splenium) with normal anterior and an anterior remnant CCA type in which the agenesis of posterior part of corpus callosum is seen.

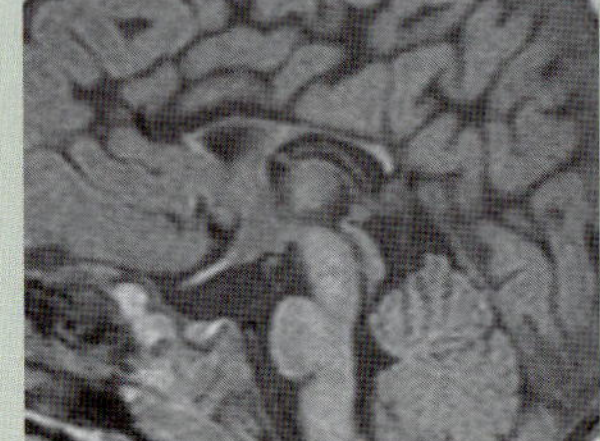
Fig. 4.3.2.71: Corpus callosum hypoplasia without dysplasia

Corpus callosum hypogenesis with dysplasia—the shape of the CC is disrupted, and it is not limited to its posterior aspect. There are two types. A) **Stripe type:** It has thin stripe that is uniform without anatomic distinction between the genu and splenium. B) **Kinked type** was the second type, which was defined by a thin, hypoplastic corpus callosum that was obviously kinked in one or more areas, either anteriorly or posteriorly.

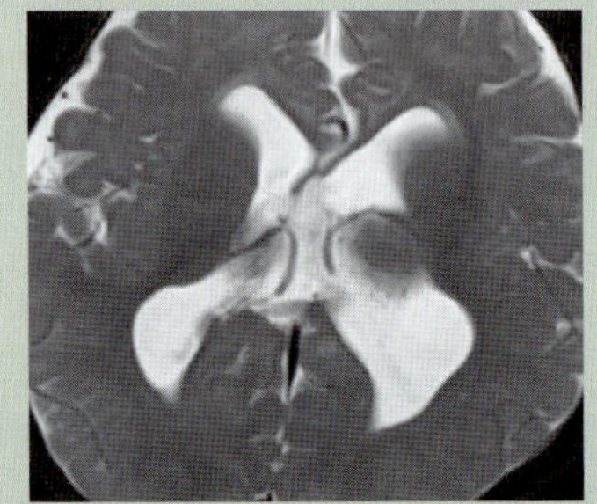
Fig. 4.3.2.72: Kinked type of CC hypogenesis with dysplasia

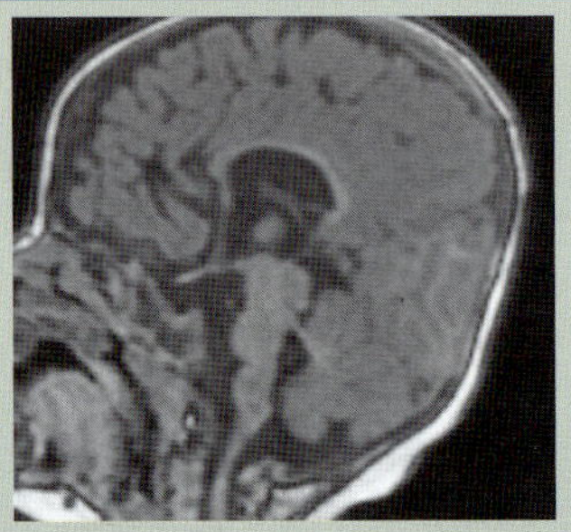
Fig. 4.3.2.73: Kinked type of CC hypogenesis with dysplasia

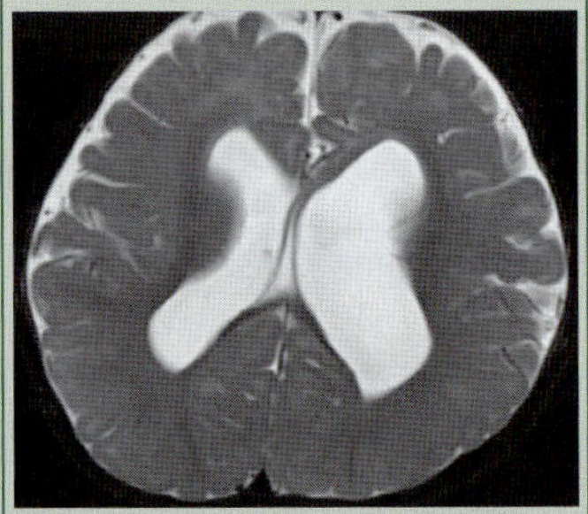
Fig. 4.3.2.74: Kinked type of CC hypogenesis with dysplasia

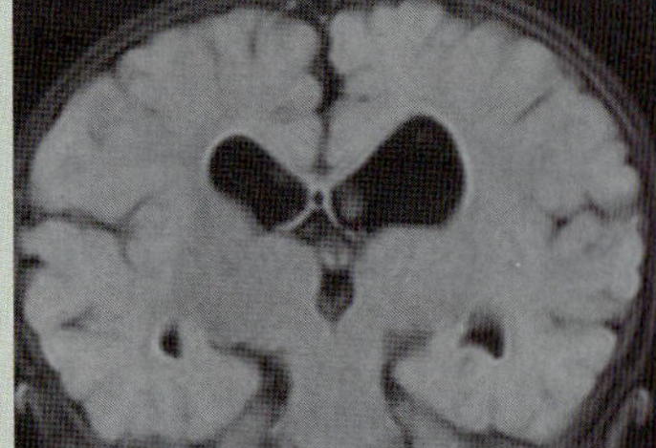
Fig. 4.3.2.75: Kinked type of CC hypogenesis with dysplasia

Kinked type of CC hypogenesis with dysplasia is seen in Figs 4.3.2.72 to 4.3.2.75

Pericallosal lipoma: An intracranial lipoma is most commonly found in pericallosal region. Lesions containing fat in the interhemispheric fissure, which are strongly connected to the corpus callosum. On imaging, there are two types: Tubulonodular and curvilinear.

Curvilinear pericallosal lipomas (Figs 4.3.2.76 to 4.3.2.81) are thin, elongated, and curvilinear lipomas that develop along the corpus callosum edge. They normally have a thickness of 1 cm and are positioned more posteriorly. corpus callosum shows mild hypoplasia.

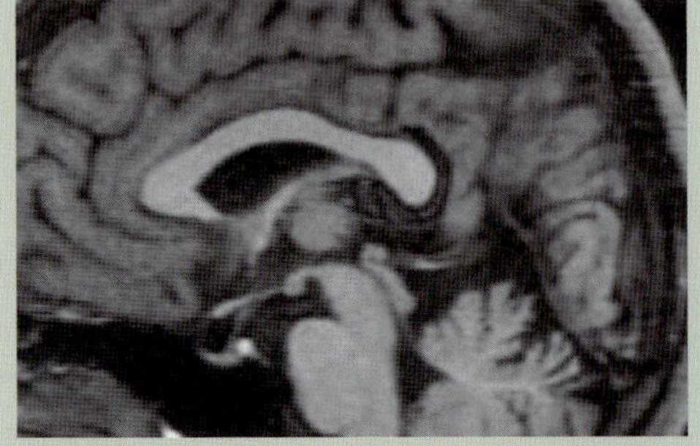
Fig. 4.3.2.76: Curvilinear pericallosal lipomas

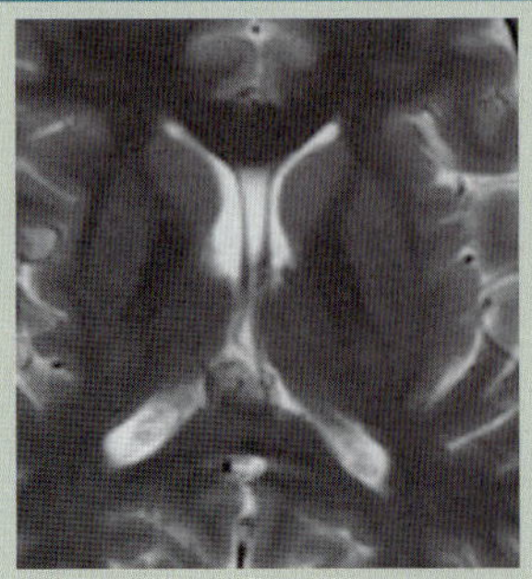
Fig. 4.3.2.77: Curvilinear pericallosal lipomas

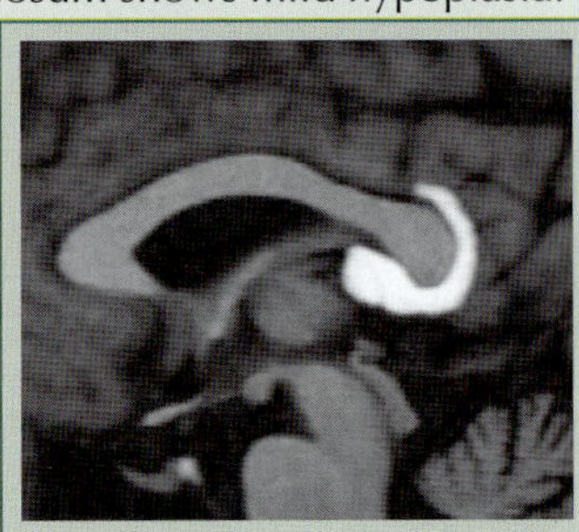
Fig. 4.3.2.78: Curvilinear pericallosal lipomas

Contd...

Table 4.3.2.1: Differential diagnosis for cortical developmental disorders *(Contd...)*

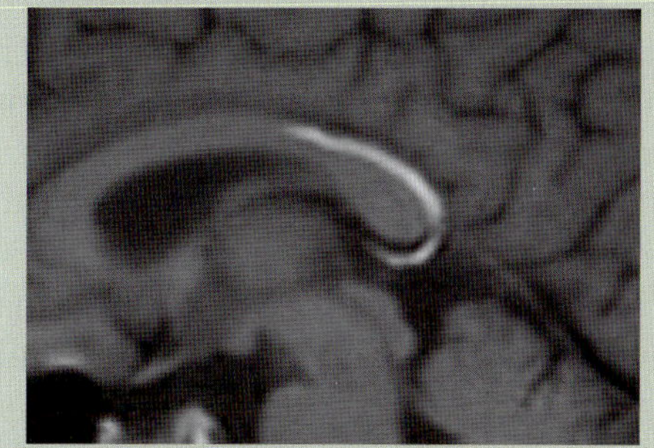

Fig. 4.3.2.79: Curvilinear pericallosal lipomas

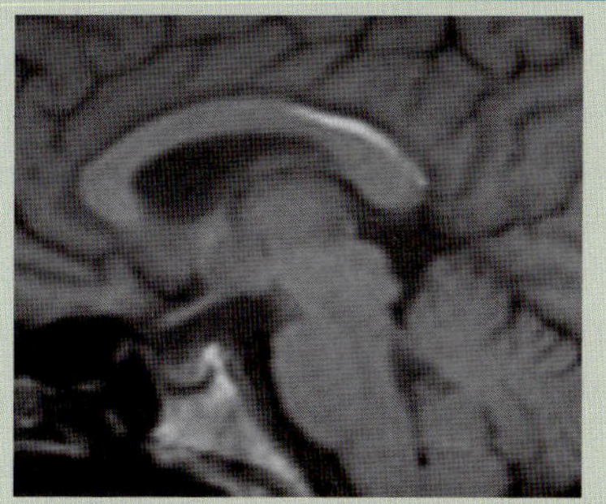

Fig. 4.3.2.80: Curvilinear pericallosal lipomas

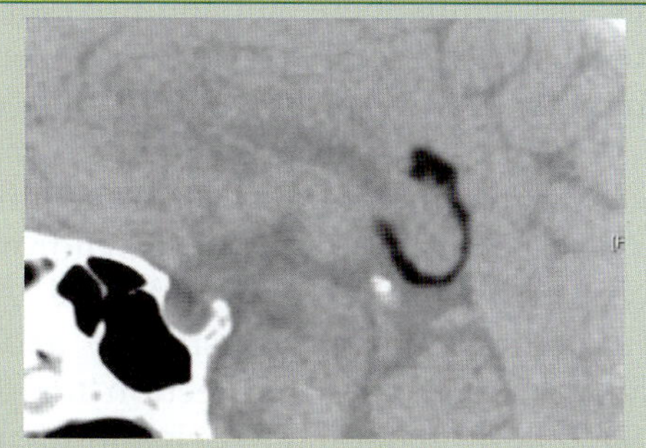

Fig. 4.3.2.81: Curvilinear pericallosal lipomas

The most prevalent type of pericallosal lipoma is **tubulonodular type** (Figs 4.3.2.82 to 4.3.2.84). They are rounded/lobular in shape and have a thickness of more than 2 cm usually. They are located anteriorly and have significant callosal and fronto-facial abnormalities. They (tubulonodular type) can spread to the choroid plexus and lateral ventricles.

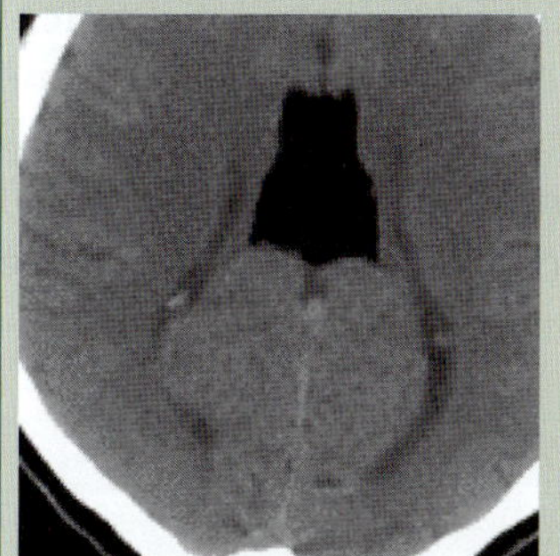

Fig. 4.3.2.82: Tubulonodular pericallosal lipoma

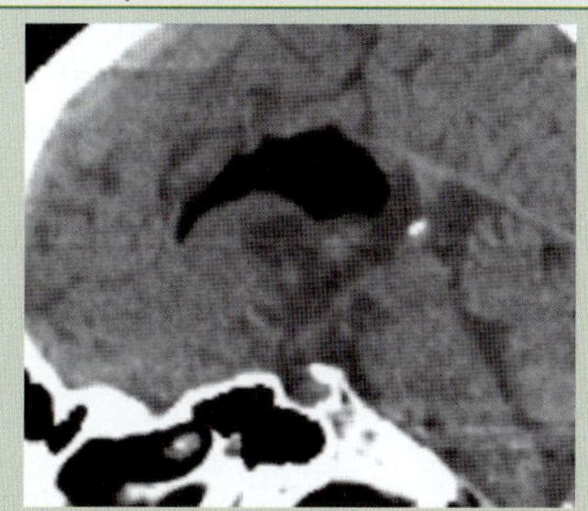

Fig. 4.3.2.83: Tubulonodular pericallosal lipoma

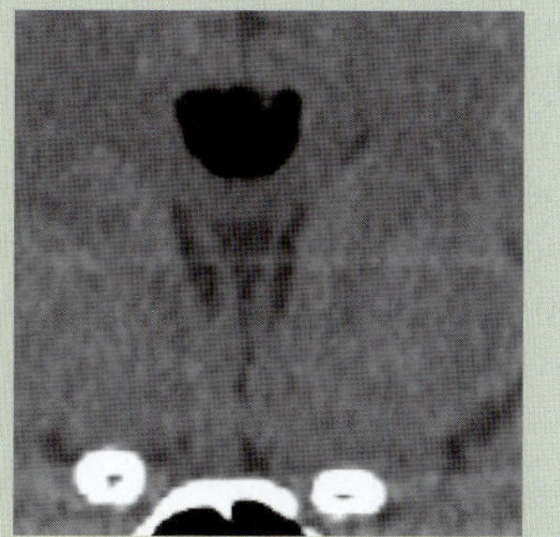

Fig. 4.3.2.84: Tubulonodular pericallosal lipoma

Table 4.3.2.2: A developmental and genetic classification for malformations of cortical development (based on 2012 update)
Group I: Abnormal cell proliferation or apoptosis Disorders of neuronal and/or glial growth or apoptosis are included in Group 1 conditions. They are divided into 3 groups: Those with aberrant brain size (A—small and B—large) and C—those with cortical dysgenesis (abnormal cells) (neoplastic or non-neoplastic) Group IA—**Microcephaly–**with normal to simplified cortical pattern / microcephaly with lissencephaly/microcephaly with extensive polymicrogyria Group IB—**Megalencephaly/macrocephaly** Group IC—There are a variety of neoplastic and non-neoplastic disorders in the cortical dysgenesis with abnormal cell proliferation group. Non-neoplastic disorders include type II focal cortical dysplasia, cortical hamartomas of tuberous sclerosis, hemi megalencephaly, cortical dysplasia with balloon cells. Neoplastic disorders include gangliocytomas, gangliogliomas, DNET
Group II: Abnormal neuronal migration Group IIA—subependymal heterotopia, marginal glioneuronal heterotopia Group IIB—lissencephaly type I: subcortical band heterotopia spectrum (band heterotopia) due to under migration; lissencephaly type II (cobblestone complex) due to over migration Group IIC—subcortical heterotopia (not including band heterotopia)
Group III: Abnormal postmigrational development Group IIIA—bilateral polymicrogyria syndromes, polymicrogyria and schizencephaly, schizencephaly; polymicrogyria or schizencephaly as part of multiple congenital anomaly/ intellectual disability syndromes Group IIIB—cortical dysgenesis secondary to inborn errors of metabolism, peroxisomal disorders, mitochondrial and pyruvate metabolic disorders. Group IIIC—type I and III focal cortical dysplasia Group IIID—post-migrational microcephaly
Not otherwise classified—malformations secondary to inborn errors of metabolism, peroxisomal disorders, mitochondrial and pyruvate metabolic disorders, sublobar dysplasia, other unclassified malformations.

resulting in several small undulating gyri forming cerebral hemisphere with multiple small sulci that shows fused appearence. Because the schizencephalic fissure is lined by polymicrogyria cortex, it is usually associated with schizencephaly. It could be sporadic or widespread. Secondary congenital CMV infection also can occur. It is associated with Zellweger syndrome, Adams-Oliver syndrome, Delleman syndrome, Arima syndrome, Fukuyama muscular dystrophy and Galoway-Mowat syndrome. It has predilection for perisylvian region (80%) and bilateral. CT helps in identifying associated anomalies like schizencephaly. NECT—altered sulcation pattern. MRI is the investigation of choice for assessing polymicrogyria. Both morphology and signal intensity may be abnormal. **T1W–irregular cortical surface appears as arc of thick (5–7 mm) cortex with irregular cortex white matter junction, without normal sulci. T2W—if age <12 months—small fine undulating cortex with normal thickness (3–4 mm); If age >18 months—thick bumpy cortex (6–8 mm) with large perivascular spaces and cortical infolding.** FLAIR helps to differentiate dilated perivascular spaces and abnormal myelination (to rule out cobblestone malformations). **Signal intensity**—polymicrogyria cortex usually has signal characteristics similar to normal gray matter. The subjacent white matter is not infrequently hyperintense on T2 weighted images (20–27%) which may relate to dilated perivascular spaces. On T2 weighted images, the inner white matter is commonly hyperintense (20–27%), which dilated perivascular spaces. The countless small gyri that can only be observed on thin-section high-resolution MRI scans. It is tough to tell the difference between it and pachygyria because both have swollen and thickened gyri. The GM-WM junction is the best place to look for the altered contour. To control epilepsy, treatment is symptomatic.

According to the basic underlying mechanism, the classification system for malformations of cortical development includes myriad disorders put into one of three broad underlying groupings: Aberrant cell proliferation or apoptosis (group 1), abnormal neuronal migration (group 2), and abnormal cortical structure (group 3).

4.4 CENTRAL NERVOUS SYSTEM

Case No. 4

Clinical history: A one-year-old male child presented with a mid-line mass over the bridge of the nose. No history of trauma/fever.

Radiological techniques and observation: Limited CT facial bone (brain and bone window) images in Figs 4.4.1 and 4.4.2 show a lytic lesion in the nasal process of frontal bone with soft tissue component isodense to the brain parenchyma situated anterior to the nasal bone near nasion (glabella) protruding anteriorly. No evidence of fat or calcifications. Bone shows well-defined sclerotic margin with scalloped border suggestive of long-standing benign process. Paranasal sinuses, bilateral orbits and other facial bones appears normal. No obvious widening of foramen caecum. Crista galli and cribriform plate appear intact. Skin covering the glabella appears intact. Serial reformatted section required to note the extent of lesion.

Mid-sagittal unenhanced T2 and unenhanced T1 weighted MRI (Figs 4.4.3 and 4.4.4) shows an extranasal lesion with signal intensity similar to the brain parenchyma, with thin stalk-like intracranial communication. No surrounding fluid/CSF intensity. Corpus callosum appears normal. No evidence of any intracranial cysts or obvious anomalies.

Interpretation: A: Young age, swelling in glabella, C: defect in fonticulus frontalis, B: Well-defined soft tissue mass in glabella with signal intensity similar to that of the brain with a stalk attaching to the brain through a defect in the nasion D: Extra nasal glioma.

Principal diagnosis is extra nasal glioma.

Differential diagnosis: Swelling in Glabella has site specific DD—1. Dermoid cyst, 2. nasofrontal cephalocele, 3. nasal glioma, 4. nasal dermal sinus; nonsite-specific DD—1. Pott's puffy tumour, 2. Haemangioma/ lymphangioma, 3. Dacryocystocele (para midline), 4. Medial angular dermoid (para midline).

Further investigations: Biopsy is contraindicated. Role of cisternography with heavily T2 weighted sequences to differentiate glioma from encephalocele.

Management: This child is referred to multidisciplinary team for surgical resection and HPE correlation. Extra nasal glioma (ENG) without intracranial connection is removed via external incision with stalk dissection.

Embryology of nasofrontal region: Nasofrontal Fontanelle, also known as fonticulus frontalis, separates the embryonic nasal and frontal bones for a short time. The transient prenasal space split up nasal bones and cartilaginous nasal capsule at the same time. A dural mater diverticulum runs from the anterior cranial fossa to the transient prenasal space via the foramen cecum. Before it retracts to cranium, it makes a short contact with the skin at the tip of the nose. The dural diverticulum's tract quickly involutes. The nasofrontal suture is formed when the nasal and frontal bones joins resulting in obliteration of the fonticulus frontalis. With the maturation of the surrounding bone structures, the prenasal space shrinks, eventually reducing to a tiny canal anterior to the crista galli known as the foramen cecum. Finally, fibrous tissue not only fills the foramen cecum, but also causes fusion of prenasal space.

Foramen cecum: It is located in front of the crista galli. Between the anterior cranial fossa and the nasal space is a primitive tract that is seen within fronto ethmoidal suture, running along the anterior cranial fossa, anterior to cribriform plate of the ethmoid bone and posterior to the frontal bone. Nasal encephalocele, dermoid/ epidermoid cyst and nasal glioma are examples of midline nasal diseases that can form along this primitive tract.

Foramen caecum closes by 5 years of age—the foramen caecum's length and width were measured only on CT scans due to their greater accuracy. The extreme length dimensions were 1.67 mm and 0.24 mm. The extreme width dimensions were 1.83 mm and 0.26 mm.

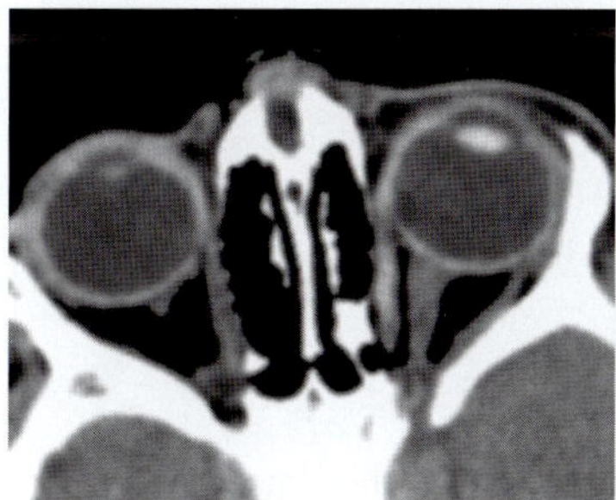
Fig. 4.4.1

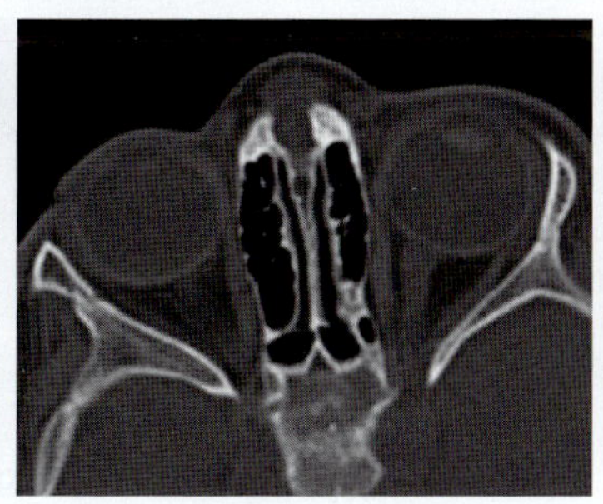
Fig. 4.4.2

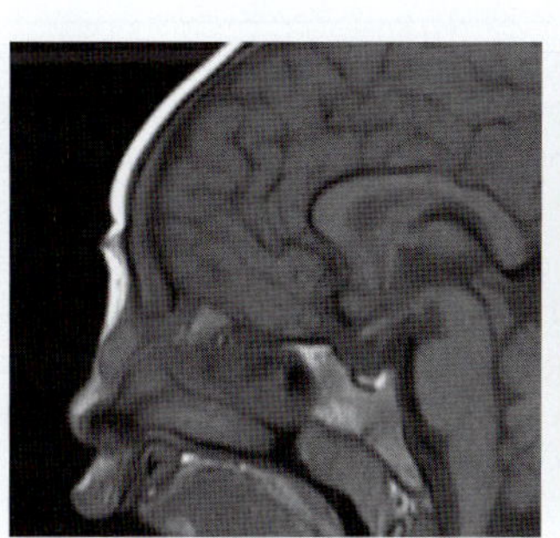
Fig. 4.4.3

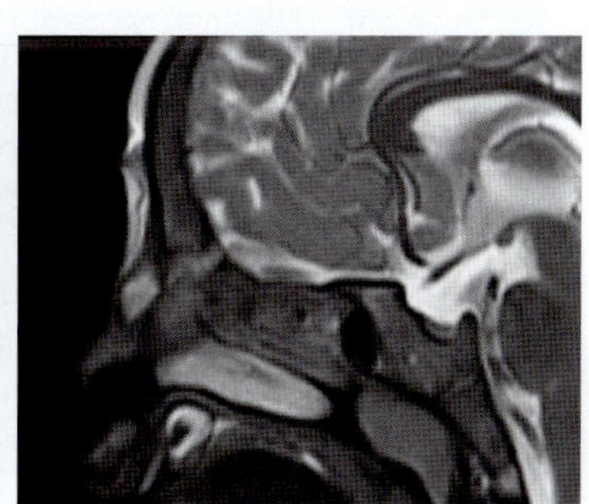
Fig. 4.4.4

4

Table 4.4.1: Differential diagnosis for glabella swelling

Dermoid cyst Dermoid are ectoderm-lined inclusion cysts that contain hair, sweat, sebaceous glands and squamous epithelium. Dermoid and epidermoid are commonly seen in the midline, frontotemporal and parietal regions. CT reveals defect in the nasal bone with a soft tissue mass protruding anteriorly. Well-defined T1 hypointense, T2 hyperintense lesion with or no intracranial extension.	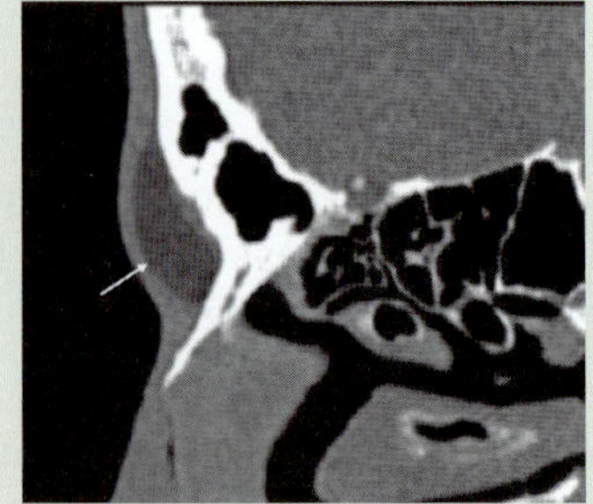 **Fig. 4.4.5:** Dermoid cyst
Pott's Puffy Tumour Swelling of the forehead caused by an underlying subperiosteal abscess with accompanying frontal osteomyelitis is most commonly a result of underlying frontal sinusitis. **Complications:** Orbital cellulitis, meningitis, parenchymal/epidural/ subdural abscess. **CT** may demonstrate frontal sinusitis, subperiosteal abscess of the frontal bone with loss of the outer table of the calvarium. **MRI** with contrast enhancement is more sensitive than CT in delineating early bony changes indicating osteomyelitis when evaluating the extent of intracranial disease and detecting small intracranial abscesses	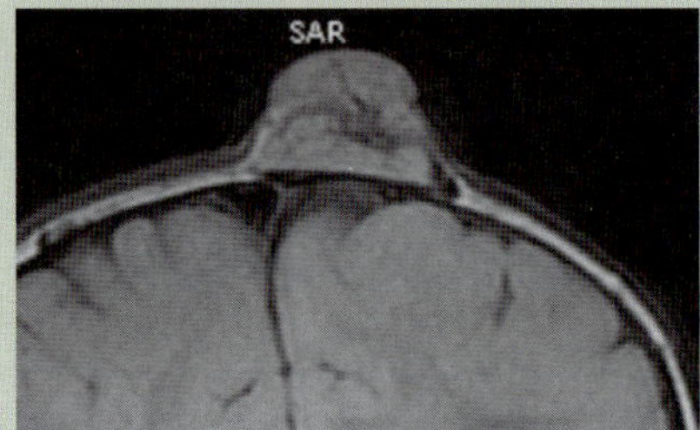 **Fig. 4.4.6:** Pott's Puffy tumour
Nasofrontal cephalocele Congenital or post-traumatic. Frontoethmoidal (sincipital) (10–15%) midface, dorsum of nose, orbits, forehead Frontonasal (40–60%): **Fonticulus frontalis** into glabella. **Naso-ethmoidal** (30%): Foramen cecum into nasal cavity. **Naso-orbital:** Maxilla, lacrimal bone into orbit. **Meningocele:** Meninges and CSF only. **Meningoencephalocele:** Brain tissue, meninges and CSF. Bone CT shows delineation of bone margins MRI: T1WI—heterogeneous signal intensity reflecting brain tissue composition, CSF T2WI- heterogeneous signal intensity reflecting brain tissue composition, CSF. Best contrast resolution, signal properties for CSF, characterizing gliosis in dysplastic brain tissue MRV–characterize venous vascular anatomy, relationship to encephalocele naso ethmoidal type of sincipital encephalocele	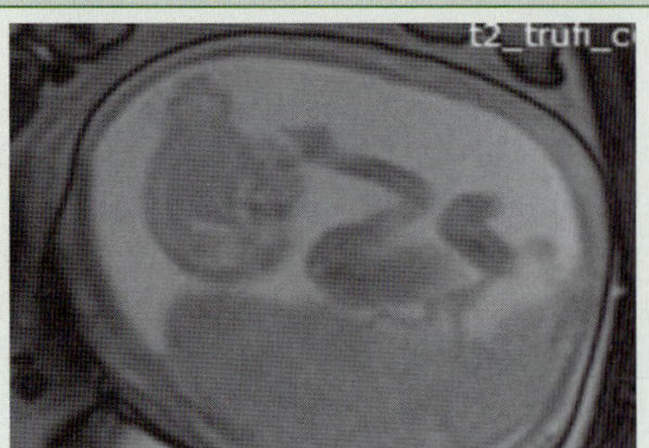 **Fig. 4.4.7:** Nasofrontal cephalocele
Dacryocystocele shows a bluish inferomedial canthus mass. Dilated nasolacrimal duct forming well-defined homogeneous thin-walled fluid dense mass involving the medial canthus or nasal cavity. The inferior turbinate bone has displaced superiorly, while the nasal septum has displaced to opposite side.	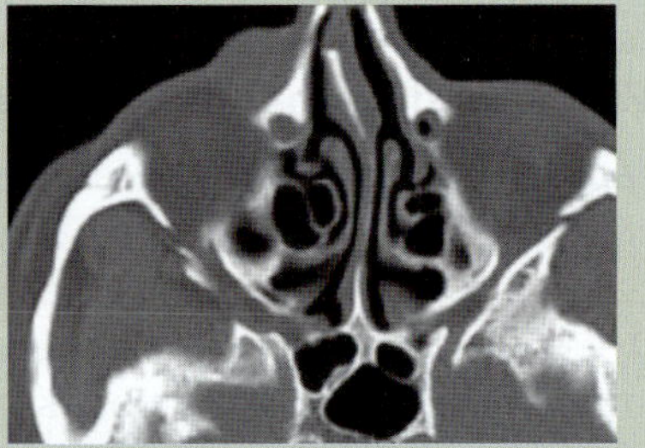 **Fig. 4.4.8:** Dacryocystocele
Nasal dermal sinus: It is a congenital abnormality that consists of an epithelial cell lined tract with an exterior opening as a small punctum along the nose's midline/off midline bridge. It occurs when the anterior neuropore fails to close during development, causing partial dura regression and the formation of a diverticulum. CT helps demonstrate the bony defect larger/ bifid crista galli and related defect in the cribriform plate. The dermal sinus tract, which extends from the base of the skull to the bridge of the nose, can be seen on MRI. It can extend superiorly with or without intracranial communication. Presence of sinus tract, rules out dermoid and epidermoid.	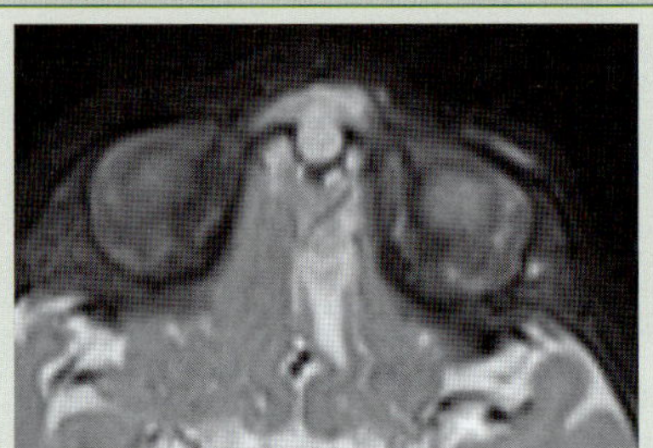 **Fig. 4.4.9:** Nasal dermal sinus

Contd...

Table 4.4.1: Differential diagnosis for glabella swelling (*Contd...*)

Internal angular dermoid cyst. These are most prevalent congenital lesions in children, which are closed sacs lined by an ectodermal epithelium.	A benign fat-containing lesion that appears near the orbit's medial or lateral angle. T1/T2 hyperintense lesion with suppression on fat-sat sequences.
Other rare causes	Osteomyelitis, LCH, Neuroblastoma metastasis
Benign fibrous histiocytoma—It is rare tumor occuring in men between 40 and 70 years. It occurs commonly in subcutaneous tissues/ orbit. They can arise from the mandible, maxilla, or pterygopalatine fossa. It is seen as homogenous T1 hypointense, T2 hyperintense mass showing intense peripheral enhancement.	

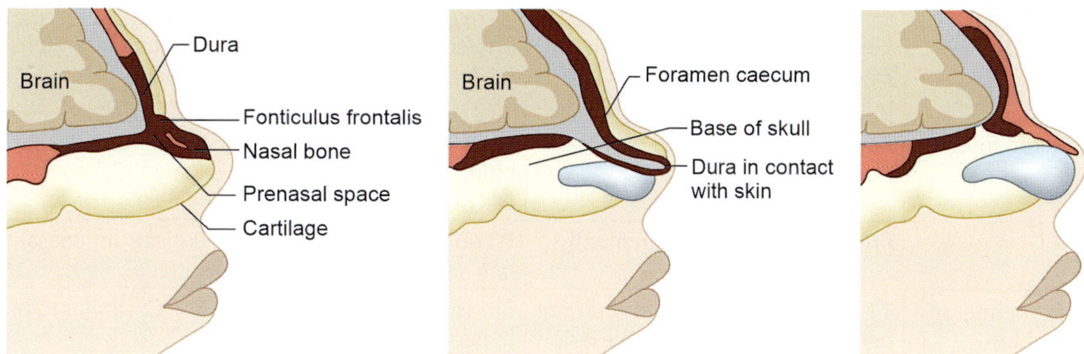

Fig. 4.4.10: Embryological development of nasofrontal region

Discussion: Nasal glioma consists of hamartomatous trapped brain tissue consisting of non-neoplastic glial cells without intracranial connection. So better termed nasal brain heterotopia or nasally trapped brain. **Extra-nasal glioma** (60%), intranasal glioma (30%), mixed (10%). Extra nasal gliomas lie external to the nasal bones and nasal cavity and most commonly they occur slightly off midline at the bridge of the nose. These represent the brain tissue that was trapped over the bridge of the nose during the closure of fonticulus frontalis. **Intranasal** glioma is found within the nasal or nasopharyngeal cavity, oral cavity or rarely in the pterygopalatine fossa. They represent the detached brain tissue which remains in the prenasal space.

CT/MRI fluid density or T1 hypo tract–sinus, fluid density or T1 hypo mass–epidermoid, fat density or T1 hyper mass–dermoid.

CT should be avoided in first 18 months of age, while investigating frontonasal masses or suspected sphenoethmoidal cephaloceles in the central skull base, as it helps to reduce both false positive and false negative examinations during a time of active ossification. The investigation of choice is MRI with a small FOV.

Imaging findings: Deep foramen cecum, small or bifid crista galli, Deformed anterior border of nasal septum. On T1W, there is an intermediate signal intensity with some contrast enhancement. Gliosis causes a high signal intensity on T2W.

Complications: Mollaret meningitis (benign recurrent aseptic meningitis), infectious meningitis, abscess, osteomyelitis, cavernous sinus thrombosis, seizures, periorbital cellulitis.

Management: Surgical resection, extranasal glioma (ENG) without intracranial connection removed via external incision with stalk dissection. Intranasal glioma (ING) via endoscopically, mixed type (rare) by combined approach.

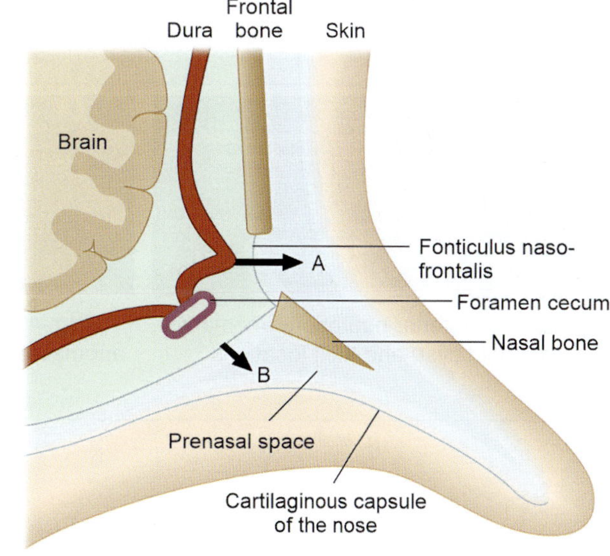

Fig. 4.4.11: Embryological basis for anterior neuropore anomalies

Table 4.4.2: Anterior neuropore anomalies

Nasal dermoid	*Nasal glioma*	*Nasal dermal sinus*	*Sinciput encephalocele*
Ectoderm-lined inclusion cysts that contain hair, sweat, sebaceous glands and squamous epithelium.	Dysplastic neurogenic tissue sequestrated and isolated from sub-arachnoid space. Extranasal–60%, intranasal 30%	Defective embryogenesis of anterior neuropore resulting in mixture of dermoid, epidermoid cyst and sinus tract in nasofrontal region.	Cerebral neuronal tissue and overlying meninges herniate out via a gap in the bony cranium in this type of neural tube defect/ cephalocele.
Midline–anywhere from the glabella to the columella. Other locations include at the anterior fontanelle, subocciput or vertex	Off midline Right >Left	Midline–anywhere from nasal tip to anterior skull base to foramen cecum	Midline. Can be nasofrontal, naso ethmoidal, naso-orbital
Can extend intracranially 20%	Usually no intracranial extension, Extension + in 15–20% attached to brain by a stalk	Intracranial extension + (20%)	Intracranial extension is always present
Patent foramen cecum in 20%	Foramen cecum fails to obliterate	Large foramen cecum with bifid or deformed crista galli or cribriform plate.	Patent foramen caecum
Projects extranasally	Projects extranasally/intranasally	Pit on skin, +/- protruding hair	Projects intranasally
Well-defined T1 hypo-intense, T2 hyperintense and fat-suppressed lesion.	T1 mixed, T2-hyperintense do not enhance, No CSF around the lesion	Sinus tract –T1 hypo, T2 hyper DWI–epidermoid	T1, T2 similar to brain tissue
Fig. 4.4.12: Nasal dermoid	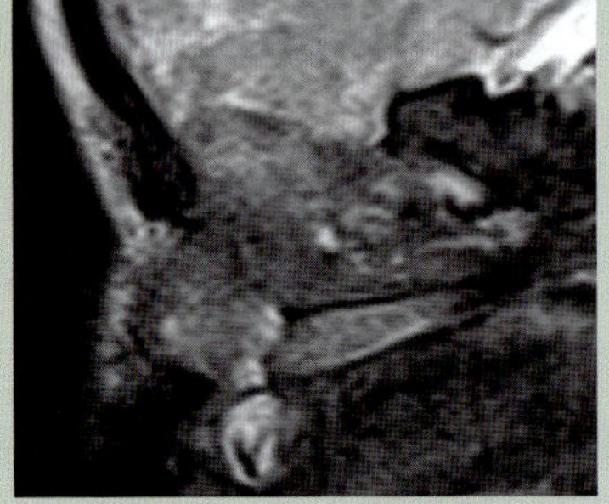 **Fig. 4.4.13:** Nasal glioma	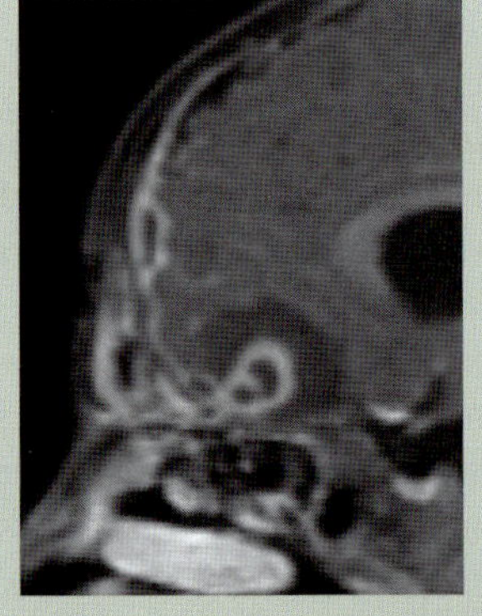 **Fig. 4.4.14:** Infected nasal dermal sinus with abscess	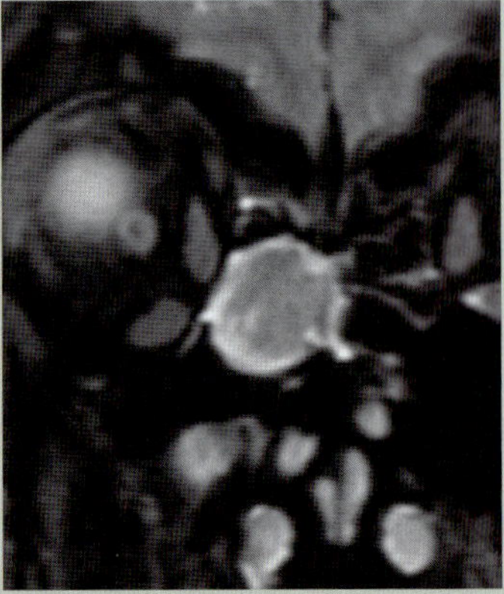 **Fig. 4.4.15:** Sinciput encephalocele

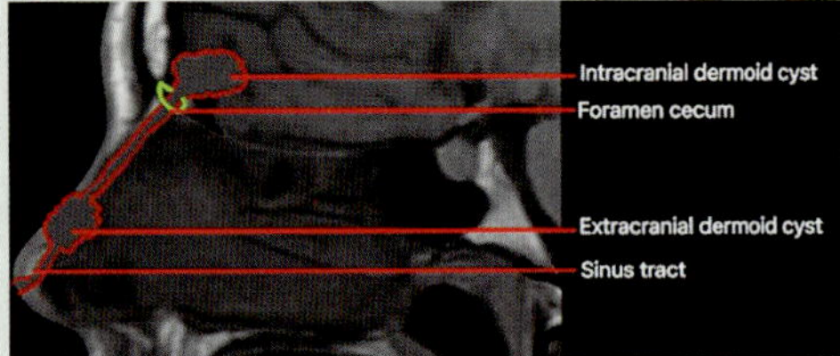

Fig. 4.4.16: Anterior neuropore anomalies (dermoid cyst) and their locations

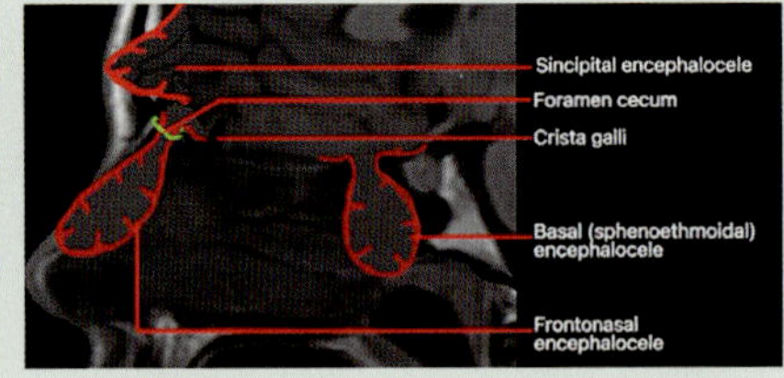

Fig. 4.4.17: Anterior neuropore anomalies (encephaloceles) and their locations

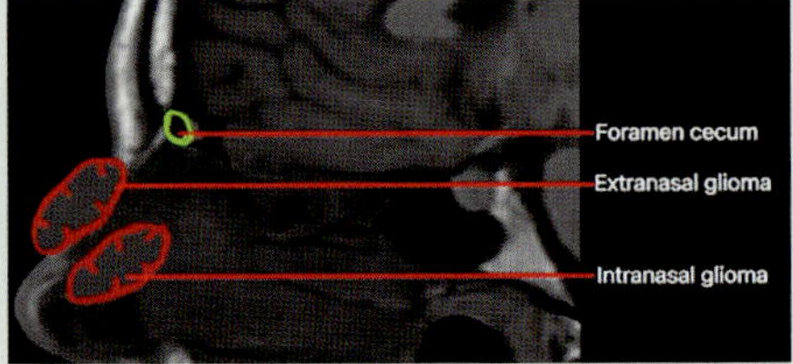

Fig. 4.4.18: Anterior neuropore anomalies (glioma) and their locations

4.5 CENTRAL NERVOUS SYSTEM

Case No. 5

Clinical history: A 1-year-old male with soft palpable mass at vertex.

Radiological techniques and observation: NECT sagittal section (Figs 4.5.1 and 4.5.2) shows a calvarial defect of parietal bone in the midline with an overlying soft tissue mass having intracranial communication. CT bone window shows a lytic lesion with wider inner table defect than outer table which suggests extension of an intracranial lesion extracranially. The lytic lesion shows well-corticated sclerotic margins which suggests benign long standing etiology. Sagittal T1 image (Fig. 4.5.3) sequence reveals a hypointense subcutaneous scalp mass with intracranial extension via a sharply marginated calvarial defect the lesion appears hyperintense on T2W (Fig. 4.5.4) with no obvious evidence of fluid signal intensity. A cigar-shaped CSF tract is noted within the interhemispheric fissure with a prominent supracerebellar cistern. There is a characteristic peaked appearance of tentorial incisura with a persistent falcine sinus seen on MR Venogram (Fig. 4.5.5). Rest of the brain appears normal. No evidence of transosseous veins.

Interpretation: A—child (<15 yrs) parietal bone lesion, C—skin covered midline bony lytic hypointense subcutaneous scalp mass with persistent falcine sinus, B—wider inner table defect than outer table, intracranial extension, corticated sclerotic margins D—parietal atretic cephalocele

Principal diagnosis: Parietal atretic cephalocele.

Discussion: Atretic cephaloceles are considered as involuted true cephalocele (meningocele or encephalocele) connected to dura mater via a fibrous tract, it originates from overdistended rhombencephalic vesicle at 7–10 weeks. Most commonly sporadic, most atretic cephaloceles

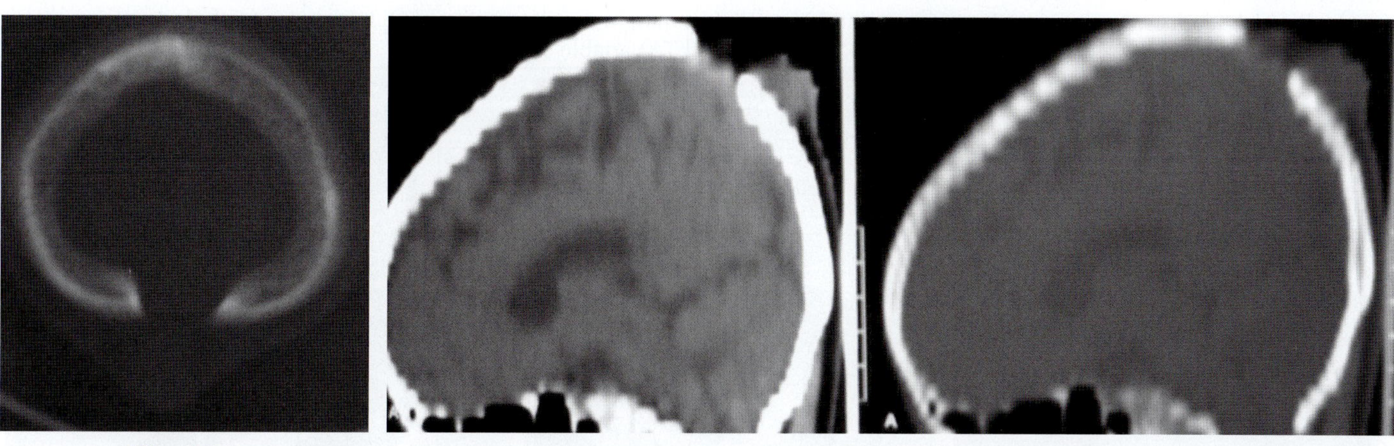

Fig. 4.5.1

Fig. 4.5.2

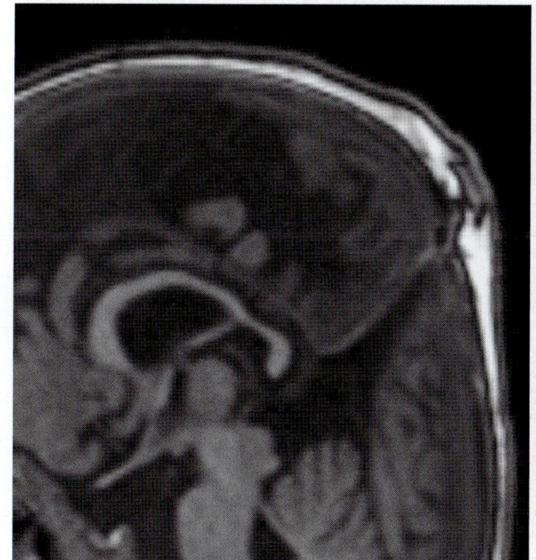

Fig. 4.5.3

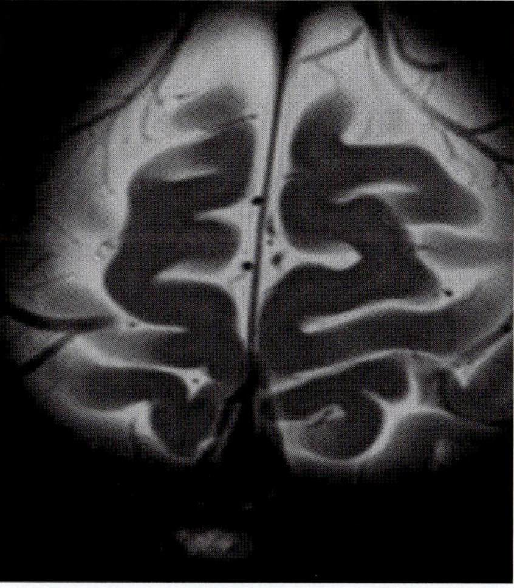

Fig. 4.5.4

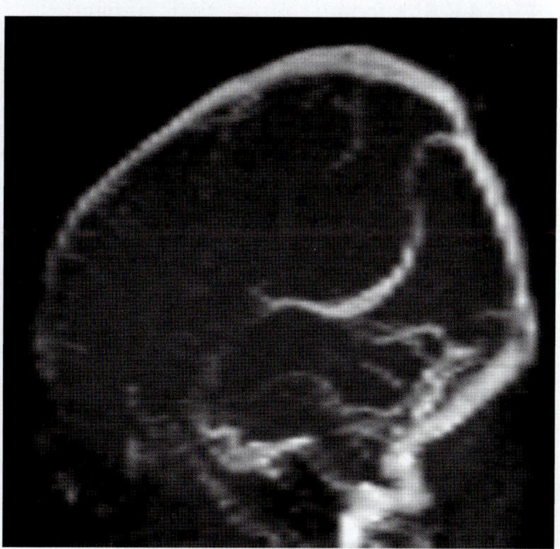

Fig. 4.5.5

are incidentally identified without additional intracranial anomalies. Holoprosencephaly, corpus callosal agenesis, eye anomalies and interhemispheric cysts are common syndromic associations. Atretic cephaloceles may enlarge with crying, overlying skin may be abnormally thin (cutis aplasia) and hairless (alopecia). Atretic cephaloceles are ten times more common than large parietal cephalocele. More common in female infants and young children of western hemisphere.

Associated with maternal folate deficiency and valproic acid use.

Occur at the obelion. Radiography: Cranium bifidum (midline defect in skull) may be difficult to appreciate. **CT:** Subgaleal soft tissue mass with small cranium bifidum superior to lambda. **CECT:** Extension of subcutaneous scalp mass through a dura delineated by enhancing veins. **CTA:** Vertical embryonic positioning of straight sinus (falcine vein). **T1W:** Heterogenous subcutaneous scalp mass with intracranial extension, cigar-shaped CSF tract within interhemispheric fissure and spinning top configuration of tentorial incisura.

T2W: Hyperintense subcutaneous scalp mass. **MRV:** Vertically positioned straight sinus equivalent (persistent falcine vein). Focal fenestration or lateral displacement of superior sagittal sinus at atretic parietal cephalocele. **Imaging recommendation:** Multiplanar MR with intravenous contrast and MRV.

Management: **Surgical** resection of cephalocele with dural repair is the treatment of choice. Prognosis depends more on associated occult brain anomalies (more common in syndromic patients) than existence of cephalocele itself. **Goals of cephalocele imaging** are to

Table 4.5.1: Differential diagnosis of vertex lesions

Dermoid/epidermoid cyst/dermal sinus: Ectodermal inclusion at sites of sutural and neural tube closure. Common location anterior fontanelle, glabella, nasion, vertex, subocciput and in intraosseous diploic space.	Midline fat (dermoid)/fluid soft tissue density (epidermoid) lesion often located near sutures, scallops outer table of calvaria, marginal enhancement. T1 hyperintense cholesterol content. T2 variable signal	
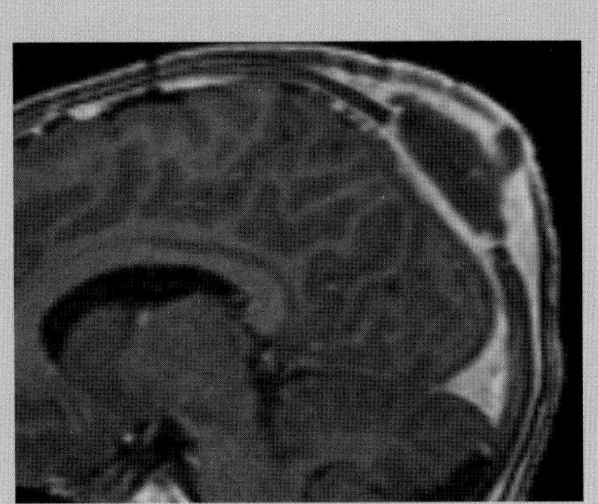 **Fig. 4.5.6:** Infected dermal sinus sagittal	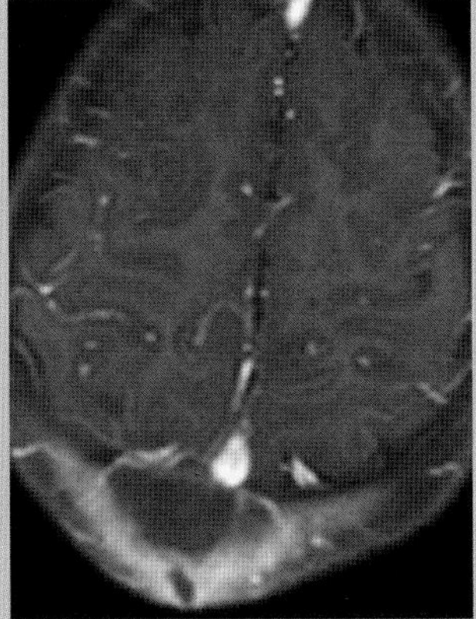 **Fig. 4.5.7:** Infected dermal sinus axial	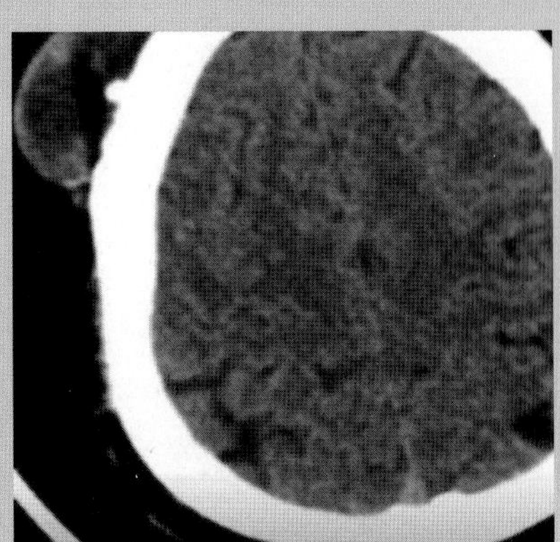 **Fig. 4.5.8:** Dermoid cyst
Proliferating hemangioma: 1–2% in neonates. Increased incidence in Caucasians and premature neonates. Proliferative growth in the first year of life followed by a stationary period. Treatment: Embolization, sclero cryotherapy/surgery.	Lobulated soft tissue mass with internal flow voids with avid contrast enhancement. T1 intermediate, T2 high signal with areas of flow voids +	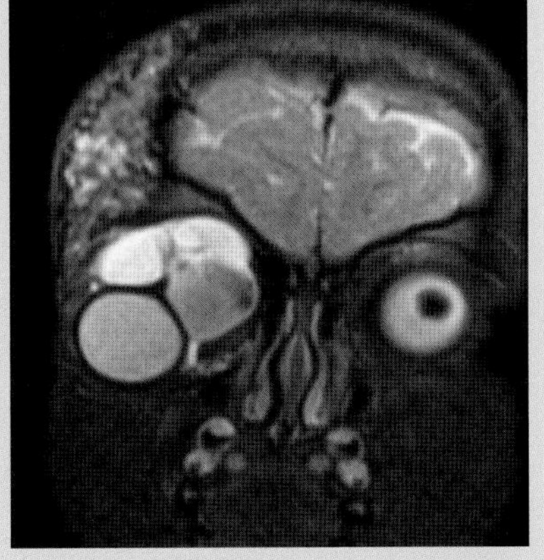 **Fig. 4.5.9:** Proliferating hemangioma

Contd...

Table 4.5.1: Differential diagnosis of vertex lesions *(Contd...)*		
Sinus pericranii: 95% midline/parasagittal. Age range 0–70 years. Usually discovered in children. Complications: Thrombosis and haemorrhage. Treatment: Evaluate DVS network, surgical ligation of transosseous emissary vein. Endovascular therapy, percutaneous embolization.	Abnormal communication between intracranial and extracranial venous system through osseous calvarial defect often associated with atretic cephalocele. Increased size on Valsalva, robust contrast enhancement to the same degree as cerebral venous structures.	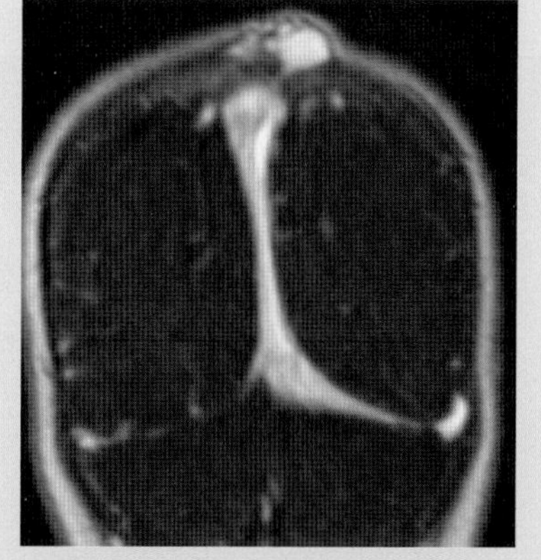 **Fig. 4.5.10:** Sinus pericranii
Subgaleal hematoma: Increased incidence with forceps extraction, more common in male infants of primiparous mothers.	Newborn following vaginal delivery/post-trauma. Fluid in subgaleal space adjacent to intact calvaria. No intracranial communication. Subgaleal hematoma crosses suture lines while **cephalhematoma do not cross suture line** as cephalhematoma lies between bone and periosteum.	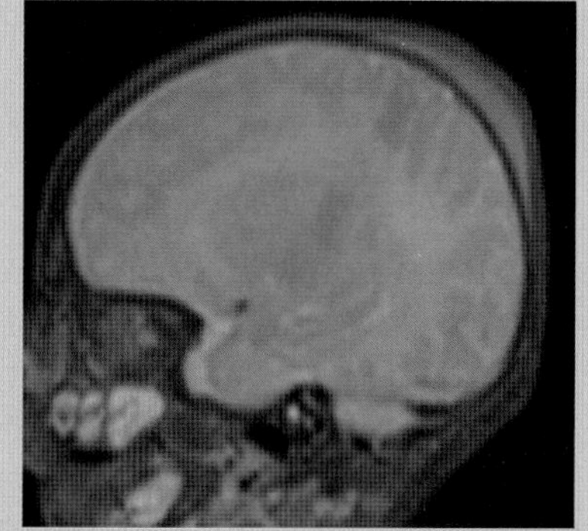 **Fig. 4.5.11:** Subgaleal hematoma
Metastasis: More common in older population. Destructive calvarial lesion with soft tissue mass. Consider neuroblastoma in infant (along the sutures, around orbit and skull bones)	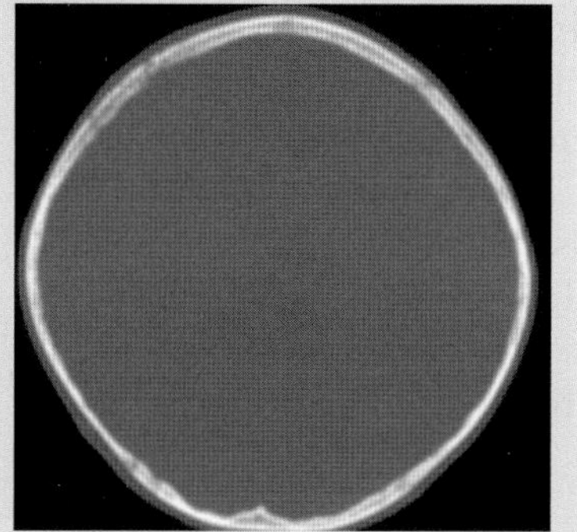 **Fig. 4.5.12:** Lytic skull metastasis in frontal bone	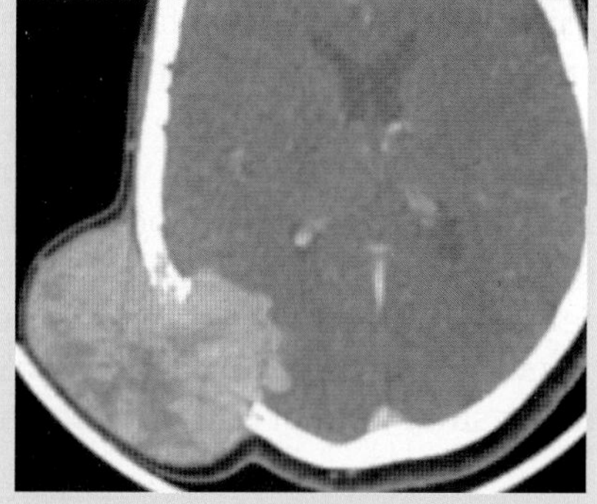 **Fig. 4.5.13:** Metastasis in parietal bone with soft tissue component
Leptomeningeal cyst: Occur in <3 years. Complicates 1% of skull fractures. Treatment: Cyst resection with surgical repair of dura.	Growing skull fractures, occurs near post-traumatic encephalomalacia. Lytic skull lesion with scalloped edges. Can be associated with brain herniation, hydrocephalus, porencephalic cyst and unilateral ventricular dilatation.	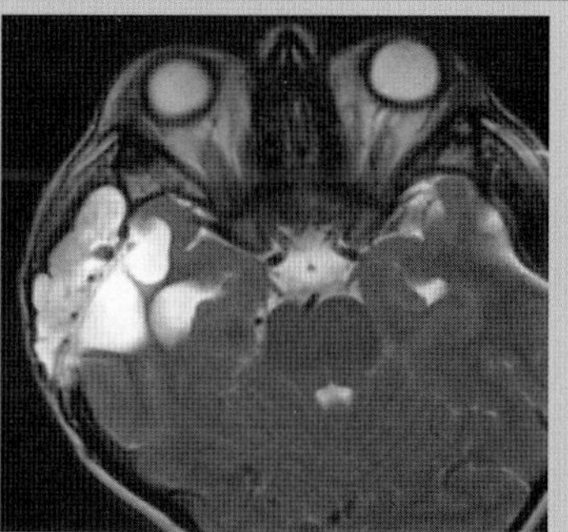 **Fig. 4.5.14:** Leptomeningeal cyst in the right anterior temporal region

Contd...

Table 4.5.1: Differential diagnosis of vertex lesions *(Contd...)*		
Pott's puffy tumor		
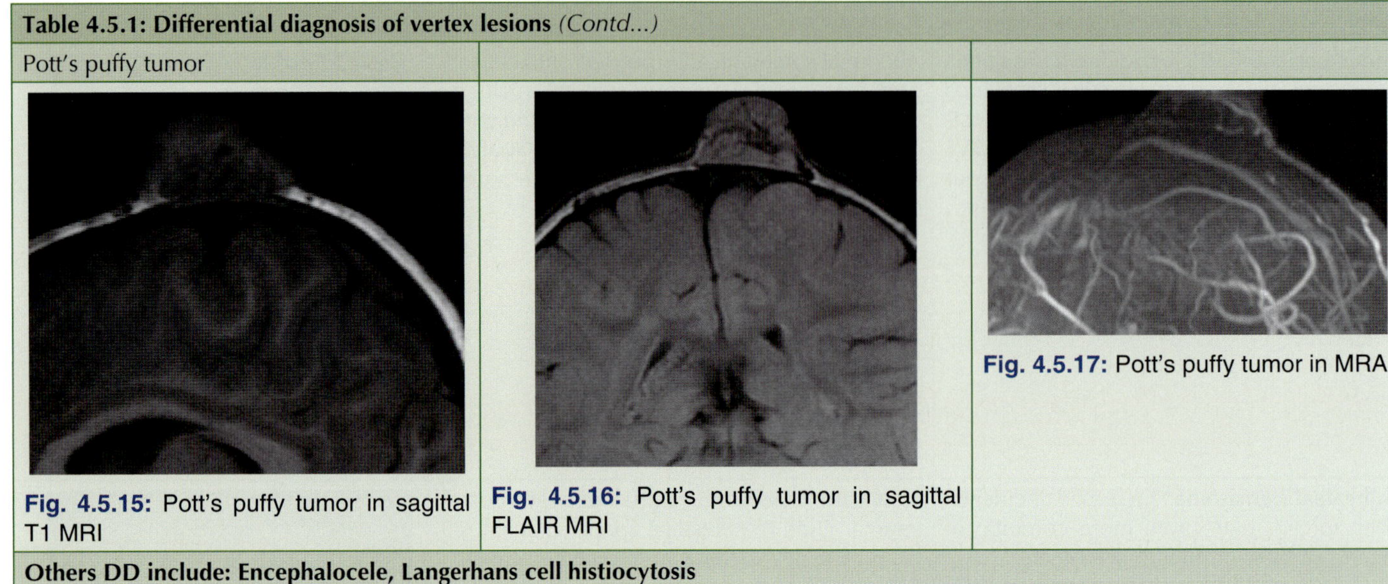 Fig. 4.5.15: Pott's puffy tumor in sagittal T1 MRI	Fig. 4.5.16: Pott's puffy tumor in sagittal FLAIR MRI	Fig. 4.5.17: Pott's puffy tumor in MRA
Others DD include: Encephalocele, Langerhans cell histiocytosis		

depict the osseous defect, to delineate the sac and define its contents, to map the course of adjacent arteries and determine the integrity of the dural venous sinuses and to identify any co-existing anomalies.

The superior sagittal sinus drains the deep cerebral venous system within the falx cerebri via falcine sinus, which is a normal part in the foetus. After birth, it typically involutes. The falcine sinus may recanalize or continue if the straight sinus is missing/thrombosed.

The front portion of the **median prosencephalic vein of Markowski** regresses when internal cerebral veins form, but the posterior portion remains as the Galen vein. Because the vein is thin-walled, lies free inside the subarachnoid space, and is subjected to increased pressure, an AV fistula balloons out to produce an aneurysmal vein of Galen malformation.

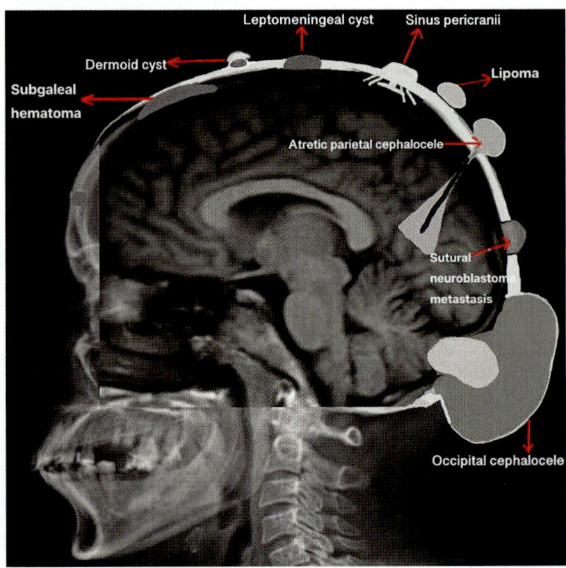

Fig. 4.5.18: Vertex lesions

4.6 CENTRAL NERVOUS SYSTEM

Case No. 6

Clinical history: A 14-year-old male, presented with complaints of progressive soft tissue swelling in the left orbit for the past 3 years.

Radiological techniques and observations

Plain radiograph skull AP view (Fig. 4.6.1)*:* The left orbit appears enlarged. Absence of the innominate line in the left orbit noted, causing **bare orbit sign**. The sphenoid ridge in the left orbit appears normal. No evidence of intraorbital calcifications. Left orbital margins appear normal. Right orbit appears normal. No lytic or sclerotic foci noted in the skull. Mild increase in soft tissue density noted. **Radiograph of right forearm with elbow joint AP view** (Fig. 4.6.2) shows lateral bowing of right ulna with resorption of a short segment of bone between mid and distal 1/3rd of the diaphysis, mimicking a joint. Proximal bone shows cupping with the absent section and sharp narrowed appearance of the distal bone is noted. No other foci of lysis, sclerosis or fracture noted in the ulna. Bowing with cortical thickening of the right radius noted at the mid-diaphysis, with no evidence of fracture. Elbow joint appears normal. No soft tissue component. **Radiograph of left leg with ankle joint AP and lateral view** (Figs 4.6.3 and 4.6.4) shows anterior bowing of left tibia with resorption of a short segment of bone between mid and distal 1/3rd of the diaphysis, mimicking a bony joint. Proximal bone shows cupping with the absent section and sharp narrowed appearance of the distal bone is noted. No other foci of lysis, sclerosis or fracture noted in the tibia. Ankle joint appears normal. No soft tissue component. **Non-enhanced CT brain** in axial section (Fig. 4.6.5) shows severe dysplasia of left greater wing of sphenoid bone. Severe degree of proptosis of the left eye (anterior sclera >18 mm from the interzygomatic line) noted. Thickening noted near the insertion site of left lateral rectus. Left anterior temporal lobe appears herniated through the bony defect in the left greater wing of sphenoid towards the left orbit. Right orbit, right greater wing of sphenoid appears normal. No evidence of cutaneous or subcutaneous soft tissue thickening to suggest neurofibromas or plexiform neurofibromatosis. Rest of the bones appears normal.

Interpretation: A—14-year-old male, pathology in sphenoid, ulna and tibia, C—shows sphenoid wing dysplasia, right ulnar pseudoarthrosis and left tibia pseudoarthrosis, B—left temporal lobe herniation through bony defect in sphenoid, D—NF1.

Principal diagnosis: Neurofibromatosis type 1.

Differential diagnosis for pseudoarthrosis: Fracture non-union, failed bone graft, neurofibromatosis type 1, Ehlers-Danlos syndrome, osteogenesis imperfecta, fibrous dysplasia, congenital pseudoarthrosis, ochronosis (alkaptonuria), ankylosing spondylitis (post-trauma), diffuse idiopathic skeletal hyperostosis (post-trauma), developmental dysplasia of the hip.

DD for bare orbit sign is metastasis (neuroblastoma in younger children) and congenital sphenoid wing dysplasia in neurofibromatosis type 1.

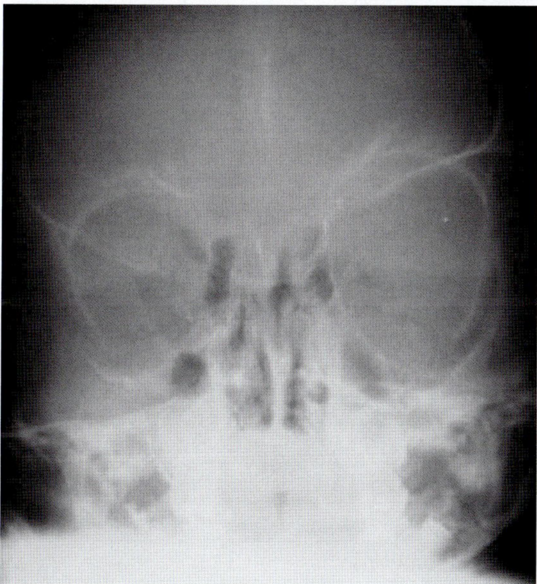

Fig. 4.6.1

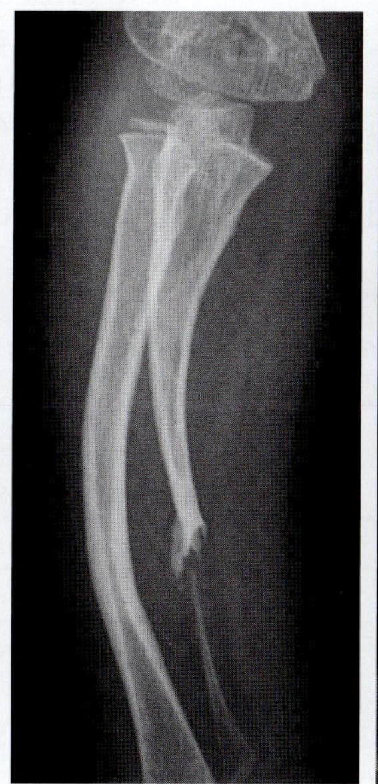

Fig. 4.6.2

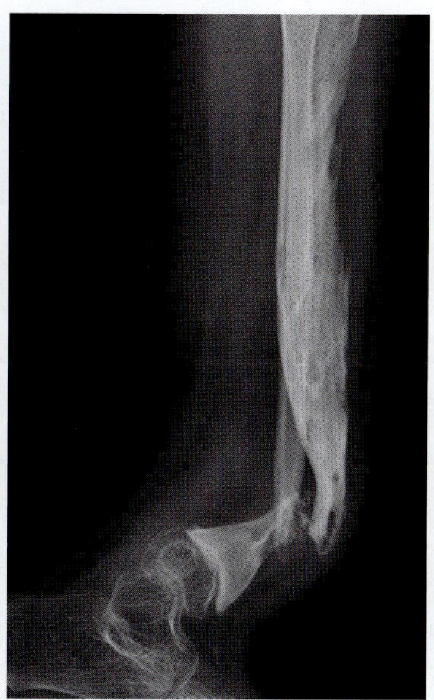

Fig. 4.6.3

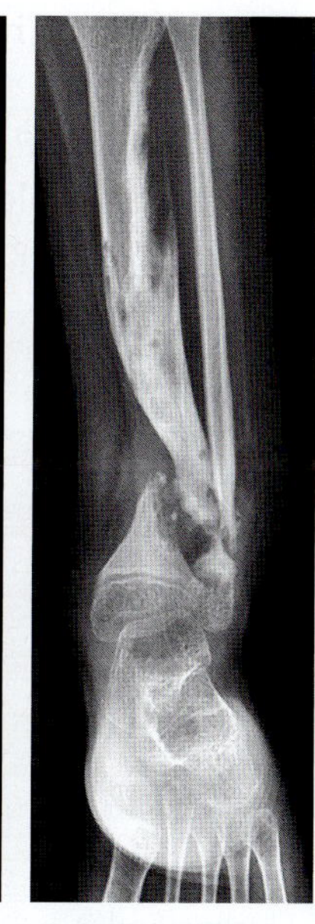

Fig. 4.6.4

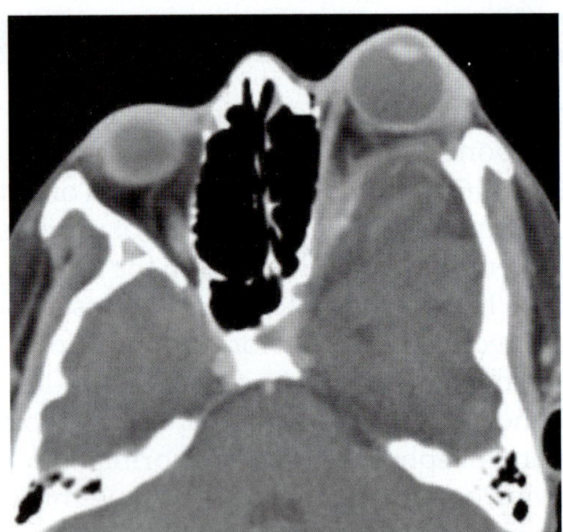

Fig. 4.6.5

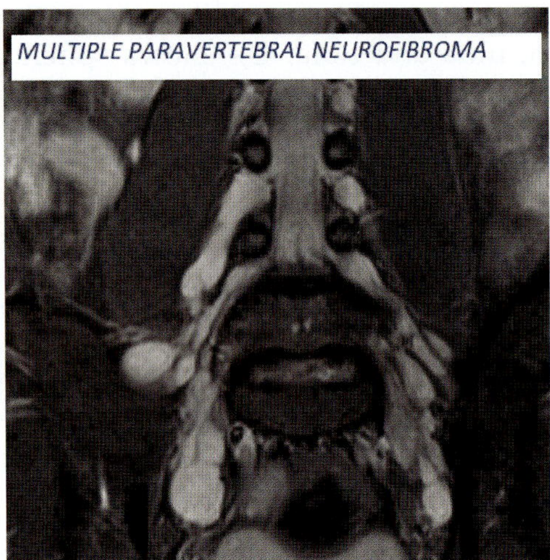

Fig. 4.6.6

DD for thickened peripheral lumbar nerve roots are AIDP/CIDP, Charcot-Marie-Tooth disorder, neuritis, NF1.

Management: Patient to be referred to neurosurgery and ophthalmology department for further evaluation. Further imaging workup with MRI brain and spine is needed to look for the presence of CNS manifestations, plexiform neurofibroma involving the nerve roots.

Treatment

1. *Medical:* Efficacy of medical treatment is unknown. Carboplatin can be used for optic nerve glioma.
2. *Surgical:* Plexiform neurofibromas has higher rate of reoccurrence. Higher risk of paraplegia in surgeries for spinal neurofibromas. Surgical removal can be done for pheochromocytomas and other tumors.

Discussion: Neurofibromatosis type 1—also known as von Recklinghausen disease, is a multisystem neurocutaneous disorder, and the most common phakomatosis. Additionally, it is also one of the most common inherited CNS disorders and inherited tumour syndromes.

Intracranial CNS manifestations include characteristic NF1 "spots" (FASI–focal areas of signal intensity/UBO–unidentified bright objects) and low-grade neoplasms. Most common sites are the globi pallidi (GP), centrum semiovale, cerebellar WM, dentate nuclei, thalamus, and brainstem. The FASI lesions may wax and wane for the first decade of life or so and then regress. After the second decade of life, they become rare. There may be optic gliomas, as well as gliomas in the brain stem, cerebellum, tectal plate, and basal ganglia (mainly pilocytic astrocytomas). Gliomas with a high grade can also occur.

Pterion and lambdoid suture defects are seen rarely in neurofibromatosis: 1. The pathological reason is still unclear. Progressive bone resorption is seen in bone defects, which may be due to overlying plexiform neurofibroma or meningioma when present in the convexity as opposed to skull base defects—"growing skull fractures". The sphenoid wing and the orbital roof defects are on the contrary, nonprogressive and congenital in origin. The calvarial defects may be of congenital origin due to primary mesenchymal hypoplasia or

Table 4.6.1: Riccardi classification of neurofibromatosis

Type	*Inheritance pattern*	*Clinical characteristics*
Peripheral neurofibromatosis (NF 1) (von Recklinghausen disease)	AD	CLS (café au lait spots) , neurofibromas, Lisch nodules, axillary freckling, neurological and bone alterations, benign and malignant neoplasms
Central neurofibromatosis (NF 2)	AD	Bilateral vestibular schwannomas, a few CLS and neurofibromas
Mixed (NF 3)	AD	Combination of 1 and 2
Variant (NF 4)	Unknown	Variations in CLS, neurofibromas, Lisch nodules, CNS neoplasms
Segmental (NF 5)	Non-heritable	Segmental neurofibromas and/or CLS
Familial CLS (NF 6)	Unknown	CLS
Late onset (NF 7)	Unknown	After the 3rd decade of life, neurofibromas, a few CLS
Unspecified (NF 8)		Variable signs

Table 4.6.2: Diagnostic clinical criteria of neurofibromatosis type 1	
Diagnostic clinical features of neurofibromatosis type 1 (at least two required)	
Cutaneous lesions	*Eye abnormalities*
≥6 cafe au lait spots (earliest manifestation) Prepubertal: ≥ 0.5 cm Post-pubertal: ≥ 1.5 cm	≥2 Lisch nodules (pigmented iris hamartomas) Optic pathway pilocytic astrocytoma
Freckling of armpits or groin ≥2 neurofibromas (any type) 1 plexiform neurofibroma	*Distinctive bone lesion* Sphenoid dysplasia/absence Long bone cortex dysplasia/thinning
	Family history First-degree relative with NF1
Café au lait spots: NF-1—smooth—coast of California McCune-Albright syndrome–irregular–coast of Maine. Segmental distribution, predominate on one side of the body and do not cross midline. Causes of Café au lait spots—Mnemonic: "MAN Bought TV Set as Present for Girl" M: MEN 1, Marfan's, McCune-Albright; A: Ataxia telangiectasia; N: NF-1, NF-2 (light brown "coffee with milk"), Noonan; B: Bloom's syndrome; TV: Tuberous sclerosis, von Hippel-Lindau; S: Silver-Russell syndrome; P: Peutz-Jegher's; F: Fanconi anemia; G: Gaucher's	

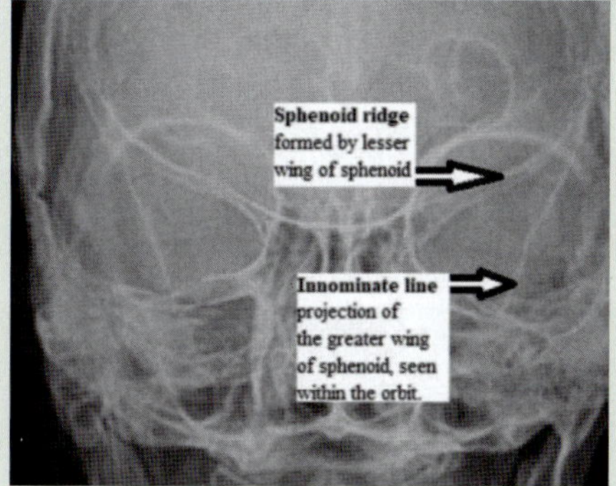

Fig. 4.6.7: Sphenoid ridge and innominate line

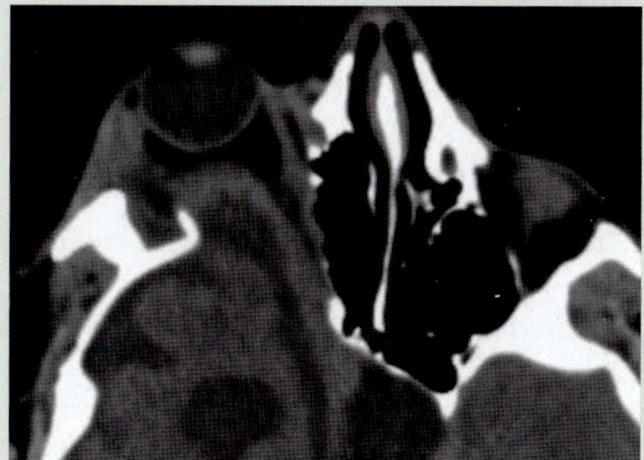

Fig. 4.6.8: Right sphenoid wing dysplasia

Table 4.6.3: Difference between neurofibroma and schwannoma		
Imaging features	*Neurofibroma*	*Schwannoma*
Situation of the parent nerve	Predominantly peripheral nerves	Predominantly cranial nerves
Target sign on T2W image (central dark due to collagen and peripheral bright due to myxoid tissue)	+++	+
Fascicular sign	+	++
Cystic necrosis/cavitations	+/-	++
Enhancement pattern	Diffuse, predominantly central	Diffuse, predominantly peripheral

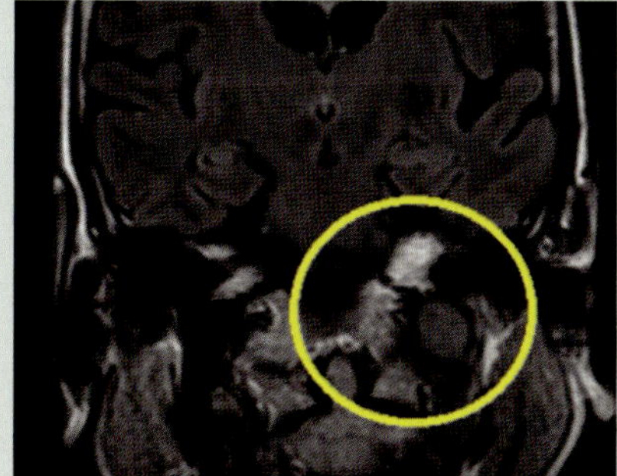

Fig. 4.6.9: Neurofibroma of hypoglossal nerve

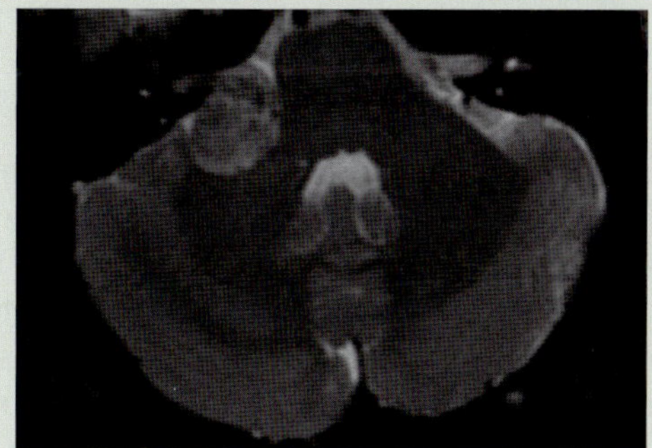

Fig. 4.6.10: Acoustic schwannoma

Table 4.6.4: Difference between neurofibromatosis type 1 and 2		
	Neurofibromatosis 1	*Neurofibromatosis 2*
Epidemiology	Incidence: 1: 3000–5000 NF1 is a tumor-suppressor gene encoded by chromosome 17q11.2	1: 50,000 (less common) NF2 is a tumor-suppressor gene encoded by chromosome 22q12.2
Clinical manifestations	**Cutaneous neurofibromas** are the most common manifestation of NF-1. Other common findings include plexiform tumors, optic gliomas, Lisch nodules (hamartomatous nodules in the iris), and cafe´ au lait macules.	The classic feature of NF 2 is **bilateral vestibular schwannomas** (95% of NF 2). Schwannomas can involve other cranial nerves, most frequently III and V. Patients with NF-2 can also have cutaneous neurofibromas, though to a much lesser extent than in NF-1.
MR brain imaging findings	Focal areas of T2 hyperintensity (FASI), most common sites are the globi pallidi (GP), centrum semiovale, cerebellar WM, dentate nuclei, thalamus, and brainstem. In T1 they appear iso to hyperintense. Pilocytic astrocytomas, brain stem gliomas, plexiform neurofibromas, and orbital gliomas.	Vestibular schwannoma "MISME lesions" Multiple intracranial schwannomas Multiple meningiomas Ependymoma
Routine MR brain imaging screening	Need for routine MR screening is controversial. May diagnose potentially debilitating tumors before they become clinically evident, but the clinical treatment is rarely affected	Always indicated for patients with NF-2, given the high prevalence of CNS tumors
Additional imaging		Cervical spine MR imaging is suggested for the evaluation of spinal tumors, most commonly ependymomas (in 95% of NF 2)

Table 4.6.5: Differential diagnosis for rib notching in inferior surface and superior surface	
Rib notching—inferior surface	*Rib notching—superior surface*
Arterial 1. Coarctation of the aorta 2. Aortic thrombosis—usually the lower ribs bilaterally 3. Subclavian obstruction—most commonly after a Blalock operation 4. Pulmonary oligaemia	*Connective tissue diseases* 1. Rheumatoid arthritis 2. Systemic lupus erythematosus 3. Scleroderma 4. Sjögren's syndrome
Venous Superior vena caval obstruction	*Metabolic* Hyperparathyroidism
Arteriovenous 1. Pulmonary arteriovenous malformation. 2. Chest wall arteriovenous malformation.	*Miscellaneous* 1. Neurofibromatosis 2. Restrictive lung disease 3. Poliomyelitis 4. Marfan's syndrome 5. Osteogenesis imperfecta 6. Progeria
Neurogenic Neurofibromatosis	

dysplasia. They may also be acquired due to secondary enlargement of small fusion defects, due to the effect of cerebrospinal fluid pulsations transmitted to the defect. Intracranial CNS manifestations: Characteristic NF1 "spots" (FASI—focal altered signal intensities/ NBO—neurofibromatosis associated bright objects/ UBO—unidentified bright objects). Optic glioma noted in the right optic nerve ('Dotted i' appearance).

Common Neurocutaneous Syndromes

1. Neurofibromatosis 1
2. Neurofibromatosis 2
3. Tuberous sclerosis
4. Sturge-Weber syndrome
5. von Hippel-Lindau syndrome

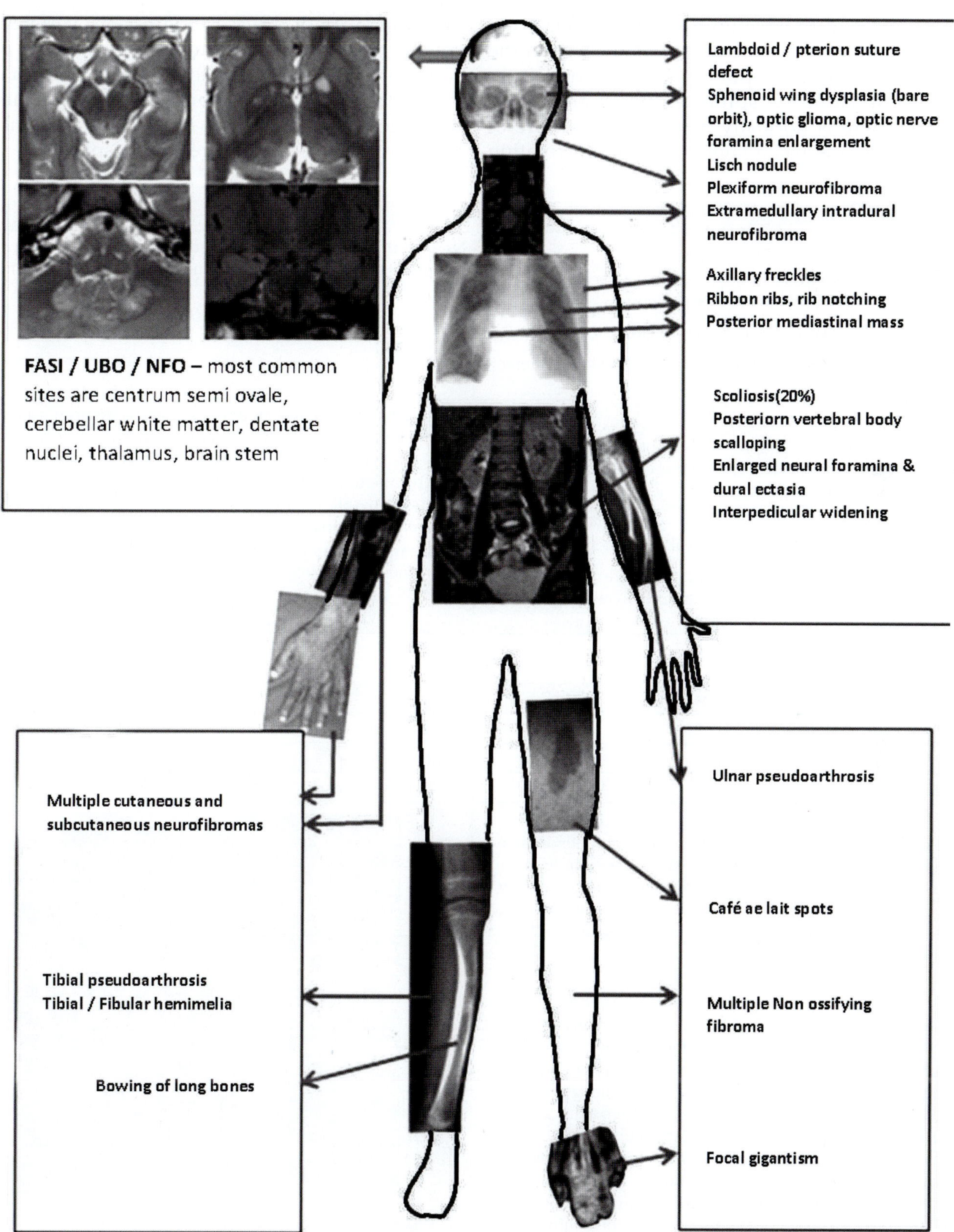

Fig. 4.6.11: Whole body illustration of neurofibromatosis type 1

Scoliosis: Normal thoracolumbar spine is relatively straight in the sagittal plane and double curve in the coronal plane. Thoracic spine in convex posteriorly (kyphosis) and lumbar spine is convex anteriorly (lordosis). There is normally no lateral curvature of the spine. Scoliosis has a lateral curve with rotation of vertebra. With disease progression, vertebrae and spinous process of major curve rotates towards curve's concavity. Ribs are close together, the height of the vertebrae and intervertebral discs are reduced on the concave side while on the convex side, ribs and intervertebral disc height are widely spaced.

Table 4.6.6: Causes of scoliosis

Idiopathic 1. **Infantile**—occurs mostly in boys less than 4 years with right thoracic concavity and resolves spontaneously. 2. Juvenile—progressive pattern occurring in girls of 4 to 9 years age 3. Adolescent—females of 10 years up to maturity with left thoracic concavity.	**Neuropathic disorders**—tethered cord, syringomyelia, Chiari malformations, diastematomyelia, meningocele/ myelomeningocele.
Congenital 1. Failure of formation—multiple hemivertebra, free hemivertebra, wedge vertebra central defect/butterfly vertebra, incarcerated hemivertebra 2. Failure of segmentation—a) Bilateral → block vertebra with a short spine (Klippel-Feil); b) Unilateral unsegmented bar 3. Mixed defects—hemivertebra with unilateral unsegmented bar, partially segmented incarcerated hemivertebra, bilateral segmentation failure forming hemivertebra.	**Mesodermal and neuroectodermal diseases:** Neurofibromatosis—severe kyphosis with short segment sharply angled scoliosis; Marfan's syndrome has 2 structural curves; Homocystinuria-2 structural curves; Other skeletal dysplasias–viz. spondylo-epiphyseal dysplasia congenita, spondyloepimetaphyseal dysplasia, pseudoachondroplasia. **Post-radiotherapy-induced discrepancies in leg length:** Neuromuscular diseases like poliomyelitis, myelomeningocele, cerebral palsy, spinal muscular atrophy, Friedreich's ataxia, muscular dystrophy.

Table 4.6.7: Classification of scoliosis

Nonstructural scoliosis	*Transient structural scoliosis*
Postural scoliosis	Sciatic scoliosis
Compensatory scoliosis	Hysterical scoliosis> inflammatory scoliosis
Radiographic assessment of the scoliosis patient: Erect anteroposterior and lateral views of the entire spine (occiput to sacrum). AP view is used to calculate the scoliotic curve, identify curve's convexity is to the right or left, with each curve measured separately. Lumbar spine—lateral view is helpful for spondylolysis or spondylolisthesis in scoliosis (5% prevalence). Scoliosis is typically assessed using the Cobb technique. The terminal vertebrae (vertebrae at each end of the curve) are chosen. These are the endplates that deviate the most from horizontal. The angle formed by a line drawn along the superior endplate of the superior terminal vertebra and a line drawn along the inferior endplate of the inferior terminal vertebra is referred to as curvature. Endplates might be difficult to notice in severe curvatures, for which, the measurement might be taken using the inferior cortex of the pedicle as a landmark. Scoliosis can also be measured using the Ferguson method, where scoliosis angle is formed by lines which are drawn from the apical vertebra's centre to the centre of each terminal vertebrae.	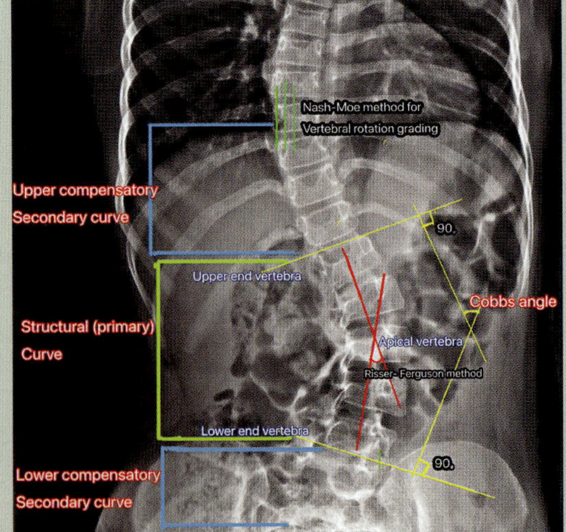 **Fig. 4.6.12:** AP dorsolumbar spine showing measurement of Cobb's angle in scoliosis

4

Table 4.6.8: Rare neurocutaneous syndromes			
Sjögren-Larsson syndrome Congenital ichthyosis, spastic diplegia, tetraplegia, and mental retardation. Pruritus is a prominent feature, is not found in other types of ichthyotic disorders. Photophobia, macular dystrophy and decreased visual acuity.	MR imaging and MRS abnormalities are confined to the cerebral white matter and corticospinal tract. Delayed myelination, periventricular gliosis, and a permanent myelin deficit seen. The lipid peak at 1.3 ppm in the MRS of cerebral white matter is characteristic of SLS.	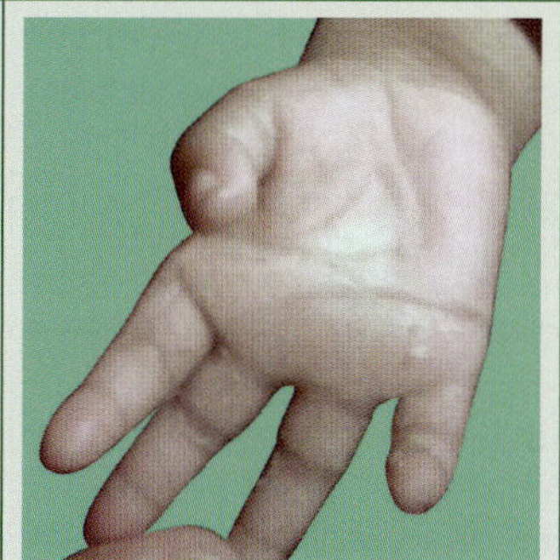 **Fig. 4.6.13** 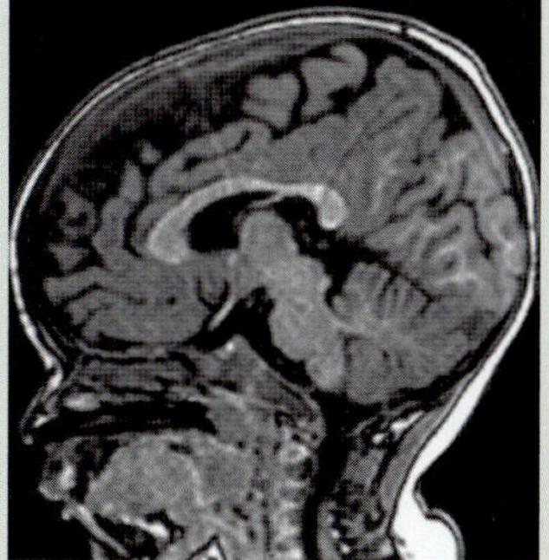 **Fig. 4.6.15:** Periventricular gliosis	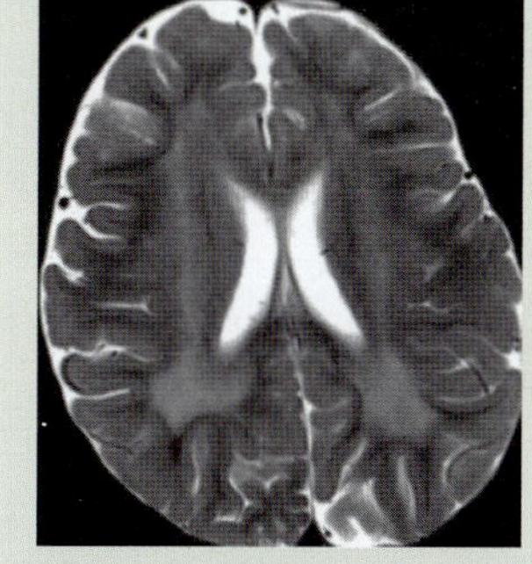 **Fig. 4.6.14:** Delayed myelination 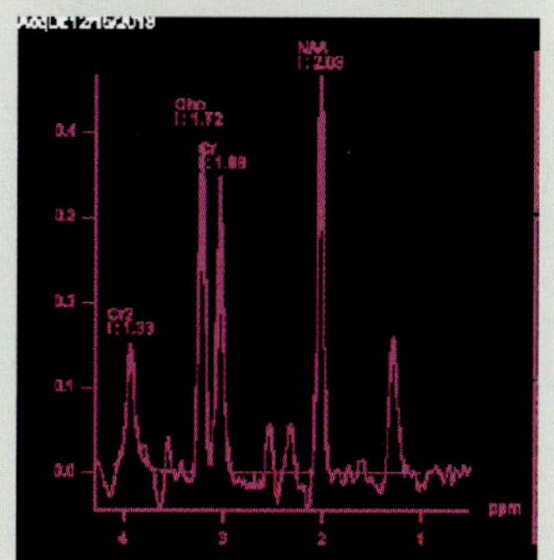 **Fig. 4.6.16:** Lipid peak at 1.3 ppm
Neurocutaneous melanosis An increase in the number of melanotic cells is seen. (Basal layer of the epidermis, pia mater, reticular formation of medulla and substantia nigra.) Types: Leptomeningeal and parenchymal melanosis.	The anterior temporal lobes, and particularly the amygdala—most frequent location for parenchymal melanocytic accumulation. T1 shortening on the MR imaging—confirm diagnosis (Figs 4.6.18 to 4.6.20). Meningeal deposits are typically benign but undergo transformation to melanoma in approx 2–3% of patients.	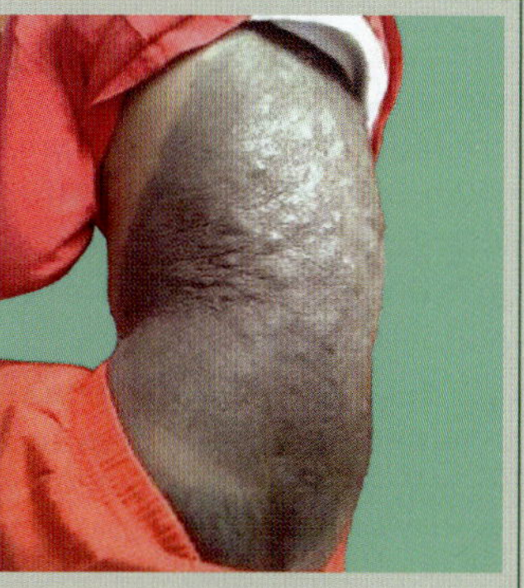 **Fig. 4.6.17:** Neurocutaneous melanosis 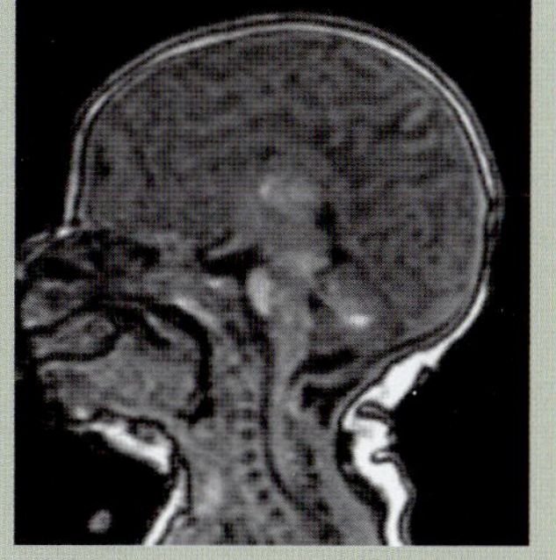 **Fig. 4.6.19:** Neurocutaneous melanosis	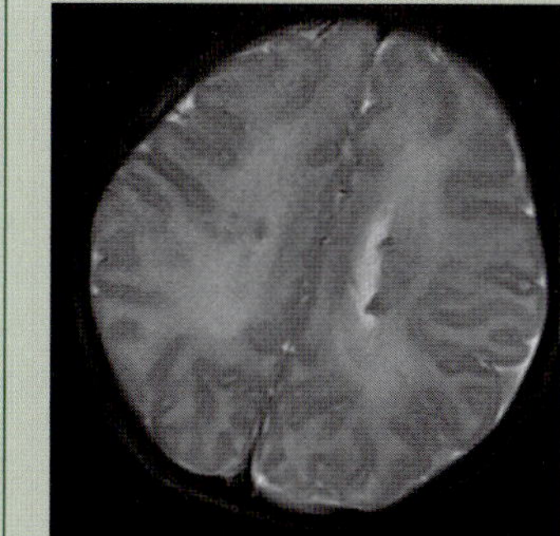 **Fig. 4.6.18:** Neurocutaneous melanosis 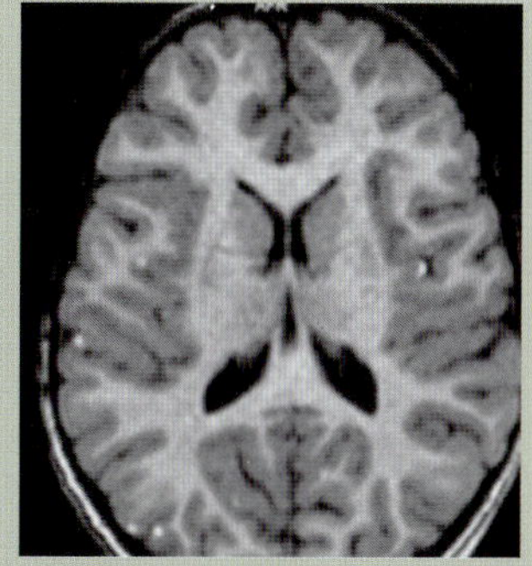 **Fig. 4.6.20:** Neurocutaneous melanosis

Contd...

Table 4.6.8: Rare neurocutaneous syndromes *(Contd...)*

Hypomelanosis of Ito with hemimegalencephaly Hypopigmented patches in face and left upper limb in a baby (Fig. 4.6.21) with multiple seizure episodes in the form of abnormal movements of both upper limbs.	Hemi megalencephaly will occur on either side of skin lesions (Fig. 4.6.22). Periventricular white matter changes. Hypoplastic corpus callosum, heterotopia, vascular malformations, medulloblastoma and choroid plexus papilloma. Straightening of the ipsilateral frontal horn of the enlarged ventricle—characteristically seen in Figs 4.6.23 and 4.6.24.	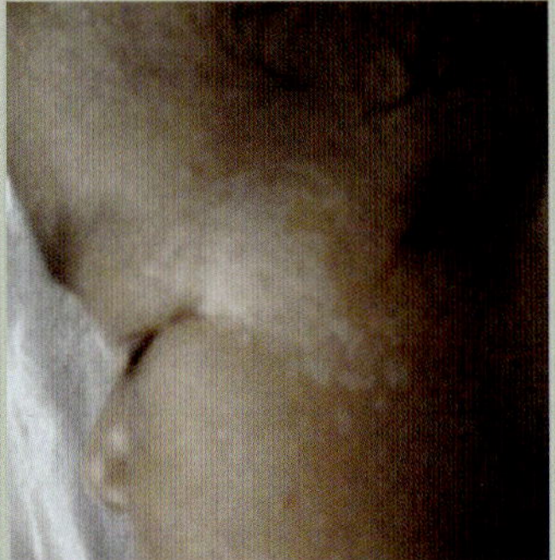 **Fig. 4.6.21:** Hypomelanosis of Ito 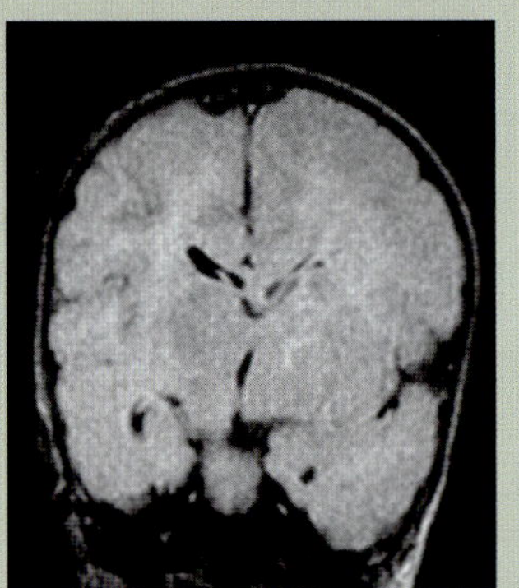 **Fig. 4.6.23:** Hemimegalencephaly	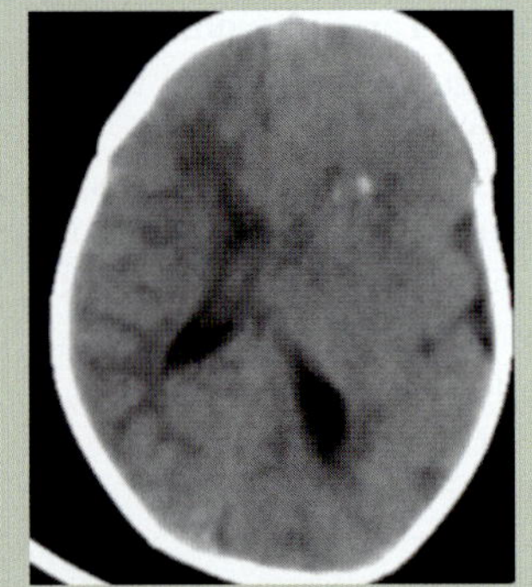 **Fig. 4.6.22:** Hemimegalencephaly 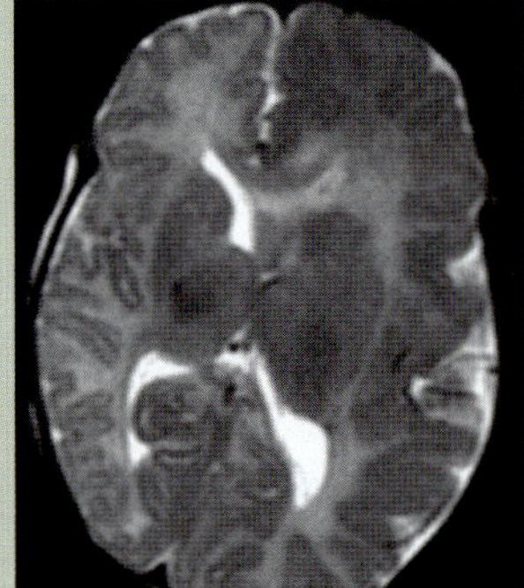 **Fig. 4.6.24:** Hemimegalencephaly
Incontinentia pigmenti Incontinentia pigmenti, also known as Bloch-Sulzberger syndrome, X-linked dominant genetic disorder, occurs much more often in females F:M 20-37:1 Vesicles at birth or during the first two months of life. Hyperkeratotic, verrucous, linear plaques that may last months.	Microcephaly, cerebral atrophy, hypoplasia of corpus callosum, periventricular white matter changes, optic atrophy, anophthalmia, microphthalmia, hypodontia. Skull deformities and hemiatrophy/shortening of the legs and arms may be seen.	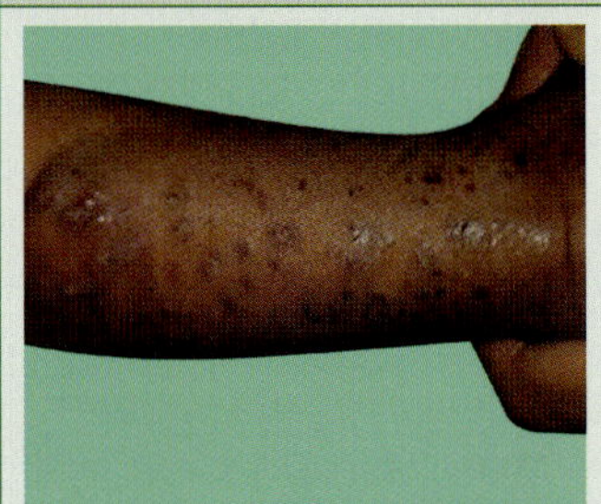 **Fig. 4.6.25:** Incontinentia pigmenti 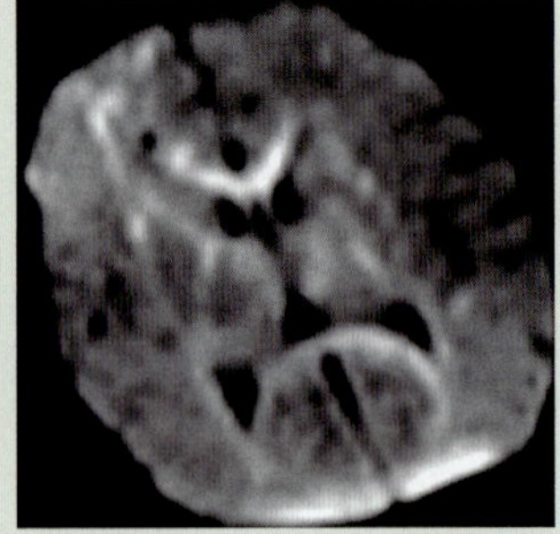 **Fig. 4.6.27:** Hypoplasia of corpus callosum	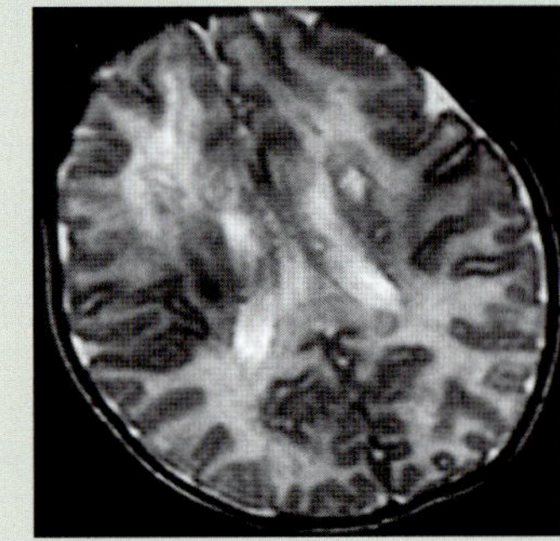 **Fig. 4.6.26:** Periventricular white matter changes 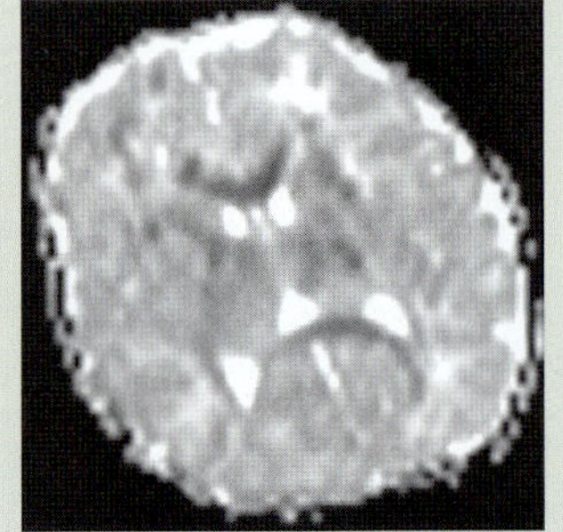 **Fig. 4.6.28:** Hypoplasia of corpus callosum with periventricular white matter showing diffusion restriction

Contd...

Table 4.6.8: Rare neurocutaneous syndromes *(Contd...)*			
Gorlin syndrome **Major criteria: Odontogenic keratocysts** >2 or 1; **Basal cell cancers** in 20 years of age; palmar pits: 3 or more **bilamellar calcification of the falx cerebri rib anomalies:** Bifid rib fused, splayed **first degree relative** with Gorlin syndrome.	**Minor criteria** Macrocephaly, frontal bossing, cleft lip or hypertelorism, Sprengel deformity, pectus excavatum or pectus carinatum, syndactyly, bridging of the sella turcica, hemivertebrae, ovarian fibroma, medulloblastoma **Diagnosis** made by either two major or, one major and two minor criteria.	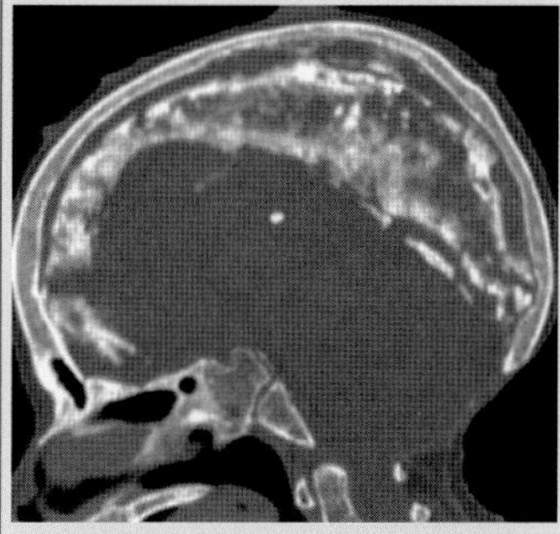 **Fig. 4.6.29:** Gorlin syndrome–dural calcification	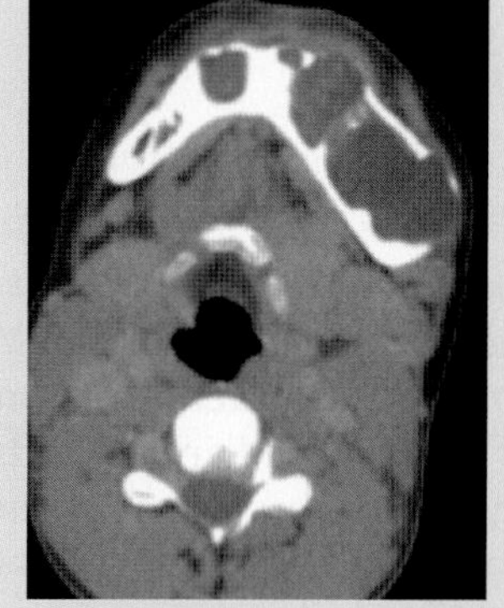 **Fig. 4.6.30:** Gorlin syndrome–odontogenic keratocyst
PHACES syndrome **P**osterior fossa malformations, **H**emangiomas (facial), **A**rterial anomalies, **C**oarctation of the aorta and cardiac defects, **E**ye abnormalities, **S**ternal clefting – 'PHACES'.	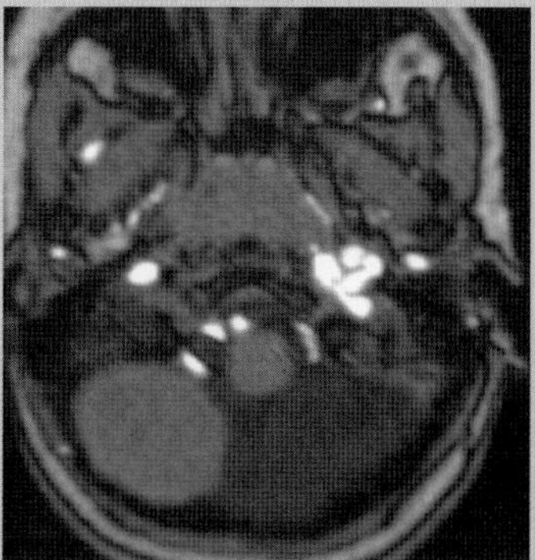 **Fig. 4.6.31:** PHACES syndrome—posterior fossa malformations	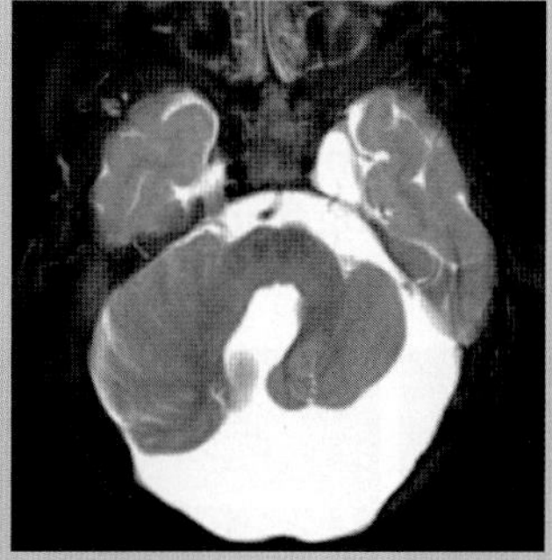 **Fig. 4.6.32:** PHACES syndrome—posterior fossa malformations	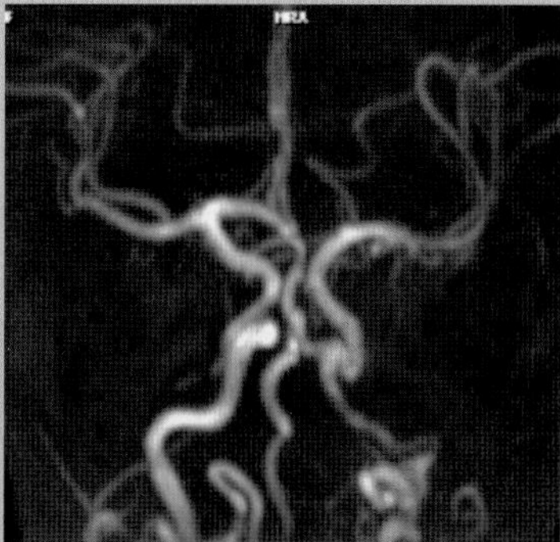 **Fig. 4.6.33:** PHACES syndrome–arterial abnormalities
		Cause is unknown. Strong female predominance, leading some to suggest an X-chromosome-linked dominant.	
Ataxia telangiectasia AR disorder Cerebellar ataxia. Telangiectasias in skin (face) and eyes. Immunodeficiency syndromes, recurrent infections and susceptibility to certain neoplastic processes. Early clinical findings: Ataxia before conjunctival telangiectasias and malignancies.	**Early MRI findings:** Cerebellar atrophy, superior vermis atrophy and bright cerebellar cortex. **Late MRI findings (more than 30 years old):** Focal and diffuse white matter signal. Brain telangiectasias. Small white matter T2 hypointensities are often seen, mostly representing tiny hemosiderin deposits from thrombosis of telangiectatic vessels.	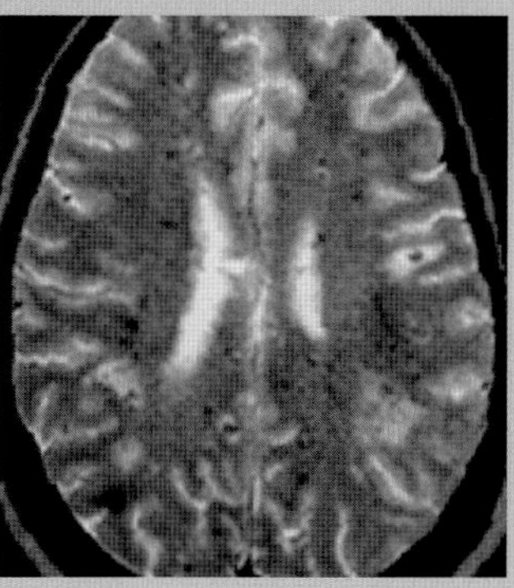 **Fig. 4.6.34:** Ataxia telangiectasia	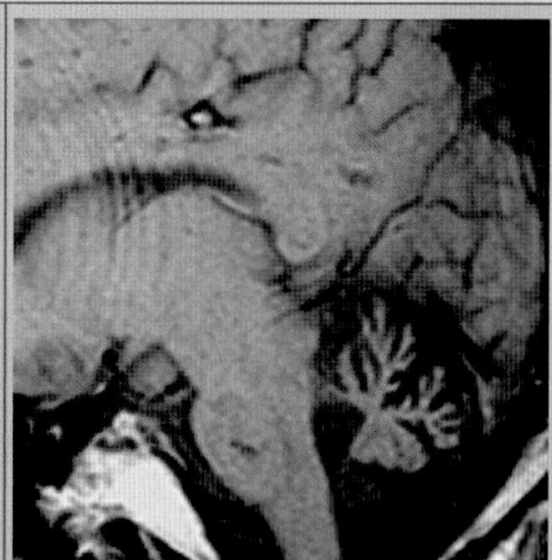 **Fig. 4.6.35:** Ataxia telangiectasia

Table 4.6.9: Differential diagnosis for localised gigantism	
Localised gigantism: Refers to focal enlargement of part of body involving both soft tissue and bone. It is always pathological.	
Neurofibromatosis type 1 Klippel-Trénaunay-Weber syndrome Lymphangiomatosis Haemangiomatosis Localised soft tissue/bone tumors	Macrodystrophia lipomatosa Fibrolipomatous hamartoma of the nerve Proteus syndrome AVM Congenital Milroy syndrome

4.7 CENTRAL NERVOUS SYSTEM

Case No. 7

Clinical presentation: A 20 years old male patient presented with seizure, for the last 3 months.

Radiologic techniques and observation: T2W axial, T1 sagittal, FLAIR coronal, SWI images (Figs 4.7.1 to 4.7.6) shows heterointense lesion approximately measuring 2 × 1 cm noted in the left lateral ventricle along the septum pellucidum in the frontal horn adjacent to foramen of Monro with evidence of blooming causing obstruction and compression of 3rd ventricle with upstream dilatation of bilateral lateral ventricles. Subependymal calcified nodule noted in left lateral ventricle in the caudothalamic groove. Multiple FLAIR hyperintensities representing cortical tubers noted in bilateral cerebral hemisphere with radial migration band of white matter hyperintensities extending from cerebral cortex. No evidence of polymicrogyria.

Interpretation: A—20 years of male, multiple lesion involving both gray and white matter, C—hetero-intense lesion in the left lateral ventricle along the septum pellucidum, subependymal calcified nodule, cortical tubers, B—radial migration band of white matter hyperintensities, D—tuberous sclerosis.

Principal diagnosis: Tuberous sclerosis with subependymal giant cell astrocytoma (SEGA).

Differential diagnosis for SEGA: **Frontal horn of lateral ventricle lesion near septum pellucidum/foramen of Monro**—central neurocytoma, subependymal giant cell astrocytoma, subependymoma, colloid cyst, neurocysticercosis, ependymoma.

Further management: Further evaluation of systemic manifestations. Surveillance MR every 1–3 years during childhood/adolescence.

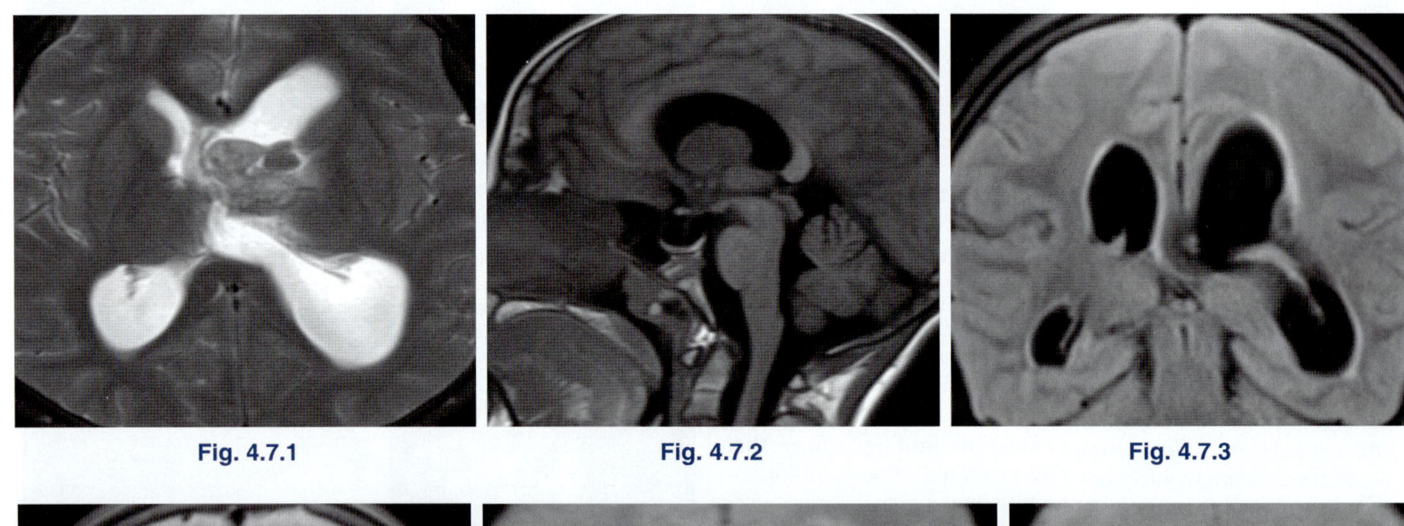

Fig. 4.7.1 Fig. 4.7.2 Fig. 4.7.3

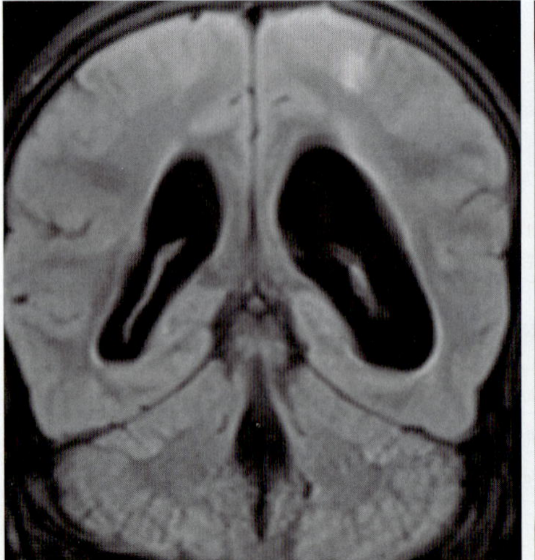

Fig. 4.7.4

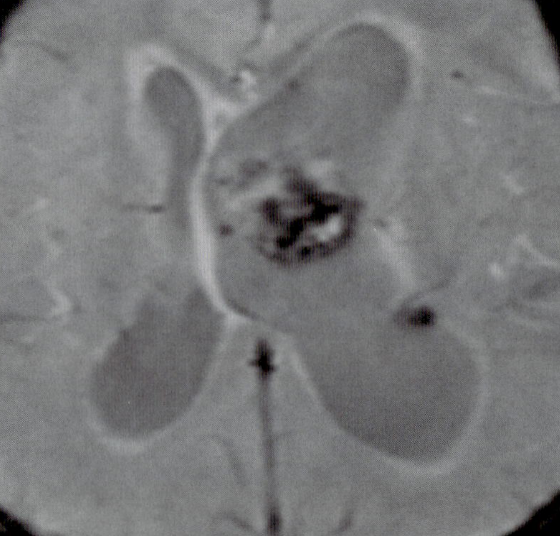

Fig. 4.7.5

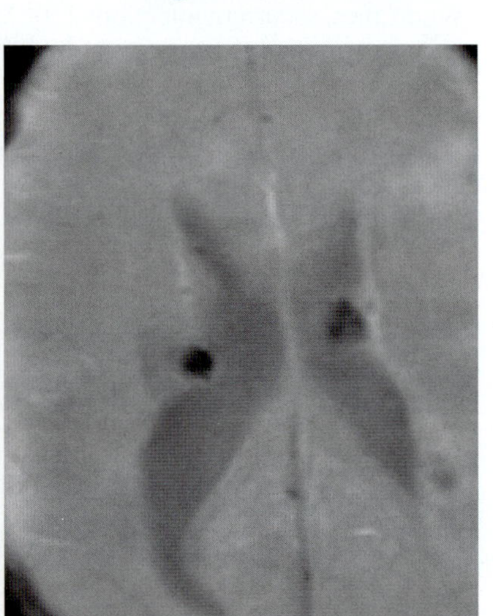

Fig. 4.7.6

Treatment: Seizures are treated symptomatically. vigabatrin is useful in infantile spasms. If there is a seizure focus or if a seizure focus can be identified amid several tubers, we have to resect isolated tubers. If a SEGA is obstructing the foramen of Monro and producing hydrocephalus, it is removed. Oral rapamycin (an inhibitor of the mTOR protein upregulation) has been observed to cause SEGA regression.

Table 4.7.1: Differential diagnosis for lesions in caudothalamic groove

Lesions in the caudothalamic groove				
Tuberous sclerosis: Bourneville disease/epiloia (**EPI**lepsy, **LO**w IQ and **A**denoma sebaceum). Multifocal systemic hamartoma and malformation. Vogt triad occurs in 29% patient, both TSC1 and TSC2 mutation.	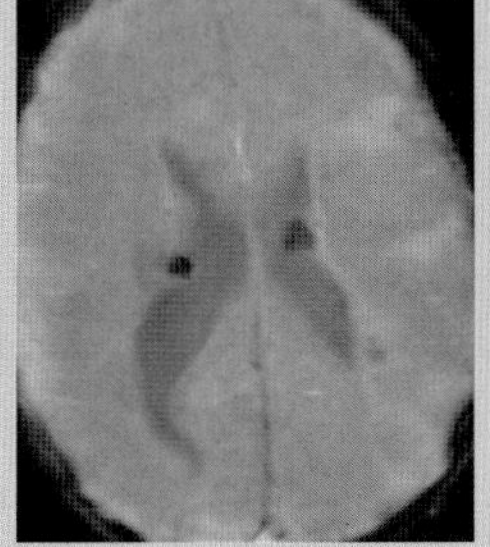 **Fig. 4.7.7:** Calcified ependymal nodules on SWI	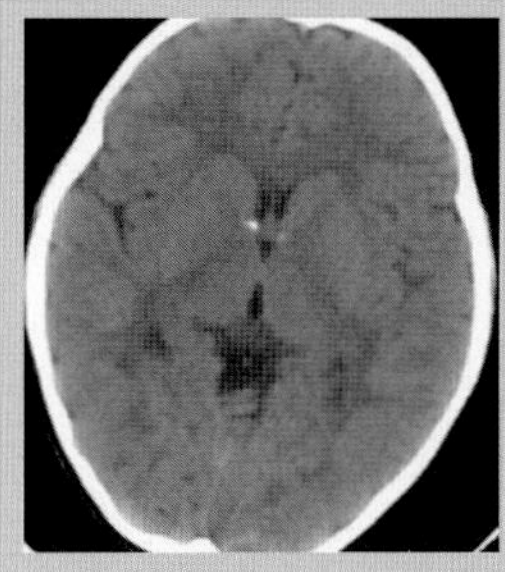 **Fig. 4.7.8:** Calcified ependymal nodules on CT	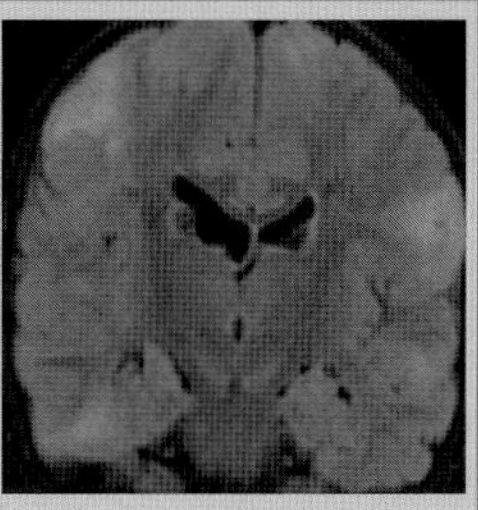 **Fig. 4.7.9:** Cortical tubers	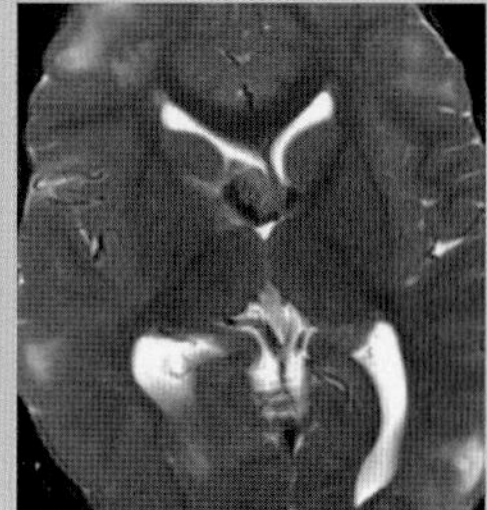 **Fig. 4.7.10:** Subcortical tubers
1. Multiple calcified ependymal nodules ("candle dripping appearance"), 2. Subependymal giant cell astrocytoma (SEGA pathognomic) located at foramen of Monro. 3. Cortical subcortical tubers, 4. White matter radial migration line.				
Congenital CMV infection: CMV neurodevelopmental sequelae including **mental retardation, cerebral palsy, sensorineural hearing loss** and **multi-organ disorders** such as hepatosplenomegaly A/W Down syndrome, foetal alcohol syndrome or spina bifida.	**CT finding:** Intracranial calcifications particularly thick and chunky in the **germinal matrix** and periventricular region with faint and punctate basal ganglia calcification. Ventriculomegaly, white matter abnormalities, neuronal migration abnormalities and extensive destructive encephalopathy.	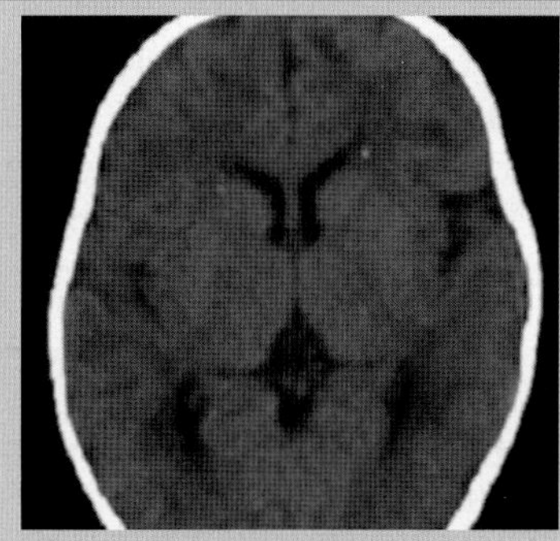 **Fig. 4.7.11:** Periventricular calcification with white matter edema in congenital CMV		
Subependymal nodular heterotopia: Also known as periventricular nodular heterotopia, most common form of heterotopia. Nodules of grey matter located immediately beneath the ependyma of lateral ventricle. It can be unilateral or bilateral associated with seizures and developmental delay.	Most frequently seen in the region of the trigones and occipital horns. Enormous subependymal nodules line the walls of the lateral ventricle. These nodules follow grey matter signal intensity on all sequences. 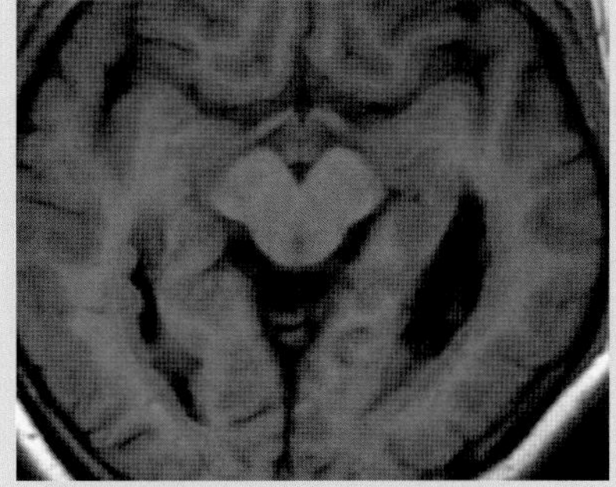 **Fig. 4.7.12:** T1W shows periventricular nodular heterotopia	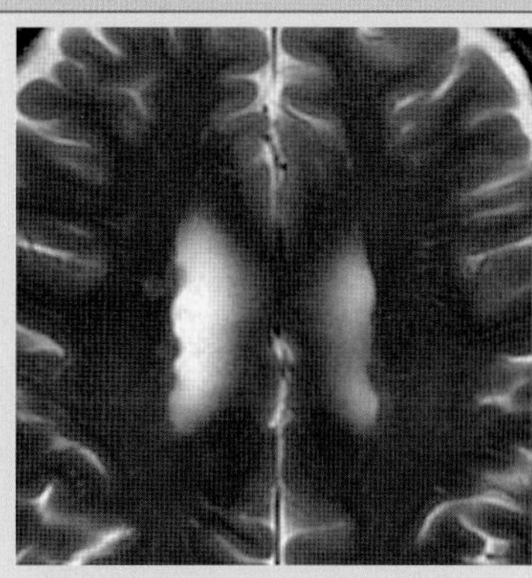 **Fig. 4.7.13:** T2W shows periventricular nodular heterotopia		

Contd...

Table 4.7.1: Differential diagnosis for lesions in caudothalamic groove *(Contd...)*		
Germinal matrix haemorrhage: Also known as peri-ventricular-intraventricular haemorrhages (PVIH)—commonest type of ICH in neonates. Related to perinatal stress affecting the highly visualised subependymal germinal matrix along the caudothalamic groove. **Refer to case 30**	At a level slightly posterior to the foramen of Monro, ultrasound will reveal a consistently echogenic mass inferolateral to the frontal horns. It might be unilateral or bilateral in nature. It may create focal compression on the lateral ventricle's inferolateral edge. The focal lesion shrinks in size and echogenicity as the hemorrhage heals, resulting in a subependymal cyst.	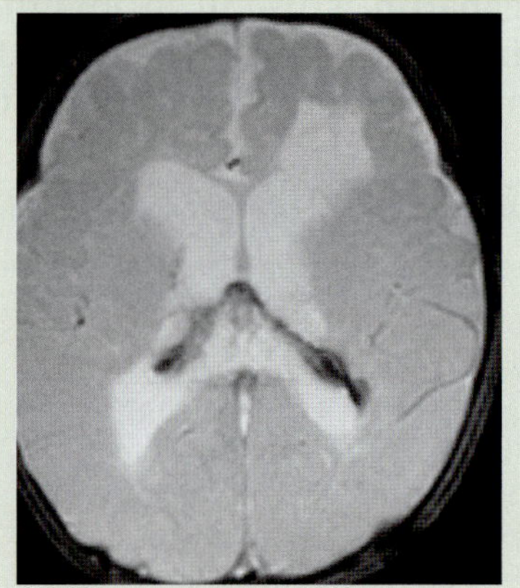 **Fig. 4.7.14:** Germinal matrix haemorrhage
Zellweger syndrome: Peroxisomal disorder, cystic spaces arise from prenatal lysis of fetal periventricular matrix tissue, rather than immature white matter, empty spaces are called "pseudocysts" or germinolytic cysts in caudothalamic groove.	Periventricular cysts are associated with cystic periventricular leukomalacia due to necrosis of periventricular unmyelinated white matter. Are located at the caudothalamic groove, tear shaped.	

Discussion: **Tuberous sclerosis complex or Bourneville-Pringle syndrome** is a neurocutaneous disorder, second most common after neurofibromatosis type 1. Characterised by development of multiple benign tumours of the embryonic ectoderm (e.g. skin, eyes, and nervous system). Classical clinical triad **"EPILOIA"—epilepsy, low IQ and angiofibroma/adenoma sebaceum.** Prevalence is 1:6000 live births. Patient with TSC2 diagnosed 9 years earlier than TSC1. Diagnosed at any age—1st year of life if infantile spasms or surveillance

Table 4.7.2: Associated other conditions in tuberous sclerosis		
Pulmonary LAM-like disease: Diffuse interstitial proliferation of smooth muscle cells and cystic change in the pulmonary parenchyma. Pneumothorax and chylous pleural effusion or ascites are two major complications of LAM. Multifocal multinodular pneumocyte hyperplasia (MMPH) is rare benign entity and non-progressive occurring in tuberous sclerosis.	Thin section CT scan demonstrates multiple lung cysts with well-defined thin wall. These cysts are found to be distributed randomly throughout the lung.	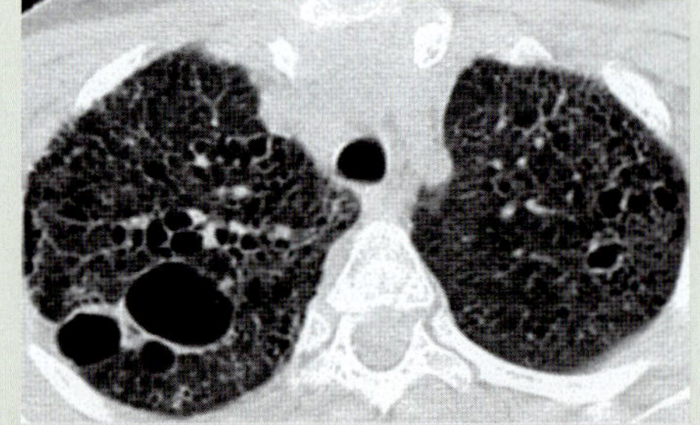 **Fig. 4.7.15:** Pulmonary LAM-like disease
Renal AML: Renal involvement of TS includes renal AML, renal cysts, and renal cell carcinoma. T2-weighted MR images, and homogeneous iso-echogenicity at USG. Lymphangiectasia and numerous ectatic lymphatic channels penetrating through the retroperitoneal angiomyolipoma can also be demonstrated.	CT: Presence of intratumoral macroscopic fat (<20 HU) without calcification. MRI—chemical shift imaging showing signal intensity loss and India ink artifact at interface of fat and no fat components.	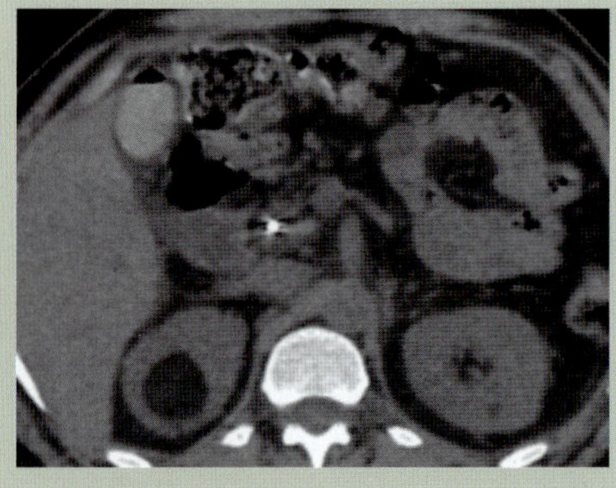 **Fig. 4.7.16:** Renal AML

Contd...

<table>
<tr><th colspan="2">Table 4.7.2: Associated other conditions in tuberous sclerosis *(Contd...)*</th></tr>
<tr><td colspan="2">**Dermatologic involvement:** Facial angiofibroma—multiple dome-shaped papules in the malar area, with a butterfly distribution. Shagreen patches are typically found as greyish-green or light brown areas in the lumbosacral region. Ash leaf macules, Koenen's periungual fibroma, confetti (café-au-lait spots), subungual fibromas are other manifestations.
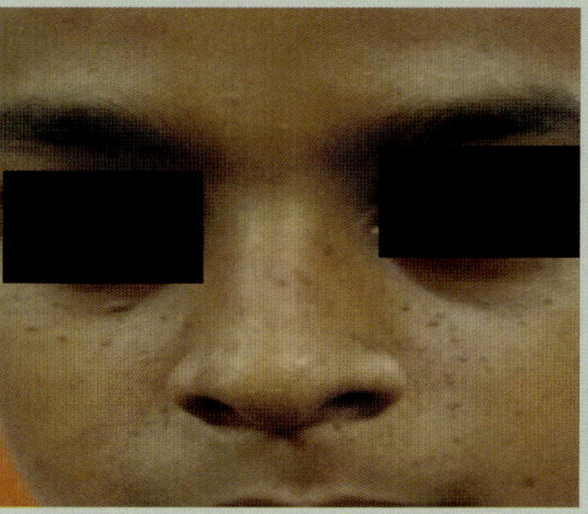
Fig. 4.7.17: Facial angiofibroma
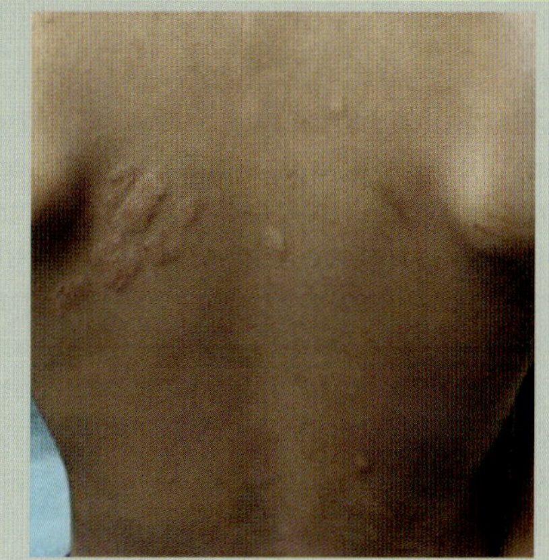
Fig. 4.7.18: Ash leaf macules</td></tr>
<tr><td>**Cardiac rhabdomyoma:** Most cardiac rhabdomyomas regress before birth and more than 80% of the tumors cause no clinical manifestations at birth.
Moreover, spontaneous regression/disappearance of the tumor can occur in 70% of children by the age of 4 years.</td><td>MRI: Cardiac rhabdomyomas multiple or single, are more commonly located on the interventricular septum.
Nodular hypointense lesion surrounded by hyperintense blood with large intraventricular mass and increased thickness of interventricular septum.</td></tr>
<tr><td>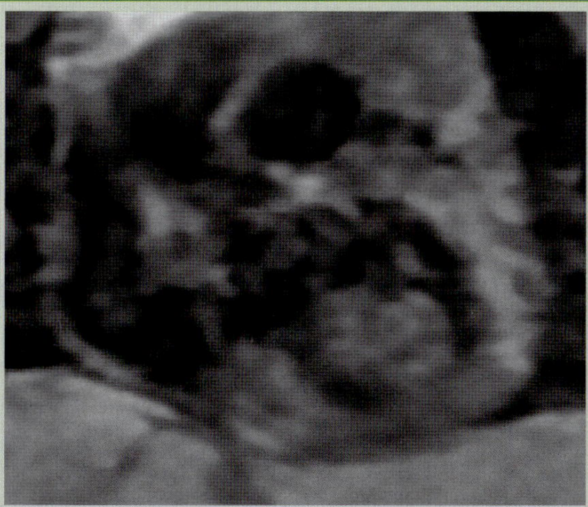
Fig. 4.7.19: Cardiac rhabdomyoma</td><td>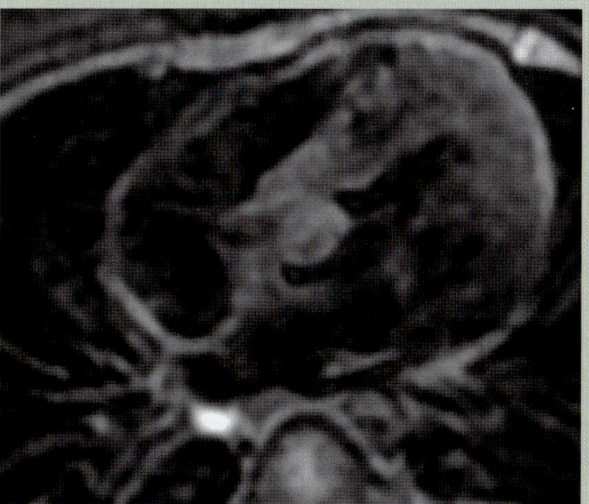
Fig. 4.7.20: Cardiac rhabdomyoma</td></tr>
<tr><td>**Intestinal polyps:** Polyps, frequently multiple and can occur anywhere from the oesophagus to the rectum.</td><td>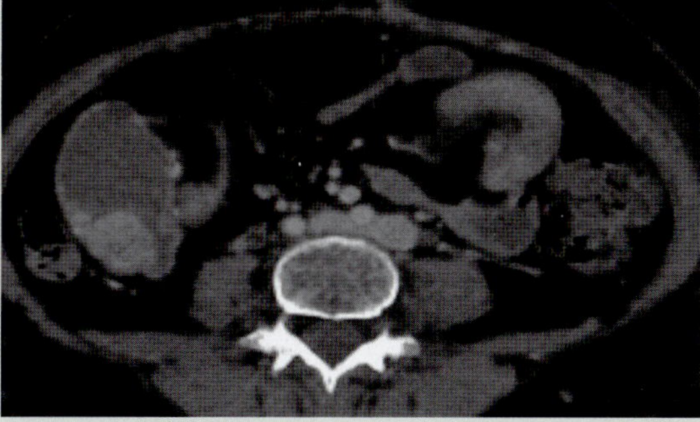
Fig. 4.7.21: Contrast-enhanced CT images of different levels demonstrate multiple high-attenuation polypoid lesions in the small intestine.</td></tr>
<tr><td>**Skeletal involvement:** Sclerotic lesion, cyst-like lesions, hyperostosis of the inner table of the calvaria, osteoblastic changes, periosteal new bone formation, and scoliosis.</td><td>Radiographs or CT images show cortical or medullary cyst-like radiolucent areas or sclerotic deposits are found focally or diffusely.</td></tr>
</table>

for positive family history. Child: Autistic-like behaviour, mental retardation, seizures, or skin lesions.

Adult: Diagnoses reported with demonstration of symptomatic subependymal giant cell astrocytoma on brain imaging. Caused by mutation in **TSC1 or TSC2 gene.** TSC2 mutation is 5 times more common than TSC1. Now considered an infantile (developmental) tauopathy—tau abnormally expressed in many of dysmorphic neurons and glial cells of TSC. Similar to focal cortical dysplasia, abnormal differentiation/proliferation of germinal matrix cells. Mutations in TSC tumour suppressor genes cause abnormal cellular differentiation, proliferation.

Cortical tubers: These are glioneuronal hamartoma. Found >90% of tuberous sclerosis patient; firm, whitish, pyramid-shaped, elevated areas of smooth gyral thickening with or without central depression. These resemble as potato, so called tubers. Tuber consists of Glial cells and dysmorphic neurons with foci of gliosis, disrupted lamination, disordered myelin. Tubers do not undergo malignant transformation.

Subependymal nodules: Located immediately beneath the ependymal lining of the lateral ventricles, along the course of caudate nucleus. These are elevated, rounded, hamartomatous lesions resemble as candle guttering or dripping. Calcify with increasing age. **Subependymal nodules along the caudothalamic groove adjacent to the foramen of Monro may undergo neoplastic transformation into subependymal giant cell astrocytoma.**

Table 4.7.3: Congenital TORCH vs tuberous sclerosis

Congenital TORCH	*Tuberous sclerosis*
Calcified lesion is from the newborn period	Subependymal nodules calcify usually after 2 years.

White matter lesion: In the subcortical white matter/fine radial lines spreading outward from the ependymal ventricular surface into the cortex, which are centres of odd dysmorphic neurons and balloon cells. Tubers are formed where the radial migration line (band) ends.

Subependymal giant cell astrocytoma: WHO grade I tumours often cause hydrocephalus but do not invade the adjacent brain. Almost exclusively seen in tuberous sclerosis in 6–9% of patients. Well-circumscribed solid intraventricular masses located near the foramen of Monro. Intratumoral calcification is common but necrosis is rare.

Imaging protocol: FLAIR and T1W-MT (magnetization transfer) is most sensitive sequences to diagnosis. Subependymal nodule (SEN) <1.3 cm while subependymal giant cell astrocytoma (SEGA) **>1.3 cm.**

Calcified subependymal nodules (hamartoma) is best clue for diagnosis, Subependymal giant cell astrocytoma typically located at foramen of Monro of caudothalamic groove. Cortical/subcortical tubers more common in frontal lobe>parietal lobe>occipital lobe>temporal lobe>cerebellum as the number of tubers increases symptoms also increase. White matter radial lines (band) is heterotopic glia with neurons along the path of cortical migration from ventricle to cortex. Cyst-like white matter

Table 4.7.4: Calcification pattern in congenital TORCH

Congenital TORCH	*Calcification pattern*	*Others*
Congenital CMV	**Caudostrial groove and periventricular** Broad sylvian fissure, cerebellar hypoplasia, polymicrogyria, microcephaly	**Fig. 4.7.22:** Caudostrial groove calcification in congenital CMV **Fig. 4.7.23:** A few calcific foci in caudostrial region in congenital CMV
Rubella	Calcification at **basal ganglia, periventricular and cortex.**	Ventriculomegaly and microcephaly
Zika	Calcification at **GM and WM junction**	Ventriculomegaly and microcephaly

Contd...

Table 4.7.4: Calcification pattern in congenital TORCH *(Contd...)*		
HIV	**Bilateral symmetrical basal ganglia calcification.** **Atrophy** and fusiform arteriopathy.	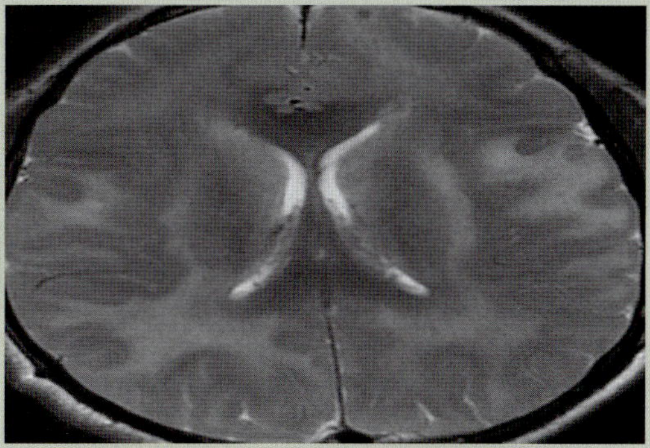 **Fig. 4.7.24:** HIV encephalopathy
Mitochondrial disease	Basal ganglia and subcortical calcification	Supratentorial and infratentorial atrophy
Toxoplasma	Scattered calcification, punctate linear (tram track) calcification in **cortical and subcortical white matter.**	Macrocephalus hydrocephalus more are common Lack of cortical malformation
Syphilis	Scattered calcification.	
Aicardi-Goutiéres syndrome Pseudo-TORCH (Baraitser-Reardon syndrome)	Basal ganglia calcification, periventricular calcification. 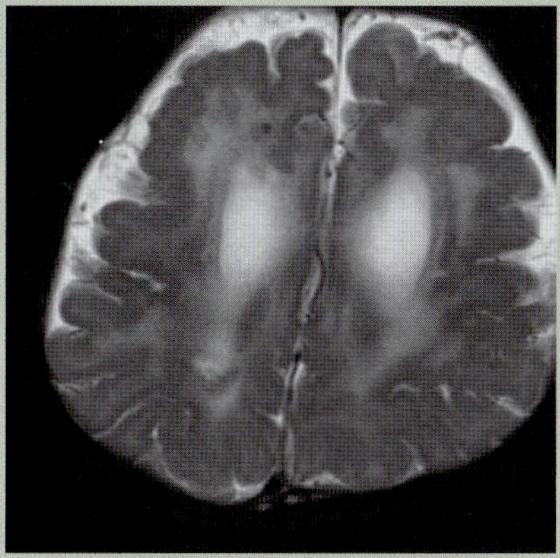 **Fig. 4.7.25:** Pseudo-TORCH	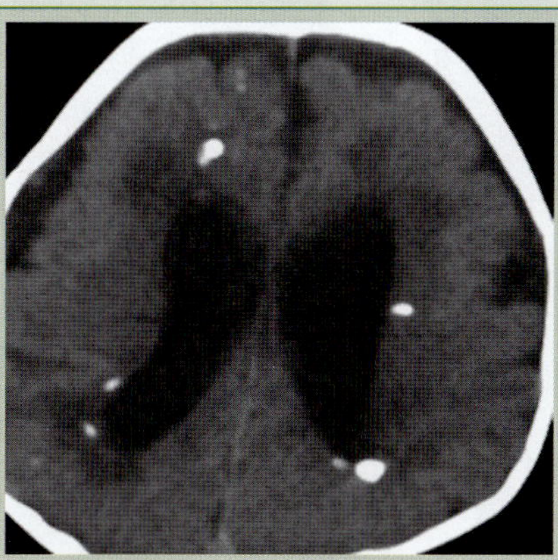 **Fig. 4.7.26:** Periventricular calcifications in pseudo-TORCH
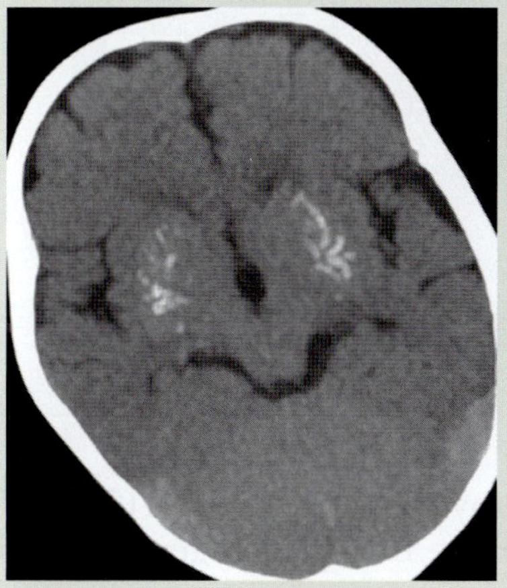 **Fig. 4.7.27:** Axial CT showing mineralising vasculopathy	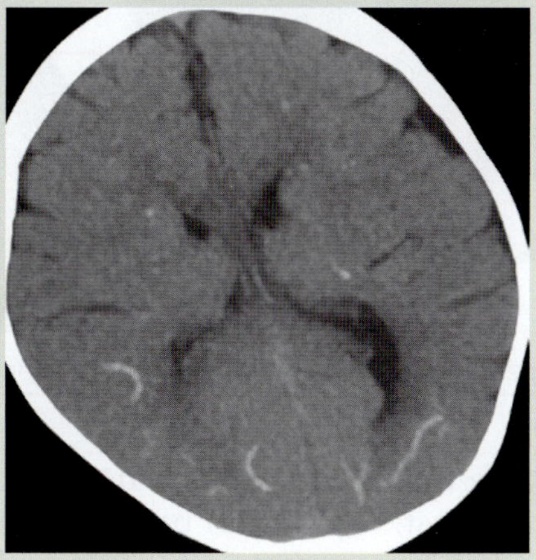 **Fig. 4.7.28:** Axial CT showing mineralising vasculopathy	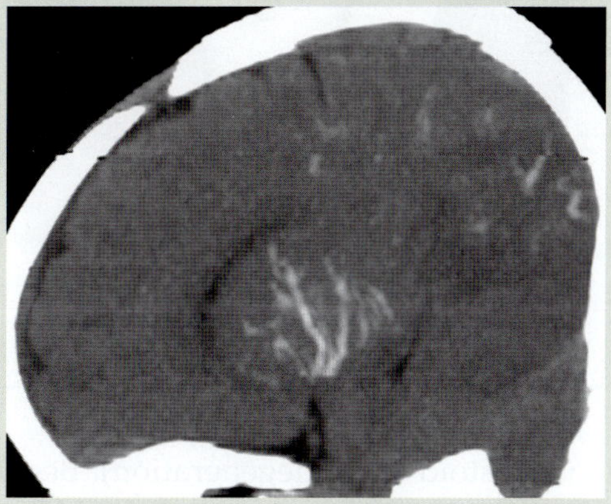 **Fig. 4.7.29:** Sagittal CT showing mineralising vasculopathy

Contd...

Table 4.7.4: Calcification pattern in congenital TORCH *(Contd...)*

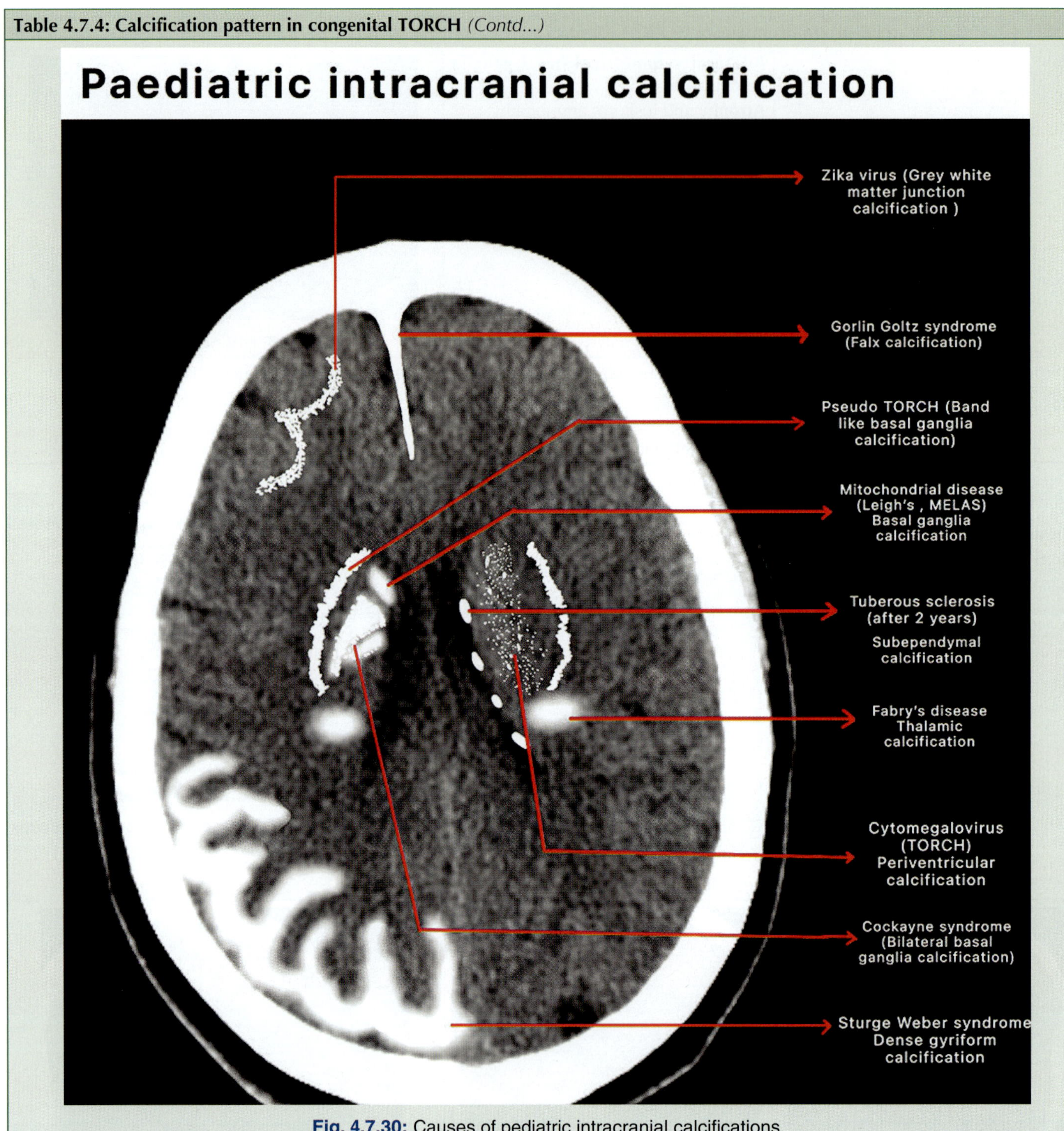

Fig. 4.7.30: Causes of pediatric intracranial calcifications

lesions (cystoid brain degeneration). Best imaging tool is MR with contrast, protocol advice MR with contrast, NECT to look for calcified subependymal nodules (SEN Ca^{++}). Yearly surveillance imaging if incompletely calcified. Subependymal giant cell astrocytoma or enhancing SEGA to look for rapid growth and ventricular obstruction. α[11C] methyl-L-tryptophan ([11C] AMT-PET) can be used to image the epileptogenic areas in pediatric patients with tuberous sclerosis as serotonin synthesis is increased between seizure episodes in epileptogenic tubers of patients with TSC.

Table 4.7.5: Subependymal nodules in tuberous sclerosis vs subependymal nodular heterotopia	
Subependymal nodules in tuberous sclerosis	*Subependymal nodular heterotopia*
Calcification (after 2 years) At 10 years 50% calcify, subsequently 85% calcify	No calcification
Tubers enhancement + varying intensity with grey matter	No enhancement
T1 hyperintensity seen.	Isointense to grey matter Follows grey matter signal on all sequences
Associated tuberous sclerosis changes	Scalloping of lateral ventricle margin
Caudothalamic groove	Scalloping of ventricular margin (more) Located along caudothalamic groove
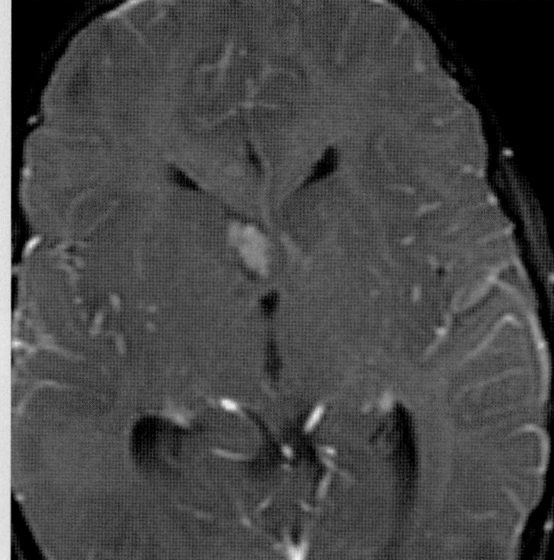 Fig. 4.7.31: Subependymal nodules in tuberous sclerosis	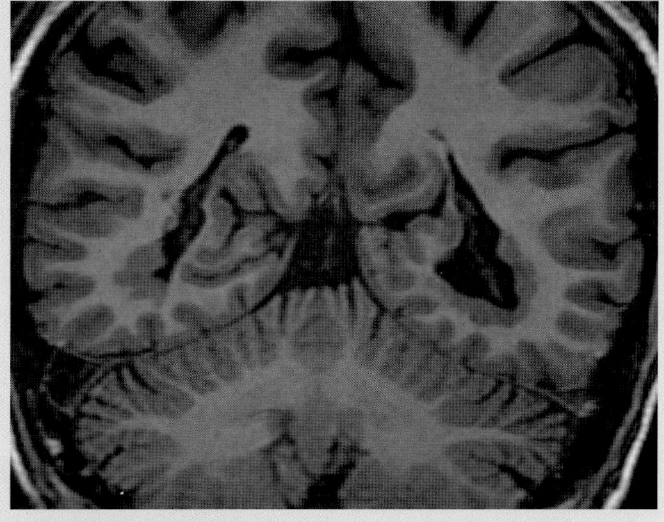 Fig. 4.7.32: Subependymal nodular heterotopia
Sturge Weber-Dimitri syndrome (encephalo-trigeminal-angiomatosis): Capillary venous angioma of the face and ipsilateral cerebral hemisphere leptomeningeal venous angioma: Parietal > occipital > frontal lobes. Enlarged and increased contrast enhancement of ipsilateral choroid plexus	**Imaging features (Figs 4.7.33 to 4.7.36):** Tram track calcifications (characteristic) that follow cortical convolutions; most common in parietal occipital lobes. Atrophic cortex with enlarged adjacent subarachnoid spaces. Ipsilateral thickening of the skull and orbit.

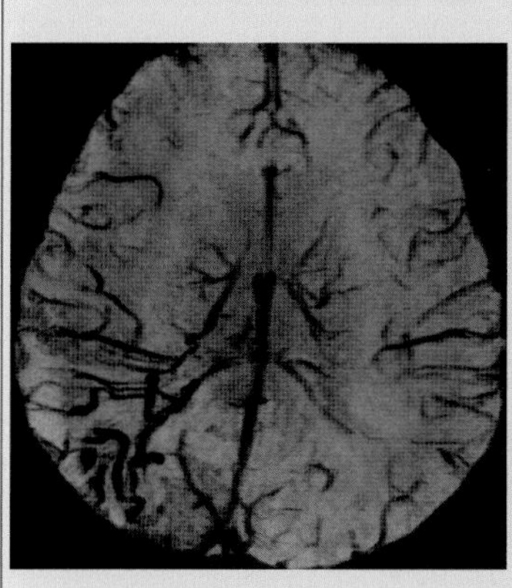 Fig. 4.7.33	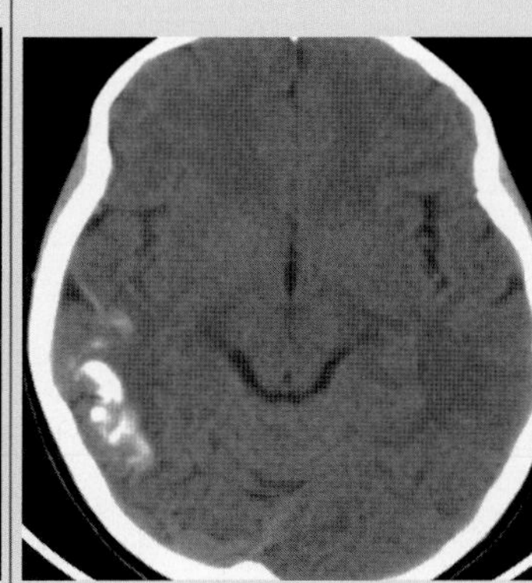 Fig. 4.7.34	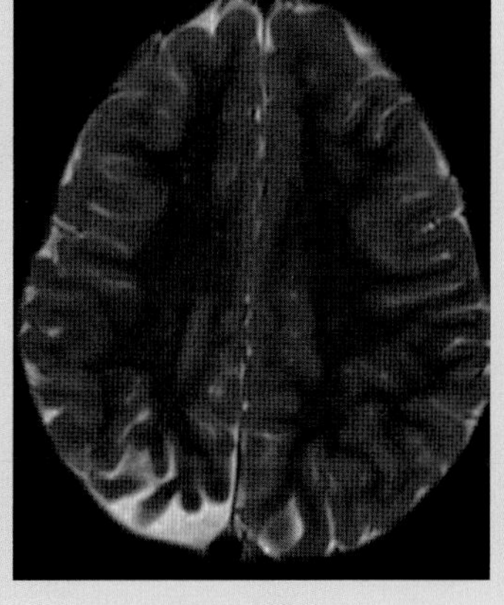 Fig. 4.7.35	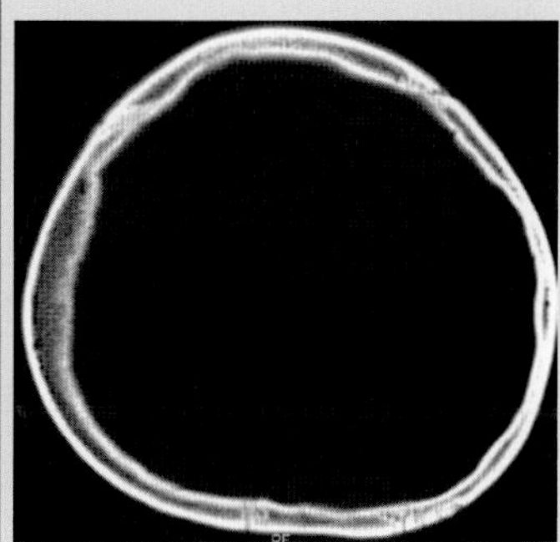 Fig. 4.7.36

Table 4.7.6: Causes for multiple focal brain T2/FLAIR hyperintensities in children

Causes for multiple focal brain T2/FLAIR hyperintensities in children:			
Tuberous sclerosis	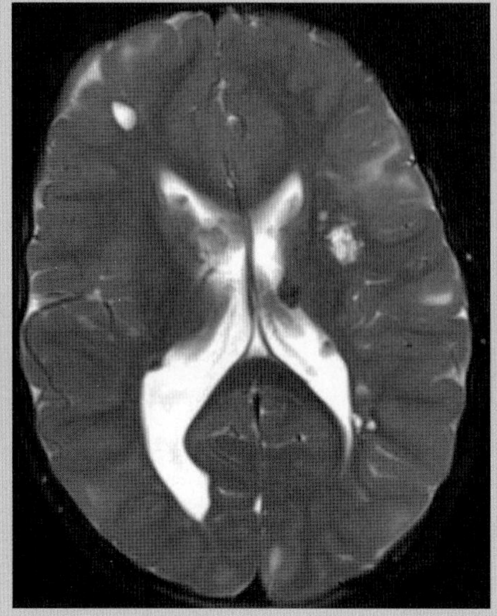 **Fig. 4.7.37:** Subependymal nodules	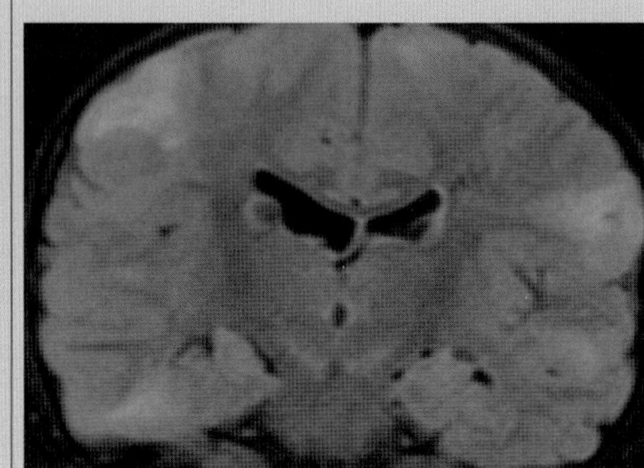 **Fig. 4.7.38:** Cortical tubers	
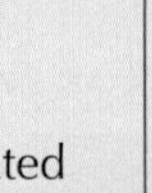 Demyelination: Acute disseminated encephalomyelitis/multiple sclerosis	**Fig. 4.7.39:** ADEM	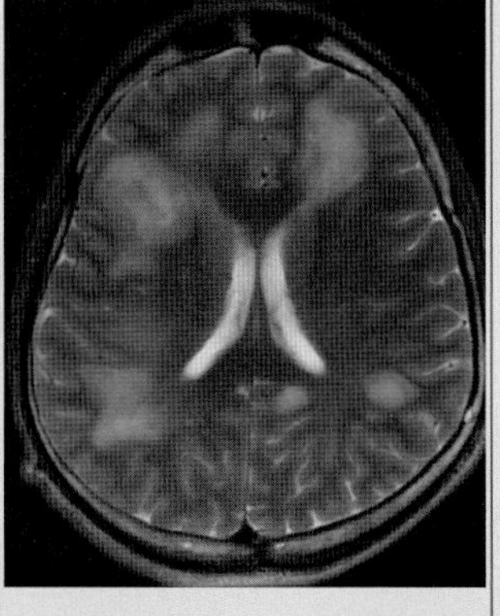 **Fig. 4.7.40:** ADEM	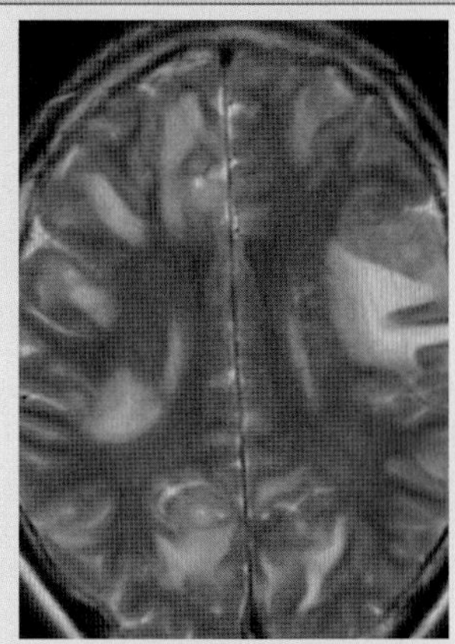 **Fig. 4.7.41:** ADEM
Multiple granuloma	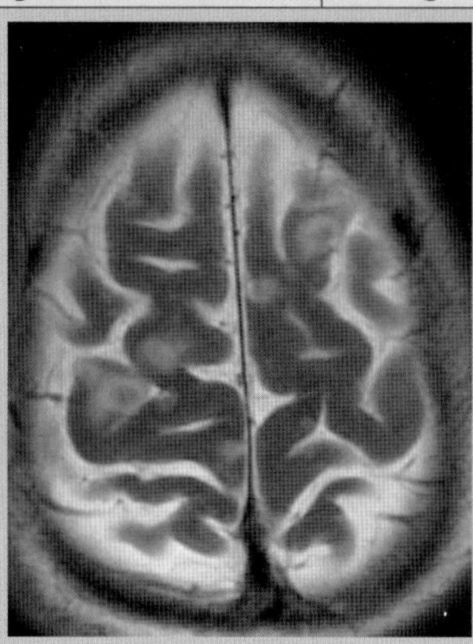 **Fig. 4.7.42** T2W image showing multiple granuloma	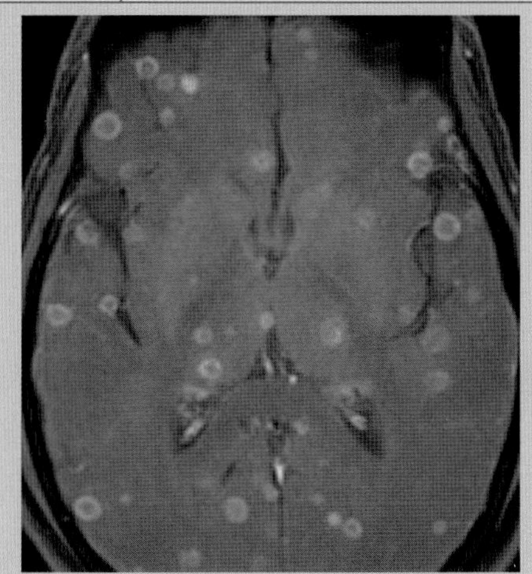 **Fig. 4.7.43:** T1+C image showing multiple granuloma	

Contd...

Table 4.7.6: Causes for multiple focal brain T2/FLAIR hyperintensities in children *(Contd...)*			
Posterior reversible leukoencephalopathy syndrome	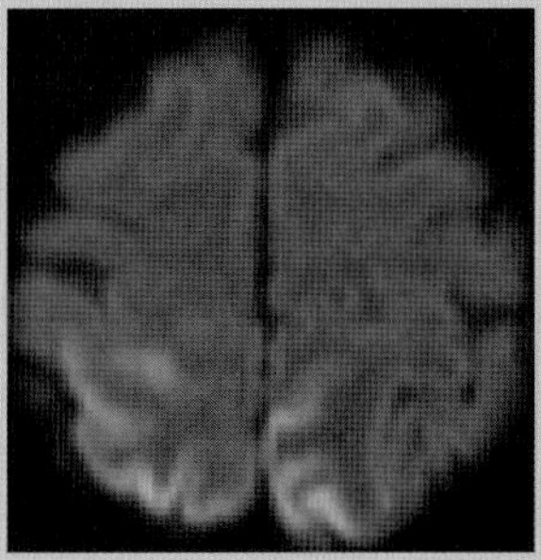 **Fig. 4.7.44:** Diffusion restriction in PRES	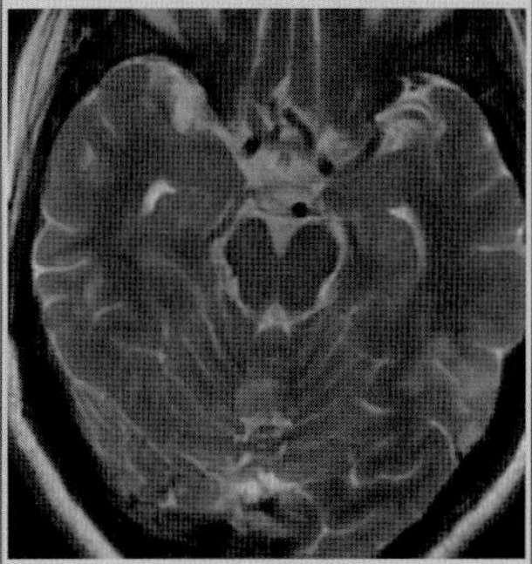 **Fig. 4.7.45:** Occipital T2 hyperintensities in PRES	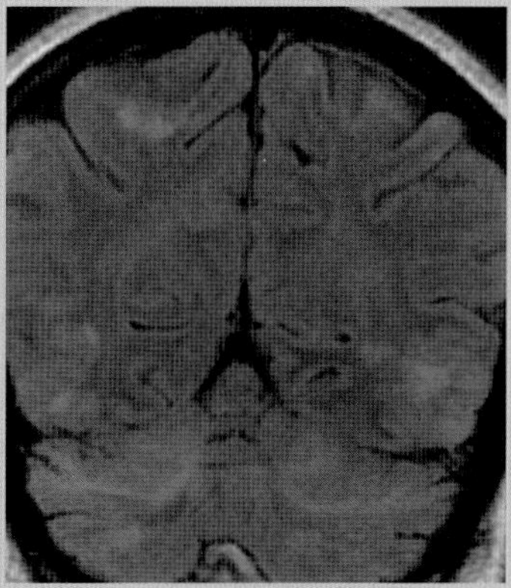 **Fig. 4.7.46:** FLAIR hyperintensities in PRES
Encephalitis/autoimmune encephalitis (Figs 4.7.47–4.7.50)			
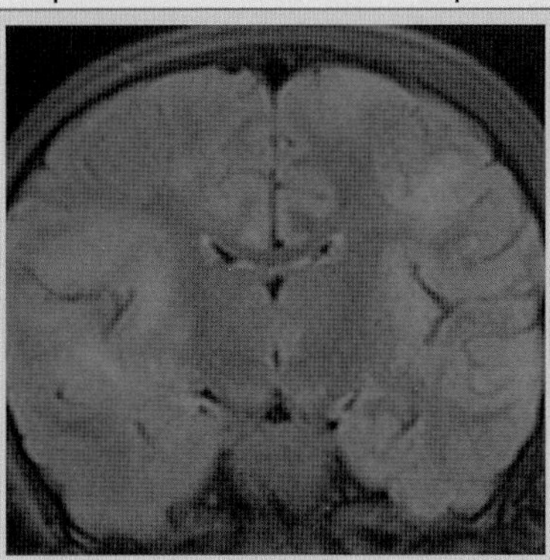 **Fig. 4.7.47**	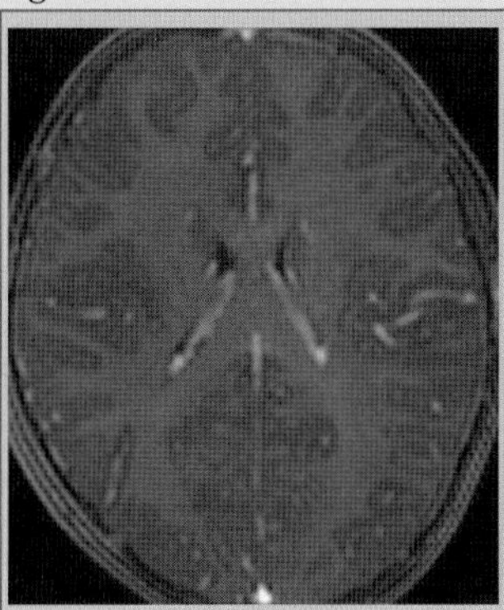 **Fig. 4.7.48**	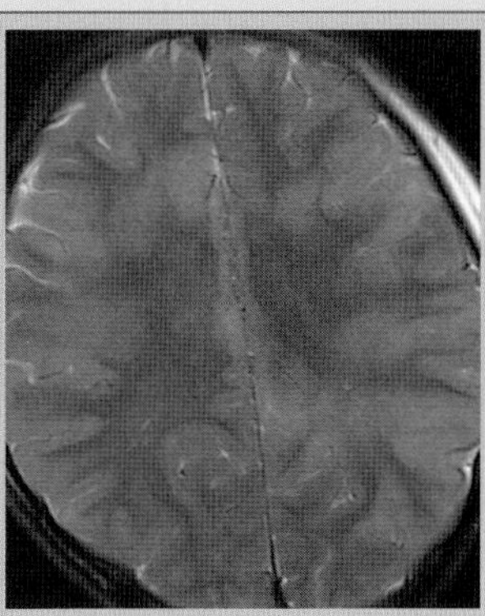 **Fig. 4.7.49**	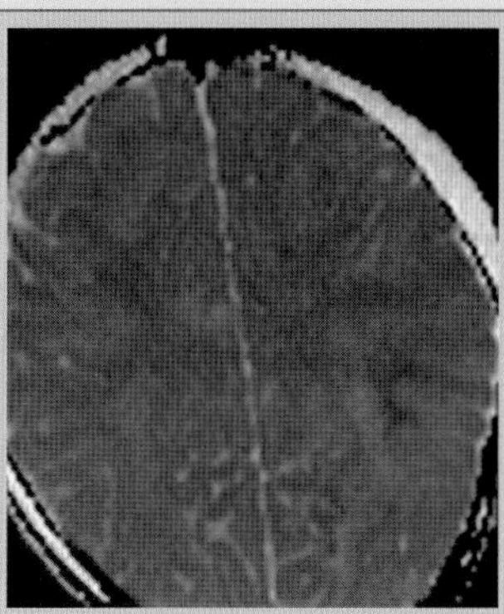 **Fig. 4.7.50**
Rarely metastasis			

Table 4.7.7: Differential diagnosis for transmantle sign		
Linear white matter hyperintensity extends from the lateral ventricle to cortex (transmantle sign)		
Tuberous sclerosis	Focal dysplasia (also in transmantle heterotopia)	Dysembryoplastic neuroepithelial tumor
Cortical tubers, subcortical tubers—present in 90–100% cases White matter changes seen as radial band	Cortical thickening with white matter hyperintensity extending to ventricular margin	Benign, supratentorial, cortical intra-axial, slow growing WHO grade I tumor. On MRI FLAIR hypointensity.
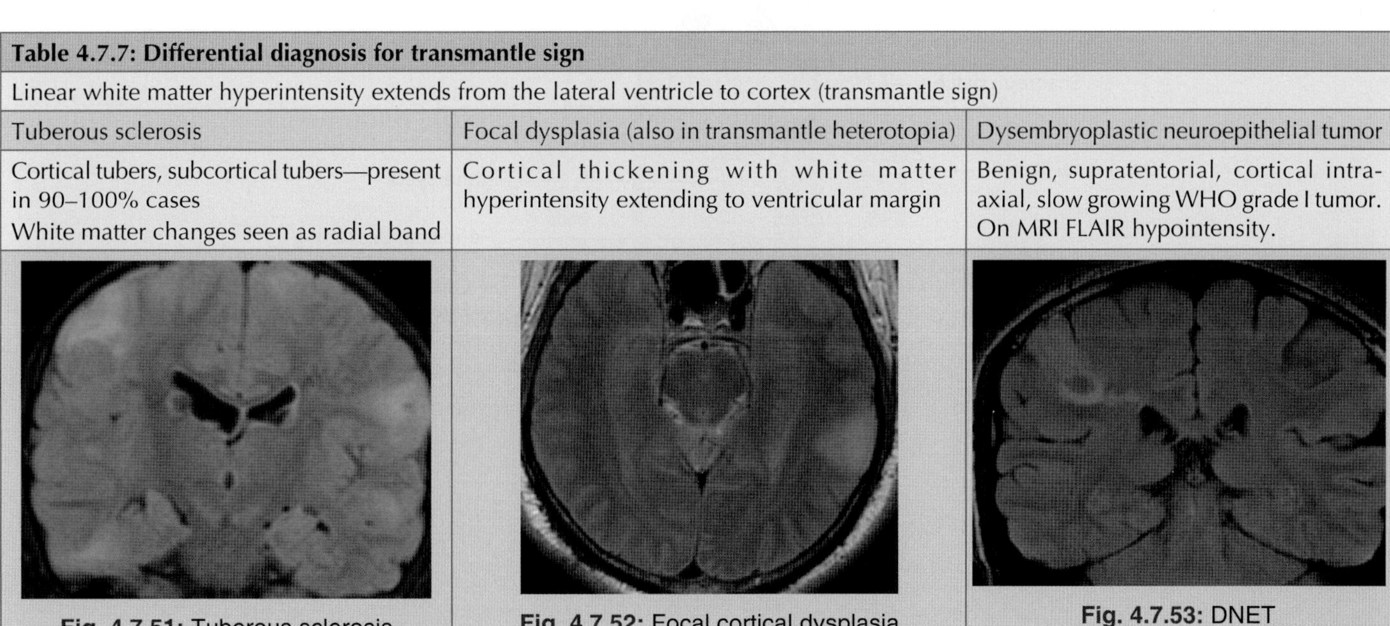 **Fig. 4.7.51:** Tuberous sclerosis	**Fig. 4.7.52:** Focal cortical dysplasia	**Fig. 4.7.53:** DNET

Table 4.7.8: Tuberous sclerosis diagnostic criteria (2012)	
Tuberous sclerosis diagnostic criteria (2012): Definite tuberous sclerosis complex: 2 major or 1major plus 2 minors. Probable tuberous sclerosis complex: 1 major plus 1 minor. Possible tuberous sclerosis complex: 1 major or 2 minors.	
Major criteria Identified clinically 3 or more hypomelanotic ('ash leaf'' macules) Facial angiofibroma or forehead plaque Shagreen patch Ungual /periungual fibroma Multiple retinal hamartoma	*Minor criteria* *Identified clinically* Gingival fibroma Affected first degree relative Pitting of dental enamel Retinal achromic patch Confetti like skin macules
Identified on imaging Subependymal nodules Cortical tubers Cardiac rhabdomyoma Renal angiomyolipoma Subependymal giant cell astrocytoma Lymphangioleiomyomatosis	*Identified on imaging* WM hamartoma, radial migration line Hamartomatous rectal polyps Nonrenal hamartoma Bone cysts Renal cysts

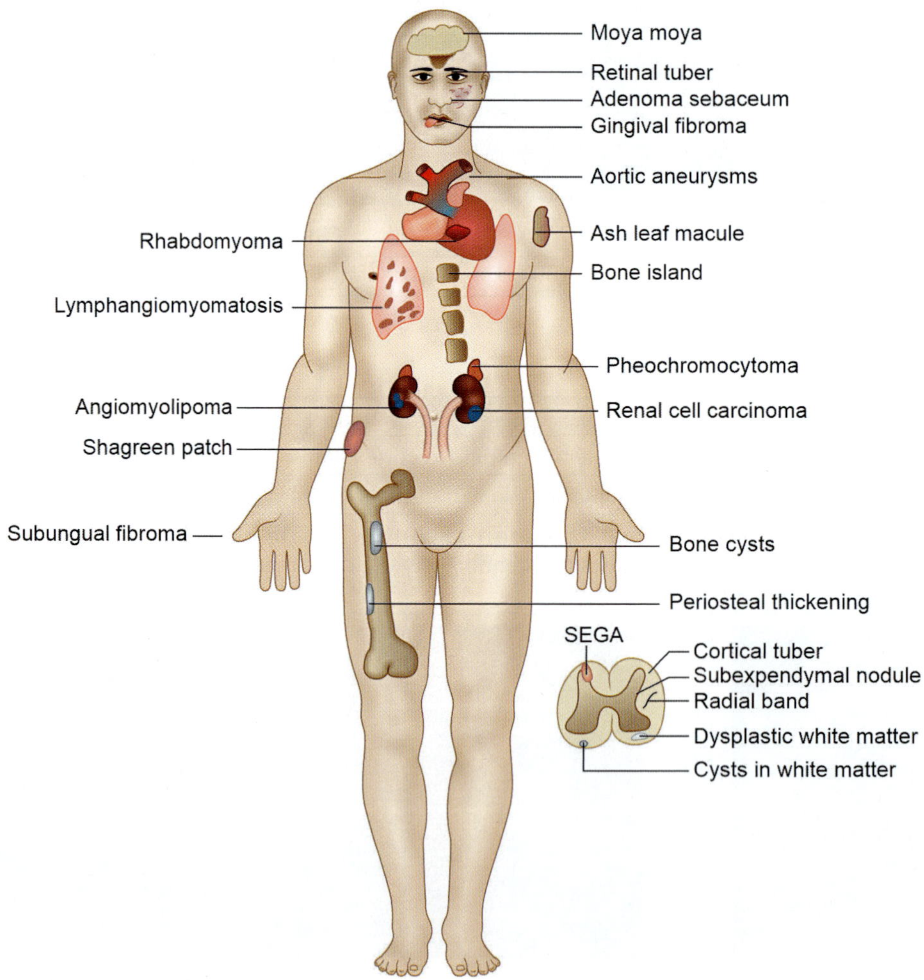

Fig. 4.7.54: Whole body illustration showing manifestations of tuberous sclerosis

4.8 CENTRAL NERVOUS SYSTEM

Case No. 8

Clinical history: A 19 years old male presented with a 6 months history of on and off headache followed by right-sided sensorineural deafness and mild gait ataxia for 1 month.

Radiological techniques and observation: Plain CT axial sections (Fig. 4.8.1) in brain and bone window (Fig. 4.8.2) with postcontrast CT in brain windows (Fig. 4.8.3) show bilateral lobulated soft tissue dense mass in the bilateral CP angle. Left side lesion is larger than right, it causes mass effect over brain stem. Bone window shows widening of the internal acoustic canals. Postcontrast there is heterogenous enhancement in the both lesions. No evidence of calcifications/bone destruction.

MR brain and spine axial T2, flair coronal, T1 sagittal, T2 sagittal of posterior fossa and C-spine and T1 axial postcontrast images (Figs 4.8.4 to 4.8.7) show bilateral lobulated soft tissue mass at CP angle which is hyperintense in T2 and isointense to grey matter in T1. The lesion in left side causes mass effect over the brain stem with compression of fourth ventricle and bilateral lateral ventricles appear enlarged. CSF cleft is seen between the lesion and brain stem. There is also T2 hetero-intense lesion in the upper cervical cord. T1 postcontrast image shows intense enhancement of the CP angle lesion and demonstrates the intracanalicular extension of the lesion giving an ice cream cone appearance.

MR T1 postcontrast of cervical, dorsal and lumbar spine in sagittal sections (Figs 4.8.8 to 4.8.11) shows multiple intramedullary and extramedullary intra-

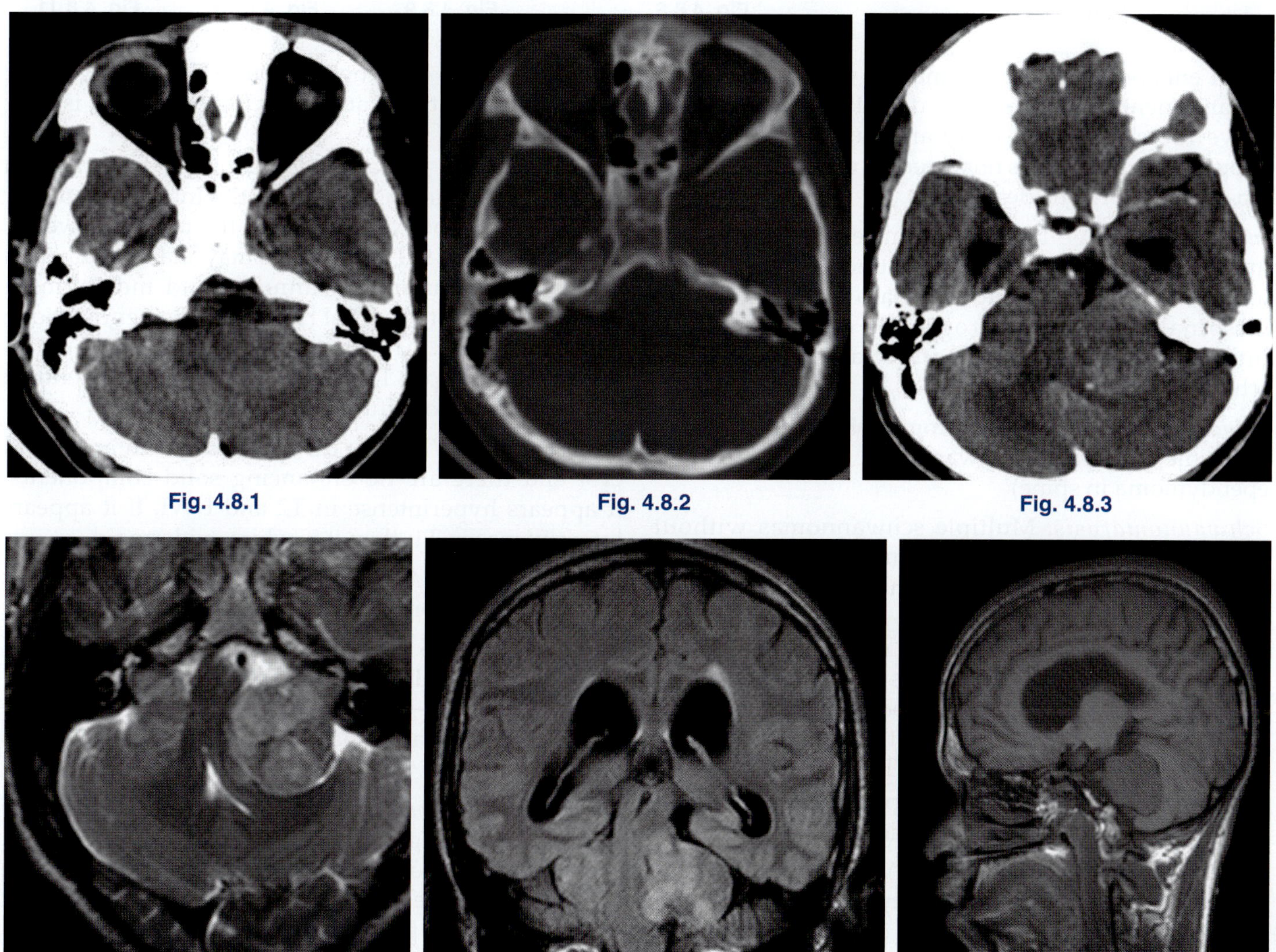

Fig. 4.8.1 Fig. 4.8.2 Fig. 4.8.3

Fig. 4.8.4 Fig. 4.8.5 Fig. 4.8.6

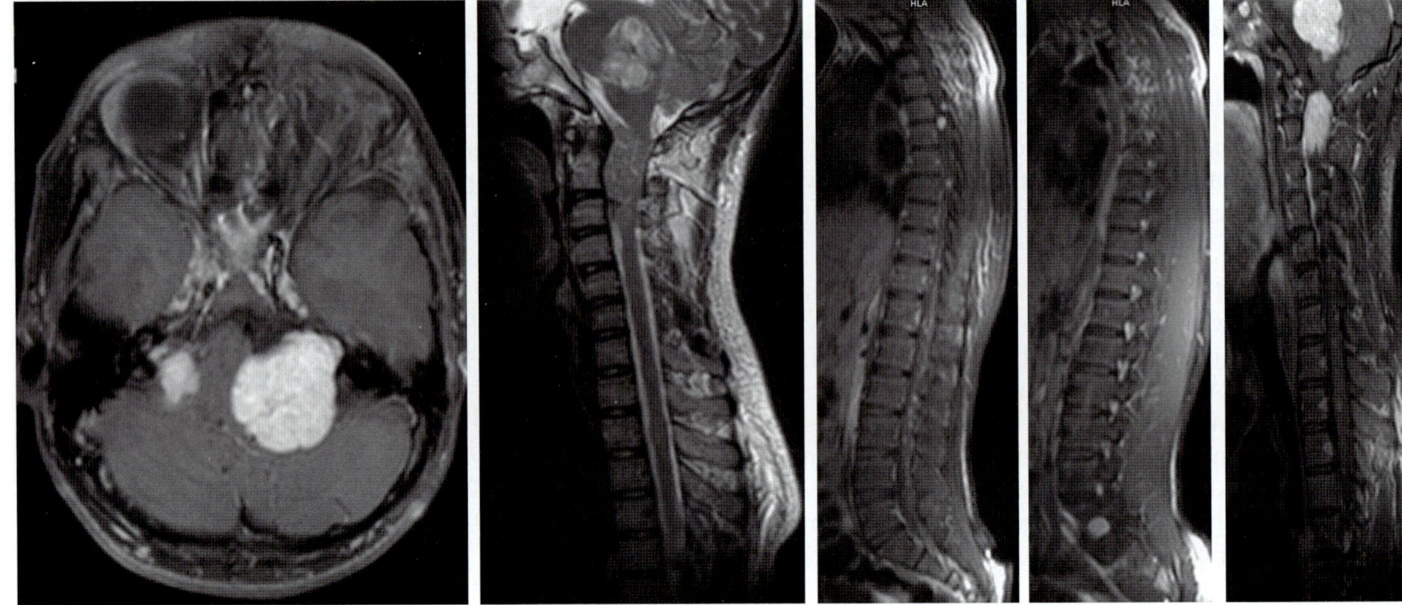

Fig. 4.8.7 Fig. 4.8.8 Fig. 4.8.9 Fig. 4.8.10 Fig. 4.8.11

dural enhancing soft tissue masses with postcontrast enhancement in cervical cord, dorsal cord and lumbar nerve roots. Vertebral body and posterior elements appear normal. There is no widening of neural formina. No evidence of bone destruction.

Interpretation: A—19 years old male, multiple lesions in brain and spine, C—multiple intracranial and spinal lesions. Multiple ependymoma and meningioma in spinal cord, B—heterogenous enhancement in intracranial lesions (indicate bilateral vestibular schwannoma), D—NF 2.

Principal diagnosis: Neurofibromatosis type II—MISME (multiple intracranial schwannoma, meningioma and ependymoma in spine).

Schwannomatosis: Multiple schwannomas without vestibular tumors. No cutaneous stigmata or meningiomas. **Facial nerve schwannoma** confined to the internal auditory canal may be difficult to distinguish it from a vestibular schwannoma. Facial nerve schwannomas are much less common and usually have a labyrinthine segment tail, look for extension along the entire labyrinthine segment of the facial nerve means the schwannoma arises from CN VII and is not a CN VIII.

The major differential diagnosis of vestibular schwannoma is CP angle meningioma.

Ependymoma: Extends into CPA from 4th ventricle. CPA masses such as **epidermoid cysts, arachnoid cysts, and aneurysms** can usually be distinguished easily from vestibular schwannoma. Vestibular schwannomas occasionally have prominent intramural cysts and enhancing solid components, but a completely cystic schwannoma without an enhancing tumor rim is very rare.

Recurrent or metastatic secondary to radiation therapy: Most meningiomas cap the Internal Auditory Canal and do not extend deep to the porus. However, a reactive dural tail in the IAC may make distinction between vestibular schwannoma and meningioma difficult unless other dural tails along the petrous ridge are also present. Arachnoid cyst: Follows CSF on all sequences. T2 hyper, T1 hypointense and no postcontrast enhancement. No diffusion restriction.

Epidermoid: DWI easily distinguishes from arachnoid cyst and there are no enhancing solid components. It appears hyperintense in T2 and DWI. If it appears hyperintense in T1, then it is white epidermoid.

Aneurysm: PICA/AICA/VA aneurysms may project into CPA. Pulsation artifact in phase-encoding direction.

Metastases: CNS primary: Glioblastoma, PNET-MB, germinoma, ependymoma metastases can coat facial and vestibulocochlear nerves within the internal auditory canal. Metastases are usually bilateral with other lesions present.

Further management: After complete evaluation of neuroaxis, management depends on symptom and disease progression. Complete resection of 8th nerve schwannoma if feasible, in difficult cases stereotactic radiosurgery is preferred. Subtotal microsurgical resection with functional cochlear nerve preservation in the last hearing ear.

Table 4.8.1: Discussion (Note—for this type of cases the diagnosis is straightforward. There is no definite differential diagnosis. So, discussion is made based on the various lesions in that location)

DD for multiple meningioma—meningiomatosis, metastasis, lymphoma, NF2

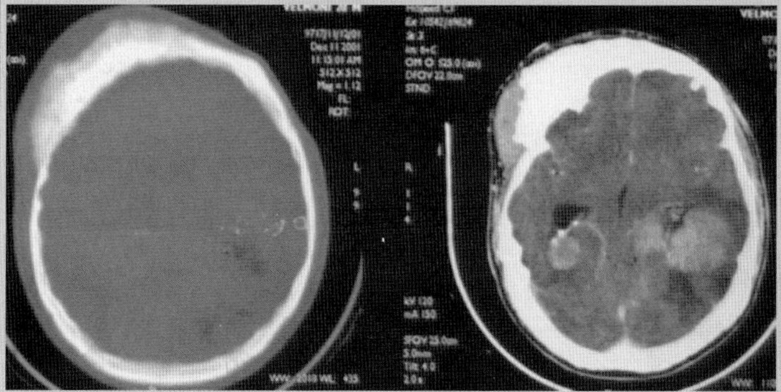

Fig. 4.8.12: Plain CT in axial-bone and brain windows showing meningiomatosis

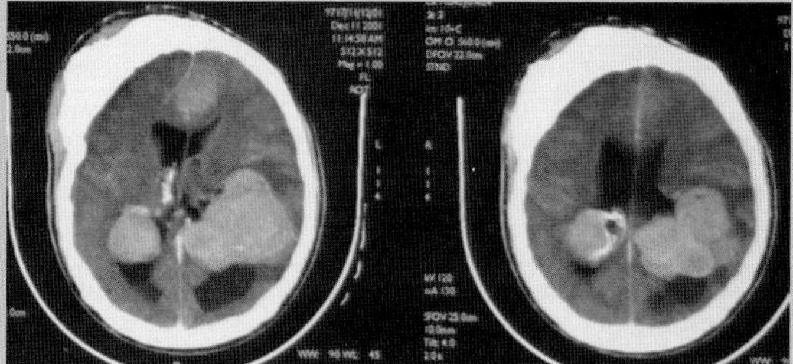

Fig. 4.8.13: Multiple meningiomatosis in a case of NF2

The important differential diagnosis for CP angle lesions includes schwannoma, metastasis, meningioma, arachnoid cyst, epidermoid, aneurysm, ependymoma, lipoma.

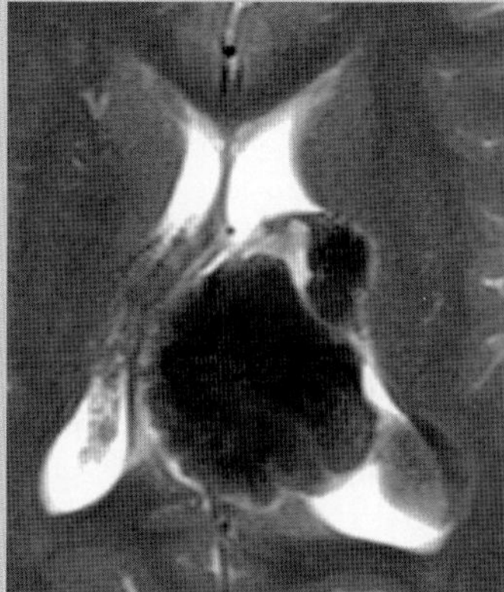

Fig. 4.8.14: A—Choroid plexus meningioma with bilateral acoustic schwannoma in NF2

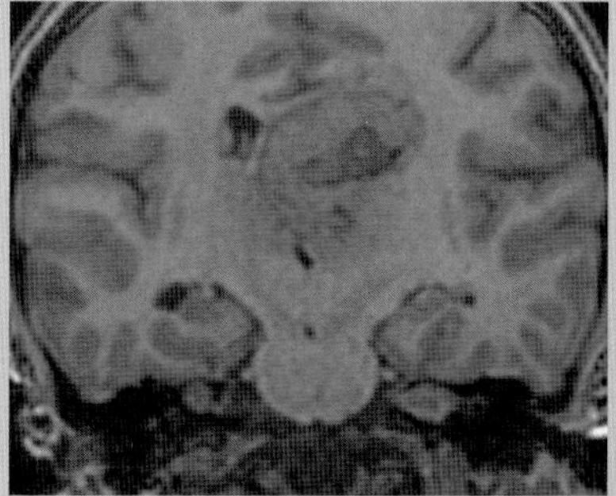

Fig. 4.8.15: B—Choroid plexus meningioma with bilateral acoustic schwannoma in NF2

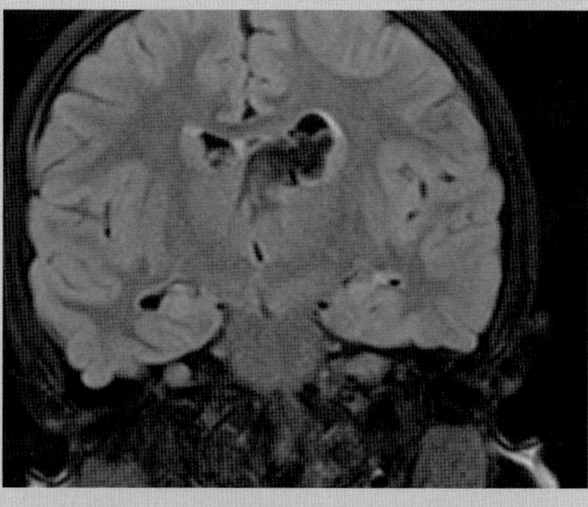

Fig. 4.8.16: C—Choroid plexus meningioma with bilateral acoustic schwannoma in NF2

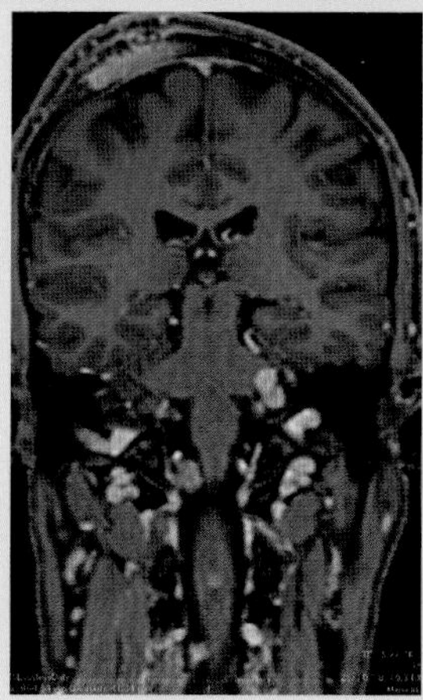

Fig. 4.8.17: Intradiploic meningioma

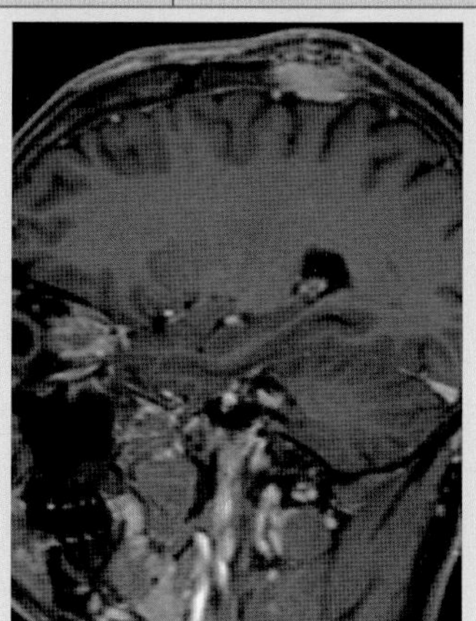

Fig. 4.8.18: Meningiomas in optic nerve and intradiploic region in NF2

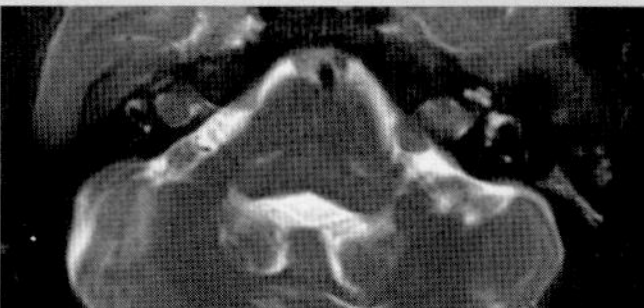

Fig. 4.8.19: Bilateral acoustic schwannoma in NF2

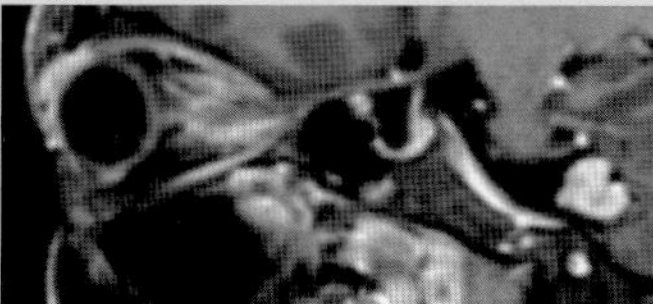

Fig. 4.8.20: Optic nerve meningioma

Optic nerve meningioma, intradiploic meningioma with bilateral acoustic schwannoma in NF2.
In case of optic nerve glioma, suspect NF1

Table 4.8.2: Differentiation between Schwannoma and neurofibroma

	Schwannoma	*Neurofibroma*	*Peripheral nerve sheath tumor*
Origin	Schwann cells	Schwann cells and fibroblasts	Schwann cells and fibroblasts
Association	NF2	NF1	50% associated with NF1
Incidence	Common, age 25–65 years, M:F-1.3:1	Uncommon, 25–65 years, M:F—1.2:1	20–65 years, M:F-1:1
Location	CN VIII > other CN	Cutaneous and spinal nerves	Seen in major nerve trunks
Malignant degeneration	No	5–10%	<5% of NF1 turns malignant
Growth	Focal	Infiltrating	Infiltrating
Mass nerve relationship	Eccentric but inseparable from nerve	Central and intimately related to nerve	Central and infiltrates along the nerve
Enhancement	+++/Central necrosis or cystic changes +/–	++/Heterogenous	Heterogeneous enhancement
T1W	70% hypointense, 30% isointense	Isointense with muscle	
T2W	Hyperintense Reverse target sign due to cystic changes in center. **Fig. 4.8.21:** T2W reverse target sign	Hyperintense Target sign seen in 50–70% **Fig. 4.8.22:** T2W target sign	Hyperintense Target sign absent
ADC	Peripheral restriction showing **reverse target sign** but **target sign** in DWI images due facilitated diffusion in central portion **Fig. 4.8.23:** Peripheral DWI restriction causing target sign	**Target sign** because of diffusion restriction due to central hypercellularity **Fig. 4.8.24:** Central DWI restriction causing target sign	Malignant changes with high cellularity show diffusion restriction.
Epicenter	Arises from the schwann cells, eccentric and displaces the fascicle **Fig. 4.8.25**	Arises from fascicle of nerve fiber. Does not displaces the fascicle **Fig. 4.8.26**	Arises from fascicle and Schwann cells.
Capsule	Seen in 70% of cases	Usually unencapsulated, but capsule seen in 30% of cases	Rare
Fascicular sign	Common	Common	Occasional focal

Contd...

Table 4.8.2: Differentiation between Schwannoma and neurofibroma *(Contd...)*			
Tail sign (continuity with parent nerve fiber)	Absent **Fig. 4.8.27:** Absent tail sign in schwannoma	Present **Fig. 4.8.28:** Positive tail sign in neurofibroma	NA
Split fat sign	Absent	Present **Fig. 4.8.29:** Split fat sign positive	NA
Intratumoral cyst	Common	Rare	NA
Margins	Well circumscribed	Well circumscribed	Often well circumscribed

Table 4.8.3: Differentiation between schwannoma and meningioma		
Imaging modality	*Schwannoma*	*Meningioma*
CT	Hypo/isodense to brain	Hyper/isodense to brain
Contrast enhancement	Homogeneous to heterogenous enhancement	Homogeneous
Calcification	Rare	Common
Location	Centred in IAC	Broad based with petrous bone
IAC	Dilated	Not dilated
T1W	Iso/hypointense to pons	Isointense to pons
T2W	Iso/hyperintense to pons	Iso/hypointense to pons
Cystic degeneration	Common	Uncommon
Involvement of other skull base foramina	Uncommon	Common (widening of spinosum)
Hyperostosis	--------	Common

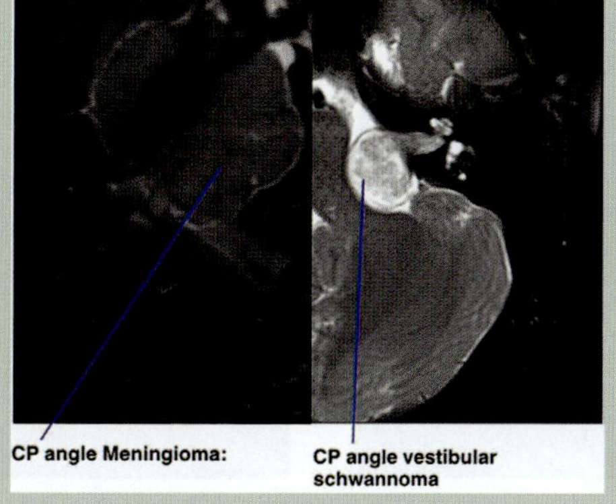

Fig. 4.8.30: CP angle meningioma vs CP angle vestibular schwannoma

Table 4.8.4: Approach to cerebellopontine angle masses			
Cisterns	Epidermoid cyst Dermoid cyst Lipoma Neuroenteric cyst Neuroepithelial cyst	Meninges	Meningioma Arachnoid cyst Miscellaneous lesions Metastasis
Arteries	Aneurysm, ectasia.	Nerves	Fifth to twelfth nerves schwannoma
Skull base	Cholesterol granuloma paraganglioma; apicitis Chordoma; chondroma Endolymphatic sac tumor Pituitary adenoma	Cerebellum and ventricles	Glioma, lymphoma, ependymoma Papilloma, hemangioblastoma, medulloblastoma DNET

Table 4.8.5: MR imaging characteristics and suggestive features of unusual lesions arising from the cerebellopontine cistern

Lesion	*T1-weighted*	*T2-weighted*	*Enhancement*	*Suggestive features*
Epidermoid cyst	Hypointense (hyper-intense–white epidermoid)	Hyperintense	No	Hyperintense on DWI
Dermoid cyst	Hyperintense	Variable hypo/hyper	No	Midline, fat and calcifications, fat fluid levels
Arachnoid cyst	Hypointense	Hyperintense	No	CSF intense, hypointense on DWI
Miscellaneous cysts	Hypointense	Hyperintense	No	Mimic arachnoid cyst except for lack of bone erosion
Lipoma	Hyperintense	Isointense to fat	No	Exactly matches signal intensity of subcutaneous fat with all sequences
Schwannoma	Hypointense	Hyperintense	Yes	Follows the anatomic course of nerve
Aneurysm	Hypointense	Hypointense	Yes	Well-circumscribed hypointense on T2
Melanoma	Hyperintense	Iso to hypointense	Yes	T1 hyperintense
Miscellaneous meningeal lesions	Hypointense	Variable	Yes	Sarcoidosis is hypointense on T2 weighted images

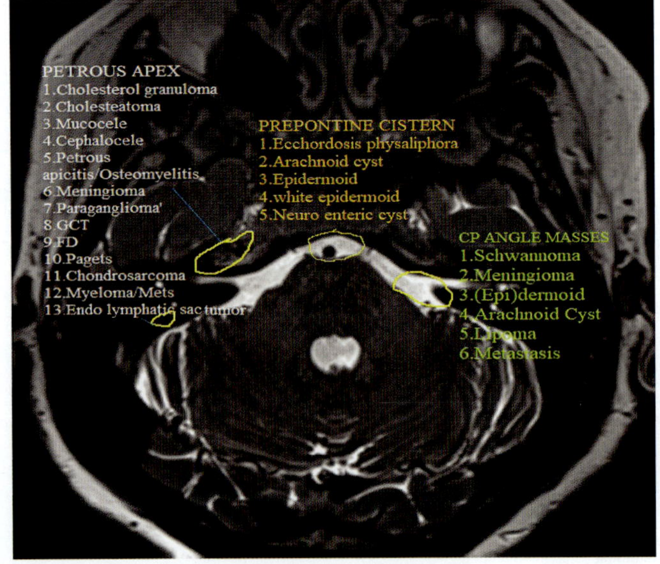

Fig. 4.8.31: Extra axial intracranial masses in petrous apex, prepontine cistern and CP angle

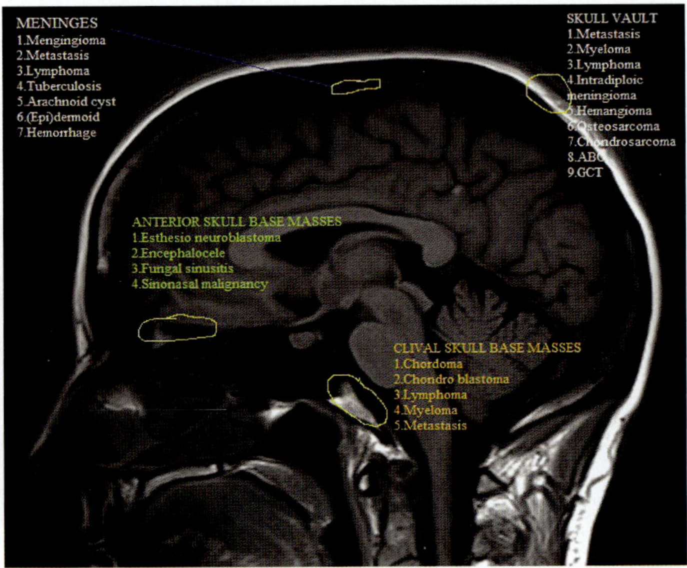

Fig. 4.8.32: Extra axial intracranial masses in meninges, anterior skull base, clival skull base and skull vault

Brief discussion about the condition—neurofibromatosis type II.

The modified criteria for definite diagnosis of NF2 are as follows: Bilateral CN VIII schwannomas on MRI or CT scan (no biopsy necessary). Any two of the following first degree relatives with NF2 and unilateral early-onset CN VIII schwannoma (age 30 years): Meningioma, glioma, schwannoma, juvenile posterior subcapsular lenticular opacity (juvenile cortical cataract)

NF 2 is otherwise called NF with bilateral acoustic schwannoma. Autosomal dominant, 50% sporadic

Caused by the mutations in a gene on the long arm of chromosome 22(22q12) that encodes protein merlin or schwannomin (a tumor suppressor).

Table 4.8.6: Imaging features of neurofibromatosis type II	
CT findings: NECT shows **hyperdense CPA mass bilaterally and multiple meningiomas.** Most schwannomas are heterogeneous on NECT scans. **Widening of IAC.** Cystic change is common. Hemorrhage is uncommon. Calcification is rare. **Strong moderately heterogeneous enhancement** after contrast administration is typical. **MR findings:** Schwannomas are generally isointense with brain on T1WI and **heterogeneously hyperintense on T2WI and FLAIR** although macroscopic intratumoral hemorrhage is rare, T2* (GRE, SWI) scans often reveal **"blooming" foci** of microbleeds. Virtually all schwannomas enhance intensely. Approximately 15% have nonenhancing intratumoral cysts. Non-neoplastic peritumoral cysts occur in 5–10% of cases, especially with larger lesions. Spinal intramedullary ependymomas will be seen. Schwannomas are benign slow-growing encapsulated tumors that are composed entirely of well-differentiated Schwann cells. Less common terms are neurinoma and neurilemmoma. Neuroimaging demonstrates a well-circumscribed extra axial mass that originates within or near a cranial nerve.	
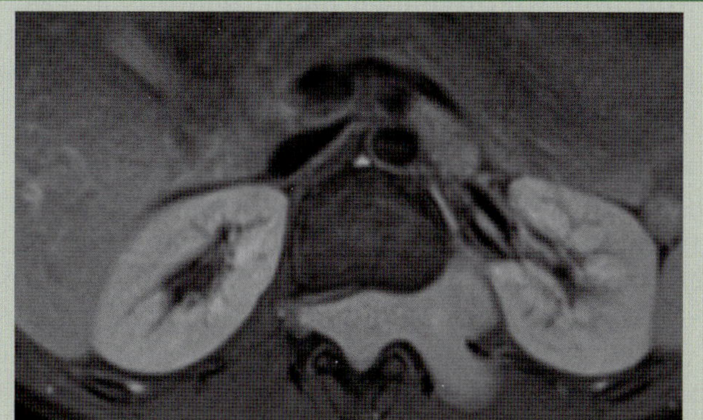 **Fig. 4.8.33:** Neurofibroma causing posterior vertebral body scalloping	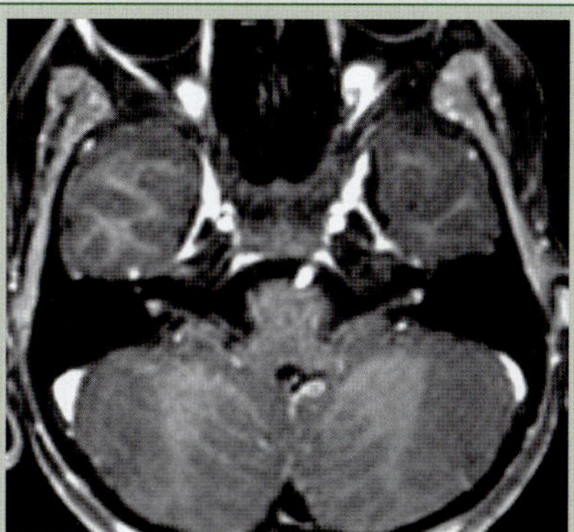 **Fig. 4.8.34:** Multiple meningioma seen anteriorly adjacent to cavernous sinus and small bilateral acoustic schwannoma

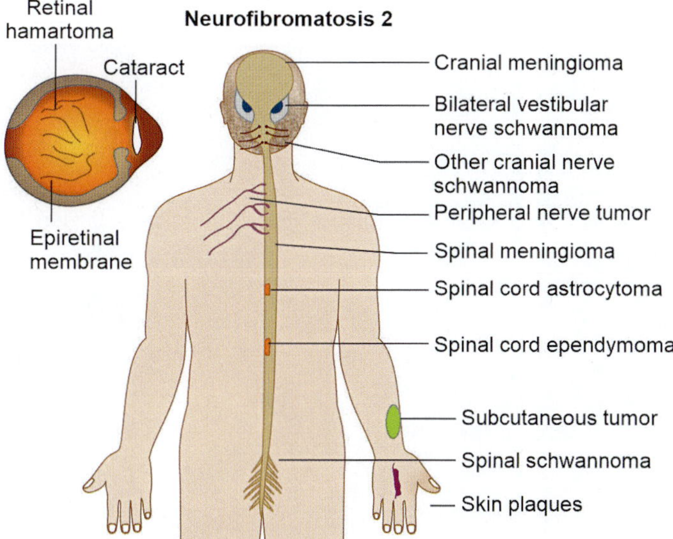

Fig. 4.8.35: Whole body illustration showing neurofibromatosis type 2 manifestations

4.9 CENTRAL NERVOUS SYSTEM

Case No. 9

Clinical history: A 20-year-old man with ataxia

Radiological techniques and observation: Postcontrast MR images of the brain (Fig. 4.9.1) show large cystic lesion with enhancing mural nodule in the superior aspect of left cerebellar hemisphere causing compression of IVth ventricle. Another similar lesion with large enhancing solid component noted in right cerebellar hemisphere. With age of the patient, this raises the possibility of hemangioblastoma in von Hippel–Lindau (VHL) syndrome.

MRI spine with contrast (Fig. 4.9.2): T2 axial images of cervical spine of same patient show hyperintense lesion in cord with multiple flow voids feeding into the lesion. Sagittal contrast enhanced T1 (Fig. 4.9.3): Shows intensely enhancing lesion in subpial location of cervical spine at C4–C5 level. Another similar enhancing lesion noted in the region of obex and also in C7–T1 level with surrounding nonenhancing syrinx in cervical and thoracic cord. There is also minimal leptomeningeal enhancement in anterior aspect of the cord.

Interpretations: A–20 years old male with lesion in cerebellum and spinal cord, C–cystic lesion with enhancing mural nodule and multiple flow void, B–syrinx, leptomeningeal enhancement, D–multiple hemangioblastoma (VHL).

Principal diagnosis: The features are consistent with von Hippel–Lindau (VHL) syndrome, with the cerebellar and spinal lesions likely representing hemangioblastomas. Further patient should be evaluated for other visceral manifestations.

Differential diagnosis: (This is a classical case, hence no differential diagnosis needed, however, the following differentials are for finer discussion)

1. **Pilocytic astrocytoma** with drop metastasis—tend to occur in children, tumor nodule lacks vascular flow voids. Tumor nodule often does not invade pial or ependymal surface.
2. **Vascular metastasis:** Irregularly thickened enhancing wall should raise the possibility of a more aggressive lesion, such as a metastasis or glioblastoma.
3. **Hemispheric medulloblastoma** with drop metastasis in teenager or young adult: Rare; occur in peripheral cerebellar hemisphere, may appear extraparenchymal, solid, gray matter intensity on T2WI.
4. **Multiple arteriovenous malformations** in vascular neurocutaneous syndrome (like Osler-Weber-Rendu syndrome) which does not show this type of enhancement.

Management: Urgent neurosurgical referral for obstructive hydrocephalus. Surgical resection of symptomatic cerebellar/spinal hemangioblastoma. Stereotactic radiosurgery provides tumor control in 70–90%. Further ultrasound abdomen/CT abdomen is indicated in this case to rule out other visceral manifestations like pancreatic cysts, renal cysts, renal cell carcinoma, pheochromocytoma.

Discussion: von Hippel tumor—retinal angiomatosis; Lindau tumor—CNS hemangioblastoma.

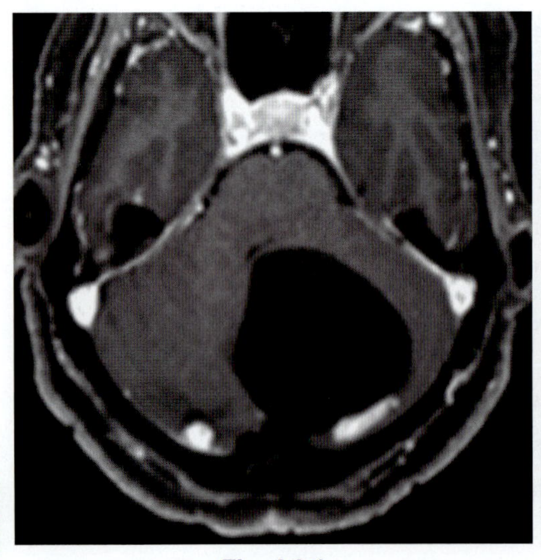

Fig. 4.9.1

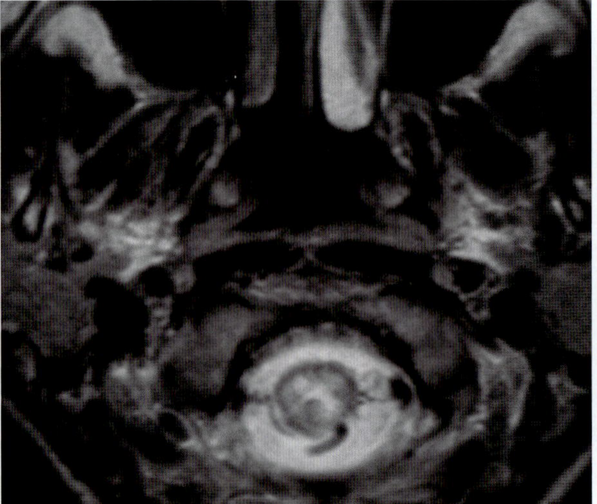

Fig. 4.9.2

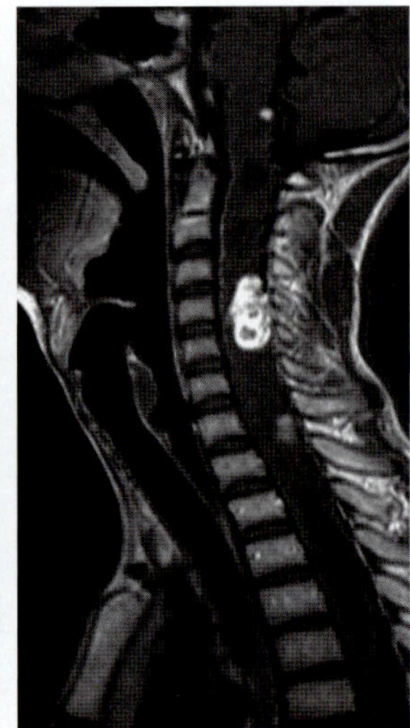

Fig. 4.9.3

Some presentations of VHL are shown below

Pancreatic neuroendocrine tumor with left renal carcinoma (Figs 4.9.7, 4.9.8, 4.9.9)

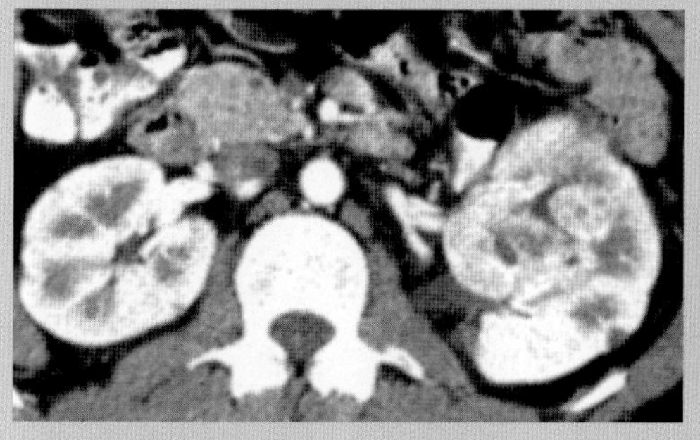

Fig. 4.9.4

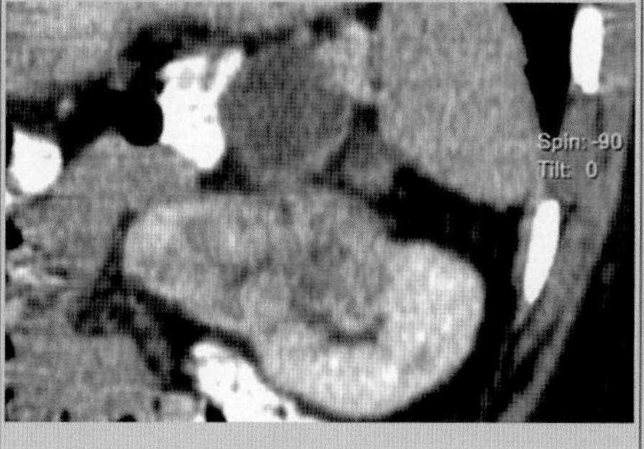

Fig. 4.9.5

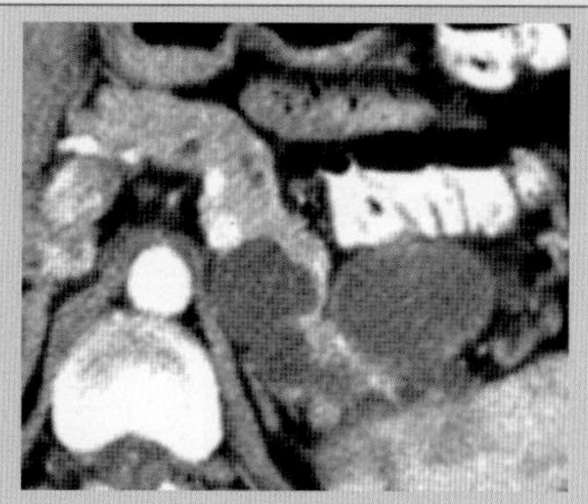

Fig. 4.9.6

In case of cases that close mimic to above VHL case, we can expect a lymphoma with both pancreas and renal involvement.

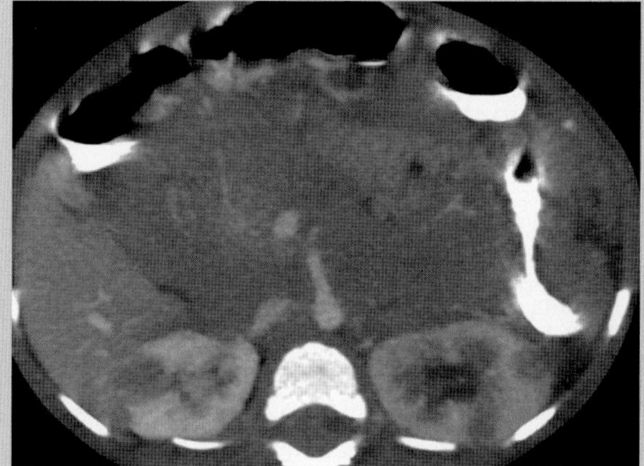
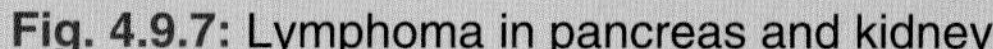

Fig. 4.9.7: Lymphoma in pancreas and kidney

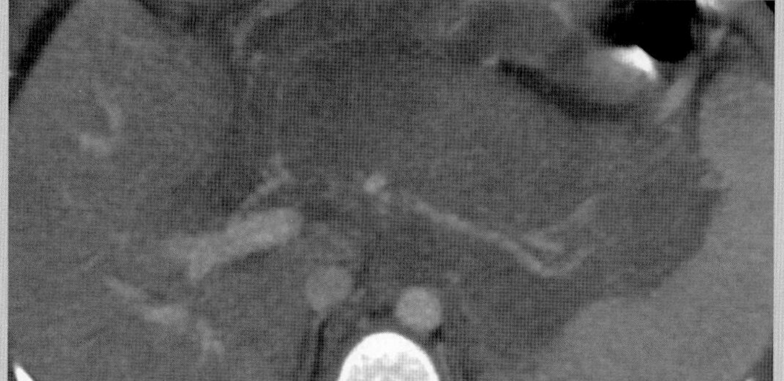

Fig. 4.9.8: Pancreatic lymphoma

Spinal hemangioblastoma with multiple renal cysts (Figs 4.9.12 and 4.9.13) in VHL. In tuberous sclerosis, think of renal AML with bony lesions.

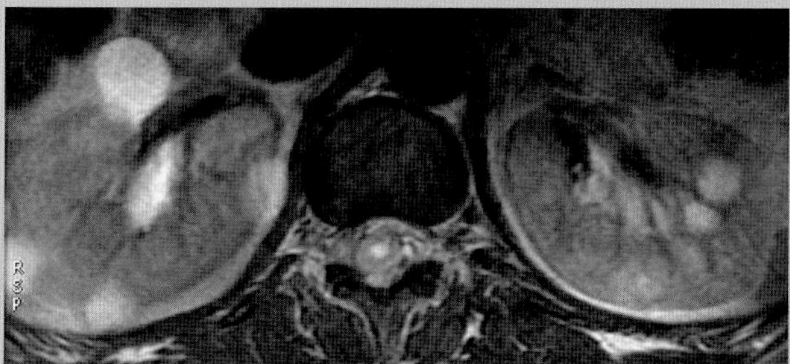

Fig. 4.9.9: Bilateral renal cortical cysts with spinal hemangioblastoma

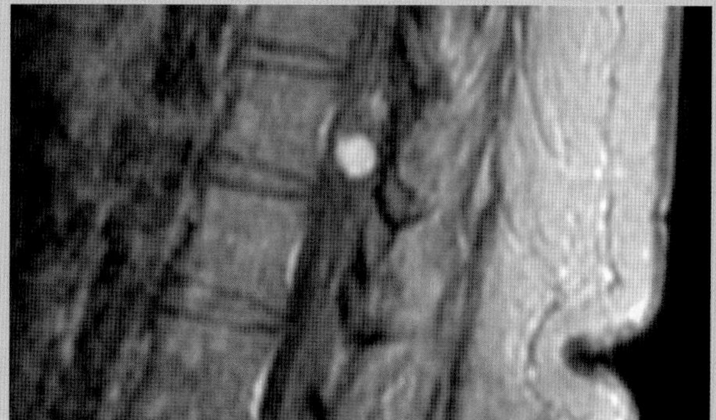

Fig. 4.9.10: Spinal hemangioblastoma in VHL

Retinal, spinal hemangioblastoma with tiny hemangioblastoma in cerebellum and pancreatic NET.

The manifestations include: 1) Retina: Retinal hemangioblastoma, 2) CNS: Cerebellar and spinal hemangioblastomas 3) Head and neck: Endolymphatic sac tumours (Heffner tumour), 4) Pancreas: Pancreatic cysts, serous cystadenoma, 5) Pancreatic: Neuroendocrine tumors (non-secretory), 6) Kidneys: Renal cysts and clear cell carcinomas, 7) Adrenal: Pheochromocytomas, 8) Reproductive organs: Epididymal cysts, papillary cystadenoma of epididymis and broad ligament in females.

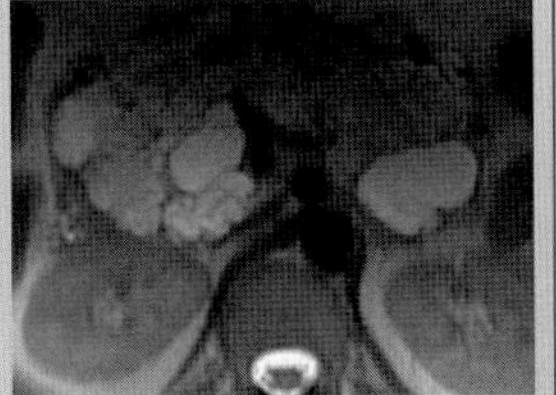

Fig. 4.9.11: Pancreatic NET in VHL

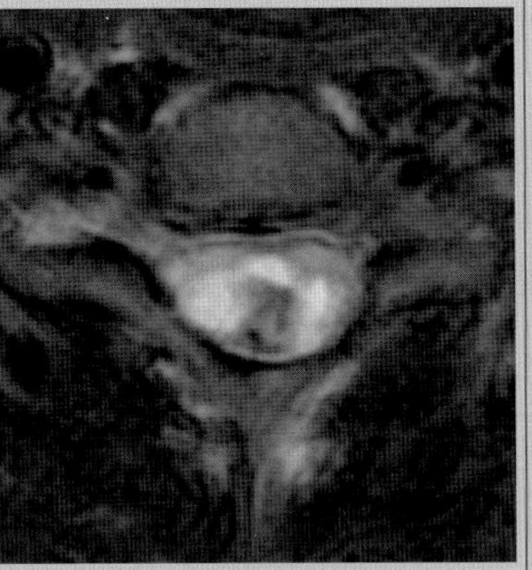

Fig. 4.9.12: Spinal hemangioblastoma in VHL

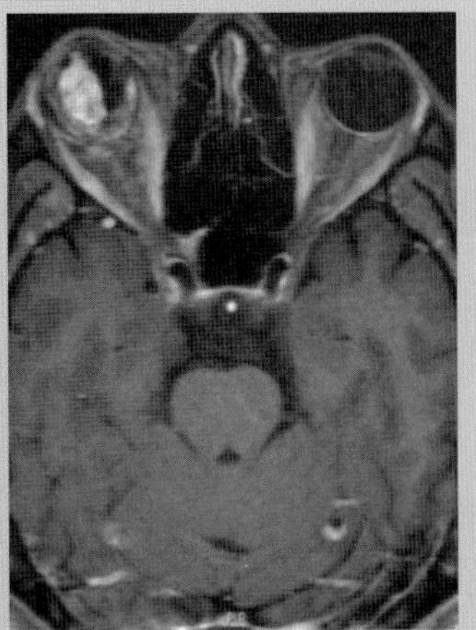

Fig. 4.9.13: Right retinal and cerebellar hemangioblastoma in VHL

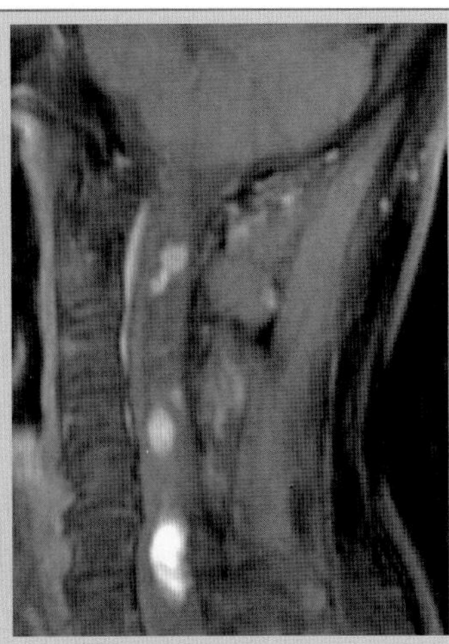

Fig. 4.9.14: Spinal hemangioblastoma in VHL

In case of NF1 we can find optic nerve glioma with FASI changes. NF2 will show optic nerve meningioma with bilateral acoustic schwannoma. In multiple sclerosis/NMO, we get optic neuritis with brain and spinal cord changes.

Table 4.9.1: Tumours associated with neurocutaneous syndromes

NF1	*NF2*	*VHL*	*Tuberous sclerosis*	*Sturge-Weber*
Neurofibroma Schwannoma Glioma: Optic nerve, diffuse brain stem glioma, spinal astrocytoma Pheochromocytoma Malignant peripheral nerve sheath tumour Carcinoid, leiomyoma, ganglioglioma leukaemia	Multiple schwannoma Meningioma Ependymoma	Retina: Retinal hemangioblastoma CNS: Cerebellar and spinal hemangioblastomas Head and neck: Endolymphatic sac tumours Pancreas: Cysts, carcinoma, hemangioblastoma, serous cystadenoma, neuroendocrine tumours Kidneys: Clear cell carcinomas Adrenal: Pheochromocytomas	Renal angiomyolipoma Subependymal giant cell astrocytoma Cardiac rhabdomyoma Renal cell carcinoma Oncocytoma Pheochromocytoma	Choroidal Haemangioma Leptomeningeal angioma

Diagnostic criteria: a) >1 hemangioblastoma of CNS, b) 1 hemangioblastoma + visceral manifestation, c) 1 manifestation with family history.

von Hippel-Lindau (VHL) syndrome is an inherited, autosomal dominant syndrome.

Phenotypic classification: Based on absence or presence of pheochromocytoma. Type 1: Low risk of pheochromocytoma; Type 2: High risk of pheochromocytoma, Type 2A (RCC low risk), Type 2B (RCC high risk), Type 2C (familial pheochromocytoma without either HGBL or RCC).

In VHL typically multiple hemangioblastoma (HGBL) occurs 40–50% in spinal cord (posterior half), 40–72% infratentorial in cerebellum (posterior > anterior). Most common site of supratentorial HGBL—pituitary infundibulum. HGBL arises from pia, if lesion is in deep white matter or center of cord, it is not HGBL.

NIH (National Institute of Health) recommendations: Contrast-enhanced MR of brain/spinal cord every 2 years from age 11 years. US of abdomen from 11 years, yearly. Abdominal CT from 20 years, yearly/every other year. MR of temporal bone if hearing loss/tinnitus/vertigo.

Syndromes associated with increased incidence of brain tumors: Basal cell nevus syndrome, or Gorlin syndrome (chromosome 9q31)—basal cell nevi and carcinomas, odontogenic keratocyst, ribbon ribs, phalangeal deformity and pitting, falcine calcification, craniofacial deformities, scoliosis, and medulloblastoma.

Cowden disease (chromosome 10q23) Multiple hamartomas, mucocutaneous tumors, fibrocystic breast disease, polyps, thyroid adenoma, Lhermitte-Duclos disease.

von Hippel-Lindau disease (chromosome 3p25) Central nervous system hemangioblastomas combine with retinal hemangioblastomas (67%); cysts of the kidney, pancreas, and liver; renal cell carcinomas; islet cell tumors; and pheochromocytomas, endolymphatic sac tumors, cystadenomas of the epididymis, and broad ligament to form von Hippel-Lindau (VHL) disease. RCC is reported to develop in 24 to 45% of patients with VHLD and is often multifocal and bilateral; **Li-Fraumeni syndrome (chromosome 17p13)** increased rate of breast cancers, soft tissue sarcomas, osteosarcomas, leukemia. Autosomal dominant with astrocytomas, PNET, choroid plexus tumors, CNS tumors in 13.5%; **Maffucci syndrome** enchondromas, soft-tissue cavernomas; **neurofibromatosis types 1 and 2; Ollier syndrome** multiple enchondromas.

Tuberous sclerosis [chromosome 9 (9q34) or 16 (16p13)] adenoma sebaceum (60 to 90% of cases), mental retardation (50%), and seizures, periventricular subependymal nodules (candle guttering) (90 to 100%), cortical and subcortical peripheral tubers (94% of patients on MR), white matter hamartomatous lesions, and subependymal giant cell astrocytomas (6 to 16%), retinal hamartomas, shagreen patches , ungual fibromas, rhabdomyomas of the heart, angiomyolipoma of the kidney (50 to 90%) and cystic skeletal lesion. **Turcot syndrome (chromosomes 5q21, 3p21, 7p22)** colonic familial polyposis, glioblastoma, rare medulloblastoma.

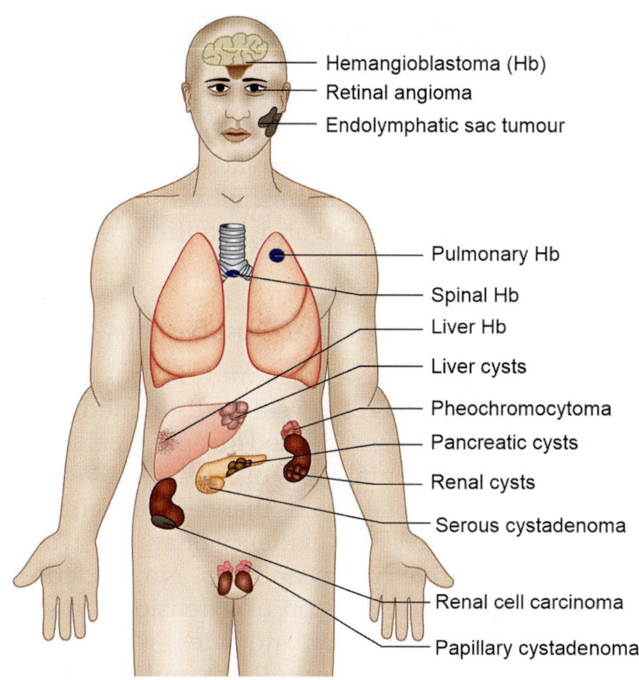

Fig. 4.9.15: Whole body illustration of VHL

4.10 CENTRAL NERVOUS SYSTEM

Case No. 10

Clinical history: A 28-year-old female with papilledema. She was complaining of diminished vision, associated with intermittent headache and vomiting for the last one year.

Radiological Techniques and Observations

MRI axial FLAIR (Fig. 4.10.1) and T1 postcontrast axial (Fig. 4.10.2) images reveal well-defined FLAIR hyperintense bubbly mass attached to septum pellucidum in anterior body—frontal horn of left lateral ventricle. Lesion shows heterogenous enhancement with non-enhancing cystic areas. No evidence of any obstructive and non-obstructive hydrocephalus. No evidence of any extraventricular extension or extension across the midline. No subependymal nodules/white matter lesions. No evidence of any other similar lesions in visualised brain parenchyma. Visualised calvarium and soft tissue appears normal. No abnormal meningeal enhancement seen.

Interpretation: A—Young adult with lesion in anterior body—frontal horn of lateral ventricle attached to septum pellucidum, C—microcystic bubbly lesion with non-enhancing cystic areas, B—without hydrocephalus, calcification, parenchymal extension, D—central neurocytoma.

Principal Diagnosis—Central Neurocytoma

Management: Complete surgical resection is the treatment of choice. If resection is incomplete, radiation therapy and radiosurgery may be helpful.

Brief discussion about the condition—central neurocytoma.

It is a well-differentiated benign neuroepithelial tumour with mature neurocytic elements.

Location: Located in the lateral ventricles, arises from septum pellucidum near foramen of Monro. It can extend through foramen of Monro and involve contralateral ventricle.

Epidemiology: Tumour of middle-aged adults accounting for nearly half of the cases. It represents 0.25 to 0.5% of all intracranial neoplasms and 10% of all intraventricular tumours.

Symptoms are due to increased intracranial pressure. Focal neurological deficits are uncommon. They are found incidentally in imaging.

Extraventricular neurocytomas: Neoplasms that resemble neurocytoma that have reported outside the ventricular system. Only distinguishing feature from central neurocytoma is location. Most common presenting symptom is epilepsy. **Imaging:** These are more commonly located in parasellar region where they resemble pituitary macroadenoma. Some of these lesions

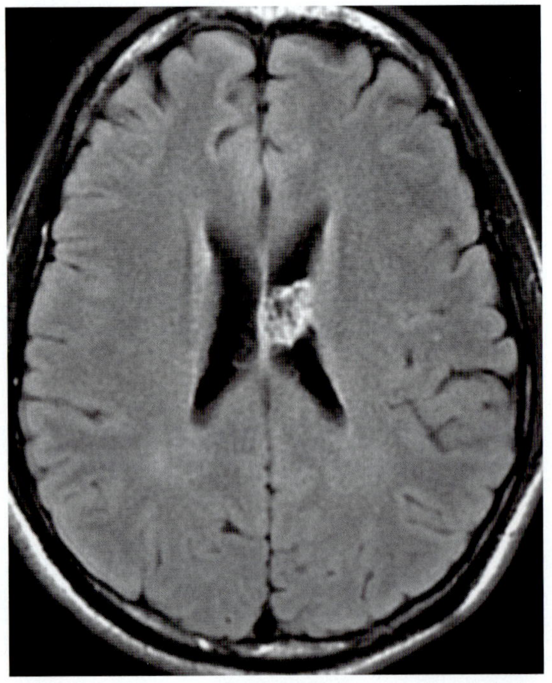

Fig. 4.10.1

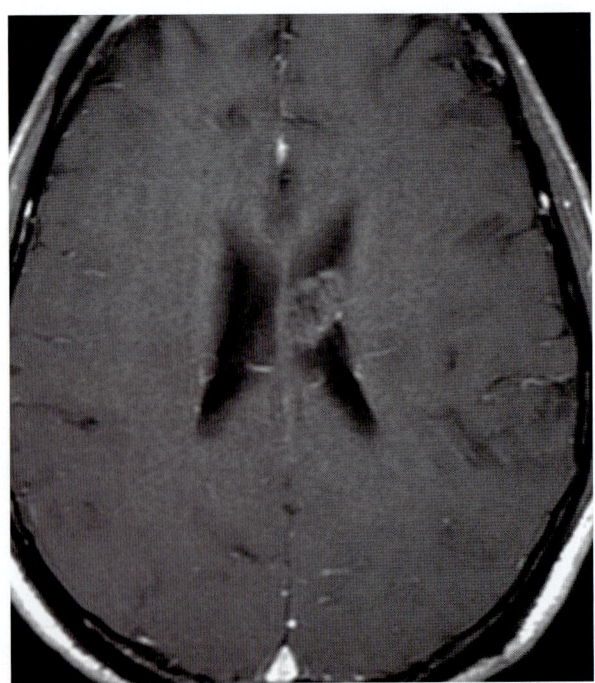

Fig. 4.10.2

Table 4.10.1: Differential diagnosis for lesions attached to septum pellucidum along anterior horn or frontal horn of lateral ventricle

1. Subependymoma Seen in older age group—5th to 6th decade. Most common site is 4th ventricle outflow tract followed by lateral and third ventricle. Central neurocytomas are tumours of young adults while subependymoma is more common in older adults.	Predominantly hyperintense solid intraventricular mass with no oedema seen in adjacent brain parenchyma. Can be indistinguishable on imaging from central neurocytoma. Usually faint or no enhancement.	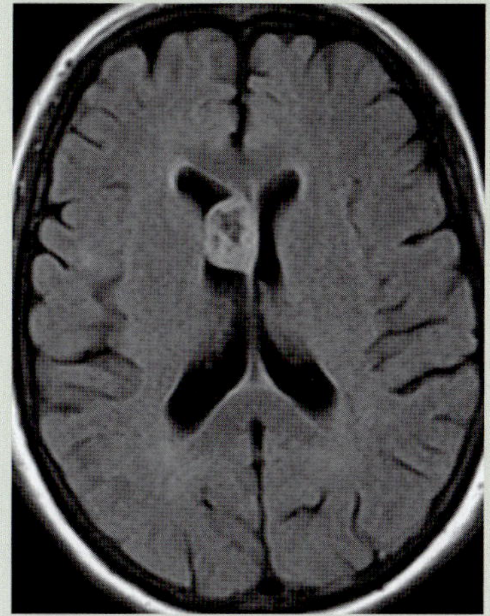 **Fig. 4.10.3:** Subependymoma
2. Subependymal giant cell astrocytoma (SEGA) Typically occurs in the first two decades, mean age of 11 years Associated with tuberous sclerosis.	Enlarging enhancing mass in foramen of Monro of size more than 1.2 cm in patients with TSC, causing obstructive hydrocephalus. Calcifications are common. Presence of interval growth suggests SEGA. Look for tuberous sclerosis changes in brain.	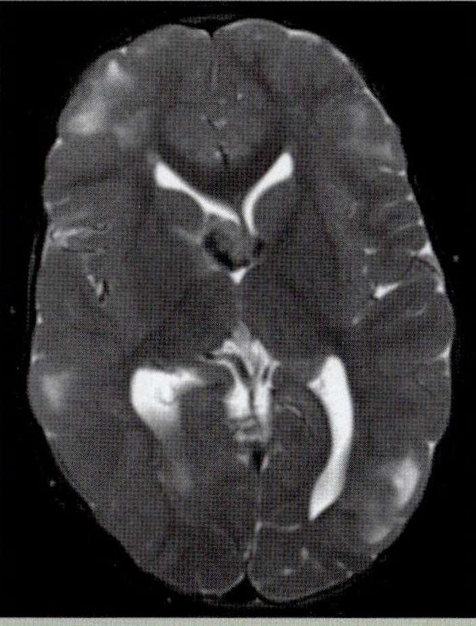 **Fig. 4.10.4:** SEGA
3. Ependymoma Children between age of 1–5 years. 2/3- infratentorial 1/3-supratentorial (50 percent shows **calcification** and 10 percent shows haemorrhage) 50 percentage of supratentorial ependymomas are **extra ventricular**. Location—cerebral hemisphere >third ventricle > lateral ventricle	CT—mixed attenuation. Large complex appearing mixed solid/cystic hemispheric mass Hyperdense—solid portion, hypodense—cystic component, calcifications—44 percentage. Lesion may show bone destruction. MR—variable morphological characters—T1-iso to hypointense. Cyst will follow CSF.T2—Variable with morphological features—cyst with mural nodule/solid mass/huge partially necrotic mass.	GRE: Blooming indicates haemorrhage or calcifications. Lesion shows diffusion restriction. On T1 postcontrast imaging lesion shows moderate enhancement 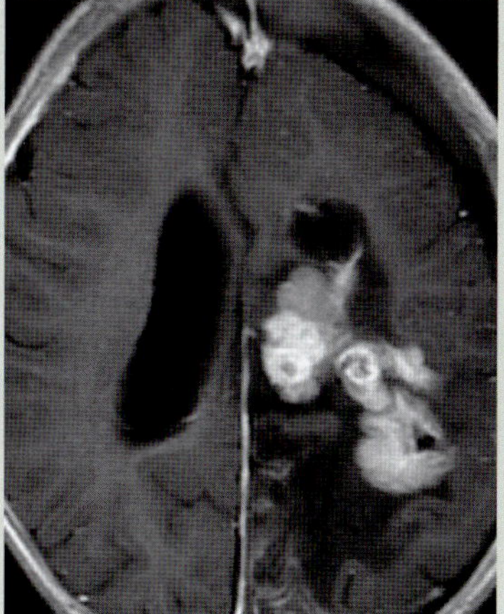 **Fig. 4.10.5:** Ependymoma

Contd...

Table 4.10.1: Differential diagnosis for lesions attached to septum pellucidum along anterior horn or frontal horn of lateral ventricle *(Contd...)*

4. Intraventricular metastasis. Uncommon, usually in older patients. Primary will be often known.	Most common site is trigone of lateral ventricle due to high vascularity of choroid plexus. Most common primary is renal cell carcinoma. Other causes are melanoma, breast carcinoma and melanoma.		
5. Colloid cyst (para-physeal cysts): Location—foramen of Monro. They are solitary lesions. Mean diameter of 1.5 cm. They can cause symptoms when it obstructs CSF flow at foramen of Monro. Most common differentials include ectatic basilar artery (NECT) and CSF flow artefact in MR	CT-Density depends on presence of haemorrhage, calcification, hemosiderin and mucin. Nearly two-thirds are hyperdense while one-third are hypo to isodense. MR—signal intensity varies with cyst contents, typically T1 hyper (T1 signal depends on cholesterol concentration) and T2 isointense. Peripheral rim enhancement+	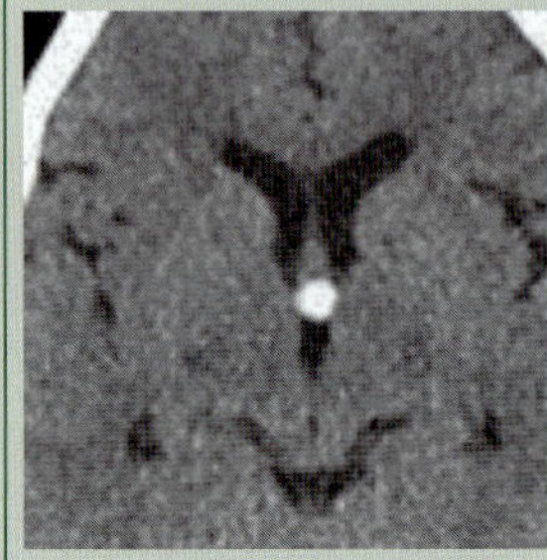 **Fig. 4.10.6:** Colloid cyst in CT	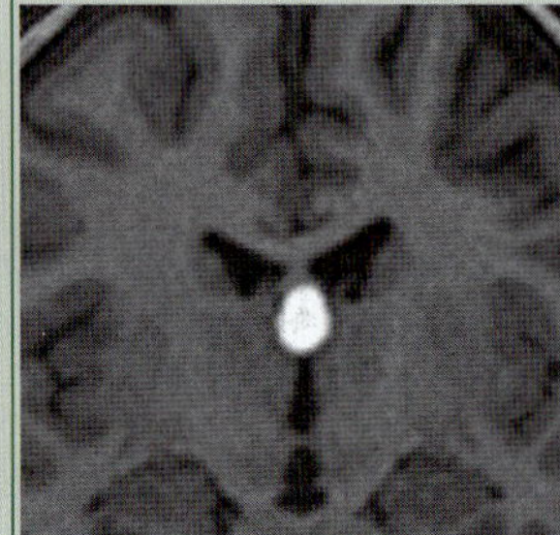 **Fig. 4.10.7:** Colloid cyst in T1W MRI
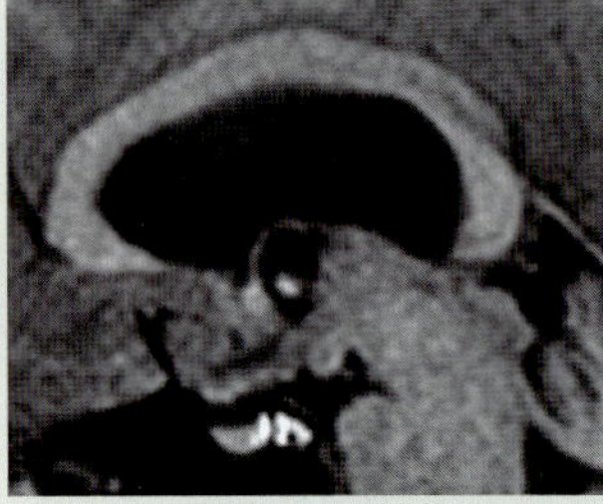 **Fig. 4.10.8** Intraventricular neurocysticercosis on T1W sagittal	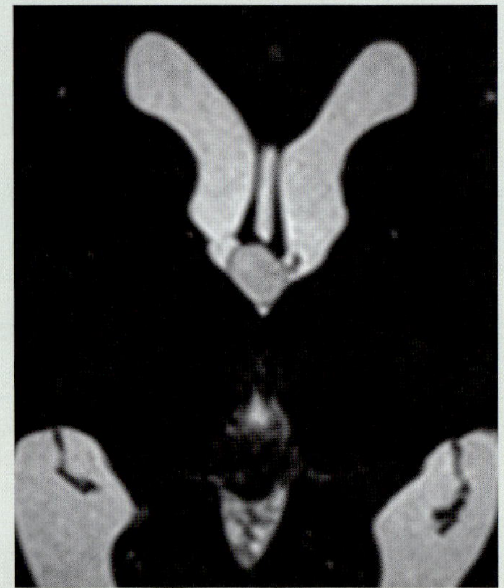 **Fig. 4.10.9** Intraventricular neurocysticercosis on CISS	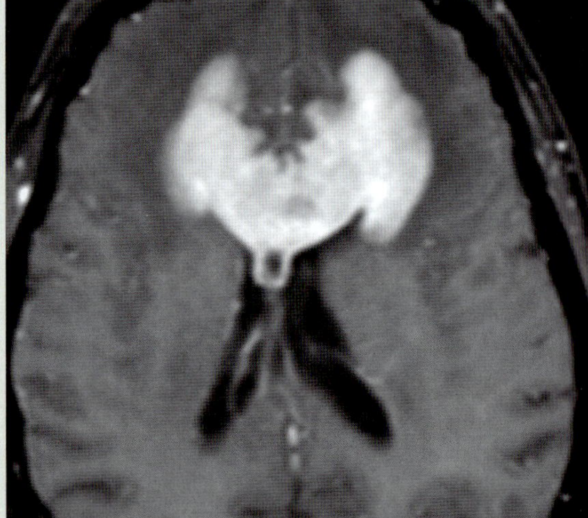 **Fig. 4.10.10:** Lymphoma arising from the frontal horns of lateral ventricle showing avid homogenous contrast enhancement in T1 + C image	
Other differentials include intraventricular gliomas, oligodendroglioma, lymphomas, intraventricular cysts and vascular malformations.			

have T2 bubbly appearance similar to DNET or central neurocytoma, while some others have cyst with mural nodule configuration similar to ganglioglioma.

Imaging features of central neurocytoma: Bubbly mass in the body or frontal horn of lateral ventricle is the classical finding. Plain CT—usually mixed solid and cystic (iso to hyperdense). Calcifications are common in 50 to 70 percent cases. Obstructive hydrocephalus is common. Rarely complicated by haemorrhage. **CECT**—moderate heterogenous enhancement is seen.

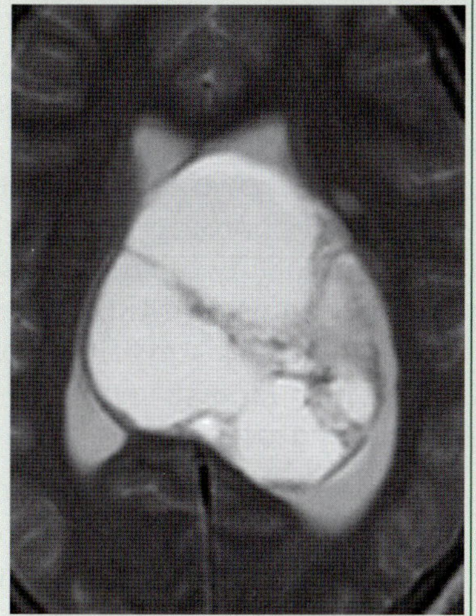

Fig. 4.10.11: Central neurocytoma seen as bubbly mass in the body of lateral ventricle in axial T2W

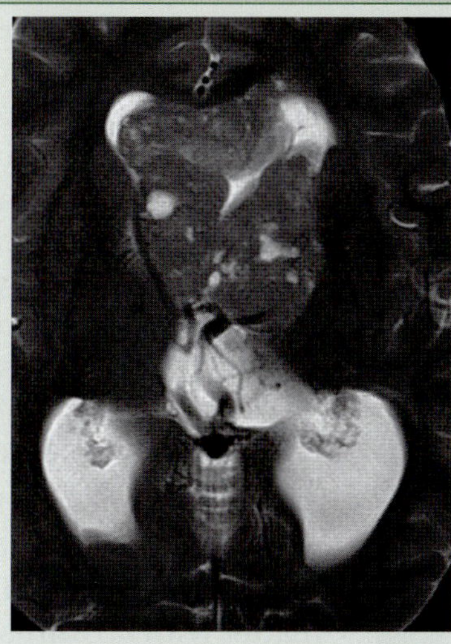

Fig. 4.10.12: Central neurocytoma seen as bubbly mass in the body of lateral ventricle in axial T2W

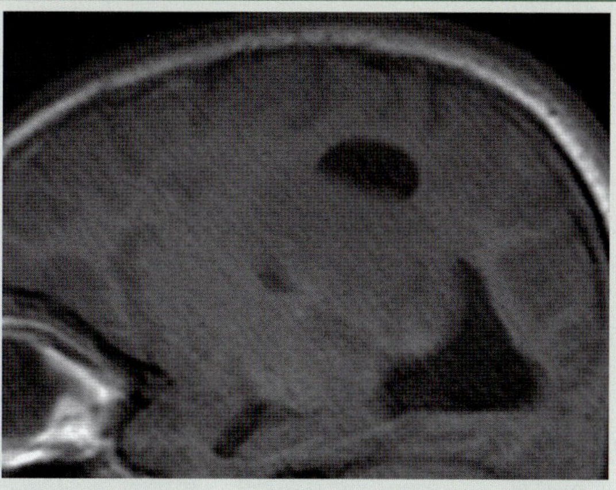

Fig. 4.10.13: C—Central neurocytoma seen as bubbly mass in the body of lateral ventricle on sagittal T1W

MRI-T1WI: Heterogeneous, mostly isointense to gray matter, cysts are hypointense. Prominent flow voids may be seen. T2WI-Heterogeneous, hyperintense **bubbly** appearance. Associated hydrocephalus is common. Calcification are hypointense. **FLAIR**-Heterogeneous, predominantly hyperintense mass

GRE: Calcification seen as areas of "blooming". **T1WI** C+T1 C -moderate heterogenous enhancement. DWI: It will show diffusion restriction in solid components due to hypercellularity. **MR spectroscopy**: Presence of some NAA and **glycine** at 3.5 ppm with a TE of 135 ms is highly suggestive of neurocytoma.

4.11 CENTRAL NERVOUS SYSTEM

Case No. 11

Clinical history: A 1-year-old female child with macrocrania and seizures.

Radiological technique: Figure 4.11.1 shows MRI brain T1 sagittal, T2 axial, T1 FS axial with contrast, diffusion weighted images with ADC map, SWI, phase images with MR spectroscopy.

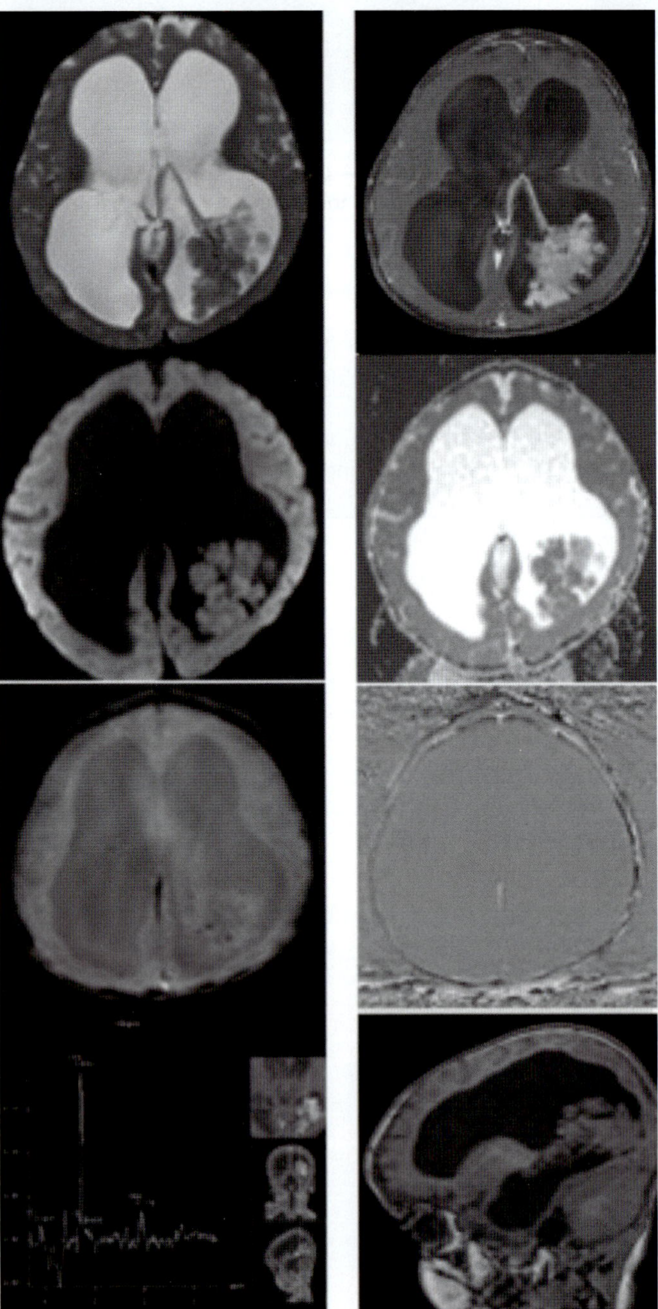

Fig. 4.11.1

Observations: T1 isointense, T2 isointense smooth lobulated cauliflower-like mass lesion noted in the atrium of left lateral ventricle. The lesion does not show any diffusion restriction. T2* image shows foci of blooming which appears bright on phase images possibly blood products. With contrast, the lesion appears to enhance intensely with contrast. Glomus of choroid plexus not visualized separately. No evidence of any calcifications. No evidence of any parenchymal extension. MRS shows a tall choline peak, short NAA peak and a myoinositol peak. Enlargement of lateral, third and fourth ventricles–nonobstructive communicating hydrocephalus.

Interpretation: A—child (<5 years) with lesion in atrium of lateral ventricle along choroid plexus, C—cauliflower like intensely enhancing T1 isointense lesion to grey matter with no diffusion restriction and tall choline peak, B—nonobstructive hydrocephalus. No parenchymal extension, D—choroid plexus papilloma.

Principal diagnosis: Choroid plexus papilloma. (typical/ atypical). Difficult to distinguish between typical and atypical based on imaging alone.

Further investigations:

1. MRA: May show enlarged choroidal arteries.
2. Contrast enhanced MR of the entire neuroaxis—to look for leptomeningeal dissemination.

Management: Total surgical excision (operative mortality: 24%). Recurrence is rare.

Discussion: Choroid plexus papilloma: Tumor of neuro-epithelial origin—subgroup of non-astrocytic gliomas. WHO grade I tumor.

Location: In children: Glomus of choroid plexus in trigone of lateral ventricles, L > R. In adults: 4th ventricle + cerebellopontine angle. Tri-ventricular CPP: 5%, Extraventricular CPP: Rare, can be seen in brainstem, cerebellum, pituitary fossa and septum pellucidi. Lobulated, frond-like configuration.

Age: Most common in children <2 years of age. Rate of CSF production from choroid plexus papilloma: 1.0 ml/ min (normal rate: 0.2 ml/min). Association: von Hippel-Lindau disease.

WHO grade I occasionally demonstrates CSF dissemination (image entire neuraxis preoperatively!)

Common fetal brain tumors: 1. Teratoma, 2. Astrocytoma, 3. Craniopharyngioma, 4. Primitive neuroectodermal tumor, 5. Choroid plexus papilloma

Table 4.11.1: Differential diagnosis for lesions in trigone of the lateral ventricle

Condition	*Radiological features*	*Image*
Choroid plexus papilloma Child < 5 years with increased prevalence less than 1 year age.	**Nonobstructive hydrocephalus** due to increased CSF secretion. Cauliflower shaped. Elevation of myoinositol in CPP may help to distinguish from choroid plexus carcinoma.	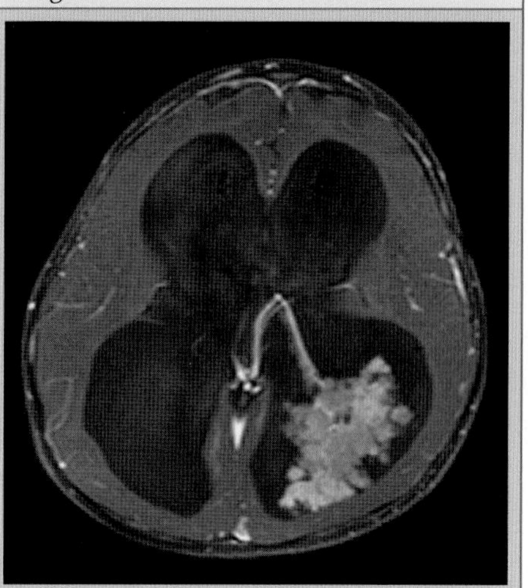 **Fig. 4.11.2:** Choroid plexus papilloma
Choroid plexus carcinoma < 3 years (80%) **Fig. 4.11.3:** Choroid plexus carcinoma 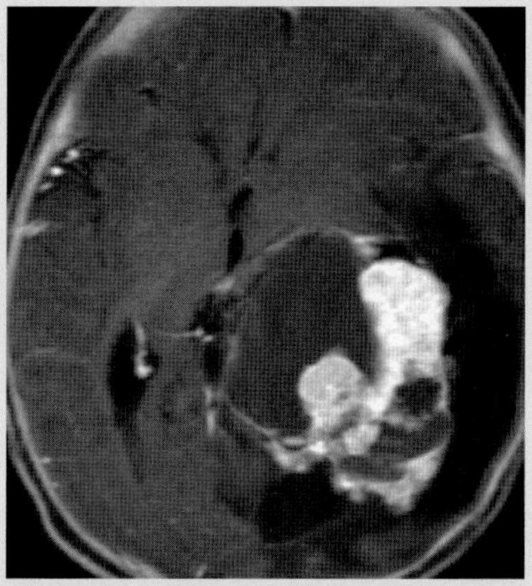	**Intraparenchymal infiltration present.** Heterogenous appearance with CSF spread. Difficult to distinguish based on imaging alone. Associated with **Li-Fraumeni and Aicardi** syndromes.	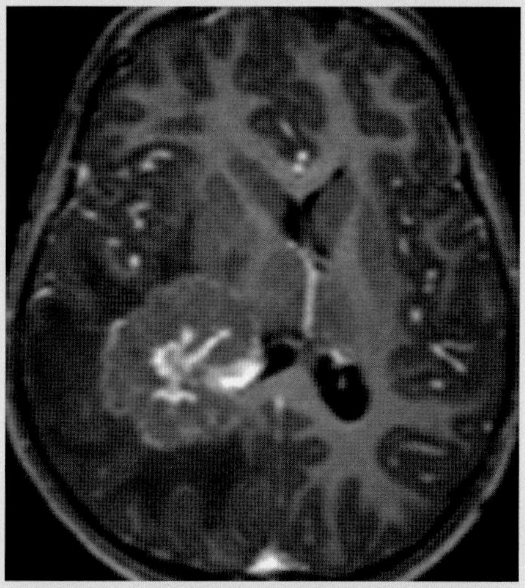 **Fig. 4.11.4** Choroid plexus carcinoma
Intraventricular meningioma >5 yrs. Occurs in older adults, associated with NF2. Well circumscribed with homogenous enhancement.	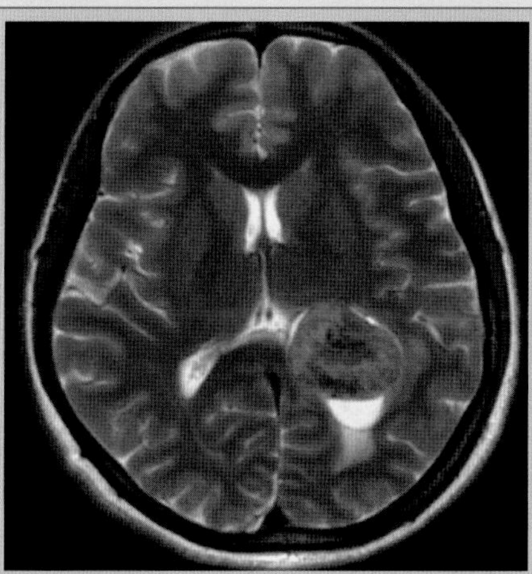 **Fig. 4.11.5:** Intraventricular meningioma on axial T2W	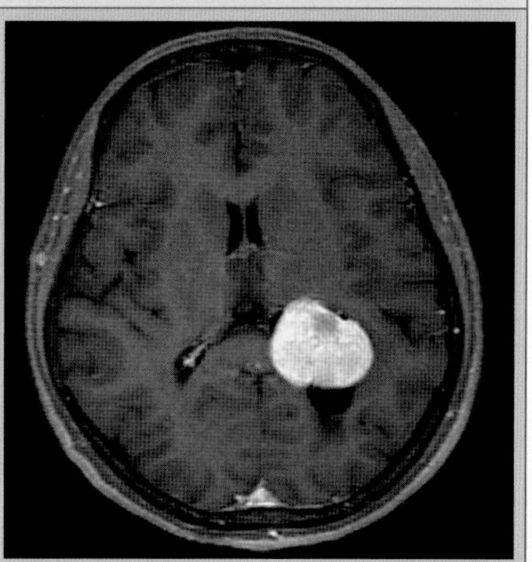 **Fig. 4.11.6:** Intraventricular meningioma on axial T1+C

Contd...

Table 4.11.1: Differential diagnosis for lesions in trigone of the lateral ventricle *(Contd...)*

Choroid plexus xanthogranuloma (adult choroid plexus cyst) usually bilateral in middle aged adults, benign incidental finding.	May show diffusion restriction. Multi-loculated cysts in enhancing choroid plexus.	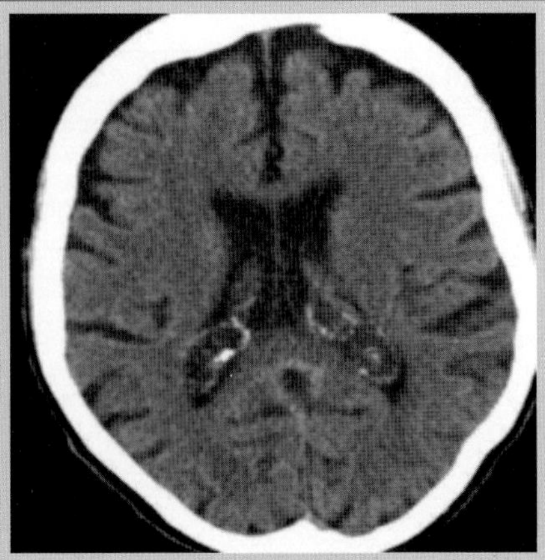 **Fig. 4.11.7:** Choroid plexus xanthogranuloma
Choroid plexitis with abscess	Shows diffusion restriction with peripheral enhancement.	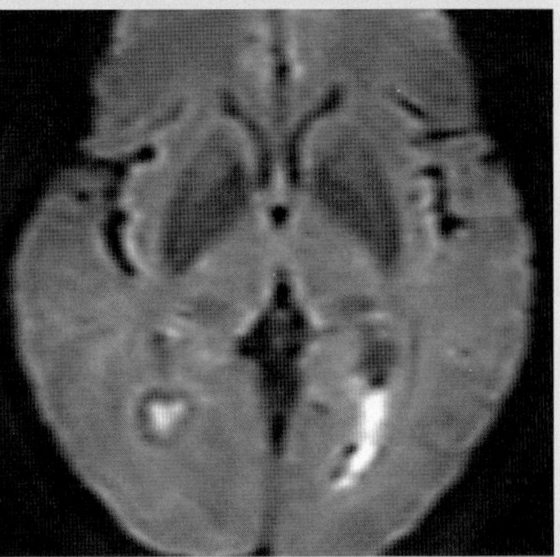 **Fig. 4.11.8:** Intraventricular abscess in case of choroid plexitis
Lymphoma Along subependymal region 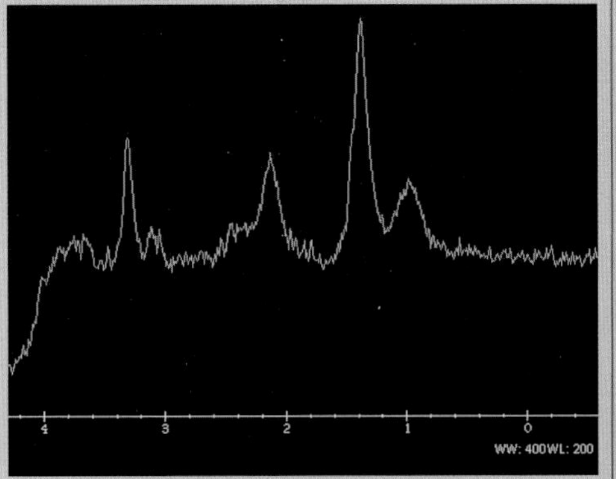 **Fig. 4.11.9:** MRS showing lipid peak in lymphoma at 1.3 ppm	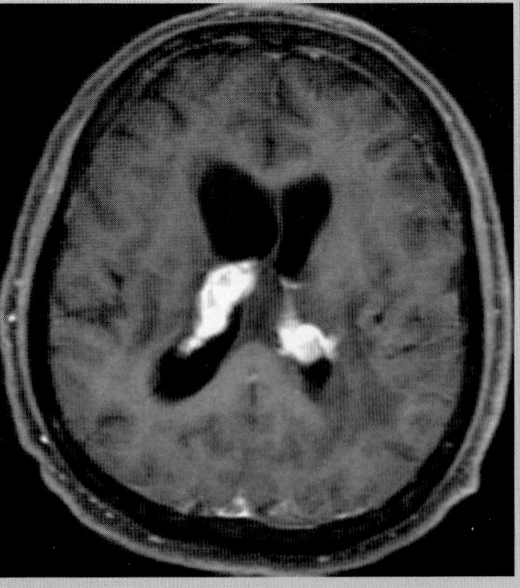 **Fig. 4.11.10:** Enhancing lateral ventricular mass-lymphoma	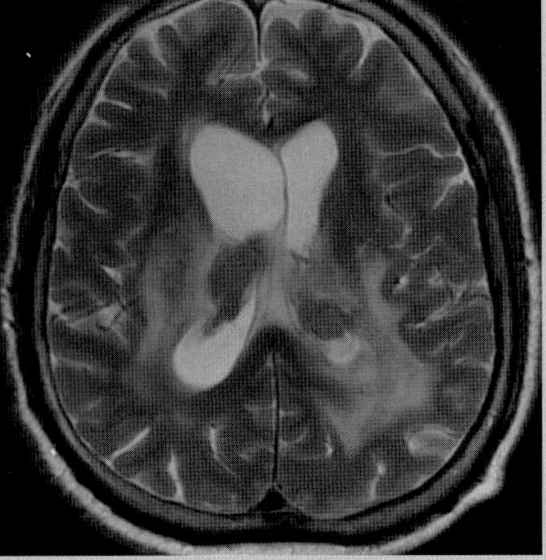 **Fig. 4.11.11:** Isointense lateral ventricle mass in T2W with adjacent edema

Contd...

Table 4.11.1: Differential diagnosis for lesions in trigone of the lateral ventricle *(Contd...)*

Fig. 4.11.12: Right lateral ventricle mass with surrounding edema in case of lymphoma	Fig. 4.11.13: Increased perfusion in case of lymphoma	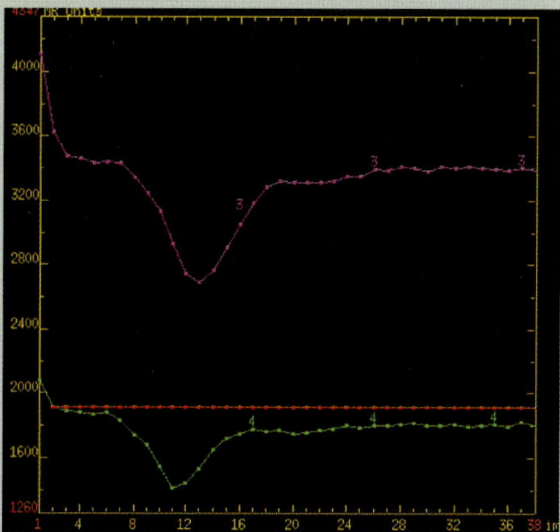 Fig. 4.11.14: Type 1 rapid upstroke curve in lymphoma
Choroid plexus epidermoid cyst 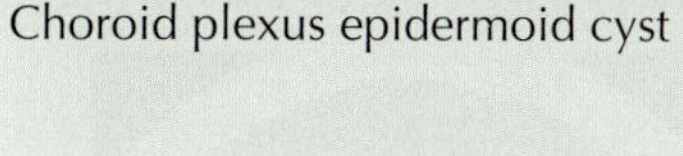	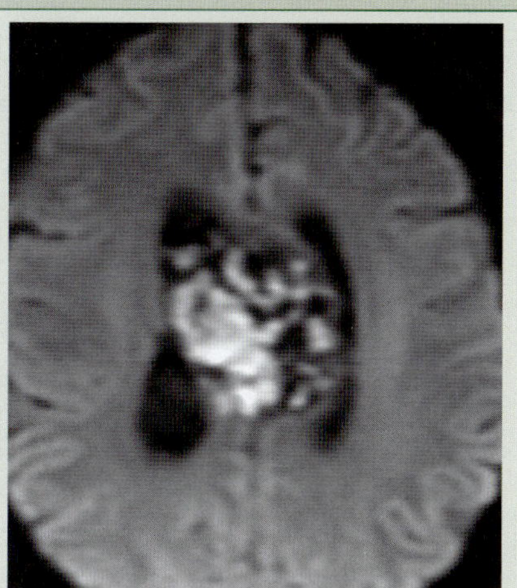 Fig. 4.11.15: Choroid plexus epidermoid cyst showing diffusion restriction	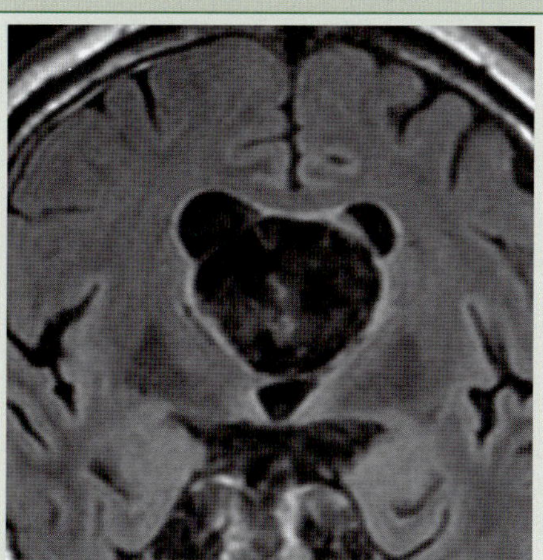 Fig. 4.11.16: T1 hypointense lesion in choroid plexus epidermoid cyst
Choroid plexus ependymoma 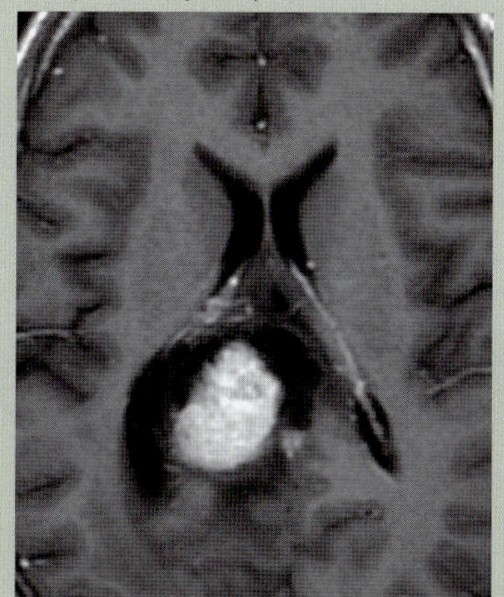 Fig. 4.11.17: Choroid plexus ependymoma	Intraventricular meningioma 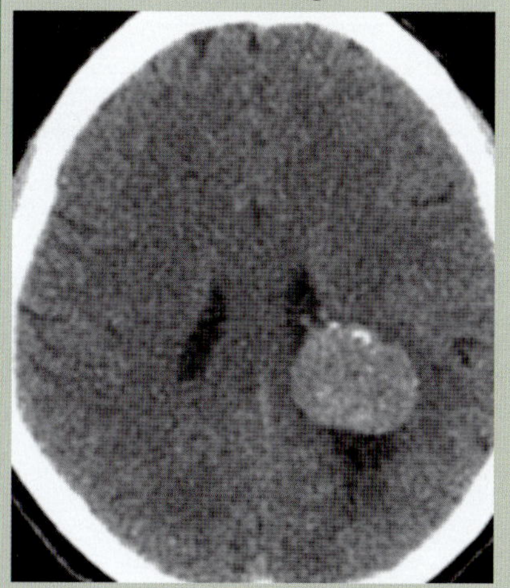 Fig. 4.11.18: Hyperdense mass in plain CT—intraventricular meningioma	Choroid plexus lipoma 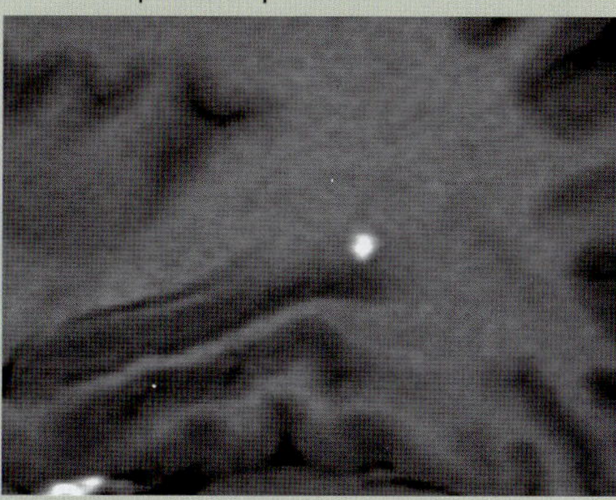 Fig. 4.11.19: T1 hyperintense lesion in temporal horn-choroid plexus lipoma

Contd...

Table 4.11.1: Differential diagnosis for lesions in trigone of the lateral ventricle *(Contd...)*

<table>
<tr><td>Choroid plexus arachnoid cyst</td><td>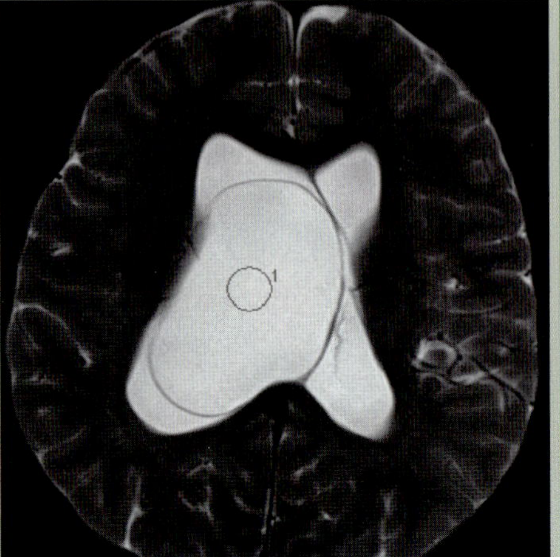
Fig. 4.11.20: T2 hyperintense lesion—choroid plexus arachnoid cyst</td><td>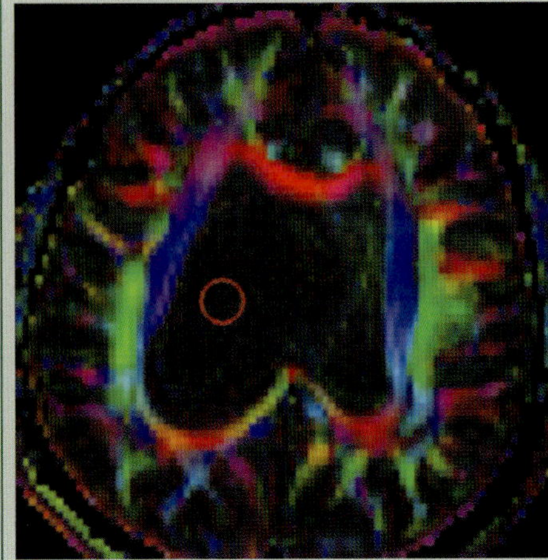
Fig. 4.11.21: DTI showing displacement of white matter tracts in choroid plexus arachnoid cyst</td></tr>
<tr><td>Bilateral enlarged choroid plexus—choroid plexus meningioma /lymphoma</td><td>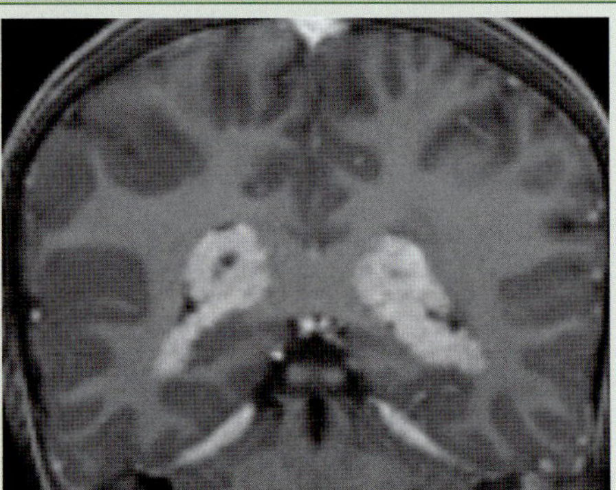
Fig. 4.11.22: Bilateral symmetrically enlarged enhancing choroid plexus—proven case of choroid plexus meningioma</td><td>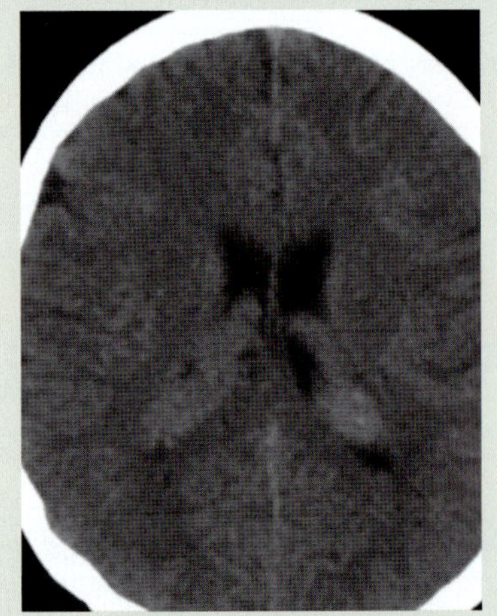
Fig. 4.11.23: Bilateral symmetrically enlarged isodense choroid plexus—proven case of choroid plexus lymphoma</td></tr>
<tr><td colspan="3">Choroid plexus hemorrhage (Figs 4.11.24 to 4.11.25)
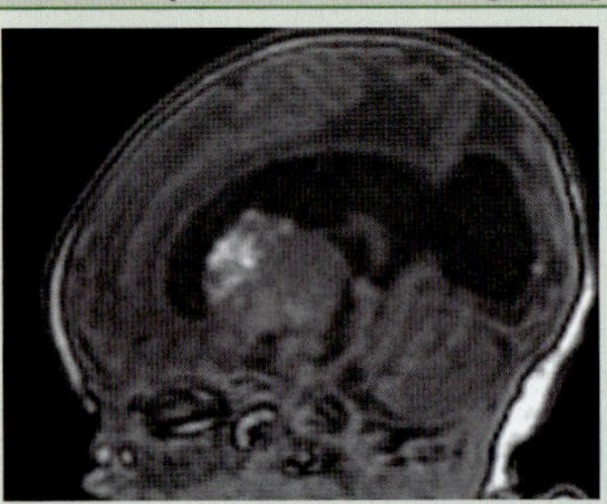
Fig. 4.11.24
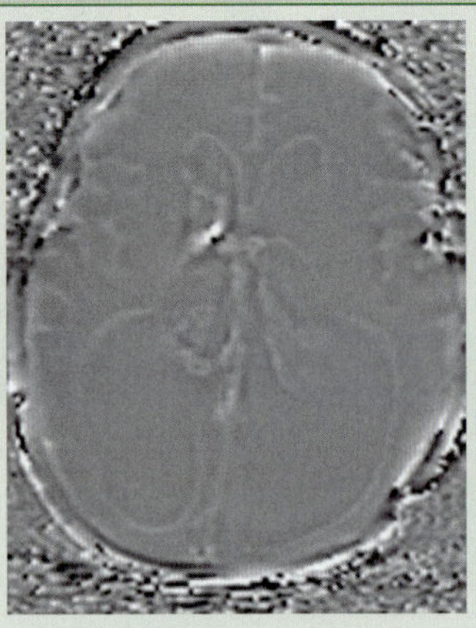
Fig. 4.11.25
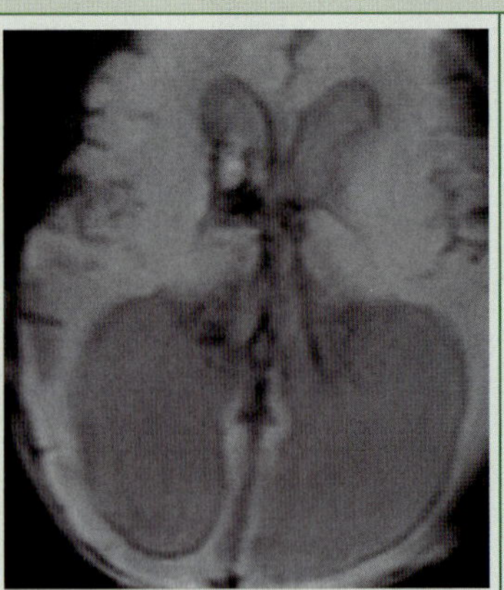
Fig. 4.11.26
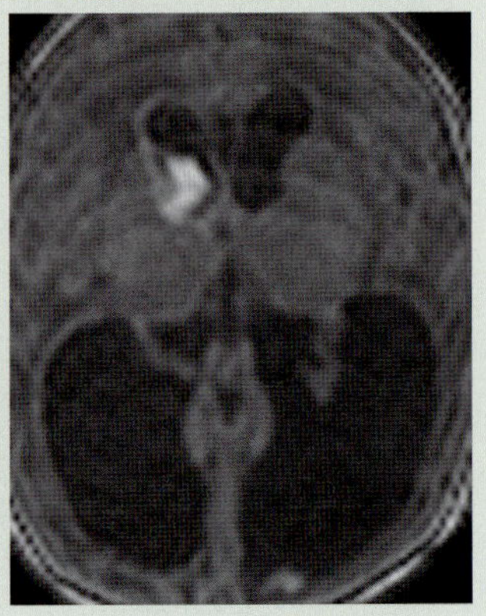
Fig. 4.11.27</td></tr>
</table>

Contd...

Table 4.11.1: Differential diagnosis for lesions in trigone of the lateral ventricle *(Contd...)*

Germinal matrix hemorrhage 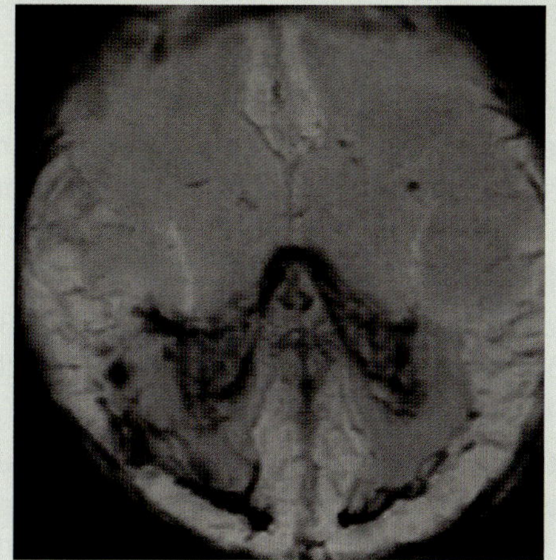 **Fig. 4.11.28:** SWI showing blooming in the areas of choroid plexus hemorrhage	Other conditions of lateral ventricular mass are astroblastoma, desmoplastic infantile ganglioglioma, metastasis, choroid plexus lipoma, intraventricular hemorrhage, ventriculitis with pyocephalus, Newborn choroid plexus cyst, AVM in choroid plexus. Enlarged choroid plexus—unilateral in Sturge-Weber and bilateral in NF2.
Antenatal choroid plexus cyst—sometimes considered as soft marker for aneuploidy (trisomy 18, 21, Klinefelter, Aicardi syndromes) typically seen in the level of atria involving the lateral ventricle. Generally, disappear by 26 to 28 weeks. They are of importance when their size >10 mm, bilateral, multiple, maternal age > 32, elevated maternal serum screening parameters. Postnatal choroid plexus cyst in absence of chromosomal abnormality has no significance.	

Approach to intraventricular mass

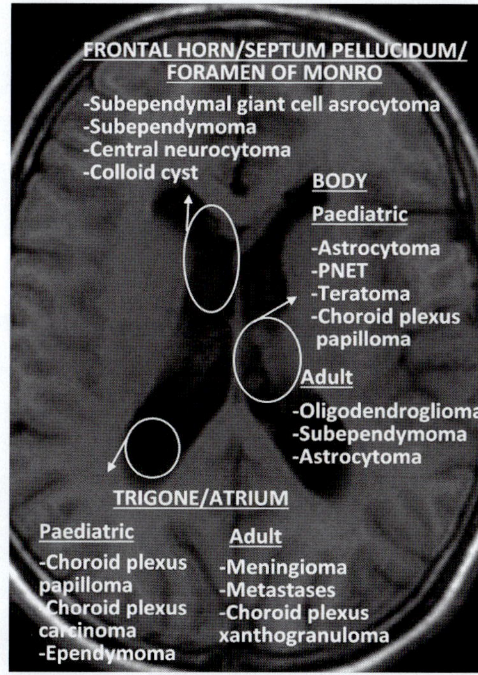

Fig. 4.11.29: Approach to intraventricular lesions—differential diagnosis for lesions in frontal horn/septum pellucidum/ foramen of Monro. Body and trigone of lateral ventricle

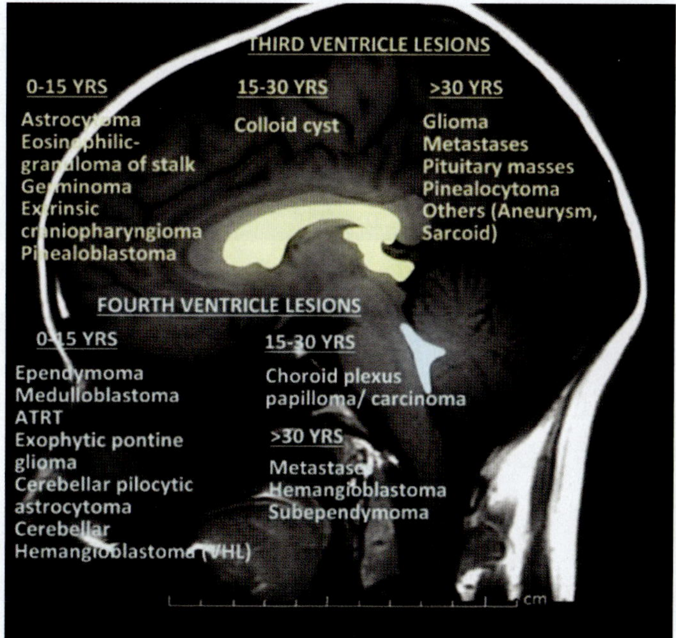

Fig. 4.11.30: Approach to intraventricular lesions—differential diagnosis for lesions in third and fourth ventricle based on age

Syndrome of the trigone: When the intracranial tumors arise in the trigone of the lateral ventricle they present with a distinctive constellation of signs and symptoms. Compression of posterior limb of the internal capsule leads to contralateral limb weakness, contralateral homonymous hemianopia and receptive dysphasia. If mass grows downward far enough to compress the superior cerebellar peduncle, then ipsilateral cerebellar signs may also be present.

4.12 CENTRAL NERVOUS SYSTEM

Case No. 12

Clinical history: 9 years old female child presented with history of headache and vomiting.

Radiological techniques and observation: MR images T2 axial, T2 sagittal, DWI, ADC, T1W+C, T1 C sagittal spine screening (Figs 4.12.7 to 4.12.8) are provided. The lesion appears T2 hypointense arising from the roof of the fourth ventricle in the vermis. It shows diffusion restriction and homogenous contrast enhancement. Clear CSF space noted between the mass and along the floor of the fourth ventricle, suggesting that the lesion arises from the roof of fourth ventricle/cerebellar vermis. No obvious extension into the foramen of Magendie/ Luschka. No evidence of tonsillar herniation. There is extensive leptomeningeal enhancement throughout the visualized spine.

Interpretation: A—young female child with mass arising from floor of 4th ventricle, C—homogenously enhancing T2 hypointense mass lesion with diffusion restriction, B—obstructive hydrocephalus, leptomeningeal enhancement in spine, D—medulloblastoma.

Principal diagnosis: Medulloblastoma (Group 3/ Group 4-midline) arising from the roof of the fourth ventricle with leptomeningeal drop metastasis.

Management: Further work up—entire neuroaxis should be screened as there is subarachnoid metastatic spread via CSF pathway to spinal cord + cauda equina **("drop metastases" in 40%)** to look into cerebral convexities,

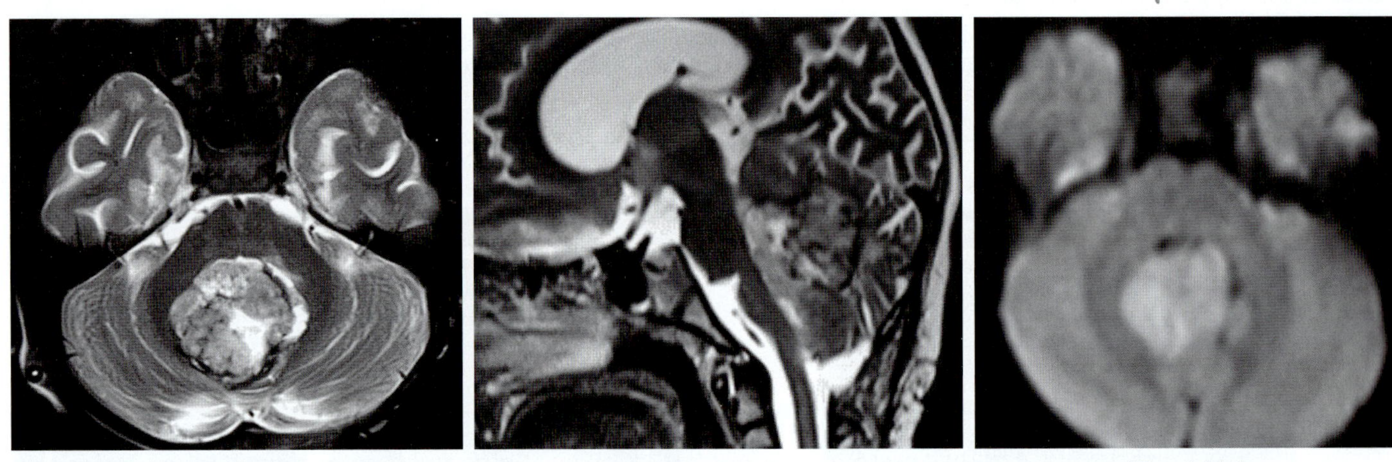

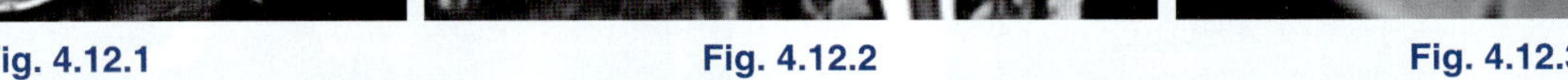

Fig. 4.12.1 Fig. 4.12.2 Fig. 4.12.3

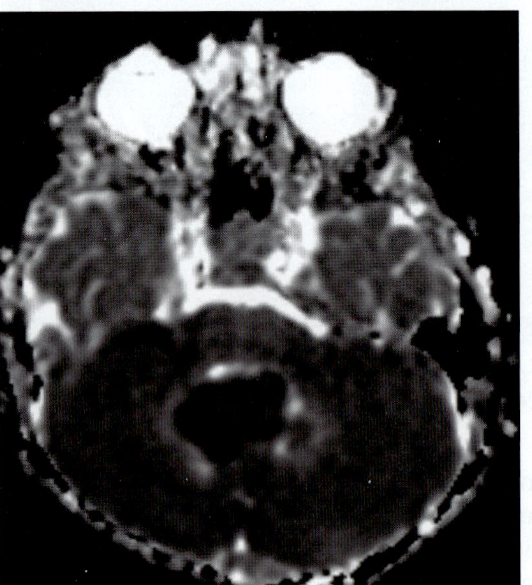

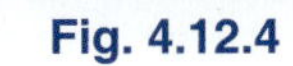

Fig. 4.12.4

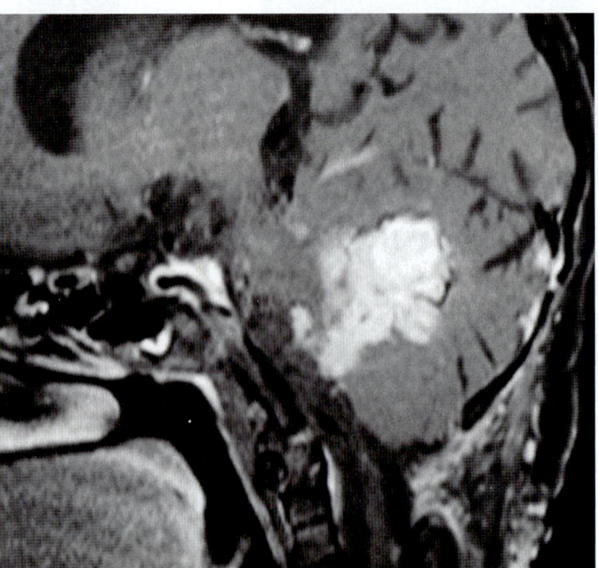

Fig. 4.12.5

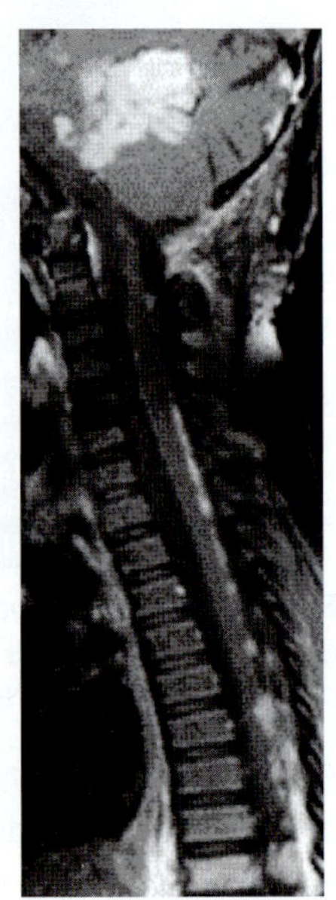

Fig. 4.12.6

<table>
<tr><th colspan="3">Table 4.12.1: Differential diagnosis for fourth ventricle mass lesion in children</th></tr>
<tr><td>1. Pilocytic astrocytoma (PA)
Age group—middle-aged" children between the ages of 5 and 15 years. The cerebellum is the most common location, accounting for nearly 60% of all PAs.</td><td colspan="2">The second most common site is in and around the optic nerve/chiasm, hypothalamus/third ventricle, the third most common location is the pons and medulla. CT scans show a mixed cystic/solid (17-8) or solid mass. Calcification occurs in 10–20% of cases. Hemispheric PAs generally present with a cyst plus an enhancing mural nodule. Cystic PAs are usually well-delineated and appear slightly hyperintense to CSF on both T1- and T2WI. They do not suppress completely on FLAIR. The mural nodule is iso-/hypointense on T1WI and iso-/hyperintense on T2WI.</td></tr>
<tr><td>2. Ependymoma
Age group—3 years (EPN-A)
60–70% posterior fossa, 30–40% supratentorial
Infratentorial ependymomas are relatively well-delineated "plastic" tumors that typically arise from the floor of the fourth ventricle and extrude through the outlet foramina.</td><td>Ependymomas are generally mixed density on NECT scans with coarse calcification occurs in approximately half of all ependymomas. Hemorrhage in 10% of cases. Ependymomas are generally heterogeneously hypointense relative to brain parenchyma on T1WI and hyperintense on T2/FLAIR. Following contrast administration, most ependymomas enhance.</td><td>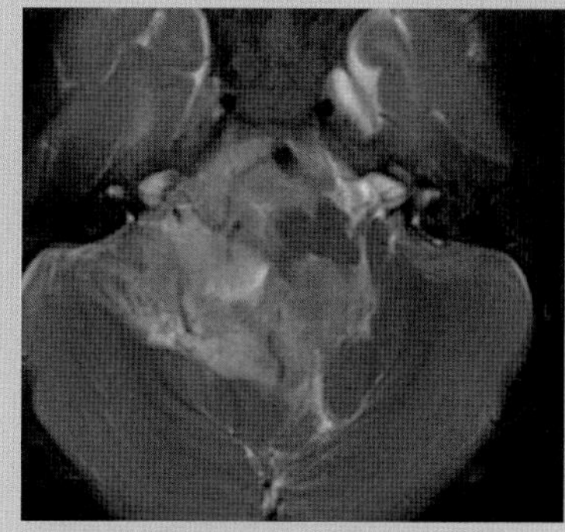
Fig. 4.12.7: Ependymoma</td></tr>
<tr><td>3. ATRT (Atypical rhabdoid teratoid tumour) Age group <3 years, infant presents with macrocephaly.
WHO-grade IV tumour, poor prognosis than medulloblastoma.
Slightly more than half supratentorial.
Infratentorial preferentially in cerebellar hemisphere.
In adults, common locations include pineal, suprasellar and spine.</td><td>T1W, T2WI: Heterointense because of cysts, haemorrhage
T1WI C+–Heterogeneous enhancement.
Leptomeningeal spread common (15–20%)
"Brain-to-brain" parenchymal metastases.
More likely to have cysts.
Teratoid: Divergent differentiation from mesenchymal, neuronal, glial and epithelial cells.</td><td>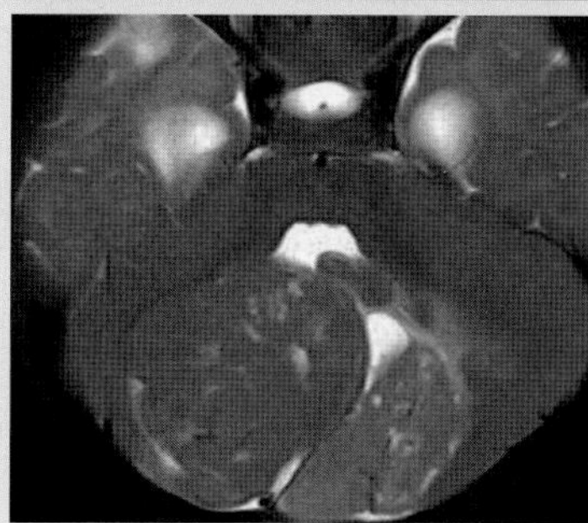
Fig. 4.12.8: T2W atypical rhabdoid teratoid tumour
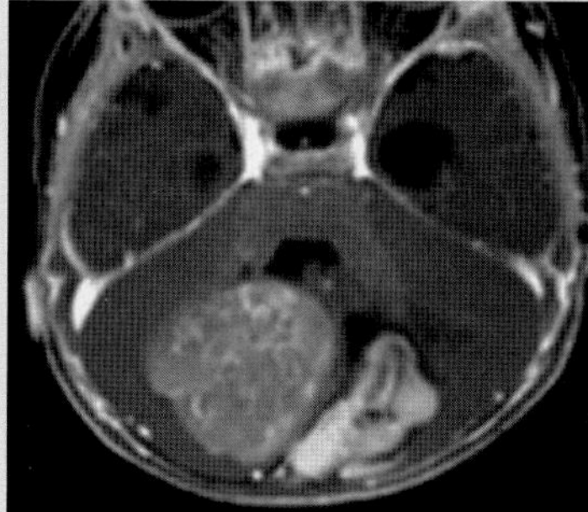
Fig. 4.12.9: Enhancing fourth ventricle mass lesion—atypical rhabdoid teratoid tumour</td></tr>
<tr><td>4. Rosette forming glioneuronal tumor—slow growing tumour of young adults. Most common site-4th ventricle.</td><td colspan="2">CT—midline cerebellar mass with solid–cystic appearance without edema.
MRI—T1 iso to hypo, T2 hyperintense lesion showing variable enhancement. Hemorrhage is common.</td></tr>
<tr><td colspan="3">5. Hemangioblastoma: Consider von Hippel-Lindau syndrome if younger age group.
Cystic lesion with mural nodule and prominent arterial feeder—Refer to case 9 for detailed explanation.</td></tr>
<tr><td colspan="3">6. Medulloblastoma</td></tr>
</table>

Table 4.12.2: Difference between medulloblastoma, ependymoma and pilocytic astrocytoma

Feature	*Medulloblastoma*	*Ependymoma*	*Pilocytic astrocytoma*
WHO grade	IV	II/III	I
NECT	Hyperdense	Isodense	Hypodense
Enhancement	Moderate	Minimal	Cyst with solid component Enhancing nodule and cyst wall
Calcification	Uncommon	Common	Uncommon
Site of origin	Vermis/roof of 4th ventricle	4th ventricle ependyma along the floor	Cerebellar hemisphere
T2WI	Hypointense	Intermediate	Hyperintense
Diffusion restriction	Present	Absent	Absent
Site	Midline/eccentric	Midline	Eccentric
Subarachnoid seeding	Common	Uncommon	rare
Age	5–12	2–10	10–20
Foraminal spread	No	Yes (foramen of Magendie and Luschka)	No
Haemorrhage and cysts	Rare	10%	Rare
NAA (MRS)	Very low. Taurine peak at 3.4 ppm specific.	Intermediate	Intermediate
Lactate (MRS)	Absent	Often present	Often present
Choline (MRS)	Very high	Mildly elevated	High

Table 4.12.3: Differential diagnosis for fourth ventricle mass lesion in adult

1. Subependymoma WHO grade I Age: Middle-aged/elderly adult (typically 5th–6th decades)	T2—Hyperintense, lobular, nonenhancing, intraventricular mass, Location—Typical: Intraventricular, **inferior 4th ventricle (60%)**: Often protrudes through foramen of **Magendie.** Heterogeneity related to cystic changes; blood products or Ca^{++} may be seen in larger lesions
2. Choroid plexus papilloma. Age group: Mean age = 1.5 years for CPPs in lateral, third ventricle, 22.5 years for fourth ventricle CPPs, and 35.5 years for CPA CPPs.	CT: Iso-/hyperdense lobulated mass, Hydrocephalus common, Ca^{++} (25%). CECT shows intense enhancement MR, iso-/hypointense on T1, iso-/hyperintense on T2/FLAIR "flow voids" common intense enhancement, no diffusion restriction.
3. Metastasis	
4. Hemangioblastoma: Cystic lesion with mural nodule and prominent arterial feeder	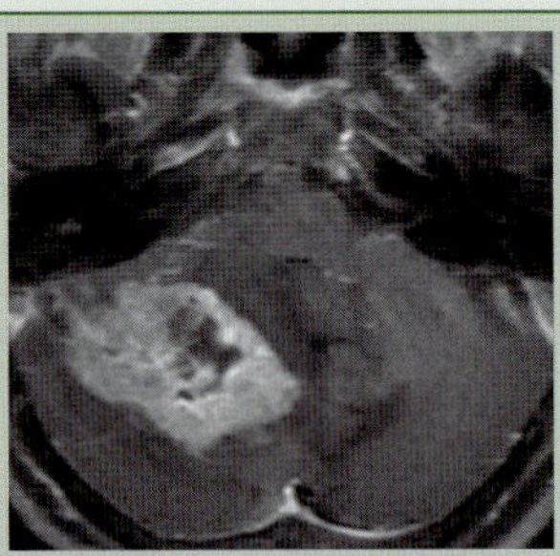 **Fig. 4.12.10:** Metastasis in fourth ventricle

Discussion: Medulloblastoma is a malignant, invasive, highly cellular embryonal tumor, WHO grade–IV tumour. Age group–75%, <10 years, Gender—M: F = 2–4:1. Most common malignant paediatric brain tumour.

sylvian fissure, suprasellar cistern, and retrograde extension into lateral and 3rd ventricle. Further screening of axial skeleton and lung should be done to rule out extracranial metastasis

Treatment: Surgery + radiation therapy (extremely radiosensitive).

Prognosis: WHO Grade—IV tumour, poor prognosis.

Table 4.12.4: Classification of medulloblastoma	
Medulloblastoma classification	
Histological	*Genetic*
Classic	WNT activated MB (10%) best prognosis
MB variants	SHH activated MB (30%)
Desmoplastic/nodular	NonWNT/NonSHH MB
MB with extensive nodularity (MBEN)	Group 3 (25%) Worst prognosis
Large cell/anaplastic	Group 4 (35%)

Four distinct MB molecular subgroups: WNT (wingless): Cerebellar peduncle/CPA cistern, children and young adults, Turcot syndrome association. SHH (sonic hedgehog): Cerebellar hemispheres **(lateral)**, infantile SHH have desmoplastic nodular and classical histology while childhood SHH have large cell anaplastic histology, Gorlin syndrome association. Group 3: Male infants, midline, metastasize in 50%. Group 4: All ages, midline (4th ventricle—predominantly but not exclusively).

Differential diagnosis: Medulloblastoma has a bimodal age distribution with second small peak in 3rd decade. The differentials in children: 1. ATRT 2. Ependymoma 3. Pilocytic astrocytoma

In adults: 1. Subependymoma, 2. choroid plexus papilloma, 3. metastasis—rarely in fourth ventricle. 4. Lhermitte-Duclos disease

Almost all WNT MBs have classic MBs histology. Most group 4 MBs have classic MBs histology. Almost all desmoplastic MBs and MBENs histology types belong to SHH group. But reverse is not true.

Imaging: NECT: 90% hyperdense (Ca^{++} uncommon, Haemorrhage rare). MR: >90% enhance (group 4 minimal/no enhancement), restricted diffusion, low ADC. T1C+ essential to detect **CSF dissemination. Extensive grape-like tumour nodules** common in desmoplastic or medulloblastoma with extensive nodularity (MBEN). MRS shows ↓↓ **NAA**, ↑↑ **choline**, lactate usually present and elevation in **Taurine** (short TE) Cr/Cho < 0.75 and myoinositol/NAA < 2.1 indicative for MB (resembles ependymoma)

Associated with **Gorlin syndrome,** Li-Fraumeni, Turcot and Cowden syndrome.

Other CNS Embryonal Tumours

1. **Embryonal tumour with multi-layered rosettes ETMR, C19MC-altered.**

   Non-MB embryonal tumours have undergone significant alterations in the classification with the **deletion of the term primitive neuroectodermal tumour (PNET)** and the recognition that they display amplification of C19MC region on chromosome 19. Features include WHO grade IV, 70% of ETMRs are supratentorial occurring in less than 2 years of life with increasing head circumference and signs of elevated intracranial pressure. Intratumoral haemorrhage and cystic components are present. Solid components show diffusion restriction. Peritumoral edema typically minimal or absent. DDs–AT/RT, RELA fusion ependymoma, astroblastoma, glioblastoma, neuroblastoma.
2. **Embryonal tumours, NOS (not otherwise specified)**

   Tumours without current molecular classification in 2016 WHO which include medulloepithelioma, CNS neuroblastoma, esthesioneuroblastoma and CNS ganglioneuroblastoma.

   New molecularly identified embryonal neoplasms. CNS NB-FOXR2 (neuroblastoma with FOXR activation), CNS EFT-CIC (Ewing sarcoma family tumour with CIC alteration), CNS HGNET-MN1 (high grade neuroepithelial tumour with MN1 alteration), CNS HGNET-BCOR (high grade neuroepithelial tumour with BCOR alteration).

Table 4.12.5: Summary of malignant rhabdoid tumours			
Malignant rhabdoid tumours: Cranial AT/RT are separated from other CNS embryonal neoplasms and non-CNS MRTs by distinct immunohistochemical, histopathologic and molecular features.			
Etiology	*Pathology*	*Clinical*	*Imaging*
Loss of expression of SMARCB1 protein required for diagnosis. Three epigenetically distinct groups – ATRT-MYC – ATRT-SHH – ATRT-TYR WHO grade IV tumour.	Poorly differentiated neuro-epithelial elements + rhabdoid cells. Supratentorial (50%) most are ATRT-MYC or SHH. Infratentorial (50%) all three subgroups. 75% of ATRT-TYR are infratentorial.	Age < 2 yrs. 10% of all CNS neoplasms in infants. Rhabdoid tumour predisposition syndrome (RTPS) Familial cancer syndrome (AD) with CNS ATR and synchronous renal or extra renal MRT +/- – Choroid plexus carcinoma – Rhabdoid meningioma.	CT: Heterogenous hyperdense, T1 T2 hetero intense, enhances strongly, restricts on DWI, CSF spread in 20% at diagnosis. Poor prognosis. DD: Supratentorial–ETMR, RELA fusion ependymoma, teratoma, malignant astrocytoma, desmo-plastic infantile astrocytoma. Infratentorial–medulloblastoma.

Table 4.12.6: Differential diagnosis for CT hyperdense /T2 hypointense/diffusion restricting masses

DD for CT hyperdense/T2 hypointense/diffusion restricting masses: Reflecting high cellularity	
CT hyperdense /T2 hypointense lesion	*Diffusion restricting lesions*
Meningioma	Abscess, subdural empyema, pyocephalus
Medulloblastoma	Acute infarct
Lymphoma	Hyperacute/late subacute hemorrhage
Pinealoblastoma	Highly cellular tumours like lymphoma, meningioma and medulloblastoma
Central neurocytoma	Encephalitis
Germinoma	Creutzfeldt-Jakob disease
ATRT (Atypical rhabdoid teratoid tumor)	Acute demyelination
PNET (Primitive neuroectodermal tumor)	Mitochondrial disease, maple syrup urine disease
Melanoma metastasis	Neonatal parechovirus/dengue encephalitis
Flow voids: Vascular malformation	Epidermoid cyst

Table 4.12.7: Approach to posterior fossa lesions near fourth ventricle

<table>
<tr>
<td>Brain stem glioma compresses fourth ventricle antero-posteriorly
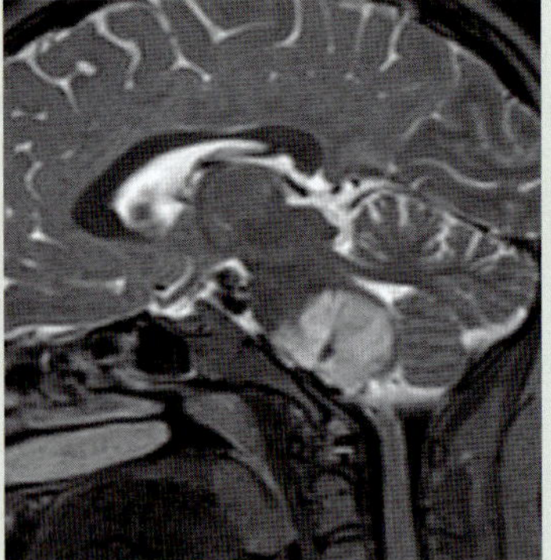
Fig. 4.12.11: Brain stem glioma
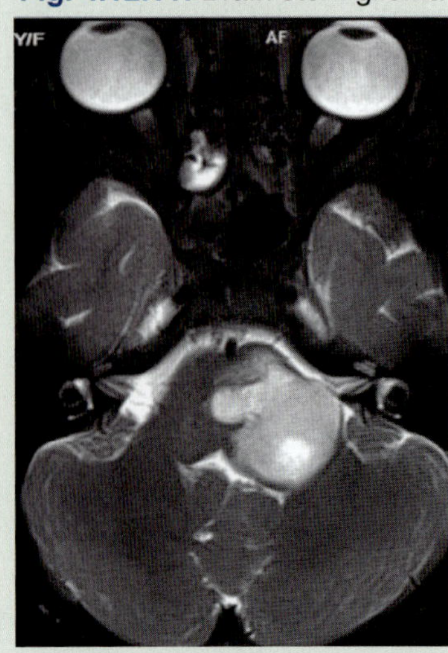
Fig. 4.12.12: Brain stem glioma</td>
<td>Ependymoma arises from floor of fourth ventricle, CSF cleft seen between the lesion and roof of fourth ventricle
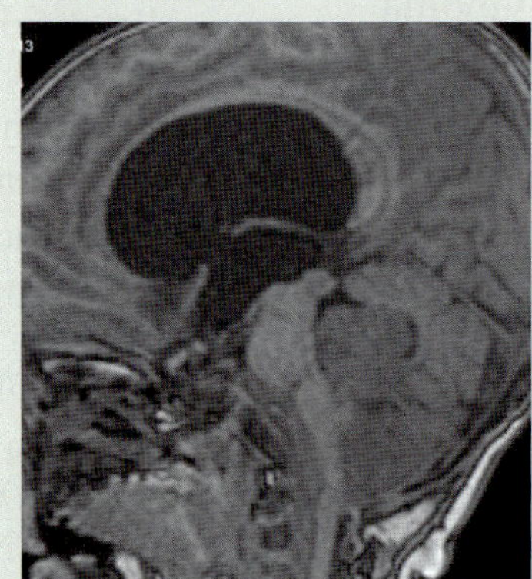
Fig. 4.12.13: Ependymoma
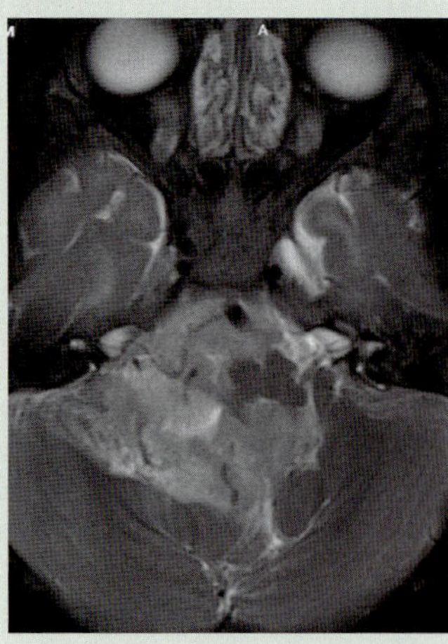
Fig. 4.12.14: Ependymoma</td>
<td>Medulloblastoma arising from roof of fourth ventricle, CSF cleft seen between the lesion and floor of fourth ventricle (pons)
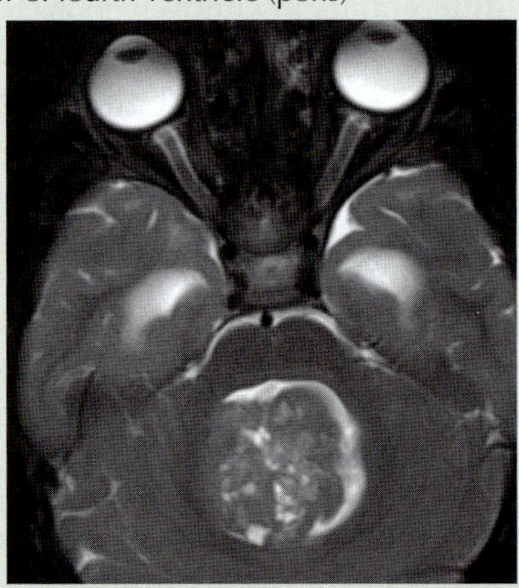
Fig. 4.12.15: Medulloblastoma
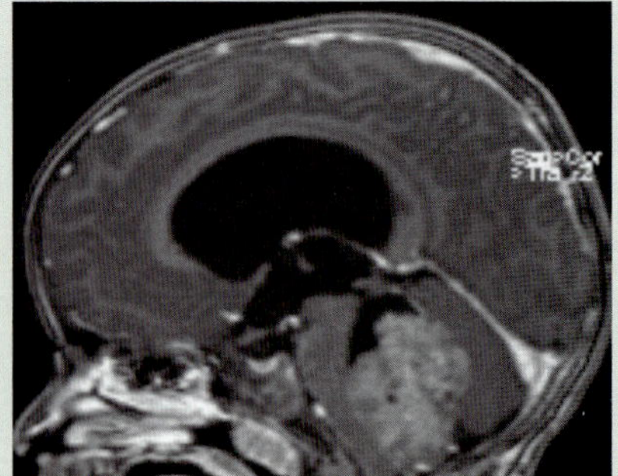
Fig. 4.12.16: Medulloblastoma</td>
</tr>
</table>

Contd...

Table 4.12.7: Approach to posterior fossa lesions near fourth ventricle *(Contd...)*

Subependymoma arises from inferior fourth ventricle in adults which compresses fourth ventricle and extrudes the foramina (Fig. 4.12.17) 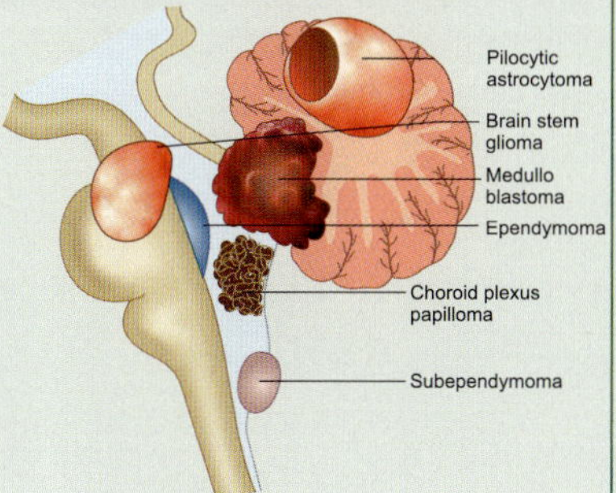 **Fig. 4.12.17:** Various brain stem lesions	Pilocytic astrocytoma/hemangioblastoma occurs in cerebellar hemispheres compresses the fourth ventricle from roof to floor. 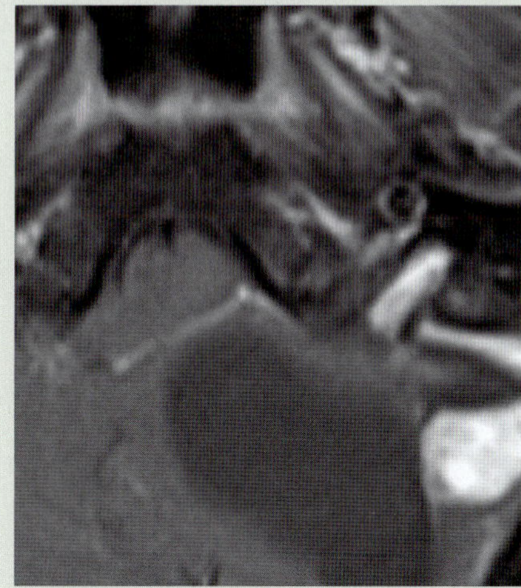 **Fig. 4.12.18:** Hemangioblastoma 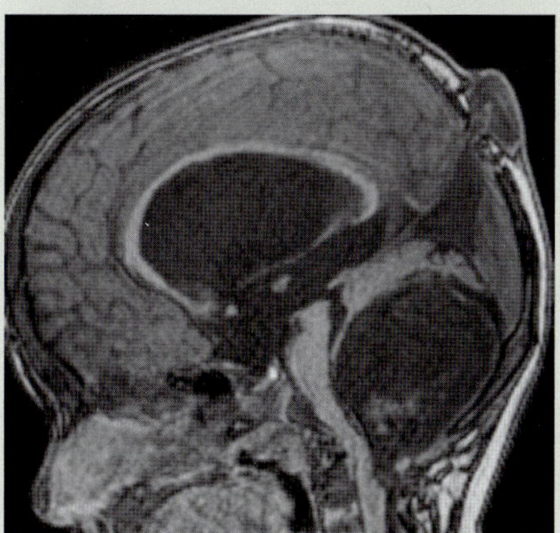 **Fig. 4.12.19:** Pilocytic astrocytoma 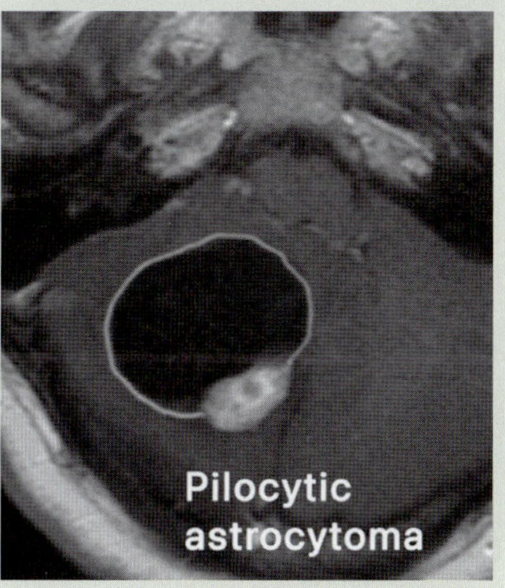 **Fig. 4.12.20:** Pilocytic astrocytoma	Retrocerebellar lesion (epidermoid, arachnoid cyst) compresses the fourth ventricle and cerebellar hemisphere. 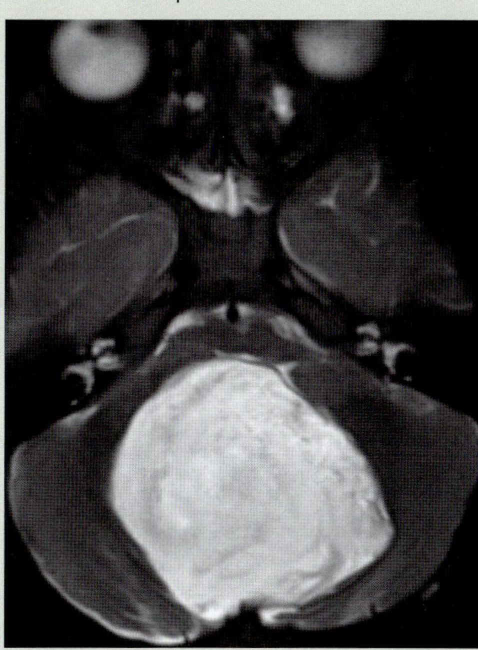 **Fig. 4.12.21:** Retrocerebellar epidermoid

Table 4.12.8: Approach to diffusion weighted imaging patterns

DWI (b1000)	*ADC*	*Interpretation and causes*
Bright 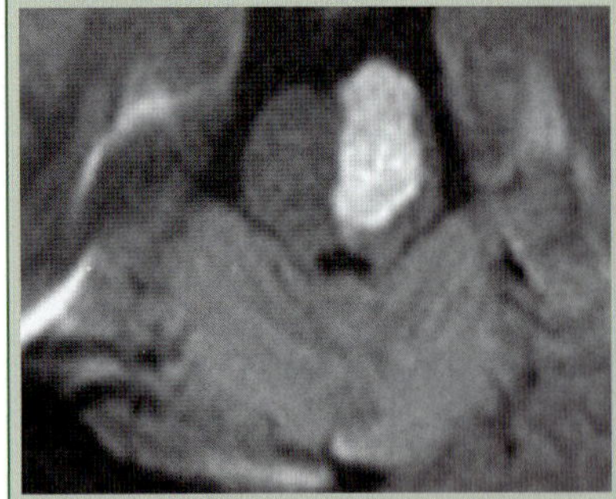 Fig. 4.12.22: DWI bright	Dark 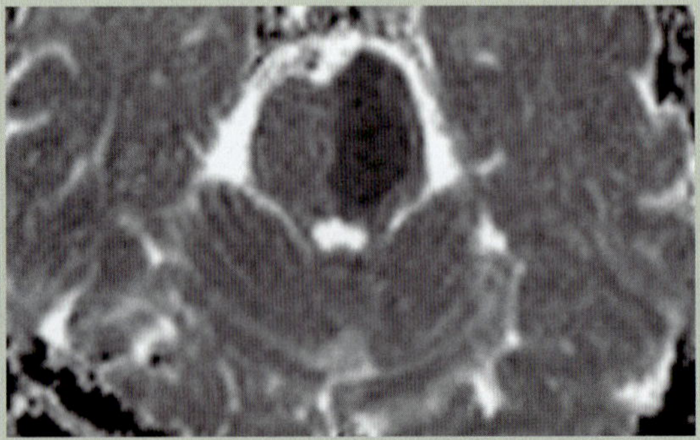 Fig. 4.12.23: ADC dark	Diffusion restriction—acute infarct (other diffusion restricting lesions)
Bright	Bright	T2 shine through vasogenic edema
Dark 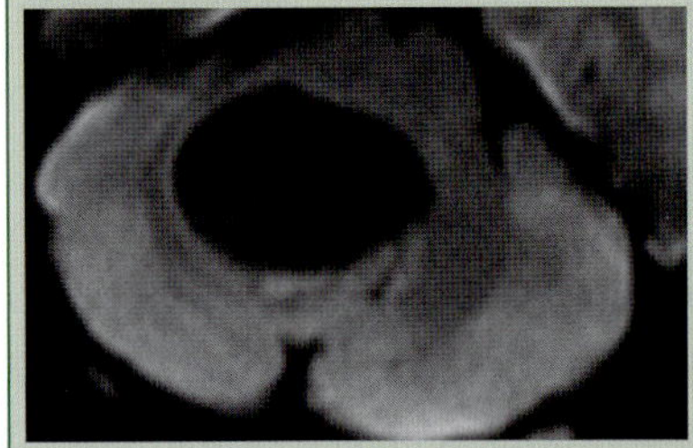 Fig. 4.12.24: DWI dark	Bright 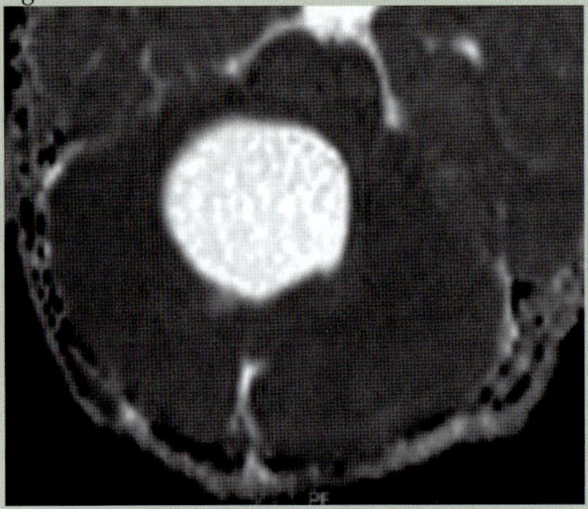 Fig. 4.12.25: ADC bright	Facilitated diffusion—cyst/gliosis
Dark 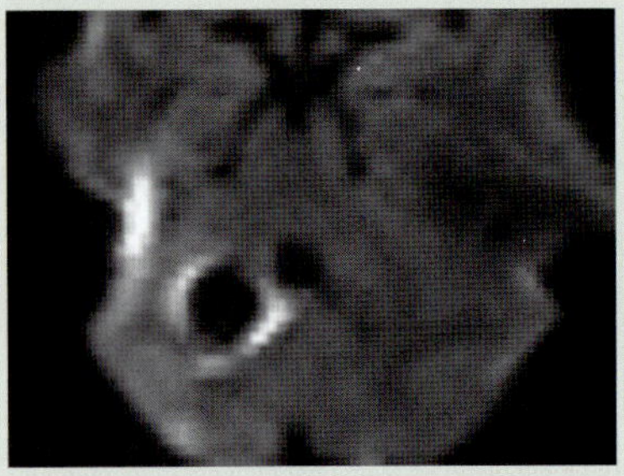 Fig. 4.12.26: DWI dark	Dark 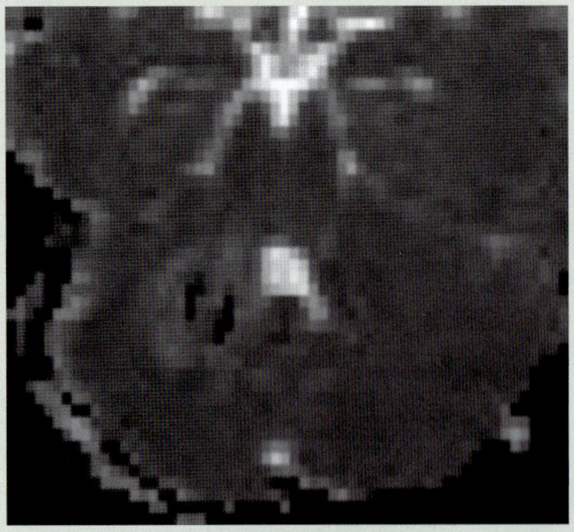 Fig. 4.12.27: ADC dark	T2 blackout—hemorrhage, calcification
Iso	Iso	Normal/pseudonormalization in subacute infarct

Table 4.12.9: Approach to SWI (susceptibility weighted imaging) patterns

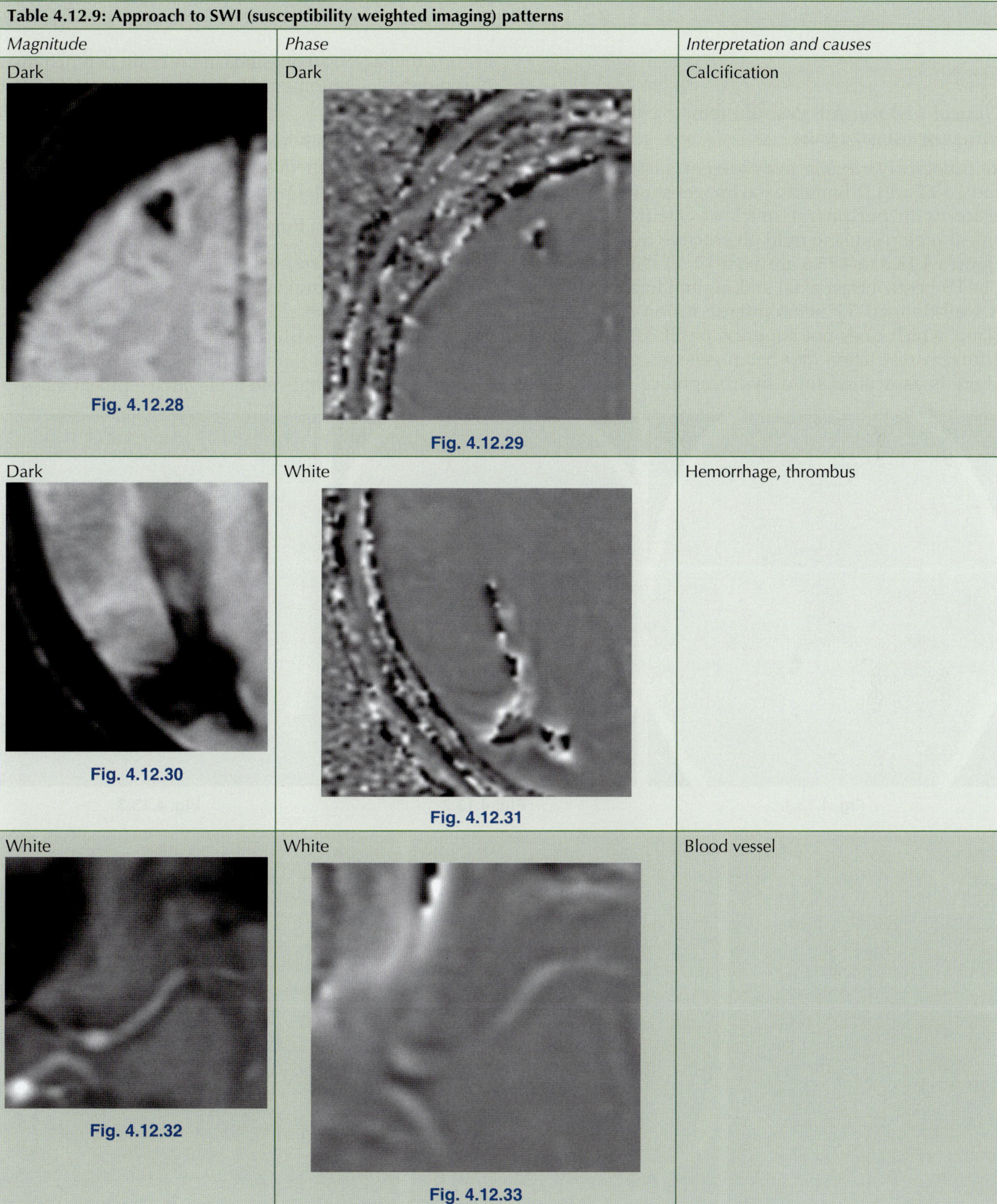

Magnitude	*Phase*	*Interpretation and causes*
Dark Fig. 4.12.28	Dark Fig. 4.12.29	Calcification
Dark Fig. 4.12.30	White Fig. 4.12.31	Hemorrhage, thrombus
White Fig. 4.12.32	White Fig. 4.12.33	Blood vessel

4.13 CENTRAL NERVOUS SYSTEM

Case No. 13

Clinical history: A 5-year-old female child presented with upward gaze palsy.

Radiological technique and observations: Figures 4.13.1 and 4.13.2 are CT limited axial images show an isodense lesion with peripheral speck of calcification in the pineal region causing mild obstructive hydrocephalus. Figures 4.13.3 to 4.13.6 are axial T2, FLAIR axial, DWI, T1+ FS postcontrast axial and sagittal images showing A well-defined T2 heterointense lesion in the pineal gland which does not suppress on FLAIR and shows diffusion restriction and heterogeneous enhancement. There is associated mild hydrocephalus noted. There are no other associated lesions in the brain parenchyma. No evidence of leptomeningeal enhancement to suggest CSF dissemination.

Interpretation: A—5-year female, pathology in pineal gland, C—heterogeneously enhancing mass, B—shows diffusion restriction, D—pineoblastoma.

Principal diagnosis: Pineoblastoma

Differential diagnosis

If the internal cerebral vein is depressed—extra pineal mass

1) Lesions of the splenium, 2) Thalamic glioma, 3) Pericallosal/callosal lipoma, 4) Subsplenial meningioma. If the internal cerebral vein is elevated—pineal mass.

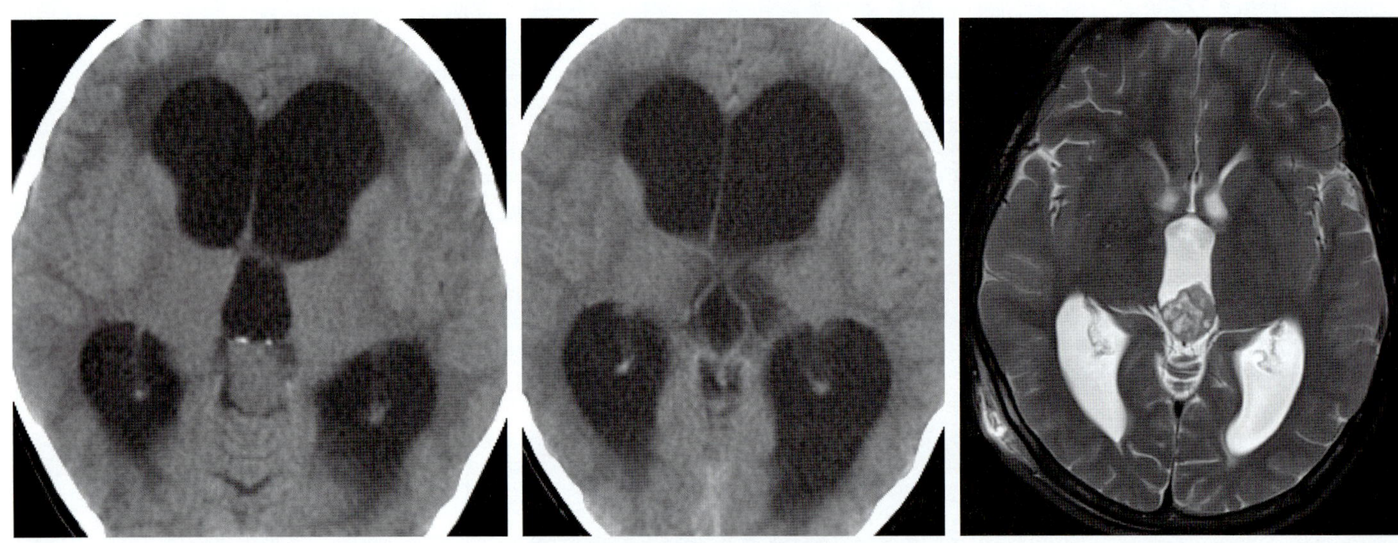

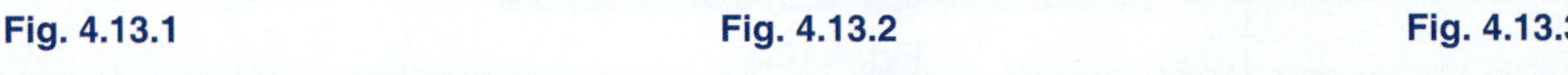

Fig. 4.13.1 Fig. 4.13.2 Fig. 4.13.3

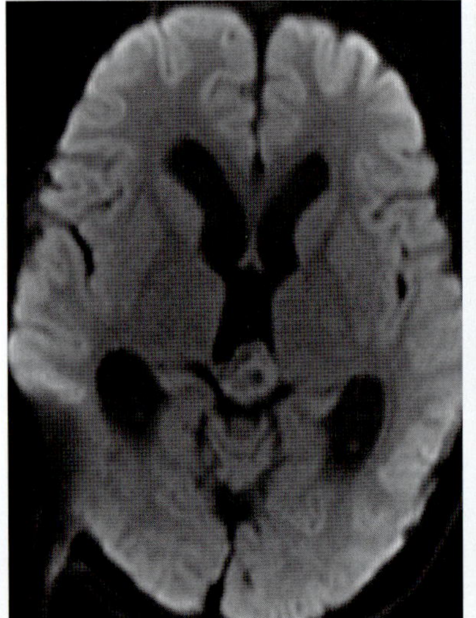

Fig. 4.13.4

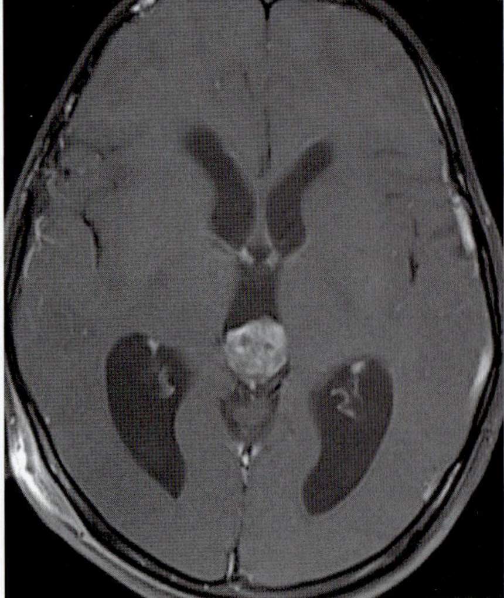

Fig. 4.13.5

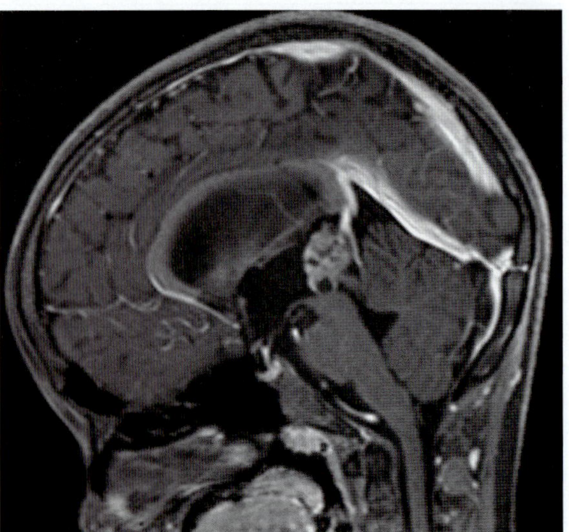

Fig. 4.13.6

Table 4.13.1: Types of germ cell tumors and nongerm cell tumors

Germ cell tumor	*Non-germ cell tumor*
1. Germinoma	1. Pineoblastoma
2. Mature teratoma	2. Pineocytoma
3. Immature teratoma	3. Glioma
4. Yolk sac tumor	
5. Embryonal carcinoma	
6. Mixed germ cell tumor	

Flowchart 4.13.1: Approach to lesions which lift internal cerebral vein

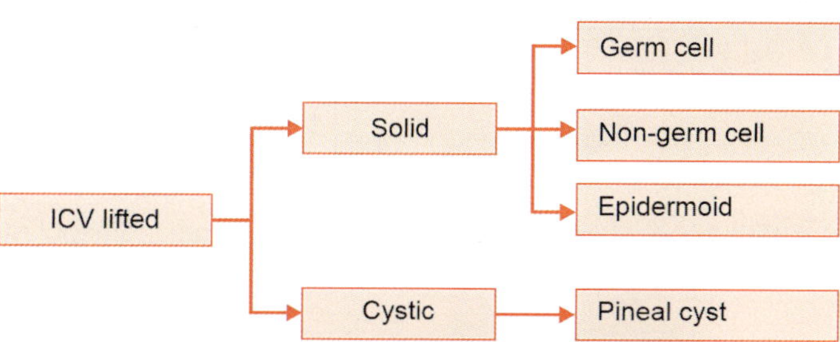

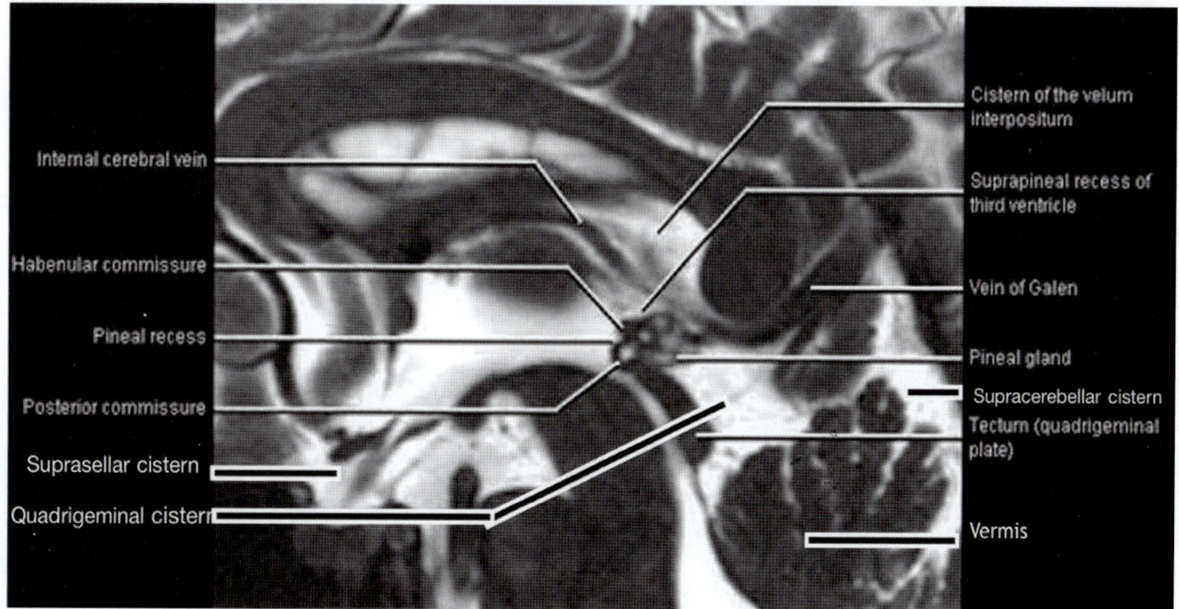

Fig. 4.13.7: Normal pineal region anatomy

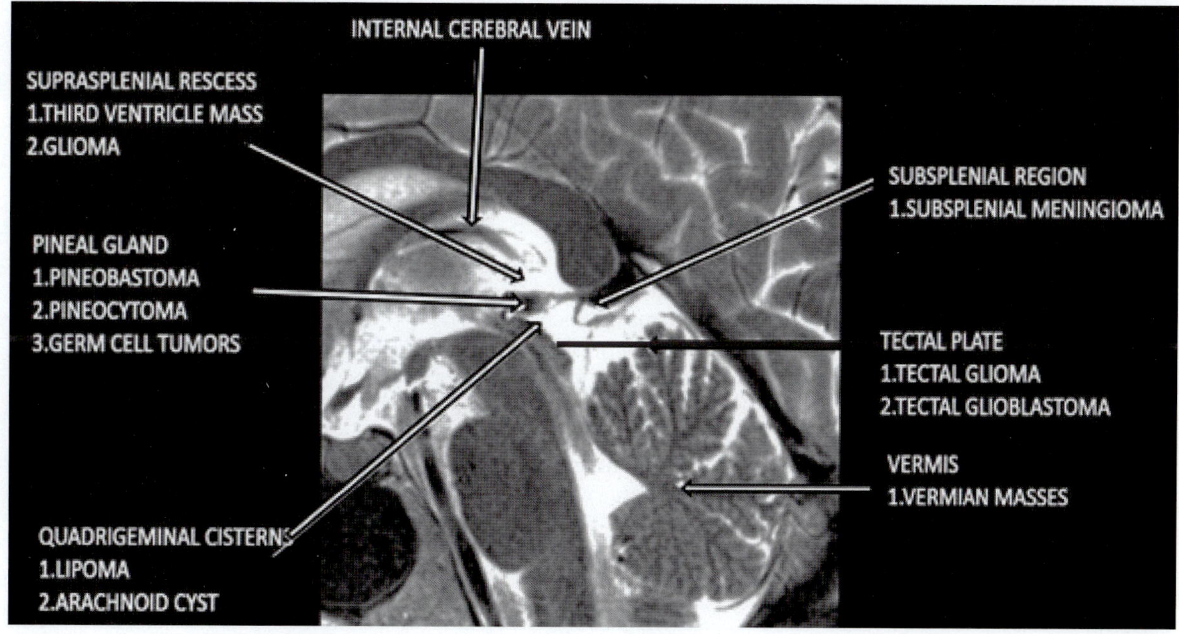

Fig. 4.13.8: Approach to diagnose pineal tumors based on site

Table 4.13.2: Approach to pineal tumors based on patterns of calcification		
"Engulfed"	*"Exploded"*	*"Irregular"*
Germinoma	Pineocytoma, pineoblastoma	Teratoma

Table 4.13.3: Biomarkers for pineal gland tumors				
Neoplasm	*Beta-HCG*	*Alpha- FP*	*Placental alkaline phosphatase*	*Immunoreactive S antigen*
Germinoma	-	-	↑	-
Yolk sac	-	↑	-	-
Choriocarcinoma	↑	-	-	-
Embryonal	↑	↑	-	-
Immature teratoma	-	↑	-	-
Pineoblastoma/cytoma	-	-		↑

Table 4.13.4: Differential diagnosis for pineal tumors		
Pineal tumors	*Features*	*Image*
Pineal parenchymal tumor of intermediate differentiation	More aggressive looking than pineocytoma, with involvement of adjacent structures (e.g. thalami/ventricles). **NECT shows engulfment of calcification within the lesion.** Solid components are isointense to grey matter and enhance heterogeneously. CSF dissemination is a feature.	Fig. 4.13.9: Pineal parenchymal tumor of intermediate differentiation
Pineoblastoma—primitive neuroectodermal tumor Affects young individuals (<20 years) Hyperdense on NECT	Hemorrhage and necrosis common leading to inhomogeneous appearance in T1/T2, with heterogenous intense enhancement. Hydrocephalus due to mass effect is common. Increased cellularity leads to diffusion restriction. peripherally exploded calcification in NECT scans. CSF dissemination is a feature. CSF analysis to demonstrate immunoreactive S-antigen.	Fig. 4.13.10: Pinealoblastoma Fig. 4.13.11: Drop metastasis in pinealoblastoma

(Contd...)

Table 4.13.4: Differential diagnosis for pineal tumors *(Contd...)*		
Pineal tumors	*Features*	*Image*
Germinoma Most of these tumors occur in young adults and mean age of onset is about 17 years (15–20). Great predilection for midline structures. 55% suprasellar, 35% pineal, 10–15% basal ganglia and thalamus. Suprasellar type produces diabetes insipidus.	Bifocal/double midline germinomas are seen in 20% (In suprasellar and pineal region). CSF dissemination and invasion is common. **Engulfs calcification in NECT scans.** Increased cellularity causes diffusion restriction. Peritumoral T2/FLAIR homogenous hyperintensity due to inflammatory response mimicking TB/sarcoid and shows intense contrast enhancement. **Abnormal accumulation of Ga-67 in scintigraphy.** ↑11-carbon-Methionine uptake in PET. Aggressive metabolic spectrum with tall choline with decreased NAA on MRS. But shows good response on chemotherapy.	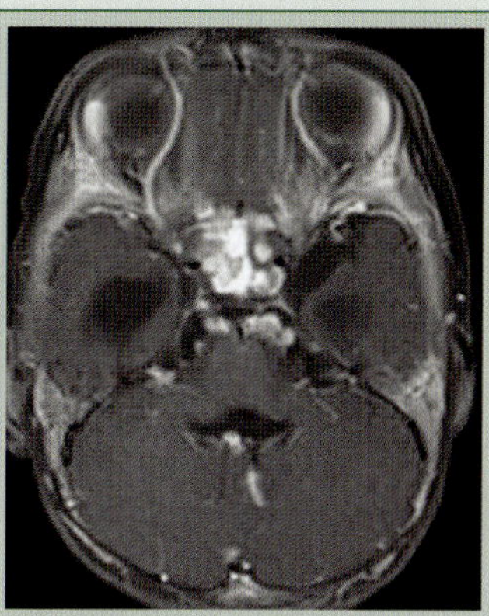 **Fig. 4.13.12:** Germinoma
Teratoma Extra-axial tridermal teratomas usually present in newborn. Second common tumor in other age group.	Heterogeneous mixture of irregular calcification, soft tissue and fat on CT. High signal from fat, which is T1 bright and suppressed by T1 FS. Perifocal edema and enhancing soft tissue components indicate immature/ malignant type. The pineal and suprasellar areas are the most common sites for teratoma to appear. They are smaller in size mostly.	
Yolk sac tumor (malignant germ cell tumor) There may be a link with Down syndrome, as with other germ cell cancers.	Rare type of extragonadal yolk sac tumor. No cystic components. Irregular, with intense homogenous enhancement The presence of high levels of alpha-fetoprotein in the CSF can be useful but not diagnostic for yolk sac cancers.	
Choriocarcinoma Pure pineal choriocarcinoma tumors secrete β-HCG.	Markedly heterogenous with haemorrhage, cyst, fibrosis and necrosis Heterogenous ring like/ nodular enhancement	
Embryonal carcinoma	Multiple cystic foci, with CSF seedling. Increased lipid, lactate and choline	
Pineal epidermoid	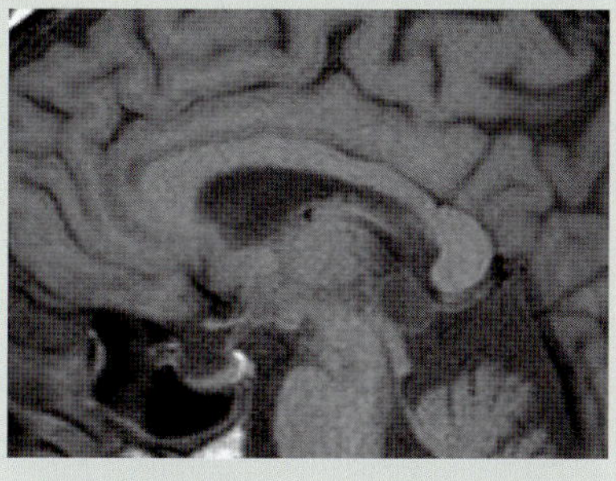 **Fig. 4.13.13:** Pineal epidermoid showing T1 hypointensity	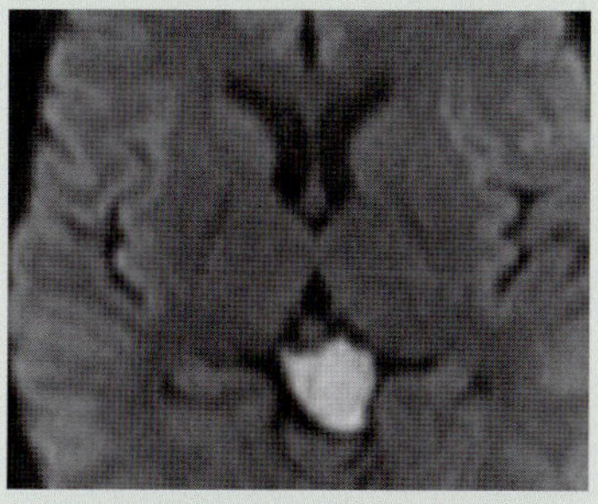 **Fig. 4.13.14:** Pineal epidermoid showing DWI hyperintensity/diffusion restriction
Pineal cyst Asymptomatic Detected usually incidental.	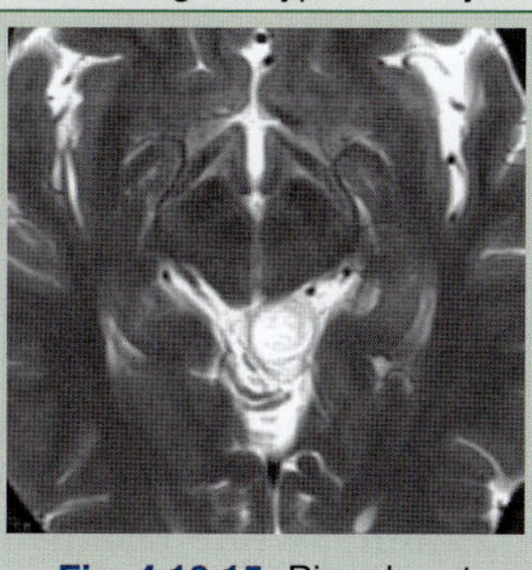 **Fig. 4.13.15:** Pineal cyst	

Table 4.13.5: Differential diagnosis for extrapineal tumors

Extrapineal tumor	*Image*	*Extrapineal tumor*	*Image*
Tectal glioblastoma Large aggressive mass with obstructive hydrocephalus Peripheral thick irregular enhancing rim with central necrosis	**Fig. 4.13.16:** Tectal glioblastoma	**Tectal glioma** Low grade, causing obstructive hydrocephalus Associated with NF1 Tectal expansion with central cystic spaces or calcification	**Fig. 4.13.17:** Tectal glioma causing obstructive hydrocephalus
Pineal region lipoma (quadrigeminal plate lipoma) Well-circumscribed mass with HU (–50 to –100) T1/T2 bright with suppression on T1 + FS Round or linear filling defects on T2 indicating flow voids	**Fig. 4.13.18:** Quadrigeminal plate lipoma	**Thalamic pilocytic astrocytoma** Well-circumscribed, WHO Grade 1, vividly enhancing mass arising from thalamus	**Fig. 4.13.19:** Thalamic pilocytic astrocytoma
Vein of Galen aneurysmal malformation AV fistula between choroidal artery and median porencephalic vein of Markowski Causes high output cardiac failure Embolization after 6 months of life		**Subsplenial meningioma:** T2 iso to hypointense extra-axial lesion arising inferior to the splenium of corpus callosum Intense enhancement on contrast Alanine and glutamine peak on MRS. Displacement of internal cerebral vein inferiorly	**Fig. 4.13.20:** Drop metastasis

Further Investigations and Management

- CSF analysis to demonstrate immunoreactive S-antigen.
- Complete surgical resection is generally curative, without recurrence or CSF dissemination. "Watchful waiting" is common with small lesions

Anatomy of the pineal region: The internal cerebral vein's displacement is critical in pinpointing the origin of the lesion in the pineal region. **Lesions of the corpus callosum at splenium cause it to be displaced inferiorly, while lesions of the pineal gland/tectum cause it to be displaced superiorly.** The pineal region includes

Flowchart 4.13.2: Pineal tumors in adults and pediatric age group

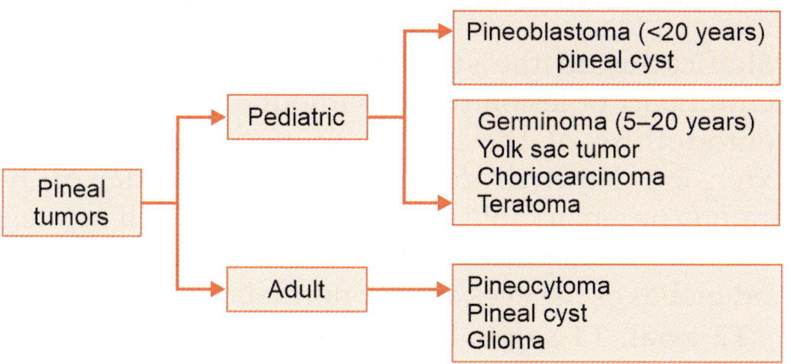

pineal gland, tectum, suprapineal recess, posterior third ventricle, vermis and superior cerebellar cistern and quadrigeminal plate cistern. The habenular commissure can be seen in the superior lamina of the pineal gland's stalk. The posterior commissure is found in the inferior stalk of the pineal gland, just inferior to the habenular commissure. Pineal recess/epiphyseal recess, is a tiny angular depression or diverticulum located at the third ventricle's posterior edge. The supra-pineal recess is found in the third ventricle's posterior portion, overlying the cerebral aqueduct.

Lesions causing CSF dissemination (drop metastasis): The lesions which are in contact with ependymal surface of the ventricle/CSF sulcal spaces cause drop metastasis. Glioblastoma and anaplastic astrocytoma, medulloblastoma, PNET, ependymoma, germinoma, choroid plexus carcinoma and pineoblastoma/pineocytoma.

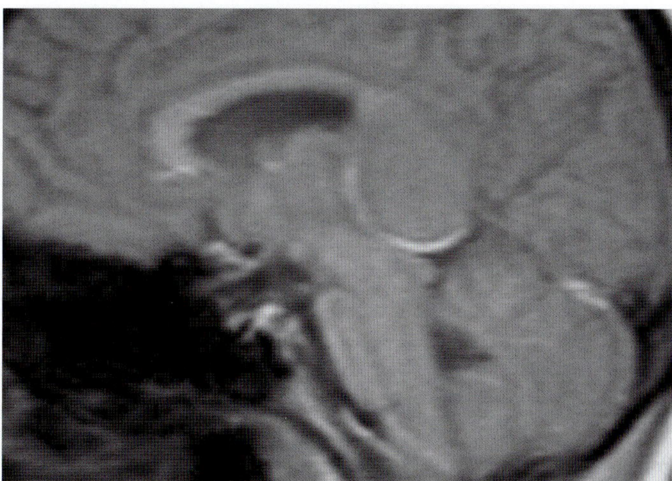

Fig. 4.13.21: Subsplenial meningioma

In individuals with leptomeningeal carcinomatosis and leptomeningeal drop metastases, sugar coating or zuckerguss (German term for sugar icing) can be found in the brain and cake icing in spinal cord. Sugar coating/zuckerguss appears as a thin linear with focal small nodularity on post-contrast CT or MRI. Cake icing are prominent nodules in spinal cord.

4.14 CENTRAL NERVOUS SYSTEM

Case No. 14

Clinical history: A 45 years old male, with the history of worsening of vision.

Radiological techniques and observation: Frontal and lateral radiograph of skull (Figs 4.14.1 to 4.14.2) shows normal sella without any expansion/widening of the sella. The orbital margins appear normal. The remainder skull is unremarkable. The patient can be further evaluated by cross sectional imaging like CT, Since there were no obvious findings in favour of any particular diagnosis.

CT brain axial and coronal reformatted image in brain (Figs 4.14.4–4.14.6) ***and bone window*** (Fig. 4.14.3) show a well-defined hypodense lesion with peripheral calcification in the suprasellar region. Hypodense central part of lesion noted without adjacent erosion/remodelling of the bone and no sphenoid sinus extension. No hydrocephalus. The remainder of the brain is unremarkable. Sphenoid sinus is well aerated. Anterior clinoid process is non-aerated. Visualised orbits and globes of the eyes appear normal.

T2 axial, T1 sagittal, T2 FLAIR coronal, diffusion and MRA MR images (Figs 4.14.7 to 4.14.11) show T1/T2 hyperintense **lobulated cystic mass which is not suppressible in FLAIR noted centred in the suprasellar region.** The lesion does not show diffusion restriction. The lesion can be seen separately from the pituitary, but not separately seen from infundibulum. The mass abuts the optic Chiasm's posterior edge superiorly, splaying and lateral displacement of optic tracts. It indents the

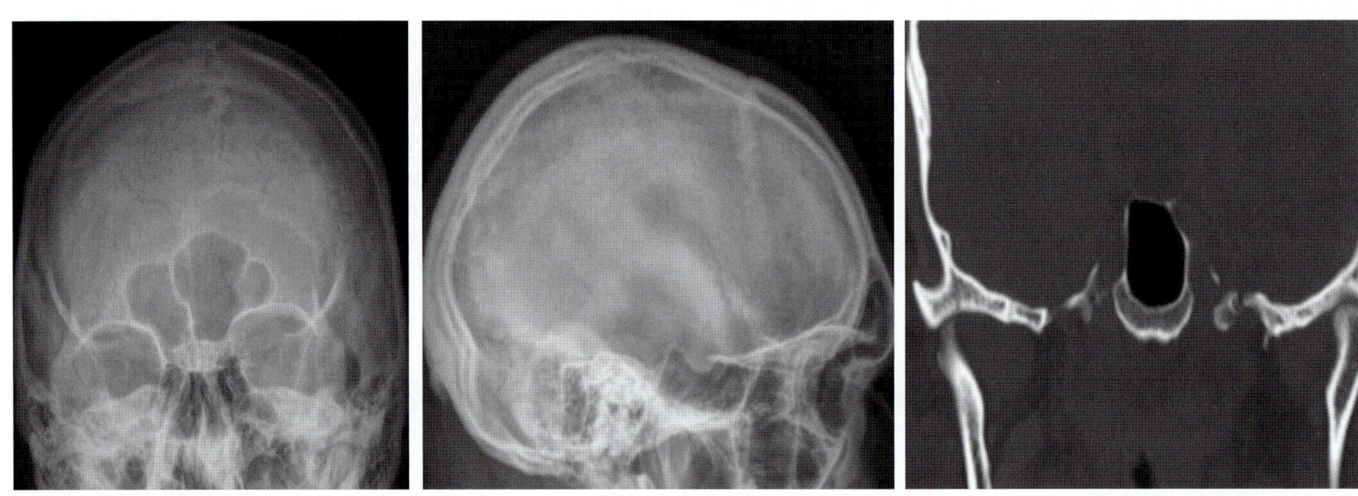

Fig. 4.14.1 Fig. 4.14.2 Fig. 4.14.3

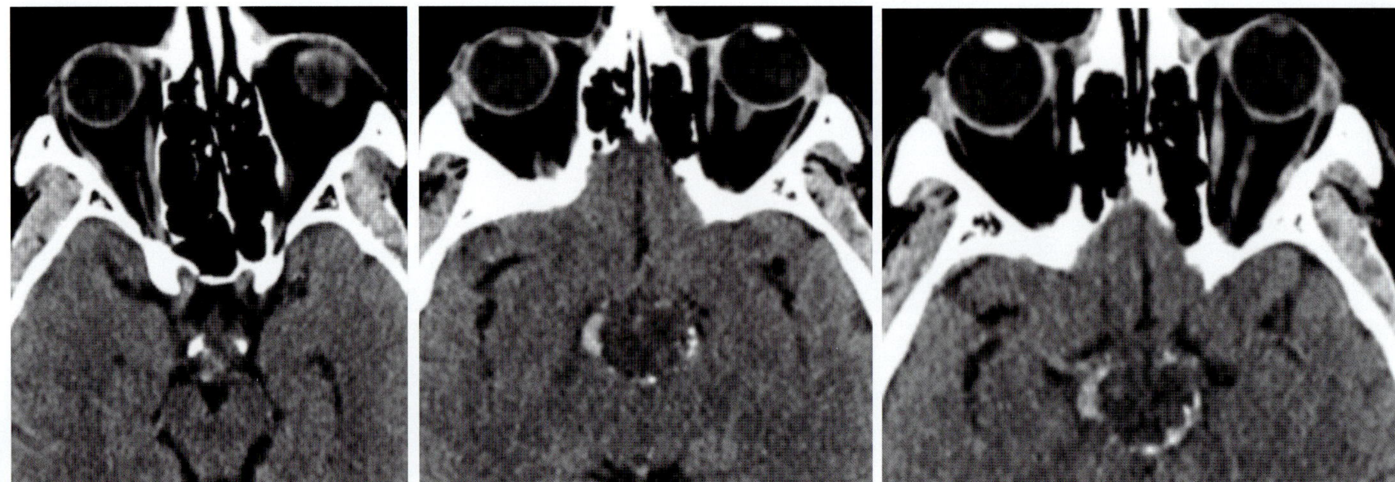

Fig. 4.14.4 Fig. 4.14.5 Fig. 4.14.6

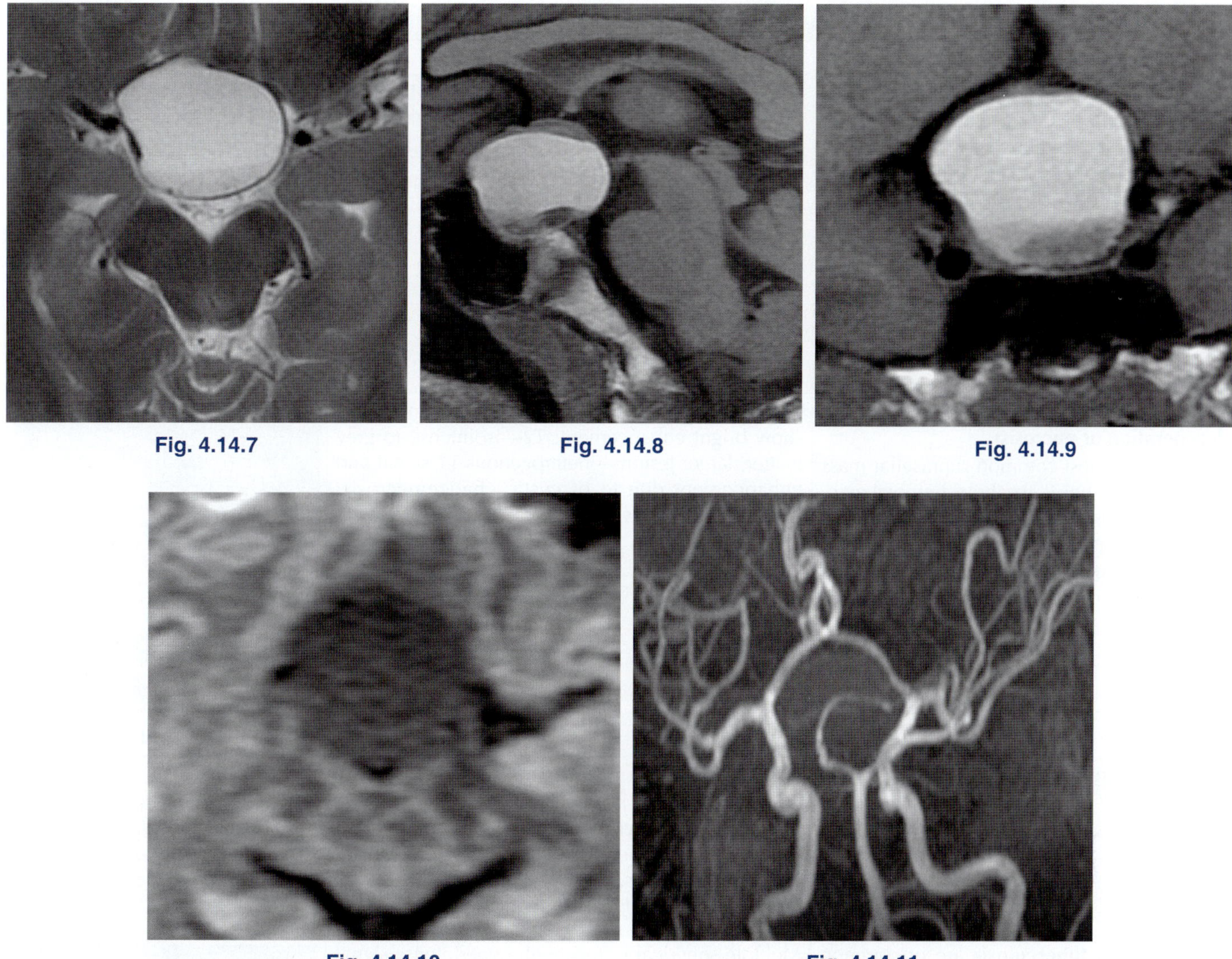

Fig. 4.14.7

Fig. 4.14.8

Fig. 4.14.9

Fig. 4.14.10

Fig. 4.14.11

third ventricle's floor and contacts the supraclinoid ICAs and basilar arteries without compressing or encasement. Splaying of the A1 segments of the bilateral ACA without pulsation artefact associated with this mass. The rest of the brain that was imaged appeared to be unremarkable.

Interpretations: A 45-year-old male, pathology in suprasellar region C-T1/T2 hyperintense lobulated cystic mass which is not suppressible on FLAIR with peripheral rim of calcification causing mass effect on optic chiasm and causing splaying of A1 segment of ACA, B—No diffusion restriction/pulsation artefact, D—suprasellar craniopharyngioma.

Principal diagnosis: The above findings are consistent with a suprasellar craniopharyngioma.

Differential diagnosis: Rathke cleft cyst, cystic pituitary macroadenoma, suprasellar teratoma.

Management: Patient referred to neurosurgeon for surgical excision and HPE correlation.

Visual symptoms, headaches, and increased intracranial pressure hormonal imbalances, short stature and delayed puberty in children, decreased libido, amenorrhea, diabetes insipidus, and behavioural changes as a result of frontal or temporal extension are all symptoms of craniopharyngioma.

Craniopharyngioma: 90% Tumor, 90% occurring in children, 90% cystic in nature, 90% shows calcification and 90% has enhancing nodule.

Causes for peripheral calcification in radiology: Cysts/pseudocysts, chronic abscess/hydatid cyst, aneurysms/atherosclerosis, craniopharyngioma, egg shell calcification in lymph node.

Table 4.14.1: Differential diagnosis for suprasellar lesions

Suprasellar lesions	*Imaging features*	*Images*
Rathke cleft cysts are non-neoplastic, sellar/suprasellar epithelium-lined cysts arising from the embryologic remnants of Rathke pouch in the pituitary gland. They are incidentally identified. Surgical treatment is indicated for symptomatic cases. MRI: T1 50% are hyperintense (high protein content), 50% are hypointense. T2 70% are hyperintense, 30% are iso or hypointense. T1 C+ (Gd) no contrast enhancement of the cyst is seen; however, a thin enhancing rim of surrounding compressed pituitary tissue may be apparent.	CT: Non-contrast typically **non-calcified and of homogenous low attenuation,** uncommonly it may contain small curvilinear calcifications in the wall (seen in 10–15% of cases). Postcontrast typically non-enhancing.	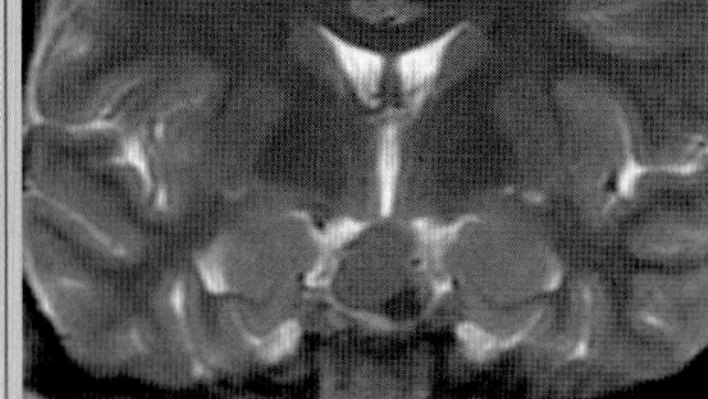 Fig. 4.14.12
Pituitary macroadenoma (with cystic degeneration or necrosis) They are the most common suprasellar mass in adults. CT helps to show hemorrhagic, cystic, or necrotic components in the lesion. GRE/SWI helps to distinguish calcification and hemorrhage. Treatment—transphenoidal hypophysectomy, gamma knife radiosurgery.	MRI—T1isointense; T1 C+ (Gd)—solid components show bright enhancement. T2—isointense to grey matter, larger lesions—heterogenous T1 signal and enhancement due to of cystic change/necrosis/haemorrhagic areas.	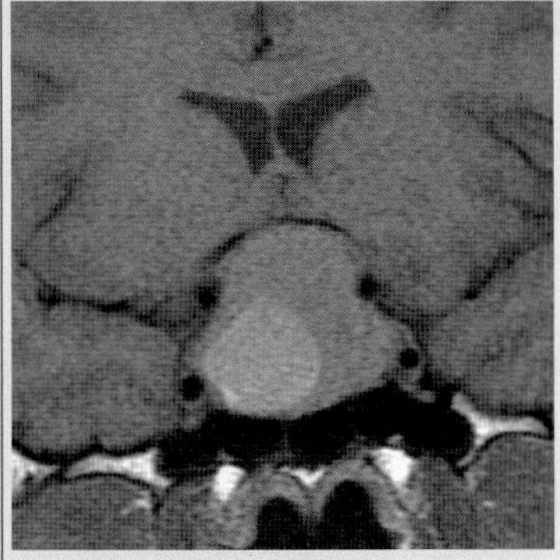 Fig. 4.14.13
Suprasellar teratoma are midline tumors which may contain calcium, soft tissue, cysts and fat. They occur from the optic chiasm to pineal regions. Treated by surgical resection.	Usually presents in younger children. CT: Demonstrate at least some fat and some calcification, which is usually solid / "clump-like". MRI: T1 **hyperintense components due to fat** and proteinaceous/lipid-rich fluid, intermediate components of soft tissue, hypointense components due to calcification and blood products. T1 C+ (Gd): Solid soft tissue components show enhancement, T2: again, mixed signal from differing components.	
Optic chiasm tuberculosis are uncommon and can be present at diagnosis of pulmonary tuberculosis or develop paradoxically during treatment. Ocular chiasmatic tuberculomas development is seen in younger age, female gender with a higher CSF protein level. Steroids will reduce inflammatory response and subsequent brain damage. Surgical decompression is done for optic chiasmatic tuberculomas with defective vision.	Multiple spherical lesions with hyperintense signal intensity wall and hypointense centre are seen on T1W MRI in the suprasellar cistern. Multiple rounding lesions can be seen on a T2W MRI. Multiple ring enhancing lesions surrounding the optic chiasma on postgadolinium-enhanced T1W MRI.	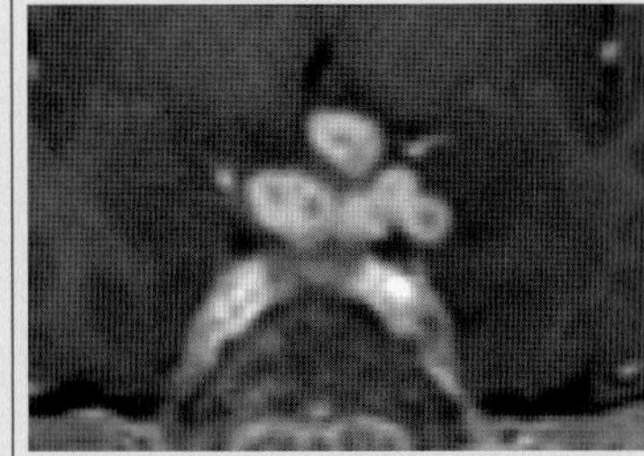 Fig. 4.14.14 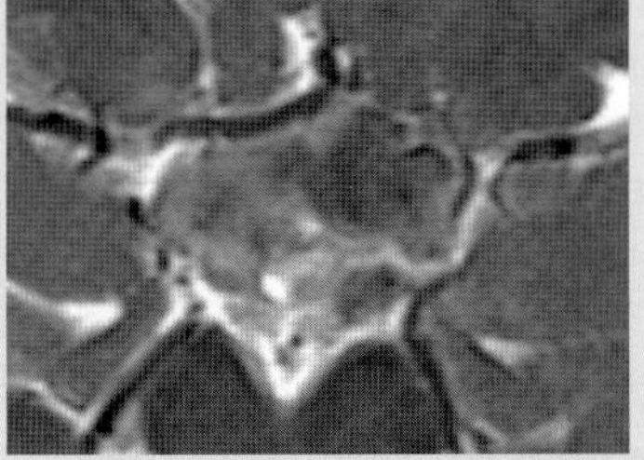 Fig. 4.14.15

Contd...

Table 4.14.1: Differential diagnosis for suprasellar lesions *(Contd...)*		
Suprasellar lesions	*Imaging features*	*Images*
Sphenoid fungal sinusitis Fig. 4.14.16: Sphenoid fungal sinusitis	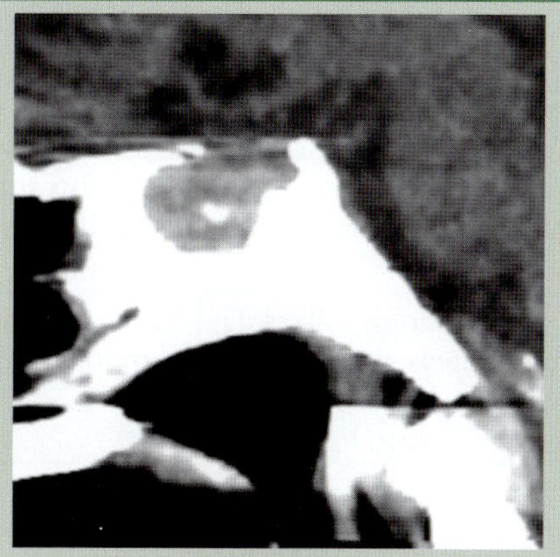 Fig. 4.14.17: Sphenoid fungal sinusitis	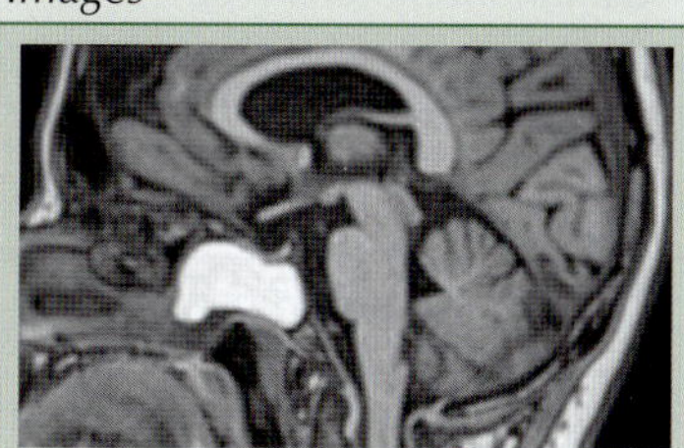 Fig. 4.14.18: Sphenoid mucocele
Suprasellar meningioma 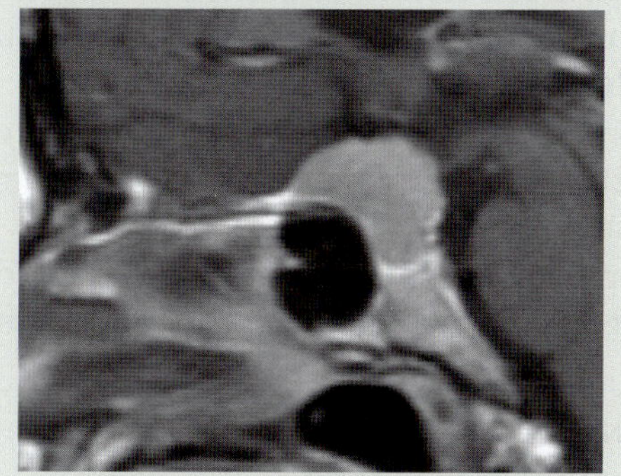 Fig. 4.14.19: Suprasellar meningioma	**Sellar and Suprasellar dermoid** 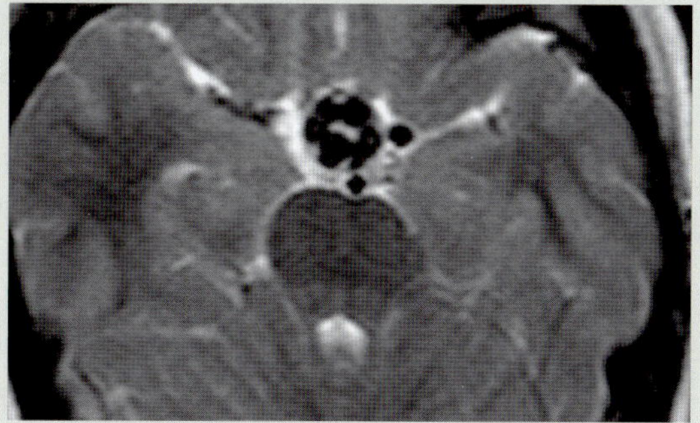 Fig. 4.14.20: Suprasellar dermoid 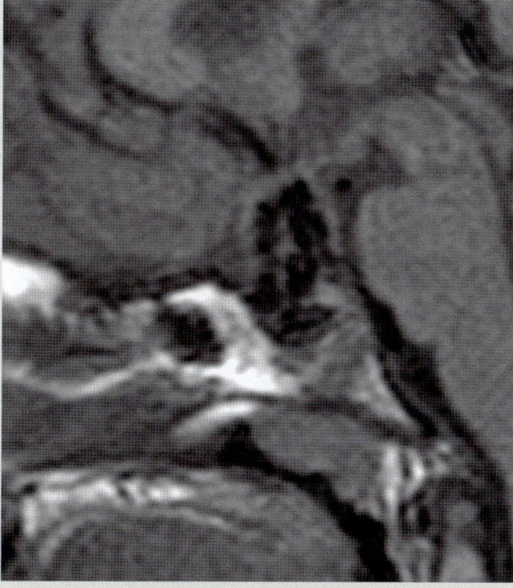 Fig. 4.14.21: Sellar dermoid	
Other DD – Sphenoid mucocele		

Discussion: Craniopharyngiomas—WHO grade I benign neoplasms in the sellar/suprasellar region with 1 to 5% prevalence among primary brain tumors. Bimodal age distribution: (5 to 15 and over 40 years old).

Table 4.14.2: Craniopharyngioma difference between adamantinomatous vs papillary type	
Adamantinomatous type	*Papillary type*
Bimodal: 5 to 15 years and over 40 years of age.	Only over 40 years of age
Uni or multilocular cysts with motor oil fluid appearance.	Solid tumor without cysts
Calcification common (90%).	Calcification rare
CT-Cysts: Near-CSF density (90%). Solid component: Soft tissue density and enhancement in 90%. Calcification (90%) typically stippled and often peripheral in location.	CT—cysts small and not a significant feature. solid component: Soft tissue density with vivid enhancement. Calcification: Uncommon, rare
T1 hyperintense cystic high protein content motor oil cysts, they are variable signal on T2W solid components show intense enhancement SWI can find calcification within the lesion MRA—A1 segment of the ACA is displaced by lesion. MRS broad lipid peak.	T1 hypointense cystic lesions, T2 variable signal intensity with solid components showing vivid enhancement. MRS—no lipid peak

Table 4.14.3: Summary of suprasellar mass lesions	
Suprasellar mass lesions	
Neoplastic	*Non-neoplastic*
Extension of pituitary macroadenoma Meningioma Craniopharyngioma Chiasmatic glioma Infundibular mass Hypothalamic hamartoma	Ectatic or aneurysmal carotid artery Arachnoid cyst Epidermoid cyst Dermoid Rathke's cleft cyst Lymphocytic histiocytosis Sarcoidosis

Infundibular lesions in children: Langerhans cell histiocytosis, Germinoma, Meningitis, lymphoma, glioma.

Suprasellar mass lesions: (SATCHMOE) S: Sarcoid, A: Aneurysm, T: Teratoma/Tuberculosis, C: Craniopharyngioma, Cleft cyst (Rathke), Chordoma, H: Hypothalamic glioma, Hamartoma of tuber cinereum, Histiocytosis, M: Meningioma, Metastasis, O: Optic nerve glioma, E: Epidermoid, Dermoid.

DD for T1 hyperintense lesions in suprasellar region: Colloid cyst, Rathke's cleft cyst, craniopharyngioma, sphenoid mucocele. white epidermoid.

Hyperdense suprasellar mass in CT includes meningioma, Rathke's cleft cyst (10%), pituitary apoplexy, aneurysm

Hyperdense suprasellar cystic lesions in CT include long standing cyst-like bronchogenic cyst, colloid cyst, white epidermoid.

Pituitary stalk imaging:

Normal: <2 mm with inferior tapering.

Uniform thickening: Langerhans cell histiocytosis and neurosarcoidosis.

V-shaped: Metastatic lymphoma. Round/diamond: Lymphocytic hypophysitis. Pyramidal: Langerhans cell histiocytosis.

Table 4.14.4: Imaging approach to suprasellar lesions

Optic chiasmatic glioma	*Hypophysitis*	*Macroadenoma*	*Craniopharyngioma*	*Hypothalamic hamartoma*
Anterior to pituitary stalk	Infundibular thickening	Figure of 8 appearance	No waist, T1 hyperintensity	Posterosuperior to optic chiasm and infundibulum
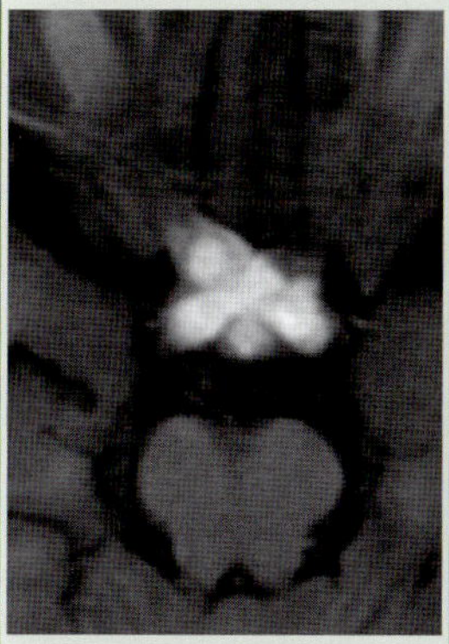 Fig. 4.14.22	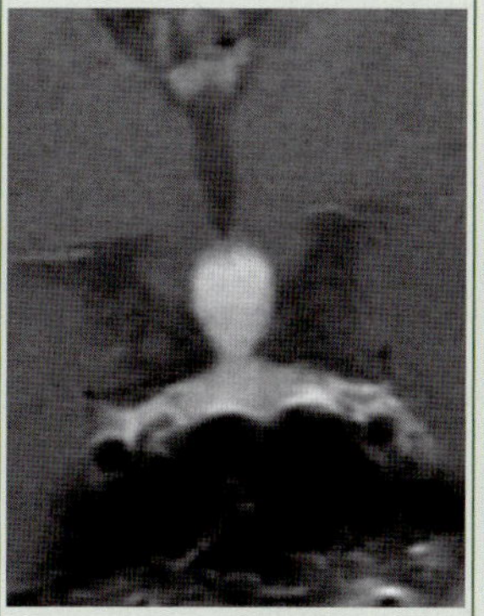 Fig. 4.14.25	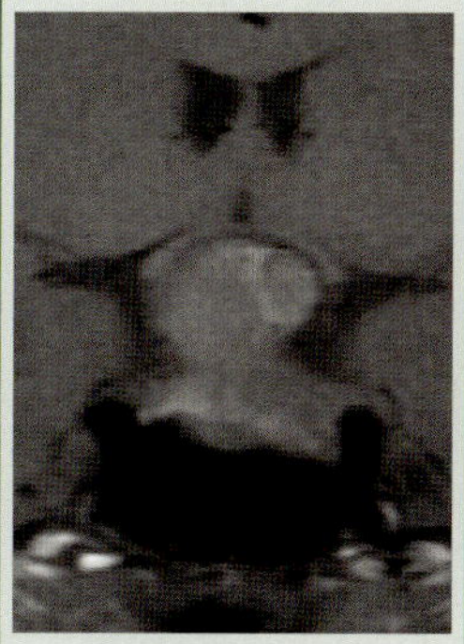 Fig. 4.14.28	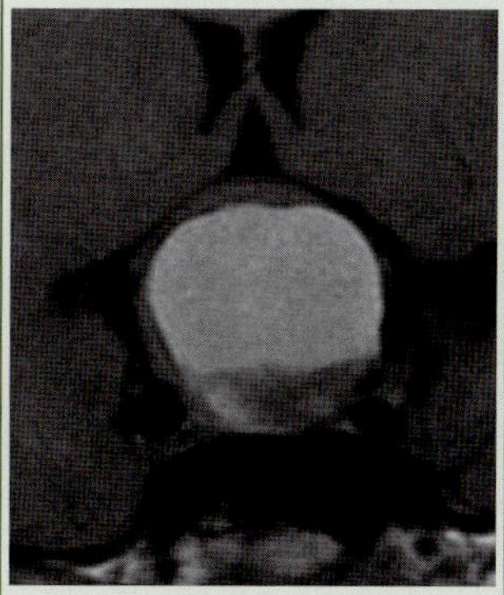 Fig. 4.14.31	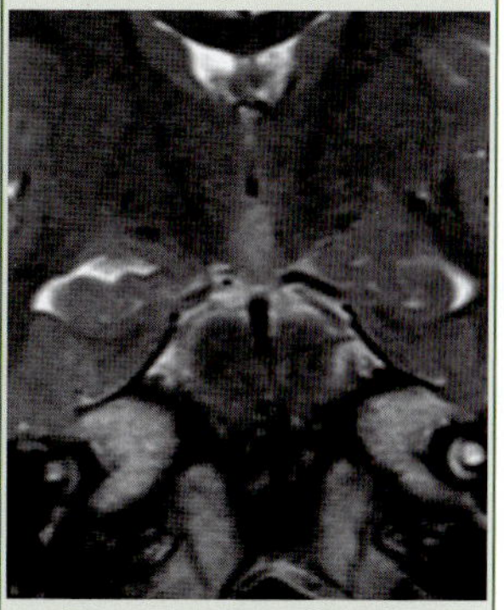 Fig. 4.14.34
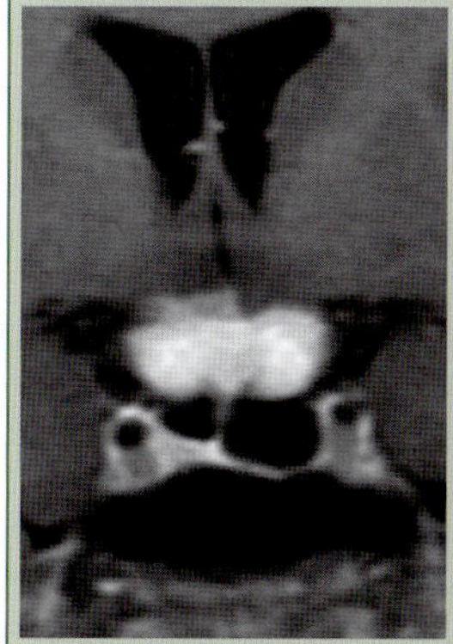 Fig. 4.14.23	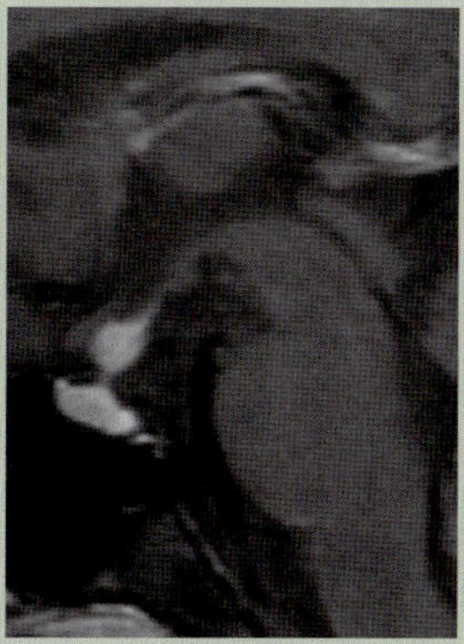 Fig. 4.14.26	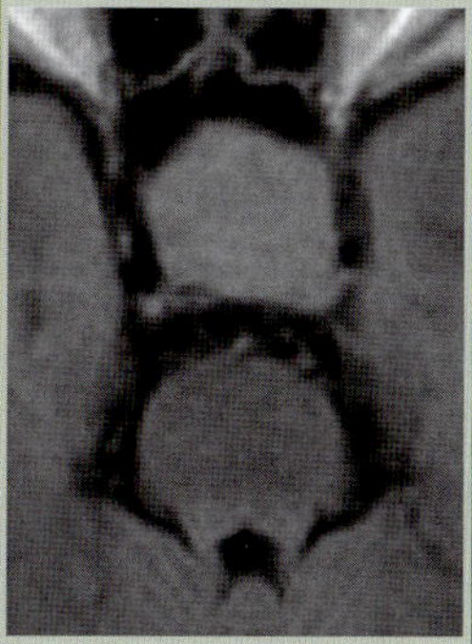 Fig. 4.14.29	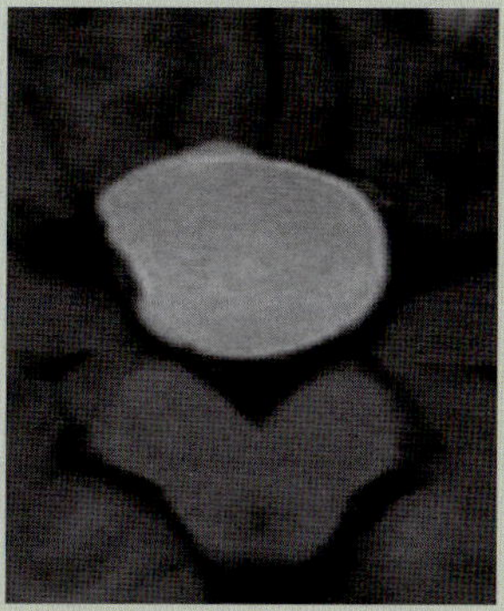 Fig. 4.14.32	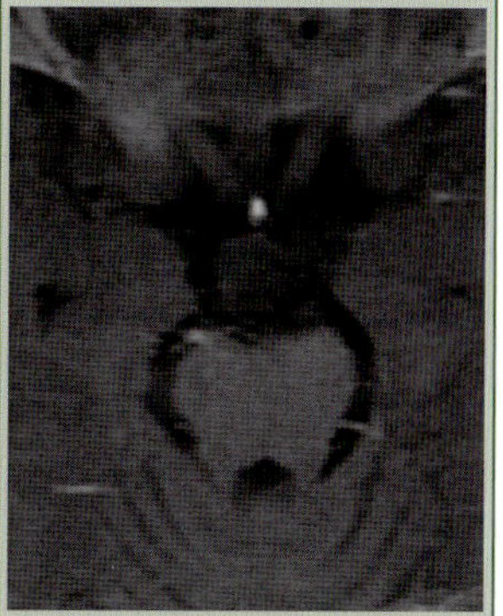 Fig. 4.14.35
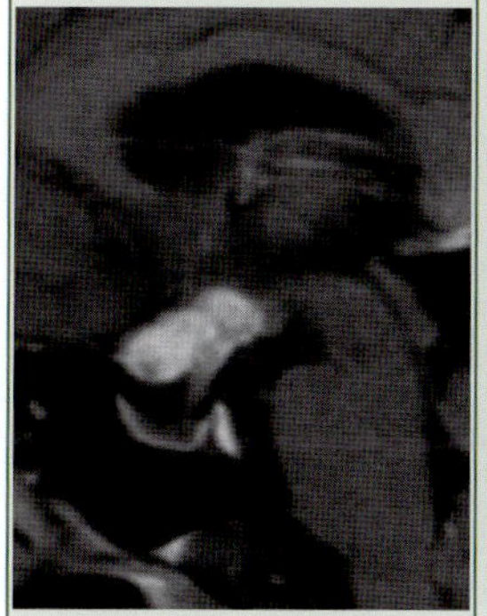 Fig. 4.14.24	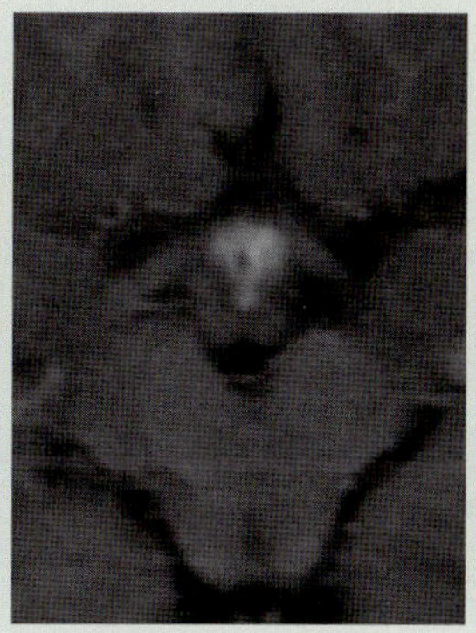 Fig. 4.14.27	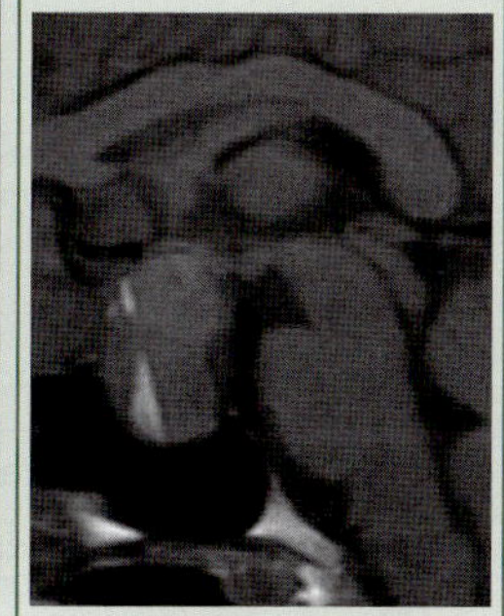 Fig. 4.14.30	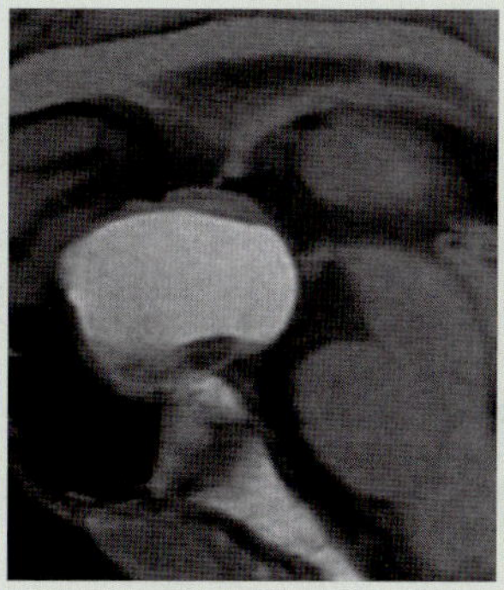 Fig. 4.14.33	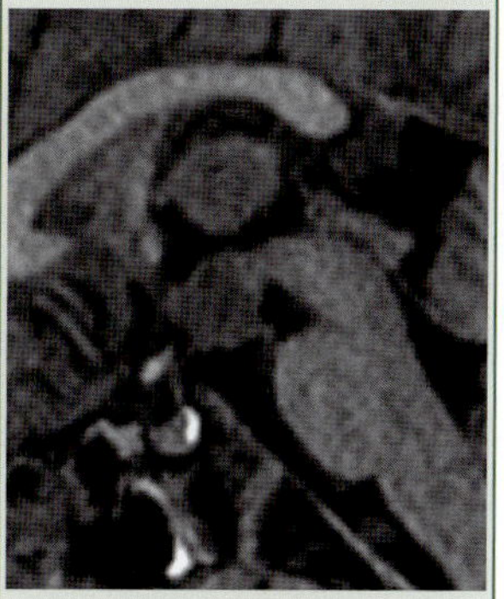 Fig. 4.14.36

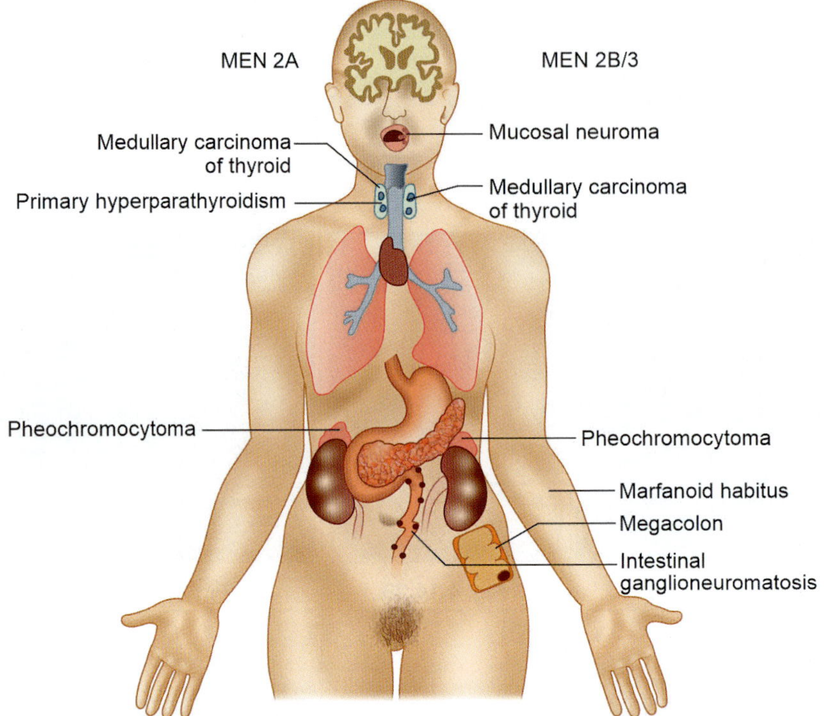

Fig. 4.14.37: Features of MEN 2A and 2B/3

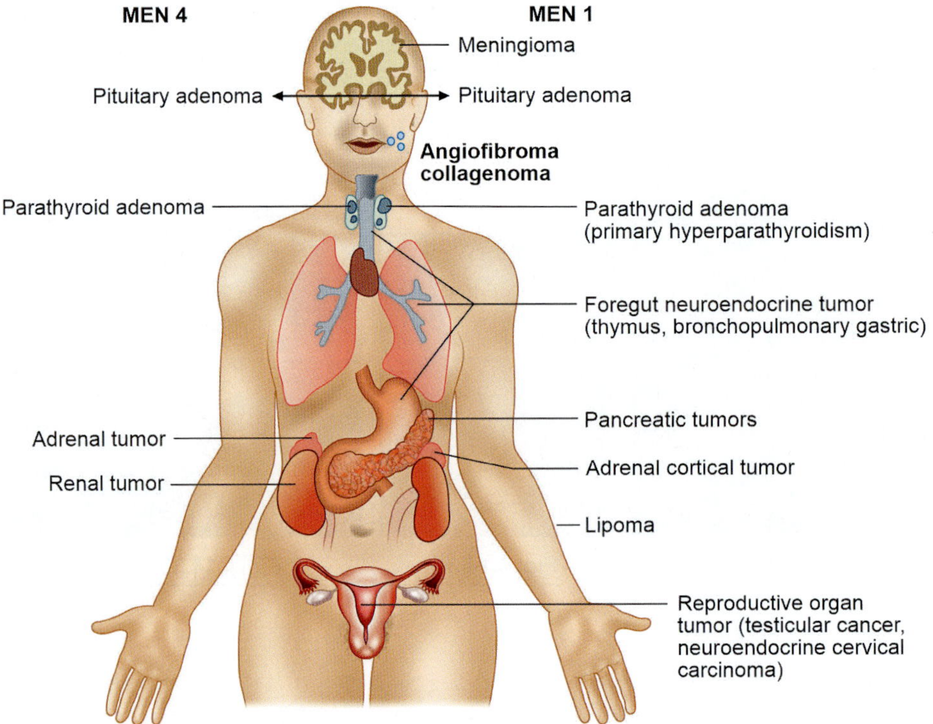

Fig. 4.14.38: Features of MEN 4 and MEN 1

4.15 CENTRAL NERVOUS SYSTEM

Case No. 15

Clinical history: 44 years old male patient with complaints of headache, diplopia and giddiness.

Radiological techniques and observation: Figures 4.15.1 and 4.15.2 are **plain radiograph** of hand in frontal view of 44 years old male patient show ungual tufting **(spade like appearance)**, widening of the bases of distal phalanges. Mild osteoporosis noted in the visualized bone. No evidence of joint space narrowing, no evidence of soft tissue swelling/soft tissue calcification. No evidence of peri-articular sclerosis or lysis. Figure 4.15.3 is **plain radiograph skull in lateral view** showing **widened sella,** thickened skull vault, pneumosinus dilatans (dilated paranasal sinuses), prominent external occipital protuberance and obtuse angled mandible (prognathism). Visualized cervical spine appears normal. No evidence of any soft tissue swelling. No evidence of dental malalignment. Figure 4.15.4 is **plain radiograph foot in lateral view** showing **increased heel pad thickness** measuring 24 mm.

Figures 4.15.5 and 4.15.6 are **plain CT brain in axial section** in bone and brain window respectively showing widened pituitary fossa with thinning of walls of sella, in brain window shows an ill-defined isodense lesion in the pituitary fossa. Sphenoid sinus shows presellar type of pneumatisation with a septum attached towards the right of roof of sphenoid. Adjacent brain parenchyma appears normal. No evidence of extension into the ethmoid sinus. Visualised optic nerve and orbit appears normal. Figures 4.15.7 and 4.15.8 are **MRI** pituitary fossa in T1 sagittal and T2 axial sections showing expanded sella with T1 iso and T2 hyperintense lesion in the sellar region with suprasellar extension. Pituitary gland and posterior pituitary bright spot not visualised separately. Pituitary infundibulum is compressed. No evidence of compression of optic chiasma. No evidence of cavernous sinus/sphenoid sinus extension. Bilateral internal carotid artery appears normal. No evidence of hemorrhage. Visualised brain parenchyma appears normal.

Interpretation: A—44 years old male patient, pathology in pituitary gland C-T1 isointense and T2 hyperintense lesion arising from the pituitary gland (pituitary gland not visualised separately), with suprasellar extension giving a "figure of 8 appearance", compressing the pituitary stalk. B—ungual tufting (spade-like appearance), widening

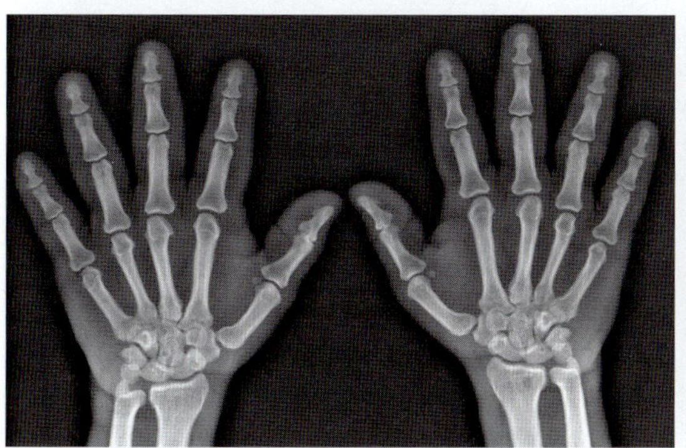

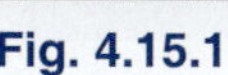

Fig. 4.15.1

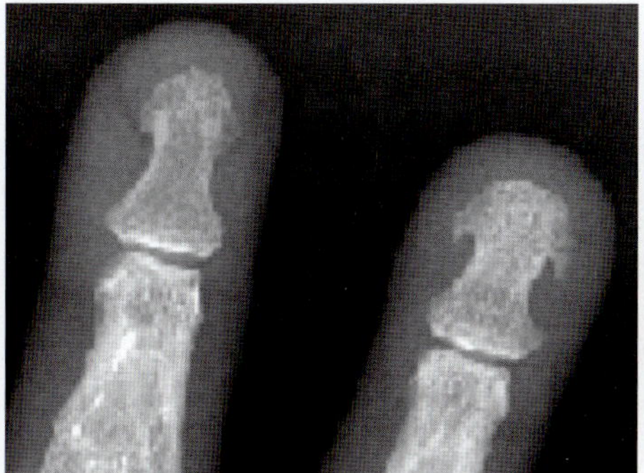

Fig. 4.15.2

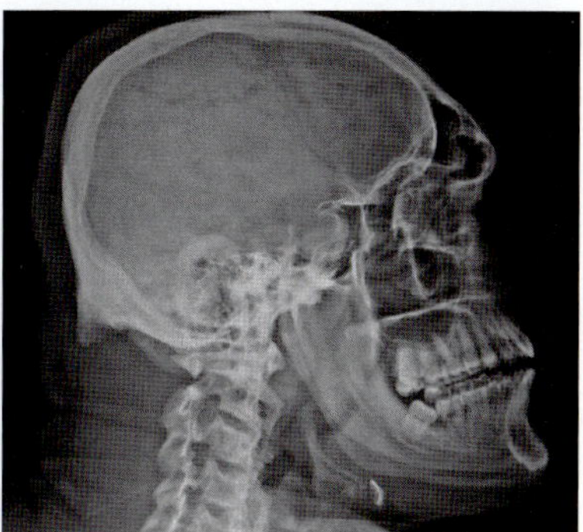

Fig. 4.15.3

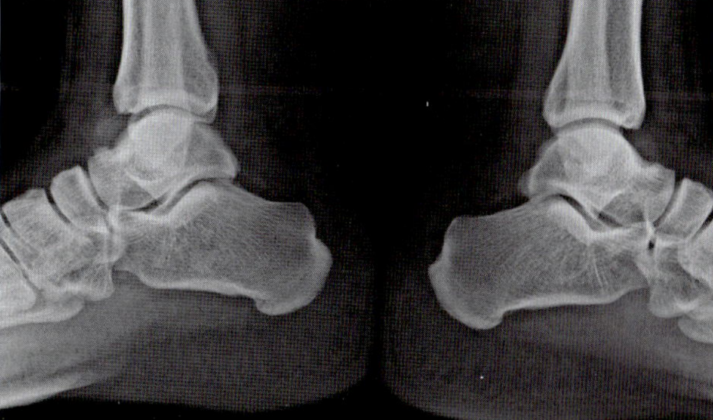

Fig. 4.15.4

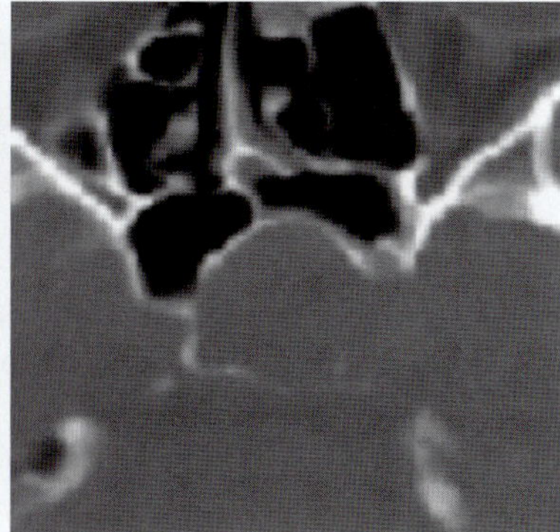

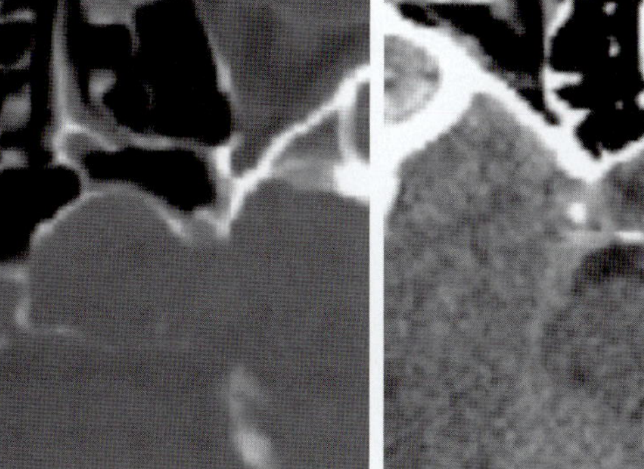

Fig. 4.15.5

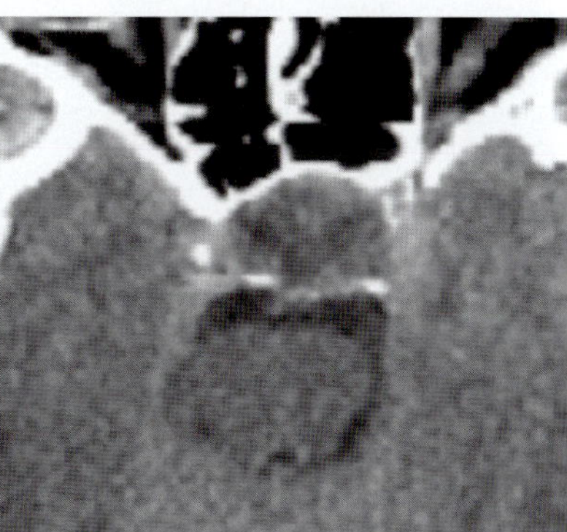

Fig. 4.15.6

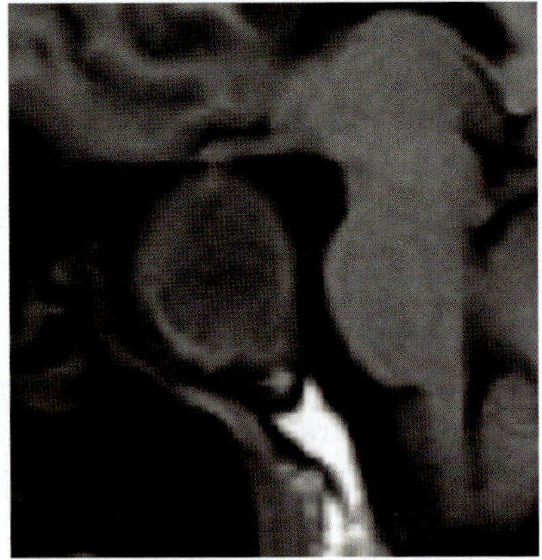
Fig. 4.15.7

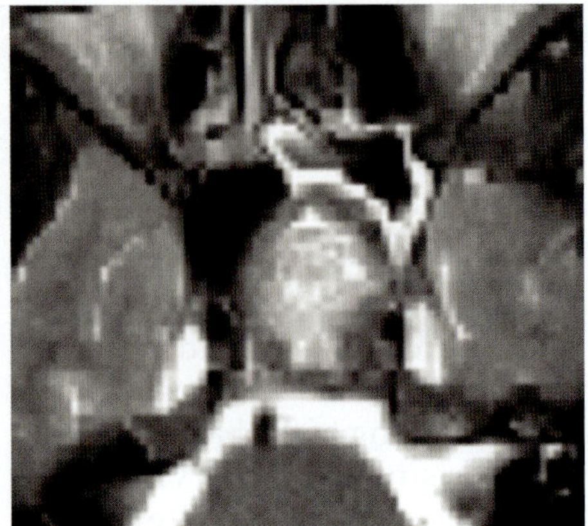
Fig. 4.15.8

Table 4.15.1: Differential diagnosis for suprasellar mass

Condition	*Radiological features*	*Image*
Pituitary hyperplasia M:F 2:1, 18–35 years, Enlarged pituitary in pre-pubscent male/ female—do hormonal work up	Convex upward margin of the gland >10 mm, usually 12–16 mm Homogenous enhancement on postcontrast. Rarely ACTH secreting tumors show focal nodular enhancement postcontrast.	Fig. 4.15.9: Pituitary hyperplasia
Saccular aneurysm Well-defined eccentric suprasellar lesion, not directly suprasellar. Pituitary gland visible separately.	**CT** hyperdense lesion which shows the vessel of origin in CTA. **MRI:** Flow void and vessel of origin identified in MRA.	Fig. 4.15.10: Saccular aneurysm
Meningioma Young adults and old age with mean age of presentation is 69 years. M:F 3.5–4:1. WHO grade I tumor	**CT:** Well-defined dural-based **hyperdense extra axial lesion** with CSF cleft and adjacent hyperostosis. **MRI:** Well-defined **T1** and **T2** iso to hypointense lesion with diaphragma sella identified as thin dark line between the mass above and the normal pituitary below. FLAIR hyperintense peritumoral edema. **On contrast shows intense homogenous enhancement with dural tail.**	Fig. 4.15.11: Meningioma

(Contd.)

Table 4.15.1: Differential diagnosis for suprasellar mass (*Contd.*)		
Condition	*Radiological features*	*Image*
Craniopharyngioma Bimodal distribution (5–15 years and >65 years) M = F **CT—adamantinous type (children)**—90% tumor—90% mixed solid and cystic, calcify and enhance. **Papillary type**—adults, solid, rarely calcifies	**MRI**—T1-hyperintense cyst with an isointense nodule that enhances on postcontrast T1 FS/ T1 isointense solid lesion showing homogenous enhancement of solid component. **T2/FLAIR** variably hyperintense cysts with hypointense areas of calcification. Variable on diffusion.	**Fig. 4.15.12:** Craniopharyngioma
Empty sella An empty sella (ES) is an **arachnoid-lined, CSF-filled protrusion** that extends from the suprasellar cistern through the diaphragma sellae into the sella turcica **Primary**—defect in diaphragm sella **Secondary**—postsurgery/ radiotherapy/ bromocriptine therapy/pituitary apoplexy/Sheehan syndrome Any age, but most common in **5th decade with M: F–4:1**	**CT**—CSF-dense fluid with normal sized or enlarged sella. The **bony floor** of the sella is intact in primary ES, but, in secondary ES, it often shows a **surgical defect caused by transsphenoidal hypophysectomy.** **CECT:** The infundibular stalk and pituitary remnant enhance normally. **In empty sella, stalk is usually at midline. In sellar/suprasellar arachnoid cyst, stalk is displaced by the lesion.** **MRI**—cyst follows CSF intensity in all sequences without any diffusion restriction	**Fig. 4.15.13:** Empty sella
Arachnoid cyst Refer to Case No 21 **Fig. 4.15.14:** Arachnoid cyst	**ICA aneurysm** **Fig. 4.15.15:** ICA aneurysm	**Fig. 4.15.16:** Pituitary cyst
Rathke's cleft cyst	**Refer to Case 14**	

(*Contd.*)

Table 4.15.1: Differential diagnosis for suprasellar mass (*Contd.*)

Condition	*Radiological features*	*Image*
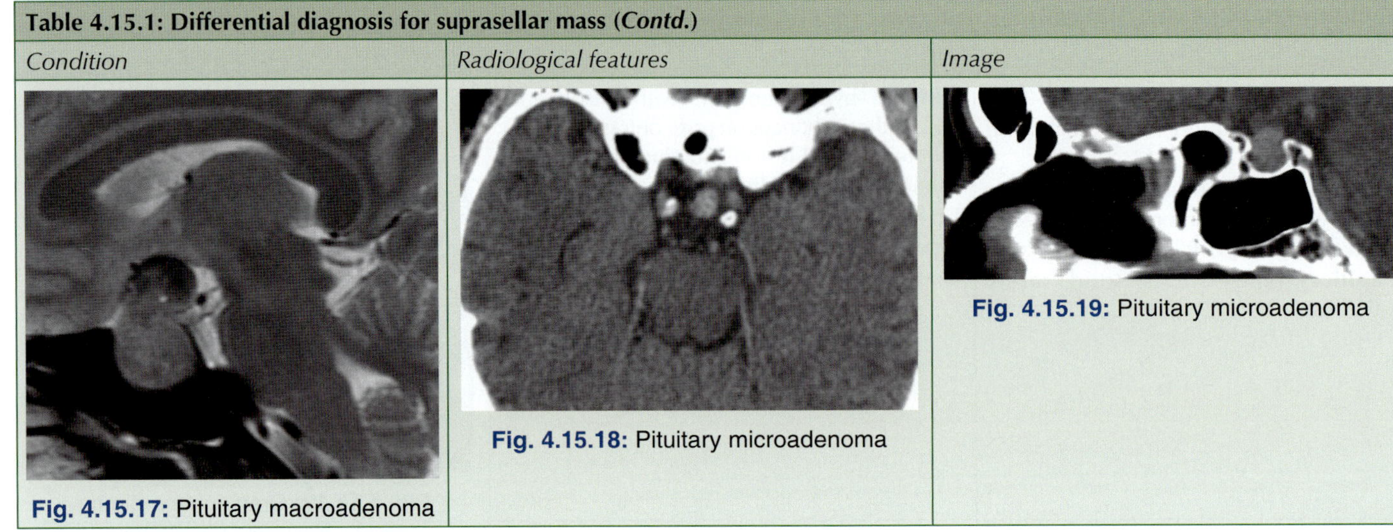 **Fig. 4.15.17:** Pituitary macroadenoma	**Fig. 4.15.18:** Pituitary microadenoma	**Fig. 4.15.19:** Pituitary microadenoma

of the bases of distal phalanges. Mild osteoporosis in the visualized bones. D—functioning pituitary macroadenoma with acromegaly.

Principal diagnosis: Functioning pituitary macroadenoma with acromegaly.

Differential Diagnosis

1. **Pituitary hyperplasia**
2. **Meningioma** of the diaphragma sella (pituitary seen separately)
3. **Metastasis**—more common in pituitary stalk from breast/lung (spread through adjacent bone/cavernous sinus)
4. **Craniopharyngioma** in adults (as solid form), here pituitary seen separately
5. **Aneurysm** from circle of Willis (usually off midline, MRI shows flow voids, flow related artefact noted, CT cerebral angio is diagnostic)

Management

1. **Biochemical investigations:** Growth hormone, prolactin, ACTH, TSH levels.
2. **Medical:** Prolactin secreting tumors—cabergoline or bromocriptine.
3. **Surgery:** Stereotactic radiosurgery, conventional transphenoidal surgery.

Discussion

Clinical features: 40–50% present with hyper prolactinemia, 10% with acromegaly, 6% with cushing syndrome/Nelson syndrome (rapid enlargement of an adenoma following bilateral adrenalectomy) and 1% with hyperthyroidism. Female patients with prolactinemia present with amenorrhoea—galactorrhoea, male patients with hypogonadism and impotence. GH secreting tumors cause acromegaly in adults and gigantism in children.

Prolactin Levels

Normal: <20 ng/ml, 30–200 ng/ml—pregnancy, postpartum, stress, hypothyroidism, renal and liver failure, 300 ng/ml—macroadenoma secretin prolactin.

X-ray features of acromegaly:

1. **Enlargement of cartilage spaces:** Widened interphalangeal, metacarpophalangeal, intervertebral disc spaces and prominent costochondral articulations.
2. **Skull:** Sella turcica enlargement from the pituitary neoplasm, sinus overgrowth (pneumosinus dilatans),

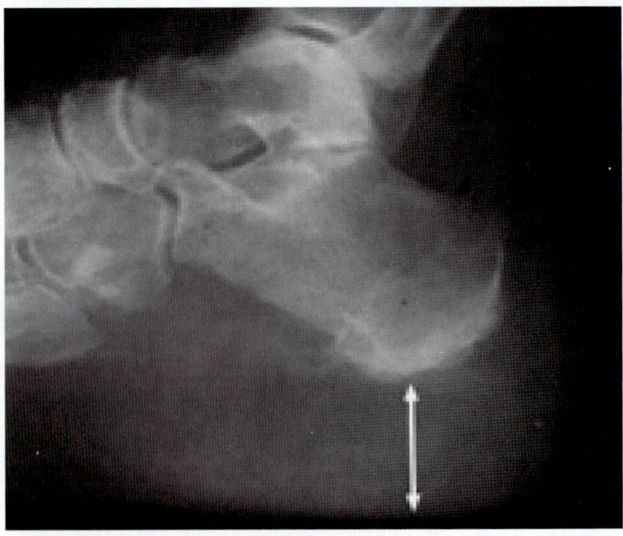

Fig. 4.15.20: Increased heel pad thickness in acromegaly

occipital protuberance overgrowth, malocclusion, and obtuse mandibular angle (prognathic jaw).

3. **Others:** Spade-like terminal tufts, squaring of metacarpal heads, thickenend diaphysis of long bones (normal cortical thickness), in vertebral body, there is increase in AP diameter than transverse diameter with posterior vertebral body scalloping, generalised osteoporosis with premature osteoarthritis.
4. **Soft tissue enlargement** especially of hand and feet with prominent muscle attachments and increased heel pad thickness. (Male >21.5 mm, female >23 mm)
   Heel pad sign: Heel pad thickness >23 mm may indicate acromegaly.
5. **Sesamoid index:** Defined as **the product of height and width (in mm) of the medial sesamoid at the metacarpophalangeal joint of the thumb**—(not a reliable criteria as there is a large overlap between the normal and acromegalic patients).

Pituitary Adenoma

Pituitary adenoma is a benign neoplasm of the adenohypophysis.

Microadenoma—<1 cm, macroadenoma >1 cm.

CT—well-defined **isodense lesion** in the sella with/without areas of necrosis and cystic changes, calcification and hemorrahge is rare.

On CECT shows heterogenous enhancement of the lesion. On bone CT the lesion causes **widening** of the sella with **erosion of floor and extension into the sphenoid sinus.**

On MRI T1 and T2 isointense lesion with absent (20%) or displaced posterior pituitary bright spot. **Pituitary gland cannot be seen separately from the lesion.**

On postcontrast imaging, the lesion shows intense homo to heterogenous enhancement. Cases showing splaying of ICA with encasement in <10–20% cases.

Pituitary Protocol

Pituitary gland **is outside the blood–brain barrier** and hence enhances rapidly and strongly than the normal brain tissue. It requires **half the normal dose of gadolinium** (normal dose—0.1 to 0.2 mmol/kg, pituitary—0.05 mmol/kg). Enhancement is slightly less than that of the venous blood in the cavernous sinus.

6 consecutive sets of 3 images taken in coronal plane every 10 s apart.

- The enhancement occurs in the pituitary stalk first, then in the pituitary tuft (the junction of stalk and gland) and finally there is a centrifugal opacification of the entire anterior lobe.

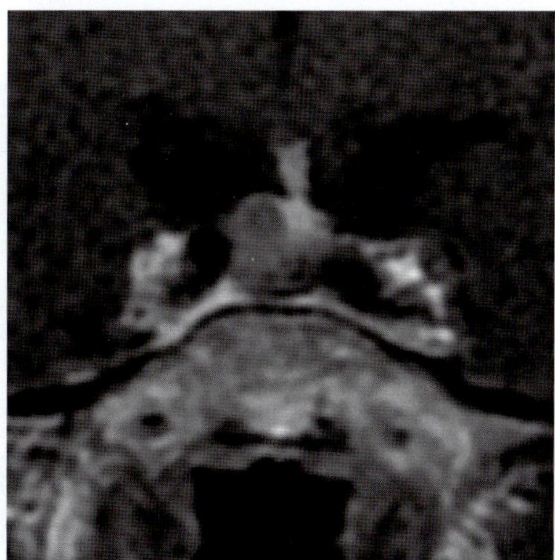

Fig. 4.15.21: Postcontrast fat suppressed coronal image showing hypoenhancing lesion in right side of pituitary gland: Microadenoma

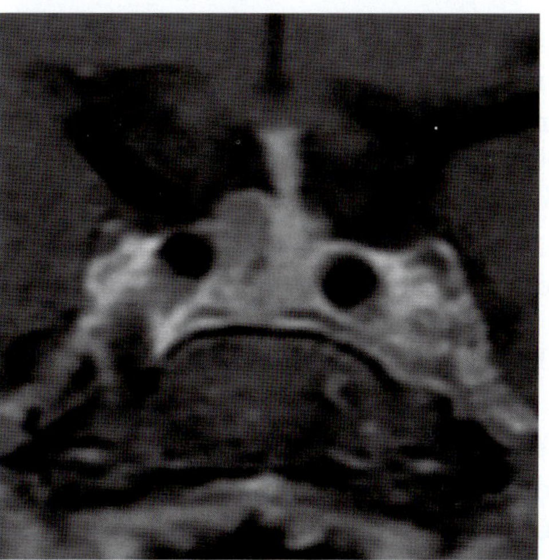

Fig. 4.15.22: Postcontrast fat suppressed coronal image showing hypoenhancing lesion in right side of pituitary gland: Microadenoma

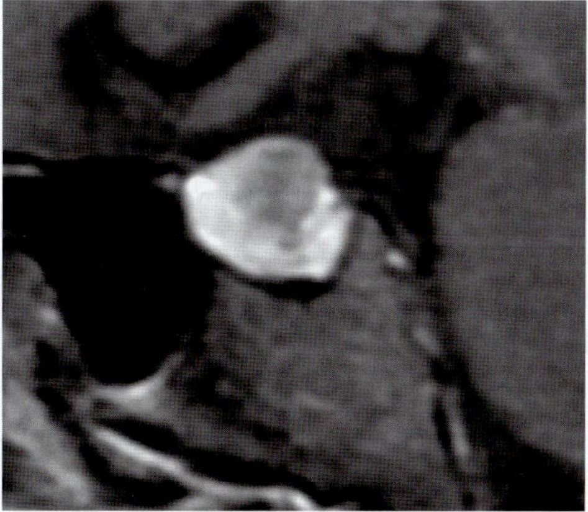

Fig. 4.15.23: Postcontrast fat sat sagittal image showing well-defined hypoenhancing lesion in the sella arising from the pituitary gland—pituitary microadenoma

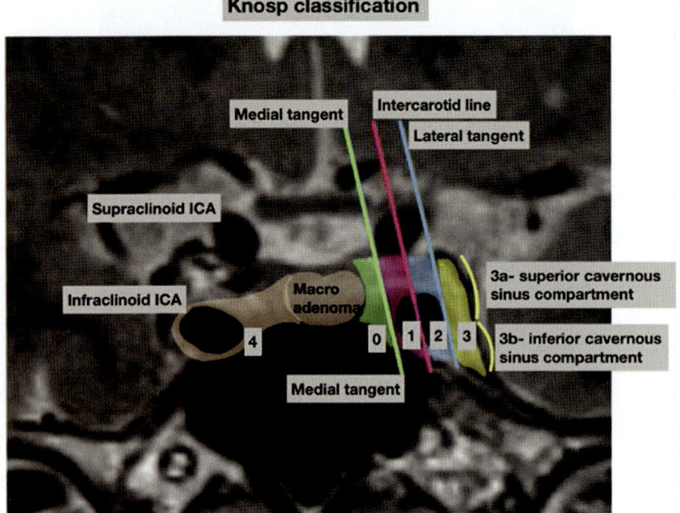

Fig. 4.15.24: Knosp classification

- Within 30–60s the entire gland shows homogenous enhancement.
- The maximum image contrast between the normal pituitary tissue and microadenoma is attained about 30–60 s after the bolus injection of the IV contrast.

Dynamic MRI: Used for the identification of pituitary microadenomas. Coronal T1 postcontrast images, in coronal plane with small FOV and 3 mm thickness taken at 0s, 30s, 60s, 90s, 120s and 180s.

Pituitary Microadenoma

Microadenoma is the lesion <10 mm.

WHO grade I tumors, occurs as a part of MEN syndrome, Carney complex or McCune-Albright syndrome.

CT—small lesions are **isodense** to adjacent normal pituitary and invisible. **On CECT—two-thirds are hypodense to normal pituitary.**

MRI—T1 heterointense, T2 isointense lesion which appears as **filling defect in the background of normal pituitary gland on immediate postcontrast T1** and **shows delayed enhancement (evident on dynamic MRI).**

Angiography supra sellar extension of macroadenoma **splaying of supraclinoid ICA** and anterior choroidal arteries with a **tumour blush.**

Treatment: 1. Surgical—resection is the primary therapy (15% recurrence); 2. Medical (bromocriptine and cabergoline); 3. Stereotaxic radiosurgery; 4. Conventional XRT.

Elster's rule in pituitary gland height: 6 mm—infants and children; 8 mm—men and postmenopausal women; 10 mm—women of childbearing age; 12 mm—women in late pregnancy or in postpartum women.

Sella dimensions: AP 5–16 mm (11 mm), CC 4–12 mm (8 mm), TR 9–19 mm (14 mm).

Criteria for cavernous sinus invasion:

1. The lesion encasing >270 degrees of the circumference of ICA.
2. Any lateral displacement of the lateral border of cavernous sinus compared to opposite side.
3. Any increased soft tissue lesion between the ICA and lateral wall of cavernous sinus

Knosp Grading of Cavernous Sinus Invasion in Pituitary Macroadenoma

Grade 0—does not cross the medial carotid line

Grade 1—between the medial and median carotid line

Grade 2—beyond median carotid line but does not cross the lateral carotid line

Grade 3—crosses the lateral carotid line.

Grade 4—involves whole of cavernous sinus.

Enlarged Pituitary Fossa

Apparent: Double floor, elevation or erosion of clinoid process, loss of lamina dura.

True enlargement: Intrasellar/parasellar mass, raised ICT, empty sella, Nelson's syndrome (postadrenalectomy for cushings syndrome).

'J'-shaped sella: Normal variant, optic chiasm glioma, neurofibroma, achondroplasia, mucopolysaccharidoses, chronic hydrocephalus.

Hyperdense cyst in CT: Colloid cyst, white epidermoid.

Cystic lesions of sellar region: Intrapituitary cyst—Rathke's cleft cyst, cystic pituitary adenoma; Empty sella; Epidermoid cyst; Arachnoid cyst.

Approach to Sellar Mass

Key structures to identify and assess in 'normal' studies include: (1) Pituitary gland including posterior pituitary bright spot and infundibulum; (2) optic nerves, chiasm and tracts; (3) diaphragma sella and boundaries of the pituitary fossa; (4) boundaries of the cavernous sinus and Meckel's cave; (5) internal carotid arteries and branches; (6) dynamic enhancement of the pituitary gland.

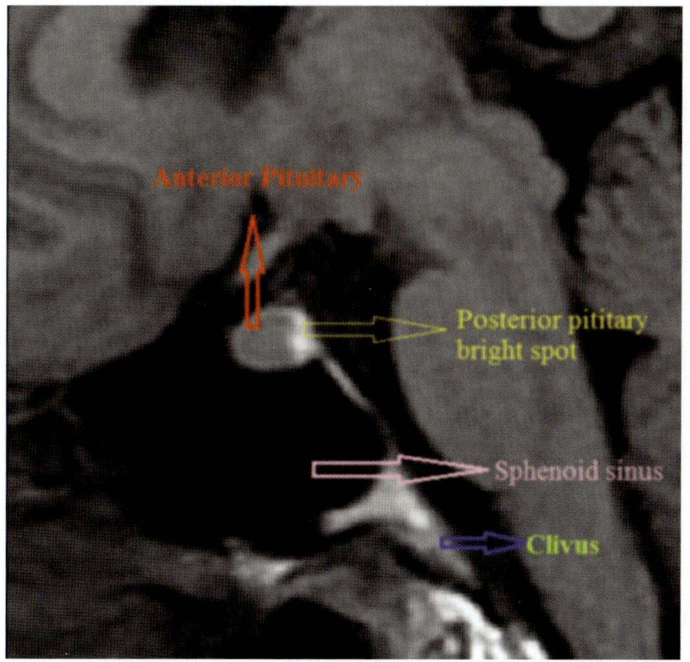

Fig. 4.15.25: Key structures for sellar mass approach

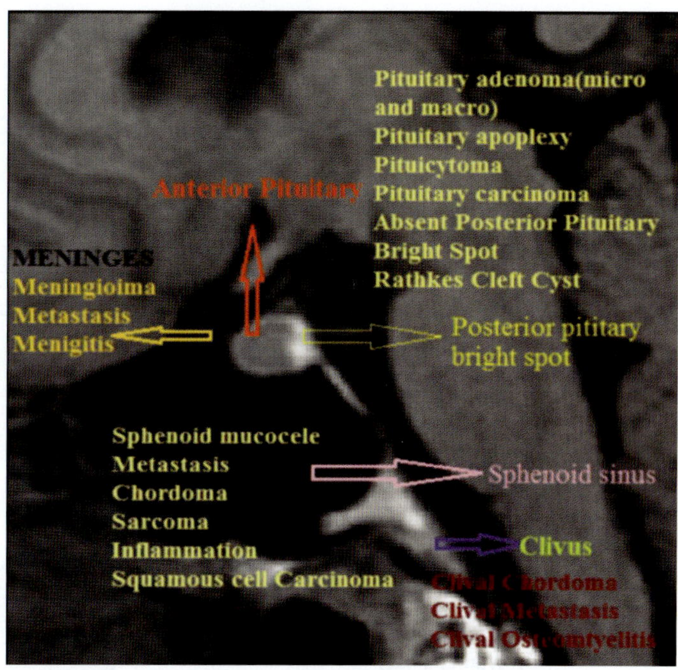

Fig. 4.15.26: Approach to sellar mass

Helpful signs: Also look for diaphragma sella displacement is either up or down.

Dural tail: Meningioma and hypophysitis and metastases.

Aunt Minnie findings: Carotid narrowing seen in meningioma, erosion of sella (rather than remodelling) is seen in metastasis; If we are able to identify pituitary as separate usually implies non-adenoma.

Specific sublocation follows the normal distribution of peptide containing cells.

Prolactinomas and growth hormone secreting tumors—the two most common pituitary. Adenomas—tend to arise laterally within the adenohypophysis thyroid-stimulating hormone (TSH) and ACTH secreting tumors are more often midline.

Table 4.15.2: Reporting a sellar lesion—essential points to be included in report

Pattern of location Purely **intrasellar** (if so, look if pituitary is seen separately or the lesion is the pituitary, diaphragm sella displaced upwards). Purely **suprasellar** (diaphragm sella displaced downwards). **Both** suprasellar and intrasellar (waist sign/narrowing at the point of diaphragm sella).	**Mass** Size in 3 dimensions Necrotic/cystic areas Size of diaphragm sella opening—narrow waist at diaphragm sella (giving figure of '8' or snowman appearance) causes difficulty in transsphenoidal surgery for removal of suprasellar component. Invasion into cavernous sinus
Age/Sex of presentation: **Adults**—meningioma, adenoma, aneurysm. **Children**—craniopharyngioma, physiological hyperplasia(male). **Postpartum female**—pituitary apoplexy, lymphocytic hypophysitis.	**Vessels** Medially located or aberrant carotid arteries Aneurysms Cavernous sinus anomalies
Pattern of morphology Solid and enhancing lesion Mixed cystic and solid lesion Cystic lesion	**Bone: Size** of sella (any widening) Degree of **sphenoid sinus pneumatization** (conchal/sellar/presellar), septum (attachment of the septum) and any normal variants (Onodi cell) **Sphenoid bone dehiscence** involving carotid arteries Any sinus disease, nasal polyps and septal spurs

Table 4.15.3: Location based differential diagnosis for lesions in and around sella

Intrasellar	*Suprasellar mass in adult*	*Suprasellar mass in children*
Pituitary hyperplasia Microadenoma Rathke's cleft cyst	Macroadenoma Meningioma Metastasis Lymphoma (Epi)dermoid cyst Aneurysm	Craniopharyngioma Astrocytoma (optic chiasm/hypothalamus) Germinoma Tuber cinerium hamartoma Arachnoid cyst
Infundibular mass—adult	*Infundibular mass—children*	*Suprasellar bright spot on T1W MRI*
Hypophysitis Sarcoidosis Metastasis Pituicytoma	Pituitary dwarfism Histiocytosis Germinoma Lymphoma	Ectopic pituitary bright spot Lipoma Dermoid Thrombosed aneurysm

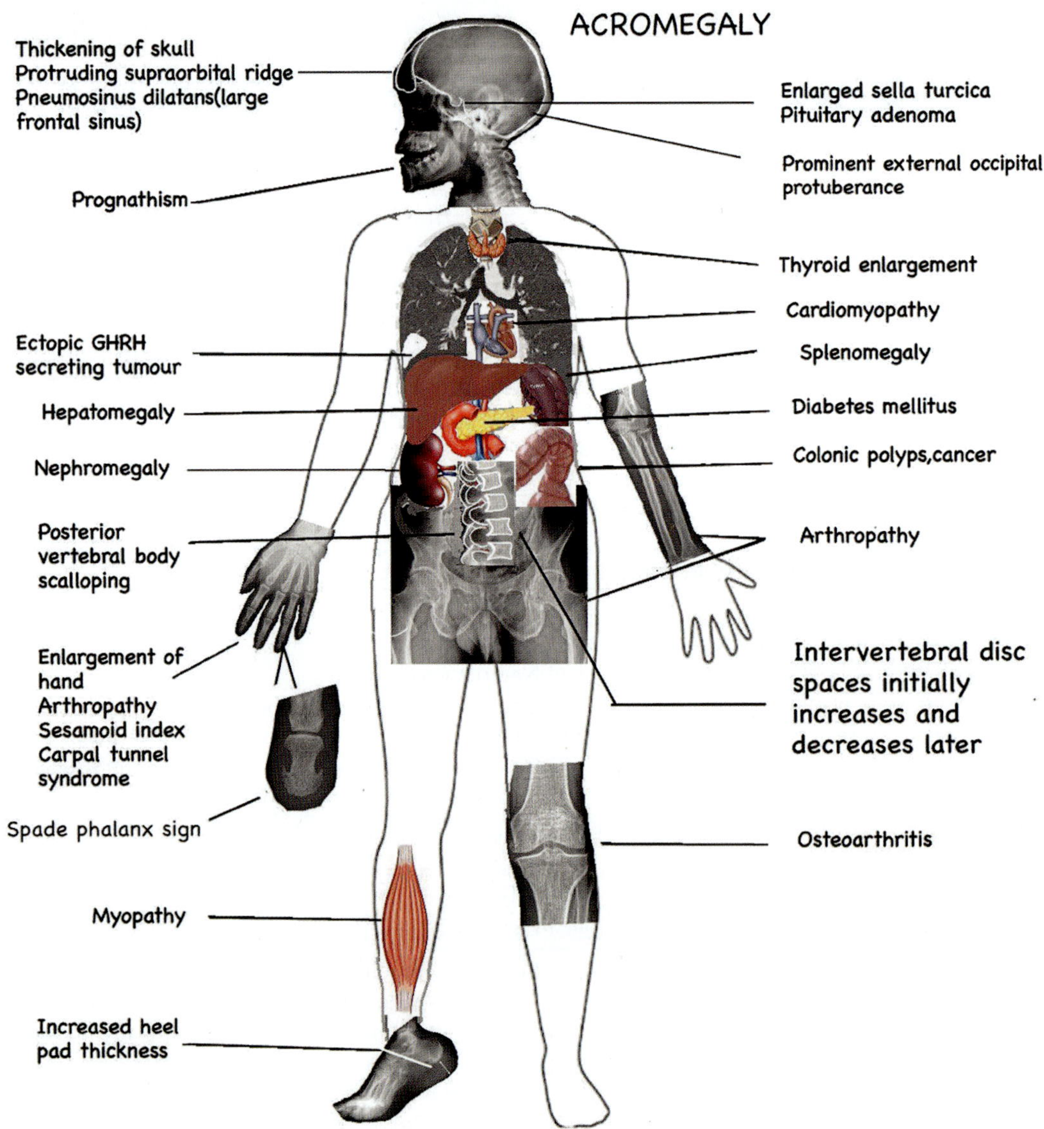

Fig. 4.15.27: Whole body illustration showing features of acromegaly

4.16 CENTRAL NERVOUS SYSTEM

Case No. 16

Clinical history: A 35-year-old male with partial ptosis on left side.

Radiological techniques and observation: Figures 4.16.1 and 4.16.2 are postcontrast T1 weighted MRI limited axial sections at the level of cavernous sinus demonstrating avidly enhancing extra-axial lesion originating from the lateral dural wall of left cavernous sinus with enhancing dural tail indenting the left anteromedial temporal lobe. There is mild constriction of the lumen of left ICA. There is no extension into the sphenoid sinus. Left 5th nerve appears normal. Right cavernous sinus and remaining visualized brain structures appear normal. No extension to orbit noted.

Interpretation: A—35 years old male, left cavernous sinus shows, C—avidly enhancing extra-axial lesion originat-ing from the lateral dural wall of left cavernous sinus, B—enhancing dural tail indenting the left antero-medial temporal lobe, D—left cavernous sinus menin-gioma.

Principal diagnosis: Left cavernous sinus menin-gioma.

Discussion: Normal lateral wall of the cavernous sinus is straight or concave, but it becomes convex in pathological conditions. Lateral dural wall give rise to majority of cavernous sinus meningiomas but also develop entirely within the cavernous sinus. Meningioma is usually hypo- to isointense on T1 and iso- to hyperintense on T2, with regard to grey matter, and enhances intensely. Calcified meningiomas are T1/T2 hypointense without enhancement. Degree of hypointensity on T2 is directly proportional to the hardness of the meningioma during surgery. A dural tail can be seen extending away from the tumor's border and into the ipsilateral tentorium. **The ICA lumen is constricted by meningiomas.** Meningiomas can grow inside the cavernous sinus, the Meckel cave, and the prepontine cistern via the porus trigeminus. Artery of Bernasconi and Cassinari arising from infra and clinoid segment of ICA supplies cavernous sinus meningioma.

Management: Since the vicinity of the tumor with vital structures shape operative strategy, Thin section CT with bone window, 3D spiral reconstruction, MRI, MRA are further investigations to be performed. Surgical resection limited to tumors with extracranial extensions is the most accepted way of management. Radiosurgery or stereotactic fractionated radiotherapy may complement surgery and reserved for growing remnants.

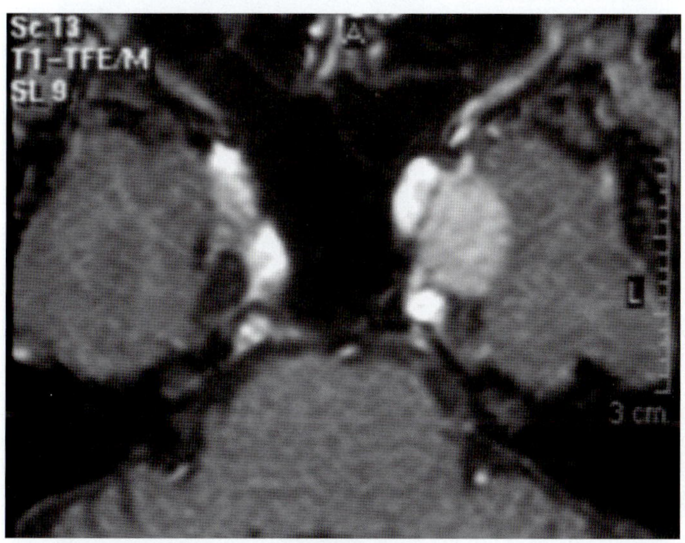

Fig. 4.16.1

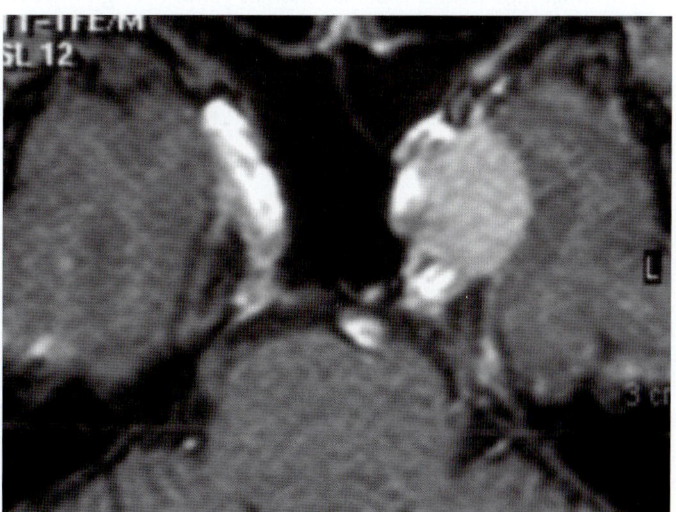

Fig. 4.16.2

Table 4.16.1: Differential diagnosis for cavernous sinus/parasellar lesions

Schwannoma: Middle aged and elderly female predilection. Surgery is the treatment of choice 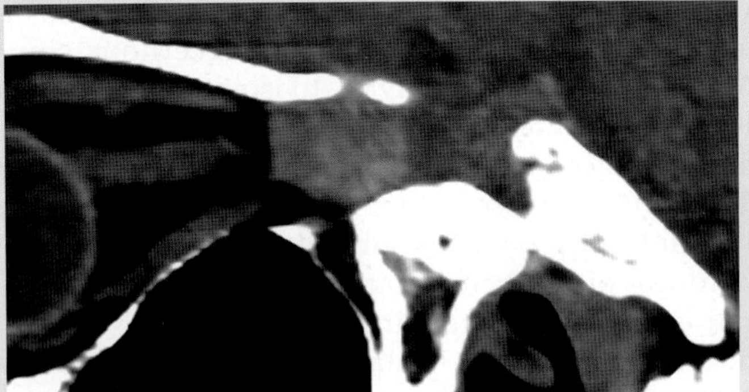 Fig. 4.16.3: Optic nerve schwannoma	Large tumors are heterogeneous. Iso to hypointense on T1W MRI hyperintense on T2. Contrast enhancement +. Follows the course of nerves from which they arise. Multiple in NF2 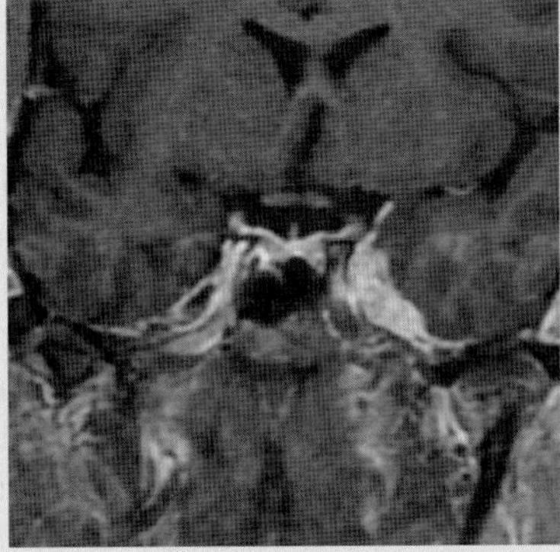 Fig. 4.16.4: Meckel's cave schwannoma	
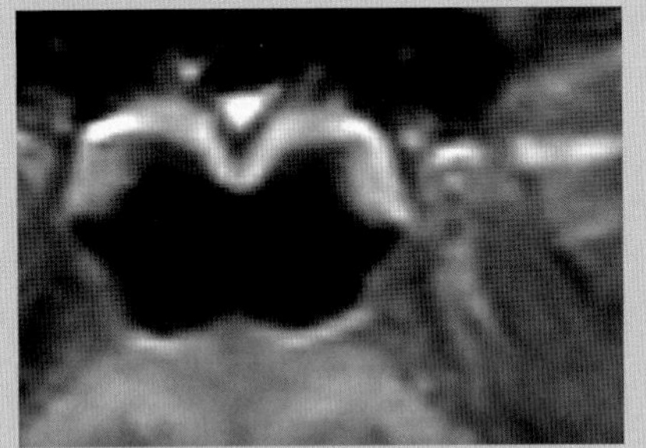 Fig. 4.16.5: Oculomotor schwannoma in cavernous sinus	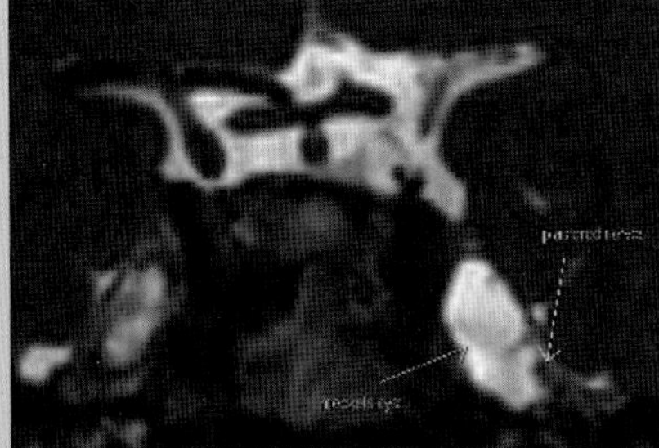 Fig. 4.16.6: Oculomotor schwannoma in cavernous sinus	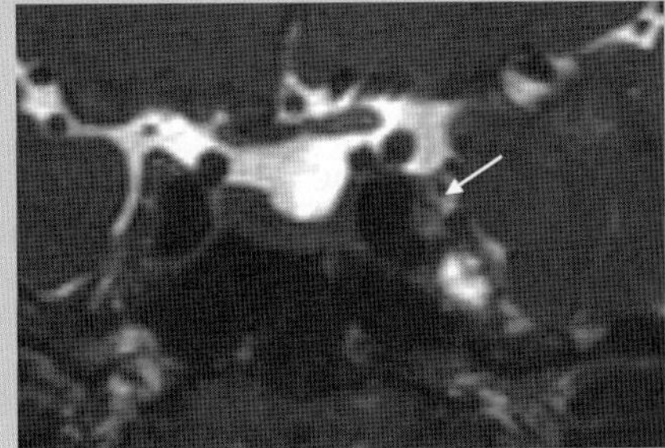 Fig. 4.16.7: Oculomotor schwannoma in cavernous sinus
Pituitary adenoma—MEN1 association. <1 cm microadenomas. Macroadenomas twice as common as microadenomas.	May grow laterally and invade the cavernous sinus. A sign of cavernous sinus invasion is encasement of intracavernous ICA by more than 270 degrees or tumor extension to top of ICA (12 o'clock). **Pituitary adenomas generally do not narrow the ICA.**	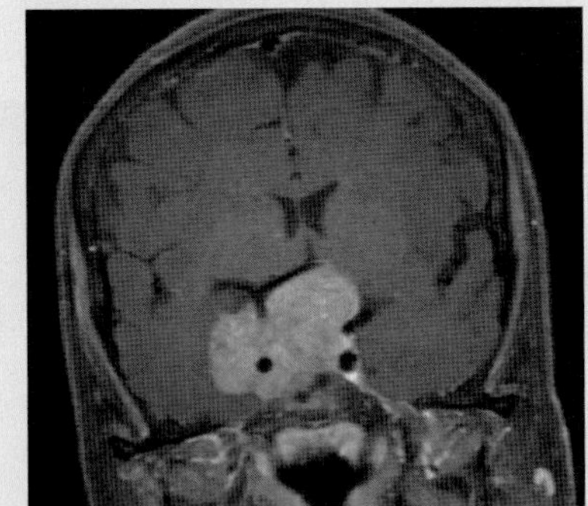 Fig. 4.16.8: Pituitary adenoma
Fungal infection: More common in immunocompromised patients. Aggressive medical and surgical debridement. Systemic antifungal with correction of diabetic ketoacidosis and neutropenia.	Invasive aspergillosis may extend to cavernous sinus, orbit, brain and carotid arteries in immunocompromised causing cavernous sinus thrombosis, **carotid occlusion**, pseudoaneurysm resulting in fatal haemorrhage. Low signal intensity on both T1 weighted and T2 weighted MRI images (ferromagnetic elements and calcium). Intense inhomogeneous contrast enhancement seen.	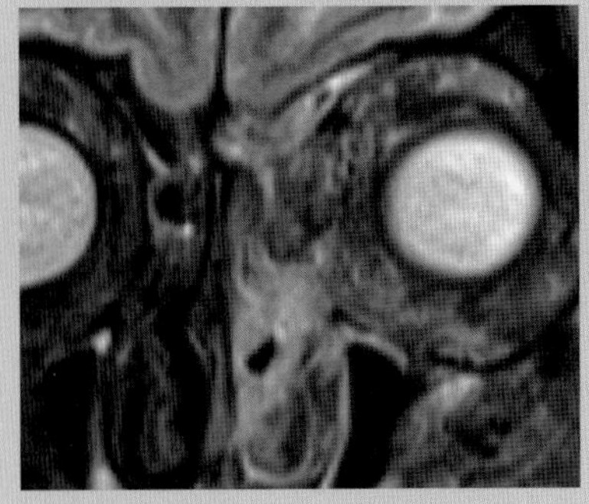 Fig. 4.16.9: Fungal sinusitis

(Contd.)

Table 4.16.1: Differential diagnosis for cavernous sinus/parasellar lesions (*Contd.*)

Plexiform neurofibroma: Diagnosed early childhood. Found in 30% patients with NF1.	Most commonly involves the first and second branches of trigeminal nerve, Tortuous fusiform enlargement of nerves with heterogeneous signal intensity. 30% seen in NF1.	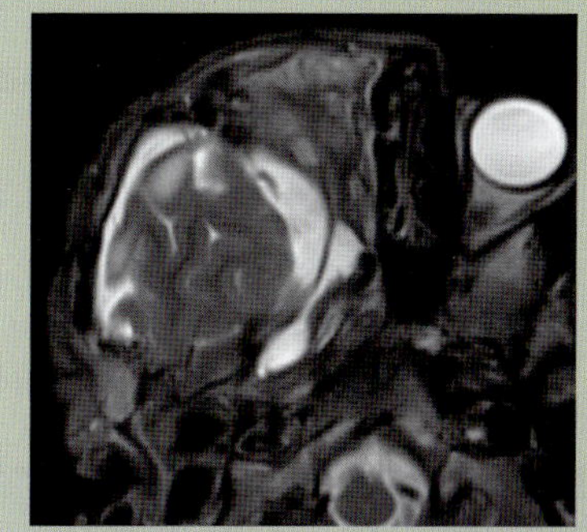 Fig. 4.16.10: Plexiform neurofibroma
Metastasis: Perineural spread common in adenoid cystic carcinoma and SCC.	Hematogenous or perineural in nature. Primary from renal, gastric, thyroid, lung and breast malignancies. MR shows CS enlargement outward bowing of lateral wall and replacement of Meckel's cave with soft tissue that homogeneously enhances.	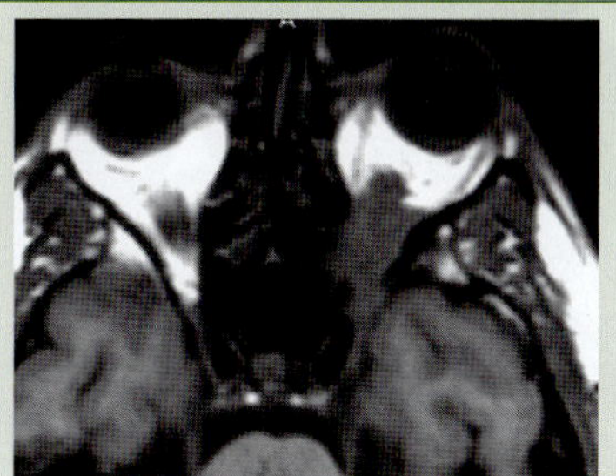 Fig. 4.16.11: Cavernous sinus metastasis
Tolosa Hunt syndrome: Painful ophthalmoplegia amenable to steroid therapy. Clinical diagnosis of exclusion. Retro-orbital pseudotumor extending to cavernous sinus. Clinical triad unilateral ophthalmoplegia, cranial nerve palsies and dramatic response to systemic corticosteroids.	MR imaging findings include an enlarged cavernous sinus containing abnormal soft tissue that is isointense to muscle on T1W, dark or bright on T2W and display contrast enhancement with focal narrowing of ICA.	
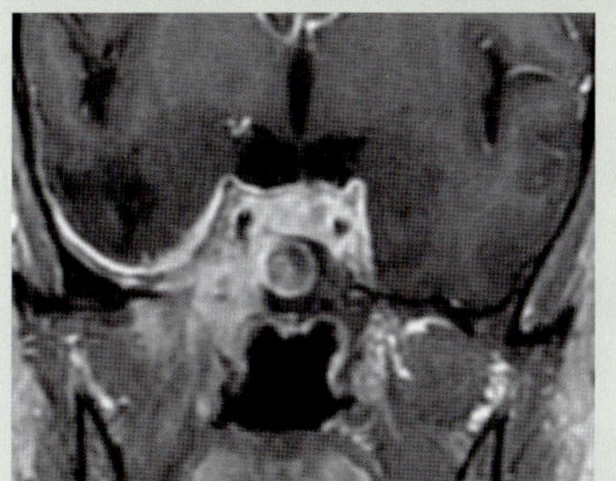 Fig. 4.16.12: Tolosa Hunt syndrome	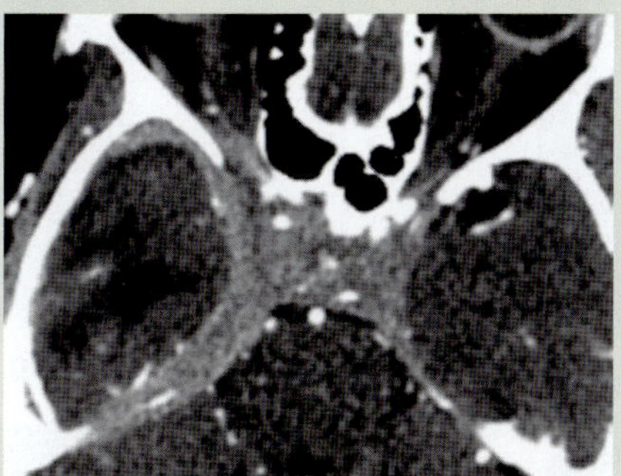 Fig. 4.16.13: Tolosa Hunt syndrome	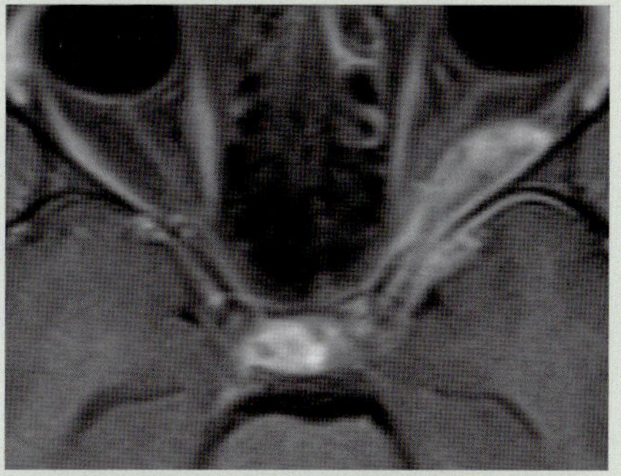 Fig. 4.16.14: Tolosa Hunt syndrome
Hemangioma: Predilection for middle aged women. Multiple cranial nerve palsies. Surgical resection challenging due to intraoperative blood loss.	Diagnostic clue—'soft' appearing mass centred on the cavernous sinus, with pronounced T2 hyperintensity and contrast enhancement. T1: Hypointense to brain **T2: Markedly high signal intensity.** T1 C+ vivid homogeneous enhancement gradual filling in on dynamic sequences	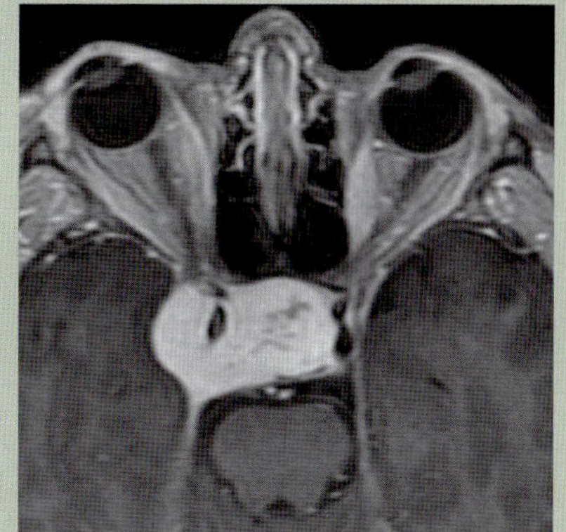 Fig. 4.16.15: Hemangioma

(Contd.)

Table 4.16.1: Differential diagnosis for cavernous sinus/parasellar lesions (*Contd.*)

<table>
<tr>
<td>Cavernous ICA aneurysm: Traumatic/ infectious/ idiopathic. <12 mm asymptomatic lesions do not require surgery. Endovascular coil embolization/ microsurgical clip placement.
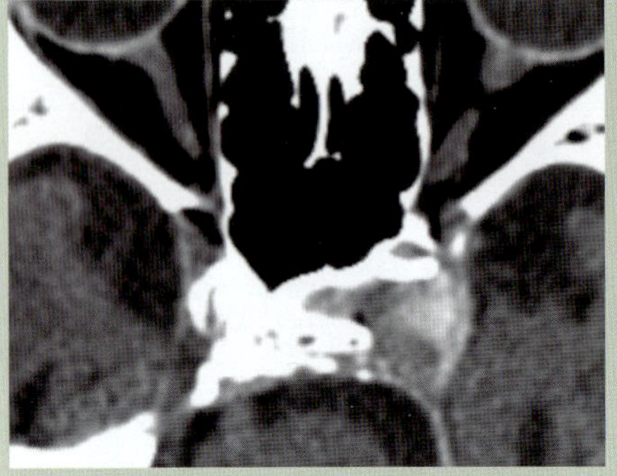
Fig. 4.16.16: Right cavernous ICA aneurysm</td>
<td>An aneurysm appears as a well-defined round, slightly hyperattenuating lesion, most apparent on maximum intensity projection reformatted images. Peripheral rim calcification can be present. Postcontrast patent aneurysm: Bright and uniform enhancement, thrombosed aneurysm: rim enhancement due to filling defect. Flow void + pulsation artefact
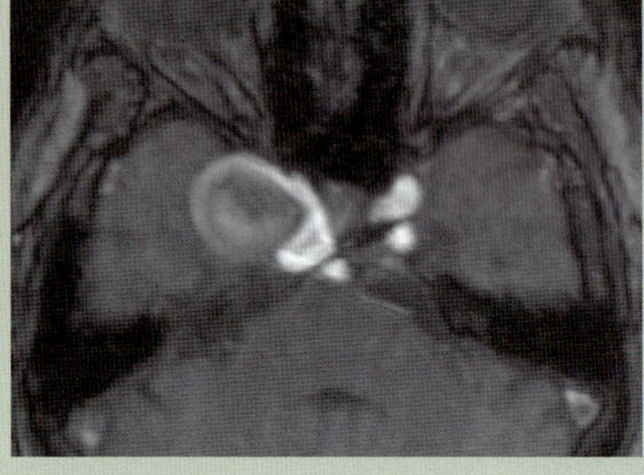
Fig. 4.16.17: Right cavernous ICA aneurysm</td>
<td>Right cavernous sinus thrombosis (also note the associated cavernous part of ICA thrombosis)
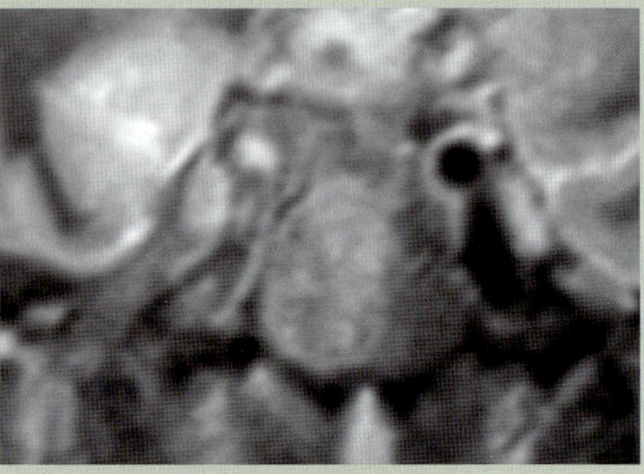
Fig. 4.16.18: Left cavernous sinus thrombosis</td>
</tr>
<tr>
<td colspan="2">Bony pathologies: Metastasis, osteomyelitis, chondrosarcoma, chordoma.
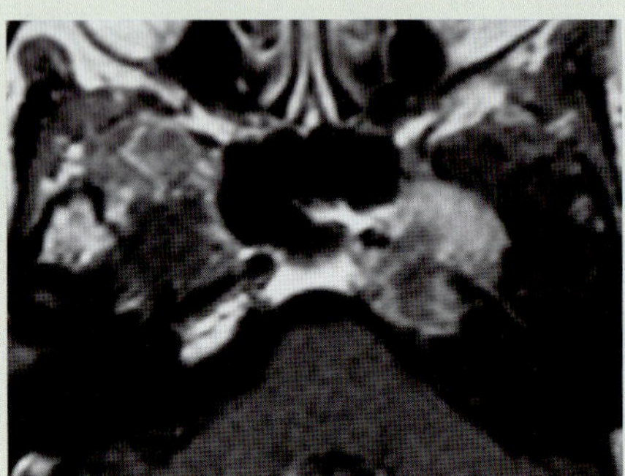
Fig. 4.16.19: Bony metastasis
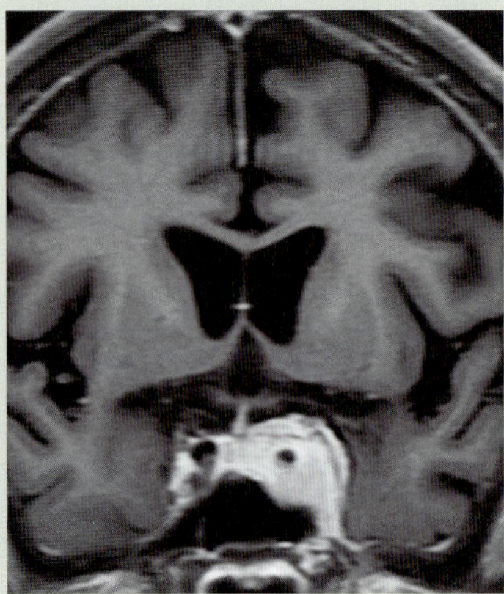
Fig. 4.16.21: Meningioma with left ICA narrowing</td>
<td>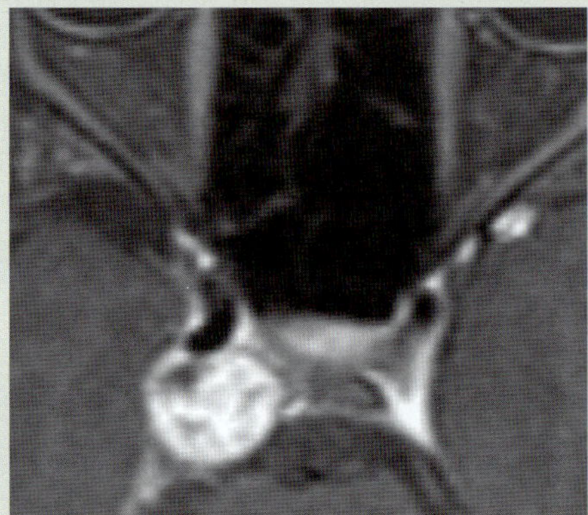
Fig. 4.16.20: Chondrosarcoma
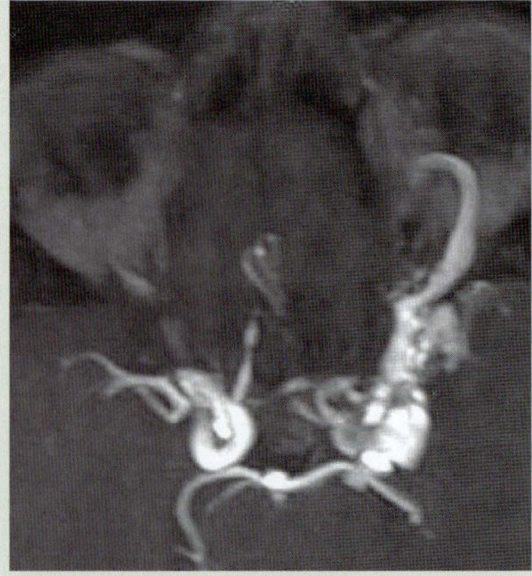
Fig. 4.16.22: Caroticocavernous fistula</td>
</tr>
</table>

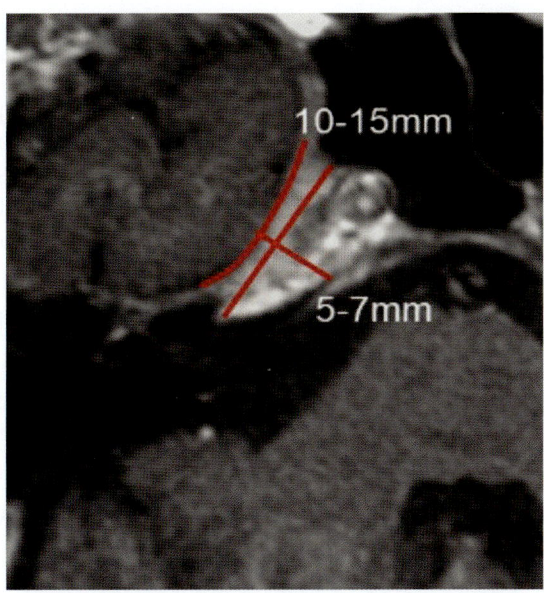

Fig. 4.16.23: Cavernous sinus measurements

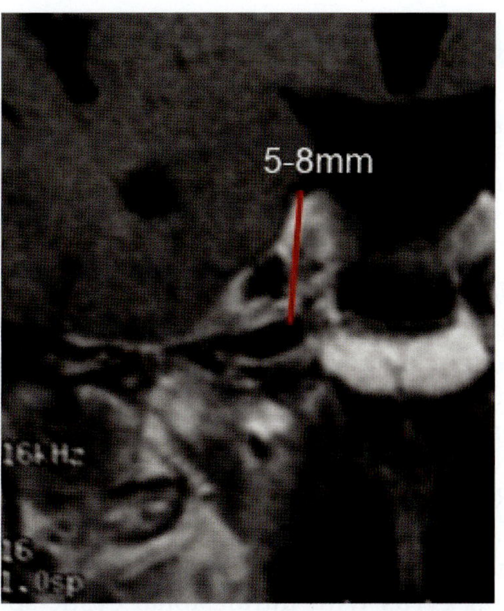

Fig. 4.16.24: Cavernous sinus measurements

Table 4.16.2: Cavernous sinus/parasellar lesions—based on location	
Cavernous sinus contents	CN 3, 4, 6, V1, V2—Neurofibroma/ schwannoma; ICA—Aneurysms
Meningeal covering	Meningioma
Adjacent bone	Metastasis, lymphoma, chondrosarcoma, osteomyelitis
Sella	Pituitary macroadenoma
Sphenoid sinus	Fungal sinusitis
Orbit	Tolosa-Hunt/pseudotumor

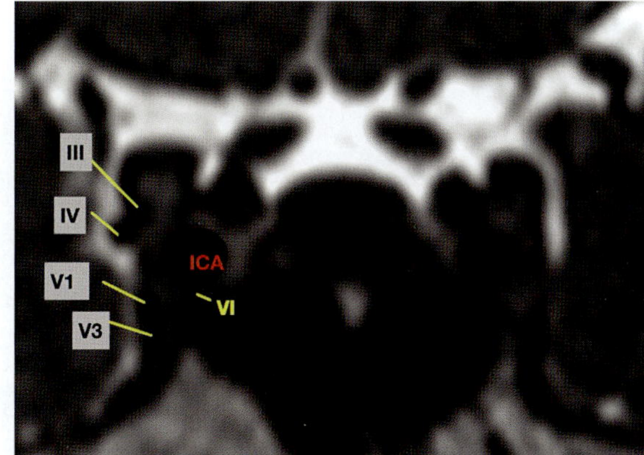

Fig. 4.16.25: Structures in cavernous sinus

Table 4.16.3: Cavernous sinus lesions based on etiology		
Neoplastic	**Origin within cavernous sinus**	Schwannoma, neurofibroma, meningioma, hemangiopericytoma, lipoma, melanoma, hemangioma
	Invasion from lesions of adjacent structures	Pituitary adenoma, chondrosarcoma, JNA, rhabdomyosarcoma, adeno cystic Ca, sinonasal CA, craniopharyngioma, germ cell tumor, chordoma, meningioma
	Systemic neoplasia	Lymphoma/multiple myeloma, histiocytosis
	Metastatic disease	
Vascular	ICA aneurysm, carotico cavernous fistula, cavernous sinus thrombosis	
Inflammatory	**Infective**	Invasive fungal sinusitis, tuberculosis, actinomycosis
	Non-infective	Sarcoidosis, IgG4 disease, granulomatosis with polyangiitis, Tolosa-Hunt syndrome
Miscellaneous	Arachnoid cyst, epidermoid cyst, dermoid cyst, pseudolesion	

4

4.17 CENTRAL NERVOUS SYSTEM

Case No. 17

Clinical history: A 15 years old female admitted with seizure for 2 months and altered behaviour for past 3 months.

Radiological techniques and observation: Figure 4.17.1 and 4.17.2 are plain CT brain showing a hypodense cleft seen in right temporoparietal region adjacent to sylvian fissure. Both lateral and third ventricle appears normal. Adjacent calvarial bone appears normal. No midline shift seen. No calcification seen. No extra axial collections seen. Rest of the brain appears normal. Figures 4.17.3 to 4.17.8 are MRI brain images showing cortical based non-enhancing T2 hyperintense lesion in right superior temporal gyrus with intralesional cystic spaces and subcortical cystic areas with facilitated diffusion. No perilesional edema. No evidence of any hemorrhage.

Interpretation: A—15 yrs old female, right superior temporal gyrus shows C—cortical based non-enhancing T2 hyperintense lesion B—with intralesional cystic spaces and subcortical cystic areas with facilitated diffusion and no perilesional edema D—dysembryoplastic neuroepithelial tumour.

Principal diagnosis: Dysembryoplastic neuroepithelial tumour.

Management: Discuss with neurologist and neurosurgeon, simple excision and removing the active epileptogenic areas around the tumour.

Differential diagnosis: 1. Ganglioglioma, 2. Pleomorphic xanthoastrocytoma, 3. Oligodendroglioma, 4. Focal cortical dysplasia, 5. Focal cerebritis, 6. Postictal oedema, 7. Vein of Labbé thrombosis, 8. Desmoplastic infantile astrocytoma.

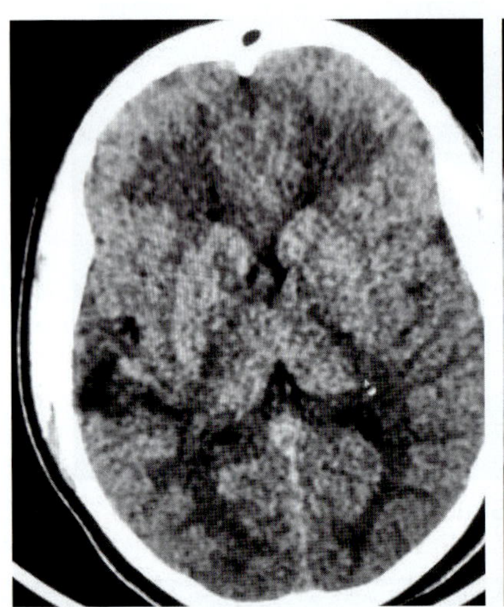

Fig. 4.17.1

Fig. 4.17.2

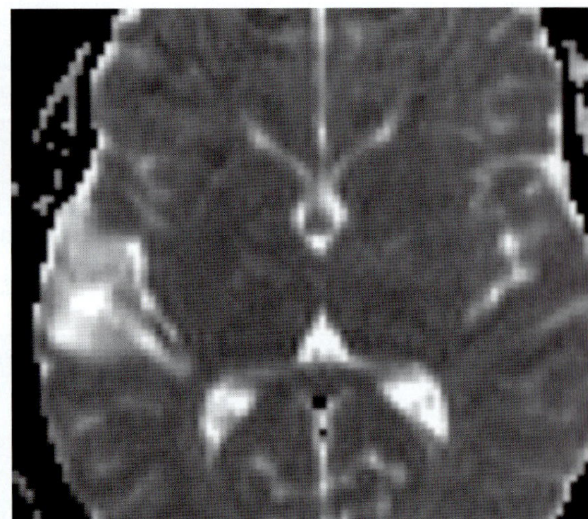

Fig. 4.17.3

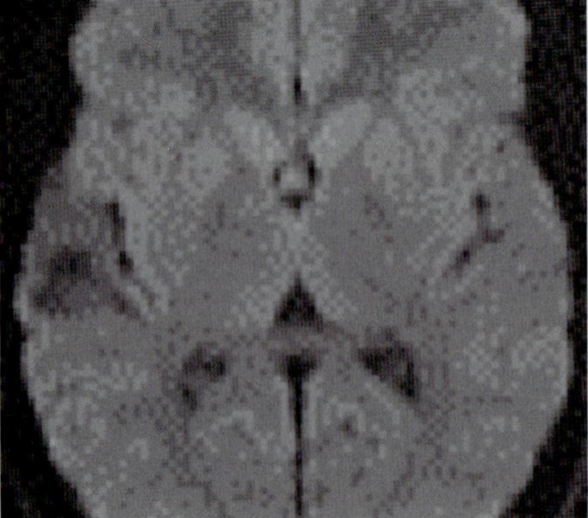

Fig. 4.17.4

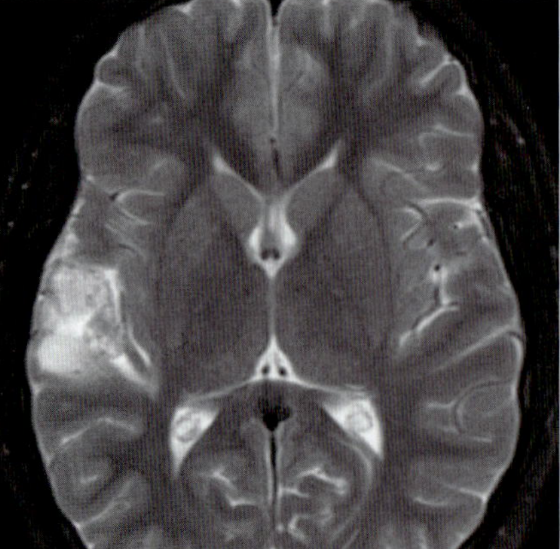

Fig. 4.17.5

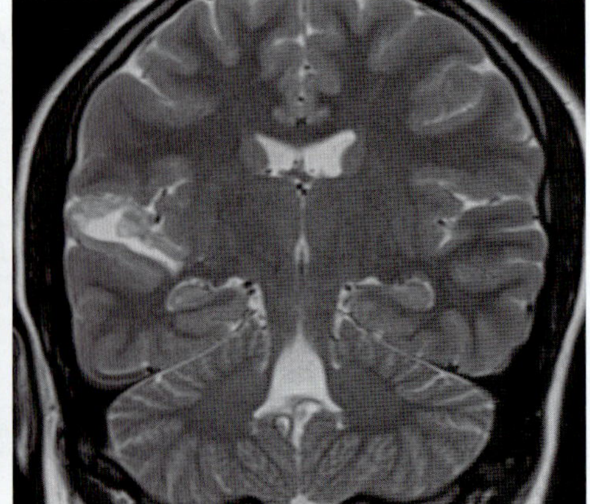

Fig. 4.17.6

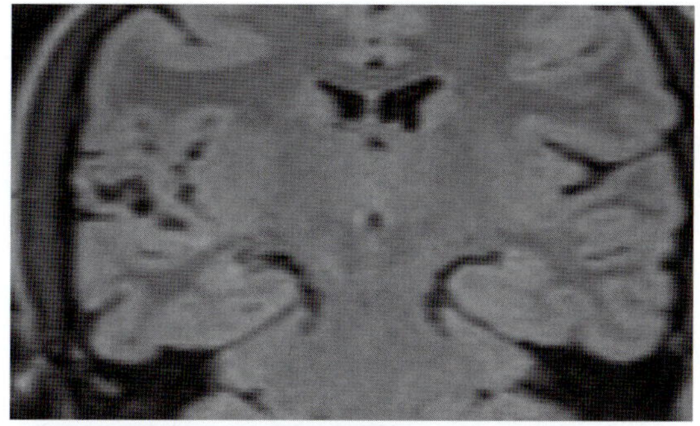
Fig. 4.17.7

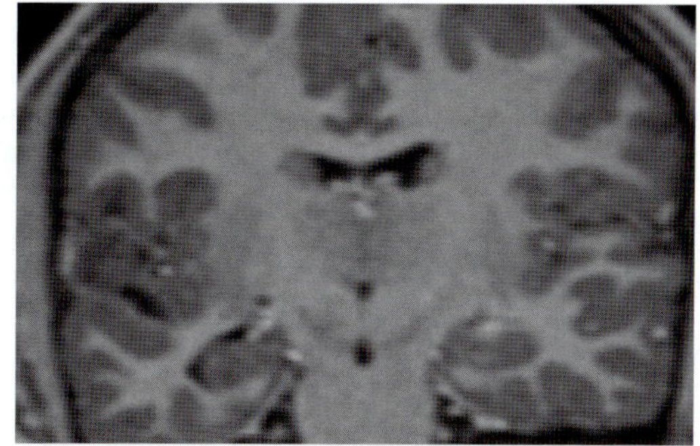
Fig. 4.17.8

<table>
<tr><td colspan="3">1. Ganglioglioma: Refer to case 19</td></tr>
<tr><td colspan="2">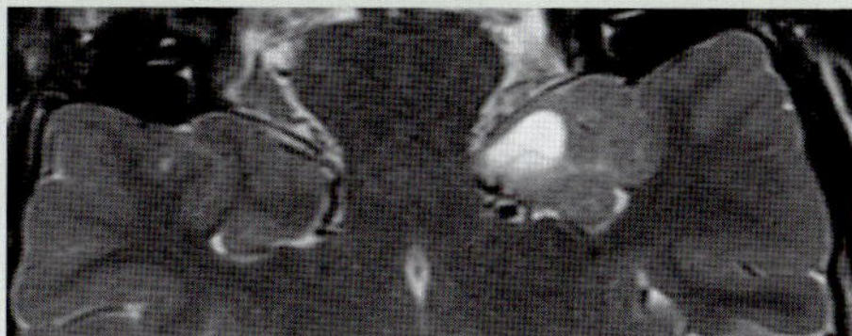
Fig. 4.17.9: Ganglioglioma</td><td>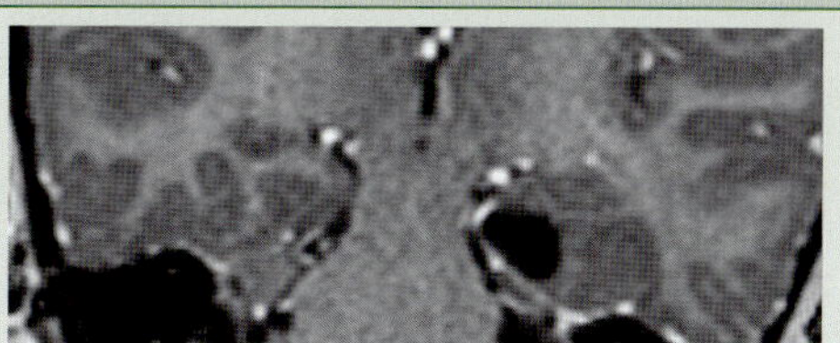
Fig. 4.17.10: Ganglioglioma</td></tr>
<tr><td>2. Pleomorphic xanthoastrocytoma WHO grade 2 tumor
Temporal lobe is most common site, seizure associated neoplasm.
Most common age group is childhood and young adult.</td><td colspan="2">Superficial cortical based with adjacent leptomeningeal involvement.
Tumour nodule shows heterogeneous hyperintensity on T2WI and FLAIR. Enhancing nodule abuts the pia with pial enhancement. Smooth remodelling of adjacent calvaria. Calcifications are present in 40% of cases. Dural tail sign was seen in 15–50% of cases.</td></tr>
<tr><td>3. Oligodendroglioma: Most common site is frontal lobe. Most common in middle aged adults. WHO grade 2 tumors. Cortical/ subcortical neoplasm. Calcification is more common.</td><td>Heterogeneous enhancing mass lesion. Calcification seen as blooming foci on gradient. Lesion does not show diffusion restriction. Calvarial erosion seen. The mass not associated with cortical dysplasia.</td><td>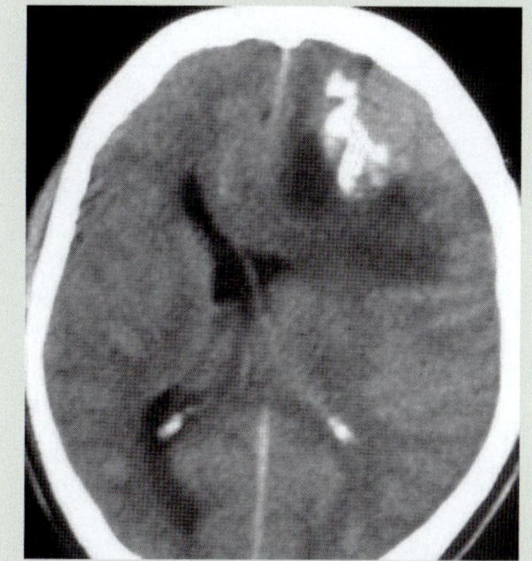
Fig. 4.17.11: Oligodendroglioma</td></tr>
<tr><td>4. Focal cortical dysplasia: Most common cause of medically refractory seizure in both children and adults. FCD type 2 is found in 15–20% of patients undergoing epilepsy surgery. Transmantle sign is seen in type 2 FCD.</td><td>In MRI shows cortical thickening, blurring of GW junction with wedge shaped area of T2/FLAIR hyperintensity extending from the bottom of sulcus into the subcortical and deep white matter and abnormal sulcal gyral pattern. Signal intensity varies with age. In neonates hyperintense on T1WI and mildly hypointense on T2WI.</td><td>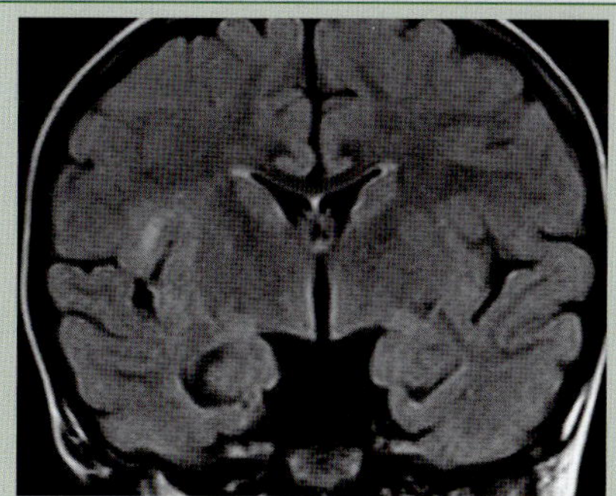
Fig. 4.17.12: Focal cortical dysplasia</td></tr>
</table>

5. Focal cerebritis: Causes are bacterial, viral, fungal and parasitic. Early prodromal symptoms are more common.	T2/FLAIR hyperintensity with diffusion restriction involving the medial aspect of left temporal lobe, T1 contrast shows patchy enhancement. Both cortical and subcortical white matter involvement seen.	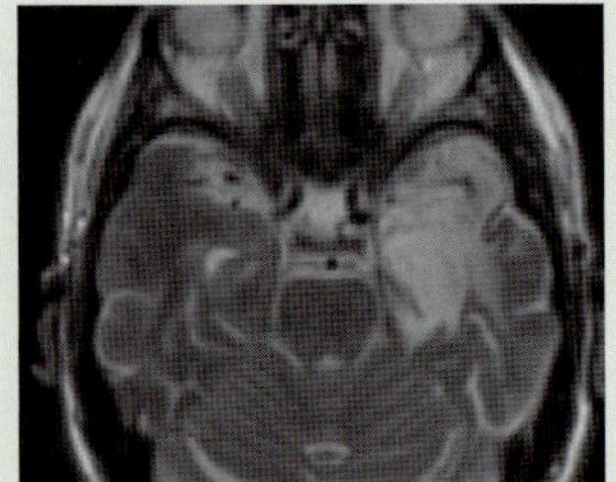 **Fig. 4.17.13:** Focal cerebritis
6. Postictal edema: Seizure precipitated by many causes like infective, metabolic, toxic and developmental. Mainly affect the temporal lobe.	Postictal MR T2/ FLAIR hyperintensity with gyral swelling and diffusion restriction involving the left inferior temporal gyrus, non-vascular distribution, subcortical and deep white matter not involved.	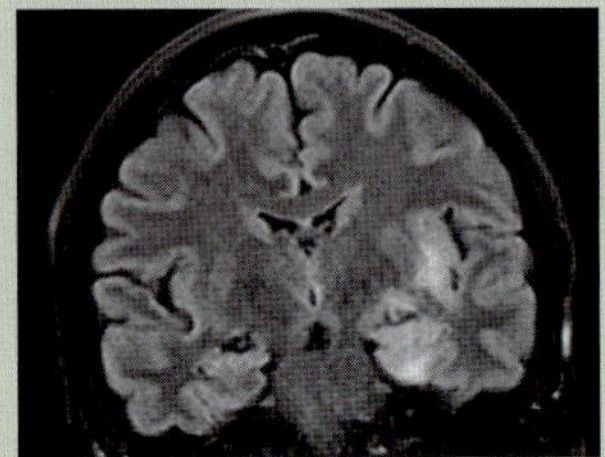 **Fig. 4.17.14:** Postictal edema
7. Vein of Labbé thrombosis: Prominent posterior anastomotic vein, vein of Labbé, courses inferolateral over the temporal lobe to drain into the transverse sinus.	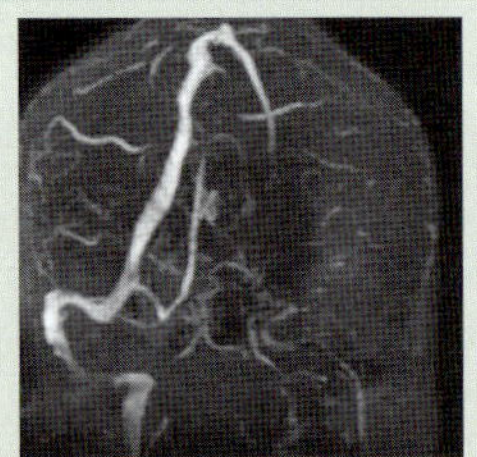 **Fig. 4.17.15:** Vein of Labbé thrombosis on MRV	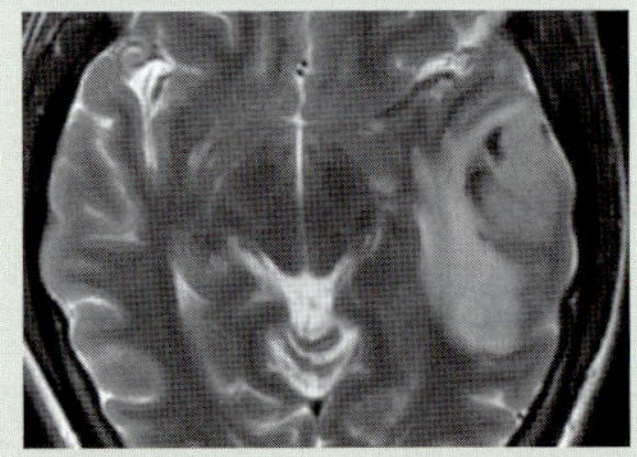 **Fig. 4.17.16:** Vein of Labbé thrombosis with hemorrhage in left temporal region

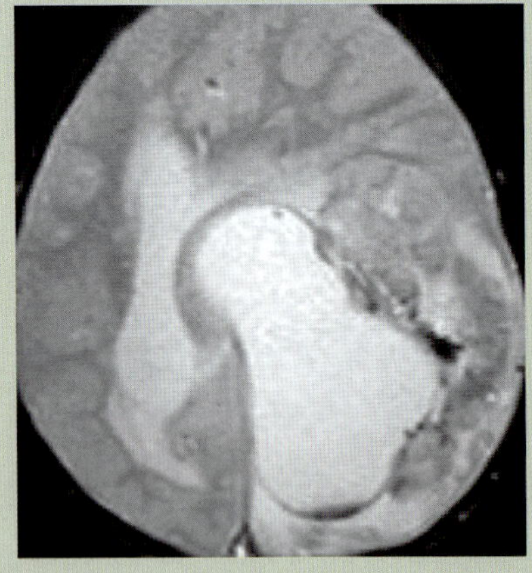

Fig. 4.17.17: Desmoplastic infantile ganglioglioma

8. Desmoplastic infantile ganglioglioma:

WHO Grade: I.

Age: 1–2 years.

Large cyst with cortical based enhancing tumor.

Desmoplastic infantile astrocytoma and desmoplastic infantile ganglioglioma are now grouped together in WHO classification of CNS tumor.

Enhancement of adjacent pia and reactive **dural thickening** are specific findings. On T1 the hypointense cyst may contain septae while the nodule is heterogeneous.

Leptomeningeal desmoplastic component:

Vimentin: Positive

GFAP: Positive

SMA: Variable

Neuroepithelial component:

GFAP: Positive

Neuronal markers (e.g. synaptophysin): Positive, if ganglion cells present

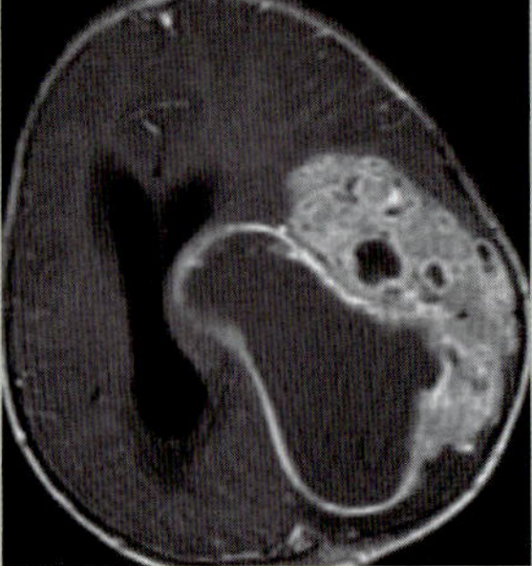

Fig. 4.17.18: Desmoplastic infantile ganglioglioma

9. Others:

a. Cortical tubers in tuberous sclerosis—Refer to case 7

b. 1p19q nonco-deleted low-grade glioma

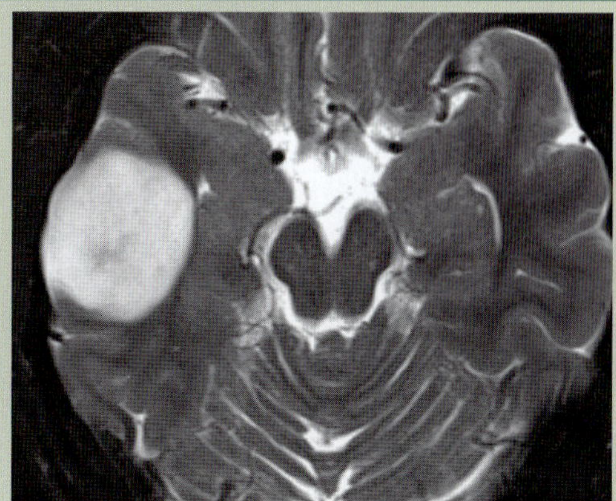

Fig. 4.17.19: T2 hyperintense mass in right temporal region—1p19q nonco-deleted low-grade glioma

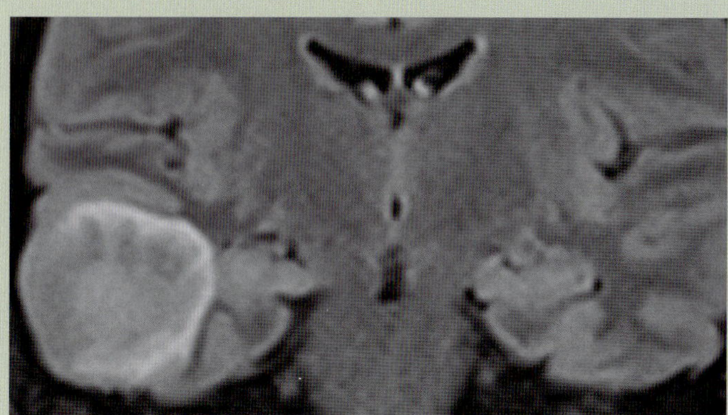

Fig. 4.17.20: T2-FLAIR mismatch hyperintense mass in right temporal region—1p19q nonco-deleted low-grade glioma

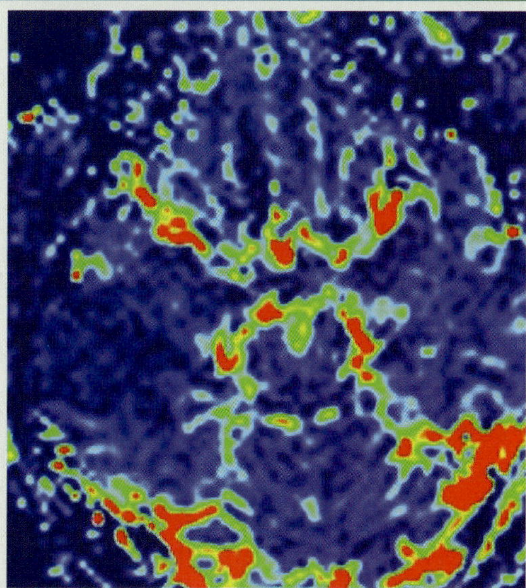

Fig. 4.17.21: Decreased perfusion in right temporal region—1p19q nonco-deleted low-grade glioma

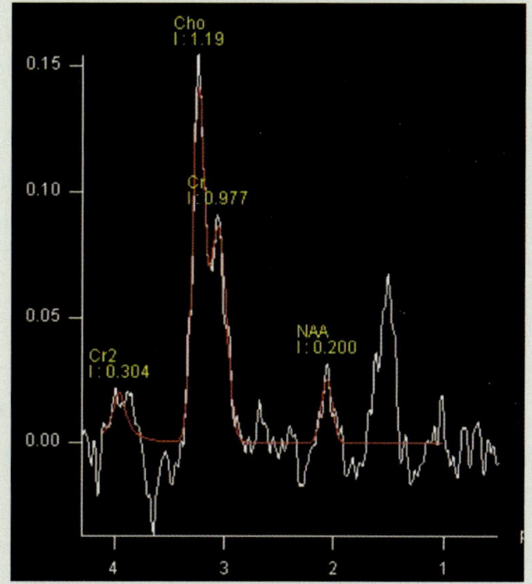

Fig. 4.17.22: MRS showing elevated choline peak in 1p19q nonco-deleted low-grade glioma

c. Cavernoma with bleed

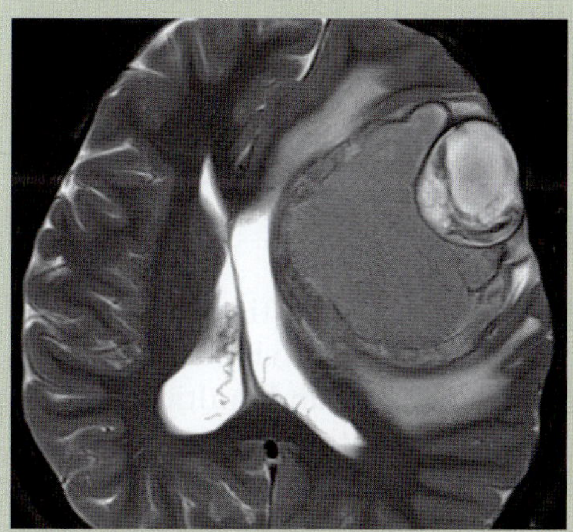

Fig. 4.17.23: Cavernoma with bleed

d. DNET

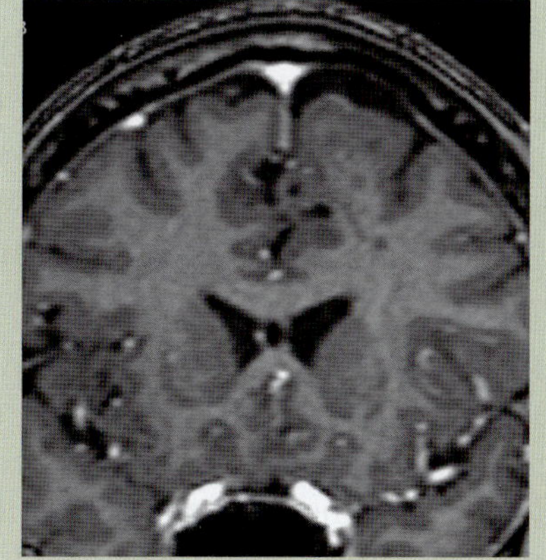

Fig. 4.17.24: DNET in left frontal region

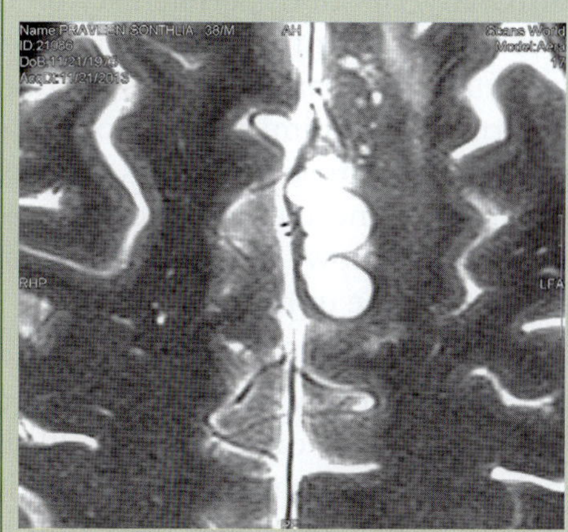

Fig. 4.17.25: DNET

e. T2/FLAIR mismatch tumor

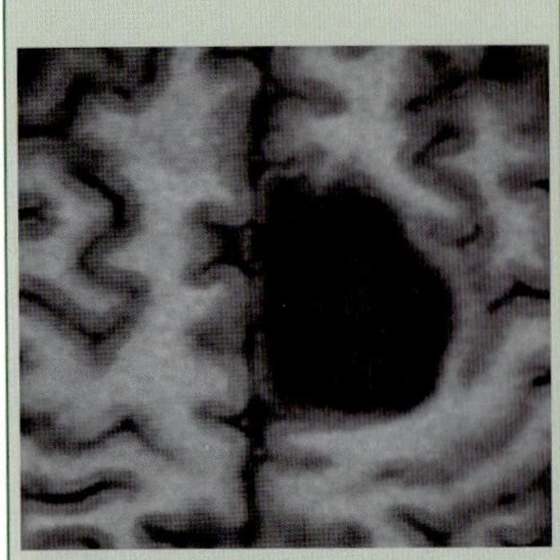

Fig. 4.17.26: T2/FLAIR mismatch tumor showing T1 hypointense mass in left high frontal region

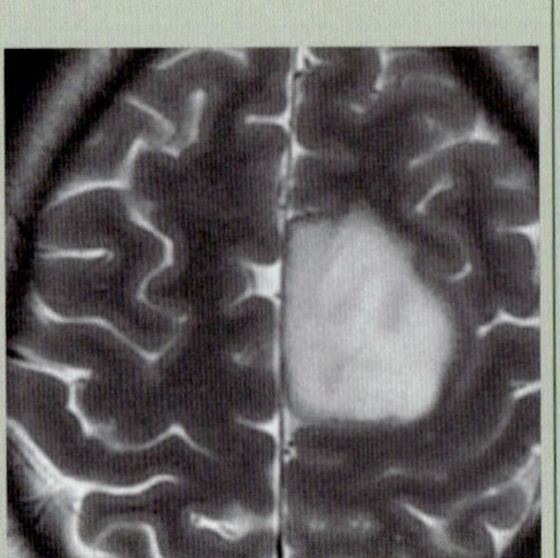

Fig. 4.17.27: T2/FLAIR mismatch tumor showing T2 hyperintense mass in left high frontal region

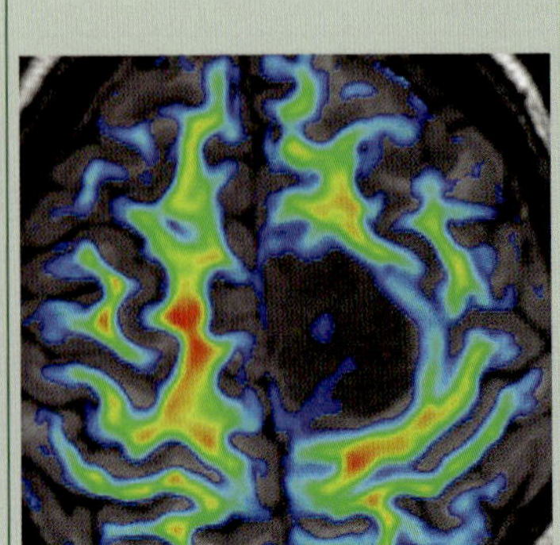

Fig. 4.17.28: T2/FLAIR mismatch tumor showing decreased perfusion in left high frontal region

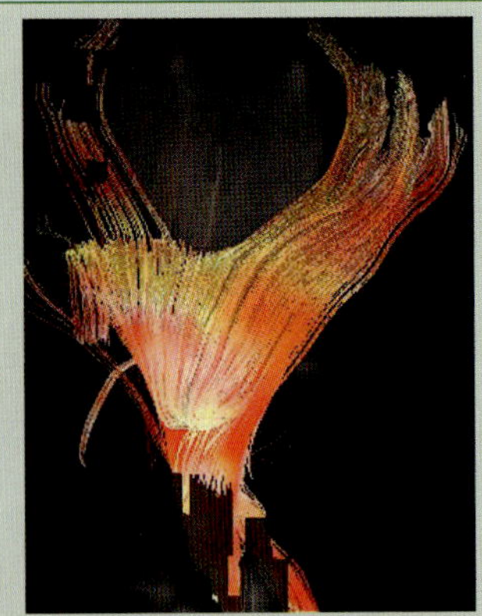

Fig. 4.17.29: Tumor in high frontal region with DTI showing displaced white matter tracts

Discussion: **Dysembryoplastic neuroepithelial tumor**—WHO grade 1 tumor. The 2021 WHO classification includes DNET in the category of neuronal and mixed neuronal glial tumor. Benign, highly epileptogenic tumor associated with cortical dysplasia.

Location: Temporal lobe is most common site followed by frontal lobe; cortical mass frequently points towards the ventricle.

Age and sex: More common age group is 2nd to 3rd decade of life, slight male predominance, patient present with drug resistant complex partial seizure.

Associations: DNET occasionally occurs in patient with neurofibromatosis type 1 or XYY syndrome.

Imaging: In contrast enhanced CT shows nonenhancing cortical-based wedge-shaped mass, higher incidence of recurrence if enhancement seen, multilobular T1 hypointense/T2 hyperintense cystic lesion with high diffusivity, rim of hyperintensity on FLAIR. The lesion does not show peritumoral edema. Bleeding into DNET is uncommon but can occur possibly due to microvascular abnormalities (mimics cavernoma) with blooming on gradient. Spectroscopy shows decreased NAA without elevated choline and nonspecific lactate peak is seen. In FDG 18 PET shows glucose hypometabolism and lower 11c methionine uptake.

Clinic radiologic criteria for the diagnosis of DNET: (a) History of having partial seizures, with/without generalization, onset before 20 years of age; (b) absence of neurologic deficit; (c) cortical location of the lesion and (d) absence of mass effect and peritumoral edema.

Treatment: Surgical resection of epileptogenic foci includes cortical dysplasia is usually curative. Recurrence rate is usually very rare.

Diagnostic Pearls of DNET

1. Cortical-based brain tumor
2. Temporal lobe more commonly involved than frontal lobe
3. Bubbly (cystic) intracortical mass
4. FLAIR rim sign: Complete or incomplete hyperintense ring surrounding the mass
5. The lesion has high diffusivity changes
6. The lesion does not enhance on contrast
7. T2W/FLAIR hyperintense band extending into ventricle (trans mantle sign)
8. Scalloping of the bone
9. With or without calcification (30%—with calcification)
10. With or without cortical dysplasia
11. MRS nearly normal
12. Epileptogenic tumour
13. FDG shows glucose hypometabolism and lower 11c methionine uptake
14. No peritumoral edema

MR spectroscopy: Spatial localization methods in spectroscopy can be divided into two broad categories, single-volume or a voxel methods and multiple-volume methods. The single-volume method obtains spectrum from an area of interest while the multiple volume method obtains a spectrum from every point in an image.

1. **Single voxel MRS:** Types of proton localization techniques **STEAM** (Stimulated Echo Acquisition Method); ISIS 3 frequency selective inversion pulses are applied in presence of orthogonal gradients. Fourth pulse is observational. Image selected in *in vivo* spectroscopy. Used in 31P spectroscopy; **PRESS** (Point-RESolved Spectroscopy); Chemically selective saturation (CHESS) is applied prior to the selected localization technique.
2. **Multivolume Spectroscopy:** Chemical shift Imaging (CSI)

Normal metabolites in MRS include NAA , creatine/GABA and choline. Other metabolites in MRS include lipids, lactate, glutamine, glutamate, myoinositol.

PPM	*Metabolite*	*Properties*	*Normal*
0.9 and 1.3	**Lipids**	**Products of brain destruction**	Not present normally
1.3	**Lactate**	**Product of anaerobic glycolysis**	Not present normally, can be seen in preterm infants
2	**NAA**	**Neuronal marker**	Present normally
2.2–2.4	**Glutamine, glutamate**	**Neurotransmitter**	Not present normally
3	**Creatine/GABA**	**Energy metabolism**	Used as standard reference
3.2	**Choline**	**Cell membrane marker**	Present normally
3.5	**Myoinositol**	**Glial cell marker, osmolyte**	Not present normally

Metabolities in MRS

1. Branched chain amino acid

(0.9 PPM)

Maple syrup urine disease, abscess

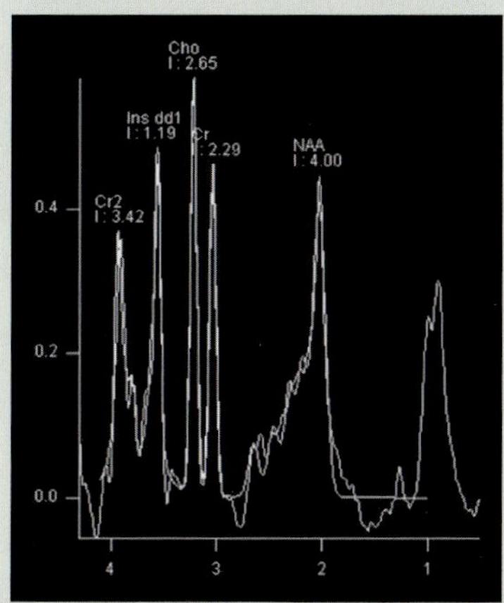

Fig. 4.17.30: Branched chain amino acid peak

2. Lipids

Multiple peaks with in 0.9 to 1.3 ppm.

Indicates necrosis and/or disruption of myelin sheath.

Contamination from scalp.

Lipid peak is seen in tumors, toxoplasmosis, PML necrosis, demyelination hypoxia, infarction, lymphoma, central pontine myelinolysis, shaken baby syndrome, active growing tumour, cryptococcoma, inflammatory diseases, lipid metabolism disorder and Sjögren's Larsson disease, TB.

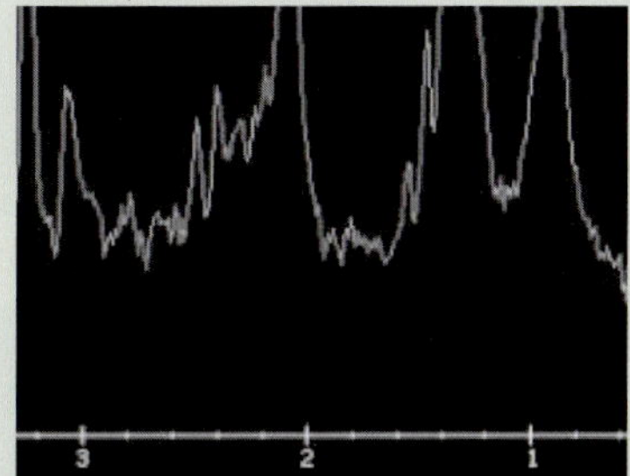

Fig. 4.17.31: Lipid peak in lymphoma

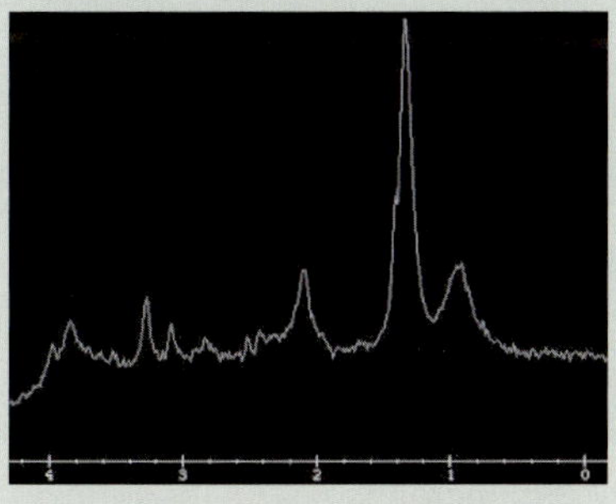

Fig. 4.17.32: Lipid peak in tuberculoma

CNS lymphoma

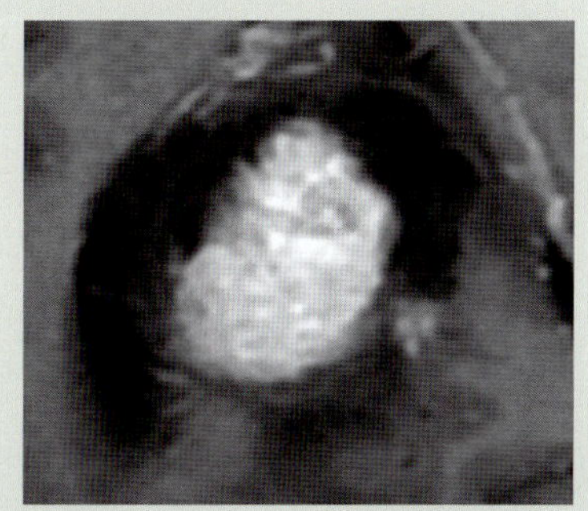

Fig. 4.17.33: Enhancing mass in CNS lymphoma

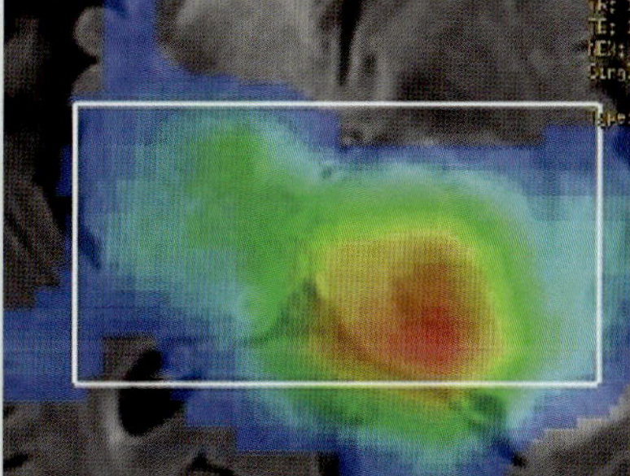

Fig. 4.17.34: Increased perfusion in lymphoma

3. Ethanol: 1.16 ppm (triplet). Ethanol peak is seen in alcohol abuse.

Tall lipid peak is also seen in a few cases of CNS lymphoma that mimics tuberculoma.

Very tall lipid-lactate peak with high choline peak—suggests tumoral spectrum.

4. Lactate (Lac): Doublet centred at 1.33 ppm, quartet at 4.11 ppm. Inverts with TE of 135. Lactate peak is seen in hydro-cephalus, hypo/hyperventilation hypoxia, anoxia, near drowning, intracranial haemorrhage, stroke, acute/subacute infarction, necrosis, cystic lesion, abscess, tumors, hyperglycemia recovery demyelination, lymphoma (lac + lipid), mitochondrial disorders, Canavan's, Alexander's

PML—small increase in lactate and lipid, toxoplasma—15–20-fold increase in lactate and lipid.

MRS showing inversion of lactate peak in TE 135

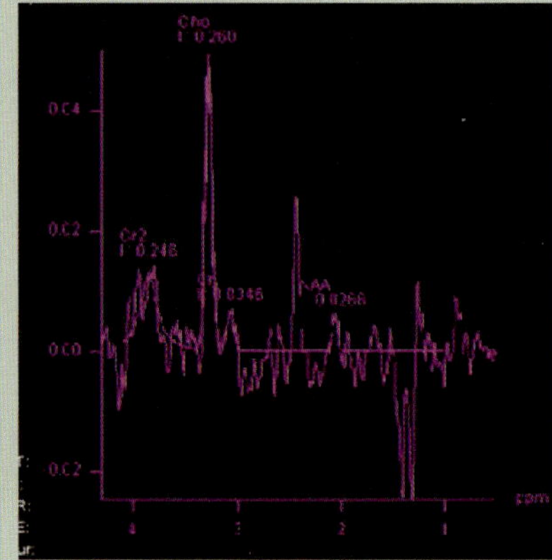

Fig. 4.17.35: Lactate peak inverted on TE 135

5. Alanine (Peak 1.48 ppm, 3.78 ppm, doublet)

Meningiomas, abscess, neurocysticercosis

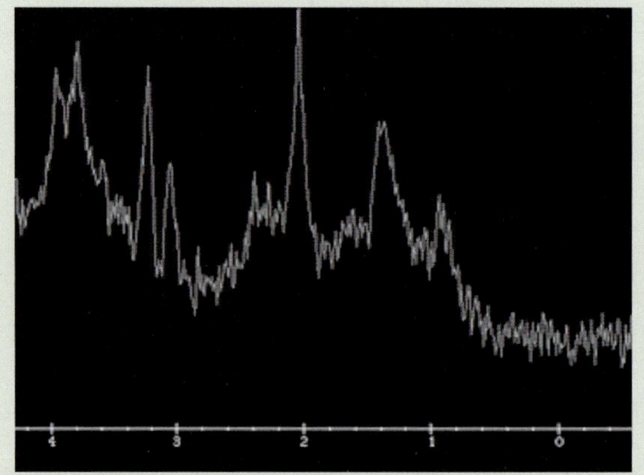

Fig. 4.17.36: Alanine peak

Fig. 4.17.37: Inverted alanine peak

6. Acetoacetate (1.99 ppm) abscess. Succinate and acetate are present in anaerobic abscess.

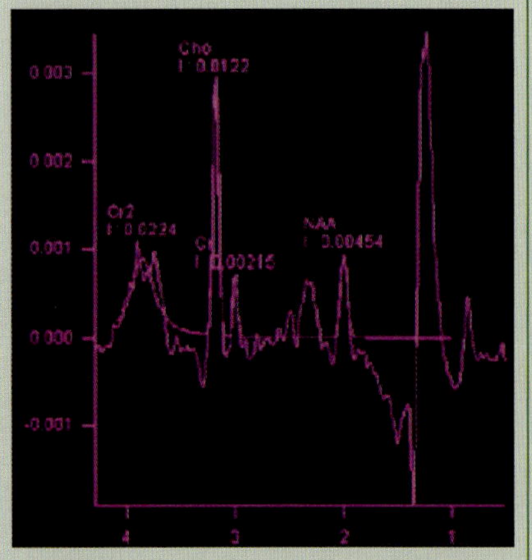

Fig. 4.17.38: Acetoacetate peak

8. NAA (Peaks—2.02, 2.5 and 2.6 ppm), marker of neuronal and axonal viability. In Salla's disease, N— acetyl muramic acid resembles and resonate as NAA. Increase in NAA is seen in Canavan's disease, neuroenteric cyst/white epidermoid, Salla's disease.

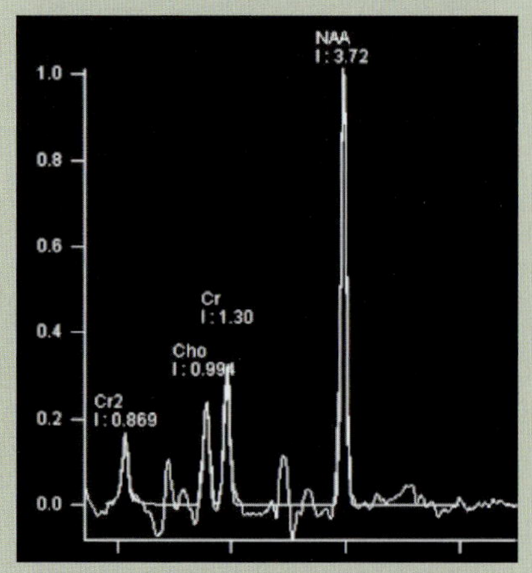

Fig. 4.17.39: Increased NAA peak in Canavan's disease

Nearly any brain insult can cause decrease in NAA.

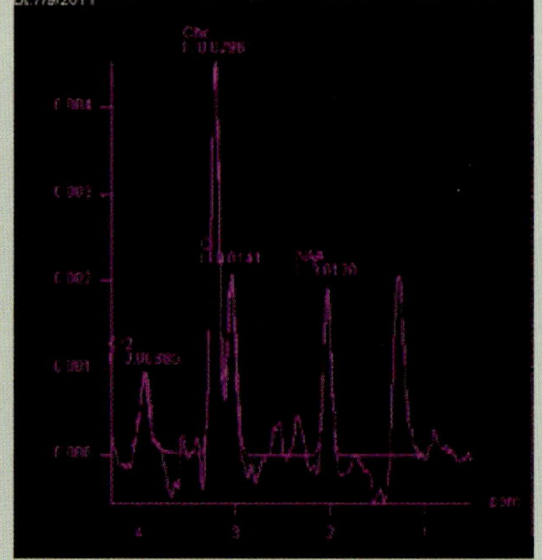

Fig. 4.17.40: Decreased NAA

4

9. G/x: Glutamine (Gln) and glutamate (Glu) Peak 2.1—2.55 ppm, complex multiplet neurotransmitters.

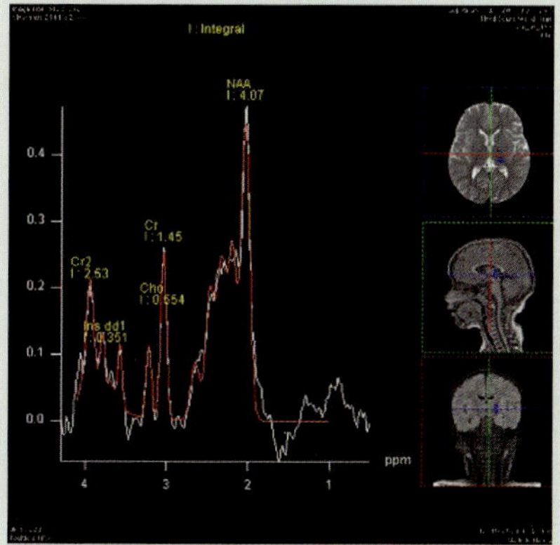

Fig. 4.17.41: Glutamate/glutamine peak

Increased peak in CHE, meningiomas, acute hepatic encephalopathy, Reye's syndrome encephalitis, hypoxia, oligodendroglioma, near drowning, OTC (ornithine transcarbamylase) deficiency.

Decreased peak in Alzheimer's, hyponatremia, SIADH, head injury

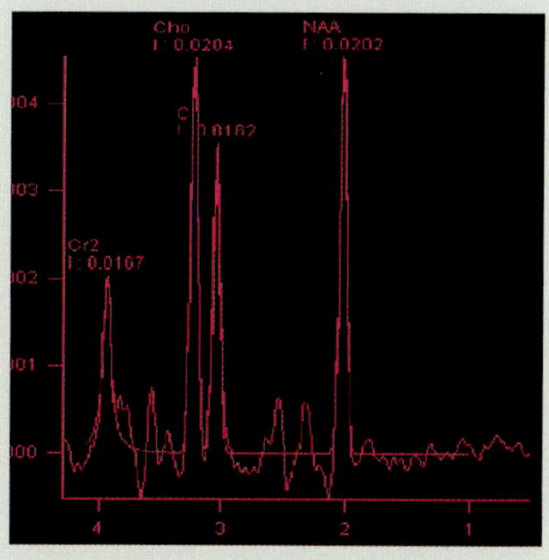

Fig. 4.17.42: Decrease in glutamine/ glutamate

10. Ketones: 2.2 ppm

Diabetic ketoacidosis will show ketone peak.

11. Succinate, pyruvate and malate (2.3–2.4 ppm)

Neurocysticercosis—lactate > succinate

Hydatid—succinate > lactate

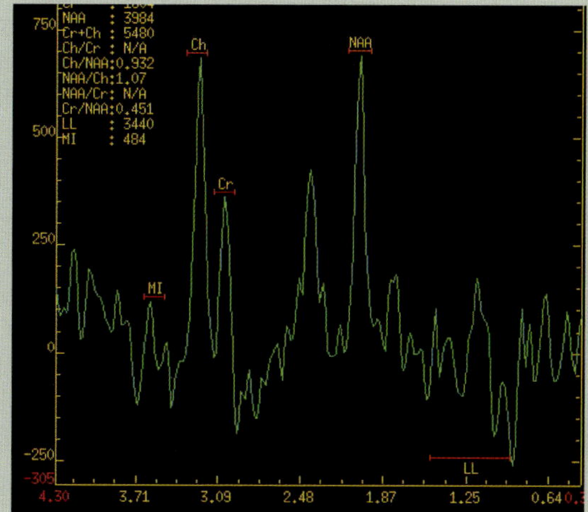

Fig. 4.17.43: Succinate peak in hydatid

12. Cr-Creatine (Peaks 3.02 and 3.94 ppm). Cerebral metabolism marker.

Absence of creatine peak is seen in creatinine deficiency. After hepatic transplant and trauma will show creatine peak. Decrease in creatine peak will be seen in tumors, toxoplasmosis PML, infections, hyponatremia, SIADH, necrosis, chronic hepatic disease, hypoxia, stroke, neonate, trauma, cryptococcoma. MRS shows decreased creatine peak.

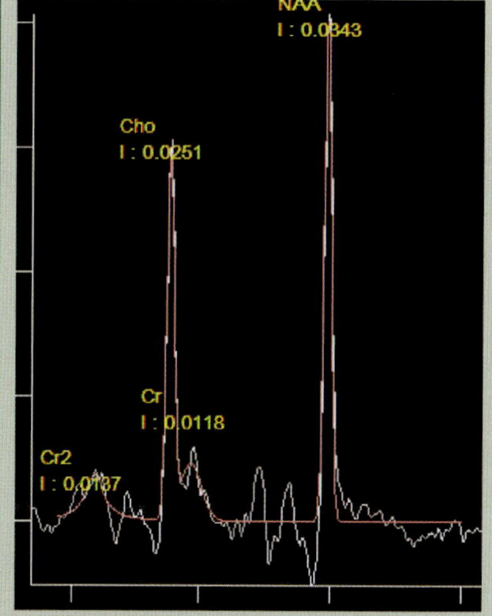

Fig. 4.17.44: Absence of creatine peak

13. Cho: Choline (peak 3.22 ppm)

Altered cell membrane turnover marker

Mild increase in choline is seen normally in most cases and hence not specific.

Tumours, trauma, DM

Encephalitis, demyelination, Alzheimer's, Down syndrome, infarction, neonates, postliver transplant, elderly, PML, chronic hypoxia, hyperosmolar will show increased choline peak

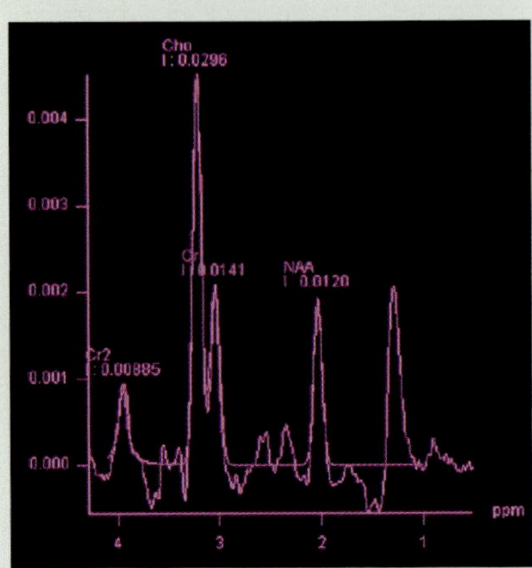

Fig. 4.17.45: Increase in choline peak

Decreased choline peak is seen in toxoplasmosis, necrosis abscess, asymptomatic hepatic disease, hepatic encephalopathy SIADH, hyponatremia, cryptococcoma nonspecific dementias

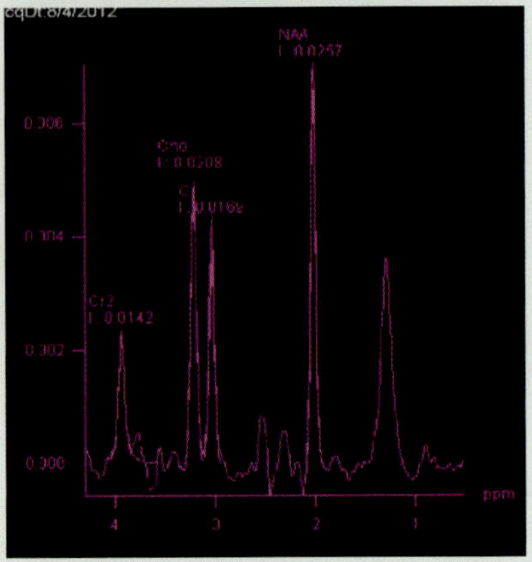

Fig. 4.17.46: Decrease in choline

14. Taurine: Tau 3.44, 3.38, 3.32, 3.27

Medulloblastoma show taurine peak

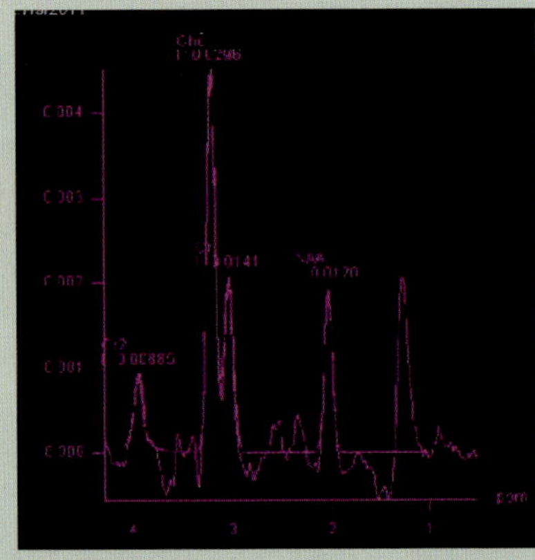

Fig. 4.17.47: Taurine peak

15. Glycine GLY 3.56

Central neurocytoma, hyperglycinaemia

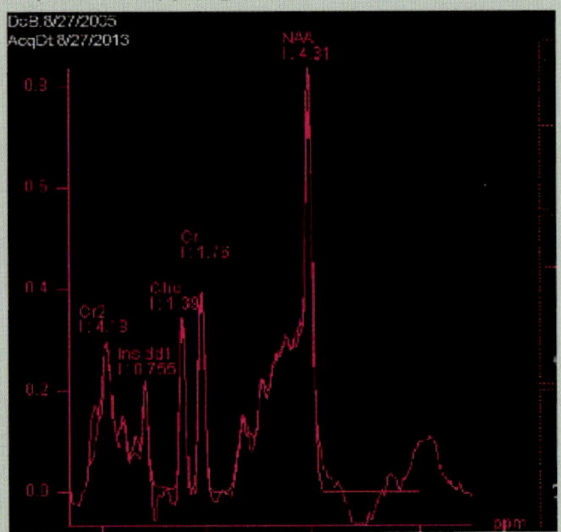

Fig. 4.17.48: Glycine peak

16. MI: Myoinositol

(Peak—3.56 and 4.06 ppm)

Glial marker located in the astrocytes

Multiple sclerosis, neonatal

Leukodystrophy, renal failure

Alzheimer's disease, diabetes, Pick's disease, Down syndrome, PML, recovered hypoxia, hyperosmolar states

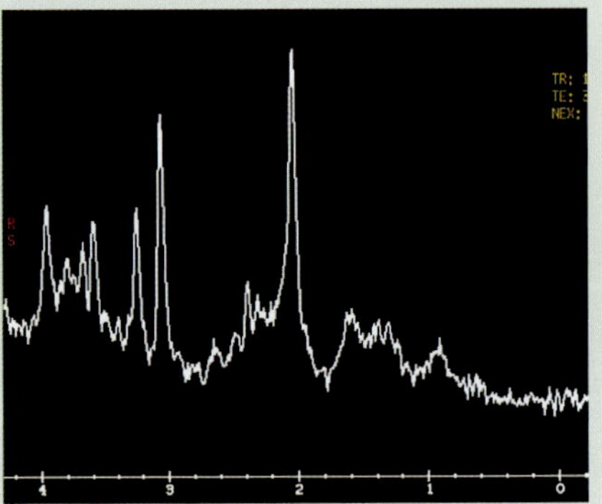

Fig. 4.17.49: Myoinositol peak

Low grade tumors, infarction, hyponatremia, SIADH

Hepatic and hypoxic

Encephalopathy, toxoplasmosis, cryptococcoma, lymphoma low-grade tumors

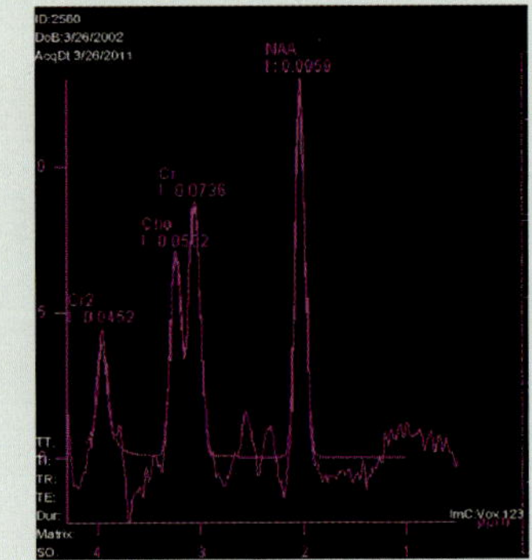

Fig. 4.17.50: Decrease in myoinositol

17. Mannitol: 3.8 ppm, complex multiple. Peak at 3.8 ppm will be seen in tumors treated with mannitol

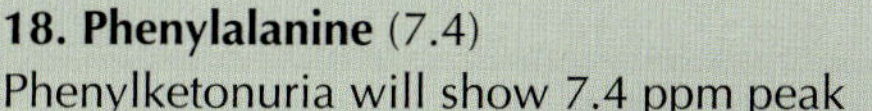

18. Phenylalanine (7.4)
Phenylketonuria will show 7.4 ppm peak

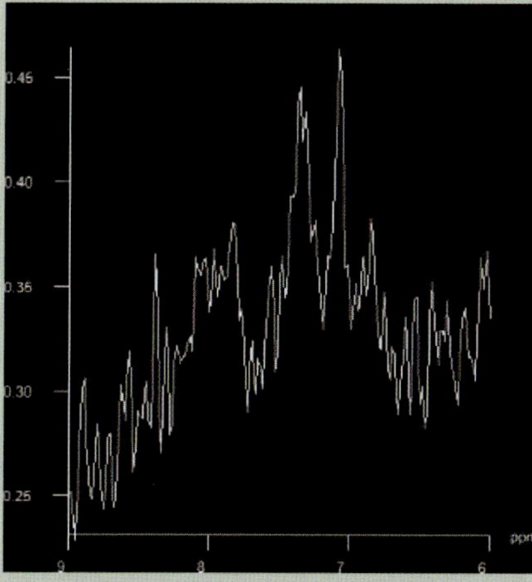

Fig. 4.17.51: Phenyl alanine peak

Hunter's angle formed by myoinositol, choline, creatine and NAA metabolites. If the angle and peaks roughly corresponded to the 45° angle, the curve was considered probably normal. If the peaks drifted from the Comb's angle, the curve was abnormal. It aids in distinguishing between normal and abnormal MRS. Hunter's angle is used in MRI brain acquired using a stimulated echo acquisition mode (STEAM) sequence with a short echo time (TE). With age, the usual spectrum shifts. NAA levels are low at birth, although choline and myoinositol levels are high. By the age of four, the spectra will be similar to that of adults. Within certain areas of the brain, the typical spectrum varies as well. Choline levels are higher in the frontal lobes than in the parietal lobes, and in the white matter than in the cortical grey matter, above the level of the ventricles.

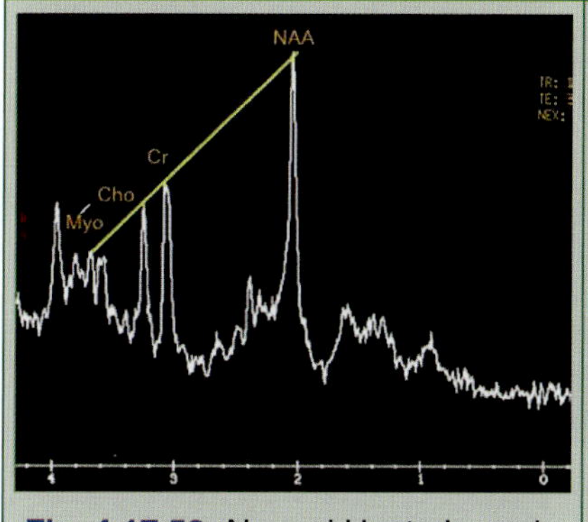

Fig. 4.17.52: Normal Hunter's angle

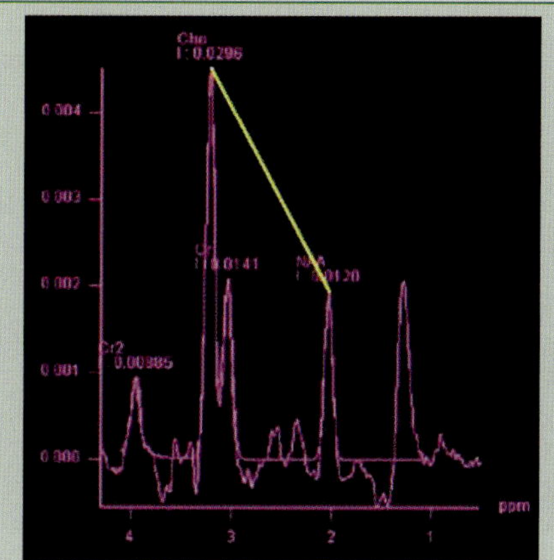

Fig. 4.17.53: Reverse Hunter's angle seen in tumors and normal newborn

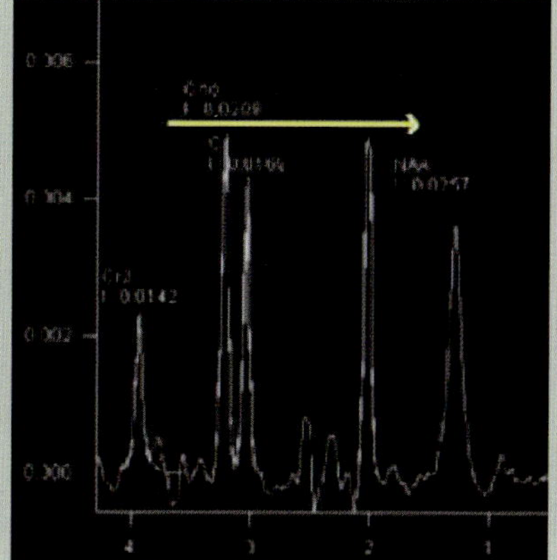

Fig. 4.17.54: Even spectral line seen normally between 2 and 4 years and Alzheimer's disease

Short TE	Short TE	Short TE
All peaks are positive	All peaks are positive	All peaks are positive

4.18 CENTRAL NERVOUS SYSTEM

Case No. 18

Clinical history: A 51-year-old male presents with a history of increasing confusion.

Radiological techniques and observation: Figures 4.18.1 to 4.18.6 shows MRI examination comprises axial T2-weighted images, susceptibility weighted image and T1-weighted images with and without contrast. These sequences show a heterogeneous T2 hyperintense lesion involving the posterior aspects of both parietal lobes, more extensive on the right, with callosal involvement. There is a cystic component in the bilateral posterior parietal white matter and an enhancing component within. There is an associated mass effect with gyral expansion and lateral ventricle effacement.

Interpretations: **A**—middle age male, lesion in both parietal lobes with callosal involvement, **C**—cystic and enhancing components, **B**—aggressive mass lesion crossing the midline, **D**—high grade glioma.

Principal diagnosis: **High grade butterfly glioma—IDH wild type glioblastoma—Grade 4.**

Management: Referral to neurophysician, neurosurgeon, medical oncologist, radiotherapist and multidisciplinary approach to manage the case. Biopsy/tumor debulking followed by radiotherapy, chemotherapy.

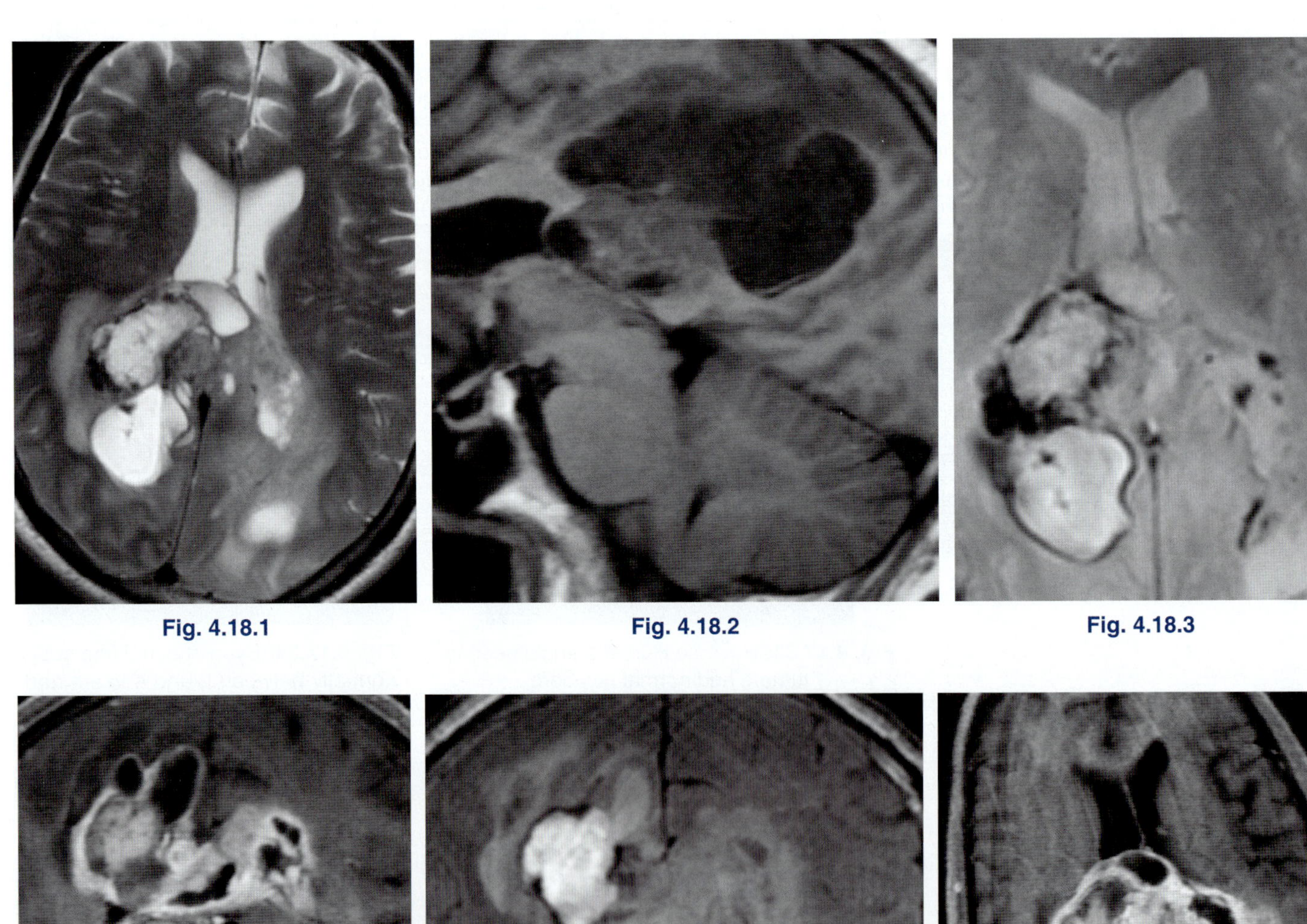

Fig. 4.18.1 Fig. 4.18.2 Fig. 4.18.3

Fig. 4.18.4 Fig. 4.18.5 Fig. 4.18.6

Table 4.18.1 Differential diagnosis for focal intracerebral tumor		
CNS lymphoma 95%—diffuse large B cell lymphoma 5%—primary CNS lymphoma	Periventricular enhancing mass often crosses corpus callosum Typically, isointense/hypointense on T2WI. Necrosis common in AIDS-related lymphoma	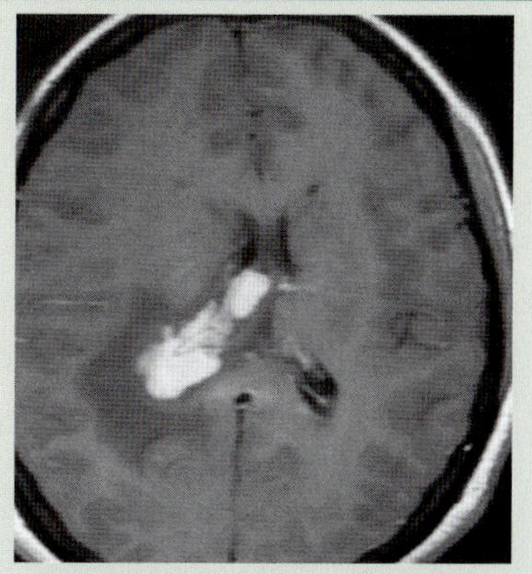 **Fig. 4.18.7:** CNS lymphoma
Metastasis Most common CNS neoplasm >50 years (5 times more common) Through haematogenous dissemination, direct geographic extension, perineural, perivascular spread	Typically, multiple lesions at gray-white junctions. Rounder than infiltrating lesion Variable edema, necrosis, haemorrhage	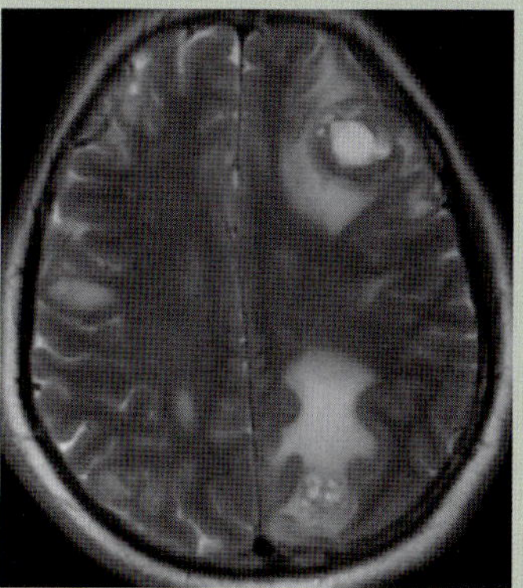 **Fig. 4.18.8:** Metastasis
Tumefactive demyelination Larger areas of demyelination mimics mass in younger patients Females more commonly affected. Can involve corpus callosum and spread to opposite cerebral hemisphere.	Large hypointense mass often incomplete, horseshoe-shaped enhancement, open towards cortex. Lesions in typical locations. MRS—decreased NAA and increased choline	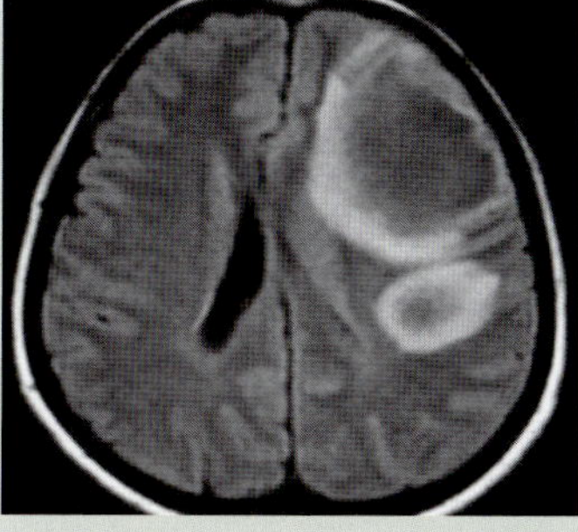 **Fig. 4.18.9:** Tumefactive demyelination
Abscess (immunocompromised) Can be pyogenic /fungal abscess Stages—early cerebritis, late cerebritis, early capsule, late capsule formation	Ring enhancement typically thinner than GBM, T2 hypointense rim, diffusion restriction is typical	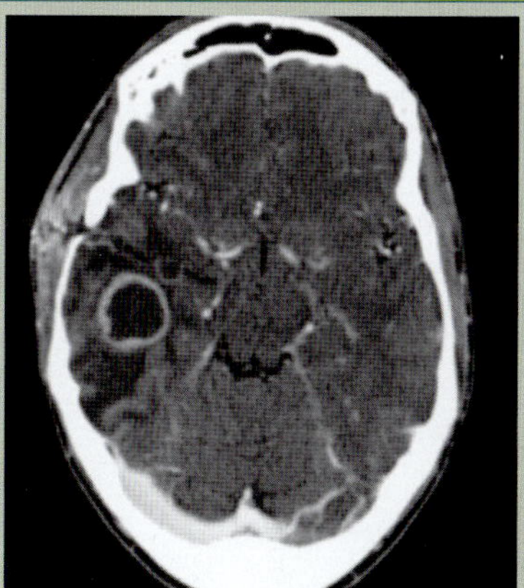 **Fig. 4.18.10:** Abscess

Table 4.18.2: Approach to differentiation of focal brain lesions

Brain tumor *vs* infarct	Infarct involves both grey and white matter, specific vascular territory (anterior, middle, and posterior cerebral arteries) and acute onset. It shows diffusion restriction (acute/early subacute)	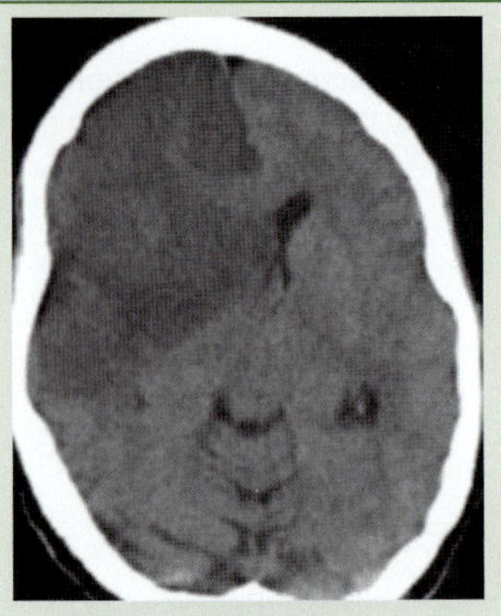 **Fig. 4.18.11:** Infarct
Status epilepticus Active seizures may cause signal abnormalities and enhancement.	T2/FLAIR transient hyperintensity of grey matter and/or subcortical white matter with mild mass effect with areas of diffusion restriction. **Perfusion:** Increased rCBF follow-up imaging may be necessary.	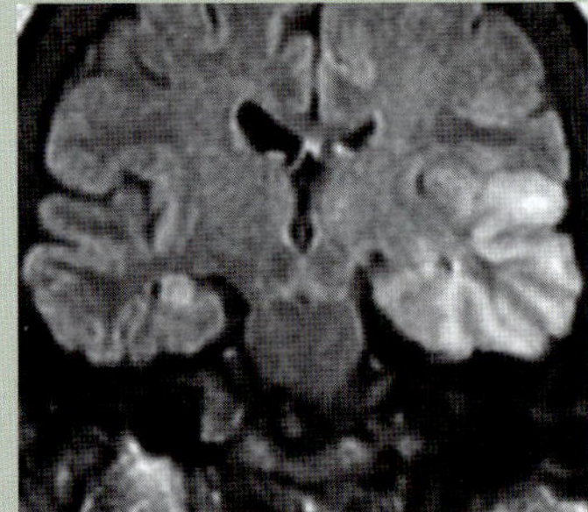 **Fig. 4.18.12:** Status epilepticus
Herpes encephalitis Occurs in limbic system, temporal lobes, cingulate gyrus. Typically, acute onset	Swollen gyri with diffusion restriction with or without enhancement. Bilateral asymmetrical Crossing the arterial territory	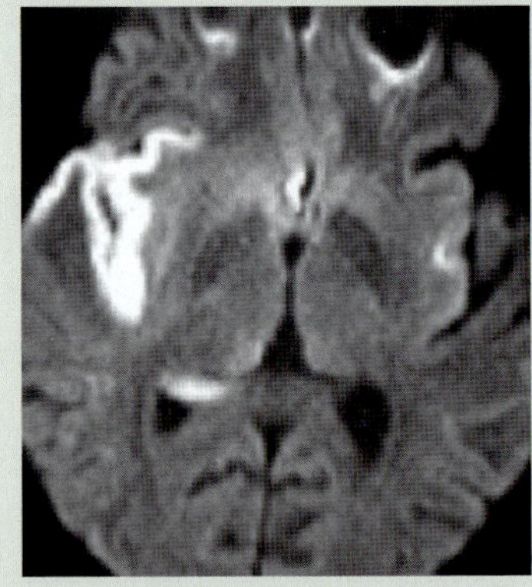 **Fig. 4.18.13:** Herpes encephalitis
Vasogenic edema Occurs due to disruption of blood–brain barrier, it is an extracellular edema which mainly affects the white matter leakage of fluid from capillaries	White matter hypodensity which extends in finger like fashion with maintained grey white differentiation. T2/FLAIR hyperintensity with no diffusion restriction in MRI	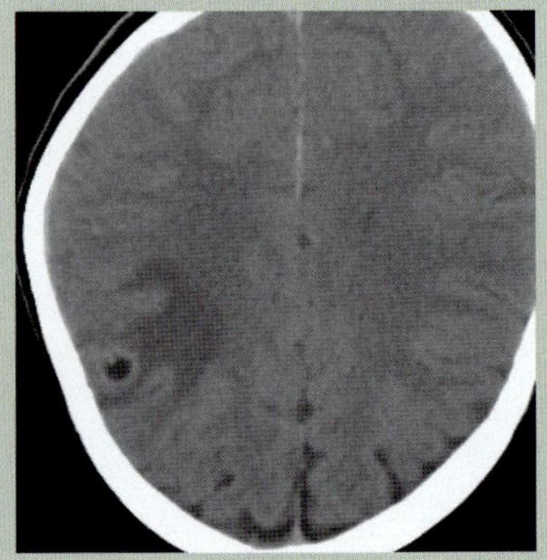 **Fig. 4.18.14:** Vasogenic edema

Table 4.18.3: Differential diagnosis for butterfly intracerebral tumor

High grade glioma, metastasis, lymphoma (hyperdense mass), gliomatosis cerebri, tumefactive demyelination, abscess, progressive multifocal leukoencephalopathy in immunocompromised and adrenoleukodystrophy (in children). Further investigations include MRI with contrast.

Adrenoleukodystrophy—frontal predominant variant	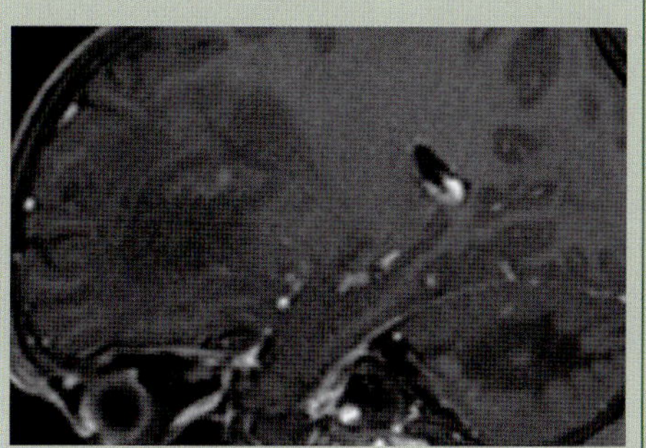 **Fig. 4.18.15:** Adrenoleukodystrophy	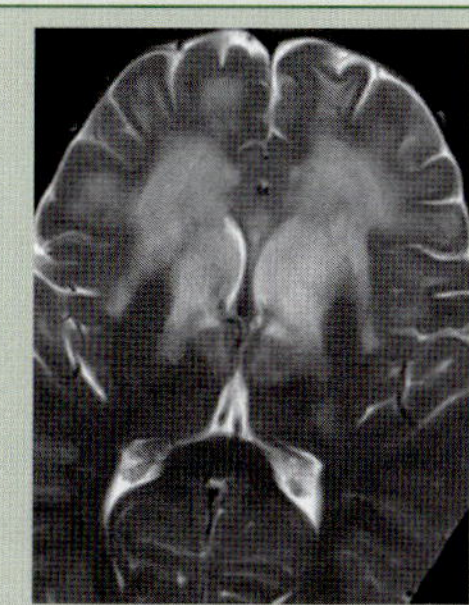 **Fig. 4.18.16:** Adrenoleukodystrophy Loes score-5
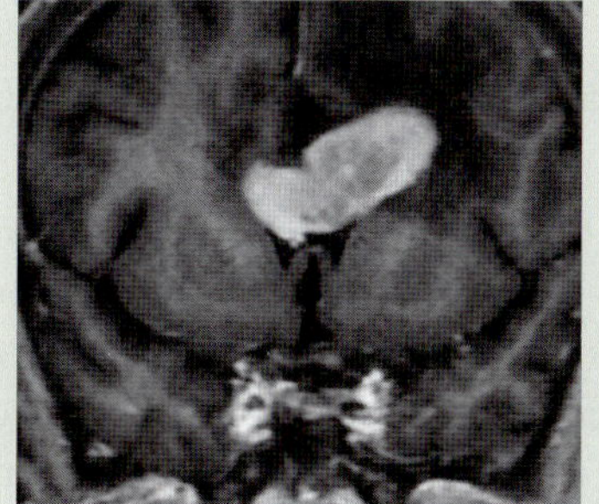 **Fig. 4.18.17:** Butterfly glioma	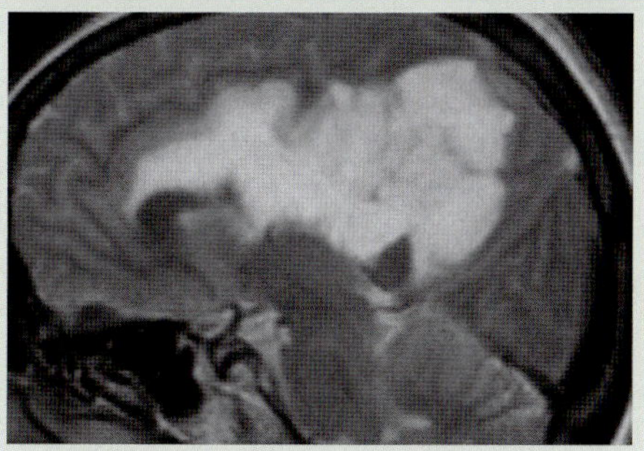 **Fig. 4.18.18:** Corpus callosal glioma	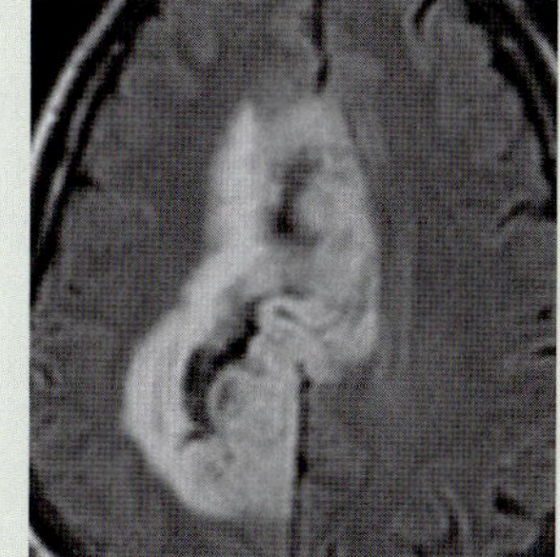 **Fig. 4.18.19:** Corpus callosal glioma
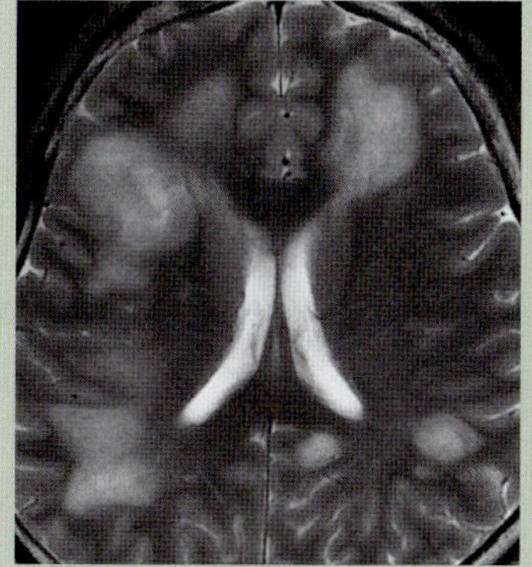 **Fig. 4.18.20:** ADEM	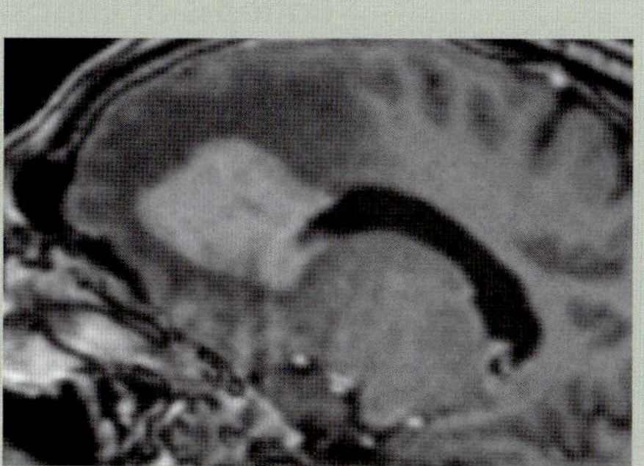 **Fig. 4.18.21:** Butterfly lymphoma	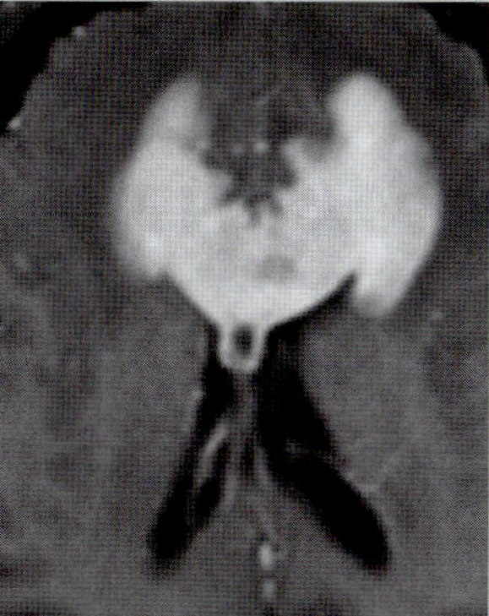 **Fig. 4.18.22:** Butterfly lymphoma
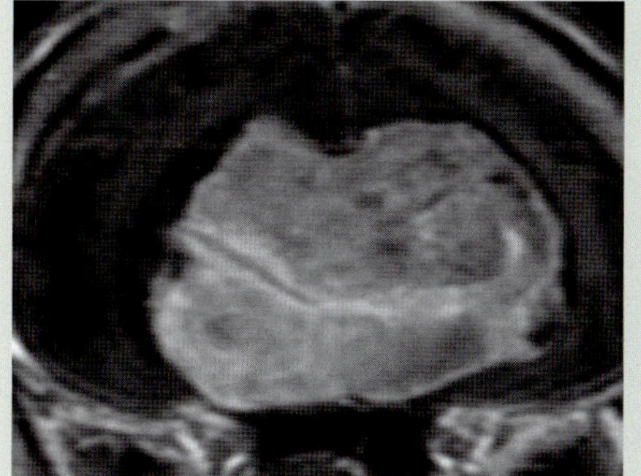 **Fig. 4.18.23:** Meningioma	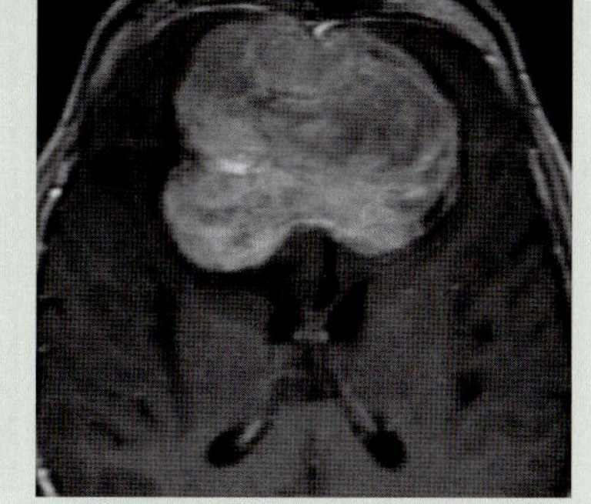 **Fig. 4.18.24:** Meningioma	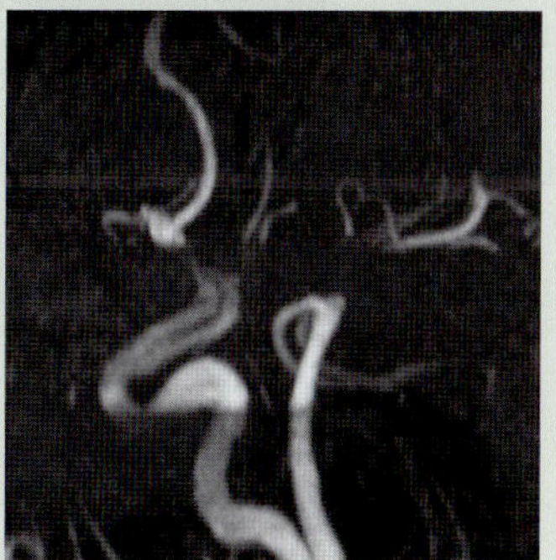 **Fig. 4.18.25:** Meningioma

(Contd.)

Table 4.18.3: Differential diagnosis for butterfly intracerebral tumor (*Contd.*)			
	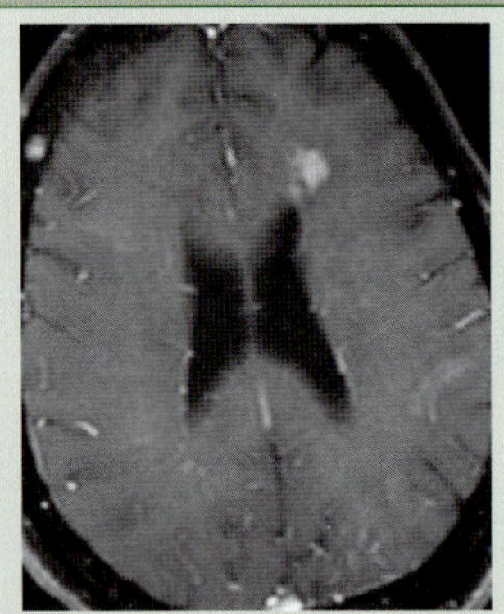	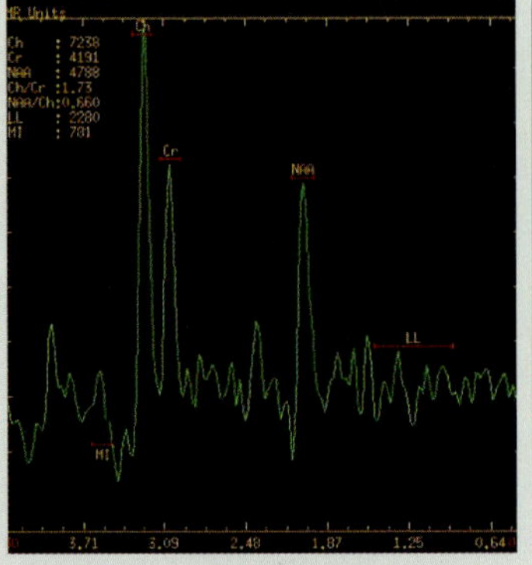	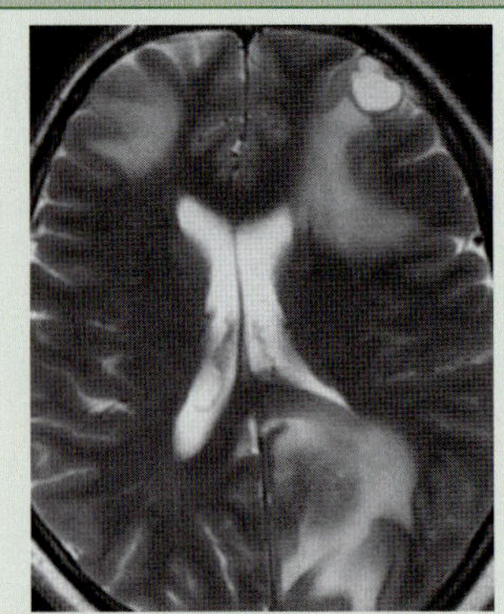
Fig. 4.18.26: Progressive multifocal leukoencephalopathy	**Fig. 4.18.27:** Progressive multifocal leukoencephalopathy	**Fig. 4.18.28:** MRS showing tall choline peak in PML	**Fig. 4.18.29:** Metastasis
Meningioma or granuloma in meninges with adjacent edema can mimic butterfly appearance.			

Discussion: Brain tumors originate from the normal constituents of the brain and its coverings (meninges). Key points in analysis of a brain tumor:

1. Age of the patient
2. Localization (intra *vs* extra-axial, what compartment, midline crossing)
3. CT and MRI characteristics (calcification, fat, cystic and T1, T2, DWI)
4. Contrast enhancement
5. Effect on surrounding structures (mass effect—edema)
6. Solitary—multiple
7. Pseudotumor

Cortical-based brain tumors: Oligodendroglioma, DNET, ganglioglioma, pleomorphic xanthoastrocytoma.

Intracranial tumors with calcification: Oligodendroglioma (90%), ependymoma (50%), ganglioglioma (40%), ATRT, pineoblastoma, intracranial lipoma, central neurocytoma, DNET (microscopic), germinoma, olfactory neuroblastoma, meningioma (25%), skull base chondrosarcoma, craniopharyngioma (90%), teratoma.

Common locations: Oligodendroglioma—frontal lobes, ganglioglioma—temporal lobe, DNET—frontal, temporal, ependymoma—supratentorial (1/3rd)—extra ventricular (45–65%)—frontal lobe, infratentorial (2/3rd)—intraventricular, pilocytic astrocytoma—cerebellum, subependymoma—inferior 4th ventricle (obex), lateral ventricle attached to septum pellucidum.

Patterns of Enhancement in Tumors

Homogeneous enhancement: Metastases, meningioma, lymphoma, germinoma and other pineal gland tumours, pituitary macroadenoma, ganglioglioma, pilocytic astrocytoma and hemangioblastoma (solid component), and schwannoma.

Patchy enhancement: Oligodendroglioma, metastases, radiation necrosis, glioblastoma multiforme.

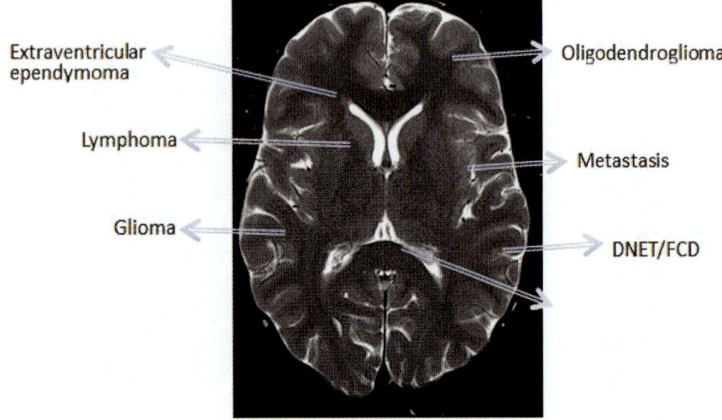

Fig. 4.18.30: Common focal intracranial tumors at the level of caudothalamic groove

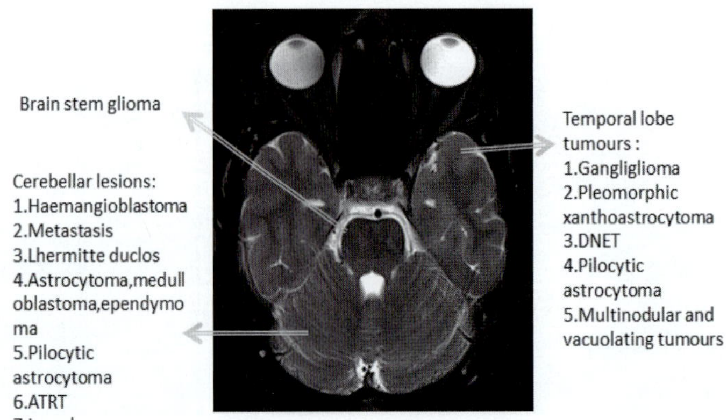

Fig. 4.18.31: Focal intracranial tumors at level of pons

Table 4.18.4: Summary of high-grade glioma	
Features of high-grade glioma: Mass lesion with surrounding disproportionate edema and areas of haemorrhage and necrosis. Non-necrotic area shows diffusion restriction. T1WI C+- Thick, irregular ring of enhancement surrounding central necrosis. MRS—shows decreased NAA and increased choline, lipid lactate peak at 1.3 ppm. Perfusion—increased rCBF (>2.5 times). PET—Malignant tumors have high glucose metabolism and avidly accumulate FDG. SUV—Tumor: WM >1.5 and tumor: gray matter (GM) >0.6	
Fig. 4.18.32	**Fig. 4.18.33:** High grade glioma in left frontal region
Fig. 4.18.34: High grade glioma in bilateral frontal region with butterfly appearance	

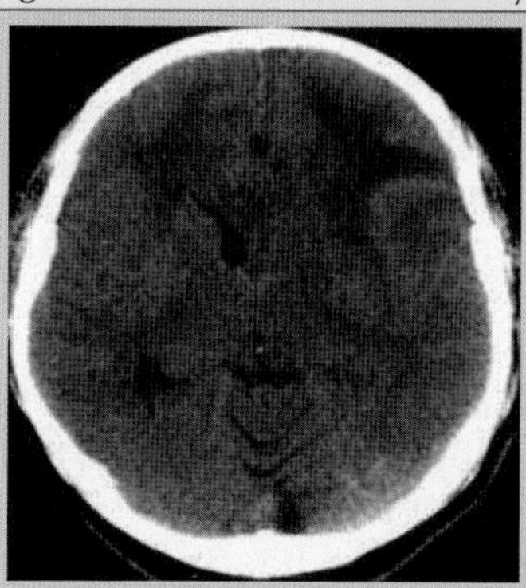

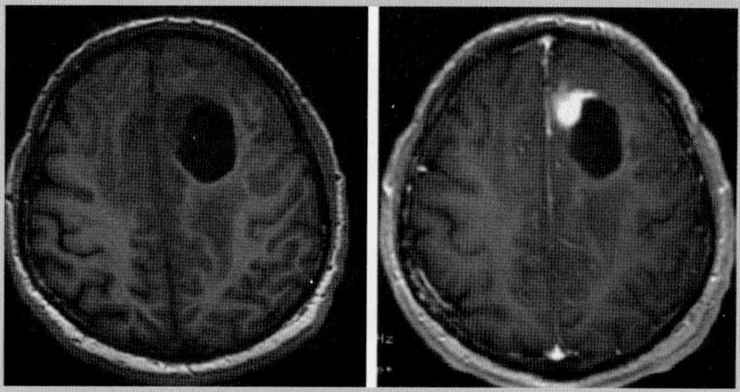

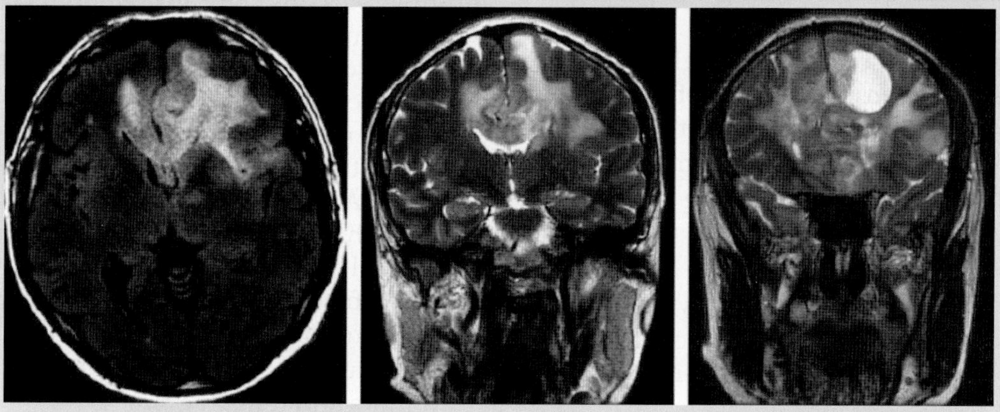

No enhancement: Nontumoral cystic lesions, dermoid cyst, astrocytomas (low grade), epidermoid cyst, arachnoid cyst.

Gliomatosis cerebri: Diffuse gliomas with unique widespread brain invasion, with three or more lobes, frequent bihemispheric, basal ganglionic involvement. Now most of these are IDH—wild type anaplastic astrocytomas.

Ring enhancement in glioma vs granuloma: Granulomas show thin smooth ring enhancement; Gliomas–thick irregular enhancement.

T2 FLAIR mismatch sign seen in diffuse astrocytoma (IDH–mutant type) T2 hyperintensity which gets suppressed on FLAIR indicative of diffuse astrocytoma.

Perfusion imaging: Can be CT perfusion/MR perfusion. MR perfusion is of three types:

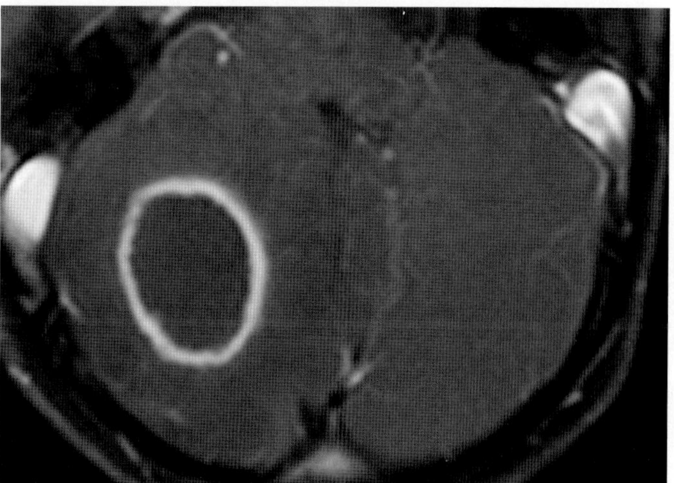

Fig. 4.18.35: Ring enhancement in granuloma

1. Dynamic susceptibility—weighted contrast enhanced (DSC) imaging exploits the susceptibility effects of the contrast gadolinium, which, because of its paramagnetic properties, causes transient signal

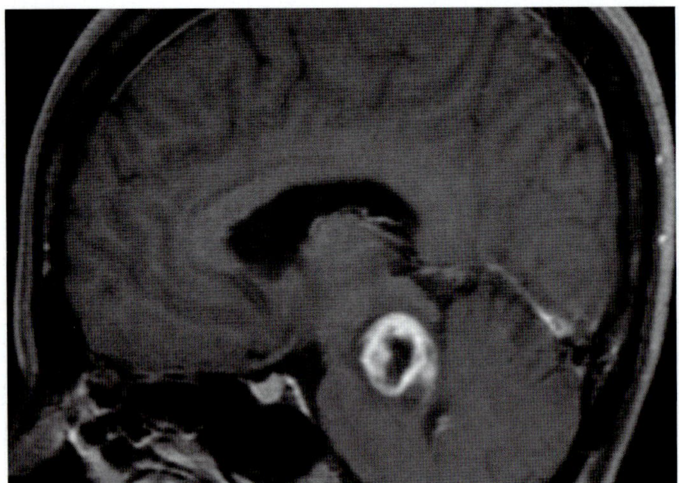

Fig. 4.18.36: Ring enhancement in glioma

loss on T2-weighted images during the passage of gadolinium bolus.

2. Dynamic contrast-enhanced (DCE) imaging measures the increase of signal intensity on a series of T1-weighted images following gadolinium administration.
3. Arterial spin labelling (ASL) uses magnetically labelled blood as endogenous tracer to assess blood flow and does not require an injection of a contrast medium.

Diffusion tensor imaging: Tractography is useful in the preoperative assessment of the brain tumors and helps to differentiate between displacement and infiltration of the white matter tracts.

The main usefulness of **fMRI** in tumor imaging lies in the preoperative localisation of eloquent cortical regions that might have been displaced, distorted or compressed by the tumour and identifying the evidence of any functional reorganisation. It will improve the safety of the surgery and allow for a little more radical resection of the tumor. If possible, an indicated fMRI should be combined with MRI tractography in order to minimise intraoperative injury to the white matter tracts connected to eloquent cortical areas.

The **WHO classification of CNS tumors, 5th edition (2021)** has greater emphasis on molecular markers both in terms of classification and grading. Layered report structure consists of Integrated diagnosis, histopathological classification, CNS WHO grade, molecular information. **Type and subtype**—type replaces "entity", subtype replaces "variant". For example, meningioma type has multiple subtypes instead of previous meningioma variant which has multiple variants. **Not elsewhere classified (NEC)**—in addition to not otherwise specified (NOS), which signifies cancers for which complete molecular classification is not available, NEC has been added to denote tumors that have been thoroughly characterised but do not fit into the current categorization system. **Grades in Arabic numerals**—to bring CNS tumor grades in line with other systems, the Roman numbers I, II, III, and IV will be replaced with the Arabic numerals 1, 2, 3, and 4. **Diffuse glioma nomenclature and grading**—the changes proposed is summarized as:

1. Glioblastoma will be reserved for IDH—wildtype tumors and remain grade 4;
2. Astrocytoma will be definitionally IDH—mutant and graded based on histological and molecular phenotype to grades 2 through 4;

Table 4.18.5: Difference between tumor recurrence and radiation necrosis

	Tumor recurrence	*Radiation necrosis*
Timing	Immediate or delayed	Months to years
Mass effect/edema	Present	Present
Enhancement	+	Soap bubbles/swiss cheese pattern
PET (18-FDG), SPECT (Thallium-201, methionine-11C)	Shows activity	No activity
MRS	Increased choline	Increased lip/lac
MR perfusion	Perfusion shows increased rCBV (>2.6)	Not increased (<0.6)

Table 4.18.6: Difference between tumor and metastasis

Tumor	*Metastasis*
High-grade gliomas showed metabolically active tumor to be present beyond the area of T2 signal abnormality in 88% of cases.	No increased choline in peritumoral area
An NAA: tCho ratio less than 1 and elevated tCho: tCr levels have been found in peritumoral regions of high-grade gliomas	
Increased rCBF and rCBV in peritumoral area	Normal MR perfusion parameters in peritumoral region

Table 4.18.7: Basic difference between the methods of MRI perfusion sequences

	*Postcontrast T2*W imaging*	*Postcontrast T1W imaging*	*Noncontrast ASL*
Quantification method used	Relative more than absolute	Relative and absolute	Relative and absolute
Kinetic parameters derived	rCBV, rCBF, MTT	K trans	CBF, arterial arrival time (AAT)—not currently in clinical use (CBV cannot be measured)
Pathological correlates	Tumour grade and microvessel	VEGF	Microvessel blood flow
Clinical applications	Non-invasive brain tumor grading	Predicting response to treatment	Brain tumor perfusion and stroke imaging
Tissue signal intensity	Darkening	Enhancement change	Darkened
Duration of effect	Seconds/sub-second	Minutes/2–25 s	1.5–2 seconds
Magnitude of effect	Small	Large	Small
Optimal contrast medium	>0.2 mmol	0.1–0.2 mmol	None
Physiological property	Perfusion/blood volume, trans endothelial permeability	Capillary surface area, lesion leakage space	Perfusion/blood volume

3. Anaplastic astrocytoma and anaplastic oligodendroglioma will be referred to as grade 3 or grade 4 astrocytomas or grade 3 oligodendrogliomas, depending on molecular features.
4. **IDH-mutant diffuse gliomas:** Previously, glioblastoma was defined as a glial tumor with necrosis or microvascular proliferation. IDH status predicted survival, and thus glioblastoma IDH wild and glioblastoma IDH mutant subtypes were defined. There has been an attempt to reclassify these tumours to make 'glioblastoma' a more homogeneous group, as IDH mutant tumours accounted for 10% of all glioblastomas, predicted significantly improved survival, and were assumed to come from de-differentiation of lower-grade astrocytoma. As a result, the revised classification system suggestions include the elimination of IDH mutant glioblastoma and the establishment of IDH mutant astrocytoma grading up to WHO grade 4. IDH mutant astrocytoma will be rated based on histology and the presence or absence of a novel genetic parameter, CDKN2A/B homozygous deletion, in the proposed grading system.

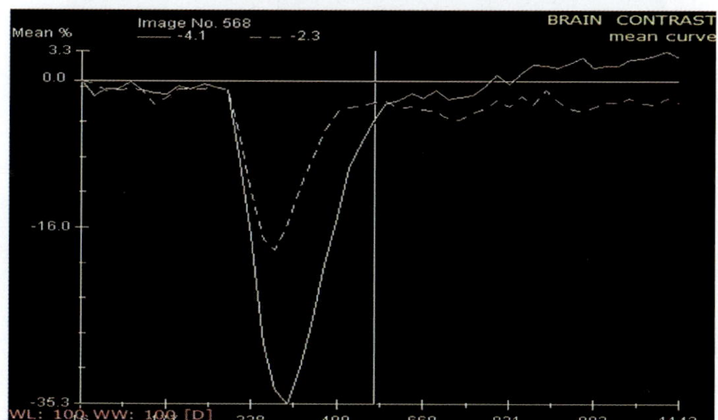

Fig. 4.18.37: High perfusion curve in high grade glioma. **Note:** Area under the curve is rCBV

5. **IDH-mutant astrocytic glioma, WHO grade 2** is a diffusely infiltrative astrocytic glioma with an IDH1 or IDH2 mutation that is well-differentiated and lacks anaplasia histological characteristics. Mitotic activity is either undetectable or very low.
6. **Astrocytoma, IDH-mutant, WHO grade 3** refers to a diffusely infiltrative astrocytic glioma with an IDH1 or IDH2 mutation that demonstrates focal or distributed anaplasia and considerable mitotic activity and lacks microvascular proliferation, necrosis, and CDKN2A/B homozygous deletions. Microvascular growth, necrosis, and homozygous CDKN2A/B deletions are all not seen.
7. A **diffusely infiltrative astrocytic glioma with an IDH1 or IDH2 mutation** that demonstrates microvascular growth or necrosis, CDKN2A/B homozygous deletion, or any combination of these symptoms is classified as an IDH-mutant astrocytoma, WHO grade 4. As a result, all (2016) IDH mutant glioblastomas (characterised by microvascular growth or necrosis) will be reclassified as IDH mutant astrocytoma (WHO grade 4) in 2020. Previous diffuse or anaplastic astrocytomas with a CDKN2A/B mutation will be reclassified as IDH mutant astrocytoma (WHO grade 4) in 2020.
8. **Diffuse gliomas with IDH wild:** The presence of IDH wild in diffuse gliomas is a poor prognostic factor. Non-diffuse glioma (and indeed normal brain) is intrinsically IDH crazy, thus this is not true. Many IDH

Table 4.18.8: Interpreting perfusion curves using rCBV

Mild increase in the rCBV, overshoots baseline—lymphoma	rCBV perfusion more than 2.5 times of the normal brain area—high grade glioma	rCBV perfusion more than 2.5 times of the normal brain area and does not reach the baseline due to leakage—meningioma

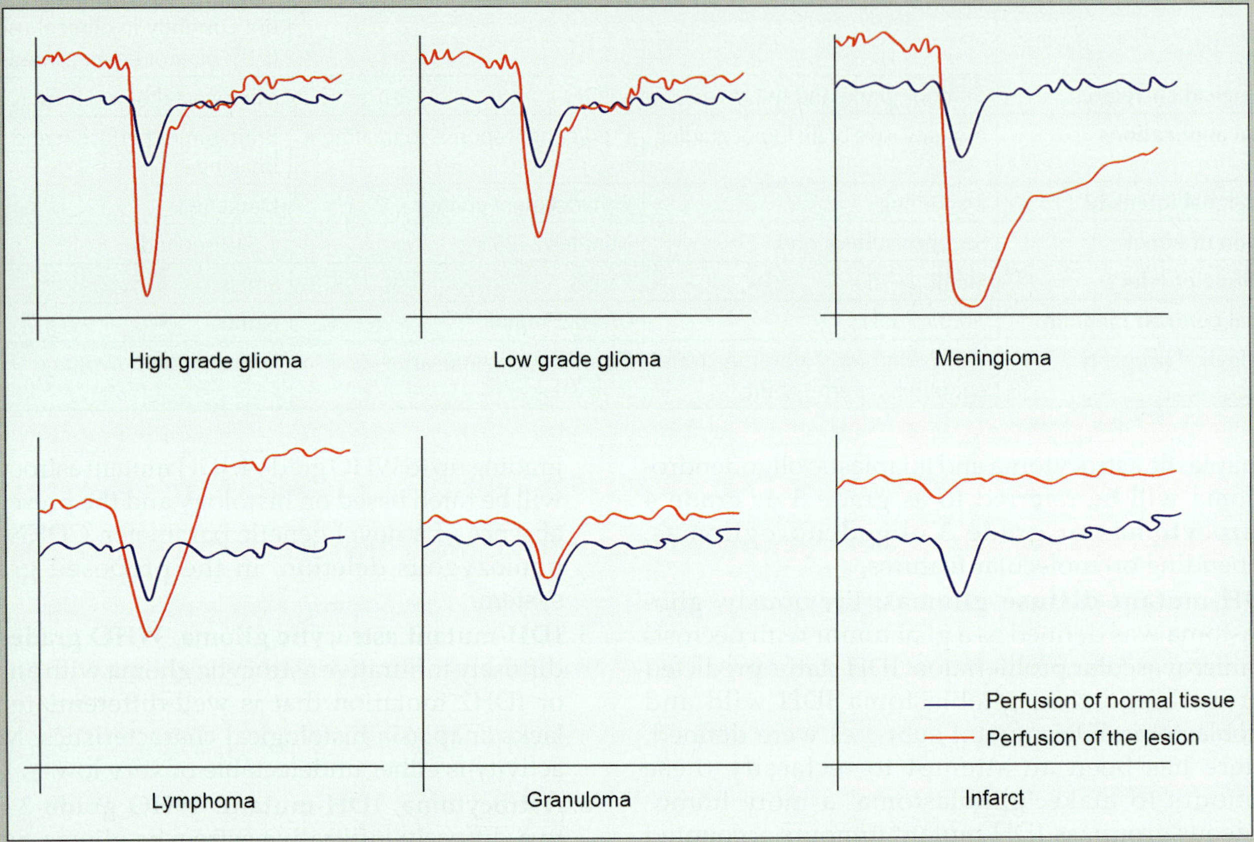

High grade glioma

Low grade glioma

Meningioma

Lymphoma

Granuloma

Infarct

Perfusion of normal tissue

Perfusion of the lesion

Fig. 4.18.38: Various perfusion curves observed in common brain tumors

wild astrocytomas, despite having a lower histological grade due to the lack of mitoses, microvascular proliferation, or necrosis, act aggressively and follow the same path as glioblastoma (IDH wild). As a result, IDH wild astrocytoma is reclassified into either more aggressive (i.e. IDH wild glioblastoma) or low-grade (non-diffuse glioma or reactive normal brain) types. IDH wild glioblastoma is now the separate kind of glioblastoma, and the diagnostic criteria for it have been expanded to include molecular characteristics that indicate a bad prognosis: IDH-wildtype glioblastoma has microvascular proliferation, necrosis, and one or more of the following molecular features: EGFR gene amplification, TERT promoter mutation, chromosome 10 loss (+7/–10) and chromosome 7 gain.

Molecular grading: For the first time, molecular characteristics have been expressly introduced to the grading system, and they may now take precedence

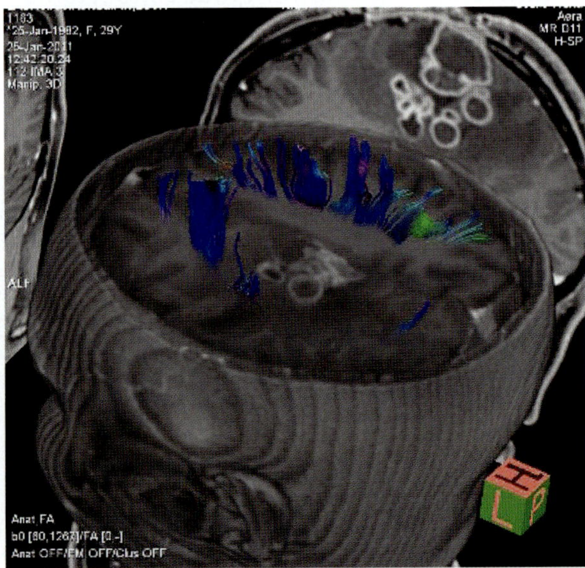

Fig. 4.18.39: DTI shows destruction of corticospinal tract by tuberculoma

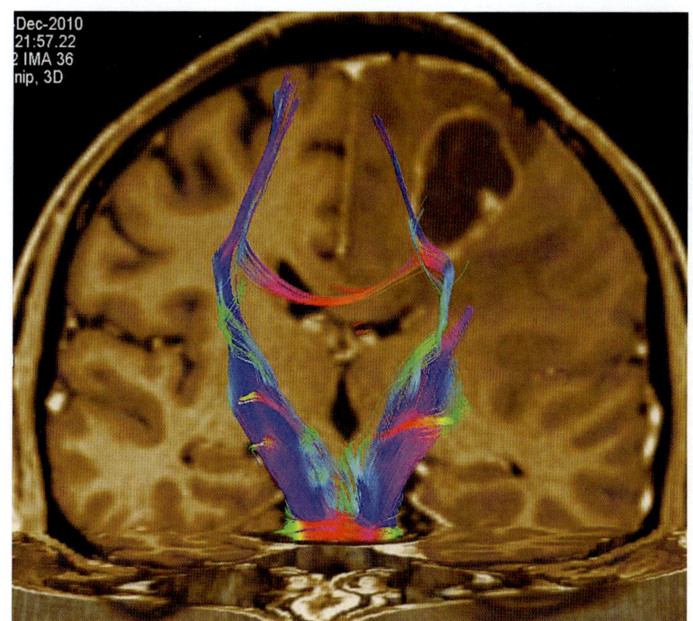

Fig. 4.18.40: DTI showing left white matter tract displacement by mass

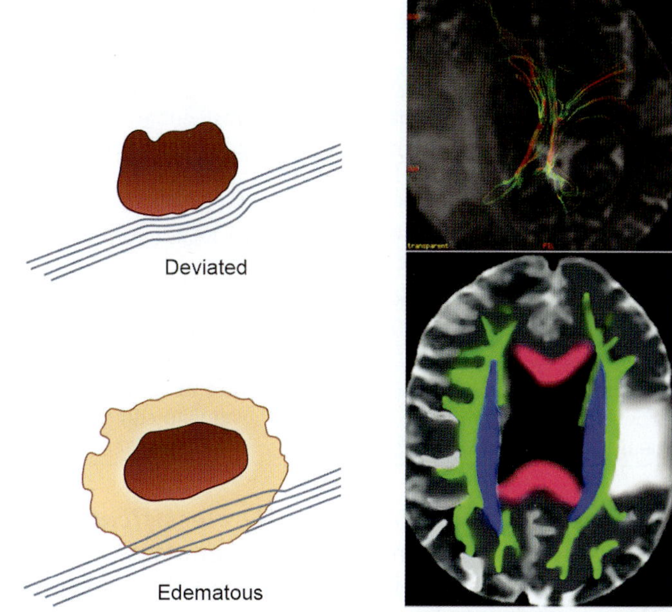

Fig. 4.18.42: Interpreting DTI in case of WM tract in case of displacement

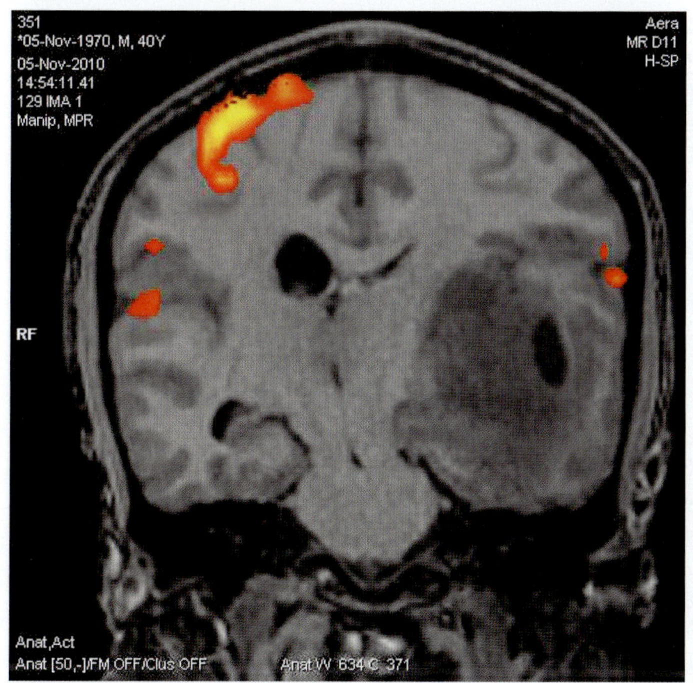

Fig. 4.18.41: Language area fMRI shows activation in both frontal and temporal lobe suggests codominant or plasticity

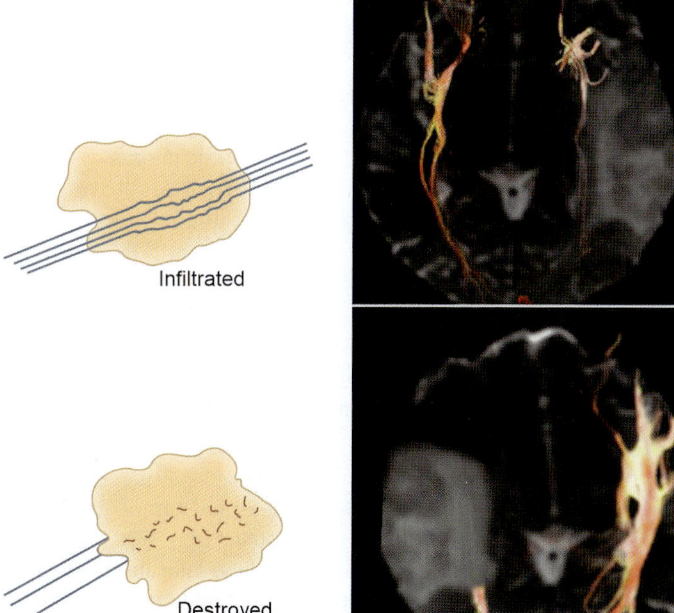

Fig. 4.18.43: Interpreting DTI in case of WM tract infiltration or destruction

over histological characteristics. In the context of EGFR amplification, TERT promoter mutation, or combined gain of chromosome 7 and loss of chromosome 10 [+7/–10], an IDH-wildtype astrocytoma with low-grade histologic characteristics can be termed grade 4 (glioblastoma). Essential and desired diagnostic criteria—each tumour type has been assigned essential diagnostic criteria for a specific diagnosis, as well as non-essential but desirable criteria.

Table 4.18.9: Difference between pseudoprogression and pseudoresponse	
Pseudoprogression	*Pseudoresponse*
Pseudoprogression is due to an inflammatory reaction, which results in a temporary increase of contrast enhancement and edema, usually within 12 weeks of chemoradiation, and subsides subsequently without additional treatment. The hallmark is increasing size of the enhancing component of a GBM **Perfusion:** Reduced cerebral blood volume (viable tumor usually has increased rCBV) **Spectroscopy:** Low choline ratio: Cho/NAA ratio ≤1.4, increased lactate peak, increased lipid peak the trace can be generally flat (hypometabolic) **ADC:** Tumors which respond to treatment and result in pseudo progression will have elevated ADC values due to cell death ADC mean values ≥1300 × 10^{-6}	Pseudoresponse is characterised by a decrease of enhancement and oedema following the administration of antiangiogenic drugs without improved survival. In pseudoresponse the tumour progresses by infiltrative patterns without neoangiogenesis, resulting in an increase of non-enhancing T2/FLAIR hyperintense tumour portions. High grade gliomas (e.g. glioblastoma) in which a rapid decrease in contrast enhancement and edema can be observed in a short period of time after administration of antiangiogenic agents (e.g. bevacizumab and cediranib), often without any significant change in actual tumor size as visualized by T2 (non-enhancing tumor) or diffusion/perfusion studies.

Changes in 4th edition of WHO classification: If the histological phenotype and genotype are not same, then genotype is used to make the diagnosis. IDH status (mutated *vs.* wildtype) and 1p19q co-deletion status for oligodendrogliomas are used to modify diffuse gliomas. Medulloblastoma molecular subgroups have been found. Solitary fibrous tumors of the dura and hemangiopericytoma have now been integrated since, despite their dissimilar appearances, they are histologically the same tumor.

Table 4.18.10: WHO classification of CNS tumors 5th edition (2021)			
Gliomas, glioneuronal tumors, and neuronal tumors			
Adult-type diffuse gliomas Astrocytoma, IDH-mutant Oligodendroglioma, IDH-mutant, and 1p/19q-codeleted Glioblastoma, IDH-wild type	**Pediatric-type diffuse low-grade gliomas** Diffuse astrocytoma, MYB- or MYBL1-altered Angiocentric glioma Polymorphous low-grade neuroepithelial tumor of the young Diffuse low-grade glioma, MAPK pathway-altered Diffuse midline glioma, H3 K27-altered	**Pediatric-type diffuse high-grade gliomas** Diffuse hemispheric glioma, H3 G34-mutant Diffuse pediatric-type high-grade glioma, H3-wildtype and IDH-wildtype Infant-type hemispheric glioma	**Circumscribed astrocytic gliomas** Pilocytic astrocytoma High-grade astrocytoma with piloid features Pleomorphic xanthoastrocytoma Subependymal giant cell astrocytoma Chordoid glioma Astroblastoma, MN1-altered
Glioneuronal and neuronal tumors ganglioglioma		**Ependymal tumors**	**Choroid plexus tumors**
Desmoplastic infantile astrocytoma/ganglioglioma (DIG) • Dysembryoplastic neuroepithelial tumor • Diffuse glioneuronal tumor with oligodendroglioma-like features and nuclear clusters • Papillary glioneuronal tumor • Rosette-forming glioneuronal tumor	• Myxoid glioneuronal tumor • Diffuse leptomeningeal glioneuronal tumor gangliocytoma • Multinodular and vacuolating neuronal tumor • Dysplastic cerebellar gangliocytoma (Lhermitte-Duclos disease) • Cerebellar liponeurocytoma • Central neurocytoma • Extraventricular neurocytoma	Supratentorial ependymoma Supratentorial ependymoma, ZFTA fusion-positive Supratentorial ependymoma, YAP1 fusion-positive Posterior fossa ependymoma Posterior fossa ependymoma, group PFA Posterior fossa ependymoma, group PFB Spinal ependymoma Spinal ependymoma, MYCN-amplified Myxopapillary ependymoma subependymoma	Choroid plexus papilloma Atypical choroid plexus papilloma Choroid plexus carcinoma

4

(Contd.)

Table 4.18.10: WHO classification of CNS tumors 5th edition (2021) *(Contd.)*

Embryonal tumors	**Other CNS embryonal tumors**	**Pineal tumors**	**Cranial and paraspinal nerve tumors**
Medulloblastoma 1. Medulloblastomas, molecularly defined: a. Medulloblastoma, WNT-activated medulloblastoma, b. SHH-activated and TP53-wildtype medulloblastoma, c. SHH-activated and TP53-mutant medulloblastoma, d. Non-WNT/non-SHH medulloblastomas, histologically defined	AT/RT Cribriform neuroepithelial tumor (provisional inclusion) embryonal tumor with multilayered rosettes (ETMR) CNS neuroblastoma, FOXR2-activated CNS tumor with BCOR internal tandem duplication CNS embryonal tumor	• Pineocytoma • Pineoblastoma papillary tumor of the pineal region. • Pineal parenchymal tumor of intermediate differentiation Desmoplastic myxoid tumor of the pineal region, SMARCB1-mutant	Schwannoma and schwannoma (intracranial) Neurofibroma Perineurioma Hybrid nerve sheath tumor Malignant melanotic nerve sheath tumor Malignant peripheral nerve sheath tumor Paraganglioma
Meningiomas			
Mesenchymal, non-meningothelial tumors			
Soft tissue tumors • Fibroblastic and myofibroblastic tumors • Solitary fibrous tumor	**Skeletal muscle tumors** • Rhabdomyosarcoma vascular tumors • Hemangiomas and vascular malformations • Hemangioblastoma	**Uncertain differentiation** • Intracranial mesenchymal tumor, FET-CREB fusion-positive • CIC—rearranged sarcoma • Primary intracranial sarcoma, DICER1-mutant • Ewing sarcoma	**Chondro-osseous tumors** • Chondrogenic tumors • Mesenchymal chondrosarcoma • Chondrosarcoma **Notochordal tumors** • Chordoma (including poorly differentiated chordoma)
Melanocytic tumors	**Hematolymphoid tumors**		
a. Diffuse meningeal melanocytic neoplasms—meningeal melanocytosis and meningeal melanomatosis b. Circumscribed meningeal melanocytic neoplasms—meningeal melanocytoma and meningeal melanoma	**Lymphomas** a. CNS lymphomas primary diffuse large B-cell lymphoma of the CNS b. Immunodeficiency—associated CNS lymphoma c. Lymphomatoid granulomatosis d. Intravascular large B-cell lymphoma	**Miscellaneous rare lymphomas in the CNS** a. MALT lymphoma of the dura b. Other low-grade B-cell lymphomas of the CNS c. Anaplastic large cell lymphoma (ALK+/ALK–) d. T-cell and NK/T-cell lymphomas	**Histiocytic tumors** Erdheim-Chester disease Rosai-Dorfman disease Juvenile xanthogranuloma Langerhans cell histiocytosis Histiocytic sarcoma
Tumors of the sellar region Pituitary adenoma (pitNET), craniopharyngioma, pituitary blastoma, pituicytoma, granular cell tumor of the sellar region, and spindle cell oncocytoma.	**Metastases to the CNS** Includes metastasis to brain spinal cord and meninges.		**Germ cell tumors** Mature teratoma Immature teratoma Teratoma with somatic-type malignancy Germinoma Embryonal carcinoma Yolk sac tumor Choriocarcinoma Mixed germ cell tumor

Structure: Despite progress toward molecular markers for some entities, classification is still organised by cell of origin (e.g. ependymal cancers) or anatomical origin (e.g. melanoma) (e.g. tumours of the sellar region).

cIMPACT (the Consortium to Inform Molecular and Practical Approaches to CNS Tumor Taxonomy): Forum under International Society of Neuropathology that proposes change to future WHO CNS tumors classification system.

Table 4.18.11: Summary of cIMPACT updates since 2016 WHO classification

Update/year	*Main topics*	*Highlights*	*Comments*
1/2018	Nomenclature, NOS vs. NEC	NOS ("not otherwise specified") and NEC ("not elsewhere classified")	NOS: Molecular testing not available NEC: Test results do not fit known tumor
2/2018	H3K27m	WHO grade 4 restricted to H3K27m diffuse midline gliomas	Other tumors harbouring the H3K27 mut, not necessarily aggressive
	Diffuse astrocytoma, IDH mutant	IDH mutant, ATRX loss, diffuse p53-positivity suffice for astrocytoma diagnosis	1p19q analysis not essential to exclude oligodendroglioma
3/2018	Diffuse astrocytoma, IDH wild	When histological criteria of GBM not fulfilled: CDKN2A/2B deletion or EGFR-amplification or TERT-promotor mutation	Prognosis similar to GBM with any of the listed molecular criteria
4/2019	Pediatric diffuse gliomas	MYB, MYBL1, or FGFR1 alterations or BRAFV600E mut	Brain tumors in children beyond the scope of this article
5/2020	Grading, Arabic numbers	Arabic in lieu of Roman numerals	—
	Grading, IDH mutant astrocytomas	Grade 2: no M, MVP, N, D Grade 3: M Grade 3: MVP and/or N and/or D	GBM refers only to IDH wild, H3wt astrocytomas
6/2020	New tumor entities and summary of earlier publications	PLNTY (polymorphous low-grade neuro-epithelial tumor) Chordoid glioma, PRKCA D463H-mut High-grade astrocytoma with piloid features	—
7/2020	Ependymomas	Myxopapillary, WHO grade 2 Classified according to location and molecular profile	*Supratentorial*[a] RELA (C11orf95)-fusion YAP-fusion *Posterior fossa* Type A Type B *Spinal* MYCN-amplified

M mitoses, *MVP* microvascular proliferation, *N* necrosis, *D* CDKN2A/B deletions, [a]Supratentorial excluding subependymoma

4.19 CENTRAL NERVOUS SYSTEM

Case No. 19

Clinical history: A 10-year-old female, complaints of headache and vomiting with seizures.

Radiological techniques and observation: Figures 4.19.1 and 4.19.2 are axial CT sections plain and with intravenous contrast respectively showing a midline cystic lesion with mural nodule in the posterior fossa which shows intense enhancement after intravenous contrast administration. Visualised sections show enlarged temporal horns of bilateral lateral ventricles and the fourth ventricle is not visualised. So, the lesion might be compressing the fourth ventricle causing obstructive hydrocephalus. No other similar lesions noted in the visualised brain parenchyma. Visualised sellar, parasellar and suprasellar regions are normal. Bilateral cerebello-pontine angles are free. Visualised bilateral MCA appears normal. No abnormal meningeal enhancement noted. Visualised calvarium and soft tissue appears normal.

Figures 4.19.3 to 4.19.5 are axial MR images in T1 sequence with intravenous contrast, T2 sequence and DWI respectively showing intra-axial lesion in the cerebellar vermis. The lesion is cystic with a small solid area, which shows intense enhancement after intravenous contrast administration. Mild enhancement of the cyst wall noted. No diffusion restriction noted. No evidence of similar lesions in other locations or retinal angioma/capillary hemangioma. No evidence of any prominent flow void or feeding vessel noted. No surrounding edema. No obvious arterial feeder to nodule noted.

Interpretation: A—10 years old female child, cerebellar vermis, C—cystic lesion with a mural nodule, B—intense contrast enhancement of the mural nodule and cyst wall

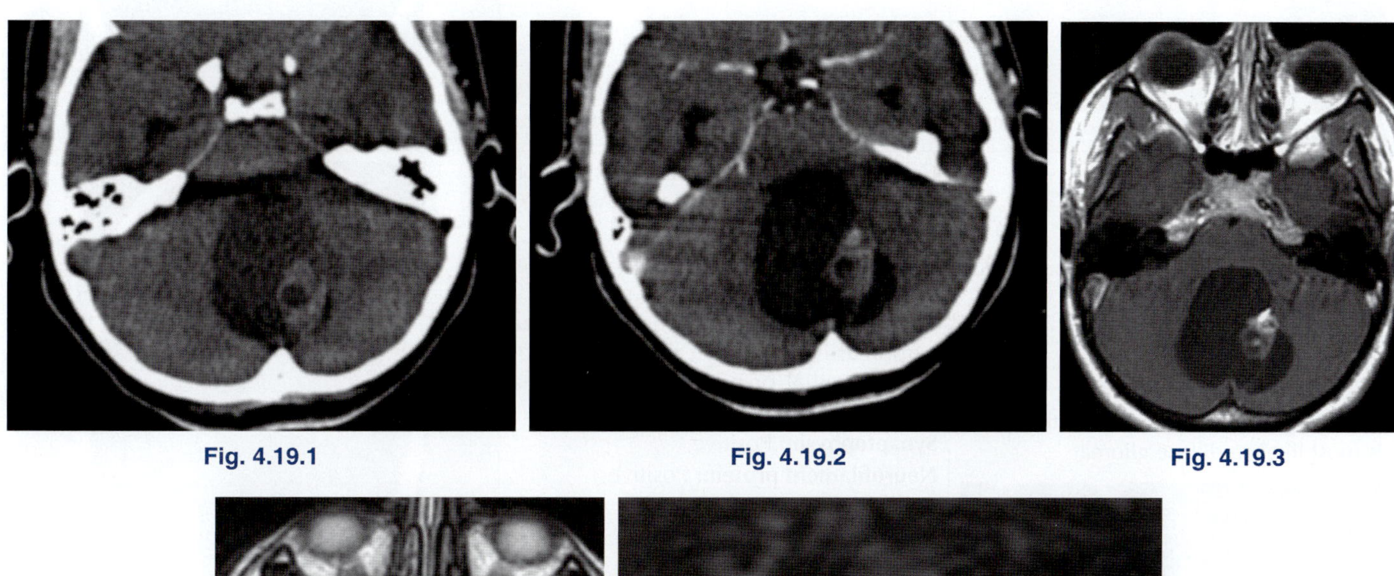

Fig. 4.19.1 Fig. 4.19.2 Fig. 4.19.3

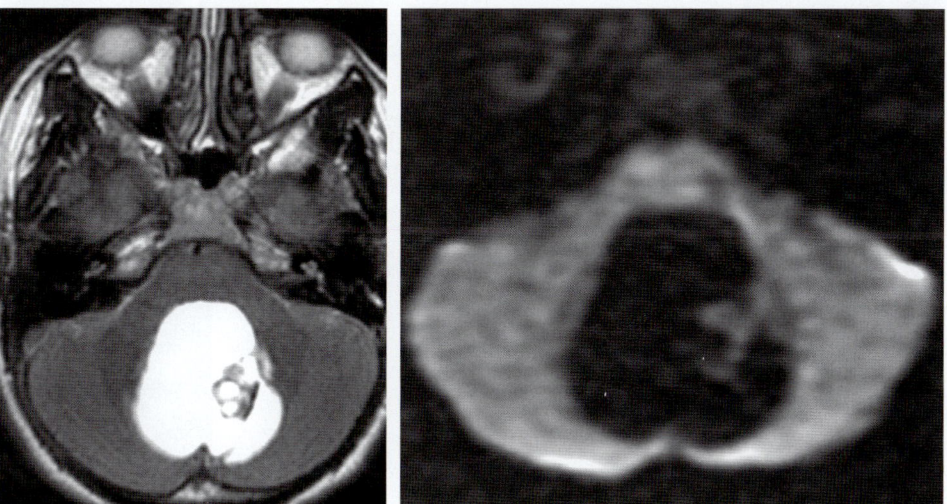

Fig. 4.19.4 Fig. 4.19.5

4

Table 4.19.1: Differential diagnosis for cyst with mural nodule

<table>
<tr>
<td>Hemangioblastoma:
WHO Grade-I.
Age: 40–60 years.
Most common in the posterior fossa.
Associations:
Pheochromocytoma
Multiple RCCs
von Hippel-Lindau (VHL) disease
Polycythemia: Due to secretion of erythropoietin from lesions</td>
<td>Flow voids visible in T1 and T2 in the nodular portion. The lesion abuts the pia. The cyst is slightly hyperintense in T1 compared with CSF. Enhancement of the walls of the cyst is very rarely found in hemangioblastoma.
MR perfusion imaging: High rCBV ratios.
Angiography (DSA): Enlarged feeding arteries and often dilated draining veins are demonstrated, with a dense tumor blush centrally.</td>
<td>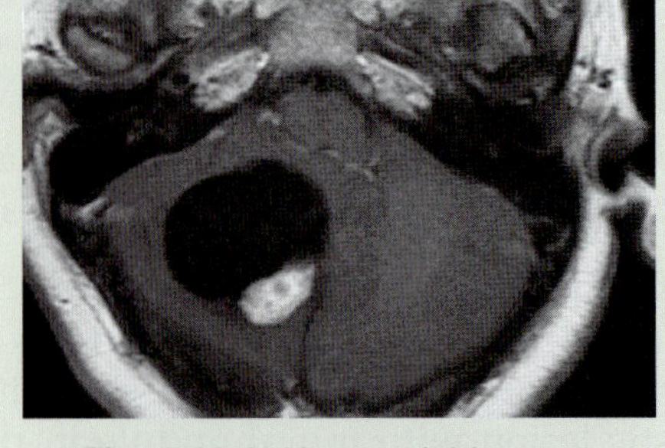
Fig. 4.19.6: Hemangioblastoma</td>
</tr>
<tr>
<td>Pleomorphic xanthoastrocytoma:
WHO Grade-II.
Age: 10–30 years.
Supratentorial, superficial cortical mass. Usually in the temporal lobe. If mitoses are more frequent (>5 mitoses per 10 high-power fields), then a diagnosis of anaplastic pleomorphic xanthoastrocytoma (WHO grade III) should be made.</td>
<td>Cystic portion is isointense to the CSF. Enhancement of the adjacent meninges, with an appearance of dural tail. Despite vivid enhancement, they are usually avascular on angiography.
GFAP: Positive, although often only weakly, S100: Positive
Neuronal markers including synaptophysin, MAP2 and neurofilament: Variable Ki-67 proliferation index: <1%</td>
<td>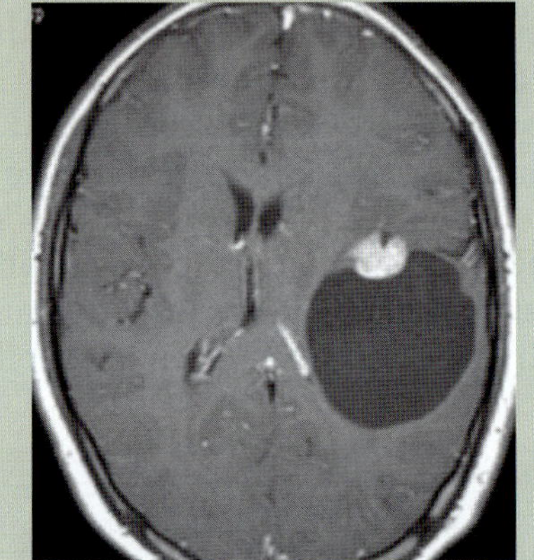
Fig. 4.19.7: Pleomorphic xanthoastrocytoma</td>
</tr>
<tr>
<td>Ganglioglioma:
WHO Grade-I/II.
Age: 10–20 years.
Cortical based mass in a child/young adult with temporal lobe epilepsy.
Genetics
BRAF-V600E mutations are encountered in 20–60% of cases.
IDH: Negative (if positive, then the tumor is most likely a diffuse glioma)
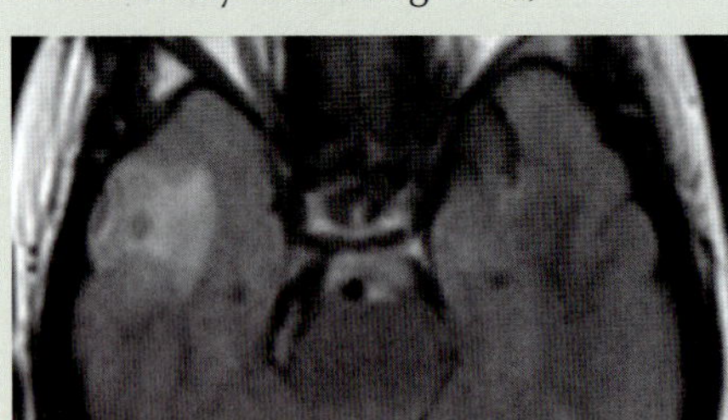
Fig. 4.19.8: Ganglioglioma</td>
<td>Calcification inside the lesion is a common finding. The cyst often expands the cortex.
Composed of:
1. Ganglion cells (large mature neuronal elements): Ganglio.
2. Neoplastic glial element: Glioma primarily astrocytic, although oligodendroglial or pilocytic astrocytoma components are also encountered.
Synaptophysin: Positive
Neurofilament protein: Positive
MAP2: Positive
Chromogranin-A: Positive (usually negative in normal neurons)
CD34: Positive in 70–80%
The glial component may also show cytoplasmic positivity for GFAP.</td>
<td>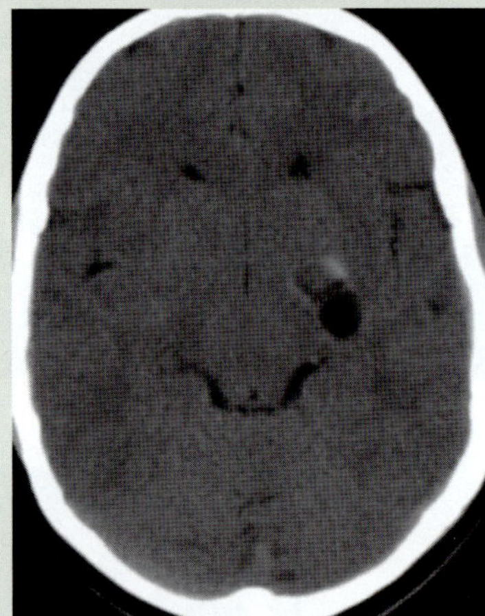
Fig. 4.19.9: Ganglioglioma
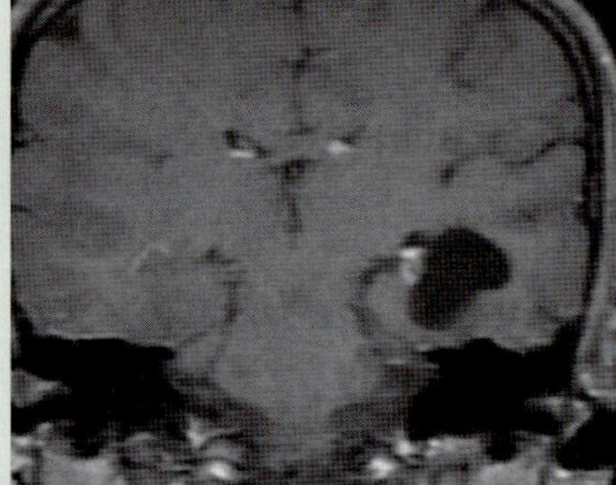
Fig. 4.19.10: Ganglioglioma</td>
</tr>
</table>

(Contd.)

Table 4.19.1: Differential diagnosis for cyst with mural nodule (*Contd.*)
Desmoplastic infantile ganglioglioma: Refer to case 17
Other causes of cystic lesions with mural nodule: **Metastases:** A frank cyst with mural nodule pattern in metastasis is rare. Cystic metastasis is much more common from lung, but also occurs in other metastatic cancers like breast, pancreas, kidney and even melanoma. **Tanycytic ependymoma:** Tanycytic ependymomas are a subtype of ependymomas. The tumor cells have morphological characteristics resembling tanycytes, a special subtype of ependymal cells. Tanycytic ependymomas arising in the cervicomedullary junction have been consistently associated with a cyst with mural nodule appearance. **Cystic meningioma:** The term "cystic meningioma" has been used to describe meningiomas with **intratumoral** or **peritumoral cysts**. The presence of an associated cyst is an uncommon imaging feature that may make it difficult to differentiate the tumor from an intra-axial primary glial neoplasm. Proposed mechanisms include cystic degeneration of the tumor, secretion of fluid from tumor cells, or loculated cerebrospinal fluid from scar tissue within or adjacent to the tumor. **Intracerebral schwannoma:** Since Schwann cells are normally not present in the cerebral parenchyma, it is little difficult to explain the origin of intracranial parenchymal schwannomas; it is suggested that they derive from Schwann cells within **perivascular nerve plexus.** **Rosette-forming glioneuronal tumor (RGNT) of the fourth ventricle:** RGNT was described as an entity in 2002. Usually it presents as a cerebellar lesion in a young adult. It originates from the roof and protrudes into the fourth ventricle and is often present with a cyst with mural nodule pattern. **Papillary glioneuronal tumor:** PGNT was described as an entity in 1998. It is a very rare lesion located usually in the temporal lobe. Many of the few PGNT described had a cyst with mural nodule pattern. **Vascular lesions: Parenchymal brain perianeurysmal cyst** is a very rare but potentially very dangerous lesion that radiologists should be aware of when facing a cyst with mural nodule. The mechanism of cyst formation is still controversial. **Cavernous angiomas** accompanied by a cyst are a rare occurrence. **Neurocysticercosis:** It is the most common parasitic disease of the CNS. The typical cyst with mural nodule pattern is very rare in neurocysticercosis and is mainly present when the lesion is in the colloidal stage.

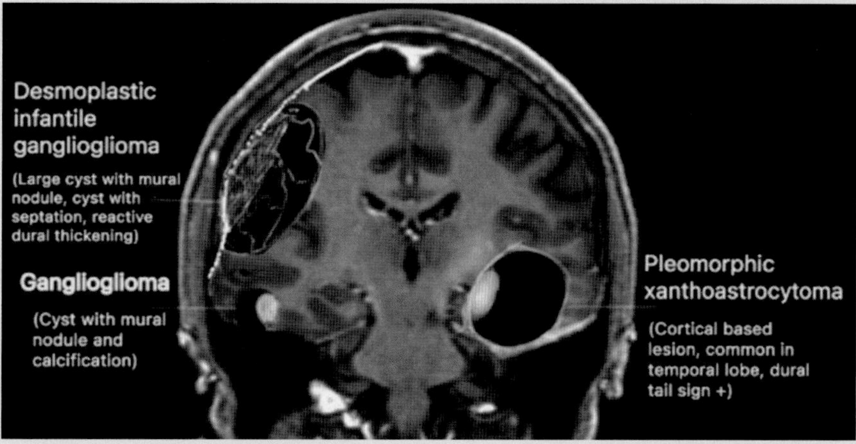

Fig. 4.19.11: Approach to cyst with mural nodules

enhancement without diffusion restriction or prominent flow voids, D—pilocytic astrocytoma.

Principal Diagnosis: Pilocytic astrocytoma.

Brief discussion about the condition: Pilocytic astrocytomas, also known as **juvenile pilocytic astrocytomas**, are low-grade, relatively well-defined astrocytomas which tend to occur in young patients. They are considered WHO grade I tumors in the current (2016) WHO classification of CNS tumors and correspondingly have a relatively good prognosis. Cerebellar astrocytoma—20–25% of posterior fossa tumours. Vermis (50%) or hemispheres (20%) or both sites (30%) ± extension into the cavity of the fourth ventricle. Calcification in 20%. CT/MRI—large lesion displacing the fourth ventricle → obstructive hydrocephalus. 80% are juvenile pilocytic astrocytomas with an **excellent prognosis**. Tumor can be cystic, solid or solid with central necrosis. 50% of all tumors are a cyst with an isodense enhancing mural nodule. The cyst contents have slightly increased CSF attenuation on CT. 40–45% are solid with central necrosis. The solid component is isodense to hypodense to white matter on CT, low signal on T1W MRI and high signal on T2W MRI. The solid component enhances on CT and MRI. Larger tumor at diagnosis than the solid type. The solid type accounts for 10%.

Table 4.19.2: Pathology of pilocytic astrocytomas	
Microscopic appearance	*Immunophenotype*
The term pilocytic refers to the **elongated hair-like projections** from the neoplastic cells. The presence of **eosinophilic Rosenthal fibres** is a characteristic feature and hyalinization of blood vessels is also common. The histological features are, however, fairly heterogeneous even within the one tumor, with some areas mimicking diffuse astrocytomas and even oligodendrogliomas.	Immunohistochemistry reflects astrocytic differentiation: GFAP: Positive S100: Positive OLIG2: Positive **IDH R132H mutation:** Negative p53 protein: Negative or weak

Table 4.19.3: Difference between hemangioblastoma and juvenile pilocytic astrocytoma		
Feature	*Hemangioblastoma*	*Juvenile pilocytic astrocytoma*
Age	30–40 yrs (In VHL 15 to 30 yrs, uncommon before 15 yrs of age)	5–15 years
Site	Periphery: Pial side	Central: Glial cells
Pial attachment and prominent flow voids	Present. Nodule abuts pial surface. Prominent arterial feeder is present.	Absent
Peritumoral edema	Significant	Variable
Mural nodule	Feeder with mural nodule	Strong enhancing mural nodule
Cyst wall enhancement	Absent—compressed non-neoplastic brain. No enhancement of cyst wall.	Present as delayed enhancement of cyst wall
Calcifications	Rare	20–25%
Flow voids	Present	Absent
Angiography	Prolonged tumor blush with early draining veins present.	Intense prolonged staining of mural nodule. But AV shunting with early draining veins uncommon.
Association	VHL	NF-1
MRS	Lipid peak may be present. Choline peak with absent NAA peak (non-neurogenic origin)	Pseudomalignant—elevated choline peak, low NAA and lactate peak.
Perfusion MR	Markedly elevated rCBV	Low to moderate rCBV

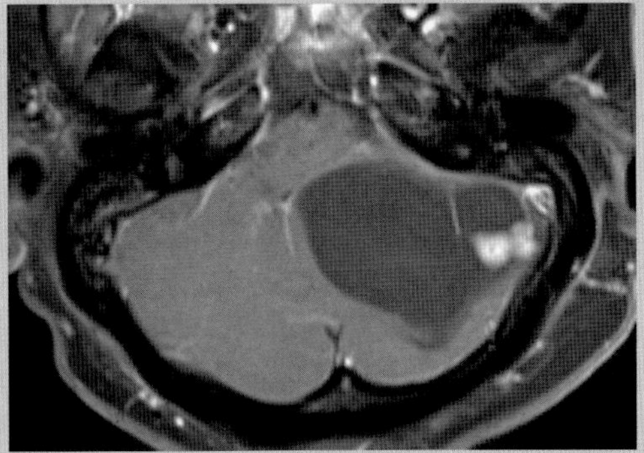

Fig. 4.19.12: Hemangioblastoma

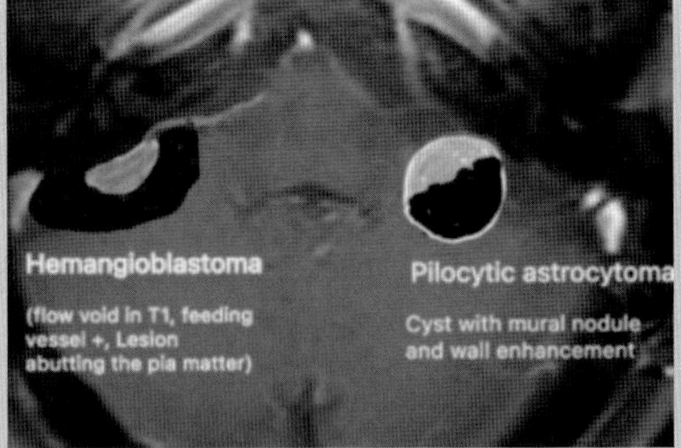

Fig. 4.19.13: Both hemangioblastoma and pilocystic astrocytoma

Associations: There has been a strong association with neurofibromatosis type 1 **(NF1)**. NF1 associated tumors have a tendency to affect the optic nerves and optic chiasma.

Treatment: Surgical resection is the treatment of choice and often curative; **radiation** therapy and **chemotherapy** reserved for tumors of the optic chiasm and hypothalamic region, recurrent tumor, and disseminated disease (rare); chemotherapy used for children younger than 5 years.

4

4.20 CENTRAL NERVOUS SYSTEM

Case No. 20

Clinical history: A 25-year-old male presented with long standing epilepsy, no history of fever, no trauma.

Radiological techniques and observation: Figures 4.20.1 to 4.20.3 are MRI brain in T2 axial, T1 axial and FLAIR coronal images showing a moderate size cyst which is intra-axial, intraparenchymal smooth walled and off midline in the right parieto-occipito-temporal junction measuring 5 × 4 × 6 cm communicating with the occipital horn of the right lateral ventricle. It follows CSF signal in all sequences, with no diffusion restriction or enhancement. Cyst appears to be lined by FLAIR hyperintense gliotic white matter. No evidence of grey matter lining. Slight remodelling of the overlying calvarium noted. No evidence of any mass effect.

Interpretation: A: 25 years old male, intraparenchymal right parieto-occipito-temporal junction, C: Well-defined smooth-walled cystic lesion which follows CSF signal in all sequences, B: Communicating with ventricle typically lined by gliotic white matter with slight remodelling of the overlying calvarium, D: Porencephalic cyst.

Principal diagnosis: Porencephalic cyst.

Management: This patient is referred to neurological team for supportive management.

Differential diagnosis: Schizencephaly, encephalomalacia, neoplastic cyst.

Discussion: **Porencephaly** is a rare congenital disorder that results in cystic degeneration and encephalomalacia and the formation of **porencephalic cysts**. Being a focal cystic area of encephalomalacia that communicates with the ventricular system and/or the subarachnoid space. Often signs and symptoms become evident in the first year of life, with spasticity and seizures being common early manifestations. Language impairment, intellectual disability, and motor deficits are also frequently encountered. The cysts are typically lined by white matter. They are thought to occur from focal encephalomalacia due to a localized cerebral insult most frequently during early gestation.

Ultrasound: On an antenatal ultrasound scan, these may be seen as one or more intracranial cysts that communicate with the ventricular system and/or subarachnoid space. There may also be asymmetrical ventricles with displacement of the midline ventricular echo.

CT: Porencephalic cysts appear as an intracranial cyst which has a well-defined border and central attenuation the same as CSF. There is usually no mass effect on the adjacent parenchyma, although occasionally enlarging cysts do **result in local mass effect**. There is no enhancement with contrast and no solid component.

MRI: The content of the cyst follows CSF signal on all sequences, DWI: No restricted diffusion.

Diffusion tensor imaging: Conventional MR does not always differentiate various cystic lesions of brain. Diffusion-weighted imaging (DWI) deals with restriction of random motion of water molecules which indirectly depicts the nature of the tissue in which these water molecules are moving.

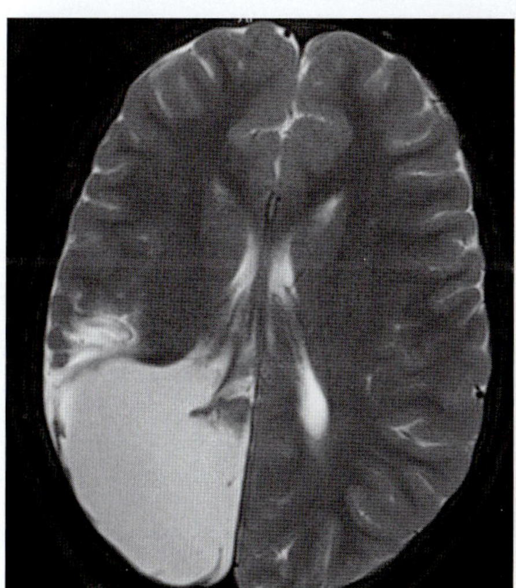

Fig. 4.20.1

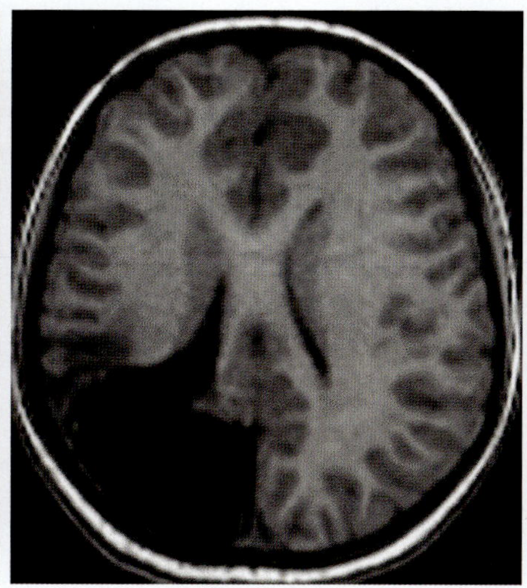

Fig. 4.20.2

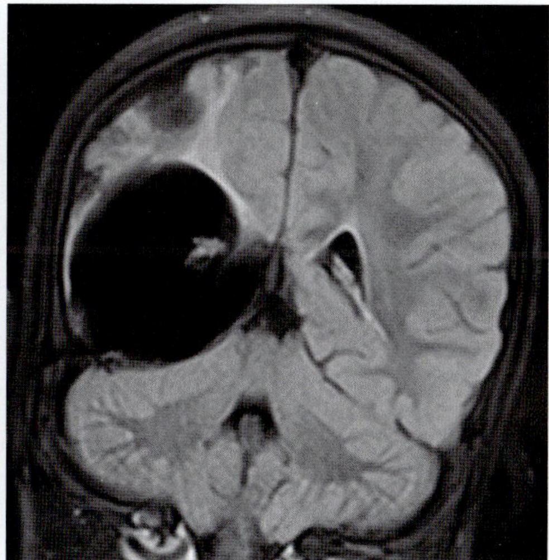

Fig. 4.20.3

Table 4.20.1: Differential diagnosis for intracranial cystic lesions		
Neuroglial cyst (glioependymal cysts, neuroepithelial cysts): Congenital lesion due to sequestration of neural tube embryonic elements that develop into a fluid-filled cavity, lined by glial cell and located within the white matter.	Follows CSF signal: Hypointense on T1 and hyperintense on T2. They do not enhance with gadolinium. They are usually suppressed on T2 FLAIR sequences. No communication with the ventricles or the subarachnoid space	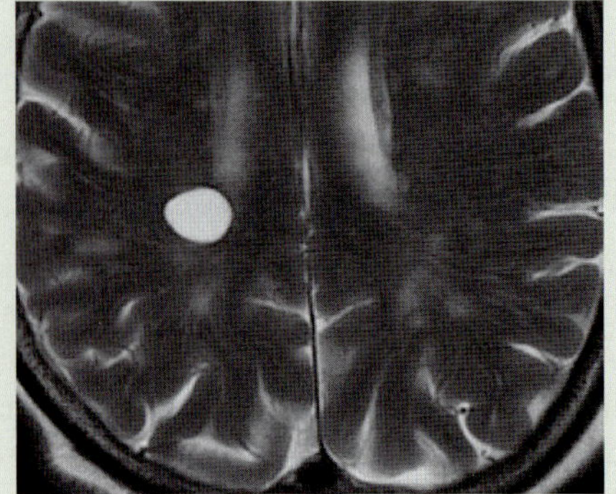 **Fig. 4.20.4:** Neuroglial cyst
Enlarged perivascular spaces (Virchow-Robin): These are pial-lined interstitial fluid-filled structures that accompany penetrating arteries and veins.	Typically, less than 5 mm in diameter and isointense to CSF at all sequences. They are common and considered a normal variant.	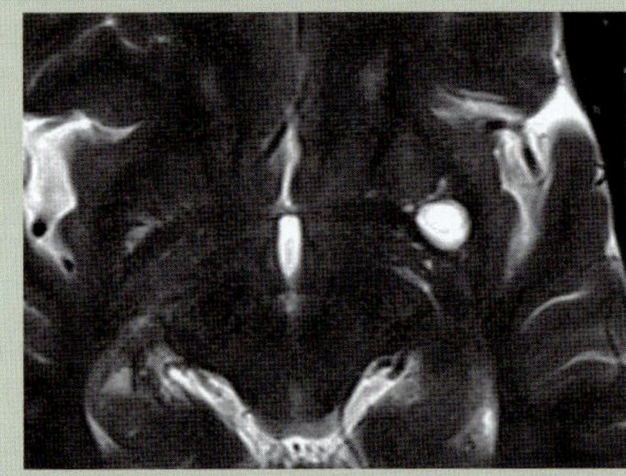 **Fig. 4.20.5:** VR space
Colloid cysts: Occur in the roof of the third ventricle immediately adjacent to the foramina of Monro on occasion results in sudden obstructive hydrocephalus	Well-delineated hyperdense mass on unenhanced CT. On MRI they usually are hyperintense on T1 and isointense to brain on T2 weighted images. Peripheral rim enhancement may be present in some cases.	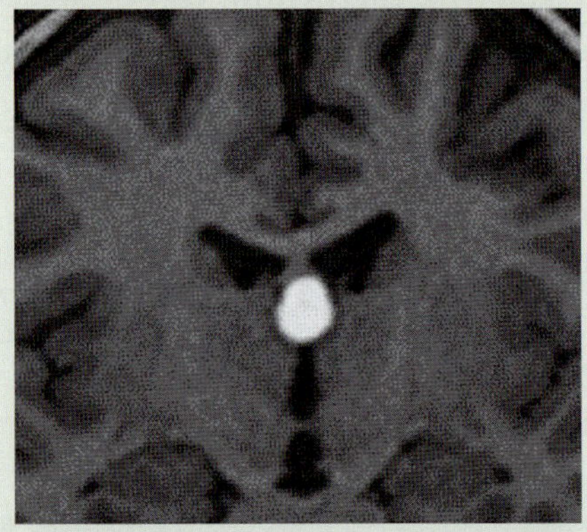 **Fig. 4.20.6:** Colloid cyst
Choroid plexus cysts: Non-neoplastic epithelial-lined cysts of the choroid plexus. Usually bilateral and commonly located in the lateral ventricular atria. They are asymptomatic and found incidentally.	Iso- to hyperdense to CSF on nonenhanced CT. Peripheral calcification is common, may enhance. Signal intensity is variable. Most are iso- or hyperintense to CSF, may show rim or nodular enhancement, do not become completely hypointense on FLAIR. Two-thirds show restriction on diffusion.	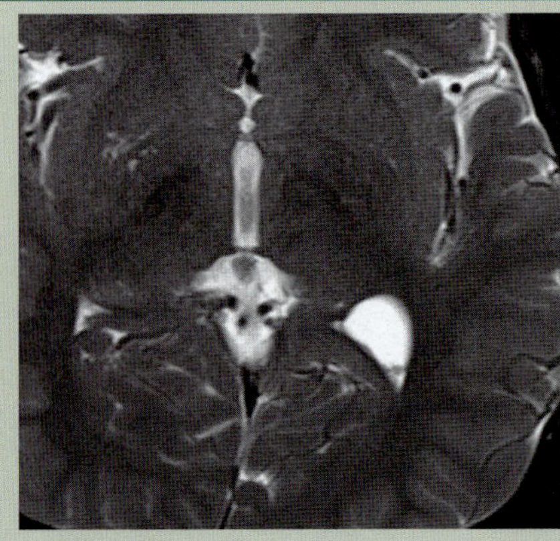 **Fig. 4.20.7:** Choroid plexus cysts

(Contd.)

4

Table 4.20.1: Differential diagnosis for intracranial cystic lesions (*Contd.*)		
Choroidal fissural cyst: Benign intracranial cysts occurring within choroidal fissure. They are usually asymptomatic and discovered incidentally. They may cause **headache and seizures (20–25%)** due to mass effect on the temporal lobe. **Bilateral in 8–10%.**	MR signal characteristics are similar to CSF on all sequences. The cyst walls are thin. Contrast enhancement, surrounding edema and gliosis are absent. 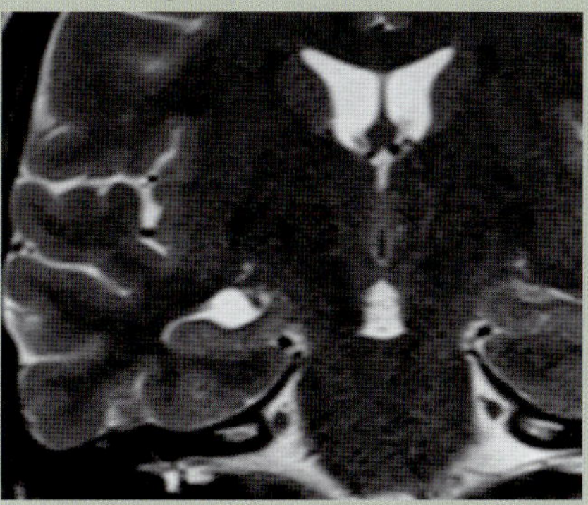 **Fig. 4.20.8:** Choroidal fissural cyst	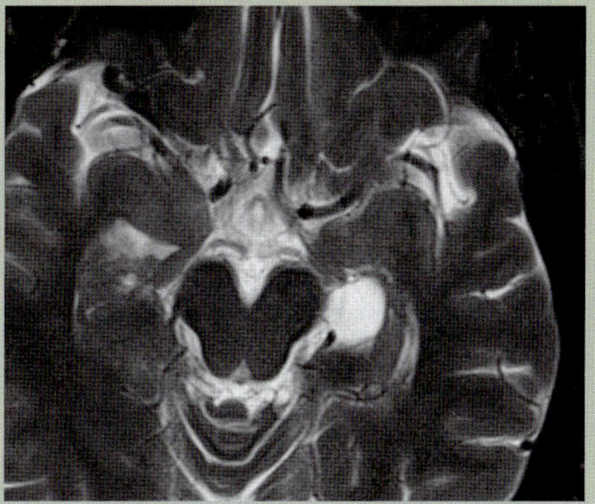 **Fig. 4.20.9:** Choroidal fissural cyst
Ependymal cyst: Rare benign neuroepithelial cysts lined by ependymal cells. Most are small and asymptomatic and only cause symptoms, if large.	Typically, periventricular in location. Follows CSF signal on all sequences and does not demonstrate diffusion restriction. Occasionally the cyst may be hyperintense to CSF if there is a high protein content. No contrast enhancement.	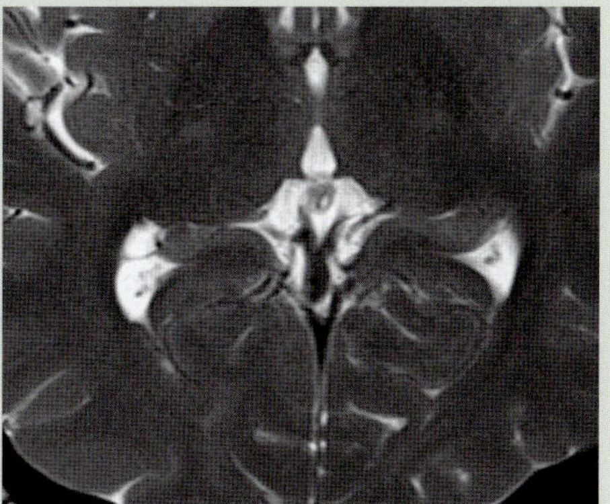 **Fig. 4.20.10:** Ependymal cyst
Hydatid cyst: Cerebral hydatid disease is a rare account for 1–2%. **Primary** hydatid cysts occur as direct invasion of larva via liver and lung to the brain, usually solitary but may be multiple. **Secondary** hydatid cysts occur as a result of rupture of primary cysts in other organs, then reaching by embolization to the brain usually multiple.	Well-defined circumscribed spherical non-enhancing intra-axial cystic lesion lies in the territory of the middle cerebral artery. Cyst fluid is isointense with CSF in all pulse sequences, no calcification or/and typically no surrounding edema. Presence of perilesional edema usually indicates complication as rupture or secondary infection. Succinate (pyruvate/malate) in 2.3 to 2.4 ppm > lactate.	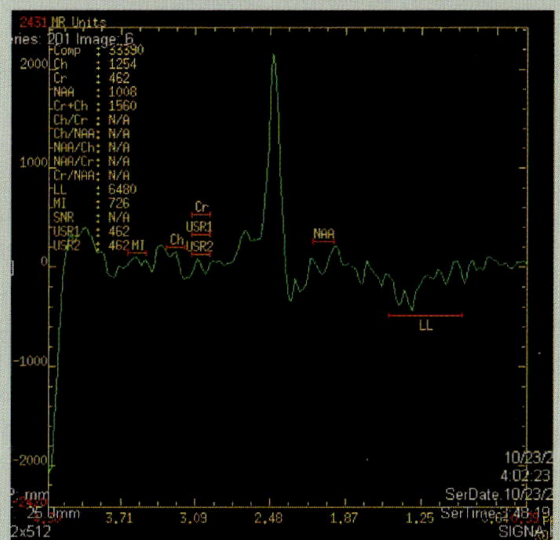 **Fig. 4.20.11:** Succinate peak in hydatid cyst

(*Contd.*)

Table 4.20.1: Differential diagnosis for intracranial cystic lesions (*Contd.*)

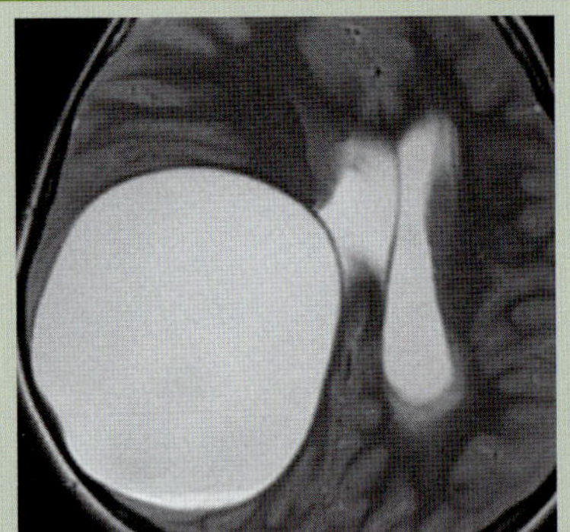 **Fig. 4.20.12:** T2 hyperintense hydatid cyst	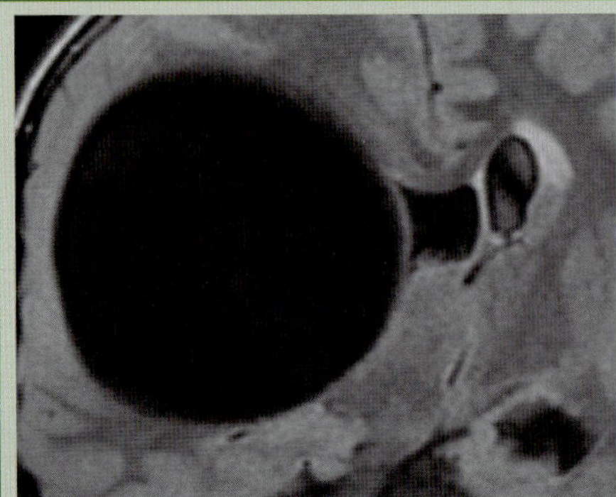 **Fig. 4.20.13:** Coronal FLAIR shows fluid suppression in hydatid cyst	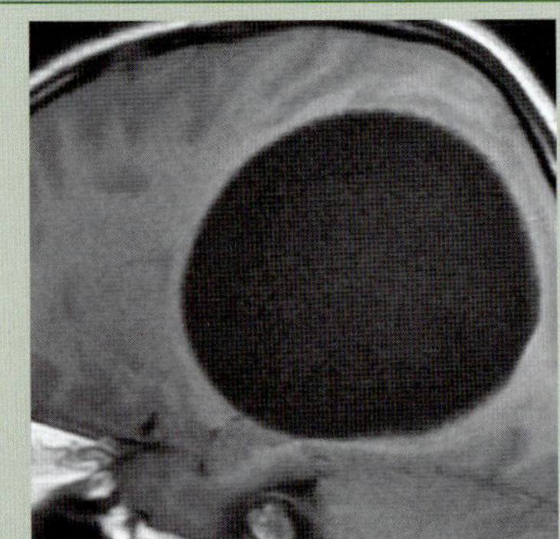 **Fig. 4.20.14:** Sagittal FLAIR shows fluid suppression in hydatid cyst
Neurocysticercosis: Succinate (pyruvate/ malate) in 2.3 to 2.4 ppm < lactate.	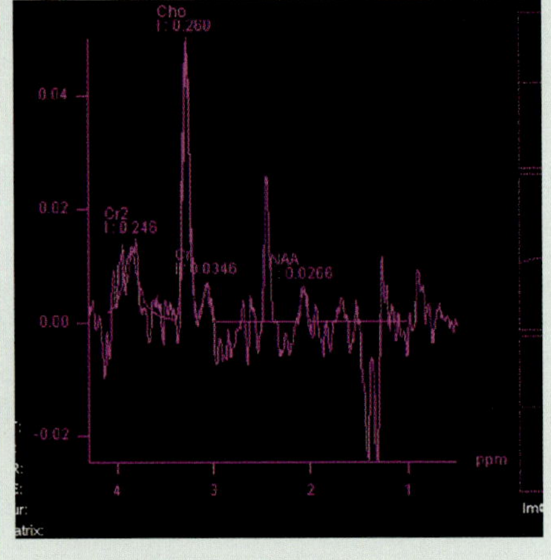 **Fig. 4.20.15:** MRS showing inverted lactated peak	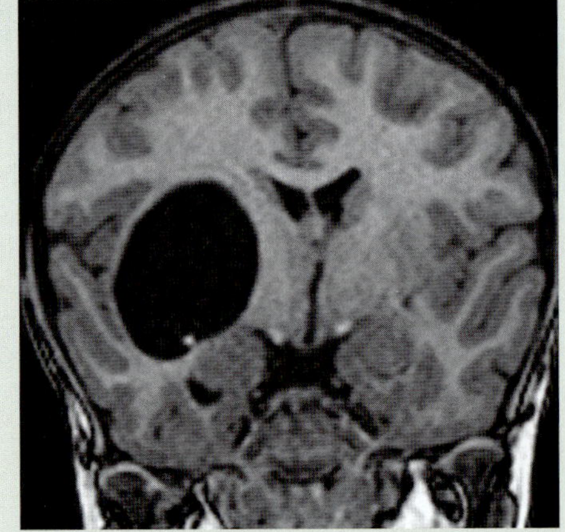 **Fig. 4.20.16:** T1 hypointense cyst with hyper-intense scolex in neurocysticercosis
Multinodular and vacuolating neuronal tumors (MVNT): Multiple bubbly T2 hyperintense cystic subcortical tumors that do not suppress on FLAIR and show no contrast enhancement. It is more common in temporal lobe and presents with seizures. **Other cystic lesions of brain include:** Cystic metastasis, necrotic tumors, abscess, T2/FLAIR mismatch tumor, DNET, connatal cyst, non-necrotic cyst of tumor, gelatinous cysts in Zellweger and cryptococcosis.		

Table 4.20.2: Analysis of intracranial cystic lesions with DTI

Fractional anisotropy (FA) and mean diffusion (MD) are two important diffusion tensor parameters, which along with other metrics measure the directional variation, and interactions between these directions provide important information about tissue connectivity. **DTI does prove useful in differentiation of intracranial cystic mass lesions.** Porencephalic cyst composed of cerebrospinal fluid (CSF) without much cellular materials, to stop the movement of water molecules which is reflected by the highest MD and **very low FA compared to all the other cysts.**	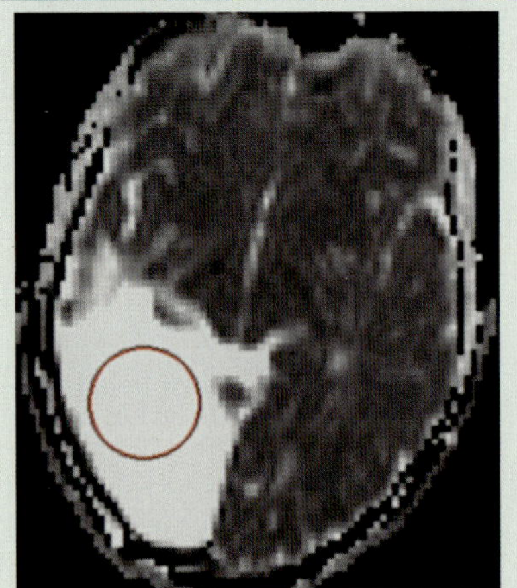 **Fig. 4.20.17:** DTI in arachnoid cyst (diffusion map)	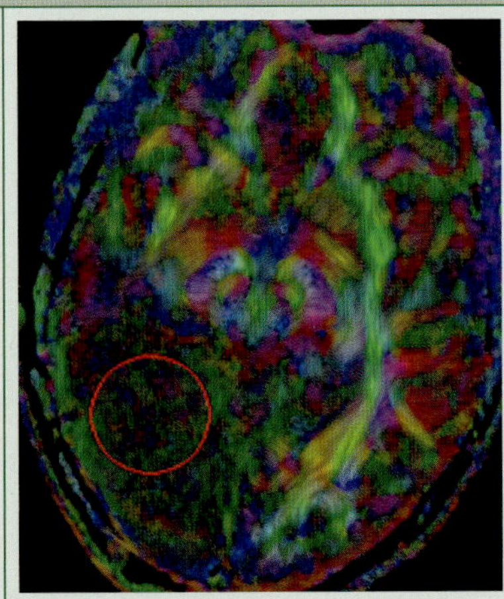 **Fig. 4.20.18:** DTI in arachnoid cyst (FA map)

Table 4.20.3: Difference between intracranial and extracranial cystic lesions				
Cystic lesions of brain	*Extra-axial*		*Intra-axial*	
	Midline	*Off midline*	*Parenchymal*	*Ventricular*
Anatomical variants	—	—	—	Cavum septi pellucidi Cavum vergae Cavum veli interpositi
Benign lesions	Pineal cyst Dermoid cyst Rathke cleft cyst Sellar, suprasellar arachnoid cyst	Arachnoid cyst Epidermoid cyst	Enlarged periventricular space, neuroglial cyst Porencephalic cyst Corpus callosum cyst (agenesis with dorsal cyst)	Choroid plexus cyst Xanthogranuloma Ependymal cyst Colloid cyst
Infectious lesions	Hydatid cyst	Neurocysticercosis	Neurocysticercosis Cystic tuberculoma Hydatid cyst Brain abscess	Neurocysticercosis
Tumoral lesions	Craniopharyngioma	Cystic meningioma Cystic schwannoma	Cystic glioblastoma Cystic metastasis Cystic lesions with mural nodule	Central neurocytoma

Approach to neurocysticercosis	*Features*	*CT*	*MRI*
Vesicular stage	Discrete, eccentrically located scolex completes the image of a parenchymal cyst.	No inflammatory response, no surrounding edema	The cyst fluid is similar to CSF in signal intensity. No contrast enhancement of the cyst wall.
Colloidal vesicular stage	Larva begins to degenerate and the scolex shows gradual shrinkage of its size. Cyst fluid becomes macroscopically turbid	Cyst fluid hyperattenuating to CSF	White matter edema, contrast enhancement +, the cyst fluid is hyperintense to CSF on T1
Granular nodular	Cyst undergoes retraction, the scolex is transformed into a coarse mineralized granule.	Surrounding edema regresses gradually	Cyst fluid is almost completely reabsorbed and the cyst seen as a nodular or a thick, small ring like enhancement
Nodular calcified stage	Shrunk to one half or one quarter of its original size and it is completely mineralized.	No surrounding edema, calcified nodule	Magnetization transfer ratio is higher in T2 hypointense lesions of cysticercus granulomas
Vesicular Fig. 4.20.19: Vesicular stage in NCC	**Colloid vesicular** Fig. 4.20.20: Colloid vesicular stage in NCC	Fig. 4.20.21: Three stages of NCC in same patient	Fig. 4.20.22: Nodular calcified stage

Virchow-Robin Space

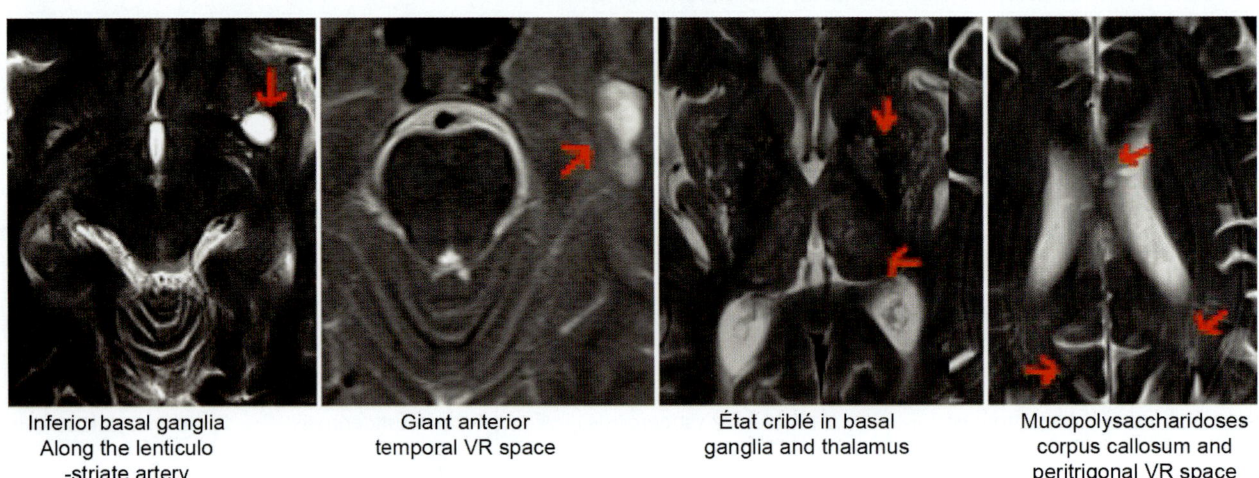

Fig. 4.20.23: Spectrum of VR spaces presentation

Treatment and prognosis: Management is essentially supportive. The extent of impairment is somewhat related to the size and location of the lesion.

The questions that may help the diagnostic approach for cystic brain lesions are:

1. Is the cyst extra-axial or intra-axial?
2. Is it supra- or infratentorial?
3. If it is extra-axial, is it midline or off-midline?
4. If it is intra-axial, is it parenchymal or intraventricular?

4.21 CENTRAL NERVOUS SYSTEM

Case No. 21

Clinical history: A 42 years old male with sudden onset headache.

Radiological techniques and observation: Figure 4.21.1 is NECT image showing a hypodense cystic lesion in the left middle cranial fossa with an imperceptible wall. The lesion displaces the adjacent temporal lobe and causes scalloping of the overlying bone. No evidence of calcifications/mural nodule. No intra- or extra-axial hemorrhage is seen. No hydrocephalus.

Figures 4.21.2 to 4.21.6 are MRI images showing that the lesion is T2 hyperintense, completely suppressed on FLAIR without diffusion restriction. T1 + contrast shows no enhancement of lesion. The lesion displaces the adjacent vessels laterally.

Interpretation: A—middle aged male with cyst in left temporal region, B—displaces the adjacent vessels laterally, C—nonenhancing T2 hyperintense cystic lesion suppressed on FLAIR without diffusion restriction, D—arachnoid cyst in left temporal region.

Principal diagnosis: Arachnoid cyst in left temporal region.

Management: 1. Endoscopic resection, 2. Open fenestration/marsupialisation, 3. Cystoperitoneal shunting with a programmed valve.

Differential diagnosis: 1. Epidermoid cyst, 2. chronic subdural haematoma, 3. porencephalic cyst, 4. dermoid cyst, 5. schizencephaly, 6. hydatid cyst, 7. neuroenteric cyst, 8. white epidermoid, 9. ecchordosis physaliphora.

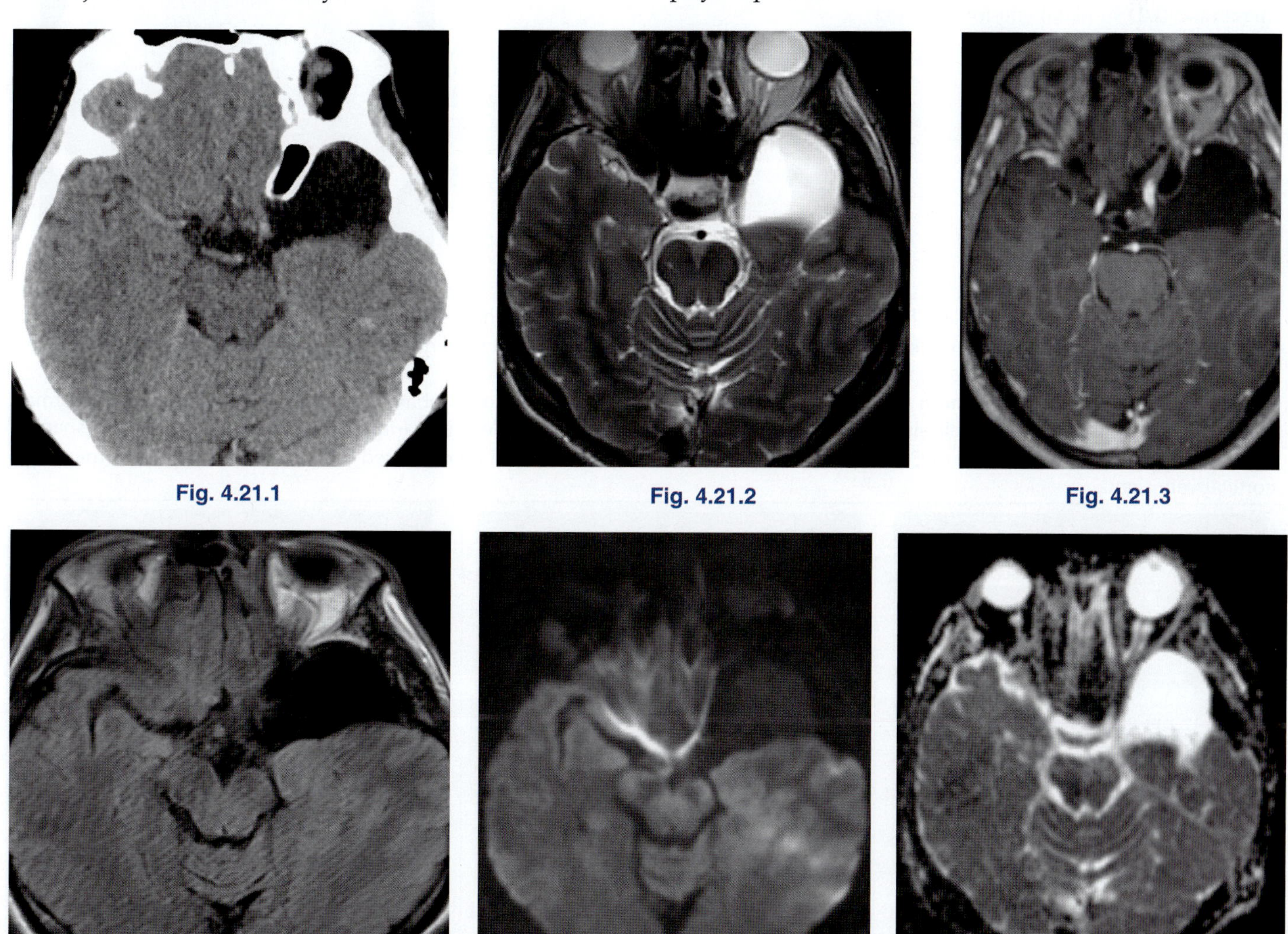

Fig. 4.21.1

Fig. 4.21.2

Fig. 4.21.3

Fig. 4.21.4

Fig. 4.21.5

Fig. 4.21.6

Table 4.21.1: Differential diagnosis for arachnoid cysts		
1. Epidermoid cyst: Also known as ectodermal inclusion cyst/intracranial epidermoid/congenital inclusion cyst. Most common symptom is headache; most common location is basal cisterns cauliflower like lobulated configuration instead of the sharply marginated borders of an arachnoid cyst. Insinuating growth pattern, extends through cistern, surrounds and **encases vessels, rather than displaces.**	The cystic lesion shows scalloped margin, Partial suppresses on FLAIR Restricted on diffusion. Iso or slightly hyperintense compared with CSF on both T1WI and T2WI.	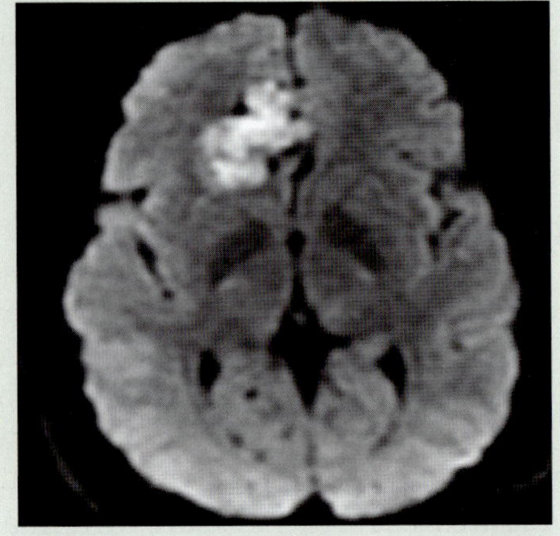 Fig. 4.21.7: Epidermoid cyst
2. Chronic subdural haematoma: Often bilateral, signal not identical to CSF, **foci of blooming on gradient** and with **enhancing membrane D/D** subdural effusion	Hypodense crescentic fluid collection seen involving the left cerebral convexity in frontoparietal region.	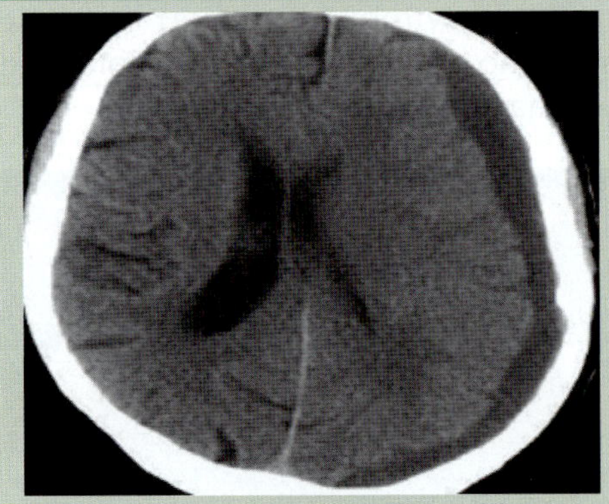 Fig. 4.21.8: Chronic subdural haematoma
Subdural effusion: Collection of clear fluid over cerebral convexities or in the interhemispheric fissure. **Subdural empyema:** Suppuration collection between dura and arachnoid mater, crescent shape, surrounding membrane enhances intensely and uniformly with diffusion restriction. **Benign enlargement of subarachnoid space in infancy:** Usually involves frontal lobe subarachnoid spaces, macrocephaly, normal ventricular size, positive cortical vein sign (cortical vein will be adjacent to inner table of calvarium, traversing the subarachnoid space). **Subdural hygroma:** Accumulation of CSF fluid in subdural space. Cortical vein will be displaced away from the inner table (negative cortical vein sign).		
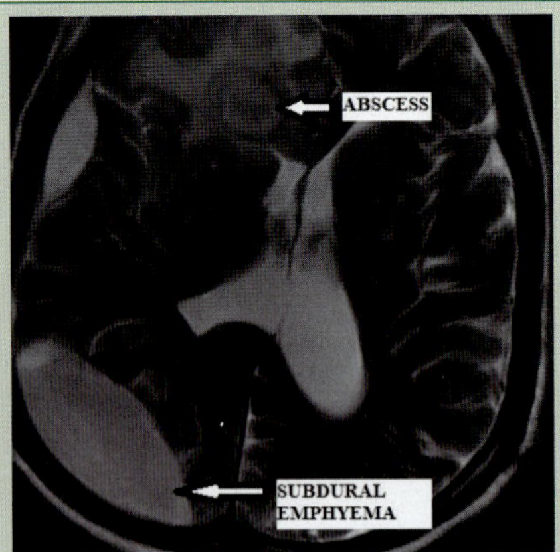 Fig. 4.21.9: Subdural emphyema and abscess	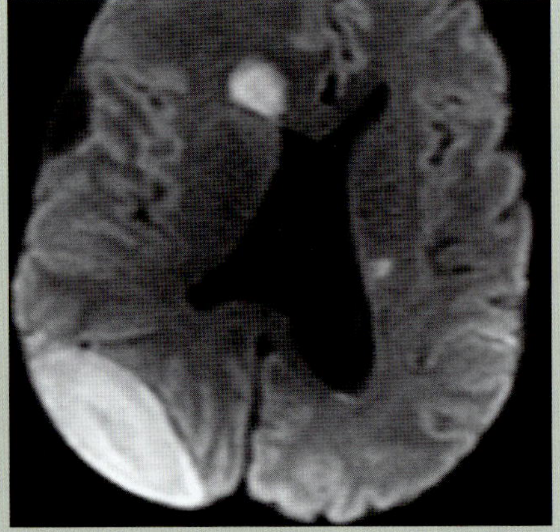 Fig. 4.21.10: DWI showing subdural emphyema and abscess	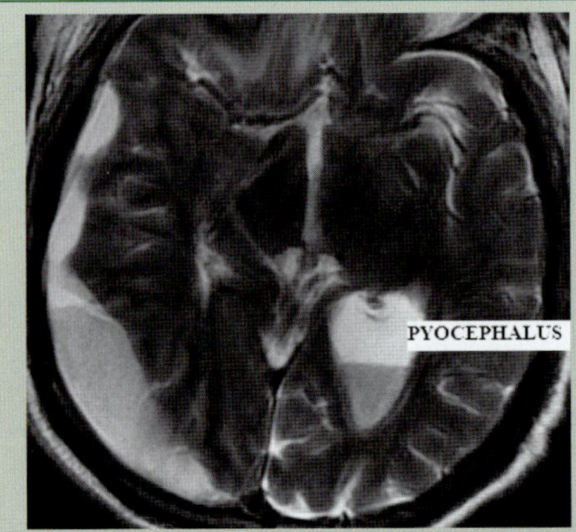 Fig. 4.21.11: Pyocephalus

(Contd.)

Table 4.21.1: Differential diagnosis for arachnoid cysts (*Contd.*)

3. Porencephalic cyst: Refer to case 20		
4. Dermoid cyst: Also known as dermoid inclusion cyst/ectopic squamous epithelial cyst containing dermal elements including hair follicles, sebaceous and sweat glands. Fat suppression sequence confirm the diagnosis.	Usually in midline. Heterogeneous intense lesion seen involving the left inferior frontal region. Confirmed by fat suppressed T1WI sequence	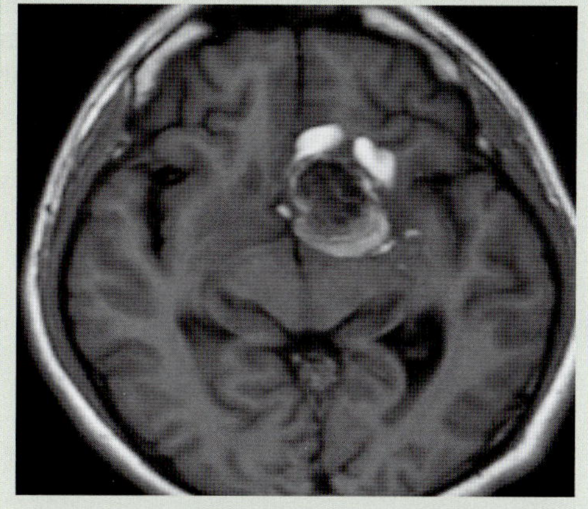 **Fig. 4.21.12:** Dermoid cyst
5. Schizencephaly: Refer to case 3		
6. Hydatid cyst: Parasitic infection caused by echinococcus tapeworms, echinococcus granulosis and echinococcus multilocularis. **Refer to case 20**	CISS image shows well-delineated cyst with detached germinal membrane seen in left cerebellopontine region. Intracystic daughter cyst seen. The cyst fluid is isointense with CSF on T1WI and T2WI.	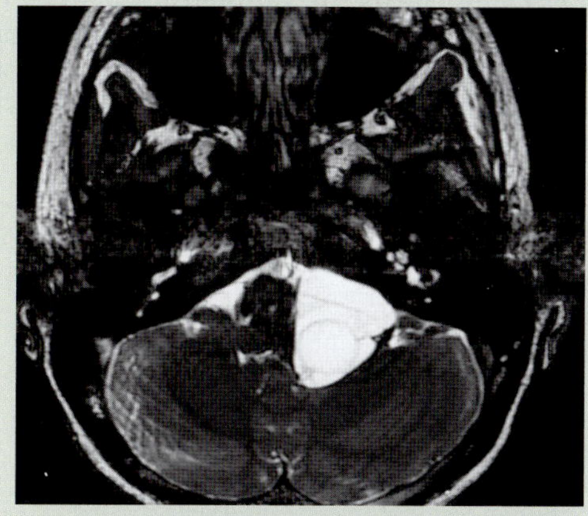 **Fig. 4.21.13:** Hydatid cyst
7. White epidermoid: See section below on prepontine cystic lesions		
8. Neurenteric cyst: Extra-axial cyst. Most commonly occur in posterior fossa, midline or off midline, just anterior to the pontomedullary junction. Age distribution is bimodal large peak in third and fourth decades and smaller peak in first decade. Slightly males more common than females.	MRI image shows cyst seen in anterior to pontomedullary junction, absent diffusion restriction. Hyperintense compared to CSF on T1WI, hyperintense to CSF on T2WI. Not suppress on FLAIR. No calcification, no haemorrhage, no enhancement on contrast. On MRS elevated NAA seen.	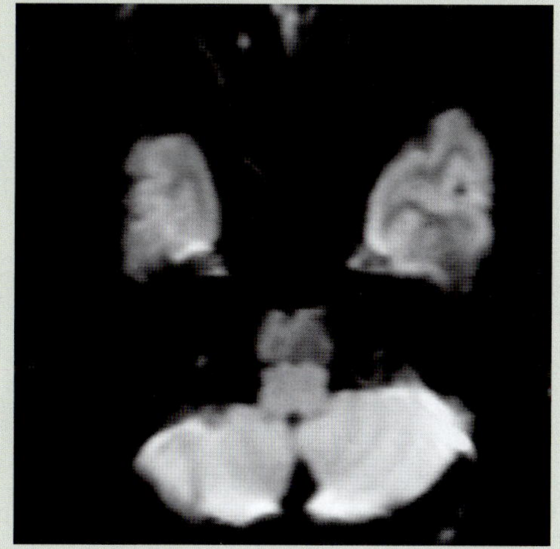 **Fig. 4.21.14:** Neurenteric cyst

(*Contd.*)

Table 4.21.1: Differential diagnosis for arachnoid cysts (*Contd.*)

9. Intraventricular neurocysticercosis: Neurocysticercosis caused by encysted larvae of pork tapeworm *Taenia solium*. Most common locations are CNS, eyes, muscle and subcutaneous tissue.	T1 contrast MRI shows ring enhancing lesion in temporal horn of left lateral ventricle/grape-like clusters of cysts lacking identifiable scolex, + hydrocephalus	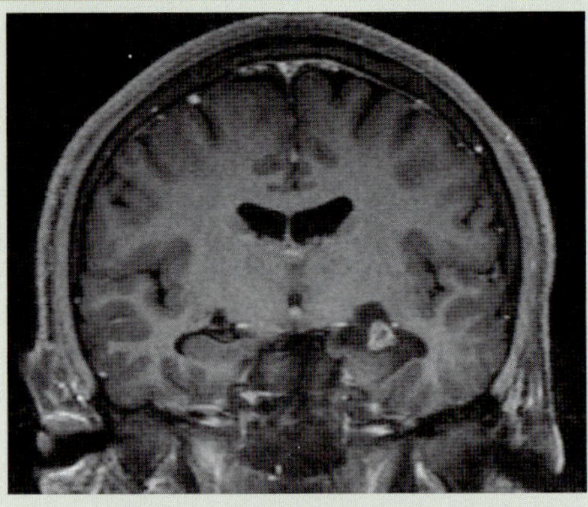 **Fig. 4.21.15:** Intraventricular neurocysticercosis
10. Cystic neoplasm like craniopharyngioma and other suprasellar cystic lesions Refer to case 14		
11. Ecchordosis physaliphora: Small <1 cm gelatinous soft tissue mass. Ectopic notochord remnant. Occur anywhere along the midline craniospinal axis from the dorsum sellae to the sacrococcygeal region. 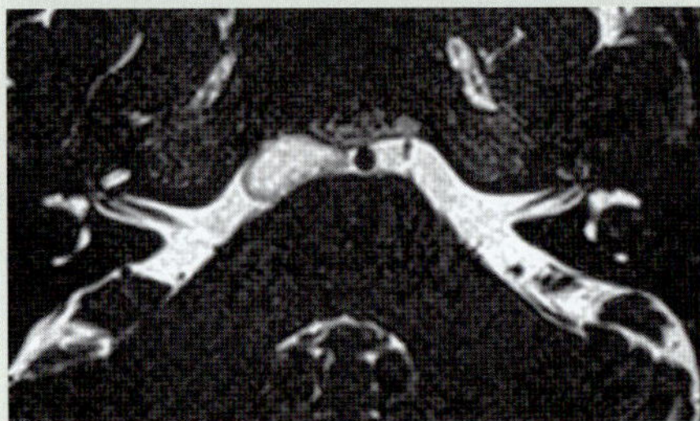 **Fig. 4.21.16:** Ecchordosis physaliphora	CT shows well-delineated hypodense, nonenhancing midline mass scalloped sclerotic margins. Presence of small stalk or pedicle that connects the clival lesion to an intradural component in prepontine cistern. The mass hypointense to brain on T1WI and hyperintense to CSF on T2WI. No enhancement, follow-up study shows no change in lesion size. 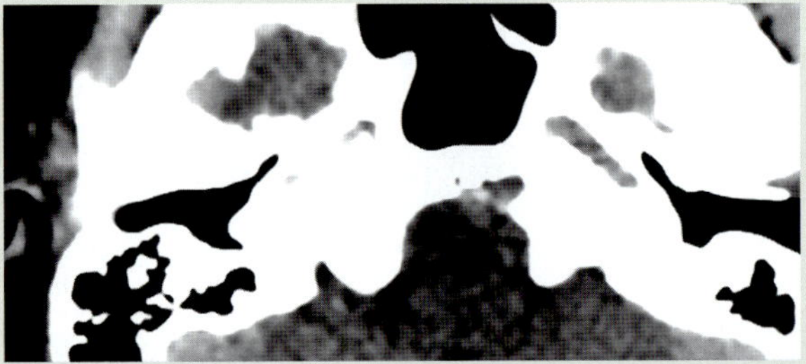 **Fig. 4.21.17:** Ecchordosis physaliphora	
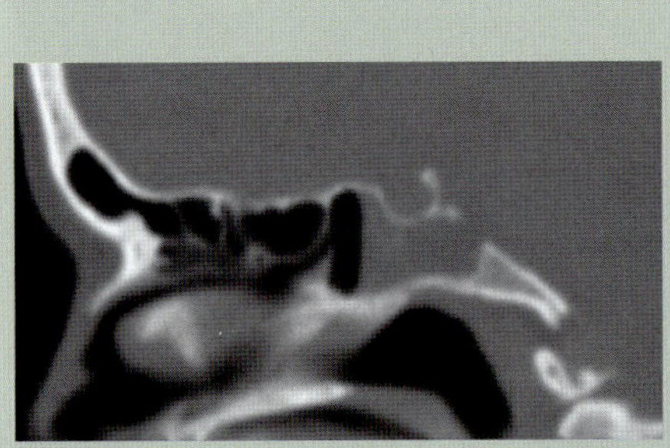 **Fig. 4.21.18:** Ecchordosis physaliphora	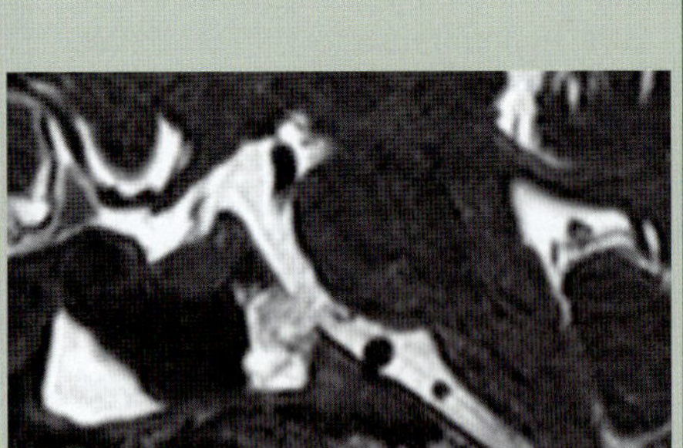 **Fig. 4.21.19:** Ecchordosis physaliphora	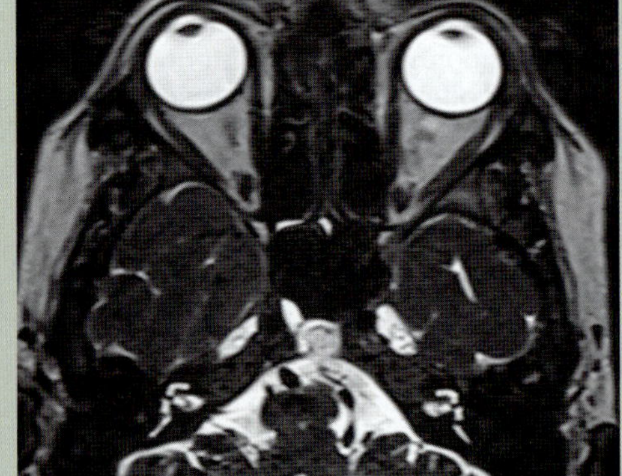 **Fig. 4.21.20:** Ecchordosis physaliphora
Other rare differential diagnosis includes non-neoplastic tumor associated cysts, choroid fissure cyst and hippocampal sulcal remnants.		
Differential diagnosis of prepontine cystic lesions: White epidermoid, neuroenteric cyst, arachnoid cyst, ecchordosis physaliphora.		
White epidermoid cyst: Rare type of epidermoid cyst that does not follow the usual near CSF density. High T1 signal on MRI due to high triglyceride and unsaturated fatty acid content. Seen in anterior to pontomedullary junction. Hypointense on T2WI, do not suppress on FLAIR, restrict on diffusion, no enhancement, no haemorrhage, calcification seen in 10–25% of cases.		

(Contd.)

Table 4.21.1: Differential diagnosis for arachnoid cysts *(Contd.)*		
DD: Intraventricular cyst is trapped fourth ventricle, choroid plexus cyst, colloid cyst, choroidal fissure cyst and ependymal cyst.		
Preponting white epidermoid: Hyperdense mass, which is T1 hyperintense in prepontine region.		
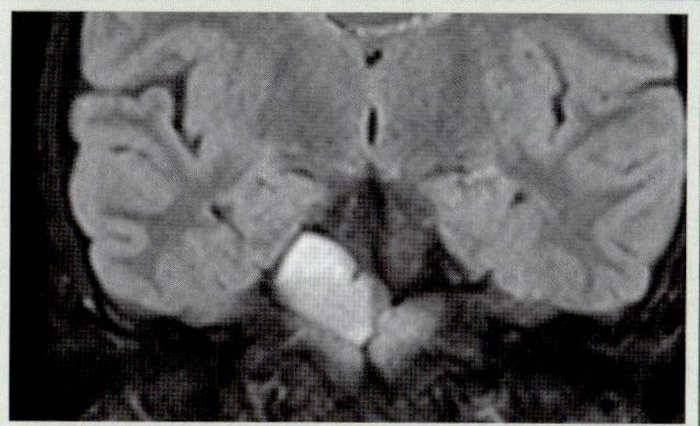 **Fig. 4.21.21:** Prepontine white epidermoid	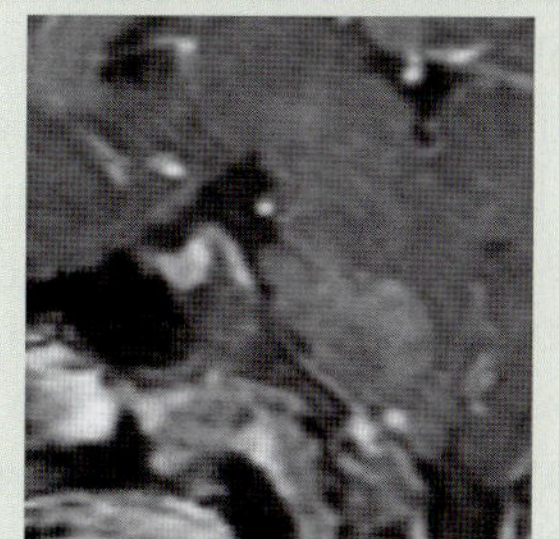 **Fig. 4.21.22:** Prepontine white epidermoid	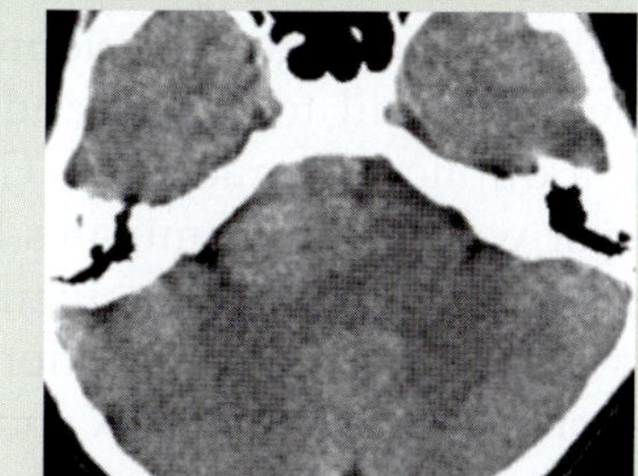 **Fig. 4.21.23:** Prepontine white epidermoid
Prepontine epidermoid		
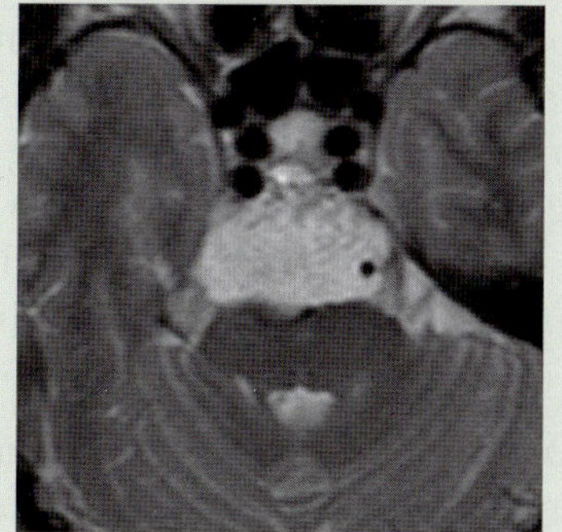 **Fig. 4.21.24:** Prepontine epidermoid	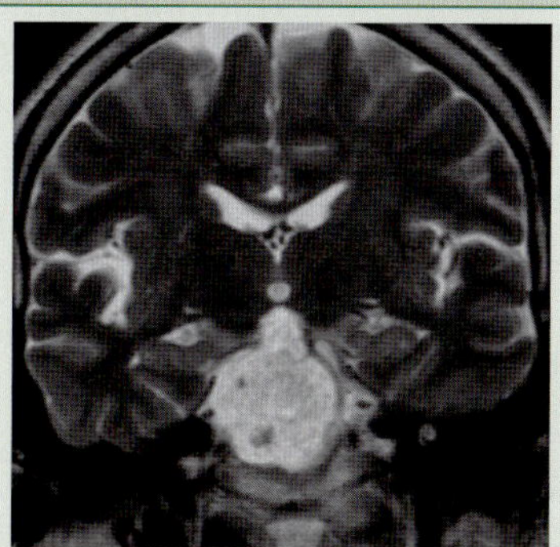 **Fig. 4.21.25:** Prepontine epidermoid	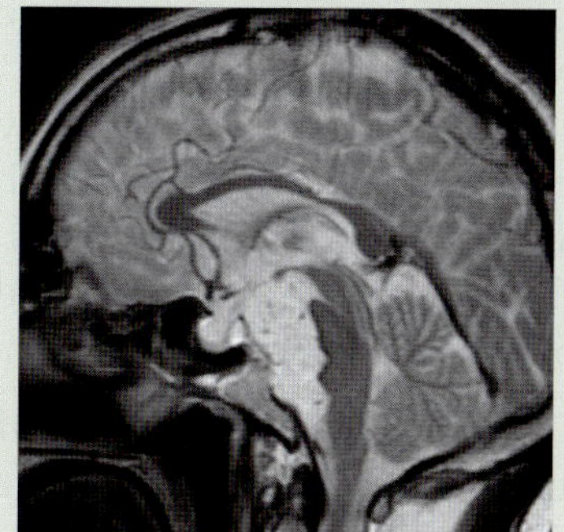 **Fig. 4.21.26:** Prepontine epidermoid
Prepontine neurenteric cyst		
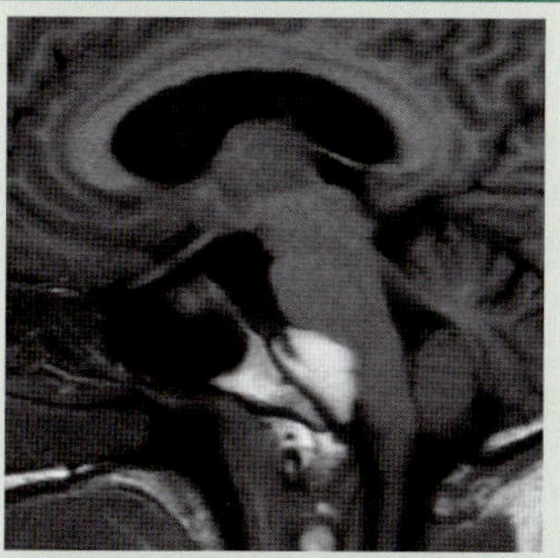 **Fig. 4.21.27:** Prepontine neurenteric cyst	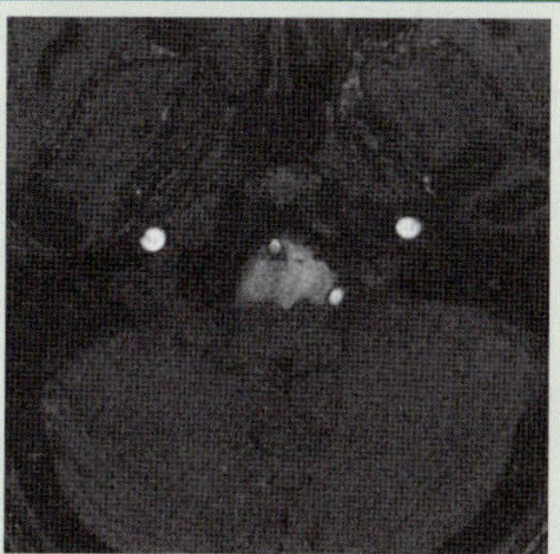 **Fig. 4.21.28:** Prepontine neurenteric cyst	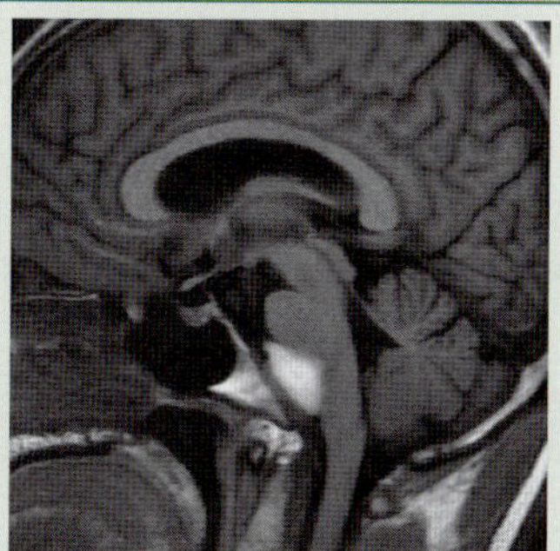 **Fig. 4.21.29:** Prepontine neurenteric cyst
Prepontine hydatid		
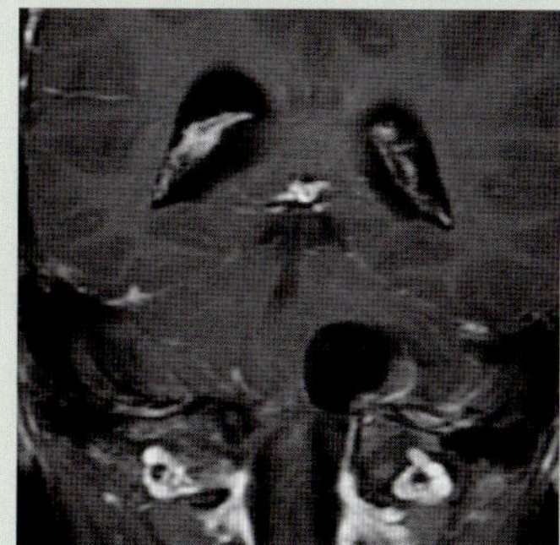 **Fig. 4.21.30:** Cerebellopontine angle hydatid	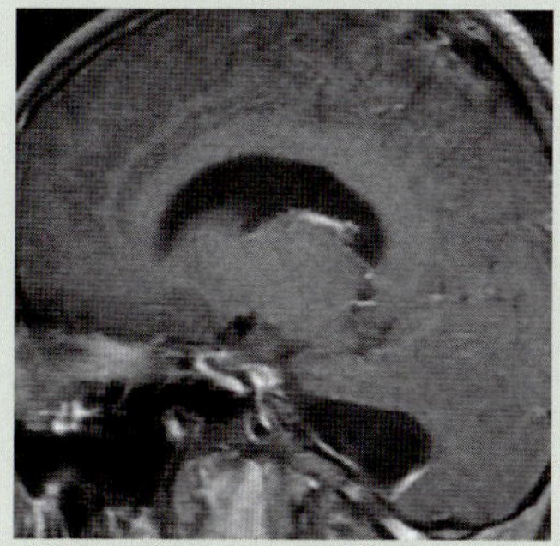 **Fig. 4.21.31:** Cerebellopontine angle hydatid	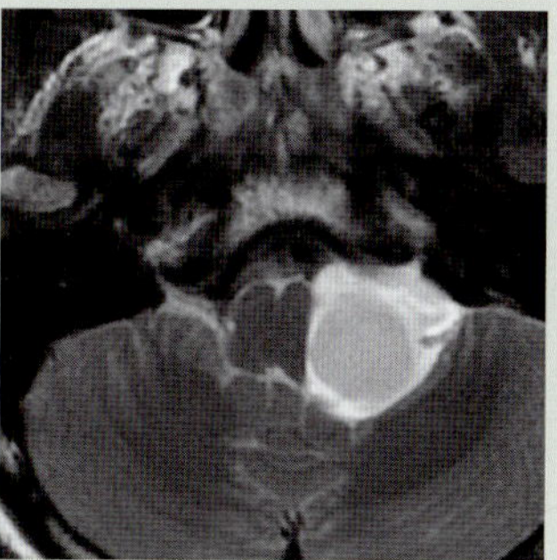 **Fig. 4.21.32:** Cerebellopontine angle hydatid

Discussion: **Arachnoid cyst:** Also called meningeal cyst. Intracranial CSF filled cyst that does not communicate with ventricular system, most common location is middle cranial fossa. The vast majority of arachnoid cyst arise as anomalies of meningeal development. The embryonic endo meninges fail to merge and remain separated, forming a duplicated arachnoid. CSF secreted by cells in the cyst wall and accumulates between the layers. Less commonly, arachnoid loculations are acquired as a result of haemorrhage, infection or surgery. Extra-axial lesion displaces the cortex and buckles gray white interface. Arachnoid cysts can be found at any age. 75% in children (symptom onset, if any, may be delayed), males are more affected, especially middle cranial fossa. Asymptomatic usually, symptoms depend upon size and location of cyst. Associated syndromes include Aicardi, acrocallosal and Pallister-Hall syndrome, associated abnormalities are temporal lobe hypoplasia, subdural haematoma. Periventricular giant arachnoid cyst may cause hydrocephalus and associated with foramen of Monro stenosis and aqueduct stenosis/occlusion.

Imaging findings: Usually CSF density on plain CT, does not enhance on contrast, in MRI sharply marginated extra-axial fluid collection isointense with CSF, completely suppress on FLAIR, no restriction on diffusion. MRA shows cortical vessels displaced away from the calvaria. Phase contrast cine MR shows flow quantification can help distinguish arachnoid cyst from enlarged subarachnoid space. Arachnoid cyst is variable types, **communicating type and noncommunicating type**. In communicating ball valve type CSF accumulates by **one-way (ball valve) flow**. Cyst arises from Liliequist membrane not communicate with subarachnoid space; it is a noncommunicating type of arachnoid cyst. Cystic dilation of interpeduncular cistern called communicating type of arachnoid cyst. CT cisternography demonstrates communication of cyst with the subarachnoid space.

CISS and FIESTA sequence help to delineate cyst wall and adjacent anatomic structure. CSF flow imaging such as 2D cine PC may demonstrate communication between cyst and adjacent arachnoid space. Patients with completely communicating arachnoid cyst may not need surgical intervention.

Treatment usually none—majority of ACs are found incidentally. Indication for surgery: 1. Symptomatic arachnoid cyst, 2. Large arachnoid cyst causing compressive symptoms, 3. Periventricular giant arachnoid cyst causing hydrocephalus. Surgeries are: 1. Resection (may be endoscopic), 2. Fenestration/marsupialization, 3. Shunt (cystoperitoneal is common option).

Galassi classification for middle cranial fossa arachnoid cysts: Increases with increase in size/mass effect and decrease in communication with basal cisterns.

Type A: Small, spindle-shaped; limited to anterior MCF.

Type B: Superiorly extent along sylvian fissure; temporal lobe displaced.

Type C: Huge, fills entire MCF; frontal/temporal/parietal lobe displacement.

Table 4.21.2: Difference between arachnoid cyst and epidermoid cyst

Features	*Arachnoid cyst*	*Epidermoid cyst*
Signal intensity	Isointense to CSF on T1W Isointense to CSF on PDW Isointense to CSF on T2W	Mildly hyperintense to CSF on T1W Hyperintense to CSF on PDW Isointense to CSF on T2W
Enhancement	No	Usually non-margin of cyst may show enhancement (25%)
Margin of lesion	Smooth	Irregular
Effect on adjacent structure	Displaces	Engulfs, insinuates
Pulsation artefact	Present	Absent
DWI	Follows CSF	Restricted diffusion
FLAIR	Suppress like CSF	Not completely suppressed
Calcification	No	May occur
MRS	Lactate peak seen—not specific	Lactate peak. No NAA/choline/lipid

(Contd.)

Table 4.21.2: Difference between arachnoid cyst and epidermoid cyst (*Contd.*)

Features	*Arachnoid cyst*	*Epidermoid cyst*

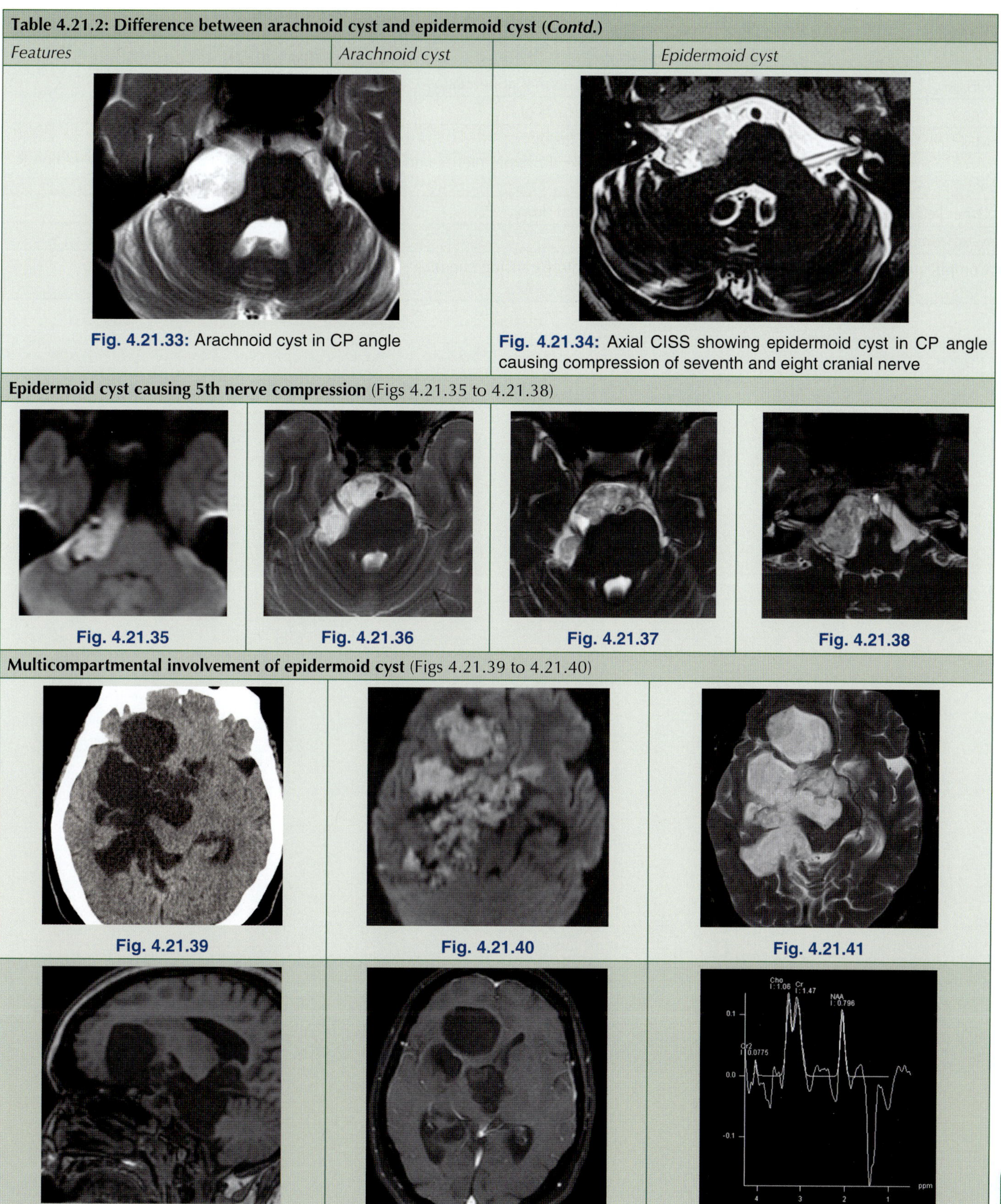

Fig. 4.21.33: Arachnoid cyst in CP angle

Fig. 4.21.34: Axial CISS showing epidermoid cyst in CP angle causing compression of seventh and eight cranial nerve

Epidermoid cyst causing 5th nerve compression (Figs 4.21.35 to 4.21.38)

Fig. 4.21.35 **Fig. 4.21.36** **Fig. 4.21.37** **Fig. 4.21.38**

Multicompartmental involvement of epidermoid cyst (Figs 4.21.39 to 4.21.40)

Fig. 4.21.39 **Fig. 4.21.40** **Fig. 4.21.41**

Fig. 4.21.42 **Fig. 4.21.43** **Fig. 4.21.44**

Table 4.21.3: Difference between dermoid cyst and epidermoid cyst		
	Dermoid cyst	*Epidermoid cyst*
Origin	Epidermal and dermal appendages	Epidermal appendages
Age	1st and 2nd decade of life	5th decade of life
MRI	Fat containing lesion T1 hyperintense, T2 hyperintense and FLAIR hyperintense	CSF like. T1 hypointense, T2 hyperintense and FLAIR hyperintense
Other sequences	T1 fat sat—signal drop	Diffusion restriction
Most common location	Suprasellar	CP angle cistern
Complications	Commonly rupture causing chemical meningitis	—

4.22 CENTRAL NERVOUS SYSTEM

Case No. 22

Clinical history: A 48-year-old male patient came with complaints of headache. Ocular examination was normal.

Radiological techniques and observation: Plain CT of brain in bone window, axial and coronal views (Figs 4.22.1 and 4.22.2) show an ill-defined midline expansile lytic lesion of the clivus and the basi-sphenoid with soft tissue component with a few areas of speckled calcification. Erosion of the petrous part of the temporal bone noted. No evidence of extension into the sphenoid sinus/internal auditory canal/carotid canal/bilateral pterygoid plates. Remaining bone appears sclerotic. Adjacent brain parenchyma appears normal.

Plain MRI brain T2 and T1 in sagittal view and T1 postcontrast in coronal view (Figs 4.22.3 to 4.22.5) show a well-defined T2 heterointense predominantly hyperintense and T1 hypointense lesion with heterogeneous contrast enhancement on T1 postcontrast image involving the clivus and no evidence of extension of lesion into the adjacent brain parenchyma. Optic tract appears normal. The visualized cervical spine appears normal. No evidence of extension of lesion into the sphenoid sinus. Pituitary gland visualized separately. The nasopharyngeal mucosa appears intact. Visualized brain stem appears normal.

Interpretation: A–48 years old male, clivus, C—ill-defined T2 hyperintense and T1 hypointense lytic heterogeneous enhancing lesion, B—midline expansile lesion with intact cortex and intratumoral calcification, D—clival chordoma.

Principal diagnosis: Clival chordoma.

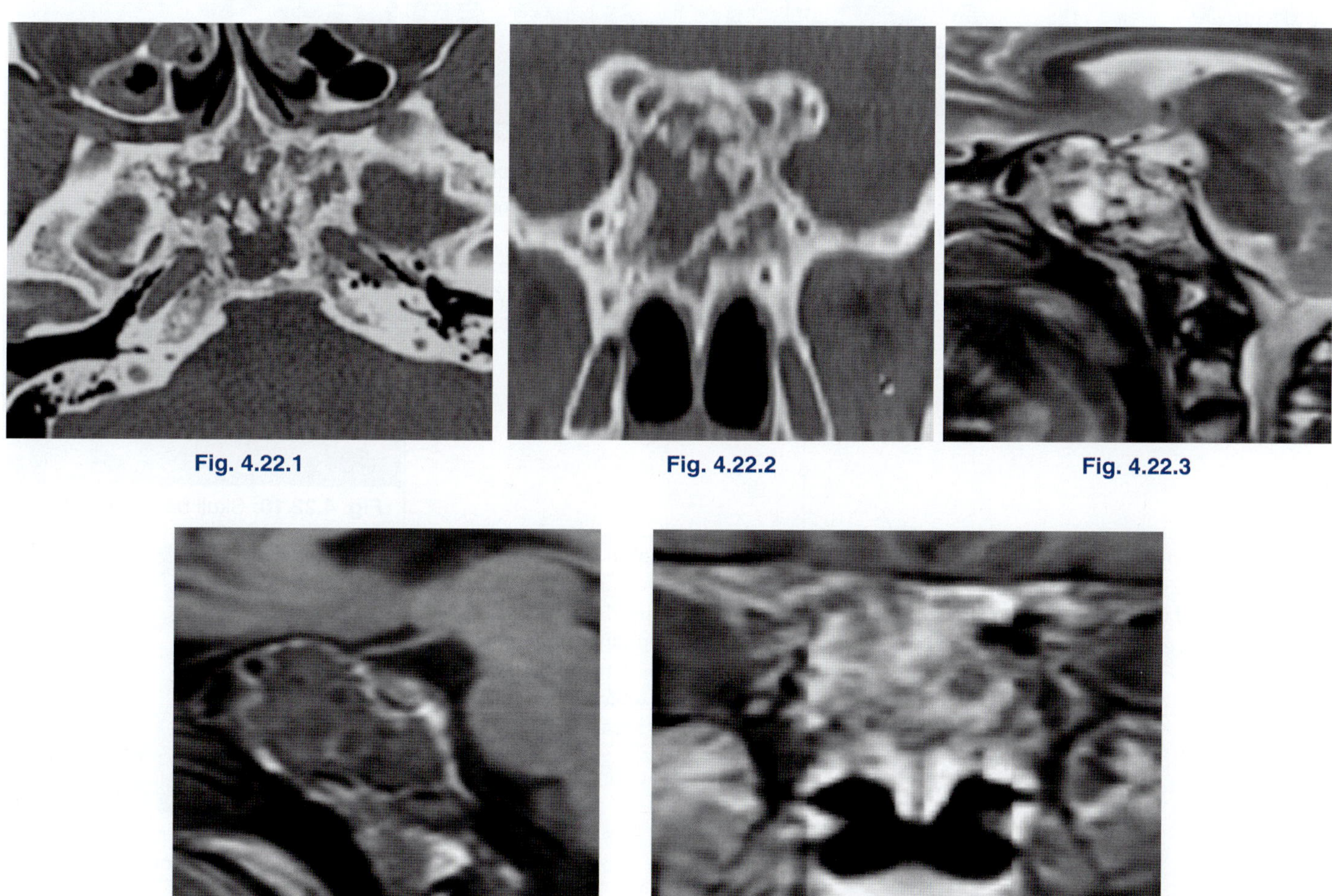

Fig. 4.22.1 Fig. 4.22.2 Fig. 4.22.3

Fig. 4.22.4 Fig. 4.22.5

Table 4.22.1: Differential diagnosis of skull base lesions

Skull base osteomyelitis: Refer to case 71 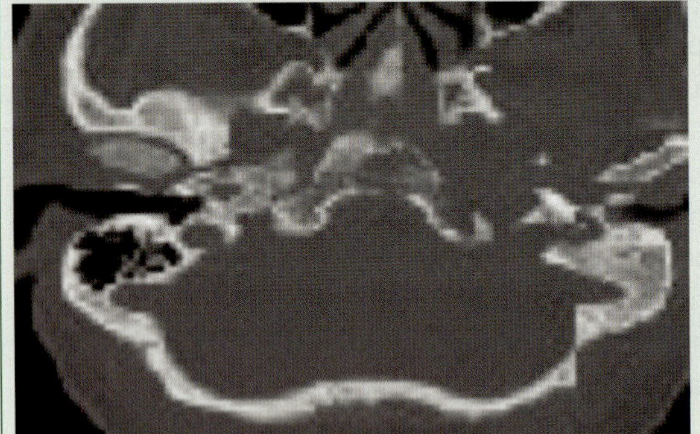 **Fig. 4.22.6:** Skull base osteomyelitis	Common presentation in elderly diabetics and immuno-compromised. Associated with middle ear infection (malignant otitis externa), retropharyngeal abscess. Presents with ear pain, ear discharge and rarely cranial neuropathies. Lysis of the skull base involving the clivus, petrous apex, sphenoid processes associated with soft tissue opacification in the middle ear. **MRI: T1 hypo- and STIR/T2 hyperintensities** with surrounding extensive edema noted. **Postcontrast MRI** shows heterogeneous enhancement.	
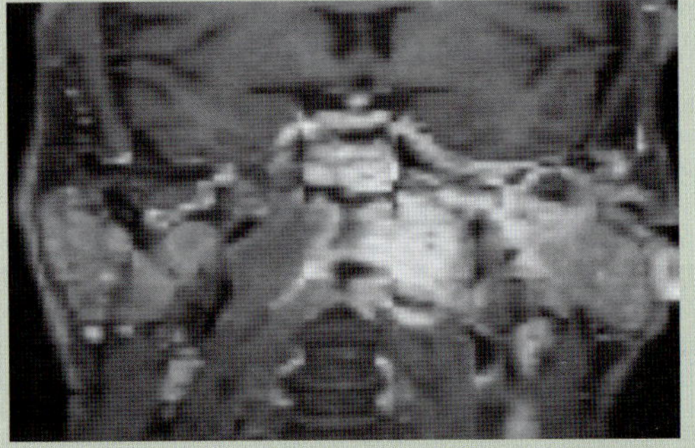 **Fig. 4.22.7:** Skull base osteomyelitis	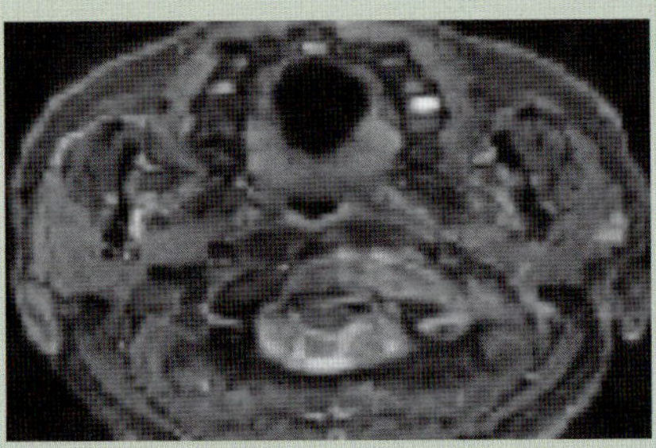 **Fig. 4.22.8:** Skull base osteomyelitis	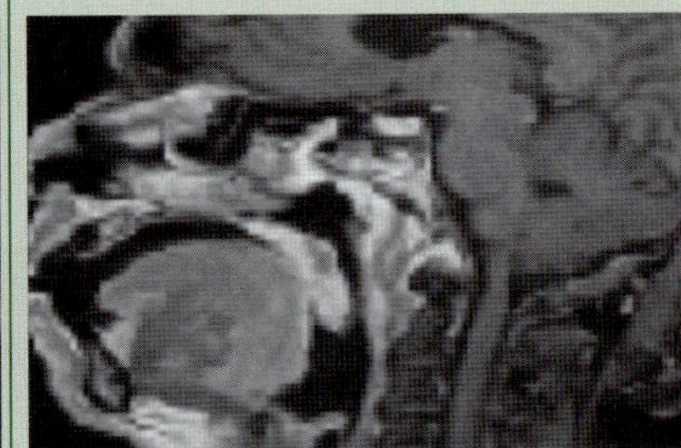 **Fig. 4.22.9:** Skull base osteomyelitis
Skull base metastasis Age >50 years with a known primary of **breast, lung** and **prostate,** or an unknown primary. Presents with complaints of mass effect on the adjacent brain stem structures.	**CT:** Destructive mass centered in the bone with no sclerotic rim. **T1** hypointense (lytic Mets) that shows variable intensity on **T2**, with + diffusion restriction and heterogeneous enhancement **postcontrast**.	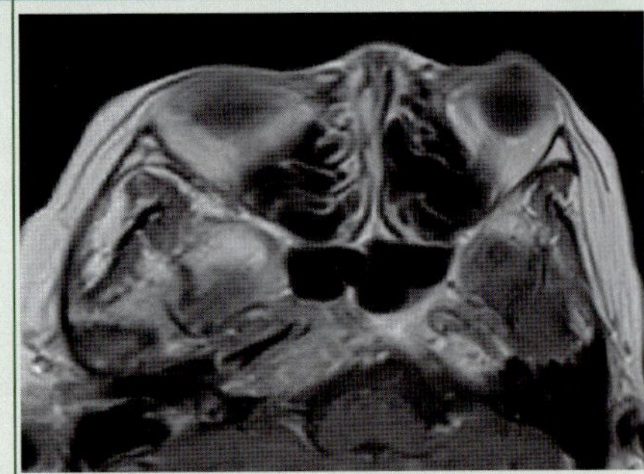 **Fig. 4.22.10:** Skull base metastasis
Solitary bone plasmacytoma Most common sites **vertebra** (thoracic > lumbar> cervical), **skull** (any bone) and **pelvis**. Usually involves the red marrow of the bone.	**X-ray**—geographic lytic lesion without any specific matrix. **CT**—well-defined soft tissue dense lesion which enhances on contrast. **MRI**—T1 hypointense, T2 intermediate intense lesion which shows enhancement on postcontrast.	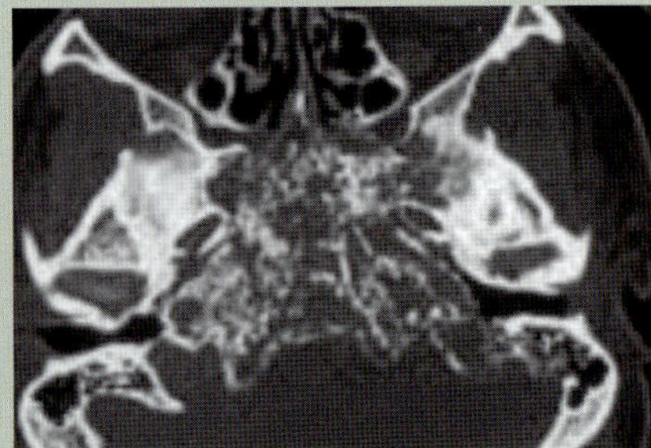 **Fig. 4.22.11:** Solitary bone plasmacytoma
Invasive pituitary macroadenoma/pituitary carcinoma: Refer to case 15		

Contd...

<table>
<tr><th colspan="3">Table 4.22.1: Differential diagnosis of skull base lesions (Contd...)</th></tr>
<tr><td>Skull base chondrosarcoma
<7% of all chondrosarcomas.
Presents with mass effect over the adjacent brain, brain stem and cranial nerves
Most common site—petro-occipital synchondrosis followed by sphenoethmoidal junction 82% of chondrosarcomas are off midline when compared to midline chordomas.</td><td>X-ray—well-defined lytic lesion with foci of calcification in the petro-occipital synchondrosis (off midline).
CT—expansile off midline lytic lesion with ring and arc calcification in the typical location.
MRI—T1 hypo, T2-hyperintense lesion with heterogenous enhancement.</td><td>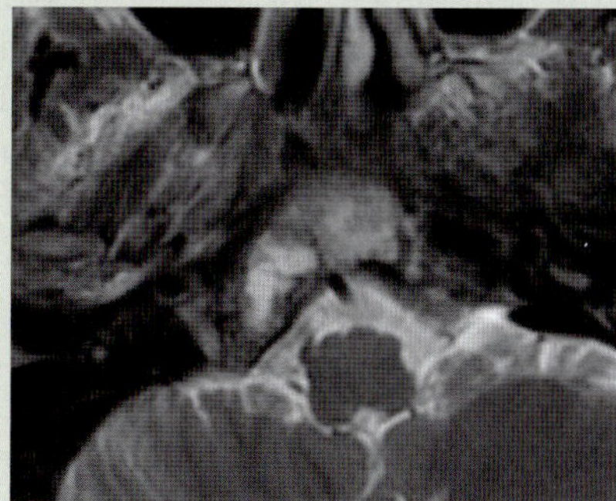
Fig. 4.22.12: Skull base chondrosarcoma</td></tr>
<tr><td>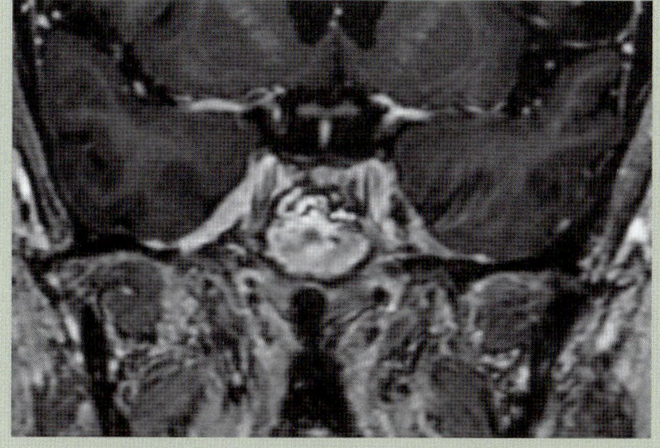
Fig. 4.22.13: Clival lymphoma</td><td>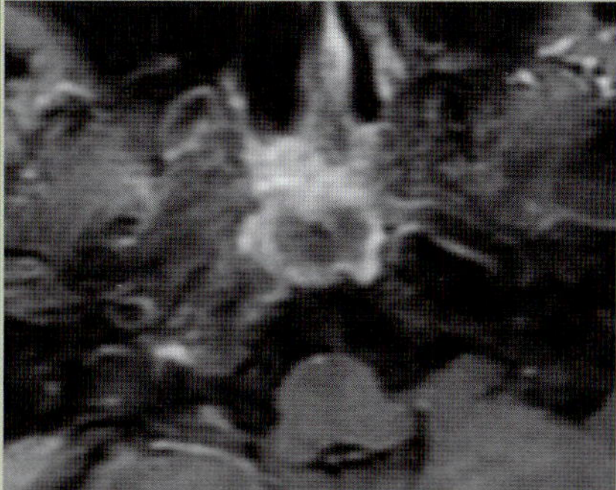
Fig. 4.22.14: Lymphoma involving clivus</td><td>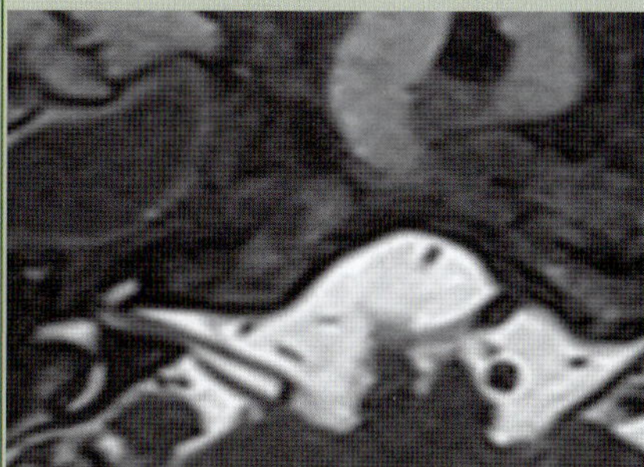
Fig. 4.22.15: Osteomyelitis involving clivus</td></tr>
<tr><td colspan="3">Other lesions include: Lymphoma, skull base GCT, meningioma, rhabdomyosarcoma, ecchordosis physaliphora, fossa navicularis magna, IgG4 disease, nasopharyngeal carcinoma infiltration.</td></tr>
</table>

Table 4.22.2: Differential diagnosis for T2 very hyperintense lesions in body and common skull base tumors in adults

T2 very hyperintense lesions in body	*Common skull base tumors in adults*
Hemangioma	Chondroma
Fluid-cyst, necrosis, abscess	Metastasis
Chondroid matrix—chordoma, chondrosarcoma	Paraganglioma
Plexiform neurofibroma, myxoma, pheochromocytoma	Chondrosarcoma
Medullary CA of thyroid and breast	Myeloma
Pleomorphic adenoma	Esthesioneuroblastoma
	Lymphoma
	Sinonasal carcinoma

Management: Complete surgical excision is difficult and hence **irradiation/trans sphenoidal surgical removal** of the tumor is the treatment of choice.

Differential diagnosis: 1. Skull base chondrosarcoma (**off midline** lesion in the sphenopetrous suture), 2. skull base osteomyelitis, 3. metastasis, 4. pituitary macro-adenoma eroding clivus, 5. contiguous spread of nasopharyngeal carcinoma.

Discussion: **Chordoma**, a rare primary malignant tumor, arising from the remnants of the notochord. More common 40–70 years, M: F = 1.8:1. It arises in the midline structures, most common being the sacrococcygeal chordoma.

Sacrococcygeal chordoma (50%): Predominantly lower segments, (S4–S5), initially asymptomatic, later, as the tumor size increases, localized pain with pressure symptoms from the bladder and rectum are common.

Basisphenoid-basioccipital chordoma (35%) presents with headaches, for years. Pressure from the enlarging midline mass may create ocular disturbances, increased intracranial pressure, ataxia, deafness, and tinnitus.

Vertebral chordoma (15%) involves anterior vertebral body sparing posterior elements and dura. In the cervical spine chordoma, dysphagia is a common presenting symptom, most commonly involves the C2 vertebrae. Sensory complaints include numbness in an arm or leg, usually followed by pain. Motor weakness may occur, with vertebral body collapse, creating paraplegia or quadriplegia as a late complication.

X-ray: Well-defined **expansile lytic** lesion with **scalloped margins**, narrow zone of transition, areas of **flocculant calcification**, soft tissue component noted without a cortical break.

MRI: The lesion appears **very hyperintense on T2** with loss of normal hypointensity in T1, on contrast, there is inhomogeneous moderate enhancement. **Thumbing of the pons sign**—thickening of pons will be seen in clival chordoma. Low ADC values $1474 +/- 117 \times 10^{-6}$ mm^2/s—less than chondrosarcoma ($2051 +/- 261 \times 10^{-6}$ mm^2/s).

Treatment: The treatment of **intracranial chordomas** is quite discouraging because the operative mortality rate is high and complete resection is rarely attainable. The same is also true for the vertebral body lesions. Irradiation has been the most commonly employed treatment for clivus and vertebral body lesions; however, recently **proton beam irradiation** has shown to improve the prognostic outcome of any lesion that has undergone incomplete resection. **Low sacrococcygeal lesions** are resected while the lesions above S2 are partially resected due to increased risk of denervation of anorectal and urogenital structures. This leads to increased risk of recurrence.

4.23 CENTRAL NERVOUS SYSTEM

Case No. 23

Clinical history: A 50 years old female presented with swelling over left side of scalp for 7 years, insidious in onset and slowly progressive. Giddiness and headache for 3 years on and off.

Radiological techniques and observation

Skull PA view: Ill-defined lytic lesion in the squamous part of left temporal and parietal bone with suspicious areas of cortical break and soft tissue thickening involving the adjacent scalp (Fig. 4.23.1).

Lateral view: Well-defined lytic lesion in the region of left temporal and parietal bone with well-delineated borders. The lesion shows irregular sclerotic border in its anterosuperior border. No specific matrix/intralesional calcification seen. No spiculations seen. Edges are not bevelled. There is narrow zone of transition. No evidence of periosteal reaction. No lesions elsewhere in the skull and visualized bones (Fig. 4.23.2).

Differential diagnosis: For solitary large lytic lesion in the skull in adult.

Metastases—breast/lung/thyroid/kidney etc., osteoporosis circumscripta, plasmacytoma, epidermoid, hemangioma, osteomyelitis, intraosseous meningioma, hemangiopericytoma, GCT, lymphoma.

CT scan in bone window (Figs 4.23.3 to 4.23.6): Expansile lytic lesion noted in the squamous part of left temporal bone with narrow zone of transition with cortical break

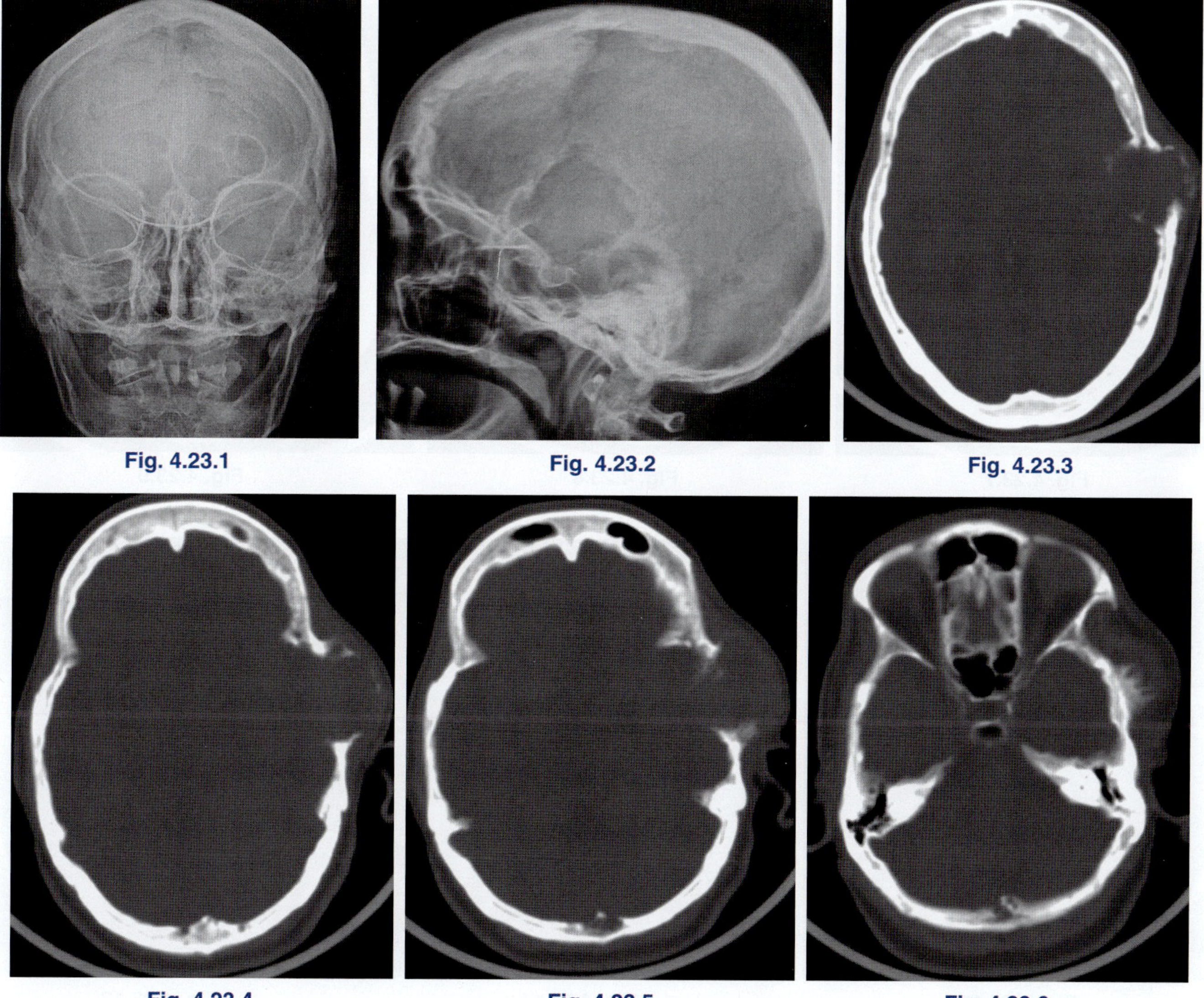

Fig. 4.23.1 Fig. 4.23.2 Fig. 4.23.3

Fig. 4.23.4 Fig. 4.23.5 Fig. 4.23.6

and extracranial extension into the scalp and intracranial extension. Bony spiculations seen in the lateral border of the lesion representing periosteal reaction. No specific matrix inside the lesion. Incidental lytic lesion involving the inner table of the occipital bone representing arachnoid granulation.

CT in brain window (Figs 4.23.7 to 4.23.9): Expansile iso to hyperdense lesion in the skull vault with adjacent edema having intracranial and extracranial extension and mass effect on the ipsilateral lateral ventricle with midline shift of 5 mm to the right.

Differential Diagnosis

1. Intraosseous meningioma
2. Hemangiopericytoma (solitary fibrous histiocytoma).
3. Expansile lytic metastases—RCC, thyroid, pheochromocytoma, melanoma.
4. Plasmacytoma.
5. Lymphoma

Further characterization can be done with MR imaging.

In MRI T2 axial sections (Figs 4.23.10 to 4.23.12) the dumbbell-shaped lesion appears isointense to the gray matter measuring 7 × 4 cm noted in the squamous part of left temporal bone with epicenter in the intra-diploic space with well-defined borders and prominent flow voids and **spoke wheel pattern** of internal vascularity. CSF cleft noted at the periphery with prominent flow voids. White matter edema noted in the left frontotemporal regions. No evidence of any intralesional necrosis.

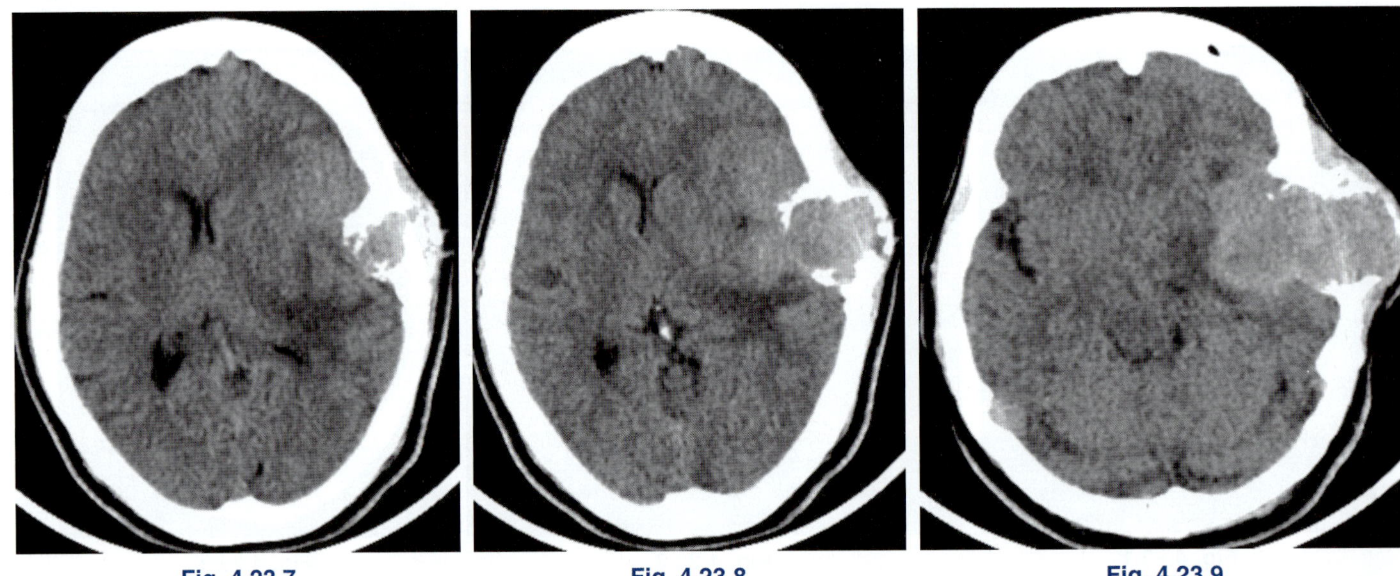

Fig. 4.23.7 Fig. 4.23.8 Fig. 4.23.9

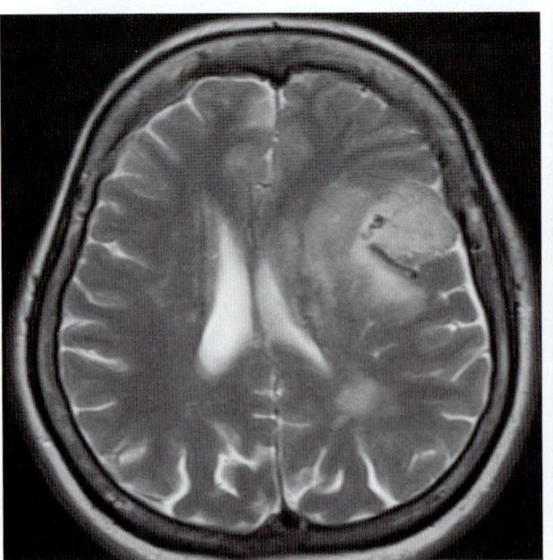

Fig. 4.23.10

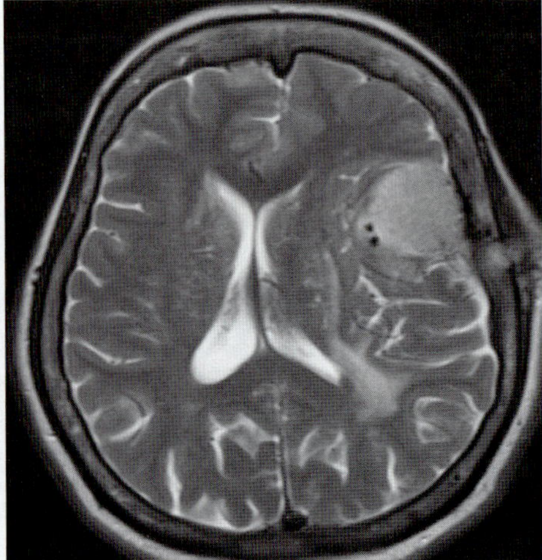

Fig. 4.23.11

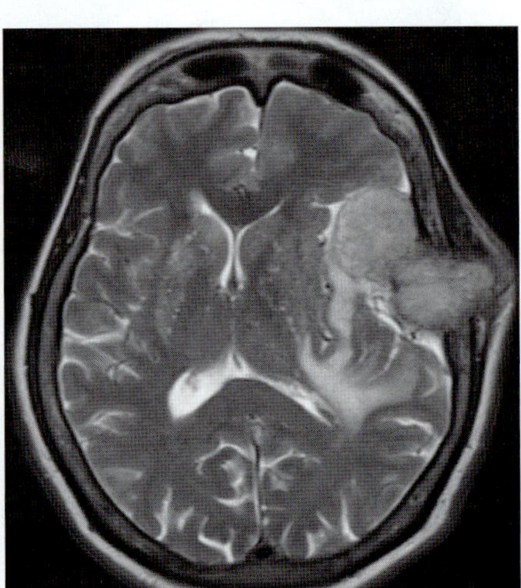

Fig. 4.23.12

<table>
<tr><th colspan="3">Table 4.23.1: DD for lytic skull lesions</th></tr>
<tr><td>1. Meningeal hemangiopericytoma
Also called solitary fibrous tumor of the dura.
Age: Younger adults (30–50 years) with up to 10% being diagnosed in children. Frequently manifests as a large aggressive dural lesion that extends through the skull vault. Mostly, they are lobulated solitary supratentorial lesions with high vascularity eroding neighbouring bone.</td><td>CT—vivid enhancement, erosion of adjacent bone. No hyperostosis. No calcification.
MRI—T1: Isointense to grey matter, T1 C+ (Gd)-vivid enhancement. Grade 2 tumors will show dural tail. T2W—isointense to grey matter with multiple flow voids and surrounding edema. MRS—high myoinositol, absent alanine peak (present in meningiomas)</td><td>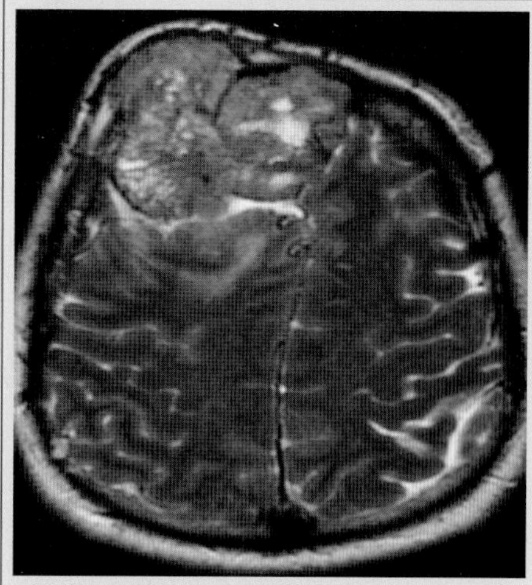
Fig. 4.23.13: Meningeal hemangiopericytoma</td></tr>
<tr><td>2. Expansile lytic metastases—RCC, thyroid, pheochromocytoma, melanoma
Age: Older population
Skull metastases has similar appearance to skeletal metastases mostly.</td><td>Even though lytic metastasis are common in skull, breast and prostate cancers present with sclerotic skull metastasis. Indistinct zones of transition, no periosteal reaction, no sclerotic margins.</td><td>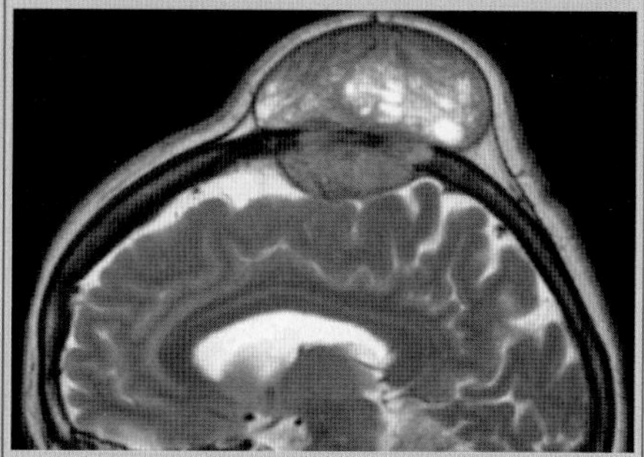
Fig. 4.23.14: Lytic skull metastasis with soft tissue component</td></tr>
<tr><td>3. Plasmacytoma. Age—55 years (10 years less than multiple myeloma). According to their location, solitary plasmacytomas can be categorised into two groups: Isolated bone plasmacytoma (70%) and extramedullary plasmacytoma (30%).</td><td colspan="2">Plasmacytoma shows well-defined, “punched-out” lytic lesion with extraosseous soft-tissue masses. The bone cortex is frequently eroded, expanded, and destroyed in advanced plasmacytoma, sometimes with extensive ridging in periphery, giving the soap bubble appearance. Absent sclerotic reaction.</td></tr>
</table>

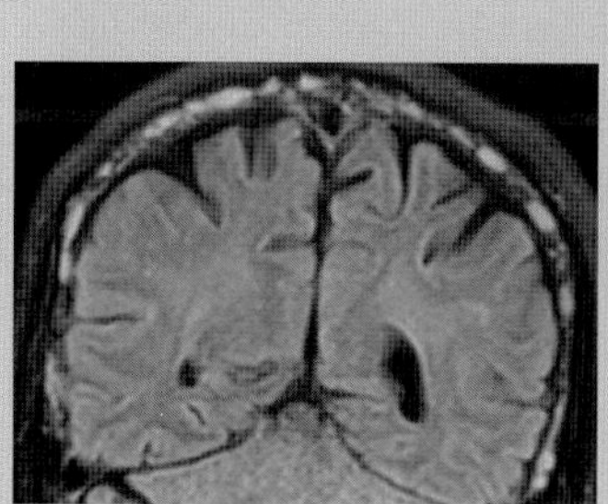 Fig. 4.23.15: Multiple myeloma involving skull	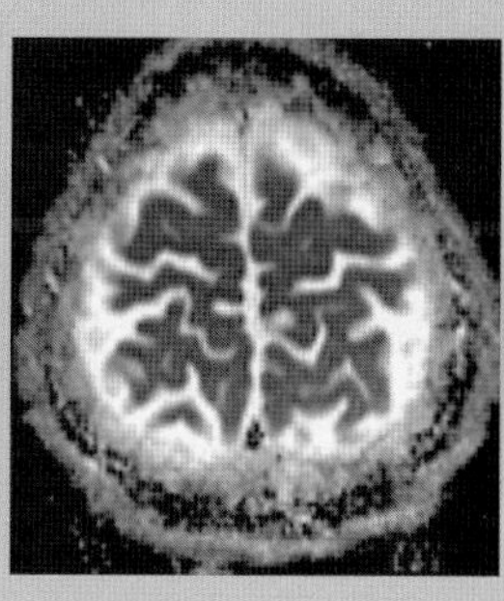 Fig. 4.23.16: Multiple myeloma involving skull	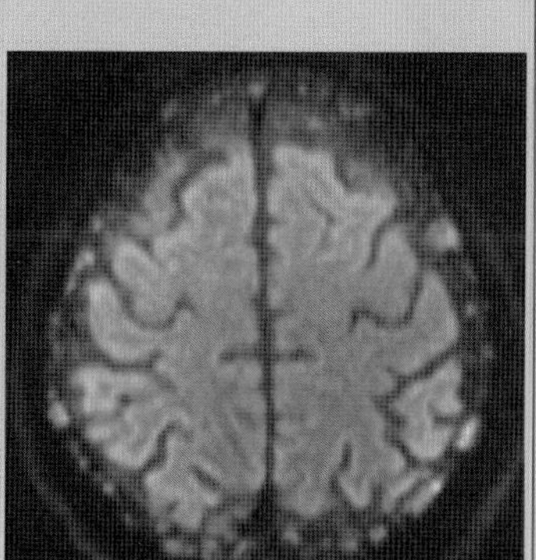 Fig. 4.23.17: Multiple myeloma involving skull	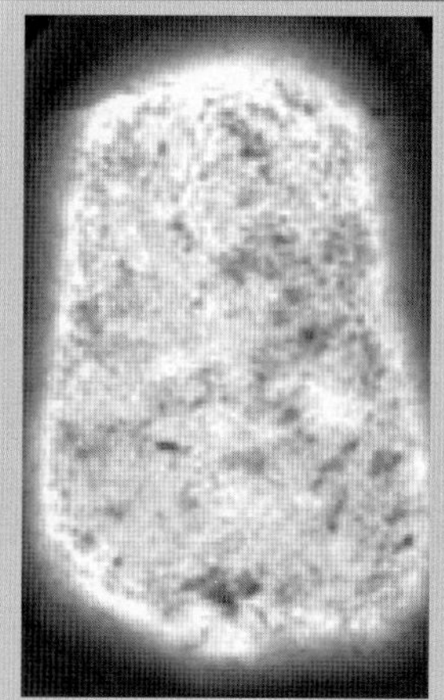 Fig. 4.23.18: Multiple myeloma involving skull

Contd...

Table 4.23.1: DD for lytic skull lesions *(Contd...)*		
4. Lymphoma **Age: 50 to 60 years** Primary bone lymphoma has lesser prevalence than secondary lymphoma, accounting for <5% bone tumors and <1% NHL.	It can present as lytic, sclerotic or mixed pattern. A lytic pattern characterised by permeative bone destruction and a large transition zone is common presentation. Diffusion restriction and rCBV with intact cortex is seen. The most prevalent subtype is diffuse large B cell lymphoma (DLBCL). The most prevalent sites are the bony pelvis and femur.	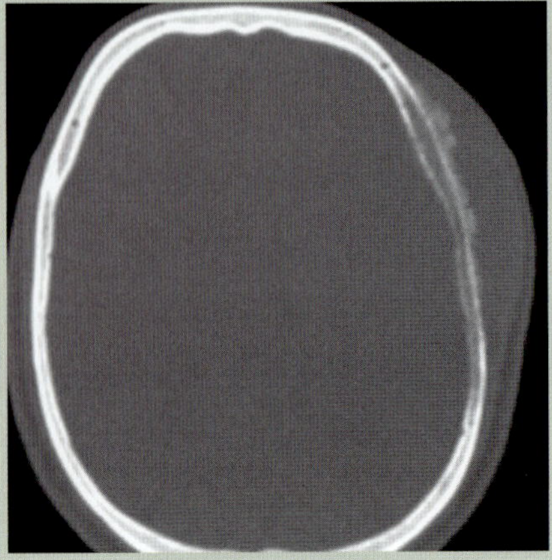 **Fig. 4.23.19:** Skull lymphoma
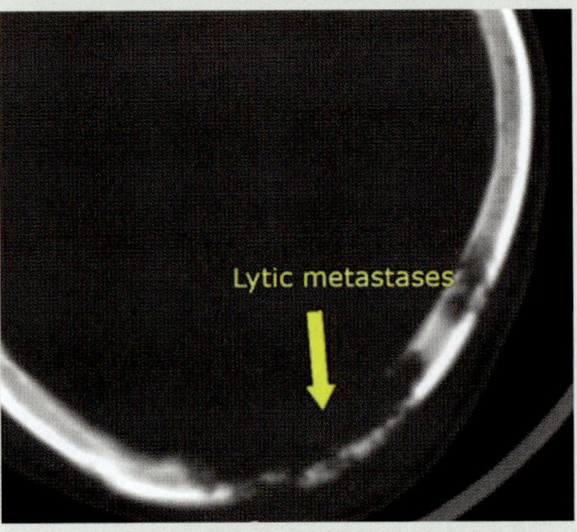 **Fig. 4.23.20:** Lytic metastasis	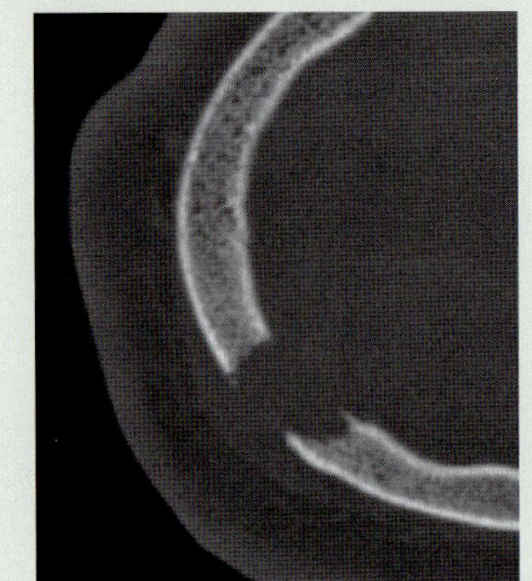 **Fig. 4.23.21:** LCH	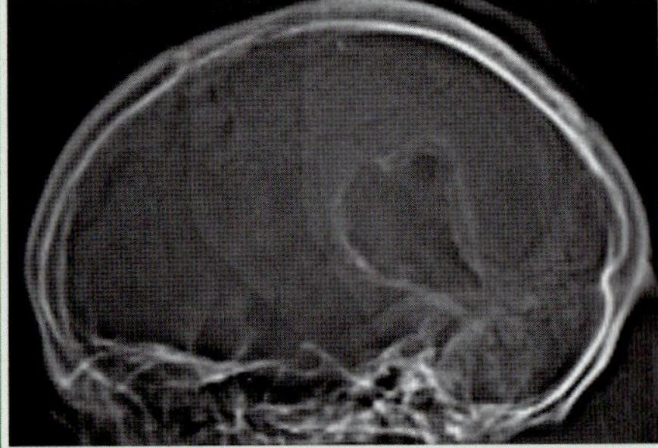 **Fig. 4.23.22:** Intra-diploic epidermoid cyst
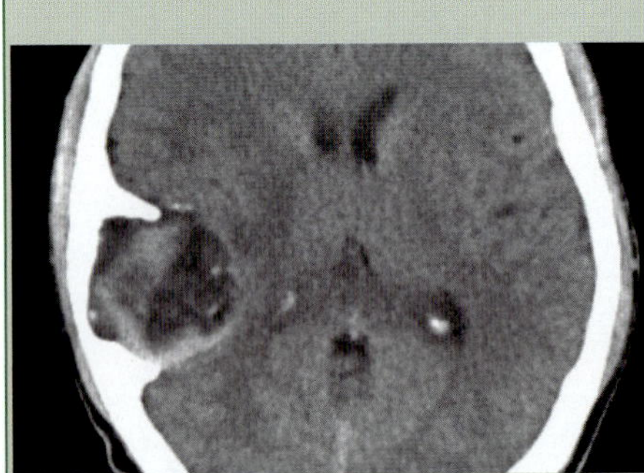 **Fig. 4.23.23:** Intra-diploic epidermoid cyst	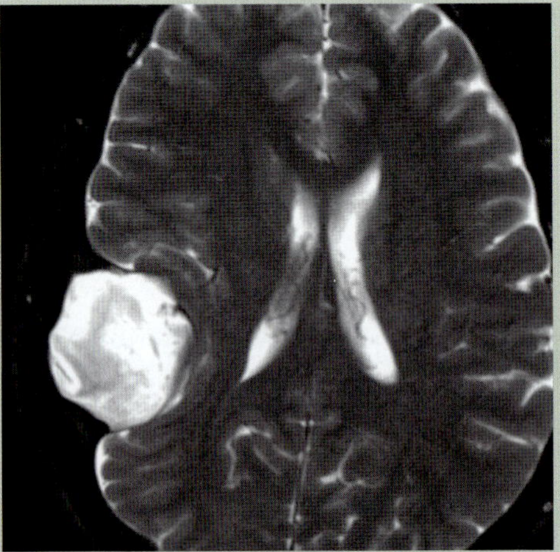 **Fig. 4.23.24:** Intra-diploic epidermoid cyst	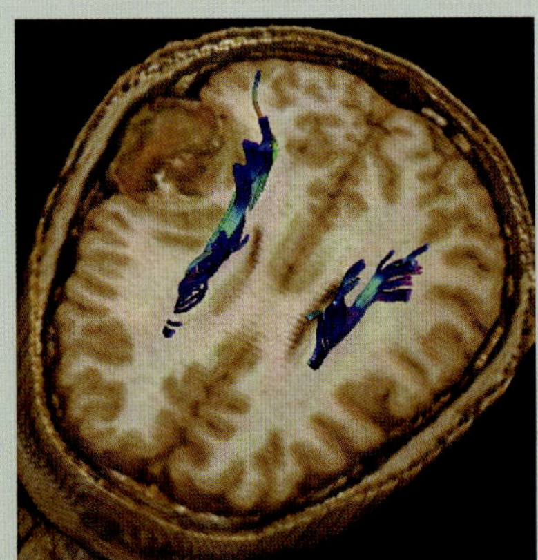 **Fig. 4.23.25:** Intra-diploic epidermoid cyst displacing the adjacent white matter tracts

Table 4.23.2: Difference between intra-axial and extra-axial lesions		
Feature	*Intra-axial lesion*	*Extra-axial leison*
Contiguity with bone or falx	Usually not present	Yes
Bony changes	Usually not present	Yes
CSF spaces, cisterns	Effaced	Often widened, CSF cleft
Cortical buckling/onion skin pattern	No	Yes
GM/WM junction	Destruction	Preservation
Vascular supply	Cerebral arteries	External (meningeal arteries)—spoke wheel pattern
Enhancement	Heterogeneous enhancement	Avid enhancement
Broad dural base	No	Yes (with dural tail sign)
Surrounding edema	+++	+
Extracranial soft tissue involvement	No	Yes

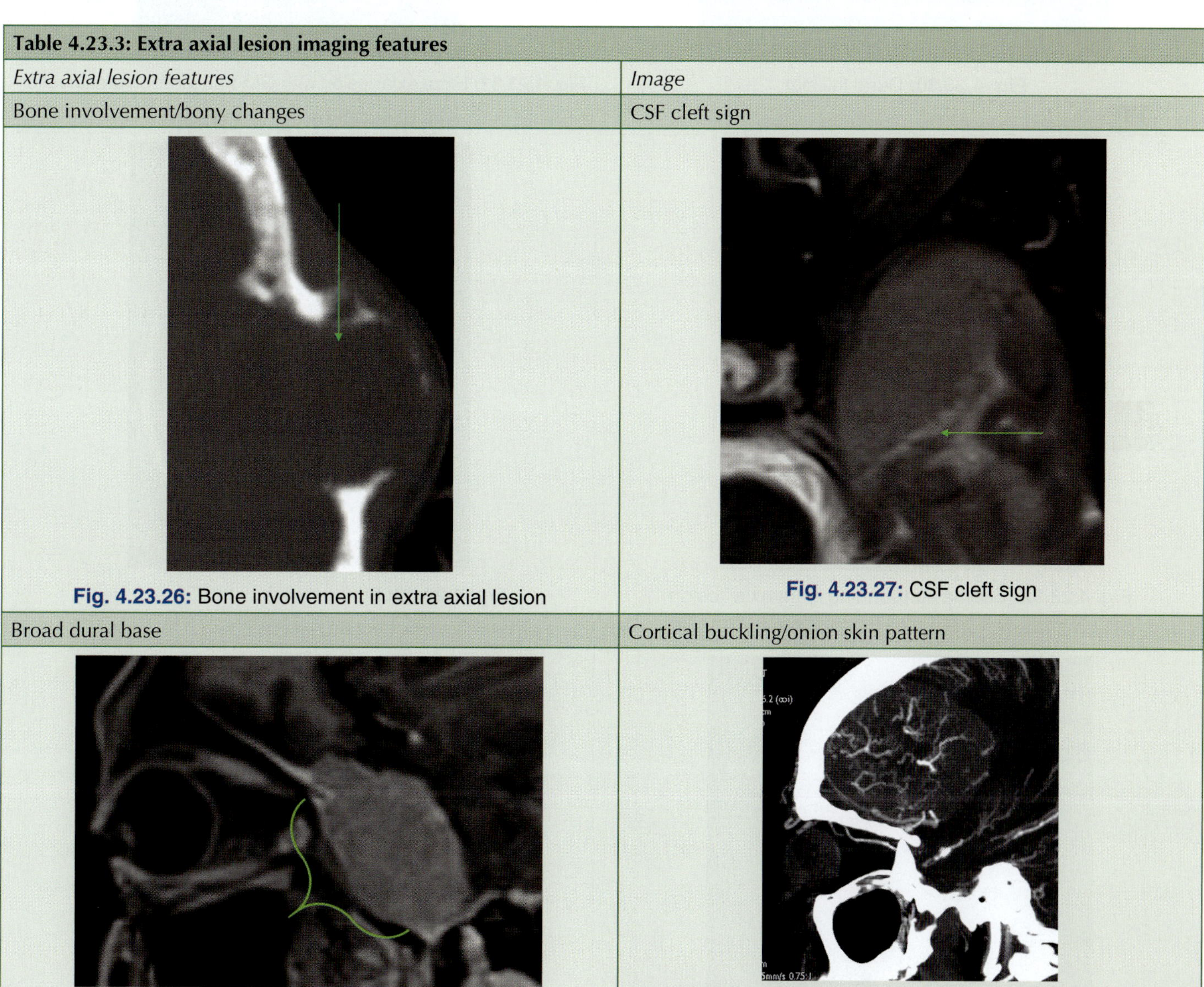

Table 4.23.3: Extra axial lesion imaging features	
Extra axial lesion features	*Image*
Bone involvement/bony changes	CSF cleft sign
Fig. 4.23.26: Bone involvement in extra axial lesion	**Fig. 4.23.27:** CSF cleft sign
Broad dural base	Cortical buckling/onion skin pattern
Fig. 4.23.28: Broad dural based extra axial lesion	**Fig. 4.23.29:** Spoke wheel pattern of vascularity, usually from middle meningeal artery

(Contd...)

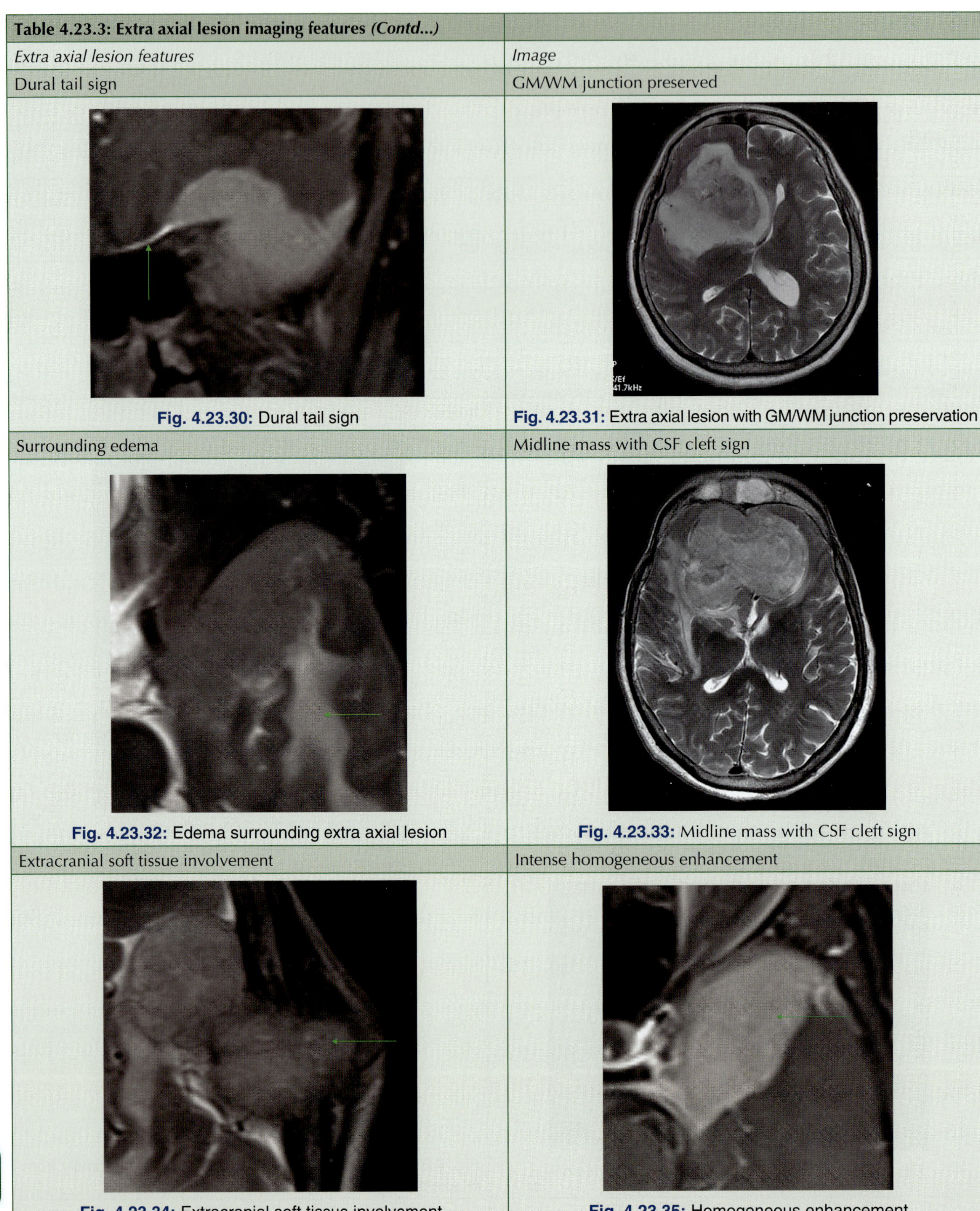

Table 4.23.3: Extra axial lesion imaging features ***(Contd...)***	
Extra axial lesion features	*Image*
Dural tail sign	GM/WM junction preserved
Fig. 4.23.30: Dural tail sign	**Fig. 4.23.31:** Extra axial lesion with GM/WM junction preservation
Surrounding edema	Midline mass with CSF cleft sign
Fig. 4.23.32: Edema surrounding extra axial lesion	**Fig. 4.23.33:** Midline mass with CSF cleft sign
Extracranial soft tissue involvement	Intense homogeneous enhancement
Fig. 4.23.34: Extracranial soft tissue involvement	**Fig. 4.23.35:** Homogeneous enhancement

Interpretation: A—50 years old female with lesion in squamous part of left temporal bone, parietal bone, B—aggressive lesion with narrow zone of transition with cortical break, bony spiculations, extracranial extension into the scalp and intracranial extension, C—ill-defined T2 isointense lytic lesion with bevelled edges and prominent flow voids, spoke wheel pattern of internal vascularity and CSF cleft sign, soft tissue extension, D—intraosseous meningioma.

Principal diagnosis: Intraosseous meningioma.

Management: Biopsy to confirm the diagnosis.

Treatment: Intraosseous meningioma are benign and slow-growing, although compared to standard meningiomas, they may have a larger proportion of malignant transformation. In symptomatic situations, surgical resection with bone grafting may be undertaken.

Brief discussion–intraosseous meningioma: The majority (65%) are osteoblastic, while the remaining (35%) are osteolytic. As a result, imaging appearances are frequently nonspecific.

The more prevalent osteosclerotic form shows widespread sclerosis and bone growth on CT. T1W shows isointense extra-axial mass component may be seen on MRI, with the expanding bony component showing low signal, T2 usually isointense to grey matter, with a tiny proportion of hyperintense meningiomas. On contrast, homogeneous avid contrast enhancement is seen.

DD for metastasis in benign lesions: Meningioma, fibroid uterus, GCT bone, primary adenoma of thyroid.

4.24.1 CENTRAL NERVOUS SYSTEM

Case No. 24.1

Clinical history: A 13-year-old male presented with history of fever for the past 5 days, 2 episodes of new onset seizure, and history of altered sensorium for 6 hours.

Radiological techniques and observations: Figures 4.24.1.1 to 4.24.1.3 are axial T2, coronal T2 images and axial DWI of MRI brain respectively showing T2/ FLAIR hyperintensity showing diffusion restriction noted in bilateral superior, middle and inferior temporal gyrus, fusiform gyrus, medial temporal lobe involving hippocampus and the insular cortex. **The lesion predominantly involves the grey matter with sparing of the white matter.** Bilateral lateral and third ventricles appears normal. No evidence of intraparenchymal/ extra-axial hemorrhage noted. Visualized brain stem and cerebellum appears normal.

Interpretation: A—13-year-old male with lesion in bilateral superior, middle and inferior temporal gyrus, fusiform gyrus, medial temporal lobe involving hippocampus and the insular cortex, C—T2/FLAIR hyperintensity, B—bilateral symmetrical hyperintensities show diffusion restriction, D—limbic encephalitis.

Principal diagnosis: Limbic encephalitis involving bilateral temporal lobe and insular cortex—possibly due to herpes simplex virus infection.

Further investigation: Contrast enhanced MRI brain—enhancement varies from none (early disease) to intense gyriform enhancement several days later. Definitive diagnosis requires PCR confirmation. CSF PCR is 96–98% sensitive.

Treatment: Antiviral therapy with IV acyclovir.

Approach to T2/FLAIR hyperintensity—bilateral medial temporal lobe involving hippocampus.

Discussion: **Anatomy of the hippocampus and limbic system:** Refer to Chapter 3.

Herpes simplex encephalitis: The most common of all causes of limbic encephalitis is the herpes simplex encephalitis. The causative agent is HSV-1. It follows bimodal age distribution: One-third occurring between 6 months and 3 years of age and one half to two-thirds occurring in patients older than 50 years.

Imaging: **CT findings:** Early cases—normal. Hypodensity in one or both temporal lobes and insula may be present. **Location:** HSE has a striking affinity for the limbic system. The anterior and medial temporal lobes, insular cortex, subfrontal area, and cingulate gyrus are most frequently affected. In extra limbic pattern which is more common in children, most often involves the parietal cortex. The basal ganglia are usually spared. Neonatal HSE involves both gray and white matter. Diffuse cerebral edema with leptomeningeal enhancement with involvement of deep gray matter is common.

CECT: Patchy or gyriform enhancement may develop after 24–48 hours.

MRI: Imaging modality of choice. **The findings are usually bilateral > unilateral; asymmetric > symmetric.**

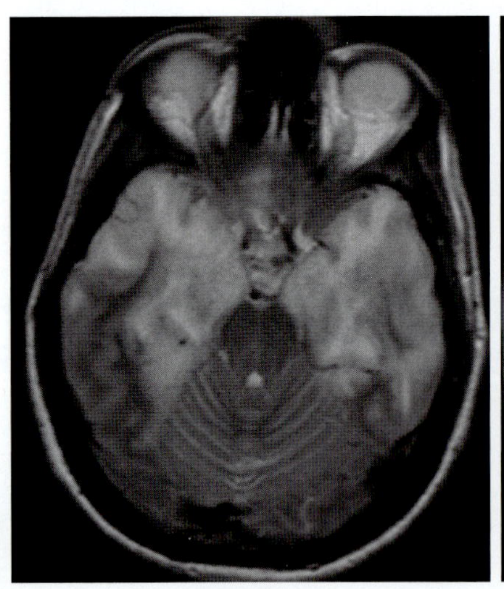
Fig. 4.24.1.1

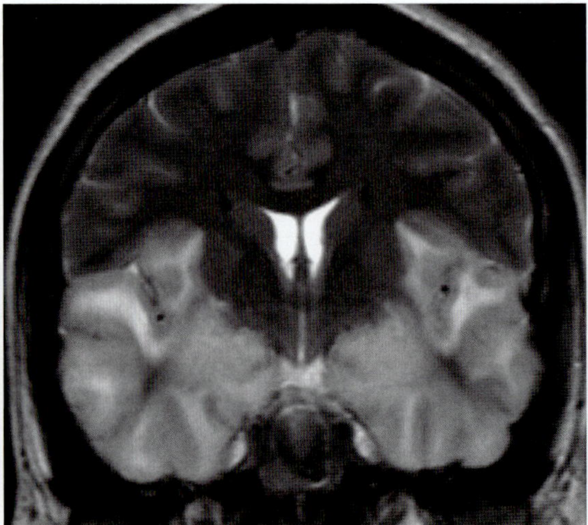
Fig. 4.24.1.2

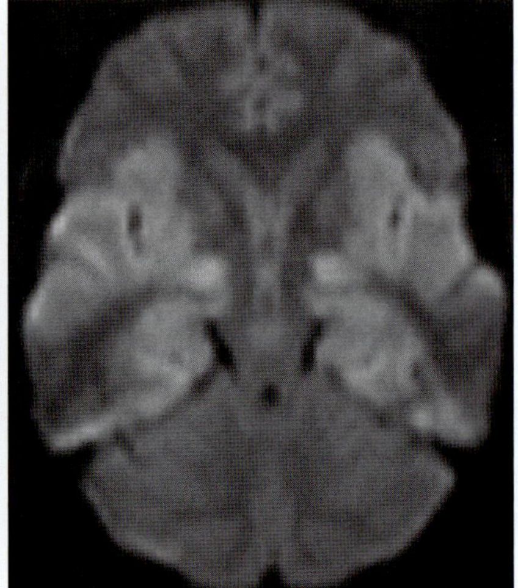
Fig. 4.24.1.3

Table 4.24.1.1: Differential diagnosis for limbic encephalitis

Condition	*Imaging findings*	*Images*
1. Other Infections: Viral infections associated with medial temporal lobe involvement include 1. Dengue virus, 2. Japanese encephalitis, 3. Rabies virus, 4. Nipah virus. Others include neurosyphilis. Typical findings in neurosyphilis include cortical and subcortical infarcts, leptomeningeal enhancement/granulomas and arteritis.	Encephalitis—T2/FLAIR hyperintensity typically involving just the cortex. Characteristic features: JE virus spares insular cortex. Nipah virus shows small punctate T2 hyperintense lesions.	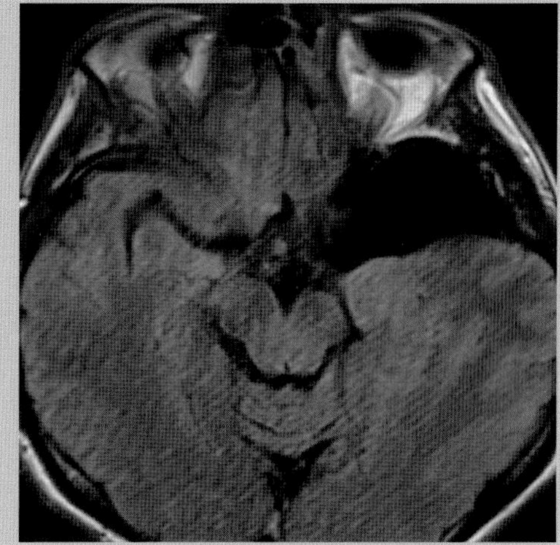 **Fig. 4.24.1.4:** Viral encephalitis with left anterior temporal pole arachnoid cyst
2. Status epilepticus/post-ictal edema: Refer to case 4.24.2		
3. Autoimmune (paraneoplastic) limbic encephalitis: Primary autoantibody is anti-HU (small cell lung carcinoma). Others include anti-Ma2 (testicular germ cell tumor). **Autoimmune (non-neoplastic) encephalitis** **Group 1-Target:** Intracellular antigen Often associated with underlying malignancy (expect anti-GAD antibody mediated type where it is usually not associated with malignancy) **Group 2-Target:** Cell surface antigen. Malignancy less common Examples: NMDAr, GABAr **Paraneoplastic encephalitis:** T2/FLAIR shows hyperintensity in one or both medial temporal lobes which are non-hemorrhagic. **Non-neoplastic encephalitis:** The most common pattern of involvement is limbic encephalitis. T2/FLAIR hyperintensity in both hippocampi and amygdala is typical. Enhancement is generally absent. Other malignancies associated: Neuroblastoma, breast cancer, Hodgkin lymphoma, thymoma and immature ovarian teratomas.		
4. Post-transplant acute limbic encephalitis (PALE) syndrome: Occurs most commonly following hematopoietic stem cell transplantation. Causative organism—human herpesvirus 6	Transient T2/FLAIR hyperintensity involving just the medial temporal lobes on both sides with restriction on DWI. T2* shows no evidence of hemorrhage.	
5. Vein of Labbé thrombosis with infarct: The inferior anastomotic vein drains the medial, anteroinferior and posteroinferior temporal lobe and is a part of superficial cerebral venous system	**CT:** Cortical based hypodensity with areas of hemorrhagic transformation involving the vein of Labbé territory. **MRI:** Loss of flow void in T2/FLAIR with areas of T2/FLAIR hyperintensity showing diffusion restriction. **CECT/CEMR:** Filling defect within the vein of Labbé.	
6. Mesial temporal sclerosis: Refer to case 4.24.2		
7. Focal cortical dysplasia: Refer to case 4.24.2		
Thickened gray matter DD: Focal encephalitis, cortical laminar necrosis		

Table 4.24.1.2: Location of various encephalitis	
Location of various encephalitis	
Herpes simplex virus type1(HSV1)	*Limbic system*
Cytomegalovirus (CMV)—pediatric and adult	Deep periventricular WM
Epstein-Barr virus (EBV)	Multifocal, diffuse involvement of brain and spinal cord. Splenium of corpus callosum
Varicella-zoster virus (VZV)	
Varicella	May affect multifocal areas of cortex
Zoster	Brainstem/cortical GM, cranial nerves
Cerebellitis	Bilateral cerebellar hemispheres
Eastern equine encephalitis (EEE)	BG and thalami
Enteroviral encephalomyelitis	
– Enterovirus (EV) 71	Posterior medulla, pons, midbrain, dentate nuclei, spinal cord
– Polio, Coxsackie	Midbrain, anterior spinal cord
Hantavirus	Pituitary gland hemorrhage
HIV-1	Cerebral WM, brainstem, thalamus, BG
Japanese encephalitis	Bilateral thalami, brainstem, cerebellum, spinal cord, cerebral cortex
Murray Valley encephalitis (MVE)	Bilateral thalami; may affect midbrain, cervical spinal cord
Nipah viral encephalitis	Multifocal WM
Rabies encephalitis	Brainstem, hippocampi, hypothalamus, WM, GM
Rhombencephalitis	Brainstem and cerebellum
St. Louis encephalitis	Substantia nigra
West Nile virus (WNV)	BG and/or thalami may affect brainstem, cerebral WM, substantia nigra, cerebellum, spinal cord
CJD encephalitis	Insula, cingulate gyrus, superior frontal gyrus
Rasmussen encephalitis	One brain hemisphere.
Chikungunya encephalitis	No basal ganglia involvement
Zika virus encephalitis	Corpus callosum hypoplasia/agenesis; pontine atrophy, hypoplastic cerebellum
Dengue encephalitis	Bilateral basal ganglia, thalami, cortical grey matter, and subcortical and deep white matter involvement
TORCH infection	Periventricular and deep white matter region
Parecho virus	Periventricular white matter, corpus callosum, deep white matter, optic radiation, internal capsule, posterior thalami, and cerebral peduncles.
Acute hemorrhagic encephalitis most commonly caused by ADEM, herpes simplex, dengue, COVID-19, cerebral vasculitis, Marburg type of MS, tumefactive demyelination.	

Flowchart 4.24.1.1: Approach to T2/FLAIR hyperintensity—bilateral medial temporal lobe involving hippocampus

- T2 /FLAIR hyperintensity
  - Associated atrophy +
    - Grey and white matter
      1. Mesial temporal sclerosis
      2. CADASIL (lacunar infarcts)
      3. Focal cortical dysplasia (unilateral)
    - White matter only
      1. Alzheimer's disease (hippocampal atrophy)
      2. Frontotemporal dementia
  - No atrophy
    - Grey and white matter
      1. MELAS
      2. Gliomatosis cerebri
      3. Wilson's disease
    - White matter only
      1. Megalencephalic leukoencephalopathy (MLC)
      2. Congential CMV infection
      3. Myotonic dystrophy
    - Grey and white matter
      - Encephalitis
        1. Herpes simplex virus
        2. Limbic (autoimmnune, paraneoplastic)
      - Hyperammonemia

Temporal horn
Hippocampal sulcus
Dentate gyrus
CA3
CA4
CA2
CA1
Sub
Parahippocampal gyrus

Fig. 4.24.1.5: Anatomy of hippocampus and limbic system illustration

T1—gyral swelling with indistinct grey–white interface. T2—cortical/subcortical hyperintensity with relative sparing of the white matter. FLAIR—most sensitive sequence and may be positive before signal changes are apparent in T1/T2.T2* (GRE, SWI)—may demonstrate petechial hemorrhages in the form of confluent blooming foci after 24–48 hours. Diffusion restriction occurs early in the course of disease.

Contrast enhanced MRI brain: Enhancement varies from none (early disease) to intense gyriform enhancement several days later. Definitive diagnosis requires PCR confirmation. CSF PCR is 96–98% sensitive.

Table 4.24.1.3: Pattern of involvement in various encephalitis

Pediatric viral encephalitis

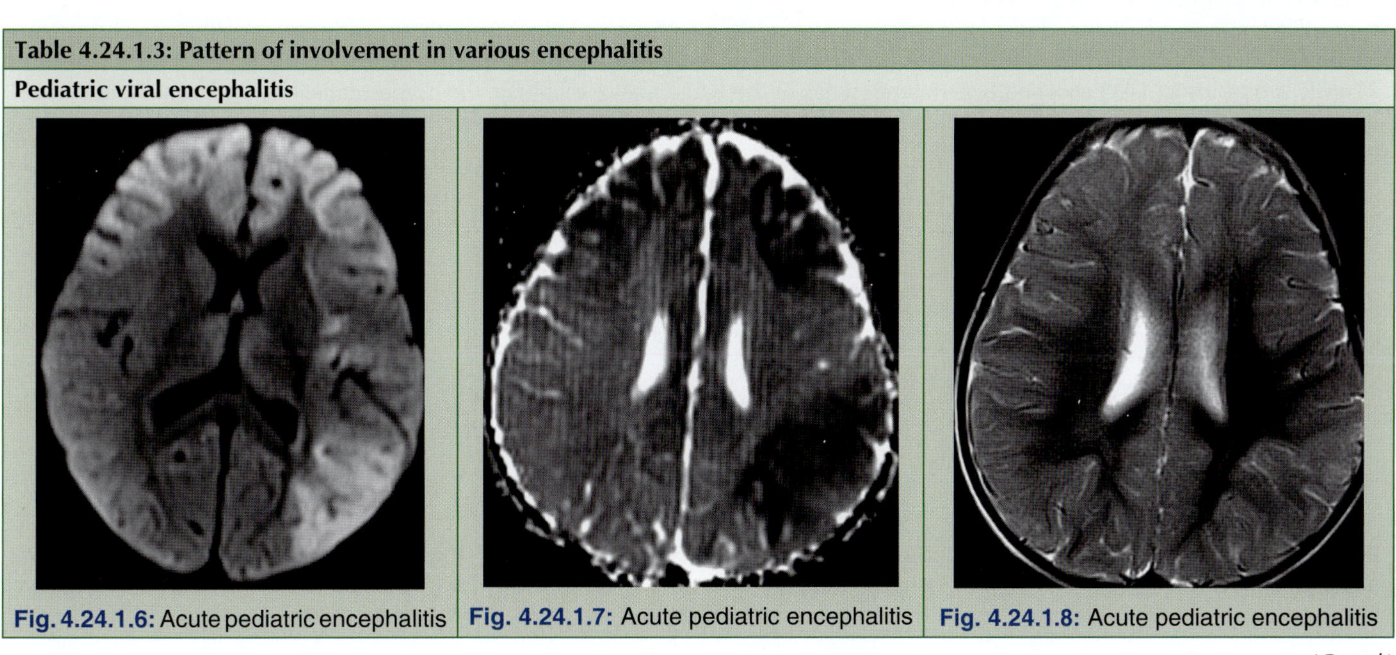

Fig. 4.24.1.6: Acute pediatric encephalitis

Fig. 4.24.1.7: Acute pediatric encephalitis

Fig. 4.24.1.8: Acute pediatric encephalitis

(Contd.)

Table 4.24.1.3: Pattern of involvement in various encephalitis (*Contd.*)

Enteroviral encephalitis

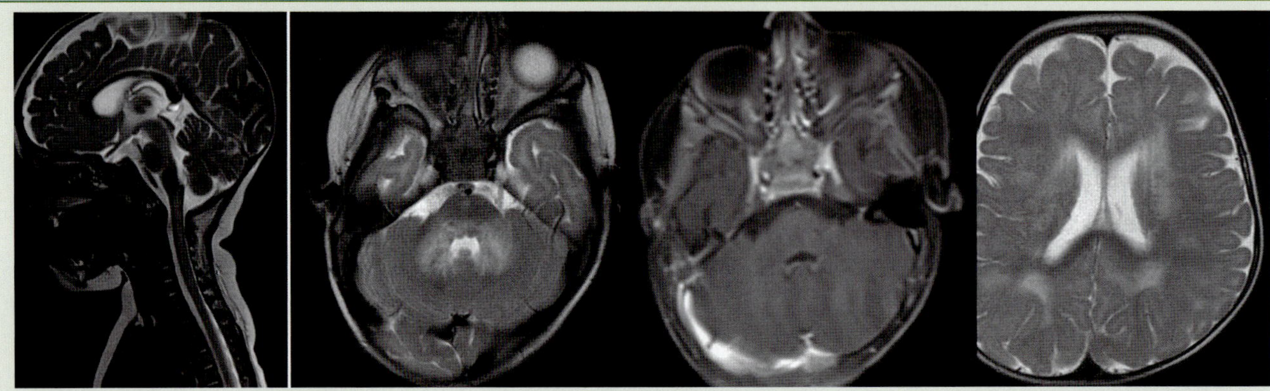

Fig. 4.24.1.9: Enteroviral encephalitis

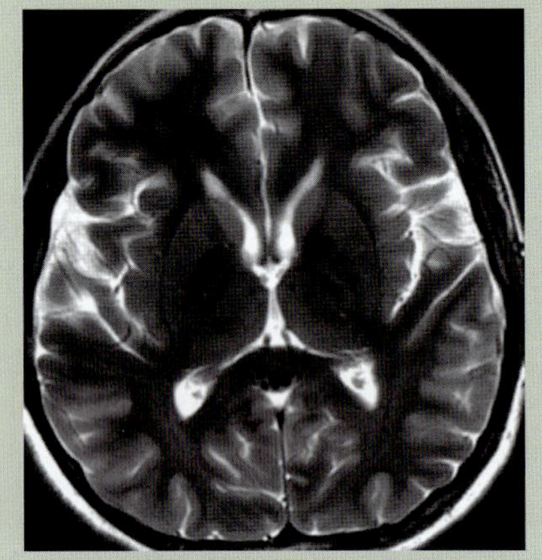

Fig. 4.24.1.10: CJD encephalitis

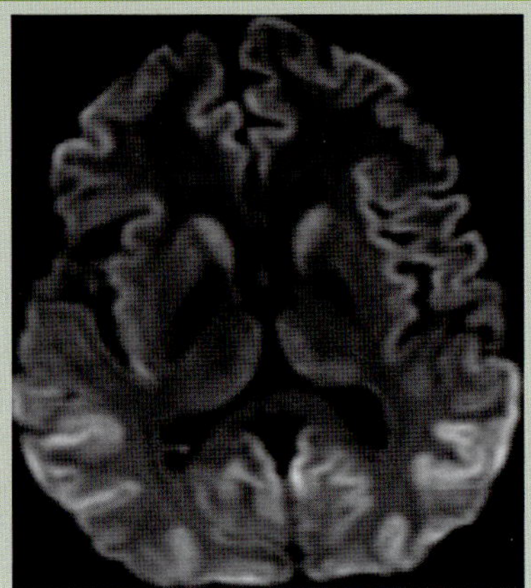

Fig. 4.24.1.11: CJD encephalitis

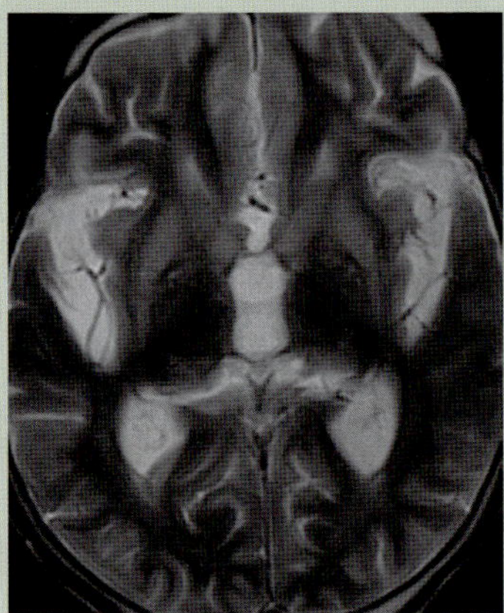

Fig. 4.24.1.12: CJD encephalitis

CJD encephalitis

NEONATAL CHIKUNGUNYA ENCEPHALOPATHY

Typically, a disease of adult and pediatric population presenting with fever, arthralgia, arthritis, rash and constitutional symptoms. Neurotropism of chikungunya is much **rarely been described in neonates.**

RT-PCR is diagnostic. DWI showing hyperintense areas of the white matter involving the corpus callosum, the frontal and parietal lobes. **Two weeks later,** frontal and parietal lobes white matter show **characteristic hypointensity**, while corpus callosum remaining hyperintense.

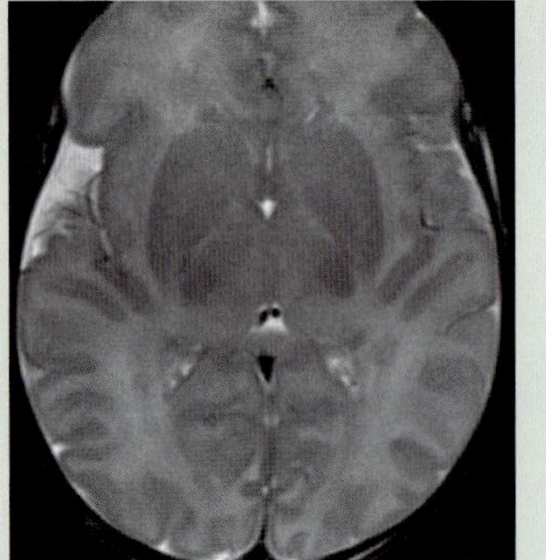

Fig. 4.24.1.13: Neonatal chikungunya encephalopathy

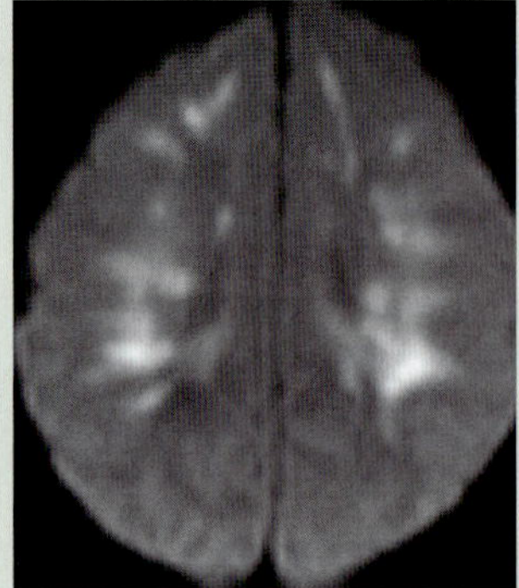

Fig. 4.24.1.14: Neonatal chikungunya encephalopathy

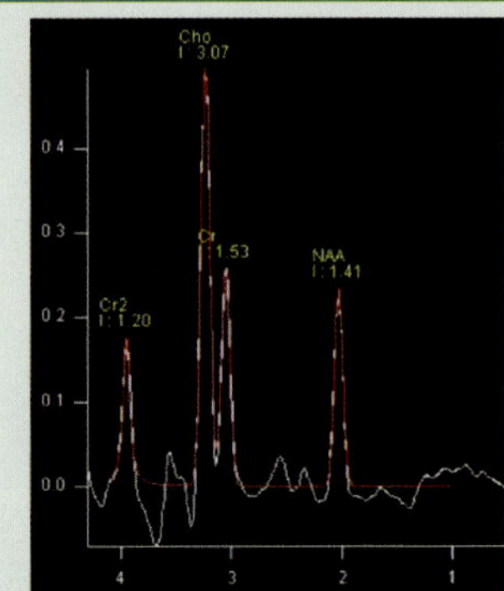

Fig. 4.24.1.15: Increased choline peak and reduced NAA in neonatal chikungunya encephalopathy

(*Contd.*)

Table 4.24.1.3: Pattern of involvement in various encephalitis (*Contd.*)

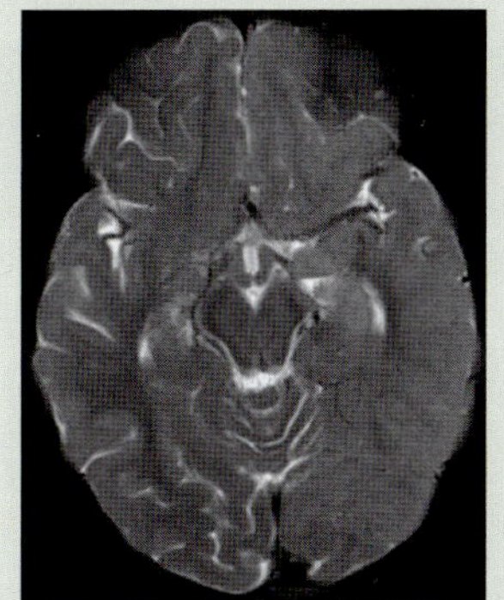 **Fig. 4.24.1.16:** Acute encephalitis	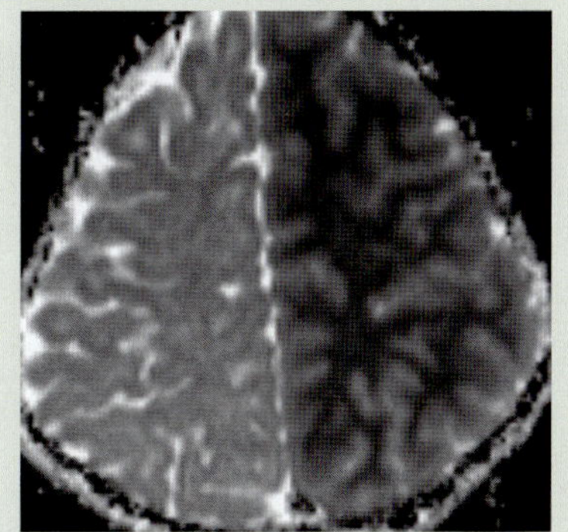 **Fig. 4.24.1.17:** Acute encephalitis	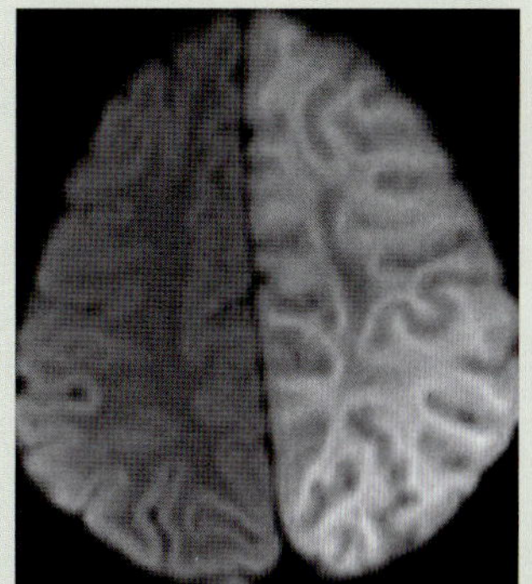 **Fig. 4.24.1.18:** Acute encephalitis
Acute encephalitis		
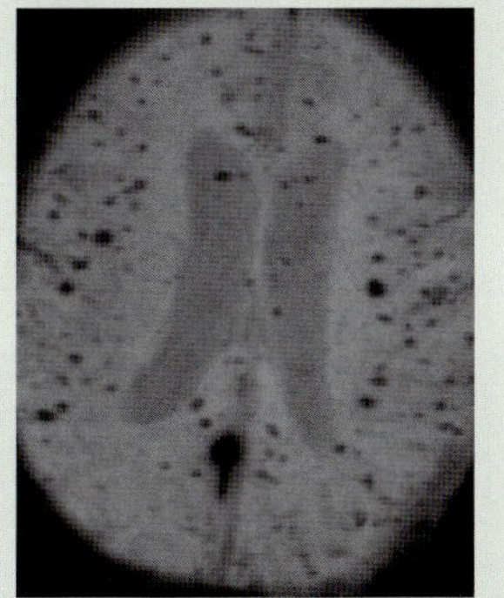 **Fig. 4.24.1.19:** Hemorrhagic encephalitis	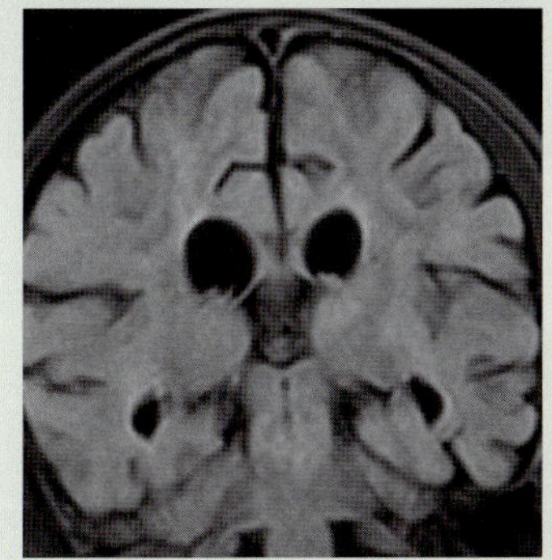 **Fig. 4.24.1.20:** Hemorrhagic encephalitis	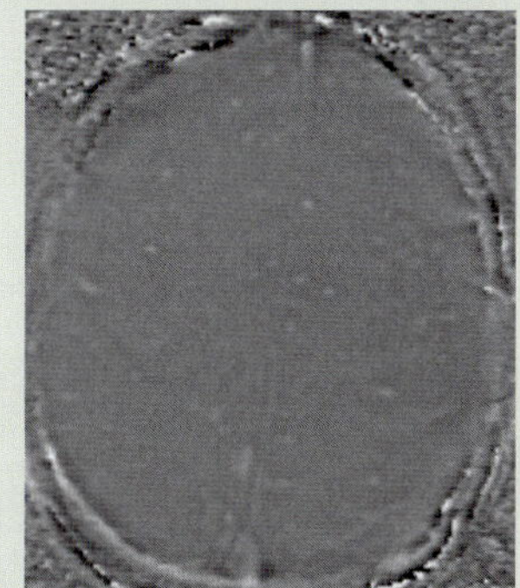 **Fig. 4.24.1.21:** Hemorrhagic encephalitis
Hemorrhagic encephalitis		
Limbic encephalitis 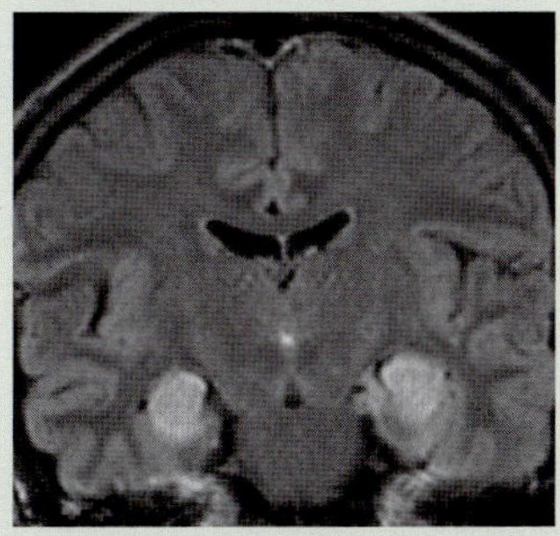 **Fig. 4.24.1.22:** Limbic encephalitis	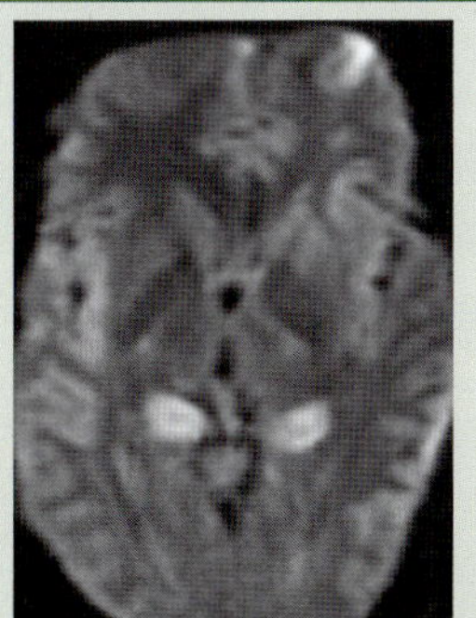 **Fig. 4.24.1.23:** Limbic encephalitis	**NEC encephalitis** 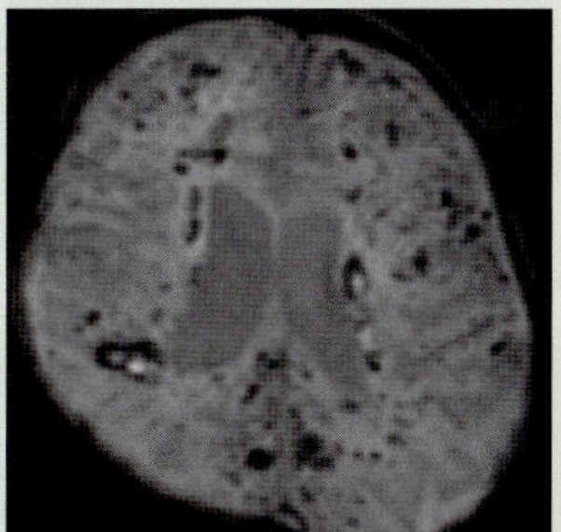 **Fig. 4.24.1.24:** NEC encephalitis
Hypoglycemic encephalitis 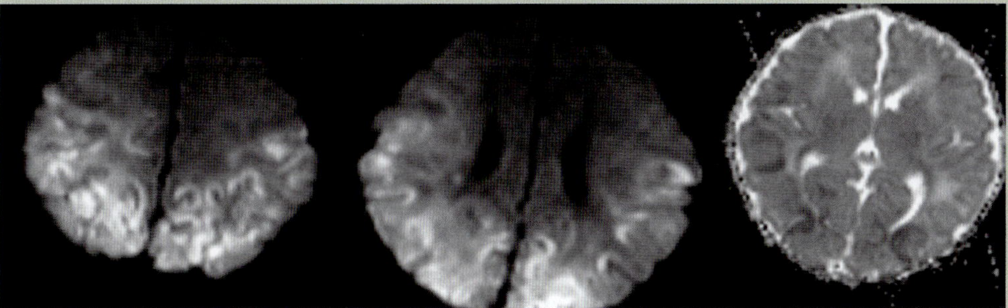 **Fig. 4.24.1.25:** Hypoglycemic encephalitis		

(*Contd.*)

Table 4.24.1.3: Pattern of involvement in various encephalitis (*Contd.*)

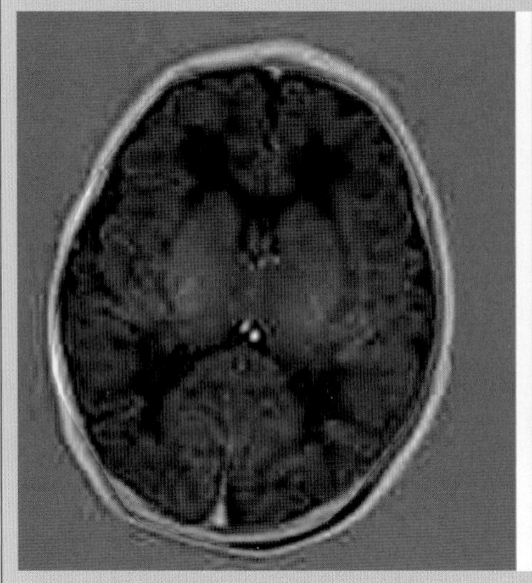
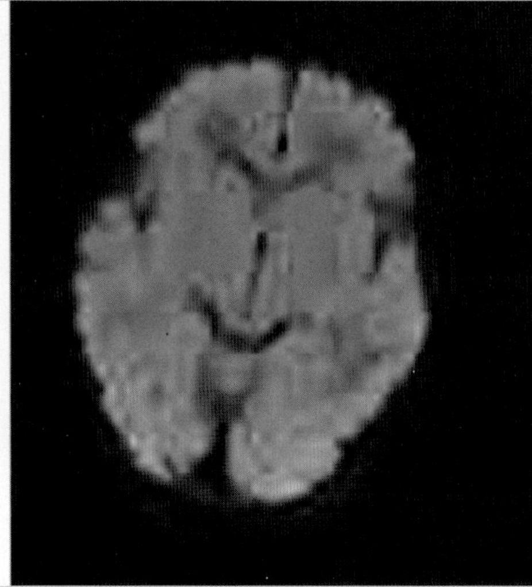
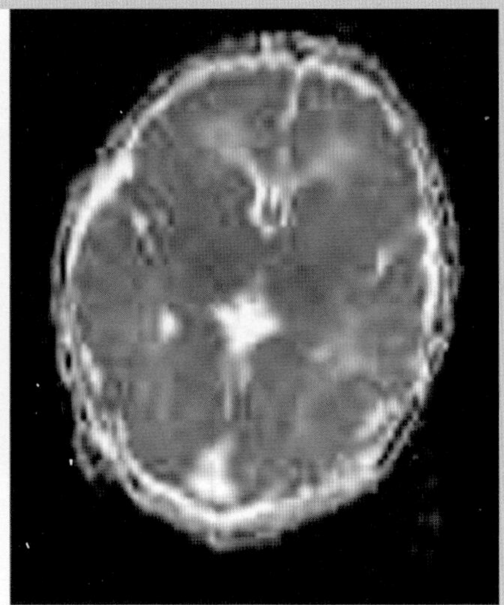

Fig. 4.24.1.26: Kernicterus

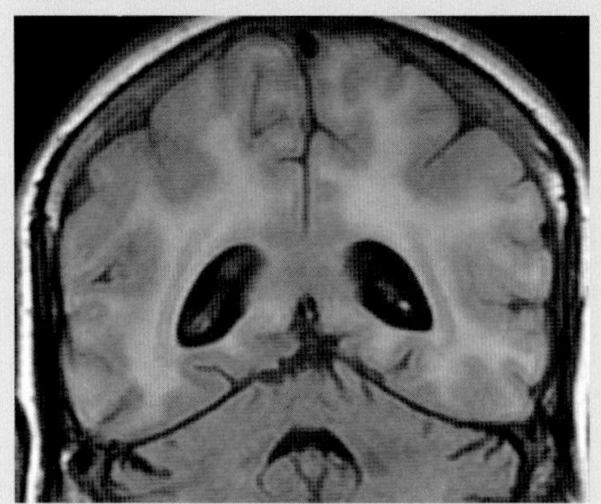

Fig. 4.24.1.27: Leukoencephalitis

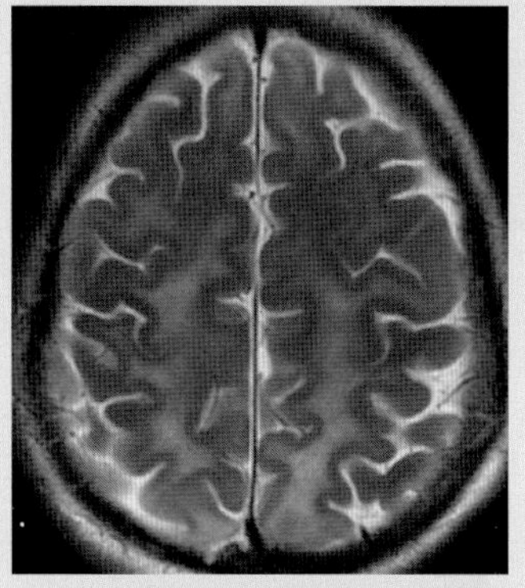

Fig. 4.24.1.28: Leukoencephalitis

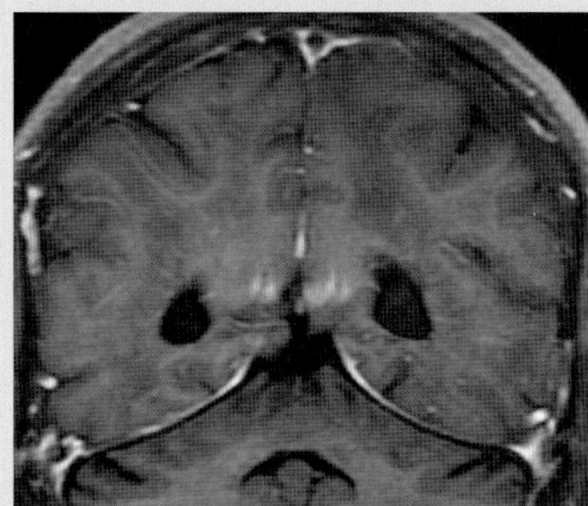

Fig. 4.24.1.29: Leukoencephalitis

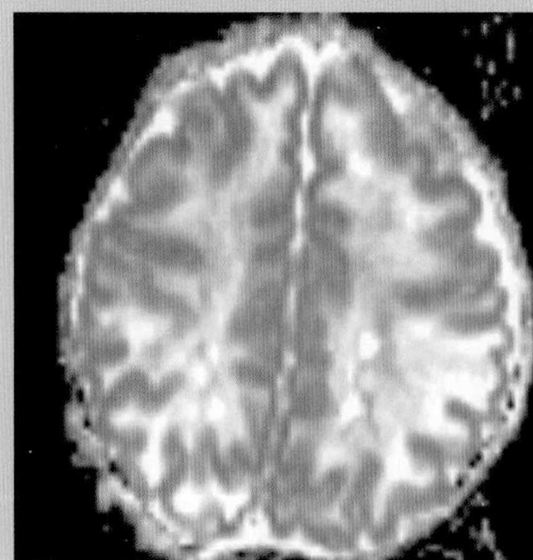

Fig. 4.24.1.30: Neonatal encephalitis

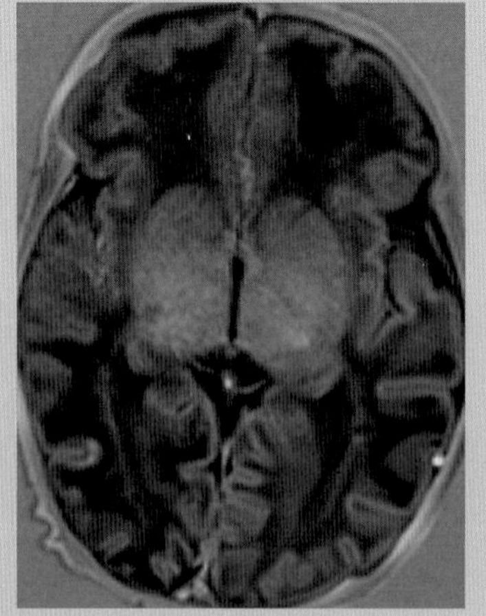

Fig. 4.24.1.31: Neonatal encephalitis

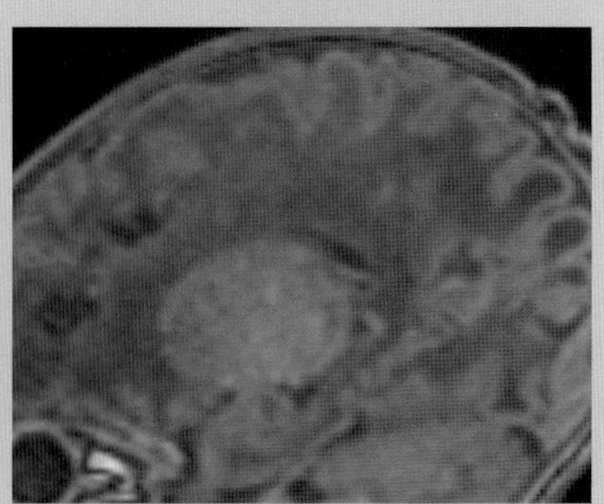

Fig. 4.24.1.32: Neonatal encephalitis

(*Contd.*)

Table 4.24.1.3: Pattern of involvement in various encephalitis (*Contd.*)

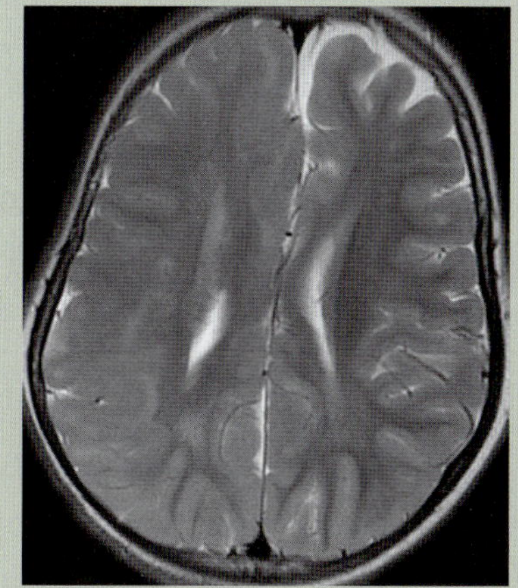

Fig. 4.24.1.33: Acute Rasmussen encephalitis involving right hemisphere which goes for atrophy later

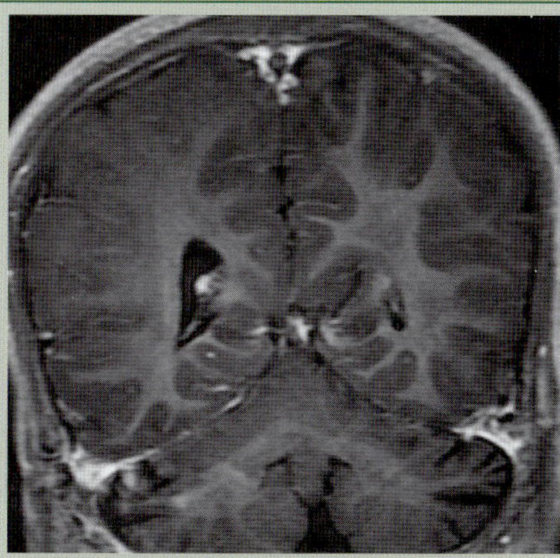

Fig. 4.24.1.34: Acute Rasmussen encephalitis involving right hemisphere which goes for atrophy later

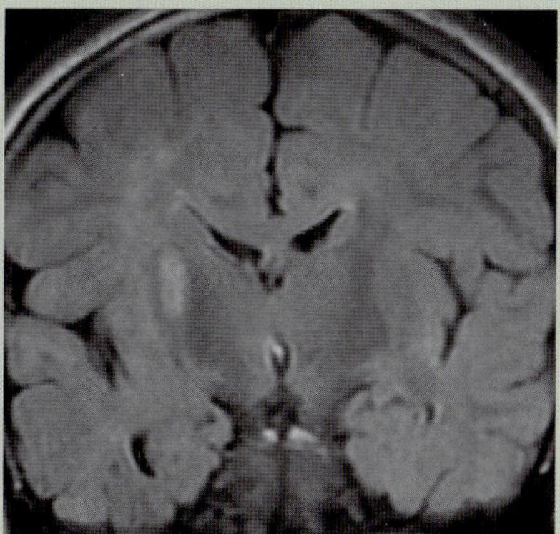

Fig. 4.24.1.35: Acute Rasmussen encephalitis involving right hemisphere which goes for atrophy later

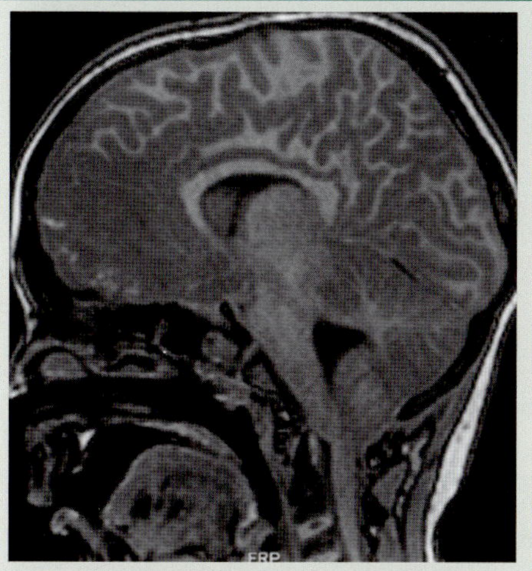

Fig. 4.24.1.36: Brain death due to encephalitis

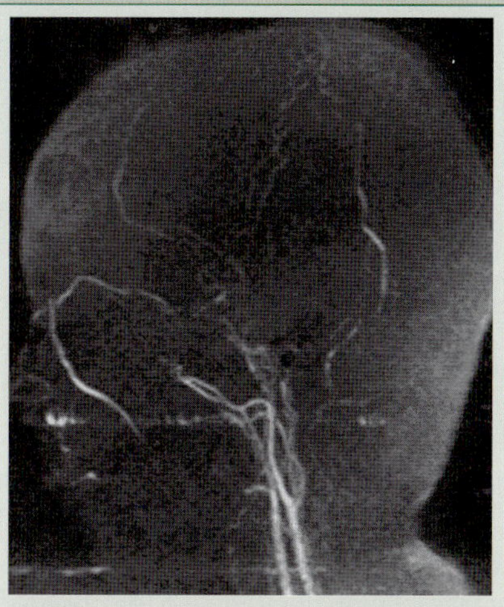

Fig. 4.24.1.37: Brain death due to encephalitis

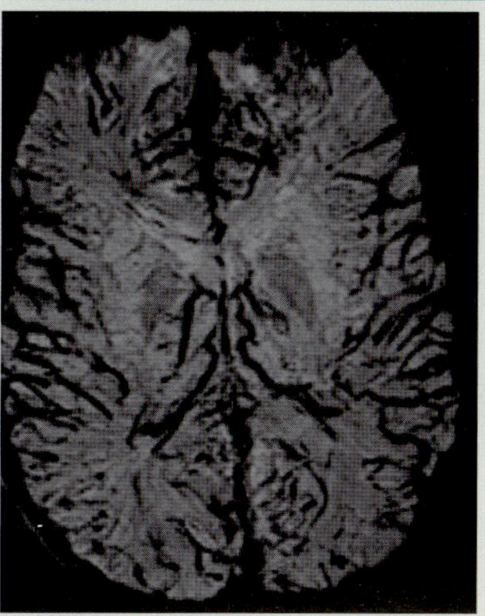

Fig. 4.24.1.38: Brain death due to encephalitis

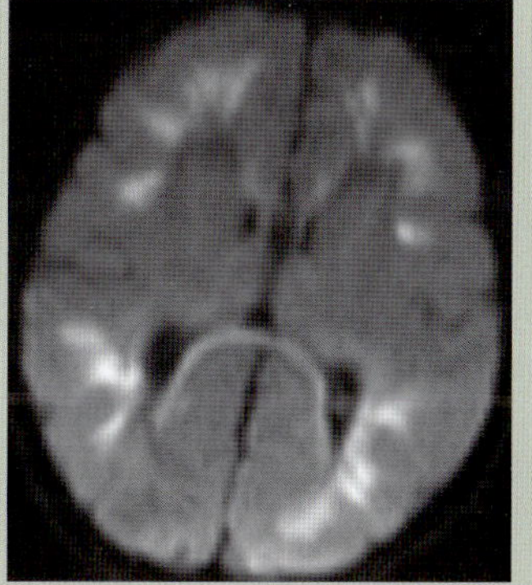

Fig. 4.24.1.39: Parechovirus encephalitis in nonketotic hyperglycemia

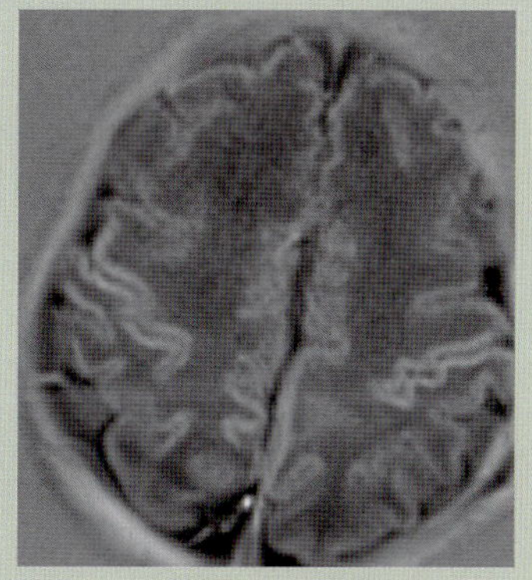

Fig. 4.24.1.40: Parechovirus encephalitis in nonketotic hyperglycemia

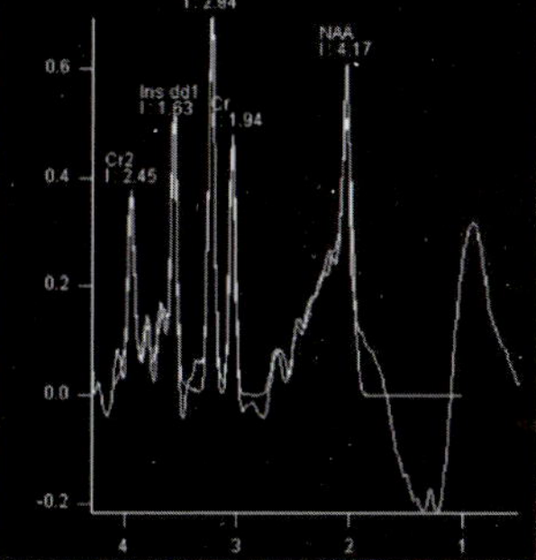

Fig. 4.24.1.41: MRS showing glycine (3.6 ppm) and choline peak in parechovirus encephalitis in nonketotic hyperglycemia

(*Contd.*)

Table 4.24.1.3: Pattern of involvement in various encephalitis (*Contd.*)

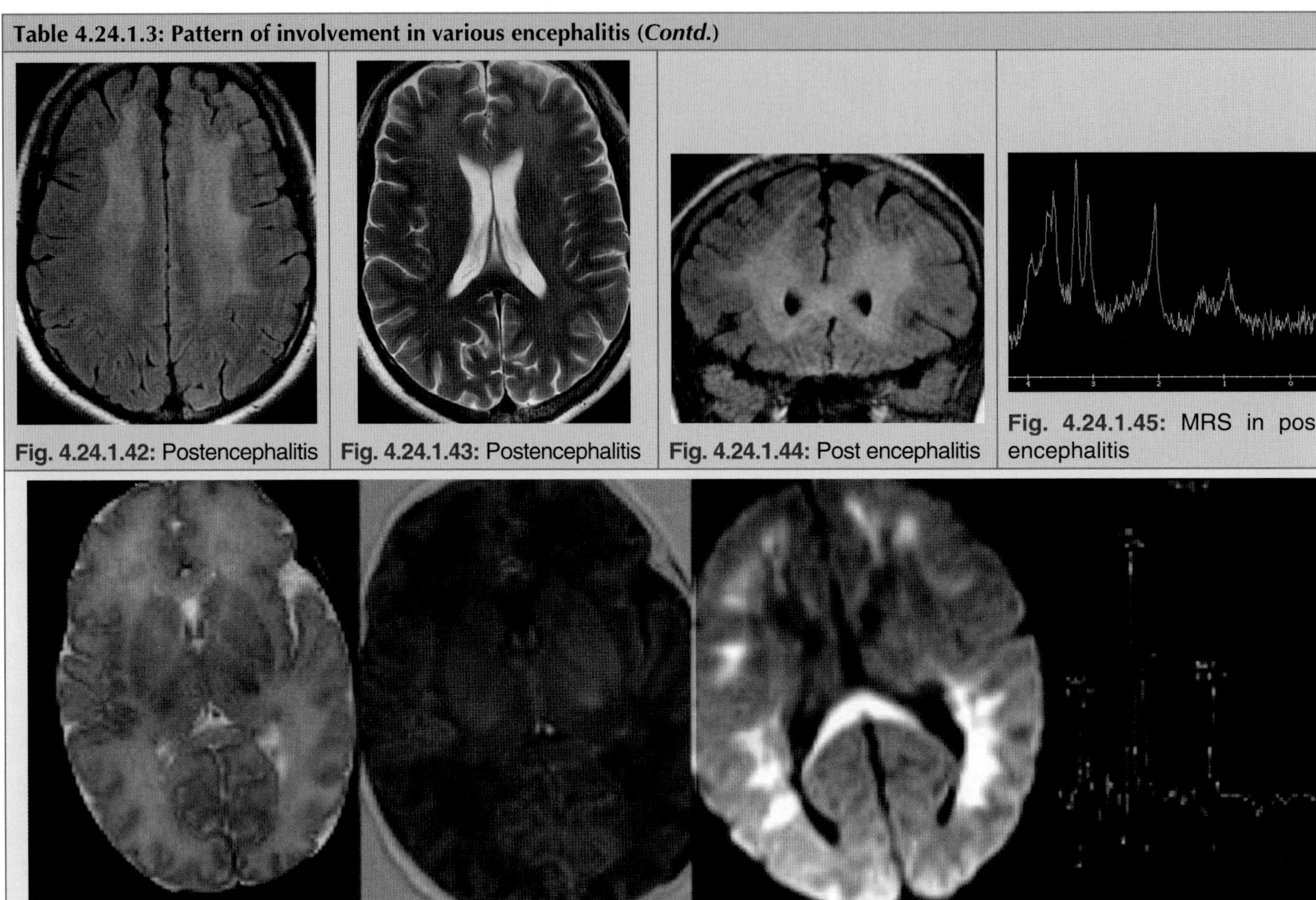

Fig. 4.24.1.42: Postencephalitis

Fig. 4.24.1.43: Postencephalitis

Fig. 4.24.1.44: Post encephalitis

Fig. 4.24.1.45: MRS in post-encephalitis

Fig. 4.24.1.46: Parechovirus encephalitis

Parechovirus causes a spectrum of diseases including aseptic meningitis, gastroenteritis, encephalitis, respiratory diseases, and neonatal sepsis-like disease. HPeV infection is **more common in full-term infants in the neonatal period**. Restricted diffusion in the periventricular and subcortical white matter, in particular the frontal white matter, but also the corpus callosum, internal capsule, part of the thalamus and pyramidal tracts of the brain stem.

Table 4.24.1.4: Clinicoradiological features for various encephalitis

Disease	*Main clinical characteristics*	*Main imaging characteristics*	*Main differential diagnosis*
Herpes encephalitis	Fever, headaches, seizures and altered mental status	Asymmetric bilateral temporal lobe disease; insular disease; stops at the lateral putaminal border. Gyral enhancement and cortical micro-bleeds on MRI	HHV-6 encephalopathy, fungal infection, adult type OTC deficiency, glioma
HHV6 encephalopathy	Change in the mental status, loss of short-term memory and seizures about 3 weeks post-transplant	Symmetric mesial temporal lobe and limbic system disease	Herpes encephalitis, limbic encephalitis
Fungal infection	Spread of paranasal sinus infection in immune-compromised patients	Brain edema, hemorrhages, irregular enhancement. Paranasal sinus infection	Herpes encephalitis
Limbic encephalitis	Subacute presentation with personality changes, irritability, depression, dementia, seizures and short-term memory loss	Unilateral or bilateral mesio-temporal disease. Enhancement can occur as well as involvement of additional limbic system components and other brain regions	HHV-6 encephalopathy, Alzheimer disease, fronto-temporal dementia
Alzheimer disease	Cognitive decline interfering with daily activities	Disproportional asymmetric volume loss in the mesial temporal structures	Fronto-temporal dementia, limbic encephalitis, remote insult (sequel of herpes encephalitis, trauma)
Fronto-temporal dementia	Changes in personality and behavior and decline in semantic performance	Asymmetric temporal lobe atrophy in semantic variant of the disease	Alzheimer disease, remote insult (sequel of herpes encephalitis, trauma)
Adult type OTC deficiency	Acute encephalopathy	Symmetric disease of the insula and cingulate gyrus with increased T2 signal and diffusion restriction, and without enhancement	Herpes encephalitis, glioma
Mesial temporal sclerosis	Complex partial seizures	Hippocampal atrophy and increased T2/FLAIR. Bilateral in 10%	Limbic encephalitis, other temporal lobe epileptogenic diseases
Glioma	Insidious course of worsening neurological deficits; new onset seizures; change in mental status	Edema, infiltration and possible enhancement (depending on tumoral grade); possible spread along nerve tracts	Herpes encephalitis, limbic encephalitis, adult type OTC deficiency
Posterior circulation ischemia	Acute visual and memory deficits and altered mental status	Ischemic lesions in PCA territory	Herpes encephalitis
CADASIL	Recurrent strokes, migraine, cognitive decline	Focal lesions of increased T2 signal in anterior temporal lobe and external capsule. Periventricular and deep white matter lesions throughout the brain; lacunar infarctions	Microangiopathy, cerebral vasculitis
Trauma	History of traumatic insult	Anterior temporal cortical contusions and/or epidural or subdural hematomas	Post-traumatic encephalomalacia may simulate atrophy
Radiation necrosis	History of prior radiation to head and neck	Edema and enhancement within the radiation port	Herpes encephalitis, glioma

4.24.2 CENTRAL NERVOUS SYSTEM

Case No. 24.2

Case history: A 14-year-old female came with complaints of recurrent seizures for 3 years.

Radiological techniques and observations:
Figures 4.24.2.1 to 4.24.2.6 are FLAIR coronal, T2 coronal, T2 axial, SPGR, magnified T2 coronal and FLAIR coronal view images respectively showing altered T2 signal intensity, loss of volume in the left hippocampus with mild prominent temporal horn of left lateral ventricle. Amygdala appears prominent showing T2/FLAIR hyperintensity. Left mamillary body and fornix show mild atrophy. Cortical gyral thickening in the left temporal and right frontal region with blurring of gray white matter junction and subcortical hyperintensity in the right frontal region on FLAIR.

Interpretation: A—14-year-old female, pathology in left hippocampus and right frontal region, C—volume loss in hippocampus, B—prominent left temporal horn and prominent amygdala, mild atrophy in left mamillary body and fornix, gyral thickening with subcortical hyperintensity in frontal region, D—left mesial temporal sclerosis with focal cortical dysplasia.

Principal diagnosis: Left mesial temporal sclerosis with focal cortical dysplasia

Treatment: Anteromedial temporal lobectomy is the treatment for MTS with drug resistant temporal lobe epilepsy.

Discussion: Epilepsy is defined as "any of various disorders marked by abnormal electrical discharges in the brain and typically manifested by sudden brief episodes of altered or diminished consciousness, involuntary movements, or convulsions". Dysfunction caused by an abnormal electrical discharge in the brain. Epilepsy is the condition of spontaneously recurrent seizures. Not all epilepsy can be controlled by drugs. Surgery is a treatment alternative in selected cases. Based on anatomical location, epilepsy can be temporal lobe epilepsy (mesial and neocortical) and extra temporal epilepsy. Seizures can be partial (focal onset) and generalised (global onset with loss of consciousness). Partial seizures without loss of consciousness is simple partial seizures and partial seizures with loss of consciousness is complex partial seizures. Partial seizures can be seen with resistance to antiepileptic drugs and surgical resection of brain provoking seizures. Causes of epilepsy can be summarised as idiopathic: epilepsy due to an underlying single gene condition or complex inheritance (seizures can be only manifestation); cryptogenic (unknown cause); provoked epilepsy,

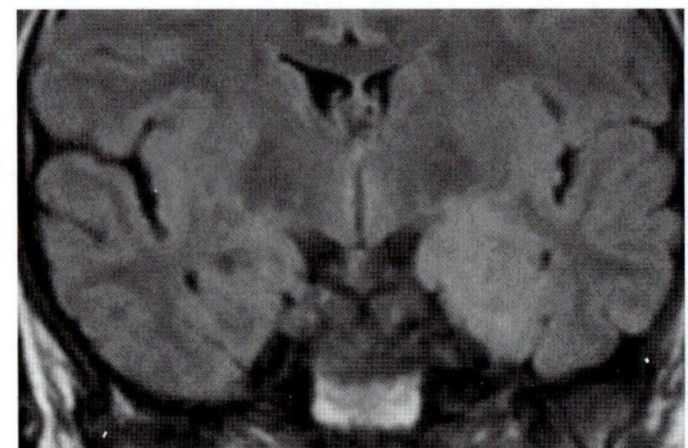
Fig. 4.24.2.1

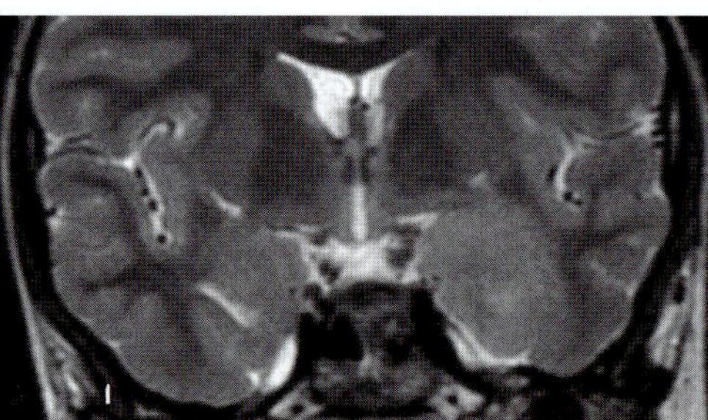
Fig. 4.24.2.2

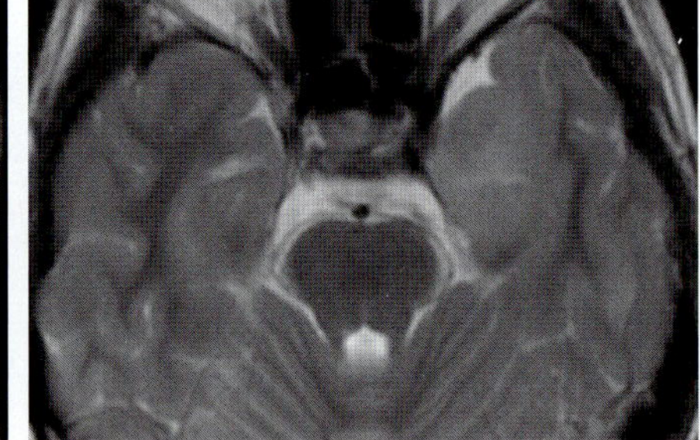
Fig. 4.24.2.3

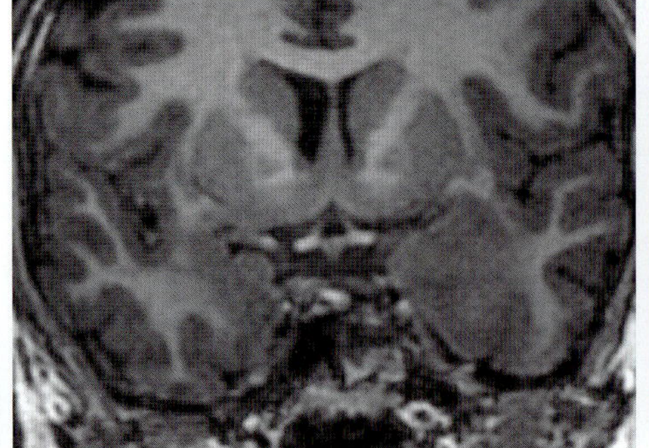
Fig. 4.24.2.4

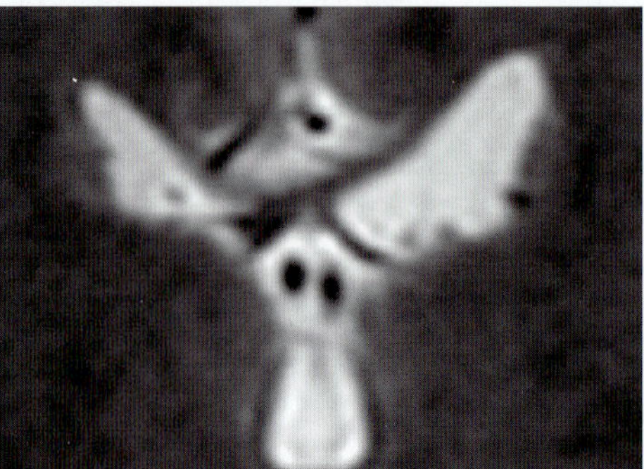
Fig. 4.24.2.5

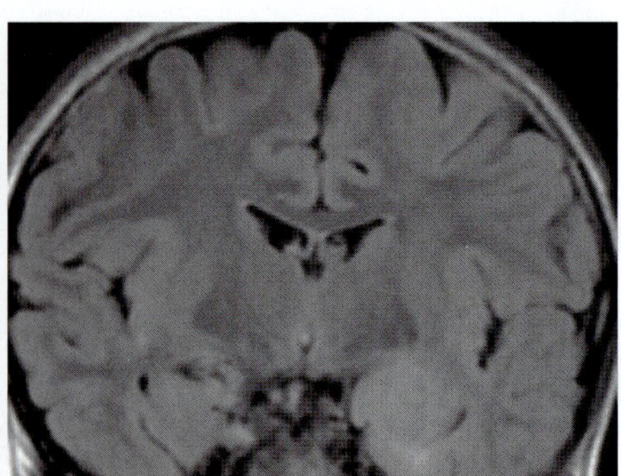
Fig. 4.24.2.6

Differential diagnosis	
Status epilepticus/Postictal edema In temporal lobe epilepsy, hyperperfusion to temporal lobes may mimic HSE. No hemorrhage is seen in status epilepticus. T2/FLAIR hyperintensity typically involving just the cortex and usually unilateral. No evidence of blooming in T2*. Diffusion restriction +	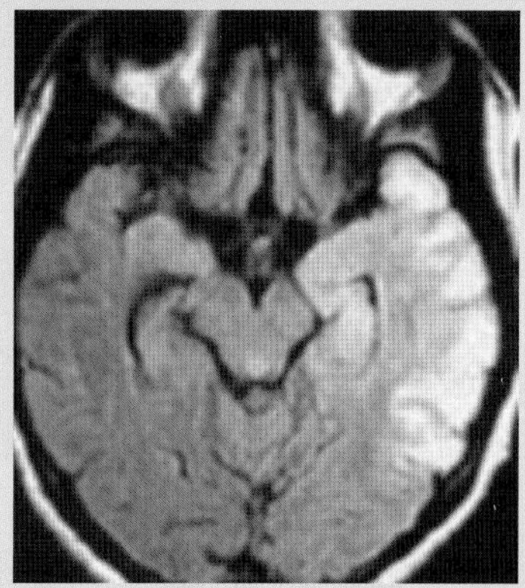 **Fig. 4.24.2.7:** Postictal edema

Status epilepticus

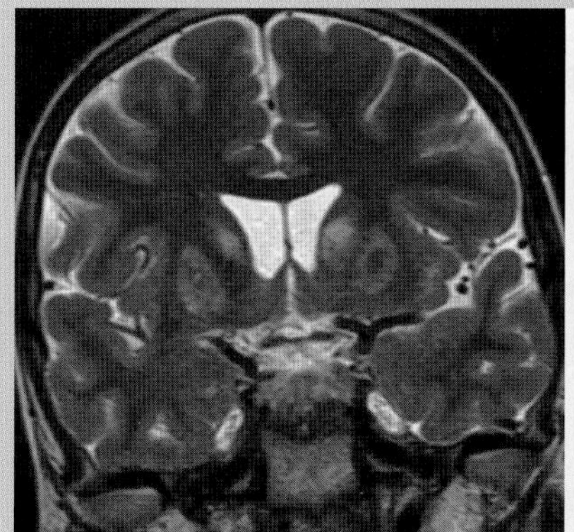
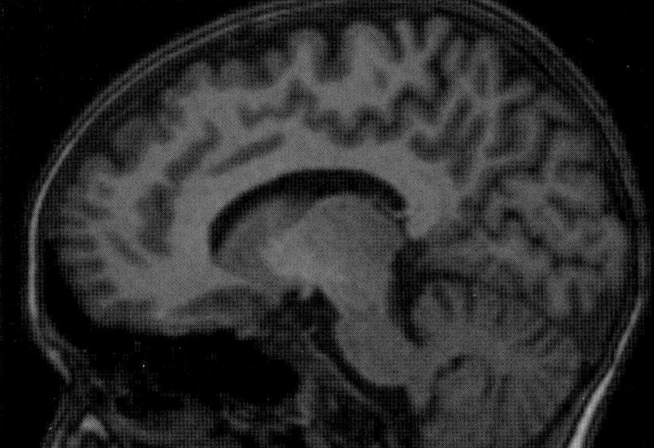
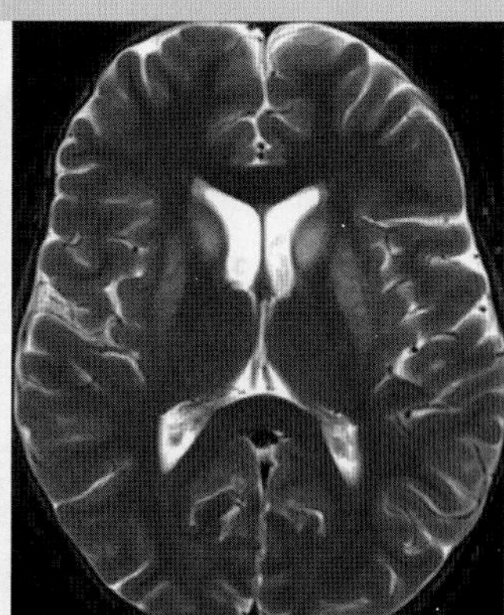

Fig. 4.24.2.8: Status epilepticus

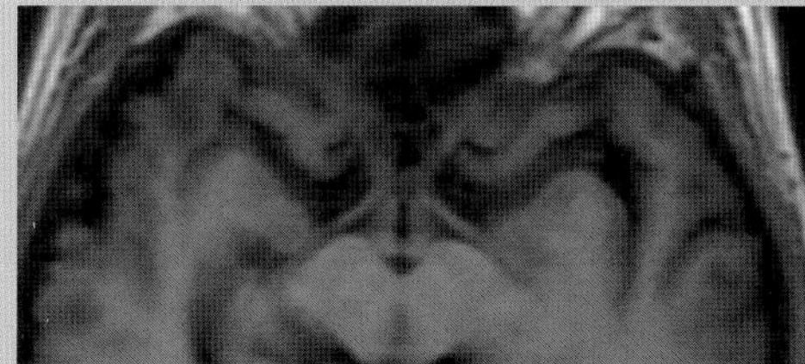
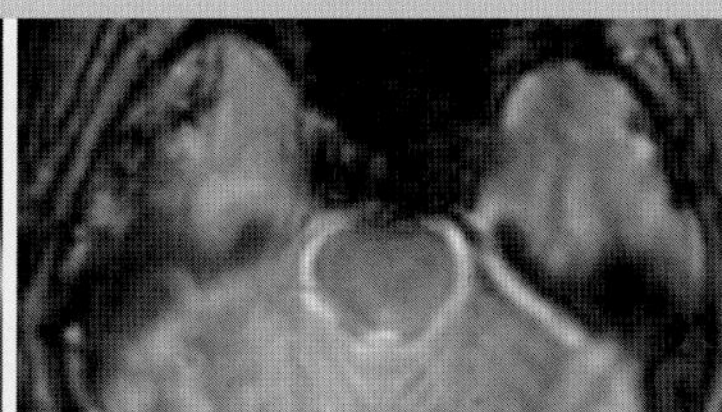
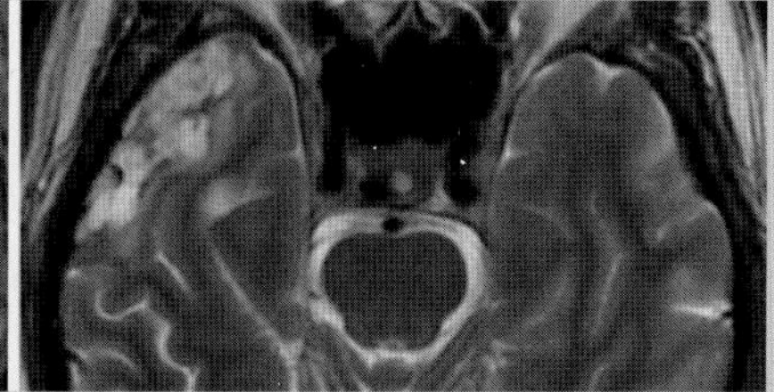

Fig. 4.24.2.9: Old trauma leading to status epilepticus

Anterior temporal lobe cortical dysplasia

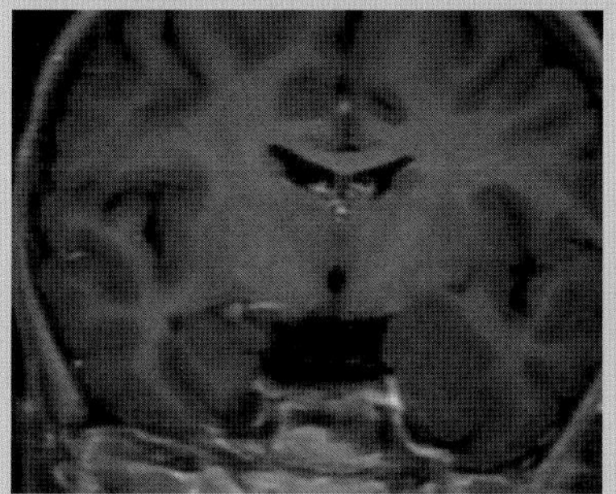 **Fig. 4.24.2.10:** Anterior temporal lobe cortical dysplasia	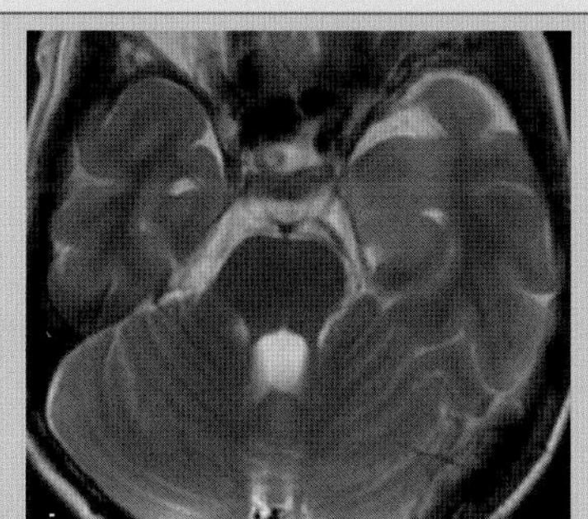 **Fig. 4.24.2.11:** Anterior temporal lobe cortical dysplasia	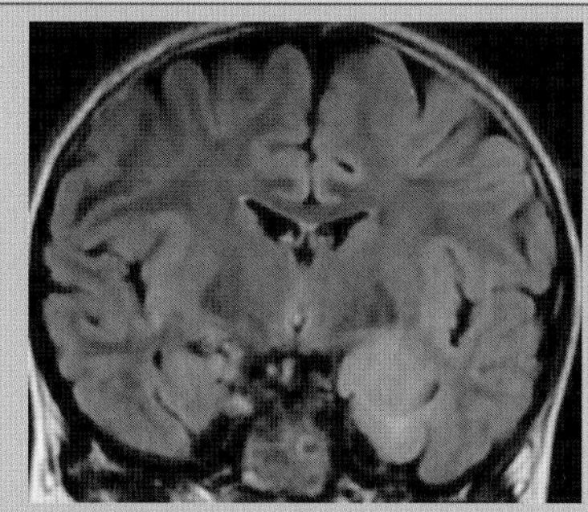 **Fig. 4.24.2.12:** Anterior temporal lobe cortical dysplasia

Contd...

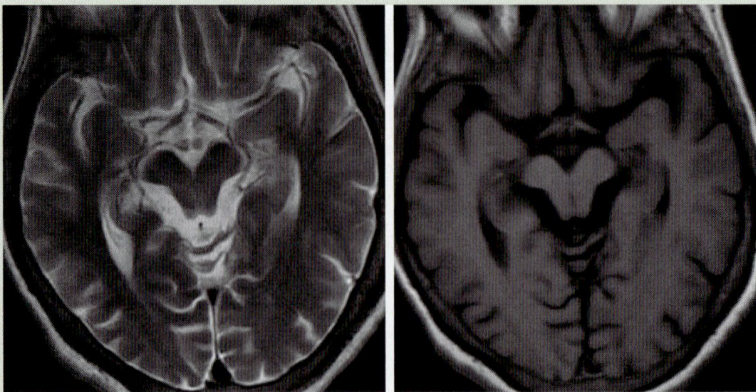

Fig. 4.24.2.13: Bilateral hippocampal atrophy

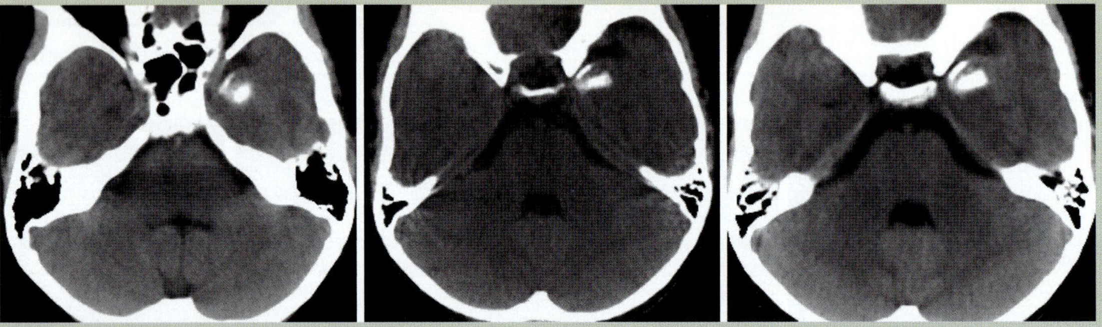

Fig. 4.24.2.14: Calcified lesion in temporal lobe

Crossed cerebellar diaschisis—refer to case 4.24.1

Focal cortical dysplasia showing cortical thickening

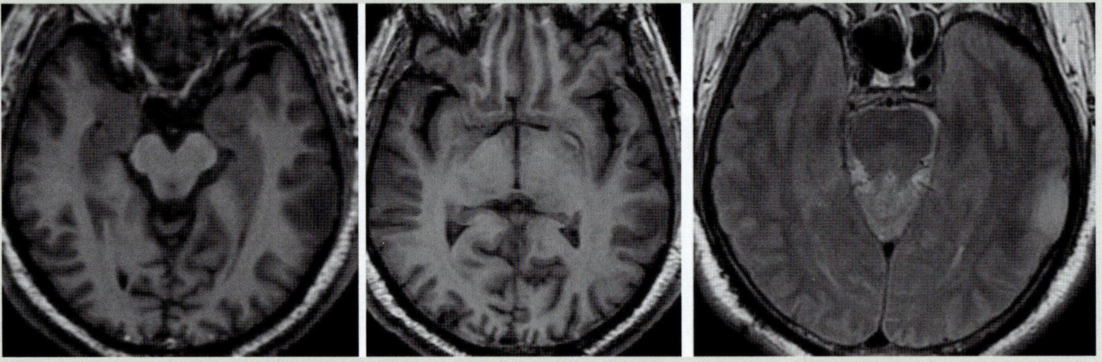

Fig. 4.24.2.15: Focal cortical dysplasia showing cortical thickening

Hemicerebral dysplasia is generally associated with seizures and hemiplegia. Changes within the brain parenchyma can demonstrate thinning of the grey matter cortex, reduced volume in underlying white matter +/– reduced/abnormal myelination, enlargement of the lateral ventricle, ipsilateral reduced size of cerebral peduncle, contralateral reduced size of cerebellar hemisphere.

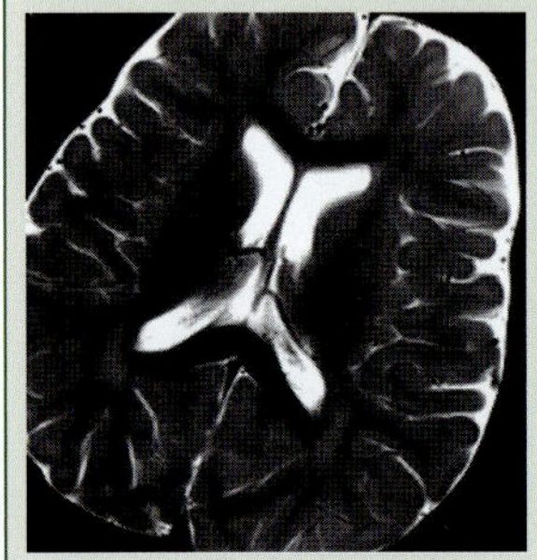

Fig. 4.24.2.16: Hemicerebral dysplasia

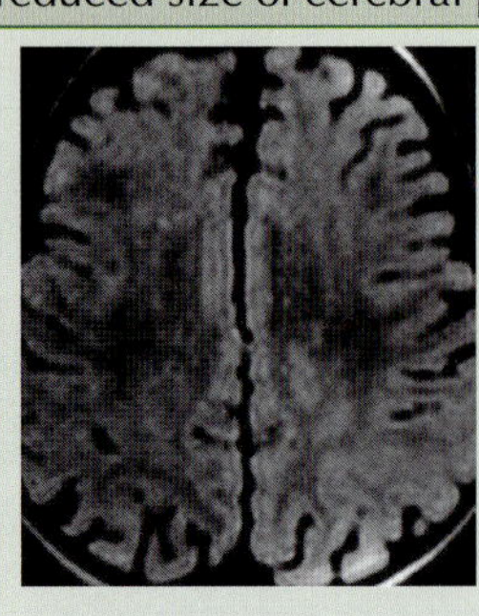

Fig. 4.24.2.17: Hemi cerebral dysplasia

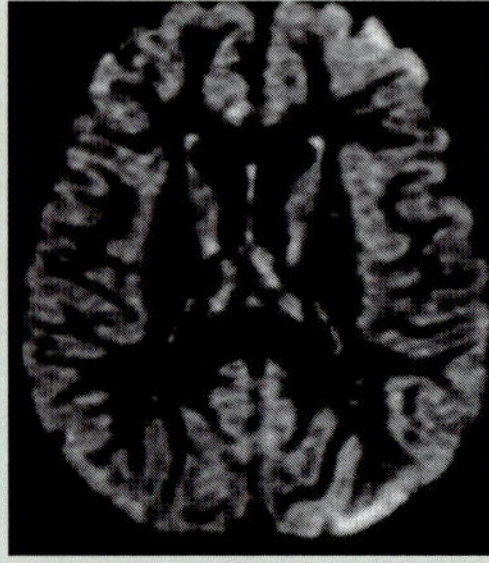

Fig. 4.24.2.18: Hemi cerebral dysplasia

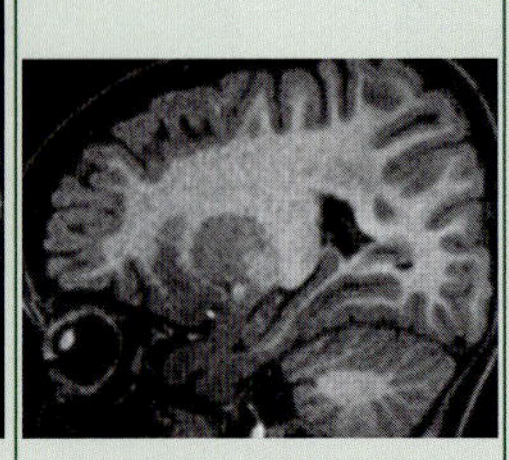

Fig. 4.24.2.19: Hemicerebral dysplasia

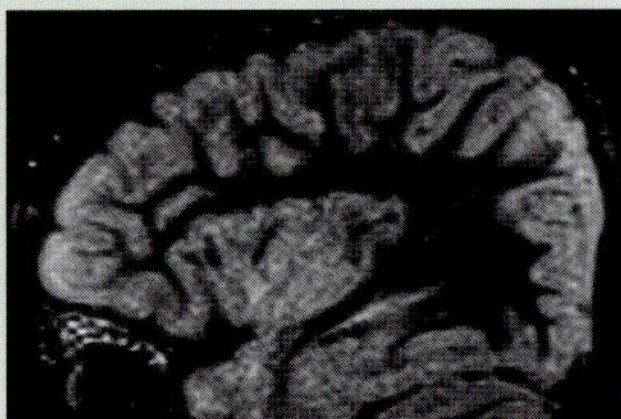

Fig. 4.24.2.20: Hemicerebral dysplasia

Postfebrile reversible claustrum damage presents as status epilepticus after an episode of febrile illness, there is bilateral reversible T2 hyperintensity without diffusion restriction. Follow-up imaging should be done 3 weeks after the onset of seizure episodes.

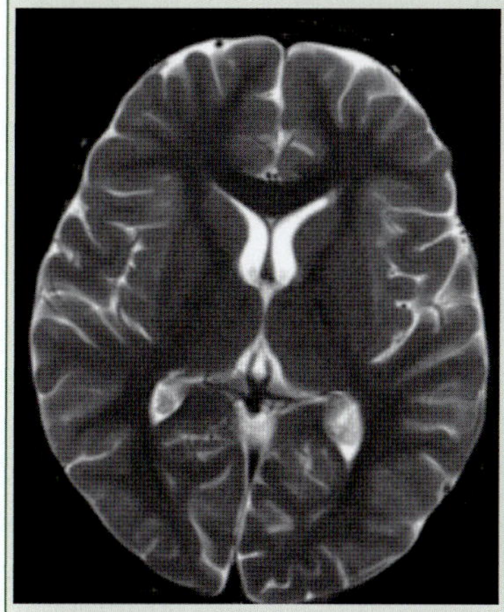

Fig. 4.24.2.21: Postfebrile reversible claustrum damage

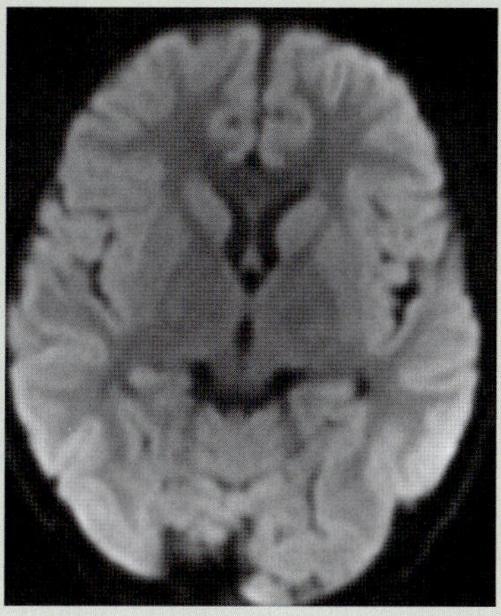

Fig. 4.24.2.22: Postfebrile reversible claustrum damage

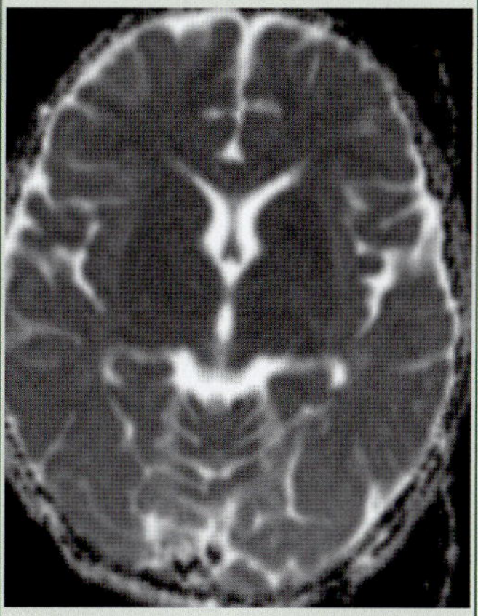

Fig. 4.24.2.23: Postfebrile reversible claustrum damage

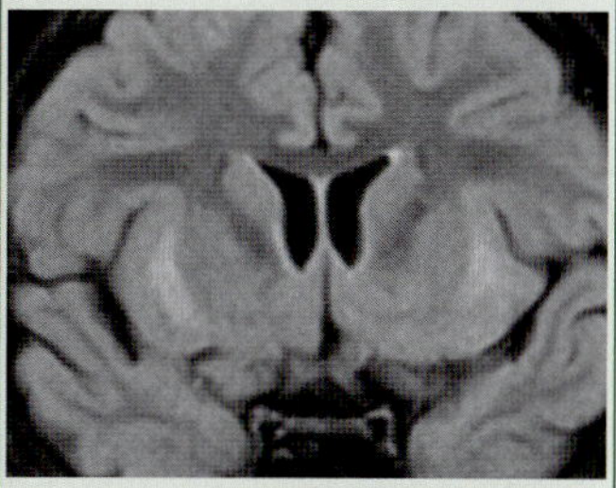

Fig. 4.24.2.24: Febrile infection related epilepsy syndrome (FIRES)

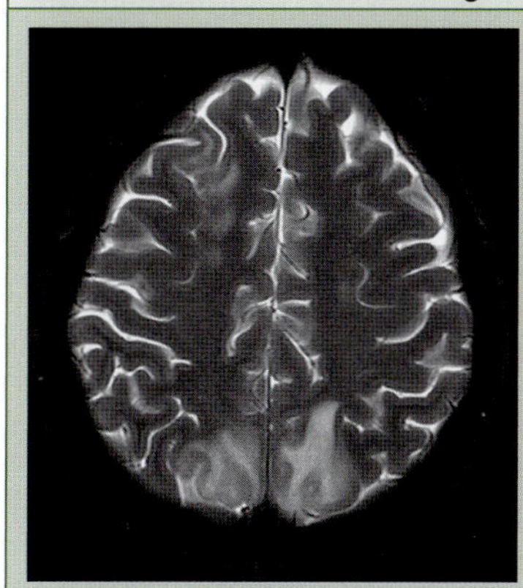

Fig. 4.24.2.25: Postpartum PRES

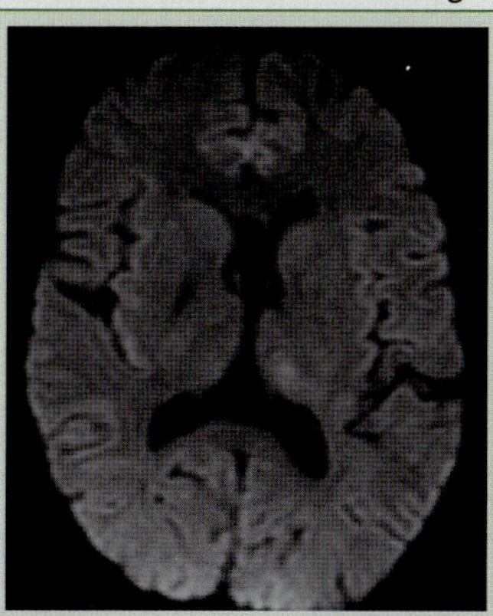

Fig. 4.24.2.26: Postpartum PRES

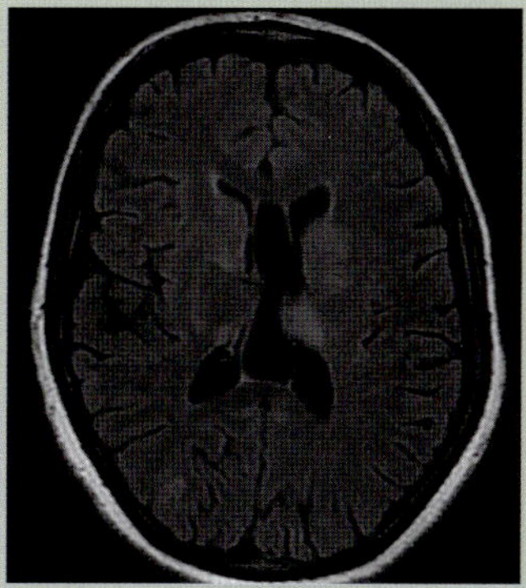

Fig. 4.24.2.27: Postpartum PRES

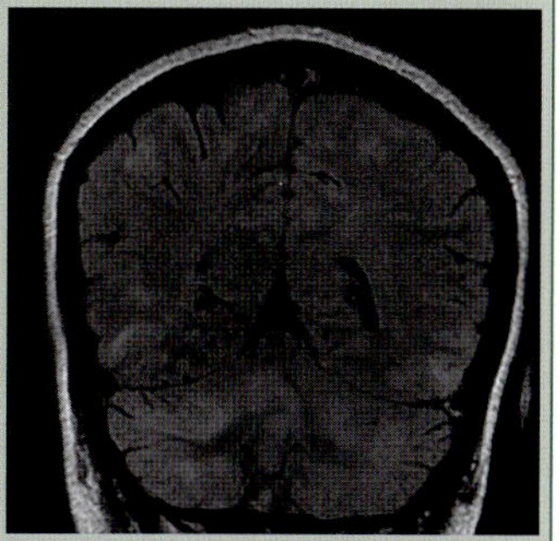

Fig. 4.24.2.28: Postpartum PRES

Rasmussen's encephalitis – Refer to case 24 A

Incomplete hippocampal inversion/vertical hippocampus:

It results from failure of hippocampal inversion during fetal development. On medical imaging, the hippocampus has normal signal intensity and volume, but an abnormal globular or pyramidal shape. The collateral sulcus has more vertical orientation than usual and is found lateral from hippocampal body. IHI is unilateral and left-sided in the majority of cases.

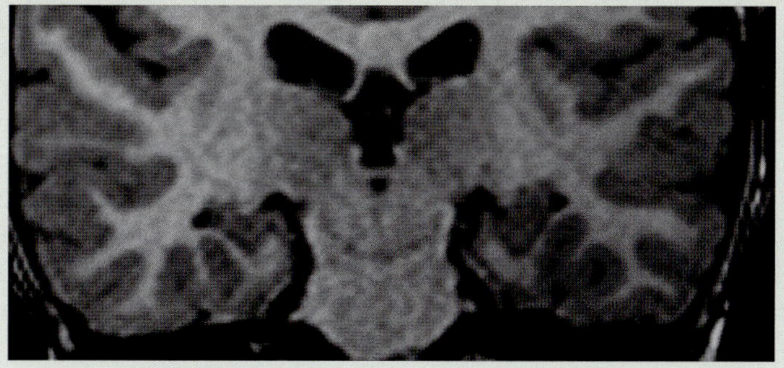

Fig. 4.24.2.29: Vertical hippocampus

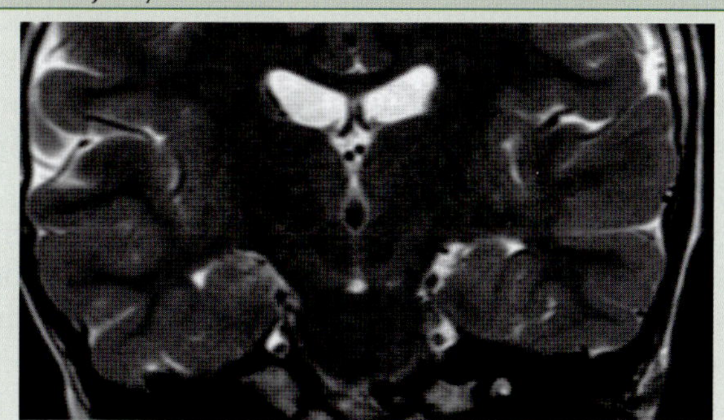

Fig. 4.24.2.30: Vertical hippocampus

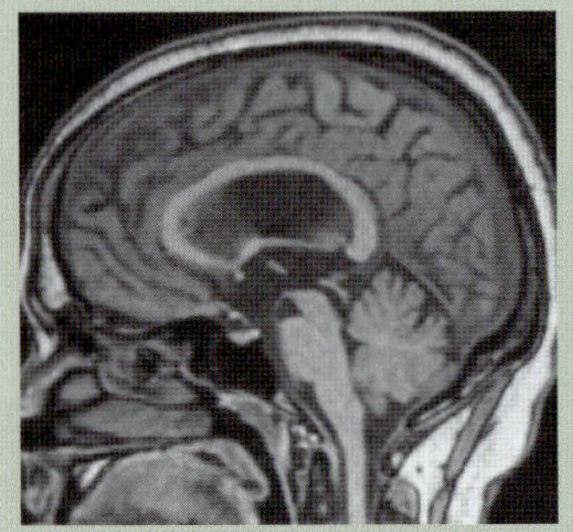 Fig. 4.24.2.31: Bilateral mesial temporal sclerosis	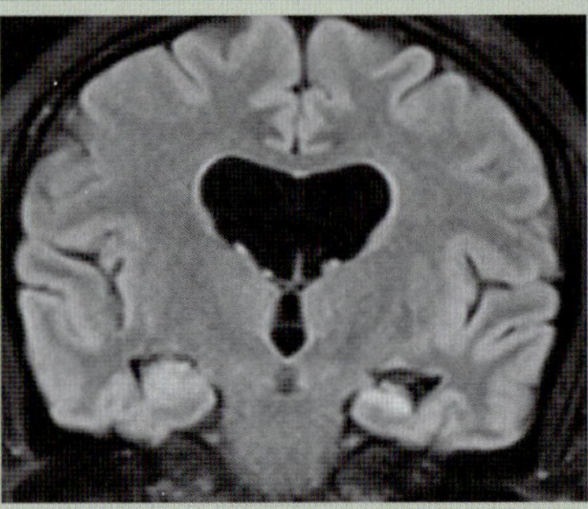 Fig. 4.24.2.32: Bilateral mesial temporal sclerosis	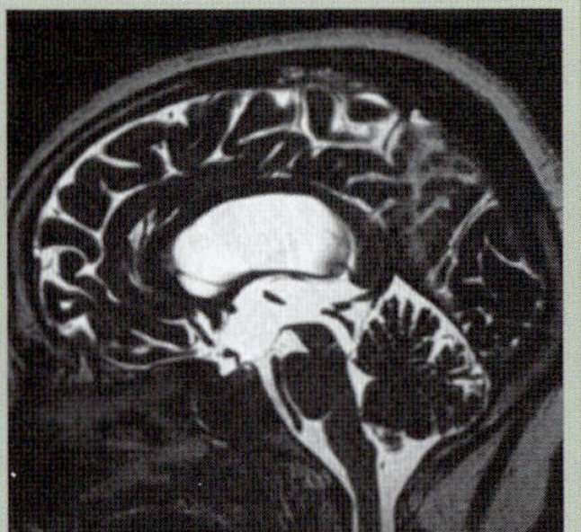 Fig. 4.24.2.33: Bilateral mesial temporal sclerosis	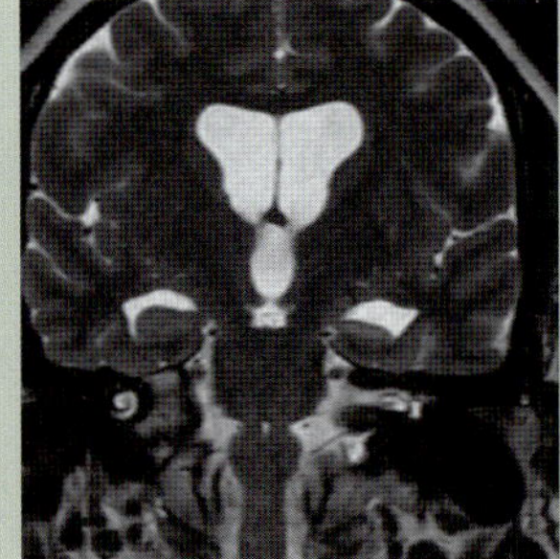 Fig. 4.24.2.34: Bilateral mesial temporal sclerosis

Other causes of epilepsy include heterotopia, polymicrogyria, hemimegalencephaly: Refer to case 3.2; Tuberous sclerosis: Refer to case 7; Leukodystrophy: Refer to case 37

Hippocampal hyperintensity without volume loss is seen in status epilepticus, low grade tumors (astrocytoma, DNET), encephalitis.

DD for microbleed in adults with epilepsy–cavernoma, cerebral amyloid angiopathy, hypertensive hemorrhage and post-trauma diffuse axonal injury.

Epilepsy associated tumors—ganglioglioma, DNET, pleomorphic xanthoastrocytoma, hypothalamic hamartoma, multinodular and vacuolating neuronal tumors (MVNT). These tumors arise in cortical location, often located in temporal lobe, may be related to developmental, malformations, typically seen in adolescents and young adults. They are characterised by benign behaviour, slow growth, sharp delineation, usually show absence of edema and signs of chronicity like bone remodelling, scalloping of adjacent skull. Ganglioglioma is the most common tumor associated with epilepsy.

DNET in a patient with epilepsy

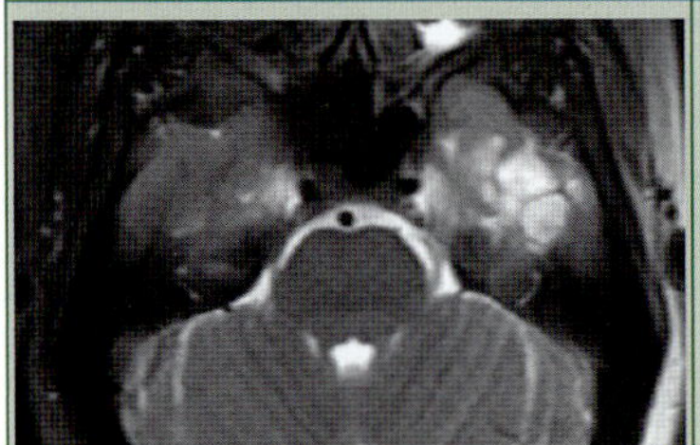 Fig. 4.24.2.35: DNET in a patient with epilepsy	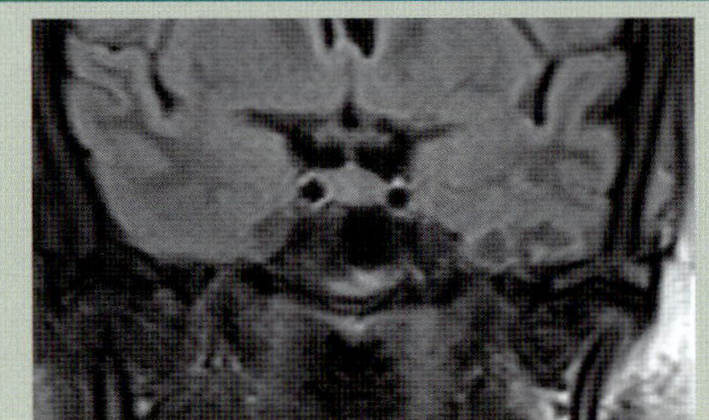 Fig. 4.24.2.36: MVNT in a patient with epilepsy	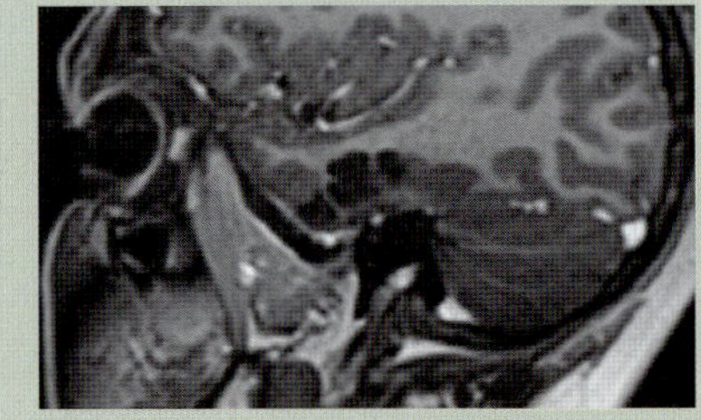 Fig. 4.24.2.37: DNET in a patient with epilepsy

e.g. secondary to fevers, bacteria/viral meningitis, head trauma, drug-induced; predominantly genetic/ developmental causation; Rasmussen encephalitis; childhood epilepsy syndromes; progressive myoclonic epilepsies; neurocutaneous syndromes (Sturge-Weber syndrome, tuberous sclerosis); chromosomal disorders; mesial temporal sclerosis; developmental cortical abnormalities (FCD, heterotopia, polymicrogyria, hemimegalencephaly; schizencephaly); stroke, cerebral palsy, vascular malformations; meningoencephaloceles; tumors (ganglioglioma, DNET, pleomorphic xantho-astrocytoma, hypothalamic hamartoma). MRI is the imaging modality of choice. SPECT perfusion brain useful for localizing the epileptogenic focus. Conditions treated by surgery: Hippocampal sclerosis— 50–70%, perinatal hypoxia—15–35%, tumors—15%, vascular malformations—3%, traumatic gliosis—2% and developmental—2%. Surgeries done for epilepsy—anterior temporal lobectomy, lesionectomy, non-lesional cortical excision, corpus callosotomy, hemispherectomy and multiple subpial transections.

Mesial temporal sclerosis: The most common type of localisation related epilepsy. It commonly affects older children and younger adults. MRI (temporal epilepsy protocol) is the modality of choice, abnormal T2/FLAIR hyperintensity with obscuration of internal hippocampal architecture. No contrast enhancement is seen. True coronal IR/3D SPGR sequence shows shrunken hippocampus with atrophy of the ipsilateral fornix and widening of the adjacent temporal horn. higher signal on ADC as a result of neuronal volume loss and increased water molecules diffusion. DWI restriction may be see following seizures. MRS—decreased NAA, NAA/Cho and NAA/Cr ratios. Decreased MI in ipsilateral temporal lobe. Increase in lipid and lactate is seen soon after seizure. MR perfusion/Tc99m HMPAO

SPECT/ECD SPECT/F18G PET—Increased perfusion in peri-ictal phase and reduced perfusion in interictal period.

Associated findings of MTS are atrophy of the ipsilateral fornix and mammillary body, increased signal and or atrophy of the anterior thalamic nucleus, atrophy of the cingulate gyrus, increased signal and/or reduction in the volume of the amygdala, reduction in the volume of the subiculum, dilatation of temporal horn and temporal lobe atrophy, collateral white matter and entorhinal cortex atrophy, thalamic and caudate atrophy, ipsilateral cerebral hypertrophy, contralateral cerebellar hemi atrophy, loss of grey-white matter interface in the anterior temporal lobe and reduced white matter volume in the parahippocampal gyrus. These are seen in chronic cases.

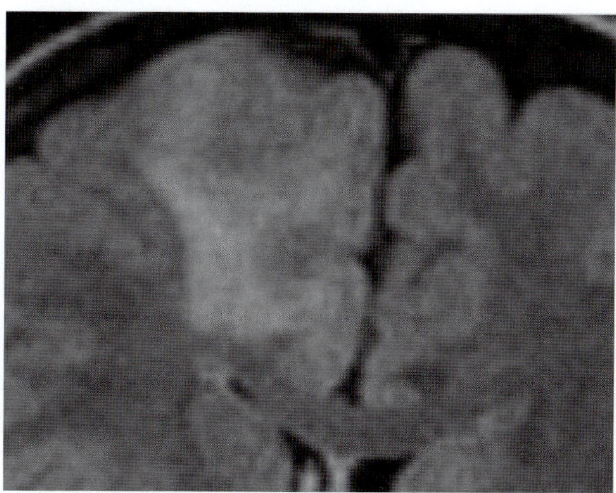

Fig. 4.24.2.38: Focal cortical dysplasia

Focal cortical dysplasia: A common cause of medically refractory epilepsy in children and adults. Mostly unilateral presentation. CT–usually normal unless the lesion is very large. MRI helps to identify general features of focal cortical dysplasia such as cortical thickening; blurring of white matter–grey matter junction with abnormal architecture of subcortical layer; T2/FLAIR signal hyperintensity of white matter with or without the **trans mantle sign (T2/FLAIR signal hyperintensity that extends from ventricles to cortex)**; abnormal sulcal or gyral pattern; segmental and/or lobar hypoplasia/atrophy.

Table 4.24.2.1: Multimodality approach for functional neuroimaging in epilepsy

Multimodality approach—functional neuroimaging: Structural MRI, SPECT—MRI, PET-MRI, functional MRI (fMRI) and diffusion MRI (DTI, tractography). Other investigations include sophisticated electrophysiological analyses based on EEG (dipole analysis, CURRY, BESA etc), MEG (megnetoencephalography), intracranial electrodes for registration and stimulation and transcranial magnetic stimulation. Six zones of epilepsy include lesion (epileptogenic area), seizure onset zone, irritative zone, symptomatogenic zone, functional deficit zone and epileptogenic zone (theoretical concept). Ideal zone of surgery is where all zones overlap. **MRI imaging protocol**

Epilepsy outpatient protocol 'Essential Six'	**Nonfocal epilepsy protocol (ideal protocol)**	**Temporal lobe epilepsy protocol**
3D T1 – 1 mm isotropic acquisition. (SPGR) T2, FLAIR 3 mm axial and coronal - hippocampus cut plane angulation; SWI 3 mm axial	T1 axial and coronal or 3D T1 isotropic acquisition (SPGR) FLAIR-axial and angled coronal or 3D FLAIR isotropic acquisition. Double inversion recovery sequences—DIR 3D isotropic acquisition DWI/ADC SWI	T1 axial and coronal or 3D T1 isotropic acquisition (SPGR) FLAIR—axial and angled coronal or 3D FLAIR isotropic acquisition. T2—angled coronal DWI/ADC SWI Fiber tracking technique

Functional imaging: Ictal SPECT– Single-photon-emission computed tompgraphy **(SPECT MRI –SISCOM)**. It is technically challenging as we watch the patient and EEG full time with isotope at hand. Isotope is injected as soon the seizure begins (10 to 20 sec). Seizures should be stereotype and last >10 sec. Increased cerebral blood flow in regions affected by seizure activity. Tc99m-labelled compounds (cysteinate dimer-HMPAO) is used followed by snapshot of blood perfusion taken in a couple of hours of injection. It takes 15–20 seconds for Tc99m to reach the brain. It has possibility to identify the seizure origin zone, reveal previously occult abnormality and guide placement of intracranial electrode placement.

Table 4.24.2.2: Classification of focal cortical dysplasia		
Palmini classification system for cortical dysplasia's—older classification system that divides cortical dysplasia into mild MCD (type 1 and 2) and FCD (types 1a/ab and 2a/ab) is now obsolete.		
	Classification system of focal cortical dysplasia by Blumcke, et al. 2011	*Radiological correlation features*
Type	*Pathological characteristic features*	
I	a. Focal cortical dysplasia with abnormal radial cortical lamination b. Focal cortical dysplasia with abnormal tangential 6-layer cortical lamination c. Focal cortical dysplasia with abnormal radial and tangential cortical lamination	a. Temporal lobe predominant, mild hemispheric hypoplasia without other visible lesions.
II	a. Focal cortical dysplasia with dysmorphic neurons b. Focal cortical dysplasia with dysmorphic neurons and balloon cells	Frontal lobe predominant Type II—cortical thickening, blurring if GWM junction, cortical signal intensity, subcortical WM hyperintensity and trans mantle sign Lesion signal intensity in FCD type IIb is hyperintense in T1W and mildly hypointense in T2W with increased diffusion, fractional anisotropy, reduced NAA: Cr ratio and increased myoinositol rates. Decreased/normal rCBV.
III	a. Architectural distortion of cortical layer in temporal lobe with hippocampal atrophy b. Architectural distortion of cortical layer adjacent to glial or glioneuronal tumor c. Architectural distortion of cortical layer adjacent to vascular malformation d. Architectural distortion of cortical layer adjacent to other lesions acquired in early childhood such as trauma, ischemic event, encephalitis	Type III–hippocampal sclerosis IIIa—volume loss in the anterior temporal lobe with abnormal white matter hyperintensity on T2 and FLAIR images, while the cortex appears normal from other views. III b/c/d—underlying cause such as glioneuronal tumour (b), vascular malformation (IIIc), gliosis due to early childhood insult (III d) can be identified.

4.25 CENTRAL NERVOUS SYSTEM

Case No. 25

Clinical history: 25-years-old female with complaints of recurrent history of focal motor and sensory deficits.

Imaging technique and observation:

Figures 4.25.1 to 4.25.7 are MRI T1 axial, T2 axial/ sagittal sections of the brain and T2 sagittal cord images respectively. It demonstrates numerous white matter T2 hyperintense lesions predominantly in a callososeptal interface, periventricular, juxtacortical and infratentorial regions. As well as T1 linear hypointensities in periventricular region—Dawson finger. No evidence of optic nerve involvement. Multiple patchy short segment T2 hyperintensiy involving the cervical and upper dorsal cord are seen.

Interpretation: A—25 years old female, callososeptal interface, periventricular, juxtacortical, infratentorial and cervical cord shows linear/ovoid T2 hyperintensities with T1 hypointensities, B—multiple tiny short segment lesions in cord, D—multiple sclerosis.

Principal diagnosis: Multiple sclerosis.

Management:

Further investigation: CSF Oligoclonal bands (80%) in multiple sclerosis.

Treatment: Acute phase: Oral or IV methylprednisolone 1 gm per day for 3 days; ***disease modifiying therapy:*** Relapsing and remitting multiple sclerosis (RRMS)–either interferon beta or Glatiramer acetate to be started. Secondary progressive multiple sclerosis (SPMS)–interferon beta to be started.

Discussion: Revised McDonald criteria (2017) for MS Diagnosis: ***Dissemination in space (DIS)*** ≥1 T2 hyperintense lesion(s). In at least 2 of the following

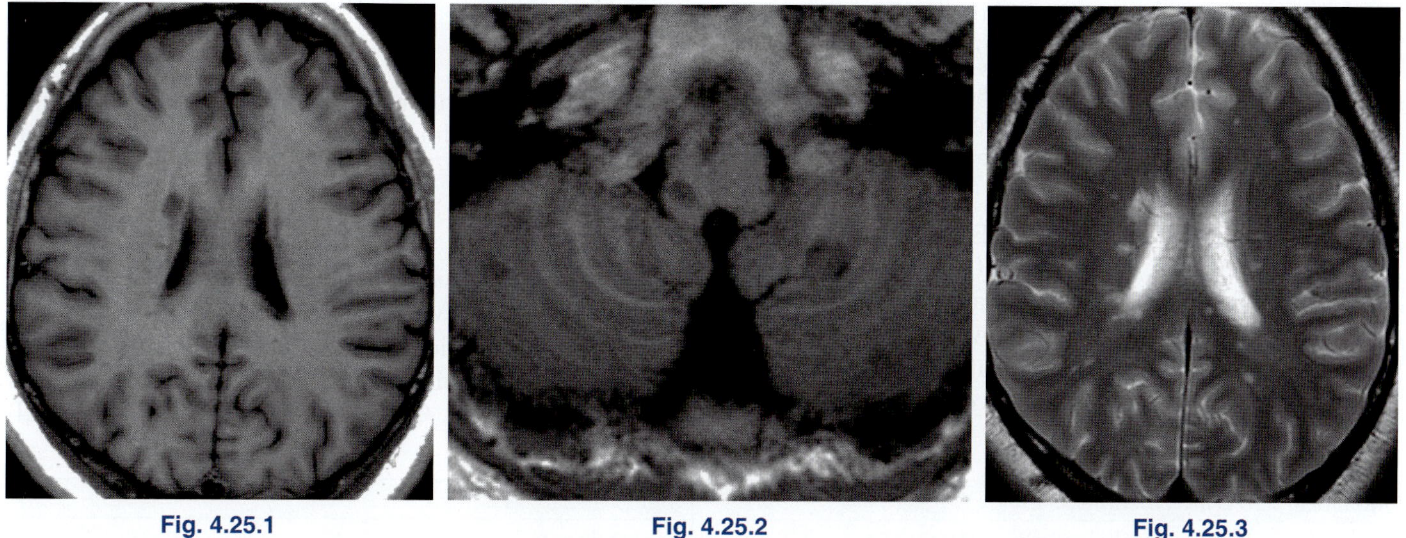

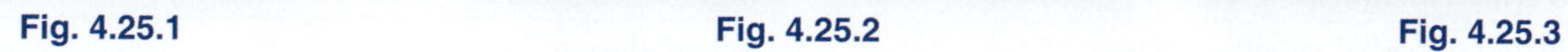

Fig. 4.25.1 Fig. 4.25.2 Fig. 4.25.3

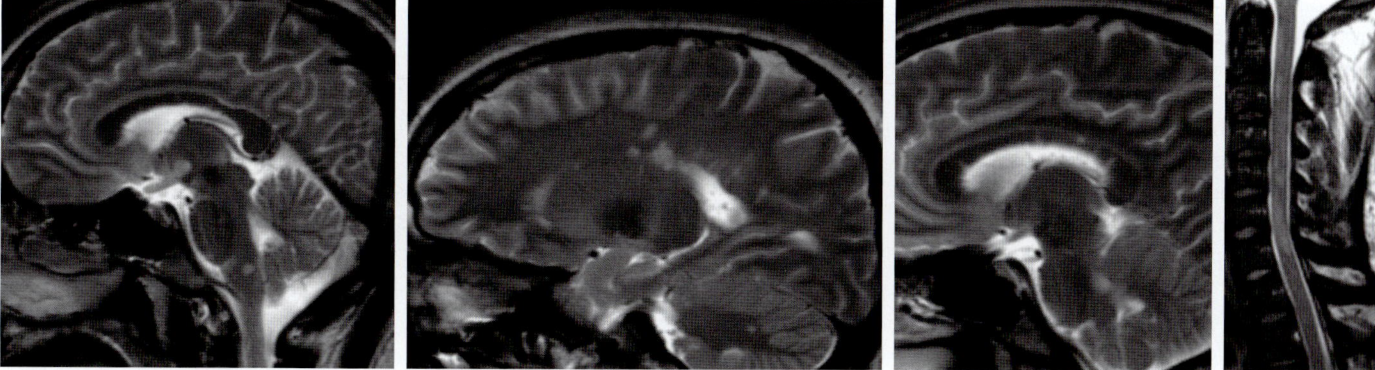

Fig. 4.25.4 Fig. 4.25.5 Fig. 4.25.6 Fig. 4.25.7

4 areas: 1. Periventricular, 2. juxtacortical/cortical, 3. infratentorial, 4. spinal cord.

Dissemination in time (DIT): Either new T2 or Gd-enhancing lesion(s) on follow-up MR or simultaneous presence of asymptomatic Gd-enhancing and nonenhancing lesions at any period of time.

Spinal cord screening: The most common site of involvement is cervical cord. Characteristic features are involvement of less than ½ cross-sectional area, <2 segments involvement, dorsolateral, peripheral involvement, associated with brain lesions with remitting and relapsing course.

Atypical acute presentations of multiple sclerosis: ***Tumefactive demyelination***—large demyelinating brain lesions that mimic primary brain tumors.

Marburg variant—rare variant of fulminant form of idiopathic inflammatory demyelination in young adults, involving the brain stem.

Baló's concentric sclerosis—rare severe acute process involving centrum semiovale and corona radiata with T2 alternating concentric rings (onion bulb).

Schilder's disease—rare acute/subacute disorder affecting children and young adults. Clinical: Psychiatric symptomatology, acute IICT, progressive in course, MRI: Large ring enhancing lesions usually over the parieto-occipital region.

Recurrent ADEM: 25 to 33% of ADEM patients will have relapses in the future. Recurrence of the initial symptoms and signs three or more months after the first ADEM event without involvement of new clinical areas. MR imaging: Lesions in same distribution. Event does not occur while on steroids. Usually occurs at least 1 month after completing therapy.

Multiphasic ADEM: ADEM followed by a new clinical event also meeting criteria for ADEM. Recurrence after recovery from the initial illness, involvement of new anatomic areas of the CNS. Event must occur at least 3 months after the onset of the initial ADEM event, at least 1 month after completing steroid therapy.

MRI shows new areas of involvement and demonstrate complete or partial resolution of those lesions associated with the first ADEM event.

Pseudo-recurrence: Recurrence of symptoms during period of corticosteroid taper or soon after discontinuing. Represents flaring up of a protracted single phase.

Idiopathic Inflammatory Demyelinating Diseases

1. **Monophasic:** Optic neuritis, internuclear ophthalmoplegia, ADEM, Marburg variant of MS, Balo's concenteric sclerosis.
2. **Primary progressive MS:** Chronic progressive myelopathy, progressive ataxic syndrome, progressive dementing syndrome
3. **Relapsing and remitting:** Multiple sclerosis, NMO

Pediatric MS

Brain lesions in younger children are typically large with poorly defined borders, and are frequently confluent at disease onset. Such T2-bright foci in younger children can vanish on repeat scans, unlike those seen in teenagers or adults.

Clinical presentation: Encephalopathy at the onset may occur in childhood MS (20–40%)

Monosymptomatic presentation is typical in adult MS, but polysymptomatic presentation is more common in pediatric MS (50%). CSF: Less chance of finding OCB

Multifocal T2/FLAIR hyperintensities	*Multiple sclerosis mimics*
Acute disseminated encephalomyelitis (ADEM).	Behçet disease
Autoimmune-mediated vasculitis.	Systemic lupus erythematous(SLE)
Lyme disease.	Sarcoidosis
Susac syndrome.	Binswanger's disease
Chronic lymphocytic inflammation with pontine perivascular enhancement responsive to steriods (CLIPPERS).	Vascular dementia
Small vessel ischemic changes	Pontine infarction
Ependymitis granularis	CADASIL
Neuromyeltits optica (NMO)	Mitochondrial encephalopathy with lactic acidosis and stroke like episodes (MELAS)
PRES	Central pontine myelinolysis (CPM)
Bickerstaff encephalitis	Progressive multifocal leucoencephalopathy (PML)
	HIV infection
	Leucodystrophy
	Radiation encephalitis
	Other demyelinating diseases like NMO, ADEM

<table>
<tr><td>Acute disseminated encephalomyelitis (ADEM)
Viral prodrome, monophasic illness, more common in children
Can mimic multiple sclerosis.</td><td>ADEM lesions tend to be larger, more edematous and often asymmetric involving white matter: Subcortical, periventricular and basal ganglia. Gray matter often involved. Affection of both CNS and PNS seen. With bilateral optic nerve involvement. Complete myelopathy and encephalopathy are common</td><td>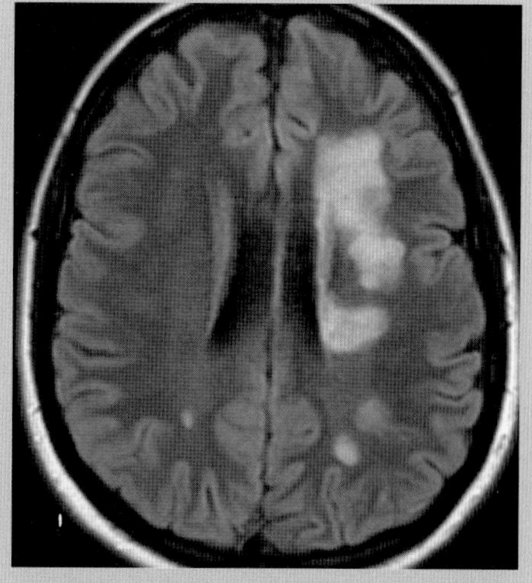
Fig. 4.25.8: ADEM</td></tr>
<tr><td>Autoimmune-mediated vasculitis
Commonly affects young females.
Black blood vessel wall imaging – helps in whole brain coverage with better evaluation of vertebral arteries, distal intracranial segments and depiction of more leptomeningeal and pachymeningeal enhancement.</td><td>Enhancing lesions spare callososeptal interface.
Multiple T2 hyperintense white matter lesions noted in bilateral cerebral hemisphere as well as corpus callosum.
"Beaded" angiogram appearance seen on contrast MR image.
Cortical, subcortical + basal ganglia, parenchymal microhaemorrhages, SAH, punctate linear enhancement in T1 + C.
Ring enhancing lesions may mimic infection.</td><td>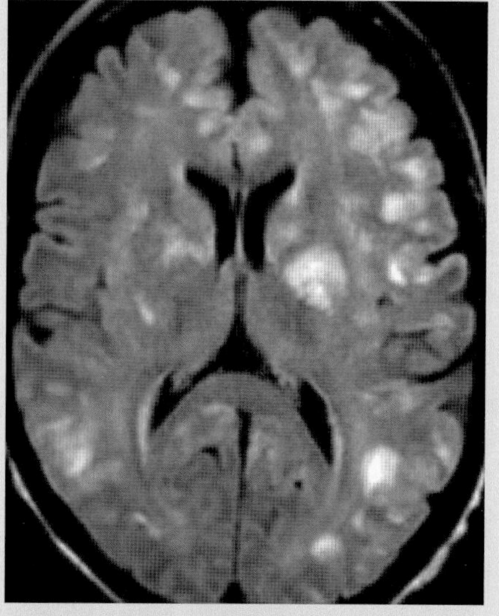
Fig. 4.25.9: Autoimmune-mediated vasculitis</td></tr>
<tr><td>Lyme disease
It is a multisystemic disease caused by Borrelia burgdorferi. It consists of nonspecific white matter chnages in brain.</td><td colspan="2">MS-like white matter lesions (may enhance) 2–8 mm (large "tumefactive" lesions rare) with or without multiple enhancing cranial nerves, with or without cauda equina, meningeal enhancement.</td></tr>
<tr><td>Susac syndrome—also known as SICRET (small infarctions of cochlear, retinal and encephalic tissue)
Commonly affects females at 2nd to 4th decades. Typically involves central fibres of callosal body and splenium. They present with skin and muscle lesions (called livedo reticularis)</td><td colspan="2">Classic triad: Encephalopathy, branch retinal artery occlusions, hearing loss
MR shows multiple T2 hyperintense 'snowball' lesions involving the entire thickness of corpus callosum. T1 punched out hypointensities in DWM. Roof of the corpus callosum is frequently involved rather than callososeptal interface.
Multiple peri ventricular and deep white matter hyperintensities in T2 and FLAIR in over 90% cases.</td></tr>
<tr><td colspan="3">Sneddon syndrome (antiphospholipid syndrome)—systemic non-inflammatory vasculopathy characterised by livedoreticularis and progressive occlusive cerebrovascular thrombosis</td></tr>
</table>

Clinical presentation	*Additional criteria to make MS as diagnosis*
In a person who has experienced typical attack/clinically isolated syndrome (CIS) at onset	
2 or more attacks and clinical evidence of 2 /more lesions; OR • 2/ more attacks and evidence of 1 lesion along with clear historical evidence of prior attack involving lesion in an alternate location	None. DIS and DIT have been met.
Evidence of 1 lesion and 2 or more attacks	One of these criteria: A second clinical attack involving a different part of the CNS—at least one MS—common T2 lesions in two or more CNS areas at spinal cord, periventricular, cortical, juxtacortical, infratentorial
Clinical evidence of 2 or more lesions and 1 attack	One of these parameters in DIT: New T2 or enhancing MR lesion compared to baseline scan—simultaneous presence of both enhancing and non-enhancing MS typical MR lesions, or new T2 or enhancing MR lesion (without regard to timing of baseline scan)— Oligoclonal bands in CSF
Clinical evidence of 1 lesion and 1 attack	One of these criteria reveals DIS: An additional attack involving a different CNS location has been discovered. At least one MS—typical T2 lesions in two or more CNS areas: Periventricular, cortical, spinal cord, juxtacortical or infratentorial and DIT shown by one of the following criteria—second clinical assault. The existence of both enhancing and non-enhancing MS at the same time as compared to a baseline scan, conventional MR lesions, or new T2 or enhanced MR lesions (without no respect to baseline scan time)—oligoclonal bands in CSF
Person with steady disease progression since onset	
Disease progression for 1 year (prospective/ retrospective)	At least two of these characteristics indicate DIS: At least one MS—common T2 lesions (periventricular, cortical, juxtacortical or infratentorial)—2 or more T2 lesions in the spinal cord—oligoclonal bands in CSF

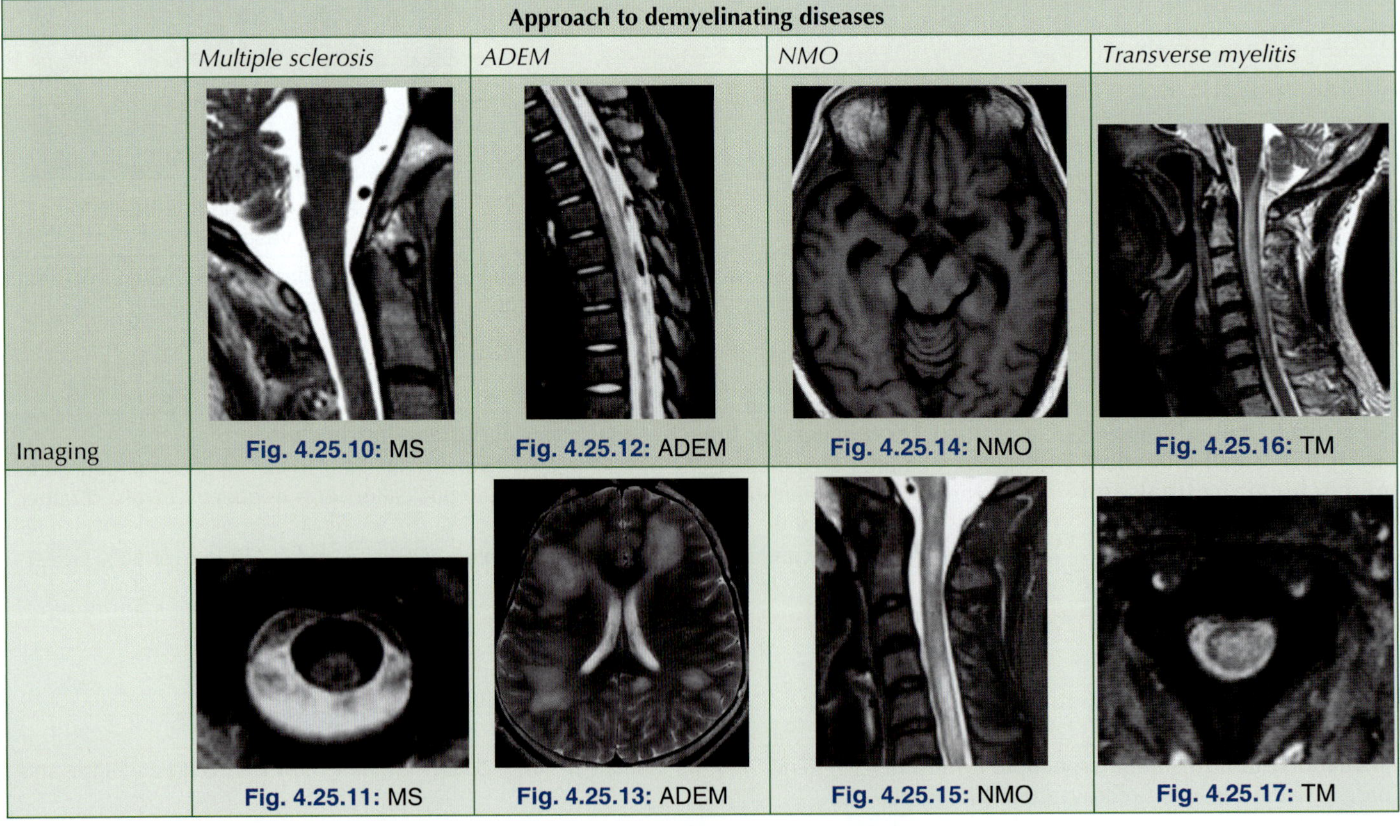

Approach to demyelinating diseases				
	Multiple sclerosis	*ADEM*	*NMO*	*Transverse myelitis*
Imaging	**Fig. 4.25.10:** MS	**Fig. 4.25.12:** ADEM	**Fig. 4.25.14:** NMO	**Fig. 4.25.16:** TM
	Fig. 4.25.11: MS	**Fig. 4.25.13:** ADEM	**Fig. 4.25.15:** NMO	**Fig. 4.25.17:** TM

Age	Peak onset: 20–40 years, common in adult female.	Typically childhood or young adult with male predominance	Mean age range: 30–40 years F > M (4:1)	Any, but peaks at 10–19 and 30–39 years
Clinical features	Cord lesions may be asymptomatic Paresthesia Muscle weakness Hyperreflexia Gait disturbance	Typically monophasic illness lasting from 2–4 weeks Encephalopathy Paresis	Recurrent optic neuritis, recurrent transverse myelitis,	Preceding viral-like illness with rapid progression to maximal neurologic deficits within days
Biochemical markers	CSF oligoclonal bands	CSF pleocytosis	NMO IgG antibodies	—
Common site in the spinal cord	Cervical cord	Anywhere in spinal cord	Spinal cord + optic nerves/ chiasm	Thoracic cord
Longitudinal involvement	<2 vertebral segments in length	Punctate to segmental	Longitudinally extensive (>3 vertebral segments)	>2 vertebral segments in length
Axial invovlement	<1/2 of cross-sectional area of spinal cord Dorsolateral aspect of cord—V sign	—	Involve entire cross section of cord	Central cord location. More than 2/3 cross sectional area of spinal cord
Cord expansion	Normal or mild focal cord expansion	Mild cord swelling	Swollen in acute conditions.	STIR -Hyperintense cord expansion
Enhancement pattern	Homogeneous, nodular, or ring enhancement during acute or subacute phase	Punctate, ring-shaped, or fluffy enhancement	Enhancement of optic nerves seen.	Eccentric enhancement
Brain involvement	Concomitant intracranial lesions in periventricular, subcallosal, brain stem, or cerebellar white matter.	Lesions in deep cerebral hemispheric and sub-cortical white matter, basal ganglia, gray-white junction, brainstem, cerebellum	MS-like lesions in 10–30% of NMO patients. Tend to cluster around 3rd and 4th ventricles and the dorsal midbrain and aqueduct of sylvius/area postrema/ brainstem.	—
Optic nerve involvement	Unilateral/bilateral optic neuritis–predominantly anterior.	Bilateral optic neuritis+	Bilateral optic neuritis +++ predominantly posterior involving optic chiasma	—
Treatment	IV and oral prednisone Plasmapheresis Interferon β Glatiramer acetate	Intravenous methylprednisolone is treatment of choice, plasmapheresis in fulminant case	Intravenous steroids Immunosuppressive medications	High-dose intravenous steroid pulse therapy Physical therapy

Tumefactive demyelination are demyelinating brain disease resembling primary brain cancers such as PCNSL and high-grade glioma. They are usually greater than 2 cm in diameter. MRI features—T2 hypointense rim, no significant mass effect, absent or moderate perilesional oedema, an open ring or incomplete rim enhancement, closed ring/complete rim augmentation. Diffusion restriction in the periphery with high ADC values, MRS–choline peak, lower NAA, lactate, and glutamine/glutamate peak, DTI—lower FA values, perfusion imaging—rCBV and rCBF decreased.

Right frontoparietal tumefactive demyelination with reduced cerebral blood flow on perfusion ASL

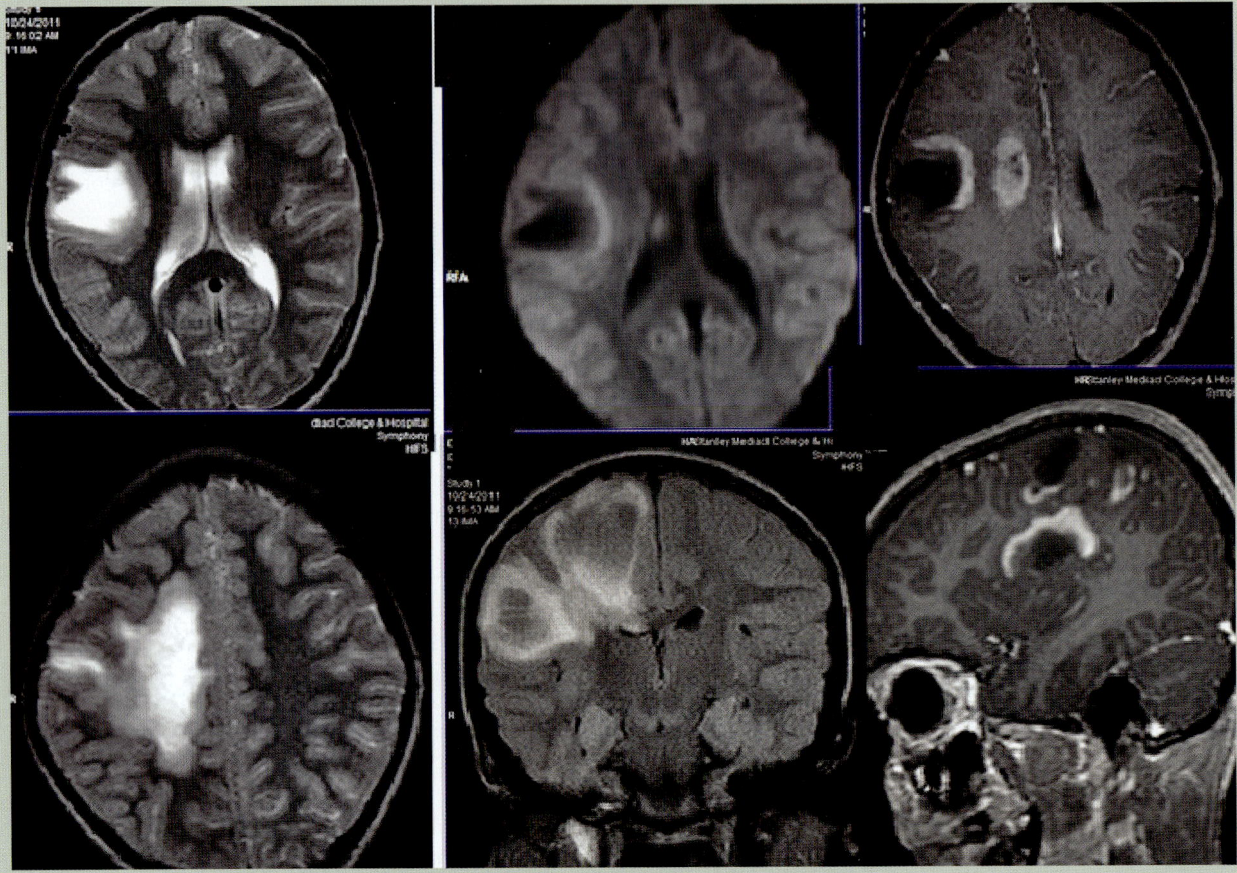

Fig. 4.25.18: Right frontoparietal tumefactive demyelination

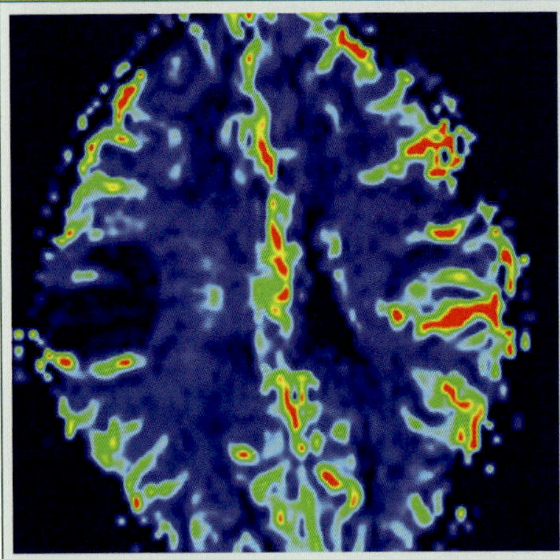

Fig. 4.25.19: Tumefactive demyelination showing reduced cerebral blood flow on perfusion

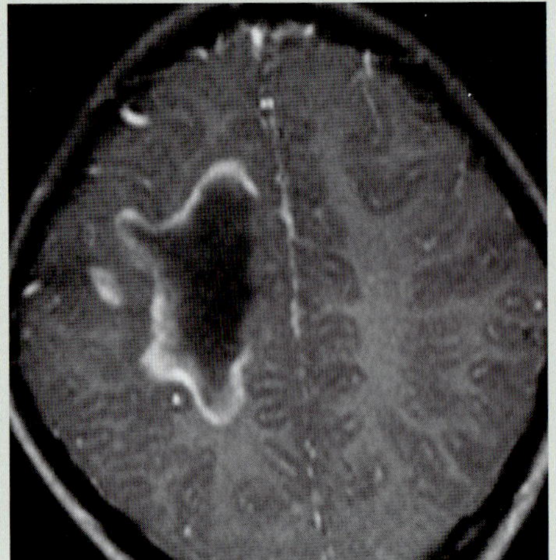

Fig. 4.25.20: Right frontoparietal tumefactive demyelination

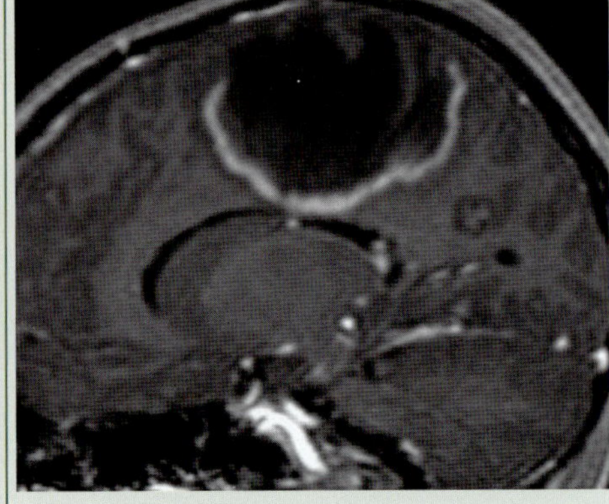

Fig. 4.25.21: Right frontoparietal tumefactive demyelination

Mimics of Solitary "Tumefactive" MS: Neoplasm (GBM, metastasis), PML/PML-IRIS in natalizumab-treated MS, Etanercept related.

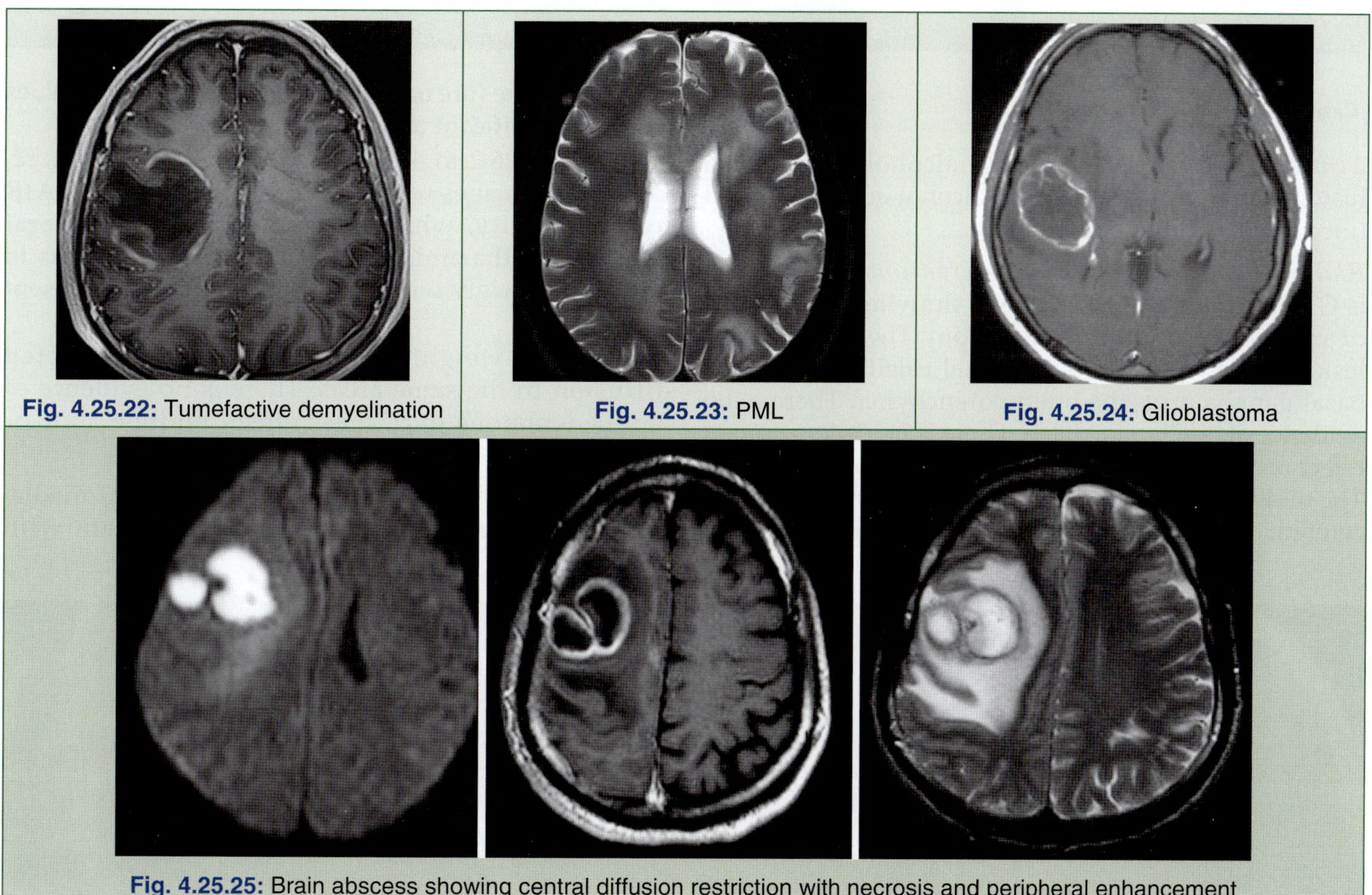

Fig. 4.25.22: Tumefactive demyelination

Fig. 4.25.23: PML

Fig. 4.25.24: Glioblastoma

Fig. 4.25.25: Brain abscess showing central diffusion restriction with necrosis and peripheral enhancement

(45%) or IgG index (35%), More pleocytic—higher percentage of neutrophil. MRI: Fewer T2—bright foci and more-frequent tumefactive MS lesions.

Ears of lynx sign
Infarct
Virchow Robin space
Multiple sclerosis
ADEM
Metastases
Fazeka's grade 1
Fazeka's grade 2
Fazeka's grade 3
PRES

Fig. 4.25.26: White matter lesions in brain

Treatment: Currently available first-line therapies for adults with MS seem to be safe and well tolerated in pediatric MS.

Etiological Classification of Demyelinating Disorders (CNS)

1. Inflammatory/immune disorders—MS, optic neuritis, paraneoplastic encephalomyelitis, rheumatoid arthritis, Behçet's disease, Sjörgen disease, NMO, GBS, tumefactive demyelination and ADEM
2. Infectious disorders—HIV, PML, Lyme disease, HTLV-1, neurosyphilis, meningitis (bacterial/viral)
3. Granulomatous disorders—sarcoidosis, Wegner granulomatosis, lymphoid granulomatosis
4. Myelin disorders—Metachromatic leukodystrophy, Adrenoleukodystrophy/adrenomyeloneuropathy Globoid cell (Krabbe's) leukodystrophy, Alexander disease, Canavan disease
5. Toxic/metabolic disorders—B12 deficiency, radiation myelitis, PRES, SLE, central pontine myelinolysis and carbon monoxide poisoning.

4.26 CENTRAL NERVOUS SYSTEM

Case No. 26

Clinical history: A 51-year-old alcoholic male with history of overconsumption of alcohol and was found unconscious and hypothermic.

Radiological techniques and observation: Figure 4.26.1 is **CT brain plain (NECT) image showing** no evidence of any volume loss or cortical atrophy. There are no focal lesions seen.There is no abnormal calcification in the basal ganglia or in the brain parenchyma. There is no evidence of any hemorrhage. There is no oedema, mass effect or herniation. The ventricles are normal in size. The midbrain, pons and cerebellum appear normal. The cerebral cortex appears normal. The visualized calvarial and facial bones are normal. The extracranial soft tissues show no significant abnormality.

Figures 4.26.2 to 4.26.5 are MRI brain—FLAIR, T2, DWI, ADC images respectively. MRI shows **T2/FLAIR hyperintensity,** which is **symmetrical in bilateral paramedian thalami.** Small tiny hypointense areas in T2/FLAIR images within the lesion probably represent hemorrhage.

Diffusion weighted imaging showed **restricted diffusion** in the same areas. There is no evidence of any oedematous gyri, mass effect, midline shift or herniation.

Interpretation: A–51-year-old male, Bilateral medial thalami, B–symmetrical, C–normal CT brain with

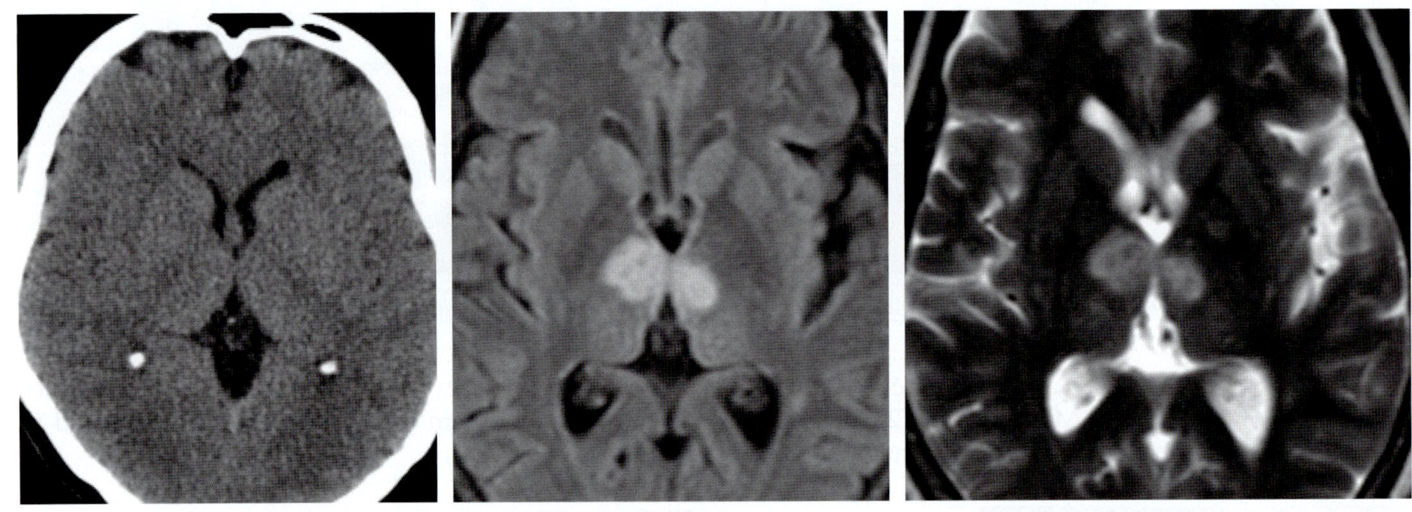

Fig. 4.26.1 Fig. 4.26.2 Fig. 4.26.3

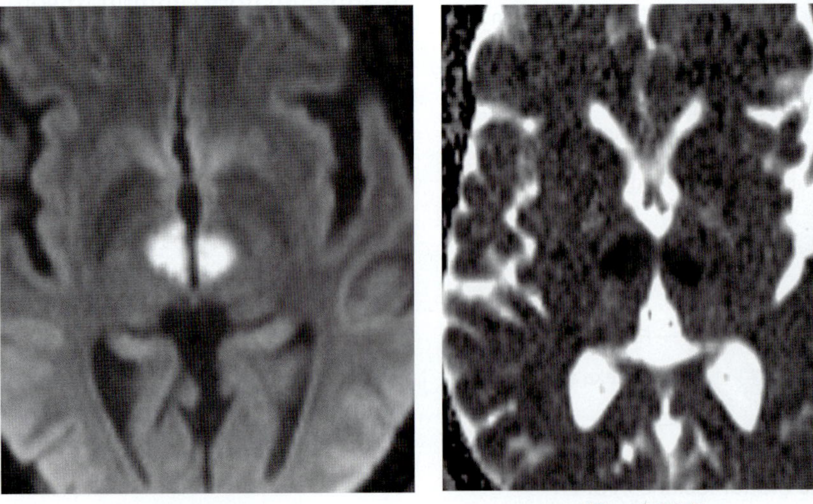

Fig. 4.26.4 Fig. 4.26.5

presence of T2/FLAIR hyperintensity with diffusion restriction, D–occlusion of a single unpaired artery of Percheron arising from the PCA.

Principal diagnosis: Unpaired artery of Percheron infarct.

The **artery of Percheron** is known anatomic variant where a **single unpaired** artery arising from P1 portion of posterior cerebral artery supplies the bilateral paramedian thalami and sometimes cranial midbrain. **Bilateral paramedian thalamic infarction is observed when this artery is occluded.**

Management: Urgent referral to neurophysician.

Discussion: The basal ganglia and thalamus are paired deep gray matter structures that can be involved by wide variety of diseases. The basal ganglia are highly metabolically active and symmetrically affected in toxic poisoning, metabolic abnormalities, and

Table 4.26.1: Differential diagnoses for bilateral thalamic lesions

Infection	*Vascular aetiology*	*Metabolic causes*	*Others*
Variant Creutzfeldt- Jacob disease. Japanese encephalitis. Cerebral malaria. Toxoplasmosis. Cryptococcosis.	Lacunar infarcts Arterial infarct Venous ischemia and infarction. Perinatal hypoxia.	Carbon monoxide poisoning Wernicke's encephalopathy Inherited metabolic conditions (Leigh, Fahr, Fabry).	Status epilepticus. Glioma

Variant CJD Bovine spongiform encephalopathy in cattle is transmitted to humans through infected beef—also known as new variant CJD (NVCJD). Seen in young patients. Rapidly progressing dementia, with death usually ensuing within months of onset. No effective treatment.	Variant CJD is associated with the bovine spongiform encephalopathy. FLAIR shows 2 signs seen in vCJD—"Pulvinar" sign: Bilateral symmetrical hyperintensity of **pulvinar** (posterior) nuclei of thalamus,**"Hockey stick" sign:** Symmetrical pulvinar and dorsomedial thalamic nuclear hyperintensity. DWI shows gyriform hyperintense areas in cerebral cortex **("cortical ribbon" sign)**	Fig. 4.26.6: Variant CJD
Japanese encephalitis Most common endemic encephalitis in Asia with high morbidity and mortality.	The most characteristic MRI imaging finding of Japanese encephalitis is T2 hyperintensity, typically with bilateral involvement of the **posteromedial thalamus.** Intralesional hemorrhages and restricted diffusion have also been described. Other sites of involvement include basal ganglia, substantia nigra, red nucleus, pons, hippocampi, cerebral cortex, and cerebellum.	Fig. 4.26.7: Japanese encephalitis
Arterial infarction The thalamus is mainly vascularised by thalamo geniculate arteries, the tubero-thalamic artery, the thalamosubthalamic arteries and the posterior choroidal arteries.	**Considering that all the arteries supplying the thalamus are terminal arteries, the thalamic infarctions have most often a lacunar aspect.** **Imaging findings:** Hypodense lesions on CT, MR shows T2/FLAIR hyperintensity with diffusion restriction.	Fig. 4.26.8: Arterial infarction

(Contd.)

Table 4.26.1: Differential diagnoses for bilateral thalamic lesions (*Contd.*)

Venous infarction Thrombus initially forms in dural sinus >Clot propagates into cortical veins >Venous drainage obstructed, venous pressure elevated >Blood–brain barrier breakdown with vasogenic edema, haemorrhage > Venous infarct with cytotoxic edema ensues	Venous thrombosis of deep venous system, vein of Galen, or the straight sinus may lead to the bilateral thalamic vasogenic edema **(hyperintense on both DWI and ADC map)**. The MRI signal intensity of venous thrombus varies according to the time of imaging from the onset of the thrombus formation. CT venography or TOF/gadolinium-enhanced MR venography is the most frequently used technique to show venous thrombosis.	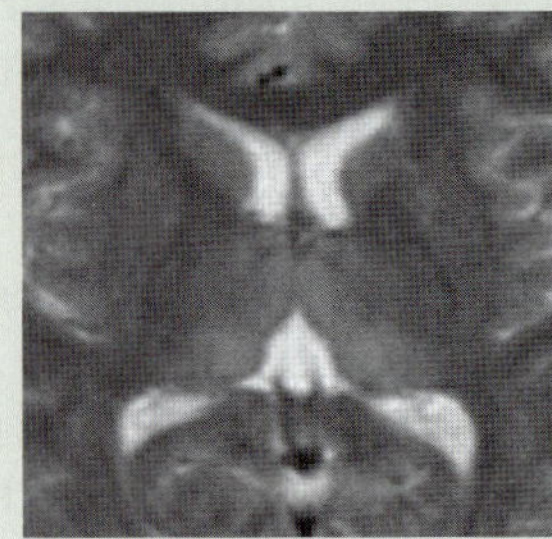 **Fig. 4.26.9:** Venous infarction 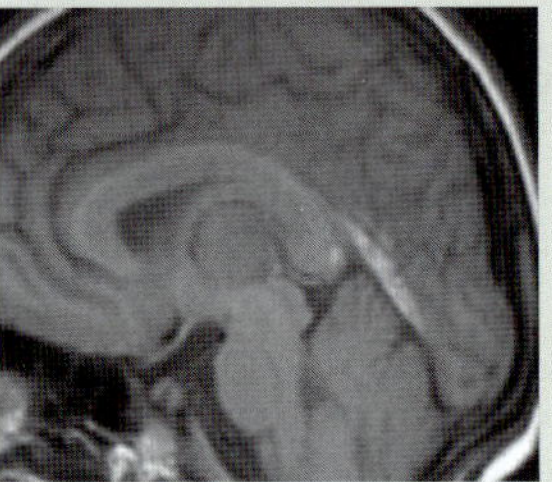 **Fig. 4.26.10:** Venous thrombosis
Perinatal hypoxia Clinical syndrome defined in term or near-term neonates. The deep gray matter structures (thalamus and basal ganglia) are the most metabolically active and hence more susceptible to oxidative stress and shows effects of hypoxia earlier.	Thalamic hyperintensity due to hypoxia is **diffuse** and can range from very subtle to overtly hyperintense. It has to be distinguished from the normal subtle increase in signal intensity in the posterolateral quadrant.	
Wernicke's encephalopathy Wernicke encephalopathy typically results from vitamin B1 (thiamine) deficiency.	Typical findings at MRI imaging include symmetric T2 prolongation in the **medial thalamus,** periaqueductal area, mamillary bodies, and tectal plate. Petechial haemorrhage, diffusion restriction, and contrast enhancement of the affected areas may be noted.	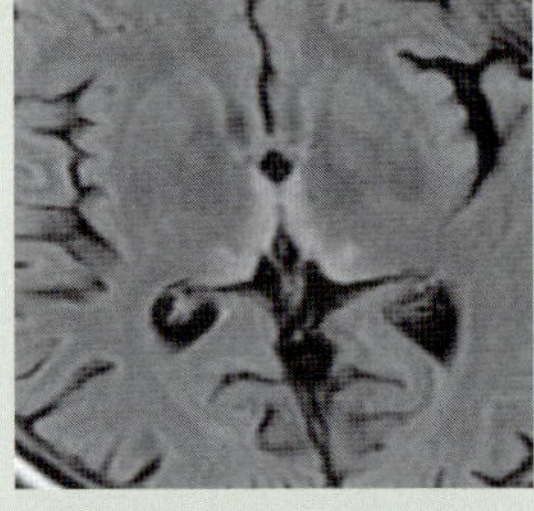 **Fig. 4.26.11:** Wernicke's encephalopathy
Fabry's disease Also known as **Anderson-Fabry disease,** is a multisystem disorder resulting from an X-linked inborn error of metabolism and is a lysosomal storage disorder.	T1 weighted images also demonstrate high signals in the deep grey matter especially that of the **pulvinar**, relating to mineralization. **Exclusive involvement of pulvinar is thought to be characteristic of the condition.** 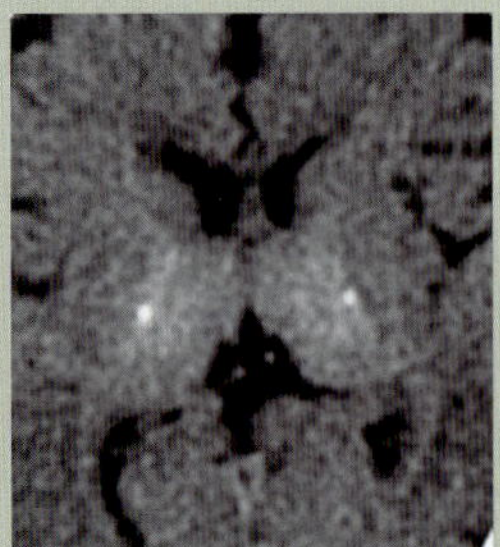 **Fig. 4.26.12:** Fabry's disease	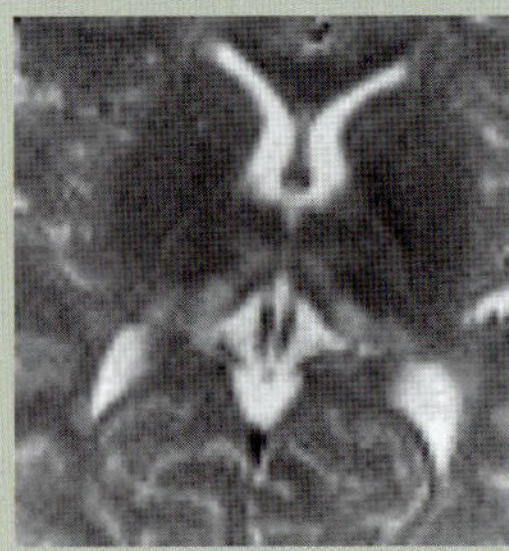 **Fig. 4.26.13:** Fabry's disease

(*Contd.*)

<table>
<tr><th colspan="4">Table 4.26.1: Differential diagnoses for bilateral thalamic lesions (Contd.)</th></tr>
<tr><td colspan="2">Bilateral thalamic gliomas
Bilateral thalamic gliomas are very rare but characteristic low-grade astrocytomas which occur in both children and young adults.</td><td colspan="2">CT and MRI typically show expansion of both thalami. Imaging findings on MRI include T2/FLAIR hyperintensity, no diffusion restriction, no contrast enhancement on T1+C images.</td></tr>
<tr><td>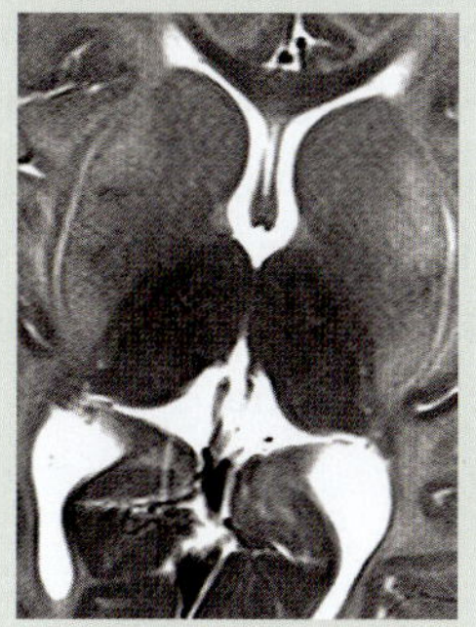
Fig. 4.26.14: Krabbe's disease</td><td>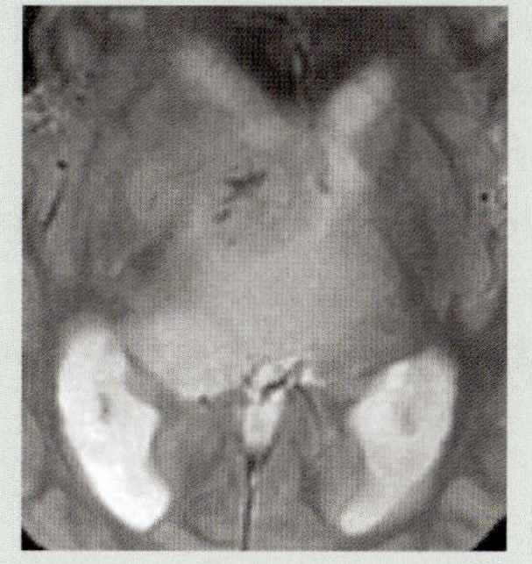
Fig. 4.26.15: Bilateral thalamic gliomas</td><td>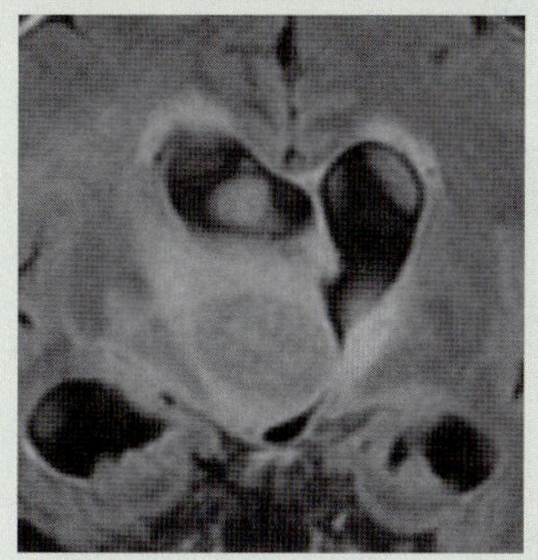
Fig. 4.26.16: Bilateral thalamic gliomas</td><td>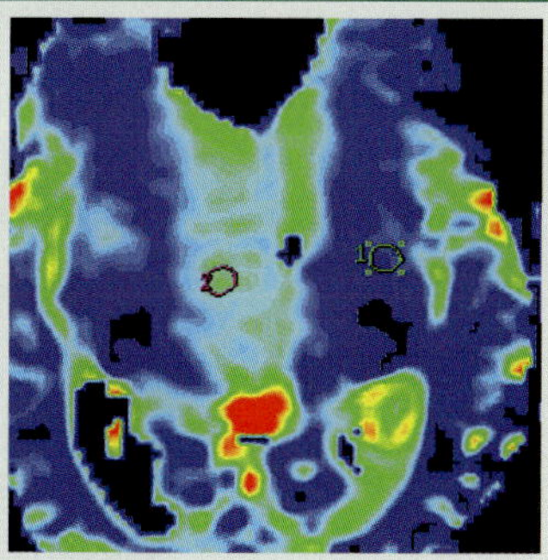
Fig. 4.26.17: Bilateral thalamic gliomas</td></tr>
</table>

<table>
<tr><th colspan="3">Table 4.26.2: Differential diagnosis for thalamic lesions</th></tr>
<tr><td colspan="3">Bithalamic lesions by age</td></tr>
<tr><td>Childhood bithalamic lesions</td><td colspan="2">Adult bithalamic lesions</td></tr>
<tr><td>• Hypoxic-ischemic encephalopathy
• ADEM
• Bithalamic astrocytoma
• Inherited metabolic disorder
• Acquired metabolic disorders
• Acute necrotizing encephalitis</td><td colspan="2">• Deep venous occlusion
• Artery of Percheron, "top of the basilar" occlusion
• Profound hypoperfusion
• ADEM
• Wernicke encephalopathy
• Osmotic demyelination
• Vasculitis
• CJD</td></tr>
<tr><td colspan="3">Bithalamic lesions</td></tr>
<tr><td>Common</td><td>Less common</td><td>Rare</td></tr>
<tr><td>Vascular lesions
• Deep venous occlusion
• Arterial ischemia
• Vasculitis
Hypoxic-ischemic encephalopathy</td><td>Infection/post-infection/inflammatory disorders
• ADEM
• CJD
Toxic/metabolic disorders
• Osmotic myelinolysis
• Wernicke encephalopathy
• Solvent inhalation
• Acute hypertensive encephalopathy (PRES)—atypical
• Status epilepticus
Neoplasms
• Bithalamic low-grade astrocytoma
• Germinoma
• Lymphoma</td><td>Infection/postinfection/inflammatory disorders
• Multiple sclerosis
• Acute necrotizing encephalopathy of childhood
• Flavivirus encephalitis
• Neuro-Behçet
Inherited disorders
• Mitochondrial disorders
• Wilson disease
• Fahr disease
Neoplasm
• Glioblastoma
• Anaplastic astrocytoma
Paraneoplastic syndromes</td></tr>
<tr><td>MR-T2 hypointense lesions in thalamus
1. Krabbe's disease
2. Status marmoratus
3. GM1/2 gangliosidoses
4. Neuronal ceroid lipofuscinosis</td><td colspan="2">CT hyperdense lesions in thalamus
1. Fahr disease
2. Leigh's disease
3. Krabbe's disease
4. Calcification in status marmoratus
5. Neuronal ceroid lipofuscinosis
6. Juvenile GM1 gangliosidoses
7. Fabry's disease</td></tr>
</table>

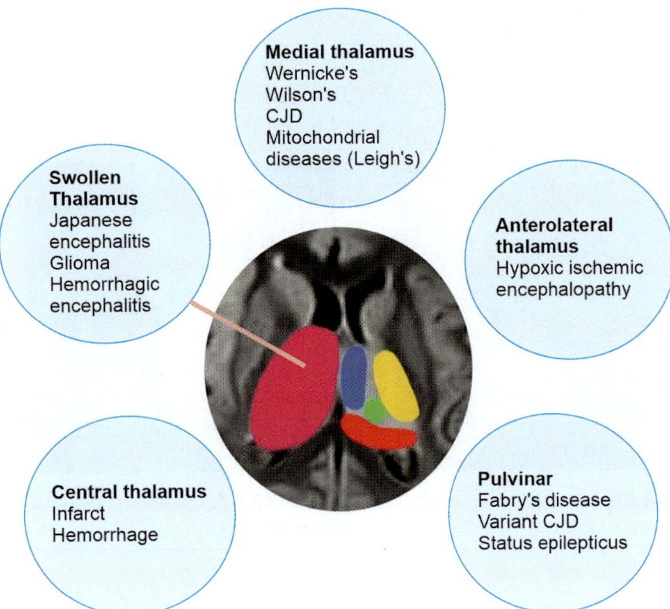

Fig. 4.26.18: Approach to lesions in thalamus

neurodegeneration with brain iron accumulation. **The thalamus is typically affected alone by focal conditions than by systemic diseases.**

It consists of multiple nuclei which are responsible for relaying sensory and motor signals to and from the cerebral cortex and are involved in regulating consciousness, sleep, and alertness. Hence, the lesions affecting the thalamus often result in disorders of consciousness and abnormalities of sensation. **Thalamic infarct is an important cause of dementia.**

4.27 CENTRAL NERVOUS SYSTEM

Case No. 27

Clinical history: A 45-year-old male patient with complaints of altered sensorium for 4 days. History of altered sleep–wake cycle, irritability for 3 months.

Radiological techniques and observations: Figure 4.27.1 **NECT shows no significant abnormality**. Figures 4.27.2 and 4.27.3 are MR images showing **bilateral T1 hyperintensity involving the globus pallidi, subthalamic nucleus and substantia nigra.** There is no evidence of any oedematous gyri, mass effect, midline shift or herniation. There is no evidence of any other lesions within the brain parenchyma. The cerebellum, pons and medulla are normal. The other regions of the basal ganglia such as the caudate, thalamus and putamen are normal. There is no evidence of any infarcts or haemorrhage.

Interpretation: A–45 years old, bilateral globus pallidus, subthalamic nucleus and substantia nigra, B–symmetrical, C–T1 hyperintensity, D–hepatic encephalopathy.

Principal diagnosis: Hepatocellular dysfunction.

Classic MR imaging abnormalities include high signal intensity in the globus pallidum on T1-weighted images, likely a reflection of **increased tissue concentrations of manganese.**

Management: Urgent referral to neuro physician.

Discussion: The **globi pallidi** are paired structures and one of the nuclei that make up the basal ganglia. The basal ganglia form the core of extrapyramidal system and regulate motor activity. The putamen and globus pallidus are rich in mitochondria, vascular supply, neurotransmitters and chemical content compared with other areas in the brain and their high metabolic activity and increased utilization of glucose and oxygen make them vulnerable to metabolic abnormalities and many systemic or generalized disease processes. Typically, abundant vascular supply to the basal ganglia make them more susceptible to toxins and infectious agents.

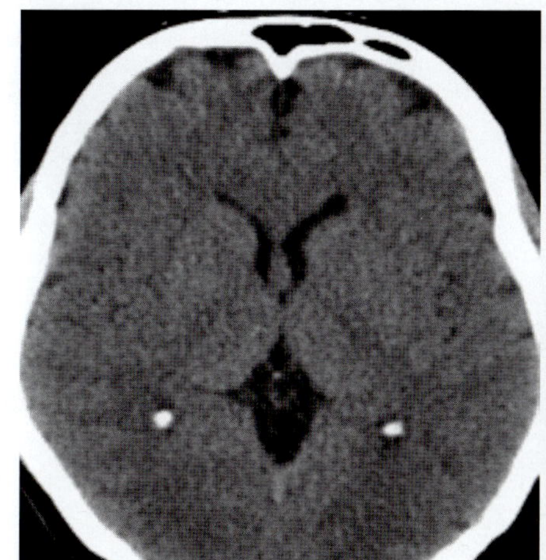

Fig. 4.27.1

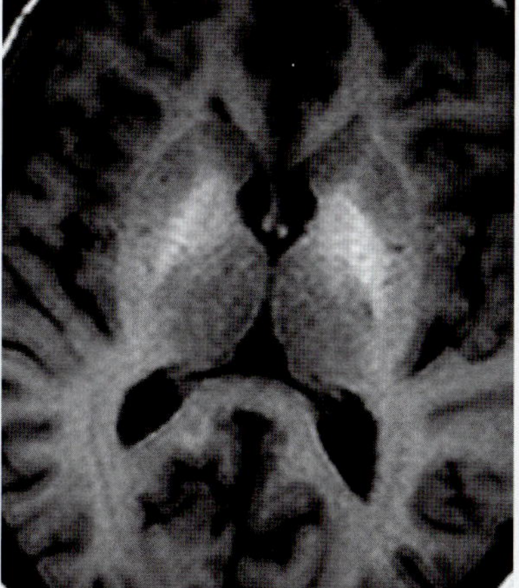

Fig. 4.27.2

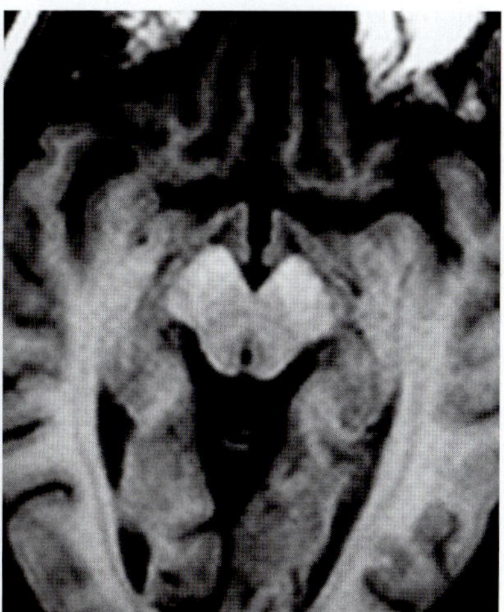

Fig. 4.27.3

Table 4.27.1: Differential diagnoses for bilateral GP lesions

Poisoning **1. Carbon monoxide poisoning:** CO toxicity decreases the delivery of oxygen by means of three proposed mechanisms which are competitive binding to haemoglobin, direct toxicity to mitochondria and shifting of the classical oxyhaemoglobin binding curve to the left.	CO poisoning causing high signal intensity typically within the globus pallidi and sometimes within the caudate or putamina on T2-weighted images. Both hyperintensity and hypointensity within the globus pallidi may be observed on T1-weighted images. **Changes within the globus pallidi are due to be most likely related to infarction resulting from poor oxygenation.**	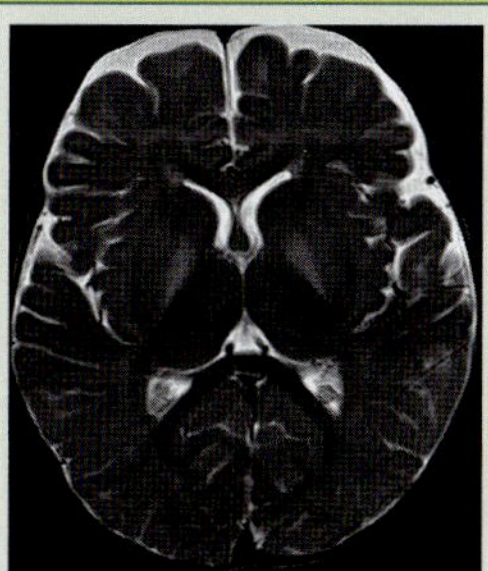 Fig. 4.27.4: Carbon monoxide poisoning

(Contd.)

<table>
<tr><th colspan="3">Table 4.27.1: Differential diagnoses for bilateral GP lesions (Contd.)</th></tr>
<tr><td colspan="2">2. Cyanide poisoning: Cyanide deactivates cytochrome oxidase which is a terminal enzyme in the cellular respiratory chain, which explains the preferential involvement of the basal ganglia.</td><td>MR findings typically show edema of the putamina and globus pallidi, and sensorimotor cortex.</td></tr>
<tr><td colspan="2">3. Heroin and MDMA abuse: Ischemic stroke is a complication of MDMA and heroin use and occur due to vasoconstriction by the serotonin release and μ-opioid receptor activation, respectively.
The distribution of serotonin receptors makes the globus pallidi and occipital cortex particularly susceptible to MDMA-induced ischemia.</td><td>Infarcts in the setting of heroin use typically involve the watershed territories as the cerebellum, hippocampus and globus pallidus.</td></tr>
<tr><td>4. Methyl malonic acidemia: Autosomal-recessive disorder caused by mutation of the gene encoding methylmalonic CoA mutase. Presents early in life with episodic ketoacidosis, lethargy, tachypnoea, progressive hypotonia, and seizures, eventually progressing to coma and death. Central hypotonia with pyramidal tract signs, dystonia and choreoathetosis are seen in survivors.</td><td>MR findings include ventricular enlargement, cortical atrophy, cerebellar volume loss, and T2/FLAIR hyperintensity involving the periventricular WM and globi pallidi. MR findings are reflective of increased water within involved tissues (therefore, reduced attenuation on NECT and T1 and T2 prolongation on MR).</td><td>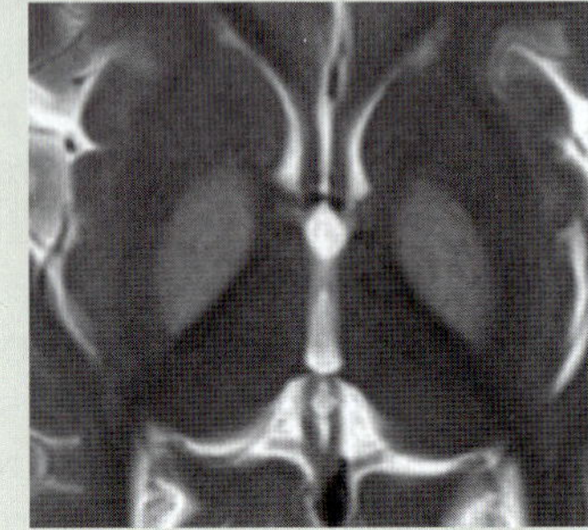
Fig. 4.27.5: Methyl malonic acidemia</td></tr>
<tr><td>5. Pantothenate kinase-associated neuro-degeneration (PKAN): Also called Hallervorden-Spatz disease. It is an autosomal recessive disorder causing involuntary spasticity and progressive dementia. It is a subset of neurodegeneration with brain iron accumulation.
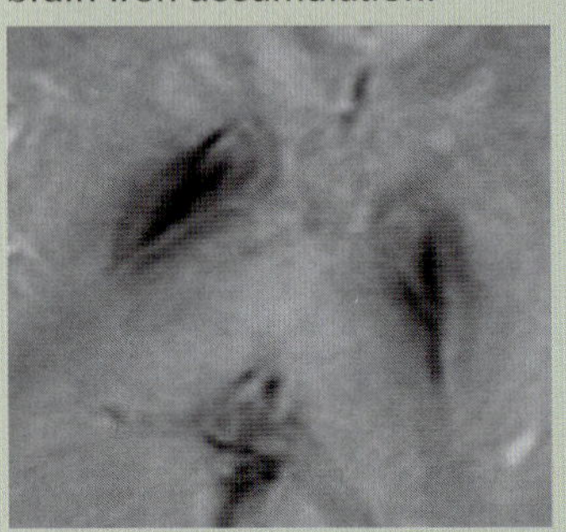
Fig. 4.27.6: Eyes of tiger in pantothenate kinase-associated neurodegeneration</td><td>T2 images often demonstrate hypointense changes in the globus pallidi and substantia nigra.
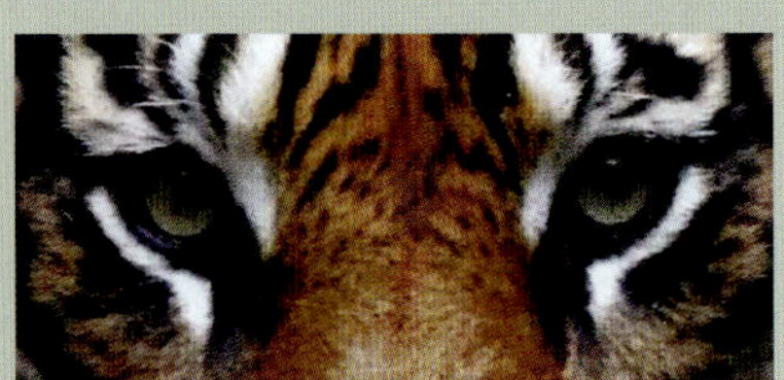
Fig. 4.27.7: Eyes of tiger</td><td>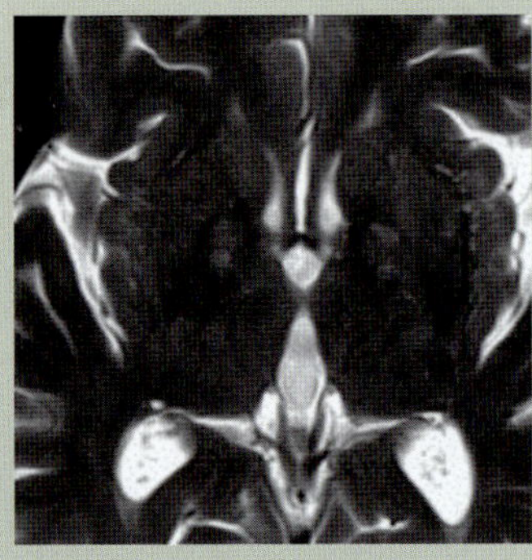
Fig. 4.27.8: Pantothenate kinase-associated neurodegeneration</td></tr>
<tr><td>6. Wilson's disease which is also known as hepatolenticular degeneration, a multisystem disease due to abnormal accumulation of copper.</td><td>MR imaging findings include T1/T2 hyperintensity of the basal ganglia and midbrain (face of the giant panda appearance).
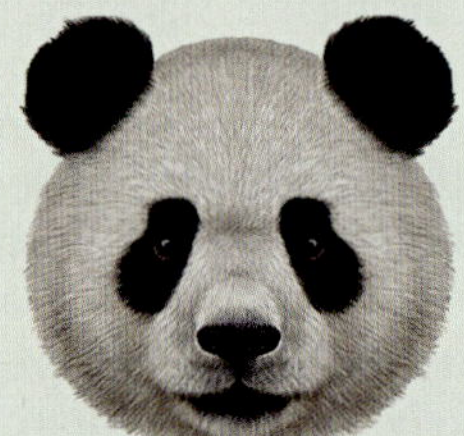
Fig. 4.27.9: Face of the giant panda</td><td>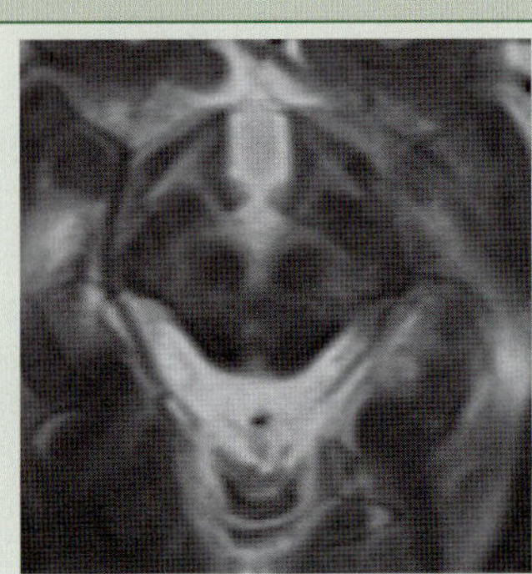
Fig. 4.27.10: Wilson disease</td></tr>
</table>

(*Contd.*)

Table 4.27.1: Differential diagnoses for bilateral GP lesions (*Contd.*)		
7. **Neurofibromatosis-1:** UBOs/ focal altered signal intensity (FASIs)/ neurofibromatosis related bright objects (NBOs) are frequently found in globus pallidi. They do not produce any clinical symptoms and **regress during adolescence**.	**Unidentified bright objects (UBOs)** are brain lesions that show up on MRI as increased T2W signal intensity area in children with neurofibromatosis type 1. (NF1).	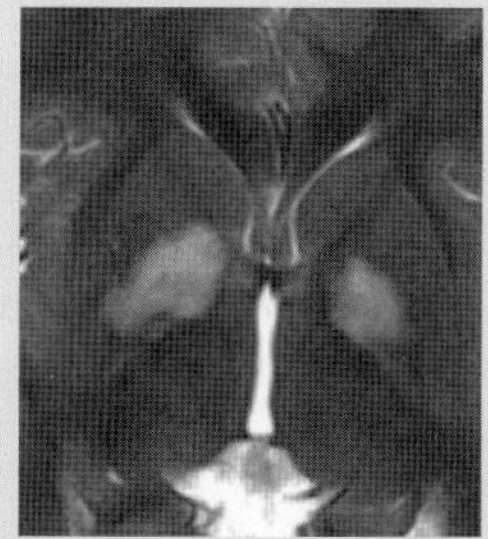 **Fig. 4.27.11:** UBO in NF1
8. Hypoglycaemia in adult: Hypoglycaemia acutely results in "brain energy failure" and in membrane ionic pump failure, the latter of which causes a prominent rise of intracellular water.	The regions of affected brain are variable mainly include the temporal–parietal–occipital cortex and hippocampus, and basal ganglia, especially the caudate and lentiform nuclei. Findings include—**T1 hypo-, T2/FLAIR hyperintensity, reversible diffusion restriction.**	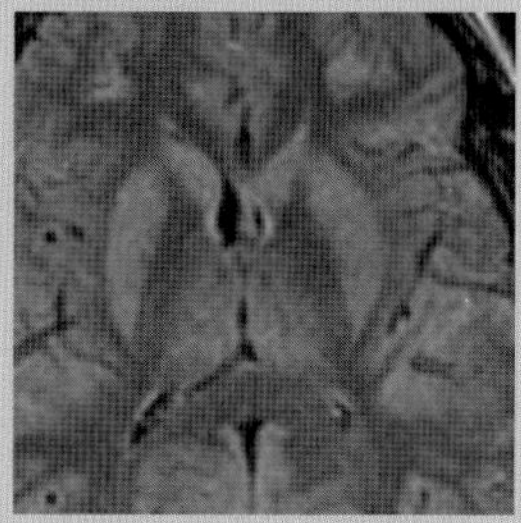 **Fig. 4.27.12:** Hypoglycemic encephalopathy
9. **Fahr disease:** There is no evident underlying cause. **It is a diagnosis of exclusion.**	It is characterized by abnormal vascular calcium deposition, particularly in the **basal ganglia, cerebellar dentate nuclei, and white matter,** with subsequent atrophy.	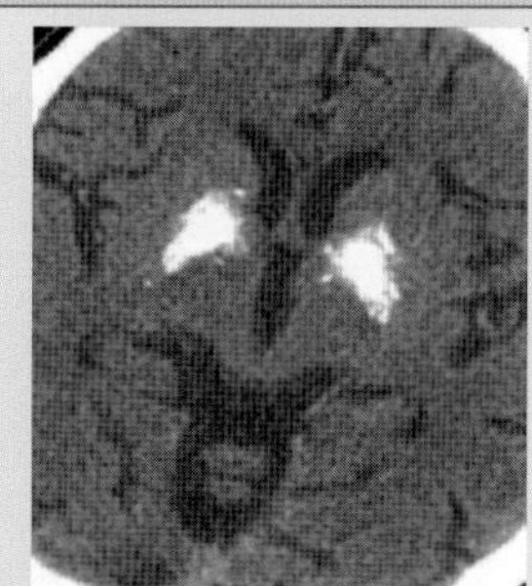 **Fig. 4.27.13:** Fahr disease

Table 4.27.2: Differential diagnosis for globus pallidus lesions		
	Globus pallidus lesions	
Common	*Less common*	*Rare*
Normal variant • Physiologic calcification: Medial GP **Hypoxic-ischemic encephalopathy** • Anoxia, hypoxia (near-drowning, cerebral hypoperfusion) • Neonatal HIE (profound acute) **Toxic/metabolic disorders** • Chronic liver disease—T1 hyperintensity, T2* hypointensity • Carbon monoxide—T2 hyperintense medial GP	**Toxic/metabolic disorders** • Postopioid toxic encephalopathy: Often combined with HIE • Hyperalimentation: Manganese deposition, short T1 • Chronic hypothyroidism: Punctate calcification, T1 hyperintensity, T2 hypointensity **Inherited disorders** • NF1 • Leigh disease	**Toxic/metabolic disorders** • Kernicterus: T1 shortening • Cyanide poisoning: Hemorrhagic GP, laminar cortical necrosis **Inherited disorders** • Fahr disease: Dense symmetric confluent calcification • Wilson disease: T2 hyperintensity in GP, putamen, "Face of giant panda" sign in midbrain • PKAN: "Eye of the tiger" (central T2 hyperintensity, peripheral hypointensity) • Neurodegeneration with brain iron accumulation (NBIA): GP, substantia nigra hypointensity ± putamen • Maple syrup urine disease: Edema (GP, brainstem, thalami, cerebellar WM) • Methylmalonic acidemia (MMA): Symmetric GP T2 hyperintensity ± WM **Degenerative diseases** • Hepatocerebral degeneration: T1 shortening • Progressive supranuclear palsy: Also affects subthalamic nucleus, substantia nigra

Table 4.27.3: Differential diagnosis for globus pallidus lesions based on age and appearance

Globus pallidus lesions by age	*Globus pallidus lesions by characteristic appearance*	
GP lesions of adulthood • Hypoxia/anoxia • Drug abuse • Carbon monoxide poisoning • Hepatic encephalopathy • Hyperalimentation • Hypothyroidism • Wilson disease • NBIA **GP Lesions of childhood** • HIE • NF1 • Leigh disease • Wilson disease • Kernicterus • NBIA, PKAN • Maple syrup urine disease • Methyl malonic aciduria	**CT–hyperdensity** • Physiologic Ca^{++} • Hypothyroidism • Fahr disease • Kearns-Sayre syndrome • Fabry's disease	**MRI–T1 hyperintensity** Chronic hepatic encephalopathy Hyperalimentation (manganese deposition) Neurofibromatosis1 Hypothyroidism Kernicterus (acute) Wilson disease Renal failure (on dialysis) Carbon monoxide poisoning Prior administration of linear gadolinium chelates Unidentified bright objects (NF1)

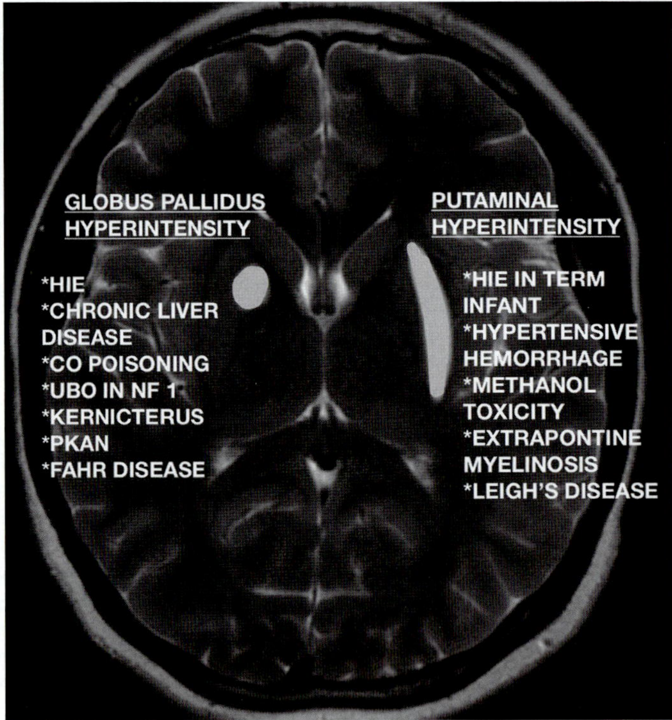

Fig. 4.27.14: Differential diagnosis for globus pallidus and putaminal hyperintensities

4.28 CENTRAL NERVOUS SYSTEM

Case No. 28

Clinical history: A 13-year-old male with history of involuntary movements. His parents give history of behavioural changes for the past two months. His liver function tests show elevated bilirubin levels.

Radiological techniques and observation: MRI brain axial sections in T1WI, T2WI, coronal FLAIR, axial sections (Fig. 4.28.1) in diffusion WI and ADC mapping, SWI sequence shows: Bilateral symmetrical putamen hyperintense signal on T2WI and FLAIR sequence with hypointense signal on DWI. Susceptibility WI sequence shows blooming in the bilateral putamen. The bilateral thalamus appears normal. No evidence of involvement of cortex or white matter. Visualized sections of lateral and third ventricles appear normal.

Interpretation: A—13-year-old male, bilateral putamen lesions, B—Symmetrical, C—T2/FLAIR hyperintensity with blooming in SWI presumably reflect a combination of edema or cystic gray matter degeneration, D—Wilson disease.

Prinicipal diagnosis: Wilson disease.

Differential diagnosis:

- Leigh syndrome
- Hypoxic ischemic encephalopathy
- Creutzfeldt-Jakob disease
- Methanol toxicity
- Extrapontine myelinolysis

Management: Further investigations: Slit lamp examination of cornea for Kayser–Fleischer rings. Serum ceruloplasmin, copper, 24-h urinary copper excretion for confirmation of diagnosis. Referral to neurophysician, Gastroenterologist. Copper chelation therapy to be started.

Discussion: Wilson disease—hepatic dysfunction is the initial manifestation in most patients. 40–60% present with neurologic/psychiatric manifestations. Neurologic symptoms usually start in the late teens, but can occur even earlier. Wilson disease is a rare autosomal-recessive disorder caused by mutations in the ATP7B gene involved in the process of copper transport by mediating the formation of ceruloplasmin and by transporting excess copper into the biliary tract. A defect in this

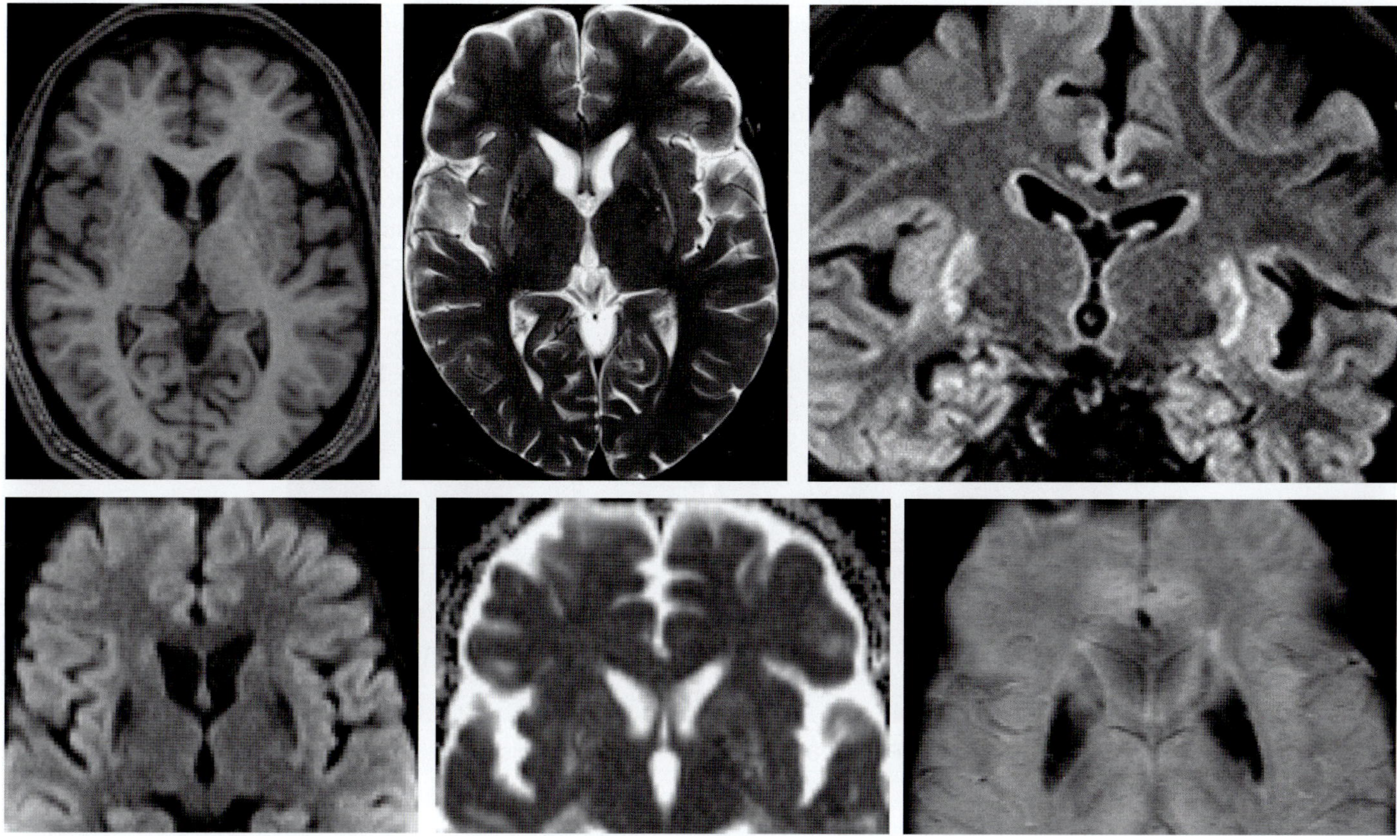

Fig. 4.28.1

Table 4.28.1: Differential diagnosis for corpus striatal hyperintensities

Condition	*Radiological findings*
Leigh syndrome: A frequently lethal disorder that usually presents during infancy, and rarely during childhood and later in life. Developmental delay, seizures, and altered consciousness are the common presenting symptoms. Elevated serum and CSF lactate levels supports the diagnosis.	MR imaging reveals bilateral symmetrical T2 hyperintense lesions of the corpus striatum. Putamen is typically involved, followed by the caudate nuclei. The globi pallidi and thalami area less frequently affected. **Acutely reduced diffusivity** on ADC maps. MRS usually reveals elevated lactate, most prominent within the lesions. Normal MRS, however, does not exclude LD.
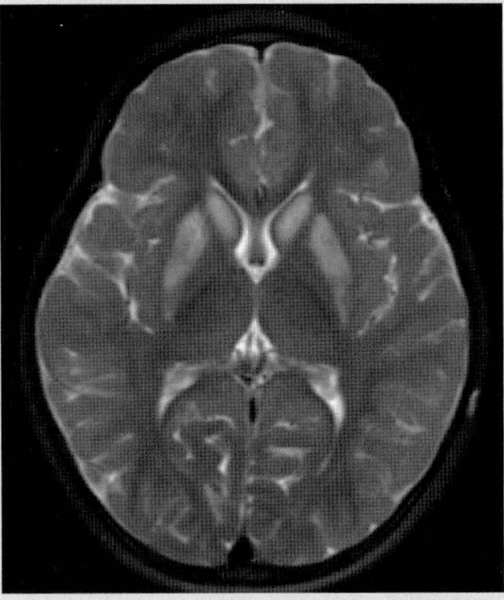 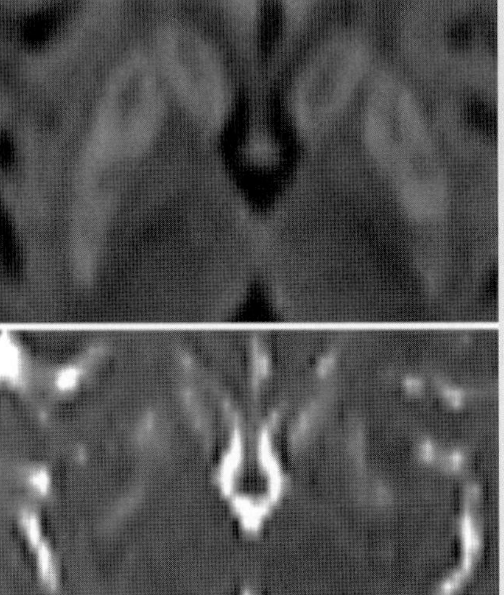 Fig. 4.28.2: Leigh syndrome	
Extrapontine myelinolysis: It most commonly occurs in chronic alcoholics, but also with debilitating illnesses, in transplant recipients, and others. It is associated with rapidly corrected hyponatremia. Symptoms include tetraplegia, bulbar and pseudobulbar palsies, altered mental status, and rapidly progressive coma.	Extrapontine myelinolysis presents as areas of high T2 signal and reduced diffusion involving the supratentorial deep gray matter and/or the corpus callosum. Involvement of the deep gray matter occurs in 10% of patients with CPM. The lesions are T1 hypointense and bright on T2 sequences. Peripheral contrast enhancement may occur during the acute to subacute periods. Reduced diffusion correlates with a worse prognosis. If the patients survive, the lesions may resolve completely or diminish in size.
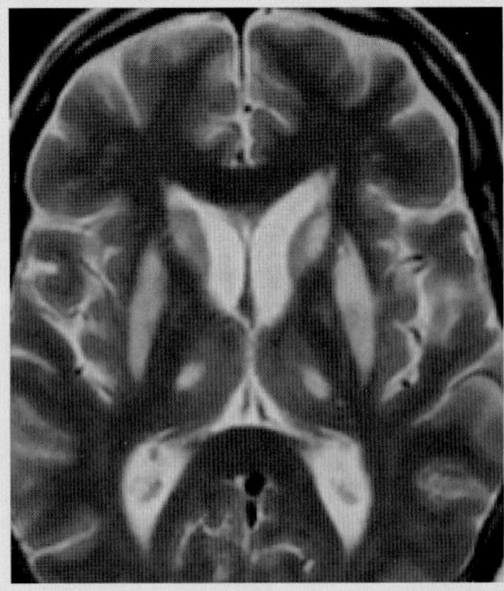 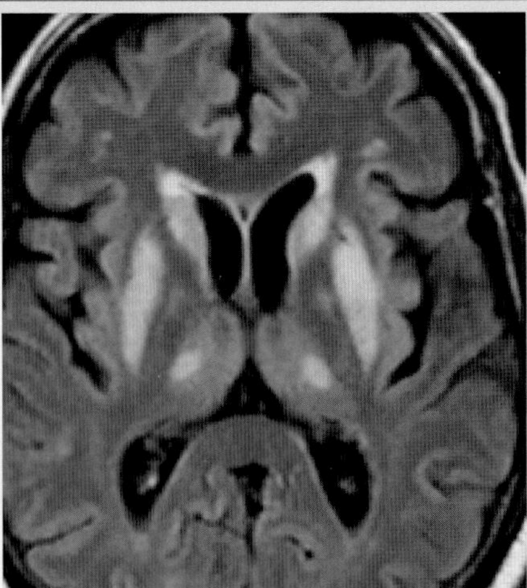 Fig. 4.28.3: Extrapontine myelinolysis	

Contd...

Table 4.28.1: Differential diagnosis for corpus striatal hyperintensities *(Contd..)*	
Condition	*Radiological findings*
Sporadic Creutzfeldt-Jakob disease is the most common form of CJD, occurring in 60 to 70 years age with rapidly progressive dementia, focal neurologic signs and visual symptoms. sharp and slow wave periodic complexes in EEG.	Symmetric high signal on DWI and FLAIR images in the corpora striata, cerebral cortex, and possibly in the thalami. In the early phase of disease, **signal changes may only be detectable on DWI**, which is the most sensitive test for diagnosing CJD. There is no contrast enhancement. A prominent symmetrical high T2 and DWI signal in the pulvinar thalami (the "pulvinar sign") is characteristic of (vCJD). Involvement of the medial thalamus is also common, and the combination has been referred to as the **"hockey stick"** sign.
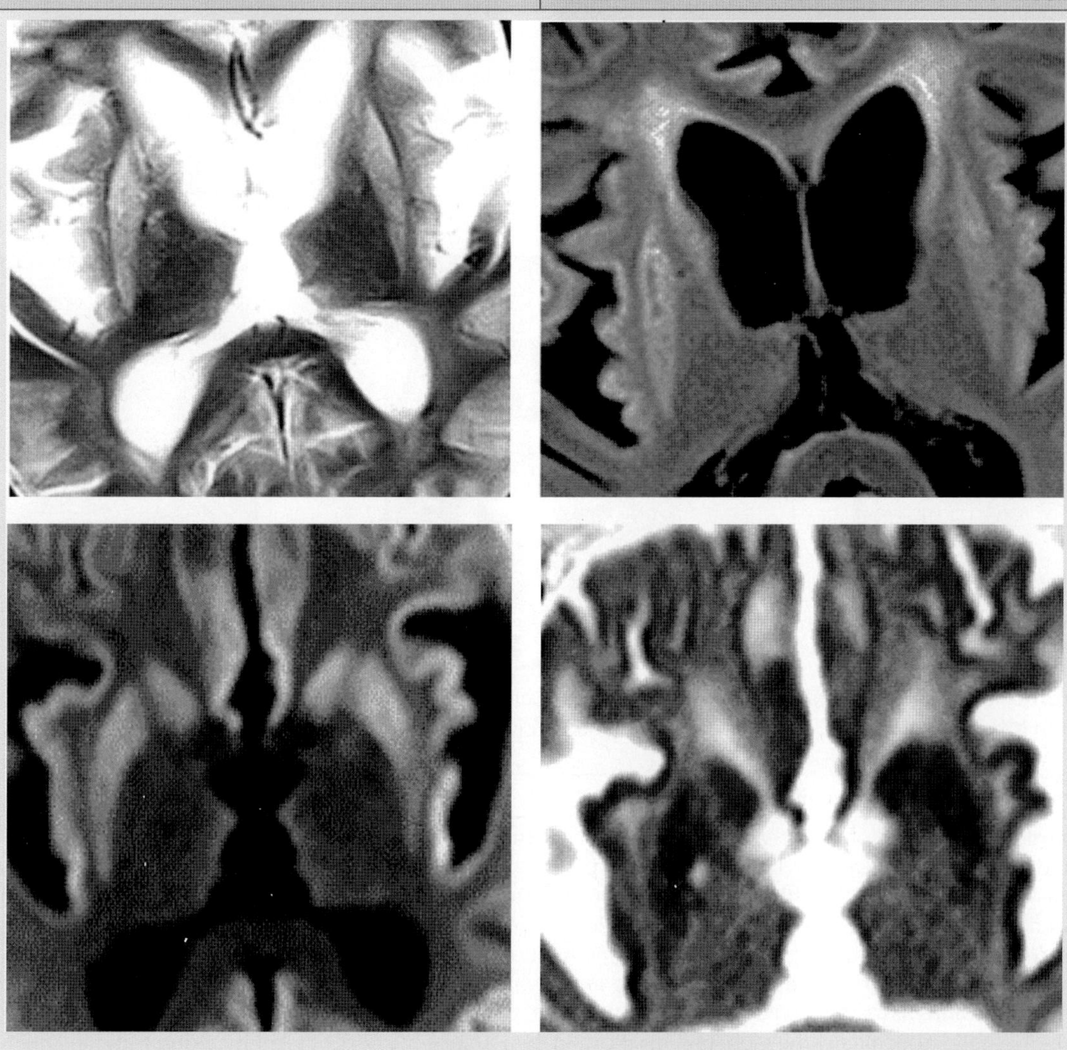 **Fig. 4.28.4:** CJD	
Hepatic encephalopathy: Refer to case 27	

Hyperosmolar hyperglycemic nonketotic syndrome—also called diabetic striatopathy or chorea-hyperglycemia-basal ganglia(C-H-BG) syndrome. It is a neurological complication of non-ketotic hyperglycemia, seen as T1 hyperintense, T2/FLAIR variable signal that shows diffusion restriction.

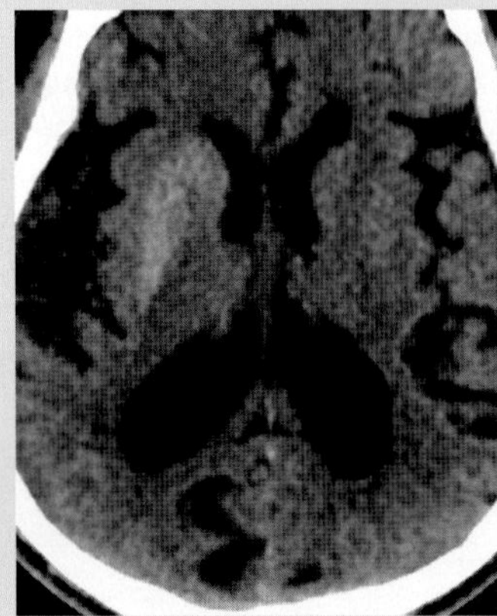

Fig. 4.28.5: Diabetic striatopathy

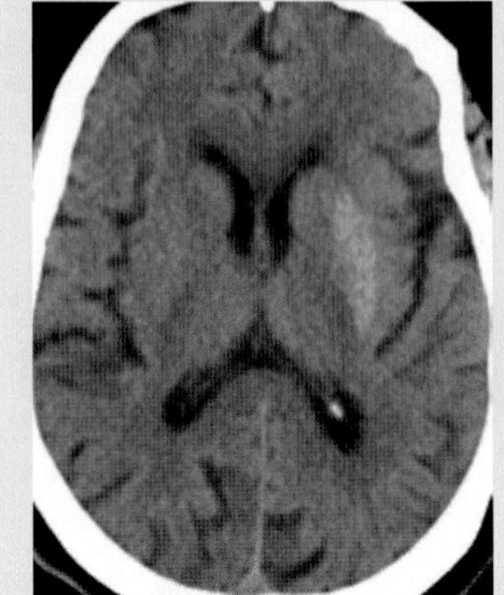

Fig. 4.28.6: Diabetic striatopathy

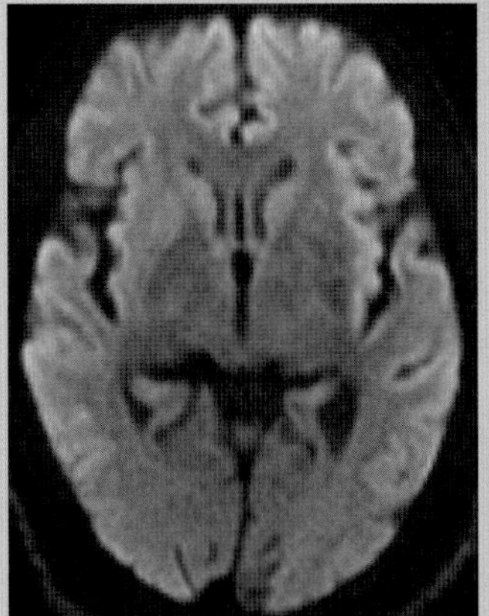

Fig. 4.28.7: Homocitrullinemia (HHH) syndrome with insula involvement syndrome

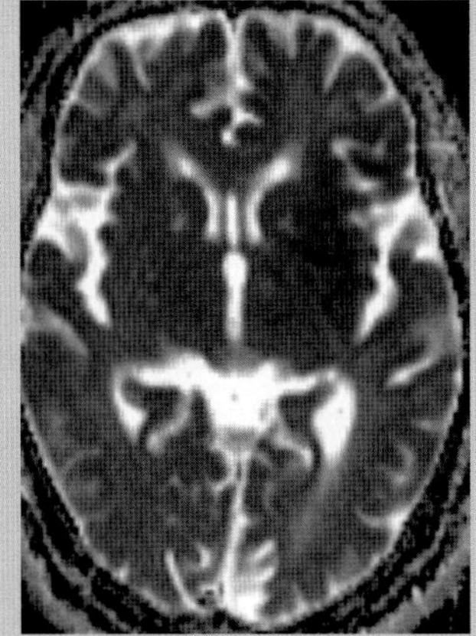

Fig. 4.28.8: Homocitrullinemia(HHH) syndrome with insula involvement syndrome

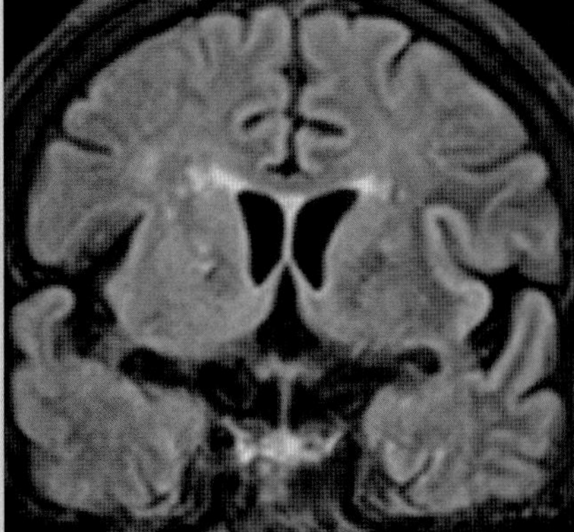

Fig.4.28.9: Homocitrullinemia(HHH) syndrome with insula involvement syndrome

Postfebrile reversible claustral damage: Refer to case 4.24.1

Urea cycle disorders—disorders of the urea cycle result from disruption of the major pathway for the excretion of nitrogen in the body; they include ornithine transcarbamylase deficiency (OTC), carbamyl phosphate synthetase deficiency, argininosuccinic aciduria (argininosuccinate lyase deficiency), citrullinemia (argininosuccinate synthetase deficiency), and hyperargininemia (arginase deficiency). OTC deficiency and citrullinemia are the commonest urea cycle disorders. All result in hyperammonemia and elevation of glutamine levels that may be worsened by high protein intake or illness. Differentiation is made by biochemical and genetic testing. The manifestation depends on the severity with more severe defects resulting in early manifestation in neonatal period with lesser severity defects seen later. CT is non-specific and may show cerebral edema in the acute phase. In MRI, The perirolandic cortex, insular cortex (posterior > anterior) and basal ganglia (specifically the globi pallidi) show T1 hypointensity and T2/FLAIR hyperintensity; In affected neonates, T1 hyperintensity of affected deep gray and cortical structures will appear within the first few days of life. In contrast to hypoxic-ischemic injury, which involves thalamus, predominant involvement of globus pallidus and putamen is seen in urea cycle disorders. In older patients, in the acute phase, the cerebral cortex shows T2 hyperintensity and edema with the frontal lobes being affected more. The perirolandic and occipital cortex seem to be specifically spared. As the disease progresses, atrophy develops; it is often severe and may be multicystic. The subcortical U fibers are involved severely and early and cerebral involvement is often mildly asymmetric. MRS in these disorders in the acute or subacute phase shows lactate doublet at 1.33 ppm and of glutamine/glutamate resonances at 2.1–2.5 ppm and at 3.75 ppm and are best seen with short echo time (20–30 ms) sequences.

The lentiform fork sign—bilateral symmetrical T2/FLAIR hyperintensities in the basal ganglia surrounded by a hyperintense rim delineating the lentiform nucleus—seen in uremic encephalopathy and end stage renal disease.

The putaminal rim sign, also known as putaminal slit sign—parkinsonism (MSA-P) – In T2/ADC map of 1.5 T MRI, linear high signal region around the lateral aspect of the putamen—seen in multiple system atrophy.

Table 4.28.2: Differential diagnosis for symmetrical putaminal/striatal hyperintensity

Symmetrical putaminal/striatal hyperintensity		*Basal ganglia anatomy*
Pediatric causes	*Adult causes*	
1. Leigh syndrome	1. Hypoxic ischemic encephalopathy	C—Head of caudate nucleus G—Globus pallidus P—Putamen
2. MELAS	2. Hypoglycaemia	
3. Wilson's disease	3. Creutzfeldt-Jakob disease (CJD)	
4. Propionic acidemia	4. Cyanide poisoning	
5. Molybdenum cofactor deficiency	5. Encephalitis	
6. Glutaric aciduria type-I	6. Wilson's disease	
7. Juvenile Huntington's disease	7. Osmotic myelinolysis	
8. Osmotic myelinolysis		
9. Hemolytic uremic syndrome		
10. Hypoxia		**Fig. 4.28.10:** Anatomy of corpus striatum Globus pallidus + Putamen = Lentiform nucleus Putamen + Caudate = Corpus striatum

protein results in progressive copper accumulation in hepatocytes, ultimately leading to hepatic dysfunction. Once the liver's capacity to store copper is exceeded, unbound copper becomes deposited in other tissues and organs, including the brain. Copper elevation induces cell death by reducing levels of XIAP, a protein that inhibits apoptosis. In addition to putamen it also involves globus pallidus, caudate nuclei, and ventrolateral thalamus. With severe liver failure, symmetric T1 hyperintensity of globi pallidi may be present, in some patients the characteristic "giant panda" sign is found in the midbrain. Cerebral and cerebellar atrophy can occur. T2 hyperintensities may improve with therapy.

Table 4.28.3: Anatomic distribution of diseases affecting basal ganglia

Anatomic distribution of diseases affecting basal ganglia

Disorder	*Caudate*	*Putamen*	*Globus pallidus*
GM2 gangliosidosis	++	-	-
Molybdenum cofactor def.	++	++	-
Propionic acidemia	++	++	-
Glutaric aciduria type I	++	++	-
Ethylmalonic encephalopathy	++	++	+
HIE-older child	++	++	+
3-hydroxyisobutyric aciduria	++	++	+
Juvenile Huntington disease	++	++	+
Glutaric aciduria type II	+	+	–
HMG-CoA lyase deficiency	+	+	–
Fried syndrome	++	+	++
3-ketothiolase deficiency	–	++	–
Wilson disease	+	++	–
Aicardi-Goutières syndrome	+	++	+
Alpha ketoglutaric aciduria	+	++	+
Cyanide intoxication	+	+	++
Carbon monoxide intoxication	+	+	++
L-2-hydroxyglutaric aciduria	+	+	++
3-methylglutaconic aciduria (type 1 and 4)	++	++	++
Hemolytic uremic syndrome	+	+	+
Uremic encephalopathy (lentiform fork sign)	+	+	+
Osmotic myelinolysis	+	+	+
Viral encephalitis	+	+	+
Leigh syndrome	+	+	+
Hypoglycemia—older child	+	+	+

Only caudate: GM2 Gangliosidosis

Putamen > caudate
Wilson disease, Alpha ketoglutaric aciduria
Aicardi-Goutières syndrome

Primarily Globus pallidus involvement
Canavan disease—NAA peak on MRS
Pantothenate kinase-associated neurodegeneration
Toxins (carbon monoxide and cyanide)
Kernicterus
Unidentified neurofibromatosis objects (NF-1)
Kearns-Sayre syndrome
Methylmalonic acidemia
Maple syrup urine disease
L-2-hydroxyglutaric aciduria
Fucosidosis (T2/FLAIR hypointensity)
Urea cycle disorders
Cree leukoencephalopathy
MSA-P

Primarily striatal involvement (caudate and putamen)
Leigh syndrome
Infantile bilateral striatal necrosis
MELAS—usually cortical involvement
Wilson disease
Alexander disease (with frontal white matter)
Ethylmalonic acidemia
Propionic acidemia
Glutaric aciduria Type I with anterior temporal lobe hypoplasia
Molybdenum co-factor deficiency
Mitochondrial ATP synthetase deficiency
3-methylglutaconic aciduria
Beta ketothiolase deficiency
Malonic acidemia
Alpha ketoglutaric aciduria
Biotin responsive basal ganglia disease
Hypoxic-ischemic injury in older child or adult
Hypoglycemic injury in older child or adult
Cockayne disease

Only anterior putamen involvement 3-methyl glutaric aciduria

Only posterior putamen HIE

Diffuse involvement of entire putamen alone 3-ketothiolase deficiency, methanol toxicity.

Table 4.28.4: Differential diagnosis for T2 hyperintensities		
Pons	*Bilateral dentate nucleus*	*Bilateral claustrum/external capsule*
Osmotic demyelination, Wilson's disease, hypoxic tegmental watershed lesions, Leigh's syndrome complex ii and iii deficiency Vigabatrin related epileptic infants	Metronidazole toxicity Krabbe's disease Canavan's disease Maple syrup urine disease Cerebro tendinous Xanthomatosis L 2 hydroxy glutaric aciduria Glutaric aciduria type 1	Wilson's disease Auto immune encephalitis Febrile infection related epilepsy syndrome Niemann-Pick syndrome
Bilateral insula	*Bilateral middle cerebellar peduncle*	*Dorsal tegmental hyperintensity*
Herpes encephalitis Adult-onset ornithine transcarbamylase (OTC) deficiency Hepatic encephalopathy, urea cycle disorders	Sporadic olivo ponto cerebellar atrophy, Spino cerebellar ataxia Hypoglycemic coma Cerebrovascular disease, Shy Drager syndrome, Adreno leukodystrophy, alcoholic liver cirrhosis, brain stem glioma, meningeal carcinomatosis, hypertensive and its related encephalopathies, AICA infarction, hypertensive encephalopathy, cyclosporin-A encephalopathy, inflammatory and demyelinating diseases, multiple sclerosis, ADEM, Behçet disease, HIV encephalopathy	Seen in child of 1 to 5 years presenting as epilepsy, cerebral palsy, neoplasm. Nonketotic hyperglycinemia, mitochondrial disorders, methionine adenosyl transferase deficiency, leukoencephalopathy with vanishing white matter, neonatal intrahepatic cholestasis due to citrin deficiency, 6-pyruvoyl-tetrahydropterin synthetase deficiency, and perinatal asphyxia are included under metabolic disorders.

4.29 CENTRAL NERVOUS SYSTEM

Case No. 29

Clinical history: A 44-day-old female baby, brought with complaints of refusal of feeds and irritability. Fever for 2 days, one episode of seizure on day 2 of admission. Full-term normal vaginal delivery/appropriate for gestational age, birth weight 2.7 kg, cried immediately after birth, APGAR score 8/10.

Radiological techniques and observations: Figures 4.29.1 to 4.29.6 are MRI brain diffusion weighted and ADC map images in axial sections with MRS images. Diffusion restriction noted in posterior limb of bilateral internal capsule, bilateral medial and ventrolateral thalamus, bilateral globus pallidus, dorsal brainstem, bilateral corticospinal tract (red arrow), bilateral dentate nuclei and middle cerebellar peduncles. Figure 4.29.4 is MRS image showing a broad peak at 0.9 ppm and another peak at 1.3 ppm, representing branched-chain amino acids and lactate, respectively. Corpus callosum, cerebral cortex and non-myelinated white matter are uninvolved. Imaging abnormalities are much more conspicuous infratentorially than supratentorially.

Interpretation: A: 44-day-old female baby, myelinated fibres of the bilateral posterior limb of internal capsule, thalamus, globus pallidus, dorsal brainstem, corticospinal tract, dentate nuclei and middle cerebellar peduncles, C: Diffusion restriction, MRS shows branched chain amino acid and lactate peak, B: Symmetrical, D: Maple syrup urine disease.

Principal diagnosis: **Inherited metabolic disease—maple syrup urine disease.**

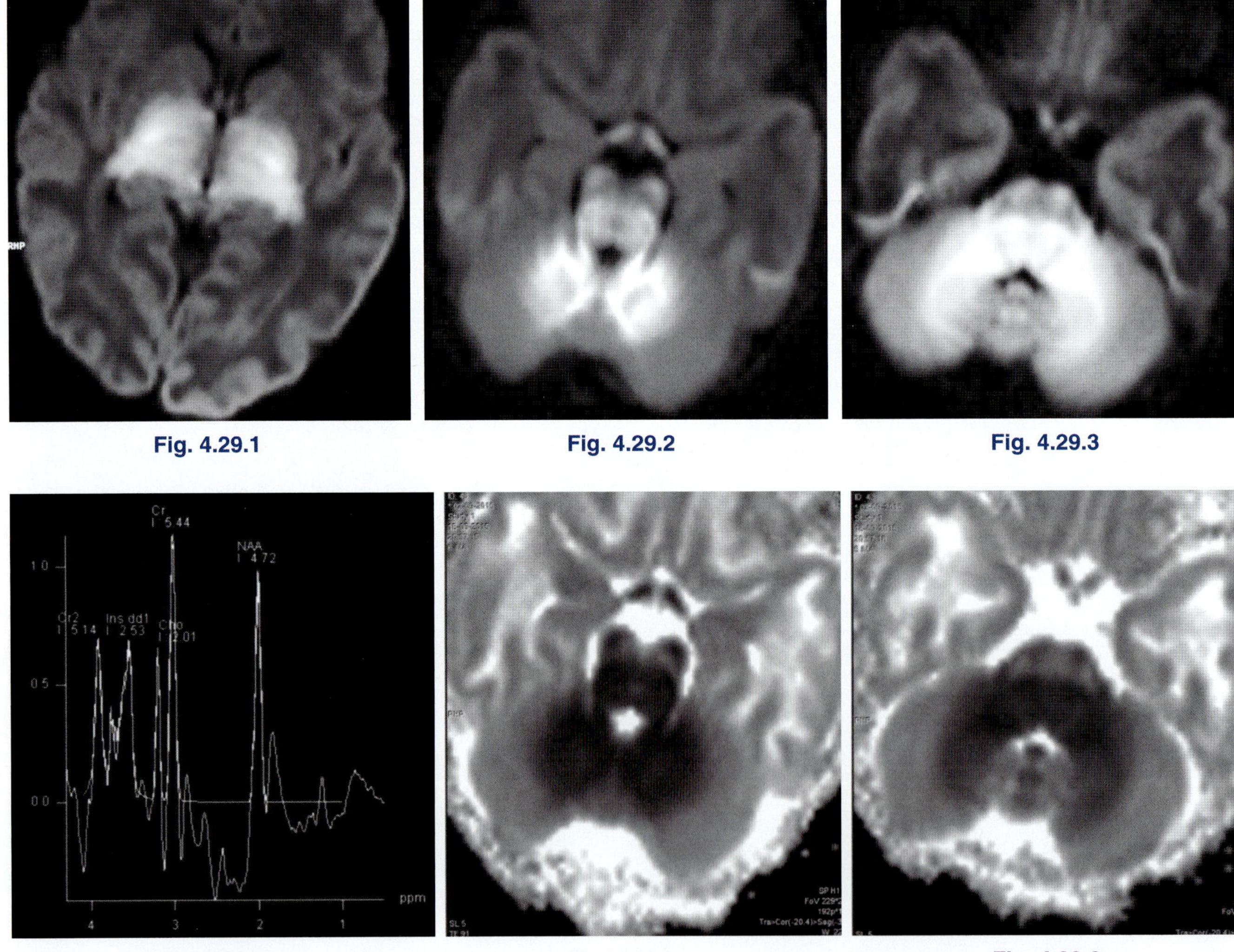

Fig. 4.29.1 Fig. 4.29.2 Fig. 4.29.3

Fig. 4.29.4 Fig. 4.29.5 Fig. 4.29.6

Table 4.29.1: Differential diagnosis of neonatal diffusion restricting lesions		
Differential diagnosis	*Imaging findings*	*Image*
Term hypoxic ischemic injury: Manifests at birth: **1 month** Affects the **early myelinating and metabolically active structures.** Thalami/basal ganglia/dorsal brainstem and cerebellum commonly involved.	Diffusion restriction, and T1 hyperintensity in globus pallidus and thalami with relative hypointensity of posterior limb of internal capsule. Elevated lactate at 1.3 ppm **(prognosticator)**	**Fig. 4.29.7:** HIE
Neonatal/infantile hypoglycemia: Most common metabolic disorder encountered in the neonatal period. Common in **2–3 months**. White matter injury common, may be predominantly periventricular in premature.	T2 hyperintensity in **bilateral parieto-occipital region.** Cortex, WM and splenium are swollen and hyperintense.	**Fig. 4.29.8:** Infantile hypoglycemia
Neonatal chikungunya encephalopathy—Refer to case 24.1		
Parecho virus (HPeV)—Refer to case 24.1		
Phenylketonuria: Occurs because of abnormal metabolism of phenylalanine. If untreated, patients may develop central nervous system impairment. Treatment is phenylalanine-restricted diet with the avoidance of foods such as breast milk, meat, nuts, dairy products and starchy foods. Reversal of CNS changes is possible with diet change.	**MRS: Phenylalanine peak at 7.37 ppm.** 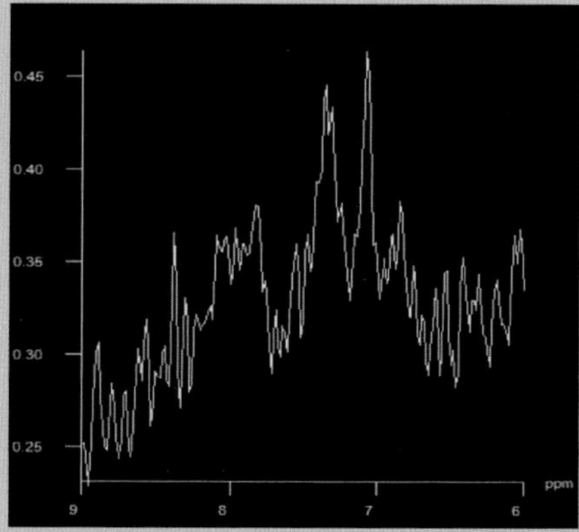 **Fig. 4.29.9: MRS:** Phenylalanine peak at 7.37 ppm	T2/FLAIR hyperintensity occurring first in the periventricular/ parieto-occipital white matter before eventually affecting the subcortical white matter. Reduced diffusion in acutely affected areas. 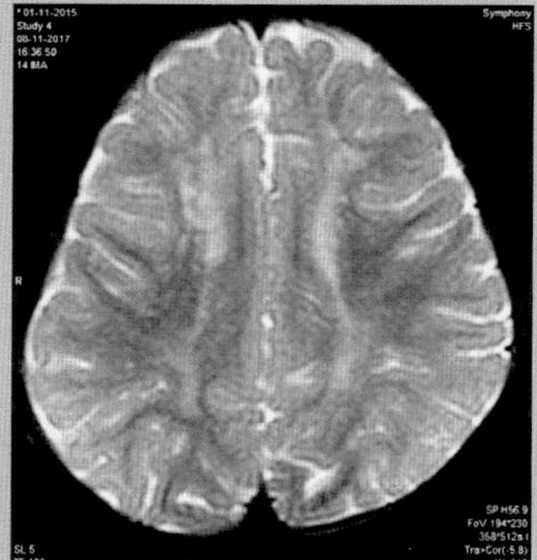 **Fig. 4.29.10:** PKU showing periventricular/ parieto-occipital white matter hyperintensity
Incontinentia pigmenti also known as Bloch-Sulzberger syndrome, X-linked dominant genetic disorder—Refer to case 6 for detailed explanation.		
Others include dengue encephalopathy		

Creatine deficiency syndrome caused by GAMT deficiency presents with neurodevelopmental delay, rarely seizures, behavioral disturbances, and mild hypotonia, posing diagnostic challenges. Metabolic investigations show low creatinine in plasma, urine and slightly elevated lactate. MRI may be normal. Correct diagnosis is possible only after MR spectroscopy. **Absence of creatine peak at 3.0 ppm is characteristic.** Normal structural MRI does not exclude a creatine deficiency syndrome. Thus, a treatable disease will not be missed (Fig. 4.29.11).

Management of MSUD: **Patient to be immediately referred to the paediatric neurology department for confirming the diagnosis and for prompt management.** Confirm the diagnosis by assessing urine and blood ketone levels. Involves dietary changes, such as life-long dietary intake restriction of foods with branched-chain amino acids (especially leucine), and early treatment of metabolic decompensation, with agents such as intravenous glucose.

Discussion: **Maple syrup urine disease (MSUD)**, also known as leucine encephalopathy, is an autosomal-recessive disorder of branched-chain amino acid (leucine, isoleucine, valine) metabolism. Transcranial US during the acute stage of MSUD oedema shows hyperechogenicity reflecting edema within the thalami and basal ganglia, periventricular white matter, brainstem and cerebellum. In fact, unexplained cerebral hemispheric, basal ganglia, thalamic, brainstem, and cerebellar edema in the newborn should provoke a consideration of MSUD in the differential diagnosis. DWI/DTI shows restricted diffusion in the T2/FLAIR hyperintense regions; look for **four-dot brainstem sign. MRS** is quite specific and shows slight reduction of N-Acetyl Asparte (NAA), elevation of lactate, a broad peak at 0.9 and 1.3 ppm representing branched-chain amino acids and lactate, respectively, and a peak at 3.6 ppm representing valine.

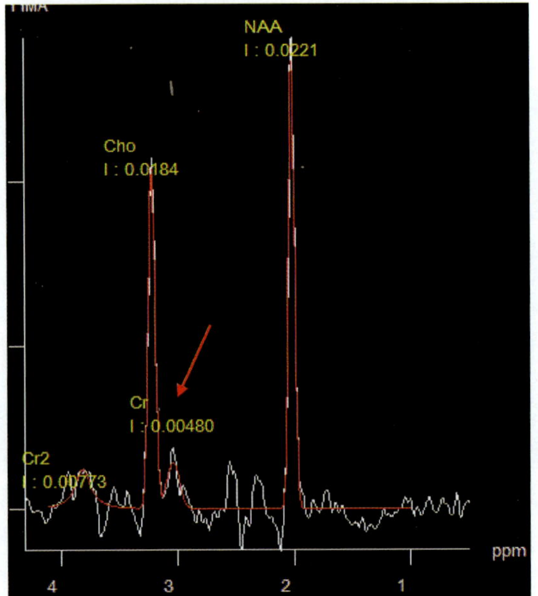

Fig. 4.29.11: Absence of creatine peak at 3.0 ppm in creatine deficiency syndrome

Table 4.29.2: Summary of neonatal metabolic diseases

Neonatal metabolic diseases	
Disorder type	*Diseases*
Amino acid metabolism disorders	Maple syrup urine disease, urea cycle defect (citrullinemia, ornithine transcarbamoylase deficiency, carbamoyl phosphate synthetase deficiency, argininosuccinic aciduria), and nonketotic hyperglycinemia.
Organic acid disorders	Canavan disease, propionic acidemia, methylmalonic acidemia, isovaleric acidemia, multiple carboxylase deficiency, and pyroglutamic aciduria.
Primary lactic acidosis	Pyruvate dehydrogenase deficiency, pyruvate carboxylase deficiency, cytochrome oxidase deficiency, complex succinate dehydrogenase (type II) deficiency.
Fatty acid oxidation disorders	Carnitine cycle defects (carnitine–palmitoyl transferase deficiency, carnitine translocase deficiency), mitochondrial β-oxidation disorders (very long-, medium-, and short-chain acyl coenzyme A dehydrogenase deficiency), and electron transfer flavoprotein dehydrogenase deficiency (glutaric aciduria type II).
Other metabolic disorders	Zellweger syndrome, neonatal adrenoleukodystrophy Krabbe disease (globoid cell leukodystrophy), Menkes disease (trichopoliodystrophy), D-bifunctional protein deficiency, sulfite oxidase deficiency, and galactosemia.

Toxic encephalopathy (adult): **1. Alcohol related toxic encephalopathy** includes: Acute alcohol poisoning, chronic alcoholic encephalopathy, Wernicke encephalopathy, Marchiafava-Bignami disease and methanol intoxication. **Acute alcohol poisoning** is rare; caused by binge drinking. Imaging shows diffuse cerebral oedema and acute demyelination. **Chronic alcoholic encephalopathy** has primary toxic effect on neurons. Secondary effects are related to liver, GI disease. Hepatic encephalopathy occurs due to malnutrition, malabsorption and electrolyte imbalance. Imaging shows atrophy (superior vermis, cerebellum, generalized) and white matter myelinolysis. **Wernicke encephalopathy** classic triad includes ocular dysfunction, ataxia and altered mental status. It can occur in children. Intravenous thiamine is imperative. In imaging MR > > CT (usually not helpful). T2/FLAIR hyperintensity, DWI restriction seen. Common location includes medial thalami (85%), periaqueductal gray matter (65%), mammillary bodies (60%), tectum (30%). Less common areas are dorsal medulla (8%), cerebellum/cranial nerve nuclei (1%), corpus callosum–splenium. SWI may show microhaemorrhages. Enhancement varies, more common in alcoholic WE; mammillary body enhancement pathognomonic. **Marchiafava-Bignami disease** known as "red wine drinkers' encephalopathy." Corpus callosum degeneration is the hallmark of MBD. CT findings may be normal in the acute stage of MBD. Chronic MBD—linear hypodensity in the genu of corpus callosum.

Methanol intoxication, bilateral basal ganglia necrosis is the most characteristic imaging feature. Selective putamina involvement with relative sparing of the globi pallidi is common. Diffuse necrosis of the subinsular and subcortical white matter occurs in severe cases. **2. Cocaine and amphetamine effects on the brain,** methamphetamine causes hemorrhagic, ischemic strokes.

MDMA (ecstasy)

It causes vasospasm and infarct. Location includes occipital cortex, globus pallidus. **Cocaine** causes delayed toxic leukoencephalopathy. **Cocaine** causes intracranial haemorrhage; hypertensive intracranial hemorrhage (50%) and "unmasked" aneurysm or arteriovenous malformation (50%). Ischemic stroke, vasospasm, vasculitis and acute hypertensive encephalopathy—posterior reversible encephalopathy syndrome (PRES). **Heroin** most commonly causes ischemic stroke in globus pallidi, white matter (resembles carbon monoxide poisoning). **Carbon monoxide poisoning:** Acute: symmetric globi pallidi necrosis. Subacute ("interval"): confluent leukoencephalopathy. In nitrous oxide abuse brain lesions rare, may result in subacute combined degeneration of the spinal cord and hyperintensities in dorsal columns. Toluene (solvent) abuse causes cerebral atrophy and white matter lesions. Cyanide poisoning causes basal ganglia haemorrhage and laminar cortical necrosis.

4.30 CENTRAL NERVOUS SYSTEM

Case No. 30

Clinical history: 20 days old female baby with birth asphyxia, in NICU, had cardiac arrest and resuscitated.

Radiological technique: Figures 4.30.1 to 4.30.6 are MRI brain of DWI, ADC map, T1, T2 and FLAIR images respectively.

T1 hyperintense symmetric altered signal intensity noted in bilateral **posterior putamen and anterolateral thalamus**. Diffusion restriction noted in bilateral posterior lentiform nucleus. Altered signal intensity also noted in anterolateral thalamus and perirolandic fronto-parietal cortex. Myelination of **posterior limb of internal capsule** is not maintained.

Interpretation: A: Neonate, lesion in posterolateral putamen and ventrolateral thalamus involvement, B: Bilateral symmetrical, C: T1 hyperintensity with diffusion restriction, D: Acute profound hypoxic ischemic encephalopathy.

Principal diagnosis: Hypoxic ischemic encephalopathy.

Differential diagnoses:

1. Venous ischemia: Asymmetrical, changes in venous distribution, gradient shows blooming.
2. Chikungunya fever.

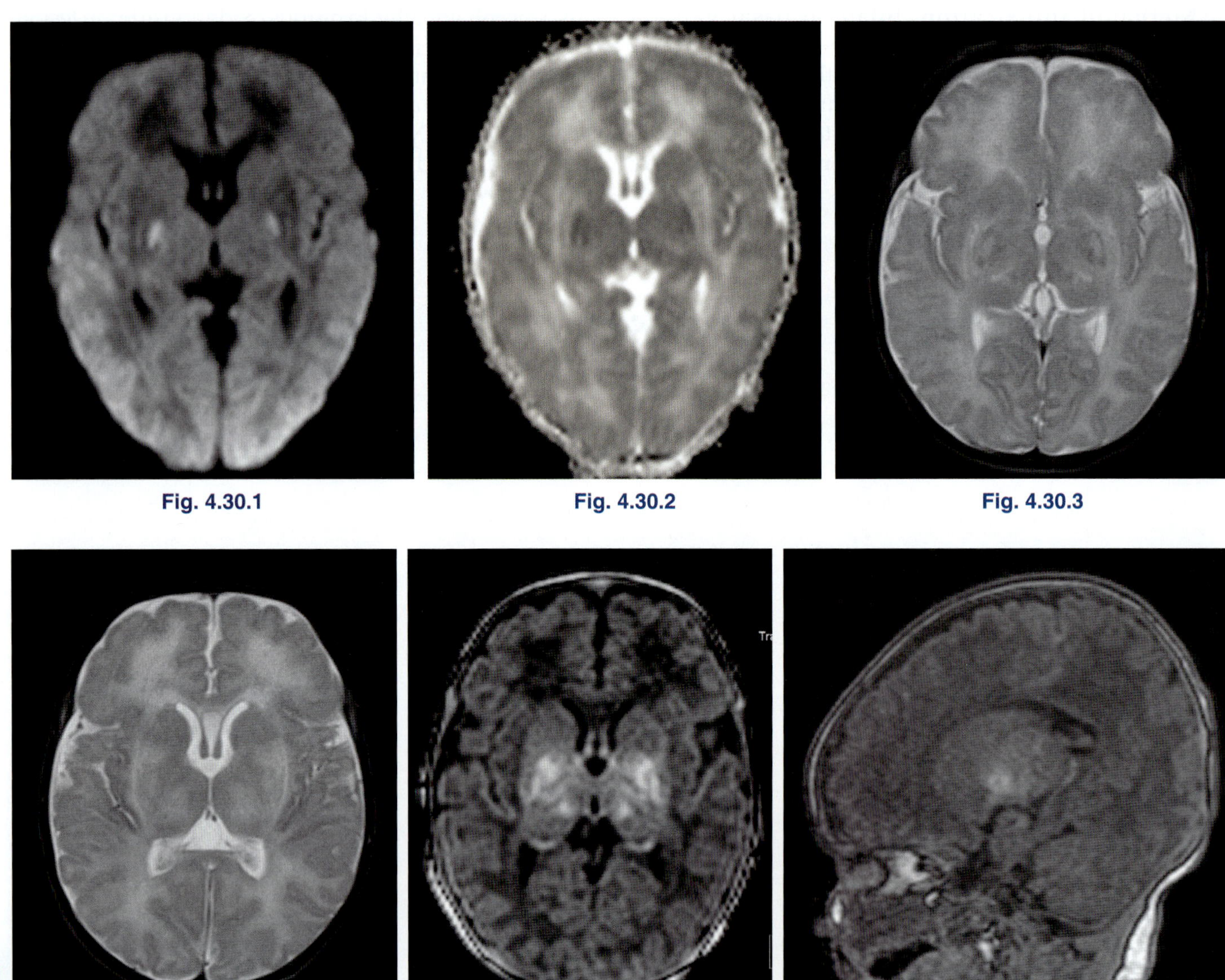

Fig. 4.30.1 Fig. 4.30.2 Fig. 4.30.3

Fig. 4.30.4 Fig. 4.30.5 Fig. 4.30.6

3. Neonatal parechovirus encephalitis.
4. Incontinentia pigmenti.
5. Mitochondrial disorders
6. Inborn errors of metabolism—MSUD, isolated sulfite oxidase deficiency and molybdenum cofactor deficiency.

Other investigations: MRS

- Increased lactate correlates with worst prognosis
- Decreased NAA correlates with worst prognosis.
- Increased alpha glutamate/glutamine peaks in basal ganglia correlates with increased severity of injury.
  US and CT: Insensitive. Useful in preterm infants.
  Doppler ultrasound: Decreased RI in severe profound HIE.

Management:

- Resuscitation, fluid correction and electrolyte imbalance.
- Therapeutic hypothermia: Cool to 33.5°C for 72 hours.

Complications:

- Spastic quadriparesis
- Extrapyramidal cerebral palsy

Brief discussion:

Neonatal hypoxic brain injuries:

1. Hydranencephaly and porencephaly
2. Periventricular—intraventricular hemorrhage
3. Periventricular and subcortical leukomalacia
4. Hypoxic ischemic encephalopathy (Tables 4.30.1, 4.30.2 and Fig 4.30.7)

Sarnat clinical staging of HIE	
I.	Hyperalert/irritable, mydriasis, tachycardia with normal EEG.
II.	Lethargy, hypotonia, miosis, bradycardia with seizure pattern.
III.	Stupor, flaccid, absent reflexes with seizure pattern.

Fig. 4.30.7: Sarnat clinical staging of HIE

Table 4.30.1: Difference between partial HIE and profound HIE

Partial HIE	*Profound HIE*
No sentinel events. Moderate lack of blood flow/O_2 Sparing of areas with high metabolic demand—redistribution.	Sentinel event like cardiopulmonary arrest. Injury to areas with high metabolic demand.

Table 4.30.2: Pattern of injury in HIE

Fetus	*Mild to moderate hypoxia*	*Profound hypoxia*	*Profound hypoxia for longer duration*
Pre-term	Watershed areas—periventricular and deep white matter (peri-ventricular leukomalacia)	Thalamus, basal ganglia and brainstem	**Multi-cystic encephalomalacia** (Figs 4.30.10 to 4.30.13)
Term	Shorter duration—perirolandic white matter involvement. Moderate—parasagittal watershed cortex and white matter. Longer duration—entire cortex and underlying white matter.	Thalamus, basal ganglia, perirolandic cortex, corticospinal tracts, dorsal brainstem and vermis.	

HII (HYPOXIC ISCHEMIC INJURY) IN TERM NEONATE

I. **Severe asphyxia in term neonates:** It results in a primarily central pattern of injury involving the deep gray matter **(putamina, ventro-lateral thalami, hippocampi, dorsal brainstem, and lateral geniculate nuclei)**.

- USG findings include a global increase in cerebral echogenicity and obliteration of the cerebrospinal fluid (CSF)—containing spaces, suggesting diffuse cerebral edema. Thalamic echogenicity suggests a more severe injury.
- **Doppler** shows **diminished resistive indexes (<0.6)** in the anterior and middle cerebral arteries—associated with a poor clinical outcome.
- **MRI**
- First 24 hours—DWI is more sensitive in early stage of the disease. T1 and T2W iamges may be normal (Fig. 4.30.9).
- DWI will demonstrate increased signal intensity in the region of the **ventro-lateral thalami and basal ganglia (particularly the posterior putamina), in the perirolandic regions, and along the corticospinal tracts,** subsequently "pseudo-normalize" by the end of the 1st week
- Day 2—hyperintensity on both T1- and T2-weighted images.
- 2nd week—T2 shortening subsequently develops in the thalami and posterior putamina.
  T1 shortening in the thalami, basal ganglia, and perirolandic cortex may persist for several months.

II. Partial asphyxia in term neonates: DWI typically demonstrates cortical and subcortical white matter restriction, most pronounced in the parasagittal **watershed territories**.

HII IN PRETERM NEONATES

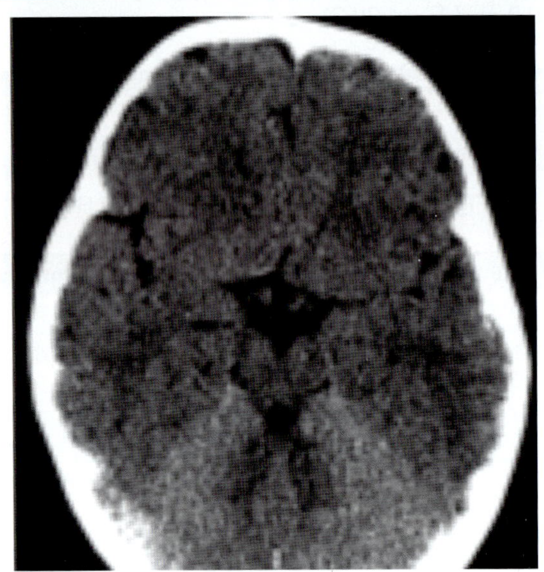

Fig. 4.30.8: Profound HIE with white cerebellum sign

HIE is more common in preterm neonates

I. Mild to moderate

1. Germinal matrix—intraventricular hemorrhages.
2. Periventricular leukomalacia and brain stem.

II. Severe: Damage to deep gray matter.

I. Mild to moderate injury in pre-term infants: Grading of germinal matrix hemorrhage (based on Burstein, Papile, et al)

1. Sub-ependymal hemorrhage with no or minimal intraventricular extension.
2. Hemorrhage extending from the germinal matrix into the ventricles without ventricular enlargement.
3. With ventricular enlargement.
4. Periventricular parenchymal hemorrhagic infarction.

Periventricular leukomalacia:

- Which is also known as white matter injury of prematurity.
- It is due to ischemia in watershed zones existing in the periventricular white matter of immature brains.
- PVL is mostly observed adjacent to the trigones of the lateral ventricles and adjacent to the foramina of Monro.
- End-stage PVL shows a reduction in the volume of periventricular white matter and centrum semiovale, ventriculomegaly with dilatation of the trigones and an irregular ventricular outline.

II. Severe injury in preterm infants:

USG: Increased echogenicity in the thalami by 48–72 hours following an insult.

MRI: Injury to the thalami, basal ganglia, hippocampi, cerebellum, and corticospinal tracts can be seen. The perirolandic cortex is spared often.

- First 24 hours: Diffusion abnormalities are usually evident in the thalami.
- 2nd day: T2 prolongation can be seen in the thalami and basal ganglia.
- 3rd day: T1 shortening will be seen in the injured areas.
- 7th day: T2 shortening develops in the injured areas.
- T1 shortening persists into the chronic stage.

HII IN POSTNATAL INFANTS AND YOUNG CHILDREN

Hypoxic-ischemic injuries in infants and young children are usually the result of drowning, severe head trauma, status epilepticus and post-cardiac arrest hypoxia or nonaccidental trauma.

Early CT—negative or may demonstrate only subtle hypoattenuation of the deep gray matter structures.

- **"Reversal sign"**—there is reversal in the normal CT attenuation of gray matter and white matter.
- **"White cerebellum sign or dense cerebellum sign"**—Diffuse decrease in density of the supratentorial brain parenchyma with relatively increased attenuation of thalami, brainstem and cerebellum. Indicates irreversible brain damage and has a very poor prognosis (Fig. 4.30.8).

  MRI—DWI in the first 12–24 hours demonstrates bright signal intensity in the posterolateral lentiform nuclei and ventrolateral thalamic nuclei. Mild to moderate asphyxia result in watershed zone injuries, involving the cortex and subcortical white matter. **HIE** in postnatal infants and young children.
- Extensive cystic gliosis involving bilateral cerebral hemisphere (frontal, parietal, temporal and occipital

Evolution of DWI in HIE

Most sensitive sequence in the first 24 hrs.

Increase in severity over days

Normalize > 1 week

Less sensitive after therapeutic hypothermia

Fig. 4.30.9: Evolution of DWI in HIE

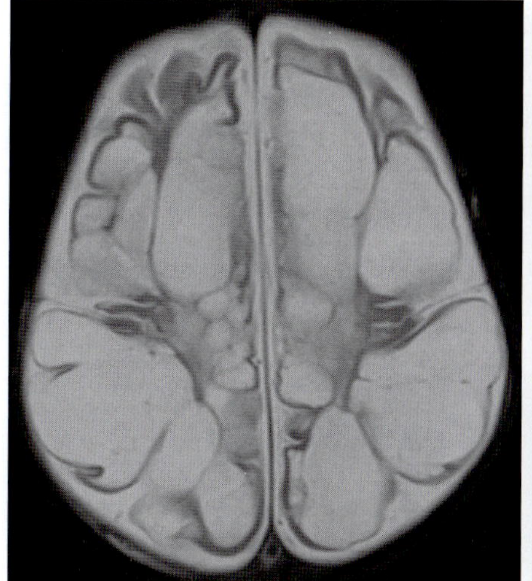
Fig. 4.30.10: Multicystic encephalomalacia

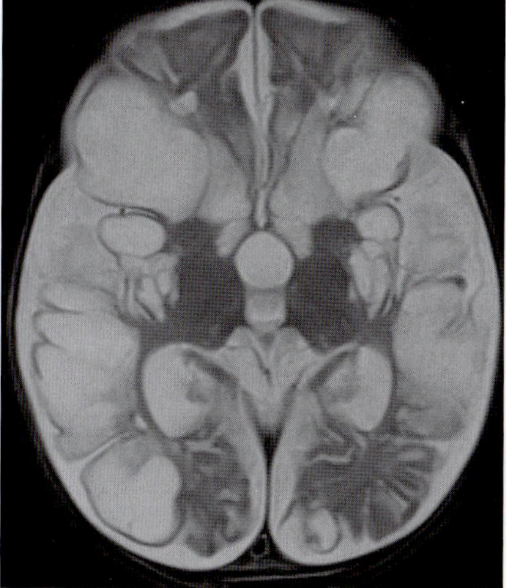
Fig. 4.30.11: Multicystic encephalomalacia

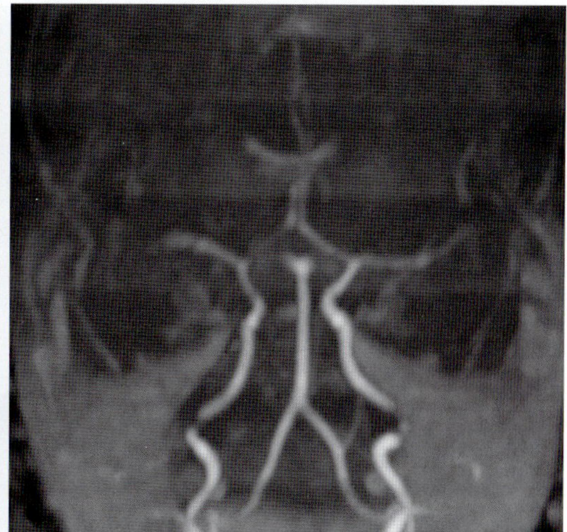
Fig. 4.30.12: Multicystic encephalomalacia

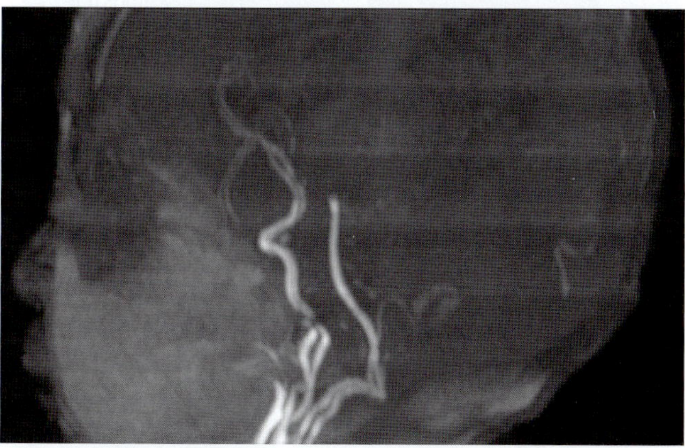
Fig. 4.30.13: Multicystic encephalomalacia

cortex with white matter), insula, basal ganglia and thalamus (Figs 4.30.10 to 4.30.13).

- Diffuse severe thinning of corpus callosum.
- Ex-vacuo dilatation of ventricles.
- MRA shows attenuated cortical branches of MCA, ACA and PCA.

Status marmoratus: Acute total asphyxia in full term infants causing bilateral basal ganglia and thalamic lesions characterized by edema, gliosis and calcifications with marbled appearance.

Role of proton MRS in the evaluation of HII: Demonstrate HII as early as **2–8 hours**.

Common sites: The deep gray nuclei, parieto-occipital region, or white matter of the parasagittal watershed zones.

Lactate elevation (appearing as a doublet centered at 1.3 ppm at 1.5T).

A glutamine-glutamate peak can be detected at 2.3 ppm.

Mean lactate: NAA ratio greater than 0.5.

Terminal zones of myelination: Differentiation between these lesions and periventricular leukomalacia (PVL) is important as the terminal zone has no clinical relevance. **Detection of normally myelinated low T2 signal white matter in-between the high signal patches** and the lateral ventricle favors the diagnosis of terminal zone (Fig. 4.30.14).

Carpus Callosal Agenesis

Imaging features: Antenatal USG (>22 weeks GA)—absence of septum pellucidum, "teardrop" ventriculomegaly, enlargement of occipital horns (colpocephaly), dilated + elevated 3rd ventricle, radial array pattern of medial cerebral sulci (Table 4.30.3).

Table 4.30.3: Corpus callosal agenesis imaging features

MRI T2/T1-IR sagittal	*MRI T2/T1-IR axial*	*MRI T2/T1-IR coronal*
• Partial or complete CC agenesis • Third ventricle appears "open" to interhemispheric fissure • Cingulate gyrus absent → gyri "radiate" outward from third ventricle	• Lateral ventricles parallel, nonconverging, widely separated • Probst bundles = WM along medial margins of lateral ventricles	• "Viking helmet" or "moose head" appearance • "High-riding" third ventricle • Pointed, upcurving lateral ventricles • Probst bundles

Table 4.30.4: Difference between hypoglycemic encephalopathy and hypoxic encephalopathy	
Hypoglycemic encephalopathy	*Hypoxic encephalopathy*
1. Bilateral symmetric areas and restricted diffusion in **occipital, parietal, medial** thalamus (hockey stick appearance). 2. White mater injury common, predominantly in periventricular in premature babies. 3. Perilesional edema +	1. T2/FLAIR hyperintensity of injured gray matter structure. 2. Earliest sign—diffusion restriction in cerebellar hemispheres, basal ganglia—perirolandic cortex, occipital cortex (due to early cytotoxic edema). After 24 hrs—pseudonormalization occurs in DWI.
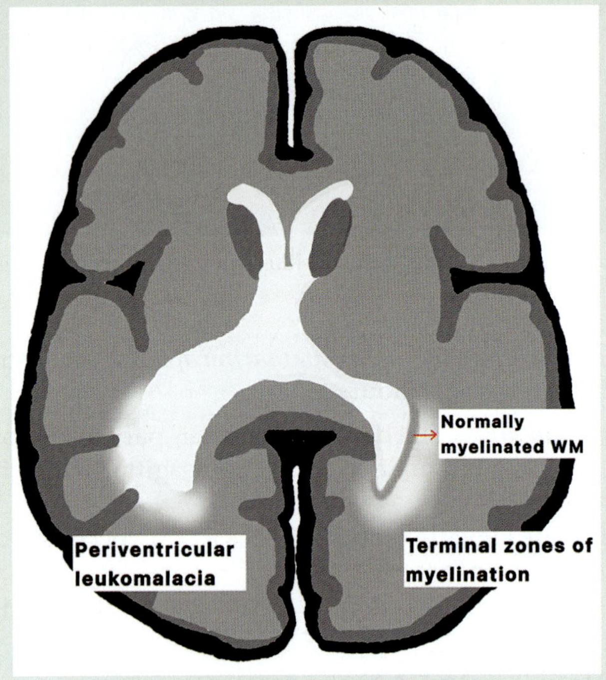 **Fig. 4.30.14:** Periventricular leukomalacia and terminal zones of myelination	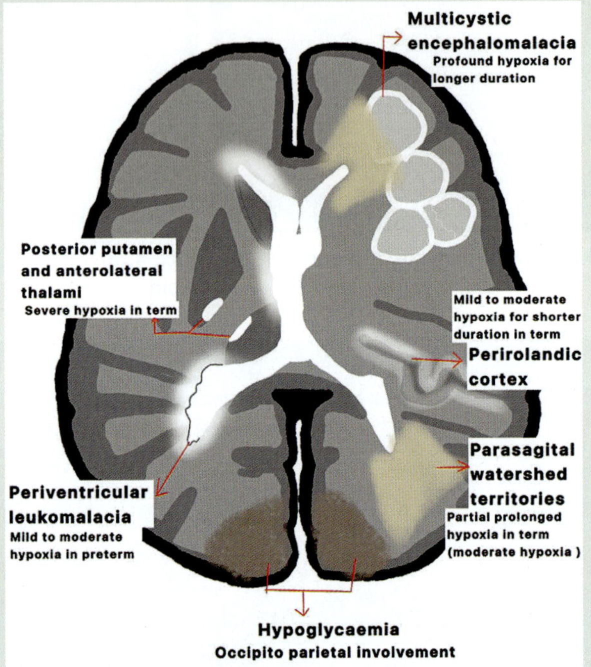 **Fig. 4.30.15:** Hypoglycemic encephalopathy/hypoxic encephalopathy

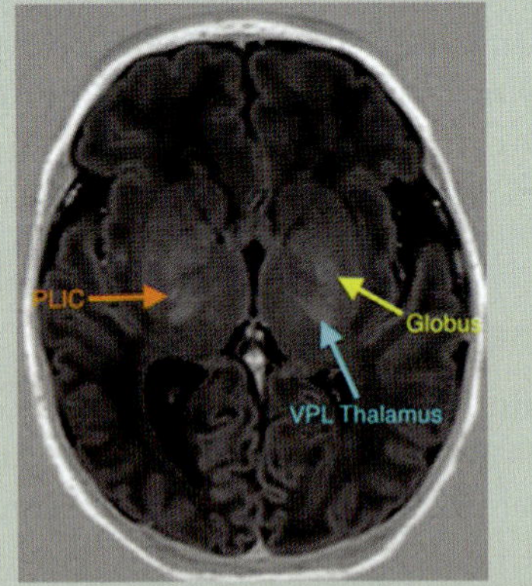 **Fig. 4.30.16:** Normal appearance of PLIC on T1 (high signal) in term child	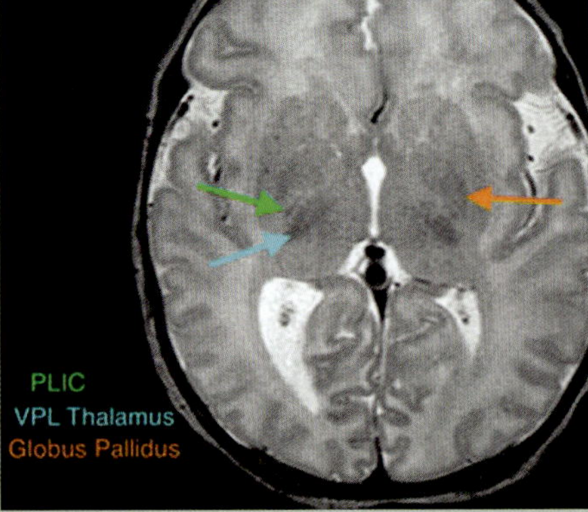 **Fig. 4.30.17:** Normal appearance of PLIC on T2 weighted images (low signal)	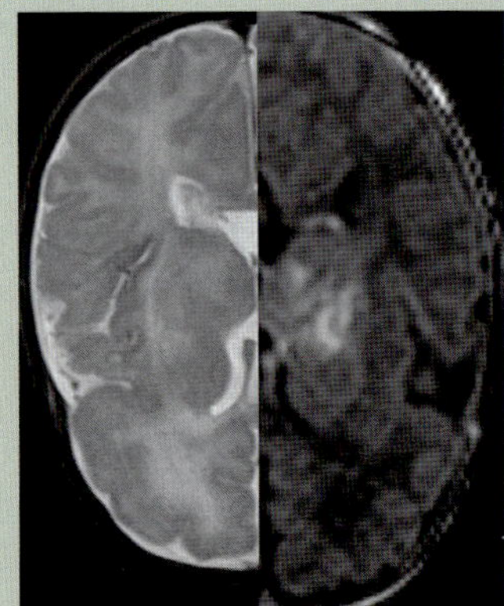 **Fig. 4.30.18:** Absence of PLIC hyperintensity in T1 and corresponding hypointensity in T2 with hyperintensity involving posterior lentiform nucleus: HIE (absent PLIC sign)

(*Contd.*)

Table 4.30.4: Difference between hypoglycemic encephalopathy and hypoxic encephalopathy (*Contd.*)

Patterns of HIE involvement		
Acute HIE 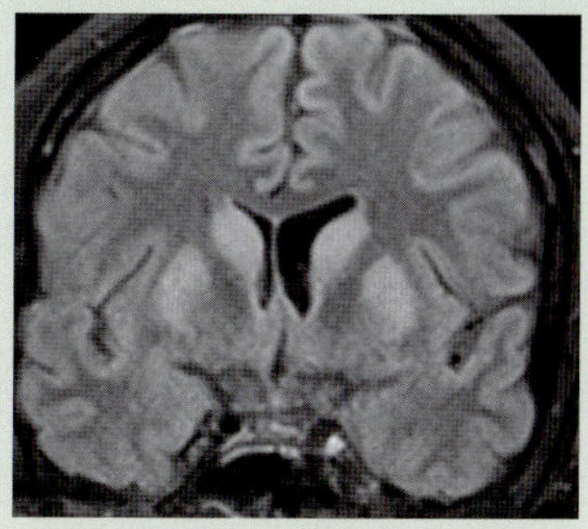 Fig. 4.30.19: Acute HIE	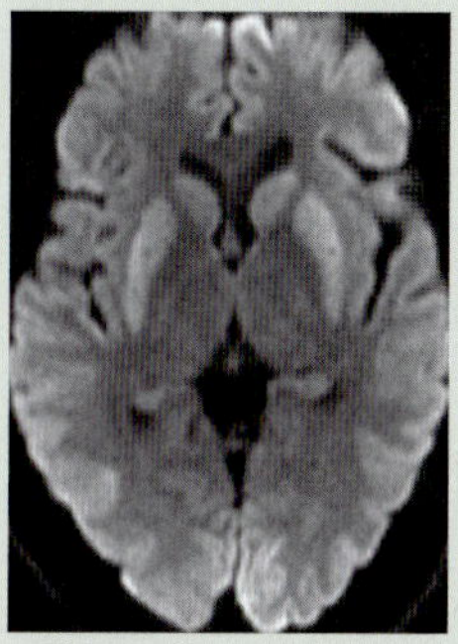 Fig. 4.30.20: Acute HIE	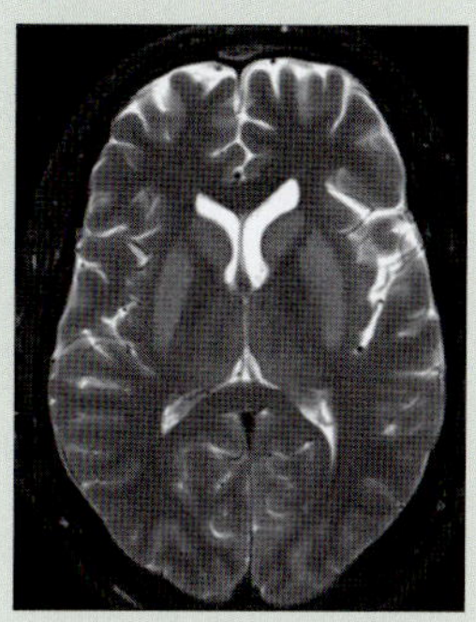 Fig. 4.30.21: Acute HIE
Acute severe HIE 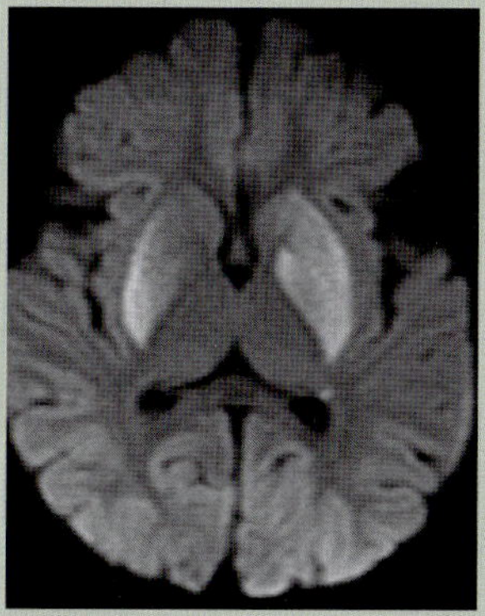 Fig. 4.30.22: Acute severe HIE	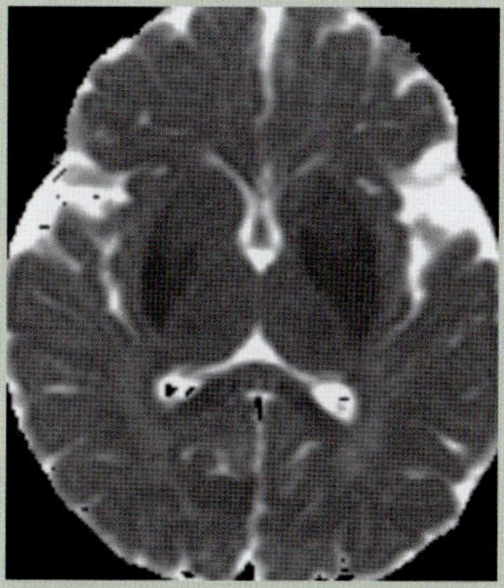 Fig. 4.30.23: Acute severe HIE	**Chronic profound HIE** 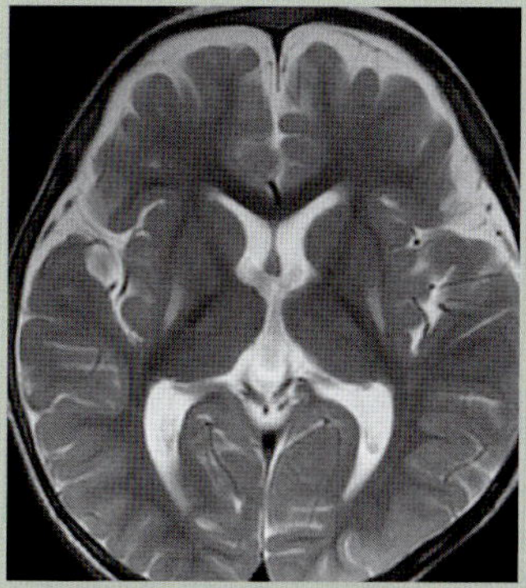 Fig. 4.30.24: Chronic profound HIE
Craniostenosis 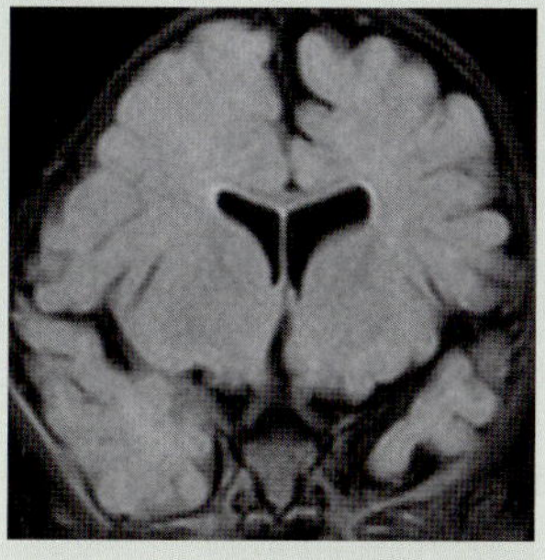 Fig. 4.30.25: Craniostenosis	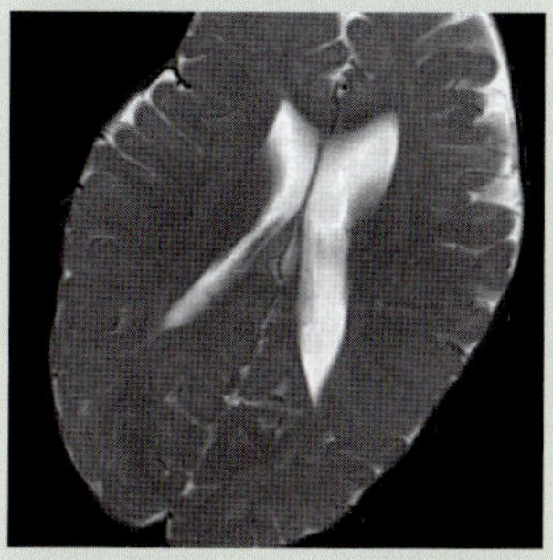 Fig. 4.30.26: Craniostenosis	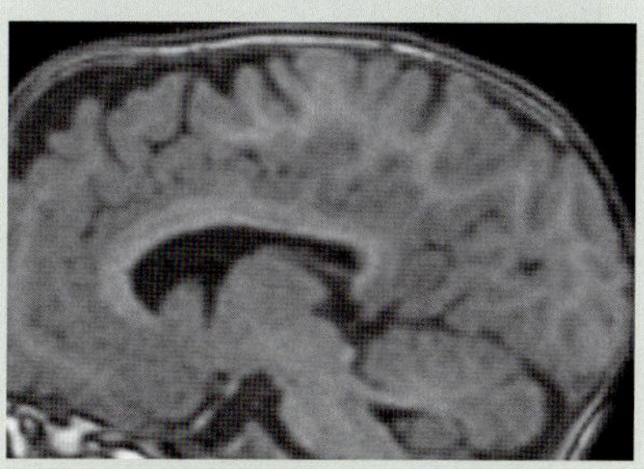 Fig. 4.30.27: Craniostenosis
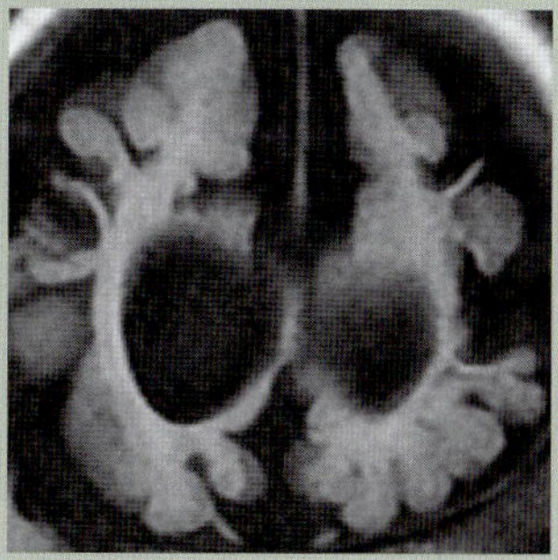 Fig. 4.30.28: Frontal predominant HIE	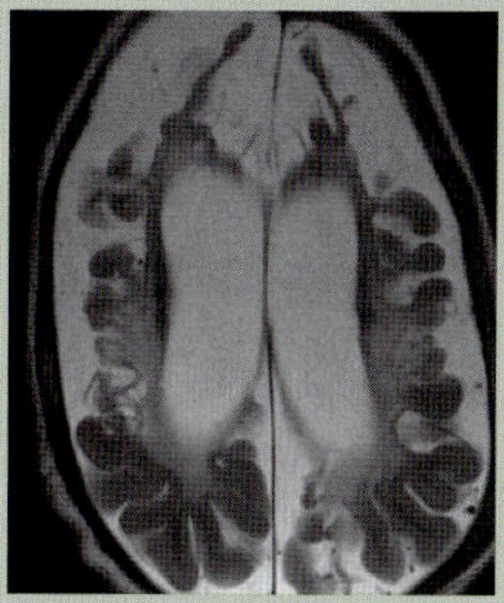 Fig. 4.30.29: Frontal predominant HIE	

(*Contd.*)

Table 4.30.4: Difference between hypoglycemic encephalopathy and hypoxic encephalopathy (*Contd.*)

<table>
<tr><td colspan="3">Hypoglycemia
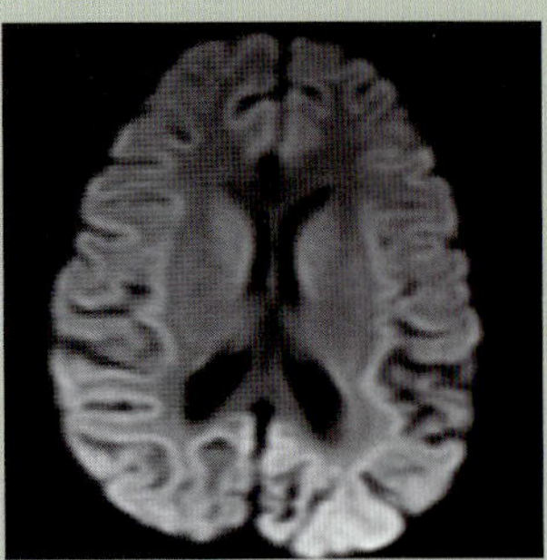
Fig. 4.30.30: Hypoglycemia</td><td colspan="3">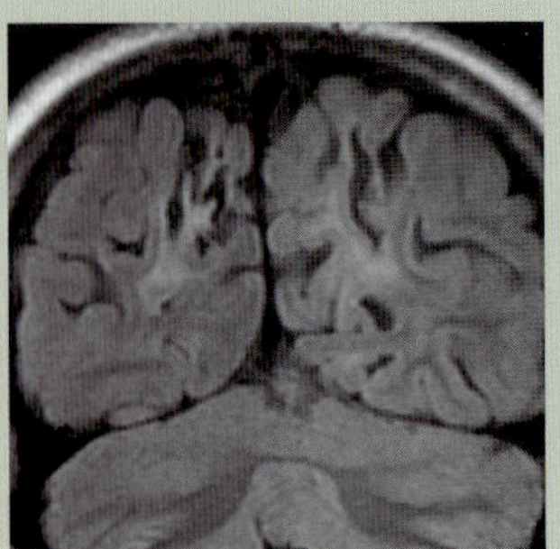
Fig. 4.30.31: Hypoglycemia</td></tr>
<tr><td colspan="2">Germinal matrix hemorrhage
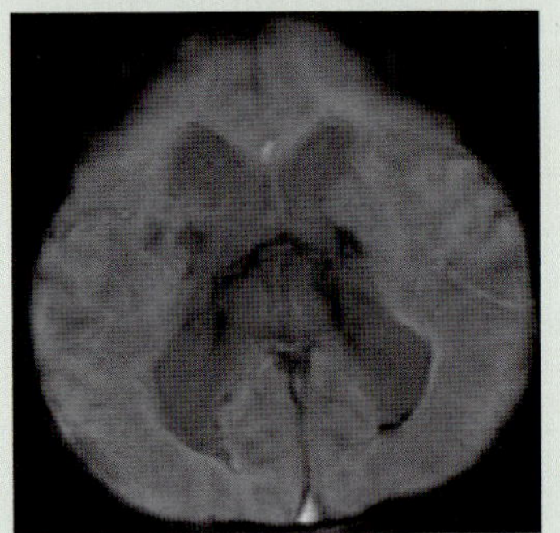
Fig. 4.30.32: Germinal matrix hemorrhage</td><td colspan="2">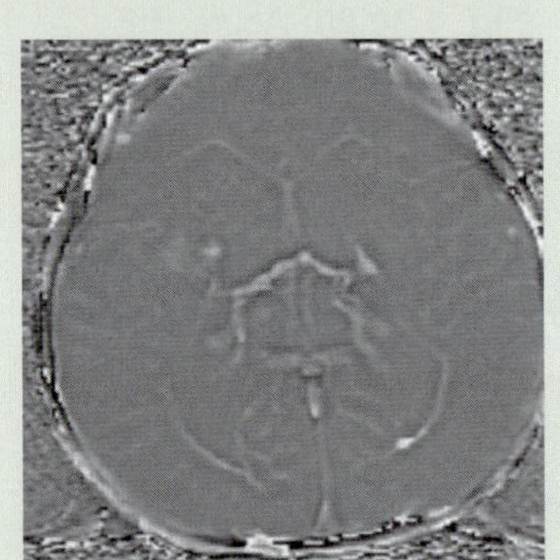
Fig. 4.30.33: Germinal matrix hemorrhage</td><td colspan="2">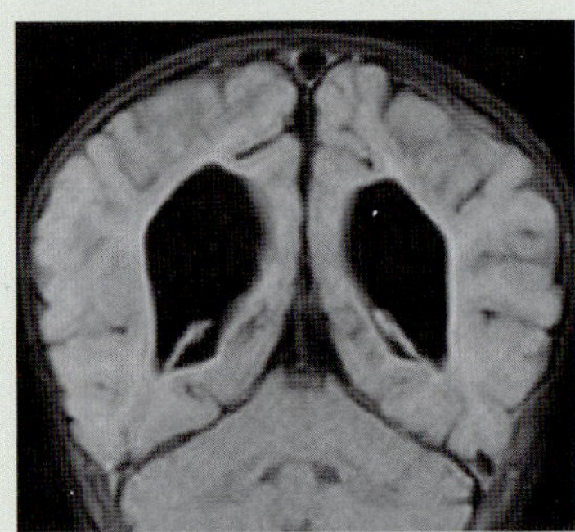
Fig. 4.30.34: Germinal matrix hemorrhage</td></tr>
<tr><td colspan="2">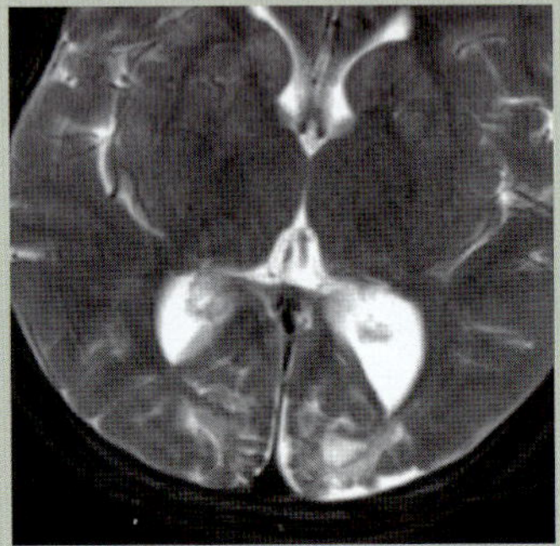
Fig. 4.30.35: Hypoglycemic encephalopathy</td><td colspan="2">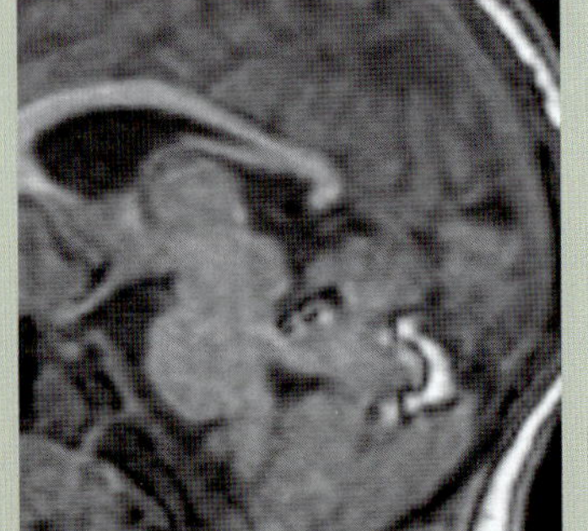
Fig. 4.30.36: Hypoglycemic encephalopathy incidental lipoma in HIE</td><td colspan="2">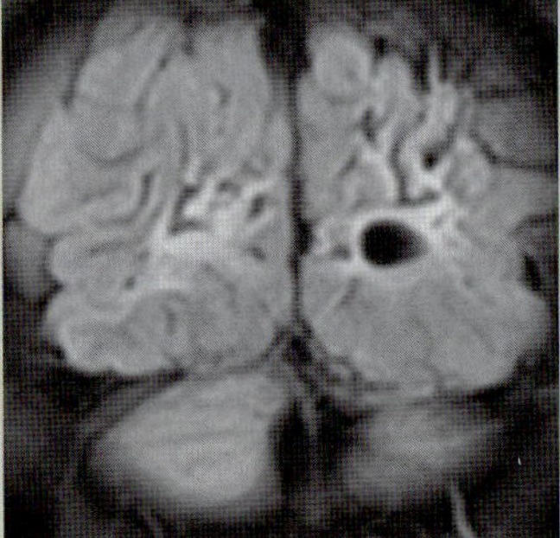
Fig. 4.30.37: Hypoglycemic encephalopathy</td></tr>
<tr><td colspan="6">CMV related HIE resulting in multicystic encephalomalacia</td></tr>
<tr><td colspan="2">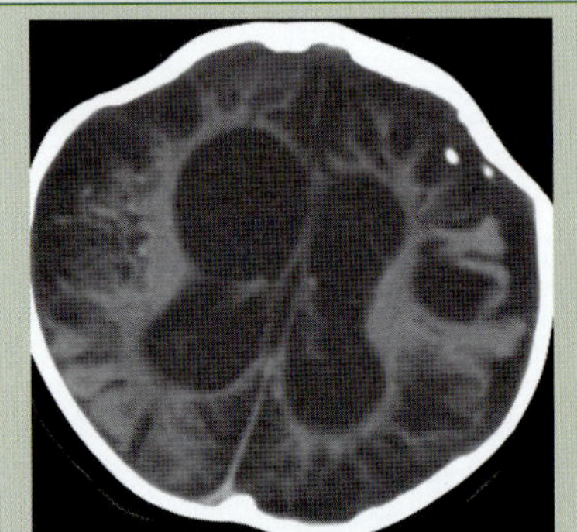
Fig. 4.30.38: CMV related HIE resulting in multicystic encephalomalacia</td><td colspan="2">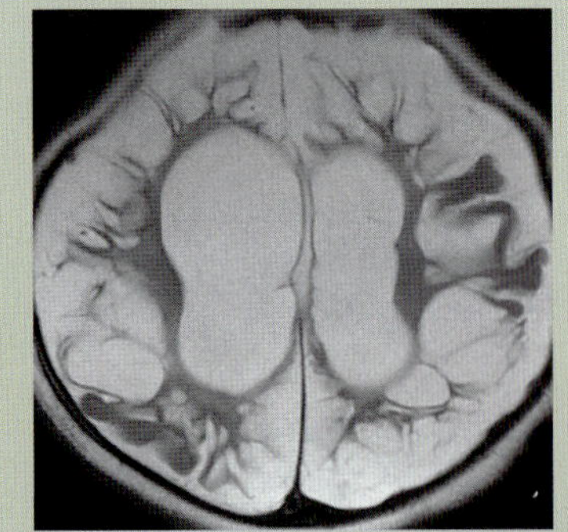
Fig. 4.30.39: CMV related HIE resulting in multicystic encephalomalacia</td><td colspan="2">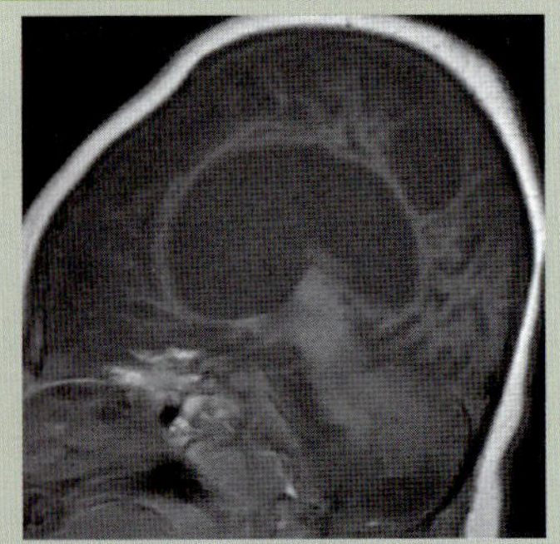
Fig. 4.30.40: CMV related HIE resulting in multicystic encephalomalacia</td></tr>
</table>

(*Contd.*)

Table 4.30.4: Difference between hypoglycemic encephalopathy and hypoxic encephalopathy (*Contd.*)

Hypoglycemia related HIE causing occipital gliosis

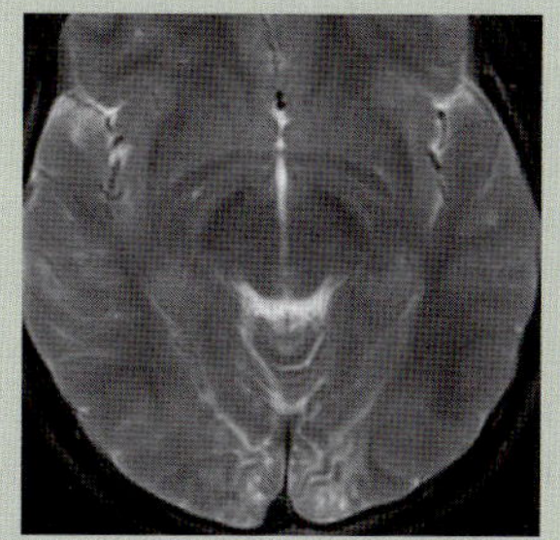

Fig. 4.30.41: Hypoglycemia related HIE causing occipital gliosis

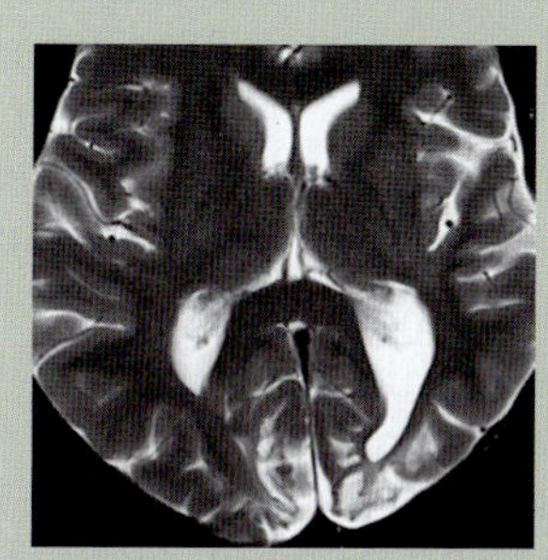

Fig. 4.30.42: Hypoglycemia related HIE causing occipital gliosis

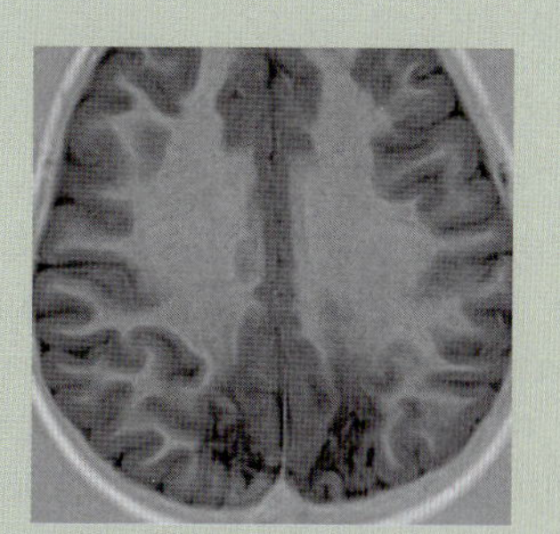

Fig. 4.30.43: Hypoglycemia related HIE causing occipital gliosis

Periventricular leukomalacia

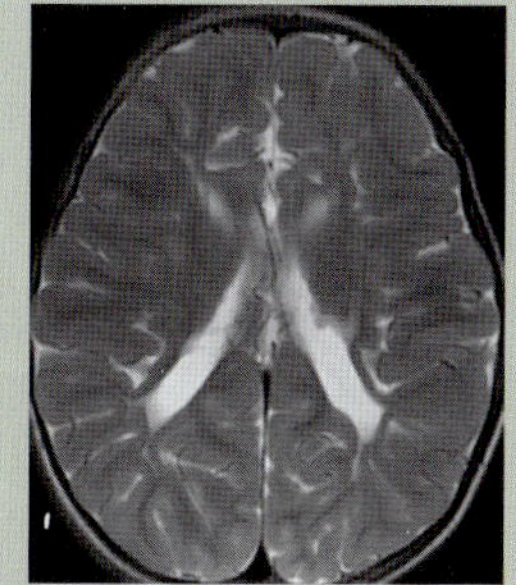

Fig. 4.30.44: Periventricular leukomalacia

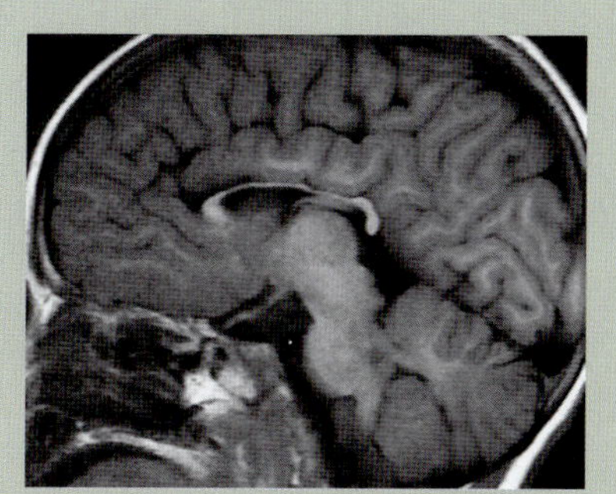

Fig. 4.30.45: Periventricular leukomalacia

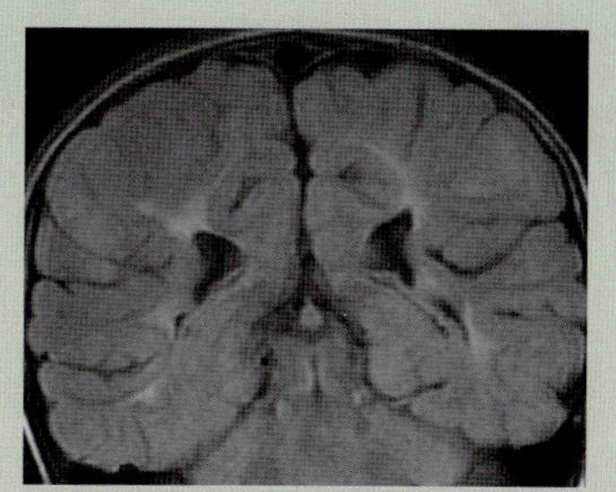

Fig. 4.30.46: Periventricular leukomalacia

PVL and terminal zones of myelination

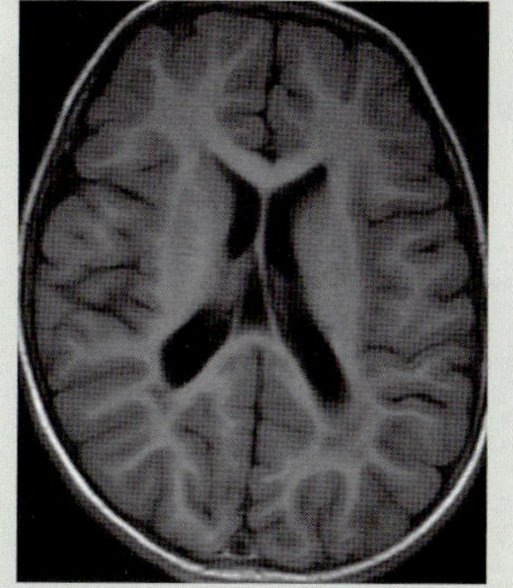

Fig. 4.30.47: Right side terminal zone of myelination with left periventricular leukomalacia

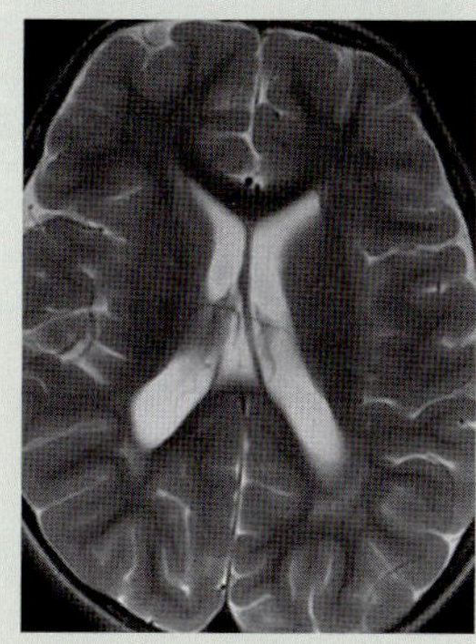

Fig. 4.30.48: Right side terminal zone of myelination with left periventricular leukomalacia

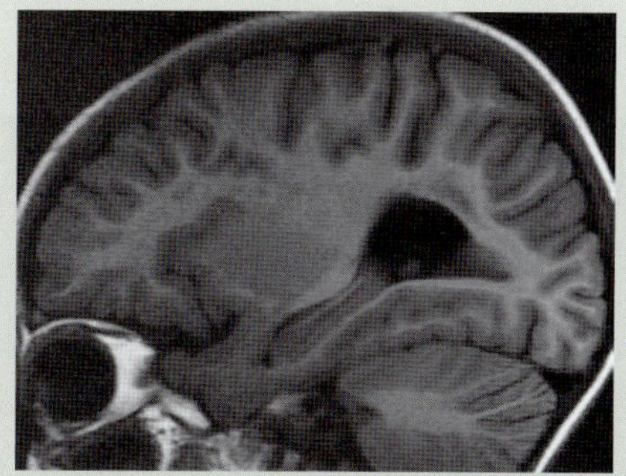

Fig. 4.30.49: Terminal zone of myelination

PVL with congenital torch

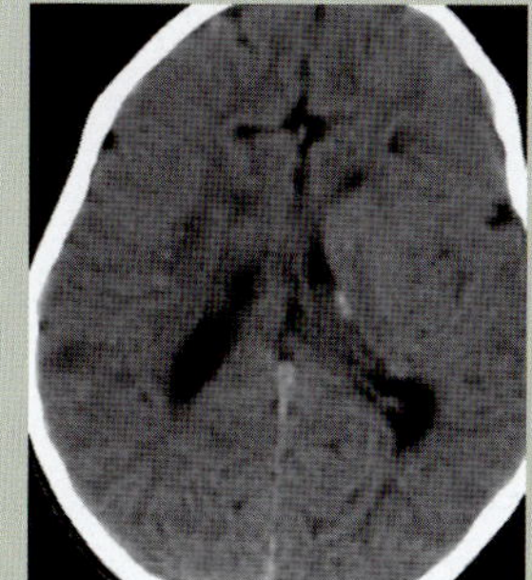

Fig. 4.30.50: PVL with congenital torch

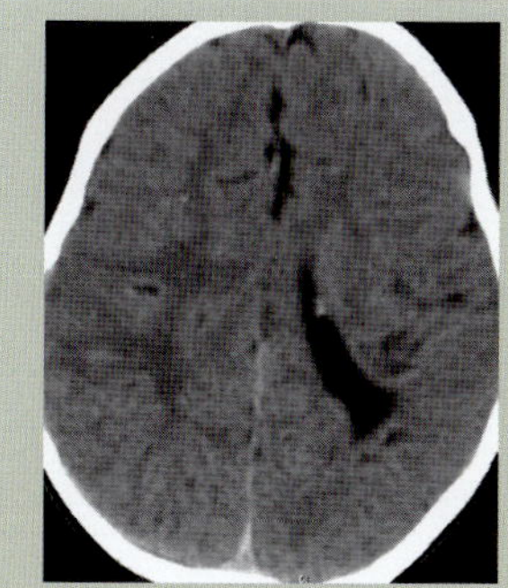

Fig. 4.30.51: PVL with congenital torch

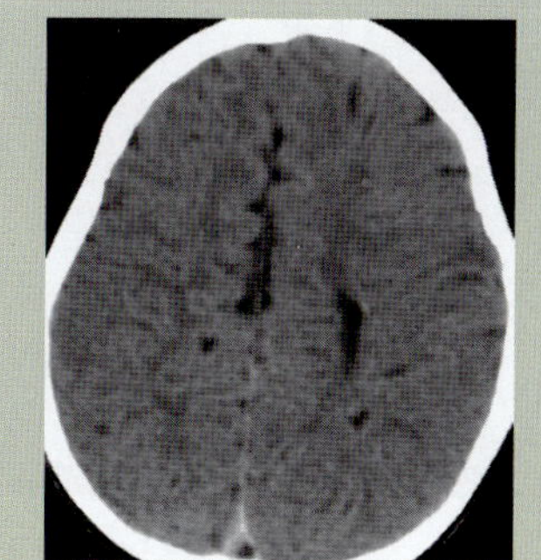

Fig. 4.30.52: PVL with congenital torch

4.31 CENTRAL NERVOUS SYSTEM

Case No. 31

Clinical history: A 54-year-old female, complaints of left sided weakness.

Radiological techniques and observation:

Figure 4.31.1 is plain CT image showing ill-defined punctuate areas of hyperdensity in the deep white matter of right frontal lobe, superior frontal gyrus and paracentral lobule junction. Causes of hyperdense lesions in CT are discussed later. Figure 4.31.2 is axial T2 MR image showing multiple serpiginous flow voids noted in the deep white matter of right frontal lobe. Figure 4.31.3 is 3D time-of-flight MRA reformatted image in antero-posterior projection showing faint arterial supply to the lesion, which is in watershed zone between anterior cerebral artery and middle cerebral artery. Figure 4.31.4 are postcontrast images, where the lesion shows intense enhancement. No evidence of surrounding edema/ thrombus/aneurysm/haemorrhage/hydrocephalus. No evidence of other similar lesion in remainder of the brain parenchyma. Figure 4.31.5, DSA image in capillary phase, shows vascular blush and nidus within the lesion

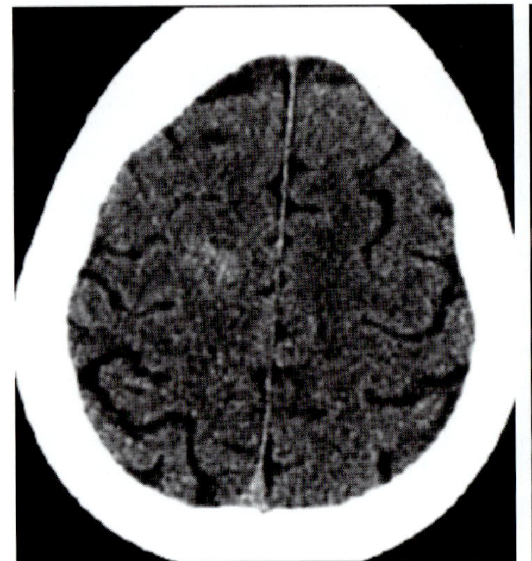

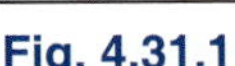

Fig. 4.31.1

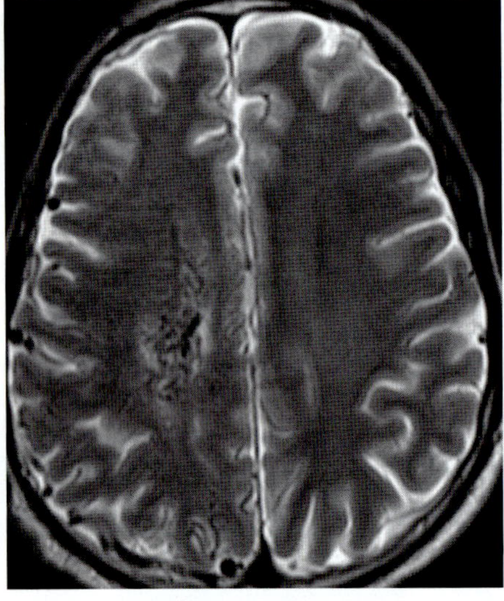

Fig. 4.31.2

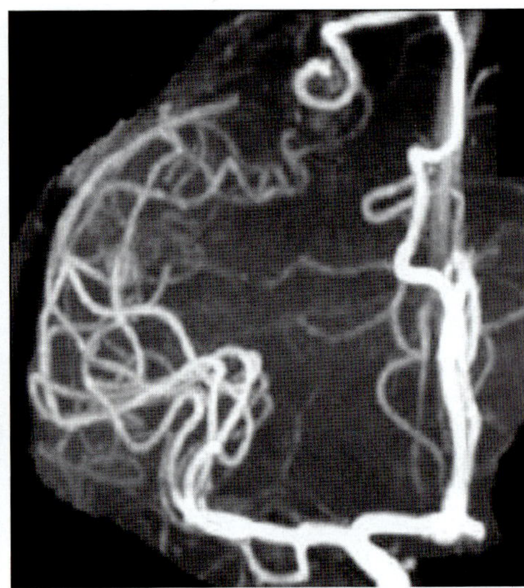

Fig. 4.31.3

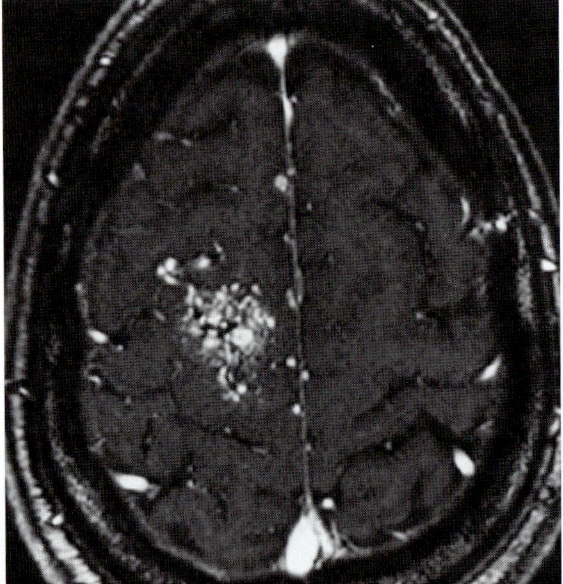

Fig. 4.31.4

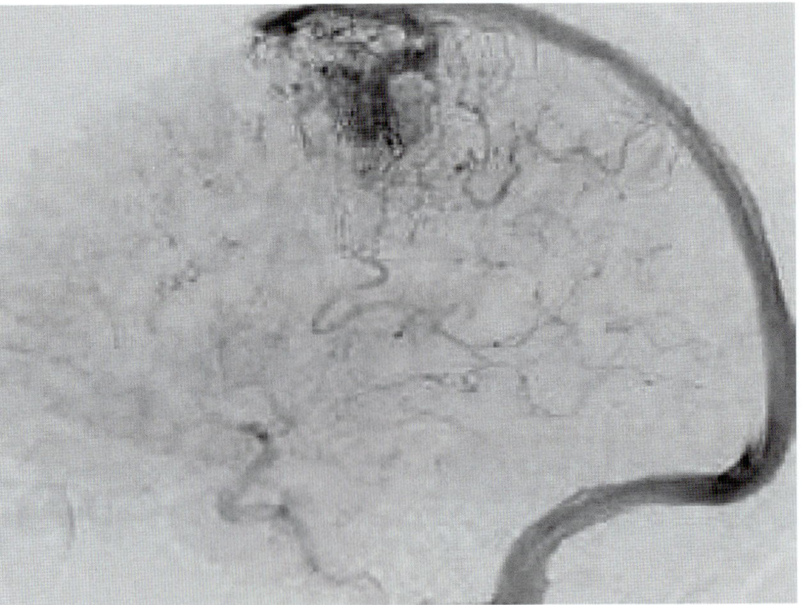

Fig. 4.31.5

Table 4.31.1: Differential diagnosis for AVM

Cerebral proliferative angiopathy Previously known as diffuse nidus type AVM. Seizures, headache, neurologic deficits > >hemorrhage Progressive course, new areas of abnormal vascularity. • Large, diffusely dispersed network of dilated vessels • Numerous arterial feeders including dural • No compact nidus; normal brain in between.	**Imaging:** The characteristic features are: • The absence of early venous drainage, which helps to differentiate CPA from a classical cerebral AVM • Large areas of parenchymal involvement, often an entire lobe or even a hemisphere is affected • Fed by multiple arteries (absence of a dominant feeder) • Feeder arteries tend to be of normal size or moderately enlarged • Associated stenosis of feeder arteries is often present • Classical appearance with scattered "puddling" of contrast which persists into the late arterial and early venous phases • The nidus usually has a fuzzy appearance, it is not well-circumscribed. • Perfusion CT and MR show hypoperfusion (steal) extending far beyond the morphologic abnormalities.	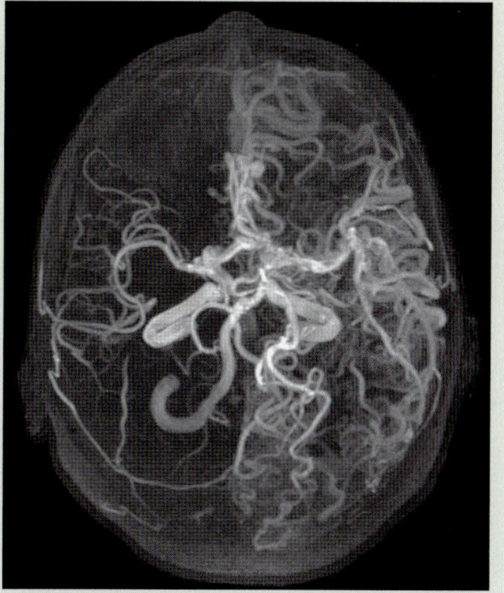 **Fig. 4.31.6:** Cerebral proliferative angiopathy 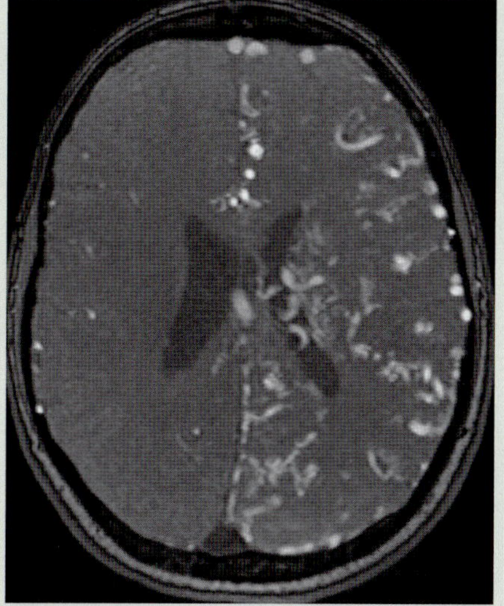 **Fig. 4.31.7:** Cerebral proliferative angiopathy

DVA (developmental venous anomaly)
Also known as venous "angioma"
• Solitary → multiple; small → large
• Enlarged white matter veins interspersed with normal brain.
• Usually found adjacent to lateral or fourth ventricle
	Imaging (MRI)
	T2/FLAIR
	• Collector vein = flow void on T2WI
	• Radicles of "Medusa head" hyperintense on FLAIR
	• **T2* (GRE/SWI)**
	  – Linear hypointensities in radicles, collector vein
	  – Blooming foci if mixed with cavernous malformation.
	  – 3T SWI may show microbleeds
	• T1 C+ **"Umbrella"** of tubular radicles → collector vein
	• pMR ↑ CBV/CBF, increased MTT
	DSA - Classic **"Medusa head"** in venous phase
		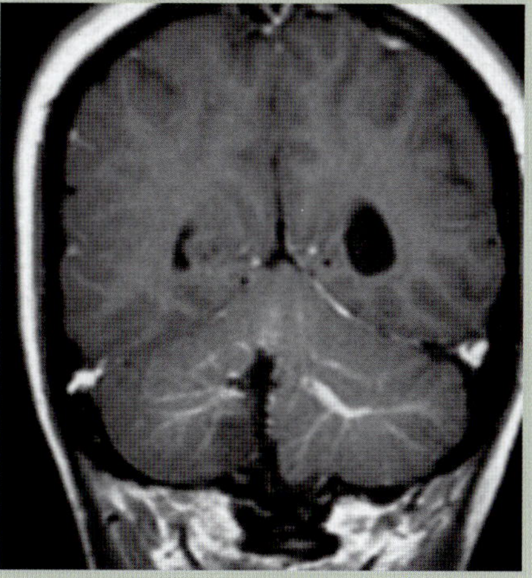
		Fig. 4.31.8: Developmental venous anomaly

Contd..

Table 4.31.1: Differential diagnosis for AVM *(Contd..)*

<table>
<tr>
<td>

AV fistula

It is a network of tiny, crack-like vessels that shunt blood between meningeal arteries and small venules within wall of a dural venous sinus.

- Common in posterior fossa and skull base

Dural AVF

- CT—none to striking. An enlarged dura sinus or draining vein can sometimes be identified on NECT
- MRI—the presence of dilated cortical veins without an identifiable nidus adjacent to normal appearing brain may suggest the presence of a dAVF.

</td>
<td>

Carotid-cavernous fistula

"Direct" CCFs are typically high-flow lesion. **"Indirect"** CCFs are usually slow-flow. CECT scans often nicely demonstrate an enlarged superior opthalmic vein and cavernous sinus

Barrow classification:

Type A: Direct ICA-CS high-flow shunt

Type B: Dural ICA branches-CS shunt

Type C: Dural ECA-CS shunt

Type D: Both ICA/ECA dural branches shunt to CS.

MR findings. T1 scans may show a prominent **"bulging"** CS and SOV as well as **"dirty"** orbital fat. T2-weighted images may show asymmetric flow-related signal loss in the affected veins. Too many **"flow voids"** in the CS are a common finding.

CT–proptosis, prominent CS with enlarged superior ophthalmic vein, enlarged EOM.

Angiography—direct CCFs show rapid flow with early opacification of the CS. Indirect CCFs show multiple dural feeders from both ICA and ECA.

</td>
<td>

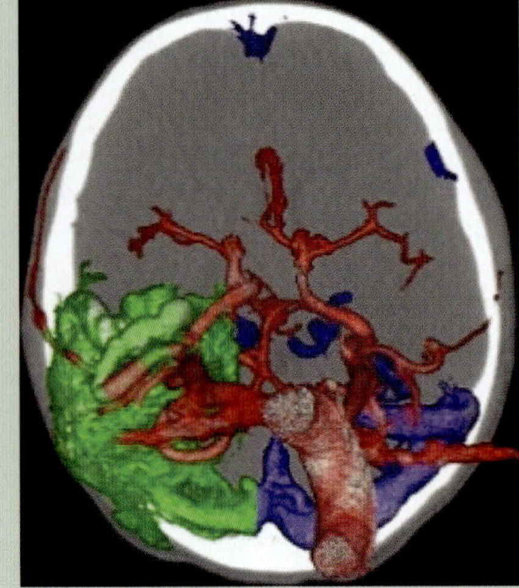

Fig. 4.31.9: dAVF

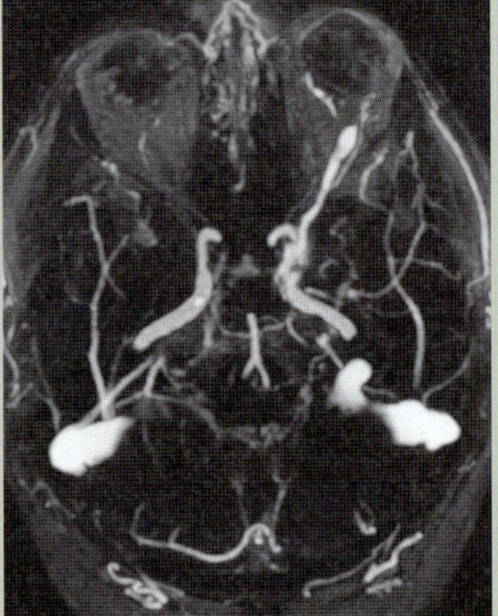

Fig. 4.31.10: CCF

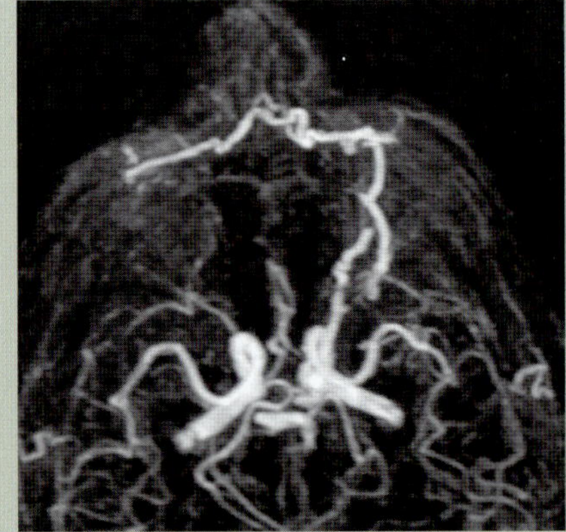

Fig. 4.31.11: CCF

</td>
</tr>
</table>

Contd...

Table 4.31.1: Differential diagnosis for AVM *(Contd..)*	
Cavernous angioma (cavernoma) Sinusoidal spaces lined with endothelium; occur anywhere in CNS, commonest pons. Often incidental findings. Multiple cavernomas may be familial.	Present with small haemorrhages (usually not associated with large haemorrhages) or seizures; (a) CT – iso/hyperdense lesion, often calcification. (b) MRI – characteristic appearance is heterogeneous signal centre with low T2 signal (hemosiderin) rim. Popcorn appearance. Gradient echo: Most sensitive sequence for detection.
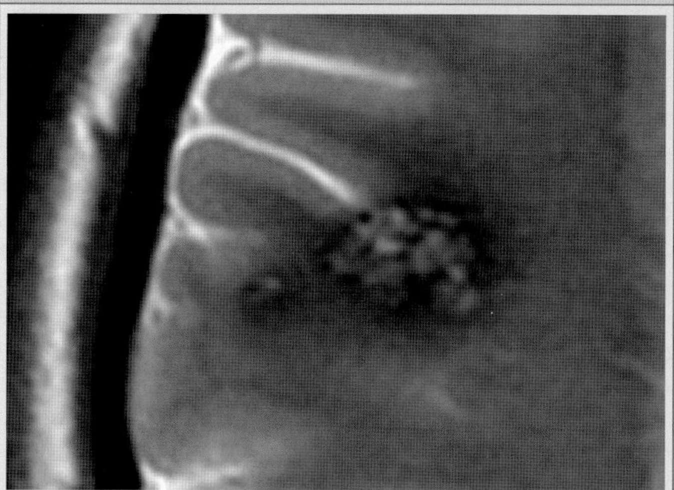 **Fig. 4.31.12:** Cavernoma	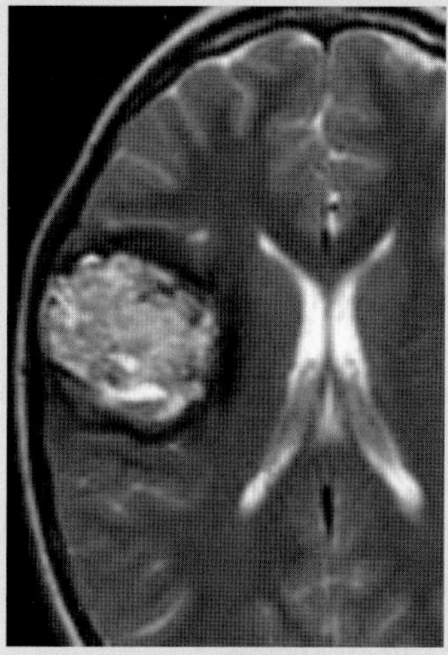 **Fig. 4.31.13:** Giant cavernoma
Capillary telangiectasia: Refer to case 4.35	

with superficial drainage into superior sagittal sinus deep drainage into internal cerebral vein.

Interpretation: A—54-year-old female with lesion in the deep white matter of right frontal lobe C—ill-defined slightly hyperdense lesion. Axial T2 multiple flow voids with intense enhancement of the lesion in the T1 post-contrast image, B—vascular blush and nidus within the lesion with superficial drainage into superior sagittal sinus and deep drainage into the internal cerebral vein on DSA D—AVM.

Principal diagnosis: Unruptured right frontal lobe arteriovenous malformation (AVM). Spetzler-Martin AVM grading scale-4.

Table 4.31.2: Classification of brain vascular malformations	
Malformations with AV shunts	*Malformations without AV shunts*
1. Arteriovenous malformations (AVMs), which may be either pial or dural.	1. Cavernous haemangiomas (or cavernomas)
2. Dural arteriovenous fistulae	2. Capillary telangiectasia
3. Vein of Galen aneurysmal malformation	3. Developmental venous anomalies
	4. Sinus pericranii

Table 4.31.3: Classification of vascular malformation		
Artery	*Capillary*	*Venous*
Aneurysm AV fistula (dural AVF, CCF) AV malformation Proliferative angiopathy	Capillary telangiectasia	Cavernoma Vein of Galen malformation Sinus pericranii Developmental venous anomaly

Differential diagnosis

- Cerebral proliferative angiopathy—absence of early venous drainage usually affecting an entire lobe or even hemisphere is affected
- Craniofacial arteriovenous metameric syndrome (CAMS)—classic locations/association with facial AVM
- Dural arteriovenous fistula (DAVF)
- Developmental venous anomaly (DVA)
- Vascular tumor/glioblastoma

Treatment: Treatment options and rate of complications are dictated in part by the Spetzler-Martin grade. In general, the management options include **microsurgical resection, endovascular occlusion and radiosurgery**.

Rarely, AVM will resolve spontaneously due to venous compression and thrombosis in a case of intracranial hemorrhage.

An untreated AVM has a 2–3% annual risk of haemorrhage due to a flow-related aneurysm, intra-nidal aneurysm, or venous thrombosis (rarely). After an episode of haemorrhage, the chance of another bleed is is up to 18% in the next year.

Arteriovenous Malformation

- Peak 20-40 years (mean = 33 years)
- 23–27% symptomatic by 15 years.

Presentation:

- Headache with intracranial hemorrhage (ICH) 55–65%
- Seizure 20–25%, neurologic deficit 25%.

Brain AVMs can be of 2 types:

A. Compact/glomerular nidus: Abnormal vessels without any interposed normal brain tissue

B. Diffuse/proliferative nidus: no well-formed nidus is present, with functional neuronal tissue interspersed amongst the anomalous vessels. When an early venous drainage is absent, this is considered a different entity, "cerebral proliferative angiopathy".

Spetzler-Martin AVM Grading Scale

In 1986, the Spetzler-Martin grading system was developed for estimating AVM surgical risk based on three AVM characteristics: Size, relationship to the eloquent brain, and presence of deep venous drainage. An eloquent brain region is one that, if injured, causes a disabling neurologic deficiency. For their grading scheme, Spetzler and Martin considered the sensorimotor, language, and visual cortexes, as well as the thalamus and hypothalamus, the internal capsule, the brainstem, the cerebellar peduncles, and the deep cerebellar nuclei. Small lesions (less than 3 cm), medium lesions (3–6 cm), and big lesions (more than 6 cm) are given 1, 2, and 3 points, respectively, with eloquent brain involvement and the presence of deep venous drainage each receiving 1 point. The Spetzler-Martin grade (range I–V) is determined by the point total, with higher grades indicating a larger surgical risk. The Spetzler-Martin system has been reduced to three categories: Class A (formerly grades I and II), class B (grade III), and class C (grade IV and V). Class A lesions are usually treated surgically. Given the prohibitive risk of surgical treatment, a conservative approach to class C lesions is now the most acceptable prescription. Mostly, they are solitary (90–95%). However, Multiple syndromic relationships, such as Wyburn-Mason syndrome/Sturge-Weber syndrome, hereditary hemorrhagic telangiectasia (Osler-Weber-Rendu syndrome), and

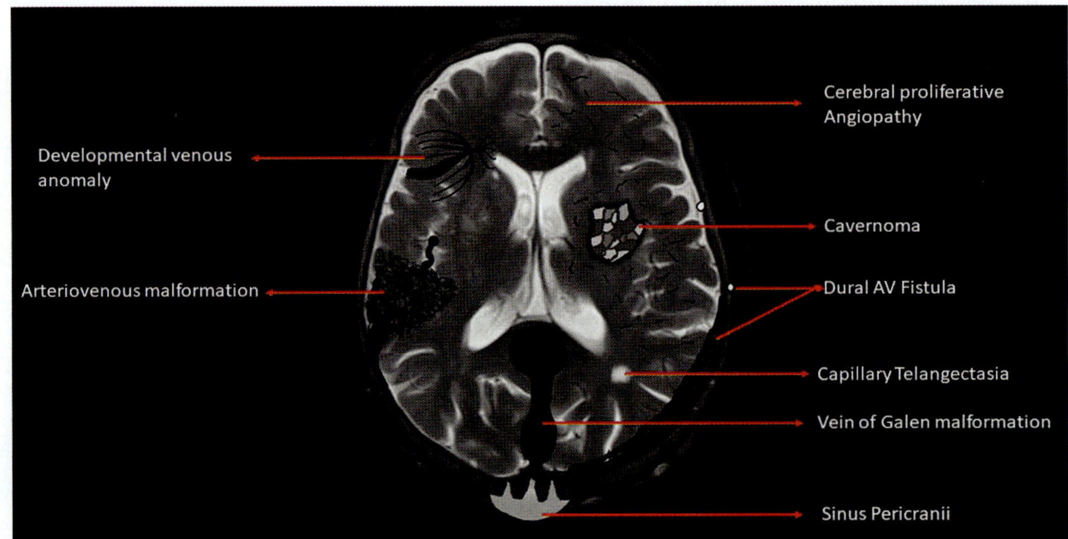

Fig. 4.31.14: Various vascular malformations

Table 4.31.4: Spetzler-Martin AVM grading scale		
Size • Small (< 3 cm) = 1 • Medium (3–6 cm) = 2 • Large (> 6 cm) = 3	**Location** • Noneloquent = 0 • Eloquent = 1	**Venous drainage** • Superficial only = 0 • Deep component = 1
General Features • Arteriovenous shunting • No intervening capillaries • 3 components – Feeding arteries – Nidus – Draining veins	**NECT** • Slightly hyperdense "bag of worms" • Tightly packed. Little/no mass effect **CECT** • Strong serpentine enhancement	**MR** • "Honeycomb" of "flow voids" • No normal brain inside

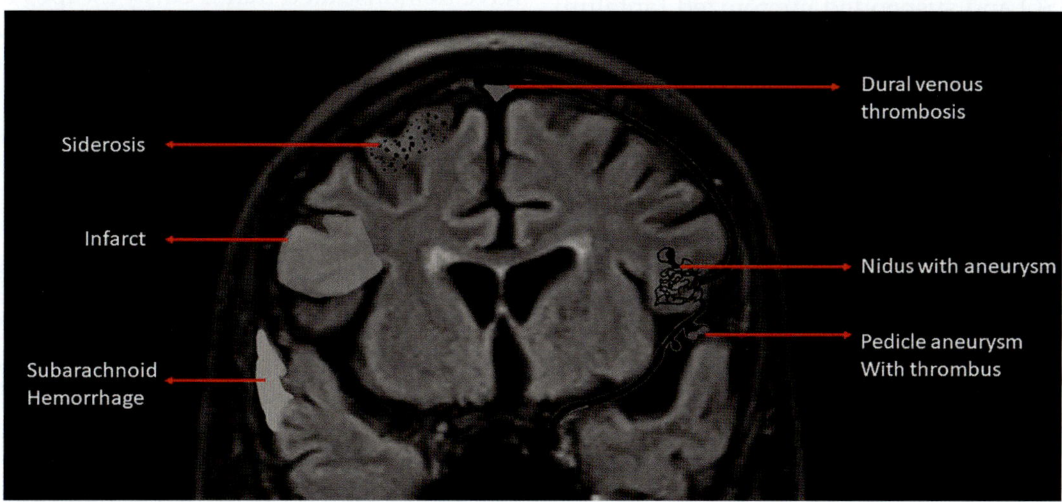

Fig. 4.31.15: Imaging features of AVM

Table 4.31.5: Angio architectural features with associated risks at endovascular treatment or radiosurgery for brain AVMs		
Angio architectural feature	*Associated risks at endovascular treatment*	*Associated risks at radiosurgery*
Arterial		
Flow-related aneurysm Indirect arterial feeder vessels (en passage type) Multiple small feeding arteries	Higher risk of intraprocedural hemorrhage Short security margin for reflux Small chance of complete cure	. . . .
Nidal		
Multiple compartments Size larger than 12 mL	Smaller chance of cure . . .	. . . Smaller chance of cure
Venous		
Venous stenosis	Higher risk of complications if embolic agent migrates	. . .
Other		
Young patient age Risk factors for future hemorrhage	. . . . . .	Increased chance of secondary malignancy Possible hemorrhage while radiation takes effect

Klippel-Trenaunay-Weber syndrome, must be evaluated in case of AVM. Complications include hemorrhage, steal phenomenon, in which blood is given to AVM at the expense of normal brain tissue, resulting in seizures, focal neurological deficit/atrophy and aneurysms can occur and cause bleeding if not treated.

Table 4.31.6: Complications of AVM	
Risk of future hemorrhage	*Risk of nonhemorrhagic neurologic deficits*
Previous hemorrhage Intranidal aneurysms Venous stenosis or ectasia (pouches) Deep venous drainage Single venous drainage Deep or posterior fossa locations	High-flow shunt Venous congestion or outflow obstruction Long pial course of draining vein Perifocal or perinidal gliosis Mass effect or hydrocephalus Arterial steal

Embolization Technique

Onyx: Onyx is a non-adhesive liquid embolic agent made up of an EVOH (ethylene vinyl alcohol) copolymer soaked in DMSO and suspended micronized tantalum powder to give contrast for fluoroscopy viewing. A 1.5 ml bottle of Onyx, a 1.5 ml vial of DMSO, and three 1 ml Onyx administration syringes make up the Onyx Liquid Embolic System. The embolization location is accessed using a DMSO compliant delivery micro catheter designed for use in the neurovasculature. Onyx comes in two different formulations: Onyx 18 (6 percent EVOH) and Onyx 34 (8 percent EVOH). Because Onyx 18 has a lower viscosity than Onyx 34, it will go further distally and enter deeper into the nidus. For both product compositions, final solidification takes less than five minutes.

Principle of operation: Onyx is injected slowly and carefully into the brain arteriovenous malformation using a tiny catheter under fluoroscopic supervision. The EVOH copolymer and suspended tantalum precipitate *in situ* as a spongy, coherent embolus when the DMSO solvent dissolves into the circulation. As the polymeric embolus hardens from the outside to the interior while going further distally in the lesion, it develops a skin.

Onyx is approved for brain arteriovenous malformations (bAVMs) embolization as presurgical procedure.

Contraindications: When any of the following situations present, the use of the Onyx Liquid Embolic System (LES) is contraindicated: A. When appropriate catheter insertion is not achievable. B. When provocative testing reveals intolerance to the occlusion technique. C. When vasospasm prevents blood flow.

Warnings: Not for use with premature newborns (under 1,500 g) or persons with serious liver and kidney function impairment. The operation of embolization to occlude blood arteries is extremely dangerous. Only clinicians with a full understanding of the pathology to be treated, angiographic procedures, and super-selective embolization should utilise this device. Blood flow patterns may be affected by AVM embolization, resulting in higher pressures in arteries involved in AVM. Hemorrhagic complication can occur at higher incidence if arterial pressure is increased. Animal studies have demonstrated that if Onyx escapes the circulatory space, as it can if the artery wall is damaged, the substance can cause a subacute inflammatory response. Brain parenchymal injury can be seen due to increased intracranial pressure caused by unresorbed Onyx material in this region. Dimethyl sulfoxide (DMSO) can cause histamine to be released, and topical dimethyl sulfoxide injection has been linked to hypersensitive reactions. One patient being treated for interstitial cystitis experienced this hypersensitivity. If anaphylactoid symptoms appear, treatment should be started immediately. Other embolic agents like polymer coated coils can interact with Onyx. When excessive blood flow prevents safe infusion of the embolic agent, therapeutic embolization should be avoided. The microcatheter tip should be positioned so that embolization of the bAVMs takes place far away from any arteries that might supply normal brain tissue or cranial nerves. If Onyx is not constantly mixed for the appropriate duration, the tantalum may not be suspended properly, leading in poor fluoroscopic visualisation during delivery. After mixing, immediately inject Onyx. Tantalum settling can occur within the syringe if Onyx injection is delayed, resulting in poor vision of Onyx during injection. Non-target vascular embolization may occur if adequate fluoroscopic visibility is not maintained during Onyx distribution. HALT Onyx delivery until appropriate visualisation is re-established if visualisation is lost at any point throughout the embolization operation.

Only utilise MTI micro catheters and MTI syringes that are indicated for use in the neurovasculature, such as Marathon, Rebar, and Ultraflow. Other micro catheters or syringes may be incompatible with DMSO, resulting in thromboembolic events due to catheter deterioration. To inject at rate of 0.16 mL/min, use only thumb pressure. The injection rate is kept at maximum of 0.3 mL/min. Rapid injection of DMSO into the vasculature has been proven in animal experiments to cause vasospasm and/or angionecrosis. In the event of a catheter occlusion, using the palm of the hand to push the plunger may result in catheter rupture owing to over pressurisation. Allow no more than one centimetre of Onyx to reflux back over the catheter tip. Excessive Onyx reflux can make catheter removal difficult. Do not try to inject any substance through a micro catheter after using Onyx as such attempts may result in an embolus or embolization of a location that was not planned. If Onyx is not visible exiting the catheter tip, STOP the injection. Over-pressurization might occur if the catheter becomes blocked. Continuously check if Onyx is exiting the catheter tip during Onyx injection. If only 0.05 ml of Onyx is injected and is not visible exiting the catheter tip, testing has revealed that over-pressurization and rupture can occur. If increasing resistance to Onyx injection is seen, STOP infusion. Determine the cause of increased resistance (e.g. Onyx obstruction in catheter lumen) and replace the catheter if necessary. Increased injection pressure should not be used to clear or overcome resistance, since this can result in catheter rupture and embolization of locations not targeted. DO NOT stop injecting Onyx for more than two minutes before restarting. Catheter occlusion can occur when Onyx solidifies at the catheter tip, and using too much pressure to clear the catheter can cause it to break.

Precautions: The following patient populations have not been examined for safety and effectiveness: a. Women who are pregnant or nursing, b. individuals under the age of 18, c. people who have aneurysms that are not connected with bAVMs nidus, or who have distal feeders to bAVMs nidus or dural AV fistulas. Wait a few seconds after the Onyx injection is finished before trying catheter removal. Failure to wait a few seconds after Onyx injection before retrieving the micro catheter may result in fragmentation of Onyx into non-target vessels.

Causes of catheter entrapment resulting in difficult catheter removal: a. Angioarchitecture: very distal bAVMs fed by afferent, lengthened, and tortuous pedicles. b. Vasospasm, c. reflux.

If catheter removal becomes difficult, the following steps will help: Pull the catheter gently to see if there is any resistance to removal, remove any "slack" in the catheter if resistance is sensed, apply gentle traction to the catheter (about 3–4 cm of stretch) and hold for a few seconds before releasing it. To reduce the danger of haemorrhage, assess the effect of traction on the vascular. This procedure can be repeated as needed until the catheter is removed.

Catheters that are difficult to remove can be removed using a different technique. Remove all slack from the catheter by applying a few centimetres of traction to the catheter system to produce a modest tension. In order to remove the catheter, grasp it firmly and pull it out with a rapid wrist snap action (from left to right) 10–15 centimetres. To reduce the possibility of catheter separation, apply no more than 20 cm of traction to the catheter. **For entrapped catheters:** In some difficult clinical settings, it may be safer to leave the micro catheter in the vascular system, as risk malformation rupture and further hemorrhagic complications by applying too much traction on an entrapped catheter. This is done by lengthening the catheter and severing the shaft near the vascular access entry point, allowing the catheter to stay in the artery. In case of catheter breakage during removal, distal migration of catheter may occur. To reduce the risk of thrombosis, same-day surgical resection should be explored.

Table 4.31.7: Differential diagnosis of cerebral metastasis

Hemorrhagic cerebral metastases	Calcified cerebral metastases	Highly cellular cerebral metastases (i.e. non-hemorrhagic, non-calcified)
Malignant melanoma (can also be hyperdense when non-hemorrhagic due to melanin)	Breast cancer	Lymphoma
Choriocarcinoma	Lung cancer	Leukemia
Colon cancer, renal cell cancer	Gastrointestinal tract cancer, e.g. Mucinous adenocarcinomas	Small cell lung cancer
Thyroid cancer	Sarcomas, e.g. osteosarcoma	
	Post-treatment, e.g. lymphoma, breast cancer	

Table 4.31.8: Hyperdense cerebral masses in plain CT

Malignant lymphomas, germinomas, and medulloblastomas show homogeneous hyperdensity on CT images because of their **hypercellularity**.	Tumorous lesions such as subependymal giant cell astrocytomas, oligodendrogliomas, ependymomas, central neurocytomas, craniopharyngiomas, and meningiomas often present with hyperdense **calcified** lesions on CT images.	**Intratumoral hemorrhage** also causes hyperdensity on CT images, and is often associated with metastatic brain tumors, glioblastomas, pituitary adenomas, and rarely with any of the other intracranial tumors.

4

Hyperdense Cerebral Masses in Plain CT

Relative to normal brain (masses with variable appearances not included).

1. Tumour

a. Meningioma (95%). Lesions mimicking meningioma, including solitary fibrous tumors, hemangiopericytoma, gliosarcoma, leiomyosarcoma, dural metastases, Hodgkin's disease, plasmocytoma, Rosai-Dorfman disease, neurosarcoidosis, melanocytic neoplasms and plasma cell granuloma.

b. Medulloblastoma (80%).

c. Metastases—hyperattenuating cerebral metastases on CT can be due to hemorrhage, calcium, or highly cellular tumors.

d. Lymphoma–highly cellular, often deep mass, does not cavitate unless on treatment or immunocompromised.

e. Pituitary adenoma (25%).

f. Craniopharyngioma (if predominantly solid).

g. Ependymoma.

h. Choroid plexus tumor.

2. **Haematoma** (up to around 7–10 days old).

3. **Giant aneurysm.**

4. **Colloid cyst** (50%).

<table>
<tr><th colspan="3">Table 4.31.9: Differential diagnosis for intracranial calcification</th></tr>
<tr><th colspan="3">Intracranial calcification</th></tr>
<tr><td>Normal variant
1. Pineal—after 10 years of age on SXR, earlier on CT.
2. Choroid plexus—trigones of lateral ventricles; unusual in third and fourth ventricles.
3. Dura—falx and tentorium.
4. Basal ganglia—globus pallidus; usually bilateral.
5. Habenular commissure—C-shaped calcification in tela choroidea of third ventricle.
6. Dentate nuclei of cerebellum.
7. Parasellar ligaments.
8. Arachnoid granulations.</td><td>Vascular
1. Vertebrobasilar and carotid vessels at skull base.
2. AVM
3. Cavernoma
4. Aneurysms—mural calcification in giant aneurysms.
5. Chronic subdural membranes.
6. Old infarct or haematoma.</td><td rowspan="2">Tumor
1. Meningioma.
2. Oligodendroglioma (50% calcify).
3. Astrocytoma (lower incidence of calcification than oligodendroglioma but higher incidence than oligodendroglioma).
4. Low-grade glioma.
5. Craniopharyngioma
6. Metastases—adenocarcinoma (gastrointestinal and breast, especially after therapy in breast).
7. Pineal region tumours—teratoma and germinoma. A pineocytoma itself does not calcify, but instead it 'explodes' the calcifications of the pineal gland.
8. Chordoma and chondrosarcoma.
9. Fatty midline tumours—dermoid and lipoma of corpus callosum.
10. Choroid plexus papilloma.
11. Dysembryoplastic neuroepithelial tumor (DNET).
12. Central neurocytoma.</td></tr>
<tr><td>Infection
1. TORCH (toxoplasmosis, other infections, rubella, cytomegalovirus, herpes simplex).
2. Cysticercosis – commonest cause of epilepsy worldwide; periventricular, cisternal and nodules at grey–white junction with nidus of calcification.
3. TB–basal cisterns, ventricles and parenchyma.</td><td>Neurocutaneous syndromes
1. Sturge-Weber syndrome—subcortical tramline calcification of pial vascular malformation with focal atrophy, ipsilateral enlargement of choroid plexus.
2. Tuberous sclerosis–periventricular and parenchymal.
3. Neurofibromatosis–choroid plexus, subependymal and basal ganglia.</td></tr>
<tr><th colspan="3">Basal Ganglia Calcification</th></tr>
<tr><td colspan="3">1. Normal variant.
2. Endocrine—hypoparathyroidism, pseudohypoparathyroidism, hypothyroidism.
3. Metabolic—mitochondrial disorders (Leigh's disease), Fahr's disease, Cockayne's syndrome.
4. Toxins—carbon monoxide, lead, post hypoxic.
5. Post-therapeutic—mineralizing angiopathy following, chemotherapy or radiation in basal ganglia, dentate nuclei of cerebellum and corticomedullary junction.</td></tr>
</table>

Contd...

Table 4.31.9: Differential diagnosis for intracranial calcification *(Contd...)*

Arteriovenous malformations seen with multiple calcifications in NCCT		
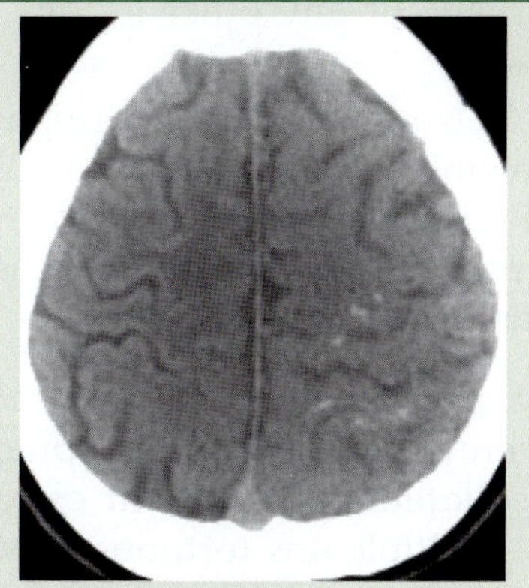 **Fig. 4.31.16:** Arteriovenous malformations seen with multiple calcifications in NCCT	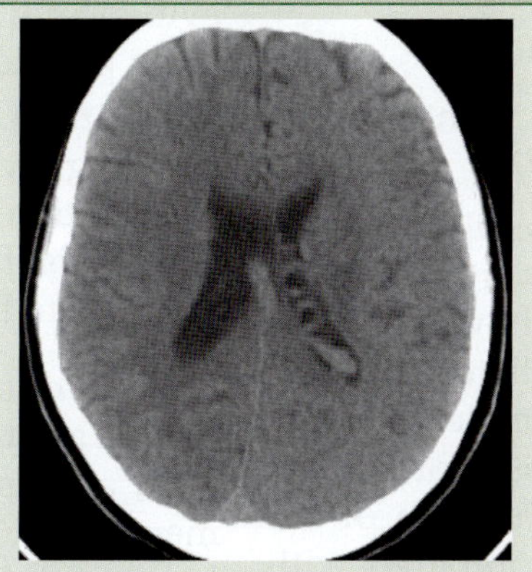 **Fig. 4.31.17:** Arteriovenous malformations seen with multiple calcifications in NCCT	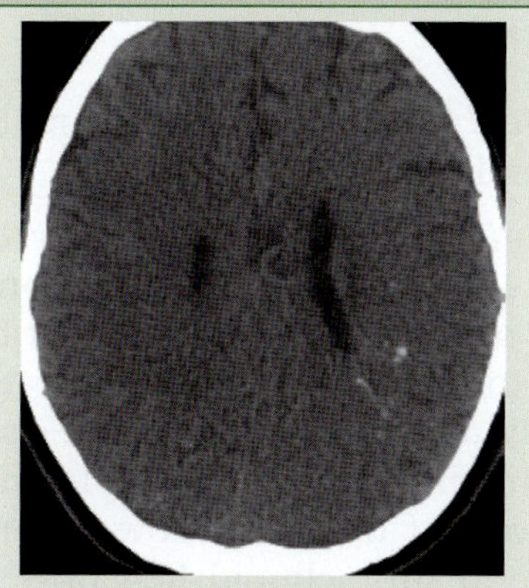 **Fig. 4.31.18:** Arteriovenous malformations seen with multiple calcifications in NCCT
Arteriovenous malformations seen with multiple calcifications and hemorrhage in NCCT		
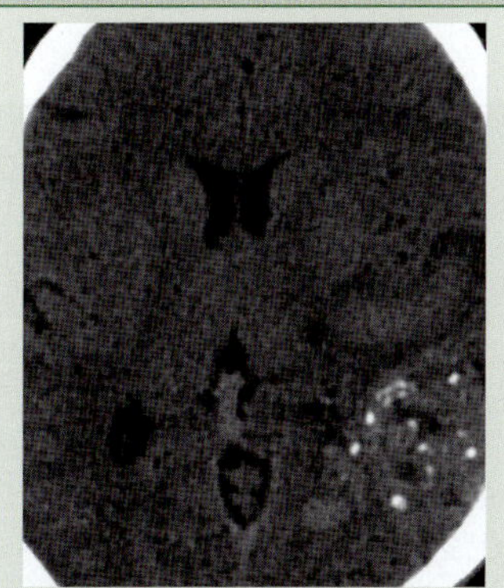 **Fig. 4.31.19:** Arteriovenous malformations seen with multiple calcifications and hemorrhage in NCCT	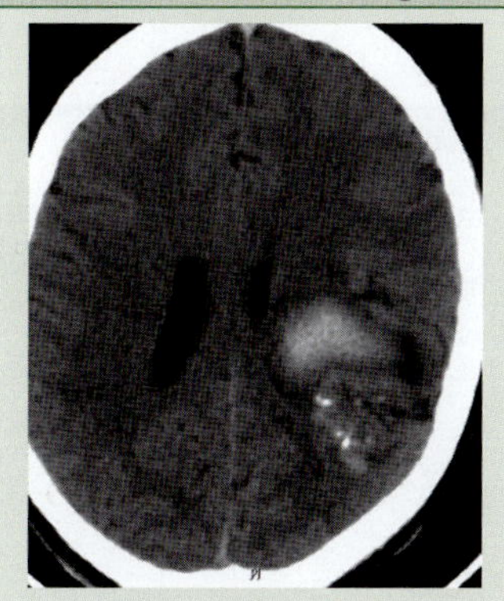 **Fig. 4.31.20:** Arteriovenous malformations seen with multiple calcifications and hemorrhage in NCCT	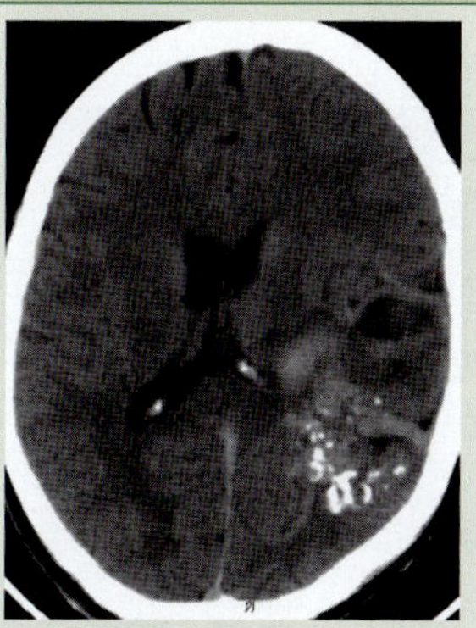 **Fig. 4.31.21:** Arteriovenous malformations seen with multiple calcifications and hemorrhage in NCCT

Flowchart 4.31.1: Approach to brain vascular malformations

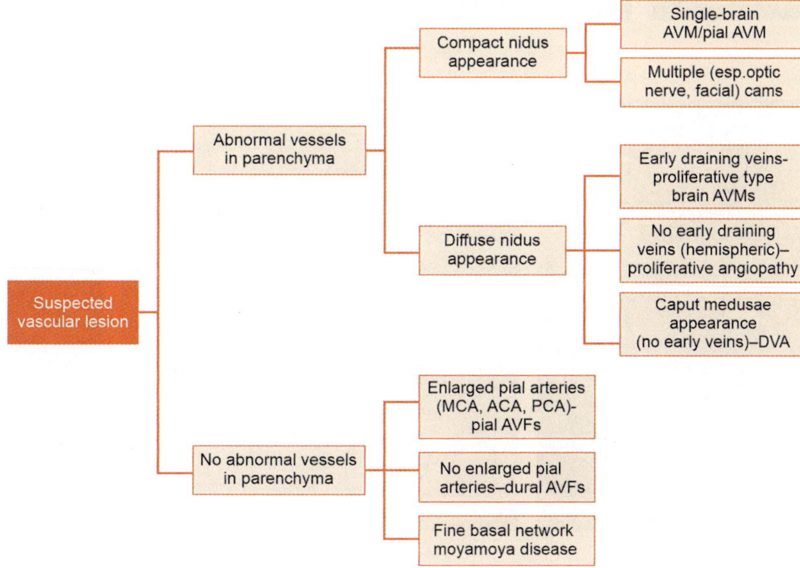

4.32 CENTRAL NERVOUS SYSTEM

Case No. 32

Clinical history: A 9-year-old male child with transient ischemic attacks and headache.

Radiological technique and observations: Figures 4.32.1 and 4.32.2 are T2 axial sections and Fig. 4.32.3 is time of flight (MRA) images of brain shows multiple tiny tortuous flow voids indicating collaterals noted involving the interpeduncular cistern, ambient cistern, quadrigeminal cistern and sylvian cisterns. More caudal sections of the scan show severe attenuation of the bilateral supraclinoid ICA flow void compared with the basilar artery. TOF image shows severe narrowing of the supraclinoid ICA with reformation of distal ICA, ACA and MCA by multiple collaterals. No evidence of any T2 hyperintense lesions suggesting infarct. No evidence of haemorrhage or any other lesions in the brain parenchyma/skull.

Figures 4.32.4 to 4.32.6 are volume rendering images showing severe narrowing of the supraclinoid ICA with reformation of distal ICA, ACA and MCA by multiple collaterals. The multiple squiggly flow voids in the brain give rise to the appearance of **"puff of smoke"**.

Interpretation: A—9 years old male, bilateral supraclinoid carotid artery, B—severe attenuation of the supraclinoid ICA, and multiple collaterals, prominent extradural meningeal artery, C—multiple tiny tortuous flow voids indicating collaterals noted involving the interpeduncular cistern, ambient cistern, quadrigeminal cistern and sylvian cisterns on T2 and MRA, D—Moyamoya disease.

Principal diagnosis: Moyamoya disease (Suzuki: Stage 3).

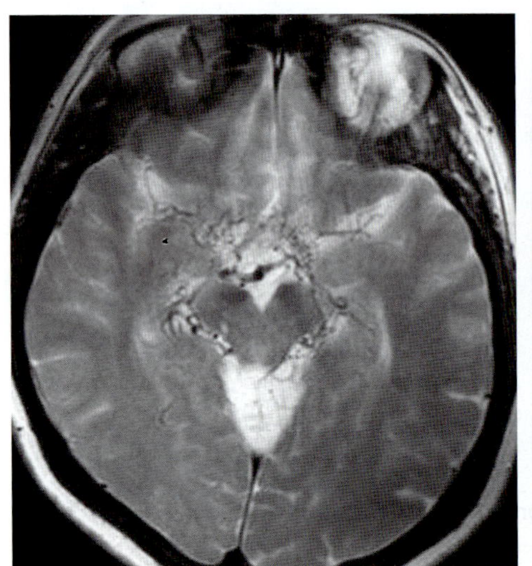

Fig. 4.32.1

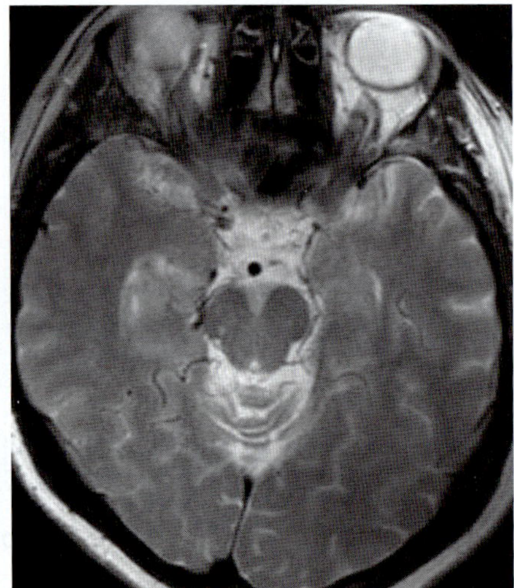

Fig. 4.32.2

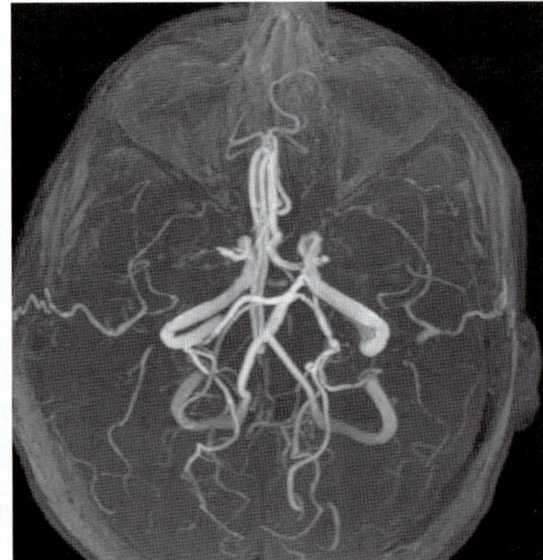

Fig. 4.32.3

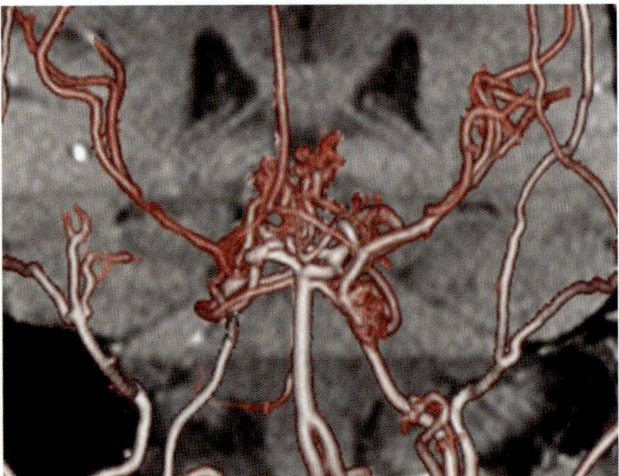

Fig. 4.32.4

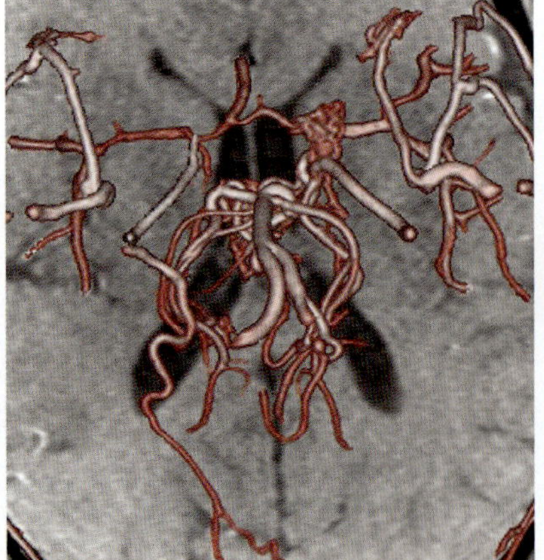

Fig. 4.32.5

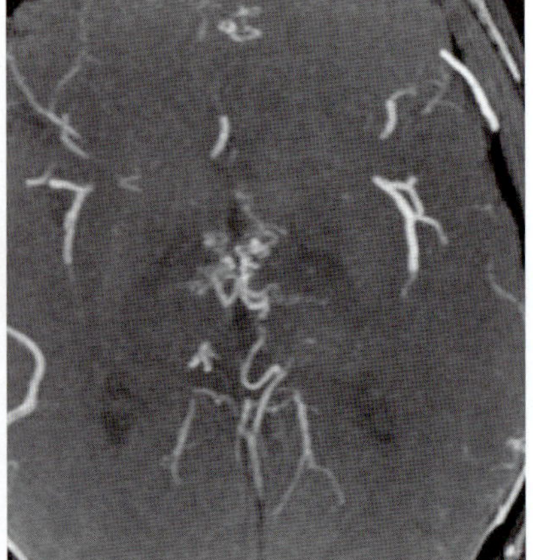

Fig. 4.32.6

Table 4.32.1: Differential diagnosis for moyamoya disease

Moyamoya disease: Progressive bilateral stenosis or occlusion of terminal internal carotid artery (ICA)/proximal circle of Willis with abnormal vascular network at base of brain.	Vessel wall imaging (VWI) in moyamoya disease typically demonstrates → concentric luminal narrowing → none or only minimal enhancement → homogeneous T2 signal → no outward remodelling	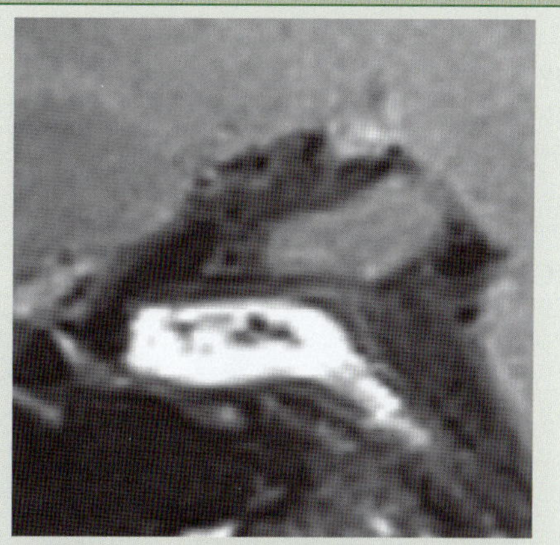 Fig. 4.32.7: Moyamoya disease
Atherosclerosis: Current treatment algorithms are based on luminal stenosis, with symptoms and 70% stenosis of the extracranial carotid artery can be used as the threshold for endovascular treatment or carotid endarterectomy.	The typical atherosclerosis plaque is **eccentric and heterogeneous and positive remodelling lesion which enhances on contrast.**	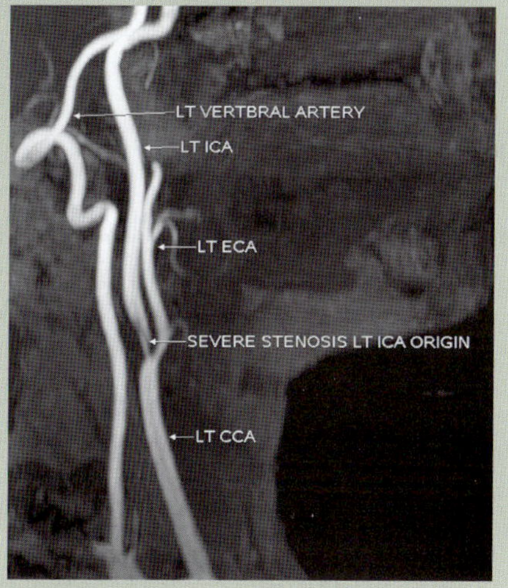 Fig. 4.32.8: Atherosclerosis
CNS vasculitis: Inflammatory vasculitis is secondary to endothelial permeability and contrast leakage	VWI **shows inflammation and edema within the vessel wall, will show thickening** and multifocal, homogeneous, and concentric enhancement.	
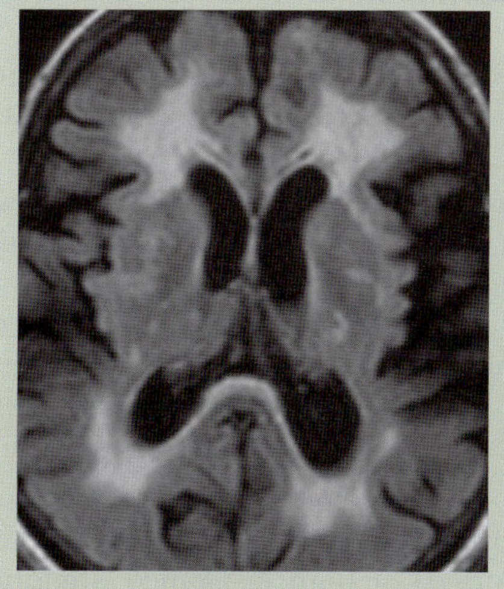 Fig. 4.32.9: CNS vasculitis	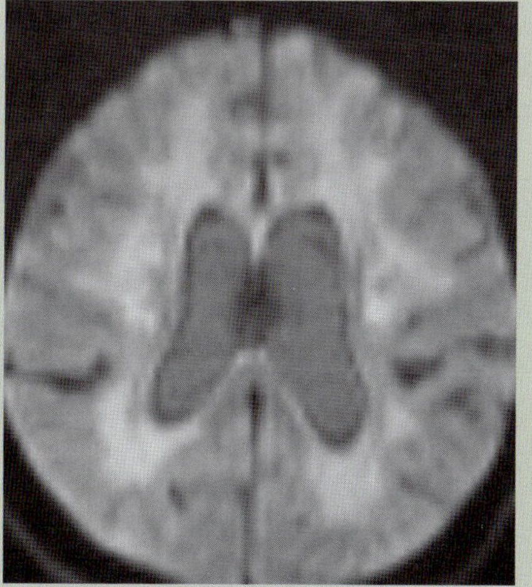 Fig. 4.32.10: CNS vasculitis	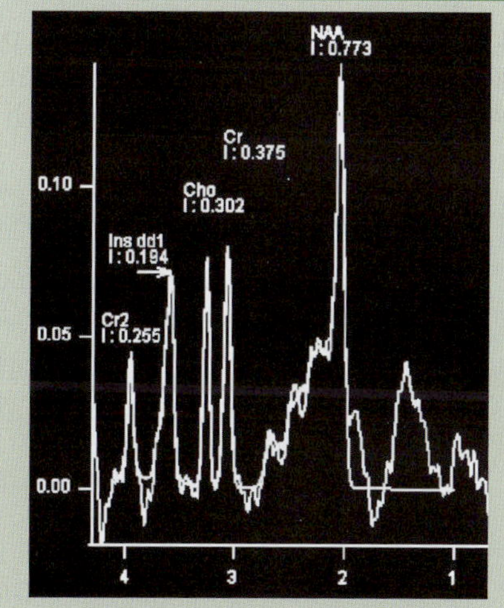 Fig. 4.32.11: CNS vasculitis

(Contd.)

Table 4.32.1: Differential diagnosis for moyamoya disease (*Contd.*)			
Reversible cerebral vasoconstriction syndrome (RCVS): RCVS presents with sudden, severe headache and concomitant neurological deficits. RCVS will show complete luminal resolution after approximately 3 months with conservative treatment	VWI shows minimal smooth, **concentric thickening with minimal diffuse** or no enhancement. Affected patients may develop infarction, SAH, edema, and intraparenchymal hemorrhage.		
ICA occlusion			
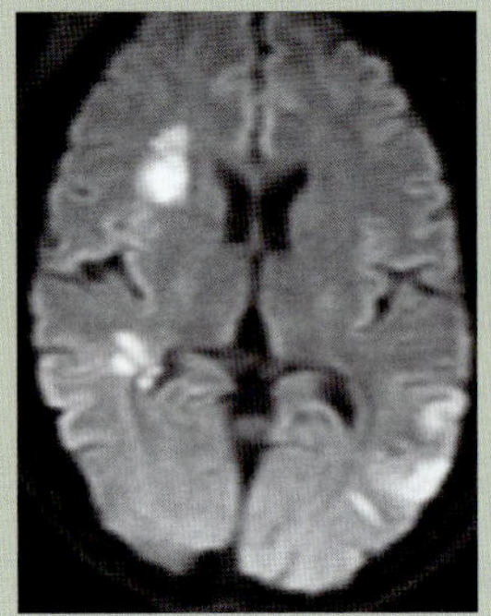 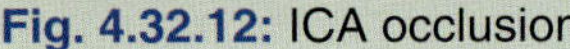 **Fig. 4.32.12:** ICA occlusion	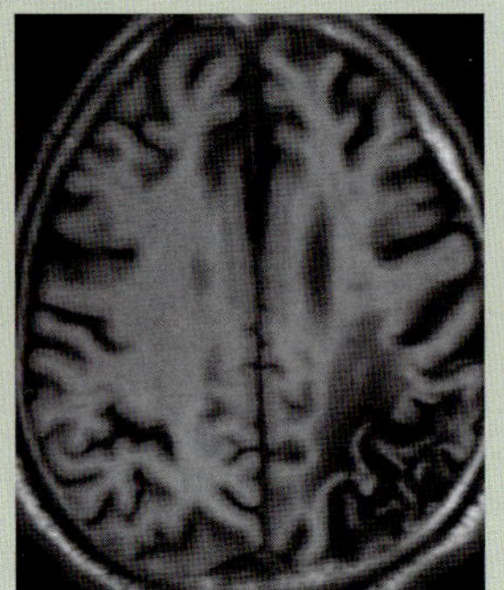 **Fig. 4.32.13:** ICA occlusion	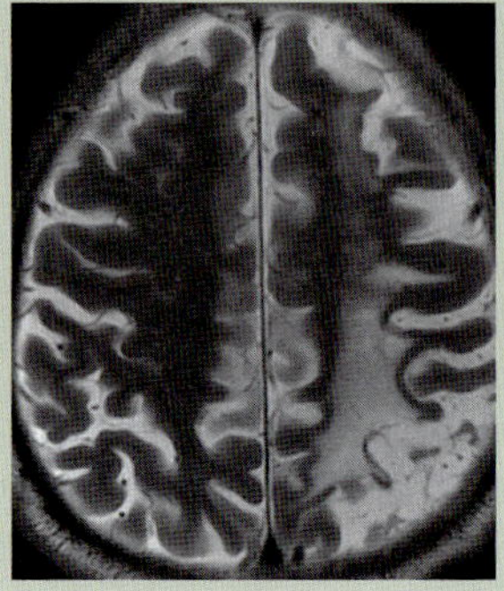 **Fig. 4.32.14:** ICA occlusion	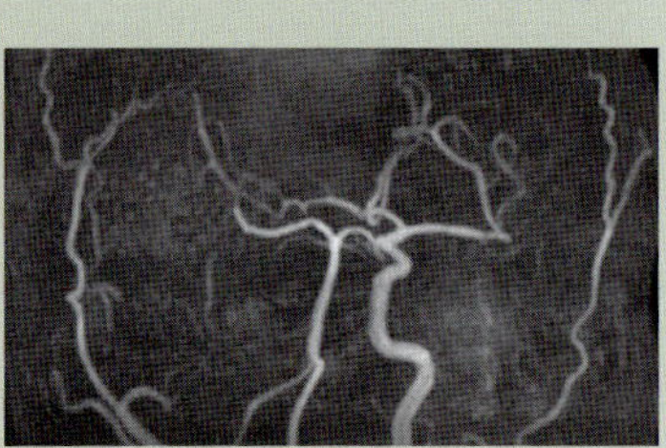 **Fig. 4.32.15:** ICA occlusion

Further investigations and management:

- **Moyamoya disease—indirect bypass: Encephalo-duro-arterio-synangiosis (EDAS)** more effective in children: Involves directly applying superficial temporal artery branches or MCA branches directly on to the pial surface of the brain. 5-year risk of ipsilateral stroke post-EDAS = 15%
- Direct bypass: Superficial temporal artery-middle cerebral artery (STA-MCA) more common in adults
- Anticoagulation; correct/control prothrombotic states and inflammatory etiologies
- Hypertransfusion for sickle cell-related moyamoya
- Perivascular sympathectomy or superior cervical ganglionectomy (adults).

Discussion: **Moyamoya disease** is progressive bilateral stenosis or occlusion of terminal internal carotid artery (ICA)/proximal circle of Willis with abnormal vascular network at base of brain.

Table 4.32.2: Causes for moyamoya appearance	
Primary moyamoya disease	*Secondary moyamoya*
RNF213 polymorphism in 95% of familial East Asian	Down syndrome, tuberous sclerosis, sickle cell disease, connective tissue disease, progeria, neurofibromatosis1, morning glory syndrome. Infections-Tuberculous meningitis Inflammatory: CNS angiitis (of childhood), basal meningitis, atherosclerosis, H and N infections. Vasculopathies and prothrombotic states: XRT, Kawasaki, anticardiolipin antibody, factor Leiden, polyarteritis nodosa, Beçhet, SLE.

Imaging: **NECT:** Children 50–60% show anterior more than posterior atrophy. Adults can present with intracranial hemorrhage. (In adults haemorrhage is more common than stroke, in children TIAs and stroke more common.)

CECT: Enhancing dots (large lenticulostriate) in BG with abnormal net-like vessels at base of brain.

CTA: Abnormal circle of Willis and net-like collaterals.

MRI findings: **T1WI:** Multiple dot-like flow voids in BG.

T2WI: Increased signal in small vessel cortical and white matter infarcts. Collateral vessels noted which appear as net-like cisternal filling defects.

FLAIR: Bright sulci giving rise to leptomeningeal **"ivy"** sign.

T2* GRE: Hemosiderin if prior haemorrhage. Asymptomatic microbleeds occasionally seen in adults.

DWI: Very useful for "acute on chronic" disease.

T1WI C+: Lenticulostriate collaterals which appear as enhancing "dots" in BG and net-like thin vessels in cisterns.

MRA: Narrowed distal ICA and proximal circle of Willis vessels, synangiosis.

PWI: Decreased perfusion in deep hemispheric white matter, relative increased perfusion in posterior circulation.

Pulsed Doppler: Doppler spectral waveforms in ICA show no flow (occluded) or high resistance (stenotic) flow pattern, increased end-diastolic flow velocity, decreased vascular resistance in external CA (ECA) collaterals.

Angiographic findings: Narrow proximal ICA and circle of Willis (earliest) "bottleneck sign". Lenticulostriate and thalamo perforator collaterals: Puff of smoke appearance (intermediate). Transdural and transosseous EC-IC collaterals (late). Dilatation and branch extension of anterior choroidal artery predicts adult hemorrhagic events.

Infarcts and hemorrhage in moyamoya: Infarcts (30%) are more common along cortical border zones. Intracranial bleed (20 %) in the form of subarachnoid bleed, intraparenchymal or intraventricular bleed common in adults. Causes of intracranial haemorrhage in MMD are rupture of dilated fragile collaterals or rupture of aneurysms along the circle of Willis and basal cerebral network of collaterals.

Staging criteria for moyamoya disease (SUZUKI-1969)

Stage 1. Narrowing of ICA bifurcation

Stage 2. ACA, MCA, PCA dilated

Stage 3. Maximal basal collaterals; small ACA/MCA

Stage 4. Fewer collaterals (vessels); small PCA

Stage 5. Further decreased collaterals; absent ACA/MCA/PCA

Stage 6. Extensive ECA—pial collaterals

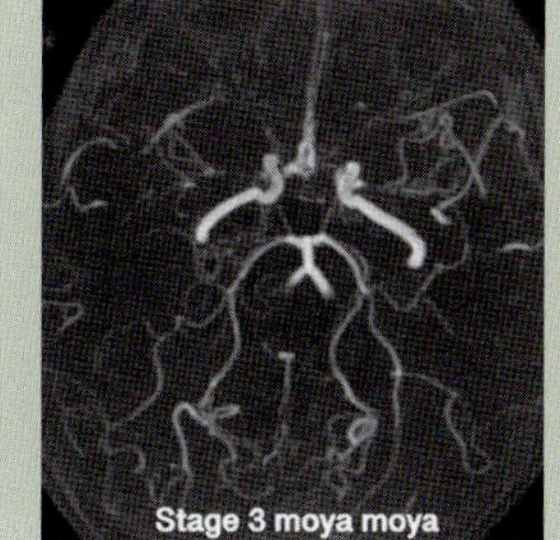

Fig. 4.32.16: Stage 3 moyamoya

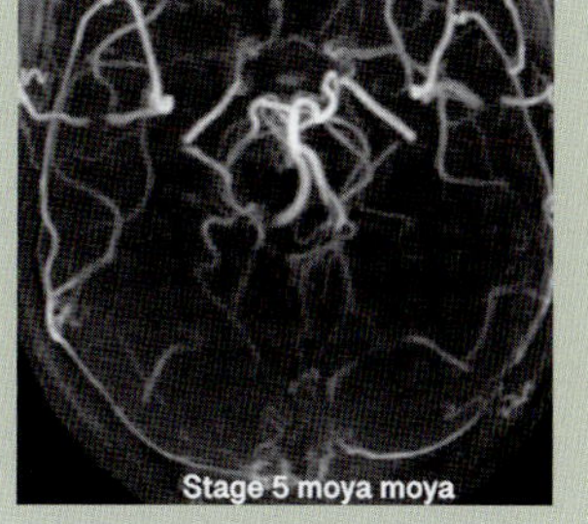

Fig. 4.32.17: Stage 5 moyamoya

Causes for Young Stroke

According to WHO, persons aged 18–35 are young adults and persons with age 35–50 are considered middle aged adults.

Table 4.32.3: Causes for young stroke

Embolic phenomena	*Arterial dissection*	*Blood disorders*
Cyanotic heart disease Cardiomyopathies Mitral valve prolapses Osler-Weber-Rendu syndrome	Trauma, spontaneous Fibromuscular dysplasia Marfan syndrome Ehlers-Danlos syndrome Homocystinuria	Sickle cell anaemia Polycythaemia Protein C deficiency Protein S deficiency
Vasculitis	*Non-inflammatory angiopathies*	*Venous thrombosis*
Neurofibromatosis type 1, 2 Beçhet disease Fibromuscular dysplasia Kawasaki disease Systemic lupus erythematosus Sarcoidosis Primary angiitis (vasculitis) of the CNS	CADASIL MELAS (mitochondrial encephalopathy, lactic acidosis and stroke-like episodes) Moyamoya disease/syndrome Divry van Bogaert syndrome Fabry disease	Pregnancy Postpartum Oral contraceptive pill use Skull base/intracranial sepsis Inflammatory bowel disease Primary antiphospholipid syndrome Eclampsia Malignancy

CNS Vasculitis

The generic terms "vasculitis" and "angiitis" denote inflammation of blood vessels affecting arteries, veins, or both. "Arteritis" is more specific and refers solely to inflammatory processes that involve arteries.

Isolated CNS vasculitis in which thorough clinical and laboratory examination does not identify another disorder causing the vascular inflammation is called primary arteritis of the CNS (PACNS). This contrasts with the many secondary causes of CNS vasculitis. Vasculitis can be caused by infection, collagen-vascular disease, immune complex deposition, drug abuse, and even neoplasms (e.g. lymphomatoid granulomatosis).

Table 4.32.4: Criteria for CNS vasculitis

American College of Rheumatology (ACR) criteria	*Chapel Hill Consensus Conference criteria*
Giant cell arteritis, Takayasu arteritis, Wegener granulomatosis, Churg-Strauss syndrome, Polyarteritis nodosa, Henoch-Schönlein purpura, and Hypersensitivity vasculitis	Immune-complex-mediated vasculitides Cryoglobulinaemic vasculitis, Recognized ANCA-associated vasculitis, and Distinguished microscopic polyangiitis

4

Primary arteritis of the CNS (PACNS) Granulomatous vasculitis—the most common histopathologic subtype of PACNS—is characterized by mononuclear infiltrates with granulomas	**Multifocal hypodensities in the basal ganglia and subcortical white matter that demonstrate patchy enhancement on CECT.** T2/FLAIR scans demonstrate hyperintensities in the same areas. T2* (GRE, SWI) may show parenchymal microhaemorrhages. Patchy enhancement with punctate and linear lesions is common on T1 C+ scans. Findings include multifocal irregularities, stenoses, and vascular occlusions	
Multiple vessel narrowing 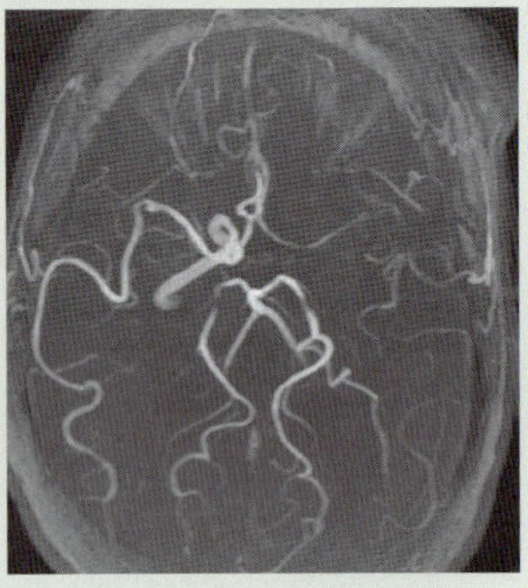 **Fig. 4.32.18:** Multiple vessel narrowing	**Left MCA occlusion** 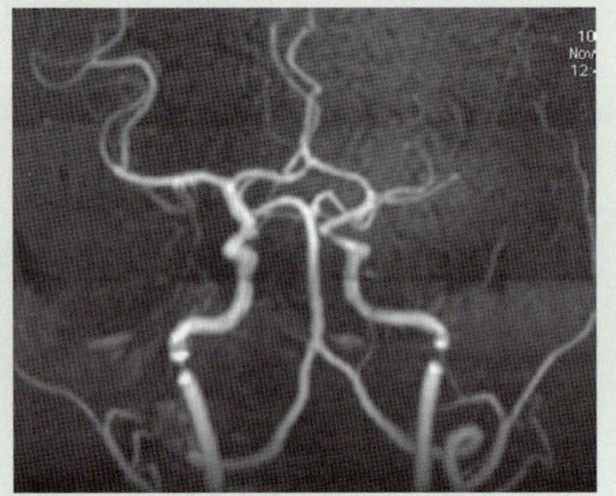 **Fig. 4.32.19:** Left MCA occlusion	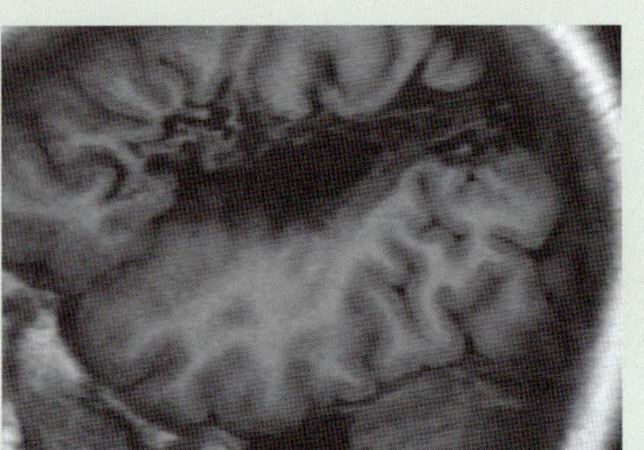 **Fig. 4.32.20:** Left MCA occlusion
Secondary Vasculitis		
Sickle cell disease (SCD) The most common worldwide cause of childhood stroke. Stroke risk is highest between the ages of 2 and 5 years.	Approximately 70–75% of SCD-related strokes are ischemic, and 20–25% are hemorrhagic. A diffusely thickened calvaria with expanded diploic space. **Subcortical and white matter hyperintensities along the deep watershed zone on T2/FLAIR.** A moyamoya-like pattern with supraclinoid ICA stenosis may develop with especially severe SCD.	
CADASIL CADASIL is the acronym for cerebral autosomal dominant arteriopathy with subcortical infarcts and leuko-encephalopathy.	Characteristic patterns may precede overt symptoms by more than a decade. Bilateral, multifocal T2 and FLAIR hyperintensities in the periventricular and deep WM. **Involvement of the anterior temporal lobe and external capsule has high sensitivity and specificity.** Lacunar infarcts in the subcortical WM, basal ganglia, thalamus, internal capsule, and brainstem. CADASIL has been identified as the most common monogenic heritable cause of lacunar stroke and vascular dementia in adults (20–40 years)	
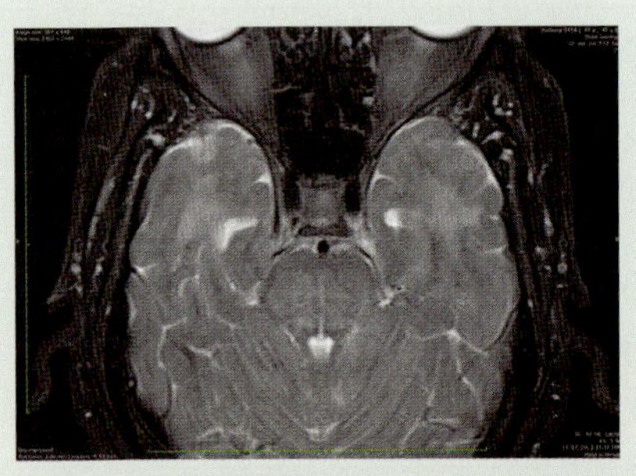 **Fig. 4.32.21:** CADASIL	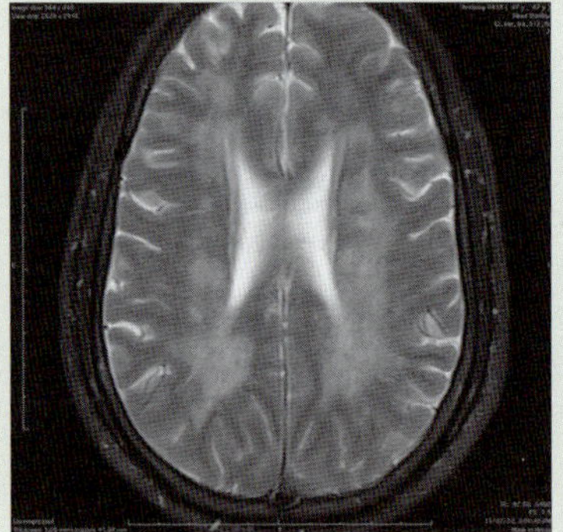 **Fig. 4.32.22:** CADASIL	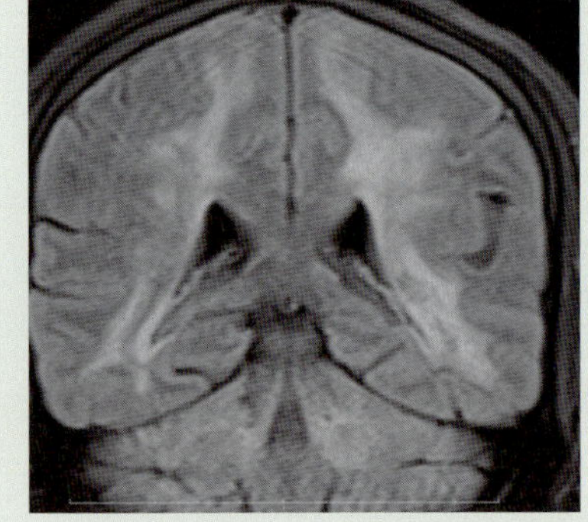 **Fig. 4.32.23:** CADASIL
Behçet disease Typically affects young adults 20 to 30 years and has a moderate male predominance. Clinical features of BD are mucocutaneous recurrent oral and genital ulcers, aphthous stomatitis, ophthalmologic lesions such as uveitis and iridocyclitis, and multiple arthralgias	Behçet disease (BD) is a chronic, idiopathic, relapsing-remitting, multisystem, inflammatory vascular disease. **Brainstem involvement—especially of the cerebral peduncles—is typical.** Thalamus and basal ganglia are the second most common sites of involvement, followed by the cerebral hemispheric white matter. Typical MR findings are small circular, linear, crescent-shaped, or irregular foci of T2/FLAIR hyperintensity in the midbrain. Primarily involves—cardiovascular system—thickening of the aorta and superior vena cava (vasculitis), venous thrombosis, arterial narrowing and aneurysmal dilatation, pericarditis. Thoracic manifestations—pulmonary arterial fusiform aneurysm, gastrointestinal manifestations	

(Contd.)

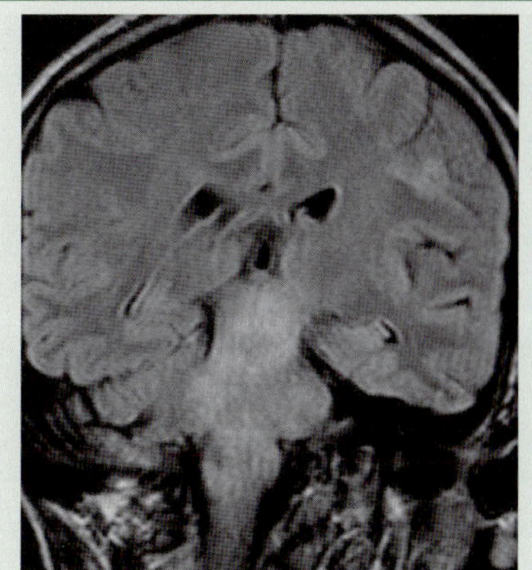 **Fig. 4.32.24:** Behçet disease	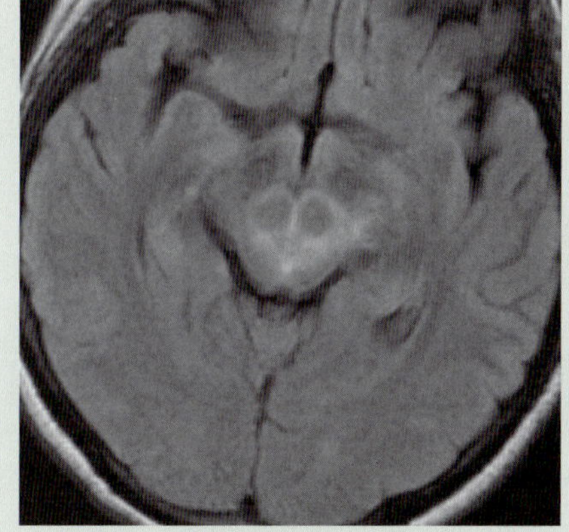 **Fig. 4.32.25:** Behçet disease	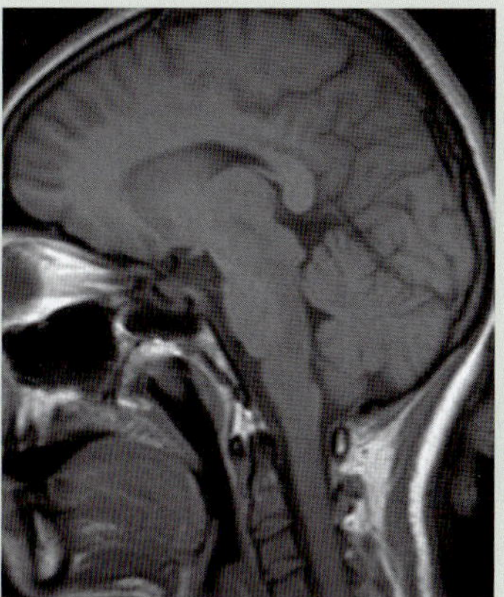 **Fig. 4.32.26:** Behçet disease
Cocaine and heroin abuse. **The complications associated with cocaine abuse include** cocaine-induced leuko-encephalopathy (rare), crack lung, septal perforation, dilated cardiomyopathy and acute reversible pulmonary hypertension.	**Cocaine: In acute setting.** **Hypertensive intracranial haemorrhage (50%), haemorrhage due to unmasked aneurysm or AV malformation** (50%), failure of cerebrovascular autoregulation at high blood pressures, resulting in hyperperfusion, disruption of the blood–brain barrier, and vasogenic edema leads to PRES via alterations in blood pressure. **In the chronic setting, ischemic leukoencephalopathy** occurs with cocaine as well as opiate use. **Heroin:** Spongiform leuko-encephalopathy with cerebellar white matter changes showing increased signal intensity. Abnormally decreased N-acetyl-aspartate peak with increased lactate peak in white matter.	
SLE (Lupus) Systemic lupus erythematosus (SLE or "lupus") is a multisystem complex autoimmune disorder. CNS SLE occurs at all ages, with peak onset between the second and fourth decades. In adults, over 90% of patients are female.	**Multiple small subcortical and deep WM hyperintensities on T2/FLAIR. Acute lesions demonstrate transient enhancement on T1 C+ studies and restricted diffusion.** Large confluent lesions that resemble acute disseminated encephalomyelitis (ADEM). Dural venous sinus and cortical/deep venous thrombosis occur in 20–30%	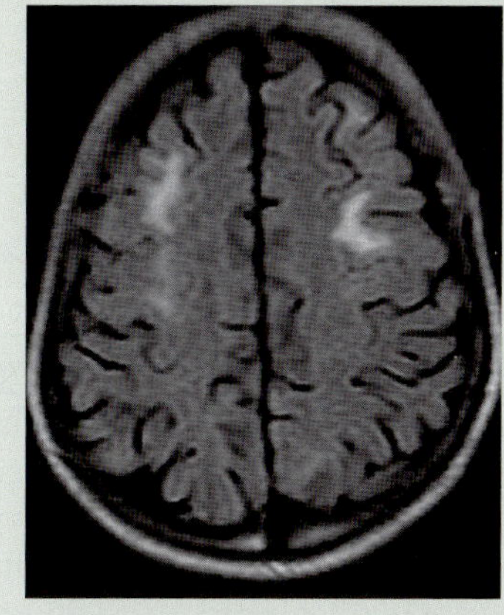 **Fig. 4.32.27:** SLE
Antiphospholipid syndrome Mean age of onset is 50 years. There is a 2:1 female predominance.	Mixed-age multifocal cortical/subcortical infarcts, parietal dominant atrophy with **relative sparing of the frontal and temporal lobes,** **"Too many for age" deep WM hyperintensities on T2/FLAIR scans are typical findings in APS. Both arterial and venous thromboses are common.** The diagnosis of APS requires the presence of at least one clinical criterion (e.g. vascular thrombosis or pregnancy morbidity) and one laboratory finding, i.e. persistently positive lupus anticoagulant, antiphospholipid antibodies, etc.	
Cerebral amyloid disease Aβ40 deposited in meningeal, cortical arterioles causing mural, perivascular inflammation. Vessel walls are thicker but weaker. CAD causes 5–20% of spontaneous intracranial haemorrhages in elderly patients (>55 years).	NCET: Lobar haemorrhages of different ages. Convexal subarachnoid haemorrhage. MRI—multifocal microbleeds; **"Blooming" hypointensities on T2*, typically cortical, meningeal (pial).** Cerebellum, brainstem, basal ganglia generally spared. Cortical superficial siderosis common. Larger, asymmetric areas of confluent WM hyperintensity on T2/FLAIR with or without microhaemorrhages are characteristic of ABRA (Aβ related angiitis). Both types may show such striking enhancement on T1 C+	

(*Contd.*)

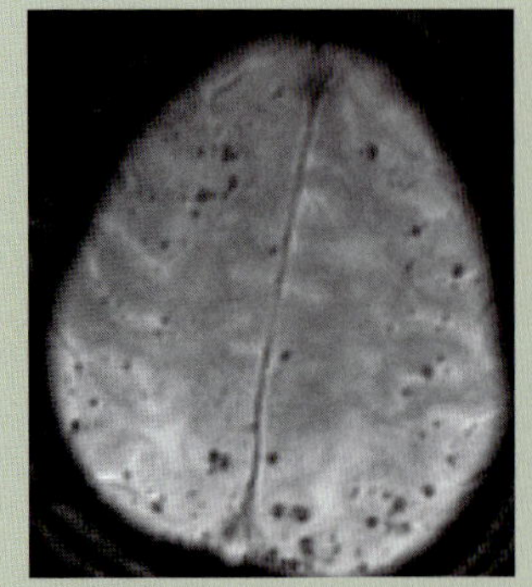
Fig. 4.32.28: Cerebral amyloid angiopathy

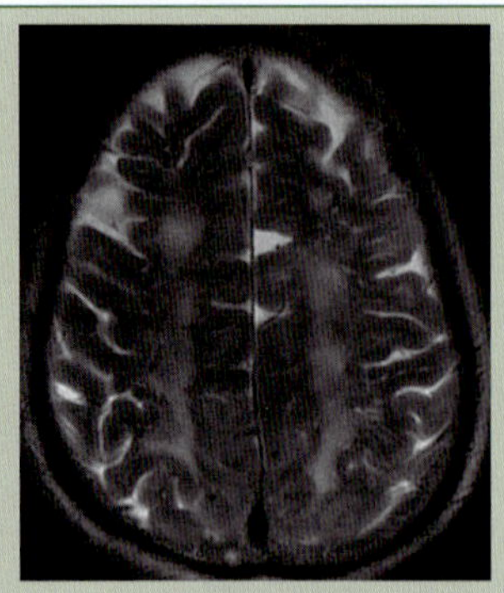
Fig. 4.32.29: Cerebral amyloid angiopathy

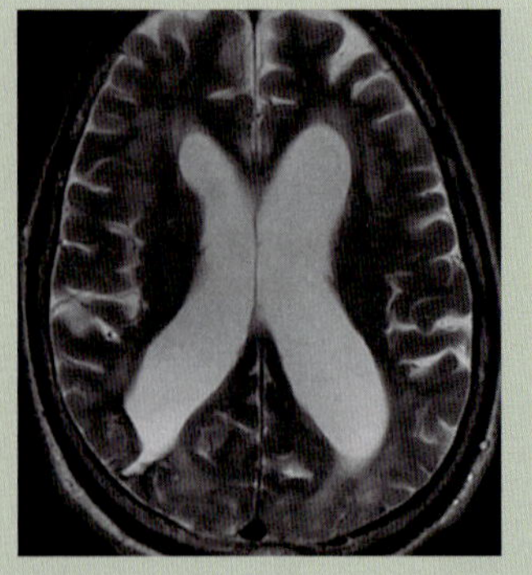
Fig. 4.32.30: Cerebral amyloid angiopathy

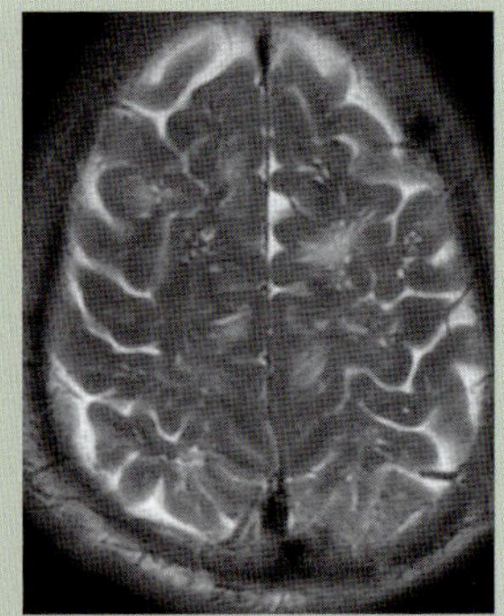
Fig. 4.32.31: Cerebral amyloid angiopathy

Thrombotic microangiopathies. Microvascular occlusive disorders with thrombocytopenia, intravascular haemolysis and ischemic organ damage	**Major types:** Disseminated intravascular coagulopathy, HUS (both Shiga-associated and complement-associated HUS) and TTP **Cortical/subcortical ischemic infarcts.** Multifocal micro-haemorrhages.
Chronic hypertensive encephalopathy (Binswanger disease)	

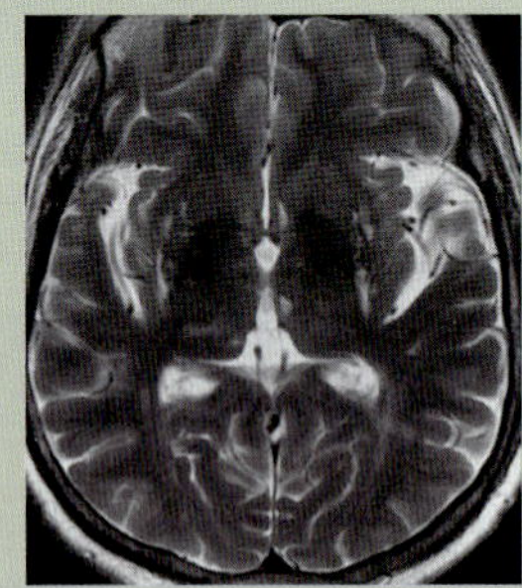
Fig. 4.32.32: Binswanger disease

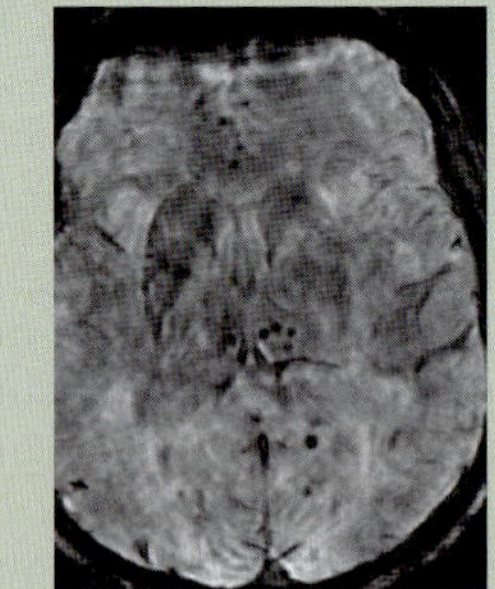
Fig. 4.32.33: Binswanger disease

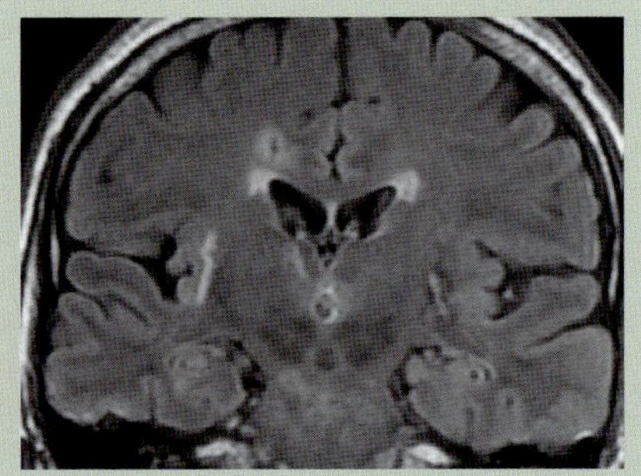
Fig. 4.32.34: Binswanger disease

Table 4.32.5: Indications of FLAIR sequence

Perilesional edema	Mesial temporal sclerosis
SAH	IVY sign
Infarction	Multiple sclerosis,
Head injuries	Basal cistern debris in TB
Syrinx/cyst in spinal cord	Post-contrast flair in meningitis

Systematic approach of VW assessment: The normal vessel wall is usually seen as a thin line surrounding the dark lumen of the vessel and is usually of the same intensity as the brain parenchyma. A wall abnormality or lesion on vessel wall imaging can be defined by either a thickening of the vessel wall >50% of the thickness of the adjacent vessel wall, and/or contrast enhancement. The thickening must then be evaluated as to whether it is circumferential (as in vasculitis) or eccentric (as in atherosclerosis). Cross correlation must be done with the opposite side (avoiding the pitfall of bilateral disease) as well as with the MRA TOF images. Stenosis and narrowing on VWI must be looked for, however the absence of stenosis on VWI does not indicate the absence of a lesion—many lesions undergo positive remodelling and thus may not show any luminal stenosis on MRA. **Contrast enhancement on VWI**—it is ideal to have both pre- and post-contrast T1 images for evaluating contrast enhancement of VW lesions. However, if only post-contrast images are available, enhancement can still be determined by either comparing it the contralateral vessel wall, or to the pituitary stalk. Enhancement can be further graded as 1 or 2 depending on whether the enhancement is greater than brain parenchyma/contralateral side but less than pituitary stalk (grade 1), or when enhancement is greater than the pituitary stalk (grade 2). Potential pitfalls to be avoided include the normal enhancement of the internal carotid wall and the vertebral artery wall at the location where they cross the dura mater, and the normal enhancement of the cavernous sinus, confounding enhancement of the cavernous part of the internal carotid artery. **Vessel wall disease—imaging findings:** Although vessel wall imaging is a recent development, there are already several clinical scenarios where VWI has proven its value. The indications for which VWI has the greatest evidence are determining the aetiology of stroke and for assessing accompanying vessel wall lesions (Table 4.32.6).

Table 4.32.6: Summary of VWI findings in various disorders

	ICAD	*Vasculitis*	*RCVS*	*Moyamoya*	*Dissection*	*Aneurysm*
Wall thickening	Eccentric	Concentric	Concentric	Concentric	Eccentric	Concentric
Distribution	Any artery	Medium/small size vessels	Medium/small size vessels	Terminal ICA, Proximal MCA	V4 vertebral artery, supra clinoid ICA, M1 MCA	Any artery
Juxta luminal T2 hyperintensity	Present	Absent	Absent	Absent	Absent	Absent
Wall enhancement	Eccentric	Concentric Grade 2	Usually absent, concentric grade 1 if present	Concentric	Absent/Mild	Concentric
Remodelling of outer wall	Positive or Negative	Negative	Negative	Negative	Positive or Negative	—
T1 hyperintensity	Intraplaque haemorrhage	—	—	—	Intramural hematoma	Intramural hematoma
Follow up	Enhancement up to 4 weeks in culprit lesion	Persists >3 months	Resolves within 3 months	Progressive	Change in morphology	

RCVS = reversible cerebral vasoconstriction syndrome, ICAD = Intracranial atherosclerotic disease

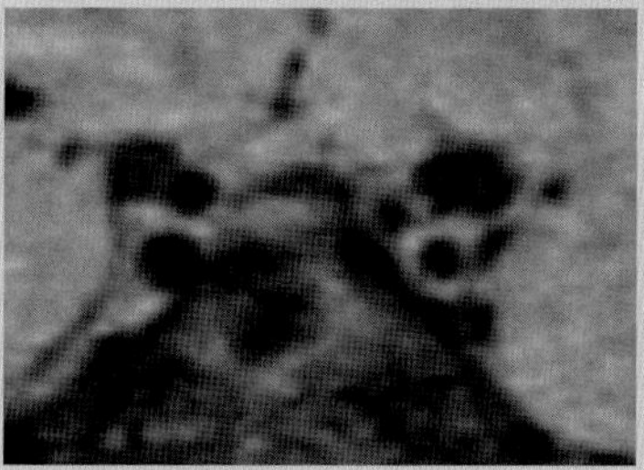

Fig. 4.32.35: Left ICA—vasculitis

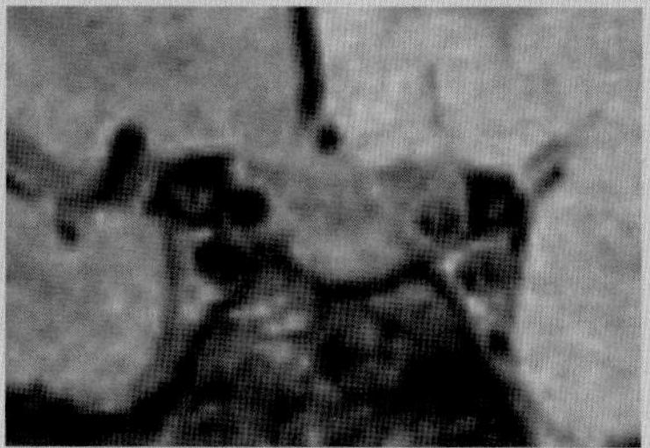

Fig. 4.32.36: Consistent with ICAD

Vasculitis vs Atherosclerosis: 3D T2 sequence (Fig. 4.32.35) **shows concentric, circumferential thickening of the vessel wall in the left ICA—Vasculitis. 3D T2 sequence** (Fig. 4.32.36) **shows eccentric, heterogenous thickening of the left ICA—consistent with ICAD.**

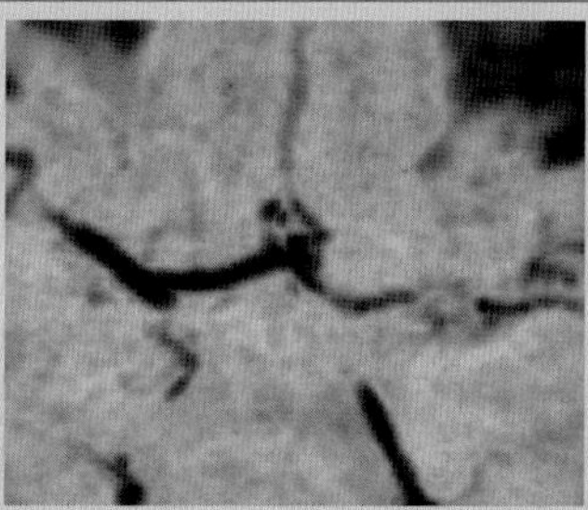

Fig. 4.32.37: Moyamoya disease

Minimum intensity projection image showing luminal narrowing of the left MCA artery without any significant vessel wall thickening in a patient with Moyamoya disease.

MRA shows attenuation of the basilar artery. Vessel wall imaging sequence shows circumferential thickening of the wall of the basilar artery—consistent with vasculitis. Patient was a case of latent neurosyphilis.

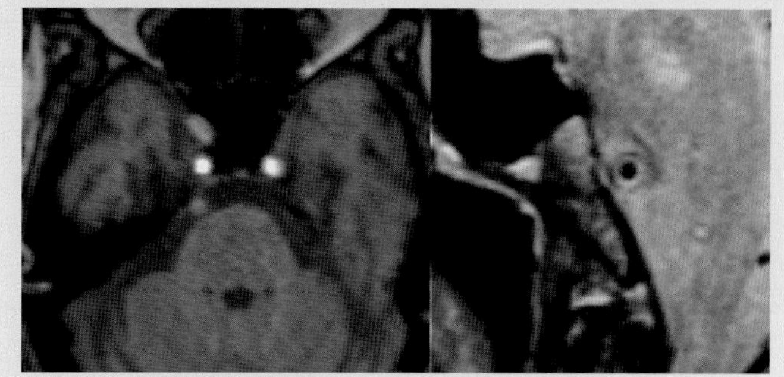

Fig. 4.32.38: Latent neurosyphilis

4.33 CENTRAL NERVOUS SYSTEM

Case No. 33

Clinical history: 55 years old female with giddiness, headache and vomiting for one day. No history of trauma or hypertension.

Radiological techniques: Figures 4.33.1 to 4.33.6 are plain CT, MR-FLAIR coronal, cerebral angiogram reformatted images respectively. NCCT images reveal a hyperdense focus anterior to the genu of the corpus callosum with hyperdensities in the pericallosal region, right sylvian fissure and the anterior interhemispheric fissure, suggestive of subarachnoid haemorrhage. No evidence of intraventricular extension/ventricular dilatation. No evidence of acute vascular territory infarct. On grounds of a non-traumatic SAH—next step would be CTA and an MRI. Contrast enhance CT shows a saccular outpouching from the anterior communicating artery. CTA shows a saccular aneurysm arising from the anterior communicating artery pointing superiorly, having a neck measuring 3 mm feeding from supply via the A1 segment. No other aneurysm is demonstrated. MR FLAIR image shows hyperintensities in the interhemispheric fissure and the right sylvian fissure. Prominent flow void noted in the pre-callosal region. No evidence of microbleeds.

Interpretation: A: 55-year-old female with hyperdensity in the pericallosal region, right sylvian fissure and the anterior interhemispheric fissure, B: Prominent flow void noted in the pre-callosal region. No evidence of microbleeds. C: CTA shows saccular aneurysm arising from anterior communicating artery (A1 segment)

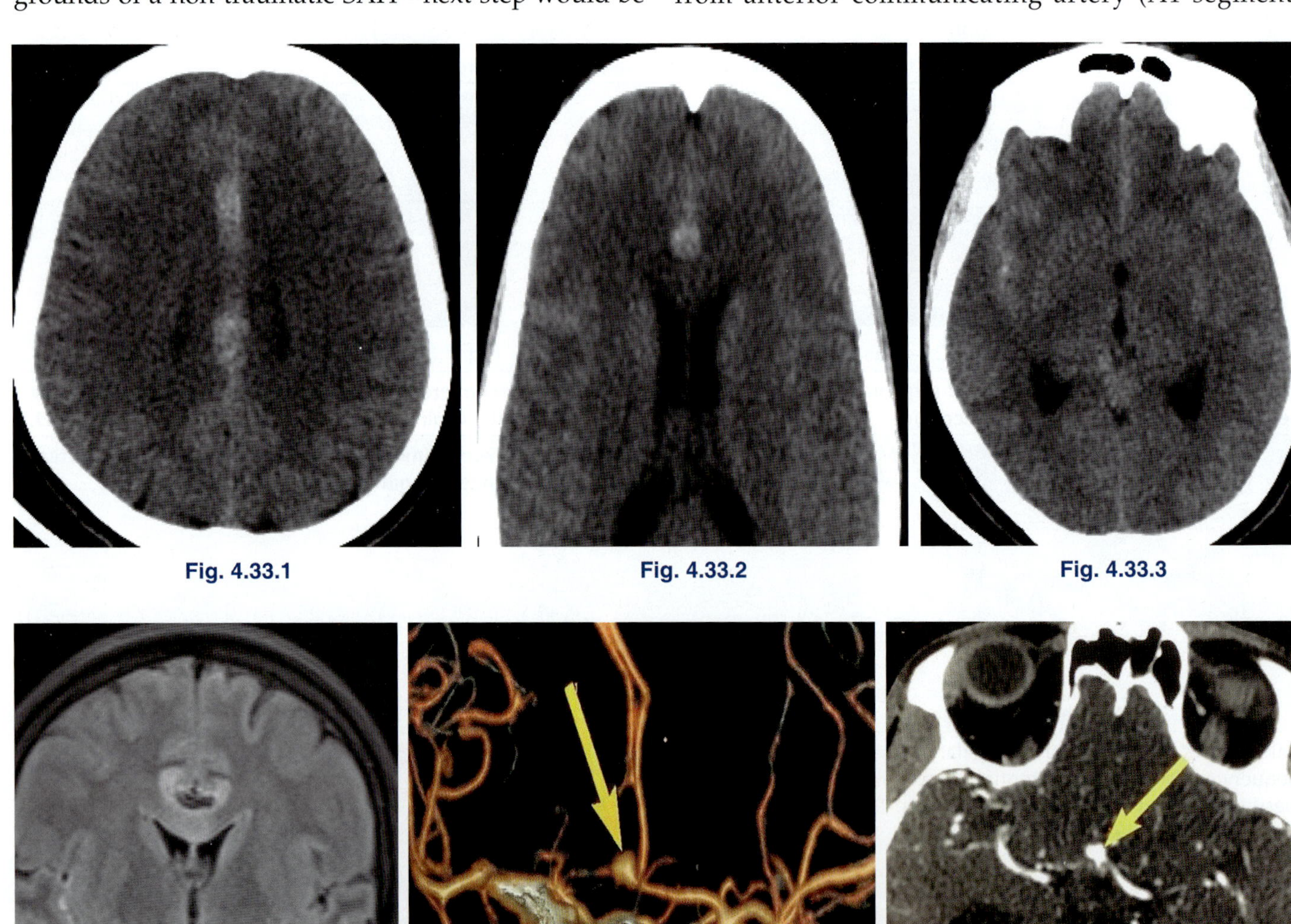

Fig. 4.33.1 Fig. 4.33.2 Fig. 4.33.3

Fig. 4.33.4 Fig. 4.33.5 Fig. 4.33.6

Table 4.33.1: Differential diagnosis for non-traumatic SAH

Peri-mesencephalic non-aneurysmal SAH **Most common cause for non-traumatic non-aneurysmal SAH,** localised to interpeduncular, ambient and prepontine cisterns, rarely. Many implicate venous rupture as the likely cause.	Criteria, which if fulfilled, in the presence of a negative CTA negates the need for DSA: SAH in peri-mesencephalic cisterns if SAH extending into the anterior interhemispheric fissure, not into all of the fissure if SAH extension into the medial sylvian fissures, not extending into the lateral fissure if interventricular extension, no frank intraventricular hemorrhage and no intraparenchymal hemorrhage. Clinically benign, complications and recurrence rare unlike aneurysmal bleed.	
Convexal SAH Causes are cortical vein or dural sinus thrombosis, AVMs, amyloid angiopathy (>60 years), vasculitis and reversible cerebral vasoconstriction syndrome (RCVS <60 years)	Unilateral, localised to superficial sulci over the cerebral convexities. Basal cisterns are typically spared.	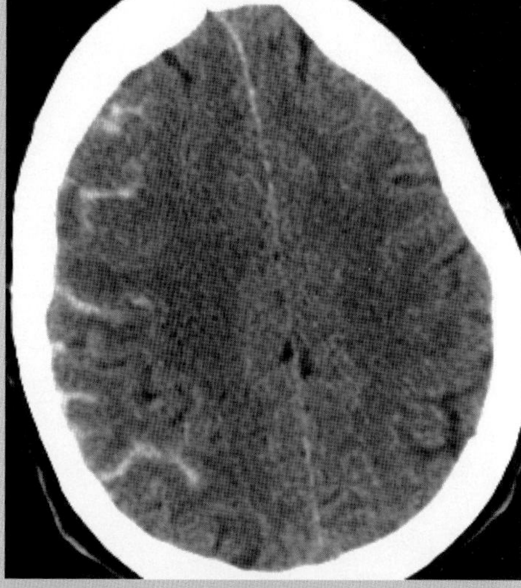 **Fig. 4.33.7:** Convexal SAH
Pseudo–SAH caused by severe cerebral oedema	Surrounding hypodensity of the brain makes blood in the cerebral arteries appear dense.	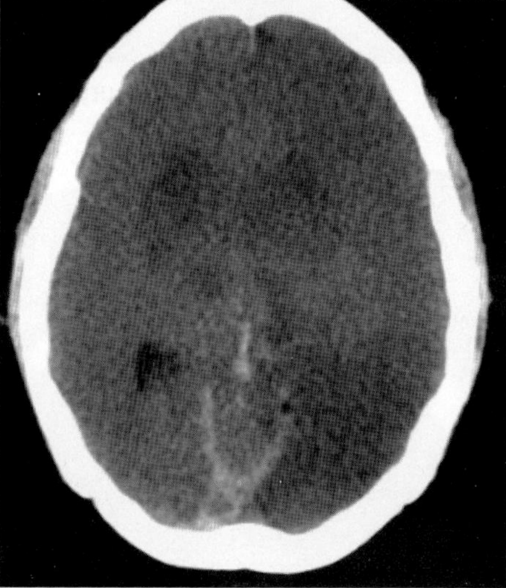 **Fig. 4.33.8:** Pseudo-SAH
Nonspecific sulcal–cisternal FLAIR hyperintensity	Occurs with meningitis, carcinomatosis, hyperoxygenation, stroke and gadolinium contrast (blood–brain barrier leakage or chronic renal failure)	
Hypertension PRES	In patients with **PRES**, occurrence of **SAH** (7–8%) is related to increased morbidity and mortality especially when the hemorrhage is diffuse or massive	

pointing superiorly, subarachnoid hemorrhage. D: Ruptured aneurysmal SAH.

Principal diagnosis: Ruptured anterior communicating artery aneurysm.

Differential diagnosis: (for non-traumatic SAH).

Above patient treated with endovascular coiling (Figs 4.33.9 to 4.33.10) and the postprocedure CT is shown.

Further investigations: The best imaging clue to aSAH is hyperdense cisterns and sulci on NECT with the

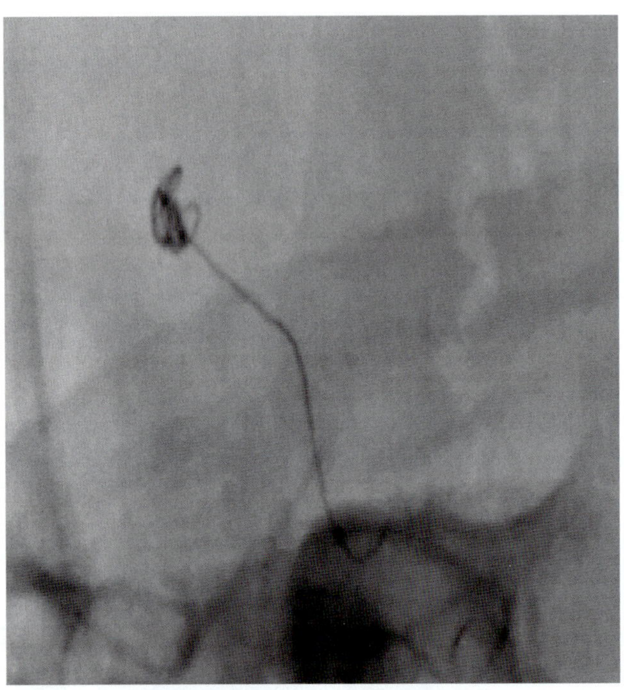

Fig. 4.33.9: Aneurysm coiling

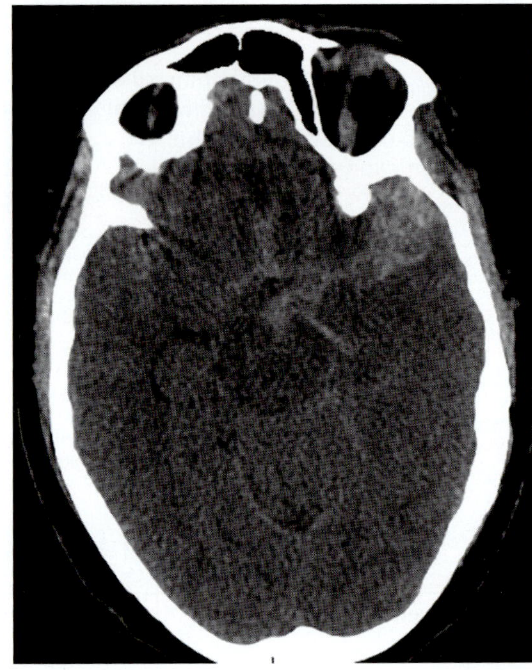

Fig. 4.33.11: Subarachnoid hemorrhage with ghost sign in left sylvian fissure

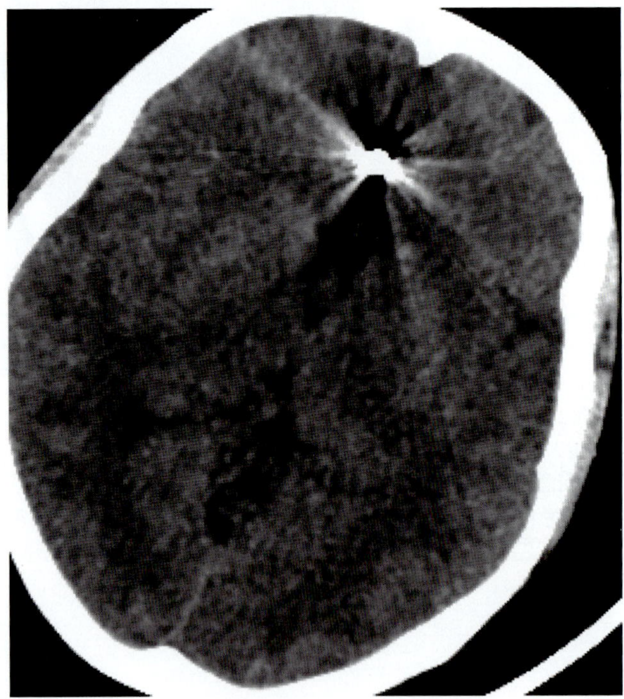

Fig. 4.33.10: Aneurysm coiling

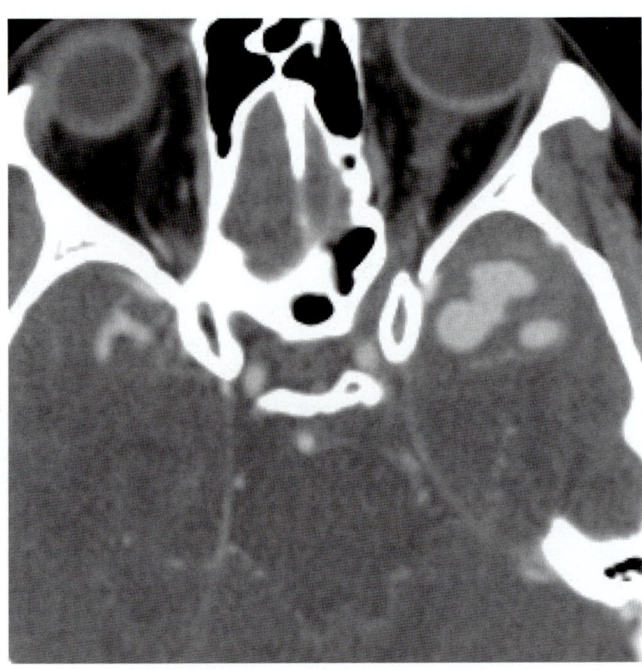

Fig. 4.33.12: Left MCA aneurysm

haemorrhage sometimes outlining the comparatively hypodense appearing aneurysmal sac.

A positive NECT for aSAH warrants a CTA. CTA is positive in 95 % cases if the culprit aneurysm is 2 mm or larger. DSA can find out the occult vascular pathology with CTA negative SAH in 13% of patients.

Sometimes an aneurysm may be seen as a hypodense region within dense subarachnoid hemorrhage, a finding often referred to as a "ghost sign" (in picture).

MRI–FLAIR is the best sequence to depict aSAH with hyperintense CSF in sulci and cisterns but is nonspecific (seen in case of meningitis, hyperoxygenation, neoplasms and as an artefact)

MR is helpful when no structural cause for non-traumatic SAH is found on screening NECT or CTA.

Repeat DSA or CTA is recommended in patients with diffuse type—SAH if initial DSA is negative.

Management: Initial management of ruptured aneurysms is administration of calcium-channel blockers (nimodipine for 21 days) to all patients which improves the outcomes after SAH. This agent is preventing cerebral vasospasm after aneurysmal SAH. Anticonvulsant is given (levetiracetam or phenytoin), particularly for patients undergoing craniotomy and those with focal cerebral hematomas in addition to the subarachnoid hemorrhage.

Blood in the subarachnoid space block the arachnoidal villi, may cause acute hydrocephalus. Blood within the ventricles may block the foramen of Monroe, also leading to hydrocephalus. When hydrocephalus leads to neurologic worsening due to raised intracranial pressure (ICP), a ventriculostomy catheter should be emergently placed for CSF diversion.

Choice of surgical technique is either obliteration of an aneurysm (ruptured or unruptured) with endovascular coiling or surgical clipping. Usually coiling is safer than clipping for both ruptured and unruptured aneurysms, at least in the acute perioperative period, clipping is slightly more durable (Figs 4.33.14 and 4.33.15).

Intraoperative angiography is used as an adjunct to clipping and permits confirmation of aneurysm occlusion and patency of nearby vessels. **A technique called near-infrared indocyanine green video angiography (ICGA) is a less invasive way of assessing aneurysm and blood-vessel patency during aneurysm surgery**. After administration of the indocyanine green dye, an operating microscope equipped with appropriate software may detect blood flow using near infrared waves. This technique is less invasive than intraoperative angiography, but one disadvantage is vessels which can be seen by the operating microscope are only evaluated.

Vasospasm: Transcranial Doppler ultrasonography (TCD) is frequently used as a non-invasive diagnostic tool and is sensitive to changes in the vessel calibre of the larger vessels of the circle of Willis. A trained technician will perform TCD daily or on alternate days during the vasospasm period (days 3–12 after SAH, depending on the extent of the haemorrhage).

So-called triple-H therapy (hypertension, haemodilution, and hypervolemia) remains the most important aspect of the medical management of vasospasm, but in refractory cases, endovascular methods are advised. Transluminal balloon angioplasty is the method of choice, but intra-arterial papaverine can be used for vasospasm in the distal vasculature, which cannot be accessible to balloons. Additionally, intra-arterial papaverine can be used to temporarily open vessels to permit passage of a balloon.

Flow diverters: Indication of flow diverters are complex aneurysms (fusiform, large and giant, wide neck, small aneurysms untreatable by conventional methods) and in the case of recurrences. The appropriateness of flow-diverting treatment must be decided on a case-by-case basis, considering experience and the relative risks against standard approaches or observation (Fig 4.33.13).

Recurrence: The overall postoperative recurrence rate of intracranial saccular aneurysms was 12.6%. The following risk factors were found to be associated with

Table 4.33.2: SAH grading

Grade	*WFNS scale for SAH*	*Modified Fisher scale: NCCT*
0	Unruptured aneurysm	No visible SAH or IVH
1	GCS = 15	</= 1 mm SAH, no IVH
2	GCS = 13–15 with no focal neurological deficit	</= 1 mm SAH +IVH
3	GCS = 13–15, with focal neurological deficit	>1 mm thick SAH, no IVH
4	GCS = 7–12	>1 mm thick SAH + IVH or parenchymal haemorrhage
5	GCS = 3–6	N/A

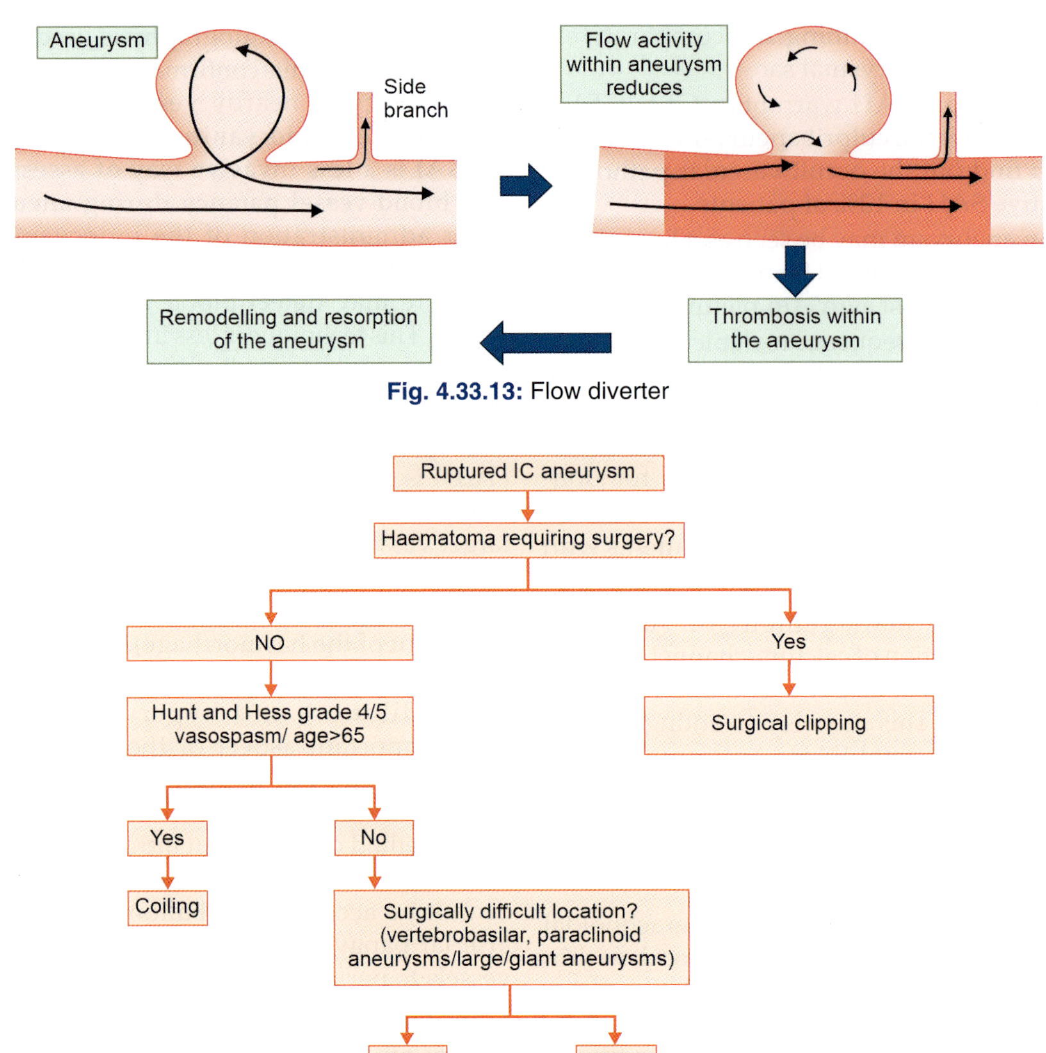

Fig. 4.33.13: Flow diverter

Fig. 4.33.14: Management of ruptured ICA aneurysm

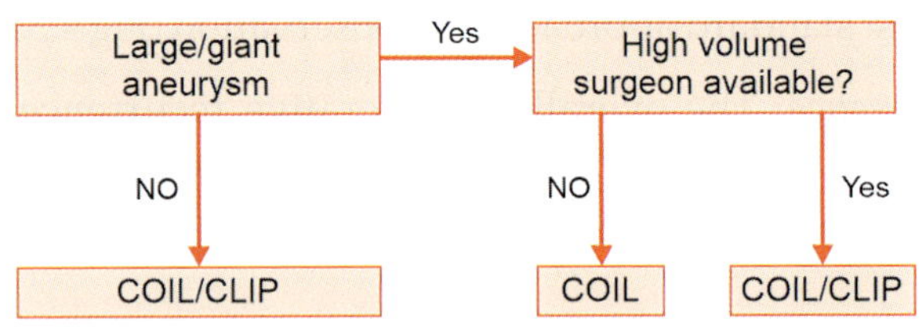

Fig. 4.33.15: Management of large/giant aneurysm

the recurrence of intracranial saccular aneurysms (ISA): Smoking, a large ISA tumor size, a wide-necked ISA, an anterior communicating or middle cerebral artery ISA, an ISA rupture, and the absence of stent assistance were risk factors for the postoperative recurrence of ISA.

Discussion: Aneurysmal SAH (aSAH)—Cause 3–5% of all strokes.

Nonspecific headache is the most common presenting complaint. Typical Thunderclap headache is seen in 4–12%. Patients who survive an aSAH develop *de novo* intracranial aneurysms at the rate of 2% per year and also carry an increased risk for other vascular diseases.

Hunt and Hess Scale for SAH

Grade 1: Asymptomatic or minimal headache and slight neck stiffness, 70% survival.

Grade 2: Moderate to severe headache; neck stiffness; no neurologic deficit except cranial nerve palsy, 60% survival.

Grade 3: Drowsy; minimal neurologic deficit, 50% survival.

Grade 4 stuporous; moderate to severe hemiparesis; possibly early decerebrate rigidity and vegetative disturbances, 20% survival.

Table 4.33.3: Stages of hemorrhage on MRI		
Haemorrhage on MRI	*T1*	*T2*
Oxy Hb (<24 hrs) Hyperacute	Isointense/hypointense	Hyperintense
Deoxy Hb (1–3 days) Acute	Isointense/hypointense	Hypointense
Intracellular Meth Hb (3-7 days) Early subacute	Hyperintense	Hypointense
Extracellular Meth Hb (1–2+ weeks) Late subacute	Hyperintense	Hyperintense
Hemosiderin Chronic	Hypointense	Hypointense

Grade 5 deep coma; decerebrate rigidity; moribund, 10% survival.

Types of aneurysms: Saccular, fusiform, blood blister – like aneurysms and pseudoaneurysms

Saccular and blood blister like aneurysms are most likely to rupture.

Family history is a risk factor for the occurrence of intracranial aneurysms. Twenty percent of patients with aneurysms have a family history of aneurysm rupture. Although the incidence of aneurysms is highest in families with two affected first-degree family members.

Bilateral aneurysms: Mirror aneurysms are generally considered as a subset of multiple aneurysms, defined as aneurysms occurring bilaterally and symmetrically on the same-named vessels. Most often involved middle cerebral artery bifurcation, followed by a para clinoid internal carotid artery and posterior communicating artery. Are rare and make up approximately 5% of all intracranial aneurysms, but they account for nearly 40% of all multiple intracranial aneurysms.

Blebs (Blood blister like) aneurysms vs Berry aneurysm: **Blood blister-like aneurysm** is a broad-based bulge at a non-branch point of a vessel, which is unlike saccular (or 'berry') aneurysms which usually occur at branch points.

Fusiform aneurysms can be atherosclerotic (common) or non-atherosclerotic (rare). In contrast to saccular aneurysms, FAs usually involve long, non-branching vessel segments and are seen as focal, circumferential outpouchings from a generally ectatic, elongated vessel.

Location of the ruptured aneurysm based on pattern of haemorrhage: In anterior communicating artery aneurysm, SAH in the interhemispheric fissure, both sylvian fissures and basal cistern is usually noted and intracerebral hemorrhage in anteroinferior frontal lobe is sometimes associated. In cases of MCA aneurysm, hemorrhage in the ipsilateral sylvian fissure, interhemispheric fissure and ipsilateral basal cistern was usual. Intracerebral hemorrhage in lateral temporal lobe was sometimes associated. Blood in lateral and 4th ventricle and parietooccipital region may indicate a ruptured PCA aneurysm. Isolated intraventricular haemorrhage may be seen in case of ruptured aneurysms in deeper cerebral arteries (4th ventricular haemorrhage with PICA aneurysm).

Imaging evaluation of an aneurysm should include: Site, size, direction, neck, number (bilaterality/multiple) presence of SAH, spasm, stealing phenomenon.

Causes of non-traumatic SAH: Aneurysmal SAH (75– 80%).

Perimesencephalic non-aneurysmal SAH (5%). Rare causes: Infectious arterial vasculitis mycotic, lyme disease, gnathostomiasis; other cerebrovascular diseases: Arterio venous angioma, dural AVF, cerebral amyloid angiopathy. Immune vasculitis: Amyloid angiopathy, cerebral venous thrombosis, moyamoya disease in adults, primary CNS angiitis, polyarteritis nodosa, Behçet's disease, Wegener's vasculitis, Churg–Strauss syndrome, primary and metastatic brain tumors (<2%), eclampsia (<2%).

Approximately 80% of cases of SAH occur in people aged 40–65 years, with 15% occurring in people aged 20–40 years. Only 5% of cases of SAH occur in people younger than 20 years. SAH is rare in children younger than 10 years, accounting for only 0.5% of all cases.

Smoking and arterial hypertension have been associated with aneurysm formation and rupture.

Average ICP in the first 48 hours is an independent predictor of mortality. Signs of raised ICP are:

CT: There is a linear association between the initial CT characteristics and the future ICP. Effacement of the ventricles, basal cisterns and other CSF spaces, brain herniation, loss of grey–white matter differentiation, Midline shift >5 mm

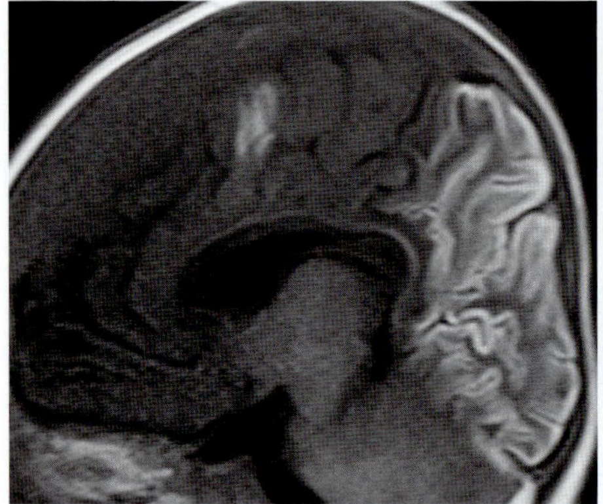
Fig. 4.33.16: Cortical laminar necrosis

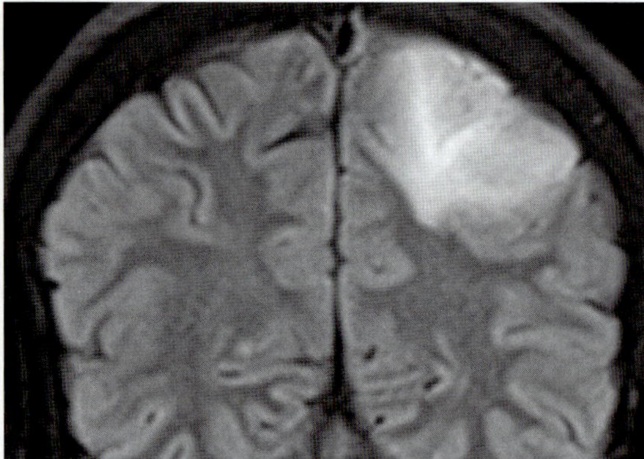
Fig. 4.33.17: Cortical laminar necrosis

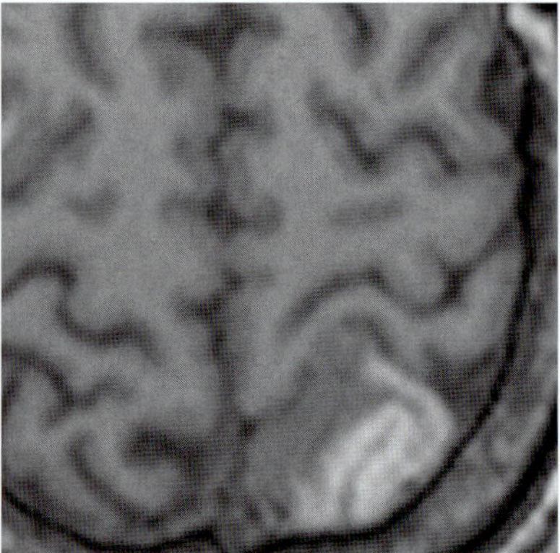
Fig. 4.33.18: Cortical laminar necrosis

Gyriform hyperintensity in T1W seen in cortical laminar necrosis, CJD.

DD for T1 hyperintensity in sulcal spaces—subarachnoid cortical laminar necrosis, meningitis, leptomeningeal carcinomatosis, FLAIR vascular hyperintensities in acute stroke, moyamoya disease, meningeal melanomatosis, meningeal melanocytosis, fat-containing lesions in subarachnoid space, lipoma, ruptured dermoid cyst, Artefactual causes like hyperoxygenation therapy and recent gadolinium administration, lasting ~2–24 hours, if there is any adjacent pathology that involves disruption of the blood–brain barrier, or neovascularization, CSF flow artefact, vascular pulsation artefact, magnetic susceptibility artefact, motion artefact. **Mirror image aneurysm defined as aneurysm developing bilaterally and symmetrically on same named vessels. Neoplastic intracranial/cerebral aneurysms/oncotic aneurysms**—are rare type of intracranial aneurysm attributed to metastatic tumor emboli. Most common cause are cardiac myxoma, choriocarcinoma. **Saccular cerebral aneurysms, known as berry** aneurysms, are intracranial aneurysms with rounded shape. They are vast majority of intracranial aneurysms and are the most common cause of non-traumatic subarachnoid hemorrhage. **Terson syndrome**—occurrence of vitreous hemorrhage of human eye in association with subarachnoid hemorrhage and elevated intracranial pressure.

4.34 CENTRAL NERVOUS SYSTEM

Case No. 34

Clinical history: A 74-year-old man with left sided hemineglect and hemiplegia.

Radiological technique and observations: Figures 4.34.1 to 4.34.4 are **NCCT, longitudinal Doppler ultrasound of the right carotid artery and reformatted CT angiography images respectively.**

NCCT: Axial images of noncontrast CT brain study showing an ill-defined hypodensity involving superior, middle, inferior frontal gyrus, paracentral lobule, precentral, postcentral gyrus and basal ganglia on right side. Area of involvement corresponds to right MCA proximal main stem territory. Surrounding edema causing mass effect on the ipsilateral lateral ventricle and midline shift to the left. No acute intra-axial or extra-axial hemorrhage.

Doppler ultrasonography: Longitudinal sections on Doppler ultrasound showing hypoechoic large soft plaque in proximal in left proximal internal carotid artery causing luminal stenosis.

MR angiography showed a cervical ostial and juxta ostial proximal ICA stenosis of approximately 90% according to NASCET criteria and a distal thrombus occupying most of the ICA diameter.

Interpretation: A—74-year-male, pathology in right proximal main stem MCA territory, Right ICA, B—mass effect, mid-line shift, cerebral edema and loss of gray white matter junction interface, C—hypodensity, no evidence of hemorrhage, right ICA plaque and 90% stenosis on Doppler and MRA (implying possible arterioarterial thromboembolism), D—malignant right MCA territory infarct.

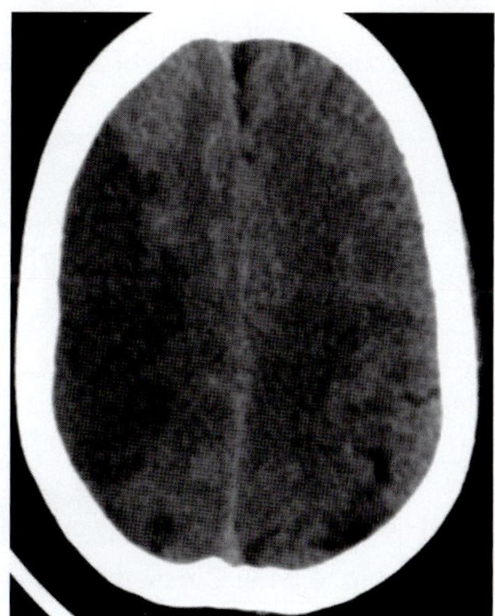

Fig. 4.34.1

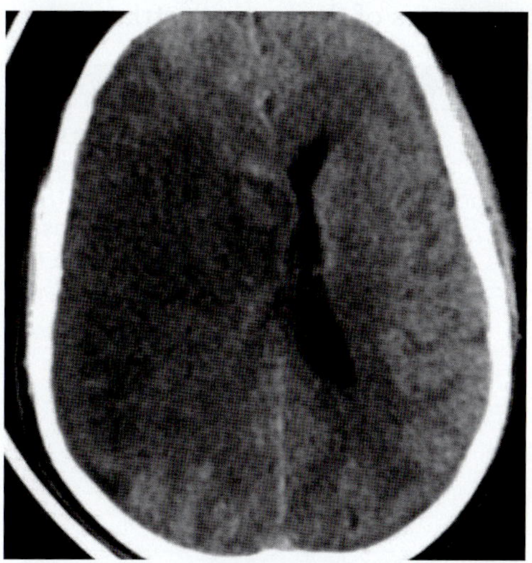

Fig. 4.34.2

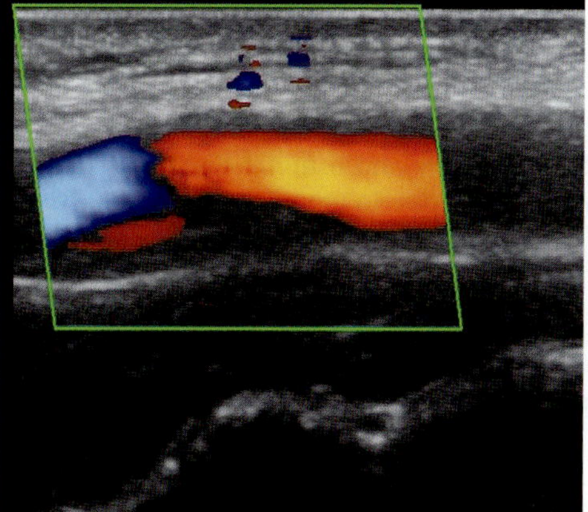

Fig. 4.34.3

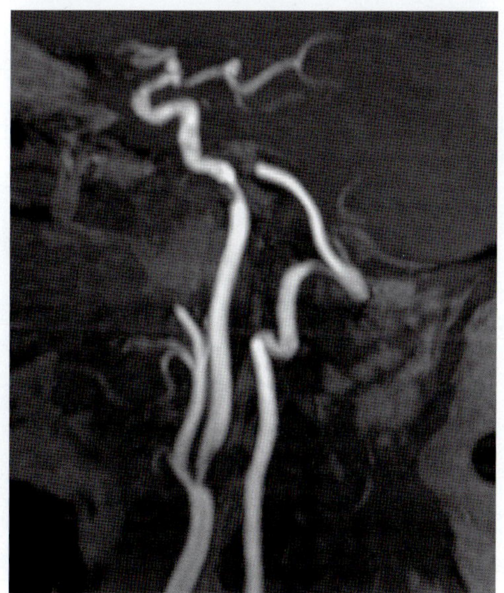

Fig. 4.34.4

Principal diagnosis: Malignant infarct in the territory of the right proximal main stem—middle cerebral artery (MCA) (territories of the lenticulostriate arteries, along with those of the superior and inferior divisions) with right proximal ICA stenosis (ASPECTS score-1).

Table 4.34.1: Stroke mimics and differential diagnosis for stroke

Seizure One-third of stroke mimics are due to seizures or postictal deficits. Sometimes, seizure may cause restricted diffusion	**The distinguishing features are nonvascular distribution, earlier edema and gyral enhancement, normal or elevated perfusion, absence of vascular occlusion,** and simultaneous restricted cortical and elevated subcortical white matter diffusion.	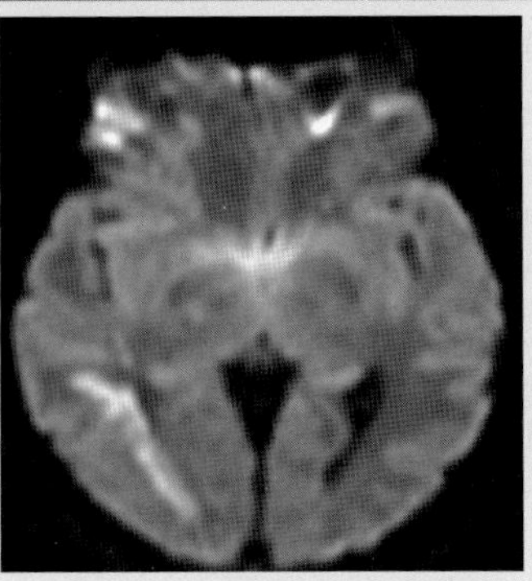 **Fig. 4.34.5:** Seizure
Hemiplegic migraine Migrainous aura and hemiplegic migraine are the causes of 5–10% of stroke mimics and may show restricted diffusion.	**The distinguishing factors are a long history of migraines, involvement of multiple arterial territories and absence of vascular occlusion.** Perfusion decreases in acute-onset aura and is normal or elevated in prolonged episodes. The lesions are usually reversible, but 15% of strokes in patients younger than 45 years of age are due to migraine.	
Hepatic encephalopathy The decrease in ADC values is attributed to the **excitotoxic injury and osmotic disturbance in astrocytes due to ammonia.**	The typical imaging finding in milder cases is symmetric T1 hyperintensity in globus pallidus. In more severe cases, MRI may show T2 hyperintensity and restricted diffusion in the cortex (especially the cingulate gyri and insula), and basal ganglia. The thalami, periventricular white matter and brainstem may also be involved.	
Moyamoya pattern In children, hemispheric ischemic strokes are most pronounced, whereas in adults hemorrhage from the abnormal vessels is more common.	Non-atherosclerotic progressive vasculo-occlusive disease involving the terminal supraclinoid internal carotid arteries and circle of Willis Moyamoya disease affects the bilateral distal ICA and circle of Willis. Up to 18% of patients with moyamoya may present with unilateral angiography-documented disease	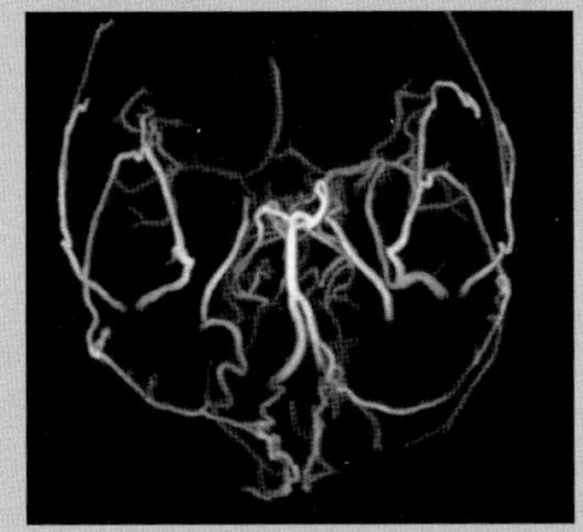 **Fig. 4.34.6:** Suzuki stage 6 moyamoya
Crossed cerebellar diaschisis Depression in function, metabolism, and perfusion affecting a cerebellar hemisphere occurring as a result of a contralateral focal supratentorial lesion (infarct)		
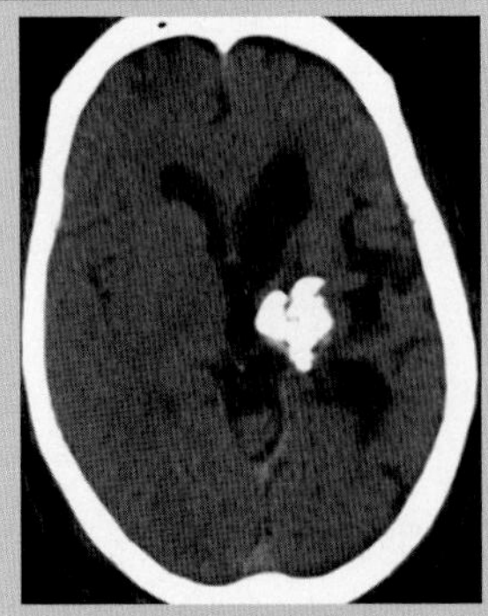 **Fig. 4.34.7:** Crossed cerebellar diaschisis	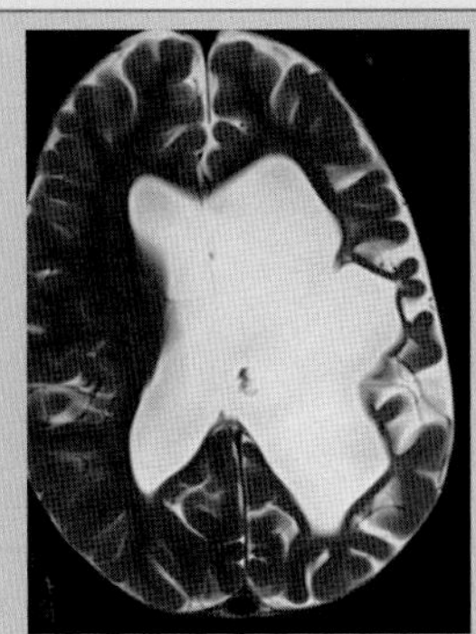 **Fig. 4.34.8:** Crossed cerebellar diaschisis	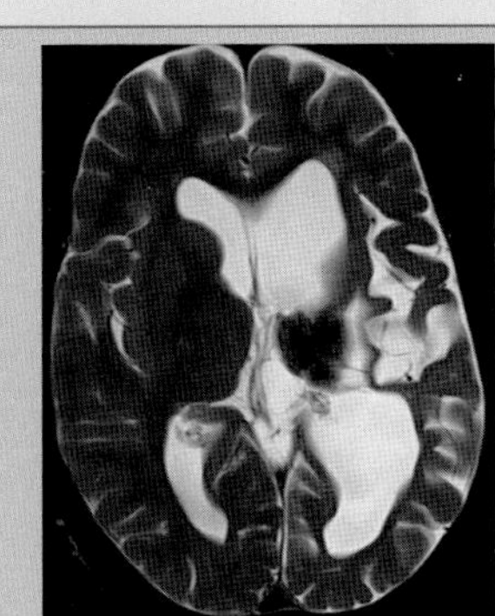 **Fig. 4.34.9:** Crossed cerebellar diaschisis

(Contd.)

Table 4.34.1: Stroke mimics and differential diagnosis for stroke (*Contd.*)

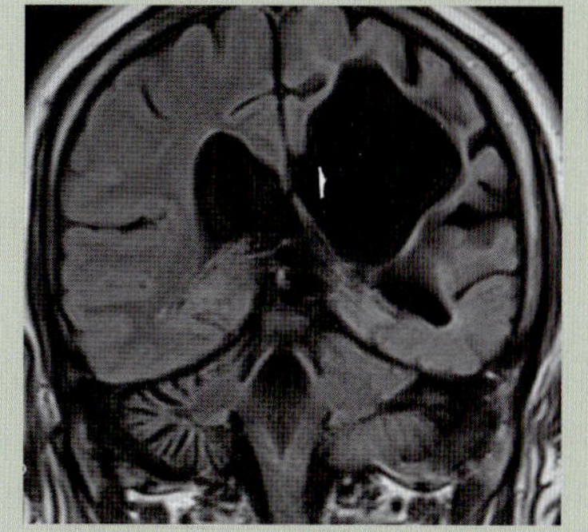 **Fig. 4.34.10:** Crossed cerebellar diaschisis	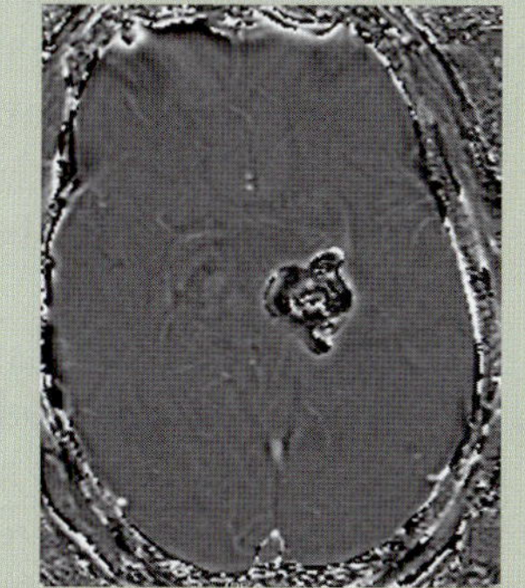 **Fig. 4.34.11:** Crossed cerebellar diaschisis	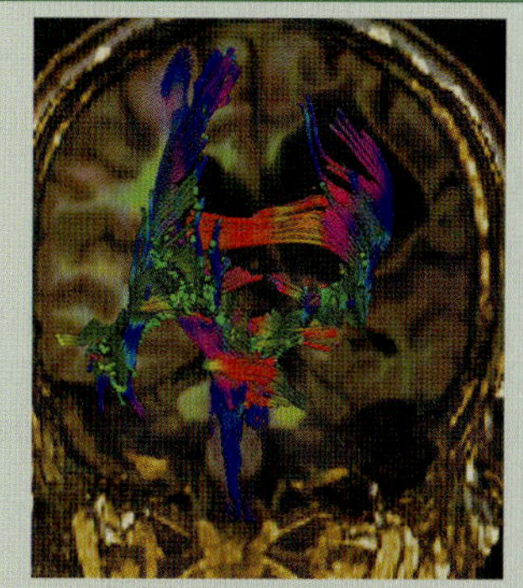 **Fig. 4.34.12:** Crossed cerebellar diaschisis
Wallerian degeneration		
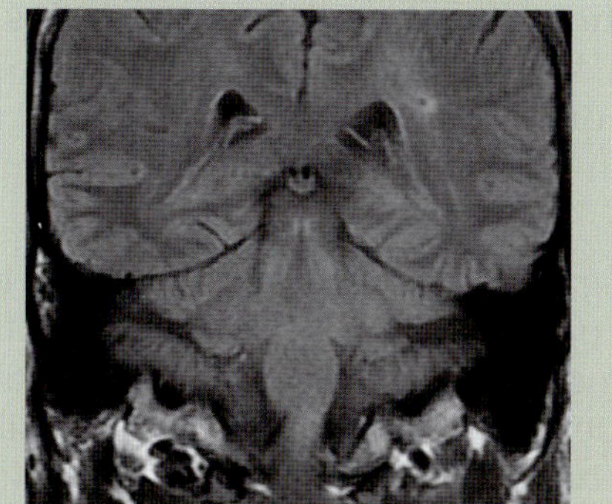 **Fig. 4.34.13:** Wallerian degeneration	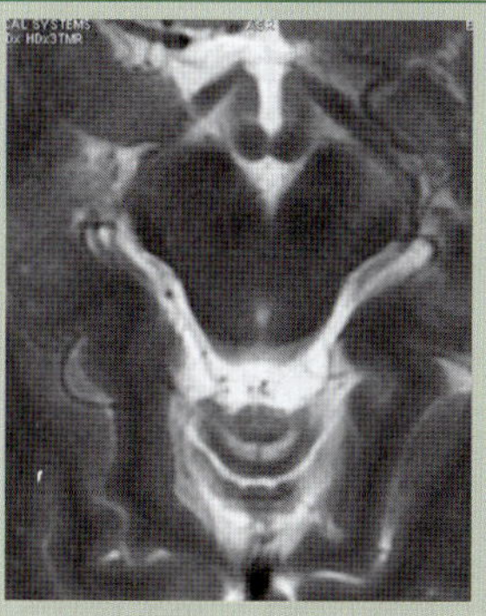 **Fig. 4.34.14:** Wallerian degeneration	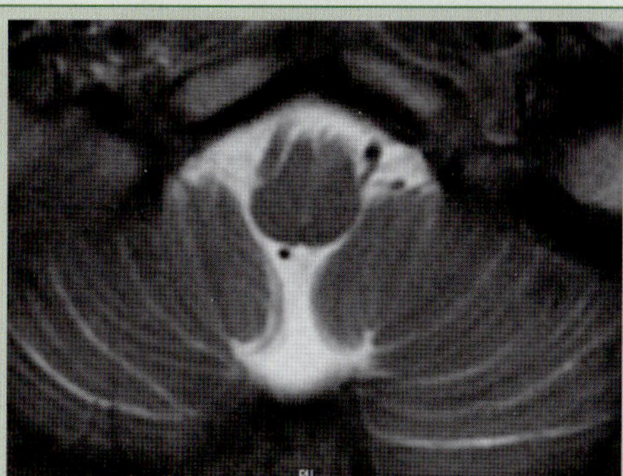 **Fig. 4.34.15:** Wallerian degeneration
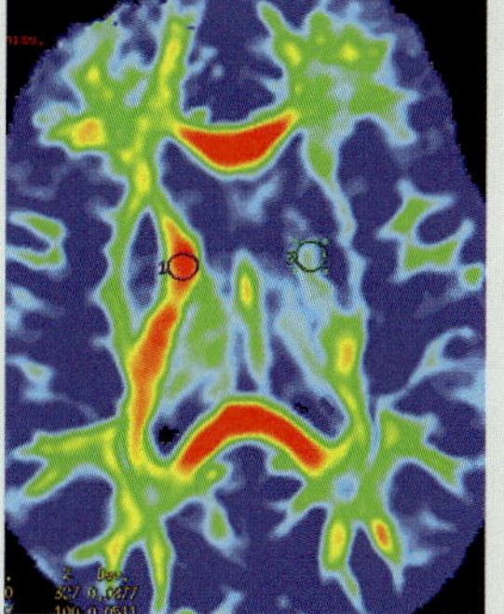 **Fig. 4.34.16:** Wallerian degeneration	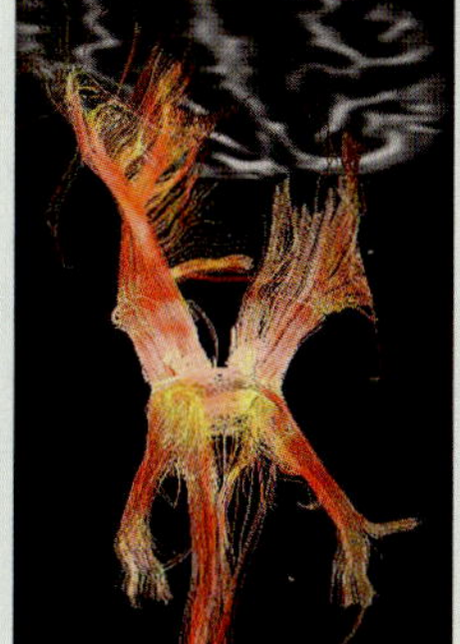 **Fig. 4.34.17:** Wallerian degeneration	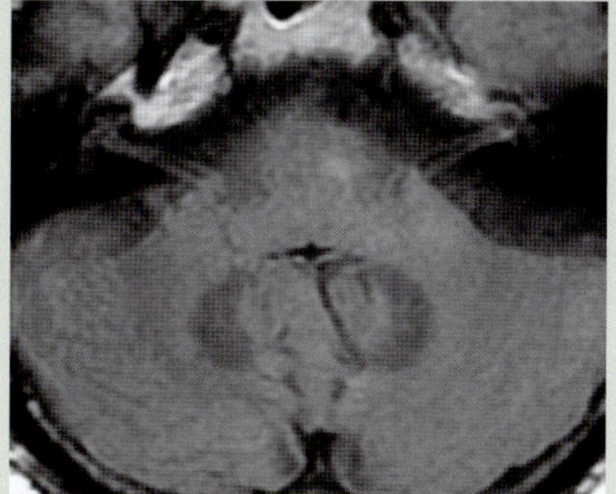 **Fig. 4.34.18:** Wallerian degeneration

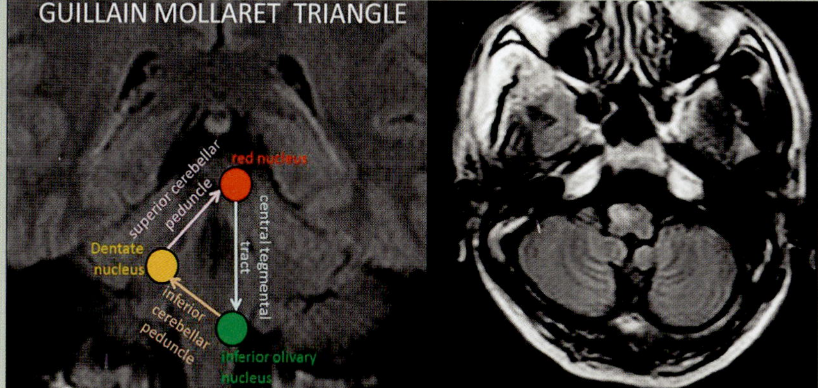

Fig. 4.34.19: Guillain-Mollaret triangle

Management: Stroke established with very low ASPECTS score. Next step of management involves pharmacologic therapy and rehabilitation followed by referral to interventional radiologist for carotid disease management.

CT: **Not to diagnose infarct**

1. To exclude intracranial hemorrhage
2. Identify early signs of ischemic stroke
3. Exclude neoplastic, inflammatory, or other processes that can mimic stroke.
4. To calculate ASPECTS score

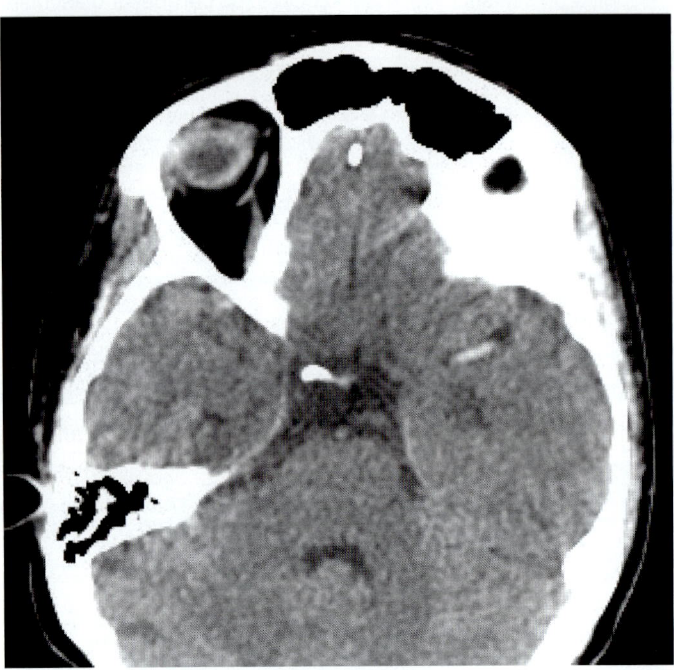

Fig. 4.34.20: Dense MCA sign

Sensitivity 45–88% (mean 55.3%)

Length of clot can again be measured by **CTA. Clot length <12 mm,** is an independent predictor for recanalization rate and good outcome.

When there is no contrast permeation through clot, it is said to be a non-permeable clot without any residual flow.

CTA can also aid in diagnosis of intracranial, extracranial dissection of vertebral and carotid arteries, vasculitis and intracranial atherosclerosis.

However, DSA and biopsy remain gold standard for diagnosing CNS vasculitis. At times it is difficult to differentiate vasculitis from intracranial atherosclerotic disease (ICAD) by CTA or DSA.

3D high-resolution vessel wall imaging helps in differentiating ICAD from vasculitis. The disease activity can be monitored by vessel wall contrast enhancement which helps in deciding the duration of treatment.

CT perfusion imaging: CTP uses the following parameters cerebral blood flow (CBF), cerebral blood volume (CBV) and mean transit time (MTT) to differentiate salvageable ischemic brain tissue (the penumbra) from irreversibly damaged infarcted brain (the infarct core) (Fig. 4.34.21, Table 4.34.2).

1. **Cerebral blood volume (CBV): Volume of blood per unit of brain tissue.** Normal 4–5 ml/100 g. When reduced to <40% of normal, is likely to indicate irreversible cell death. It reflects completed infarct volume on CBV map.
2. **Cerebral blood flow (CBF): Volume of blood flow per unit of brain tissue per minute.** Normal for grey matter = 50–60 ml/100 g/min. When reduced to <20% (16 to 18 ml/100 g/min) normal, is likely to indicate

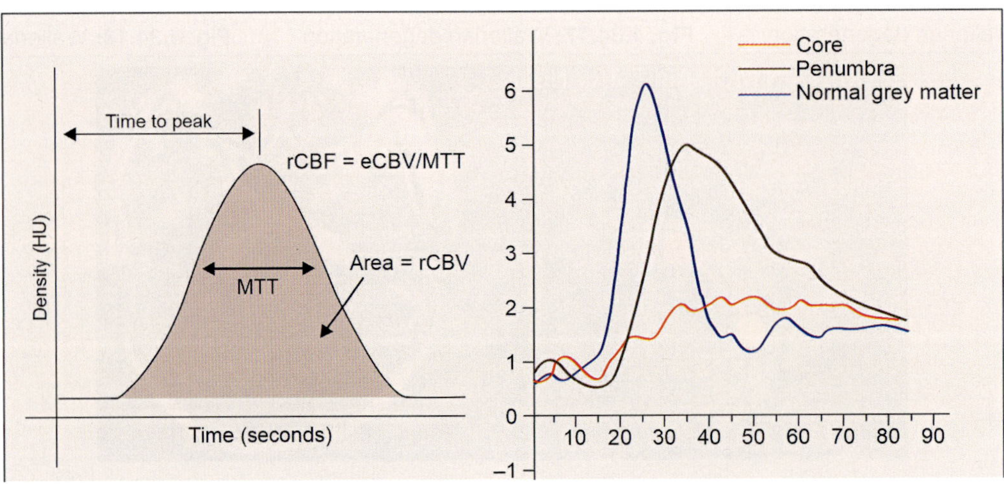

Fig. 4.34.21: CT perfusion curve analysis

Table 4.34.2: CT perfusion parameters

	MTT	*CBV ml/min*	*CBF ml/100 g/min*	*TTP*
Normal	Normal	Normal—4–5 ml/min	Normal—50–60	Normal
Infarct	Increased	Decreased—<40% of normal	Decreased <20% within an hour, <30% after that	Increased
Penumbra	Increased	Increased/ normal	Decreased (12–20 ml/100 g/min)	Increased
Reperfusion (NCCT-hypodensity/loss of G-W differentiation)	Increased	Increased/normal	Increased/normal	Increased
Oligemic tissue	Increased	Moderately reduced (60%)	Normal or slightly reduced (80%)	Increased

irreversible cell death. When area of reduced CBF is larger than area of reduced CBV on respective maps, is likely to indicate ischaemic penumbra or salvageable brain. CBF = CBV/MTT.

3. **Mean transit time (MTT): Time difference between arterial inflow and venous outflow.**
4. **Time to peak enhancement (TTP)**

Perfusion features of penumbra

↑ MTT, ↓ CBF, ↔ CBV (↑)

Perfusion features of infarcted tissue

↑ MTT, ↓ CBF, ↓ CBV

CT perfusion imaging shows increased mean transit time in the right MCA territory (Fig. 4.34.22).

Pitfalls of CT perfusion imaging: Slice selection: Large volume of brain tissue can be excluded (e.g. posterior fossa and brainstem), but more accurate. Chronic white matter changes and old infarcts—especially if severe and asymmetrical (-> look at pre-contrast). Arterial vascular stenosis. Extracranial carotid stenosis, intracranial carotid stenosis or proximal cerebral artery stenosis (-> importance of CT angio). Vasospasm. Seizure mimicking stroke. Increased perfusion of ictal regions, suggesting ischemia in contralateral hemisphere.

MR imaging: During the first week, the infarcted parenchyma continues to demonstrate high DWI signal and low ADC signal, although by the end of the first week ADC values have started to increase. Absence of normally visualised flow void in the affected vessel. The infarct remains hyperintense on T2 and FLAIR, with T2 signal progressively increasing during the first 4 days. T1 signal remains low, although some cortical intrinsic high T1 signal may be seen as early as 3 days after infarction. After day 5 the cortex usually demonstrates contrast enhancement on T1 C+. Less common patterns of enhancement include arterial enhancement, encountered in approximately half of strokes and becomes evident after 3 days, and meningeal enhancement which is uncommon and is usually seen between 2 and 6 days.

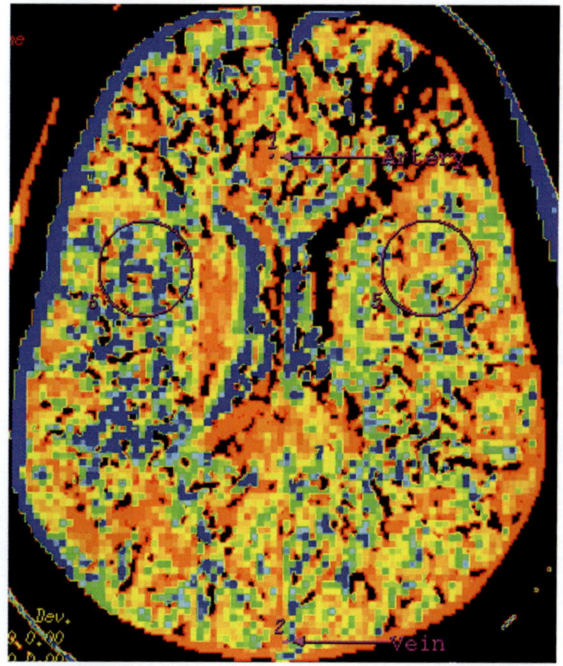

Fig. 4.34.22: CT perfusion post-processed image

Subacute phase: **T2 shortening—"fogging effect". Chronic phase:** Encephalomalacia develops and is seen as a focal area of altered signal associated with loss of volume.

MR perfusion techniques(pMR): Endogenous spin arterial labelling, Exogenous tracer-commonly used; Signal loss due to T2* shortening. Restriction on DWI reflects the densely ischemic core of the infarct, whereas **pMR depicts the surrounding—'at risk' penumbra. A DWI-PWI mismatch is one of the criteria used in determining suitability for intra-arterial thrombolysis** (Table 4.34.5).

Angiography to determine collaterals. The extent of collateral flow does not only predict final infarct volume and functional outcome, but is also associated with recanalization/reperfusion rates both in IV-tPA and endovascular treatment. In addition, it may help to

Table 4.34.3: Difference between MR perfusion and CT perfusion	
MR perfusion	*CT perfusion*
It diagnoses infarct in hyperacute stage. DWI-pMR mismatch used for identifying ischemic penumbra in hyperacute stage itself	Better availability, quick study (10 minutes); it excludes hemorrhage and aids quick planning of treatment strategy. It aids exact quantification of ischemic core and penumbra.
CT perfusion is more useful than MR perfusion in acute stroke imaging	

identify patients who benefit from recanalizing treatment beyond the current time window for intravenous and intra-arterial treatment.

4 Ps of Stroke Imaging

Parenchyma: Assess early signs of acute stroke, initial CT to rule out hemorrhage, less than 1/3rd involvement?

Pipes: Assess circulation (carotids and vertebral arteries of the neck and intracranial circulation for evidence of intravascular thrombus.)

Perfusion: Assess cerebral blood volume, cerebral blood flow and mean transit time.

Penumbra: Assess tissue at risk of dying if ischemia continues without recanalization of thrombus.

Thrombolysis and thrombectomy if no hemorrhage, involvement of <1/3rd MCA territory, ASPECTS score >7 and Penumbra >20% infarct.

Intima–media thickness measured between the two parallel lines produced between the Lumen–intima interface and the intima–media interface. **Normally measures less than 0.9 mm.**

Sonographic NASCET (The North American Symptomatic Carotid Endarterectomy Trial) Index

This study proposed the incorporation of distal ICA flow velocity on the conventional carotid Doppler study improving the diagnostic accuracy of PSV.

- **<15% stenosis** deceleration spectral broadening with a peak systolic velocity (PSV) <125 cm/s.
- **16–49% stenosis:** Pansystolic spectral broadening with a PSV <125 cm/s.
- **50–69% stenosis** a systolic spectral broadening with a PSV of >125 cm/s and end diastolic velocity (EDV) <110 cm/s or ICA/CCA PSV ratio >2 but <4.
- **70–79% stenosis**—pansystolic spectral broadening with PSV >270 cm/s or EDV >110 cm/s or ICA/CCA PSV ratio >4.

Table 4.34.4: Role of DTI in stroke		
Diffusion tensor imaging can be used to predict motor recovery, as patients with preserved tracts on DTI at the time of lesion have shown greater recovery than their counterparts with compromised tracts	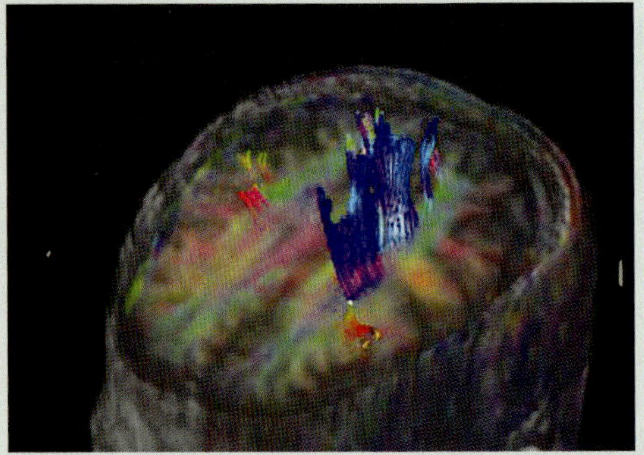 **Fig. 4.34.23:** DTI postprocessing image	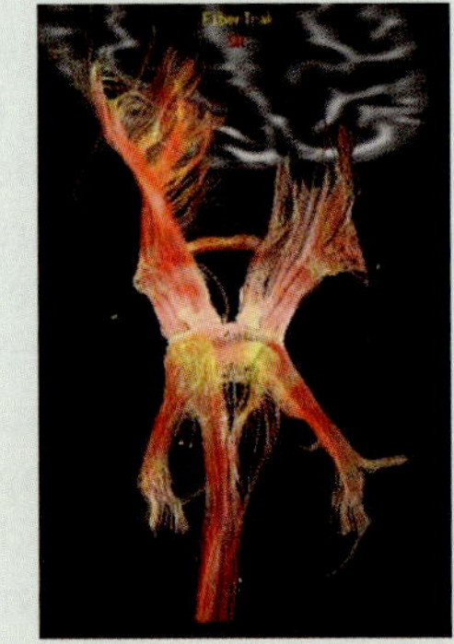 **Fig. 4.34.24:** DTI tractography shows destruction of left corticospinal tract due to infarct

Table 4.34.5: Using MR perfusion in stroke
PWI-DWI disconcordance:
Type 1: PWI >>> DWI—Ischemic penumbra present, Greater efficacy of thrombolytic treatment.
Type 2: PWI = DWI—No tissue to salvage, no use of thrombolysis.
Type 3: PWI <<< DWI—No tissue to salvage, no use of thrombolysis.
Type 4: Isolated DWI—Indicates reperfusion, initial thrombus has been lysed.
Type 5: Isolated PWI—Represents tissue at risk, TIA may progress to infarct; immediate pharmacological interventions and carotid evaluation indicated.
Type 6: Normal PWI and DWI.

- **80–99% stenosis:** EDV >140 cm/s.
- **Complete occlusion:** No flow; terminal thump.

One may also use the **society of radiologists in ultrasound (SRU) consensus,** which adds the grey scale finding of a plaque and thickening of the carotid intima to the criteria.

Methodology of plaque characterization:

Location (CCA and /ICA)

Extent (length)

Severity (thickness—in transverse view and degree of luminal narrowing in conjunction with pulsed Doppler velocity criteria)

Texture (degree of sonolucency within the plaque)

Table 4.34.6: International plaque classification

Plaque Classification (International)	
Type I	Uniformly sonolucent
Type II	Predominantly sonolucent (>50%)
Type III	Predominantly echogenic (>50%)
Type IV	Uniformly echogenic
Type V	Unclassified due to poor visualization, calcifications causing inadequate visualization

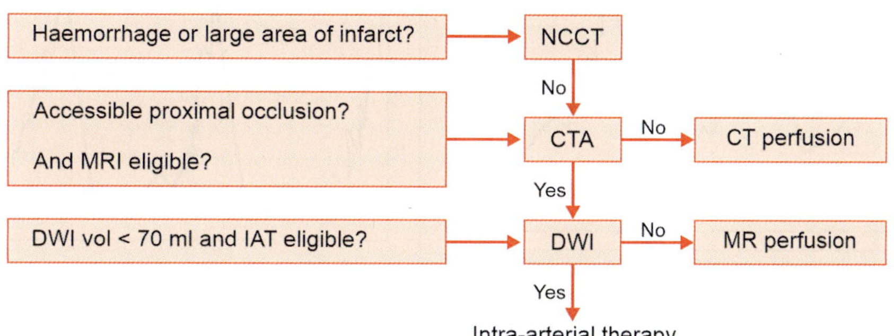

Fig. 4.34.25: Stroke imaging protocol

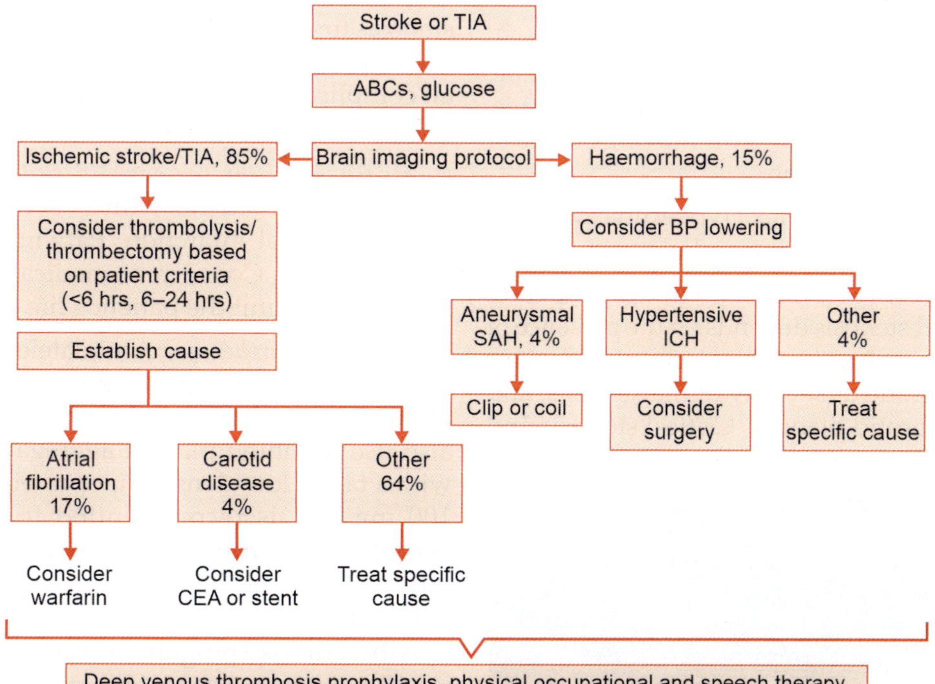

Fig. 4.34.26: Algorithm for stroke and TIA management

4

Table 4.34.7: Doppler evaluation and management of carotid artery disease	
Internal carotid artery	*External carotid artery*
Located more superficially and laterally on a posterolateral imaging approach.	Located deeper, medially on a posterolateral imaging approach.
Larger in diameter.	Smaller in diameter.
Proceeds posteriorly towards the mastoid.	Proceeds anteriorly towards the face.
No cervical branches.	Branches visualized.
No/slight oscillations on Doppler tracing with temporal tap maneuver.	Oscillations on Doppler tracing with temporal tap maneuver.
Mean PSV 100–150 cm/s.	Mean PSV 70–80 cm/s.
Low resistance Doppler flow, low pulsatile, broad peak with relatively more diastolic flow	High resistance Doppler flow, high pulsatile, sharp peak with relatively lesser diastolic flow

Plaques type 1 and 2 tend to be **unstable** and subject to abrupt increase in size following hemorrhage or embolization. **Plaques type 3 and 4** are generally composed of fibrous tissue and calcification—**benign, stable** (Table 4.34.6).

Features of ulcerated plaque: Focal depression/break in the plaque that causes an irregular surface/anechoic area within the plaque that extends to the plaque surface. Color Doppler may demonstrate slow moving eddies of color within the anechoic region.

Appearance of vulnerable plaque: Hypoechoic, without calcification, presence of fissuring and ulceration.

Management of carotid disease: The appropriate treatment for carotid stenosis depends on the presence of ongoing symptoms such as transient ischemic attack or small infarcts, the grade or severity of the stenosis, and the complexity of carotid plaques. Critical stenosis and complex plaques with suspected hemorrhage are often treated in an urgent or emergent manner. The traditional surgical treatment has been carotid endarterectomy, but endovascular repair by carotid stenting has also been applied. In cases of bilateral stenosis, carotid stenting is generally performed within the most symptomatic stenosis first. Simultaneous bilateral carotid stenting has been reported to be feasible with acceptable risks. The overall complication rate for carotid artery stenting in high-risk patients has been reported to be approximately 8%.

Fig. 4.34.27: Thick intima of ICA with hypoechoic plaque

Contraindications for carotid endarterectomy include the following: Patients with a severe neurologic deficit after a cerebral infarction. Patients with an occluded carotid artery. Concurrent medical illness that would significantly limit the patient's life expectancy.

Pharmacologic therapy: Antiplatelet therapy (cilostazol) may reduce the progression of carotid artery stenosis after stent implantation. Aspirin and Ticlopidine are also use to inhibit platelet aggregation. Statin therapy, with a target low-density lipoprotein (LDL) level below 100 mg/dL, is recommended for all patients with extracranial carotid atherosclerotic disease. A lower target LDL level, 70 mg/dL, is recommended in high-risk patients.

Alberta stroke programme early CT score (ASPECTS) is a 10-point quantitative topographic CT scan score used in hyperacute middle cerebral artery (MCA) stroke, **scored at the ganglionic and supraganglionic level.**

ASPECTS of 10 points is given to a normal CT with no early ischemic changes (EIC). One point is subtracted from 10 for any evidence of EIC for each of the below defined regions. Low ASPECTS <7 is associated with poor clinical outcome and increased risk for ICH following IV tPA.

Less than 3 hours: For eligible patients with acute ischemic stroke causing a potentially disabling neurologic deficit, **we recommend intravenous alteplase therapy when treatment is initiated within 3 hours of clearly defined symptom onset.**

3–4.5 hours: Intravenous alteplase therapy if treatment is initiated within 3 to 4.5 hours of clearly defined symptom onset. Patients in this time window should also be evaluated to determine if they are candidates for mechanical thrombectomy.

4.5 to 6 hours: **Patients within 4.5 to 6 hours from stroke symptom onset should not receive intravenous alteplase because harm may exceed benefit, but they should be evaluated to determine if they are candidates for mechanical thrombectomy.**

6 to 24 hours: Patients beyond 6 hours from ischemic stroke symptom onset are not eligible for treatment with intravenous alteplase. However, mechanical thrombectomy is an option at specialized stroke centers using imaging-based selection of patients, with anterior circulation stroke who have were last known to be normal or at neurologic baseline 6 to 24 hours before treatment.

Golden hour of stroke is first 60 minutes after the onset of symptoms.

Intra-arterial vs intravenous thrombolysis: Reperfusion can be attained by intravenous thrombolysis (IVT) or by intra-arterial thrombolysis (IAT). It is recommended that **IVT be given as first-line therapy for acute ischemic stroke within 4.5 hours of the onset of symptoms;** however, approximately 50% of patients treated with IVT do not recover and die. In addition, although **overall recanalization rates are approximately 40–50%, those of IVT are low when the occlusion is in a large artery.**

Intra-arterial thrombolysis has greater recanalization rates, customized locoregional therapy with angiographic planning. Disadvantage is delay in time to treatment.

Mechanical revascularization of clot: Clot disruption, clot removal.

Distal techniques: Retrieval devices are Goose neck snare, alligator, MERCI (mechanical embolus removal in cerebral ischemia), stent-like retrievers.

Table 4.34.8: Doppler assessment in stenotic plaques

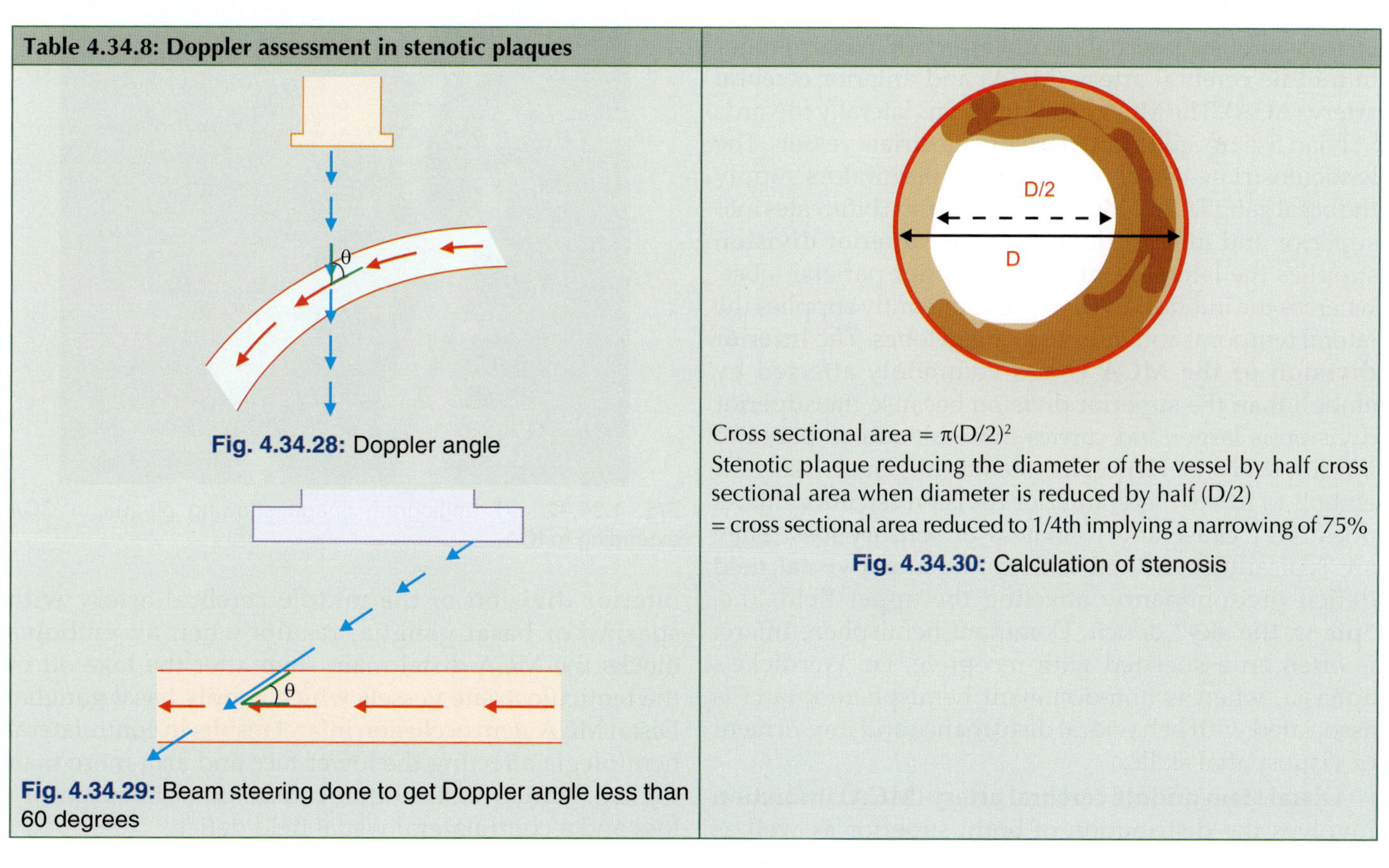

Fig. 4.34.28: Doppler angle

Fig. 4.34.29: Beam steering done to get Doppler angle less than 60 degrees

Cross sectional area = $\pi(D/2)^2$

Stenotic plaque reducing the diameter of the vessel by half cross sectional area when diameter is reduced by half (D/2)

= cross sectional area reduced to 1/4th implying a narrowing of 75%

Fig. 4.34.30: Calculation of stenosis

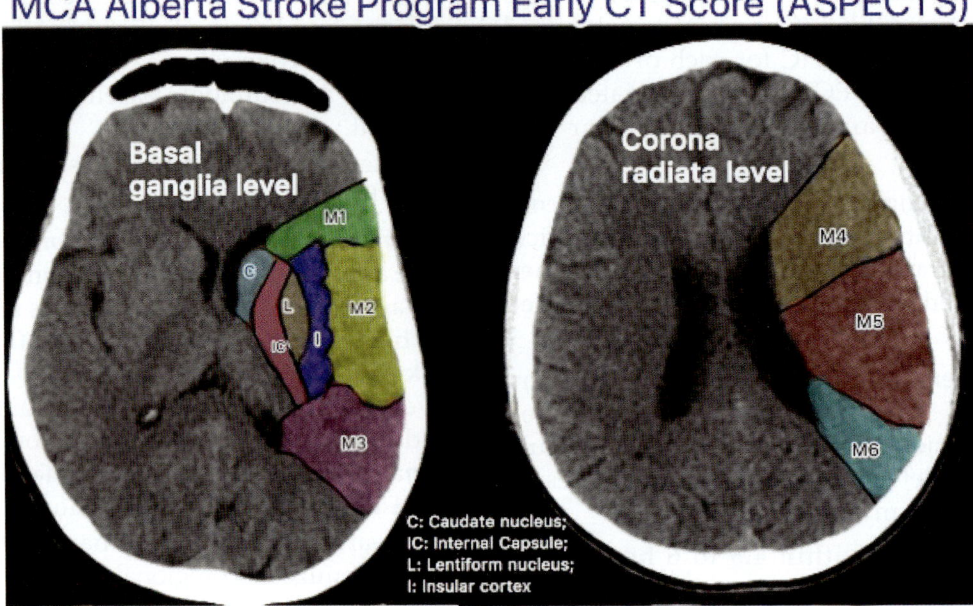

Fig. 4.34.31: ASPECTS

Proximal techniques are clot aspiration using large lumen microcatheters, thrombaspiration system: AngioJet.

Proximal techniques have low efficacy but have lesser risk of fragmentation.

Discussion: The internal carotid artery (ICA) terminates in middle cerebral artery (MCA) and anterior cerebral artery (ACA). The MCA main stem runs laterally towards Sylvian fissure, giving off the lenticulostriate vessels. The lenticulostriate vessels are the small perforators supply the basal ganglia. The MCA main stem then bifurcates into superior and inferior divisions. **The superior division** supplies the lateral frontal and superior parietal lobes, whereas the inferior division predominantly supplies the lateral temporal and inferior parietal lobes. The **inferior division of the MCA** is less commonly affected by emboli than the superior division because the superior division is larger and carries more blood compared to inferior division. Hence, it is statistically more likely for emboli to travel there. Inferior division territory infarct does NOT cause any weakness or sensory loss. They are typically associated with contralateral visual field deficit predominantly affecting the upper fields, i.e. **"pie in the sky"** deficit. Dominant hemisphere infarct is often an associated with receptive, i.e. Wernicke's aphasia, whereas non-dominant hemisphere infarct is associated with behavioral disturbance and impairment of visuospatial skills.

Distal stem middle cerebral artery (MCA) infarction involves the distribution of both, superior as well as

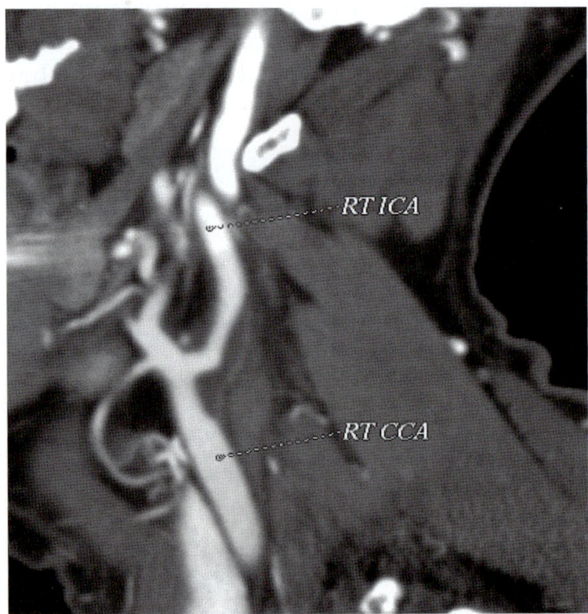

Fig. 4.34.32: CT angiogram image showing plaque in CCA extending to ICA

inferior division of the middle cerebral artery with sparing of basal ganglia, results when an embolus blocks the MCA distal main stem after the take-off of the lenticulostriate vessels which supply basal ganglia. Distal MCA stem occlusion infarct results in contralateral hemiplegia affecting the lower face and arm more than the leg, similar distribution contralateral hemisensory loss and a contralateral visual field deficit.

The earliest finding of MCA occlusion is early parenchymal signs which include blurring, decreased attenuation and swelling of the grey–white matter junction of affected regions. In proximal main stem occlusion, Lentiform nucleus and caudate nucleus appear hypodense/isodense in 70–75% of patients at 3 hours **(vanishing basal ganglia). Insular ribbon sign:** Loss of normal grey–white differentiation at the insular cortex. **Hyperdense middle cerebral artery sign (HAS):** Seen immediately and represents direct visualization of the thromboembolism. Presence of calcification is important as it is a contraindication to angioplasty (Fig. 4.34.20).

Rich red clots have a higher Hounsfield unit (45 to 70 HU) than platelet rich white clots (around 20 HU). Red clots presenting as HAS in NCCT are more likely to recanalize with IV tPA. HAS length >8 mm is associated with poor clinical outcome (less than 1%).

However, false positive HAS can occur due to high hematocrit (polycythemia), dehydration and calcified atherosclerosis.

Table 4.34.9: Difference between stroke and tumor

Stroke	*Tumor*
Sudden onset Grey and white matter involved Wedge shaped Typical distribution	Gradual onset Preferentially involves white matter Round/infiltrating Not confined to any vascular territory

Stroke in the young: Dissections involving the carotid or vertebral arteries alone cause about 15–20% of ischemic stroke in young people (Debette and Leys, 2009). Other causes seen relatively often among young patients but rarely among elderly patients are Fabry disease, systemic vasculitides, Migrainous infarction, primary angiitis (vasculitis) of the central nervous system, Systemic lupus erythematosus, primary antiphospholipid syndrome, eclampsia, sickle cell disease, genetic thrombophilic diseases (protein C, protein S, and antithrombin III deficiency; Factor V Leiden and prothrombin

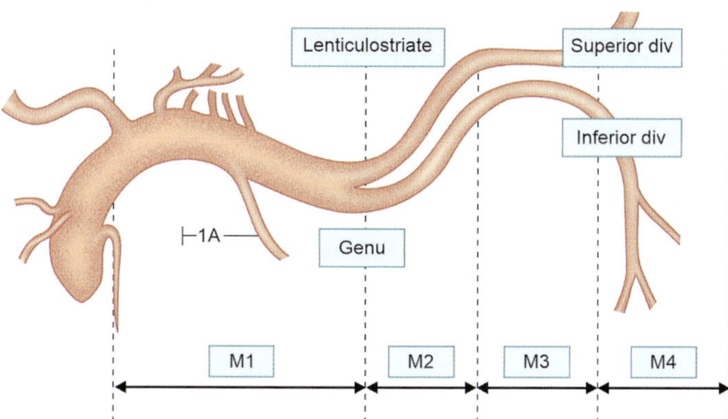

Fig. 4.34.33: Normal MCA branches illustration

Table 4.34.10: Causes of ischemic stroke

Common causes	*Uncommon causes*
Thrombosis Lacunar Large vessel Dehydration	Hypercoagulable disorders (Protein C/Protein S deficiency, anti-thrombin III deficiency, antiphospholipid syndrome Factor V Leiden mutation, SLE, sickle cell anemia)
Thromboembolism Artery to artery Carotid bifurcation Aortic arch Arterial dissection Cardiac emboli	Venous sinus thrombosis Vasculitis SAH-induced vasospasm Non-inflammatory Vasculopathy (reversible vasoconstriction syndrome, Fabry's disease)
Paradoxical embolism	Moya Moya disease
Stimulant drugs—amphetamine, cocaine	Eclampsia

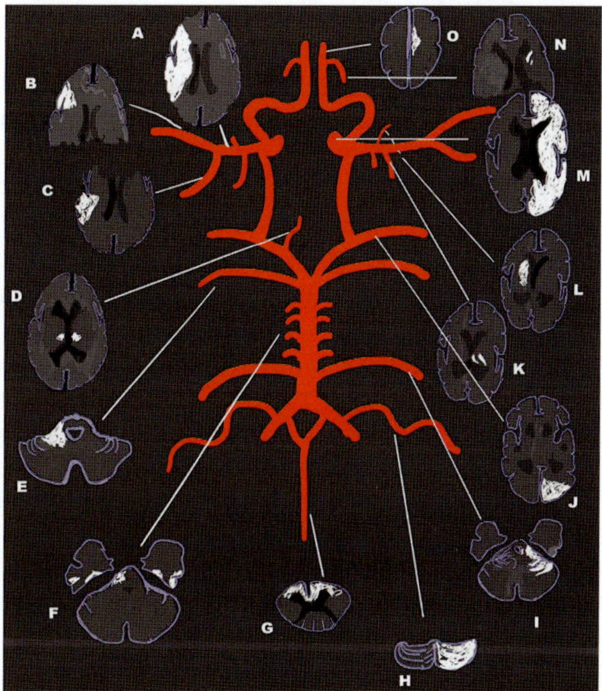

Fig. 4.34.34: Arterial stroke territories: A—main stem middle cerebral artery, B and C—insular segments of MCA, D—thalamogeniculate artery branch of p2 segment of PCA, E—superior cerebellar artery, F—basilar perforating arteries, G—anterior spinal artery, H—posterior inferior cerebellar artery, I—anterior inferior cerebellar artery, J—posterior cerebral artery, K and L—lenticulostriate branches, M—intra cavernosal part of ICA, N—recurrent artery of heubner, O—anterior cerebral artery

4

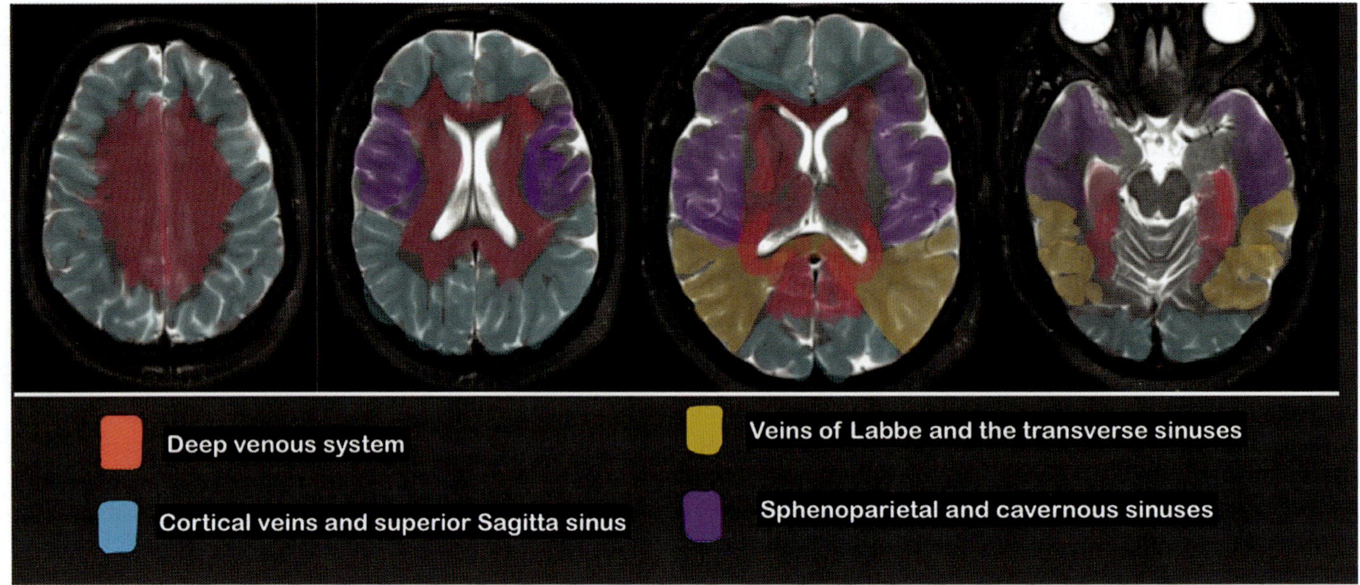

Fig. 4.34.35: Venous infarcts

gene mutations), Sneddon's syndrome, moyamoya disease or syndrome, CADASIL (cerebral autosomal—dominant arteriopathy with subcortical infarcts and leukoencephalopathy) RCVS.

Malignant MCA infarction, a term which is used to describe the rapid aggravation of neurological symptoms following an MCA infarction that are attributed to space-occupying vasogenic edema and/or hemorrhagic transformation with consecutive raised intracranial pressure. Malignant infarction has, if left untreated, a very high mortality due to compression of vital brain structures.

MRI protocol for stroke: **A good protocol involves at least:**

1. **Sagittal T1 weighted sequence: Fast-spin echo (T1 FSE) or gradient (e.g. T1 MPRAGE) purpose:** An anatomical evaluation. Cortical laminar necrosis or pseudolaminar necrosis may be seen as a ribbon of intrinsic high T1 signal, usually after 2 weeks (although it can be seen earlier).
2. **Axial T2 weighted, sequence:** T2 FSE purpose: Loss of normal signal void in large arteries may be visible immediately after 6–12 hours infarcted tissue becomes high signal. sulcal effacement and mass effect develop and become maximal in the first few days.
3. **Axial FLAIR purpose:** After 6–12 hours infarcted tissue becomes high signal, sulcal effacement and mass effect develop and become maximal in the first few days.

Axial diffusion-weighted imaging (DWI), sequence: DWI: B = 0, B = 1000 and ADC.

Axial susceptibility-weighted imaging (SWI): Highly sensitive in the detection of hemorrhage.

MR angiography (MRA), plane: Axial with reconstructions, sequence: time of flight angiography purpose: Assess for luminal diameter and occlusions.

Quick stroke protocol consists of **diffusion-weighted imaging (DWI), FLAIR and TOF to image circle of Willis. Plane:** Axial, total duration 6 to 7 minutes. Purpose: Early identification of ischemic stroke: Diffusion restriction may be seen within minutes following the onset of ischemia, DWI-FLAIR mismatch helps in estimation of infarct core correlates well with infarct core, differentiation of acute from chronic stroke.

4.35 CENTRAL NERVOUS SYSTEM

Case No. 35

Clinical history: A 56-year-old male, with history of headache for 4 months.

Radiological techniques and observation: Figures 4.35.1–4.35.4 are limited axial sections T2 axial, MR venography, T1 sagittal MR images and time of flight MR angiography respectively showing multiple linear flow voids noted within the cerebral and cerebellar hemispheres. On MRV, there is partial recanalization of chronic thrombus noted in the right transverse sinus and the anterior one-third of superior sagittal sinus. Multiple intracranial vessels communicating with prominent extracranial vessels noted. Prominent superficial temporal arteries noted, giving trans osseous branches. No evidence of nidus.

On T1 sagittal, there is sagging of the pons and midbrain with obliteration of the pontomedullary angle and the mamillopontine distance (suggestive of intracranial hypotension).

Interpretation: A—56-years-old male, pathology in the right transverse sinus and anterior one-third of superior sagittal sinus, C—partial recanalization of chronic thrombus in right transverse sinus and anterior third of superior sagittal sinus, multiple communicating vessels signify communication between the dural vessels and the vessels of the scalp with features of intracranial hypotension. B—no evidence of any nidus within the brain parenchyma. There is no evidence of any altered parenchymal signal, D—dural AV fistula.

Principal diagnosis: Dural AV fistula.

The possible differential diagnosis includes:

1. Dural AV fistula
2. Acute/chronic dural venous sinus thrombosis
3. Dural sinus stenosis
4. Pial arteriovenous malformation or other vascular malformations.

Dural AVFs are abnormal connections between arteries which normally supply the meninges, bone, or muscles, and small venules within the dura mater. Classified to group them into those with and those without cortical venous reflux. The latter are benign fistulas (Borden type 1) that never lead to neurologic deficits, whereas the former is regarded as malignant fistulas (Borden types 2 and 3). The presence of cortical venous drainage (CVD) puts a dAVF into a higher risk category. Malignant dural AVFs have an aggressive clinical course, including intracranial hemorrhage, seizure, dementia, altered consciousness, and focal nonhemorrhagic neurologic symptoms due to venous congestion or rupture of the venous pouches. Dural AVFs with cortical venous reflux will manifest with abnormal vessels which are present outside the brain parenchyma and should be differentiated from other vascular shunts.

CT—CT findings vary from none to striking. Hemorrhage is uncommon in the absence of cortical venous drainage or dysplastic venous dilatation. An enlarged dural sinus or draining vein can sometimes be identified on NECT scans. Time-resolved (4D) CTA acquires consecutive volumetric scans and can demonstrate flow dynamics in vascular malformations. **MR**—the presence of dilated cortical veins without an identifiable nidus adjacent to normal appearing brain may suggest the presence of a dAVF. The most common finding of a dAVF itself is a thrombosed dural venous sinus containing vascular-appearing "flow voids". DSA is "gold standard" in evaluating AVFs. Complete visualization of all carotid and vertebral branches, in combination with selective catheterization of dural and transosseous feeders, is usually required to identify all arterial feeders, define the fistula site, delineate venous drainage, and identify pedicle aneurysms.

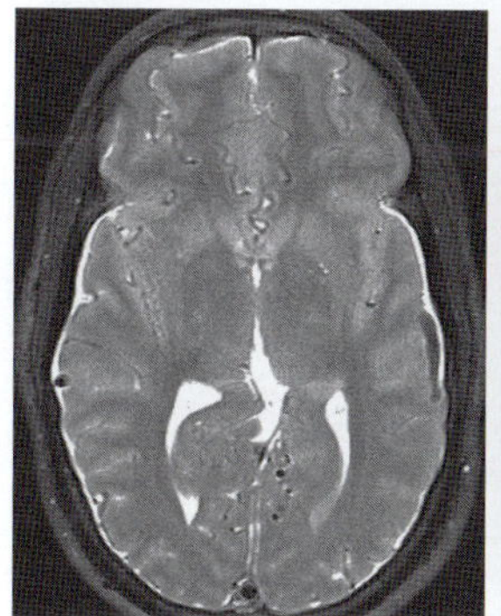
Fig. 4.35.1

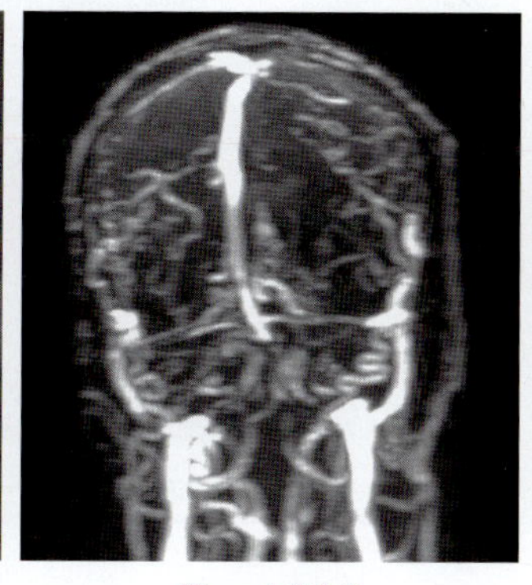
Fig. 4.35.2

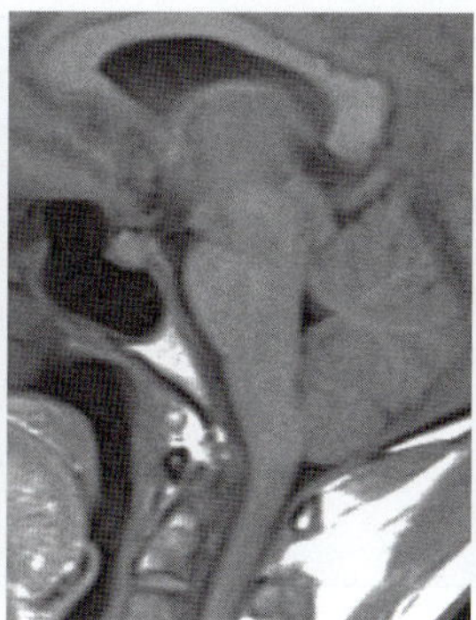
Fig. 4.35.3

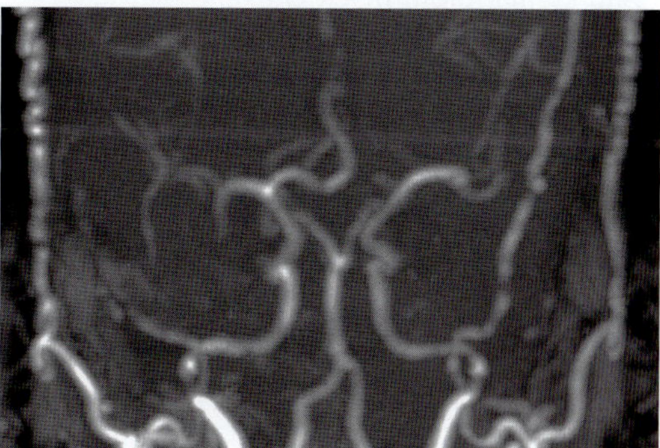
Fig. 4.35.4

Table 4.35.1: Classification of cerebrovascular malformations		
CVMs with arteriovenous shunts		
AV malformations 85% are supratentorial. Almost all are sporadic and solitary. Most are congenital and peak age of presentation occurs between 20–40 years. Most common presentation is headache associated with parenchymal haemorrhage. Seizure and focal neurological deficits also possible.	Bag of worms/flow voids on MR with nidus. NECT—numerous serpentine vessels with a little or no mass effect. Calcification is common. MRI—honeycomb of flow voids with gliotic T2 hyperintense brain parenchyma.	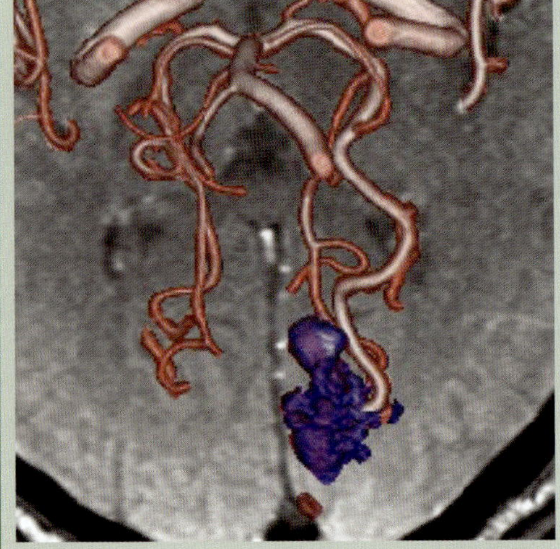 **Fig. 4.35.5:** AV malformation in left occipital lobe
Dural AV Fistula Acquired due to hypoperfusion in a thrombosed dural venous sinus. Peak age is 40–60 years. Uncomplicated lesions present with bruit or tinnitus, whereas lesions with cortical venous drainage cause seizures, dementia, ICH.	Enlarged meningeal arteries with network of tiny vessels in wall of thrombosed dural venous sinus. Thrombus is typically isointense and blooms on T2* sequences.	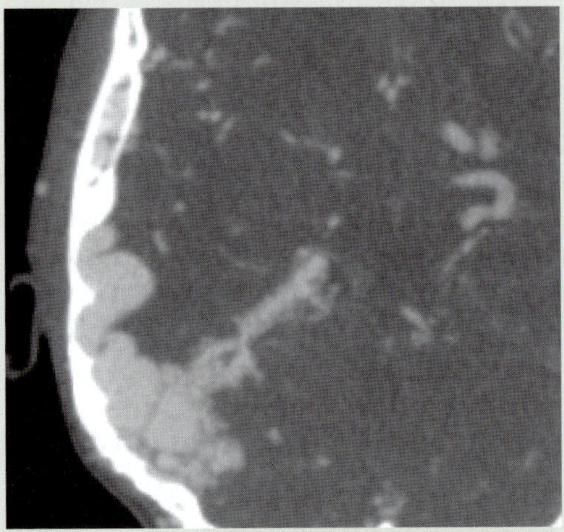 **Fig. 4.35.6:** Dural AV fistula
Vein of Galen malformation Most common extracardiac cause of high output cardiac failure in newborn. There is a male predominance. There may be a loud cranial bruit, macrocrania, hydrocephalus.	A large rounded venous pouch drains into a persistent falcine sinus or straight sinus. CT—enlarged hyperdense mass at tentorial apex. MRI—flow voids with thrombus.	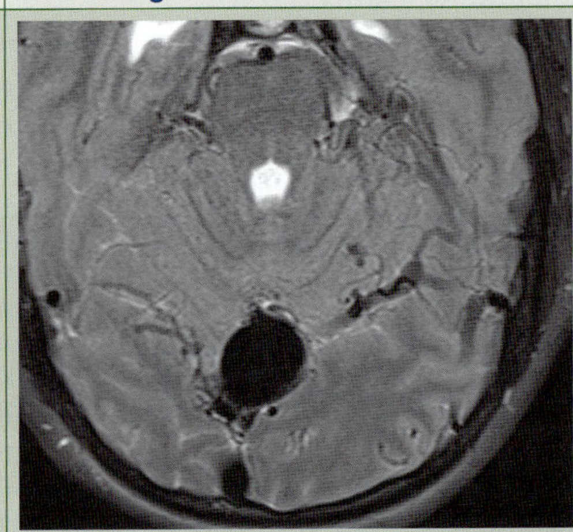 **Fig. 4.35.7:** Vein of Galen malformation

Contd...

Table 4.35.1: Classification of cerebrovascular malformations *(Contd...)*		
CVMs without arteriovenous shunts		
Developmental venous anomaly/ angioma Majority are asymptomatic incidental findings. Mostly solitary, but multiple DVAs are associated with blue rubber bleb nevus syndrome. No age or sex prediction.	DVAs are composed of radially arranged medullary veins that converge on a transcortical or subependymal large collector vein. Classical appearance—medusa head / upside down umbrella.	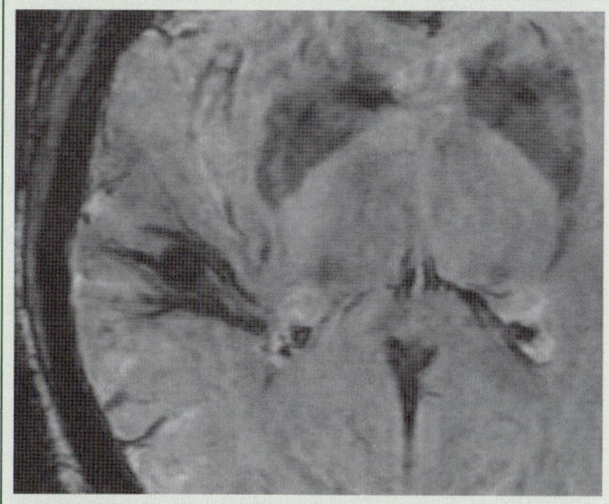 **Fig. 4.35.8:** Developmental venous anomaly
Sinus pericrania–Refer to case 5		
Cavernous malformation–Refer to case 31		
Capillary telangiectasia They are small, asymptomatic low flow vascular lesions of the brain. Can be associated with Osler-Weber-Rendu syndrome. Mostly solitary lesions affect middle aged population.Can be associated with intracranial hemorrhage (20%). Associated with HHT and cranial irradiation. Mostly asymptomatic.	Collection of enlarged thin-walled vessels resembling capillaries. Pons, cerebellum and spinal cord are the most common sites. They are inconspicuous on non-contrast MRI. May show stippled appearance on T2. Faint brush-like enhancement becomes hypointense on T2*. No oedema, calcification, haemorrhage, gliosis.	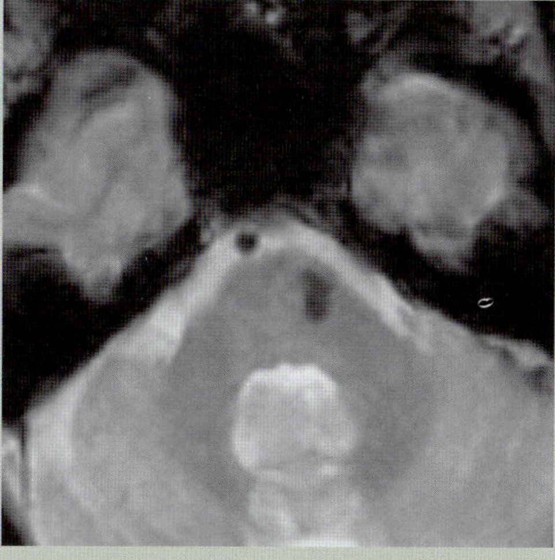 **Fig. 4.35.9:** Capillary telangiectasia in pons
Carotico-cavernous fistula	Carotid artery communicates with dural veins or its branches causing prominent superior ophthalmic vein.	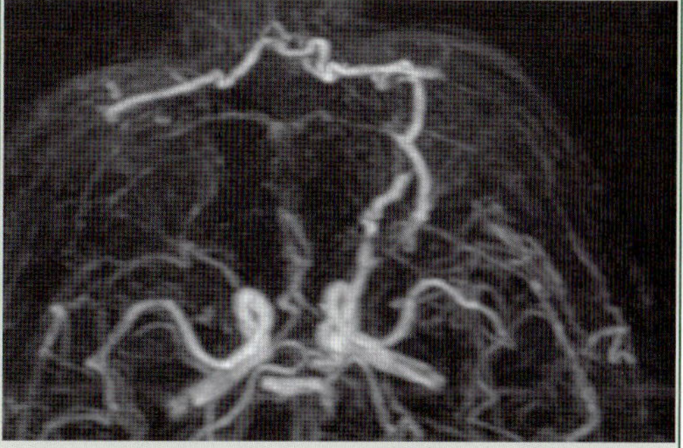 **Fig. 4.35.10:** Caroticocavernous fistula (left)

Treatment: Higher grades (Borden types II / III, Cognard types IIb-V) have an annual mortality rate of ~10% and an annual risk of intracranial hemorrhage of ~8%, so treatment should be considered: endovascular, surgical resection and Stereotactic radiosurgery.

Idiopathic intracranial hypertension (IIH), is known as pseudotumor cerebri and benign intracranial hypertension, is a syndrome characterized by increased CSF pressure and papilledema in patients without focal neurologic findings, except for occasional CN VI palsy.

Table 4.35.2: Cognard classification of dAVF	
Grade 1	In sinus wall, normal antegrade venous drainage (low risk)
Grade 2A	In sinus, reflux to sinus, not cortical veins
Grade 2B	Reflux into cortical veins (10–20% haemorrhage)
Grade 3	Direct cortical venous drainage, no venous ectasia (40% hemorrhage)
Grade 4	Direct cortical venous drainage + venous ectasia (65% haemorrhage).
Grade 5	Spinal perimedullary venous drainage
Borden classification of dAVF	
Type 1	Dural arterial supply with antegrade drainage into venous sinus
	Type 1a: Simple dAVF with single meningeal arterial supply
	Type 1b: Complex dAVF with multiple meningeal arteries
Type II	Dural supply + increased intrasinus pressure → antegrade sinus, retrograde cortical venous drainage.
Type III	Dural arteries drain into cortical veins

Table 4.35.3: Types of spinal dAV fistula

Type I	*Type II*	*Type III*	*Type IV*
Spinal arteriovenous (AV) fistula, present within dura, with intradural distended draining veins	• Glomus-type AVM • Plexiform AVM • Direct arterial/venous communications forming compact nidus within cord	Juvenile AVM	Perimedullary fistula
Imaging	*Imaging*	*Imaging*	*Imaging*
• Cord enlarged, T2WI hyperintense, vessel flow voids on cord surface • Multiple enhancing serpentine veins on cord surface	• Multiple, well-defined serpentine flow voids within substance of cord • Large cord, heterogeneous signal (blood products), flow voids • Supplied by anterior spinal artery and/or posterior spinal artery • Nidus drains to coronal venous plexus (on cord surface), which drains anterograde to extradural space	• Large complex nidus, multiple feeding vessels; may be intramedullary and extramedullary, and even extraspinal	• Hyperintense cord + flow voids • Intradural location for fistula, adjacent to cord • Draining veins may be pronounced on dorsal or ventral surface of cord • Feeding vessel from ASA or PSA connects directly with spinal vein (no nidus)

It is a diagnosis of exclusion. Imaging features which support the diagnosis of IIH include: Optic nerves—prominent subarachnoid space around the optic nerves, vertical tortuosity of the optic nerves, enhancement of the prelaminar (intra-ocular) optic nerves; papilledema-flattening of the posterior sclera, intraocular protrusion of the optic nerve; enlarged arachnoid outpouchings; partially empty sella turcica; enlarged Meckel cave; bilateral venous sinus stenosis—lateral segments of the transverse sinuses; acquired tonsillar ectopia (mimicking Chiari I malformation); increased subcutaneous fat thickness in the region of scalp and neck. **T2 multiple flow voids** occurs in dural AVF, moyamoya, cerebral multiple proliferative microangiopathy and multiple AVM.

4.36 CENTRAL NERVOUS SYSTEM

Case No. 36

Clinical features: 6 years old male child with developmental delay and seizures.

Imaging techniques and observations: Figures 4.36.1–4.36.3 are MRI brain—FLAIR coronal, T2 axial and T1 sagittal images respectively showing moderate diffuse bilateral symmetric cerebellar atrophy with enlargement of interfoveal spaces and ex-vacuo prominence of 4th ventricle noted. There is FLAIR hyperintensity of the cerebellar cortex noted. Pons shows mild atrophy. No evidence of changes in the white matter/brain stem/basal ganglia. Clava appears normal. Rest of the visualized structures appear normal.

Interpretation: A—6-year-old male child, bilateral cerebellum, C—FLAIR hyperintensity of the cerebellar cortex, B—symmetrical atrophy, fourth ventricle dilated, without any basal ganglia/brainstem/white matter abnormalities, D—bilateral cerebellar atrophy with bright cerebellar cortex.

Principal diagnosis: Bilateral cerebellar atrophy with bright cerebellar cortex.

Management: Biochemical and genetic analysis.

Unilateral vs bilateral cerebellar atrophy: Rule is congenital and metabolic causes always bilateral symmetric involvement of the cerebellar hemispheres.

Unilateral cerebellar atrophy indicates acquired causes like unilateral cerebellitis, unilateral ischemic stroke, unilateral traumatic brain injury, following posterior fossa surgery and crossed cerebro-cerebellar diaschisis.

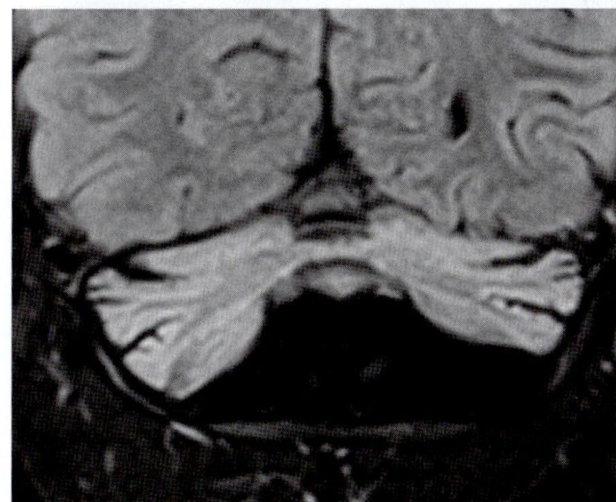

Fig. 4.36.1

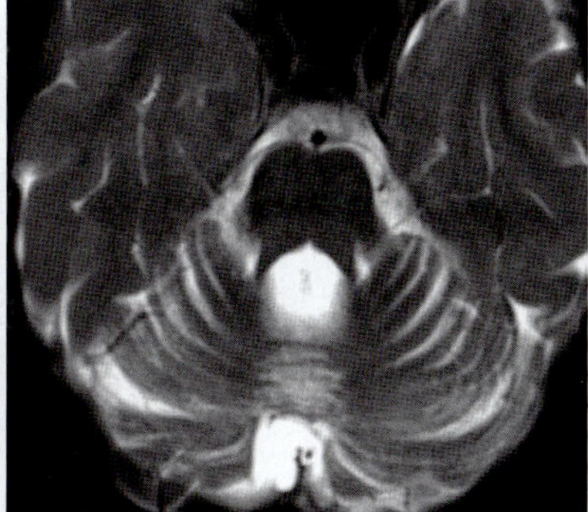

Fig. 4.36.2

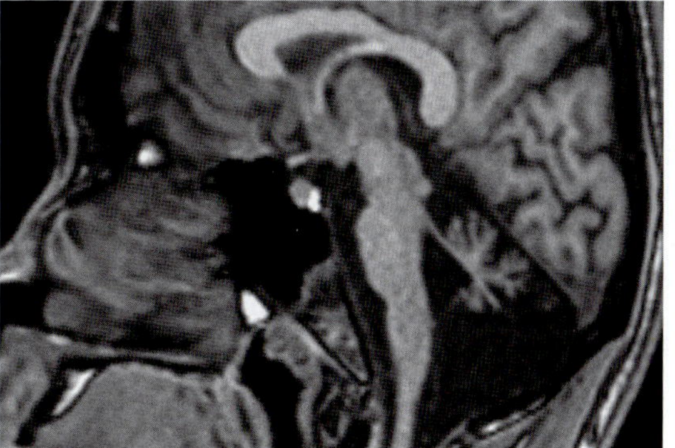

Fig. 4.36.3

Table 4.36.1: Poretti, et al. approach to cerebellar atrophy

I	Pure cerebellar atrophy	Ataxia telangiectasia and ataxia telangiectasia like disorders, late onset GM2, ataxia, oculomotor praxias.
II	Cerebellar atrophy and hypomyelination	Pelizaeus–Merzbacher disease, Salla disease, Hypomyelination and atrophy of basal ganglia and cerebellum, leukoencephalopathy with ataxia, hypodontia and hypomyelination.
III	Cerebellar atrophy and progressive white matter disorders	Periventricular: Neuronal ceroid lipofuscinosis, Niemann-Pick type C, dentatorubral pallidoluysian atrophy. Occipital: Peroxisomal disorders Diffuse: Vanishing white matter disease. Subcortical cerebellar atrophy: L-2 hydroxy glutaric aciduria.
IV	Cerebellar atrophy and cerebellar cortex T2-hyperintensity	Infantile neuroaxonal dystrophy, Marinesco- Sjögren syndrome, mitochondrial disorders.
V	Cerebellar atrophy and basal ganglia involvement	Calcification: Cockayne syndrome, Kearns-Sayre syndrome, mitochondrial disorders. ATROPHY: Hypomyelination and atrophy of basal ganglia and cerebellum. Signal changes: Mitochondrial disorders, Wilson disease, 3-methyl glutaconic aciduria.
VI	Cerebellar atrophy and brainstem involvement	Pons appears flat—congenital disorder of glycosylation Clava hypertrophied: Infantile neuroaxonal atrophy Clava atrophied: Friedrich ataxia

Important cerebellar atrophy plus syndromes			
Infantile neuroaxonal dystrophy: Rare autosomal recessive disorder. Mutation in PLA2G6. Presence of spheroid bodies in peripheral nerve biopsy C/F—psychomotor regression, hypotonia evolving into spasticity.	Imaging findings; cerebellar atrophy with cortical FLAIR hyperintensity. **CLAVA hypertrophied** increased iron deposition in basal ganglia	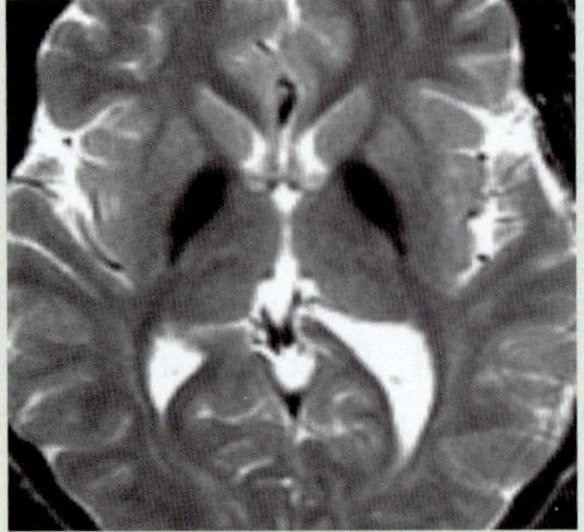 **Fig. 4.36.4:** Bilateral T2 hypointensity in infantile neuroaxonal dystrophy	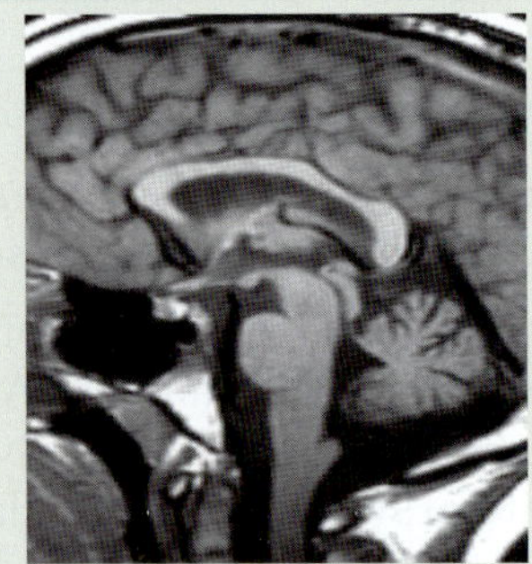 **Fig. 4.36.5:** Infantile neuroaxonal dystrophy
Congenital disorder of glycosylation Clinical clues 'earlier' Fat pads Inverted nipples	Imaging findings Cerebellar atrophy Flat pons Bright cortex	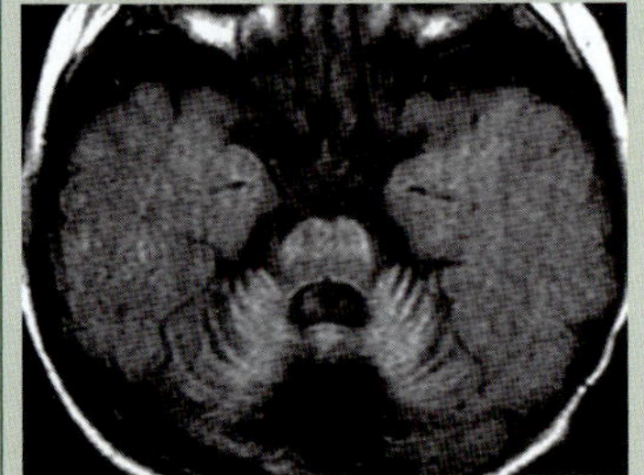 **Fig. 4.36.6:** Bright cortex with flat pons and bilateral cerebellar atrophy in glucosylation disorder	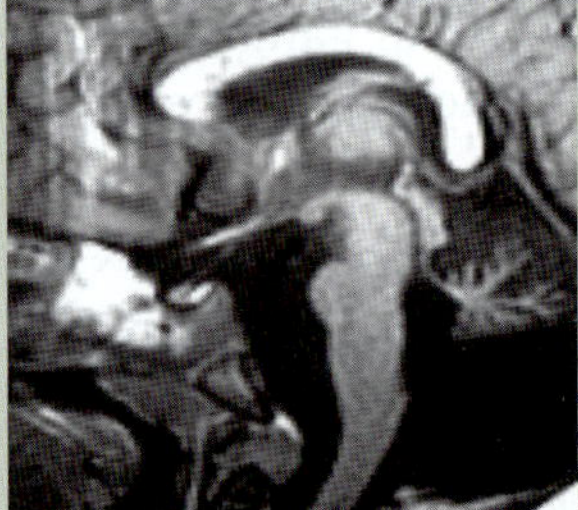 **Fig. 4.36.7:** Glycosylation disorder with vermis atrophy and flat pons
Neuronal ceroid lipofuscinosis Neurodegenerative disorder Excessive accumulation of lipofuscin. Brain atrophy with significant cerebellar atrophy and diffuse white matter changes. **Diagnostic:** Skin punch biopsy.	**Imaging findings:** Cerebellar atrophy Nonspecific T2/FLAIR hyperintense white matter changes. **Infantile subtype:** Thin periventricular hyperintense bands. **Late infantile subtype:** Hypointense thalami/basal ganglia. **Spectroscopy:** Reduced NAA, elevated MI.	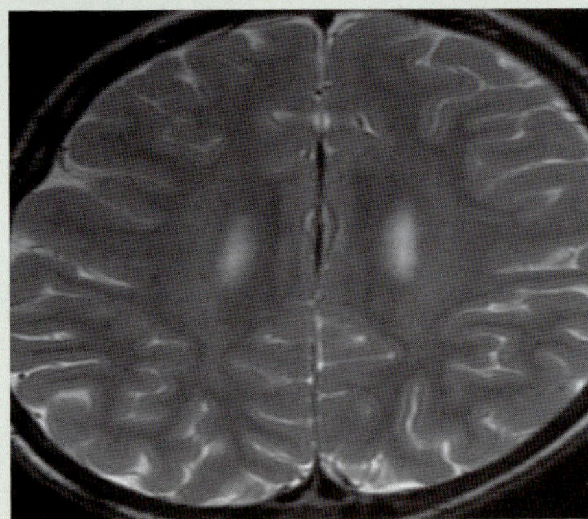 **Fig. 4.36.8:** Nonspecific T2/FLAIR hyperintensities in neuronal ceroid lipofuscinosis	
Marinesco-Sjögren syndrome Rare autosomal recessive disorder. Clinical clues Early cataracts Short stature Hypogonadism Delayed development Ataxia	Imaging findings: Cerebellar atrophy, Bright cortex	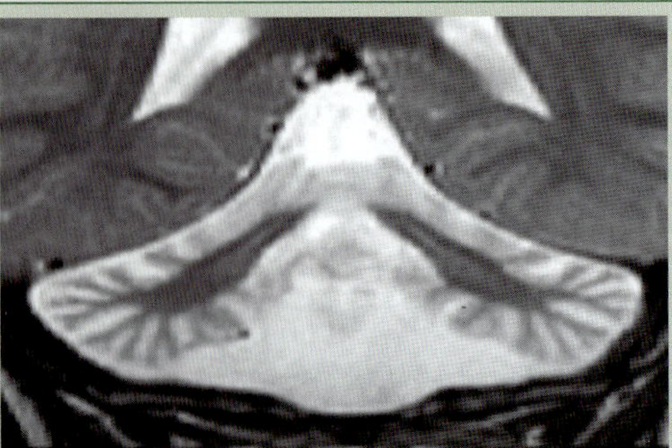 **Fig. 4.36.9:** Marinesco-Sjögren syndrome	

Other acquired causes:

- Extreme prematurity.
- Neonatal hypoxic ischemic encephalopathy
- Postinflammatory
- Multiple sclerosis
- *Neurodegenerative:* Olivopontocerebellar degeneration (MSA-C)
- Cerebro-tendinous xanthomatosis
- Post-traumatic brain injury
- Paraneoplastic (e.g. lung, ovary, Hodgkin's, LCH, opsoclonus myoclonus syndrome in neuroblastoma)
- Chronic epilepsy
- Radiation therapy
- Post-posterior fossa surgery
- Vitamin B_{12} deficiency
- *Toxins:* Phenytoin and other AED, tacrolimus, alcohol.
- Gluten sensitivity.
- JC virus granule cell neuronopathy.
- Superficial siderosis.
- Normal ageing.
- Idiopathic.

Hereditary cerebellar ataxias: Spino-cerebellar ataxia—Freidrich ataxia, ataxia telangiectasia.

Dragon fly appearance: Atrophy of cerebellar hemispheres with preserved vermis. Seen in pontocerebellar hypoplasia.

4.37 CENTRAL NERVOUS SYSTEM

Case No. 37

Clinical history: 9-year-old-male child presenting with seizures, skin changes and delayed developmental milestones.

Radiologiacal technique and observation: Figures 4.37.1–4.37.3 are MRI of T2 axial, T1 post-contrast axial and coronal views respectively showing diffuse, bilaterally symmetric T2 hyperintensities in subcortical and deep white matter—predominantly in the temporal, parietal, occipital lobes, and posterior body and splenium of corpus callosum. T1 contrast shows a thin peripheral/ leading edge enhancement. The involved cerebral area shows trizonal distribution with marked T1 hypo/T2 hyperintensity in central zone, less intense signal changes in intermediate zone and enhancement in peripheral zone. The cerebellum shows normal signal intensity. No evidence of infarct/hemorrhage/hemosiderin deposition/hydrocephalus/migrational anomaly/ cortical dysplasia. Normal cerebral sulci and ventricles noted without any abnormal extra-axial fluid collection. Intracranial vessels appear as normal flow voids. Figure 4.37.4 is MRS showing mildly elevated choline peak at 3.3 ppm and very long chain fatty acids (VLCFA) peaks at 0.9 and 1.4 ppm.

Interpretation: A—9-year-old male child, lesion in subcortical and deep white matter, C—abnormal, bilateral diffuse symmetric butterfly shaped T2 high signal involving the posterior and inferior cerebral hemispheres, corpus callosum, and with B—peripheral leading edge enhancement (representing Schaumberg zones) and mild elevation of choline and VLCFA D-X linked adrenoleukodystrophy.

Principal diagnosis: X-linked adrenoleukodystrophy.

Discussion: X-linked adrenoleukodystrophy (X-ALD) is also known as childhood cerebral X-ALD (CCALD). Also known as "bronze" Schilder disease and "melanodermic type leukodystrophy" before its adrenal involvement was recognized. Five variants other than CCALD have been described, including presymptomatic X-ALD, adolescent (AdolCALD), adult (ACALD), adrenomyeloneuropathy (AMN), and Addison—only symptomatic female carriers. **Etiology:** ALD is an inherited disorder of peroxisomal metabolism. Altered peroxisome metabolism in ALD results from absent or deficient acyl-CoA synthetase leading to impaired β-oxidation of very-long-chain fatty acids (VLCFAs). VLCFAs accumulate in the WM, causing a severe inflammatory demyelination ("brittle" myelin). Axonal degeneration in the posterior fossa and spinal cord are also typical of the disease. **Pathology:** There are two distinctive active pathophysiologic processes in ALD. The first is axonal degeneration that predominates in the posterior fossa and spinal cord, and the second is a severe inflammatory demyelination. Three distinct zones of myelin loss are seen in ALD. The innermost zone consists of a necrotic core of demyelination with astrogliosis, ± Ca^{++}. An intermediate zone of active demyelination and perivascular inflammation lies just outside the necrotic, "burned out" core of the lesion. The most peripheral zone consists of ongoing demyelination without inflammatory changes. **Classic X-linked ALD** is the most common form (45%) and is seen almost exclusively in boys 5–12 years of age. Behavioral difficulties and deteriorating school performance are common. **Hearing loss and skin** bronzing may be seen.

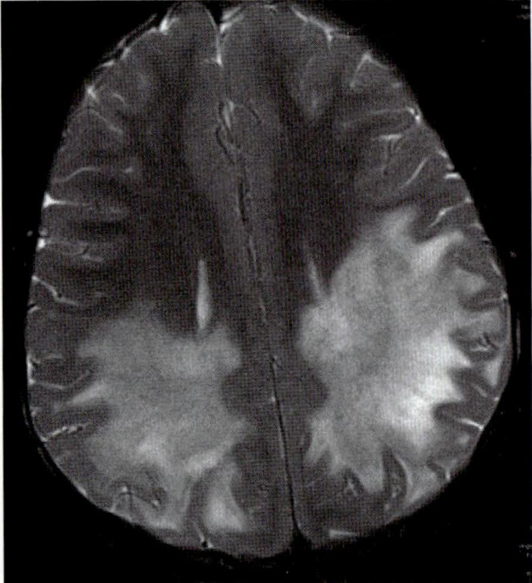
Fig. 4.37.1

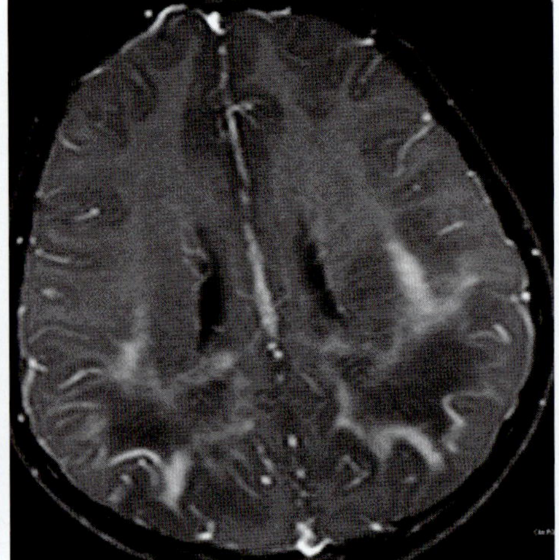
Fig. 4.37.2

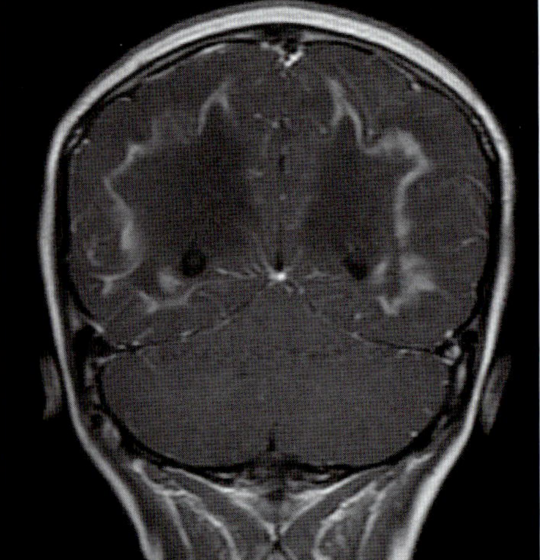
Fig. 4.37.3

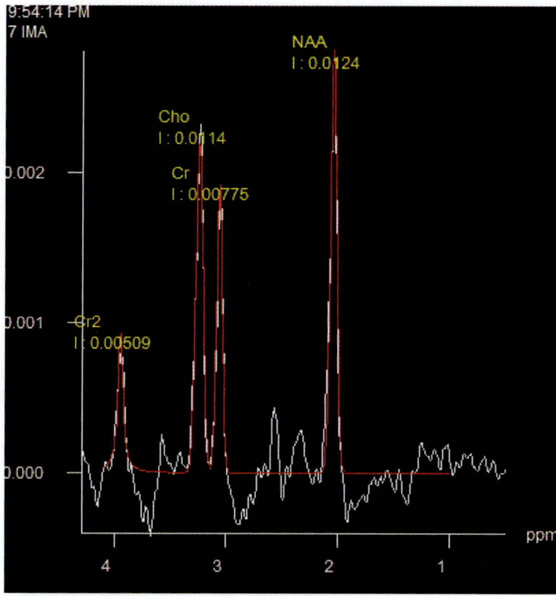

Fig. 4.37.4

Approximately 10% of affected patients present acutely with seizures, adrenal crisis, acute encephalopathy, or coma. **Adrenomyeloneuropathy (AMN)** is the second most common type (30–35%). It is another X-linked disorder that occurs primarily in male patients. It presents between 14 and 60 years, thus presenting later than classic X-ALD. AMN is characterized by axonal degeneration in the spinal cord more than the brain and peripheral nerves. Approximately 20–25% of X-ALD patients exhibit isolated adrenal insufficiency **(Addison disease)**. Neurologic involvement is absent. Other less common forms of ALD include adolescent and adult-onset ALD and mild symptomatic disease in female carriers. **CT:** NECT scans demonstrate hypoattenuation involving the corpus callosum splenium and WM around the atria and occipital horns. Calcification in the affected white matter may be seen. CECT typically shows enhancement around the central hypoattenuating white matter.

Table 4.37.1: Differential diagnosis for X-linked adrenoleukodystrophy		
Metachromatic leukodystrophy Lysosomal enzyme arylsulfatase A. Late infantile, juvenile, and adult onset	Symmetric confluent areas of high signal intensity in the **periventricular white matter**. Centrifugal spread of demyelination: Starts in corpus callosum splenium, deep parieto-occipital WM. Frontal, temporal WM affected later. Spares subcortical U-fibers, cerebellum No enhancement. The tigroid and "leopard skin" patterns of demyelination, which suggest sparing of the perivascular white matter, can be seen in the periventricular white matter and centrum semiovale	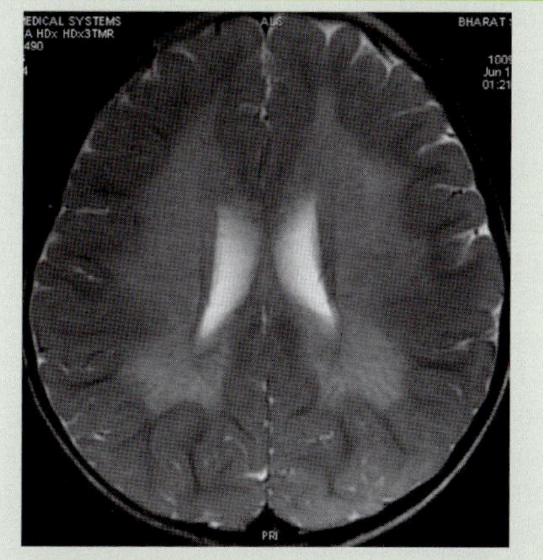 Fig. 4.37.5: Metachromatic leukodystrophy
Krabbe disease or globoid cell leukodystrophy Galactocerebroside B-galactosidase. Infantile, late infantile, juvenile, and adult forms. Typically, Krabbe disease is rapidly progressive and fatal	NECT—symmetric high-attenuation foci in the thalami The subcortical U fibers are spared until late in the disease course. Optic nerve hypertrophy The centrum semiovale, periventricular white matter, and deep gray matter demonstrate high signal intensity at T2-weighted MR imaging	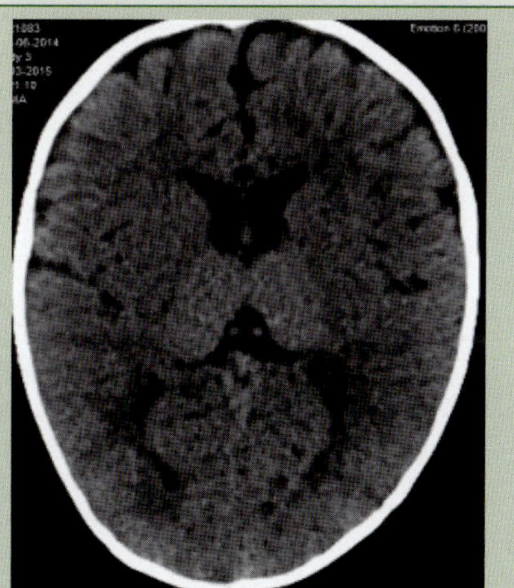 Fig. 4.37.6: Krabbe disease

Contd..

Table 4.37.1: Differential diagnosis for X-linked adrenoleukodystrophy *(Contd...)*		
Mucopolysaccharidosis lysosomal enzymes involved in the degradation of glycosaminoglycans	Focal and diffuse areas of low signal intensity on T1-weighted MR images and high signal intensity on T2-weighted images The sharply defined foci are commonly present in the corpus callosum, basal ganglia, and cerebral white matter. They are isointense relative to cerebrospinal fluid with all imaging sequences and probably represent mucopolysaccharide-filled perivascular spaces	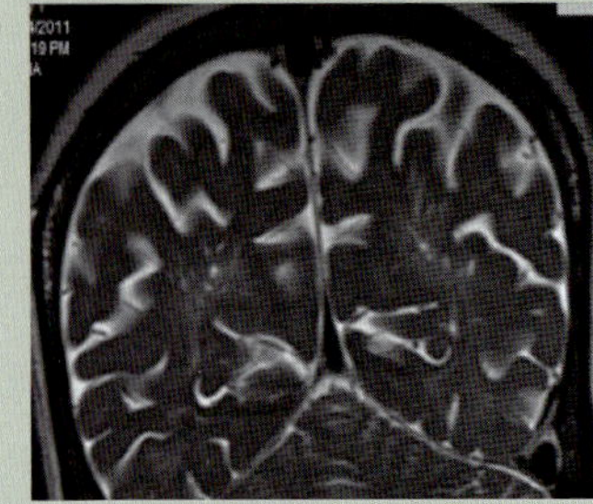 **Fig. 4.37.7:** Mucopolysaccharidosis-Prominent VR space
Zellweger syndrome—cerebro-hepatorenal syndrome	MR imaging reveals diffuse demyelination with abnormal gyration that is most severe in the peri-sylvian and perirolandic regions. Microgyria and pachygyria, Subependymal (caudothalamic) germinolytic cysts. Small renal cortical cysts.	
MELAS syndrome MELAS usually has a relapsing-remitting course. Clinical presentation is characterized by most common stroke-like episodes, Seizures, lactic acidosis, encephalopathy, dementia, muscle weakness, deafness.	Serum and cerebrospinal fluid lactate levels are usually elevated. MR imaging demonstrates multiple cortical and subcortical infarct-like lesions that cross vascular boundaries, along with varying degrees of generalized cerebral and cerebellar atrophy. The parietal and occipital lobes and the basal ganglia are frequently involved MRS—nearly two-thirds of cases with MELAS show a prominent lactate "doublet" at 1.3 ppm in otherwise normal-appearing brain. One-third of cases show no evidence for elevated lactate levels in the brain parenchyma but may demonstrate a lactate peak in the ventricular CSF.	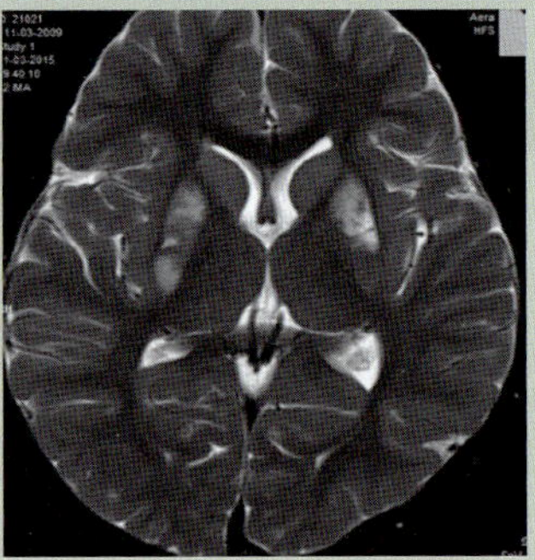 **Fig. 4.37.8** MELAS syndrome
Leigh disease or subacute necrotizing encephalomyelopathy. Typically, symptoms become evident before the age of 2, with the presentation in later childhood (juvenile form) or adulthood (adult form) being uncommon. Symptoms include psychomotor delay/regression superimposed signs of basal ganglia and brainstem dysfunction – ataxia, ophthalmoplegia, dystonia, respiratory rhythm disturbance, cranial nerve palsies	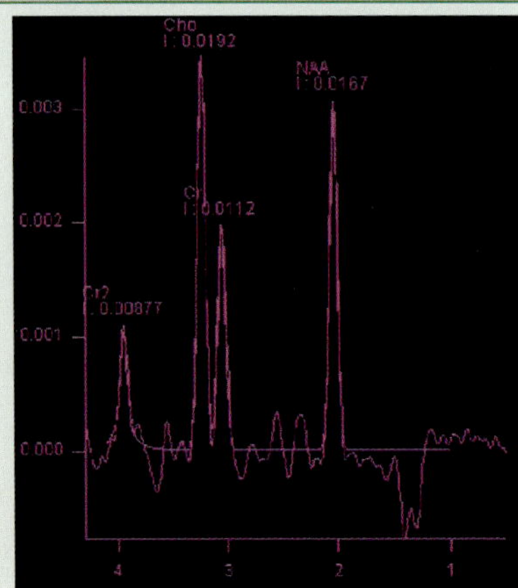 **Fig. 4.37.9:** Leigh disease Symmetric putaminal involvement, which may be associated with abnormalities of the caudate nuclei, globus pallidi, thalami, and brainstem and, less frequently, of the cerebral cortex. The cerebral white matter is rarely affected. Enhancement may be seen at MR imaging and may correspond to the onset of acute necrosis. In the acute setting some restricted diffusion may be evident MR spectroscopy shows elevated choline, occasionally elevated lactate and reduced NAA.	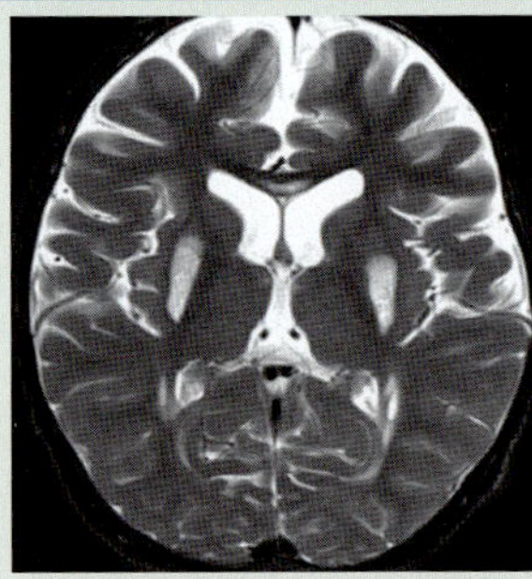 **Fig. 4.37.10:** Leigh disease 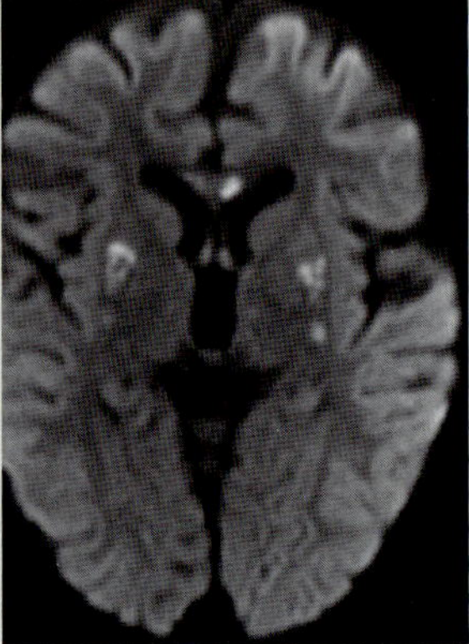 **Fig. 4.37.11:** Leigh disease

Contd...

Table 4.37.1: Differential diagnosis for X-linked adrenoleukodystrophy *(Contd...)*		
Canavan disease or spongiform leukodystrophy Deficiency of N-acetylaspartylase. 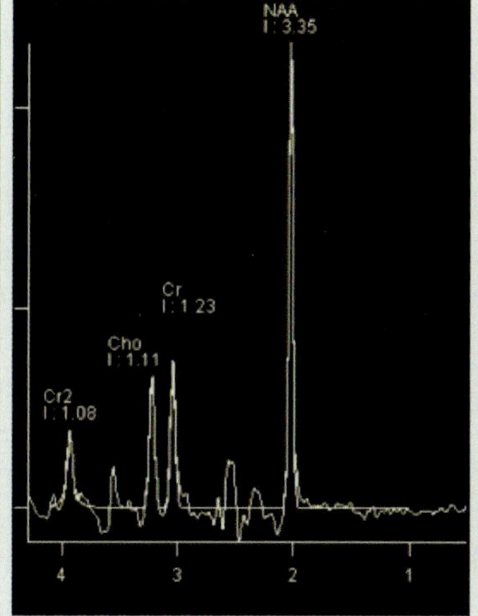 **Fig. 4.37.12:** Marked elevation of NAA in Canavan's disease	T1-weighted MR imaging demonstrates symmetric areas of homogeneous, diffuse low signal intensity throughout the white matter, whereas T2-weighted imaging shows nearly homogeneous high signal intensity throughout the white matter. The subcortical U fibers are preferentially affected early in the course of the disease. MR eventually shows virtually complete absence of myelination with confluent T2/FLAIR hyperintensity throughout the WM and globi pallidi. MRS is the key to the definitive imaging diagnosis of CD. Markedly elevated NAA is seen in virtually all cases.	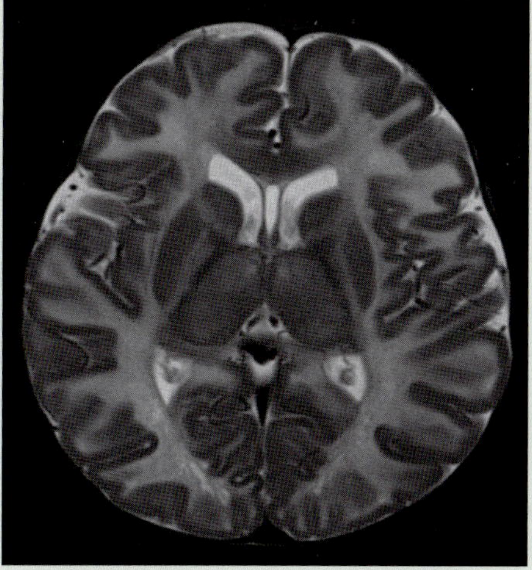 **Fig. 4.37.13:** Subcortical U fibers hyperintensities in Canavan's disease
Alexander disease, or fibrinoid leukodystrophy	Macrocephaly. CT demonstrates low attenuation in the deep **frontal lobe white matter**. Enhancement is often seen near the tips of the frontal horns early in the disease course. The characteristic frontal lobe areas of hyperintensity are seen at T2-weighted MR imaging. These hyperintense areas progress posteriorly to the parietal white matter and internal and external capsules. The subcortical white matter is affected early in the disease course. In the late stages of the disease, cysts may develop in affected regions of the brain.	
Megalencephalic leukoencephalopathy with subcortical cysts (van der Knaap) Patients typically present with megalencephaly during the first year of life associated with mild motor developmental delay and seizures.	**Types:** 1. Megalencephalic leukoencephalopathy with subcortical cysts: Swollen WM and subcortical cysts 2. Leukoencephalopathy with vanishing WM: WM replaced by CSF intensity 3. WM disease with lactate: Brain lactate and spinal involvement Hypomyelination with atrophy of BG and cerebellum (H-ABC)	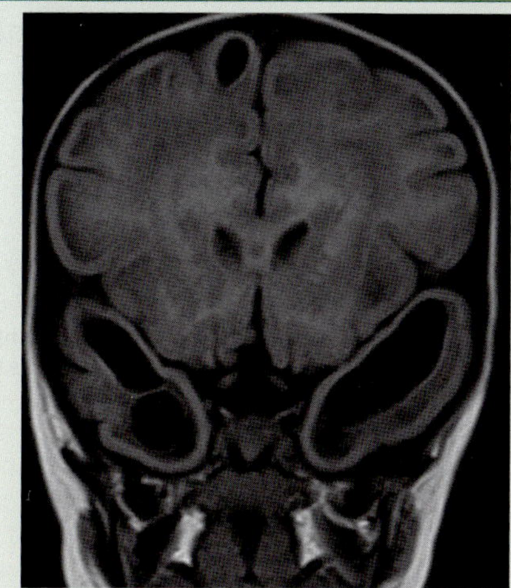 **Fig. 4.37.14:** van der Knaap

Table 4.37.2: Imaging features of myelination disorders			
Delayed myelination	*Dysmyelination*	*Demyelination*	*Hypomyelination*
T2 hyperintense	T2 hyperintense	T2 hyperintense	T2 mild hyperintensity
T1 hypointense	T1 hypointense	T1 black holes	T1 normal
Increase in myelination in serial scans	Accumulation of abnormal myelin	Breakdown of normally formed myelin	Unchanged pattern in 2 scans, 6 months apart, but one should be after 1 year of age

MR: A posterior-predominant pattern is seen in 75–80% of patients with X-ALD. The earliest finding is T2/FLAIR hyperintensity in the middle of the corpus callosum splenium. As the disease progresses, hyperintensity spreads from posterior to anterior and from the center to the periphery. The peritrigonal WM, corticospinal tracts, fornix, commissural fibers, plus the visual and auditory pathways can all eventually become involved. The leading edge of demyelination appears hyperintense on T1WI but does not enhance. The intermediate zone of active inflammatory demyelination typically enhances T1 C+. Approximately 10–15% of all patients with classic X-ALD have an anterior predominant demyelination; T2WI/FLAIR hyperintensity initially appears in the corpus callosum genu (not the splenium) and spreads into the frontal lobe white matter. DWI/DTI shows reduced diffusivity in active zones of demyelination and increased diffusivity in regions of "burnt-out" demyelination. DTI shows reduced connectivity (i.e., loss of fractional anisotropy) in white matter that MR demonstrates as abnormal and in "normal" white matter. **MRS shows, at TE of 35 ms, peaks at 0.8–1.4 (i.e. cytosolic amino acids and VLCFA macromolecules)**. Reduced NAA may be detected prior to observed MR abnormality and predicts progression. Increased choline is noted.

Bone marrow transplantation: Boys without neurological deficits should be monitored closely for radiological signs of cerebral ALD. Childhood cerebral ALD (CCALD) has not been reported before the age of 2.5 years. MRI of the brain should be done every 6 months in boys aged 3 to 12 years old to screen for early signs of CCALD. If symptoms occur suggestive of cerebral ALD (for instance, declining school performance) the MRI should be performed at the earliest available opportunity, but the detection of brain MRI abnormalities precedes any detectable cognitive dysfunction by at least 6 months to 1 year. Allogeneic hematopoetic stem cell transplantation (HCT) should be done as soon as brain MRI abnormalities typical of cerebral ALD are detected. After a successful transplant, the lesions on MRI stabilize and even regress. Treatment results are better the earlier treatment is started.

Menkes disease, or trichopoliodystrophy, is an X chromosome-linked recessive disorder that is characterized by a defect in copper transporting protein in the mitochondria and disturbed absorption of copper from the gastrointestinal tract. Patients present with hypotonia, hypothermia, and seizures. MR imaging performed during the early postnatal period may be unremarkable except for the presence of tortuous cerebral vessels. Later images typically show a progressive white matter lesion predominantly involving the frontal and temporal areas and progressive brain atrophy with subdural hemorrhage that may mimic injuries related to child abuse. MR angiography depicts characteristic tortuous cerebral vessels. Skeletal manifestations include Wormian bones, osteopenia, flared metaphysis, and rib fractures.

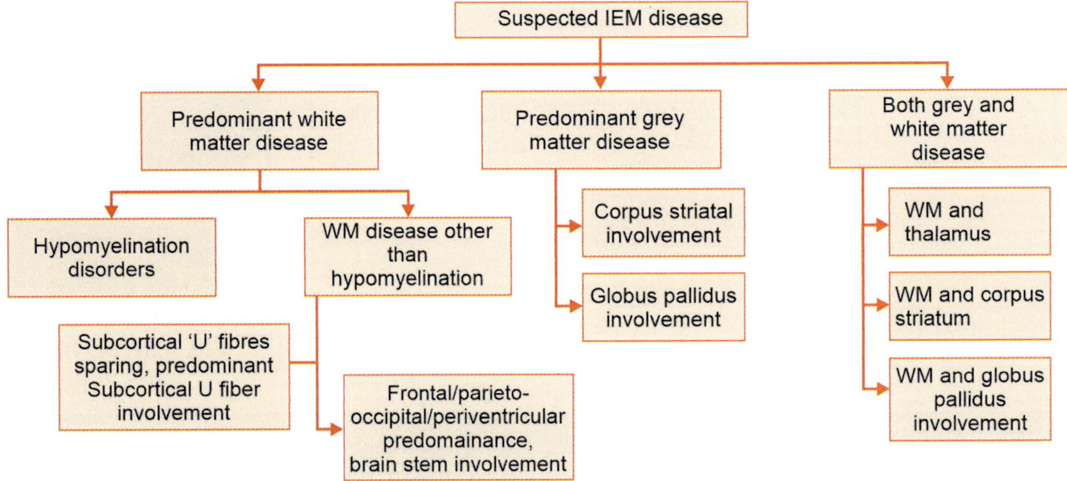

Fig. 4.37.15: Basic approach to leukodystrophies (IEM—inborn errors of metabolism)

Table 4.37.3: Differential diagnosis based on pattern of involvement in patient with myelination disorders			
Predominant white matter disease other than hypomyelination disorders			
1. *Frontal predominance*	2. *Parieto-occipital*	3. *Periventricular*	4. *Brainstem*
Alexander disease Metachromatic leukodystrophy Frontal variant X-ALD Neuroaxonal leukodystrophy with spheroids	Krabbe X-linked ALD Early onset peroxisomal disorders Late infantile MLD	Metachromatic leukodystrophy Krabbe Sjögren-Larsson syndrome	Leukoencephalopathy with brainstem and spinal cord involvement and lactate elevation (LBSL) Peroxisomal disorders Wilson disease Alexander disease Leigh syndrome
Predominant white matter disease other than hypomyelination disorders with variable subcortical U fibre involvement		**Predominant white matter disease—hypomyelination disorders**	**Mixed grey and white matter disease**
Progressive centripetal or centrifugal: Subcortical 'U' fibers spared.	Predominant involvement of subcortical 'U' fibers.	Pelizaeus-Merzbacher disease Pelizaeus-Merzbacher-like disease 18q deletion syndrome Hypomyelination with atrophy of the basal ganglia and cerebellum Salla disease	1. WM and thalamus involvement—Krabbe disease 2. WM and corpus striatum involvement—glutaric aciduria type 1, propionic acidemia Leigh, MELAS 3. WM and globus pallidus involvement–Canavan, methylmalonic acidemia, MSUD, urea cycle disorders
MLD, Krabbe`s, adrenoleukodystrophy, Pelizaeus-Merzbacher disease	Canavan's, alexander's, Van der Knaap, Kearns-Sayre, propionic acidemia, L-2 hydroxy glutaric aciduria, galactosemia, Cockayne's syndrome Urea cycle disorders		
Predominant grey matter involvement		**Macrocephaly**	**CT–high density basal ganglia/ thalamus, calcification**
Globus pallidus	**Striatal**		
Canavan's, Kearns-Sayre, methylmalonic acidemia, maple syrup urine disease, L-2-hydroxyglutaric aciduria	Leigh, MELAS, Wilson's, Glutaric aciduria type I, biotinidase deficiency, Cockayne's syndrome, Propionic academia	Alexander disease, Canavan disease, mucopolysaccharidosis type I (Hurler), Mucopolysaccharidosis type II (hunter), Van der Knaap, MLC, glutaric aciduria -1, L-2 hydroxy glutaric aciduria, GM-2 Gangliosidosis, Zellweger's	Aicardi, Krabbe, mitochondrial, TORCH
Complete/near complete lack of myelination	**Stroke-like episodes**	**Migration abnormalities**	**Enhancement following contrast enhancement**
Canavan disease, Pelizaeus-Merzbacher disease	Leigh syndrome, MELAS, MERRF, homocystinuria	Congenital muscular dystrophy, Zellweger's, congenital cytomegalovirus infection	Alexander disease, ALD, Krabbe's
High grade myelin edema (diffusion restriction)	**Medium grade myelin edema**	**Low grade or no myelin edema**	**Thick meninges**
Krabbe disease, Canavan disease, maple syrup urine disease, LBSL, mitochondrial disease	Metachromatic leukodystrophy, adrenoleukodystrophy	Mucopolysaccharidoses, GM gangliosidosis, van der Knaap disease, phenylketonuria, adrenomyeloneuropathy, vanishing white matter disease, Zellweger disease	Hurler syndrome
Deep white matter involvement with normal thalami—metachromatic leukodystrophy			
Deep white matter involvement with corticospinal tract extension—adrenoleukodystrophy, Krabbe's, infantile Refsum disease			
Global involvement of white matter—MLC, vanishing white matter, end stage of all progressive white matter disorder			

Contd...

Table 4.37.3: Differential diagnosis based on pattern of involvement in patient with myelination disorders *(Contd...)*

Multifocal white matter abnormalities: Mitochondrial defects, Zellweger syndrome, mucopolysaccharidosis

Opercular atrophy–glutaric aciduria

Dentate nucleus—l2 hydroxyglutaric aciduria, Canavan, Krabbe's

Causes for dilated Virchow-Robin spaces—normal variant, Rat criblé, MPS, Cryptococcosis, Lowe's syndrome, '**malo myocardial' with 'velo cardio-facial syndrome'**

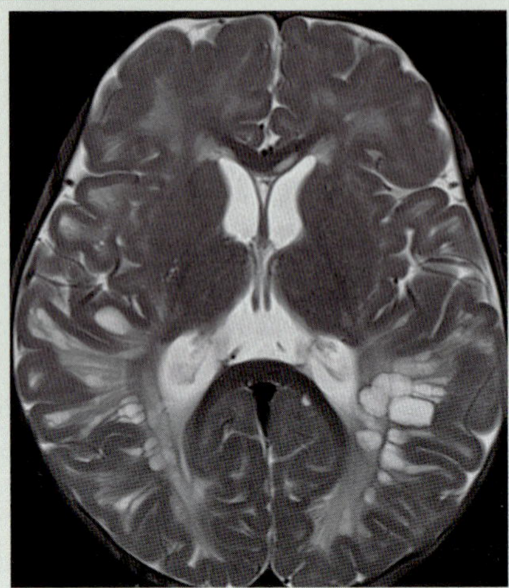

Fig. 4.37.16: Enlarged VR spaces

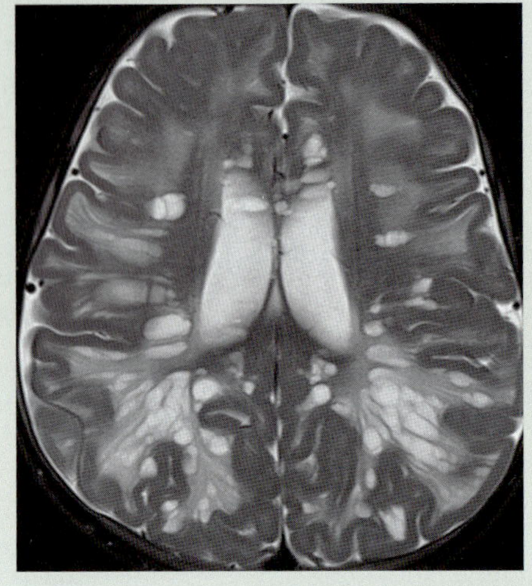

Fig. 4.37.17: Enlarged VR spaces

Vacuolating myelinopathy—Anterior neonatal maple syrup urine disease, nonketotic hyperglycinemia, and Canavan disease. (In active vacuolating myelinopathy, water is trapped in vacuoles between myelin sheets, resulting in intramyelinic edema, which leads to restricted diffusion)

Cystic changes in brain—Ant temporal brain cysts—van der Knapp, leukoencephalopathy with calcifications and cysts, congenital muscular dystrophy, CMV, Pseudo-TORCH, non-megalencephalic leukoencephalopathy with subcortical cysts; cerebellar cysts—congenital muscular dystrophy; caudothalamic cysts–Zellweger's

Batwing arachnoid cysts—glutaric aciduria; **subdural effusions**—Menkes, glutaric aciduria

Diffuse white matter involvement (vanishing white matter/childhood ataxia with CNS hypomyelination): Chronic and progressive neurologic deterioration, often exacerbated by infection, minor head trauma, or acute fright. It is caused by mutations of the translation e-IF gene. MRI shows diffuse T2 and FLAIR hyperintensity throughout the cerebral WM. Later, the MRI signal on FLAIR and T1-weighted sequences is low because of the progressive cystic degeneration ("vanishing") of the cerebral WM with residual meshwork of strands in the abnormal WM. MRS shows stage-dependent loss of the NAA, choline, and creatine signals in the cerebral WM. No contrast enhancement seen.

Fukuyama congenital muscular dystrophy—pachygyria, polymicrogyria

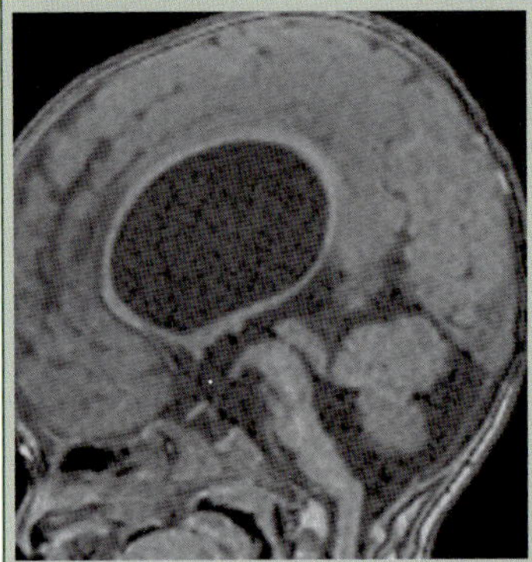

Fig. 4.37.18: Fukuyama congenital muscular dystrophy

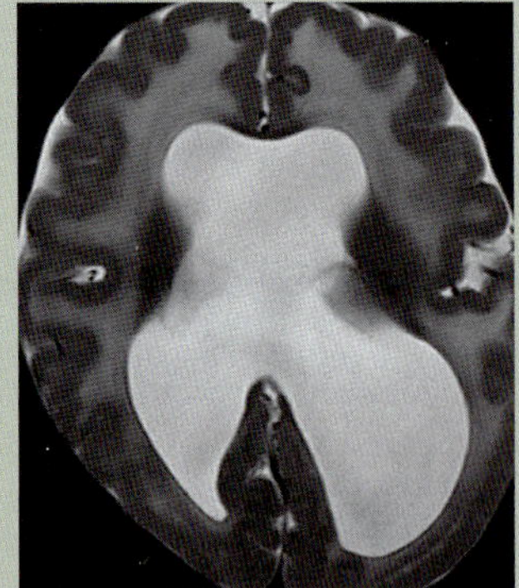

Fig. 4.37.19: Fukuyama congenital muscular dystrophy

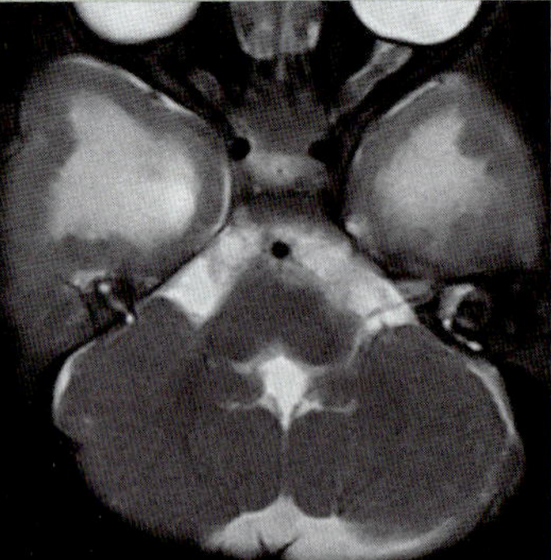

Fig. 4.37.20: Fukuyama congenital muscular dystrophy

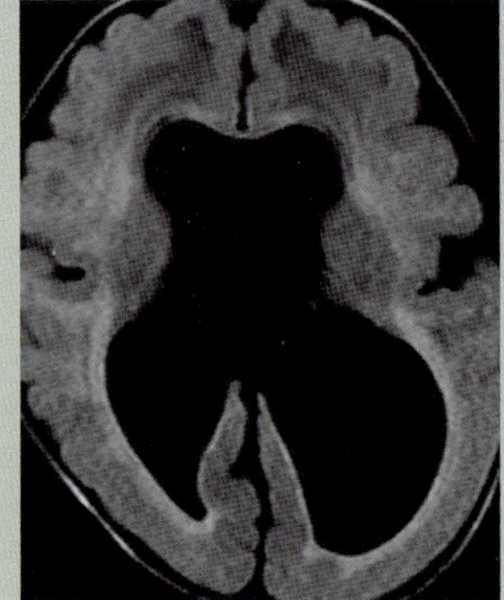

Fig. 4.37.21: Fukuyama congenital muscular dystrophy

Merosin deficient congenital muscular dystrophy

Contd...

Table 4.37.3: Differential diagnosis based on pattern of involvement in patient with myelination disorders *(Contd...)*

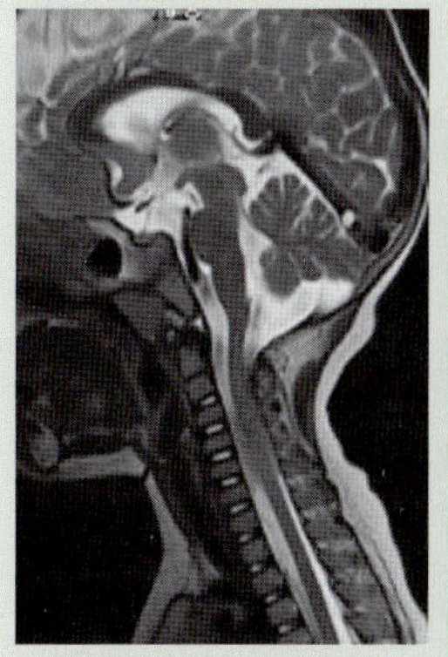 **Fig. 4.37.22:** Merosin deficient congenital muscular dystrophy	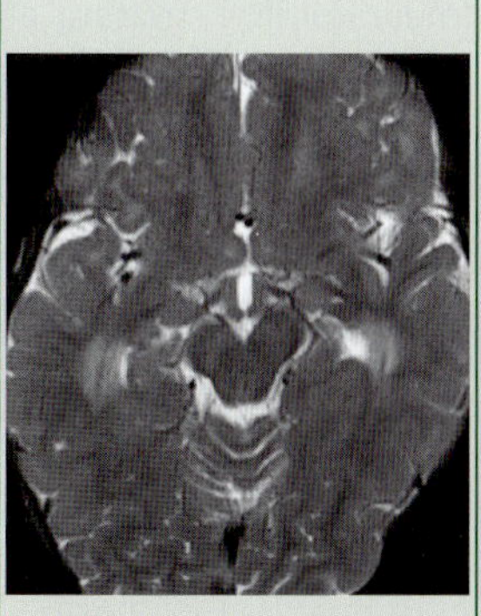 **Fig. 4.37.23:** Merosin deficient congenital muscular dystrophy	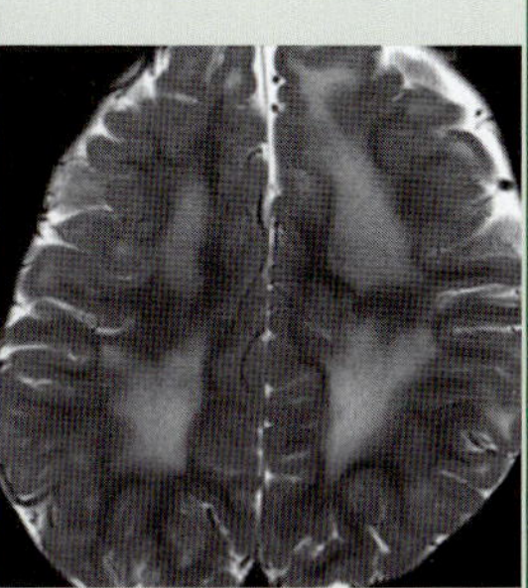 **Fig. 4.37.24:** Merosin deficient congenital muscular dystrophy	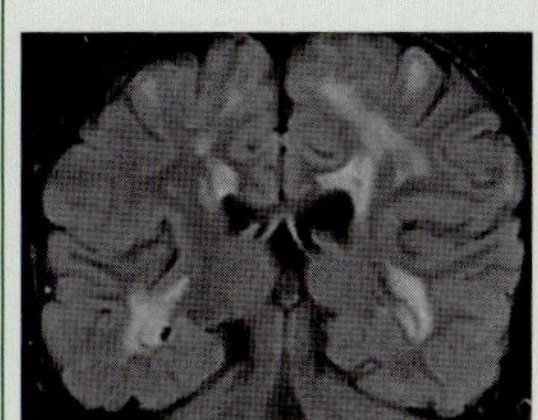 **Fig. 4.37.25:** Merosin deficient congenital muscular dystrophy	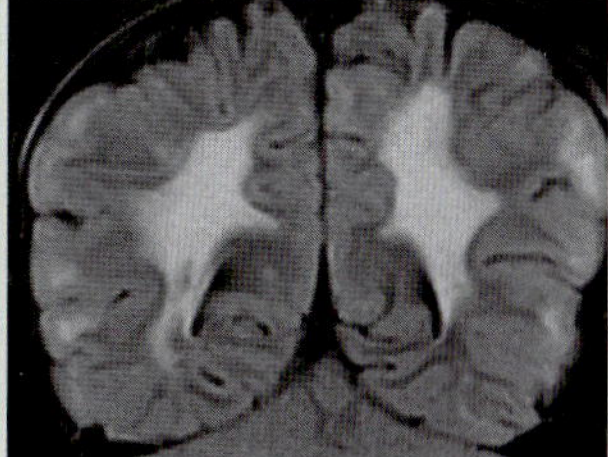 **Fig. 4.37.26:** Merosin deficient congenital muscular dystrophy
Anterior temporal pole cyst with white matter changes				
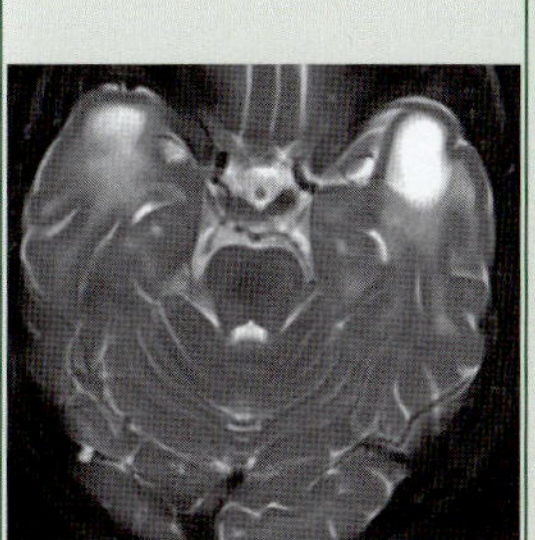 **Fig. 4.37.27:** Anterior temporal pole cyst with white matter changes	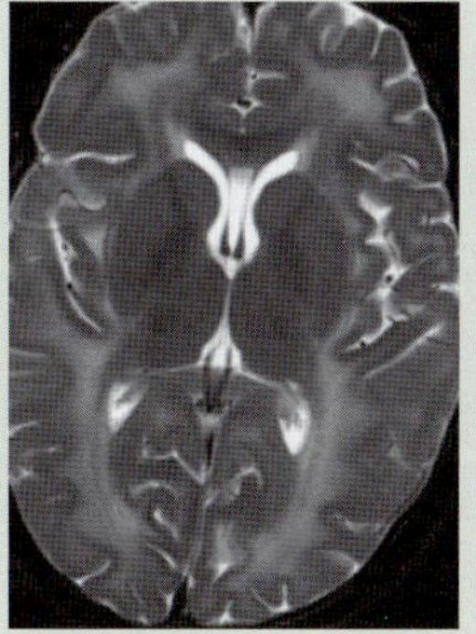 **Fig. 4.37.28:** Anterior temporal pole cyst with white matter changes	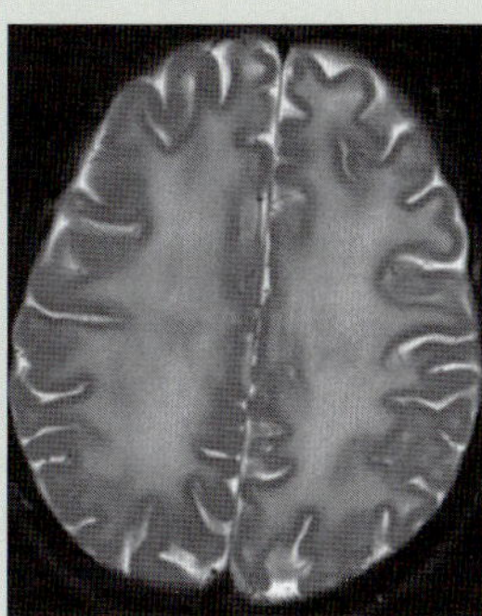 **Fig. 4.37.29:** Anterior temporal pole cyst with white matter changes	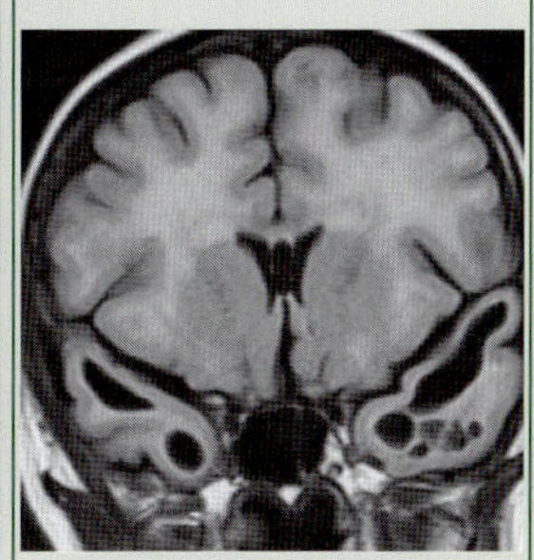 **Fig. 4.37.30:** Anterior temporal pole cyst with white matter changes	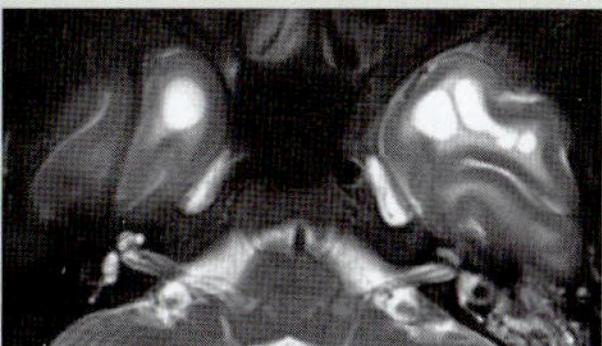 **Fig. 4.37.31:** Anterior temporal pole cyst with white matter changes

Table 4.37.4: Summary of myelination disorders with clinical and radiological correlation

Category, disorder	*Primary classification*	*Cause*	*Metabolic consequence*	*Key points and imaging features*
Predominant white matter disease Hypomyelination disorders				
Pelizaeus-Merzbacher disease	Hypomyelination	Proteolipid protein-1 deletion	Decreased proteolipid protein	Minimal or slow myelination with diffuse T2 hyperintensity and variable T1 changes
Pelizaeus-Merzbacher-like disease	Hypomyelination	No proteolipid protein-1 deletion	Hypomyelination	Minimal or slow myelination with diffuse T2 hyperintensity and variable T1 changes along with brainstem involvement
18q deletion syndrome	Hypomyelination	18q deletion	Unknown	Symmetric deep white matter abnormality, with sparing of brainstem and cerebellum

Contd...

Table 4.37.4: Summary of myelination disorders with clinical and radiological correlation *(Contd...)*				
Hypomyelination with atrophy of the basal ganglia and cerebellum Salla disease	Leukoencephalopathy Lysosomal	Unknown defect in sialic acid transport	Unknown elevated N-acetyl neuraminic acid	Partial hypomyelination with corpus striatum atrophy and preservation of globus pallidus and thalamus Scandinavian ancestry, minimal or slow myelination with diffuse T2 hyperintensity and variable T1 changes
Leukoencephalopathies with macrocrania				
Alexander disease (fibrinoid leukodystrophy)	Leukoencephalopathy	Presence of Rosenthal fibers, glial fibrillary acidic proteins in astrocytes	Failure of myelin deposition due to astrocyte dysfunction	Macrocephaly, frontal predominance with involvement of the basal ganglia, thalami, and brainstem; abnormal enhancement
Canavan disease (spongiform leukodystrophy)	Leukoencephalopathy	Inability to metabolize N-acetyl aspartate into aspartate and acetate	N-acetyl aspartate accumulation	Macrocephaly, diffuse white matter abnormality with basal ganglia involvement; lack of abnormal enhancement
Megalencephalic leukoencephalopathy with sub-cortical cysts (van der Knaap disease)	Leukoencephalopathy	Mutations in the MLC1 and HEPACAM genes	Unknown	Macrocephaly with diffuse white matter abnormalities and subcortical cysts
Chronic leukoencephalopathy				
Globoid cell leukodystrophy (Krabbe disease)	Lysosomal	Decreased galacto cerebro-side activity	Accumulation of globoid cells in brain tissue	Symmetric deep white matter abnormality with dark thalami
Metachromatic leukodystrophy Mucopolysaccharidosis	Lysosomal	Decreased arylsulfatase A activity Multifactorial	Metachromatic sulfatide deposits Mucopolysaccharide accumulation	Symmetric deep white matter abnormality, with sparing of subcortical U fibers Symmetric deep white matter abnormality with dilated Virchow-Robin spaces
Zellweger syndrome (cerebrohepatorenal syndrome)	Peroxisomal	Abnormalities of peroxisome biogenesis genes	Elevated long chain fatty acids, aminoaciduria, albuminuria	Diffuse white matter abnormality, cortical migration anomalies, and germinolytic cysts
Refsum disease and neonatal adrenoleukodystrophy	Peroxisomal	Abnormalities of peroxisome biogenesis genes	Accumulation of long-chain fatty acids	Similar features as in Zellweger syndrome with less severe cortical malformation
X-linked adrenoleukodystrophy	Peroxisomal	Deficiency in oxidizing very long-chain fatty acids	Accumulation of long-chain fatty acids	Symmetric peritrigonal abnormality with involvement of the splenium of the corpus callosum; abnormal peripheral enhancement
Acute leukoencephalopathy				
Leigh disease (subacute necrotizing encephalopathy)	Mitochondrial	Mutation in mitochondrial or nuclear DNA	Disorders of oxidative phosphorylation	Symmetric abnormalities of the basal ganglia
Mitochondrial encephalopathy, lactic acidosis, and stroke-like episodes	Mitochondrial	Mutations in mitochondrial DNA genes	Impaired mitochondrial ability to synthesize protein and produce energy	Nonterritorial and basal ganglia infarcts

Contd...

Table 4.37.4: Summary of myelination disorders with clinical and radiological correlation *(Contd...)*

Urea cycle disorders	Urea cycle	Deficiency in detoxification of ammonia to urea	Glutamine and ammonia accumulation	Extensive cortical and subcortical abnormalities; thalami sparing
Glutaric aciduria	Organic aciduria	Glutaryl-coenzyme A dehydrogenase deficiency	Glutaric acid accumulation	Frontotemporal atrophy, widening of sylvian fissures, and basal ganglia abnormalities
Maple syrup urine disease	Organic aciduria	Defect in branched-chain dehydrogenase blocking oxidative decarboxylation	Elevation of branched- chain amino acids, leucine, isoleucine, and valine	Maple syrup urine disease edema (cytotoxic edema of myelinated white matter) and vasogenic edema of unmyelinated white matter
Methylmalonic acidemia	Organic aciduria	Defect in methylmalonyl-coenzyme A mutase	Elevation of methylmalonic acid, glycine, and ammonia	Abnormalities of the cerebral white matter and bilateral globus pallidus
Propionic acidemia	Organic aciduria	Defect in propionyl-coenzyme A carboxylase	Elevated propionic acid, glycine	Abnormalities of the cerebral white matter and the corpus striatum

Disease	*Neonatal conventional MRI*	*Neonatal 1H-MRS*	*Neonatal DWI*	*MRI in older children*
Urea cycle disorders	Diffuse generalized cytotoxic edema (cerebral cortex, subcortical WM); abnormal signal of BG (T1-/T2-hyper of the globi pallidi, T2-hyper of putamen and caudate nuclei)	Prominent glutamine/ glutamate peaks	Scalloped ribbon of restriction at the depth of sulci	Ulegyria, sparing of occipital and peri-rolandic cortex
Maple syrup urine disease	Increased signal of myelinated structures (cerebellar and peri-rolandic, dorsal brainstem, cerebral peduncles, PLIC, thalami and globi pallidi)	Branched-chain amino and keto acids (0.9 ppm)	Diffusion restriction of myelinated structures, superimposed vasogenic edema of unmyelinated WM	Profound lack of myelination
Glutaric aciduria type 1	Enlarged fronto-temporal CSF spaces, wide sylvian fissures	Probably normal (if no acute encephalopathy)	Probably normal (if no acute encephalopathy)	Increased signal of BG (mostly putamen and caudate), caudate atrophy
Pyruvate dehydrogenase complex deficiency	CC dysgenesis, MCM, subcortical heterotopias, pachygyria, cortical atrophy, T2-hyper lesions BG (putamen) and WM (cerebellum, PLIC and occipital lobes), subependymal cysts	Lactate doublet	Diffusion restriction of BG and WM (cerebellum, PLIC and occipitally)	Leigh-like findings, delayed myelination, atrophy
Mitochondriopathies	Cerebral atrophy, T2-hyper lesions (dorsal midbrain, cerebral peduncles, pontine corticospinal tracts, central tegmental tracts, dorsal medulla, subcortical WM), subependymal cysts	Lactate doublet	Restriction of dorsal midbrain, cerebral peduncles, pontine, corticospinal tracts, central tegmental tracts, dorsal medulla, subcortical WM	Leigh-like changes of the basal ganglia, atrophy of BG and WM

Contd...

Disease	*Neonatal conventional MRI*	*Neonatal 1H-MRS*	*Neonatal DWI*	*MRI in older children*
Sulfite oxidase deficiency: Extensive generalized edema cerebellar hypoplasia	S-sulocysteine (3.61 ppm), taurine (3.42 and 3.24 ppm), cysteine (2.92 and 2.97 ppm)	Generalized diffusion restriction (frontal and temporal cortex and thalami may be spared)	Rapid evolution to extensive cystic lesions in the cerebral WM and global cortical atrophy	Frontal and temporal cortex and thalami may be spared
Zellweger syndrome	Polymicro-/pachygyria (particularly peri-sylvian and parieto-temporo-occipital lobes), hypomyelination, subependymal cysts	Increased lactate and lipids (0.9–1.33 ppm), decreased NAA	Normal	WM signal abnormality (generalized, cerebellum), atrophy, polymicro-/pachygyria
Congenital disorder of glycosylation type 1a	Early maybe normal or ponto-cerebellar hypoplasia, abnormal signal cerebellar WM, intracranial hemorrhages	Probably normal	Probably normal	Superimposed cerebellar atrophy, supratentorial atrophy, stroke-like lesions
Smith-Lemli-Opitz syndrome	Ventriculomegaly, hypoplastic frontal lobes and cerebellum, CC dysgenesis, holoprosencephaly	Lipid peak (0.8–1.5 ppm)	Normal	Similar to the neonatal findings
Krabbe disease	Thick optic nerve and chiasm may be first clue, T2-hyper lesions in cerebellar WM	Increased myo-inositol and choline, decreased NAA	Reduction of subcortical WM, caudate, ALIC	T2-hyper lesions in cortical spinal tracts and thalami
Pyridoxine-dependent epilepsy, isthmus of the CC, MCM, findings similar to HIE	Usually normal; thinning of the unknown	May be abnormal (findings similar to HIE)	WM abnormalities, ventriculomegaly	
Nonketotic hyperglycinemia	T2-hyperlesions of the myelinated WM tracts, CC agenesis, vermian hypoplasia	Glycine peak	Restricted diffusion of myelinated WM tracts	Delayed myelination, ventriculomegaly, enlarged subarachnoid spaces
Creatine deficiency syndromes	Normal	Absent or severely deficiency creatine peak	Probably normal	Probably normal
GLUT1 deficiency	Normal	Probably normal	Probably normal	Probably normal

Table 4.37.5: Normal myelination pictorial representation

Age	*Normal myelination*
At birth (T1W high signal, T2W low signal)	Medulla, dorsal midbrain, inferior and superior cerebellar peduncles, post-limb of internal capsule, ventrolateral thalamus

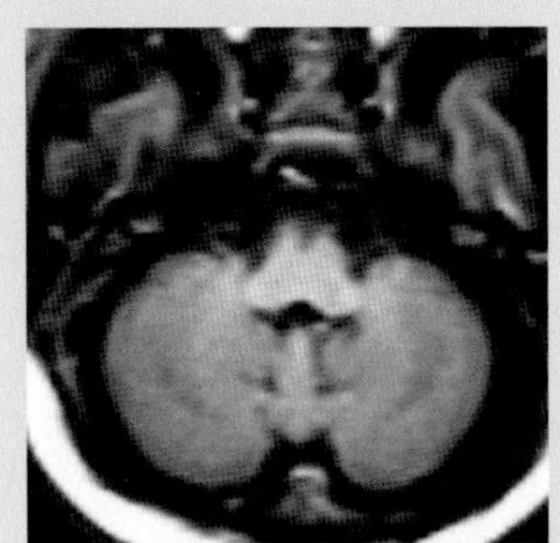

Fig. 4.37.32: Normal myelination T1 hyperintensity at birth in medulla

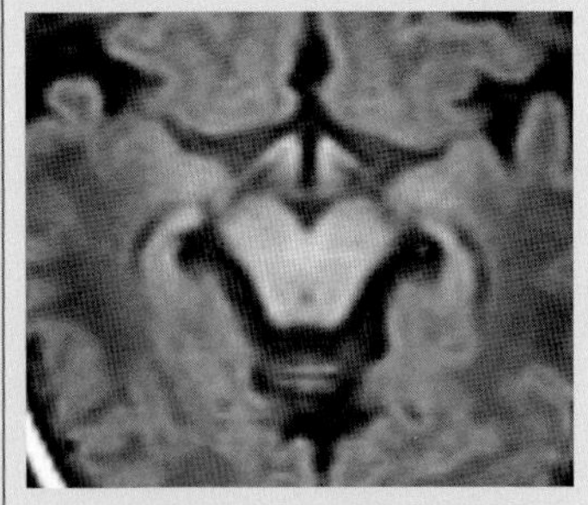

Fig. 4.37.33: Normal myelination T1 hyperintensity at birth in dorsal midbrain

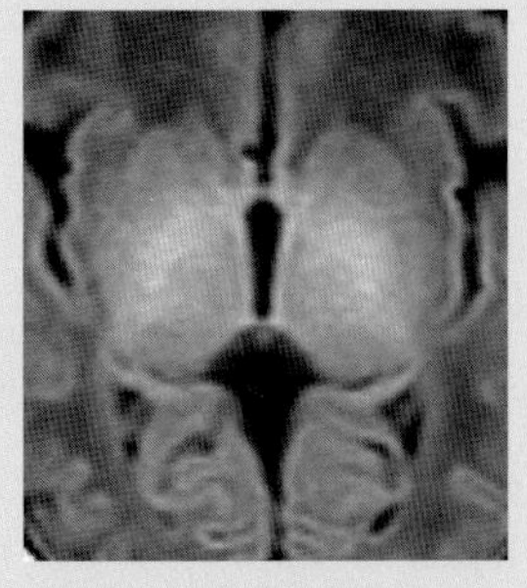

Fig. 4.37.34: Normal myelination T1 hyperintensity at birth in PLIC

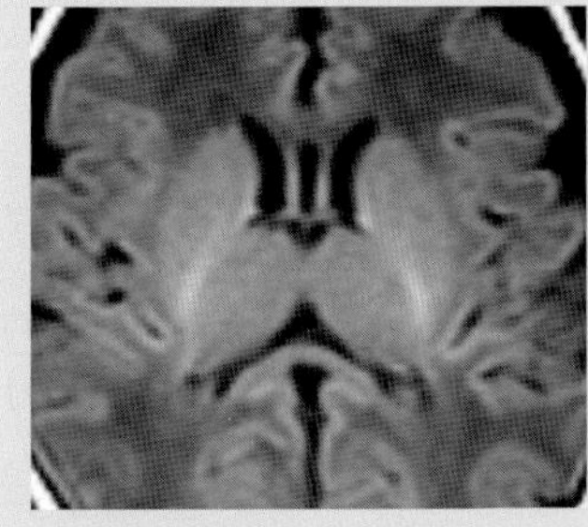

Fig. 4.37.35: Normal myelination T1 hyperintensity at birth in ventrolateral thalamus

Contd...

<table>
<tr><th colspan="4">Table 4.37.5: Normal myelination pictorial representation (Contd...)</th></tr>
<tr><td colspan="2">Age</td><td colspan="2">Normal myelination</td></tr>
<tr><td colspan="2">3 months (T1W–high signal, T2W–low signal)</td><td colspan="2">Deep cerebellar white matter, cerebellar folia, middle cerebellar peduncles, ventral brainstem, optic nerves, optic tracts, optic radiations, anterior limb of internal capsule, occipital subcortical white matter</td></tr>
<tr><td>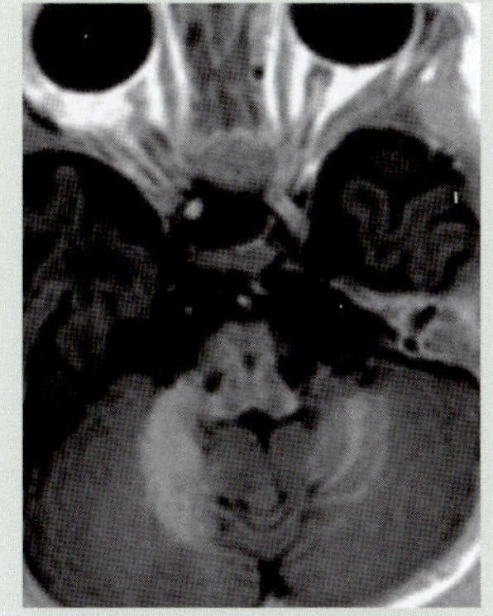
Fig. 4.37.36: Normal myelination T1 hyperintensity at 3 months in bilateral deep cerebellar white matter</td><td>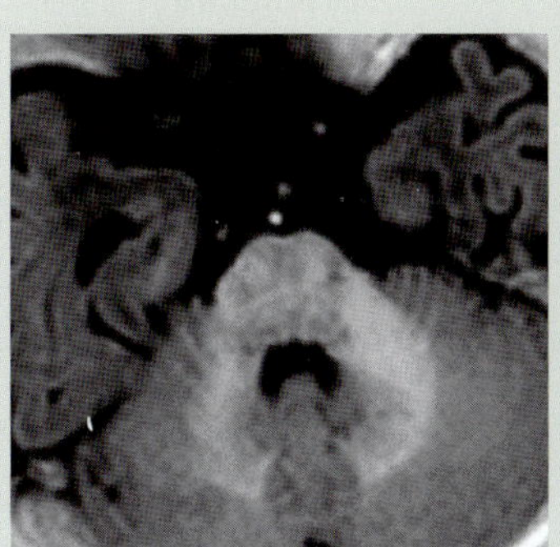
Fig. 4.37.37: Normal myelination T1 hyperintensity at 3 months in bilateral deep cerebellar white matter</td><td>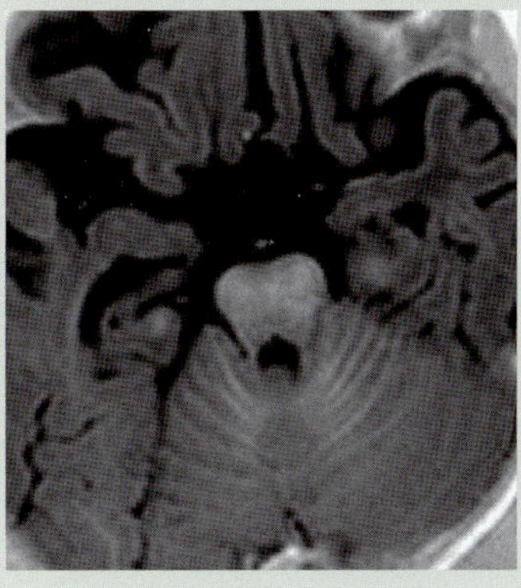
Fig. 4.37.38: Normal myelination T1 hyperintensity at 3 months in ventral brain stem and cerebellar folia</td><td>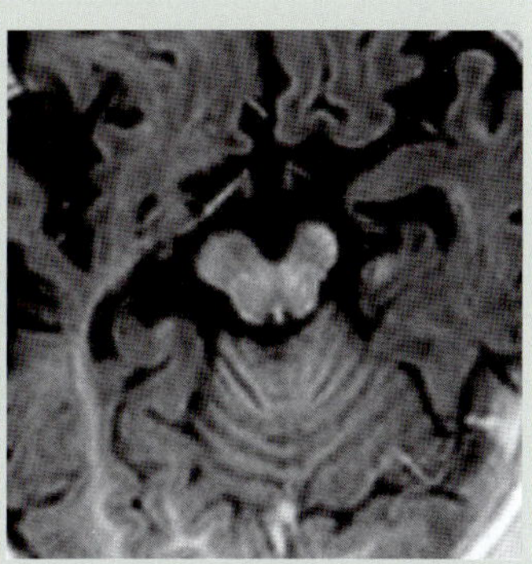
Fig. 4.37.39: Normal myelination T1 hyperintensity at 3 months ventral brain stem</td></tr>
<tr><td colspan="2">Normal myelination at 6 months
Splenium (4 months), genu (6 months), centrum semiovale, rostral subcortical white matter
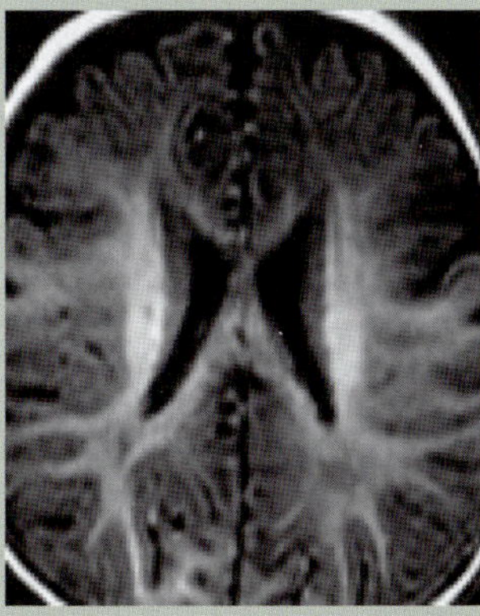
Fig. 4.37.40: Normal myelination at 6 months showing T1 hyperintensity in centrum semiovale, rostral subcortical WM</td><td colspan="2">Normal myelination at 10–12 months: Most of the central structures (dark centre and bright periphery on T2WI)
Subcortical U fibres (parietal and occipital fibres)
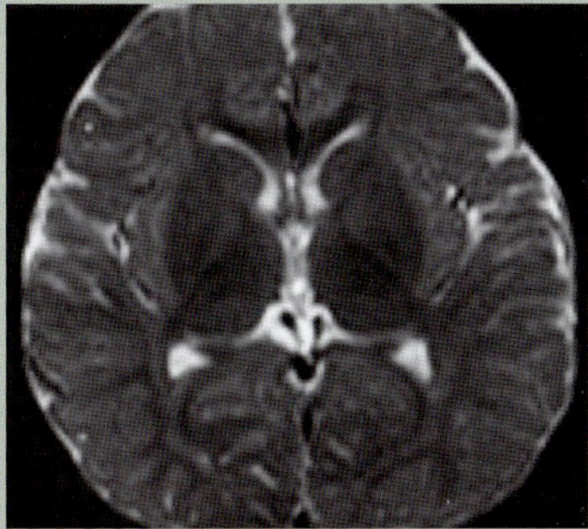
Fig. 4.37.41: Normal myelination at 12 months showing T2 hypointensity in subcortical U fibres</td></tr>
<tr><td>18–24 months—progressive myelination in internal capsule, corpus callosum, forceps minor, forceps major, subcortical white. By 24 months – essentially complete, identical to adult, terminal zones of myelination—occipital parietal periventricular white matter</td><td colspan="2">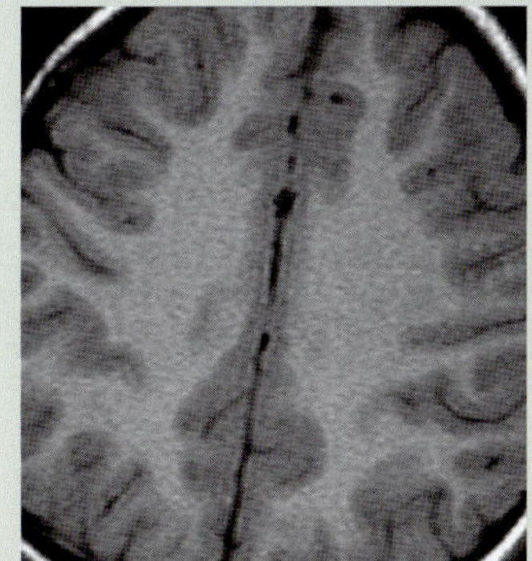
Fig. 4.37.42: Normal myelination at 24 months</td><td>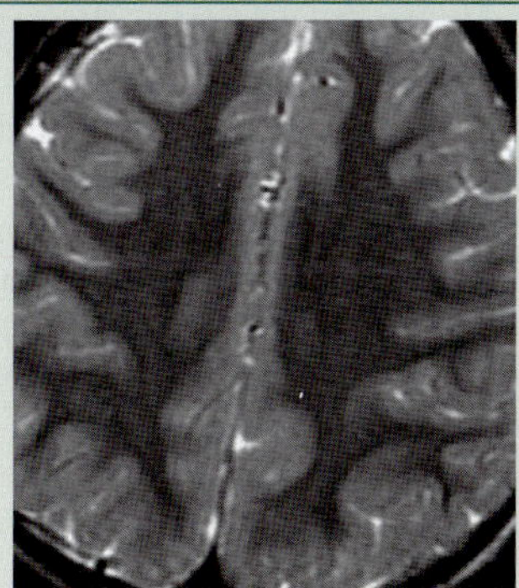
Fig. 4.37.43: Normal myelination at 18 months</td></tr>
</table>

Table 4.37.6: Normal myelination chart			
Area	*T1 (high signal)*	*T2 (low signal)*	*Flair (low signal)*
Dorsal brainstem (dorsal pons, midbrain and medulla)	Term birth	Term birth	4 months
Posterior limb internal capsule	Term birth	Term birth (only partial), completed by 3–4 months	4 months
Superior and inferior cerebellar peduncles	Term birth	Term birth	2 months
Ventrolateral thalamus	Term birth	Term birth	2 months
Perirolandic gyri	Term birth	Term birth	2 months
Brachium pontis	Term birth	2 months	4 months
Optic nerve	Term birth	2 months	6 months
Optic tract	Term birth	2 months	6 months
Optic radiation	Term birth	4 months	6 months
Ventral brainstem	3–4 months	6 months	6 months
Anterior limb of internal capsule	3–4 months	6 months	8 months
Splenium of corpus callosum	3–4 months	6 months	7 months
Central and posterior corona radiata	3–4 months	3–4 months	-
Deep occipital white matter	3–5 months	9–14 months	12 months
Subcortical occipital white matter	4–7 months	11–15 months	14 months
Deep midfrontal white matter	3–6 months	11–16 months	14 months
Subcortical midfrontal white matter	7–11 months	14–18 months	20 months
Deep anterior frontal white matter	5–8 months	12–18 months	14 months
Subcortical anterior frontal white matter	10–15 months	24–30 months	20 months
Centrum semiovale	3–4 months	7–11 months	6 months
Cerebellar white matter	6 months	12 months	
Genu of carpous callosum	6 months	7 months (starts)	6–8 months
Parietal and occipital white matter	6 months	6 months	-
Most of corona radiata	12 months	12 months	-
Posterior subcortical white matter	12 months	12 months	-
All white matter except temporal, frontal U-fibers	18 months	18 months	-
Anterior temporal, frontal U-fibers	24 months	24 months	22–25 months
Note: FLAIR has same pattern as T2 but lags behind somewhat. The exception is deep cerebral white matter, which begins as heterogeneously hypointense during the first few months of life.			
Approach to myelination disorders based on type of myelination disorder			
A. Arrested or highly delayed myelination: Pelizaeus-Merzbacher disease, Infantile-onset neuronal degenerative disorders; Infantile GM1 and GM2 gangliosidosis, infantile neuronal ceroid lipofuscinosis, Alpers disease, Menkes disease **B. Abnormal and irregular myelination:** Amino organic acidopathies, phenylketonuria, propionicacidemia, maple syrup urine disease, non-ketotic hyperglycemia, chromosomal abnormalities (e.g.,18q syndrome) **C. Hypomyelinating disorders most common:** Hypomyelination of unknown cause; 4H syndrome, Pelizaeus-Merzbacher disease, Pelizaeus-Merzbacher-like diseases, less common include hypomyelination with congenital cataract, GM2 gangliosidosis, Salla disease (sialuria), fucosidosis, Cockayne syndrome, GM1gangliosidosis, hypomyelination with atrophy of the basal ganglia and cerebellum. Rare-18q-syndrome; Cockayne syndrome, trichothiodystrophies (brittle, sulfur-deficient hair)			

4.38 CENTRAL NERVOUS SYSTEM

Case No. 38

Clinical history: A 7-years-old male child presented with history of fever for 2 days and seizure 2 episodes. On examination, neck stiffness seen. No previous history of seizure. Normal developmental milestones up to age. Birth history normal. No history of open contact with tuberculosis.

Radiographic technique and observation: Figures 4.38.1 to 4.38.3 are T1W post-contrast axial and sagittal images showing conglomerate ring enhancing lesions in the suprasellar and left sylvian cisterns. Wall of the lesion appears irregular with no evidence of mural nodule or perilesional edema.

Leptomeningeal enhancement involving the chiasmatic and sylvian cisterns predominantly in the basal cisterns. No evidence of hydrocephalus and no features of vasculitis—infarcts or haemorrhage. Pituitary stalk not clearly visualised. No evidence of abnormal cranial nerve enhancement.

Interpretation: A—7-year-old male child, lesion in suprasellar and left sylvian cistern, C—ring enhancing lesion with B—leptomeningeal enhancement, D— tuberculous meningitis with meningeal granuloma.

Diagnosis: Tuberculous meningitis with meningeal granuloma.

Differential diagnosis: Leptomeningeal metastasis and neurosarcoidosis.

Discussion: Meningeal enhancement can be Pachy meningeal (dural) and leptomeningeal (pia and arachnoid). Normally some degree of dural enhancement is seen in falx, tentorium and cavernous sinus. Normal dura mater, which is extra axial nonneural connective tissue, does not have blood–brain barrier. The arachnoid matter provides the layer with barrier function that prevents the movement of fluid across it. The pia is highly vascular, connective tissue envelope surrounding the brain and spinal cord. The dura mater formed by fusion of the periosteum of the inner table of the skull and a meningeal layer, is called pachymeninges (thick meninges). The dural reflections of the tentorium cerebelli, falx cerebri, cavernous sinus and falx cerebelli is seen as pachy meningeal enhancement. The pia and arachnoid are leptomeninges (thin meninges). Leptomeningeal enhancement is seen in subarachnoid region. The pachy meningeal pattern of enhancement is also known as dura-arachnoid enhancement because the usual, thin arachnoid membrane is connected to the inner surface of the dura mater. Pial or pia-arachnoid enhancement, on the other hand, refers to enhancement on the brain's surface. The enhancement can be seen along the pial surface of the brain, filling the sulci and cisterns' subarachnoid spaces. This pattern is known as leptomeningeal augmentation and is often described as "gyriform" or "serpentine" in appearance. **Normal meningeal enhancement pattern** is thin (maximum 2 mm), smooth, discontinuous. Best detected on coronal MR sequences, marked in the anterior portion of temporal lobe, parasagittal, and at sites of dural reflection of the superior sagittal sinus.

Tuberculous meningitis caused by mycobacterium tuberculosis, most common clinical manifestation is fever, headache, vomiting and neck stiffness. Cranial nerve palsies of 3rd, 4th and 6th nerves are seen, seizure, focal neurological deficit, stupor and coma seen in late

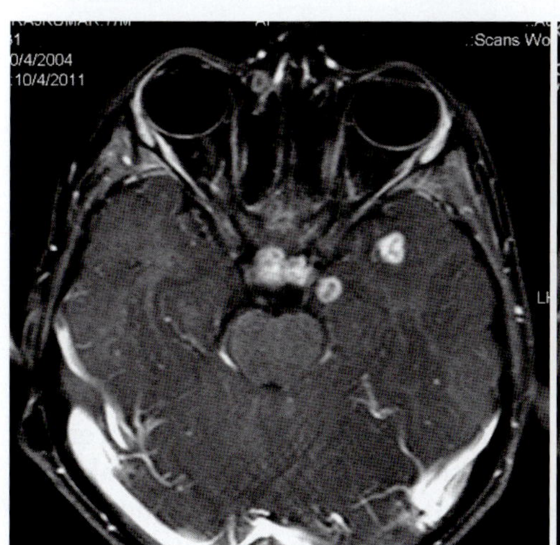

Fig. 4.38.1

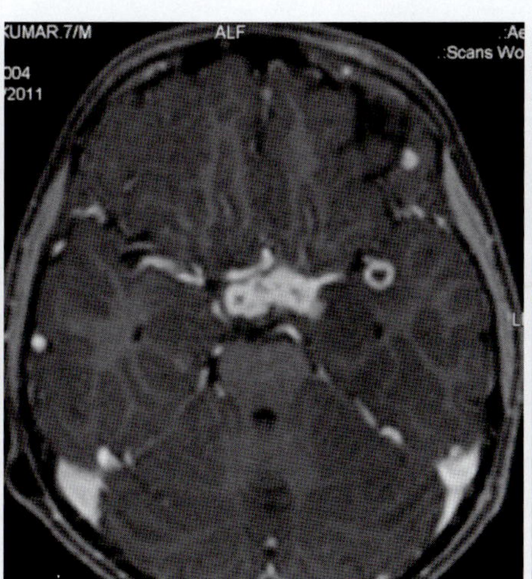

Fig. 4.38.2

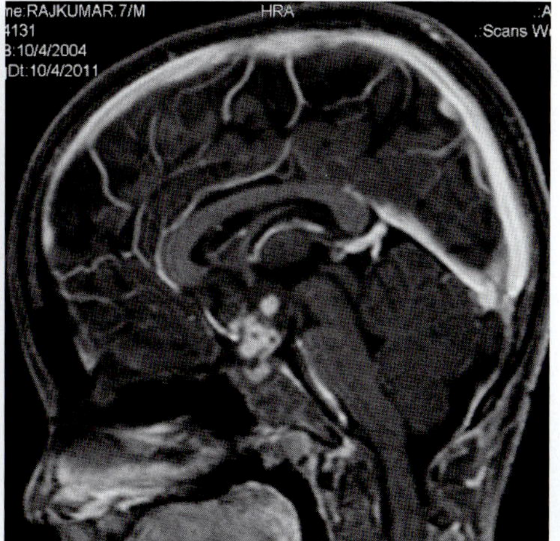

Fig. 4.38.3

Table 4.38.1: Differential diagnosis of leptomeningeal enhancement		
Leptomeningeal metastasis: Other synonyms include meningeal carcinomatosis, neoplastic meningitis and carcinomatous meningitis, most common extra cranial primary tumor causing leptomeningeal enhancement are breast and small cell carcinoma of lung.	Patient known case of lung cancer. Gadolinium enhanced T1W MRI shows thick and lumpy enhancement of bilateral cerebellar folia	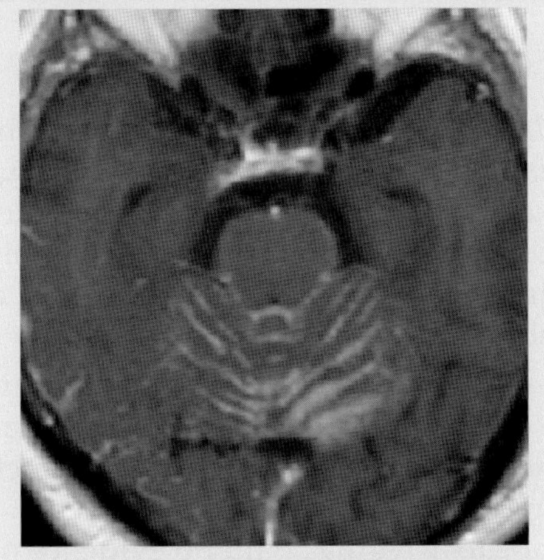 Fig. 4.38.4: Leptomeningeal metastasis
Neurosarcoidosis: Central nervous system involvement is usually seen in 20% of patient with systemic sarcoidosis. More common age group is 30–40 years of age with a female predilection. Infiltration of pituitary gland, infundibulum and hypothalamus is common. The most common presentation is cranial nerve deficit mainly optic and facial nerves are affected.	Chiasmatic and sylvian cistern enhancement with pituitary stalk enhancement. Linear/nodular leptomeningeal enhancement, cranial nerve enhancement most commonly seen.	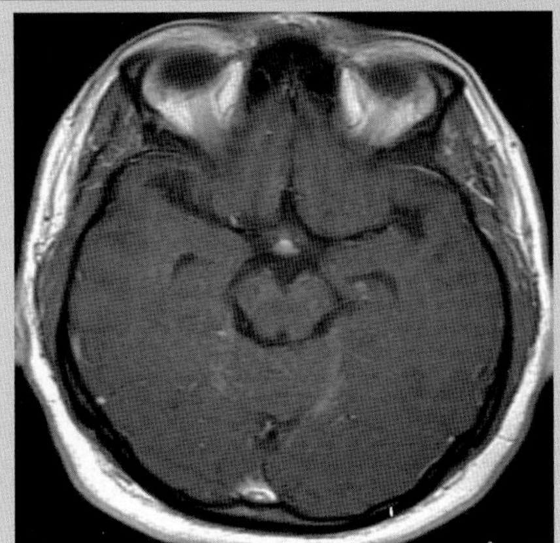 Fig. 4.38.5: Neurosarcoidosis
Other DD: Racemose type of NCC	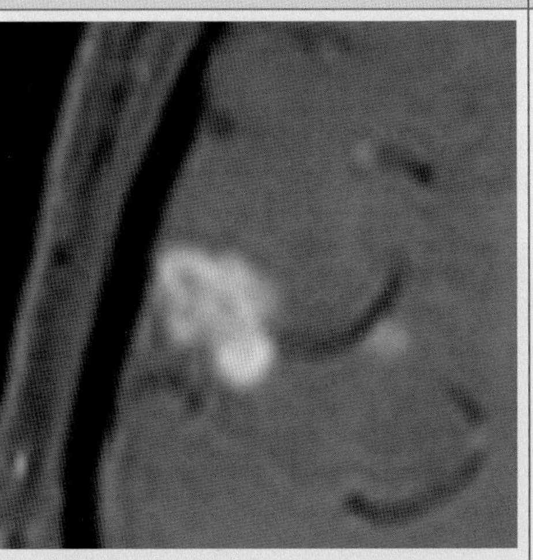 Fig. 4.38.6: Racemose type of NCC	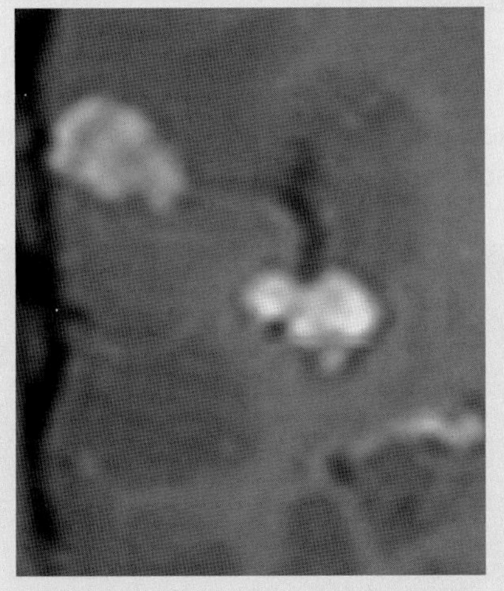 Fig. 4.38.7: Racemose type of NCC

stages. CSF analysis reveals lymphocytosis, increased protein level and decreased glucose levels. Nonspecific hydrocephalus is the most frequent finding on non-contrast CT. Contrast-enhanced CT shows intense enhancement of basilar meninges and subarachnoid space. Marked nodular leptomeningeal enhancement seen on T1 post-contrast. **CT criteria of abnormal basal meningeal enhancement** Y-shaped enhancement at the junction of the suprasellar and middle cerebral artery cisterns, obliteration by contrast of the CSF spaces

Table 4.38.2: Causes of abnormal meningeal enhancement	
Diffuse	*Focal*
Post-operative, meningeal infections, carcinomatous meningitis, subarachnoid haemorrhage, sarcoidosis, histiocytosis, idiopathic pachymeningitis, dural thrombosis, intracranial hypotension.	Meningioma, postoperative, metastasis, sarcoidosis, histiocytosis, rheumatoid nodules, arteriovenous malformation, lymphoma. Post-ictal, post-op scar, neurosyphilis, Sturge-Weber

Table 4.38.3: Causes of patterns of enhancement in brain coverings		
Pachy meningeal enhancement (dural arachnoid enhancement)	*Leptomeningeal enhancement (pia-arachnoid enhancement)*	*Ependymal enhancement*
1. Skull base osteomyelitis 2. Meningioma and lymphoma Metastasis (especially breast in women and prostate in men) 3. Following lumbar puncture 4. Intracranial hypotension (venous congestion), intracranial inflammatory pseudotumors—idiopathic, chronic DST, IgG4 related 5. Hypertrophic pachymeningitis show Eiffel-by-night sign due to falco-tentorial dura enhancement 6. Venous thrombosis—chronic DST 7. Granulomatosis with polyangiitis (Wegener's) Chronic granulomatous diseases 8. Extramedullary haematopoiesis 9. Rheumatoid arthritis 10. Sarcoidosis	1. All types of infection 2. Metastasis—breast and small cell lung cancer Diffuse leptomeningeal glioneuronal tumour 3. Meningeal carcinomatosis Meningeal seeding of primary brain tumour 4. Leukaemia and lymphoma Infarct–surface enhancement 5. Subarachnoid haemorrhage in subacute phase 6. Pial angioma of Sturge weber syndrome 7. Sarcoidosis (most common lepto around base of brain) 8. Rheumatoid arthritis 9. Neurocutaneous melanosis-meningeal melanomatosis - mimic	1. Infection—ventriculitis (early sign of bacterial ventriculitis), CMV, VZV, immunocompromised 2. Neoplastic-nodular—lymphoma, glioblastoma, metastasis Mass like-ependymoma, giant cell astrocytoma 3. Granulomatous–TB (basal meningitis), sarcoidosis (cranial nerve and dura) 4. Intraventricular hemorrhage 5. Subependymal venous congestion a) deep CVT, b) AVM, c) Sturge-Weber syndrome
Fig. 4.38.8: Pachymeningeal enhancement	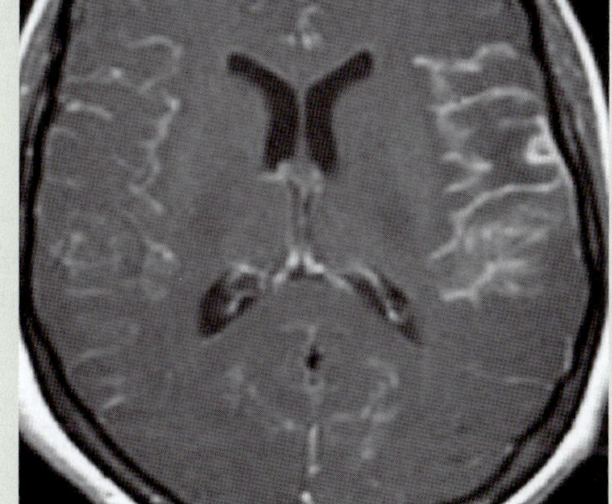 **Fig. 4.38.9:** Leptomeningeal enhancement	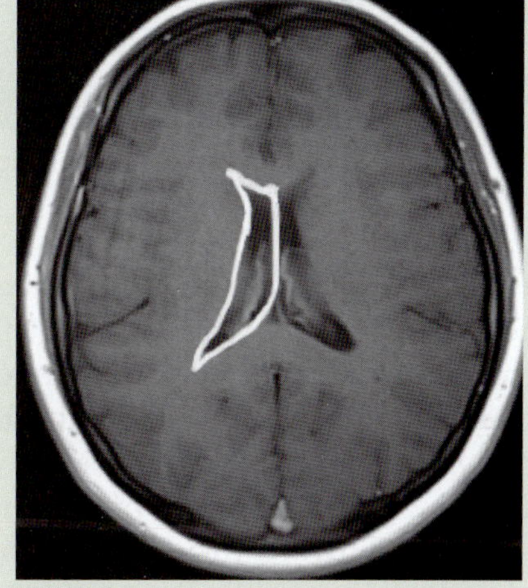 **Fig. 4.38.10:** Ependymal enhancement

around normal/vascular enhancement and linear contrast enhancement of the middle cerebral artery cisterns.

Treatment of tuberculous meningitis is rifampicin and isoniazid for 12 months and ethambutol and pyrazinamide for 2 months.

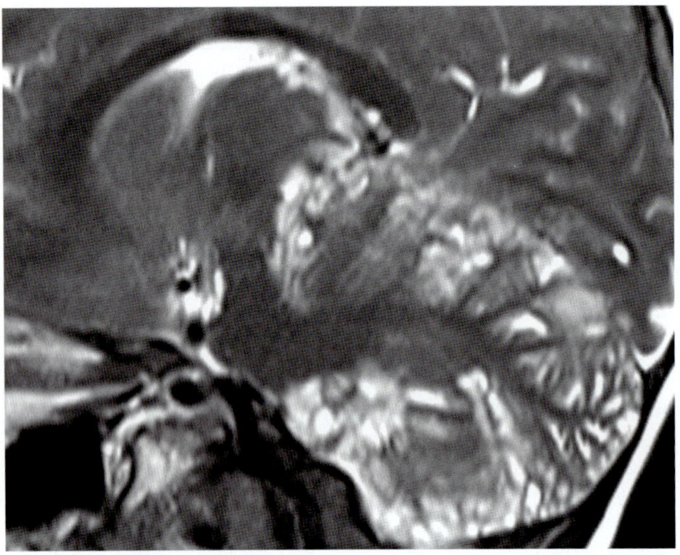

Fig. 4.38.11: Leptomeningeal oligodendroglioma

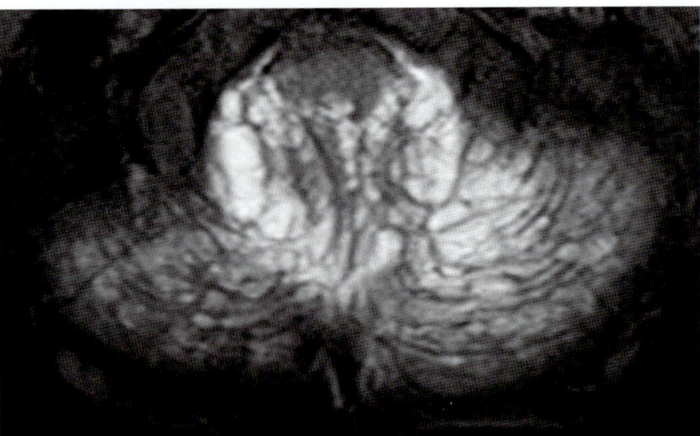

Fig. 4.38.13: Leptomeningeal oligodendroglioma

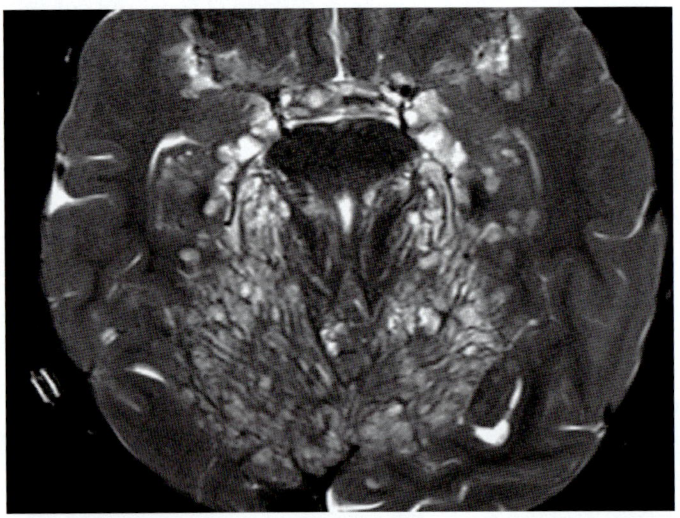

Fig. 4.38.12: Leptomeningeal oligodendroglioma

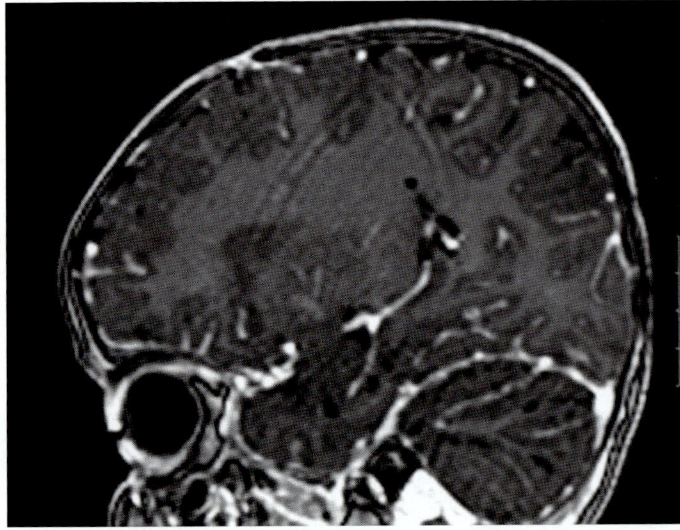

Fig. 4.38.14: Leptomeningeal oligodendroglioma

Idiopathic intracranial hypotension: The findings include, postural headache that worsens when upright, thick linear pachymeningeal enhancement, no enhancement of the sulci or brain surface, enhancement above and below the tentorium, enlargement of the pituitary gland, descent of the brain (low cerebellar tonsils, downward displacement of the third ventricle below the incisural line), and subdural effusions/SDH.

Leptomeningeal oligodendroglioma—also called diffuse leptomeningeal glioneuronal tumor thick nodular leptomeningeal enhancement in Basal cisterns and over brain surface.

Rosai-Dorfman disease: Sinus histiocytosis with massive lymphadenopathy, bilateral cervical lymphadenopathy and intracranial intensely enhancing dural-based mass.

Table 4.38.4: Causes of pachymeningeal and leptomeningeal enhancement with their various enhancement patterns

Meningeal enhancement			
Pachymeningeal		Leptomeningeal	
Pattern		Pattern	
1. *Smooth linear*	2. *Irregular and Nodular*	1. *Linear/curvilinear*	2. *Ring/nodular*
Intracranial hypotension (postlumbar puncture, over shunting, skull base leak, spinal leak), chronic subdural haematoma, post-operative status, Idiopathic Hypertrophic pachymeningitis	Metastasis, lymphoma skull base osteomyelitis Solitary fibrous tumor of dura Granulomatous diseases–TB/ sarcoidosis/syphilis, fungal disease	Thin linear–meningoencephalitis: TB, viral meningitis, breast cancer Thick linear: Bacterial meningitis AIDP, CIDP Pial angioma of Sturge-Weber	Carcinomatosis—metastatic (breast, lung), lymphoma, ependymoma, germinoma, medulloblastoma, glioblastoma, pineoblastoma. Rheumatoid nodule, Wegner's, TB
Fig. 4.38.15: Smooth linear pachymeningeal enhancement	**Fig. 4.38.16:** Irregular and nodular pachymeningeal enhancement	**Fig. 4.38.17:** Linear leptomeningeal enhancement	**Fig. 4.38.18:** Nodular leptomeningeal enhancement

Table 4.38.5: Causes of abnormal meninges enhancement in spinal cord

Spinal cord						
Leptomeningeal metastasis		*Ependymoma*	*Subdural abscess*	*Epidural abscess*	*Nerve root*	
Zuckerguss	*Ice caking*	Intense nodular enhancement	Diffuse dural and subdural enhancement	Diffuse dural enhancement	*AIDP*	*CIDP*
Linear sheet like enhancement	Diffuse enhancement				Smooth pial enhancement	Diffuse pial enhancement

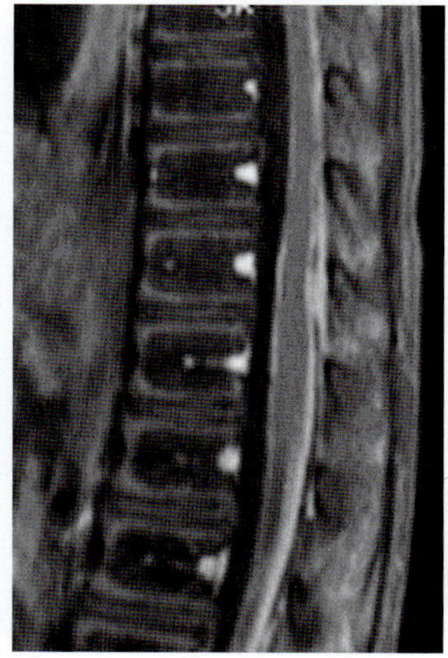

Fig. 4.38.19: Zuckerguss appearance—leptomeningeal metastasis

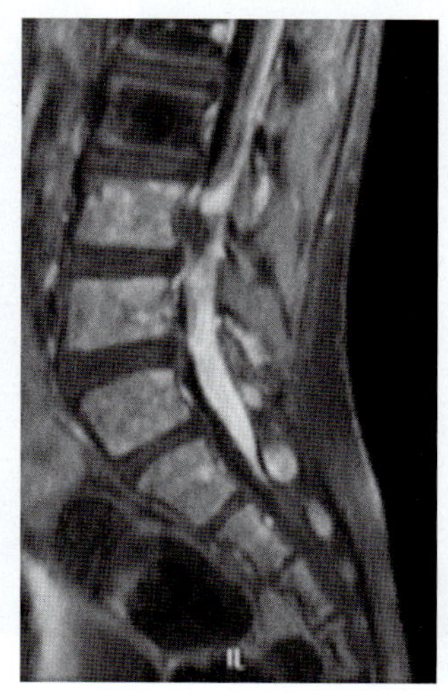

Fig. 4.38.20: Ice caking appearance—leptomeningeal metastasis

4.39 CENTRAL NERVOUS SYSTEM

Case No. 39

Clinical history: A 38-year-old male with history of headache, vomiting, low grade fever and one episode of seizure.

Radiological techniques and observations: Figures 4.39.1 to 4.39.4 are MRI plain and contrast study of brain with selected axial images in T2, DWI, and coronal FLAIR sequence images respectively showing well-defined round T2/FLAIR hypointense lesion (>2 cm) in the right cerebellar hemisphere with surrounding edema causing mass effect over the fourth ventricle. The margins appear smooth. No evidence of fluid intensity in the lesion. Similar T2/FLAIR hypointense lesions seen in right posterior parietal lobe and right anterior temporal lobe. No DWI restriction noted. Further MR contrast study shows thin **smooth complete ring enhancement** of the lesion in right cerebellar hemisphere. No evidence of nodular or internal enhancing component. No evidence of prominent feeding vessel. No lepto/pachy meningeal enhancement. Figure 4.39.5 is MRS intermediate TE (TE-135 ms) study showing **elevated** peak at **0.9 and 1.3 ppm.**

Interpretation: A: 38 years old male, lesion in right cerebellum C: Multiple T2 hypointense lesions with B: Smooth ring enhancement in the right cerebellar hemisphere, right posterior parietal and right anterior temporal lobe likely to be granulomatous lesion. In MRS there is lipid peak which favours tuberculous etiology, D: CNS tuberculoma.

Principal diagnosis: **CNS tuberculoma.**

Ring enhancing lesions in brain may be single, multiple, unilocular or multilocular.

Differentials for ring enhancing CNS lesions include infection: Parasitic—neurocysticercosis, toxoplasmosis; Bacterial—tuberculoma, pyogenic abscess; Fungal—histoplasma, aspergillosis, nocardiosis

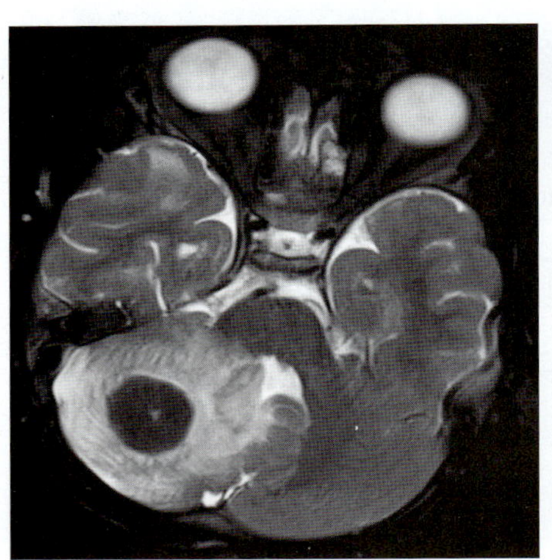

Fig. 4.39.1

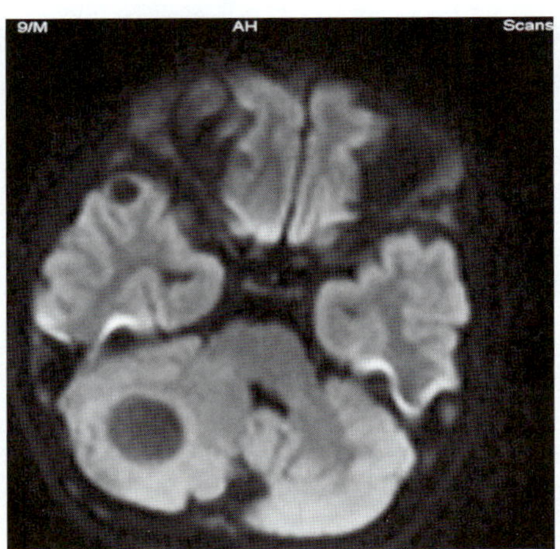

Fig. 4.39.2

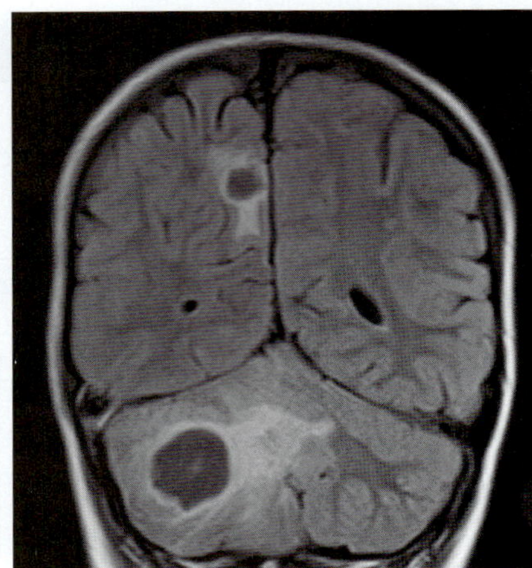

Fig. 4.39.3

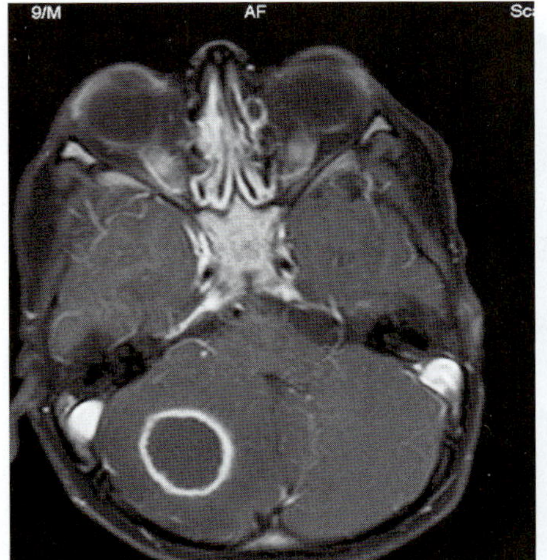

Fig. 4.39.4

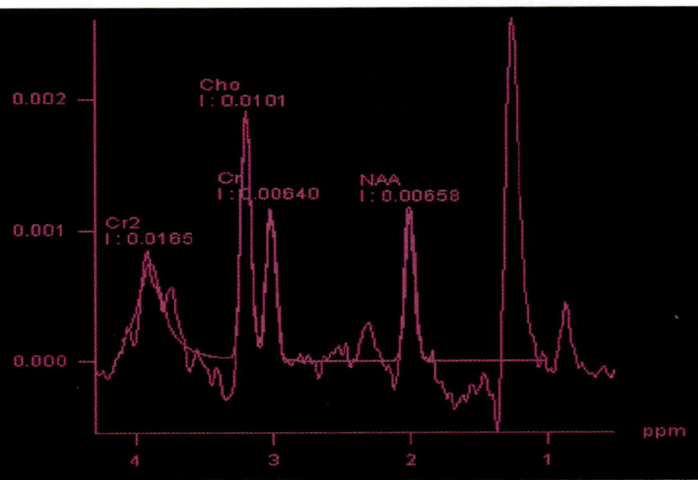

Fig. 4.39.5

1. Neoplastic—primary brain tumors, metastasis, primary CNS lymphoma in HIV
2. Demyelination—multiple sclerosis, tumefactive demyelination (incomplete rings)

Others—subacute infarct, resolving hematoma, cavernous haemangioma, radiation necrosis, aneurysm with central thrombus, postoperative, ADEM, sarcoidosis.

Table 4.39.1: Differential diagnosis for ring enhancing lesions

Neurocysticercosis caused by the CNS infection with the pork tapeworm *Taenia solium*. There is no gender or race predilection and most symptomatic patients are aged 15–40 years. Most common symptom and the most common cause of seizures in young adults. Infection can be both intra- and extra-axial. Albendazole and praziquantel, the two antiparasitic with steroids are commonly used for treatment.	On MRI, the wall of the cysticercus granuloma (a colloid cyst stage) becomes **thick and hypointense and there is marked perilesional edema on T2 weighted images.** The lesion shows a ring pattern of enhancement. Usually, the lesions are <20 mm in diameter. **Calcified eccentric scolex** is also often seen. The lesions are often multiple and most often do not have peri lesional oedema. Most common location, frequently seen near the **grey matter–white matter junction.**	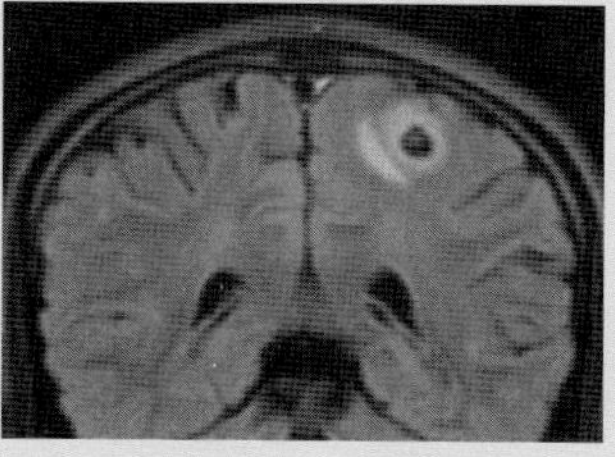 **Fig. 4.39.6:** Neurocysticercosis 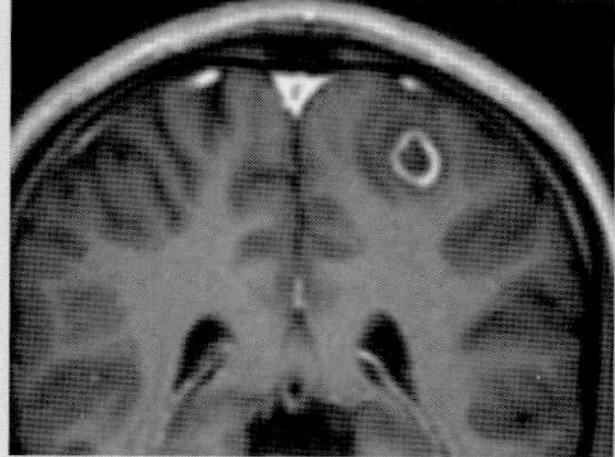 **Fig. 4.39.7:** Neurocysticercosis
Pyogenic abscess: Can occur in all age groups. Early cerebritis, late cerebritis, early abscess/ encapsulation may occur 10 days after infection, late abscess/ encapsulation may occur >14 days after infection. Focal neurological deficit seizures, raised ICT are common clinical features. Neurosurgical intervention and decompression craniotomy is mainstay of treatment along with IV antibiotics. 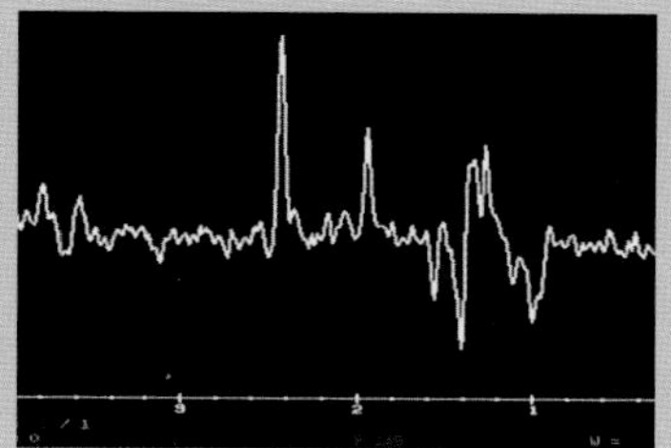 **Fig. 4.39.8:** MRS in anaerobic pyogenic abscess	The lesions are commonly located at the grey–white matter junction. Non-contrast MRI shows an isointense to slightly hyper-intense capsule on T1 weighted images. The ring enhancement on post-contrast images is usually **thin and smooth** and often thinner along the medial margin. The lesion appears **very bright in T2 and shows diffusion restriction.** Marked perilesional edema is seen. **MRS:** Cytosolic amino acids (0.9 ppm), lactate and lipids (1.3 ppm), acetate (1.9 ppm), succinate (2.4 ppm). Only anaerobic abscesses have succinate and acetate.	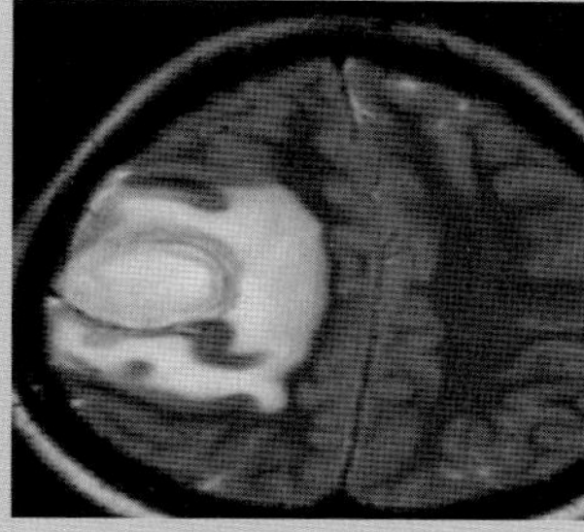 **Fig. 4.39.9:** Pyogenic abscess 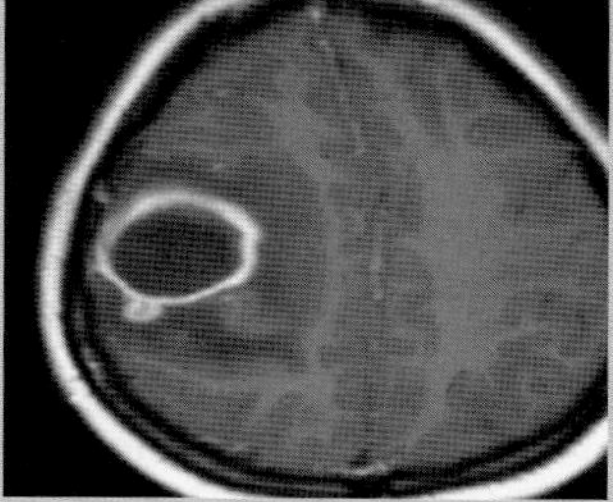 **Fig. 4.39.10:** Pyogenic abscess 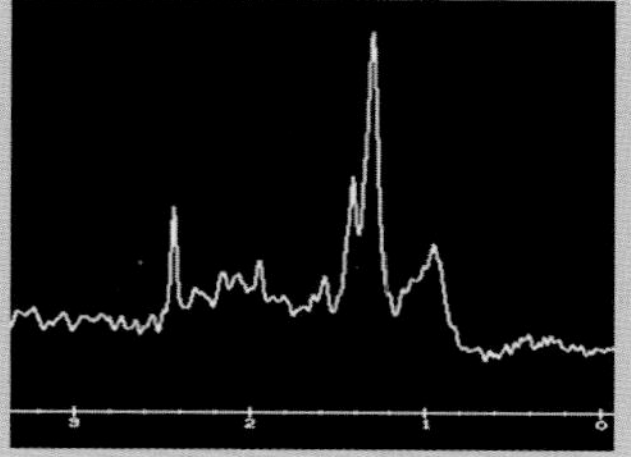 **Fig. 4.39.11:** MRS in pyogenic abscess

(Contd.)

<table>
<tr><th colspan="6">Table 4.39.1: Differential diagnosis for ring enhancing lesions (Contd.)</th></tr>
<tr><td colspan="3">CNS lymphoma: Primary CNS lymphomas (PCNSL) are relatively uncommon tumors, accounting for 2.5% of all brain tumors. By definition, there is no co-existing systemic disease at the time of diagnosis, distinguishing it from CNS involvement from systemic lymphoma (secondary CNS lymphoma). Symptoms and signs of raised intracranial pressure, focal neurological disorders and seizures. Treatment is predominantly with steroids (which can dramatically shrink a tumor due to combined anti-edema and cytotoxic effects) and methotrexate-based chemotherapy, whole brain irradiation.</td><td colspan="3">MRI shows typically hypointense to grey matter in T1 weighted images. In T1 post-contrast, typical high-grade tumours show intense homogeneous enhancement while low-grade tumours have absent to moderate enhancement. Peripheral ring enhancement may be seen in immunocompromised patients (HIV/AIDS). Thallium-201 scintigraphy. PET 18 FDG PET, carbon-11 methionine. PET shows increased uptake. Present as solitary (60–70%) or multiple (30–40%) lesions with a predilection for the periventricular white matter.
Tall lipid peak is also seen in a few cases of CNS lymphoma that mimics tuberculoma. DWI is problem solving in such cases.</td></tr>
<tr><td colspan="2">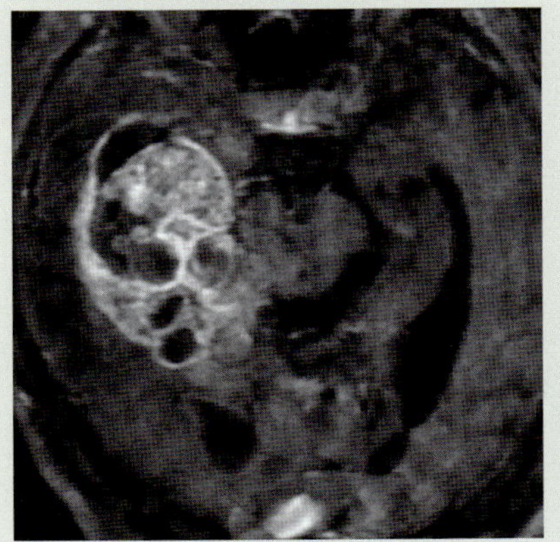
Fig. 4.39.12: Peripheral enhancement in lymphoma</td><td colspan="2">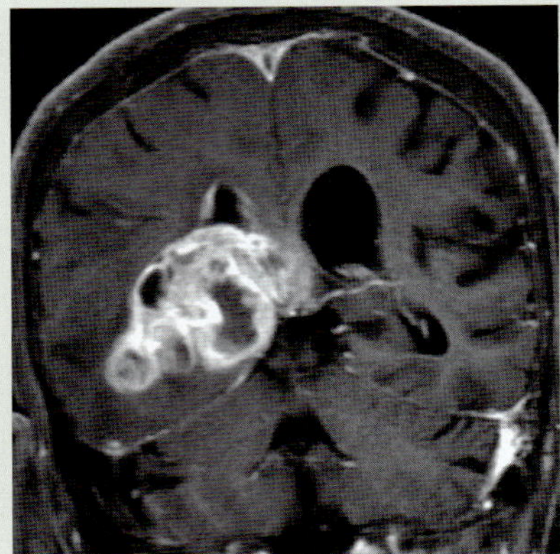
Fig. 4.39.13: Peripheral enhancement in lymphoma</td><td colspan="2">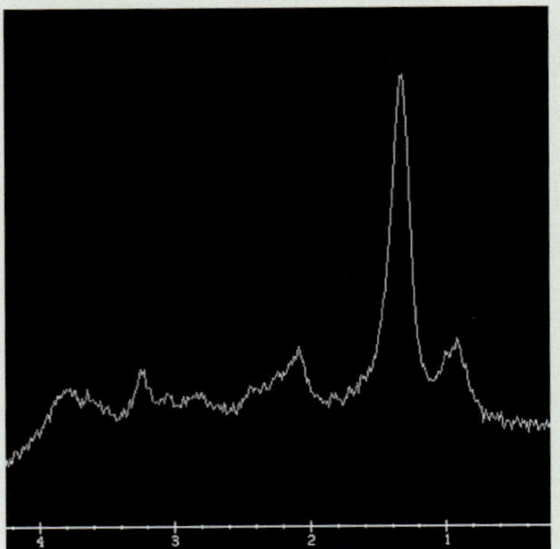

Fig. 4.39.14: Tall lipid peak in CNS lymphoma</td></tr>
<tr><td colspan="2">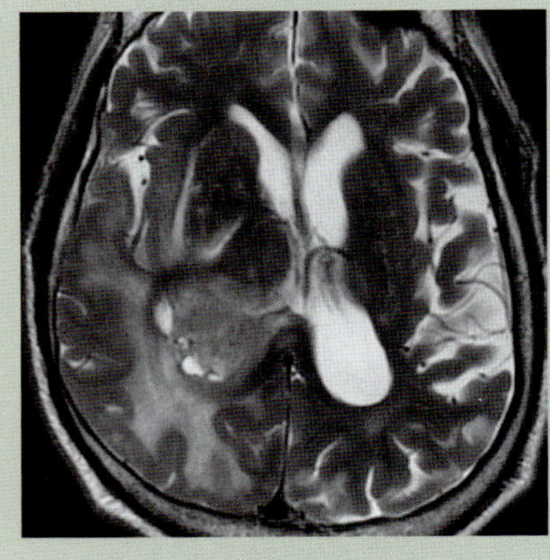
Fig. 4.39.15: CNS lymphoma</td><td colspan="2">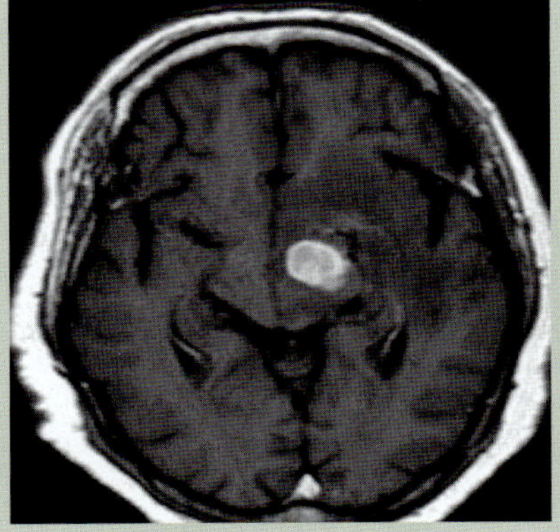
Fig. 4.39.16: CNS lymphoma</td><td colspan="2">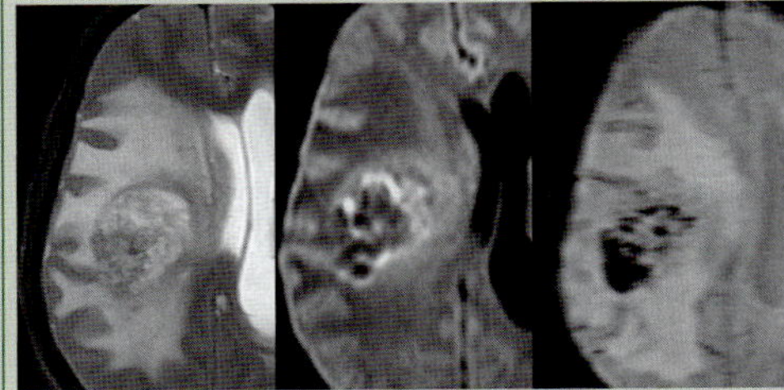
Fig. 4.39.17: Fungal abscess</td></tr>
<tr><td colspan="6">Demyelination—multiple sclerosis, tumefactive demyelination—also sometimes referred to as mono focal acute inflammatory demyelination (MAID)—Refer to case 25 for detailed explanation</td></tr>
<tr><td colspan="3">Neurotoxoplasmosis: Neurotoxoplasmosis is a common cerebral opportunistic infection in patients with HIV.
Immunocompromised patient is presented with headache and altered sensorium. Pathologically a central avascular zone of coagulative necrosis, an intermediate vascular zone containing numerous organisms and an outermost zone of encysted organisms. Toxoplasma lesions do not have a capsule. Treatment consists of sulfadiazine with pyrimethamine.</td><td colspan="3">Predilection for the basal ganglia, thalami, and corticomedullary junction. MRI of brain shows multiple T2 hyperintense lesions in bilateral frontoparietal regions and basal ganglia with minimal surrounding edema. Post-gadolinium MRI shows multiple ring enhancing rings with "eccentric target sign" (pea in pod sign) consisting of an eccentric nodule along the rim of an enhancing lesion which is considered pathognomonic. In MR spectroscopy elevated lipid-lactate at 1.3 ppm and choline peak at 3.2 ppm is seen.</td></tr>
</table>

(Contd.)

Table 4.39.1: Differential diagnosis for ring enhancing lesions (*Contd.*)

<table>
<tr><td>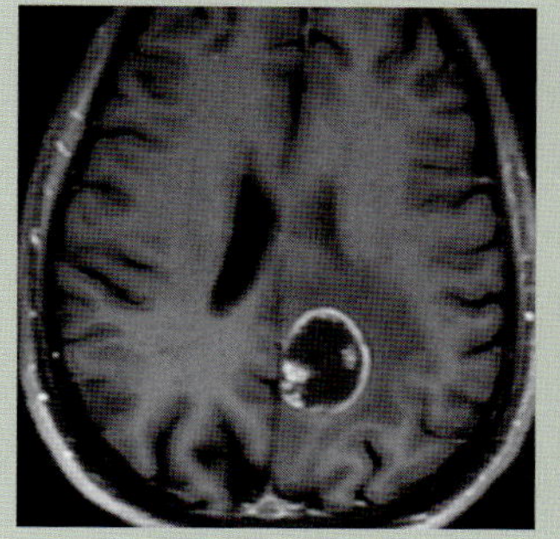
Fig. 4.39.18: Neuro-toxoplasmosis</td><td>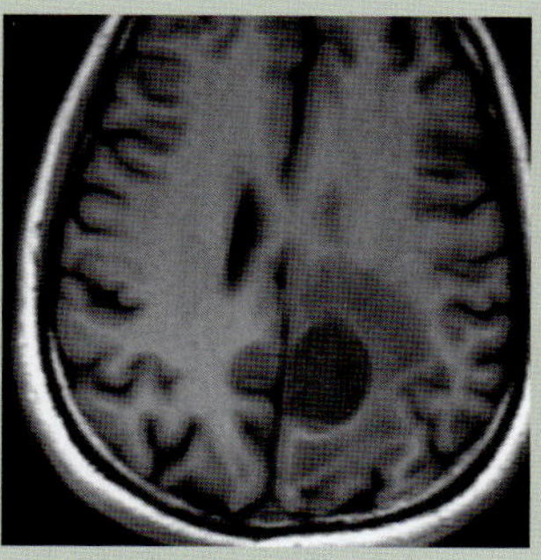
Fig. 4.39.19: Neuro-toxoplasmosis</td><td>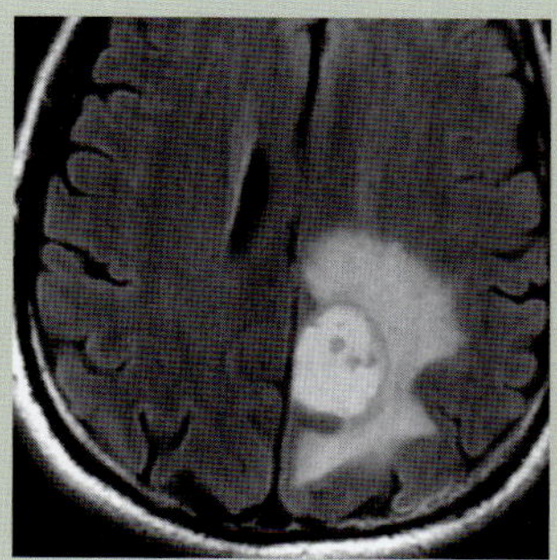
Fig. 4.39.20: Neuro-toxoplasmosis</td><td>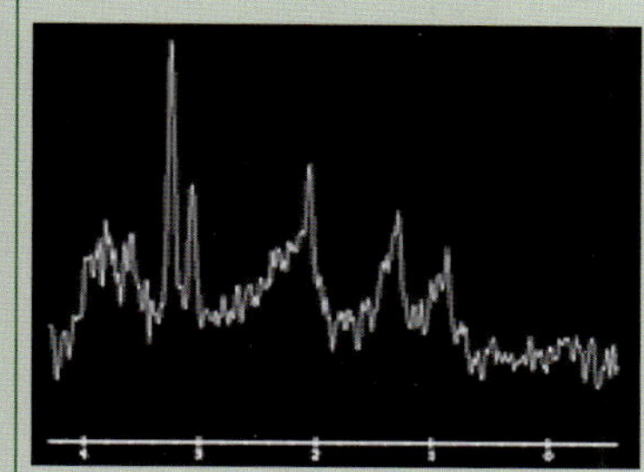
Fig. 4.39.21: MRS showing choline and lipid lactate peak in neurotoxoplasmosis</td></tr>
<tr><td>Brain metastasis: Intracranial metastasis can occur in up to 15–40% of cancer patients. It is most commonly associated with cancers of the lung, breast, kidney, thyroid, melanoma, colon, etc. They may be solitary or multiple. Solitary brain metastasis occurs in approximately 40–50% of the cases.</td><td>MRI of brain showed a solitary T2 hyper-intense lesion with a hypointense periphery in right parietal region at the GM-WM junction with significant disproportionate surrounding edema. Post-gadolinium administration, the lesion showed ring enhancement. MR spectroscopy shows elevated choline at 3.2 ppm</td><td colspan="2">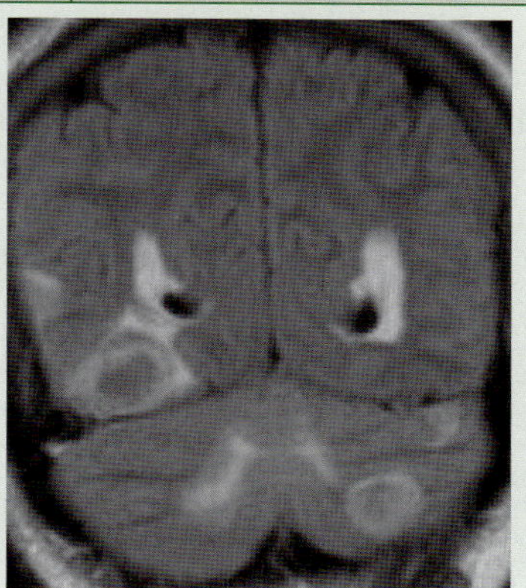
Fig. 4.39.22: Brain metastasis</td></tr>
<tr><td>Glioblastoma multiforme: Most glioblastomas arise without evidence of any precursor lesion after a short clinical course of approximately 3 months. 9–11% of the GBM are secondary (progressing from a low grade tumor, IDH mutated). The mean age of patients with primary glioblastoma is 55 years, whereas secondary GBM are found in a younger population.</td><td>MRI of brain showed a strong T2 hyperintense lesion in right parietal region with significant surrounding edema. Post-gadolinium MR shows irregular nodular ring enhancement in the lesion with central necrotic area was noted. GRE sequence showed areas of hemorrhage at the periphery with increased rCBV at the periphery of the lesion on MR perfusion. MR spectroscopy showed elevated choline peak at 3.2 ppm.</td><td colspan="2">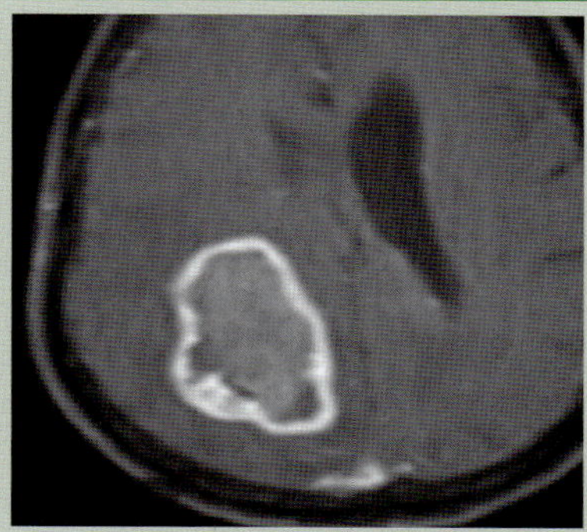
Fig. 4.39.23: Glioblastoma multiforme
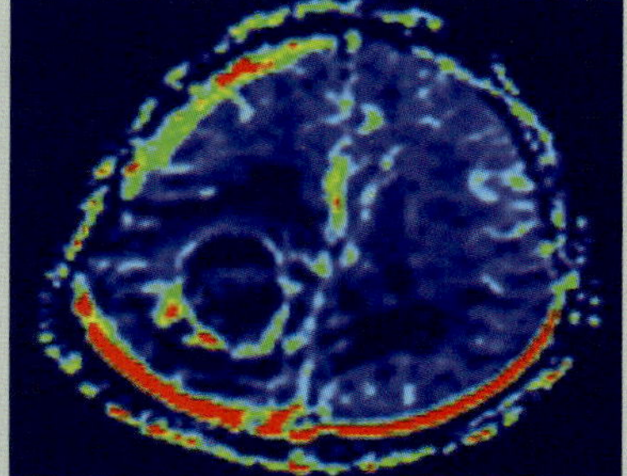
Fig. 4.39.24: Glioblastoma multiforme–Grade 4 astrocytoma</td></tr>
</table>

(*Contd.*)

Table 4.39.1: Differential diagnosis for ring enhancing lesions (*Contd.*)

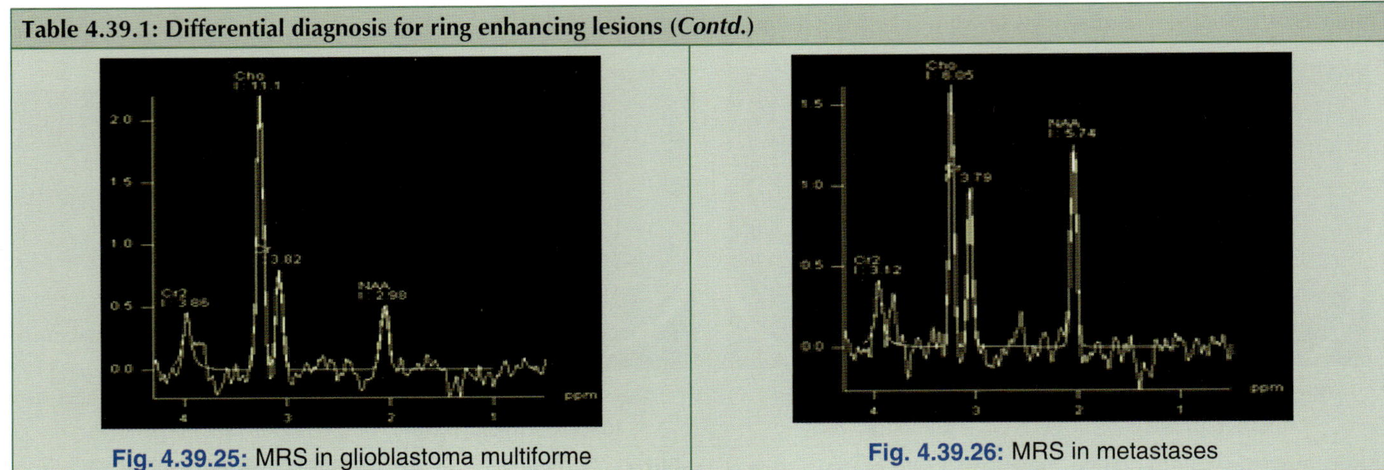

Fig. 4.39.25: MRS in glioblastoma multiforme

Fig. 4.39.26: MRS in metastases

Both MRS in GBM and metastasis shows elevation of choline peak at 3.2 ppm and decreased NAA at 2.0 ppm, the difference is GBM which shows choline peak and decreased NAA at perilesional edema but metastasis will not show.

Table 4.39.2: Difference between neurocysticercosis and tuberculoma

Neurocysticercosis	*Tuberculoma*
Lesions are smaller (<20 mm)—may be single or multiple. May be conglomerate	Often larger (>20 mm) because of coalescence/conglomeration. Single or multiple
Less edema	More edema
Smooth margin	Irregular margin
Mural nodule present **(scolex)**	Mural nodule absent
Midline shift uncommon	Midline shift more common
Meningitis is not a feature	**Meningitis** is usually associated
Present at grey white matter junction	More common in posterior fossa
Diffusion restriction +	No diffusion restriction
Muscles, orbits or subcutaneous tissues may be involved	Spread is mostly secondary to infection somewhere else in body. Enlarged cervical nodes may be seen.
MT ratio: Higher, mean MTR of 32 ± 1.2	MT ratio: Lower, mean MTR 16.6 +/– 3.1
Progressive focal neurological deficit absent	Progressive focal neurological deficit present
Raised ICP: Transient (<24 hours)	Raised ICP: Common
Constitutional symptoms absent	**Constitutional symptoms** present
MRS shows multiple amino acid peak. **Lactate** is predominantly elevated than succinate and pyruvate peak	MRS shows **lipid peak**
Fig. 4.39.27: Neurocysticercosis	**Fig. 4.39.28:** Tuberculoma

(*Contd.*)

Table 4.39.2: Difference between neurocysticercosis and tuberculoma (*Contd.*)

Neurocysticercosis	*Tuberculoma*
Fig. 4.39.29: Stages of NCC	**Fig. 4.39.30:** Imaging findings in CNS tuberculosis

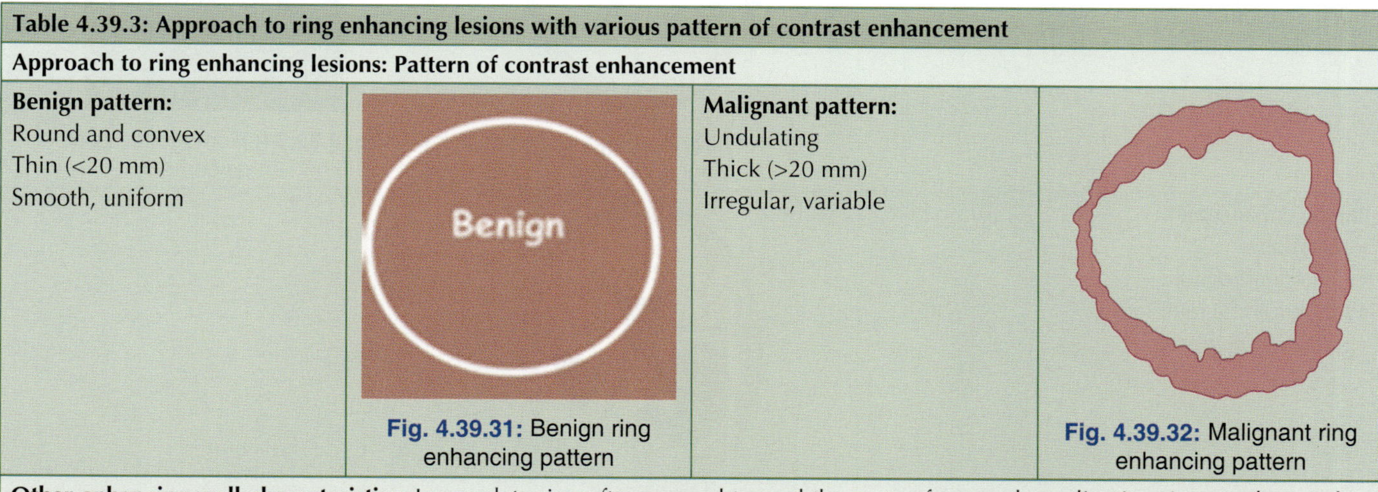

Table 4.39.3: Approach to ring enhancing lesions with various pattern of contrast enhancement

Approach to ring enhancing lesions: Pattern of contrast enhancement			
Benign pattern: Round and convex Thin (<20 mm) Smooth, uniform	**Fig. 4.39.31:** Benign ring enhancing pattern	**Malignant pattern:** Undulating Thick (>20 mm) Irregular, variable	**Fig. 4.39.32:** Malignant ring enhancing pattern
Other enhancing wall characteristics: Incomplete ring often opened toward the cortex favours demyelination, intermediate to low T2 signal capsule favours abscess, restricted diffusion of enhancing wall favours GBM or demyelination.			
Surrounding oedema: Extensive oedema relative to lesion size favours abscess increased perfusion favours neoplasm (metastases or primary cerebral malignancy). **Central fluid content:** Restricted diffusion favours abscess, an absence of diffusion restriction favours tumour with a central necrotic component (classically metastases).		**Number of lesions:** Similar sized rounded lesions at grey-white matter junction favours metastases or abscesses irregular mass with adjacent secondary lesions embedded in the same region of 'oedema' favours GBM. Small (<1–2 cm) lesions with thin walls, especially if other calcific foci are present, suggest neurocysticercosis.	

Further management: Management depends upon the diagnosis, further biochemical investigations and chest screening should be suggested. Primary management is medical by giving anti-tubercular regimen drugs for 18 to 24 months and interval imaging is required to assess the progression of the disease. Other complications like meningitis, hydrocephalus should be assessed before treating, spinal screening also done if there is clinical relevance.

Table 4.39.4: Causes of ring enhancing lesions

Bacterial	*Fungal*	*Parasitic*	*Inflammatory and demyelinating disorders*	*Neoplastic*
• Pyogenic abscess • Tuberculous abscess • *Mycobacterium avium* intracellulare • Listeriosis	• Nocardiosis • Actinomycosis • Rhodococcosis • Zygomycosis • Coccidiomycosis • Paracoccidiodomycosis • Mucormycosis • Aspergillosis • Cryptococcosis • Histoplasmosis	• Neurocysticercosis • Amoebic abscess • Toxoplasmosis • Chagas' disease	• Multiple sclerosis • Acute disseminated encephalomyelitis • Sarcoidosis • Vasculitis and Behçet disease	• Metastases • Primary brain tumor

Table 4.39.5: Other patterns of CNS enhancing lesions

Homogeneous solid enhancement • Lymphoma • Meningioma • Pituitary macroadenoma • Pilocytic macroadenoma • Germinoma • Schwannoma • Gumma	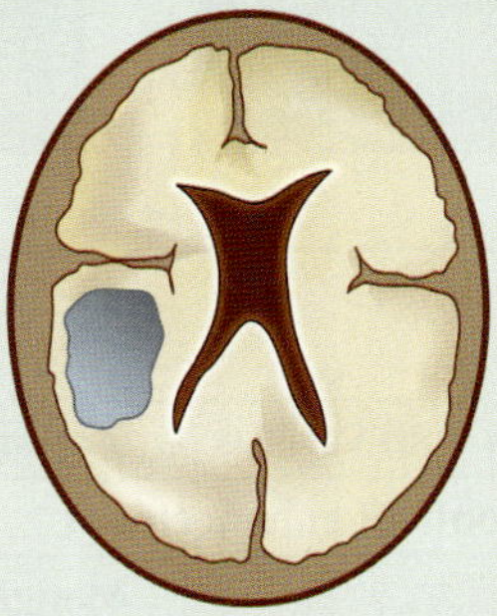 **Fig. 4.39.33:** Homogeneous solid enhancement	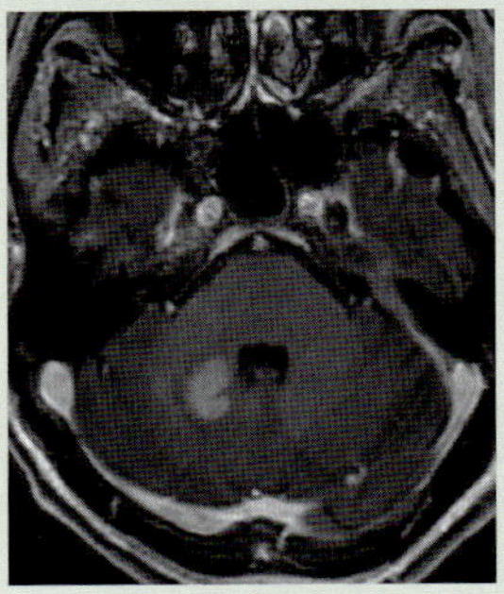 **Fig. 4.39.34:** Homogeneous solid enhancement
Patchy enhancement • Metastasis • Oligodendroglioma • Glioblastoma multiforme • Radiation necrosis	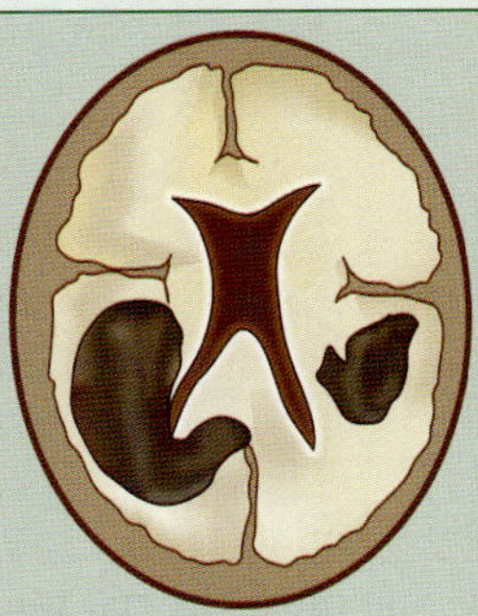 **Fig. 4.39.35:** Patchy enhancement	
Gyriform enhancement • Subacute infarct • Encephalitis • Leptomeningeal metastasis • Sturge-Weber • PRES	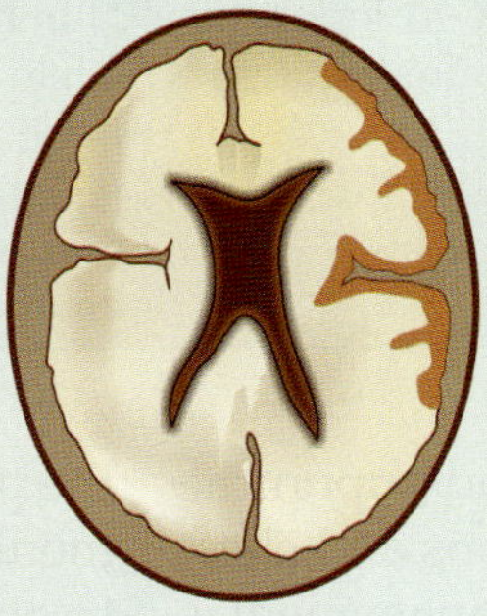 **Fig. 4.39.36:** Gyriform enhancement	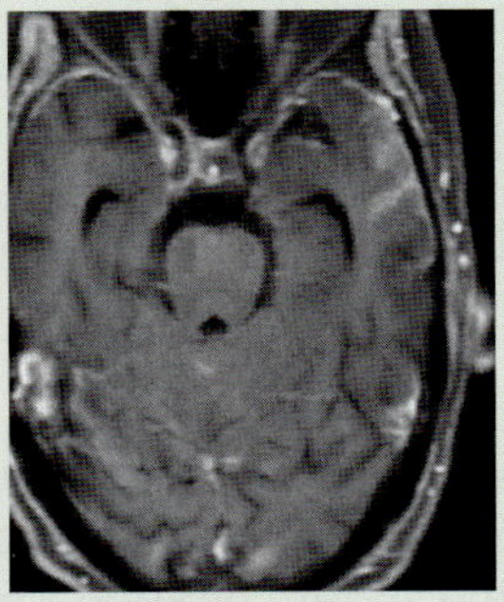 **Fig. 4.39.37:** Gyriform enhancement

(Contd.)

Table 4.39.5: Other patterns of CNS enhancing lesions (*Contd.*)

Punctuate enhancement • Lymphomatoid granulomatosis • Demyelination • CLIPPERS • Susac syndrome • Posterior reversible encephalopathy syndrome • MOG associated demyelination	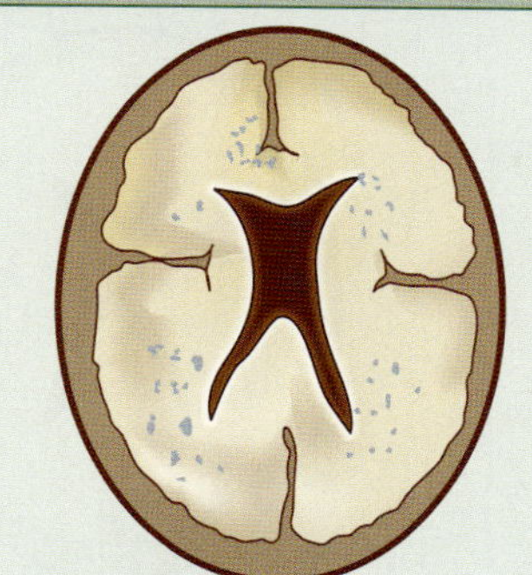 **Fig. 4.39.38:** Punctuate enhancement	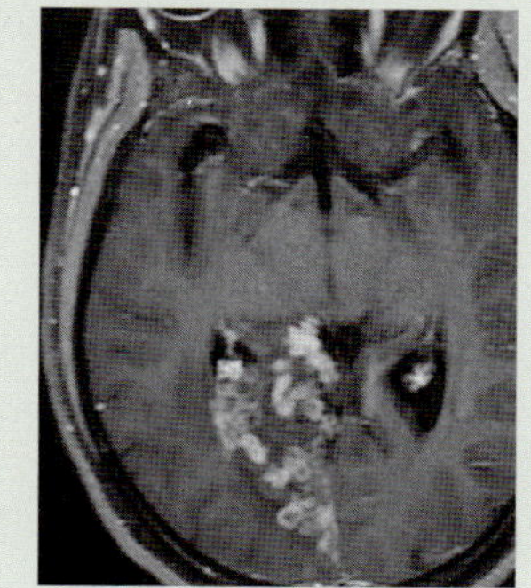 **Fig. 4.39.39:** Punctuate enhancement
Nodular subcortical enhancement • Metastasis • Miliary tuberculosis	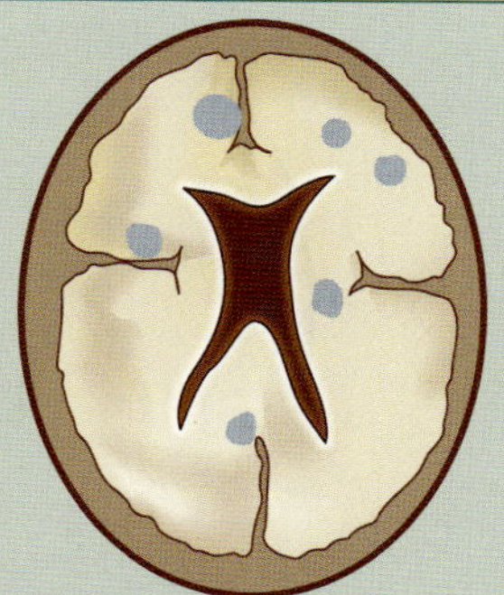 **Fig. 4.39.40:** Nodular subcortical enhancement	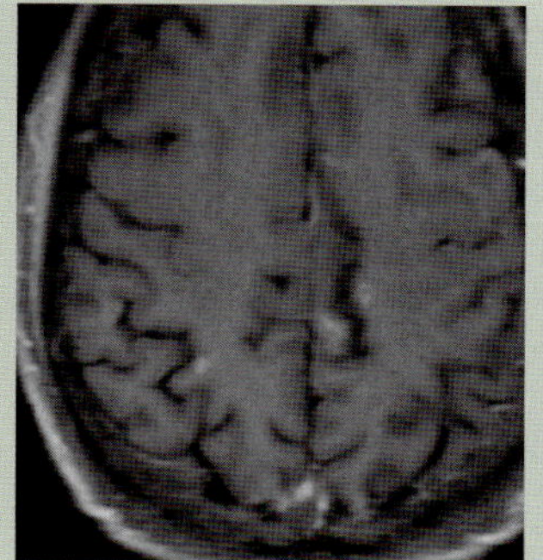 **Fig. 4.39.41:** Nodular subcortical enhancement
Periventricular enhancement • Infectious ependymitis (most commonly CMV) • Primary high grade glial tumor • Multiple sclerosis • Thick periventricular nodular enhancement—primary CNS lymphoma (in HIV)	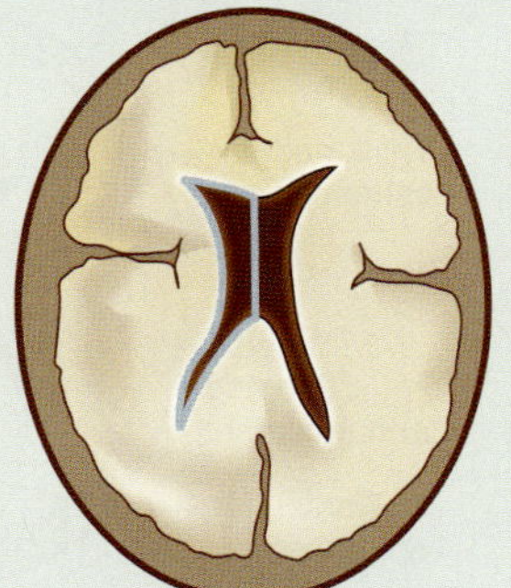 **Fig. 4.39.42:** Periventricular enhancement	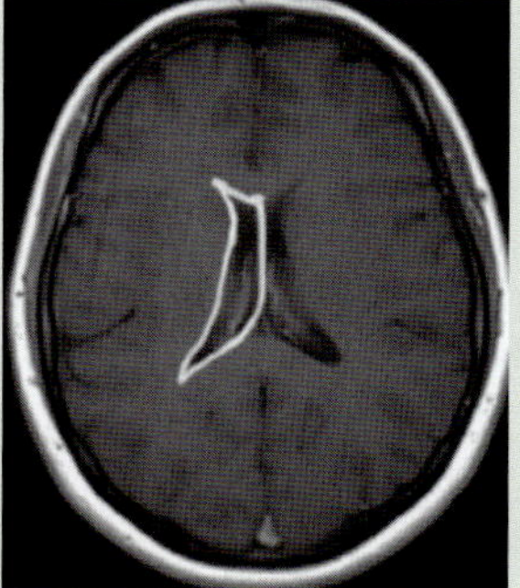 **Fig. 4.39.43:** Periventricular enhancement
Cyst with mural nodular enhancement • Pilocytic astrocytoma • Ganglioglioma • Hemangioblastoma • Pleomorphic xanthoastrocytoma	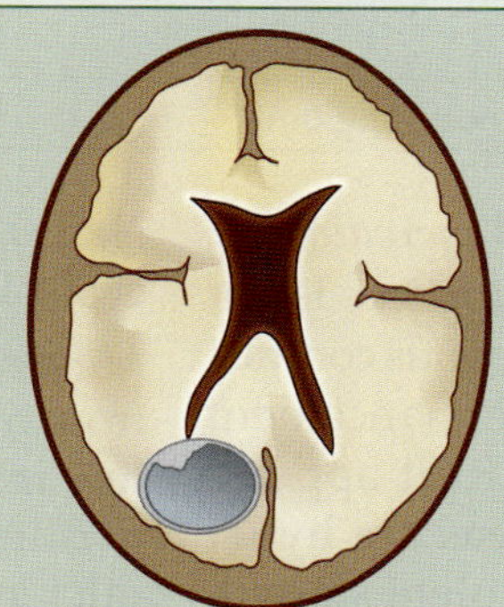 **Fig. 4.39.44:** Cyst with mural nodular enhancement	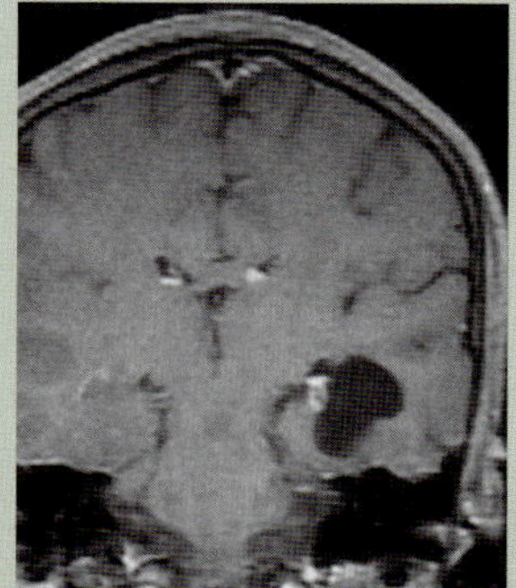 **Fig. 4.39.45:** Cyst with mural nodular enhancement

(*Contd.*)

Table 4.39.5: Other patterns of CNS enhancing lesions (*Contd.*)

Cyst with eccentric dot sign—toxoplasmosis **NCC**	**Fig. 4.39.46:** Cyst with eccentric dot sign	**Fig. 4.39.47:** Cyst with eccentric dot sign
Lesions without enhancement • Low grade astrocytoma • Non-tumoral cystic lesions – Epidermoid cyst – Dermoid cyst – Arachnoid cyst • Acute infarct	**Fig. 4.39.48:** Lesions without enhancement	**Fig. 4.39.49:** Lesions without enhancement
Ring enhancement • Complete ring • Thin smooth: Tuberculosis and other infections • Thick nodular: High grade neoplasm with necrotic core • Incomplete ring: Tumefactive demyelination, ADEM, multiple sclerosis	Thick nodular enhancement Smooth thin ring enhancement Partial ring enhancement **Fig. 4.39.50:** Ring enhancement	**Fig. 4.39.51:** Complete ring enhancement
Other rare conditions include caput medusa, venous angioma		

Brief discussion about the condition–CNS Tuberculomas: Most common site is grey–white matter junction. Iso or hypodense to normal brain in CT. Homogeneous contrast enhancement in solid lesions and rim enhancement when central liquefaction occurs. On MRI it appears hypointense on T1 and T2. **Liquefied areas are hyper on T2.** Variable oedema. In contrast **complete smooth rim enhancement.** Dural-based masses. MRS shows prominent **lipid lactate peak at 1.3 ppm** and there is no amino acid peak.

Miliary TB appears T2 bright.

Newer sequences: DTI differentiates NCC from other cysts. DTI high fractional anisotropy in NCC.

Magnetisation transfer factor: Differentiate tuberculomas from pyogenic abscess and NCC. **MT ratio high in NCC, low in TB, very low in pyogenic abscess.** It is difficult to differentiate between granular nodular and nodular calcified stages, except in some cases of multiple NCC in nodular calcified stage where they produce starry sky appearance.

Tuberculous meningitis: The most useful CT criteria of abnormal **basal meningeal enhancement,** cisterns of the

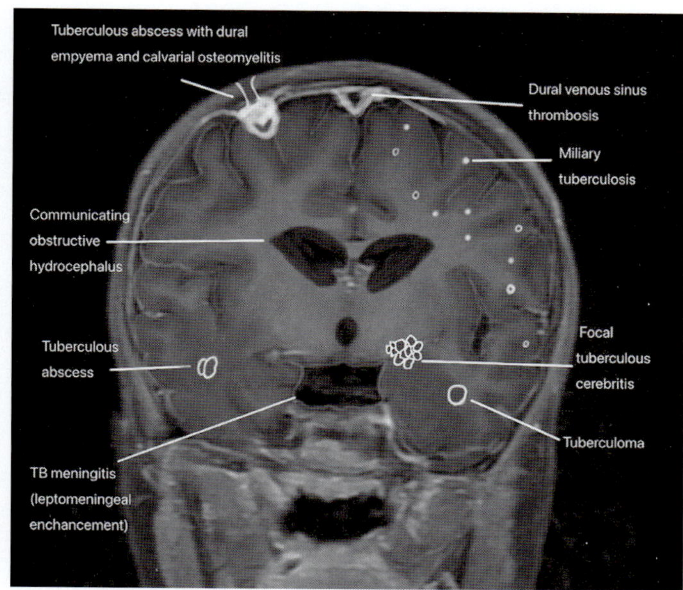

Fig. 4.39.52: CNS tuberculosis imaging findings

middle cerebral artery have been enhanced in a linear fashion. CSF voids around normal vascular enhancement are obliterated by contrast. At the intersection of the suprasellar and middle cerebral artery cisterns, there is a Y-shaped augmentation. **Asymmetry** of enhancement.

Causes of low T2 signal: Normal-flowing blood, bone, calcification, air, CSF flow—especially foramina of Monro and cerebral aqueduct, metallic prosthesis, gadolinium contrast; pathological—cerebral aneurysms—small aneurysms show flow void, giant aneurysms may show complex flow signal ± mural thrombus, arteriovenous malformations—enlarged feeding vessels and draining veins, blood–acute: Deoxyhaemoglobin and intracellular methaemoglobin; chronic: Haemosiderin, highly cellular tumors–medulloblastoma, lymphoma, high glioma; proteinaceous material–colloid cyst, Rathke's cleft cyst, sinus secretions; melanin–melanoma metastasis, meningeal melanocytosis, minerals deposition (calcium, copper, iron), invasive fungal sinusitis.

Patterns of CNS tuberculosis: **Meningeal**—TB meningitis, leptomeningeal granuloma; **Parenchymal**—granuloma, abscess, meningitis, ascites, cerebritis, miliary, caseation necrosis; **Complication**—IRIS, cranial TB, vasculitis and infarction, cranial neuropathy, subdural empyema, epidural abscess.

Table 4.39.6: Spectrum of CNS tuberculosis presentation

TB meningitis 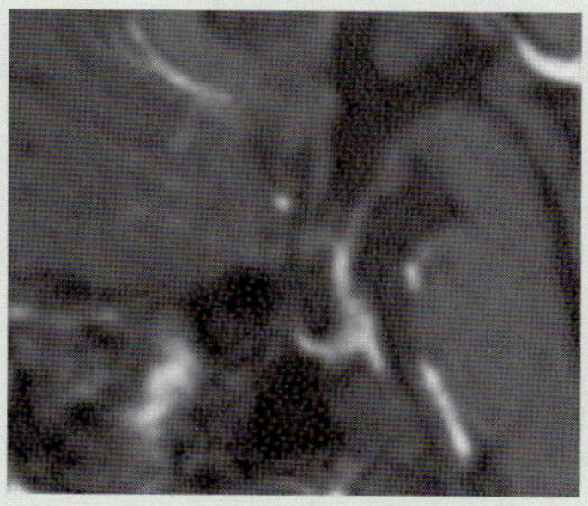 **Fig. 4.39.53:** TB meningitis	**Double and triple line sign** Linear enhancement of middle cerebral artery cistern 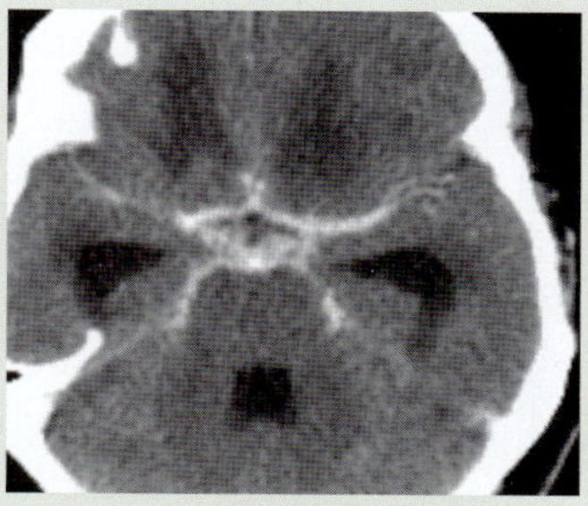 **Fig. 4.39.54:** Triple line sign	The **'Y' sign** at the junction of the suprasellar cistern and middle cerebral artery cistern 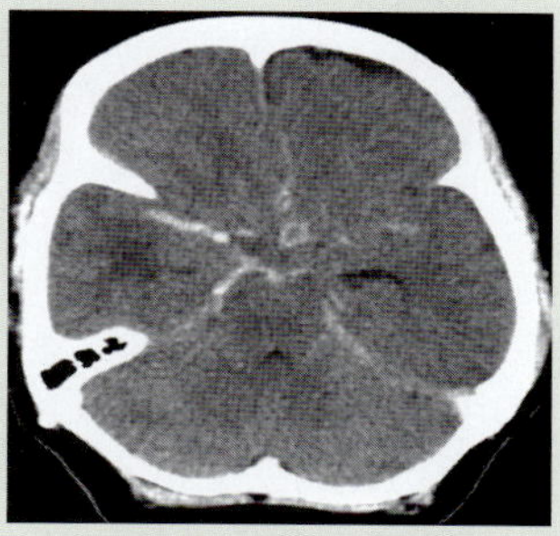 **Fig. 4.39.55:** Y sign
Leptomeningeal granuloma 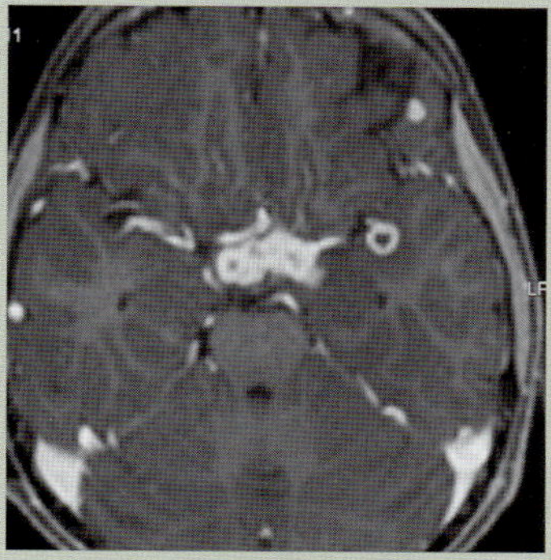 **Fig. 4.39.56:** Leptomeningeal granuloma	**Cranial nerve involvement** 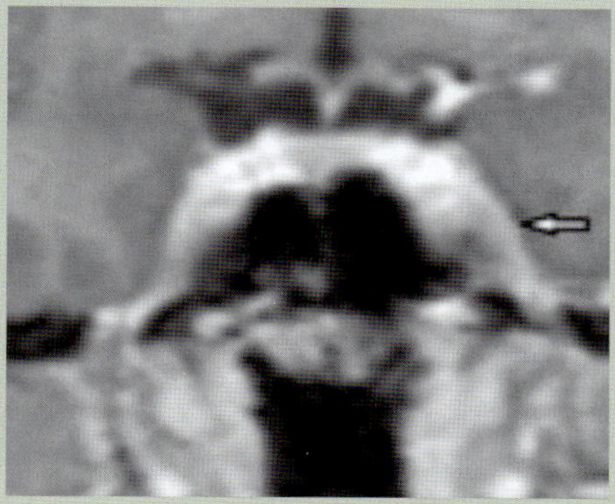 **Fig. 4.39.57:** Cranial nerve involvement	**Cortical vein thrombosis** 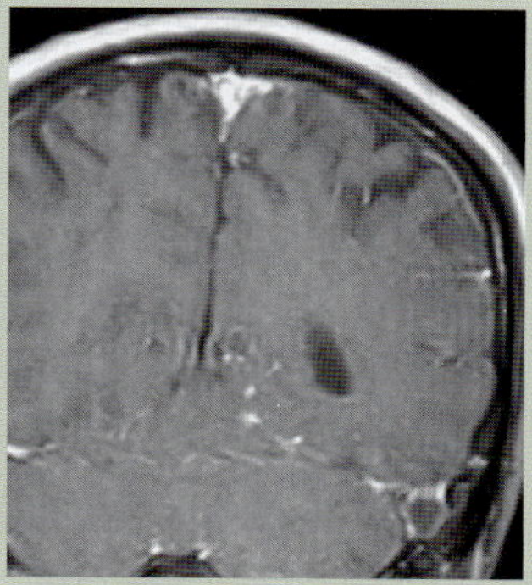 **Fig. 4.39.58:** Cortical vein thrombosis

(Contd.)

Table 4.39.6: Spectrum of CNS tuberculosis presentation (*Contd.*)

Fig. 4.39.59: Tuberculoma

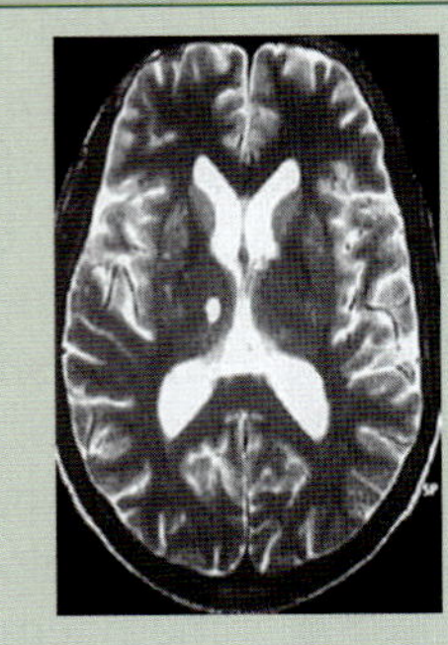

Fig. 4.39.60: Non-caseating granuloma

Fig. 4.39.61: Granuloma with liquid centre

Fig. 4.39.62: Tubercular cerebritis

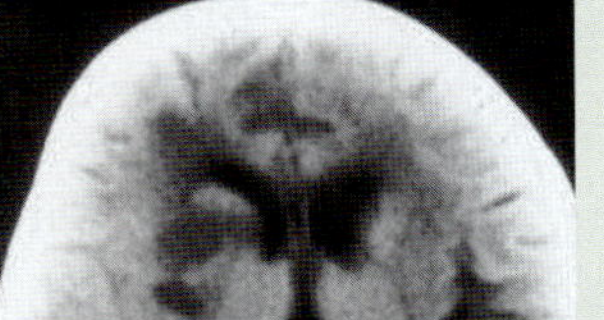

Fig. 4.39.63: Ischemic infarcts

Fig. 4.39.64: Subdural and epidural abscess

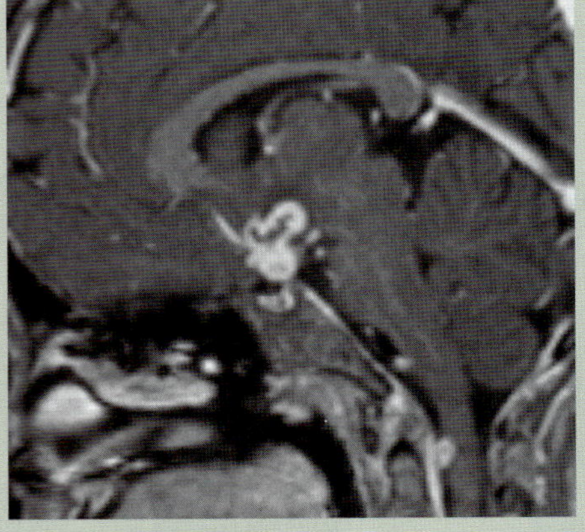

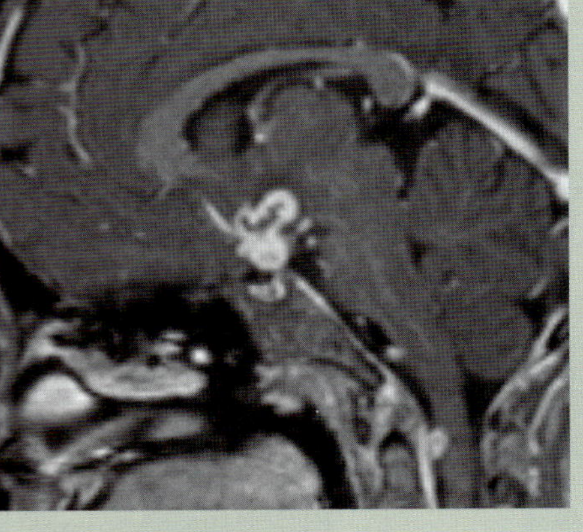

Fig. 4.39.65: Optochiasmatic meningeal granuloma

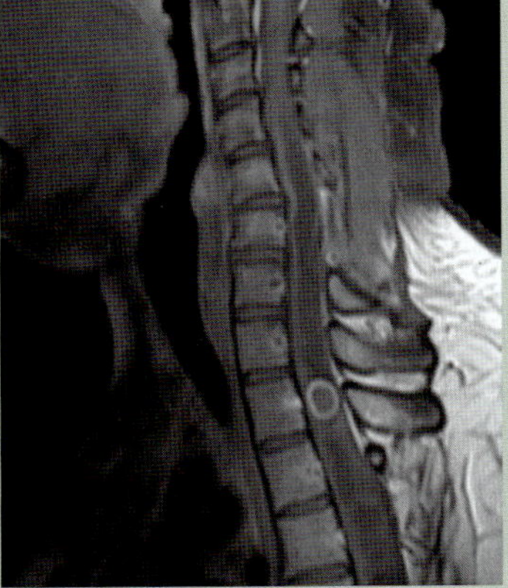

Fig. 4.39.66: Cord granuloma

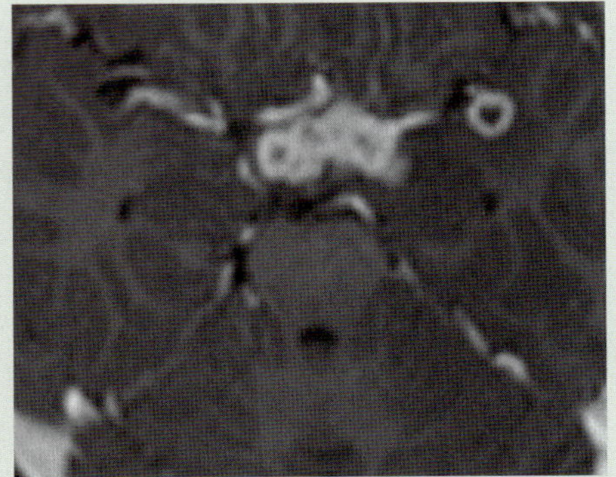

Fig. 4.39.67: Optochiasmatic meningeal granuloma

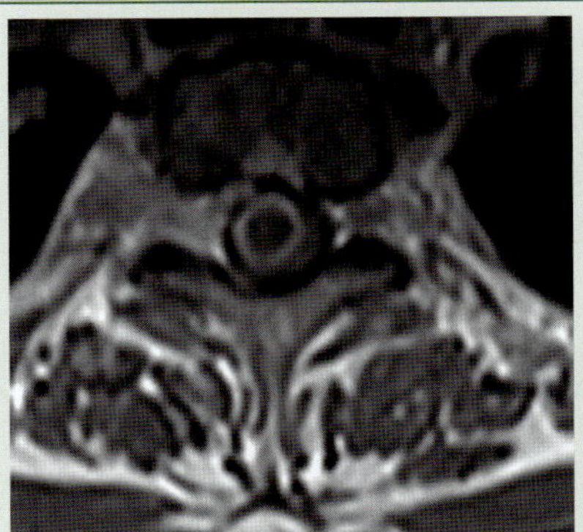

Fig. 4.39.68: Cord granuloma

(*Contd.*)

Table 4.39.6: Spectrum of CNS tuberculosis presentation (*Contd.*)

Basal meningitis with hydrocephalus			**Dural exudates**
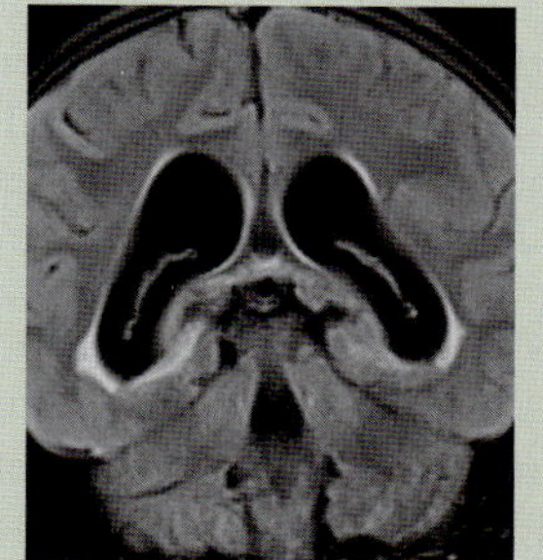 **Fig. 4.39.69:** Basal meningitis with hydrocephalus	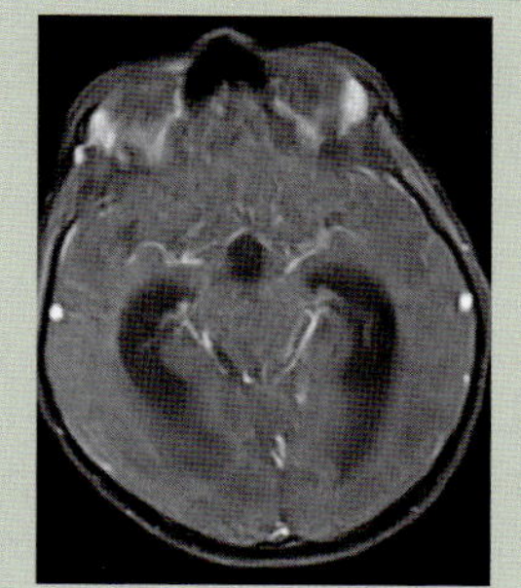 **Fig. 4.39.70:** Basal meningitis with hydrocephalus	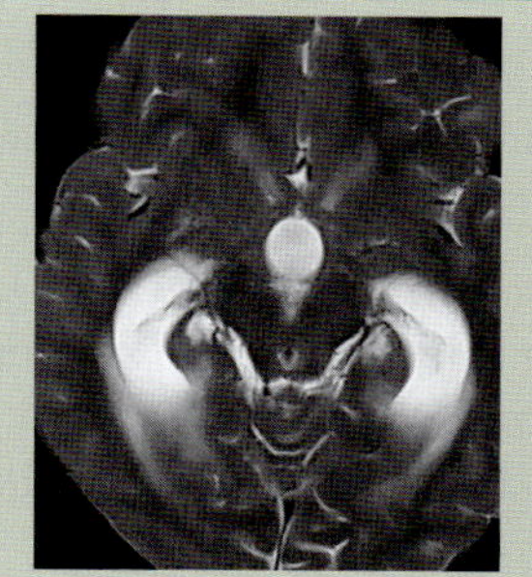 **Fig. 4.39.71:** Basal meningitis with hydrocephalus	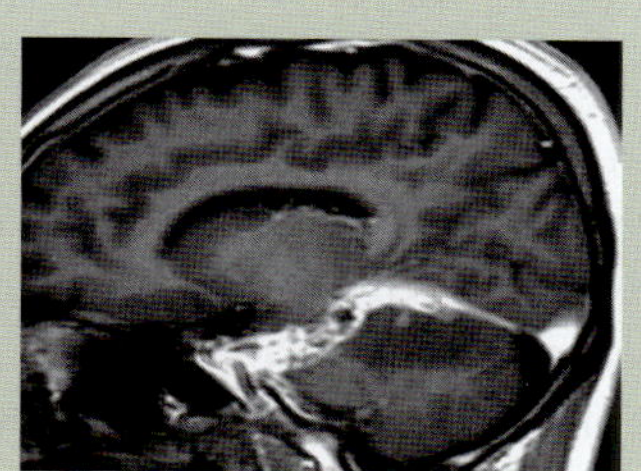 **Fig. 4.39.72:** Basal meningitis
Granulomatous meningitis		**Meningeal granuloma**	
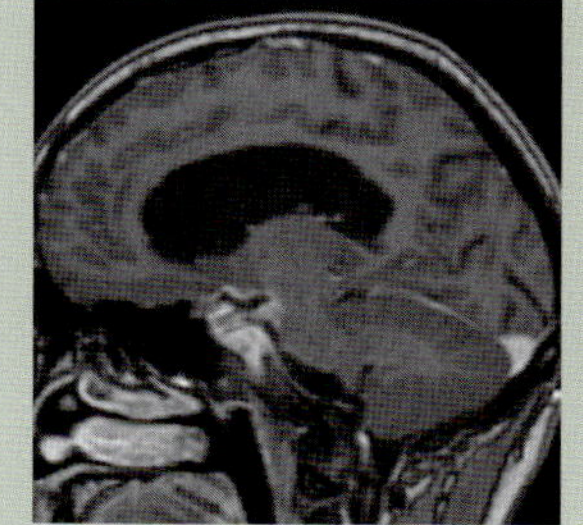 **Fig. 4.39.73:** Granulomatous meningitis	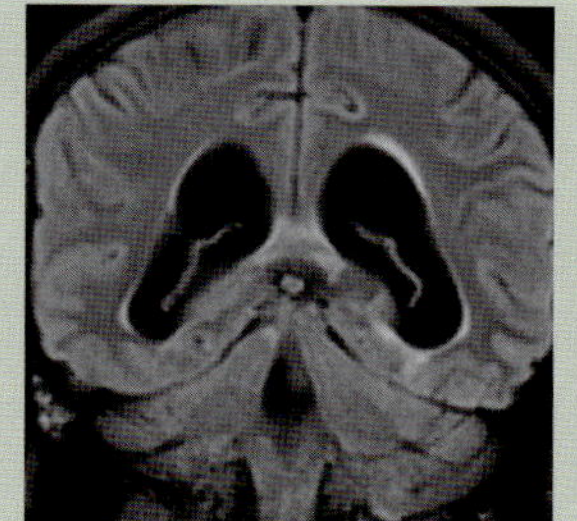 **Fig. 4.39.74:** Granulomatous meningitis	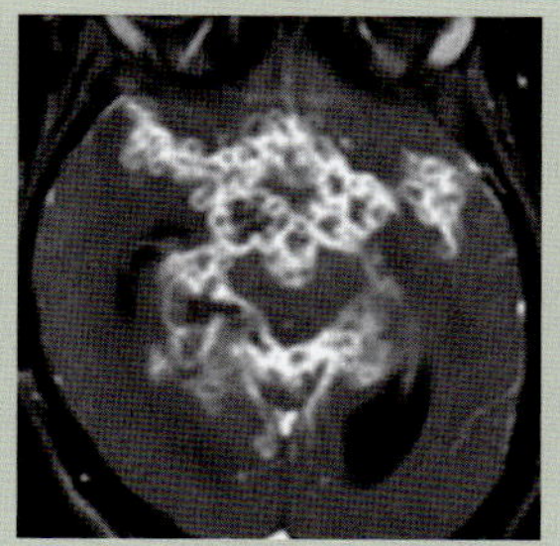 **Fig. 4.39.75:** Meningeal granuloma	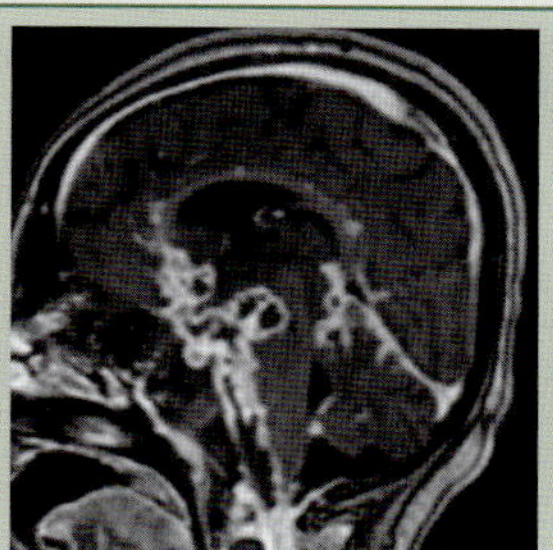 **Fig. 4.39.76:** Meningeal granuloma
TB meningitis with granuloma convexity			
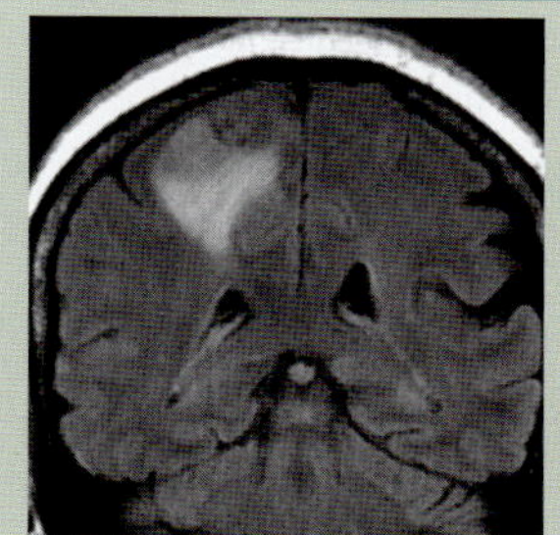 **Fig. 4.39.77:** TB meningitis with granuloma convexity	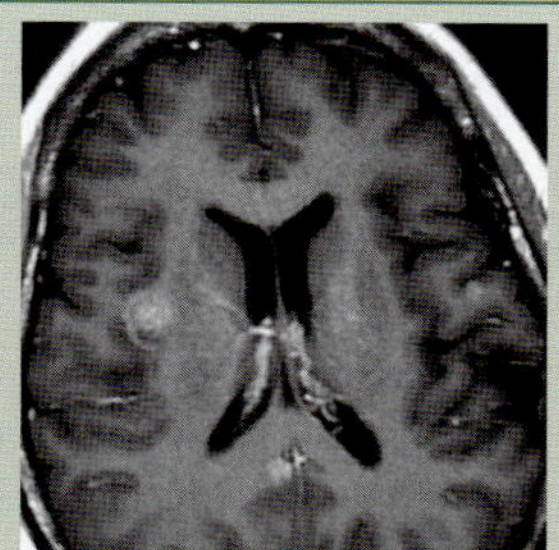 **Fig. 4.39.78:** TB meningitis with granuloma convexity	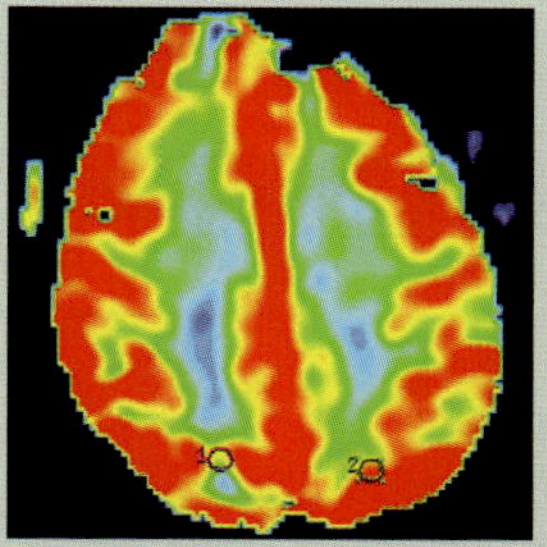 **Fig. 4.39.79:** TB meningitis with incresed peripheral perfusion than central	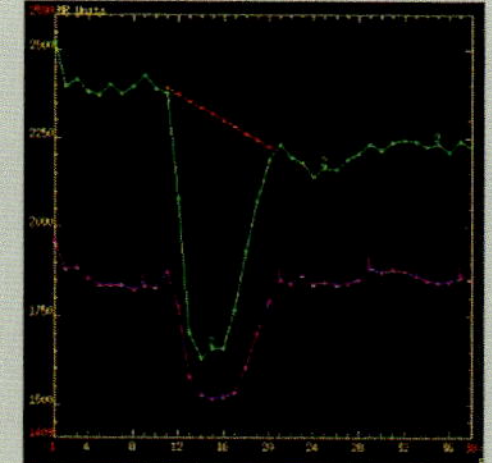 **Fig. 4.39.80:** Type 2 time intensity curve showing mildly incresed perfusion in TB meningitis
Caseating granuloma			
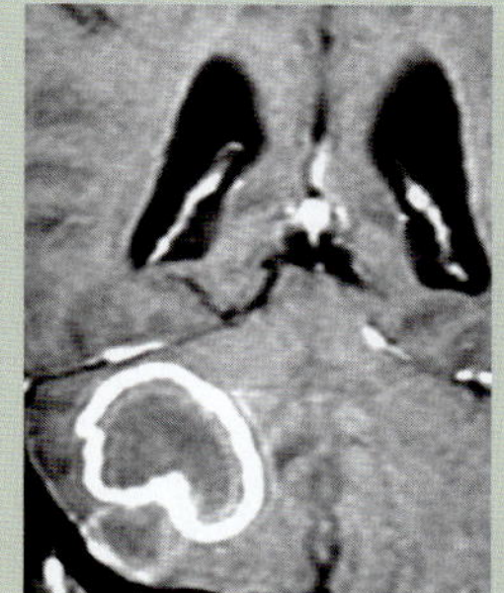 **Fig. 4.39.81:** Caseating granuloma	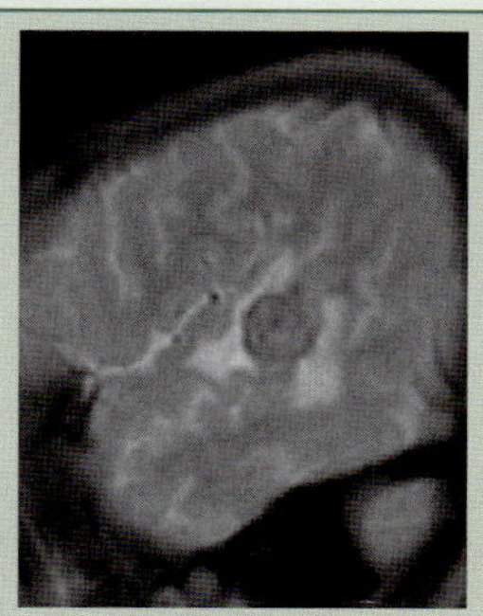 **Fig. 4.39.82:** Caseating granuloma	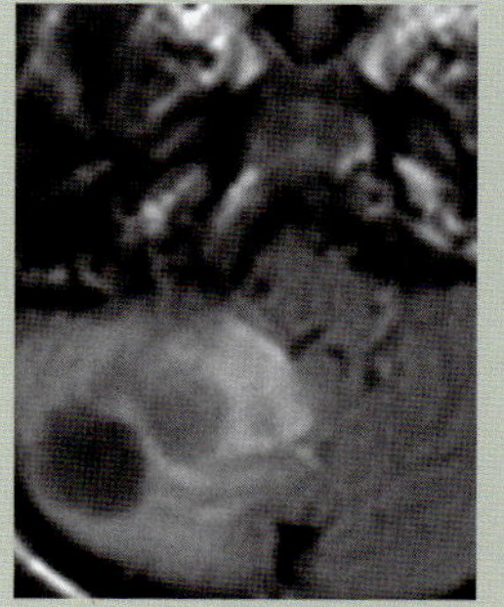 **Fig. 4.39.83:** Caseating granuloma	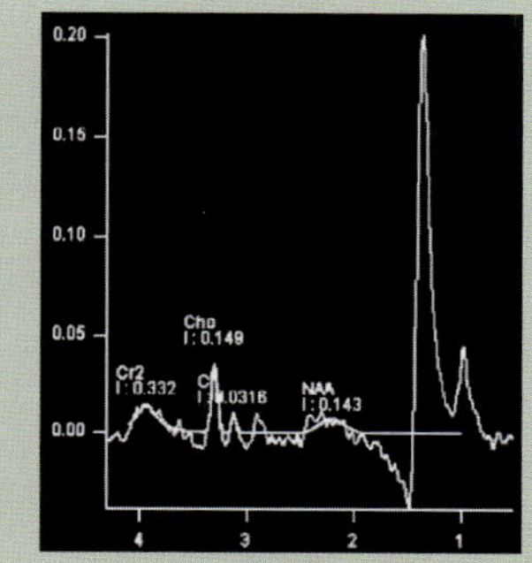 **Fig. 4.39.84:** MRS showing lipid peak in caseating granuloma
Others: IRIS, spinal tuberculosis			

4

4.40 CENTRAL NERVOUS SYSTEM

Case No. 40

Clinical history: 34-years-old male patient, known case of HIV presented with altered sensorium.

Radiological technique and observations: Figure 4.40.1 is plain CT brain image showing widened sulcal spaces, dilated ventricles (indicating mild cerebral atrophy), symmetrical hypodensity in bilateral periventricular regions. No focal lesions/hemorrhage.

Figures 4.40.2 and 4.40.3 are MRI brain—T2 axial and FLAIR—coronal images showing cerebral atrophy, widened sulcal spaces, mild dilation of ventricles, bilateral symmetrical T2/FLAIR periventricular white matter hyperintensities with sparing of subcortical U fibers. Figure 4.40.4 is MRS showing elevated choline and decreased NAA.

Interpretation: A—34 years old male PLHA patient, Bilateral periventricular regions, C—mild cerebral atrophy, T2/FLAIR periventricular white matter hyperintensity sparing subcortical U fibres, B—symmetrical, D—HIV encephalitis.

Principal diagnosis: HIV encephalitis.

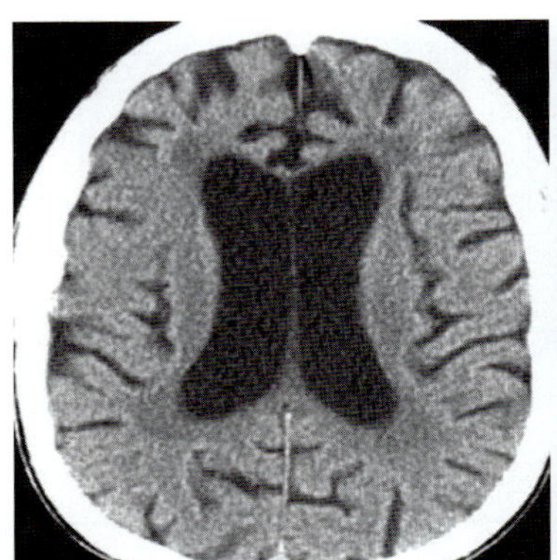

Fig. 4.40.1

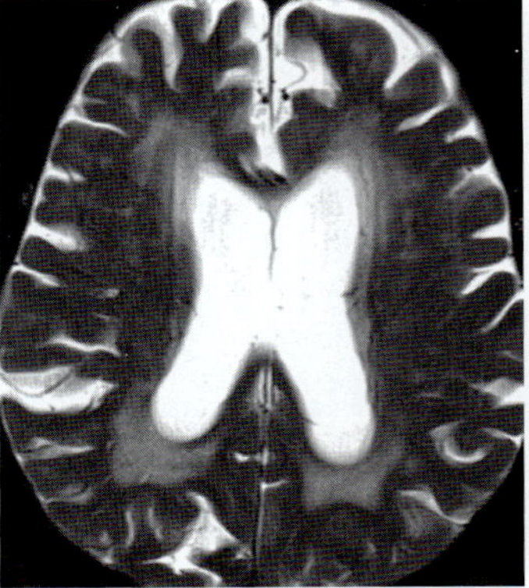

Fig. 4.40.2

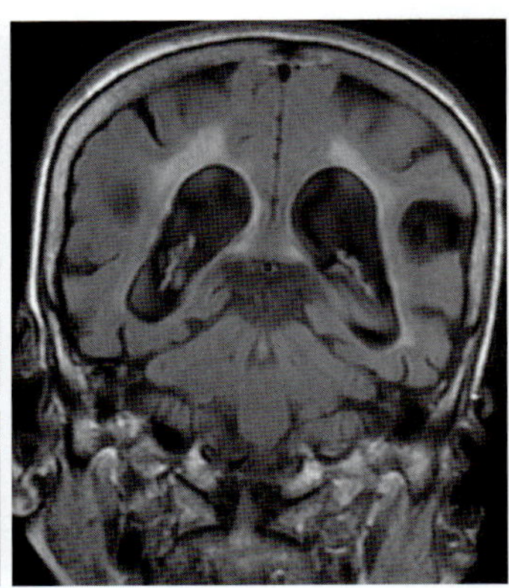

Fig. 4.40.3

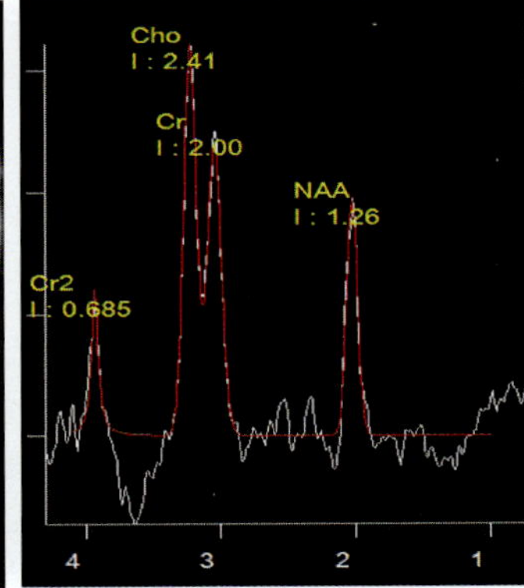

Fig. 4.40.4

Table 4.40.1: Difference between PML and HIV encephalitis

Progressive multifocal leukoencephalopathy (PML)	*HIV encephalitis*
Occur in CD4 count <50–100 Lack of significant cortical or deep atrophy Bilateral asymmetrical, multiple foci white matter involvement Typically involve subcortical white matter. No enhancement	Occur in CD4 count <200 Significant cortical and deep atrophy Bilateral, symmetrical periventricular white matter involvement Subcortical white matter spared No enhancement
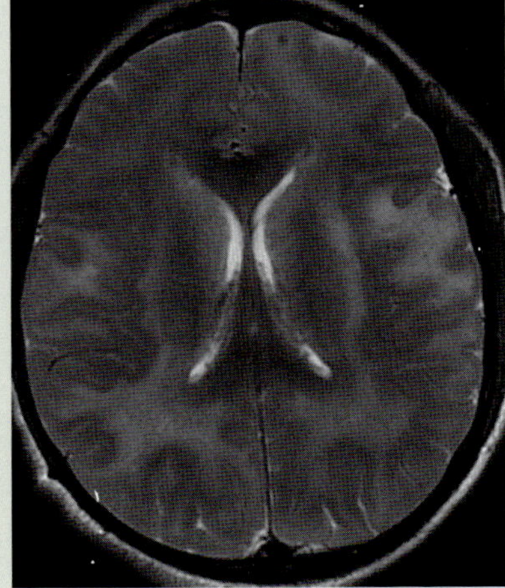 **Fig. 4.40.5:** PML	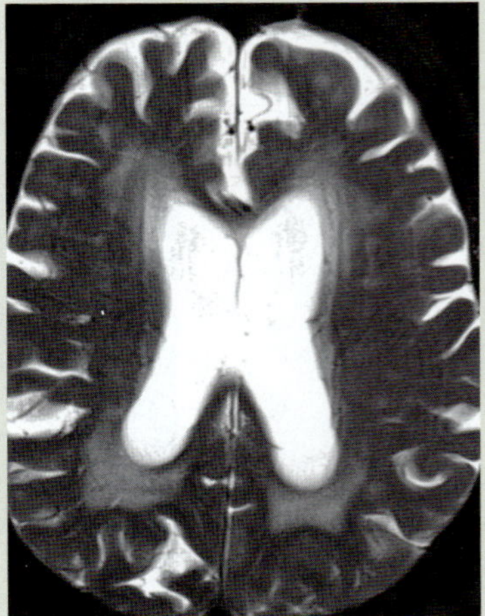 **Fig. 4.40.6:** HIV encephalitis

Table 4.40.2: Other manifestations in HIV

HIV virus itself	*Drugs*	*Malignancy*	*Opportunistic infections*
HIV encephalitis HIV dementia complex HIV myelopathy	HAART therapy IRIS following treatment	Lymphoma Kaposi sarcoma	Bacterial–tuberculosis Viral JC Virus, PML, herpes Encephalitis, cytomegalovirus Fungal: Cryptococcus Parasitic—toxoplasmosis

Table 4.40.3: Opportunistic infections and lesions occurring in HIV patients with respect to CD4 count

CD4 count cells/cubic mm	*Opportunistic infections and lesions*
>500	Nil
200 to 500	Thrush (oral candidiasis), skin infections, bacterial sinus and lung infections, and TB.
<200	PCP pneumonia, HANDS—HIV associated neurocognitive disorders
<100	Toxoplasmosis, Kaposi sarcoma, lymphoma, oesophageal candidiasis, herpes, cryptococcosis
<50	CMV

Table 4.40.4: Difference between toxoplasmosis and primary CNS lymphoma

Toxoplasmosis	*Primary CNS lymphoma*
• More common • Smaller size • Often multiple... but may be single • Basal ganglia and thalamus, corticomedullary location • More edema, Haemorrhagic lesion • DWI-restriction sometime • MRS-increased lipid, lactate and decreased naa, choline • After treatment lesion size decrease (pyrimethamine sulfadiazine folic)	• Less common • Large lesion size (>4 cm) • Often single, but may be multiple • Periventricular location, subependymal spread • Extension across or involvement of corpus callosum • DWI—restriction always • MRS—increased choline • PET-CT/ Thallium 201 SPECT +ve • MR perfusion mild increased blood volume • Response to steroids/radiotherapy

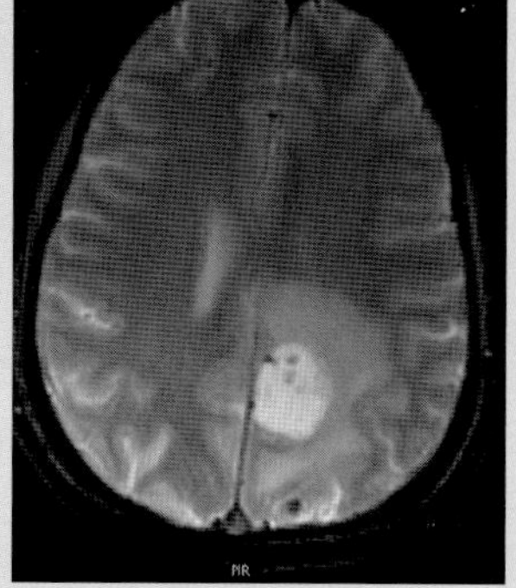
Fig. 4.40.7: Toxoplasmosis

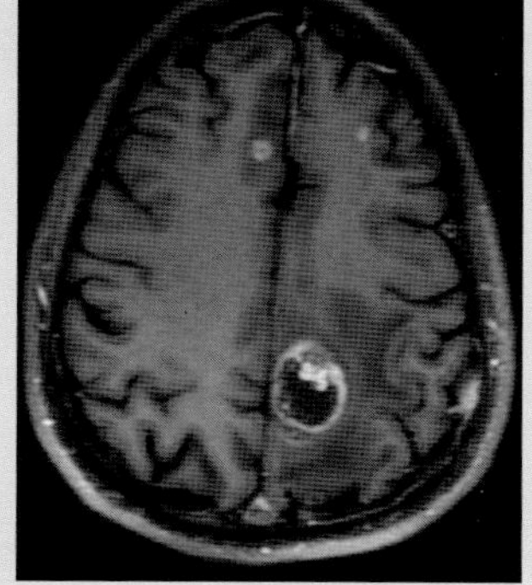
Fig. 4.40.8: Toxoplasmosis

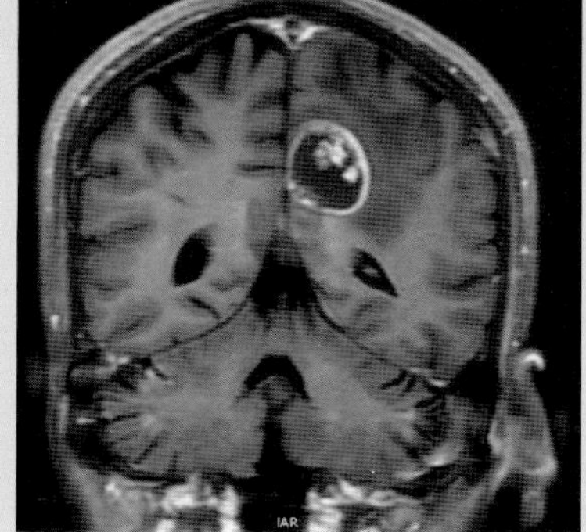
Fig. 4.40.9: Toxoplasmosis

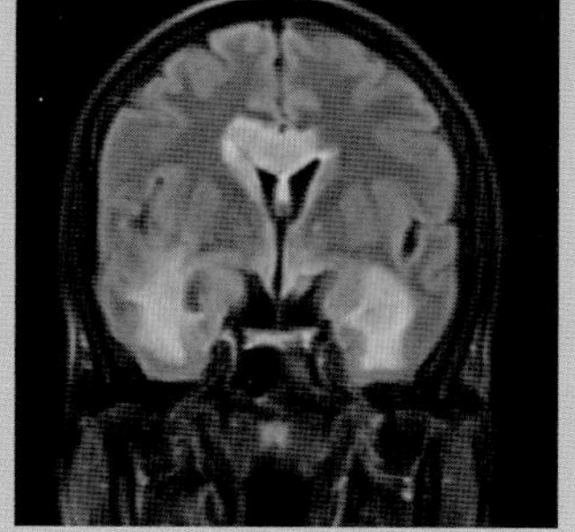
Fig. 4.40.10: Primary CNS lymphoma

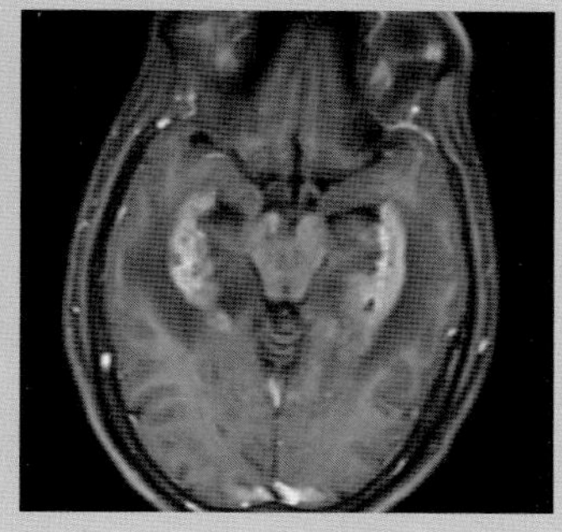
Fig. 4.40.11: Primary CNS lymphoma

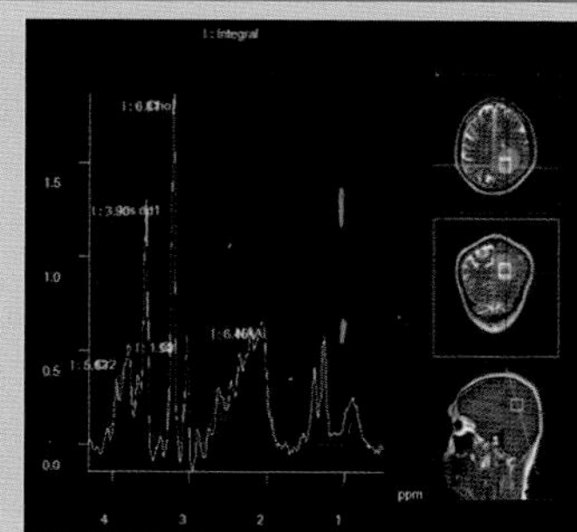
Fig. 4.40.12: Primary CNS lymphoma

Table 4.40.5: Opportunistic infections associated with HIV			
Tuberculosis			
A total of 5–9% of AIDS patients may develop tuberculosis and of these, 2–18% will have CNS infection 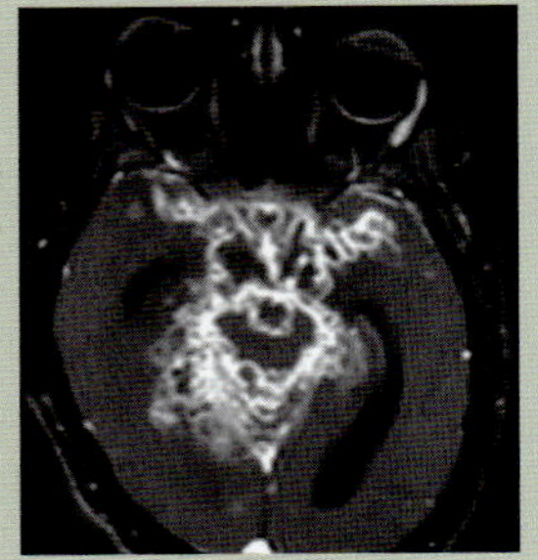 **Fig. 4.40.13:** CNS tuberculosis in HIV patient	1. Meningitis and hydrocephalus. (Basal exudates with enhancement producing 'Y' sign at the junction of the suprasellar cistern and middle cerebral artery cistern) 2. Cerebral abscesses 3. Tuberculomas 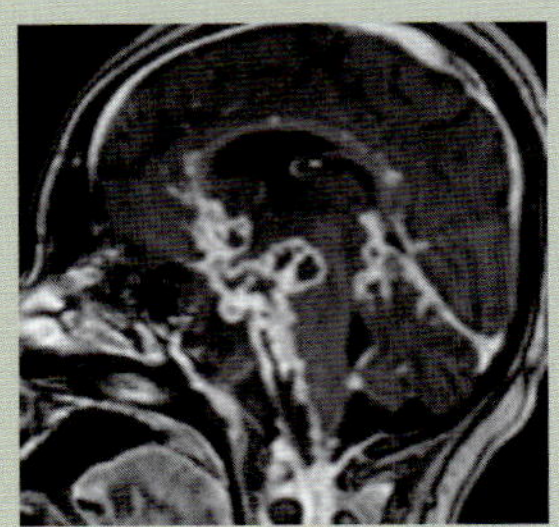 **Fig. 4.40.14:** CNS tuberculosis in HIV patient	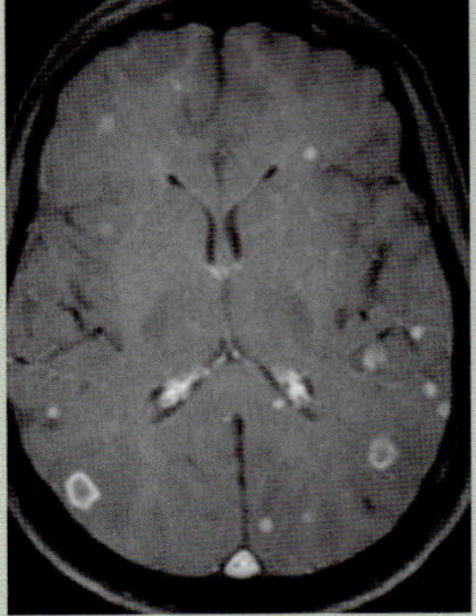 **Fig. 4.40.15:** CNS tuberculosis in HIV patient	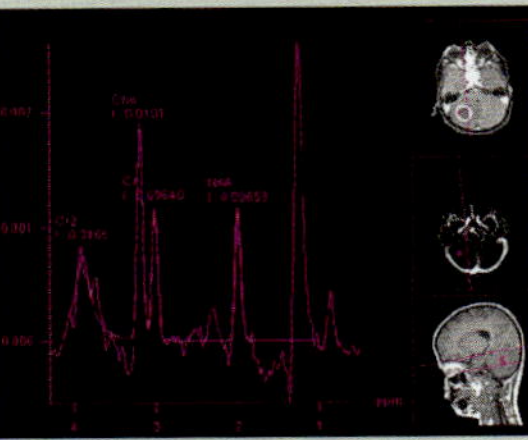 **Fig. 4.40.16:** CNS tuberculosis in HIV patient
Cryptococcus infection. CD4-<100 cells/cu.mm	Normal—40% Cryptococcal meningitis—MC CNS manifestation **Gelatinous pseudocysts in basal ganglia** (enhancement uncommon). **Cryptococcoma**—hyperintense on T2 (nodular enhancement common). Other findings—diffuse atrophy, hydrocephalus and diffuse cerebral edema.		
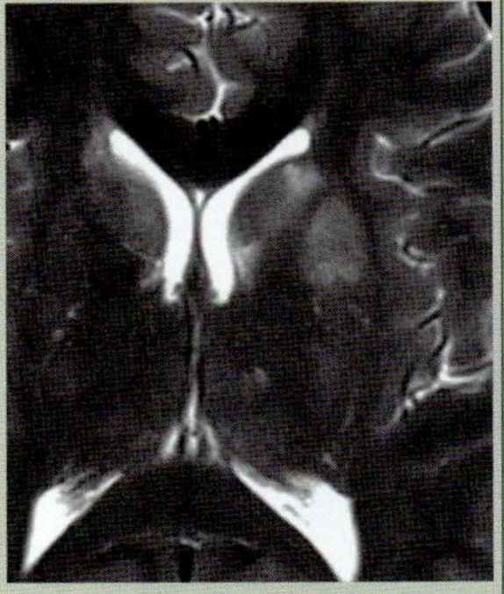 **Fig. 4.40.17:** Cryptococcus infection in patient with HIV	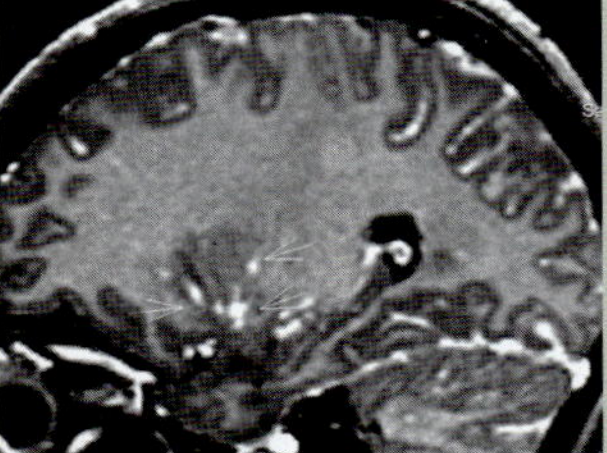 **Fig. 4.40.18:** Cryptococcus infection in patient with HIV	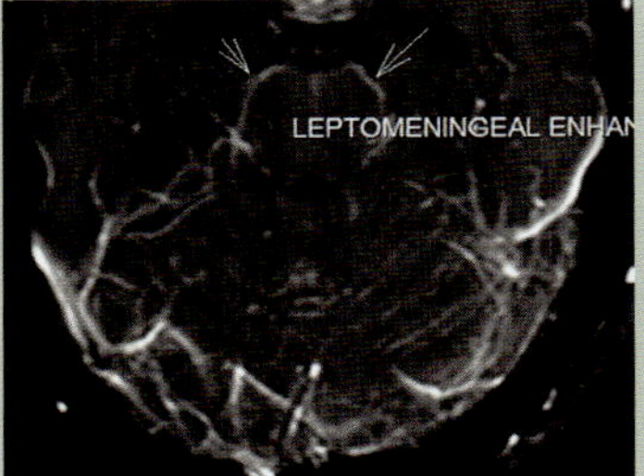 **Fig. 4.40.19:** Cryptococcus infection in patient with HIV	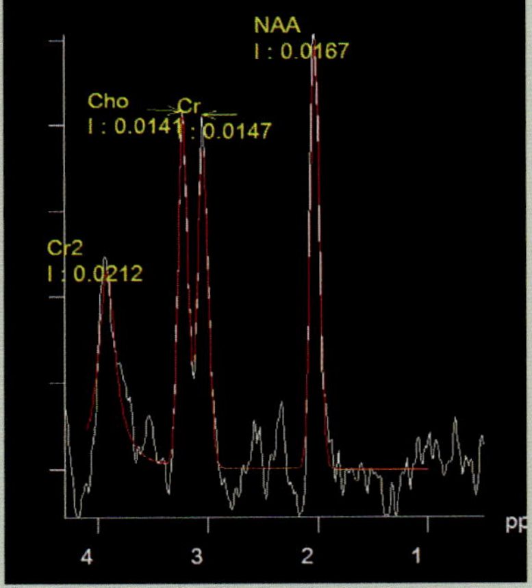 **Fig. 4.40.20:** Cryptococcus infection in patient with HIV
Cytomegalovirus CD4-<50 cells/cu.mm	Imaging—nonspecific, may be normal. Ependymitis, meningoencephalitis or ventriculitis (circumferential hyperintensity around the lateral ventricle without enhancement)	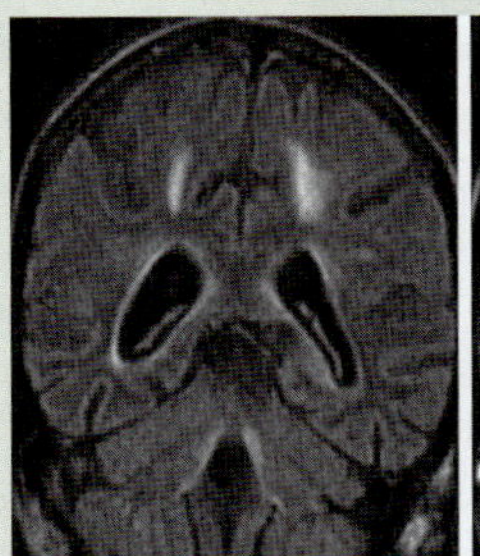 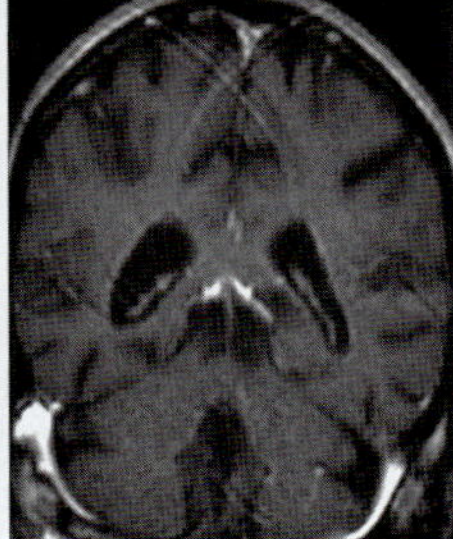 **Fig. 4.40.21:** CMV infection in patient with HIV (ependymitis)	

Contd...

Table 4.40.5: Opportunistic infections associated with HIV *(Contd...)*

Aspergilloma Hemorrhage associated with lesions in HIV-possibility of aspergillosis.	• Multiple cortical and subcortical regions of low attenuation on CT images, T2 hyperintensity on MRI • Multiple ring-enhancing lesions • Dural enhancement is seen adjacent to enhancing lesions of the paranasal sinuses and calvaria	**Fig. 4.40.22:** Aspergilloma infection in patient with HIV
HIV vacuolar myelopathy	Bilateral symmetric signal intensity abnormality within the dorsal columns characteristic of SACD of the spinal cord.	**Fig. 4.40.23:** HIV vacuolar myelopathy
Fig. 4.40.24: Spectrum of lesions in HIV		

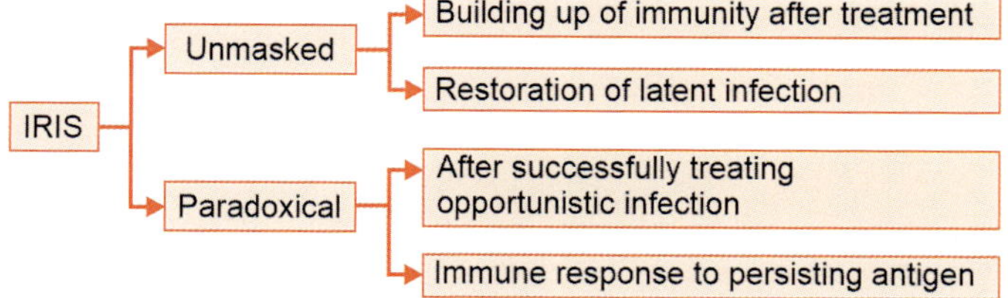

Fig. 4.40.25: Pathogenesis of IRIS

Iris-immune reconstitution inflammatory syndrome: IRIS is related to reconstitution of immunity, which leads to abnormal immune response to either specific infectious or non-infectious antigens. Paradoxical deterioration in their clinical status when their CD4 counts rise and viral replication decreases.

Imaging: Increase in parenchymal high FLAIR signal abnormalities, contrast enhancement of the leptomeningeal spaces and/or of the parenchymal lesions, mass effect, and restricted diffusion are the features predominate in CNS-IRIS.

Treatment: Steroids.

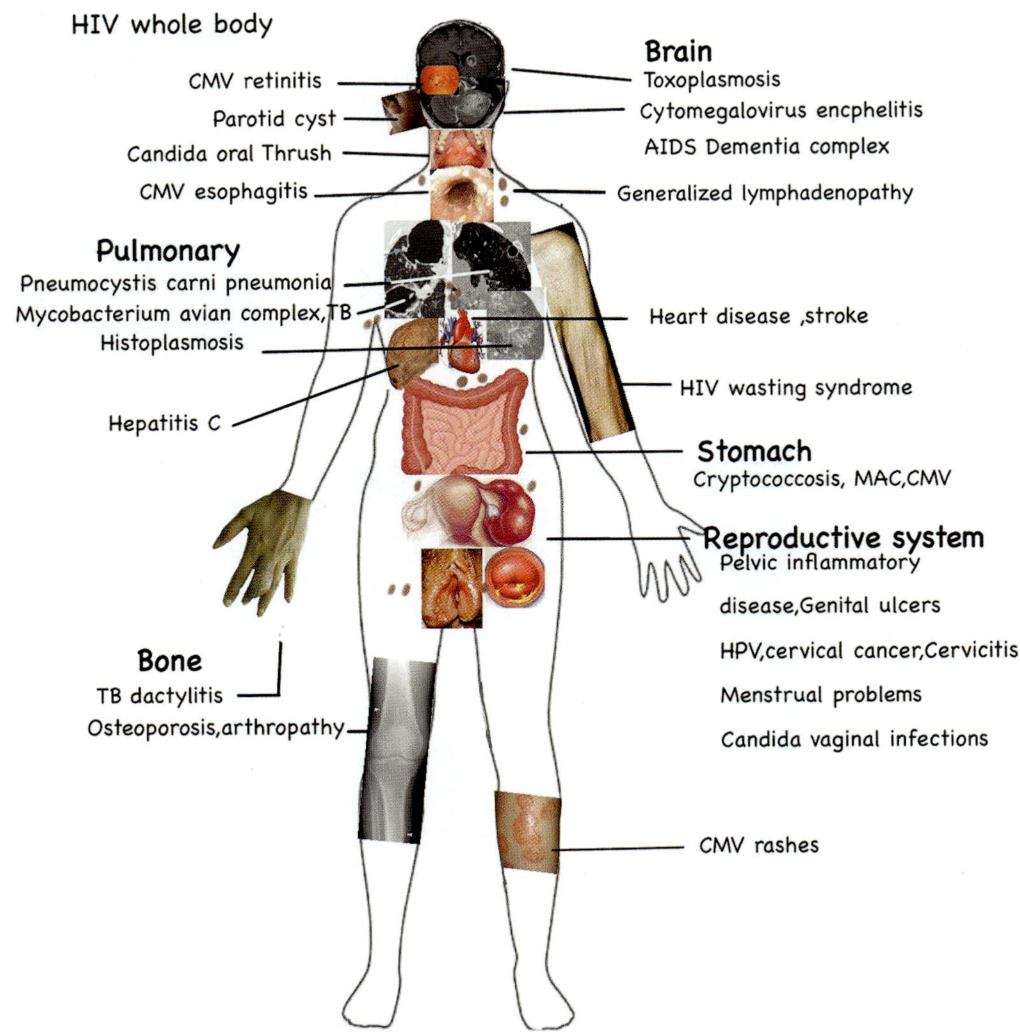

Fig. 4.40.26: Whole body illustration showing various manifestations of HIV

4.41 CENTRAL NERVOUS SYSTEM

Case no. 41

Clinical history: A 55-year-old male presented with history of road traffic accident and altered sensorium to the emergency department with a GCS of 6/15.

Radiological techniques: Figure 4.41.1 is plain CT image of brain.

Observations: Axial plain CT images reveal crescent shaped subdural hemorrhage crossing the suture lines along the left fronto-temporal convexity of maximum thickness 5 mm, causing mass effect on the ipsilateral lateral ventricles with subfalcine herniation of the brain parenchyma to the right and midline shift of 7 mm to the right. Hemorrhagic contusion measuring 5 × 3.5 mm noted in the left frontal lobe (posterolateral orbitofrontal gyrus) with surrounding edema. Subarachnoid hemorrhage seen in the right frontal region. Subdural/subarachnoid hemorrhage seen in the anterior interhemispheric fissure.

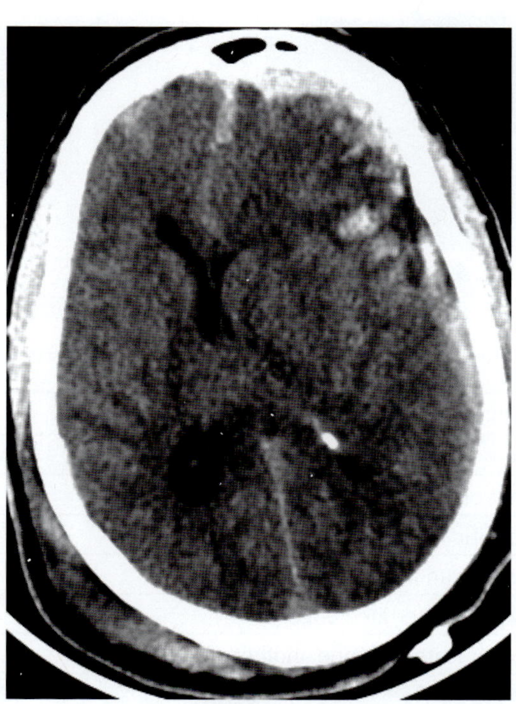

Fig. 4.41.1

Interpretation: A—55-years-old male, pathology in bilateral frontal region, C—hemorrhagic contusion in the left frontal lobe, subarachnoid hemorrhage seen in the right frontal region. Subdural hemorrhage along the left fronto-temporal convexity causing, B—mass effect on the left lateral ventricles with subfalcine herniation and midline shift to the right, D—traumatic brain injury.

Principal diagnosis: Traumatic brain injury—left subdural hemorrhage with subarachnoid hemorrhage in the right frontal region and hemorrhagic contusion in the left frontal lobe causing significant mass effect and midline shift.

Treatment: Urgent call over to neurosurgery team for immediate evacuation of subdural hemorrhage.

Traumatic brain injury (TBI): Classification of traumatic brain injury is based on the clinical scale—Glasgow Coma Scale as severe (3–8), moderate (9–12) and mild (13–15). Correlation with morbidity on the mild end of the spectrum is poor, whereas at moderate to severe levels of traumatic brain injury it correlates well with morbidity and mortality rates.

Imaging protocol: Non-enhanced head CT is a class 1 recommendation for patients with moderate to severe TBI. MRI has substantially higher sensitivity than CT for the detection of EDH, SDH, non-hemorrhagic cortical contusions, brainstem injuries and white matter axonal injuries. Scout image: Look for cervical spine abnormalities such as fracture or dislocation, jaw and/facial trauma, and the presence of foreign objects. The presence of fracture or mal-alignment of the cervical spine mandates MDCT of the cervical spine. CT or MR angiography is recommended when a fracture traverses the carotid canal, posterior arch of C1, foramina transversarium of C1 to C7 in cases of penetrating injury, post-traumatic vasospasm and when the intracranial hemorrhagic pattern is atypical for trauma. Atypical

Classification of head trauma	
Primary effects	*Secondary effects*
• Scalp and skull injuries • Extra-axial hemorrhage/hematoma • Parenchymal injuries—contusion and lacerations, axonal injury, deep cerebral gray matter injury • Miscellaneous injuries—intraventricular hemorrhage, pneumocephalus.	• Herniation syndromes • Diffuse cerebral edema • Cerebral ischemia—hypoxic brain injury • Vascular injury (can be primary or secondary)

Primary effects		
Scalp and skull injuries: Skull fractures can be caused by blunt or penetrating injury and frequently tear the underlying meninges if depressed. Fractures extending to a suture can be associated with diastasis, especially in children.	Anterior cranial fossa fractures are frequently associated with a CSF leak, especially when comminuted or oblique. Fractures that traverse a dural venous sinus or the jugular bulb are associated with injury to the underlying vein.	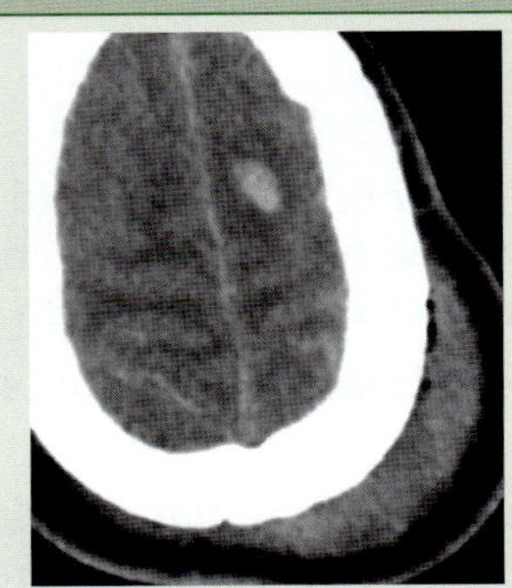 **Fig. 4.41.2:** Hemorrhagic contusion in left high frontal lobe with left occipital region scalp injury

Types of skull fracture			
Linear skull fracture	*Comminuted skull fracture*	*Depressed skull fracture*	*Ping pong fracture*
Fig. 4.41.3: Linear skull fracture in right temporal bone	**Fig. 4.41.4:** Base of skull comminuted fracture	**Fig. 4.41.5:** Depressed skull fracture	*Refer to Chapter 7 for further explanation

Fracture	*Suture*
Greater than 3 mm in width	Less than 3 mm in width
Widest at the center and narrow at the ends	Same width throughout
Runs through both outer and inner lamina of bone, hence appears darker	Lighter on X-rays compared with fracture lines
Usually over temporo-parietal area	At specific anatomic sites
Usually runs in a straight line	Does not run in a straight line
Angular turns	Curvaceous, serrated edges
Blind ending	Communicate with one another

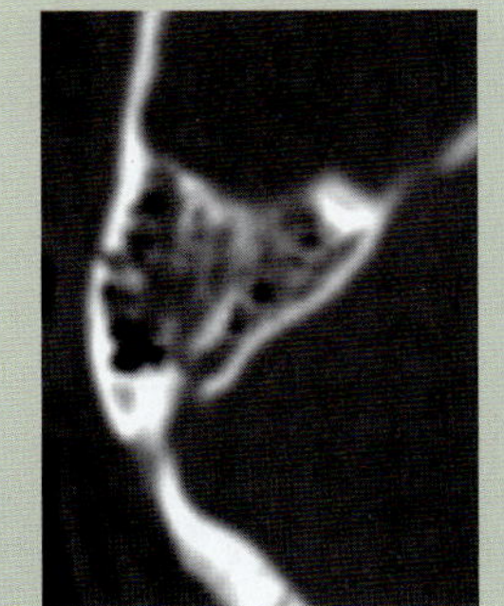
Fig. 4.41.6: Right temporal bone fracture

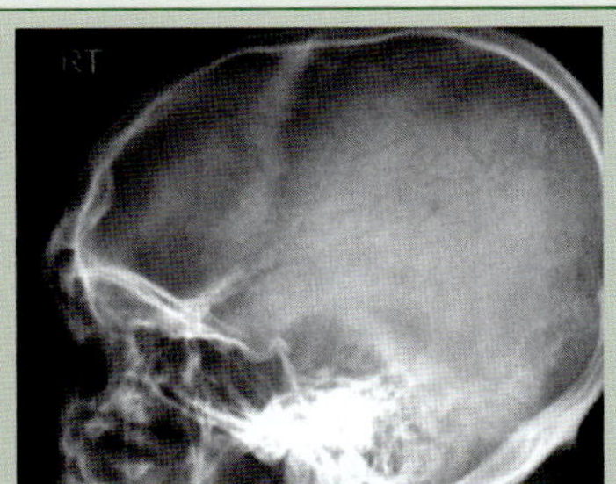

Fig. 4.41.7: Depressed frontal bone fracture

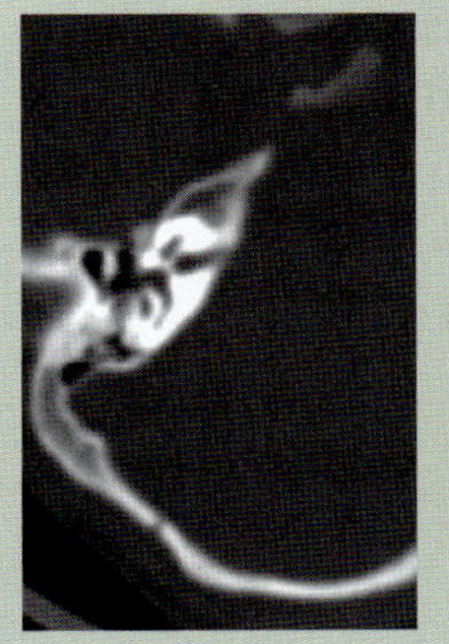
Fig. 4.41.8: Normal suture (occipito mastoid suture)

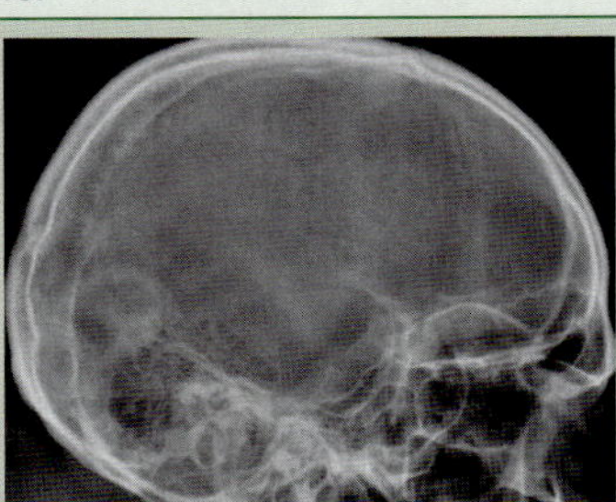
Fig. 4.41.9: Normal suture

Condition	Imaging features	Images
Extradural hemorrhage—occurs between the inner table of skull and superficial layer of the dura. In pterional region—source of EDH is middle meningeal artery. **Indication for surgical intervention:** EDH > 30 cc irrespective of GCS. EDH < 30 cc with 1) GCS <8 or 2) Midline shift >5 mm or 3) Presence of focal neurological deficit or 4) > 15 mm thickness.	Lenticular (biconvex) shaped. **Most common location is temporoparietal convexity.** May have a hypoattenuating center—indicating hyperacute active bleed **(swirl sign).** Crosses midline does not cross sutures. Venous EDH occurs when the fracture line crosses the dural venous sinuses. **Lucid interval**–period of consciousness between two unconscious period, after trauma.	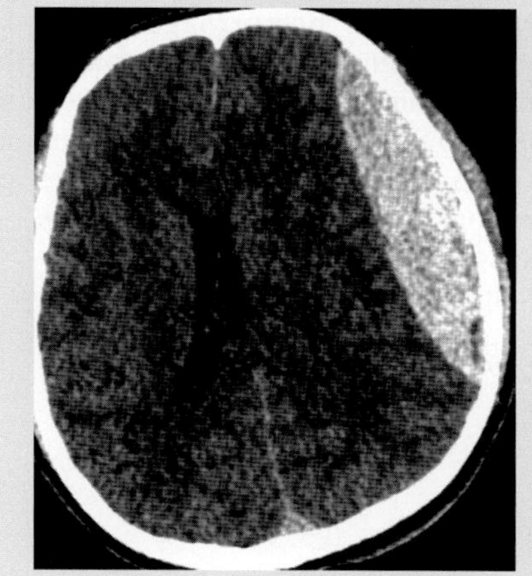 **Fig. 4.41.10:** Extradural hemorrahge
Subdural hemorrhage: Occurs between the dura and arachnoid mater. Crosses suture line does not cross midline. Source of the bleed—tear in bridging cortical veins as it crosses the dura. **Indication for surgical intervention:** Acute SDH with a thickness >10 mm or midline shift >5 mm regardless of GCS. Acute SDH with a thickness <10 mm and shift <5 mm if there is a decrease in GCS of 2 or more, worsening pupillary exam, and/or ICP greater than 20 mmHg.	Crescentic (sickle) shaped. Most common location is frontoparietal convexity. Appearance in various stages: Acute hyperdense. Subacute—iso to hypodense. Chronic—calcifications can form. Reasons for mixed attenuation of SDH 1. Acute on chronic SDH (swirl sign—NECT showing hyperacute active bleed into a hematoma) 2. Hypoattenuating areas due to hyperacute bleed or unclotted blood products in patients with coagulopathy.	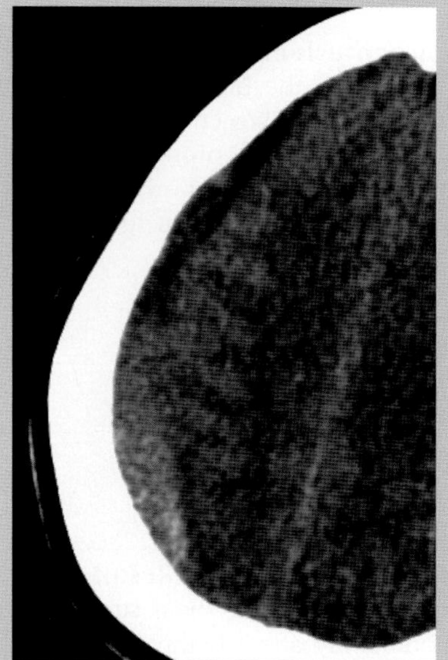 **Fig. 4.41.11:** Subdural hemorrhage
Subarachnoid hemorrhage: It occurs between the arachnoid and pia mater and is usually small volume sulcal SAH that commonly occurs at the site of impact (coup) or opposite the site of impact (countercoup). Isolated SAH in the basilar cisterns should prompt consideration of aneurysmal SAH, even in the setting of trauma.	Hyperdensity filling the sulcal spaces and gyri. Midline traumatic SAH (in the inter-hemispheric fissure or peri-mesencephalic cisterns) on initial head CT images is a marker of diffuse axonal injury at subsequent MRI. The risk of post-traumatic vasospasm is highest in severe TBI, where it occurs in up to 30–40% of patients.	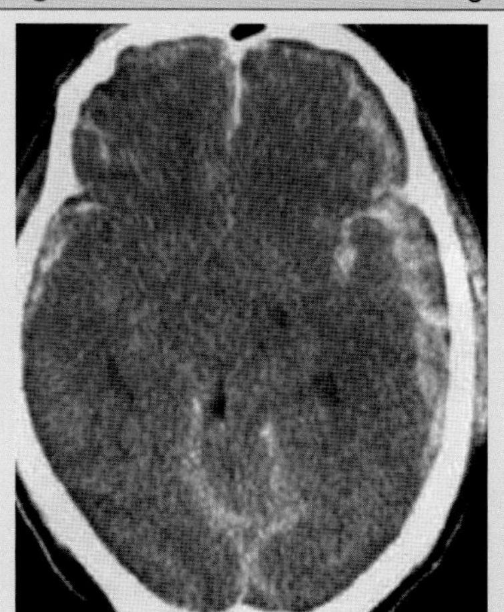 **Fig. 4.41.12:** Subarachnoid and subdural hemorrhage

Contd...

Condition	*Imaging features*	*Images*
Intraventricular hemorrhage: Intraventricular hemorrhage in the setting of trauma can originate from a ruptured subependymal vein, extension from an intra-parenchymal hematoma, or retrograde redistribution from the subarachnoid space.	Hyperdensity filling the ventricles. The clotted blood may cause occlusion causing obstructive hydrocephalus. Intraventricular hemorrhage on initial head CT images is correlated with DAI on subsequent MR images.	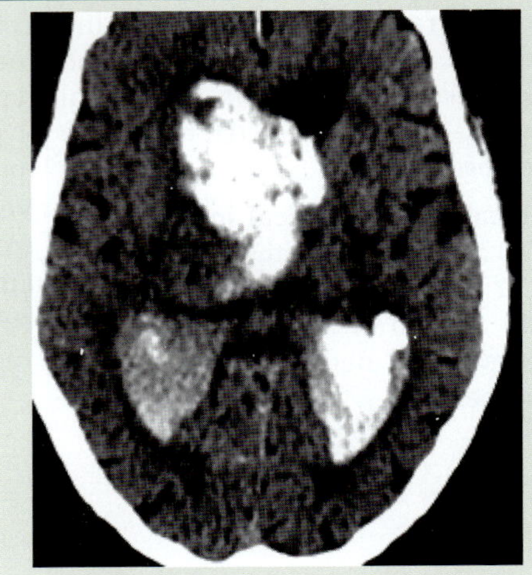 **Fig. 4.41.13:** Intraventricular hemorrhage
Brain contusion: Brain contusions are bruises of the brain parenchyma owing to impact. They characteristically occur at coup and contrecoup sites. Temporal lobe contusions on CT images are associated with worse functional outcome.	Most common location is in the inferior frontal lobes and anterior–**inferior temporal lobes.** Hyperdensity in the brain parenchyma surrounded by edema. MRI is more sensitive than CT for the detection of contusions, especially for small or non-hemorrhagic contusions.	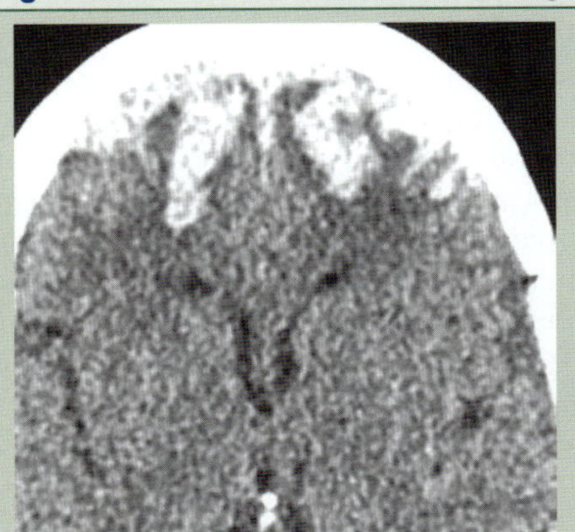 **Fig. 4.41.14:** Hemorrhagic contusions
Diffuse axonal injury: Result from axonal stretch and/or shear stress and predominantly affect highly organized white matter tracts and interfaces between brain tissues of different densities (i.e., gray-white junction). 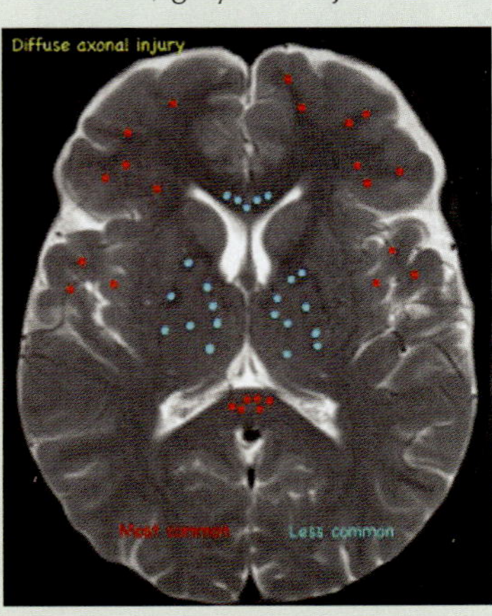 **Fig. 4.41.15:** Locations of diffuse axonal injury	Axonal injuries can result in focal T2-hyperintense white matter lesions. DAI is graded in order of increasing severity. Grade 1 involves the subcortical white matter, Grade 2 involves the corpus callosum, and Grade 3 involves the brainstem. However, these lesions are nonspecific.	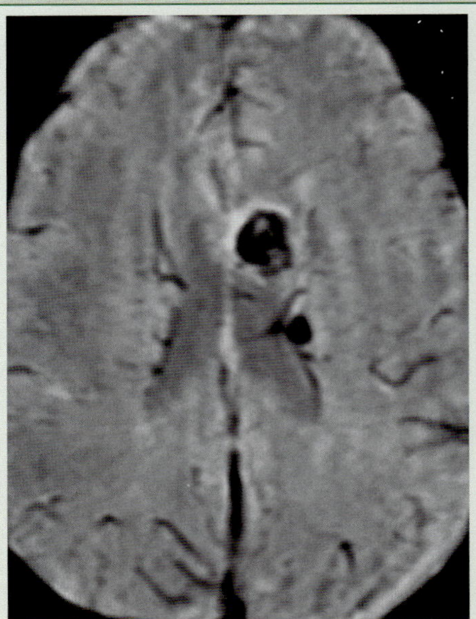 **Fig. 4.41.16:** Diffuse axonal injury

Contd...

Condition	Imaging features	Images	
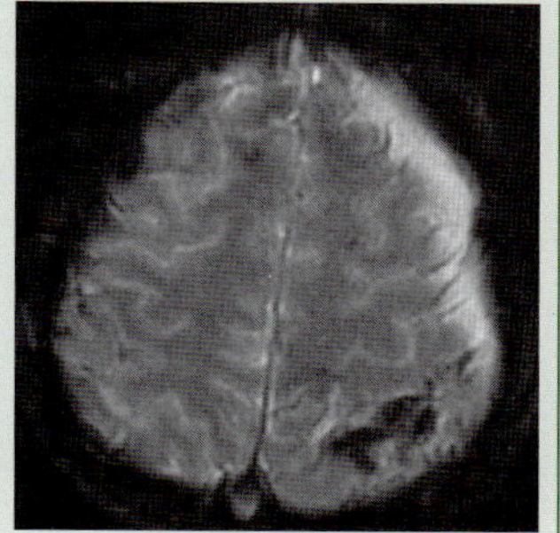 Fig. 4.41.17: Diffuse axonal injury	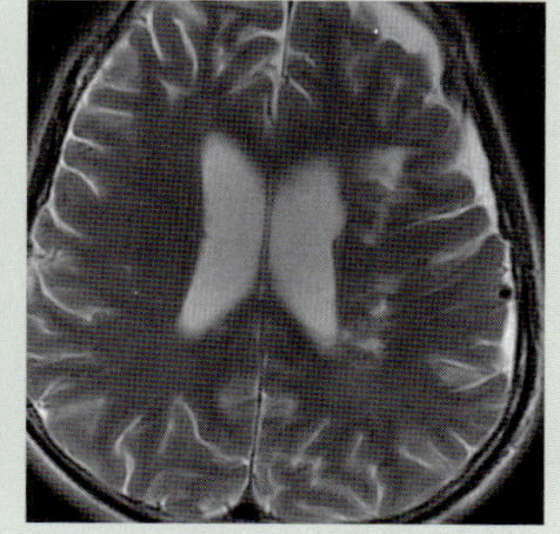 Fig. 4.41.18: Left subdural hemorrage with diffuse axonal injury	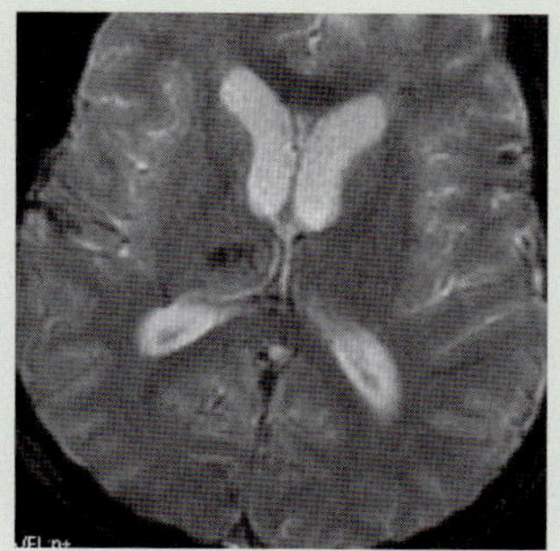 Fig. 4.41.19: Diffuse axonal injury in right thalamus	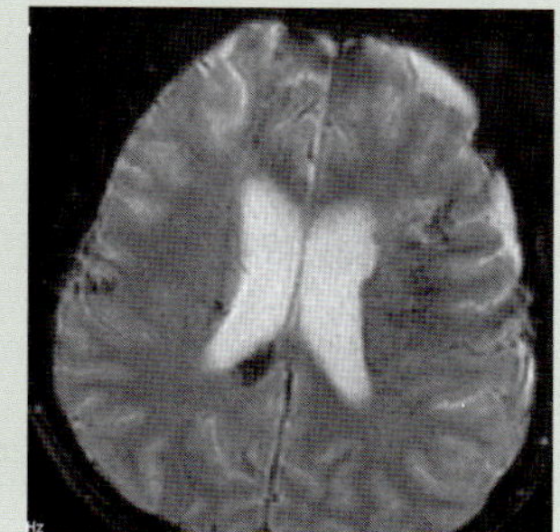 Fig. 4.41.20: Diffuse axonal injury in splenium of corpus callosum
Subdural hygroma: Subdural hygromas are caused by traumatic tears in the arachnoid membrane with resulting CSF accumulation in the subdural space. Subdural hygromas can occur in the first day, but the mean time to appearance is 9 days after injury. Common causes of subdural hygromas include trauma, post-meningitis or a component of intracranial hypotension. The fluid will be iso attenuating and isointense relative to CSF on CT and MR images, respectively. Hygromas displace vessels in the subarachnoid space from the inner table of the calvarium. A pure subdural hygroma will not have internal membranes as can subacute SDHs.	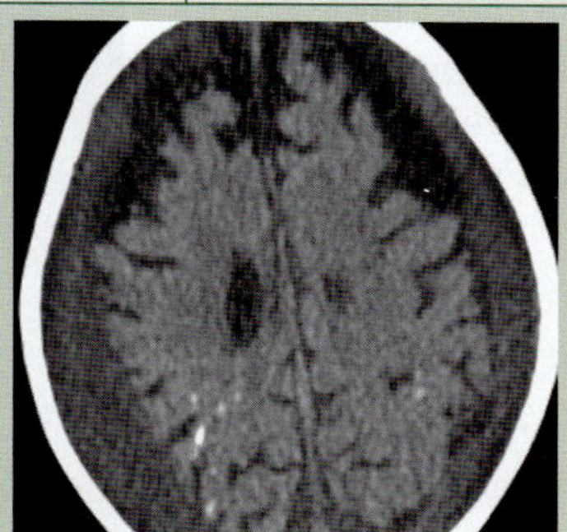 Fig. 4.41.21: Subdural hygromas	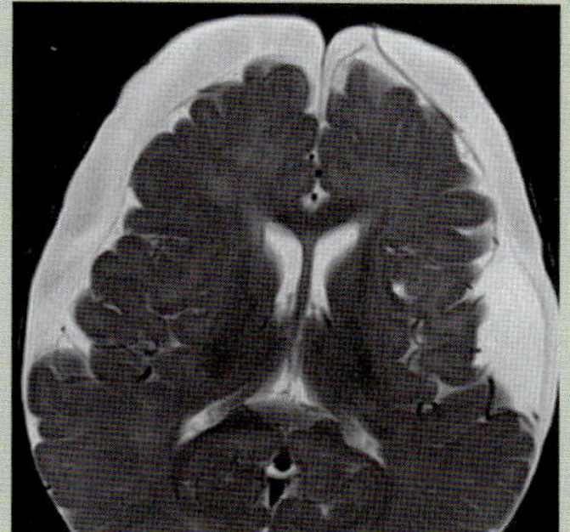 Fig. 4.41.22: Subdural hygromas	
Pneumocephalus The presence of intracranial air is caused by any breach in the calvarium, central skull base, mastoid or paranasal sinus. **Tension pneumocephalus** is the presence of intracranial air under pressure leading to neurological deterioration which also demonstrates - "**Mount Fuji Sign**" **Mimics:** Ruptured dermoid	Depending on the location: Epidural- unilateral, biconvex, does not change with head position. Subdural-confluent, crescentic, bilateral, shows crossing cortical veins, changes with head position. Subarachnoid—discrete spots and dots in sulci and cistern. Intraventricular—in frontal horn with air fluid level.	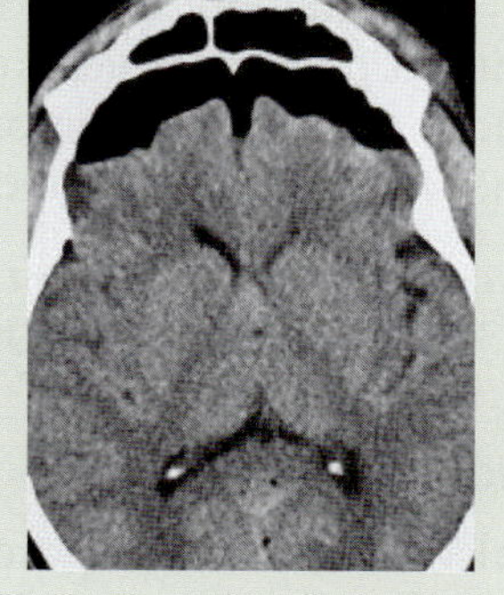 Fig. 4.41.23: Pneumocephalus	
Secondary effects			
Condition	*Imaging features*	*Images*	
Diffuse cerebral edema: Result from head injury, possibly due to dysfunctional cerebral autoregulation and blood–brain barrier disruption. The onset of cerebral edema is variable but is thought to be related to the release of various mediators that can increase blood–brain barrier permeability and result in vasogenic and cytotoxic edema	Effacement of sulcal and gyral spaces, loss of grey white mater differentiation , slit-like lateral ventricles and tonsillar herniation	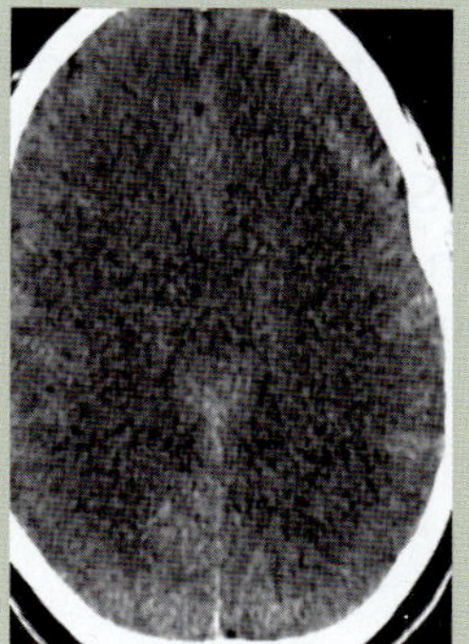 Fig. 4.41.24: Diffuse cerebral edema	

Condition	Imaging features	Images
Vascular injuries: Vascular injuries include arterial dissection (especially when a fracture traverses the skull base), pseudoaneurysm (most commonly involving the vertebral artery, followed by the anterior cerebral artery), traumatic carotid-cavernous fistula. Cervical spine fractures have the strongest association with blunt cerebrovascular injury.	Contrast enhanced CT may reveal active extravasation, vascular occlusion, traumatic dural arteriovenous fistula, and venous thrombosis (especially when a fracture traverses the dural venous sinus)	

hemorrhagic patterns include isolated SAH in the basilar cistern, isolated large volume SAH in the sylvian fissure and isolated SAH in the anterior interhemispheric fissure. Angiography in these cases to be considered to evaluate for a ruptured aneurysm. A large hematoma with associated calcification or prominent veins should raise suspicion for vascular malformation and CT/MR angiography is indicated.

Indication for Taking Head CT in Minor Degree Injury

American College of Radiology (ACR) criteria: 1. The presence of a focal neurologic deficit. 2. Children under 2 years of age.

New Orleans criteria in minor head injury: CT indicated if GCS = 15 plus any of the following: 1. Headache, 2. vomiting, 3. patient >60 years old, 4. intoxication (drugs, alcohol), 5. short-term memory deficits (anterograde amnesia), 6. visible trauma above clavicles, 7. seizure.

Canadian head CT rule in minor head injury: CT, if GCS = 13–15 and witnessed LOC, amnesia, or confusion.

Secondary Brain Herniation

Cerebral herniation is a potentially life-threatening condition that needs to be diagnosed promptly. The imaging spectrum can range from subtle changes to clear displacement of brain structures.

Brain herniation can be classified into two broad categories: intracranial and extracranial. Furthermore, intracranial hernias can be subdivided into three basic types: (a) Subfalcine hernia; (b) transtentorial hernia, which can be ascending or descending (lateral and central); and (c) tonsillar hernia.

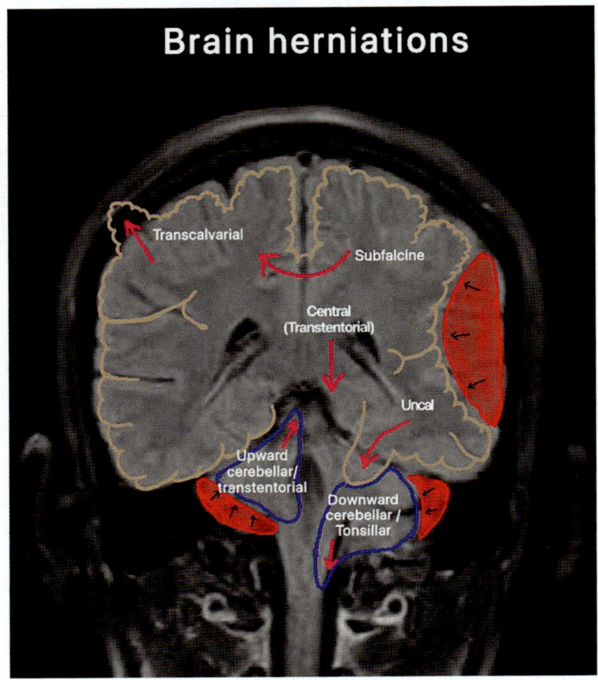

Fig. 4.41.25: Various brain herniations

Six-point approach to diagnose brain herniation syndromes

1. Clinical information (neurologic syndrome, history).
2. Anatomic landmarks (falx cerebri, septum pellucidum, tentorium and foramen magnum).
3. Direction of mass effect.
4. Displaced structure.
5. Indirect signs (other involved structures—cistern, brain stem, ventricles).
6. Herniation-related complications (stroke—ACA, PCA and PICA, cranial nerve syndromes and hydrocephalus).

Condition	*Imaging features*	*Images*
Subfalcine herniation (midline shift/ cingulate hernia): The most common type of cerebral hernia. It is generally caused by unilateral frontal, parietal, or temporal lobe disease. The degree of midline shift correlates with the prognosis; less than 5 mm deviation has a good prognosis, whereas a shift of more than 15 mm is related to a poor outcome.	Cingulate gyrus and corpus callosum gets displaced medial and anteriorly, beneath **falx cerebri**. Lateral ventriculomegaly on the side that the midline is shifting toward. Ischemic complication includes ACA infarction on the side of the mass effect.	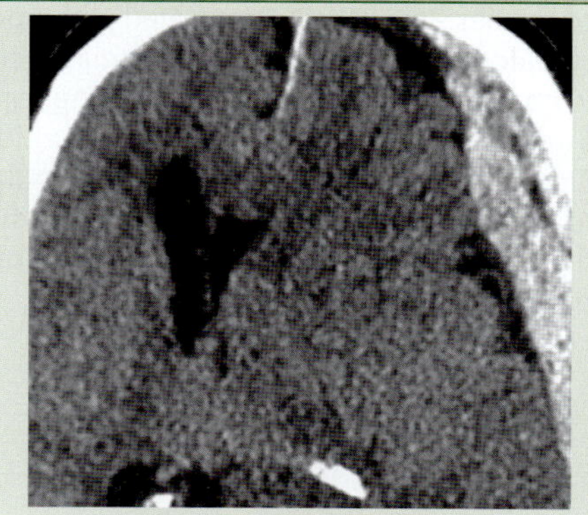 **Fig. 4.41.26:** Subfalcine herniation
Descending transtentorial herniation: The second most common type. It occurs when brain tissue is displaced downward through the tentorial notch. DTH may be divided into two types: Lateral (anterior and posterior) and central hernias. Complications include compromise of the third cranial nerve, posterior cerebral artery, and midbrain. Hydrocephalus develops because of the compression of the cerebral aqueduct. With severe and abrupt downward displacement of the brainstem—Duret hemorrhages occur at Ponto mesencephalic junction.	Structures involved—medial temporal lobe. Anterior subtype **(uncal herniation)**—uncus herniates into the ipsilateral crural cistern. Posterior subtype—the parahippocampal gyrus herniates into the posterolateral part of the tentorial incisura. In central hernias, there is descent of the diencephalon, midbrain, and pons. The initial displacement of the uncus results in effacement of the suprasellar cistern. With more advanced herniation, the midbrain and opposite cerebral peduncle are compressed against the tentorial edge—Kernohan's notch phenomenon (false localizing sign).	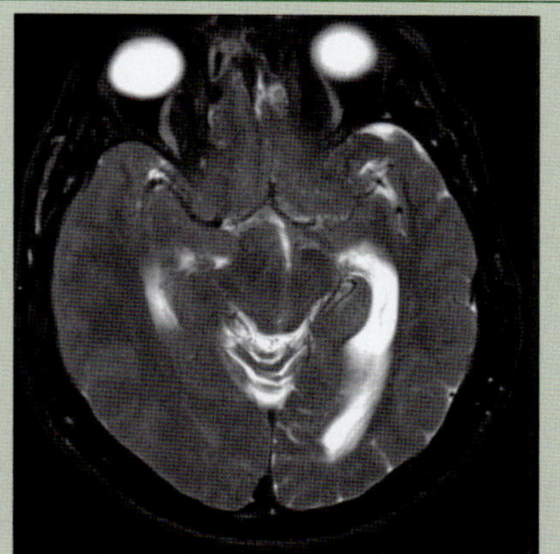 **Fig. 4.41.27:** Descending transtentorial herniation
Ascending transtentorial hernia: It occurs when a mass effect, coming from the posterior cranial fossa with an upward direction, displaces the cerebellar vermis and hemispheres superiorly through the tentorial incisura. Another possible cause is sudden relief of supratentorial intracranial hypertension.	As there is upward herniation of the cerebellar vermis, anterior displacement of the midbrain and cerebral aqueduct takes place. The normal concave configuration of the quadrigeminal plate cistern is distorted, taking on a flat or convex morphology. Ischemic infarction of the superior portion of the cerebellar hemispheres and occipital cerebral lobe may occur in severe cases.	
Cerebellar tonsillar herniation: Tonsillar hernia is inferior displacement of the cerebellar tonsils through the foramen magnum into the cervical spinal canal. The McRae line is used as a reference. The most common cause is an infratentorial mass creating a downward mass effect.	Visualization of tonsils extending below the foramen magnum, anterior brainstem displacement, and loss of CSF surrounding it. The fourth ventricle may be compressed, producing obstructive supratentorial hydrocephalus. Compression of the posterior inferior cerebellar artery can lead to cerebellar infarcts.	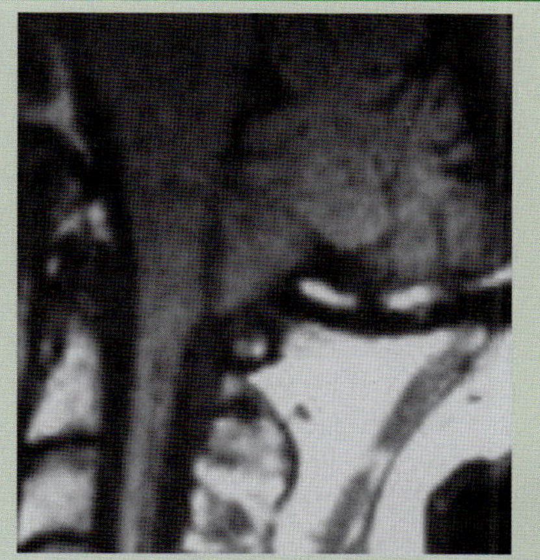 **Fig. 4.41.28:** Cerebellar tonsillar herniation

<table>
<tr>
<td>Transalar herniation: Uncommon type of hernias. It is usually associated with subfalcine and transtentorial hernias. It can be divided into descending and ascending transalar hernias. Descending type manifests secondary to frontal lobe disease. Ascending type manifests secondary to temporal lobe disease causing mass effect in middle cranial fossa.</td>
<td>In descending type—the frontal lobe is displaced posteriorly and inferiorly over the sphenoid wing, causing compression of the MCA against the sphenoid ridge. In ascending type—the temporal lobe is displaced superiorly and anteriorly across the sphenoid ridge causing compression of the supraclinoid ICA against the anterior clinoid process with infarction of the ACA and MCA.</td>
<td>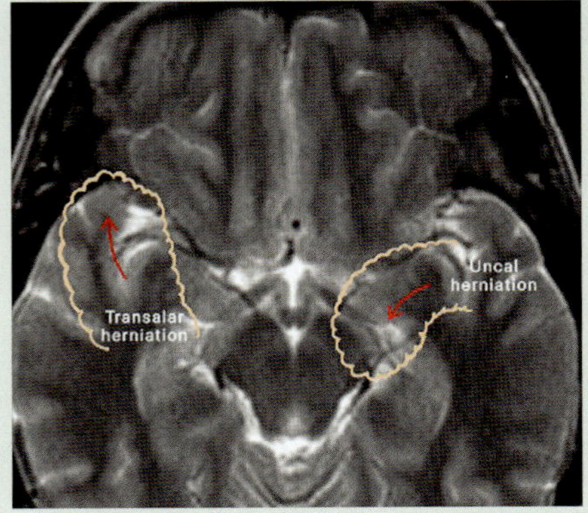

Fig. 4.41.29: Transalar herniation</td>
</tr>
<tr>
<td>Transcalvarial (extracranial) herniation: Most frequently caused by postsurgical and post-traumatic cranial defects that allow brain tissue to pass through.
Paradoxical hernia is a rare and potentially fatal complication of decompressive craniectomy. It is a neurosurgical emergency. Atmospheric pressure exceeding ICP at the site of the craniectomy causes a pressure imbalance and consequent subfalcine and/or transtentorial hernia.</td>
<td>A large craniectomy defect allows the brain to expand without constriction. If the defect is too small, swollen brain may herniate with a "mushroom cap" appearance. This can result in compression of cortical veins and lead to venous infarction and contusion of the brain at the craniectomy margins. In paradoxical hernia, the brain tissue is displaced away from the craniectomy defect—skin flap depression deep to calvarium creating S-shaped configuration—sinking skin flap syndrome.</td>
<td>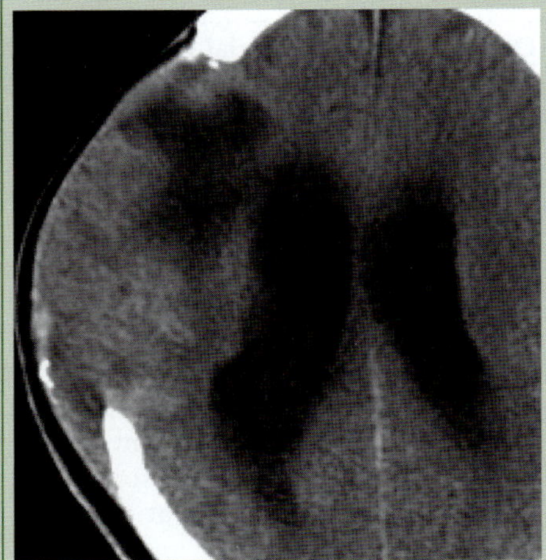
Fig. 4.41.30: Transcalvarial (extracranial) herniation</td>
</tr>
<tr>
<td colspan="3">Chronic secondary changes</td>
</tr>
<tr>
<td>Condition</td>
<td>Imaging features</td>
<td>Images</td>
</tr>
<tr>
<td>Traumatic hydrocephalus: This occurs secondary to impaired CSF resorption at the level of arachnoid villi or secondary to obstruction of the cerebral aqueduct and 4th ventricle.
Mass effect from cerebral herniation or hematoma can also cause non-communicating hydrocephalus.</td>
<td>Dilated lateral and third ventricle with periventricular seepage in case of obstruction of the cerebral aqueduct.
Dilated bilateral, third and fourth ventricle in case of impaired CSF resorption at the level of arachnoid villi.</td>
<td>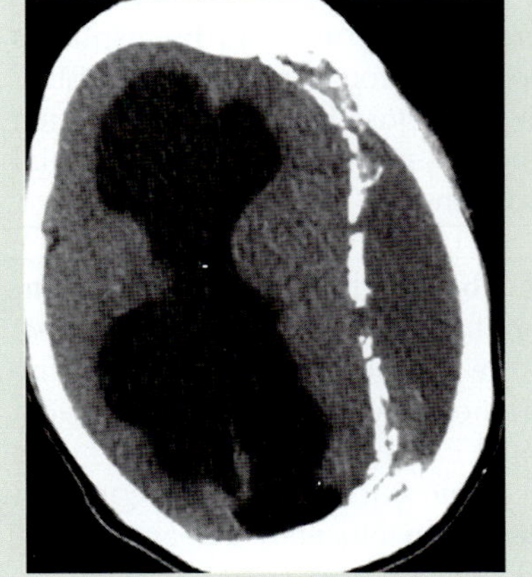
Fig. 4.41.31: Traumatic hydrocephalus</td>
</tr>
</table>

<table>
<tr>
<td colspan="2">Post-traumatic gliosis/encephalomalacia: Characteristically involves orbitofrontal (especially the gyrus rectus) and anteroinferior temporal lobes. CT shows an area of low attenuation with volume loss. Areas of gliosis appear low intensity on T1 and high intensity on T2.</td>
<td>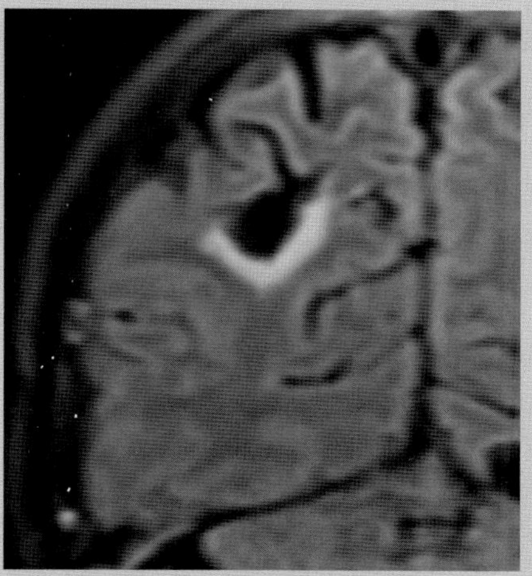
Fig. 4.41.32: Post-traumatic gliosis</td>
</tr>
<tr>
<td>Leptomeningeal cyst or growing fracture: Usually seen in children (3 years) and are associated with dural tear and a calvarial defect. Depressed fractures can lacerate the dura with herniation of pia arachnoid through the tear.
CSF pulsation fill and enlarge the subarachnoid pouch with erosion of the inner table more than outer table giving rise to beveled edges.</td>
<td>CT shows CSF-filled subarachnoid pouch in the scalp with underlying skull fracture showing beveled edges.
Other associated findings include post-traumatic encephalomalacia, focal ventricular enlargement and porencephaly.</td>
<td>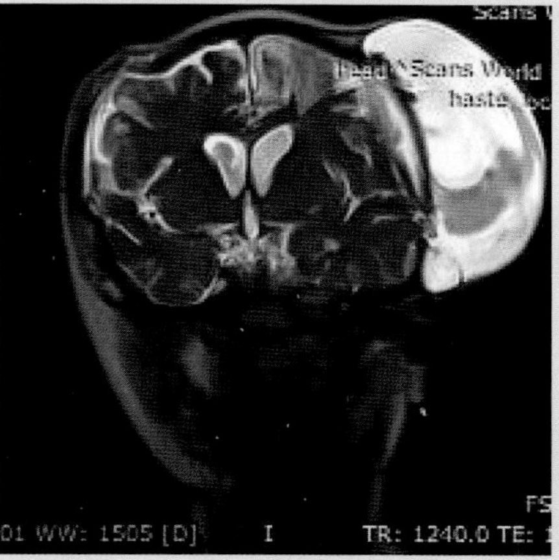

Fig. 4.41.33: Growing skull fracture</td>
</tr>
</table>

4.42 CENTRAL NERVOUS SYSTEM

Case No. 42

Clinical history: A 68-year-old female with history of progressive memory loss for the past 1 year. No gait disturbances.

CT brain (Figs 4.42.1 and 4.42.2) shows **marked volume loss in bilateral parietal lobe, hippocampi and parahippocampal** gyri with relative sparing of rest of temporal lobe. No evidence of intracranial haemorrhage. No evidence of infarction. Periventricular and deep white matter hypodensity noted suggestive of small vessel ischemic changes. Ventricles are enlarged suggestive of age-related changes. No calvarial fracture or suspicious bony abnormality noted. Imaged para nasal sinus and mastoid cells appear normal.

MRI brain flair coronal (Figs 4.42.3 and 4.42.4), T1 sagittal section demonstrates atrophy of bilateral parietal lobes associated with **volume loss of bilateral hippocampi and medial temporal lobe.** The interuncal distance at level of anterior commissure is 32. Sulcal spaces, basal cisterns, ventricles appear prominent. **MTA scale** for medial temporal atrophy—scale 3. A few small discrete T2/FLAIR hyperintensity without restricted diffusion noted in bilateral periventricular region-Fazekas scale for white matter lesion—score 1. No feature suggestive of micro-hemorrhages. **MR spectroscopy** (Fig. 4.42.5) **shows decrease in NAA, increase in myoinositol.**

Interpretation: A: 68 years old female, bilateral parietal lobe and bilateral hippocampal and medial temporal lobe, C: Volume loss with decrease in NAA, increase in myoinositol, B: Sulcal spaces, basal cisterns, ventricles appear prominent. D: Alzheimer's disease.

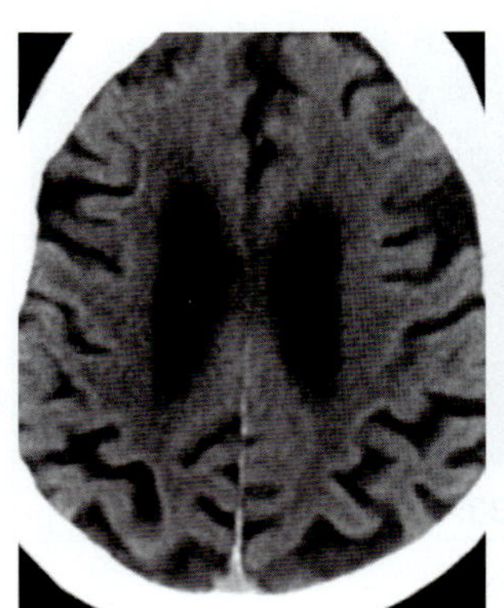

Fig. 4.42.1

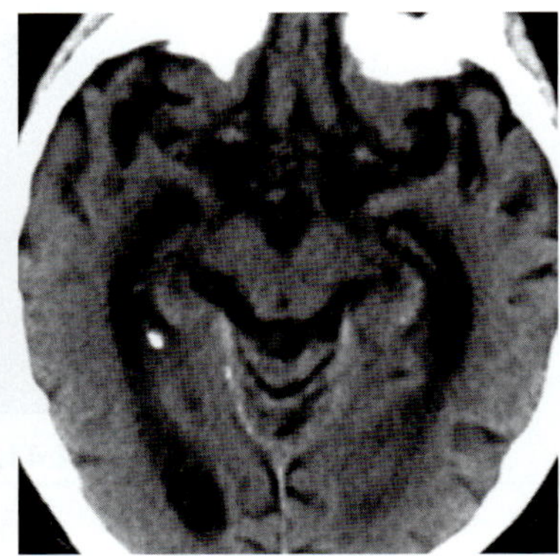

Fig. 4.42.2

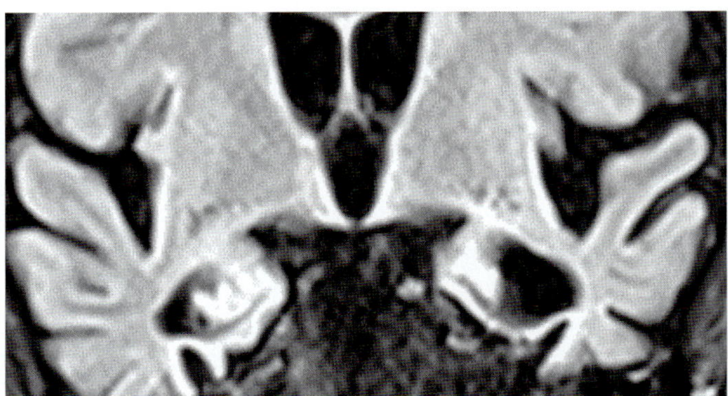

Fig. 4.42.3

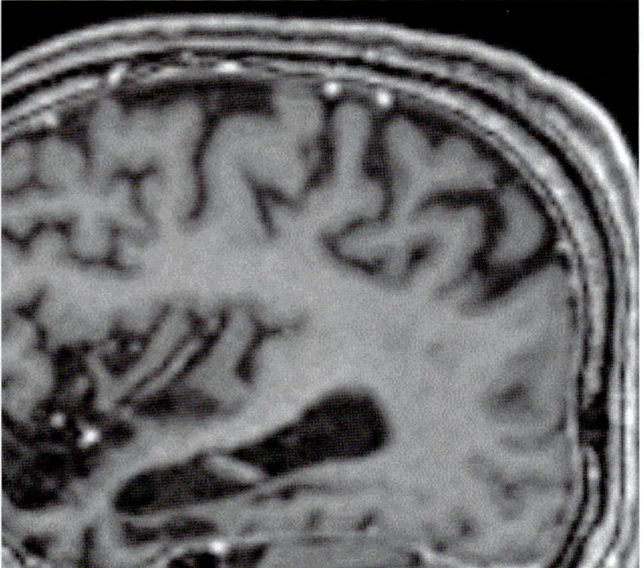

Fig. 4.42.4

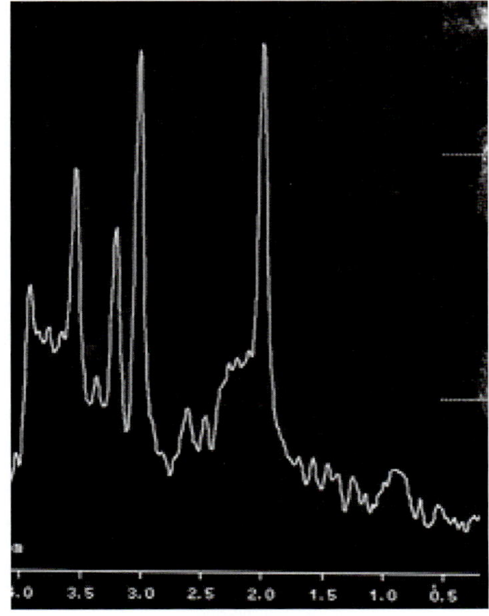

Fig. 4.42.5

Principal diagnosis: Alzheimer's disease.

Differential diagnosis: (1) Normal age-related degenerative process, (2) vascular dementia, (3) Lewy body dementia, (4) frontotemporal lobar degeneration, (5) normal pressure hydrocephalus, (6) infections–HIV related dementia, (7) Creutzfeldt Jakob disease.

Table 4.42.1: Differential diagnosis for suspected dementia case		
Vascular dementia: The 2nd most common cause. MC cause is deep white matter changes over a number of years; other cause is large vessel strategic and cortical infarcts leading to acute onset of vascular dementia. 1. Chronic small vessel ischemic changes 2. Binswanger's disease (chronic hypertensive encephalopathy) 3. Amyloid angiopathy 4. Strategic infarcts	**Small vessel (Binswanger's):** Multiple basal ganglia and white matter lesions. Extensive periventricular white matter lesions (Fazekas grade 3). B/L thalamic lesions **large vessel strategic infarcts:** B/L ACA, PCA: Paramedian thalamus, mesial temporal lobe, MCA: Parieto-temporal, temporo-occipital angular gyrus, Watershed infarcts. The appearance will be similar in chronic small vessel ischemic changes, Binswanger disease and amyloid angiopathy (Refer to case 4.32)	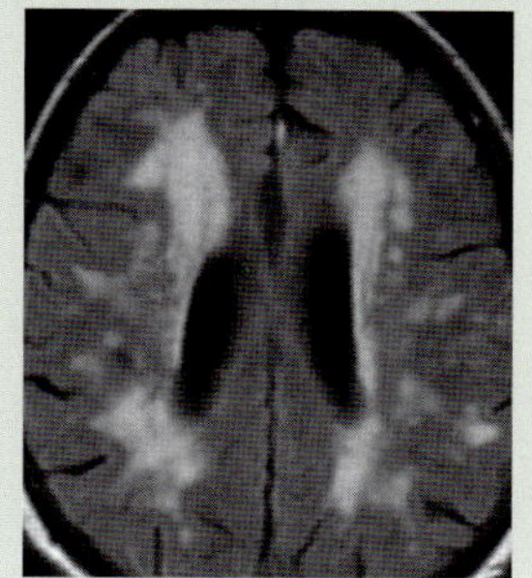 **Fig. 4.42.6:** Chronic small vessel ischemic changes
Amyloid angiopathy 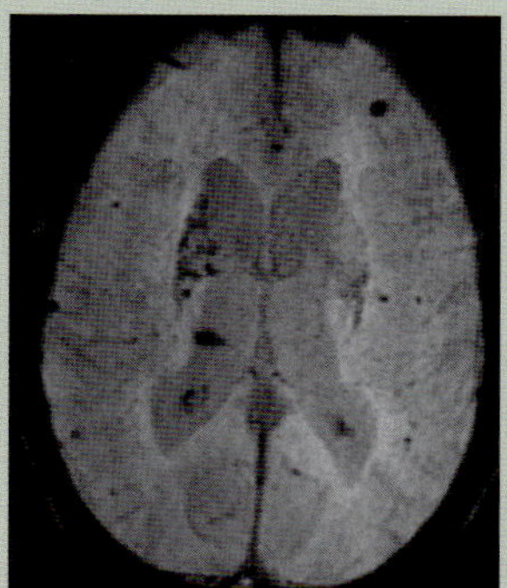 **Fig. 4.42.7:** Amyloid angiopathy	**Binswanger disease** 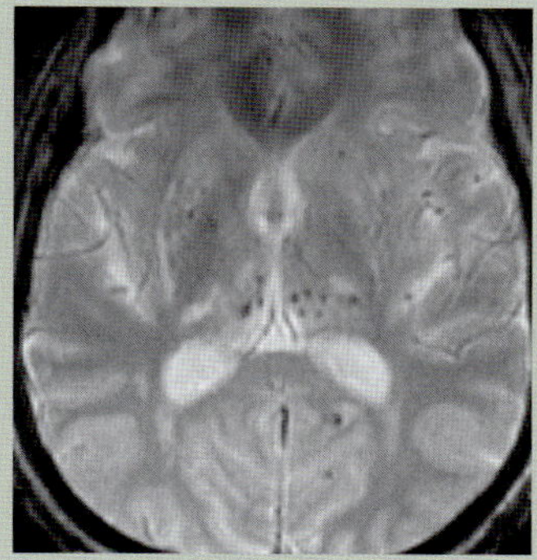 **Fig. 4.42.8:** Binswanger disease	**Strategic infarct** 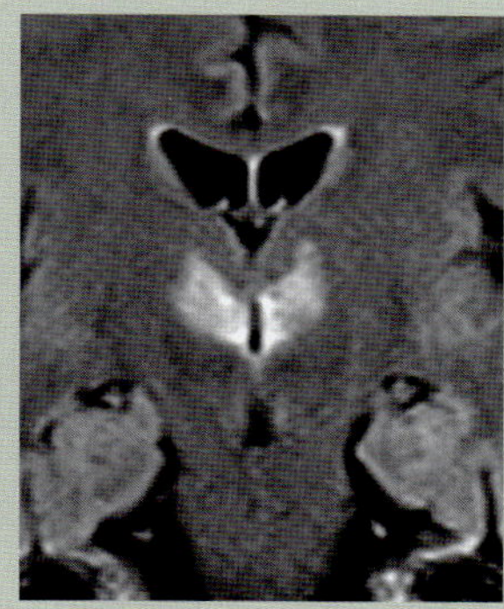 **Fig. 4.42.9:** Strategic infarct
Dementia with Lewy bodies (25%): Patient present with one among three: (1) Visual hallucinations, (2) Parkinson-like symptoms, (3) fluctuation in alertness and attention. 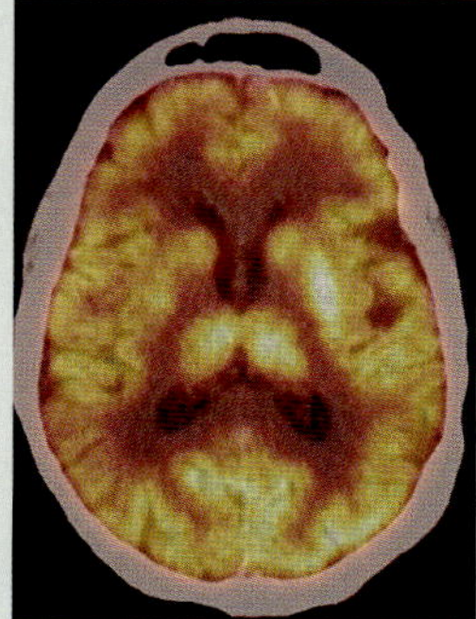 **Fig. 4.42.10:** Right corpus striatum shows reduction in uptake	Usually the MRI imaging is normal including the hippocampus—age-related changes like mild generalised atrophy without lobar predominance, nonspecific white matter hyperintensities found in normal aging patients in T2/FLAIR. DaT scan shows reduced uptake in putamen and caudate. **Cingulate island** sign—occipital hypometabolism with relative sparing of posterior cingulate cortex.	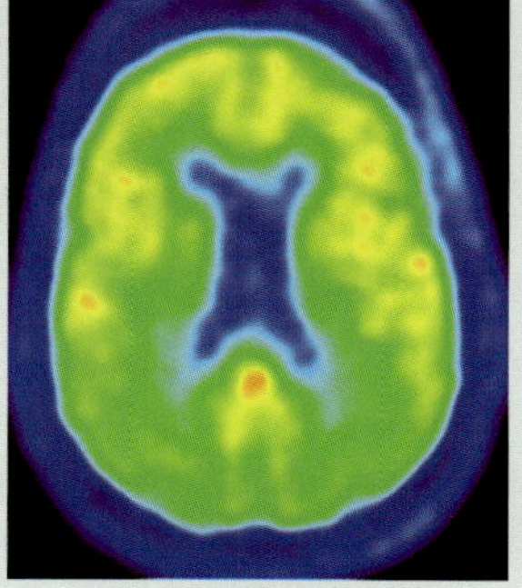 **Fig. 4.42.11:** Dementia with Lewy bodies 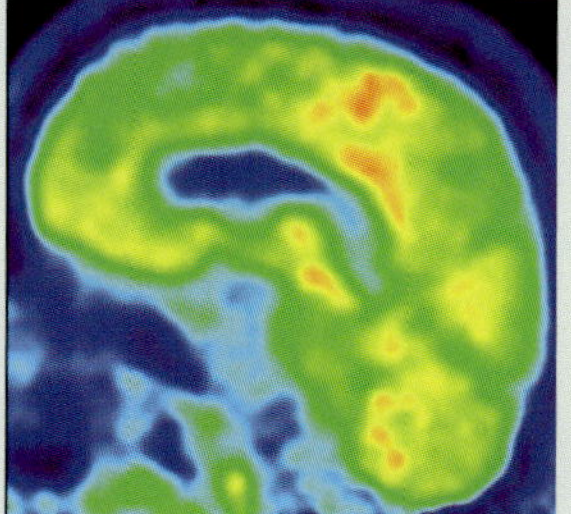 **Fig. 4.42.12:** Dementia with Lewy bodies

(Contd.)

<table>
<tr><th colspan="3">Table 4.42.1: Differential diagnosis for suspected dementia case (Contd.)</th></tr>
<tr>
<td>Frontotemporal lobar degeneration—characterised by asymmetric atrophy of frontal and temporal lobes
Fronto-temporal dementia
Behavioral and personality changes. Bifrontal/temporal atrophy.</td>
<td>Primary progressive aphasia: Non-fluent aphasia/asymmetric atrophy lateral part temporal lobe (left) progressive atrophy hemispheres (FTD)
Semantic dementia: Fluent aphasia asymmetric atrophy anterior part of medial temporal lobe.
Prosopagnosia: Asymmetric atrophy of right temporal lobe.</td>
<td>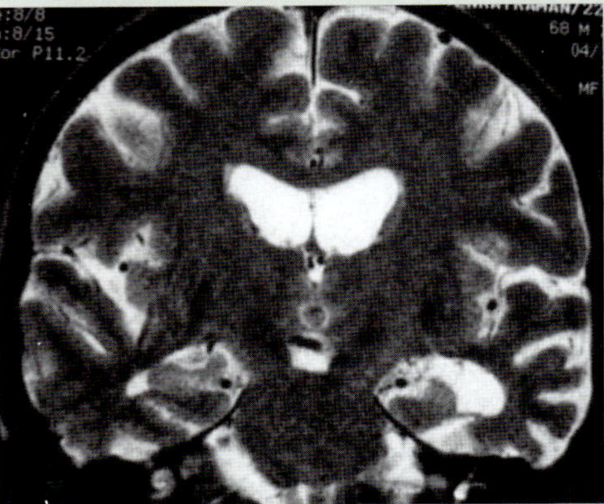
Fig. 4.42.13: Frontotemporal lobar degeneration</td>
</tr>
<tr>
<td colspan="2">Normal pressure hydrocephalus
Complaints—unstable gait, dementia, urinary urgency. Disproportionately enlarged subarachnoid space hydrocephalus (DESH)—Disproportionately dilated lateral and third ventricles with crowding of sulci superiority near the vertex and enlargement of CSF spaces in the sylvian fissure and basal brain region.
Dilated ventricles with upward bowing of corpus callosum.
Relative absence of sulcal widening. Patient with increased CSF flow voids–surgical candidate. "Cingulate sulcus sign"—posterior part of cingulate sulcus being narrower than the anterior part.
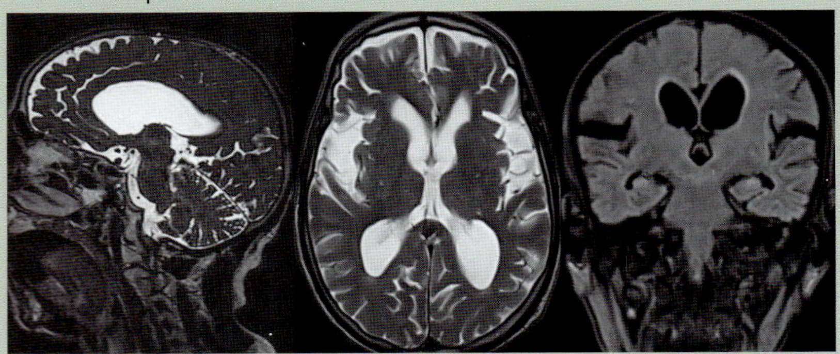
Fig. 4.42.14: Disproportionately enlarged subarachnoid hydrocephalus (DESH)</td>
<td>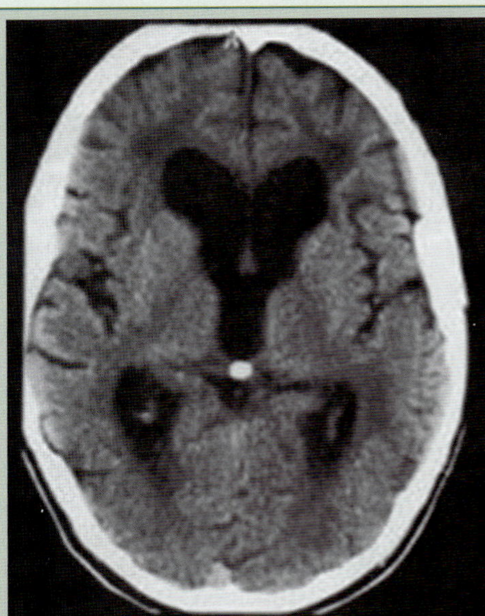
Fig. 4.42.15: Normal pressure hydrocephalus</td>
</tr>
<tr>
<td>Creutzfeldt-Jakob disease (mad cow disease) Prion disease causing dementia
Classical: Focal/diffuse/symmetric/asymmetric involvement of cortex and basal ganglia</td>
<td>Variant: Pulvinar sign
Bilateral and symmetrical high signal in the pulvinar nuclei of the thalamus
Hockey stick sign: Symmetrical hyperintensity of pulvinar and dorsomedial thalamic nuclei</td>
<td>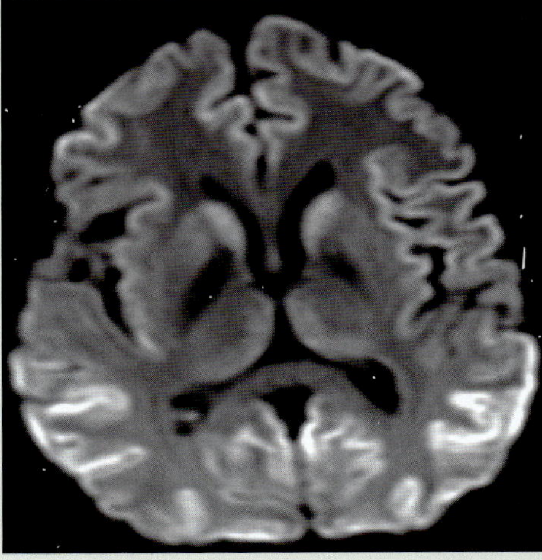
Fig. 4.42.16: Creutzfeldt-Jakob disease</td>
</tr>
</table>

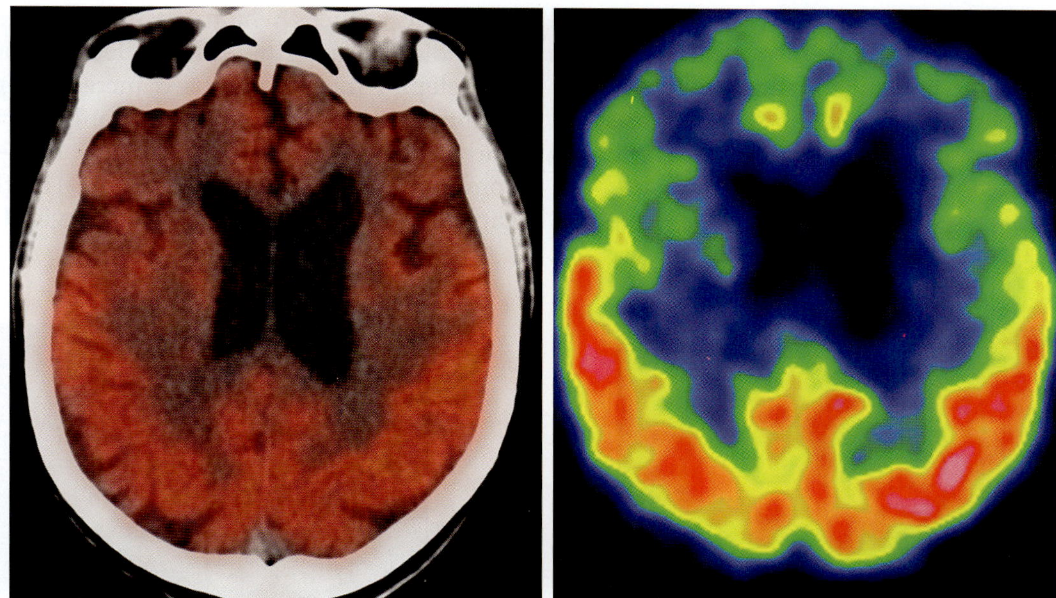

Fig. 4.42.17: Frontotemporal dementia

Brief discussion about condition: Most common dementia. Prevalence increases 15–25% per decade after 65 years. Alzheimer's disease is a progressive neurodegenerative condition that leads to cognitive decline and impaired ability to perform activities of daily living.

Pathophysiology: Macroscopic: Atrophy, widened ventricles/sulci, Weight brain is reduced (sometimes <1000 g); microscopic: Accumulation of amyloid Aβ42, neurofibrillary tangles causing neuronal death.

Imaging: **CT–medial temporal lobe atrophy** is an early sign on CT. Late findings include generalised cortical atrophy. **MRI**—common morphologic changes include thinned gyri, widened sulci, enlarged lateral ventricles.

Sparing of sensory motor cortex, basal ganglia, thalamus and primary visual cortex noted.

Table 4.42.2: Difference between presenile and senile dementia

Early onset Alzheimer's disease (presenile): <65 years	Late onset Alzheimer's disease >65 years (senile)
Posterior cortical atrophy, mainly parietal atrophy, precuneus (sagittal T1), posterior cingulate.	Disproportionate medial temporal atrophy. Focal cortical atrophy—mainly temporal/parietal, WMH and microbleeds may occur with, sparing of basal ganglia.
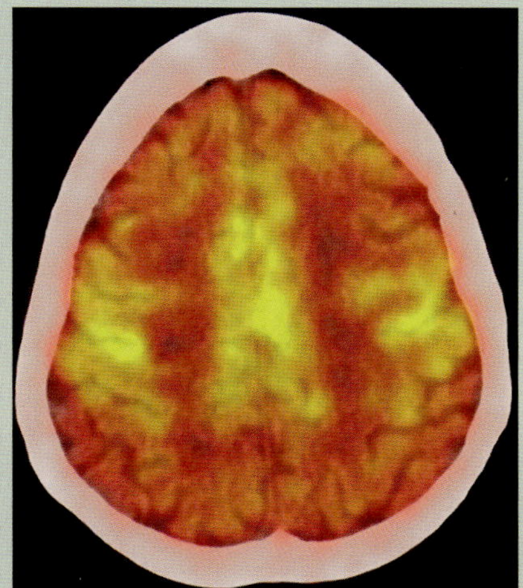 **Fig. 4.42.18:** Presenile Alzheimer's disease	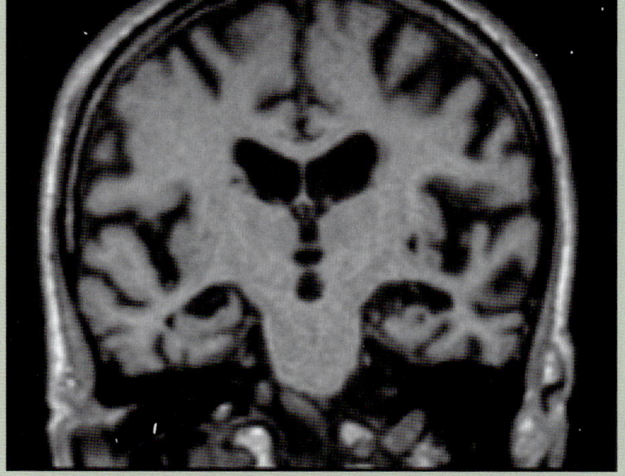 **Fig. 4.42.19:** Senile Alzheimer's disease

MRS shows **decreased NAA and increased myoinositol, decreased glutamine** in patients with Alzheimer's disease even during early stages, DTI in patients with Alzheimer's disease shows **decreased FA** in multiple regions which reflects early microstructural white matter changes.

Nuclear medicine: **18F FDG PET** shows areas of **regional hypometabolism** of parietotemporal and posterior cingulate cortices which are bilaterally symmetrical. Amyloid PET imaging: 18F labelled amyloid tracers like florbetapir is more widely used, **increased uptake in areas of amyloid deposition**—commonly parietotemporal and posterior cingulate cortices. **PIB—Pittsburgh compound B:** A radioactive analog of Thioflavin T which can be used in PET to image beta amyloid plaque.

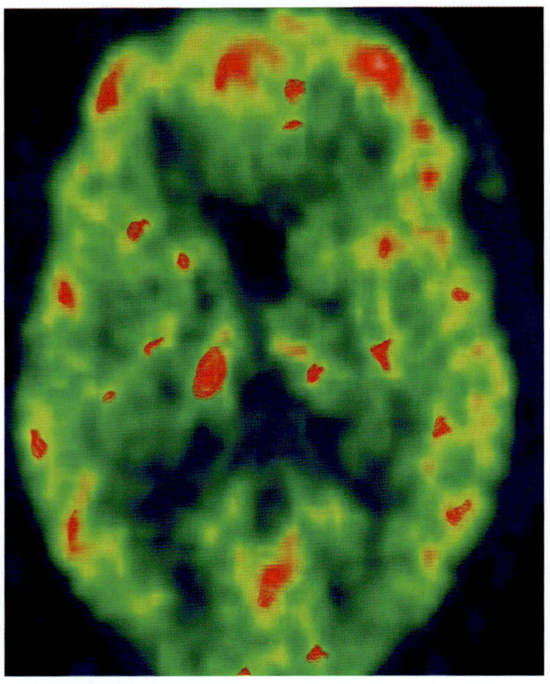

Fig. 4.42.20: Alzheimer's in amyloid imaging

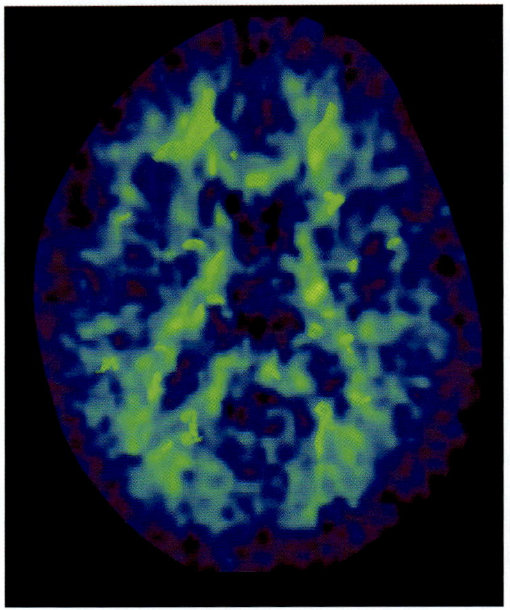

Fig. 4.42.21: Normal 11C-PIB PET

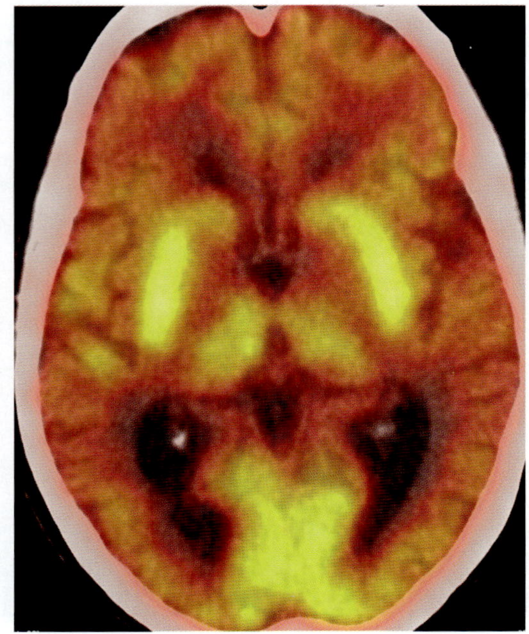

Fig. 4.42.22: Alzheimer's in 18-FDG PET

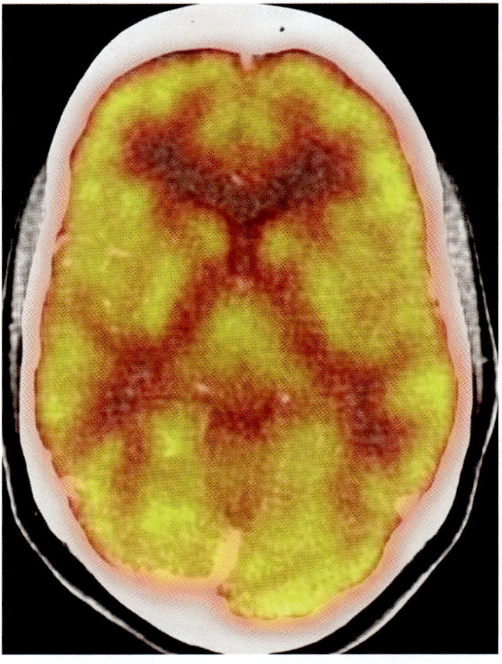

Fig. 4.42.23: Normal 18-FDG PET

Approach to Dementia

Imaging modalities:

CT: NECT is a screening procedure to r/o subdural hematoma/tumor/normal pressure hydrocephalus.

MRI: For demonstration of specific pathology like hippocampal atrophy **(hippocampal atrophy in young age—mesial temporal sclerosis).**

Nuclear imaging for demonstration of metabolic changes in structures affected

MRI protocol in analysis of dementia: No contrast media necessary!

Coronal T1-weighted: Evaluation of the medial temporal lobe

Axial FLAIR and T2 TSE: Vascular "white matter" pathology

Axial T2* gradient-echo (or SWI): Detection of (micro) bleeds.

Optional: DWI (Creutzfeldt-Jakob disease).

MRS: Voxel box should be kept in posterior cingulate gyrus.

Normal aging phenomena: Periventricular caps and bands—mild ependymal loss, subependymal gliosis, widened extracellular space

Pencil-thin lining seen in >40–50 years of age

Regular caps/bands seen in >65 years of age

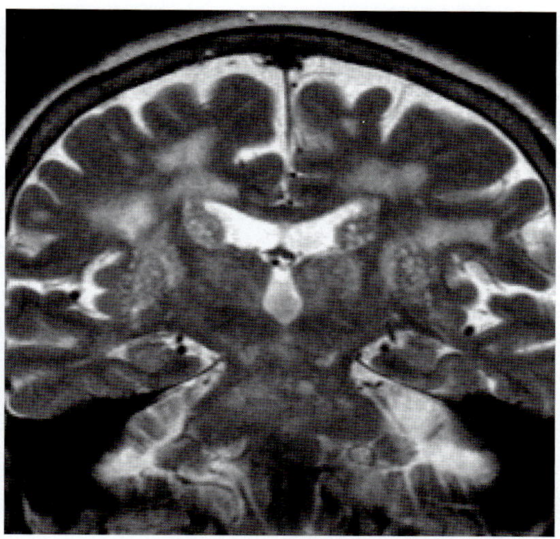

Fig. 4.42.24: Normal old age changes

Virchow-Robin spaces (VRS): Widened Virchow-Robin spaces (VRS)—perivascular extension of subarachnoid space, **around anterior commissure**—normal in early adulthood, **at the vertex**—normal in old age, incidentally giant VRS, État criblé–widening of VRS in basal ganglia is always abnormal.

Cortical atrophy: Selective atrophy of white matter (frontal and parietal regions most susceptible, occipital regions typically spared).

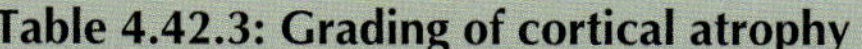

Table 4.42.3: Grading of cortical atrophy

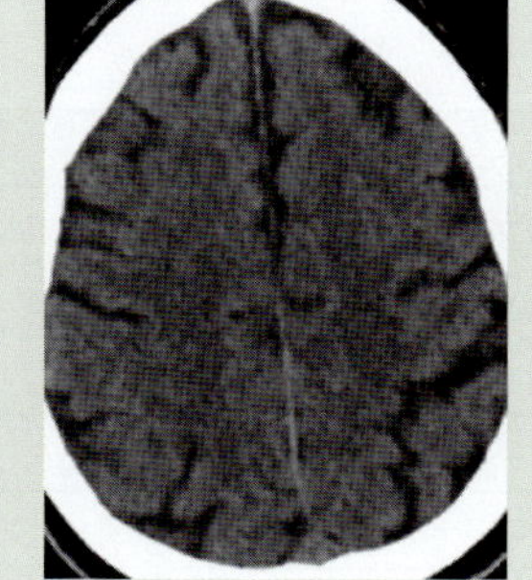	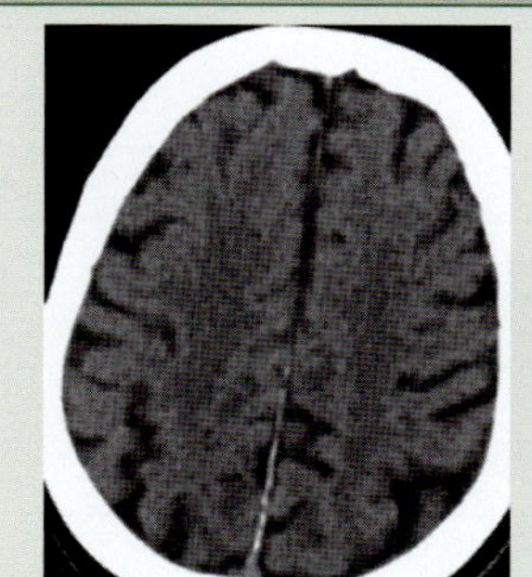	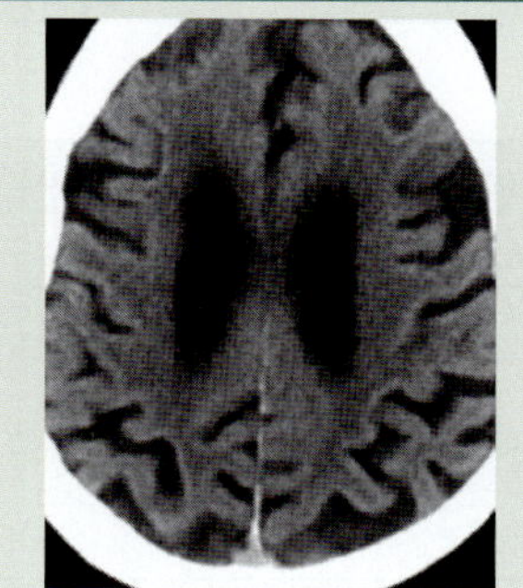	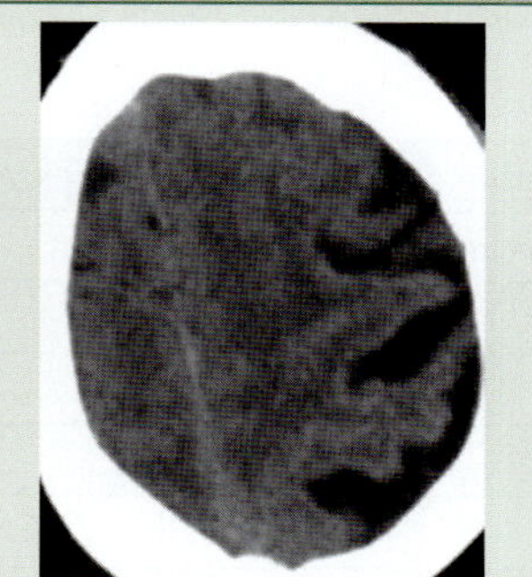
Fig. 4.42.25: Grade 0: Normal	**Fig. 4.42.26:** Grade 1: Opening of sulci	**Fig. 4.42.27:** Grade 2: Volume loss of gyri	**Fig. 4.42.28:** Grade 3: Knife blade atrophy

Medial temporal lobe atrophy (MTA), white matter lesions (WML), cerebral microbleeds (MBs), iron accumulation basal nuclei are other normal aging phenomena.

Table 4.42.4: Fazekas grading of white matter hyperintensities

Deep white matter hyperintensities	*Periventricular white matter hyperintensities*
0 = normal, no focal lesions	0 = normal, no focal lesions
1 = punctiform lesions	1= caps or pencil thin lining

(Contd.)

Table 4.42.4: Fazekas grading of white matter hyperintensities (*Contd.*)	
Deep white matter hyperintensities	*Periventricular white matter hyperintensities*
2 = early confluent lesions	2 = smooth halo
3 = confluent lesions	3 = irregular periventricular signal extending to deep white matter

Deep white matter hyperintensities

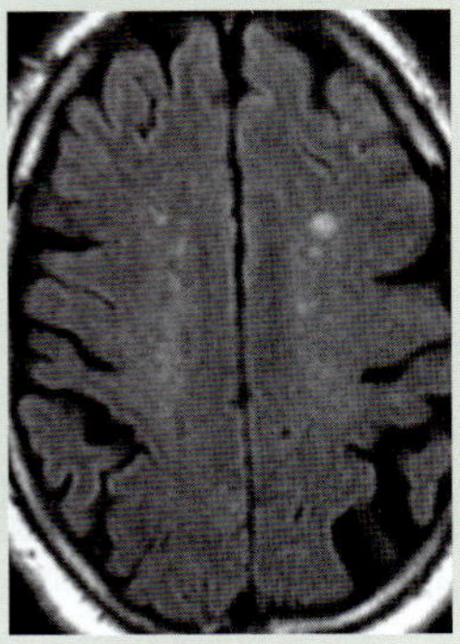

Fig. 4.42.29: Grade 1

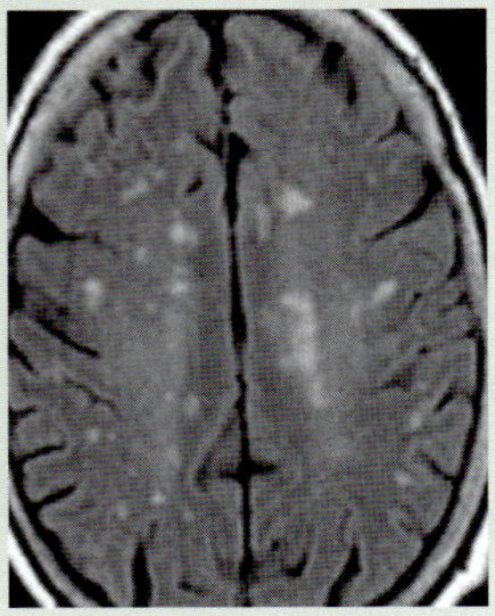

Fig. 4.42.30: Grade 2

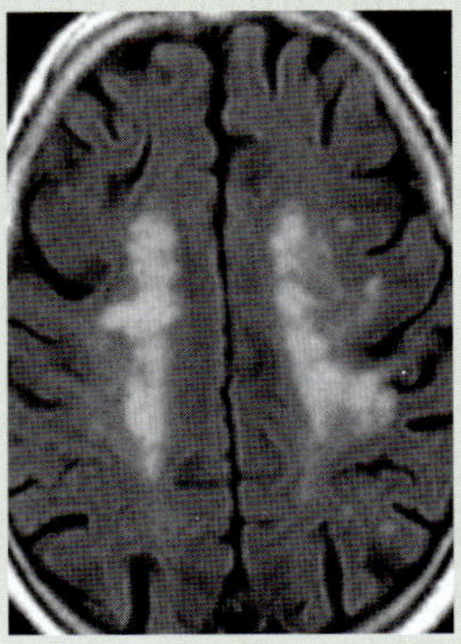

Fig. 4.42.31: Grade 3

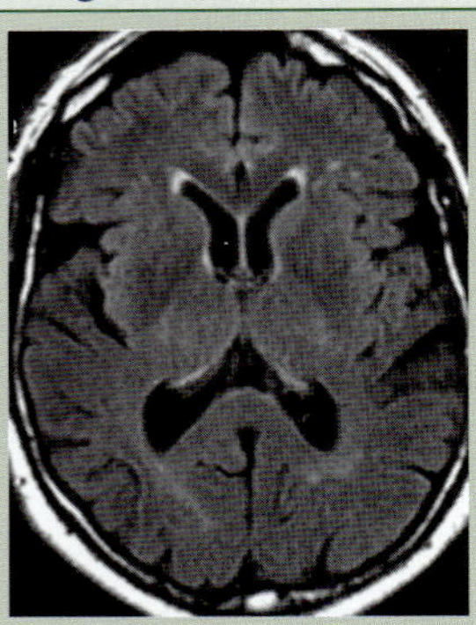

Fig. 4.42.32: Grade 1

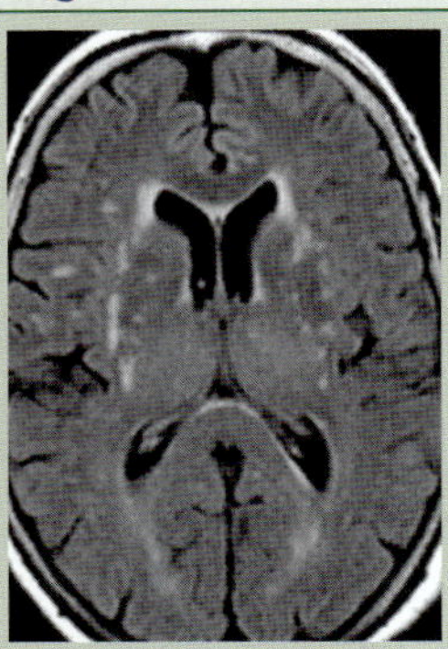

Fig. 4.42.33: Grade 2

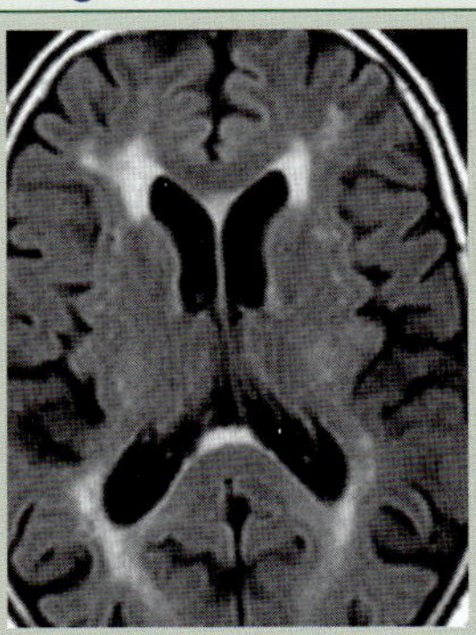

Fig. 4.42.34: Grade 3

Table 4.42.5: Visual rating scale for medial temporal atrophy			
Score	*Width of choroid fissure*	*Width of temporal horn*	*Height of hippocampal formation*
0	N	N	N
1	↑	N	N
2	↑↑	↑	↓
3	↑↑↑	↑↑	↓↓
4	↑↑↑↑	↑↑↑	↓↓↓

<75 years score >1 abnormal; >75 years score >2 abnormal

Table 4.42.6: Dementia prevalence agewise	
>65 years	*<65 years*
VaD—29% Alzheimer—39% Lewy body dementia—9% Frontotemporal dementia—3% Others—20%	VaD—18% Alzheimer—34% Lewy body dementia—7% Frontotemporal dementia—12% Others—19% Alcohol—10%

4

Table 4.42.7: Causes of dementia and areas of involvement

Various causes of dementia	*Areas of involvement*
Mild cognitive impairment Phase between dementia and expected cognitive decline of normal aging	Reduction in volume of entorhinal cortex, hippocampus (CA1 region), superior temporal and cingulate cortex
Presenile Alzheimer (<65 years)	Posterior cortical atrophy, mainly parietal atrophy, precuneus, posterior cingulate
Senile Alzheimer	Disproportionate medial temporal atrophy.
FTLD **Fronto-temporal dementia**	Bifrontal/temporal atrophy
Semantic	**Asymmetric** atrophy anterior part MTL
Prosopagnosia	**Asymmetric** atrophy of right temporal lobe
Progressive aphasia	**Asymmetric** atrophy lateral part temporal lobe (left)
Lewy body dementia	Age-related changes. **No** specific features in MRI. **^{123}I-beta-CIT SPECT** striate reduction 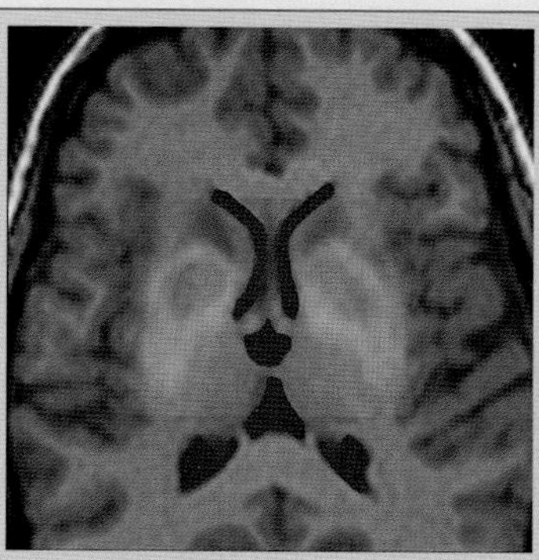 **Fig. 4.42.35:** Normal ^{123}I-beta-CIT SPECT 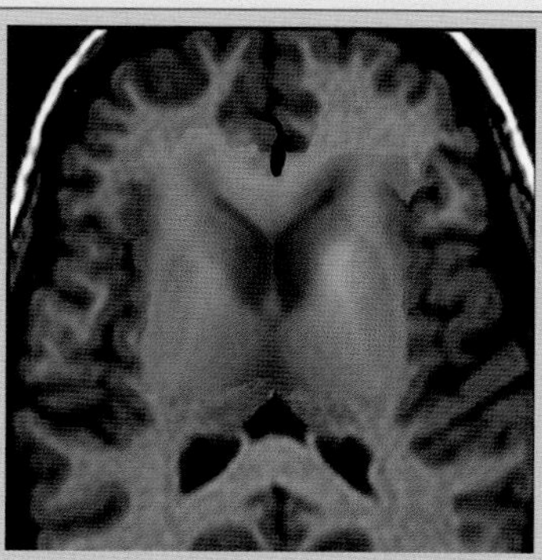 **Fig.4.42.36:** ^{123}I-beta-CIT SPECT striate reduction in Lewy body dementia
Creutzfeld-Jacob	Focal/diffuse/symmetric/asymmetric involvement of cerebral cortex/basal
Classical variant	Involvement of perirolandic cortex hockey stick sign, pulvinar sign, DWI—hyperintensity in cerebellum
HIV related	Diffuse **symmetric** cortical atrophy, periventricular white matter hypodensity
Vascular dementia	White matter lesion/stratergic infarcts
Amyloid angiopathy (accumulation of cerebral amyloid in the tunica media and adventitia of leptomeningeal and cortical vessel)	Normotensive demented patient with lobar hemorrhages and multifocal black dots on T2 and GRE.
CADASIL	**Inherited disease—NOTCH 3 mutation;** extensive white matter changes deep WM, external capsule, temporal lobes
Normal pressure hydrocephalus 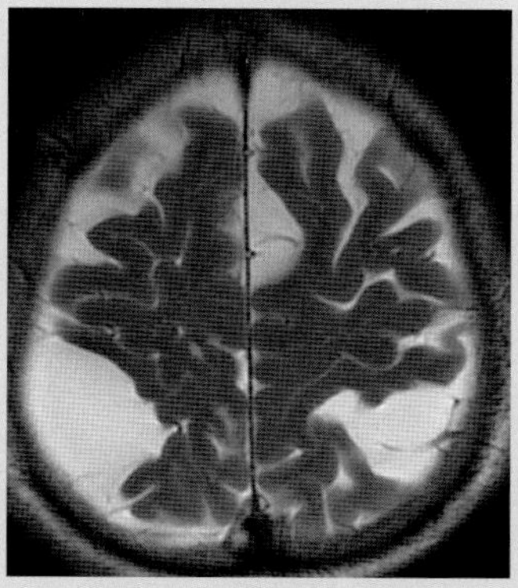 **Fig. 4.42.37:** Presenile parietal atrophy	Dilated ventricles with upward bowing of corpus callosum. Relative absence of sulcal widening

4.43 CENTRAL NERVOUS SYSTEM

Case No. 43

Clinical history: A 50-year-old male patient presents with progressive ataxia gait dysfunction, dysarthria, and dysphagia.

Radiological techniques and observation: Figures 4.43.1 to 4.43.4 are MRI T2 axial, FLAIR axial, T1 and T2 sagittal sequence images showing linear cruciform hyperintensity is evident in the pons which is seen on T2/FLAIR, creating the hot-cross bun appearance. Significant volume loss was demonstrated involving the middle cerebellar peduncles (<0.8 mm), with severe atrophy and flattening of the pons and medulla. There is prominent prepontine cistern and enlargement of the fourth ventricle and cerebello-pontine angle cisterns. Mild reduction in visualized cerebral volume with prominence of the cerebral sulci. Midbrain appears normal.

Interpretations: A—50 years old male, C—cerebellar atrophy, thinning of middle cerebellar peduncles, and pons, B—hot cross bun sign, D—MSA-C

Principal diagnosis: Multiple system atrophy-cerebellar (MSA-C) type.

Differential diagnosis: 1) Idiopathic Parkinson disease, 2) Progressive supranuclear palsy, 3) Corticobasal degeneration and 4) Spinocerebellar ataxia

Treatment and prognosis: No effective treatment is currently available, death usually within 10 years of diagnosis.

Discussion: Parkinson-plus syndrome refers to a group of neurodegenerative disorders which are characterized by features of Parkinson disease but with other neurological symptoms/signs. They have a poor response to levodopa. Conditions included in Parkinson-plus syndrome include progressive supranuclear palsy (PSP), multisystem atrophy (MSA), dementia with Lewy bodies (DLB), cortical-basal ganglionic degeneration (CBGD), frontotemporal dementia with chromosome 17 (FTDP-17), Pick disease.

Multiple system atrophy (MSA) is a neurodegenerative disease characterized by varying degrees of cerebellar ataxia, autonomic dysfunction, parkinsonism and corticospinal dysfunction.

Epidemiology: Typically, symptoms begin between 40 and 60 years of age.

Radiographic features: MRI is the modality of choice for imaging patients with suspected multiple system atrophy (MSA).

MRI: MSA-C disproportionate atrophy of the cerebellum and brainstem (especially olivary nuclei and middle cerebellar peduncle) and ADC values: Higher in the pons, cerebellum, and putamen than in Parkinson disease and fractional anisotropy (FA): Lower in the pons, cerebellum, and putamen than in Parkinson disease.

T2: Hyperintensities typically present in the pontocerebellar tracts, pons (hot cross bun sign), middle cerebellar peduncles, cerebellum

Treatment and prognosis: Unfortunately, no effective treatment is currently available. The disease progresses relentlessly culminating in death usually within 10 years of diagnosis.

MR imaging protocol for Parkinson disease: Three-dimensional (3-D) T1-weighted gradient echo and axial T2-weighted turbo spin echo imaging. Three-dimensional fluid-attenuated inversion recovery. Neuromelanin-sensitive, T1-weighted fast spin-echo sequence. Iron-sensitive susceptibility-weighted imaging, diffusion tensor imaging.

Types of PSP: 1) Classic—PSP-Richardson's syndrome, 2) brainstem variants—PSP-predominant parkinsonism (PSP-P), PSP-pure akinesia with gait freezing (PSP-PAGF) and 3) cortical variant—PSP-corticobasal syndrome (PSP-CBS), PSP-behavioral variant of frontotemporal dementia (PSP-by FTD), PSP-progressive non-fluent aphasia (PSP-PNFA).

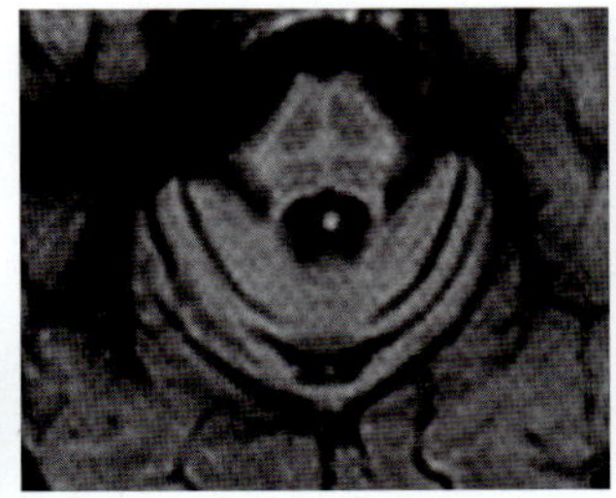

Fig. 4.43.1

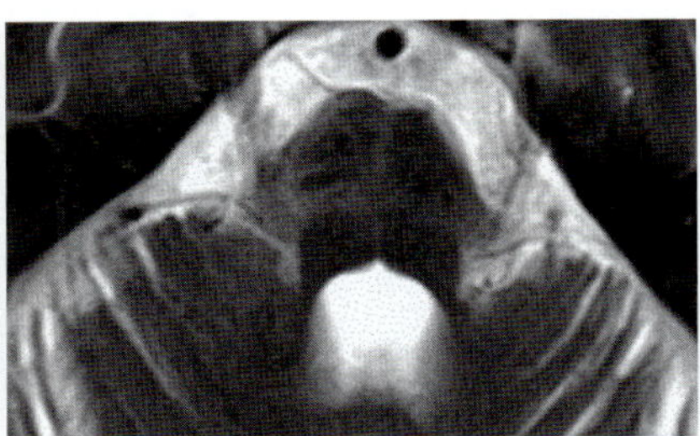

Fig. 4.43.2

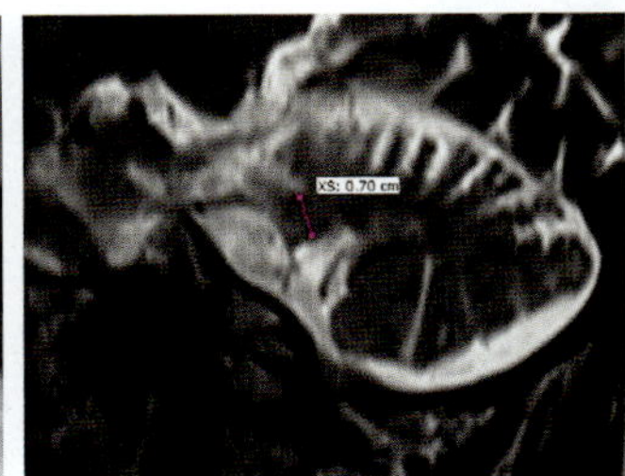

Fig. 4.43.3

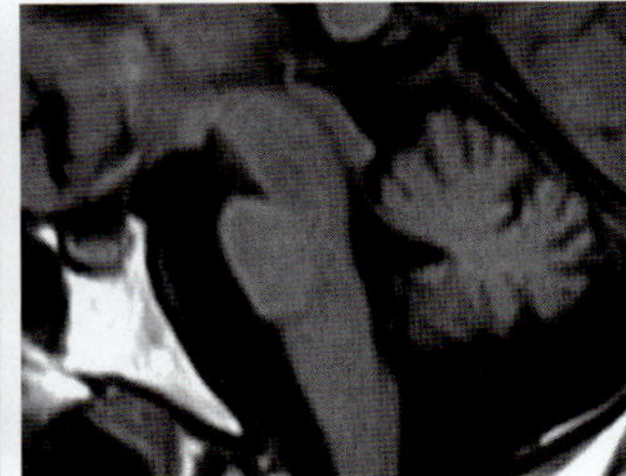

Fig. 4.43.4

Table 4.43.1: Approach to Parkinson plus syndrome

Idiopathic Parkinson disease	*Progressive supranuclear palsy*	*MSA-C*	*MSA-P*	*Corticobasal degeneration*
Because to progressive degeneration of dopaminergic neurons in the substantia nigra. Peak age—60 years. Three cardinal features Resting tremor, rigidity hypokinesia	Considered neurodegenerative disease. Insidious onset in the 6th-7th decade of life, and progresses to death usually within a decade (2–17 years from diagnosis).	Most common Parkinson plus syndrome. Clinical presentation is usually variable, but typically presents in one of three patterns: Mean age of onset: 58 MSA-P-parkinsonian symptoms predominate, MSA-C-cerebellar symptoms predominate, MSA-A-autonomic symptoms predominate		In 50–70 years of age tend to have atrophy in posterolateral and medial frontal cortical regions, but relatively preserved brainstem anatomy compared to PSP
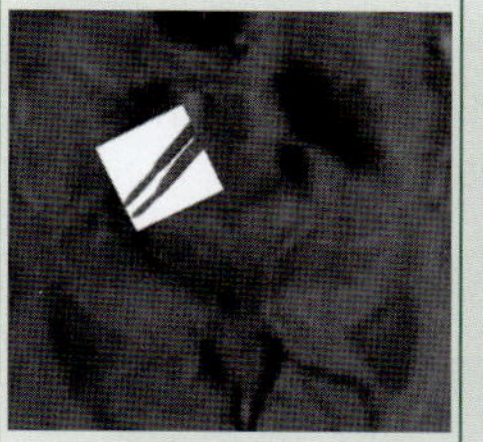 **Fig. 4.43.5:** Absent swallow tail sign in Parkinson disease	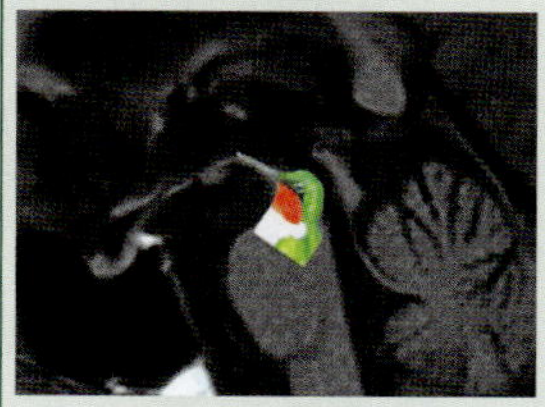 **Fig. 4.43.6:** PSP 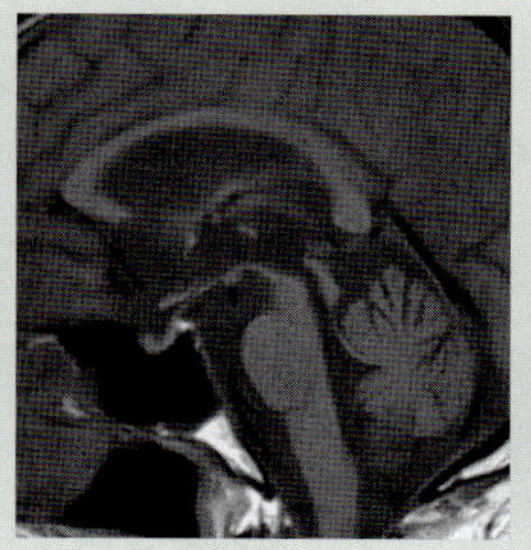 **Fig. 4.43.7:** PSP	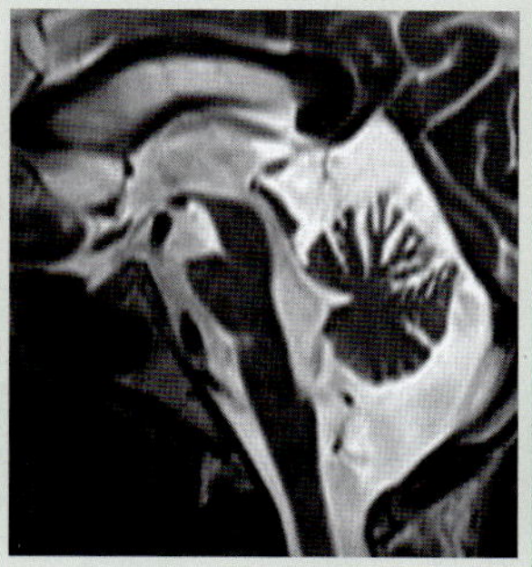 **Fig. 4.43.8** MSA-C	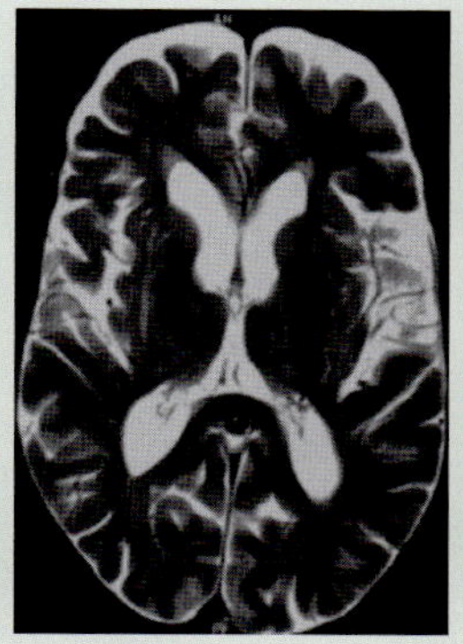 **Fig. 4.43.9:** MSA-P	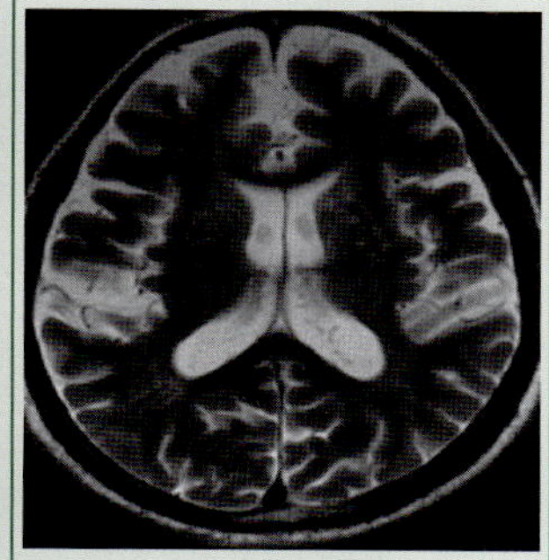 **Fig. 4.43.10:** Corticobasal degeneration
MRI: T1 may show mild hyperintensity of compact and reticular parts of the substantia nigra and red nuclei (due to iron accumulation) and loss of normal slight hyperintensity in substantia nigra due to loss of neuro-melanin. T2* (GRE/SWI) Absent swallow tail sign (nigrosome-1 is usually SWI hyper intense, but this is lost in Parkinson disease).	**Midbrain volume loss** **Hummingbird sign** sagittal midbrain less than 70 mm^3 and midbrain: Pons ratio less than 0.15 Mickey mouse appearance and morning glory sign 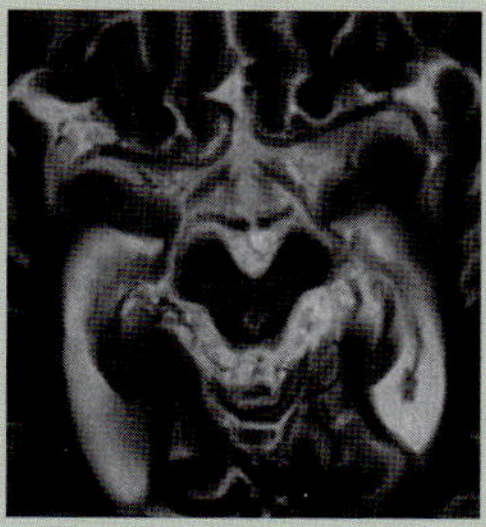 **Fig. 4.43.11:** PSP Morning glory sign	Cerebellar atrophy Small, concave middle cerebellar peduncles, shrunken, beaked pons Hot cross bun sign. 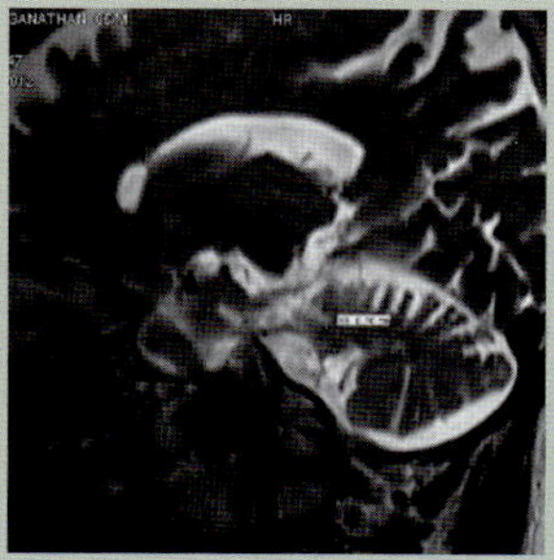 **Fig. 4.43.12:** MSA-C	Small, shrunken, hypo-intense putamen on T2/FLAIR T2/FLAIR hyperintense lateral rim (putaminal rim sign) on 1.5 T MRI Increased putaminal iron deposition	**Asymmetric cortical atrophy** Superior parietal lobule: Most constant feature bilateral atrophy of the basal ganglia and atrophy of the corpus callosum T2 hyperintensity in sub-cortical white matter of affected gyri.
	MCP width >8 mm	MCP width <8 mm		

Contd...

Table 4.43.1: Approach to Parkinson plus syndrome *(Contd...)*				
Idiopathic Parkinson disease	*Progressive supranuclear palsy*	*MSA-C*	*MSA-P*	*Corticobasal degeneration*
Imaging with I-123 ioflupane (DaT scan) Decreased striatal activity, usually asymmetrical	Symmetrical or asymmetrical decreased striatal activity.	Symmetrical or asymmetrical decreased striatal activity.		Decreased striatal activity, usually asymmetrical
FDG-PET scan: Usually normal. Preserved putaminal activity.	Decreased uptake in posterior frontal lobes, midbrain and basal ganglia.	Decreased putaminal/cerebellar uptake. Usually subtype dependent.		Asymmetrical decreased uptake in frontal and/or parietal lobe.
Hydrocephalic Parkinson disease				
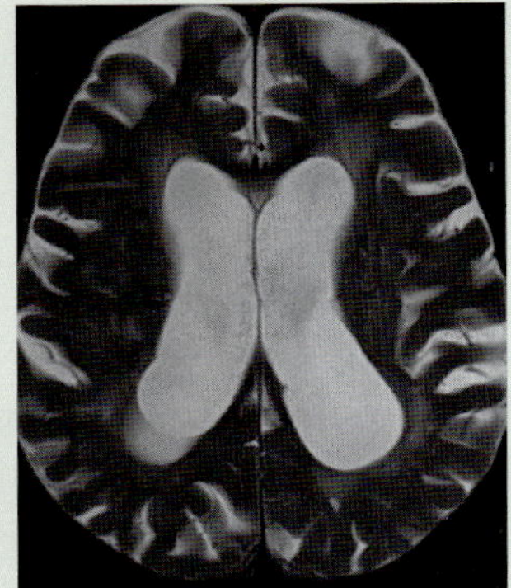 Fig. 4.43.13: Hydrocephalic Parkinson disease	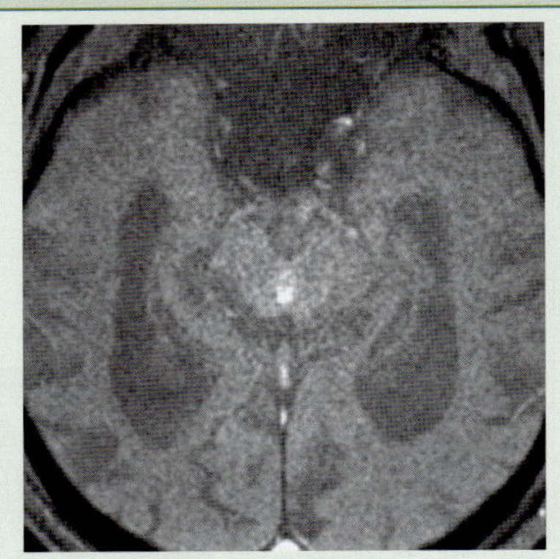 Fig. 4.43.14: Hydrocephalic Parkinson disease	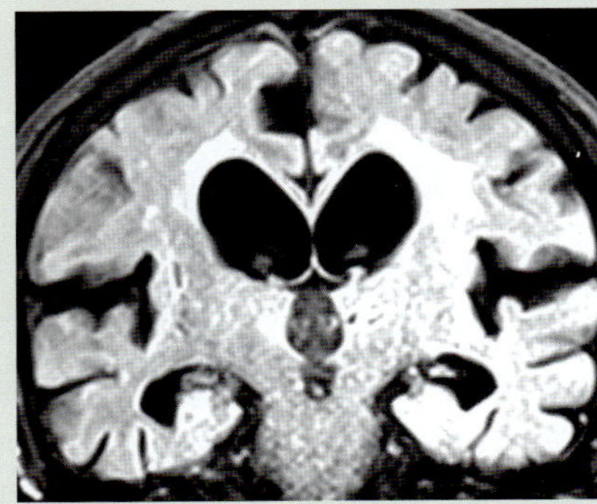 Fig. 4.43.15: Hydrocephalic Parkinson disease		
Spinocerebellar ataxia				
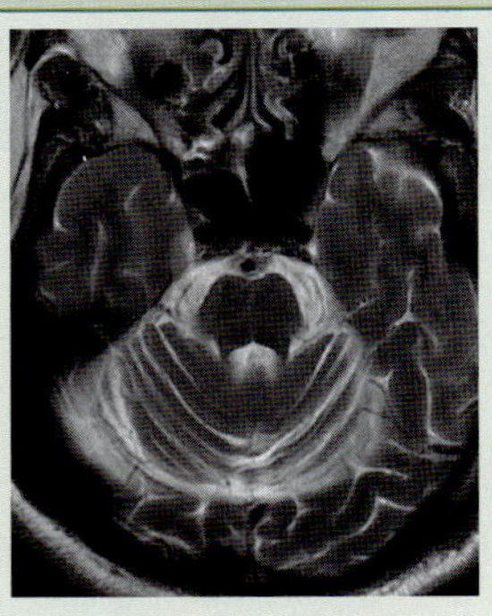 Fig. 4.43.16: Spinocerebellar ataxia	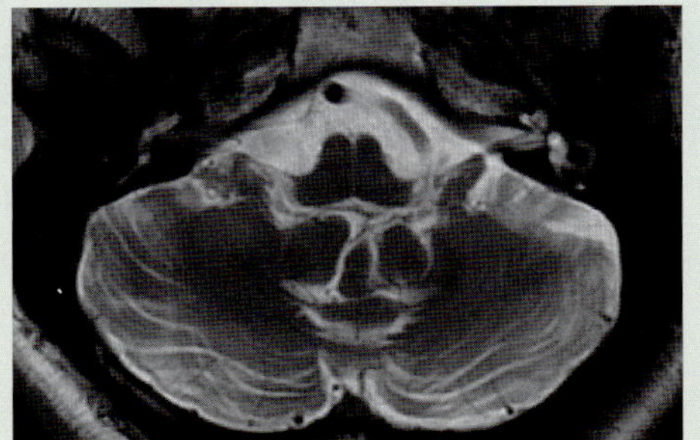 Fig. 4.43.17: Spinocerebellar ataxia	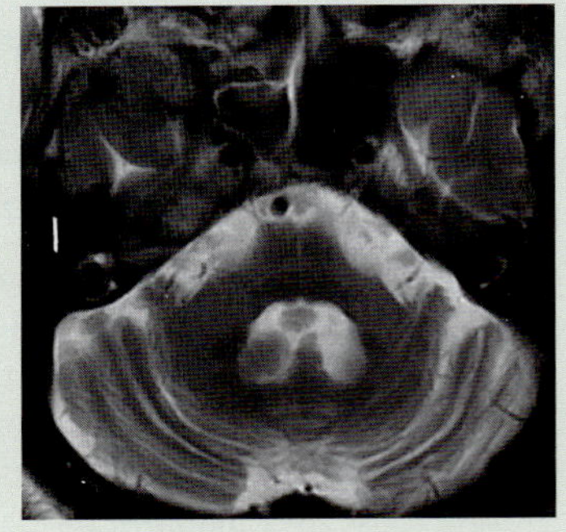 Fig. 4.43.18: Spinocerebellar ataxia		
Iron deposition in dementia				
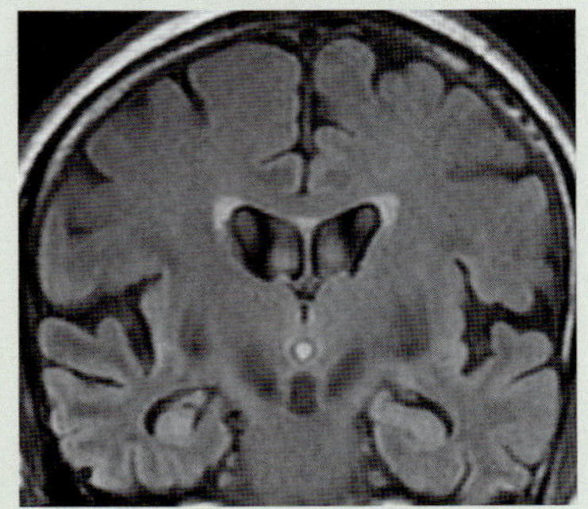 Fig. 4.43.19: Iron deposition in dementia	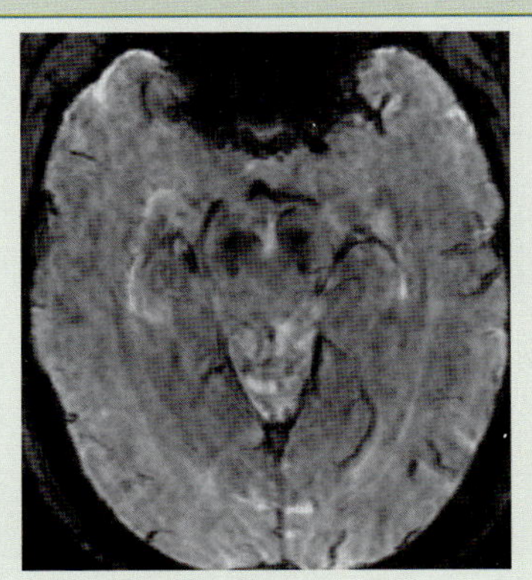 Fig. 4.43.20: Iron deposition in dementia	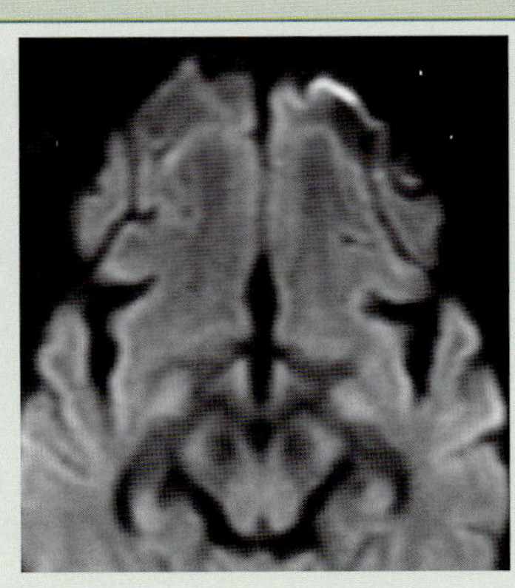 Fig. 4.43.21: Iron deposition in dementia		

MR Parkinsonism Index 2.0: Refer to OSCE

Normal pressure hydrocephalus: It is classically characterized by the triad of gait apraxia/ataxia, urinary incontinence and dementia. On imaging, it is characterized both on CT and MRI by enlarged lateral and third ventricles out of proportion to the cortical sulcal enlargement.

Hydrocephalic Parkinson disease: Communicating and non-communicating hydrocephalus can produce parkinsonism that may be relieved with ventricular shunt placement. Clinical features include bradykinesia, rest and postural tremor, loss of postural reflexes, rigidity, and bradyphrenia. Signs of dorsal midbrain impairment such as lid retraction, convergence-retraction nystagmus, light-near dissociation, and forced downgaze may be present. These atypical features suggest that parkinsonism due to hydrocephalus is pathophysiologically distinct from Parkinson's disease (PD).

4.44 SPINE

Case No. 44

Clinical history: 9-year-old-child presented with the complaints of bilateral lower limb weakness and bilateral lower limb numbness.

Radiological techniques and observation: Figure 4.44.1 is **X-ray—thoracolumbar spine–AP view** image showing non-visualization of spinous process in D12 and L1 vertebral level with linear midline vertical bony bar noted in D12, L1 vertebral level in the midline—probably osseous bar with split notochordal malformation. There is widened interpedicular distance noted in the visualized lumbar spine. There is a reduction in the vertebral disc height in the dorsolumbar vertebral level—suggestive of block vertebra. No evidence of soft tissue/cystic lesions noted.

Principal diagnosis: Formation and segmentation anomaly of the vertebrae with diastematomyelia.

Further management: **CT to confirm the presence of bony bar and MRI to assess for** 1. Extension of the diastematomyelia, 2. To look for the type, 3. To look for tethering of the cord, 4. To assess for associated spinal dysraphism and anomalies, 5. To look for the origin of nerve roots from the hemicords.

Figures 4.44.2 and 4.44.3 are CT axial and sagittal sections of dorsolumbar spine confirms the presence of midline bony bar at D12, L1 level vertebral level, dividing the hemicords.

Figures 4.44.4 to 4.44.7 are T1 sagittal, T2 axial images. T1W sagittal image shows bony bar at the level of upper lumbar vertebra level, with syrinx noted in dorsal cord. In axial images, there are two hemicords noted, each of them having a separate dural sac.

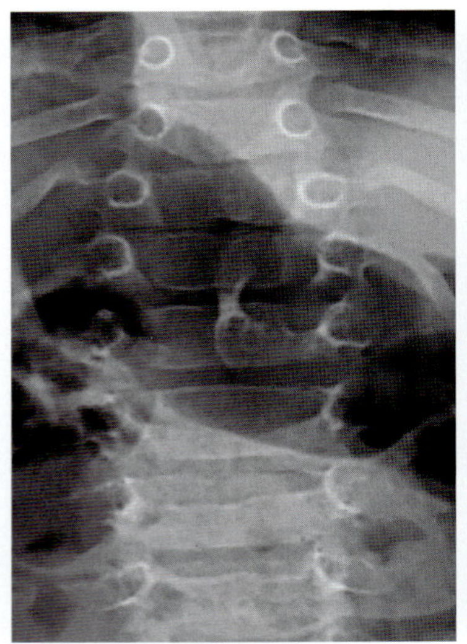
Fig. 4.44.1

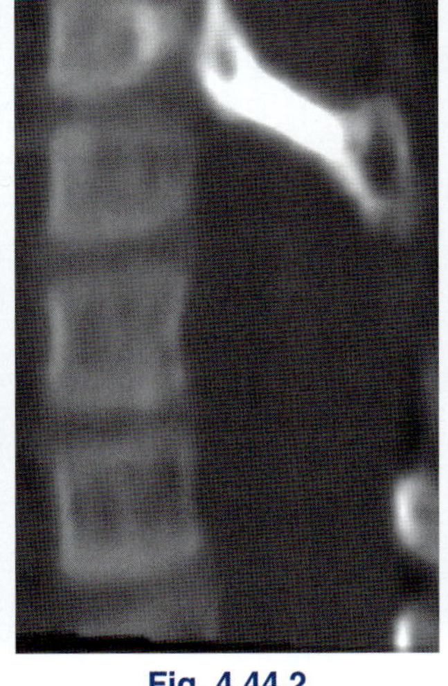
Fig. 4.44.2

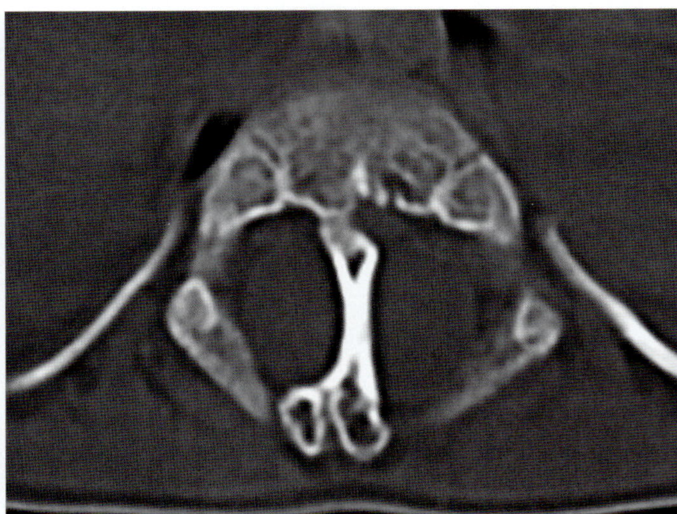
Fig. 4.44.3

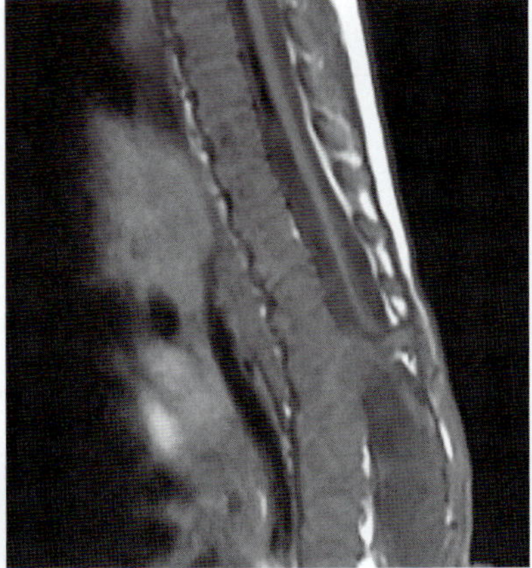
Fig. 4.44.4

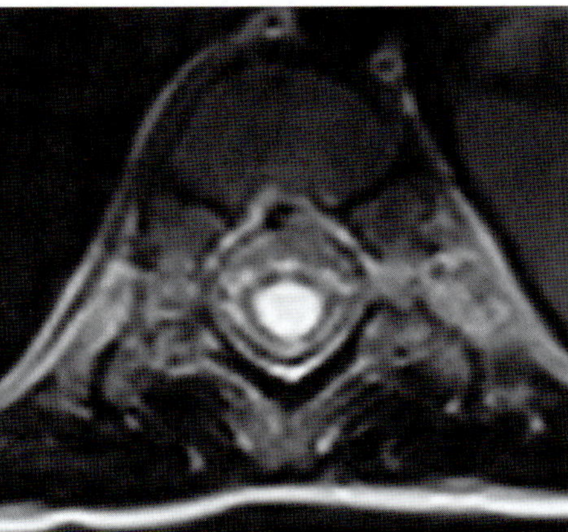
Fig. 4.44.5

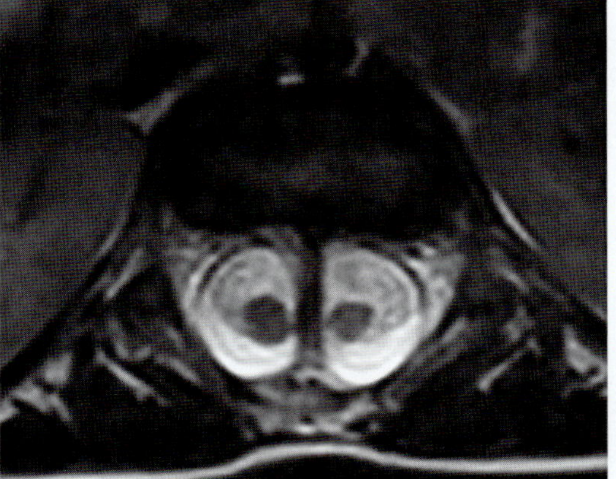
Fig. 4.44.6

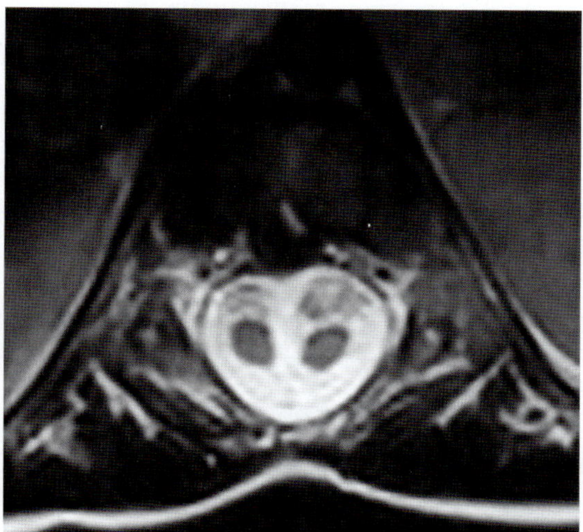

Fig. 4.44.7

Interpretation: A–9 years old child, dorsolumbar vertebra, C—non-visualization of spinous process in D12 and L1 vertebra with osseous bar in D12, L1 vertebral level in the midline and two hemicords on MRI, B—widened interpedicular distance in the lumbar spine and reduction in the vertebral disc height, D—diastematomyelia.

Principal diagnosis: **Formation and segmentation vertebral anomaly with diastematomyelia—type I.**

Further management: Surgical tethered cord release, spur (bony bar) resection, and dural reconstruction.

Differential diagnosis: **Duplicated spinal cord (diplomelia)**—2 complete spinal cords, each with 2 anterior and 2 posterior horns and roots. Diplomelia term is considered redundant now as both type 1 and type 2 diastematomyelia can have paramedian nerve roots along a spectrum of abnormalities.

Brief discussion: **Diastematomyelia**—each hemicord has a single set of anterior and posterior nerve horns and roots, resulting in segmental partial duplication of the spinal cord. Diastematomyelia is currently a part of the split cord malformations spectrum.

Embryology: Splitting of spinal canal around a persistent accessory neuroenteric canal (which becomes the septum) results in split cord malformations. The precursor mesangial cells inside becomes the medial aspect of thecal sac.

Type I: Duplicated thecal sac containing a hemicord with septum. A bony spur–sag/oblique, with hydromyelia, is more symptomatic than a type 2 fibrous non-rigid septum. Type II: Single dural sac enveloping both the hemicord without a rigid septum.

Most common location to see the defect is in the thoracolumbar region (lumbar spine 50%) T9-S1

Table 4.44.1: Classification of spinal dysraphism
1. Posterior spinal dysraphism Posterior: Open spinal dysraphism: • Myelomeningocele • Myelocele • Hemimyelomeningocele • Hemimyelocele Posterior: Closed spinal dysraphism *With subcutaneous mass:* • Meningocele • Saccular limited dorsal myeloschisis • Myelocystocele • Posterior lipomyelocele (spinal lipoma types IB, IIB, IIIB) • Posterior lipomyelomeningocele (spinal lipoma type VB) *Without subcutaneous mass:* • With cutaneous stigmata • Other than a dermal sinus: Non-saccular limited dorsal myeloschisis • Post-vertebral: Neuroenteric cysts • With dermal sinus: Dorsal dermal sinus
2. Anterior spinal dysraphism: • Anterior myelomeningocele • Anterior meningocele • Anterior myelocele • Anterior myelocystocele • Anterior lipomyelocele (spinal lipoma type IC, IIC, IIIC) • Anterior lipomyelomeningocele (spinal lipoma type VA) • Intrasacral meningocele • Pre-vertebral: Neuroenteric cysts
3. Dysraphism confined to the spinal canal: • Intramedullary spinal lipoma • Intradural lipomas – Type Ia, – Type IIa, IId – Type IIIa – Type IV: IVA–apical, IVB–mid-filar and IVC–filar tip lipomas • Tight filum terminale (Type IVD) • Intrasacral meningocele • Persistent terminal ventricle • Retained medullary cord • Split cord malformations – Type 1 and 2 diastematomyelia – Composite type diastematomyelia – Partial type diastematomyelia • Neuroenteric cysts • (Epi) dermoid/dermoid • Segmental spinal dysgenesis: Type 1
4. Dysraphism involving multiple anatomical compartments • Dorsal enteric fistula • Vertebral duplication • Caudal regression syndrome • Segmental spinal dysgenesis: Type 2 • OEIS, VACTERL, and Currarino's triad associations
5. Non-dysraphic masses of the spinal region: Sacrococcygeal teratoma, sacral chordoma

common 85% TS-20%, CS-15%. Split spinal canal malformation (SSCM) is more common in girls/women than in men/boys. Overlying skin findings are common, with hypertrichosis, hair patch (high–fawns tail hair patch)—being most frequent, nevi, lipomas, dermoid cyst, club foot, leg weakness, neurogenic bladder. Can be seen in association with vertebral body anomalies, hemivertebra, block vertebra, butterfly vertebra, kyphoscoliosis, rib abnormalities, tethered cord (75%), thick filum, hydromelia and Chiari type 2 malformation.

Diastematomyelia occurs in 5% of patients with congenital scoliosis.

Treatment is surgical with laminectomy, excision of septum and dural repair for patients with progressive clinical symptoms.

Table 4.44.2: Difference between types of diastematomyelia	
Type I: Diastematomyelia 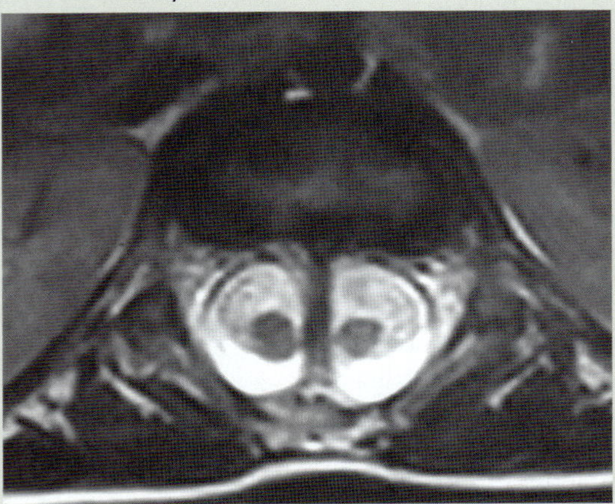 **Fig. 4.44.8:** Type I: Diastematomyelia	**Type II: Diastematomyelia** 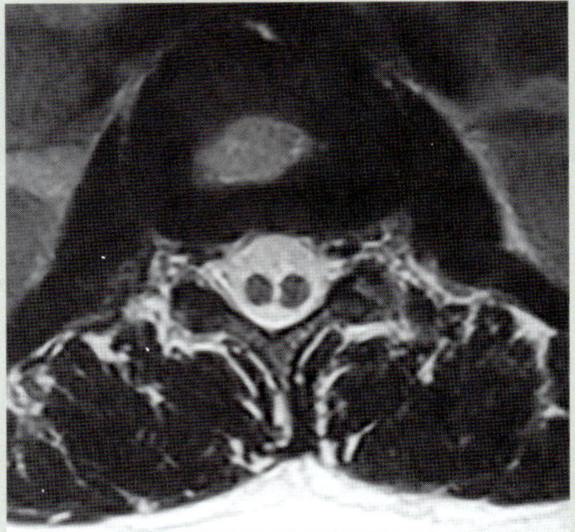 **Fig. 4.44.9:** Type II: Diastematomyelia
Presence of spur = type I SCM; more severe symptoms and anomalies, worse prognosis Two dural tubes are seen with each containing hemi cords. Early treatment will be necessary Intervening septum ("spur") may be osseous or cartilaginous, symmetric or asymmetric, complete or incomplete Tethering present due to rigid osseocartilaginous septum transfixing the cord. Tethering is also present in all type 2 SCMs due to attachment of the hemicord to the fibrous septum which in turm inserts into the dural sac	One dural sac is seen containing two hemicords. Two hemicords separated by fibrous septum. The incidence of paramedian nerve roots is nearly equal in both type I and type II SCM. 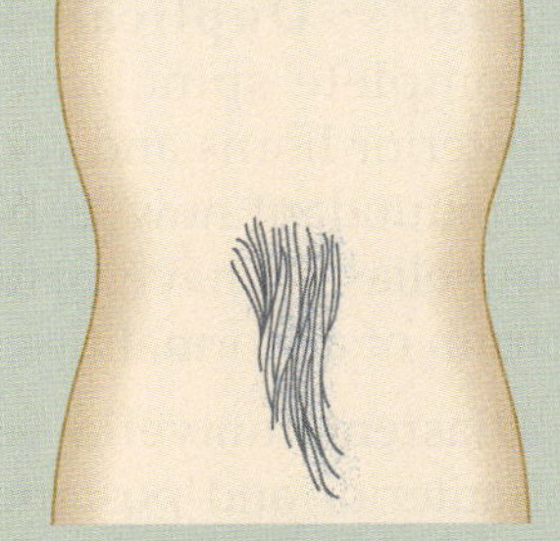 **Fig. 4.44.10:** Fawns tail hair patch

Table 4.44.3: Formation and segmentation vertebral anomalies		
Failure of formation	*Failure of segmentation*	*Mixed defects*
Incarcerated hemivertebra, is deformed vertebrae balance out each other with less change of progression. **Free hemivertebra** can be progressive. **Wedge vertebra** has better prognosis than a free hemivertebra. **Multiple hemivertebrae** can occur due to failure of formation on the same side resulting in a severe curve. Hemivertebrae on opposite sides compensate each other. **Central defect** is seen in butterfly vertebra	**A. Bilateral**—block vertebra and a short spine, e.g. Klippel-Feil. **B. Unilateral unsegmented bar**—severely progressive curve with varying degrees of kyphosis or lordosis depending on the position of the bar.	**Agenesis:** Despite the presence of the posterior parts, a vertebra's body may be completely absent. Vertebral body's ossification centres would not appear in this condition. It is possible that one or more vertebral segments are implicated. **Coronal cleft:** This anomaly results from a failure of fusion of the anterior and posterior ossification centers, which remain separated by a cartilage plate.

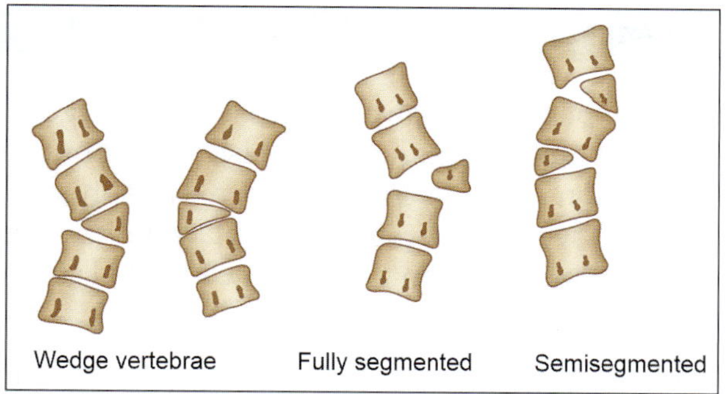

Fig. 4.44.11: Failure of formation

The sclerotome migrates around the neural tube to form a sort of model of the vertebrae that will be developing soon.

Neurons from the neural tube extend through the von Ebner's fissures in the developing sclerotome to innervate the surrounding mytome and dermatome.

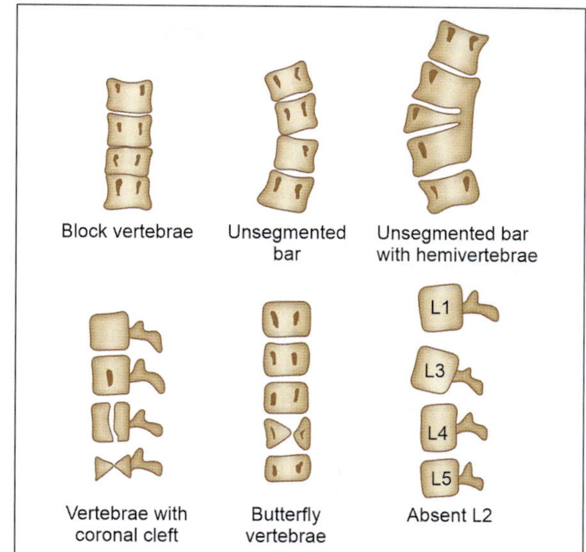

Fig. 4.44.12: Failure of segmentation

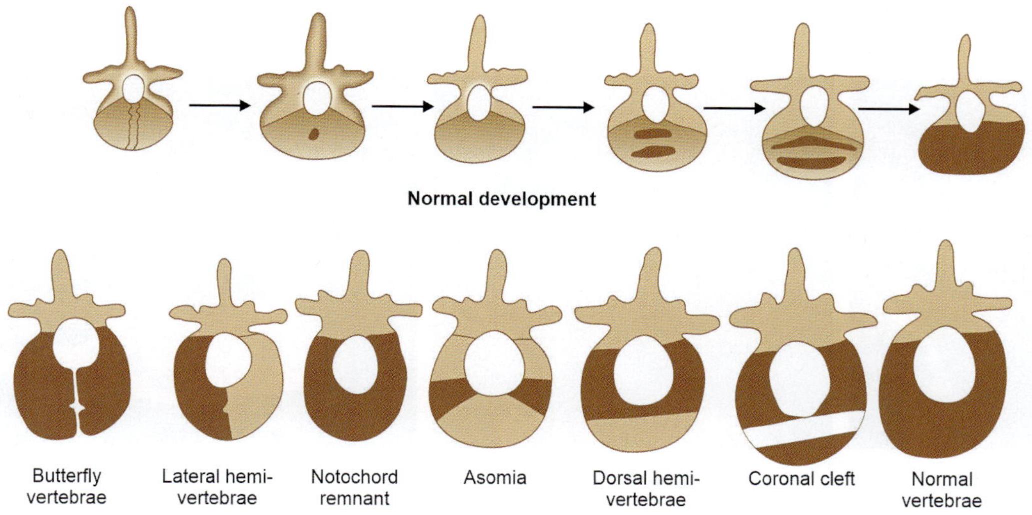

Fig. 4.44.13: Embryology of the bony spine and their abnormalities

Two adjacent sclerotomes fuse to produce one vertebra with intervertebral discs being formed at the site of von Ebner's fissures—failure in this process results in segmentation anomalies.

Chondrification centers form within the mesenchyme of the sclerotome and begin to replace the soft mesenchyme with cartilage by 6th week. By the 7th week, primary ossification centers form in the vertebral body *(by the 9th week of pregnancy, two ossification centres will be formed, one for the ventral half of the body and the other for the dorsal half. By the 12th week, these centres will have fully ossified, which quickly fuse together forming a large centre)* and the two pedicles. Any faults in this process results in formation anomalies. Bone gradually replaces the cartilage except in synovial joints and the process is not complete untill after adolescence when the sceondary ossification centres (transverse process, spinous process and the annular epiphyses) fuse to form the rest of the vertebra.

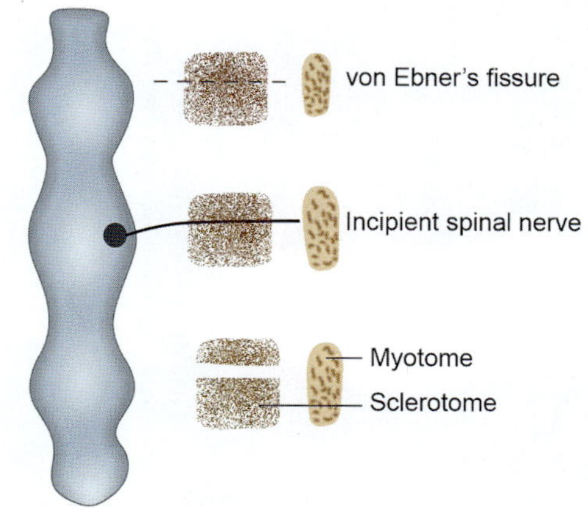

Fig. 4.44.14: Neural tube (in blue) with surrounding sclerotome

4.45 SPINE

Case No. 45

Clinical history: 1-week-old newborn with complaints of swelling in the lower back.

Imaging technique and observation: Figures 4.45.1 to 4.45.6 are MRI brain T2 sagittal, lumbar spine T2 axial, and whole spine T2 sagittal images. It shows small posterior fossa with a low attachment of the tentorium and low torcula. The brainstem appears pulled down with an elongated and low-lying fourth ventricle.The tectal plate appears beaked, the inferior colliculus is elongated and points posteriorly, with resulting angulation of the aqueduct which result in aqueductal stenosis and hydrocephalus. The cerebellar vermis is displaced inferiorly through the foramen magnum.

MRI spine shows myelomeningocele at lumbar level with the nerve roots traversing a large meningocele sac from the exposed neural placode, which merges into adjacent cutaneous fat and skin. Also, it demonstrates nondisjunction—characterized by open dysraphism with lack of skin covering over the neural placode. The neural elements are in direct contact with the external surface/skin.

Interpretation: A: 1-week-old newborn, posterior fossa and lumbar spine, C: Cerebellar tonsil and vermis downward herniation with hydrocephalus and concurrent lumbar myelomeningocele. B: Lack of skin covering over the neural placode, D: Type II Arnold-Chiari malformation.

Principle diagnosis: Type II Arnold-Chiari malformation.

Differential diagnosis:

- Arnold-Chiari I
- Arnold-Chiari III

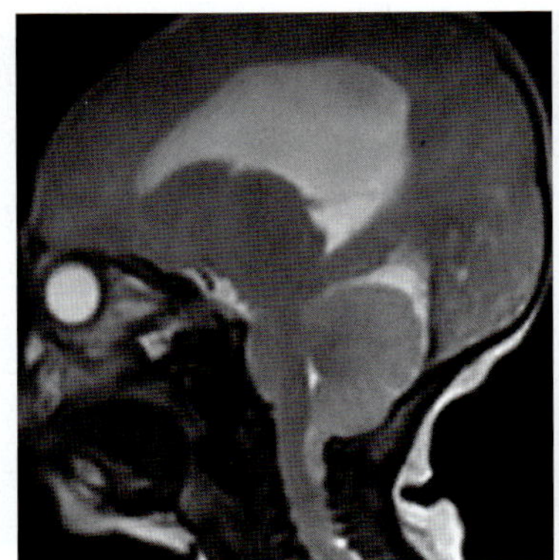

Fig. 4.45.1

Fig. 4.45.2

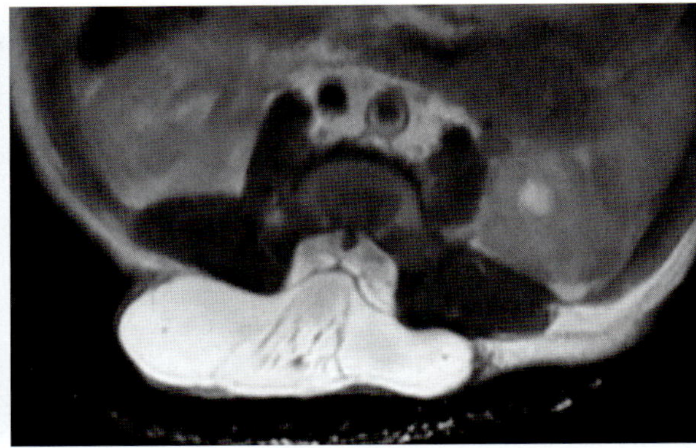

Fig. 4.45.3

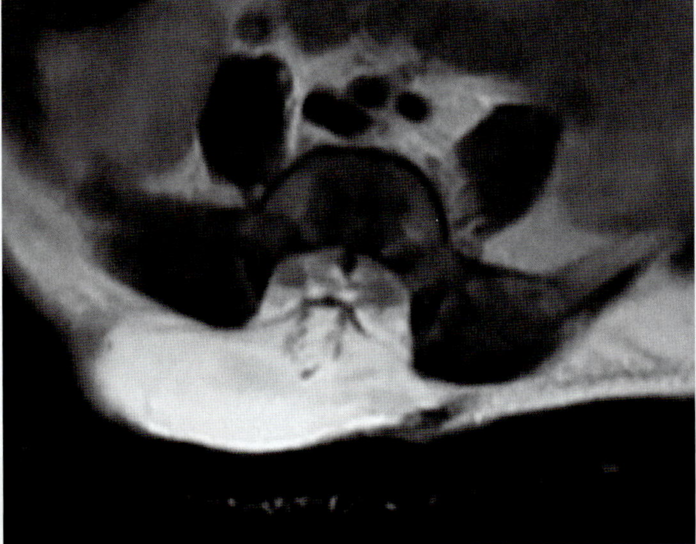

Fig. 4.45.4

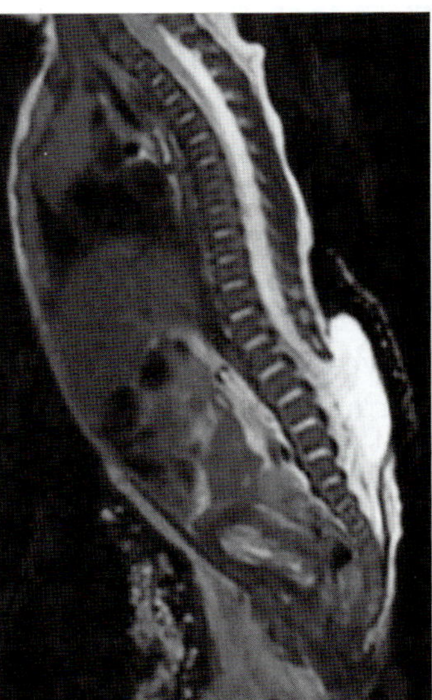

Fig. 4.45.5

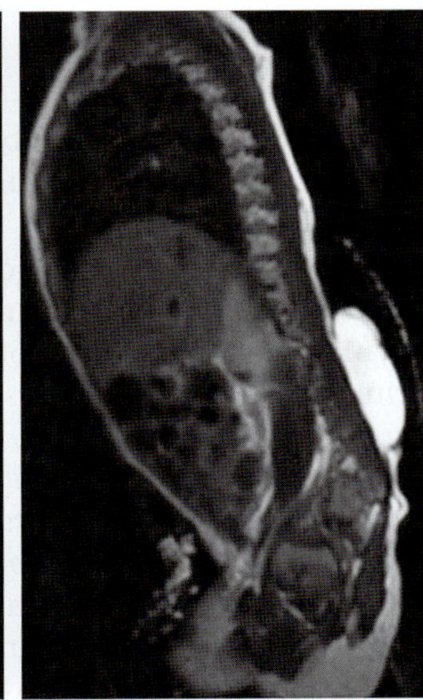

Fig. 4.45.6

Arnold-Chiari I CM1 patients with syrinx nearly always present with symptoms referable to syrinx; if syrinx extends into the medulla, bulbar symptoms predominate	Herniation of both tonsils (not vermis) ≥ 3–5 mm below foramen magnum + syrinx, cervicomedullary kinking, 4th ventricular elongation, or pointed tonsils. Not associated with myelomeningocele.	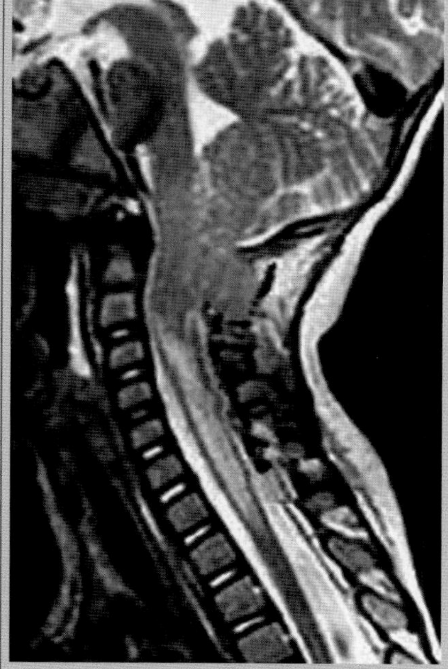 **Fig. 4.45.7:** Arnold-Chiari I
Arnold-Chiari III Microcephaly, severe developmental delay, spasticity, hypotonia, seizures.	Occipitocervical cephalocele containing cerebellum with or without brainstem in conjunction with C1–C2 spina bifida. Midline bone defect within supraoccipital bone, opisthion.	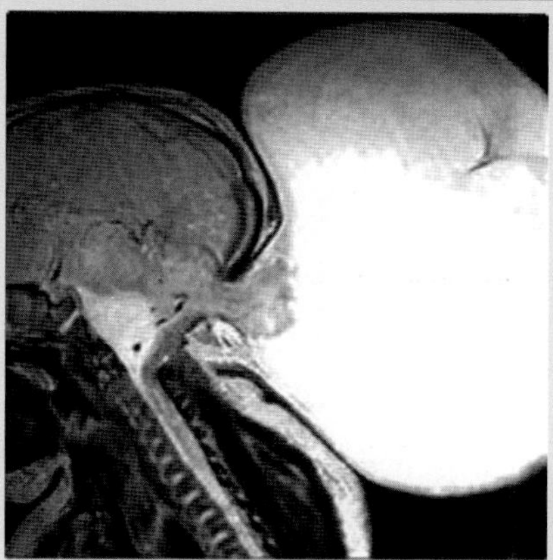 **Fig. 4.45.8:** Arnold-Chiari III
Intracranial hypotension Postural headache, nausea, vomiting, neck pain, visual and hearing disturbances. Commonly seen in middle-aged women.	Radiological features are—slumping posterior fossa with pons compressed against clivus, tonsillar ectopia, dural thickening / enhancement, Subdural collection, dural venous sinus distension and enlargement of pituitary gland.	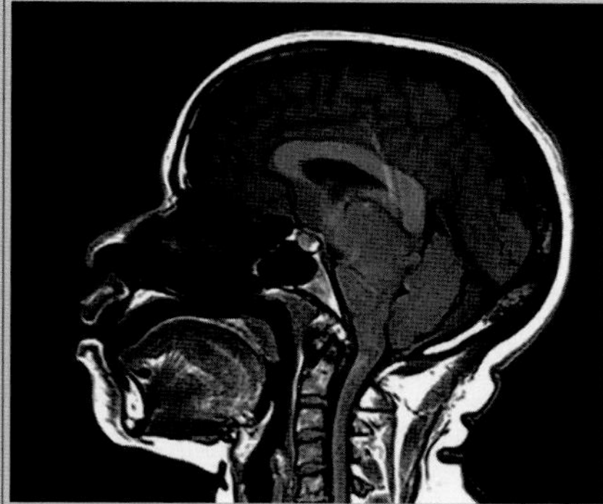 **Fig. 4.45.9:** Intracranial hypotension
Severe, chronic shunted hydrocephalus (congenital)	May cause collapsed brain, upwardly herniated cerebellum. Development of tonsillar herniation (acquired Chiari malformation) is rare but associated with lumboperitoneal shunt. Sometimes malfunctioning of VP shunt may cause tonsillar descent.	

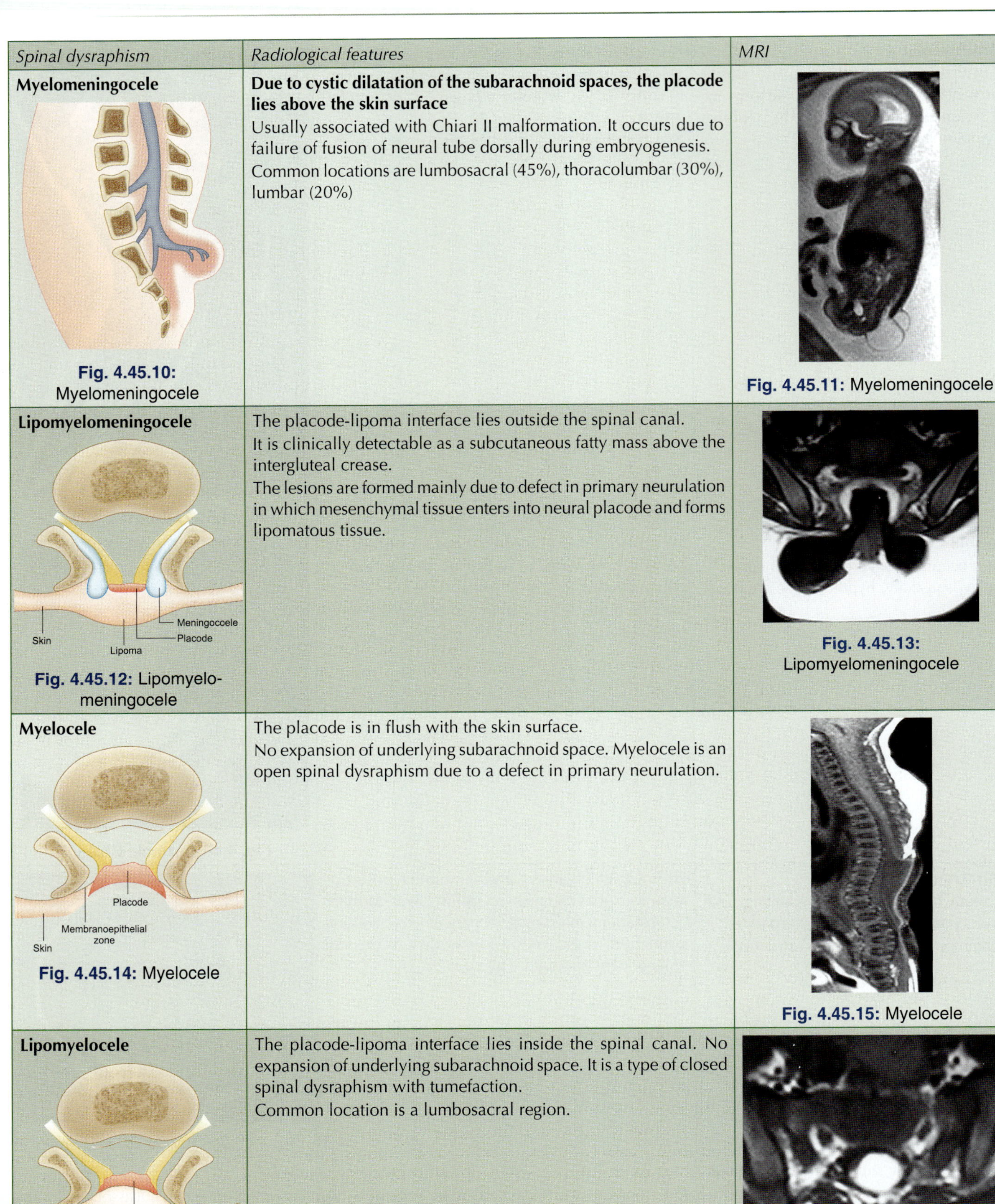

Spinal dysraphism	*Radiological features*	*MRI*
Myelomeningocele Fig. 4.45.10: Myelomeningocele	**Due to cystic dilatation of the subarachnoid spaces, the placode lies above the skin surface** Usually associated with Chiari II malformation. It occurs due to failure of fusion of neural tube dorsally during embryogenesis. Common locations are lumbosacral (45%), thoracolumbar (30%), lumbar (20%)	Fig. 4.45.11: Myelomeningocele
Lipomyelomeningocele Skin, Lipoma, Placode, Meningocoele Fig. 4.45.12: Lipomyelo-meningocele	The placode-lipoma interface lies outside the spinal canal. It is clinically detectable as a subcutaneous fatty mass above the intergluteal crease. The lesions are formed mainly due to defect in primary neurulation in which mesenchymal tissue enters into neural placode and forms lipomatous tissue.	Fig. 4.45.13: Lipomyelomeningocele
Myelocele Placode, Membranoepithelial zone, Skin Fig. 4.45.14: Myelocele	The placode is in flush with the skin surface. No expansion of underlying subarachnoid space. Myelocele is an open spinal dysraphism due to a defect in primary neurulation.	Fig. 4.45.15: Myelocele
Lipomyelocele Skin, Lipoma, Placode Fig. 4.45.16: Lipomyelocele	The placode-lipoma interface lies inside the spinal canal. No expansion of underlying subarachnoid space. It is a type of closed spinal dysraphism with tumefaction. Common location is a lumbosacral region.	Fig. 4.45.17: Lipomyelocele

- Intracranial hypotension
- Severe, chronic shunted hydrocephalus (congenital)

Management

CSF flow MRI

1. To assess hydrocephalus whether communicating or non-communicating and useful in post-operative shunt assessment.
2. Assessment of flow in the cervical CSF space to predict risk of syringomyelia formation.

Surgical management:

- Chiari decompression with resection of posterior foramen magnum, C1 ring
- CSF diversion/shunting
- Fetal myelomeningocoele repair in selected patients may ameliorate Chiari 2 severity

Types of open spinal dysraphism are: Myelomeningocele Myelocele Hemimyelocele, Hemimyelomeningocele	Open spinal dysraphisms (i.e., myelomeningocele) are typically associated with the Chiari II malformation. CSF leakage → Failure to expand the rhombencephalic vesicle → Small posterior cranial fossa with tonsillar herniations	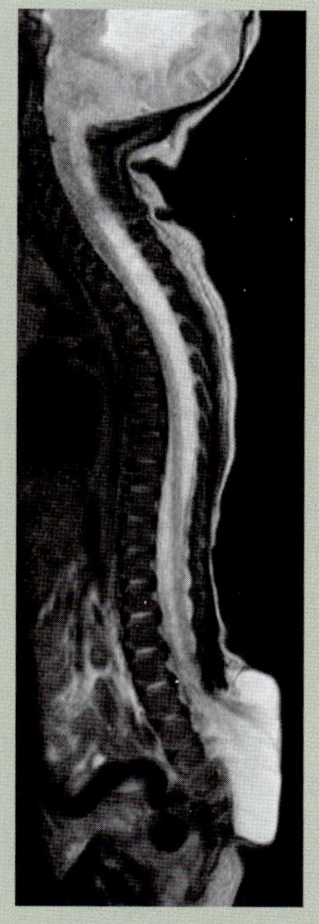 **Fig. 4.45.18:** Myelomeningocele

Syringomyelia	
Hydromyelia = cystic central canal dilatation Syringomyelia = cystic spinal cord cavity not contiguous with central cord canal Associations: Hydrocephalus, Chiari I or II malformation, myelomeningocele or other spinal dysraphism, tethered cord, congenital scoliosis, spinal cord injury. Clinical features: Cloak-like pain and temperature/sensory loss with preservation of position sense, proprioception, light touch. Differential diagnosis: • Ventriculus terminalis • Cystic spinal cord tumor • Myelomalacia	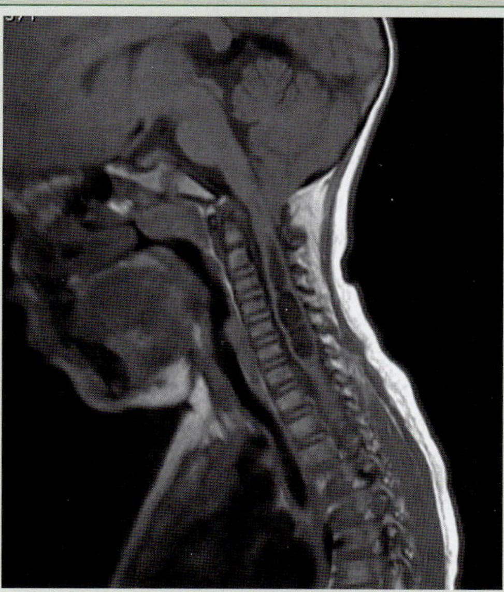 **Fig. 4.45.19:** Syringomyelia-metameric haustration seen in 20–40%—Chiari I

Prognosis

Most common cause of death in myelomenigocele are:
- Brainstem compression/hydrocephalus, intrinsic brainstem "wiring" defects
- Progression of spinal neurological deficits is rare; then suspect hydrocephalus, associated undiagnosed spinal deformity (diastematomyelia), tethered cord. Cerebellar tonsil/vermian ectopia may "improve" (ascend) following postnatal repair

Prophylaxis: Folate supplement for pregnant mothers (preconception → 6 weeks post-conception) significantly decreases myelomeningocele risk.

Discussion

Types of Chiari malformations

Chiari I: It involves inferior dislocation of the cerebellar tonsils.

Chiari II: It is always associated with myelodysplasia and involves herniation of the medulla and vermis. Supratentorial involvement—disorders of cortical and dural development is a rule, not an exception.

Chiari III: It is classically characterized as herniation of posterior fossa contents through a low occipito-cervical bony defect.

Chiari 0: Syrinx without frank tonsillar herniation.

Chiari 1.5: Caudal protrusion of brainstem in addition to the tonsils.

Chiari IV: Recognized as primary cerebellar agenesis, not a hindbrain herniation.

Chiari V: Chiari II plus occipital or high cervical myelomeningocele.

Open Spinal Dysraphism (OSD)

It is dorsal herniation of all or part of the contents of the spine with constantly exposed. All OSDs are anomalies of **primary neurulation**.

Undifferentiated neural tissue (placode). Placode is a segment of non-neurulated embryonic neural tissue (frozen at neural plate stage).

Age-wise criteria for ectopia of the cerebellar tonsils: 1st decade of life—6 mm; 2nd and 3rd decades—5 mm; 4th to 8th decades—4 mm; 9th decade, 3 mm.

Cerebellar tonsillar position (TP) is the straight line drawn from the tip of the cerebellar tonsils to the McRae line (a line drawn between the anterior and posterior margins of the foramen magnum).

Role of CSF flow study: Phase-contrast MRI technique using VENC (velocity encoding) is a commonly used method for CSF flow study.

Images of magnitude and phase were developed for anatomy and velocity data, respectively. As a result, each pixel's greyscale intensity is proportional to the CSF velocity.

CSF flow is usually depicted on phase images as shades of white, whereas cranial flow is depicted as shades of black.

For conventional CSF flow imaging, the usual VENC value is 5–8 cm/s. Low VENC values (2–4 cm/s) can help distinguish between communicating and non-communicating arachnoid cysts, as well as determine the patency of the ventriculoperitoneal shunt. In NPH, significantly higher VENC values (20–25 cm/s) should be chosen due to hyperdynamic CSF flow within the cerebral aqueduct.

Clinical application: Flow of CSF MRI can be used to distinguish between non-communicating and communicating hydrocephalus, to localise the level of obstruction in obstructive hydrocephalus, to determine whether arachnoid cysts communicate with the subarachnoid space, to differentiate between arachnoid cysts and the subarachnoid space, to distinguish between syringomyelia and cystic myelomalacia, and to assess flow. This imaging modality can also be useful in the pre-operative evaluation of NPH and Chiari I malformations, as well as the post-operative monitoring of patients who have had a neuroendoscopic 3rd ventriculostomy (NTV) and VP shunt.

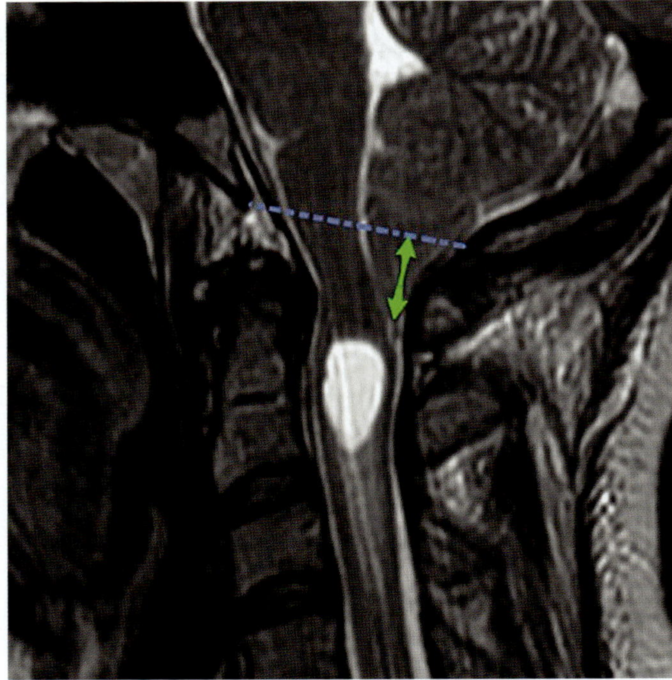

Fig. 4.45.20: Cerebellar tonsillar position

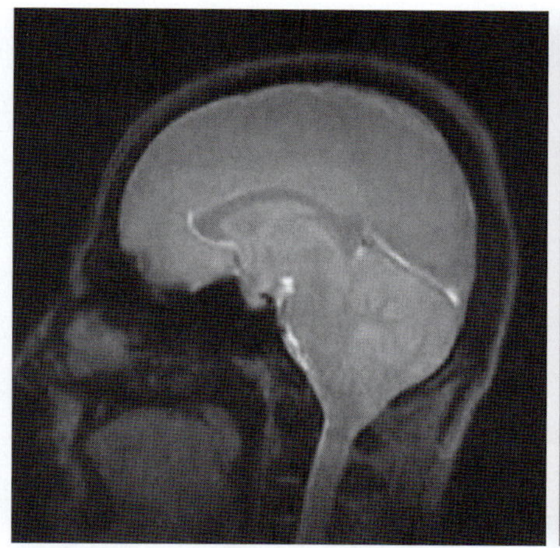

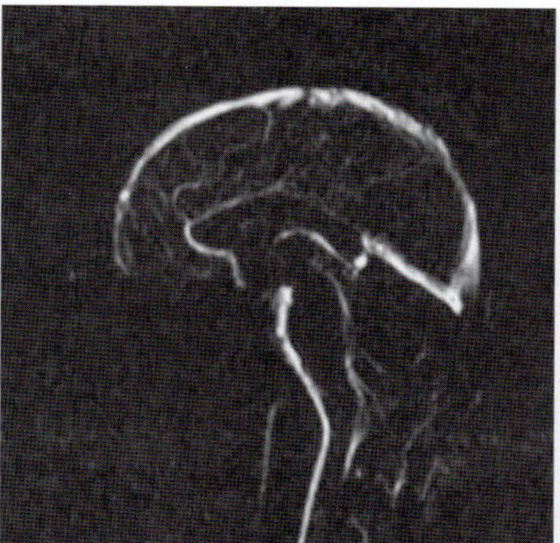

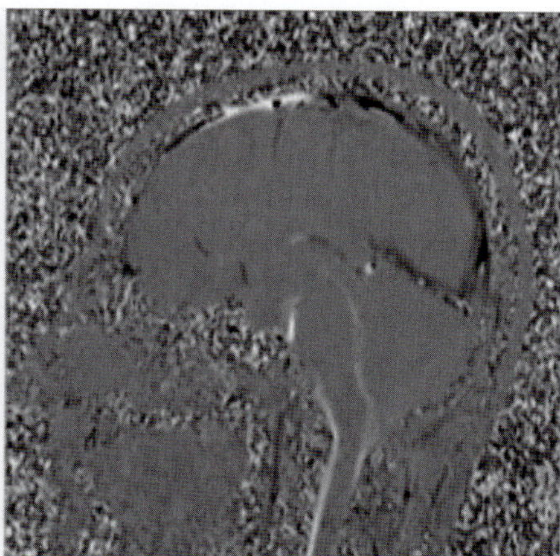

Fig. 4.45.21: Re-phased image (Magnitude of flow compensated signal) Magnitude image (magnitude of difference signal) Phase image (phase of difference signal)

Antenatal USG signs of Chiari malformation		
Lemon sign Associated with Chiari II, Spina bifida, encephalocele, Dandy-Walker malformation, thanatophoric dysplasia, cystic hygroma, corpus callosal agenesis.	Inward scalloping of the frontal bones. This sign usually appears >24 weeks which may be due to the reduced pliability of the fetal calvaria or increased intracranial pressure with associated hydrocephalus	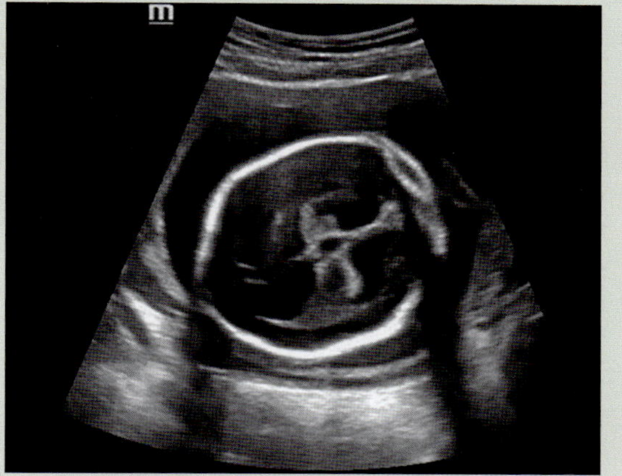 **Fig. 4.45.22:** Lemon sign
Hydrocephalus Fetal ventriculomegaly is defined as >10 mm across the atria of posterior or anterior horn of lateral ventricle at any point of gestation.	Dilated lateral ventricles with free-hanging choroid plexus known as dangling choroid sign.	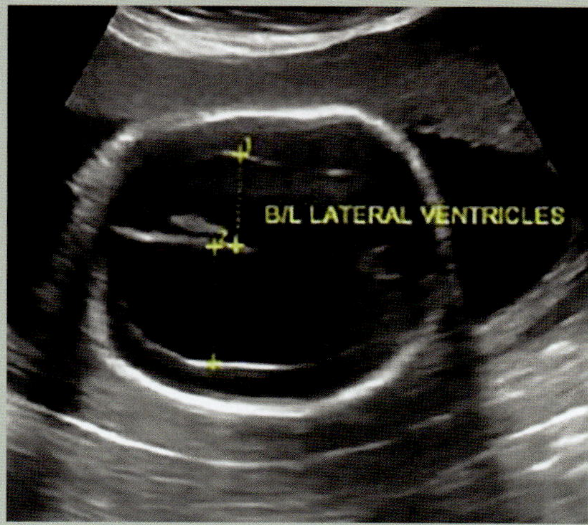 **Fig. 4.45.23:** Hydrocephalus

Banana sign Associated with Chiari II/spina bifida. Frequently associated with hydrocephalus.	Shallow posterior fossa with effacement of cisterna magna and abnormal curvature of the cerebellar hemispheres (banana sign) with downward displacement	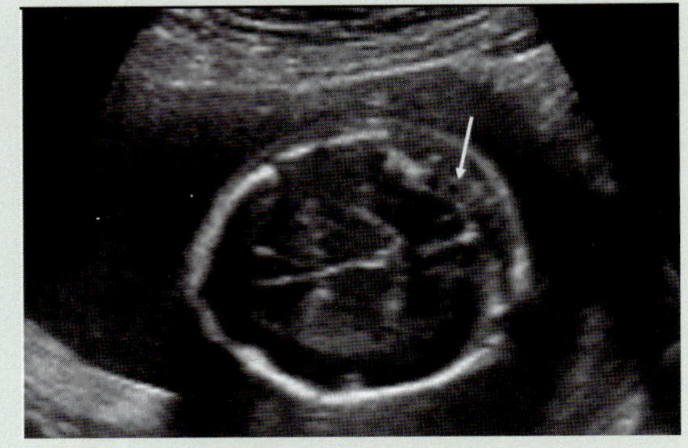 **Fig. 4.45.24:** Banana sign
Spina bifida Most common location lumbosacral (90%) followed by cervical region (2–3%). Types—spina bifida aperta and spina bifida occculta.	Dorsal ossification centres/lateral pedicles as being splayed apart (which can give a V-shaped appearance to the posterior elements).	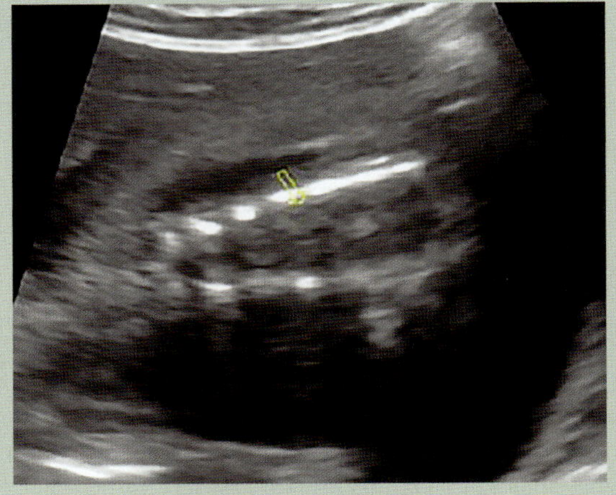 **Fig. 4.45.25:** Spina bifida
Meningocele/ Myelomeningocele Cystic herniation from defect in spina bifida noted at lumbar level.	Anechoic cystic lesion in lower lumbar region through defect dorsal ossification centres.	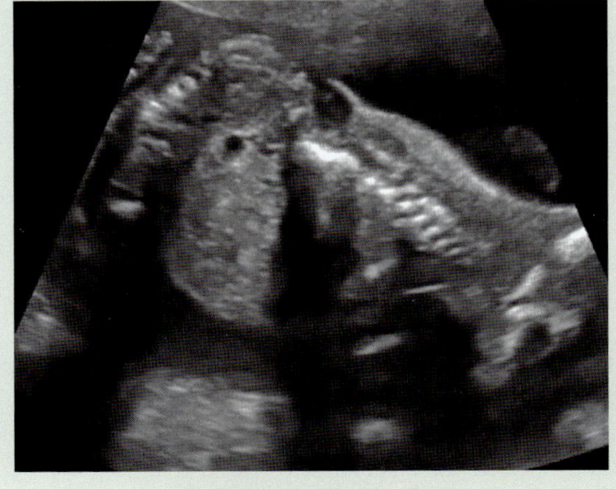 **Fig. 4.45.26:** Meningocele

4.46 SPINE

Case No. 46

Relevant clinical history: A 2-year-old female with complaints of mass in the back (skin- covered) since birth. No evidence of neurological deficit at present.

Radiological techniques and observation: Figures 4.46.1 to 4.46.3 are MR images in T1 sagittal and T2 axial and coronal sections respectively. T2WI shows a low ending cord—spinal cord. There is a large T2 hyperintense cystic region in the posterior lumbosacral region herniating through a defect in the posterior spinal elements. The cystic lesion shows multiple septations. The dilated terminal ventricle appears to herniate into the cyst through a defect in the posterior elements of the overlying vertebrae.

Interpretation: A: 2 years old female child, lumbar spine, C: A large syrinx passing through T2 hyperintense dilated subarachnoid space (meningocele), terminating in a cord cyst. Fibrolipomatous tissue surrounds both sacs. B: The overlying skin appears intact. The anterior vertebral elements, the intervertebral discs appear normal. The spinal cord shows normal signal intensity. D: Terminal myelocystocele.

Diagnosis: Terminal myelocystocele (also known as sacrococcygeal ependymal cyst.)

Differential diagnoses: Terminal myelocystocele is a **closed spinal dysraphism with tumefaction.** The other conditions are as follows.

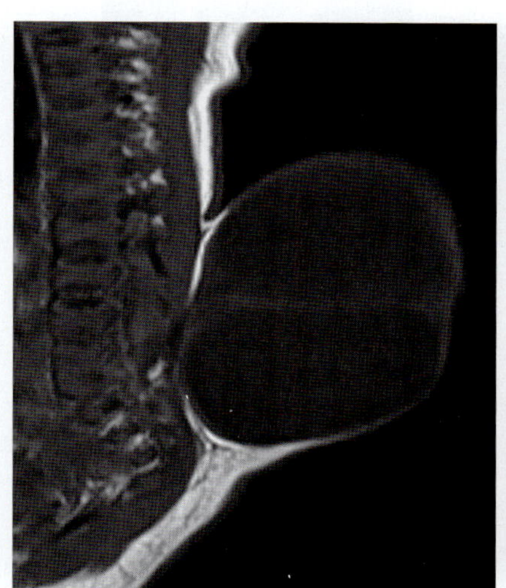

Fig. 4.46.1

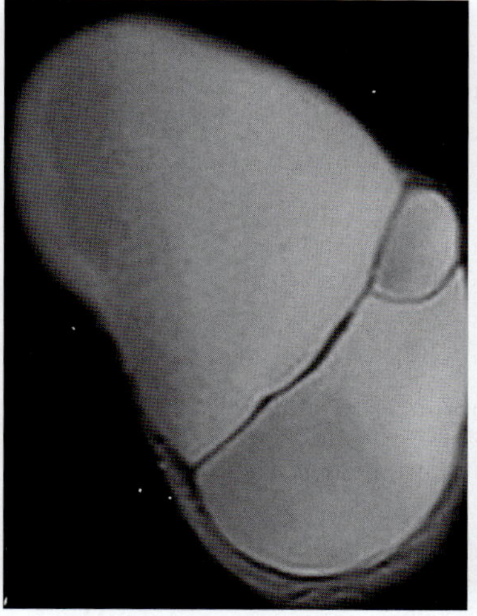

Fig. 4.46.2

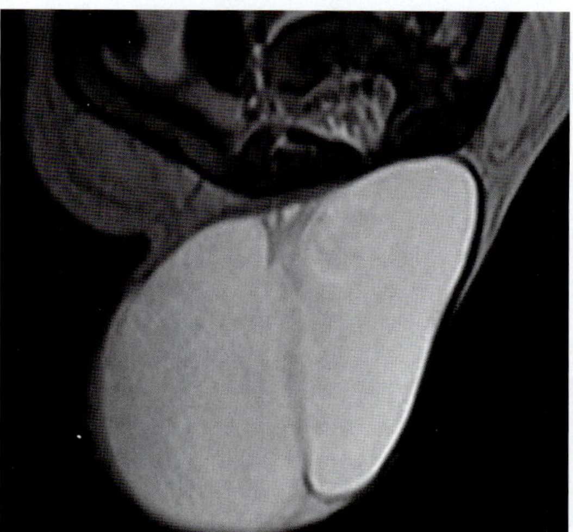

Fig. 4.46.3

Table 4.46.1: Differential diagnosis for closed spinal dysraphism		
Diagnosis	*Imaging features*	*Image*
Saccular limited dorsal myeloschisis: To refer in the discussion section		
Sacrococcygeal teratoma Congenital sacral tumor arising from toti-potential cell rests at caudal spine characterised by exophytic back masses in newborn with **mass/dimple below intergluteal cleft.** Spinal dysraphisms have dimple above the cleft.	**CECT:** Complex mixed attenuation cystic/ solid pelvic mass with enhancement of solid portions +/– calcification. **MRI:** T1/T2 heterointense sharply demarcated tumor.	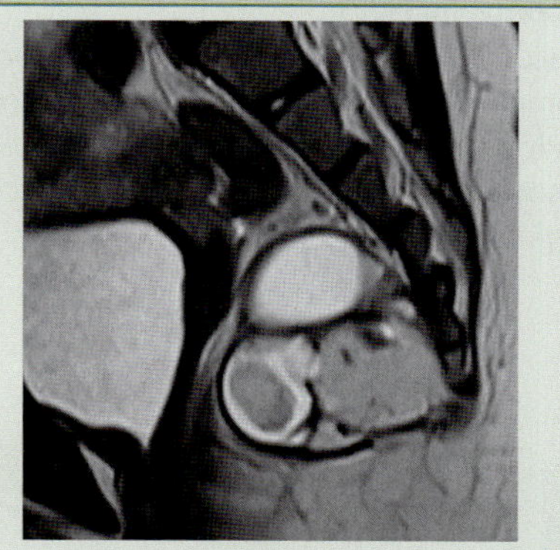 **Fig. 4.46.4:** Sacrococcygeal teratoma

(Contd.)

Table 4.46.1: Differential diagnosis for closed spinal dysraphism (*Contd.*)

Diagnosis	*Imaging features*	*Image*
Anterior sacral meningocele Sacral meninges herniating anteriorly into pelvis through focal erosion or hypogenesis of sacral +/– coccygeal vertebral elements. Onset of symptoms: 2nd–3rd decade **Currarino triad** 1. Anorectal malformation 2. Sacrococcygeal osseous defect 3. Presacral mass	Plain radiograph shows widened sacral foramina and scimitar sacrum. **CT:** Deficient sacrum with variably sized anterior cyst. **MR:** T2 hyperintense, homogeneous presacral cyst +/– cord tethering, lipoma/dermoid.	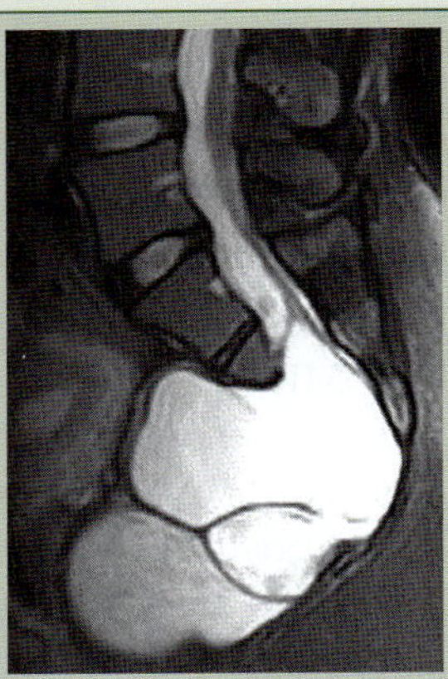 **Fig. 4.46.5:** Anterior sacral meningocele
Meningocele Protrusion of meninges through a spinal defect. Skin covered, does not contain neural elements.	NECT shows hypodense CSF dural sac-lateral thoracic meningocele. **MRI:** T1 hypointense/T2 hyperintense skin covered dural sac, conus medullaris low or normal in position.	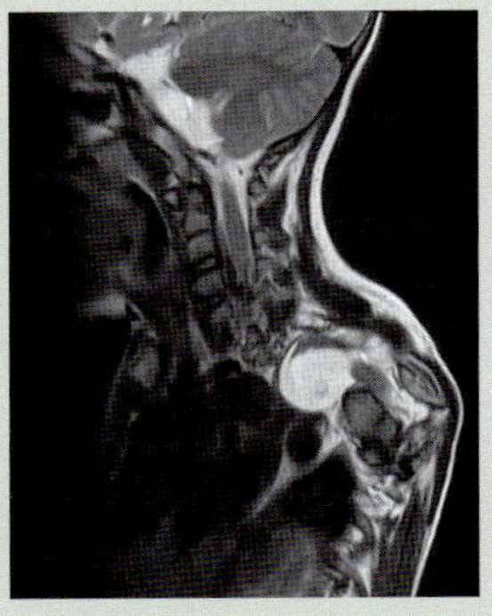 **Fig. 4.46.6:** Meningocele
Lipomyelomeningocele Lipomyelomeningoceles may be clinically detectable as a subcutaneous fatty mass above the intergluteal crease. These lesions are formed due to a defect in primary neurulation in which mesenchymal tissue enters the neural placode and forms lipomatous tissue.	**CT:** Enlargement of the canal at the placode level with fat-attenuated mass in continuity with the subcutaneous fat. **MRI:** Defect with lipomatous tissue, covered with skin. Neural placode-lipoma interface lies outside the spinal canal. A low-lying cord is present.	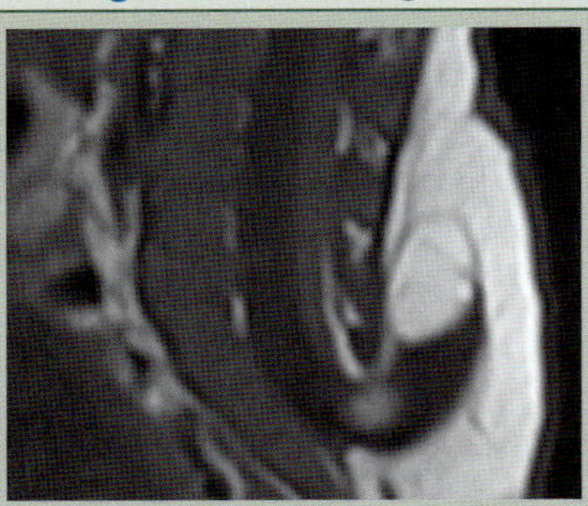 **Fig. 4.46.7:** Lipomyelomeningocele
Lipomyelocele Also known as lipomyeloschisis. It is twice as common as lipomyelomeningocele and is a closed spinal dysraphism. Over 50% are associated with cutaneous markers such as hypertrichosis or dimples.	**MRI:** Posterior spinal defect noted, which is covered by skin and interspersed lipomatous tissue. The neural placode lipoma interface lies within the spinal canal or at its edge with normal subarachnoid space.	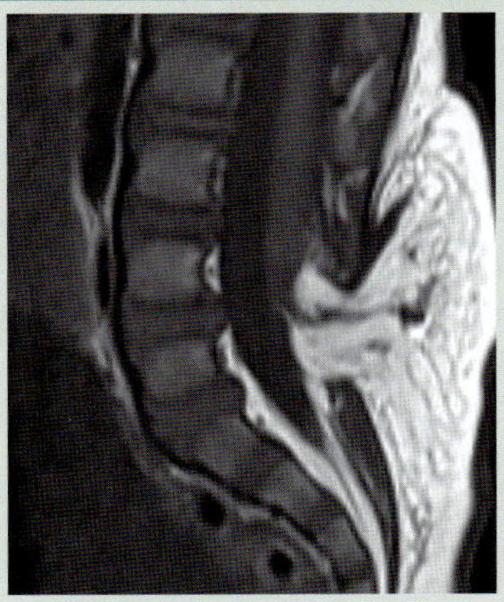 **Fig. 4.46.8:** Lipomyelocele

Discussion: Terminal myelocystocele is type of closed spinal dysraphism (complex spinal malformation) characterised by large, skin-covered back mass with hydromelic, low lying tethered spinal cord traversing dorsal meningocele and terminates in a dilated terminal cyst. Results from deranged secondary neurulation of caudal cell mass, hence associated with other caudal tail-fold malformations.

Demography: Females > males. Presents at birth.

Associations: Cloacal exstrophy, imperforate anus, omphalocele, pelvic deformities.

Syndromes: Caudal regression syndrome, OEIS syndrome constellation.

A sagittal spinal USG scan shows the spinal cord surrounded dorsally and ventrally by dilated sub-arachnoid space, the nerve roots leave the canal ventrally.

Treatment: Early diagnosis and surgical repair maximises the probability of normal neurological outcome.

Delayed recognition and operation increase odds of onset, progression of lower extremity palsy.

OEIS complex: Omphalocele, bladder exstrophy/cloacal exstrophy, imperforate anus and spinal anomalies, e.g kyphoscoliosis, hemivertebrae.

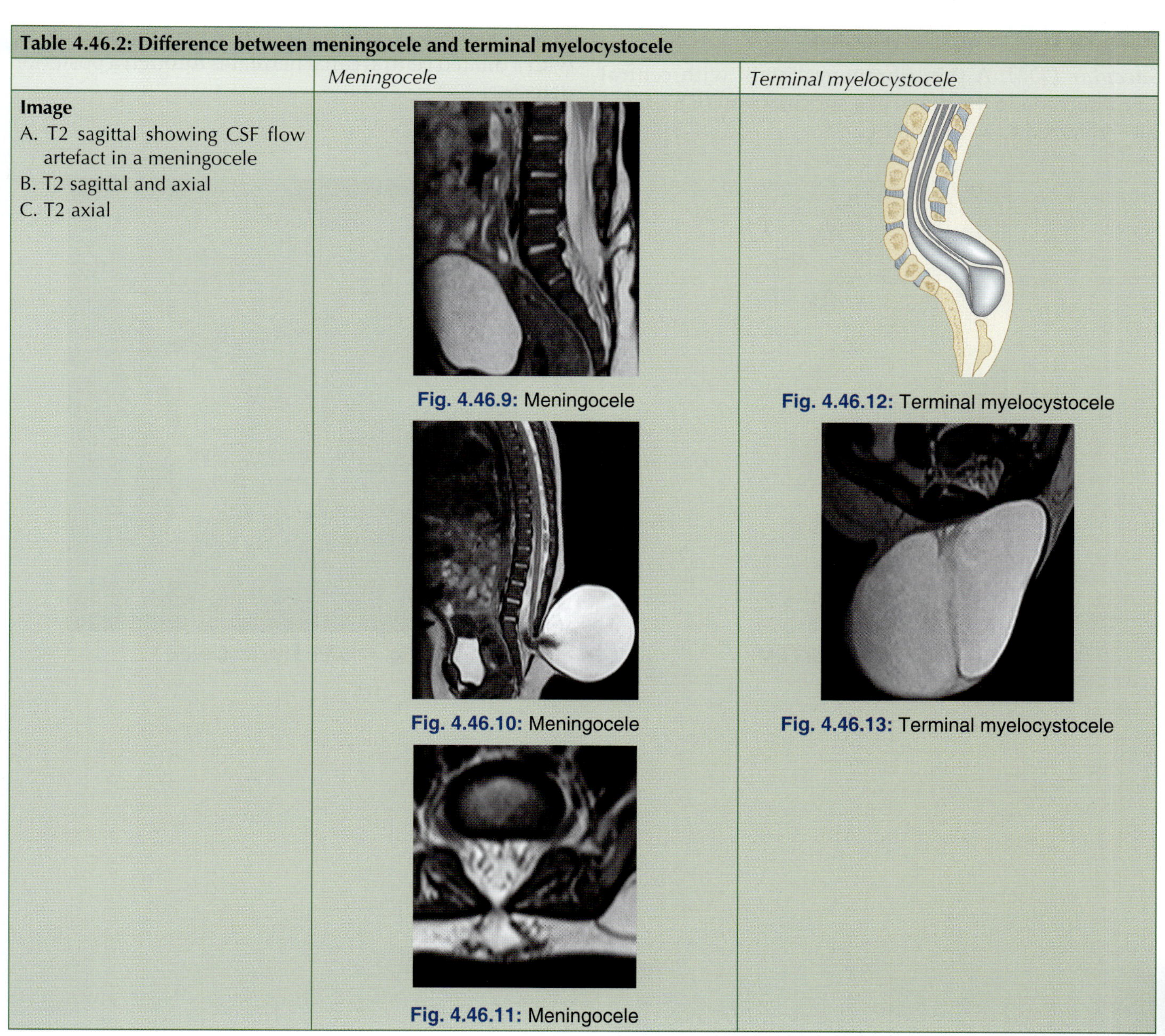

Table 4.46.2: Difference between meningocele and terminal myelocystocele

	Meningocele	*Terminal myelocystocele*
Image A. T2 sagittal showing CSF flow artefact in a meningocele B. T2 sagittal and axial C. T2 axial	**Fig. 4.46.9:** Meningocele **Fig. 4.46.10:** Meningocele **Fig. 4.46.11:** Meningocele	**Fig. 4.46.12:** Terminal myelocystocele **Fig. 4.46.13:** Terminal myelocystocele

(Contd.)

Table 4.46.2: Difference between meningocele and terminal myelocystocele (*Contd.*)		
	Meningocele	*Terminal myelocystocele*
Pathology	Skin covered, containing CSF, usually does not contain any neural elements—closed spinal dysraphism.	Complex spinal malformation where the hydromelic, low lying, tethered spinal cord traverses a meningocele to terminate in myelocystocele.
Location	Lumbosacral junction > sacrum >> cervical, thoracic	Sacrum/coccyx
Imaging	Sessile or pedunculated CSF intensity sac with a spinal dysraphism. May contain filum or nerve roots (complex meningocele)	Large CSF intensity sac through which cord traverses to terminate in a dilated terminal ventricle cyst
Associations	Hydromelia, tethered cord, diastematomyelia. Chiari 2 is associated but much less common.	Cloacal exstrophy, imperforate anus, omphalocele, equinovarus, ambiguous genitalia, renal abnormalities.

Saccular LDM vs Myelocystocele

Saccular LDM: A thin fibroneural stalk with central CSF attaching to the dome of a subcutaneous CSF-filled sac—referred to as saccular LDM.

Myelocystocele: A different entity where the cord along with a dilated central canal herniates through a posterior defect.

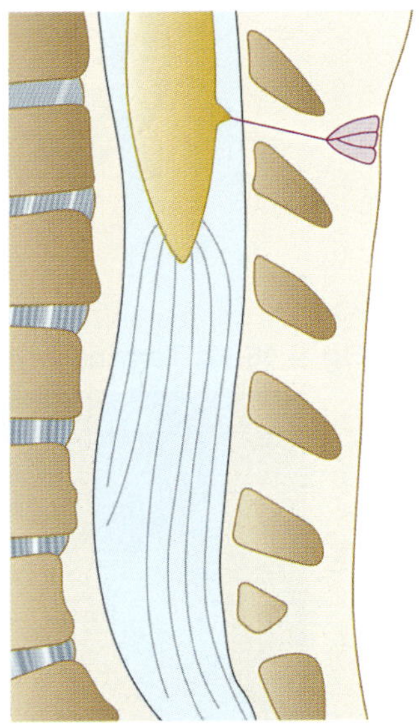

Fig. 4.46.14: Saccular LDM

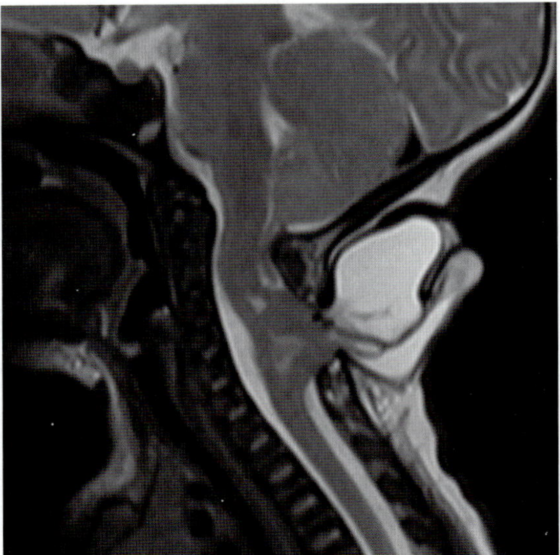

Fig. 4.46.15: Myelocystocele

4.47 SPINE

Case No. 47

Clinical details: Newborn child with imperforate anus and malformed genitalia.

Radiological technique and observation: Figures 4.47.1 and 4.47.2 are MRI-spine—sagittal and coronal images showing agenesis lower sacrum and coccyx with abrupt blind ending of the conus at T12 level. No evidence of internal fat components.

Interpretation: A—newborn child, lumbar spine, C—high abrupt blind ending spinal cord, B—no evidence of internal fat components/myelo/meningocele, D—caudal regression syndrome.

With clinical history of imperforate anus and malformed genitalia, the most likely diagnosis is caudal regression syndrome (CRS).

Discussion

Embryology (3 stages)—gastrulation (2–3 weeks)-conversion of bilaminar disc to trilaminar disc.

- **Primary neurulation** (3–4 weeks)–formation of neural tube from neural plate = brain and spinal cord portion up to S2. The neural plate's lateral boundaries elevate into neural folds, which eventually fuse in the middle to form the neural tube. Proliferation of the underlying mesoderm and hyaluronic acid causes elevation. The neural folds furrow to produce a neural groove, which finally closes to form a cord after elevation. This is accomplished by utilizing microfilaments and microtubules to produce hinge points. In 5th somite level, at intersection of the hindbrain and spinal cord, neural tube closes. It then advances cranially and caudally in zipper form. The anterior (cranial) and posterior (caudal) neuropores are the open areas of the neural tube. On day 25, the cranial neuropore closes, while the caudal neuropore closes on day 28. Overlying nonneural epidermal cells create the ectodermal layer of the skin as the neural tube closes, while neuroectoderm cells reorganise to form the roof of the neural tube.
- Secondary neurulation (5–6 weeks)—retrogressive differentiation—spinal cord portion distal to S2 developing from the caudal cell mass. CRS is due to disturbed development of caudal cell mass. Genital and anorectal structures develop simultaneously in close anatomic proximity. Insult (toxic, ischemic, infectious) occurs prior to the 4th week of gestation. Increased risk is seen with infants of diabetic mothers.

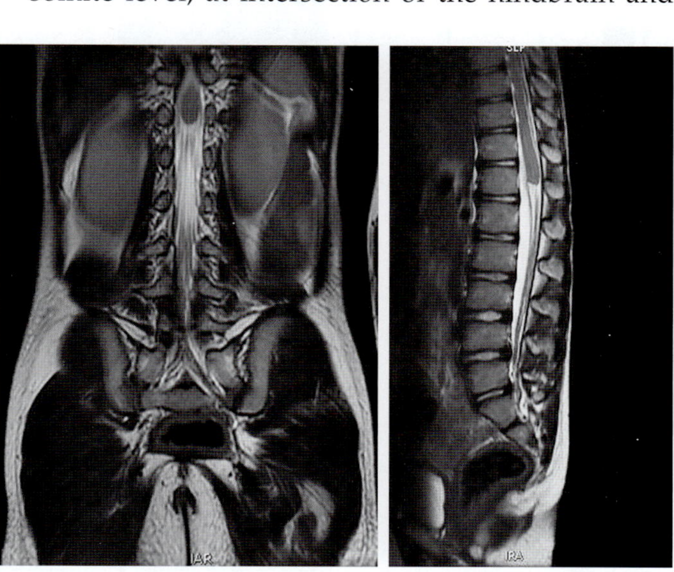

Fig. 4.47.1 Fig. 4.47.2

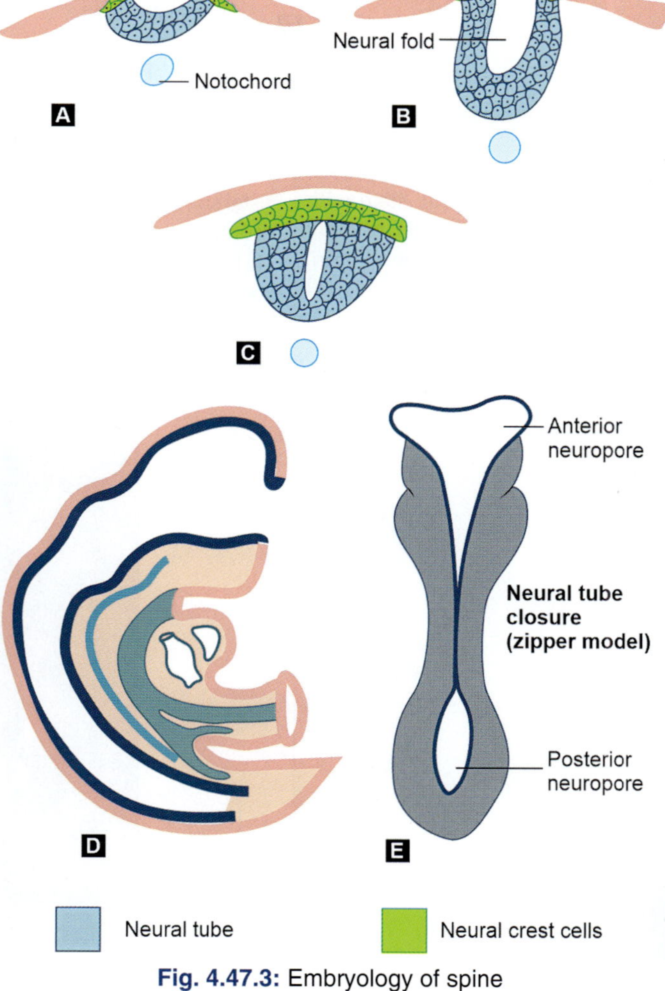

Fig. 4.47.3: Embryology of spine

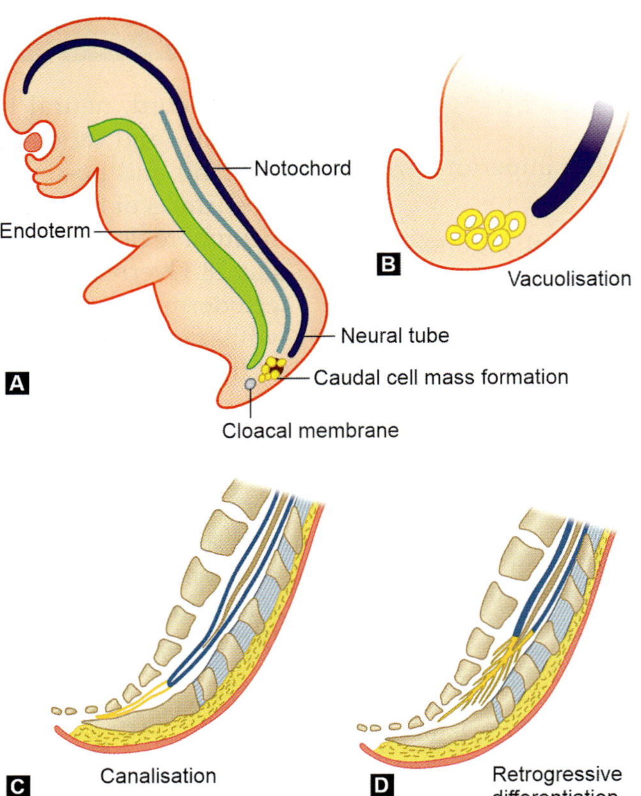

Fig. 4.47.4: Embryology of spine

Table 4.47.1: Summary of caudal regression syndrome

Caudal regression syndrome (CRS)	Group 1 (more severe)	Group 2 (less severe)
Caudal regression syndrome (CRS) is a complex dysraphic state with aberrations in gastrulation, primary as well as secondary neurulation. Midline closure defect of neural tube seen.	**Group 1 (more severe)** Distal spinal cord hypoplasia with severe visceral and osseous anomalies. High-lying wedge-shaped conus termination (decreased number of anterior horn cells) Termination of conus above L1. Neurologically asymptomatic. 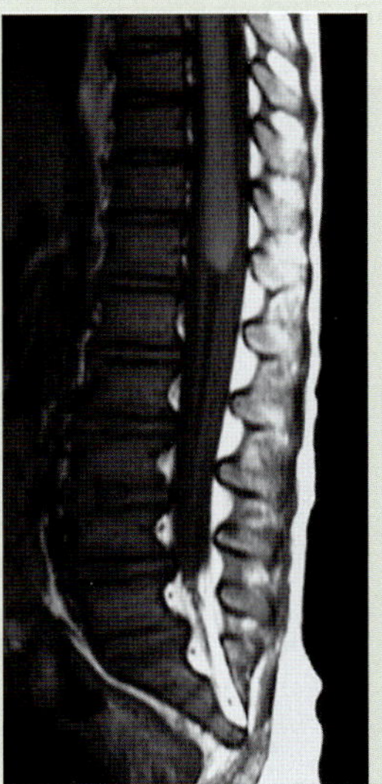 **Fig. 4.47.5:** Group 1 CRS	**Group 2 (less severe)** Has a tapered low-lying tethered spinal cord with distal cord elongation Milder associated sacral malformation Sensorimotor paresis + In general, the higher the termination of cord, the more severe is the sacral anomalies 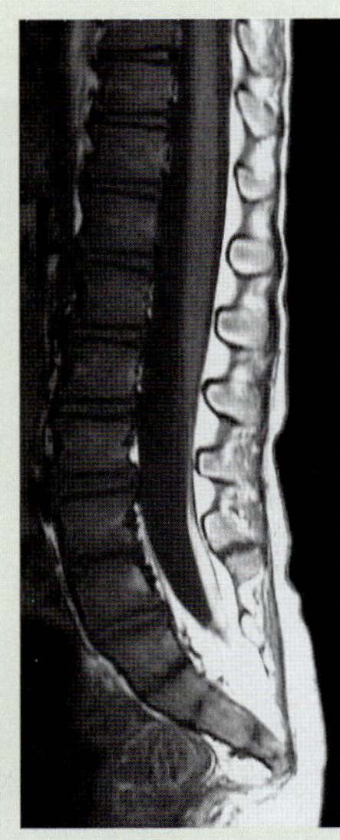 **Fig. 4.47.6:** Group 2 CRS

Contd...

Table 4.47.1: Summary of caudal regression syndrome *(Contd...)*

Segmental spinal dysgenesis		
	Segmental thoracolumbar or only lumbar vertebral and spinal cord dysgenesis or agenesis Distal spinal osseous structures are usually normal Associated with kyphoscoliosis Upper spinal cord appears normal Spinal cord atretic at the level of dysgenesis. Cord below dysgenetic level thickened and low lying.	**Fig. 4.47.7:** Segmental spinal dysgenesis
Occult sacral meningocele	Sacrum is thinned and remodelled, sometimes imitating caudal regression. Currently considered an extradural arachnoid cyst	

Table 4.47.2: Difference between types of caudal regression syndrome

Type 1:	**Type 2:**
• A club-shaped or wedge-shaped conus medullaris abruptly ending above the lower border of the L1 vertebra • Associations: Major sacral dysgenesis; in severe cases, the last intact vertebra is at T11 or T12 level • Usually presents with motor weakness and/or urinary and bowel symptoms	• A low-lying tethered cord in which the conus ends caudally to the lower border of L1 • Sacral agenesis is usually less severe • Associated with severe neurological disturbances with deterioration

Spinal Dysraphism

Spinal dysraphism refers to the congenital abnormalities of the spine and the spinal cord.

Caudal regression spectrum ranges from absent coccyx to lumbosacral agenesis.

Clinical presentation: Neurogenic urinary bladder dysfunction, sensorimotor paresis (more common in type 2), sacral sensory sparing. Narrow hips, hypoplastic gluteal muscles and shallow intergluteal cleft.

Radiography: To detect lumbar osseous hypogenesis.

The level of vertebral aplasia correlates with the motor level of involvement. Hypoplastic ilial wings seen. On MRI, CRS can be classified into 2 types.

Anorectal malformations: Anorectal abnormalities and sacral agenesis are frequently related with caudal regression syndrome. Higher levels of anal atresia, in particular, indicate more severe lumbosacral dysgenesis. The abnormal anteroposterior septation of the cloaca and deficient closure of the abdominal wall and cloacal membrane area are caused by hypoplasia and inadequate ventral and caudal push of caudal mesenchymal tissue. Rectal stenosis and imperforate anus are caused by a weak ventral push of the caudal mesenchyme, which causes posterocaudal deviation of the urorectal septum (which is an inward growth of caudal mesenchymal tissue from both lateral walls of the cloaca).

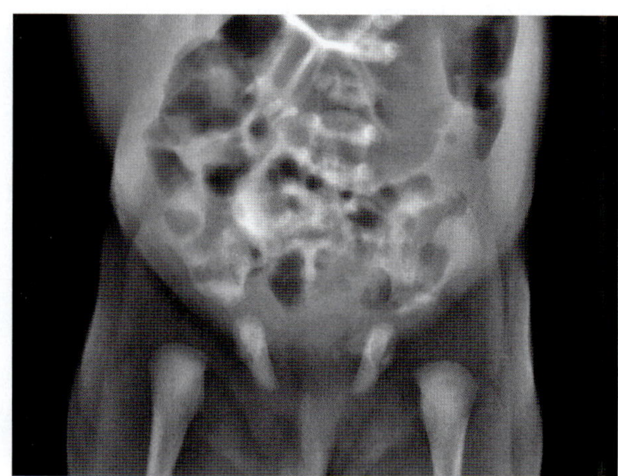

Fig. 4.47.8: Caudal regression syndrome

Table 4.47.3: Anorectal malformation		
Wingspread classification—level	*Male*	*Female*
High anomalies	1. Anorectal agenesis: a. Without fistula b. With recto-prostatic urethral fistula 2. Rectal atresia	1. Anorectal agenesis: a. Without fistula b. With rectovaginal fistula 2. Rectal atresia
Intermediate anomalies	1. Anal agenesis without fistula 2. Rectobulbar urethral fistula	1. Anal agenesis without fistula 2. Rectovaginal fistula 3. Rectovestibular fistula
Low anomalies	1. Anocutaneous fistula 2. Anal stenosis	1. Anovestibular fistula 2. Anocutaneous fistula 3. Anal stenosis
Rare malformations		Cloaca

Genitourinary anomalies: Malformed external genitalia, neurogenic bladder (if more than two segments are absent). Renal agenesis and horseshoe or low-lying kidneys can result from caudal mesenchymal hypoplasia, which affects the formation and migration of the kidneys.

Obstetric USG: Imperforate anus, short crown-rump length, mildly dilated urinary system, increased amniotic fluid, 2 hypoplastic non-fused lower extremities in a characteristic frog-like position, pelvic bone fusion, sacral agenesis.

Table 4.47.4: Currarino triad and classification of anal anomaly

Three lines are: (i) PC (pubococcygeal) line, (ii) the I (ischial) line or I point, and (iii) the anal pit

A gas bubble situated:
- Above the PC line – "high" anomaly,
- Between the PC and I line or point "intermediate" anomaly
- Below the I line (point), then it is called "low" anomaly

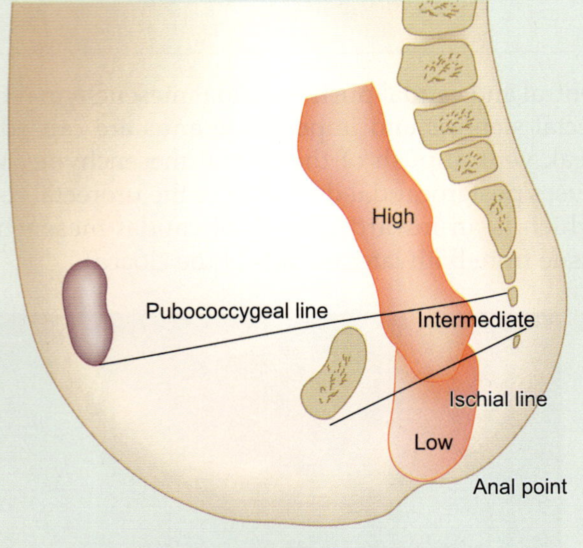

Fig. 4.47.9: Anorectal malformation

Currarino triad

1. Partial sacral agenesis (or sometimes a 'scimitar'-shaped sacrum)
2. Anorectal malformation
3. Presacral mass which may be a teratoma or anterior meningocele

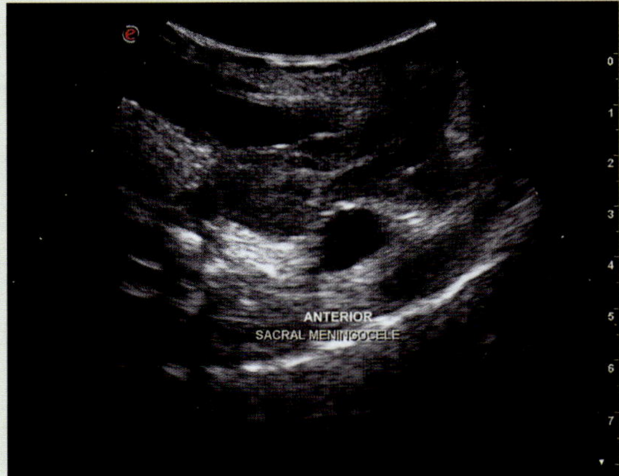

Fig. 4.47.10: Currarino triad

Treatment: Surgical untethering/surgical release/duroplasty for distal spinal canal stenosis.

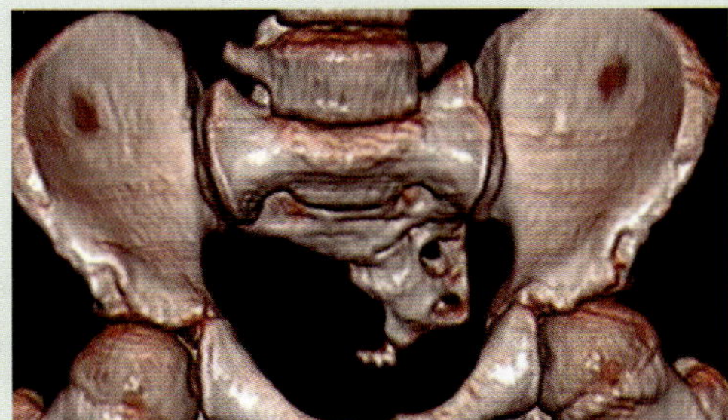

Fig. 4.47.11: Scimitar sacrum

4.48 SPINE

Case No. 48

Clinical information: 35 years old male with complaints of progressive paraesthesia and sensory abnormalities.

Radiological technique and observation: Figures 4.48.1 to 4.48.3 are MRI T2 axial without and with fat saturation sections and T1 sagittal sections showing well-defined fat containing intradural lesion seen within the spinal canal extending from L2-3 to L5-S1 level. A possible intramedullary extension of the lesion is seen with symmetrical splaying of conus medullaris. Splaying of surrounding cauda equina roots is seen. The cord appears low lying with conus ending at L3-4 level. No obvious posterior vertebral fusion anomaly is seen. Straightening of lumbar lordosis is seen. Posterocentral protrusion of L4-5 disc is seen with mild facet arthropathy indenting the thecal sac.

Interpretation: A: 35 years old male, lumbar spine, C: Intradural fat intensity lesion within the spinal canal, showing suppression on fat saturation sequences and low-lying spinal cord, B: No obvious posterior vertebral fusion anomaly seen, D: Tethered cord with dorsal intraspinal lipoma (type IIA).

Principal diagnosis: Tethered cord with dorsal intraspinal lipoma (type IIA).

Tethered cord: It is a clinical syndrome due to anchoring of the spinal cord/neural placode or filum terminale to the surrounding tissues occurring primarily or secondary to scarring or formation of a dermoid post-surgery and not just due to a low-lying cord or a thick filum terminale, usually associated with closed

Table 4.48.1: Types of spinal lipoma

Type I	**Intradural lipomas above the level of conus (Lipoma–placode interface within the dura)** **IA:** Those lipomas that are dorsal to the cord or extend cranially/caudally/around the spinal cord; entirely confined to the intradural space **IB:** Dorsal extension as a lipomyelocele **IC:** Ventral extension as a lipomyelocele
Type II	**Transitional and chaotic lipomas** **IIA:** Transitional lipoma above the last dorsal root entry zone of the conus **IIB:** Dorsal extension as a lipomyelocele **IIC:** Ventral extension as a lipomyelocele **IID:** Involving ventral fat and entangling the nerve roots—chaotic lipoma
Type III	**Conal lipomas: Arising from the level of conus medullaris below the level of last dorsal root entry zone** **IIIA:** Confined to intradural space **IIIB:** Dorsal extension as a lipomyelocele **IIIC:** Ventral extension as a lipomyelocele
Type IV	**Filar lipomas: Lipomas of the filum terminale** **IVA:** Apical lipoma **IVB:** Mid-filar lipoma **IVC:** Filar tip lipoma **IVD:** Tight filum terminale
Type V	**Lipomyelomeningocele: Lipoma–placode interface outside the spinal canal** **VA:** Anterior lipomyelomeningocele **VB:** Posterior lipomyelomeningocele
Type VI	**Intramedullary lipoma**

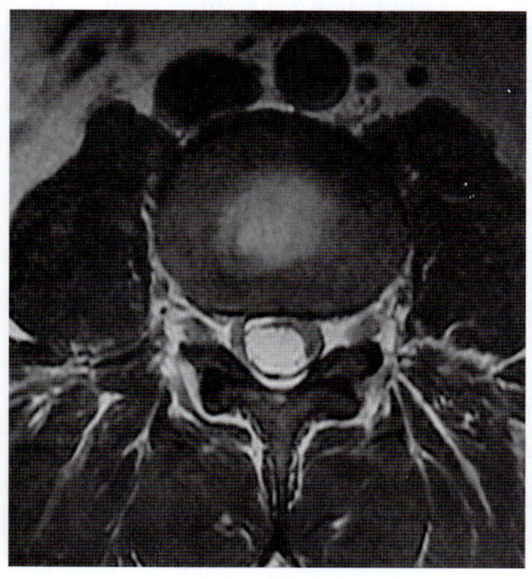

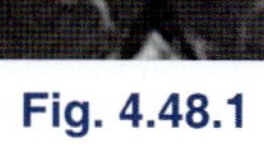

Fig. 4.48.1

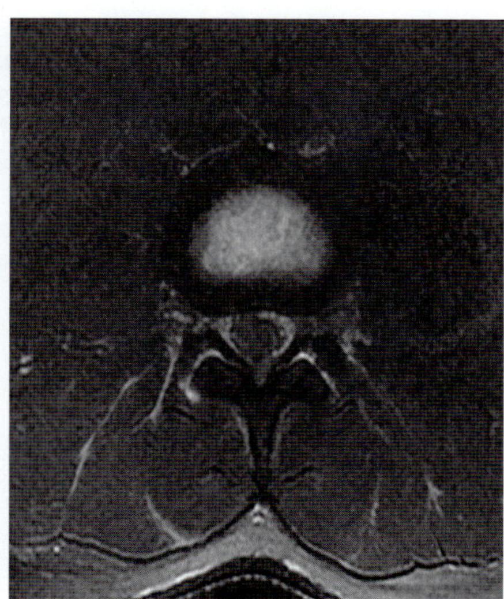

Fig. 4.48.2

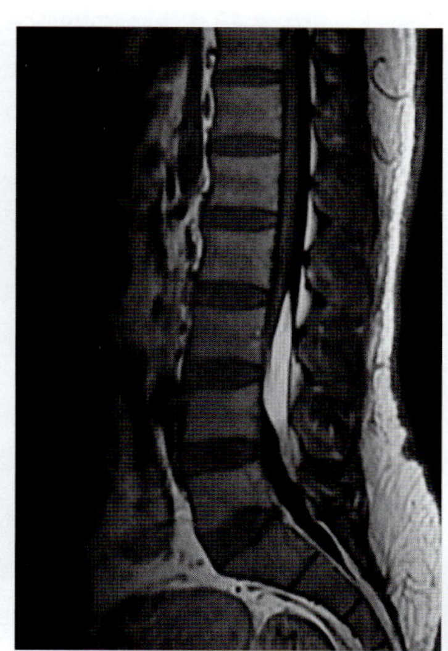

Fig. 4.48.3

spinal dysraphism like spinal lipomas, the tight filum terminale, split cord malformations, limited dorsal myeloschisis, meningoceles/meningomyeloceles. As a result of the mass effect, patients have neurological impairments.When there is no vertebral or cutaneous defects seen, they appear 10 to 30 years. Numbness or spastic weakness in the extremities is the most common clinical manifestation. Intradural lipomas can develop

Table 4.48.2: Differential diagnosis for spinal dysraphism		
Filum terminale lipoma (Type IVD) Incidentally found in 4–6% of autopsies. Surgical intervention for tethered cord and low lying conus. 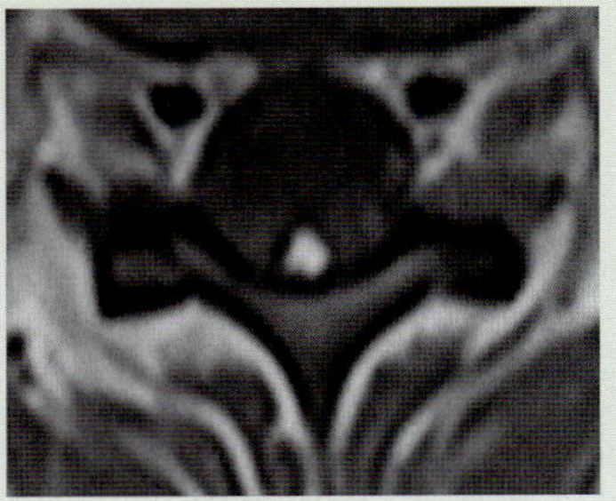 Fig. 4.48.4: Filum terminale lipoma (Type IVD)	Thin filum (diameter is <2 mm at the L5/S1 level) is not much symptomatic. When the filum is thickened (with or without fat), it is much more likely to be associated with a low lying, cord (tip of the conus at or below the midpoint of L2) and cord tethering. **Symptomatic filum >2 mm thickness.**	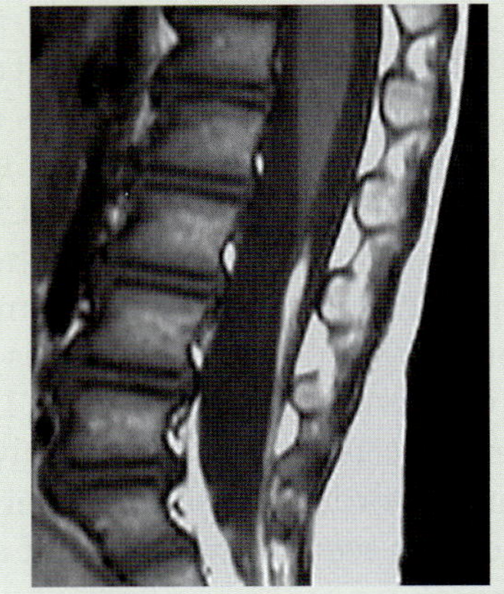 Fig. 4.48.5: Filum terminale lipoma (Type IVD)
Lipomyelocele Defect in primary neurulation. Early prophylactic surgery <1 year. To untether cord, resect lipoma and reconstruct dura. 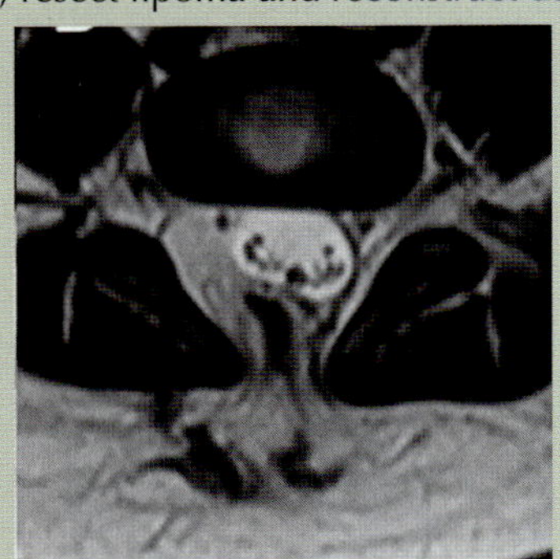 Fig. 4.48.6: Lipomyelocele	Skin covered (closed) neural placode-lipoma complex contiguous with subcutaneous fat through dysraphic defect. Lipomyelocele: The placode-lipoma interface lies within the spinal canal.	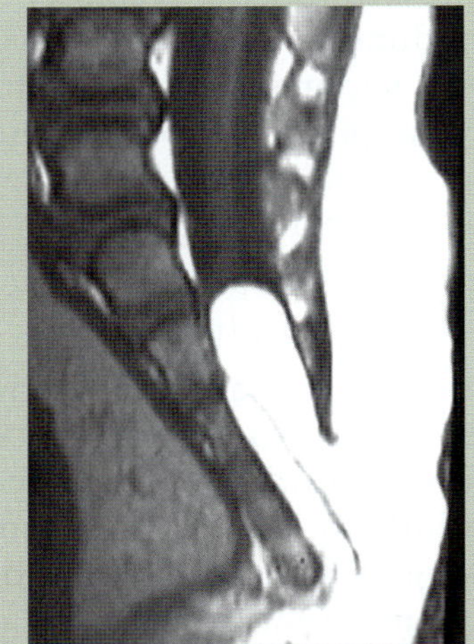 Fig. 4.48.7: Lipomyelocele
Lipomyelomeningocele (Type V) <1 year prophylactic surgery to untether cord, resect lipoma and reconstruct dura. 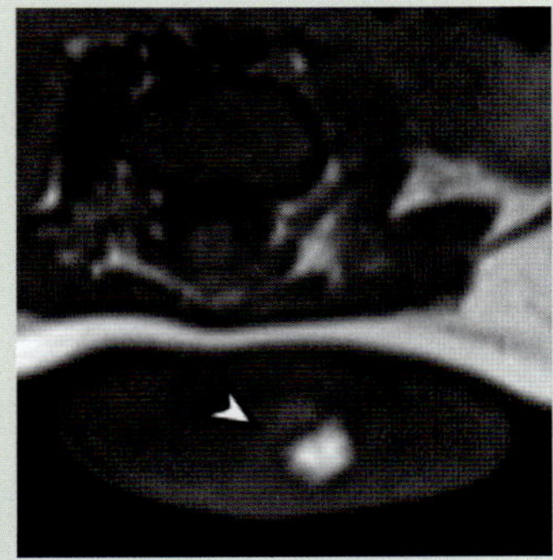 Fig. 4.48.8: Lipomyelomeningocele (Type V)	Subcutaneous fatty mass contiguous with lipoma and placode through posterior dysraphism. The placode-lipoma interface lies outside the spinal canal. Associated meningeal herniation, enlarged canal noted at the level of neural placode. May be associated with tethered/ low lying cord.	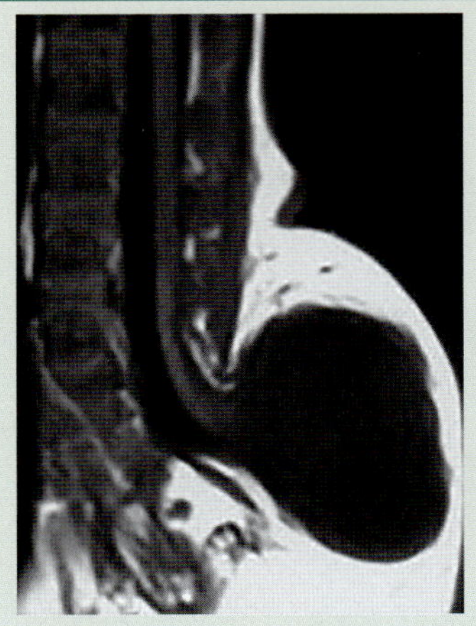 Fig. 4.48.9: Lipomyelomeningocele (Type V)

(*Contd.*)

Table 4.48.2: Differential diagnosis for spinal dysraphism (*Contd.*)		
(Epi) dermoid cyst Common in children. Mostly acquired. Although present since birth, most congenital epidermoids present at 2nd–4th decade. Males commonly affected 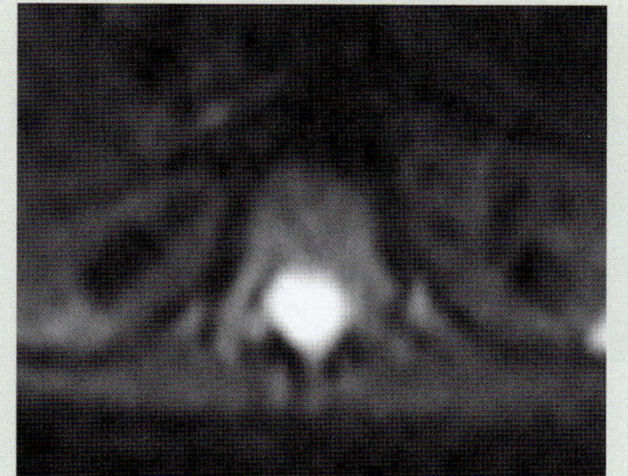 **Fig. 4.48.10:** Epidermoid cyst	Low T1 signal, similar or mildly increased signal relative to CSF. Lumbar canal / cauda equina common location. Spinal canal widening +. 40% intramedullary 60% extramedullary epidermoids. Acquired epidermoid almost always occurs at cauda equina. Epidermoid – Diffusion restriction + 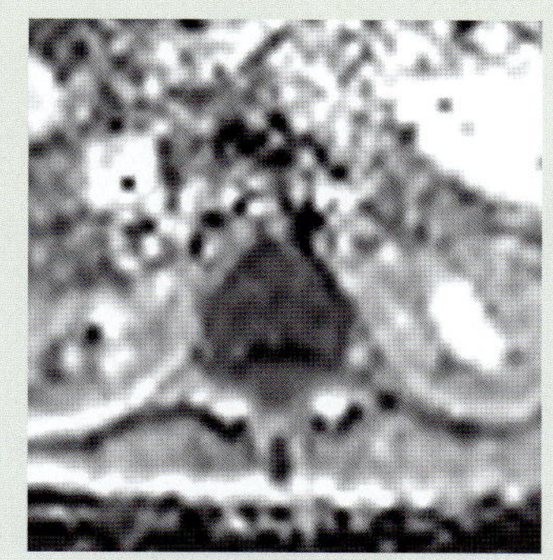 **Fig. 4.48.11:** Epidermoid cyst	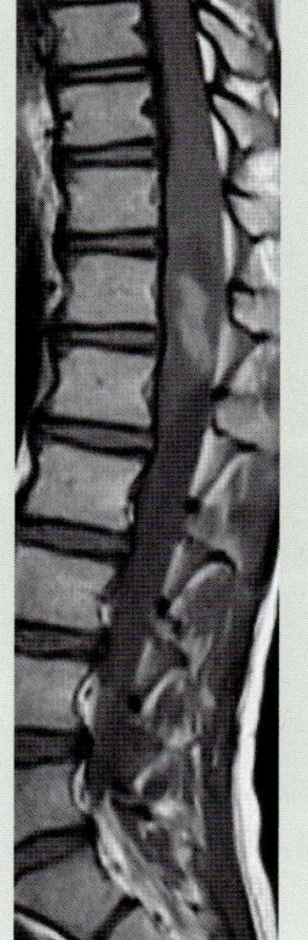 **Fig. 4.48.12:** Epidermoid cyst 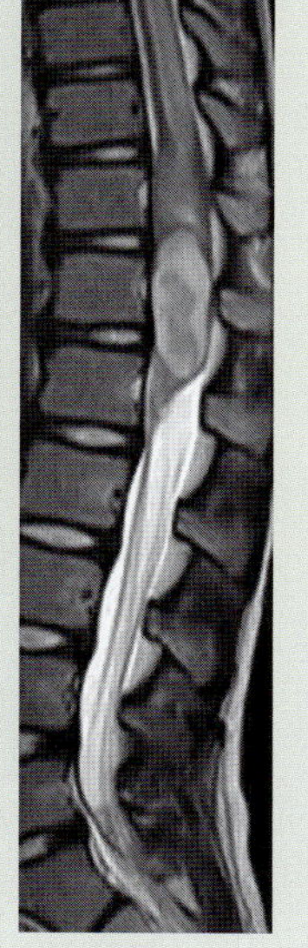 **Fig. 4.48.13:** Epidermoid cyst
Epidural lipomatosis Associated with glucocorticoid excess, obesity, idiopathic, Scheuermann's disease and following spinal surgery	The dural sac might appear narrower or even resemble a "Y"-shaped structure of the thecal sac due to excess of fat deposition within the spinal epidural space.	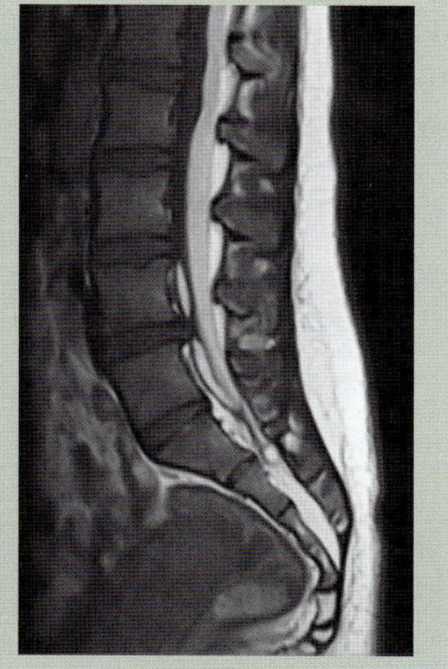 **Fig. 4.48.14:** Epidural lipomatosis

anywhere throughout the spinal canal's length. In children, cervical spine is affected, but the thoracic spine is the most common site in adults. They commonly occur dorsally, near the midline of the spinal cord. The ventral surface of the spinal cord is flattened. The tethering causes functional neurological deterioration resulting in motor and sensory dysfunction, muscle atrophy, urinary incontinence, decreased or hyperactive reflexes, spastic gait, and other deformities. Triangular tented thecal sac (pulled by filum). Exiting nerve roots have lateral or uphill course reduced/absent spinal cord movement (phase contrast MRI) absent anterior movement of cord in prone position and absent transmitted pulsations.

Retained medullary cord: Defective apoptosis during late secondary neurulation results in a persistent medullary cord. An absent filum terminale is characteristic of most RMCs. They appear as a robust cord-like structure attached from the conus to the cul-de-sac. An altered shape of the conus is visible.

They are often misread as a low-lying conus or a tight filum terminale. Although, MRI signal intensity characteristics are the same as a low-lying conus making preoperative diagnosis difficult, intra-operative neuromonitoring helps distinguish between the two as an RMC is non-functional with no electrical activity.

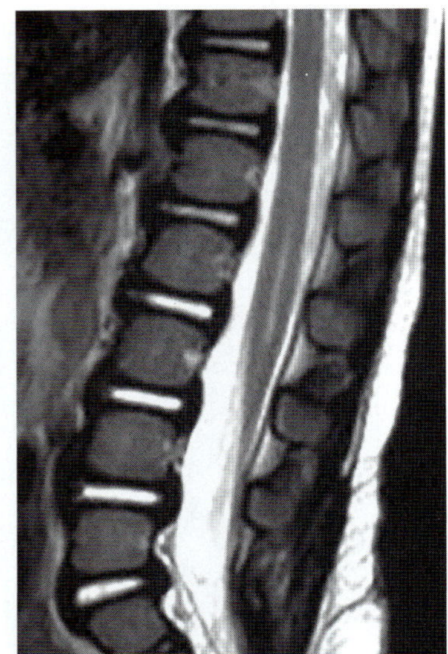
Fig. 4.48.15: Tethered cord

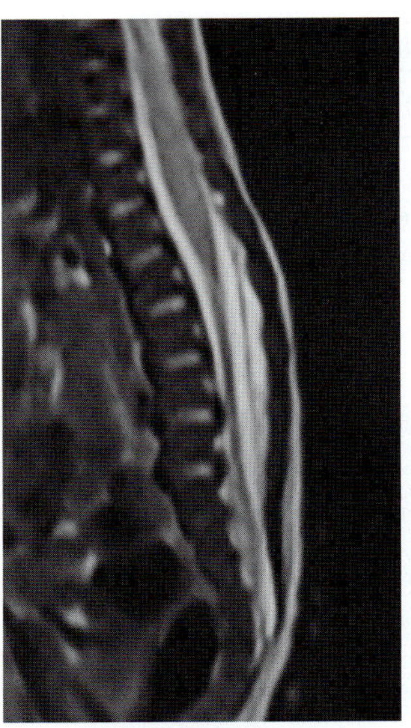
Fig. 4.48.16: Retained medullary cord

Spinal lipoma: Plain film will show thin pedicles with spinal canal widening. CT: Homogeneously fat dense lesion with no solid components. MRI–circumscribed dural masses distorting the cord. They follow fat signal on all sequences; T1 and T2: Hyperintense, fat suppressed sequences—hypointensity. T1 C+ (Gd): Will show no enhancement.

Treatment and prognosis: The treatment of choice is surgical resection. As the lipomas adhere closely to the adjacent parenchyma of the spine, they generally cannot be completely resected and the aim of surgery is to decompress. Because these lesions are typically very slow growing, a very satisfactory and long-lasting clinical effect may be obtained after achieving a subtotal excision.

Table 4.48.3: Difference between retained medullary cord and tight filum terminale

Retained medullary cord		*Tight filum terminale*	
Shape of the conus altered/not clearly demarcated		Conus shape unaffected	
Low-lying conus		Low lying/normal conus	
Usually associated with tethered cord syndrome		Usually associated with tethered cord syndrome	
Histological findings of RMCs include a dense glioneuronal core along with of fibrofatty elements, an ependymal-lined central cavity and vestigial nerve roots	**Fig. 4.48.17:** Retained medullary cord	No evidence of glioneuronal elements on histopathology	**Fig. 4.48.18.** Tight filum terminale

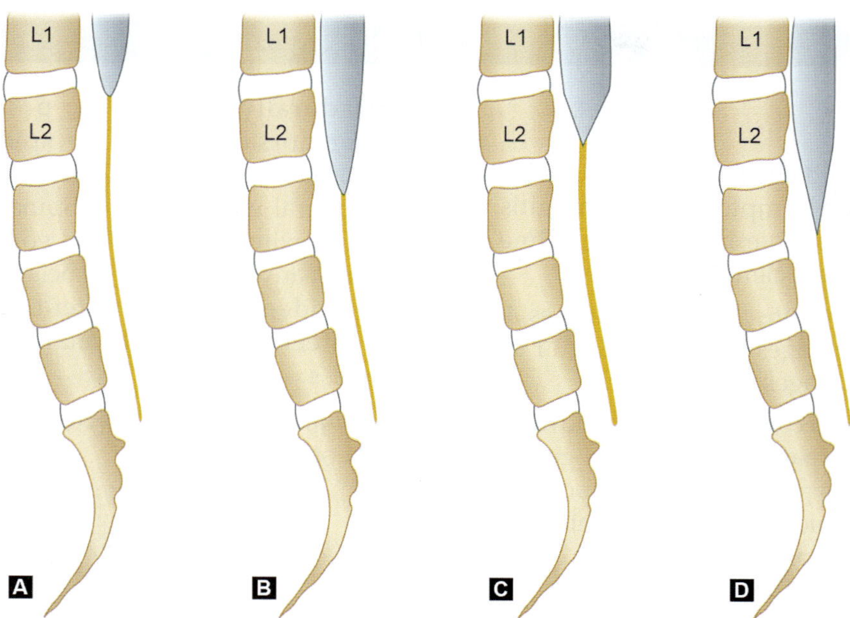

Fig. 4.48.19A to D: (A) The conus lies at a normal level; (B) Conus lies at an abnormally low level with a normal appearing filum; (C) Conus under excessive tension because of dysplastic thick and fatty filum that exhibits high signal on T1 (filum thickness >2 mm at L5-S1) and (D) Conus lies at an abnormally low level with a dysplastic appearing filum.

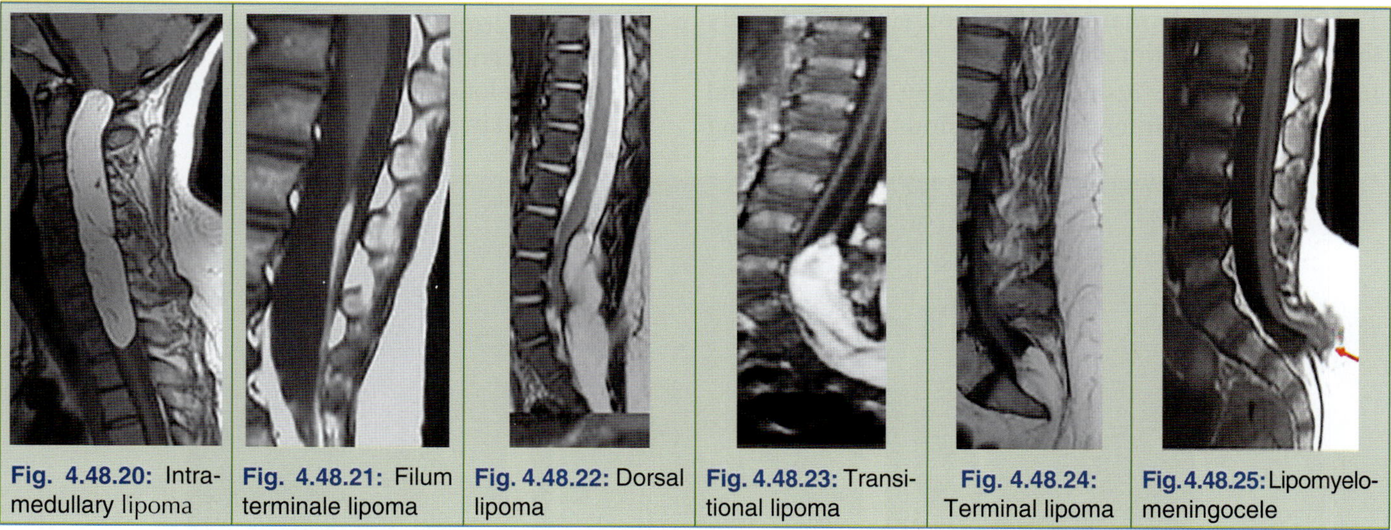

Fig. 4.48.20: Intramedullary lipoma

Fig. 4.48.21: Filum terminale lipoma

Fig. 4.48.22: Dorsal lipoma

Fig. 4.48.23: Transitional lipoma

Fig. 4.48.24: Terminal lipoma

Fig. 4.48.25: Lipomyelomeningocele

4.49 SPINE

Case No. 49

Clinical features: A child aged 12 months, was brought with clinical signs and symptoms of meningitis. The mother also gave a positive history of midline skin dimple above intergluteal cleft.

Imaging techniques and observations: Figures 4.49.1–4.49.3 are MRI spine images in T2 sagittal, T1 sagittal and T1 post-contrast images respectively.

Observations: The spinal cord at the level of lower dorsal and lumbar levels is expanded with heterogeneous T2 hyperintensity which is predominantly hypointense on T1 and demonstrates thick peripheral enhancement on T1 post-contrast. MultipleT1 hypointense collections with peripheral enhancement noted from S1 to L2 vertebral levels within the spinal canal. Tethering of spinal cord is noted. There is increased signal intensity in the proximal cord representing cord edema. No evidence to suggest any presence of associated (epi)dermoid tumor. No evidence of dorsal tenting of the spinal cord. T2 hypointense dermal sinus tract coursing intradurally through the posterior elements.

Interpretation: A: 12-month-old baby, lumbar spinal cord, C: T2 hypointense dermal sinus tract coursing intradurally through the posterior elements. The lower dorsal and lumbar spinal cord is expanded with heterogeneously T2 hyperintense showing thick peripheral enhancement. Spinal cord tethering noted with proximal myelitis and edema. B: No evidence to suggest any presence of associated (epi) dermoid tumor. No evidence of dorsal tenting of the spinal cord, D: Infected dorsal dermal sinus with intraspinal abscess.

Principal diagnosis: Infected dorsal dermal sinus with intra-spinal abscess.

Differential diagnosis: Limited dorsal myeloschisis.

Management: Surgical resection of the sinus tract, tethered cord release. IV antibiotics.

Dorsal dermal sinus: Epithelium-lined fistulous tract that extends inward from the skin surface for varying distances and frequently connects the body surface with the CNS or its coverings

- Focal incomplete disjunction of neuroectoderm from cutanectoderm, focal segmental adhesion is created when it ascends relative to spinal column, adhesion persists as elongated epithelial lined tube connecting cord with skin.

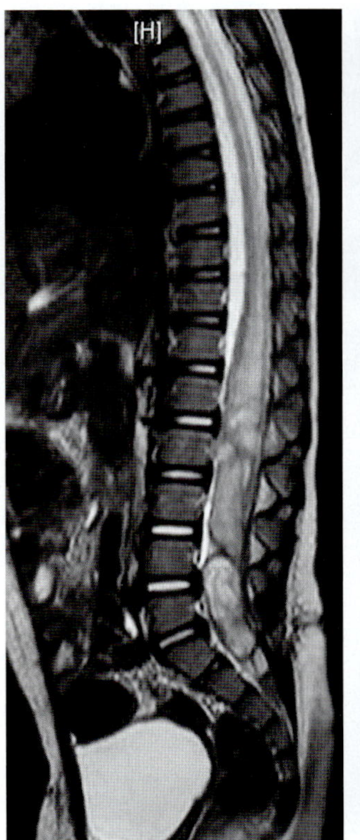

Fig. 4.49.1

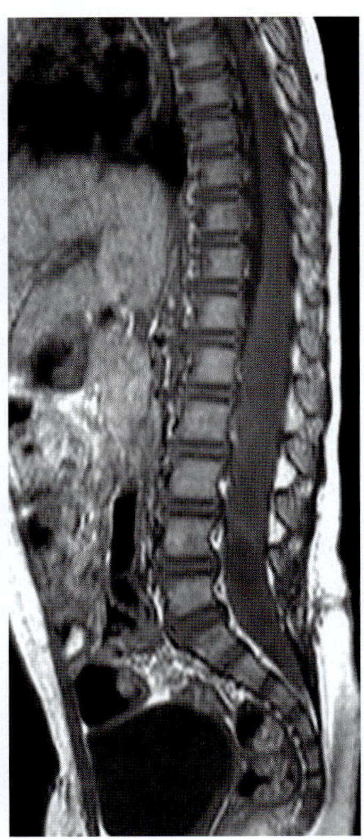

Fig. 4.49.2

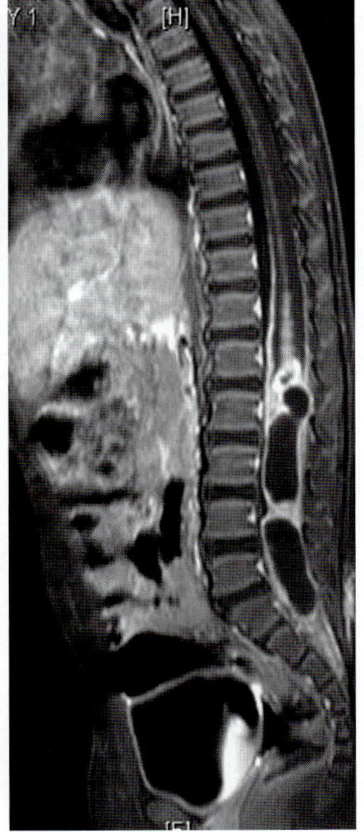

Fig. 4.49.3

Table 4.49.1: Difference between non-saccular LDM and CDS	
Non-saccular limited dorsal myeloschisis (LDM)	*Congenital dorsal dermal sinus (CDS)*
Closed skin defect	Tract with lumen communicating with the skin opening
Less chances of infection	More chances of infection
Less number of neurological defects	More number of neurological defects
Surgery only needed in cases of tethering	Surgery even in asymptomatic cases in view of ascending infections
Tract: Intrathecal tracts clearly visible	*Tract:* Intrathecal tracts not clearly visible
Attachment site: Clearly seen as hypointense round structure adhering to the dorsal aspect of spinal cord above conus medullaris	*Attachment site:* Variable and not clearly visible
Dorsal tenting of spinal cord seen in nearly all patients	Dorsal tenting of spinal cord is rare
Tethering is more common	Tethering is less common
Dermoid and (epi)dermoids are very rare	Dermoid and (epi)dermoids are more common

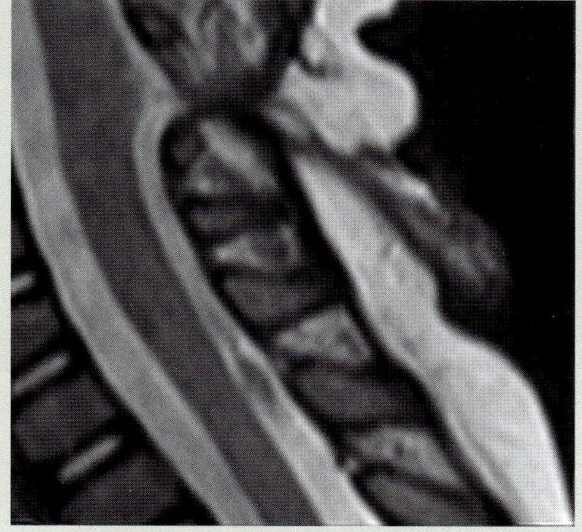

Fig. 4.49.4: Non-saccular limited dorsal myeloschisis

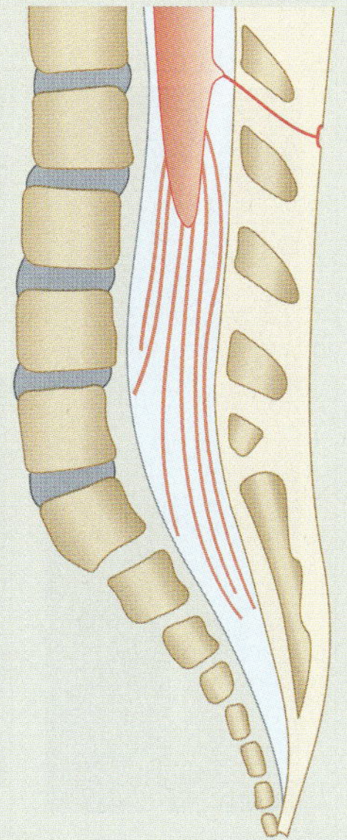

Fig. 4.49.5: Non-saccular limited dorsal myeloschisis

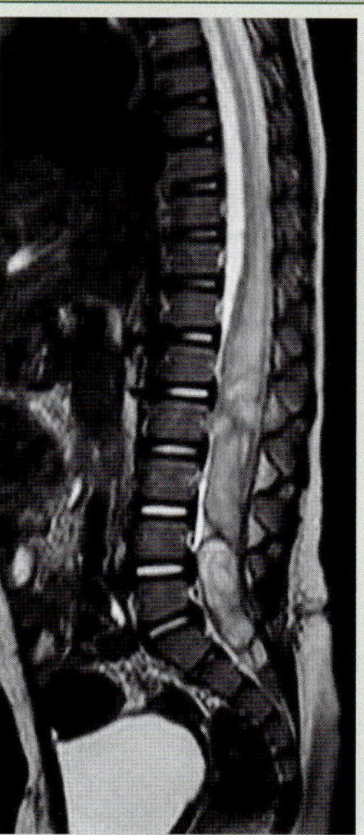

Fig. 4.49.6: Congenital dorsal dermal sinus

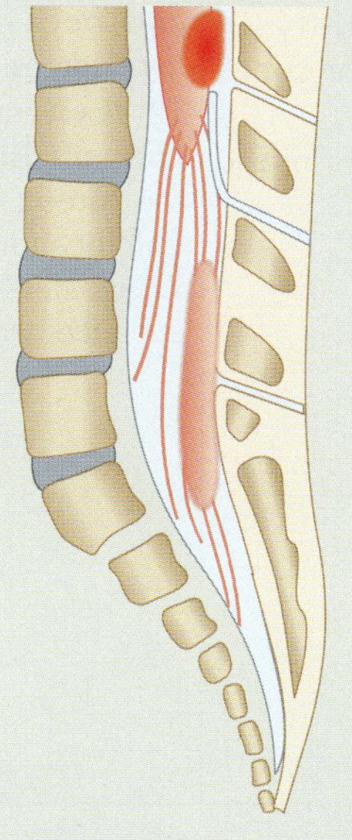

Fig. 4.49.7: Congenital dorsal dermal sinus

Low coccygeal midline dimple **Sacral dimple** Usually incidental finding. Low dimple opening in the intergluteal cleft: Sacral dimple. High dimple with leaking of fluid: Dorsal dermal sinus	Low sacral dimple connecting to coccyx by fibrous tract. Usually within the intergluteal cleft. Tract usually atretic may occasionally be filled with minimal fluid			
Spinal dermoid cyst Congenital uni/multilocular cystic tumors lined by squamous epithelium containing skin appendages. 60% extramedullary; 40% intramedullary. Age: <20 years; [M = F]. Location: Lumbosacral (60%)	Commonly appears as mass of CSF density /intensity with fat density/intensity components. CT: Well-defined mass isodense to CSF with hypodense fat. Calcification may be present. Minimal enhancement MRI: T1-Hypo/hyperintense; T2/FLAIR: Hyperintense; T1+C: Mild rim /no enhancement DWI: Less likely to show diffusion restriction than epidermoid	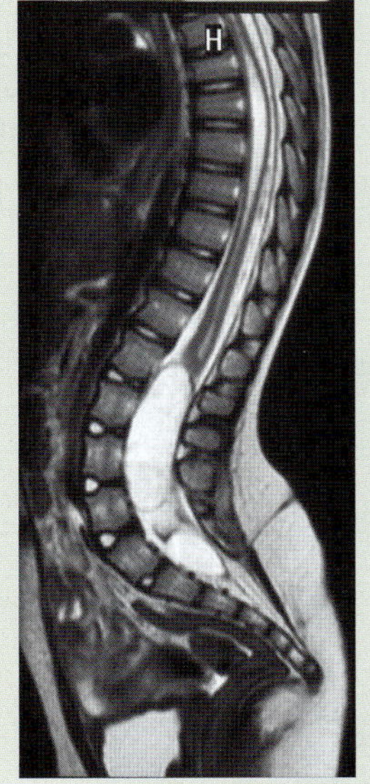 **Fig. 4.49.8:** Dorsal dermal sinus with dermoid cyst	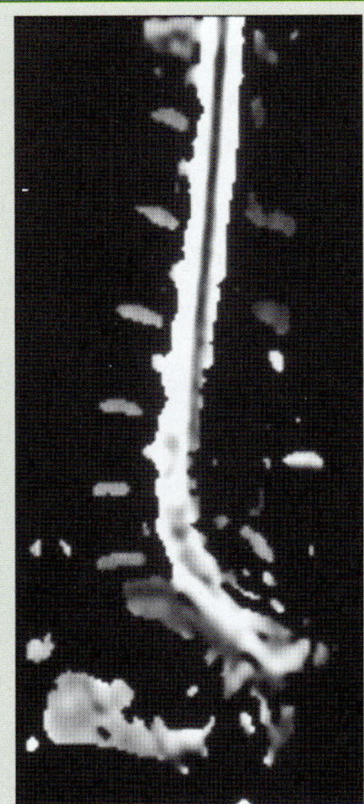 **Fig. 4.49.9:** Dorsal dermal sinus with dermoid cyst	
Pilonidal sinus Skin and subcutaneous tissue infections at the upper part of intergluteal cleft Age; >45 yrs. M > F	USG: Shows sinus anatomy to a reasonable degree MRI: Allows visualization of tract and its associated complications Fluoroscopy: Contrast injected into the opening to delineate the extent of sinus and any fistulous tract			
Myxopapillary ependymoma Variant of ependymoma that occurs predominantly in filum terminale and/or conus medullaris. Most common tumors of the cauda equina region. Age: 35 years.	T1: Usually isointense; prominent mucinous content can occasionally result in hyperintensity. T2WI: Overall it is high intensity. Low intensity can be seen at the tumor margin: Cap sign. Calcification may lead to low T2 signal; T1+C: Homogeneous enhancement	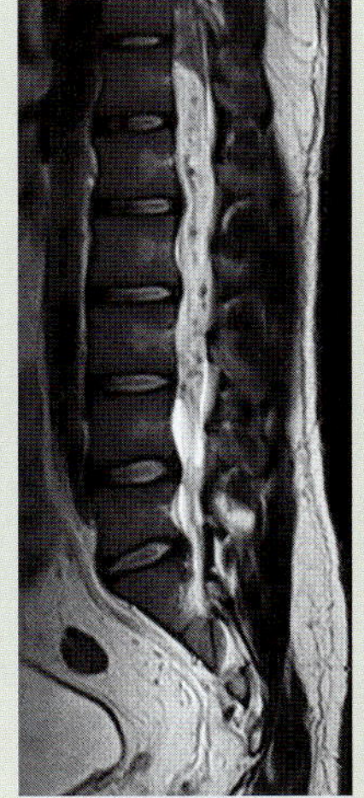 **Fig. 4.49.10:** Myxopapillary ependymoma	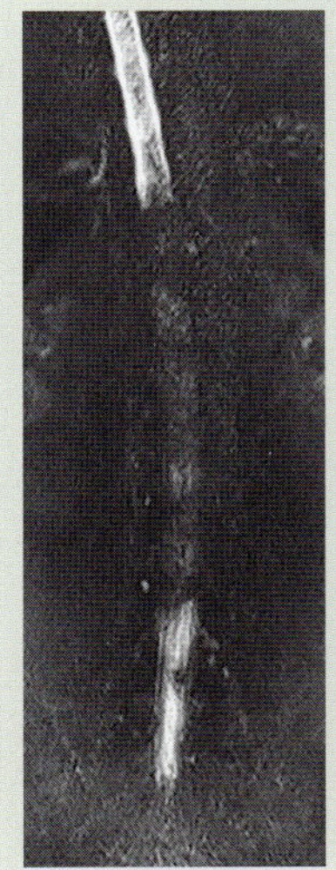 **Fig. 4.49.11:** Myxopapillary ependymoma	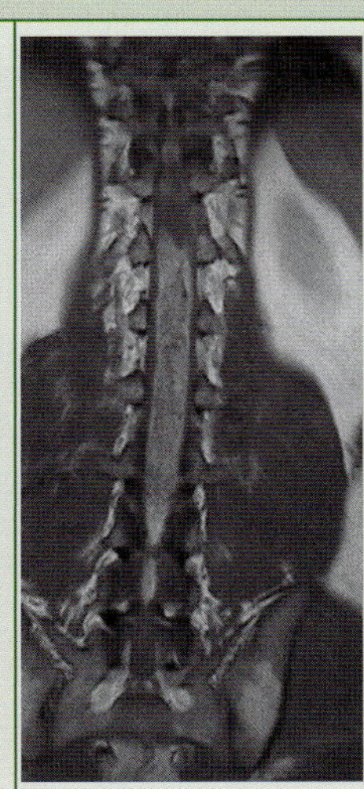 **Fig. 4.49.12:** Myxopapillary ependymoma

Intraspinal abscess ISCAs (intramedullary spinal cord abscesses) are a rare infection. It might be a primary or secondary complication of an infected epidural abscess.	MRI: T2 heterogeneously hyperintense lesion that expands the cord. Predominantly hypointense on T1. Post-contrast, Peripheral enhancement. Look for evidence of discitis/ vertebral osteomyelitis/ extradural collections. In patients with recurrent meningitis, a congenital dermal sinus with intramedullary abscess should be suspected	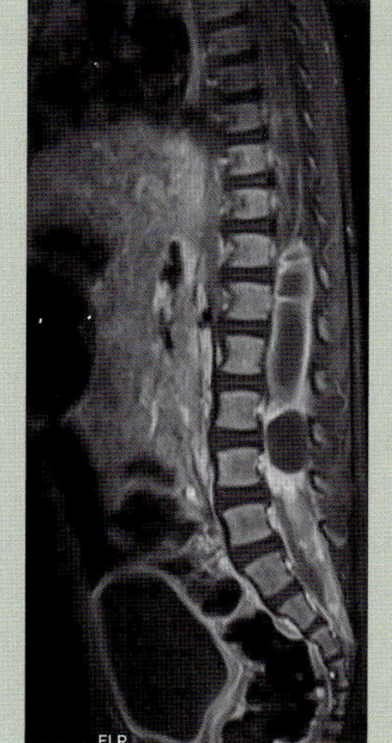 **Fig. 4.49.13:** Dorsal dermal sinus with intraspinal abscess	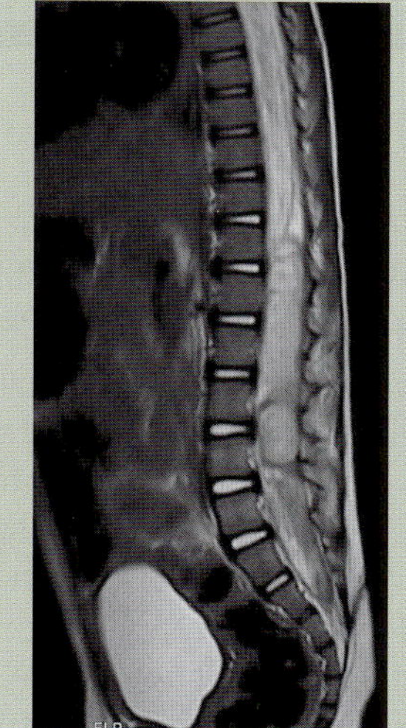 **Fig. 4.49.14:** Dorsal dermal sinus with intraspinal abscess
Leptomeningeal drop metastases CNS primary neoplasm spread inferiorly along the CSF spaces Causes: Medulloblastoma Ependymoma Choroid plexus carcinoma Pineoblastoma/pineocytoma Germinoma Glioblastoma multiforme Anaplastic astrocytoma sPNET	Solitary focal mass Diffuse thin sheet-like coating of cords Rope-like thickening of cord Multifocal discrete nodules along the cord/ roots MR: T1: Usually isointense T2: Thickened nerve roots, Cord edema T1+C: Single/multiple enhancing nodular masses like sugar coating of the cord and roots	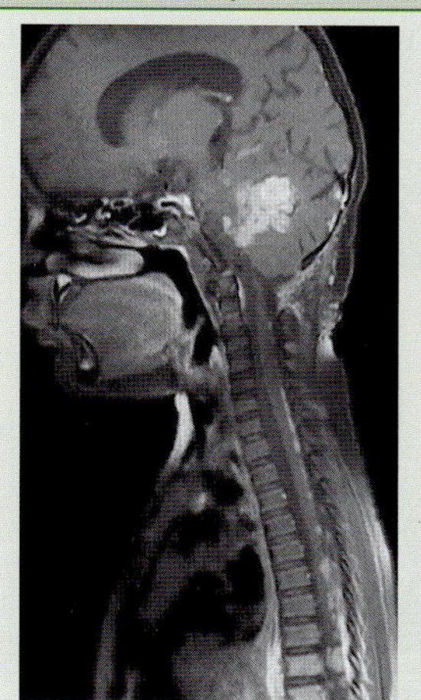 **Fig. 4.49.15:** Medulloblastoma with drop metastasis	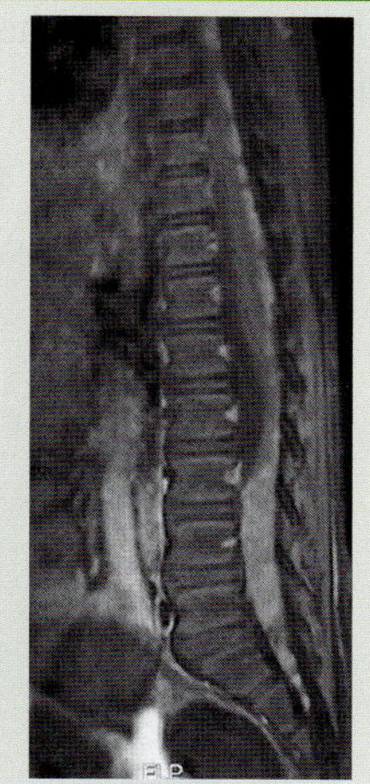 **Fig. 4.49.16:** Medulloblastoma with drop metastasis

- Sinus may terminate with subcutaneous tissue or pass through median raphe or bifid lamina towards the dura, may merge with dura; terminate into SA space/ Conus medullaris/filum/nerve root or a concomitant dermoid or (epi)dermoid.
- One-half to two-thirds extend to spinal canal; 50% end in dermoid or (epi)dermoid

Location: Lumbosacral (60%) > occipital (25 %) > thoracic (10%) > cervical (1%)

Size: Thin tract (several mm); variable length.

Morphology: Subcutaneous tract, which may extend to conus medullaris (lumbosacral) or central spinal canal (cervical, thoracic) with or without spinal dysraphism.

Radiography/CT: ±Dysraphism/laminar defect.

USG: Subcutaneous tract, is slightly hypoechoic ± low lying conus/intrathecal mass.

MR: T1WI: Sinus tract hypointense to subcutaneous fat. Dorsal dural tenting indicates dural penetration. ± Dermoid Cyst: Hypo to hyperintense (fat)/ ±(epi) dermoid cyst: Hypointense ±Tethered cord (lumbosacral sinus).

T2WI: Sinus tract hypointense to fat±(epi)dermoid cyst: Hyperintense ± Nerve root clumping (adhesive arachnoiditis)

Swelling over the spine: Relation to intergluteal cleft–above the cleft-spinal dysraphism, below the cleft-sacrococcygeal teratoma.

Skin dimple: Relation to intergluteal cleft—above the cleft—communicates with spinal cord/canal—dorsal dermal sinus. Below the cleft—does not communicate with spinal cord—pilonidal sinus. Small spinal lesions causing holocord syrinx—tuberculoma, dorsal dermal sinus, arachnoid cyst, haemangioblastoma.

4.50 SPINE

Case No. 50

Clinical history: This 59-year-old patient had visual disturbances of the left eye followed by weakness and sensory disturbances of the lower and upper extremities.

Radiological techniques and observations: Figures 4.50.1 and 4.50.2 are **MRI cervical spine sagittal sections** respectively revealing T2 weighted confluent intramedullary hyperintensity noted in spinal cord from C2–C5 level and D2–D4 levels with mild cord expansion. No evidence of any cystic or haemorrhagic components in the lesion—suggestive of **longitudinally extensive spinal cord demyelination (LETM)**. The visualised cervical vertebrae appear normal. No abnormal flow voids seen in epidural space. No evidence of herniation of cerebellar tonsils. No evidence of epidural collections.

Coronal section of MRI orbit in STIR sequence shows hyperintensity of intraorbital part of left optic nerve with mild enlargement. Mild thinning of right optic nerve noted. No evidence of any mass lesions noted in intraconal, conal and extraconal spaces of bilateral orbits. The visualised paranasal sinuses and brain parenchyma appears normal. Mild deviation of nasal septum to the right is seen.

Interpretation: A: 59 yrs old, cervical spinal cord, C: Multilevel spinal cord confluent intramedullary T2 hyperintensity with cord expansion and STIR hyperintensity of left intraorbital optic nerve. B: No evidence of any cystic or haemorrhagic components, D: Neuromyelitis optica.

Principal diagnosis: Neuromyelitis optica, however contrast study and biochemical studies are further needed to confirm the diagnosis.

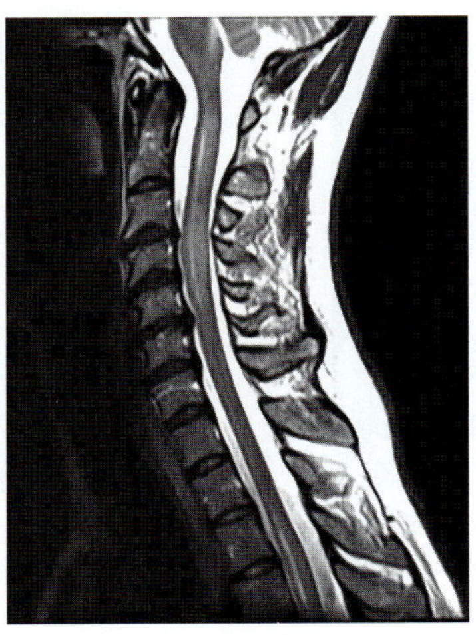

Fig. 4.50.1

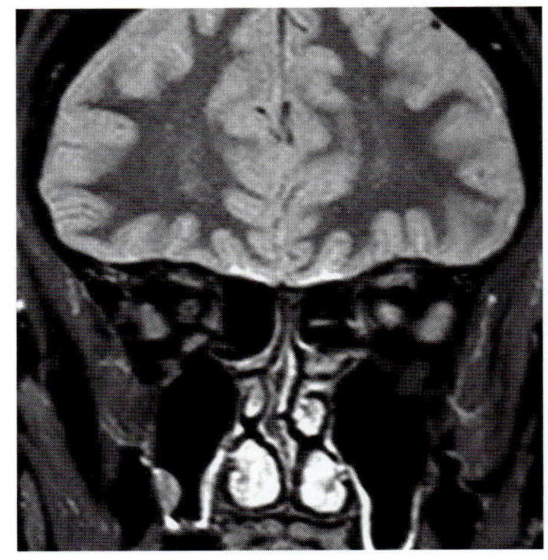

Fig. 4.50.2

Table 4.50.1: Differential diagnosis based on optic nerve findings

Condition	*Representation*	*T2 coronal MRI image*
Normal optic nerve—target sign positive	**Fig. 4.50.3:** Right—normal optic nerve	**Fig. 4.50.4:** Right—normal optic nerve
Optic neuritis—absent target sign	**Fig. 4.50.5:** Left—optic neuritis	**Fig. 4.50.6:** Left—optic neuritis

(Contd.)

Table 4.50.1: Differential diagnosis based on optic nerve findings (*Contd.*)

Condition	*Representation*	*T2 coronal MRI image*
Papilloedema—bulging of optic nerve head, cuff of CSF signal surrounding optic nerve.	**Fig. 4.50.7:** Papilloedema	**Fig. 4.50.8:** Papilloedema **Fig. 4.50.9:** Papilloedema

Table 4.50.2: Differential diagnosis based on spine imaging: (1) Multiple sclerosis, (2) transverse myelitis, (3) neuromyelitis optica, (4) ADEM

Multiple sclerosis Primary demyelinating diseases of central nervous system with multiple lesions disseminated over time and space. Peak onset: 20 to 40 years. • **Relapsing remitting** • **Secondary progressive** • **Primary progressive** • **Progressive relapsing** Oligoclonal immunoglobulin bands can be identified in CSF of MS patients with electrophoresis.	Less than half of cross sectional area of spinal cord. **Less than 2 vertebral segments in length.** Sagittal-oval, peripheral and asymmetrical patchy lesions. **Cervical** segment is most commonly involved. Concomittant intracranial lesions in periventricular, subcallosal or cerebellar white matter. The segment of optic nerve involvement is usually short, unilateral and confined to the optic disc and **anterior intraorbital segment of optic nerve.**	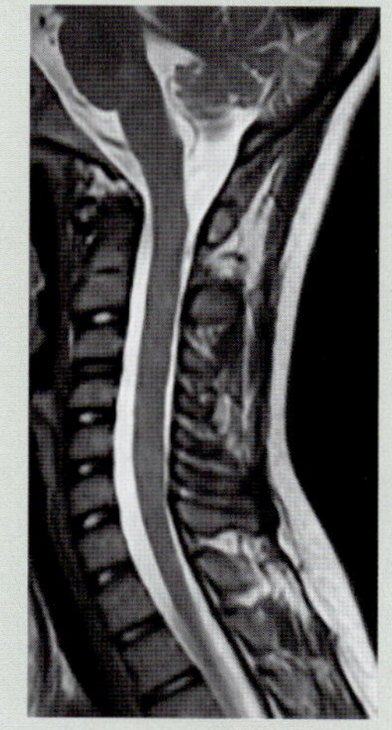 **Fig. 4.50.10:** Multiple sclerosis
Transverse myelitis Clinical features include weakness in arms and legs, sensory symptoms such as numbness and bladder and bowel symptoms. Focal inflammatory disorders of spinal cord resulting in motor, sensory and autonomic dysfunction. 1. Acute partial transverse myelitis (APTM)—lesion extending to less than 2 segments. 2. Acute complete transverse myelitis (ACTM)—lesion extending more than two segments.	Lesions are centrally located. 3 to 4 segments in length. **Involving more than two-thirds of cord cross sectional area.** Central dot sign of hyperintensity in axial MR sections may be seen. Very rarely, in up to 5% cases brain involvement can be seen. A person with TM who also has an abnormal brain MR with more than 2 lesions has an increased chance of developing MS 90%)	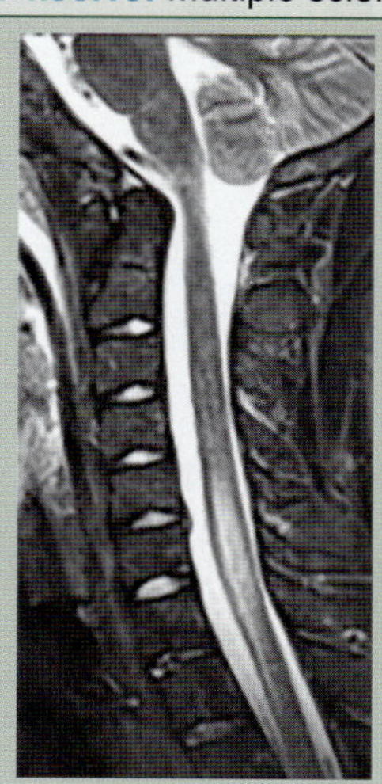 **Fig. 4.50.11:** Transverse myelitis

Table 4.50.3: Pattern of involvement in demyelination disorders

Posterior column	*Posterolateral/lateral column*	*Central cord*	*Anterior column*
• Multiple sclerosis • Vitamin B_{12} deficiency • HIV vacuolar myelopathy • HZV and CMV myelitis • Transverse myelitis • Tabes dorsalis • Tropical spastic paraparesis • Copper deficiency • Spinal dural AV fistula • Nitrous oxide (N_2O) toxicity/ abuse • Lyme disease 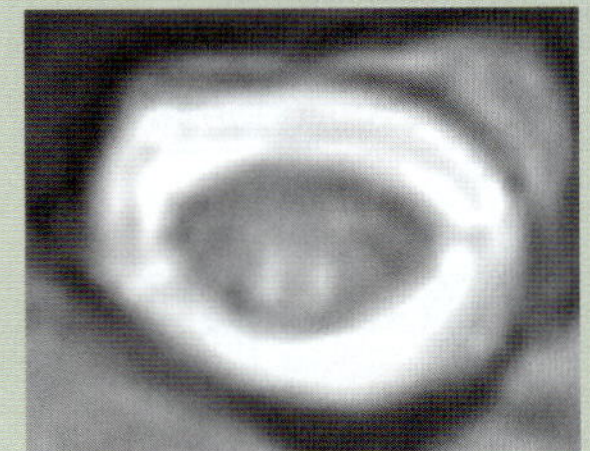 **Fig. 4.50.12:** Inverted V pattern in vitamin B_{12} deficiency 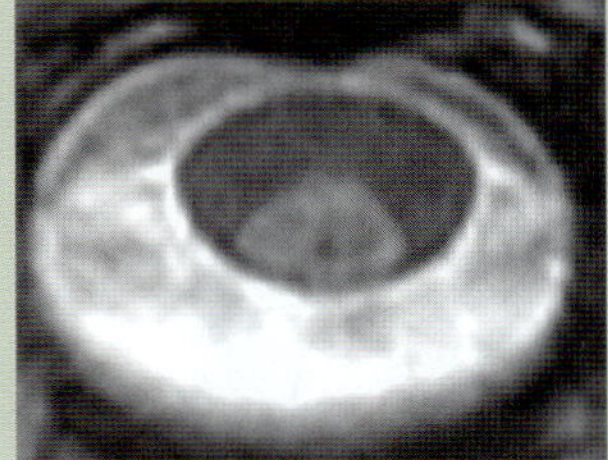 **Fig. 4.50.13:** Triangular involvement in ADEM 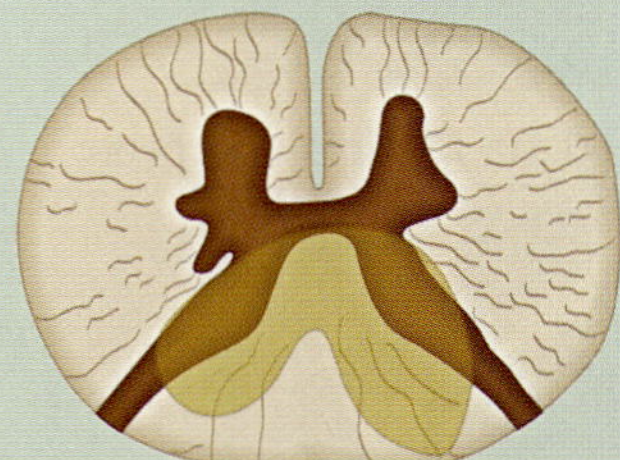 **Fig. 4.50.14:** Inverted V pattern 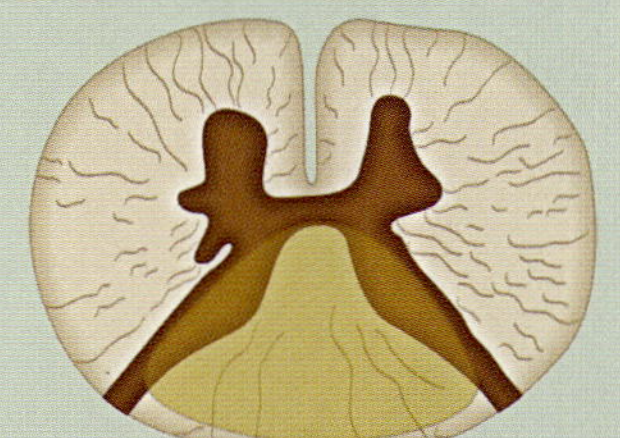 **Fig. 4.50.15:** Triangular involvement	• Multiple sclerosis • HZV and CMV myelitis • Transverse myelitis • Herpes myelitis • Paraneoplastic syndrome 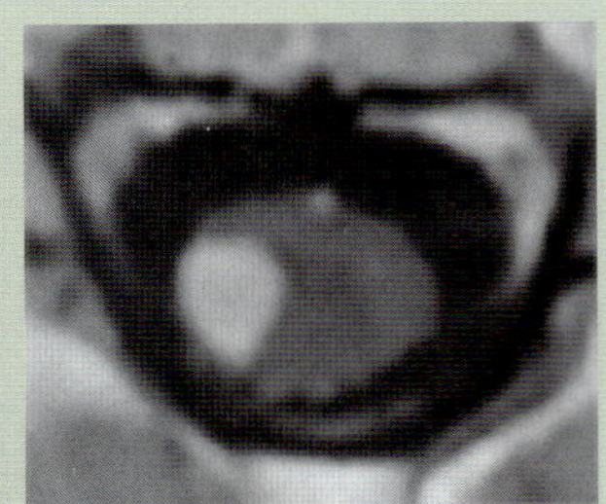 **Fig. 4.50.16:** Lateral column is affected 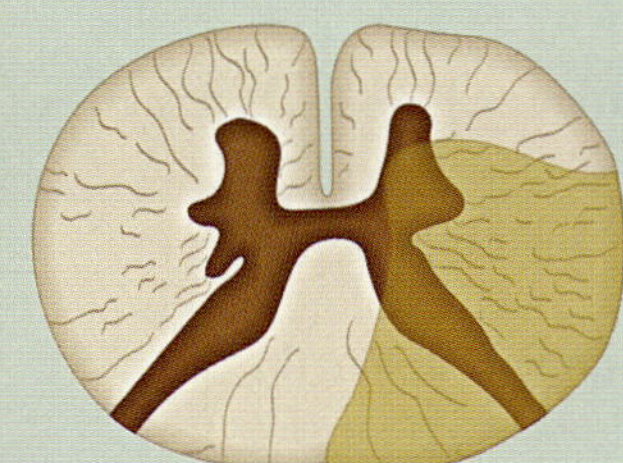 **Fig. 4.50.17:** Lateral column is affected	• Transverse myelitis • Acute disseminated encephalomyelitis • Multiple sclerosis • Devic optic neuromyelitis • Infectious disorders • Gougerot-Sjögren • Lupus • Coeliac disease • Toxic disorders • Radiation therapy • Spinal cord infarction • Syringomyelia 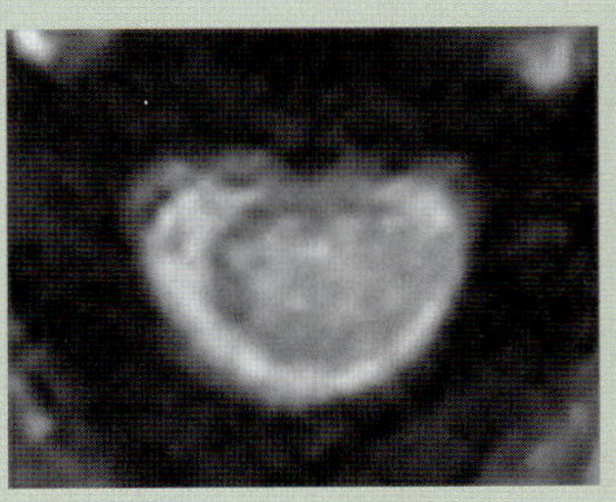 **Fig. 4.50.18:** Central cord is affected 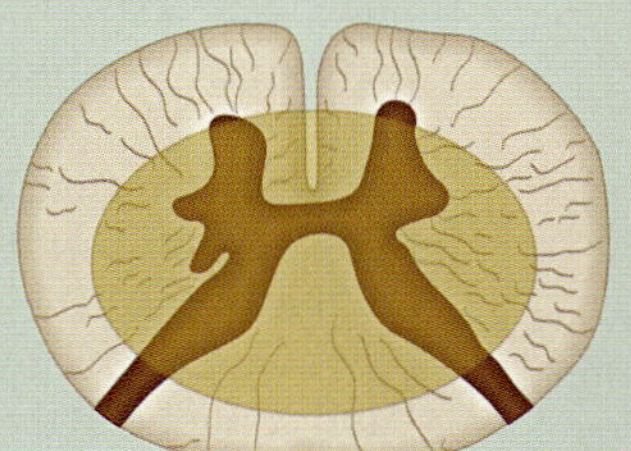 **Fig. 4.50.19:** Central cord is affected	• Spinal cord ischemia • Post-vaccination • Poliomyelitis • Neuromyelitis optica • Hirayama disease • Electric shock • Motor neuron disease 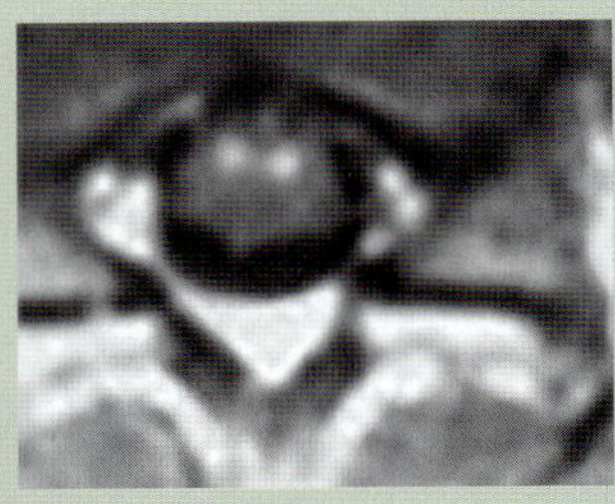 **Fig. 4.50.20:** Snake eye appearance in anterior horn cell disease 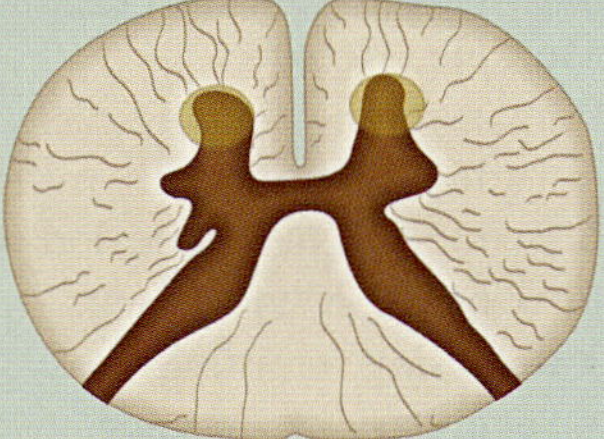 **Fig. 4.50.21:** Snake eye appearance 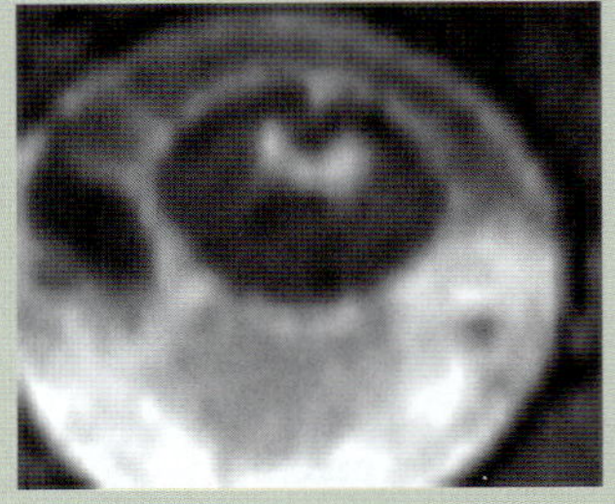 **Fig. 4.50.22:** Anterior U-shaped lesion in spinal cord ischemia 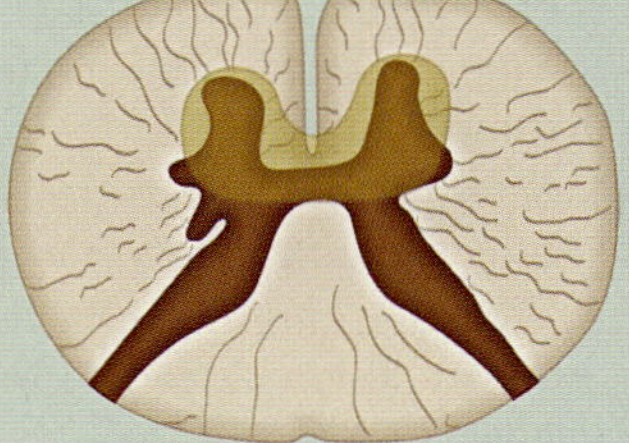 **Fig. 4.50.23:** U-shaped lesion

Causes of spinal cord demyelination:

- Demyelinating diseases
- Acute ischaemia
- Inflammatory vasculitis
- Infection

Approach to spinal cord hyperintensity:

1. **Short segment or long segment:** Short segment is less than 2 segments involvement and long segment is more than 2 segments involvement. MS is typically short segment. TM, NMO and ischaemia are long segment.
2. **How much cord is involved in transverse images:** Partial involvement is seen. In MS while involvement of both halves of cord is seen in TM and NMO.
3. **Location:** Anterior—spinal cord ischaemia (cobra head appearance or rabbit ear appearance), polio and motor neuron disease.
   Posterior—MS, vitamin B_{12} deficiency, HIV myelopathy, copper deficiency and nitrous oxide poisoning, carbon monoxide poisoning and HIV vaculopathy.
4. **Is the cord swollen:** TM and tumor—cord is swollen, MS and ADEM—cord is not swollen.
5. **Is there enhancement:** Many diseases may show enhancement, but astrocytoma has to be included in differentials.

Brief discussion about the condition: Neuromyelitis optica.

Idiopathic inflammatory demyelinating disorder of CNS characterised by severe attacks of optic neuritis and myelitis.

Clinical features: Hallmark clinical features of NMOSD include acute attacks of optic neuritis (leading to severe visual loss) and longitudinally extensive transverse myelitis (LETM) (often causing limb weakness, sensory loss, and bladder dysfunction) with a typically relapsing course. Attacks often evolve over days, with variable degrees of recovery over weeks to months. Age of onset is usually later than that of multiple sclerosis, around 39 years. Bright spotty lesions on axial T2W imaging with lentiform enhancement in contrast studies. **Core clinical features** of neuromyelitis optica involves optic neuritis, acute myelitis, area postrema syndrome (unexplained hiccups/nausea/vomiting), acute brainstem syndrome, symptomatic narcolepsy or diencephalic clinical syndrome (with NMOSD—typical diencephalic MR lesions), symptomatic cerebral syndrome (with NMSOD typical brain lesions). In NMO optic nerve involvement is typically bilateral, longitudinally extensive (>50% of the nerve) with involvement of optic chiasma and posterior optic nerve.There is often also enhancement of the optic nerve sheath.

Lesion follow the distribution of AQP 4, which is found in **periependymal region surrounding third ventricle, cerebral aqueduct and fourth ventricle.** Spinal cord atrophy in chronic phases.

Diagnostic pearls:

- No single clinical manifestation establishes a diagnosis of NMOSD.
- Beware of making the diagnosis exclusively based on serology—always need compatible symptoms/ MRI findings.

Etiopathogenesis: The discovery of a disease-specific serum **NMO—immunoglobulin G (IgG) antibody that selectively binds aquaporin-4 (AQP4)** has led to increased understanding of a diverse spectrum of disorders. Multiple sclerosis is mostly a cell-mediated disorder, whereas the pathophysiology of NMOSD is primarily mediated by the humoral immune system.In NMOSD, florid demyelination and inflammation involve multiple spinal cord segments and the optic nerves with associated axonal loss, perivascular lymphocytic infiltration, and vascular proliferation. Unlike multiple sclerosis, necrosis and cavitation typically involve both gray and white matter. The neuropathologic features of NMOSD at autopsy are those of a much more severe necrotic lesion of the cord rather than incomplete demyelination. NMOSD is frequently associated with systemic autoimmune disorders and some cases may be associated with neoplasms. NMOSD is usually sporadic, though a few familial cases have been reported. Pathologically, astrocytes are selectively targeted in NMOSD with a perivascular deposition of immunoglobulins, and complement activation. Myelin and neurons are relatively less damaged than astrocytes and hence NMOSD is pathologically an astrocytopathy. Antibodies to myelin oligodendrocyte protein **(MOGAD)** are more common in children

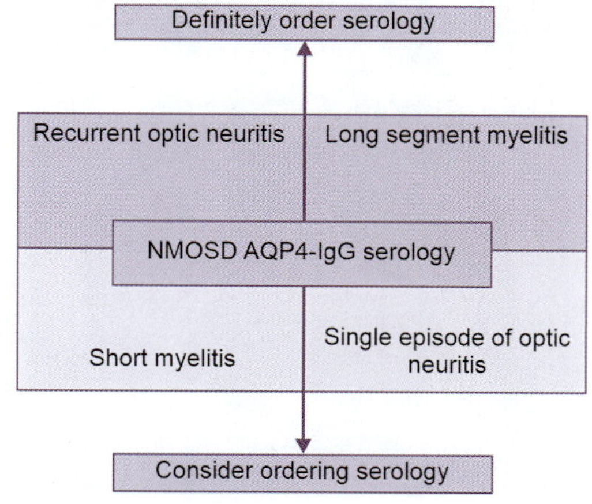

Fig. 4.50.24: IgG4 disease spectrum of spinal involvement

presenting with optic neuritis, with or without LETM and encephalitis like in ADEM. These children do not have aquaporin 4 antibodies.

Lab investigations and diagnostic criterion: Ideally, testing for AQP4 antibody status should be performed during attacks and before immunotherapy, since conversion to seronegative status may occur with immunotherapy.

Table 4.50.4: 2015 International panel of neuromyelitis optica diagnosis (IPND)

Aquaporin-4 positive	*Aquaporin4 negative/MOG+* (MOG—mylien oligodendrocyte glycoprotein)
1. Atleast one core clinical feature 2. Aquaporin4-IgG positivity 3. Exclusion of alternative diagnosis	1. Atleast 2 core clinical features occurring as a result of one or more clinical attacks and meeting all of the following requirements. a. Atleast one attack of optic neuritis/TM/area postrema syndrome. b. Dissemination in space c. Fulfilment of additional MRI requirements 2. Aquaporin4-IgG negativity 3. Exclusion of alternative diagnosis

Role of MRI in diagnosis of NMOSD: Confirming sites of disease involvement. Evaluating extent and sequelae of disease. Differentiating NMOSD from other alternative

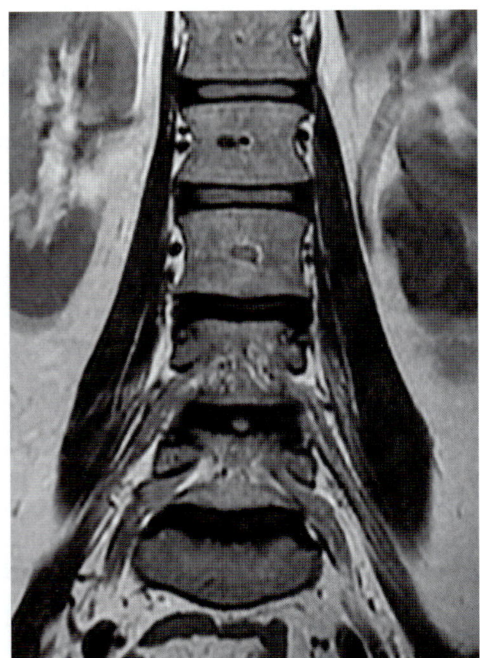

Fig. 4.50.25: CIDP

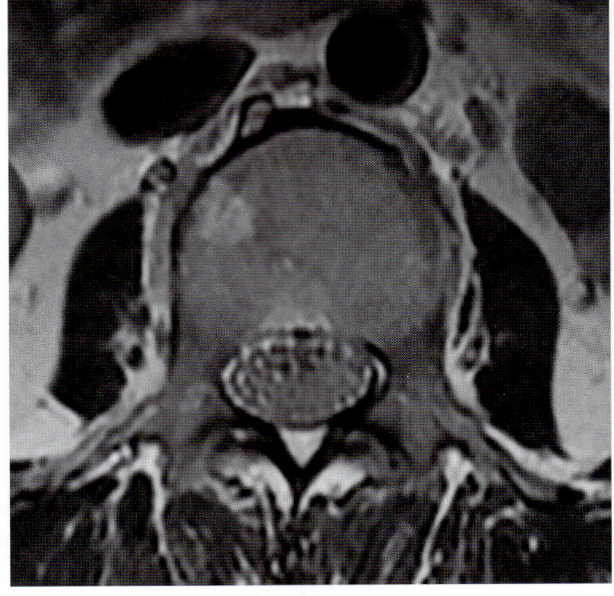

Fig. 4.50.26: CIDP

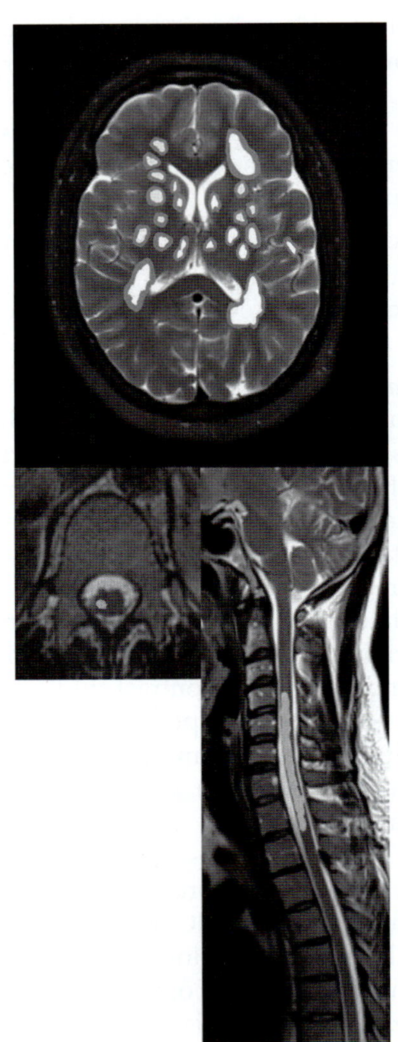

Fig. 4.50.27: Distribution of lesions in ADEM

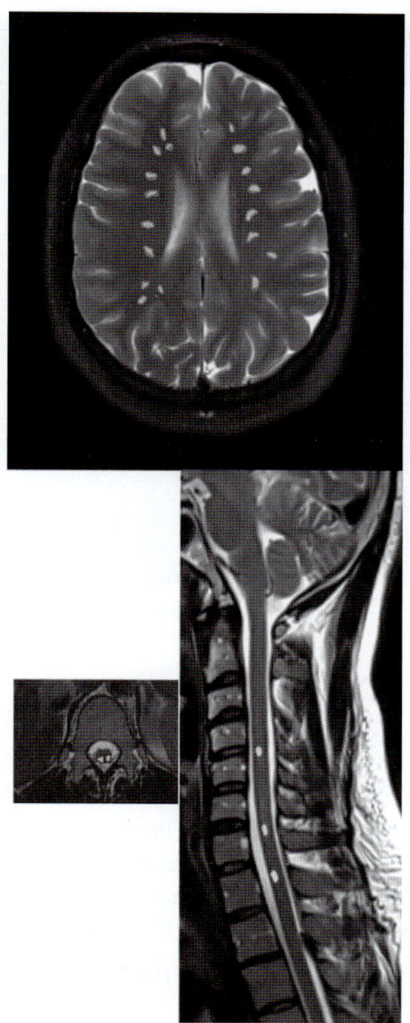

Fig. 4.50.28: Distributions of lesions in multiple sclerosis

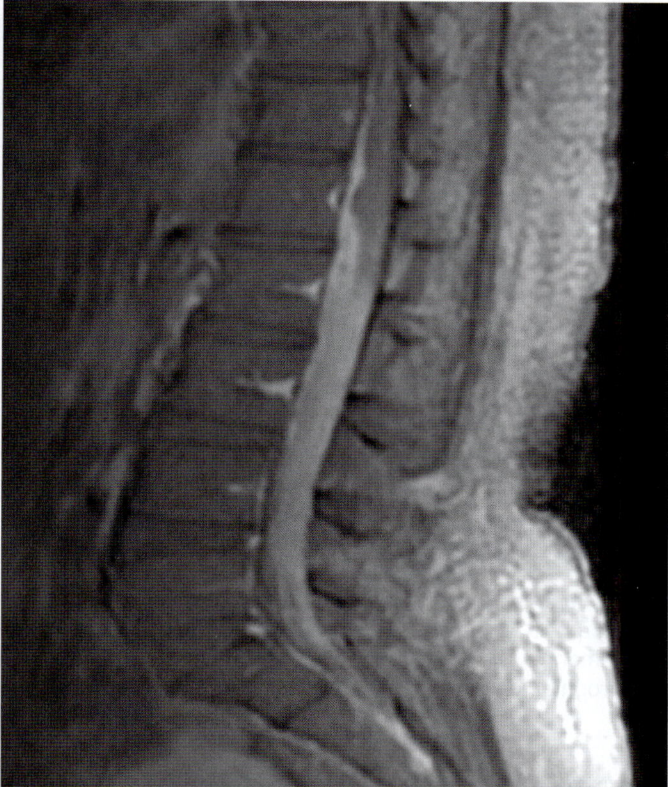

Fig. 4.50.29: CIDP

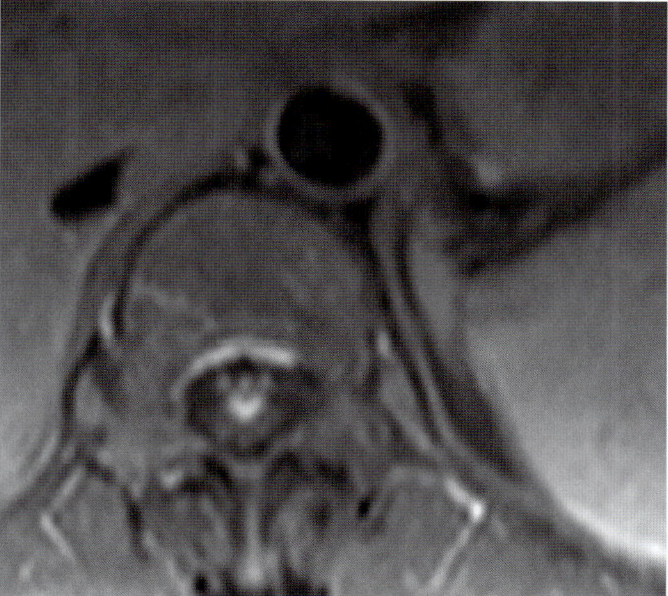

Fig. 4.50.30: Cauda equina nerve roots enhancement in GBS

diagnoses, particularly MS, ADEM and sarcoidosis. Acute callosal lesions with heterogeneous marbled appearance, arch bridge appearance with involvement of entire corpus callosum, cloud like/pencil thin enhancement pattern.

Treatment: It is important to differentiate NMO from multiple sclerosis early so that appropriate managemenmt could be started, if misdiagnosed, some drugs such as beta interferon can exacerbate the disease in NMO. Treatment of acute attacks includes high-dose methylprednisolone, plasma exchange, and IVIG, depending on the severity of the presentation and the response. Various drugs used for prevention of relapses in NMOSD are prednisone, azathioprine and rituximab (first line drugs), mycophenolate mofetil, eculizumab, satralizumab and inebilizumab.

Chronic inflammatory demyelinating polyneuropathy (CIDP): Refers to inflammation of nerve roots/ peripheral nerves characterised by mononuclear cell infiltrates and edema along with segmental demyelination and remyelination resulting in hypertrophic nerves with abnormal enhancement on MRI. Biopsy of the involved nerve along with nerve conduction studies confirms diagnosis.

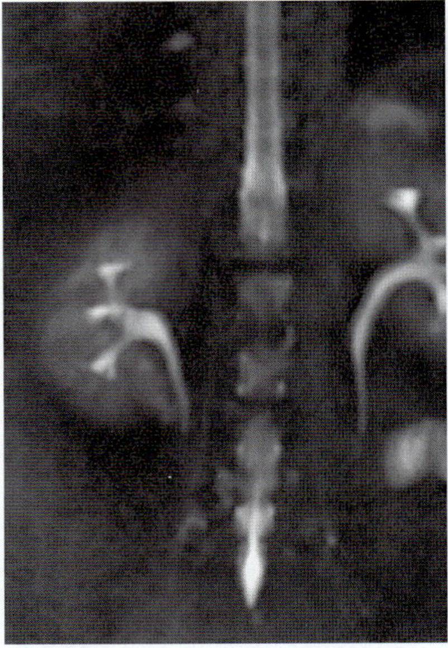

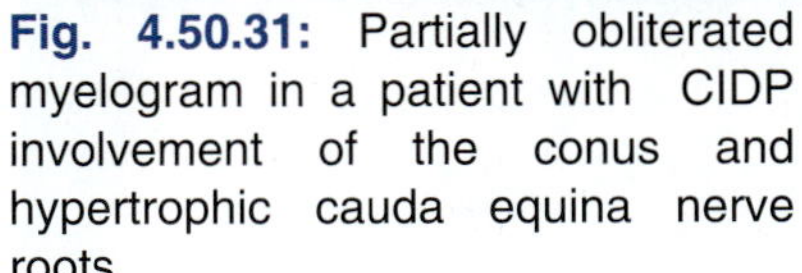

Fig. 4.50.31: Partially obliterated myelogram in a patient with CIDP involvement of the conus and hypertrophic cauda equina nerve roots

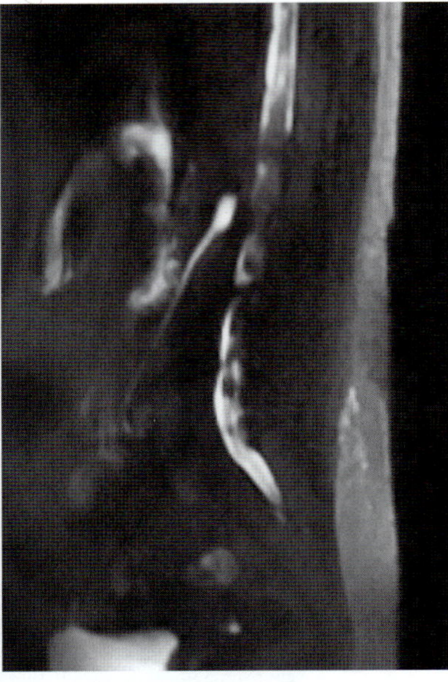

Fig. 4.50.32: Partially obliterated myelogram in a patient with CIDP involvement of the conus and hypertrophic cauda equina nerve roots

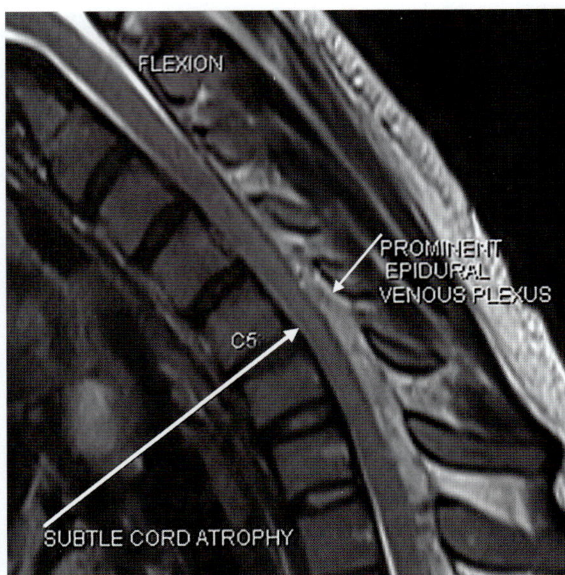

Fig. 4.50.33: Hirayama's disease

The spinal cord remains unremarkable. An 8-week temporal delineation although indicated to designate a CIDP versus AIDP, CIDP may sometimes present acutely and AIDP otherwise. Posterior column sensory signs (ataxia, vibratory or proprioceptive loss) or relapse/progression may favour CIDP, whereas autonomic involvement, facial weakness, preceding infection, and mechanical ventilation favour AIDP.

Rare new entity: **Glial fibrillary acid protein astrocytopathy**—caused by autoimmune attack in middle aged adults, with a slight female preponderance. There may be an association with ovarian teratoma and small cell lung cancer.

Presentation: Headache, delirium. Myelopathy, cerebellar ataxia, movement disorders. A flu-like prodrome is a common clinical feature.

MRI: Longitudinally extensive spinal cord involvement, T2/FLAIR confluent hyperintensities in the periventricular region extending into the brain stem. T1 C+–perivascular pattern of enhancement extending radially from the periventricular surface. **MARKER—anti-GFAP antibody, coexisting NMDA-r Abs and AQP-4 Abs may be present.**

Causes for hypertrophic neuropathy:

- AIDP
- CIDP
- Plexiform neurofibromatosis
- Leprosy
- Charcot-Marie-Tooth disease.

Causes for spinal cord thinning:

- Compressive myelomalacia—due to tumors, subdural/epidural collections
- Syringomyelia/hydromyelia/spinal cord cysts
- Hirayama's disease
- Post-operative myelomalacia
- Hereditary spastic paraparesis.

4.51 SPINE

Case No. 51

Clinical history: 20-year-old male patient with complaints of few days of paraparesis.

Radiologic technique and observation: Figures 4.51.1 to 4.51.4 are T2W sagittal and axial, T1W axial and sagittal images respectively.

Increased T2 signal and expansion of the cord is seen extending between C7 and T12. The T2 signal abnormality involves central grey matter and dorsal columns. No evidence of fluid signal intensity. The lesion is isointense on T1. No evidence of hemorrhage. The abnormality involves the intramedullary cord with no abnormality of the extra dural space. No flow-voids or vascular anomalies are noted. No blood products are present within or outside the cord. No syrinx.

Interpretation: A: 20 years old, cervical and dorsal spinal cord, B: Long segment T2 increased signal involving central grey matter and dorsal columns in cervicothoracic spinal cord with cord expansion. C: No evidence of fluid signal intensity/hemorrhage/flow voids/syrinx, D: Acute transverse myelitis.

Principal diagnosis: Acute transverse myelitis.

Differential diagnosis: Longitudinally extensive transverse myelitis (LETM).

Discussion

Acute transverse myelitis (ATM) is an inflammatory disorder affecting both halves of the spinal cord and associated with rapidly progressive motor, sensory, and autonomic dysfunction.

It affects individuals of all ages with peaks at ages 10–19 years and 30–39 years with no sex or familial predisposition and usually no prior history of neurologic abnormality.

The clinical course is highly variable but typically evolves over hours or days. Symptoms and signs are bilateral and include para- or tetraparesis, sensory impairment level with band-like dysesthesia at lesion level and sphincter dysfunction preceded by viral-like illness or prodrome of generalized body aches.

Typically monophasic. If recurrent, must consider MS, SLE, antiphospholipid syndrome, vascular malformation.

One-third of patients experience good to complete recovery Children have slightly better prognosis than adults.

One-third of patients experience fair recovery with residual spasticity and urinary dysfunction.

One-third of patients experience poor recovery with persistent complete deficits and assistance required in activities of daily living.

At least 13% of patients who fulfill the criteria for definite and possible idiopathic ATM will convert to multiple sclerosis.

Etiology

- Idiopathic ATM
- Acute infection (most commonly viral)
- Post-vaccination
- Autoimmune (SLE, MS)
- Systemic malignancy (paraneoplastic—most common small cell lung carcinoma)

Imaging: Up to 40% of cases have no findings on MRI

Further management: Treatment is with high-dose intravenous steroid pulse therapy and physical therapy.

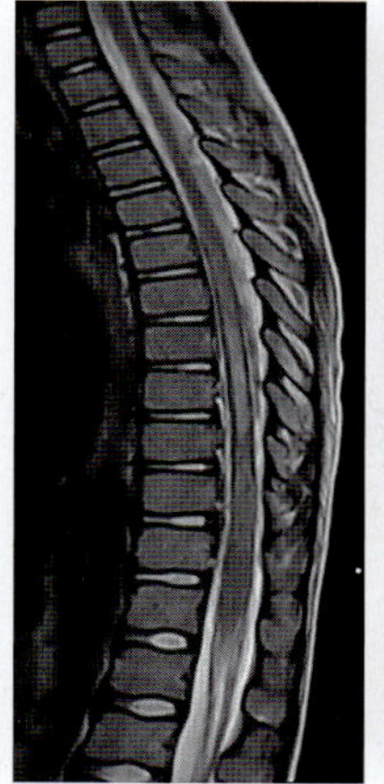

Fig. 4.51.1

Fig. 4.51.2

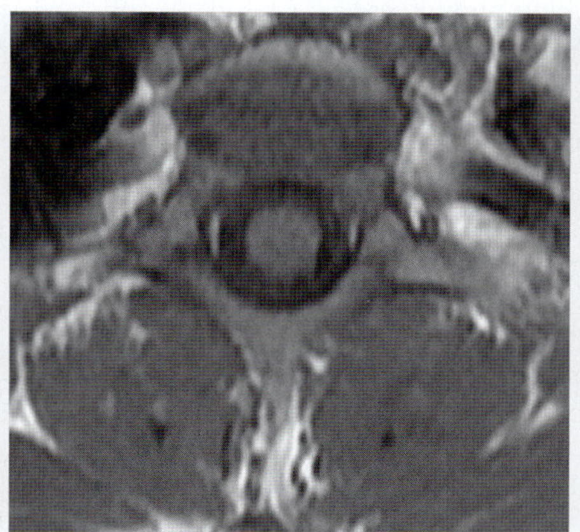

Fig. 4.51.3

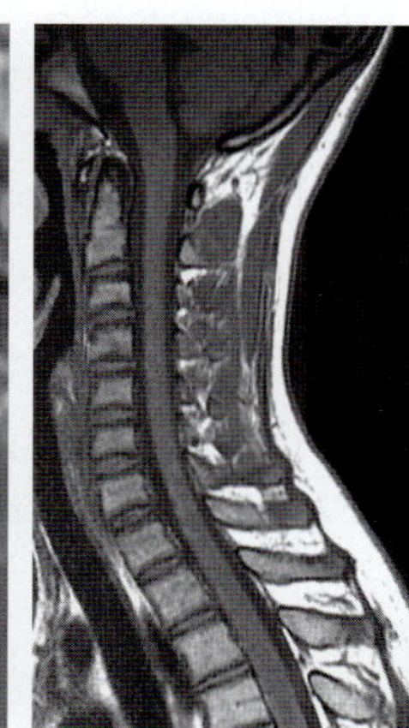

Fig. 4.51.4

Table 4.51.1: Differential diagnosis for demyelination disorders of spinal cord

Multiple sclerosis Characteristically, and by definition, multiple sclerosis is disseminated not only in space (i.e. multiple lesions in different regions of the brain) but also in time (i.e. lesions occur at different times). Peak onset—20 to 40 years. *Types* Relapsing remitting Secondary progressive Primary progressive Progressive relapsing Oligoclonal immunoglobulin bands can be identified in CSF of MS patients with electrophoresis.	• <2 vertebral segments in length • Peripheral location • <1/2 of cord cross-sectional area • 90% have associated intracranial lesions • Relapsing and remitting clinical course • Typical for MS is involvement of corpus callosum, U-fibers, temporal lobes, brainstem, cerebellum and spinal cord. • Juxtacortical lesions and temporal lobe involvement are specific 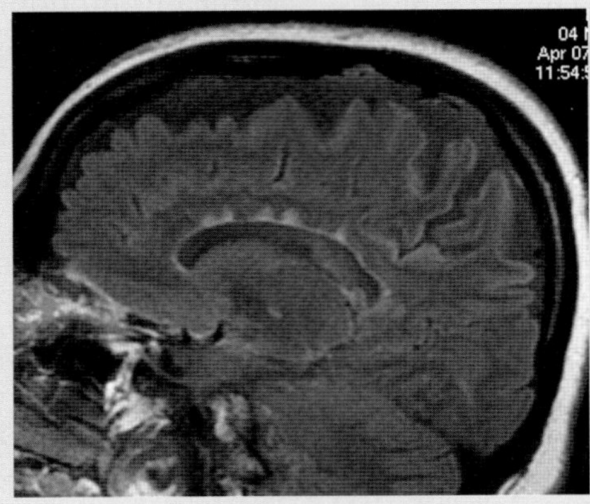 **Fig. 4.51.5:** Dawson fingers and callososeptal interface involvement	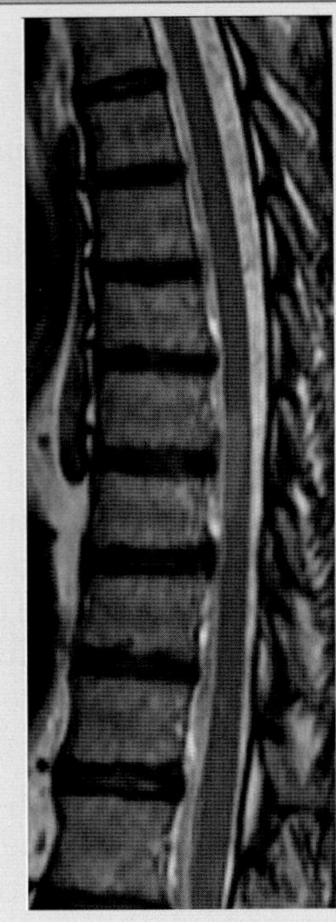 **Fig. 4.51.6:** Short segment T2 hyperintensity on sagittal image in multiple sclerosis
Neuromyelitis Optica **Devic's disease** 1. Pediatric-onset NMO: Pediatric-onset NMO is classified as onset of first NMO symptoms before 18 years of age. It represents 3–5% of all NMO cases, and the first clinical events are usually optic neuritis (50–75%) or longitudinally extensive transverse myelitis (LETM) (30–50%) 2. Late-onset NMOSD: Late-onset NMO is usually characterized by clinical onset after 50 years of age. A higher rate of myelitis and lower frequency of optic nerve and brain involvement	• Autoimmune inflammatory disorder involving neuronal myelin of optic nerves and spinal cord • Extensive (>3 vertebral segments) cord T2 hyperintensity + optic nerve enhancement • Cord swelling is usually present in the acute phase. • Limited brain involvement	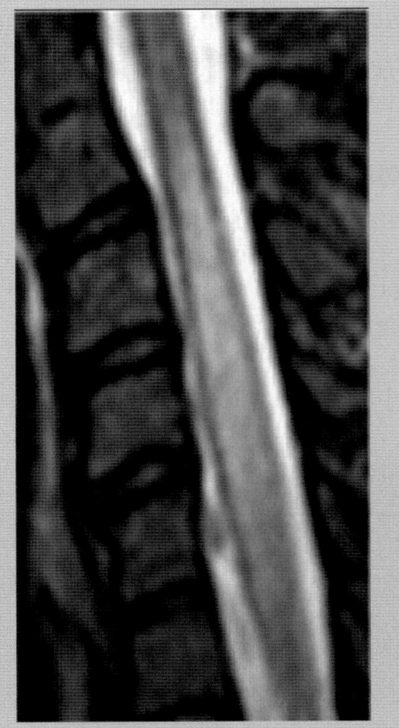 **Fig. 4.51.7:** NMO

(Contd...)

Table 4.51.1: Differential diagnosis for demyelination disorders of spinal cord *(Contd...)*

Transverse myelitis: Clinical features include weakness in arms and legs, sensory symptoms such as numbness and bladder and bowel symptoms. Focal inflammatory disorders of spinal cord resulting in motor, sensory and autonomic dysfunction. 1. Acute partial transverse myelitis (APTM)—lesion tending less than 2 segments. 2. Acute complete transverse myelitis (ACTM)—lesion extending more than two segments.	Lesions are centrally located. 3 to 4 segments in length. Involving more than two-thirds of cord cross sectional area with cord swelling. Very rarely in up to five percent cases brain involvement can be seen. A person with TM who also has an abnormal brain MR with more than 2 lesions has an increased chance of going to develop MS (90%)	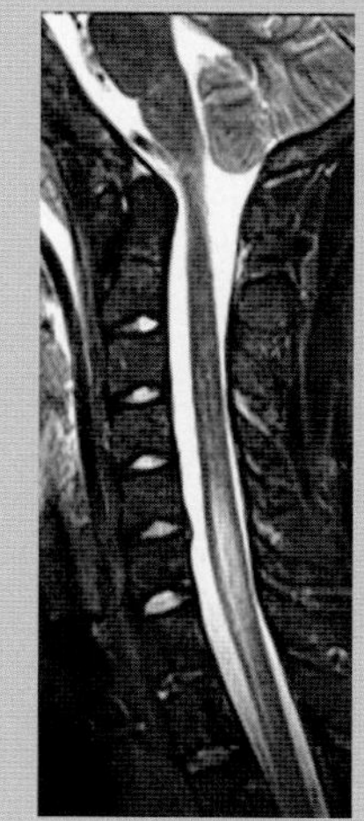 **Fig. 4.51.8:** Transverse myelitis
Spinal cord neoplasm • Cord expansion and extensive peritumoral edema invariably present • Cystic ± hemorrhage components • Diffuse or nodular contrast enhancement • Slower clinical progression	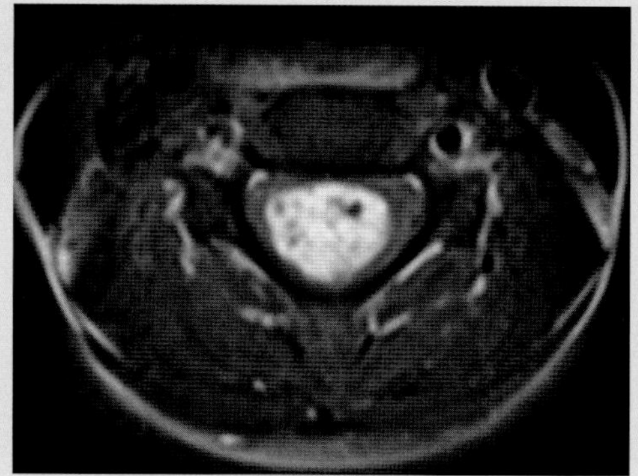 **Fig. 4.51.9:** Ependymoma	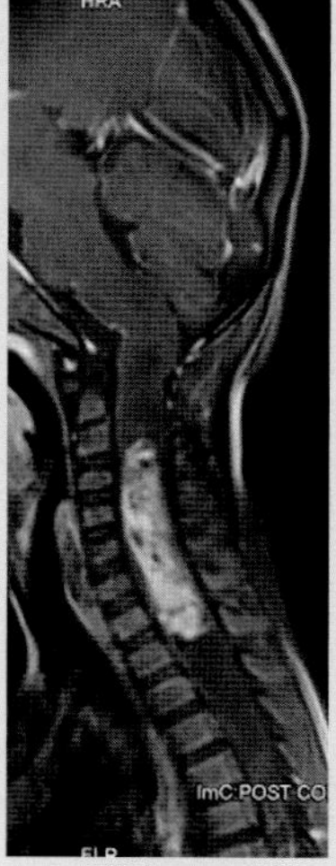 **Fig. 4.51.10:** Ependymoma
Spinal cord infarction • Ventral or central cord location, less mass effect initially • Patients present more often with motor signs than sensory signs • Immediate onset (minutes, rather than hours, days)	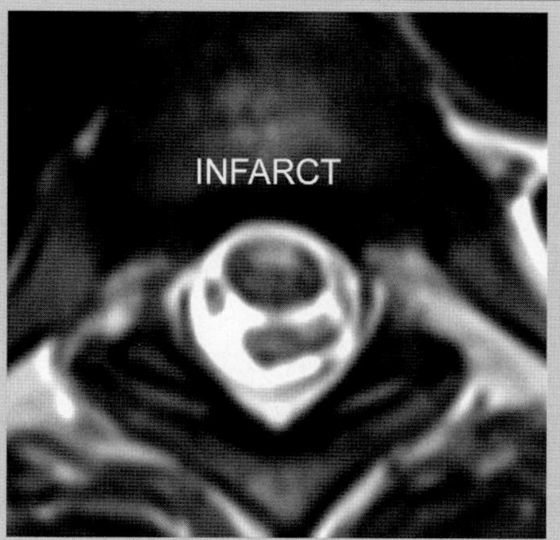 **Fig. 4.51.11:** "Snake eye" appearance on axial T2WI	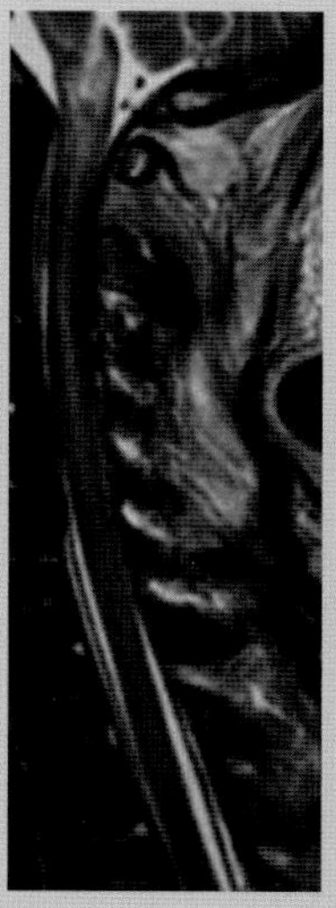 **Fig. 4.51.12:** Long segment T2 hyperintensity on sagittal image

Contd...

Table 4.51.1: Differential diagnosis for demyelination disorders of spinal cord *(Contd...)*		
B_{12} deficiency	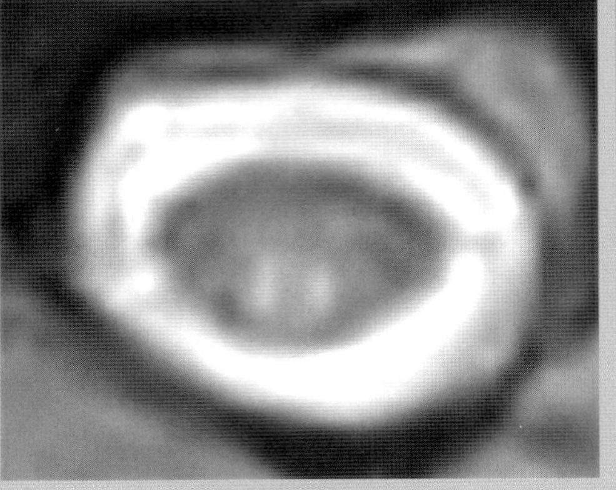 **Fig. 4.51.13:** Inverted V sign	
Spinal dural fistula SDAVFs cause symptoms through venous hypertension and congestion of the cord with edema. The most common clinical presentations are progressive pain, lower extremity weakness or sensory changes. Sphincter dysfunction may also occur.	• T2-diffuse multilevel intramedullary hyperintensity (edema)—most sensitive finding • Prominent flow voids (dilated veins) on cord surface • Lower dorsal cord 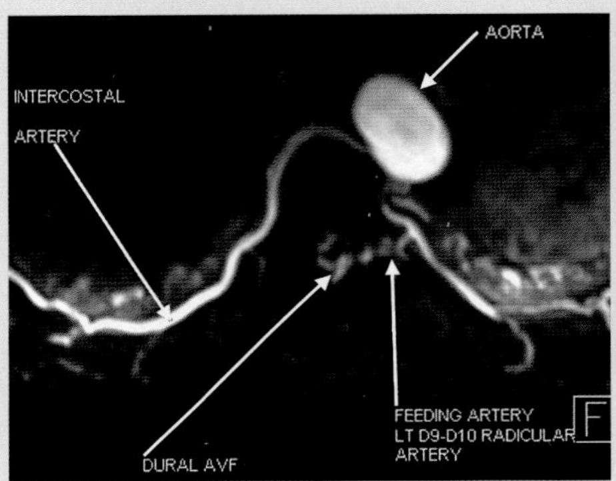 **Fig. 4.51.14:** Spinal dural fistula 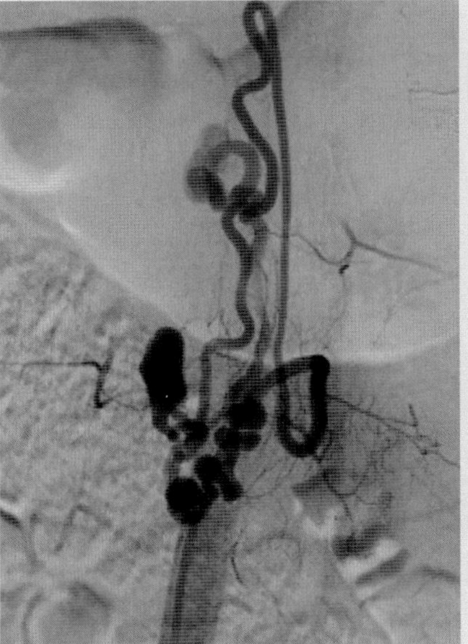 **Fig. 4.51.15:** Spinal dural fistula	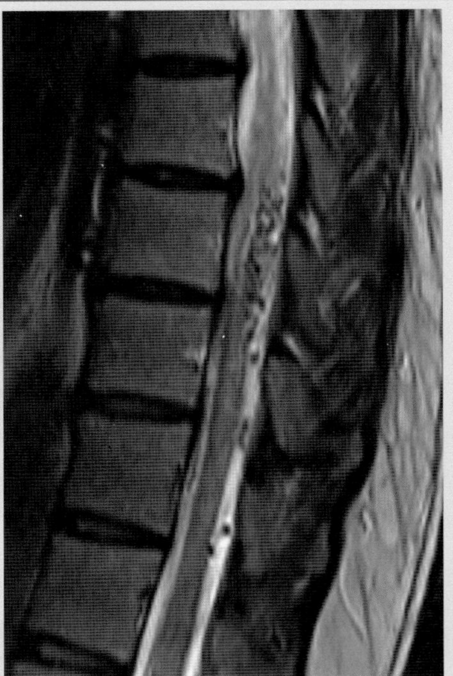 **Fig. 4.51.16:** Spinal dural fistula

Contd...

Table 4.51.1: Differential diagnosis for demyelination disorders of spinal cord *(Contd...)*		
ADEM (Acute disseminated encephalomyelitis) Slight male predominance Variants: Recurrent ADEM Hemorrhagic ADEM	Monophasic acute inflammation followed by demyelination of white matter typically following a recent (1–2 weeks prior) viral infection or vaccination. Grey matter of the basal ganglia and the spinal cord, are also often involved but to a lesser extent. Spinal cord may show confluent intramedullary lesions with variable enhancement, but these are only seen in approximately one-third of cases	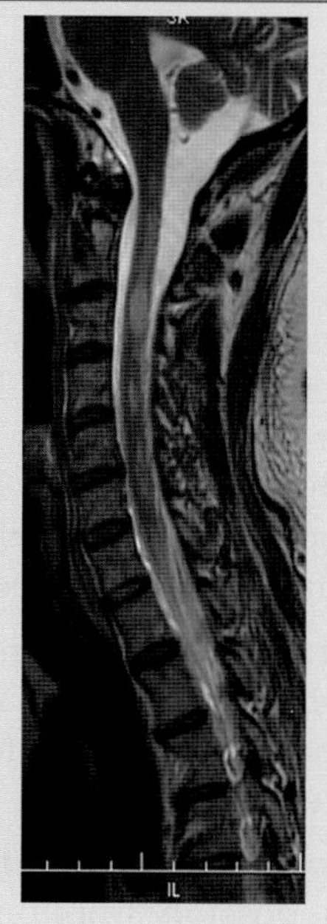 **Fig. 4.51.17:** ADEM

Table 4.51.2: Imaging features of transverse myelitis	
General	Well-circumscribed central cord lesion >2 vertebral segments in length and >2/3 of cross-sectional area of cord on axial imaging with eccentric enhancement. Thoracic cord most common
T1WI	Smooth cord expansion in acute phase; cord atrophy in late stage Iso- to hypointense
T2WI	Hyperintense cord expansion Central "dot" sign—central gray matter surrounded by edema
STIR	Hyperintense cord expansion
DWI	Significantly ↓ fractional anisotropy (FA) in lesions and distal (normal-appearing) spinal cord
T1WI C+	Variable enhancement—solitary or multifocal, focal, nodular, subtle, or patchy peripheral lesion enhancement No enhancement in up to 40–50% cases

Table 4.51.3: Criteria for acute transverse myelitis—transverse myelitis consortium working group: 2002	
Inclusion criteria	*Exclusion criteria*
Sensory, motor, or autonomic dysfunction attributable to the spinal cord Bilateral signs and/or symptoms (though not necessarily symmetric) Clearly defined sensory level Exclusion of extra-axial compressive cause by neuroimaging (MRI or myelography; CT is not adequate) Inflammation within the spinal cord demonstrated by CSF pleocytosis or elevated IgG index or gadolinium enhancement Progression to nadir between 4 hours and 21 days following the onset of symptoms	Radiation to the spine within the last 10 years Arterial distribution clinical deficit consistent with thrombosis of the anterior spinal artery Abnormal flow voids on the surface of the spinal cord indicating a dural AVF **Exclusion criteria for idiopathic ATM** Connective tissue disease CNS infection Brain MRI abnormalities suggestive of MS Optic neuritis

4.52 SPINE

Case No. 52

Clinical history: A 80 years old male, history of back pain for 1 month.

Radiological techniques and observation: Figure 4.52.1 is AP lumbar spine radiograph showing a uniformly increased opacity of entire L4 vertebra. The vertebral body shows no alteration in size and contour. This finding represents ivory vertebra, due to osteoblastic bone metastasis. There is an increased opacity of left sacroiliac joint territory and slightly sclerotic left sacral ala is noted.

Interpretation: **A: 80 years old, L4 vertebral body,** C: Uniform increased opacity of vertebrae, B: The vertebral body shows no alteration in size and contour, D: **Ivory vertebral body.**

Diagnosis: **Ivory vertebral body** due to osteoblastic metastasis, possibly from prostate cancer.

Further evaluation: 1. CECT abdomen and USG abdomen used to detect the primary tumor and to assess the spread into nearby lymph nodes and for follow-up after treatment, 2. Prostate-specific antigen blood test is used to screen for prostate cancer, if the PSA is more than 10 ng/ml, the chance of having prostate cancer is over 50%, 3. Digital rectal examination, 4. Prostate biopsy—core needle biopsy is the main method used to diagnosis prostate cancer, 5. MRI/ultrasound fusion-guided prostate biopsy: Here, MRI is done before biopsy to look for abnormal areas in the prostate. During the biopsy, TRUS helps to view prostate. A postprocessing software is used to fuse the MRI and TRUS image on a computer screen. This can help to ensure the doctor gets biopsy samples from any suspicious areas seen on the image, 6. Bone scan helps to detect the spreads to distant parts of the body, 7. Lymph node biopsy/dissection.

Fig. 4.52.1

Discussion: Ivory vertebra defined as homogeneous diffuse increase in opacity of a vertebral body without change in the size and adjacent intervertebral disc size.

The 5-year survival for CA prostate patients in case of metastasis decreases from 100 to 28%. Bone metastases are frequently seen in axial and proximal appendicular skeleton. Higher incidence of metastasis found in lumbar

Table 4.52.1: Causes of ivory vertebrae

Paediatric	*Adult*
Lymphoma: Hodgkin's	Osteoblastic metastases: Prostate cancer, breast cancer
Osteosarcoma	Lymphoma (patchy–generalized–ivory vertebra) may be associated with invading soft tissue mass
Osteoblastoma	Tuberculous spondylitis, osteomyelitis (rarely found in single vertebral body, associated erosive changes at disk margins)
Blastic metastatic disease, neuroblastoma, medullo-blastoma, Ewing's sarcoma	Haemangioma, SAPHO syndrome, sarcoidosis
	Paget's disease of bone: Vertebral body expansion and coarsened trabeculae, picture frame appearance with a relatively lucent centre

Table 4.52.2: Difference between blastic metastasis, Paget's disease and Hodgkin's lymphoma

Features	*Blastic metastases*	*Paget's*	*Hodgkin's lymphoma*
Age	>45	>50	20-40
Density	+++	+++	+++
Expansion	–	+++	–
Scalloping	–	–	+++

(Contd.)

Table 4.52.2: Difference between blastic metastasis, Paget's disease and Hodgkin's lymphoma (*Contd.*)

Features	*Blastic metastases*	*Paget's*	*Hodgkin's lymphoma*
Acid phosphatase	+++ (when arising from a primary prostate carcinoma)	–	–
Alkaline phosphatase	++	+++	++
Vertebrae	Unaltered	Picture frame	
		Also known as osteitis deformans. Hypermetabolic bone disease that affects one or more bones.Typically affects the skull, spine, pelvis and long bones. Thickening and homogenous hyperdensity of trabecular bone and bone expansion seen.	Para-aortic lymph node involvement results in formation of paraspinal masses may cause erosions of anterior and lateral margins of the vertebral body cortex. Increase in trabecular size and density.

spine as compared to cervical spine. Vertebral metastasis occurs in prostate cancer via Batson venous plexus which is a valveless network of deep pelvic veins which connect to internal vertebral venous plexus. Radionuclide bone scanning is most widely used imaging modality for diagnosis of osseous metastasis.

Management: Main aim of treatment for bone metastasis is to help to relieve the pain and prevent complication. Treatment options include: 1. Bisphosphonates—zoledronic acid, 2. Denosumab—monoclonal antibody, 3. External radiation therapy, 4. Radiopharmaceuticals—strontium-89, samarium-153 and radium—223,

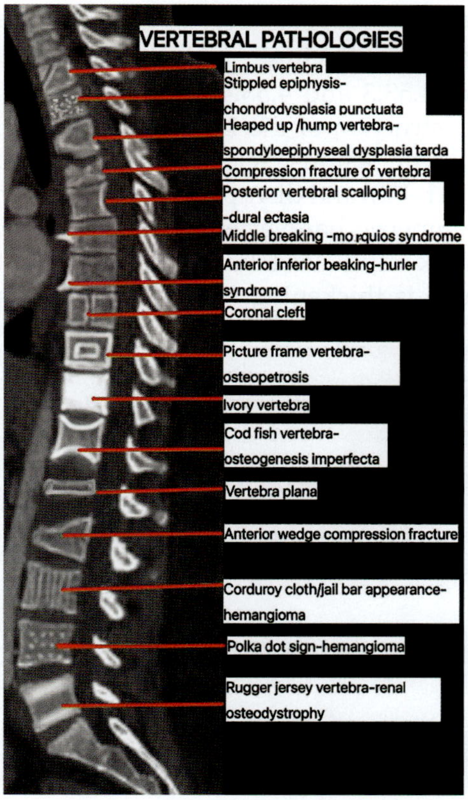

Fig. 4.52.2: Spectrum of findings in vertebral body pathologies

5. Kyphoplasty: It is a minor surgery to stabilise a painful collapsed bone in a spine weakened by a prostate cancer. A small incision done at midback during the treatment to insert balloon into the weak spinal bone. To stabilise the bone and spine, the balloon is first filled with air and then with a cement-like substance.

Diffuse sclerotic lesion	*Focal sclerotic lesion*
Familial Osteopoikilosis, osteopathia striata, osteopetrosis, pyknodysostosis, melorheostosis, multiple osteoma, multiple epiphyseal dysplasia	**Infection/inflammation** Osteoid osteoma. chronic/healed osteomyelitis, sclerosing osteomyelitis of Garre's, granuloma and Brodie abscess
Systemic disease Mastocytosis, fluorosis, bone infarcts and tuberous sclerosis	**Benign tumour** Osteoma, osteoblastoma, ossifying fibroma, healed fibrous cortical defect.
Metastasis, lymphoma, healed or healing malignant bone lesions, multiple osteosarcoma	**Malignant tumour** Osteoblastic metastasis—breast and prostate, lymphoma and Ewing sarcoma **Others** Sclerotic phase of Paget's disease, fibrous dysplasia, bone island and old bony infarct

Cause of a solitary dense pedicle of the vertebra:

- Osteoid osteoma
- Osteoblastoma (lucent nidus larger than 2 cm—presents as a lucency with a sclerotic margin)
- Congenitally absent/hypoplastic contralateral posterior elements
- Other sclerotic bone lesions—Paget's disease, fibrous dysplasia, sarcoidosis, tuberous sclerosis
- Secondary to unilateral spondylolysis—stress-induced sclerosis of contralateral pedicle
- Bone island
- Osteoblastic metastases to pedicle.

4.53 SPINE

Case No. 53

Clinical history: 40 years old male with history of chronic back pain and difficulty in moving the right lower limb with low grade fever for 5 months.

Radiological techniques and observation: Figures 4.53.1 and 4.53.2 are plain radiographs in AP and lateral view respectively showing a compression fracture of L1 vertebral body with marked inferior end plate irregularity and sclerotic changes, along with anterior deformity (Gibbus). Superior end plate irregularity with sclerotic changes and reduction in height of L2 vertebral body. Interspinous distance altered, with widening of interpedicular distance. Mild anterior wedge compression noted in D12 vertebra. There is obliteration of the disc space. Pre- and para-vertebral soft tissue opacities are also noted with obliteration of psoas shadow, extending inferiorly up to L4 level. The inferior most extent of prevertebral soft tissue forms a ill-defined radio-opacity, possibly a prevertebral collection. Posterior elements appear normal. Other bones appear normal.

What to see in spinal X-ray?

1. Vertebral body height
2. Interpedicular distance (widened in collapse vertebrae–burst fracture)
3. Spinous process alignment
4. Inter-spinous distance
5. Disc space
6. Cortical outline of vertebral body.

Causes for solitary collapse of the vertebral body are:

1. Neoplastic disease: Plasmacytoma, lymphoma and metastasis
2. Osteoporosis
3. Trauma
4. Infection
5. Langerhans cell histiocytosis
6. Benign bone tumors, e.g. haemangioma, giant cell tumor and aneurysmal bone cyst.
7. Paget's disease: Sclerosis and expansion seen.

Causes for deviation of thoracic para-spinal line:

1. Right-sided aortic arch
2. Systemic hypertension
3. Para-aortic/mediastinal lymph adenopathy
4. Para-vertebral abscess/granuloma
5. Metastasis

Causes for widened interpedicular distance:

- Spinal dysraphism: Myelomeningocele, lipomyelo-meningocele
- Intraspinal mass
- Diastematomyelia: Split cord malformations
- Trauma: Burst fracture

Figures 4.53.3 and 4.53.4 are CT in bone window reveals destruction of the L1 vertebral body showing irregular lytic lesions, sclerosis, inter-vertebral disc collapse (L1–L2), and disruption of bone circumference with asymmetric paravertebral and prevertebral soft tissue thickening. Vertebral body fragmentation is seen. There is thickening of right psoas muscle with

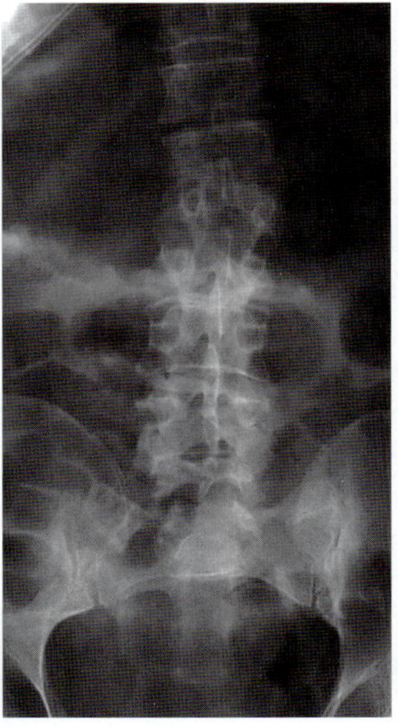

Fig. 4.53.1

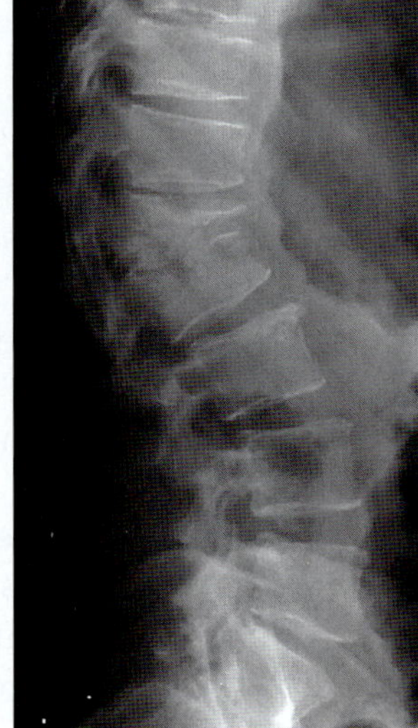

Fig. 4.53.2

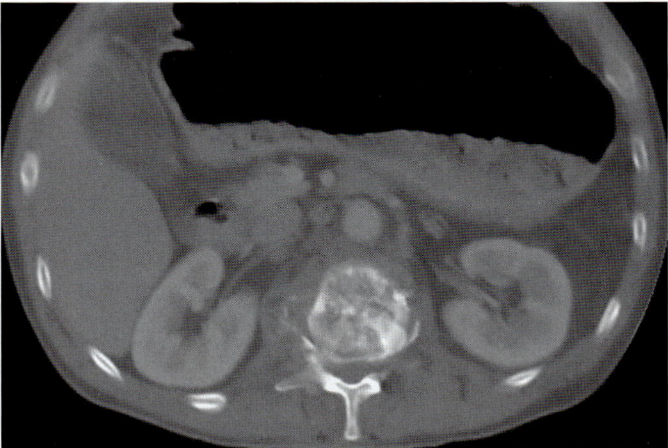

Fig. 4.53.3

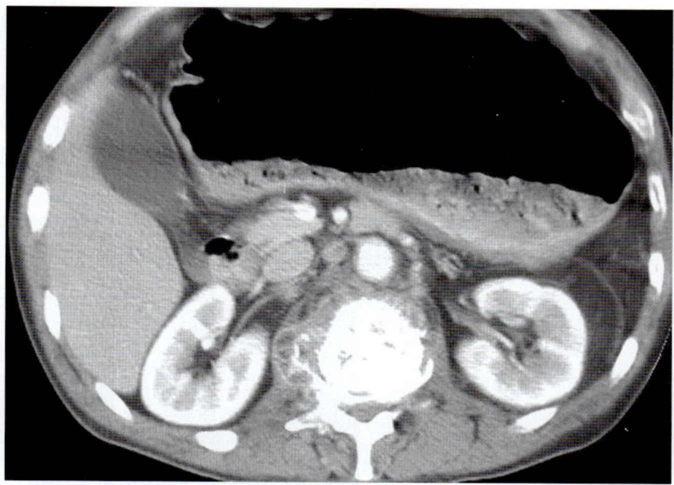

Fig. 4.53.4

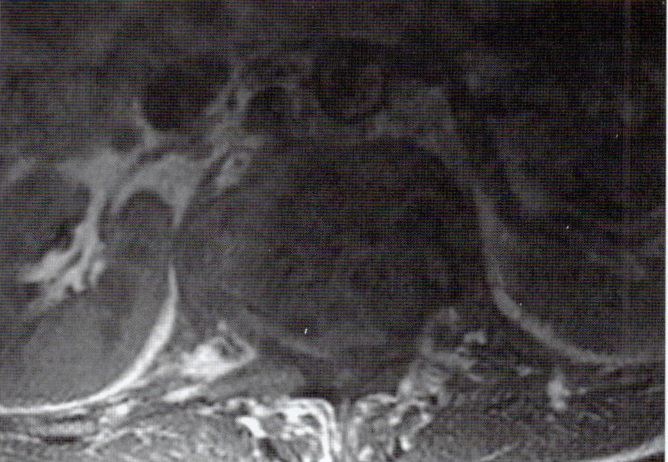

Fig. 4.53.6

calcification seen. In post-contrast CT there is peripheral enhancement of the para-vertebral soft tissue seen.

Figures 4.53.5 to 4.53.8 are MRI T1 and T2 sequence in axial sections demonstrating the extension of para vertebral soft tissue around the L1–L2 vertebral level. There is mild canal narrowing due to retropulsion of the posterior cortex. There is an epidural soft tissue component.

Post-T1 contrast MRI demonstrates focal kyphosis at the level of L1-2 secondary to destruction of both L-1 and L-2. There is edema and enhancement within L-1 and L-2 vertebral body. The prevertebral soft tissue shows the subligamentous extension of the soft tissue inferiorly and superiorly with a peripherally enhancing collection inferiorly seen in sagittal section. The right psoas muscle appears enlarged and shows post contrast enhancement.

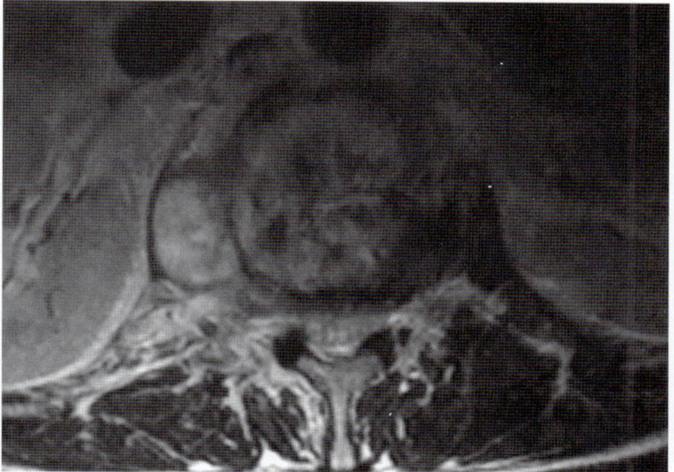

Fig. 4.53.7

Interpretation: A–40 years old, L1, L2 vertebra, bony destruction with sclerosis and fragmentation of L1 vertebral body and superior endplate erosions in L2 vertebral body. B–Obliteration of disc space. Pre- and

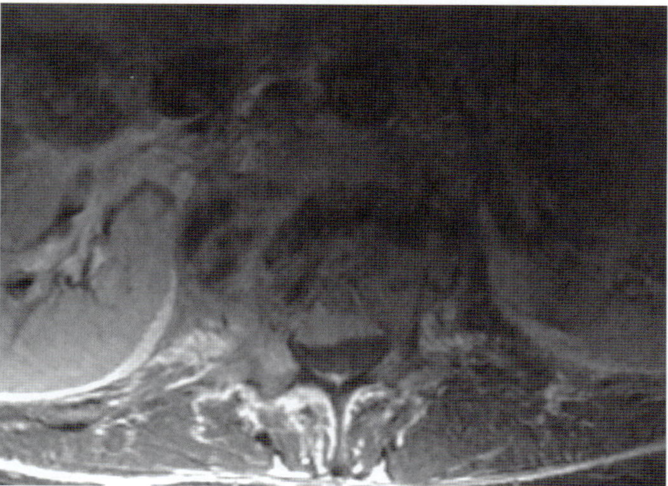

Fig. 4.53.5

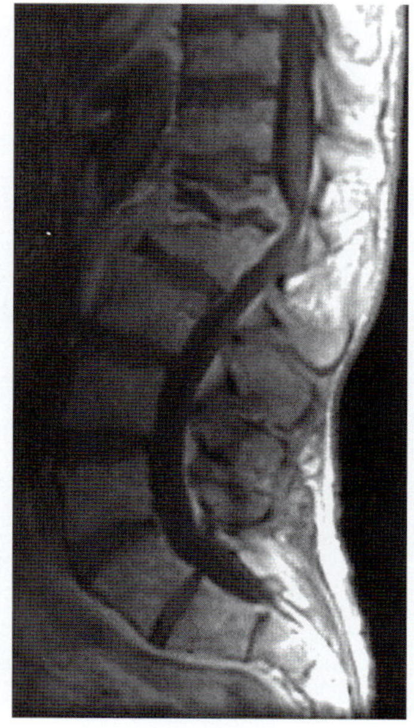

Fig. 4.53.8

paravertebral soft tissue thickening with post-contrast enhancement and calcification. Prevertebral soft tissue with subligamentous extension both superiorly and inferiorly with enhancement. Right psoas muscle enlargement with calcification and enhancement.

D: **Tuberculous spondylitis with vertebral collapse and right psoas abscess.**

Prinicipal diagnosis: **Tuberculous spondylitis with vertebral collapse and right psoas abscess** (Pott's spine) (Vertebral collapse +, Gibbus deformity+, destruction

Table 4.53.1: Differential diagnosis for TB spondylitis/spondylodiscitis

Differential diagnosis	*Radiological features*	*Imaging findings*
Pyogenic osteomyelitis Peak incidence in older patients. Predilection for lower lumbar spine. Initial infection in subchondral bone adjacent to endplate, the intervertebral discs are typically affected. Posterior element involvement is less common.	Lumbar spine commonly involved. Posterior element involvement is less common. **CT:** Pyogenic spondylitis **walls are thick and irregular.** Soft tissue calcifications and spinal deformity are infrequent. Moderate to complete destruction of the disc. **CT/MR:** Post-contrast **rim enhancement** is typically seen in disc.	**Fig. 4.53.9:** Pyogenic osteomyelitis
Brucellar spondylitis Common age group affected are 50–60 years.	Lower lumbar spine usually involved. **CT** shows **end plate spondylitis** mimicking Schmorl's nodule, moderate para-vertebral soft tissue. Nuclear medicine imaging demonstrates **maintained intra-vertebral architecture with increased uptake.** MRI shows anterosuperior epiphysitis at L4 with associated sacroiliitis. May be difficult to distinguishable from tuberculous spondylitis.	**Fig. 4.53.10:** Brucellar spondylitis
Lytic and sclerotic vertebral metastases Vertebral secondaries from primary malignancy may be sclerotic or lytic, usually seen in age more than 50 years. Extraosseous epidural or paraspinal extension and pathologic compression fractures may be seen. Disc space preserved. May be difficult to distinguish from isolated tuberculous, fungal, or brucellar spondylitis.	**MRI:** Hypointense in T1 and hyperintense on T2 signal with post-gadolinium enhancement is seen. **Posterior elements** are typically involved.	**Fig. 4.53.11:** Metastasis

(Contd.)

Table 4.53.1: Differential diagnosis for TB spondylitis/spondylodiscitis (*Contd.*)

Differential diagnosis	*Radiological features*	*Imaging findings*
Degenerative disc disease (modic type I) Modic type 1 degenerative changes represent early stages of degeneration may mimic infection. Recently Modic type I has received renewed attention due to the possibility of it representing low-grade indolent infection	**MRI: Hypointense in T1 and hyperintense T2 signal** and inflammatory marrow change is seen. Also T1 post-contrast shows enhancement.	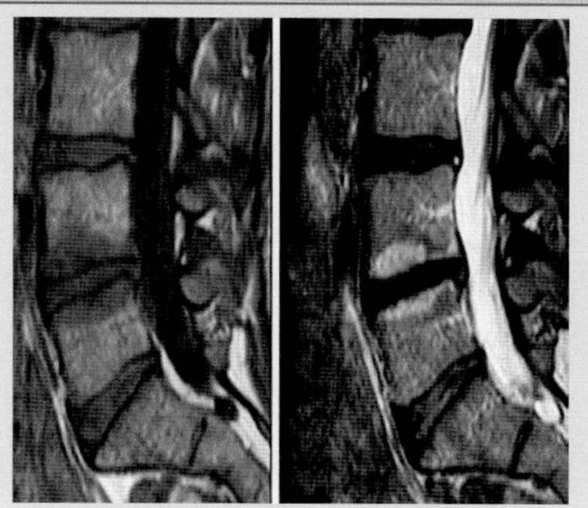 **Fig. 4.53.12:** Degenerative disc disease
Erosive osteochondritis: Erosive intervertebral osteochondritis is the destructive form of intervertebral osteochondrosis with inflammatory degeneration of the intervertebral disc	The radiographic features are characterized by **disc space narrowing, severe disc fissuring, vacuum phenomenon,** endplate cartilage erosions, and vertebral body reactive changes. The main difference of erosive intervertebral osteochondritis with Modic I changes is that there is a **hyperintensity in the disc** itself in T2, STIR, and in T1 post-contrast sequences, in addition to the characteristic changes of Modic I.	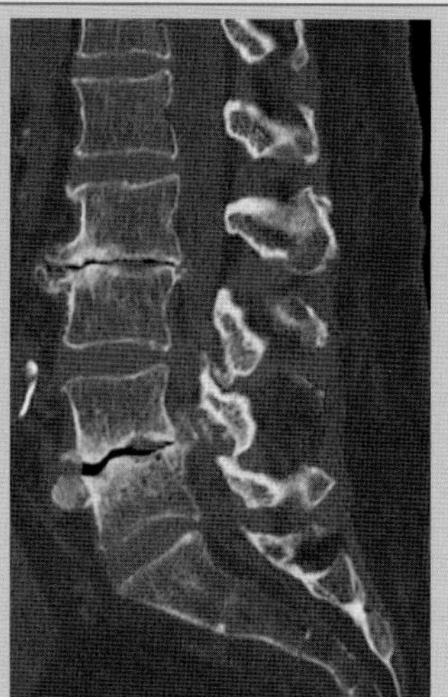 **Fig. 4.53.13:** Erosive osteochondritis
Fungal spondylitis Occurs in immune compromised individuals. Similar to TB it shows subligamentous spread. Actinomyces infection shows para vertebral soft tissue. Disc involvement is uncommon.	In MRI there is **absence of T2 hyperintensity even in disc involvement,** paramagnetic and ferromagnetic elements within the fungi contribute to the absence of signal hyperintensity in discs, e.g.—aspergillus spondylitis	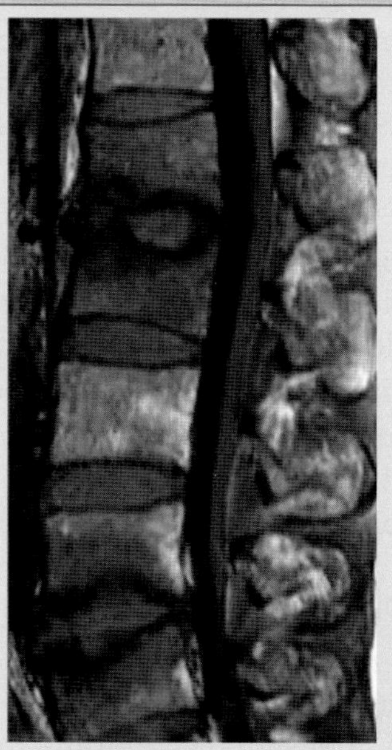 **Fig. 4.53.14:** Fungal spondylitis
Ankylosing spondylitis: Refer to case no. 63		

Table 4.53.2: Difference between brucellar spondylitis, tuberculous spondylitis and pyogenic spondylitis

	Brucellar spondylitis	*Tuberculous spondylitis*	*Pyogenic spondylitis*
Location	Lower lumbar spine	Midthoracic and upper lumbar spine	Lumbar spine more common
Bone destruction	Limited to end plates in localised disease. Less bone destruction than TB	Start at anterior vertebrae at end plates with extensive destruction, severe vertebral collapse and Gibbus deformity	Less severe destruction than that of TB. Usually involves less than two vertebral bodies
Disc	Disc collapse present	Disc collapse present	More severe disc destruction than that of TB
Extension	Localised peri-vertebral soft tissue involvement	Out of proportion para-vertebral soft tissue involvement than the bone may be seen. Subligamentous spread more than three vertebral levels	Subligamentous spread less than three vertebral levels
Calcification in para vertebral soft tissue	Less common	Para vertebral soft tissue calcification common	Less common
Age	Elderly man	Young male or female	Adults after 5th decade
Disc gas	Present	Uncommon	Uncommon
CT, MRI	End plate spondylitis mimicking Schmorl's nodule, moderate para-vertebral soft tissue	Large para vertebral abscess with enhancing thin and smooth rim and extends subligamentously and also involves spinal canal	Thick irregular rim enhancement of abscess in disc. Intra-osseous abscess less frequent than TB
Nuclear imaging	Maintained intra-vertebral architecture with increased uptake	Loss of intra-vertebral architecture with increased uptake	Increased uptake with loss of architecture

of intervertebral discs+, epidural soft tissue mass and psoas abscess+).

Further Management

Prognosis: Proper treatment leads to favourable outcome with resolution of symptoms and is particularly favourable if it is an early presentation with no neurologic deficits or spinal deformity. Delay in treatment leads to progressive vertebral collapse, irreversible neurologic deficits and death.

Treatment: Long-term anti-tuberculous medication for at least 1 year. Surgical decompression in setting of neurologic deficits ± spinal deformity.

- Indicated in 10–25% of TB spondylitis
- Laminectomy and debridement in absence of vertebral destruction
- Debridement and fusion if spinal deformity present.

Brief Discussion on TB Spondylitis/Spondylodiscitis

Clinical presentation: Most common symptom is chronic back pain (~95%), sign is focal tenderness and fever. Other signs/symptoms are paraparesis, kyphosis, sensory disturbance. Bladder and bowel dysfunction. Osseo-ligamentous destruction at cranio-vertebral junction leads to atlantoaxial instability and compression of cervico-medullary junction causing quadriparesis, bulbar dysfunction, and respiratory insufficiency. Clinical profile shows gradual, insidious onset of symptoms results in diagnostic delay. Fever relatively infrequent in TS. Neurologic deficits more common with TS than other granulomatous infections, such as bacterial spondylitis. Quantiferon assay: Interferon-γ release assay has sensitivity (84%), specificity (95%). Combination of radiological criteria, bone scan, ELISA, QuantiFERON assay is 90% predictive.

Demographics age: Most prevalent in 5th decade. Gender—male and female are equally affected in tuberculous spondylitis. **Epidemiology**—spinal TB accounts for 2% of all TB cases—rising incidence of tuberculosis in past 2 decades. Trend toward increased incidence in parallel with growing number of immunocompromised patients. Concomitant pulmonary tuberculosis in ~10% of patients. Reactivation of latent tuberculosis with anti-TNF therapies. Tuberculosis-associated immune reconstitution inflammatory syndrome (TB-IRIS) complication in HIV-type I infected TB patients on antiretroviral treatment. Neurological manifestations occur in more than 10% of TB-IRIS cases. Evidence for increased risk of serious local infections after kyphoplasty in patients with history of systemic infection. TS more aggressive in children. Kyphosis, cord compression more common.

Pathological features: Infectious organisms pass through the bloodstream as emboli and lodge in the turbulent flow of endplate arterioles. The anterior subchondral end plate is the first location of spinal pathology. After endplate degradation, disc involvement occurs. The infective centre is subligamentously dissected down either the anterior longitudinal ligament or the posterior longitudinal ligament. Scalping of the anterior vertebral body occurs, resulting in indentation. Soft tissue swelling is out of proportion to the degree of bone and discal damage when an abscess forms. The most common presentations are retropharyngeal, paravertebral (thoracic spine), and psoas abscess. Psoas abscesses usually calcify in a snowflake, thick pattern; psoas abscesses affect 5% of people with spinal TB.

Imaging: Best diagnostic clue is **gibbus vertebrae with relatively intact intervertebral discs, large paraspinal abscesses.** Early signs are lytic endplate destruction, loss of disc height, paraspinal swelling (retropharyngeal, retrotracheal, paraspinal line, psoas). Advanced signs are vertebral body collapse, gibbus formation, and obliteration of the disc.

Location: Midthoracic or thoracolumbar is greater than lumbar, cervical. Anterior vertebral body involved early. Isolated posterior element involvement possible: Laminae > pedicles > spinous process > transverse process. Multiple contiguous and non-contiguous vertebrae.

Morphology: Vertebral collapse, gibbus deformity with or without destruction of intervertebral discs. Epidural soft tissue mass. Large dissecting paraspinal abscesses over considerable distance.

Tuberculous spondylitis has higher rate of psoas abscess and involvement of posterior elements compared to brucellar spondylitis.

Radiography: Endplate irregularity, osteolysis and diffuse vertebral sclerosis, fusion across disc space in late TS. Findings may not be present until weeks after onset of infection.

NECT: Endplate destruction with vertebral body fragmentation. Calcified chronic paravertebral abscesses is common in TS than brucellar spondylitis (BS).

CECT: Diffuse or peripherally enhancing epidural and paraspinal soft tissue.

MRI: **T1WI**—hypointense marrow in contiguous vertebrae. Hypointense intraosseous, extradural, paraspinal abscesses. **T2WI**—hyperintense marrow, disc, phlegmon/abscess.

STIR: Hyperintense marrow, disc, phlegmon/abscess DWI sequence at vertebral bodies, endplates, and discs show hyperintensity in the acute phase and hypointensity in the chronic stage.

T1WI: Contrast sequence shows enhancement of marrow, subligamentous, discal, dura. Diffusely enhancing soft tissue (phlegmon) is seen. Peripheral enhancement indicates an abscess. Epidural abscess causes cord displacement or compression. Extradural infection can occur without bone destruction. Isolated vertebral body or posterior element involvement in 3–5% of tuberculous spondylitis.

Nuclear medicine findings: Bone scan shows increased spinal radionuclide uptake. Sensitive but not specific. Gallium scan shows increased radionuclide uptake in spine and paraspinal soft tissue. Highly sensitive and specific for vertebral osteomyelitis.

4.54 SPINE

Case No. 54

Clinical details: 6-year-old child presenting with back pain.

Radiological technique and observation: Lateral radiograph of lumbar spine (Fig. 4.54.1) showing complete collapse of a body of lumbar vertebra with relative sparing of posterior elements.

No evidence of sclerotic/lytic lesions in visualised vertebral bodies.

No evidence of soft tissue component.

Interpretation: A—6 years old, lumbar spine, C—complete collapse of vertebral body. B—pancake or silver dollar or coin-on-edge vertebra, D—Langerhans cell histiocytosis.

Principal diagnosis: Considering the age of the child, the most likely diagnosis is Langerhans cell histiocytosis.

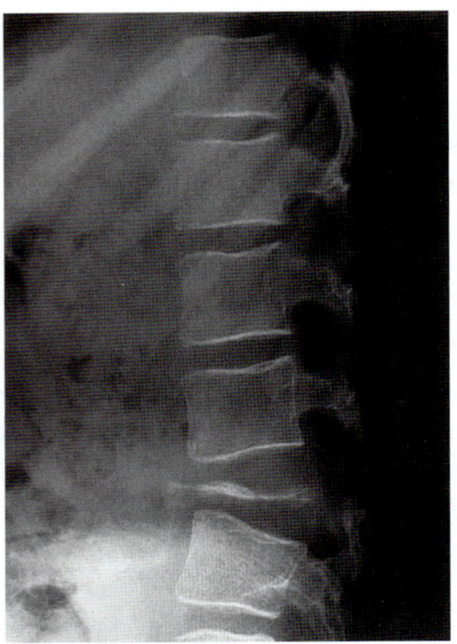

Fig. 4.54.1

Lymphoma

1. Radiological involvement in 10–20% of patients with Hodgkin's disease (50% at autopsy).
2. Involvement arises from either direct spread from contiguous lymph nodes or infiltration of bone marrow (spine, pelvis, major long bones, thoracic cage and skull are sites of predilection).
3. Patterns of bone involvement are
   a. Predominantly osteolytic.
   b. Mixed lytic and sclerotic.
   c. Predominantly sclerotic—*de novo* or following radiotherapy to a lytic lesion.
   d. 'Moth-eaten'—characteristic of round cell malignancies.

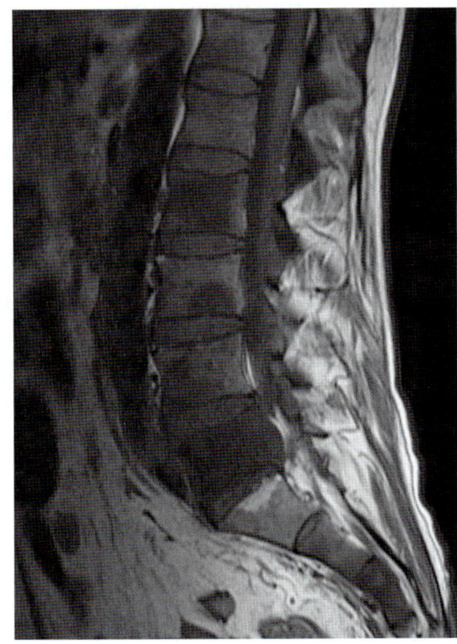

Fig. 4.54.2: Lymphoma involving spine

Table 4.54.1: Causes of vertebra plana	
Vertebra plana (coin vertebra)	
Pediatrics	*Adult*
Mnemonic: FETISH **F**racture—Trauma /osteogenesis imperfecta **E**osinophilic granuloma (Langerhans cell histiocytosis) **T**umor—metastatic neuroblastoma, leukemia, lymphoma, Ewing's sarcoma **I**nfection—Tuberculosis **S**teroids (avascular necrosis) **H**emangioma	Trauma/osteoporotic collapse Paget disease Metastasis Multiple myeloma Lymphoma Aneurysmal bone cyst Tuberculosis Steroids (avascular necrosis) Hemangioma

<table>
<tr><th colspan="2">Table 4.54.2: Differential diagnosis of LCH</th></tr>
<tr><td colspan="2">Ewing sarcoma (Refer to case 149)</td></tr>
<tr><td colspan="2">Metastasis (Refer to case 52)</td></tr>
<tr><td colspan="2">Osteomyelitis: Spinal tuberculosis spondylitis commonly causes bone destruction with somewhat relative disc preservation, which can cause vertebra plana, however, some form of vertebral endplate change is usually present. Bacterial infection commonly causes disc destruction and vertebral body endplate erosions (Refer to case 53)</td></tr>
<tr><td>Hematopoietic malignancies
Most common primary pediatric malignancy is leukemia.</td><td>Loss of vertebral height and increased sclerosis are common in the vertebral body.
B-symptoms and multiple levels involvement is seen in lymphoma.</td></tr>
<tr><td colspan="2">Other DDs include Neuroblastic tumors, non-Langerhans cell histiocytosis, Kimura disease, Kikuchi disease, IgG4 disease, Erdheim-Chester disease, Rosai-Dorfman disease</td></tr>
</table>

4. In addition, the spine may show
   a. Anterior erosion of a vertebral body caused by involvement of an adjacent paravertebral lymph node.
   b. Solitary dense vertebral body (ivory vertebra).
5. Hypertrophic osteoarthropathy.
6. Plain film may be negative with extensive disease on MRI.

Langerhans Cell Histiocytosis

Multisystemic disorder occurring due to uncontrolled monoclonal proliferation of Langerhans cells (distinctive cells of monocyte-macrophage lineage) and should be considered a malignancy although its biological behavior is very variable.

Common presentation: Child presenting with vertebra plana sparing the disk . 75% of cases occur under the age of 20 years. Male predilection 2:1. Regional pain is often the presenting symptom, a palpable tender mass may be noted on examination.

Divided based on number of lesions and systems involved.

1. Unifocal form—70% (eosinophilic granuloma)–benign condition with favourable prognosis, typically affects children
2. Multifocal unisystem—20% (Hand-Schüller-Christian disease) diabetes insipidus, exophthalmos, one or multiple bony lesions
3. Multifocal multisystem (fulminant form)—10% (Letterer–Siwe disease) affects children less than 3 years old. Most severe disease.

Skeletal manifestations

Skull

- Solitary or multiple punched out lytic lesions without sclerotic rim
- Double contour or beveled edge appearance may be seen due to asymmetrical involvement of the inner and outer tables with a hole within a hole appearance.
- Residual bone represented by a button sequestrum

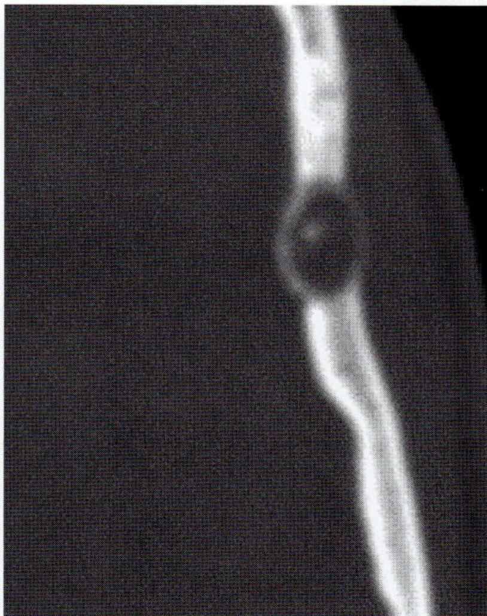

Fig. 4.54.3: Solitary punched out lytic lesions without sclerotic rim: LCH

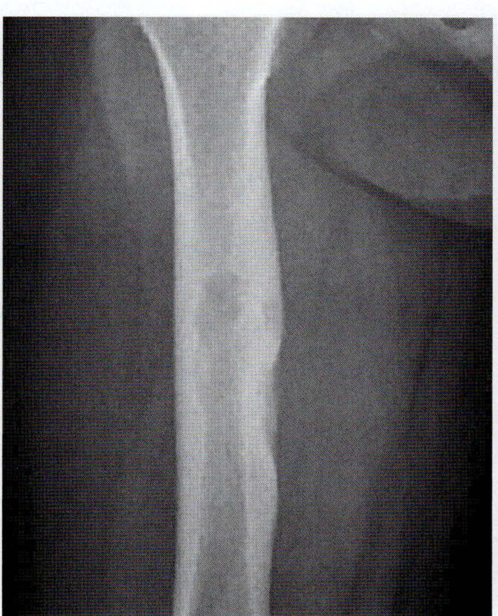

Fig. 4.54.4: LCH

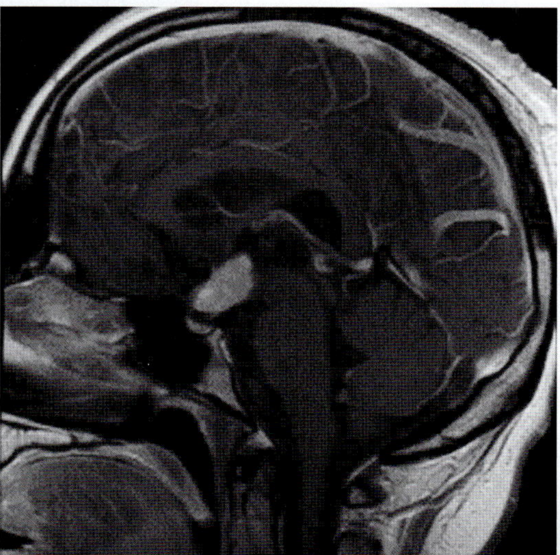

Fig. 4.54.5

Mandible—irregular radiolucent areas mostly involving superficial alveolar bone, floating tooth appearance: Loss of lamina dura and resorption of alveolar bone of the jaw.

Spine—lytic lesions can result in symmetric uniform collapse of the vertebral body with preservation of the intervertebral disc spaces. Pedicles usually involved and posterior elements spared.

Long bones—early lesions often appear lytic, expansile, and aggressive.

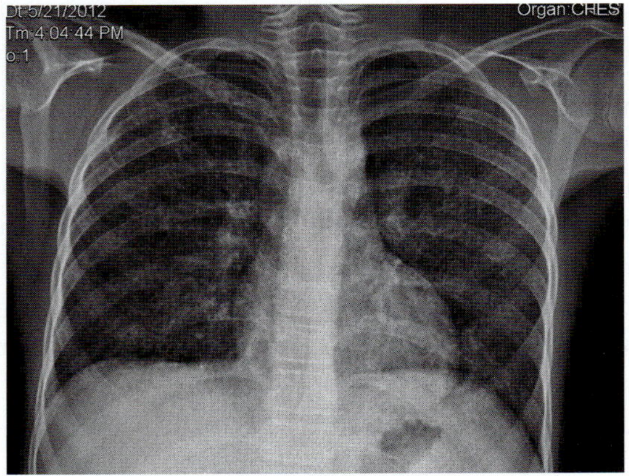

Fig. 4.54.6: Symmetrical bilateral reticular and reticulonodular opacities in LCH

Mainly involves diaphysis or meta-diaphysis.

Causes endosteal scalloping, cortical thinning and periosteal reaction.

Intracortical tunneling, and associated soft tissue mass.

CNS manifestation—thickening of pituitary stalk with loss of posterior pituitary bright spot presenting as diabetes insipidus.

Lungs—LCH is characterized by centrilobular micronodules with a predominantly bilateral symmetric upper- to mid-lung distribution.

Costophrenic angles are usually spared.

Abdomen—Hepatomegaly, splenomegaly. Mesenteric lymphadenopathy.

Treatment

Solitary lesion—good prognosis—majority heals spontaneously. Chemotherapy, radiofrequency ablation and steroids if conservative management fails.

Variable vertebral body restoration/reconstitution occurs over months to years with conservative orthopedic treatment. Reconstitution of vertebral height results from endochondral ossification at the apophyseal plate.

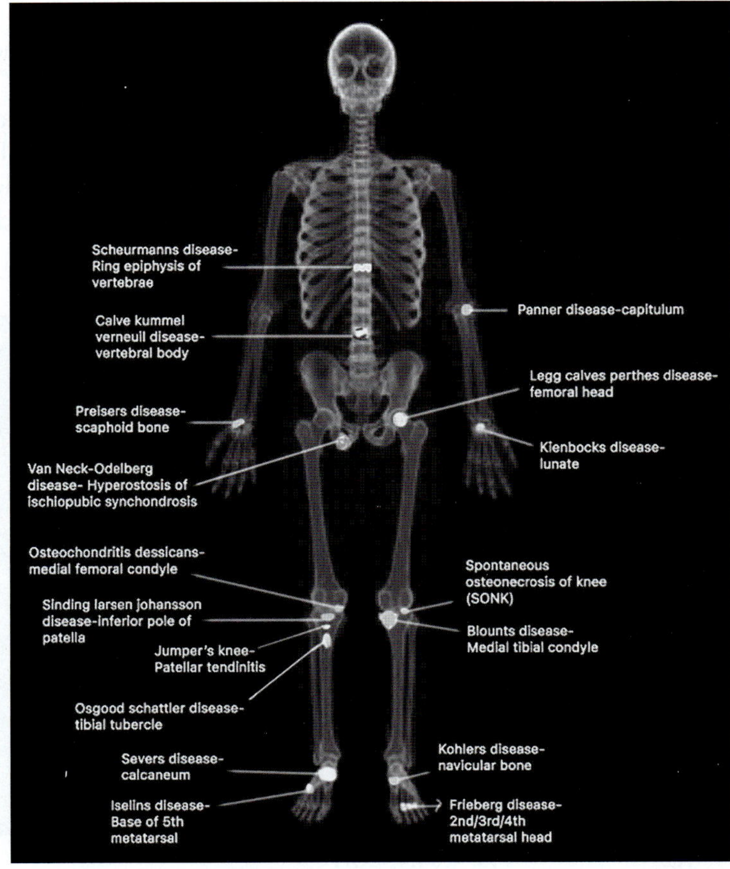

Fig. 4.54.7: Schematic representation of a vascular necrosis in various parts of the body

4.55 SPINE

Case No. 55

Clinical history: A case of 48 years old male, with complaints of vague lower abdominal pain.

Radiological techniques and observation: Figure 4.55.1 is plain radiograph pelvis (AP view) of 48-year-old male shows a well-defined radio-opacity noted in the pelvis, overlying the lower sacral segments. There are suspicious lytic areas noted in the adjacent lower sacral segments. No evidence of calcification/fat density noted within the lesion. Visualised bowel gas pattern appears normal. Bilateral sacro-iliac joint appears normal. Visualised bilateral pelvic bones, bilateral femur and lower lumbar vertebra appears normal. The patient can be further evaluated by cross sectional imaging like CT and MRI to narrow down the diagnosis.

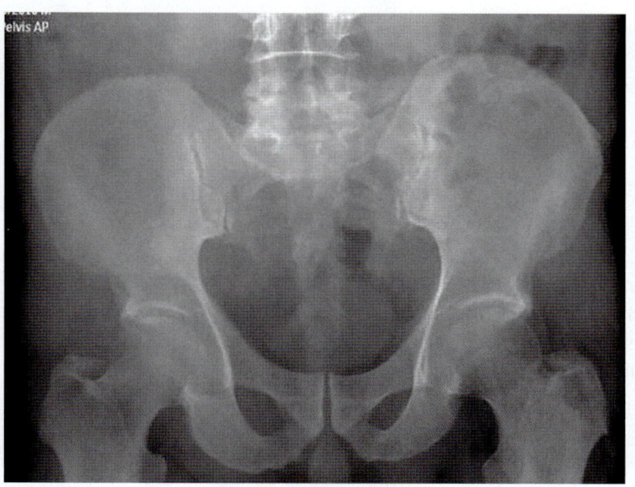

Fig. 4.55.1

Figures 4.55.2 to 4.55.5 are sagittal T1-weighted MR image of the pelvis showing a large, predominantly low-signal-intensity presacral mass involving the S4–S5 vertebra. Sagittal T2-weighted MR image shows hyperintense signal within the mass, which has a lobular growth pattern. Sagittal contrast-enhanced T1-weighted MR image shows mild heterogeneous enhancement within the mass.

Interpretation: A—48-year-old male, sacrum, C—large well-defined soft tissue mass which is T2 hyperintense with heterogeneous enhancement on T1 post-contrast imaging: Sacral chordoma.

Principal diagnosis: Sacral chordoma—the large anterior and smaller posterior soft-tissue components of the mass, are suggestive of its osseous origin.

Treatment: Surgical resection, with radiotherapy offered for recurrent cases. As an adjunct therapy, percutaneous radiofrequency ablation can be tried. Recurrence is prevalent, as it is seeding along the surgical tract. Chordomas spread metastatically in 7–14 percent of patients, with nodal, lung, bone, brain, or abdominal visceral involvement, mostly due to large tumors. Due to the highly aggressive character of these tumors, the prognosis is often poor, with a 10-year survival rate of around 40%.

Brief discussion about the condition: Chordomas appear like hard masses under the microscope. These tumors

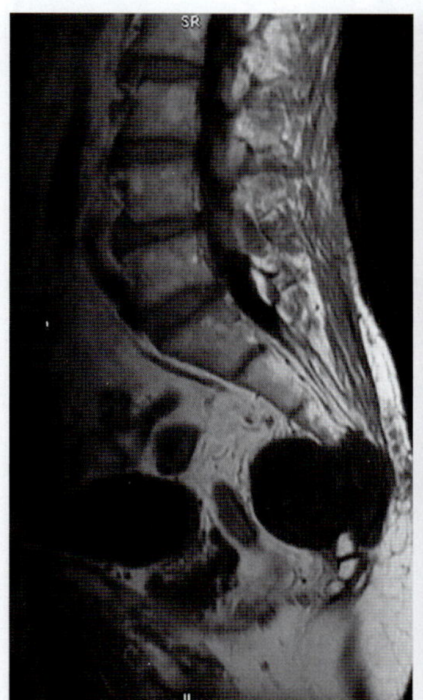

Fig. 4.55.2

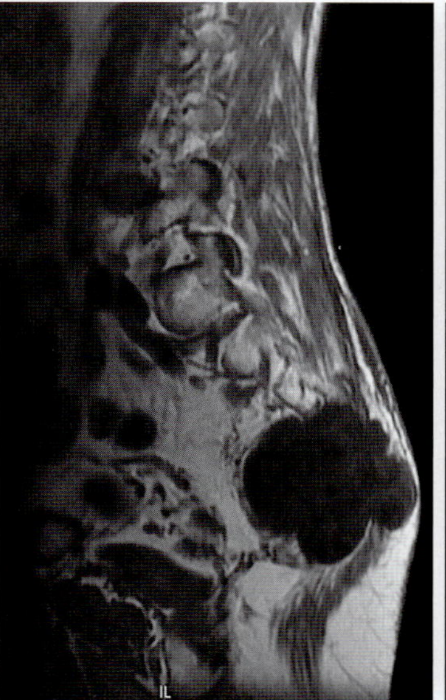

Fig. 4.55.3

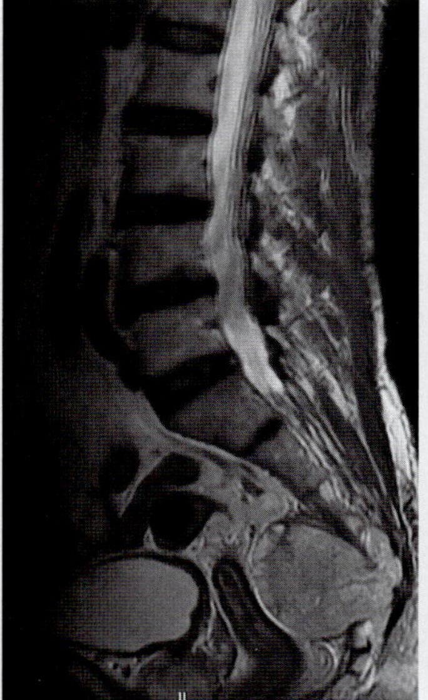

Fig. 4.55.4

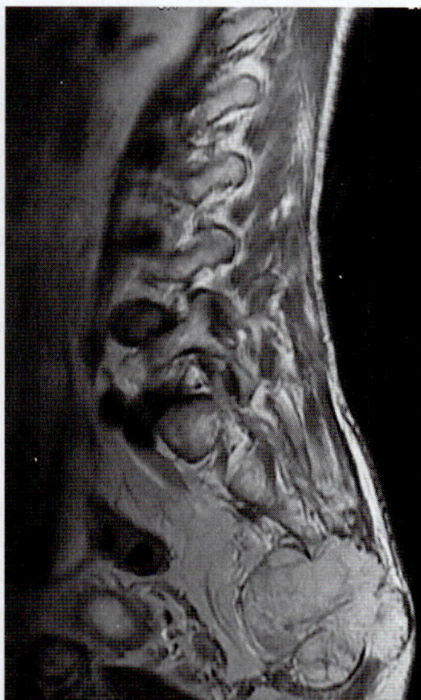

Fig. 4.55.5

Differential diagnosis		
Chondrosarcoma: Involves neural arch than vertebral body and most commonly seen in thoracic spine.	Chondroid matrix (contains rings and arcs), T1 low to intermediate signal intensity, T2 hyperintense on T2, enhances, higher ADC values (about 2050 × 10–6 mm²/s)	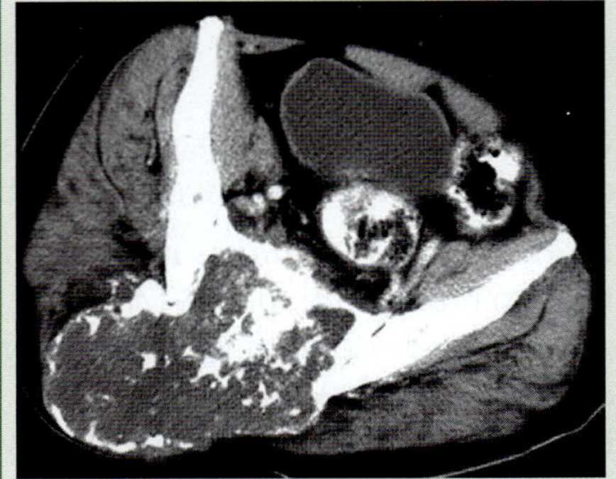 Fig. 4.55.6: Chondrosarcoma
Giant cell tumor—Sacrum > thoracic spine > cervical spine > lumbar spine,	T2 heterogeneous to hyperintense signal involving the first and second sacral segments with fluid level	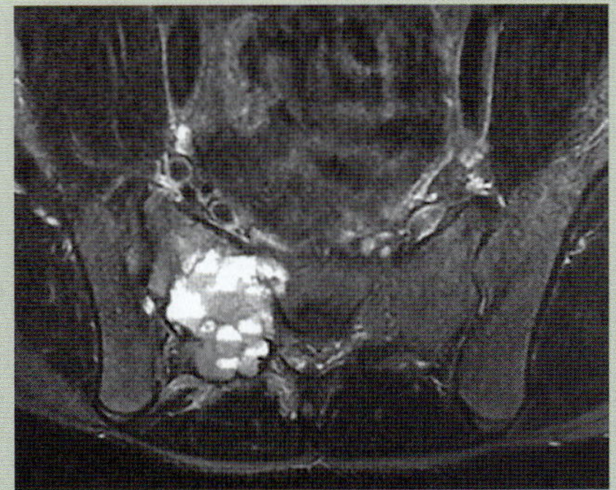 Fig. 4.55.7: GCT
Spinal metastases–Usually they are multiple, involving posterior elements than vertebral bodies. 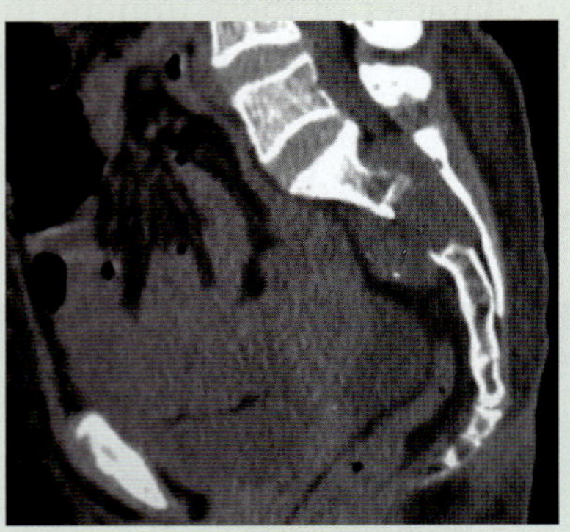 Fig. 4.55.8: Spinal metastases	Hypointense on T1; variably hyperintense on T2, In cases of spinal metastasis, spinal instability neoplastic score helps to assess spinal stability. A score of 7–18 warrants surgical consultation.	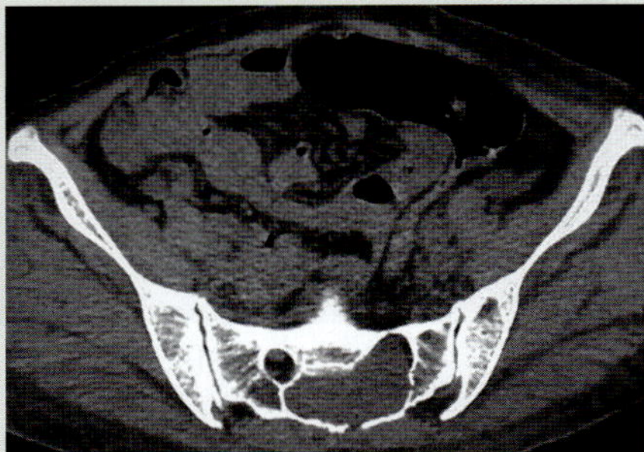 Fig. 4.55.9: Spinal metastases
Plasmacytoma–3% of all plasma cell tumors. Most commonly, in the spine, pelvis or ribs.	A well-defined, grossly expansile bone lesion. It may also exhibit soft-tissue extension, internal septa or pathological fracture. Extramedullary plasmacytomas rare. Absence of hypercalcaemia, renal insufficiency, anaemia; normal skeletal survey and normal paraprotein levels.	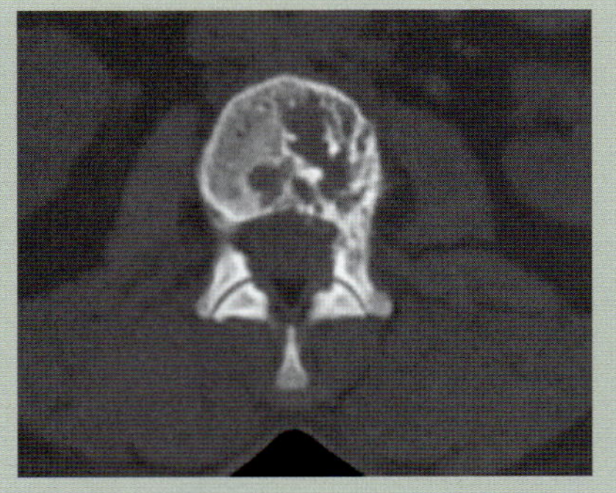 Fig. 4.55.10: Plasmacytoma

Spinal lymphoma—multifocal disease. Less than 5% of all primary bone tumors.	Heterogeneous T2 signal. Lytic: Destructive pattern Blastic: Sclerotic pattern Subtle or "near-normal" findings	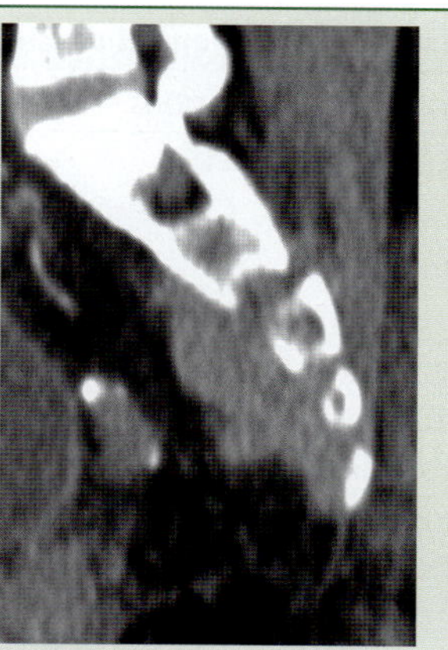 **Fig. 4.55.11:** Lymphoma

contain fluid and gelatinous mucoid substance (related with recent and old haemorrhage) as well as necrotic regions. Calcification and sequestered bone fragments are also seen in some patients. Chordomas are distinguished by physaliphorous cells under the microscope. The frequent recurrence of these malignancies is likely due to inadequate margination and microscopic distant expansion of malignant cells. The subtypes are chondroid chordoma (best prognosis), conventional chordoma (most common) and dedifferentiated chordoma (least common, worst prognosis).

Table 4.55.1: Differential diagnosis for sacral lesions
Congenital and developmental • Germ cell tumors—sacrococcygeal teratoma. • Anterior sacral meningocele • Developmental cysts (epidermoid, dermoid, enteric cysts like rectal duplication cyst, tail gut cyst) • Cystic lymphangioma and Lipoma
Extension of sacral bone tumors • Giant cell tumor/ABC • Chordoma • Osteoblastoma • Ewing sarcoma family • Osteogenic sarcoma
Mesenchymal masses • Rhabdomyo-sarcoma • Undifferentiated sarcoma • Vascular mass • Fibroma
Neurogenic masses • Neuroblastoma • Ganglioneuro-blastoma • Ganglioneuroma • Neurofibroma • Schwannoma
Inflammatory masses • IBD (UC and Crohn's) • Peri-rectal abscess/granuloma
Lymphomatous masses • Lymphoma(non-Hodgkin's) • Post-transplantation lymphomatous disorder
Other pre-sacral masses • Hematoma • Extension or metastasis to the pre-sacral space from another site

Location

- *Sacrococcygeal:* The most common location, accounting for approximately 30–50% of all chordomas and commonly involving 4th and 5th sacral segments. M:F = 2:1.
- *Spheno-occipital:* The second most common location, accounts for 30–35% of cases. The mass usually protrude posteriorly at midline, indenting the pons; this distinctive appearance is known as the "thumb sign." There is no gender difference, unlike sacrococcygeal tumors.
- *Vertebral body:* 15–30%, Although rare, they are common in the C2 vertebrae and are the 2nd most common adult primary spine malignancy, behind lymphoproliferative tumors. Variable intralesional hemorrhage can be seen as blooming on SWI.

DWI/ADC: Diffusion restriction with ADC values: Conventional chordoma: $1474 \pm 117 \times 10^{-6}$ mm^2/s; Dedifferentiated chordoma: $875 \pm 100 \times 10^{-6}$ mm^2/s; Bone scan—variable.

- S3 vertebra–radiological landmark for rectum.

T2 very bright lesions
- Cysts
- Pleomorphic adenoma
- Chordoma
- Chondrosarcoma

Table 4.55.2: Differential diagnosis for multiple vertebral lesions and contiguous vertebral lesions

Multiple vertebral lesions	*Contiguous vertebral lesions*
Metastatic disease	Osteosarcoma
Myeloma	Ewing's sarcoma
Lymphoma	Chondrosarcoma
Angiosarcoma	Osteochondroma
Hemangioma	Chordoma
Enostosis	Lymphoma
Paget's disease	Aneurysmal bone cyst
Eosinophilic granuloma.	Giant cell tumor
	Myeloma
	Plasmacytoma
	Tuberculosis

- Hemangioma
- Neurofibroma
- Myxoma
- Pheochromocytoma

Infectious Lesions of Sacrum

They could be the result of contiguous spread from a nearby infection; hematogenous spread through the bladder, intestines, or genitourinary system, or via intravenous injections in drug addicts (via the Batson plexus); Pelvic soft-tissue infections (decubitus ulcers, traumatic traumas); Iatrogenic injury from gluteal injections, sacral biopsy. Sacral osteomyelitis presents on as lytic lesion with a ill-defined borders and soft-tissue swelling.

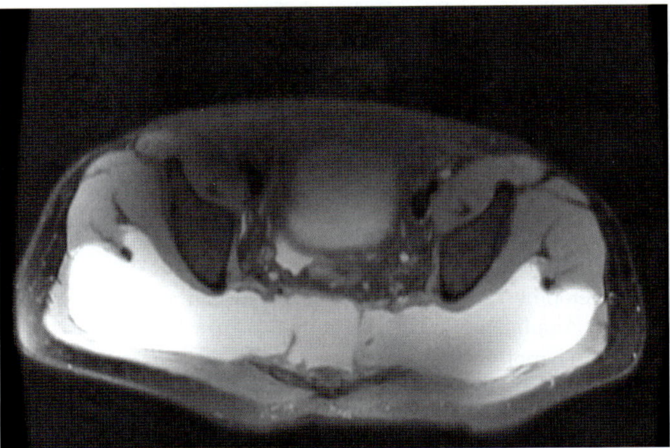

Fig. 4.55.12: Sacral osteomyelitis with collection

Noninfectious Arthropathies of Sacrum

The sacrum can be affected by a number of inflammatory disorders that impact the sacroiliac joints. They are all characterised by SI joint involvement. The involvement pattern might be unilateral or bilateral, and the intensity of the inflammation can range from mild to severe, leading in partial or total ankylosis.

a. Bilateral symmetric sacroiliac joint involvement is caused by **ankylosing spondylitis and inflammatory bowel disease**. The initial erosive alterations are followed by repair, resulting in subchondral sclerosis and ankylosis.
b. Bilateral symmetric, bilateral asymmetric (more common), or unilateral sacroiliac joint involvement can occur in **psoriatic arthritis and Reiter syndrome**, where erosions with subsequent healing, results in subchondral sclerosis.
c. Sacroiliac joint involvement might be bilateral symmetric, bilateral asymmetric, or unilateral due to osteoarthritis. Joint space narrowing, subchondral sclerosis, and osteophyte development are among the findings.
d. **Rheumatoid arthritis**
e. **Crystal deposition arthropathy** (gout, calcium pyrophosphate deposition disease). The existence or absence of symmetry, the condition of the joint space, the presence or absence of periarticular erosions or subchondral sclerosis, and the presence or absence of joint ankylosis allow sacroiliac joint arthropathies to be distinguished.

4.56 SPINE

Case No. 56

Clinical history: 2 years old boy presented with complaints of constipation.

Radiological technique and observation: Figure 4.56.1 is barium enema spot film showing pre-sacral space widening with destruction of sacrum noted. Normal contrast opacification of rectum and large bowel noted.

Figures 4.56.2 to 4.56.5 are MRI pelvis T2, T1 sagittal and T2 axial images respectively showing herniation of meninges through the defect in sacrum and coccyx forming a large cystic lesion in the presacral region. Low lying tethered cord attached to posterior thecal sac. The cystic lesion appears to displace urinary bladder and rectum anteriorly. No evidence of spina bifida/dorsal myelomeningocele. No evidence of filum terminale lipoma.

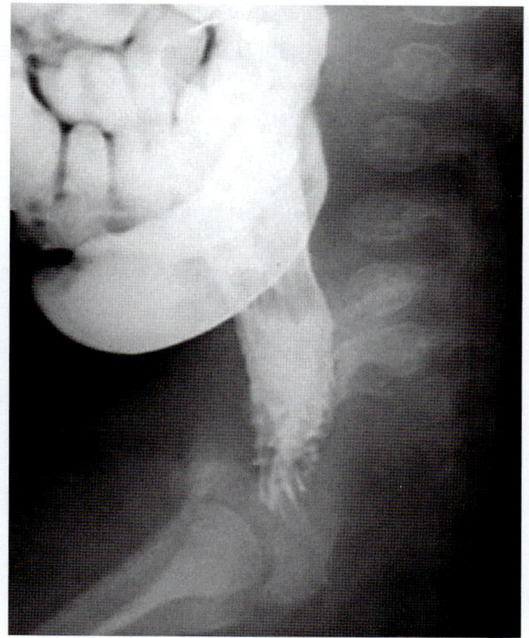

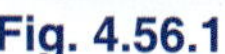

Fig. 4.56.1

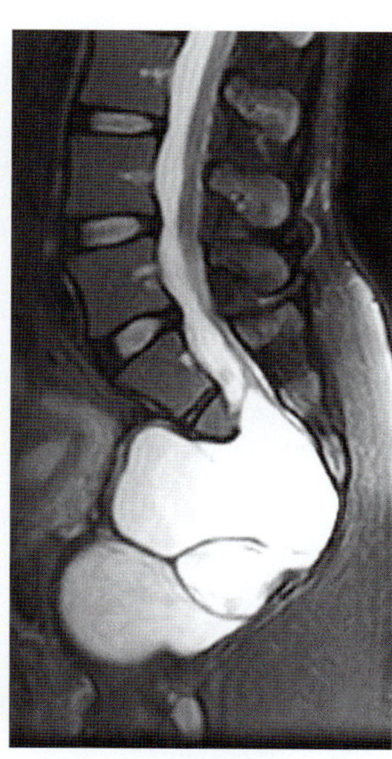

Fig. 4.56.2

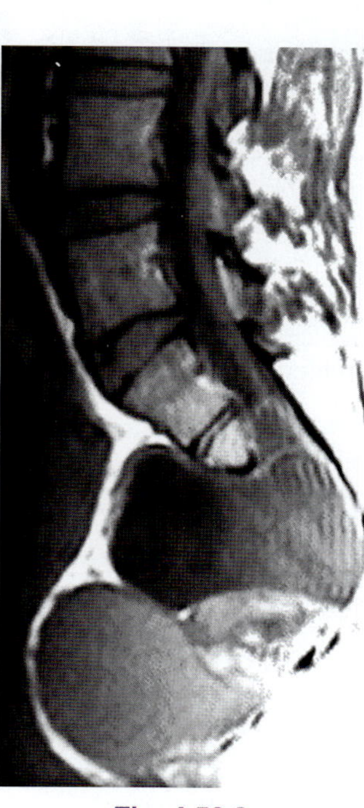

Fig. 4.56.3

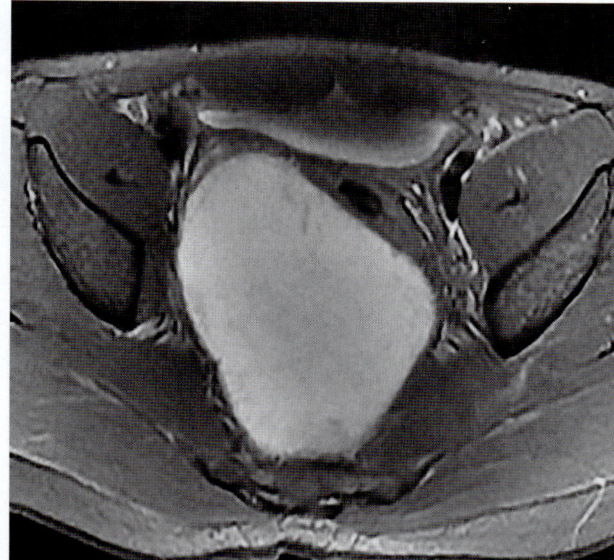

Fig. 4.56.4

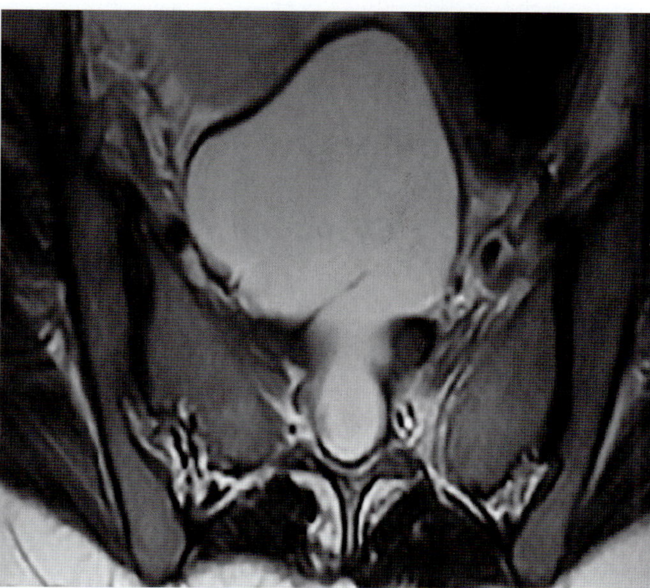

Fig. 4.56.5

Table 4.56.1: Differential diagnosis for presacral cyst

Cystic sacrococcygeal teratoma 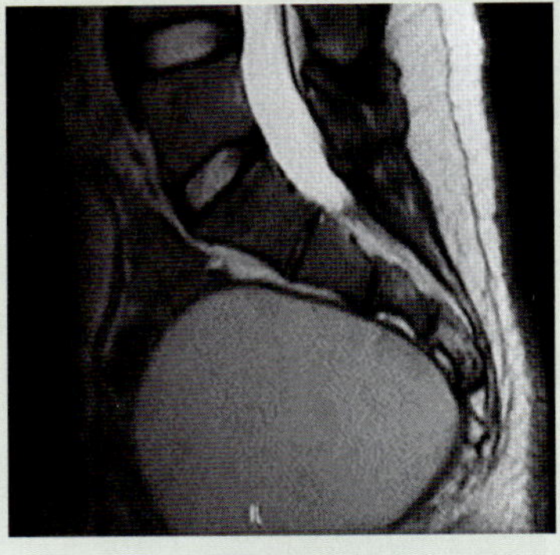 **Fig. 4.56.6:** Cystic sacrococcygeal teratoma	Large, heterogeneous sacral mass in infant variable amount of calcifications, mixed solid and cystic components, fat-debris levels, bone, hair, teeth, or cartilage. It is the most common presacral germ cell tumor in children and most common solid tumor in neonates. Monitoring—alpha1 fetoprotein	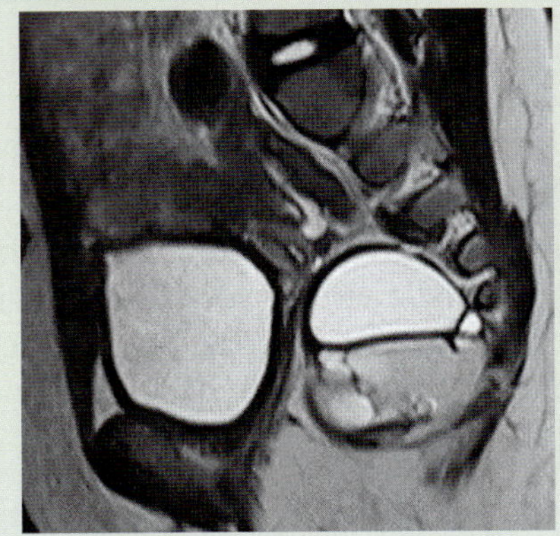 **Fig. 4.56.7:** Cystic sacrococcygeal teratoma
Cystic lymphangioma	The macrocystic variety of lymphatic malformation is also referred to as cystic lymphangioma or cystic hygroma. They present as sharply marginated unilocular or multilocular cystic lesion with attenuation similar to that of water and with thin, often contrast-enhanced walls and septa. Fluid level seen in the setting of hemorrhage.	
Neurenteric cyst	Cyst usually within spinal canal with or without rachischisis, vertebral formation anomalies. Often proteinaceous as T1 hyperintense. MRI–prevertebral cyst with spinal defect.	**Fig. 4.56.8:** Neurenteric cyst
Cystic neuroblastoma	Heterodense mass with calcifications and metastatic lesions. Presacral tumors may extend into spinal space through neural foramina. It may associated with areas of hemorrhage and necrosis and do not contain fat. Calcifications seen in 80% of neuroblastoma in CT.	
Rectal duplication cyst	Communication between the cyst and the intestinal lumen may be observed during a barium enema study. MRI clearly delineates the duplication and relation with adjacent structures.	
Rectal GIST	T1 hypointense, T2 iso-hyperintense lobulated well-defined exophytic mass lesion, no surrounding lymphadenopathy and lack of bowel luminal constriction	
Other differentials	Ovarian cyst—variable appearance, pelvic abscess—collection with diffusion restriction	

Interpretation: A—2 years old boy, presacral region, C—cystic lesion, contiguous with thecal sac through anterior osseous defect, B—no evidence of spina bifida/dorsal myelomeningocele/filum terminale lipoma. D—anterior sacral meningocele with tethered cord and partial sacral agenesis.

Principle diagnosis: Anterior sacral meningocele with tethered cord and partial sacral agenesis

Differential diagnosis:

- Cystic sacrococcygeal teratoma
- Cystic lymphangioma
- Neurenteric cyst
- Cystic neuroblastoma
- Rectal duplication cyst
- Gastrointestinal stromal tumor
- Cystic schwannoma
- Pelvic abscess/prevertebral abscess

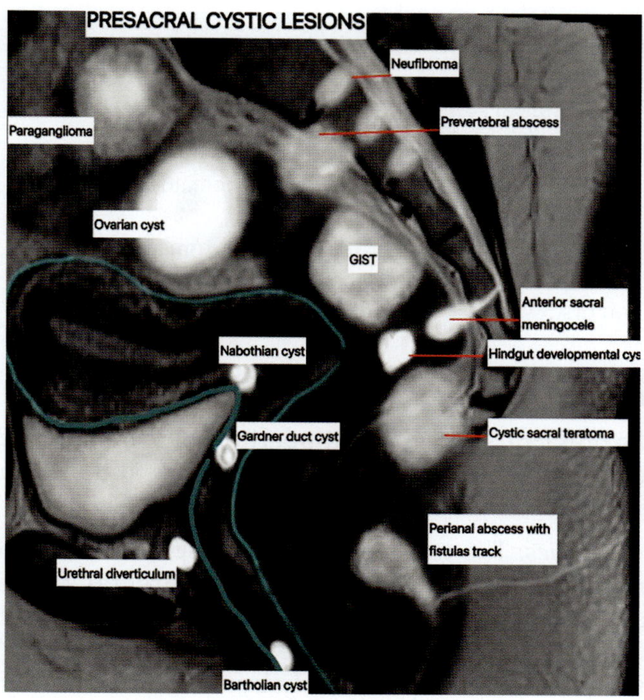

Fig. 4.56.9: Presacral soft tissue lesions

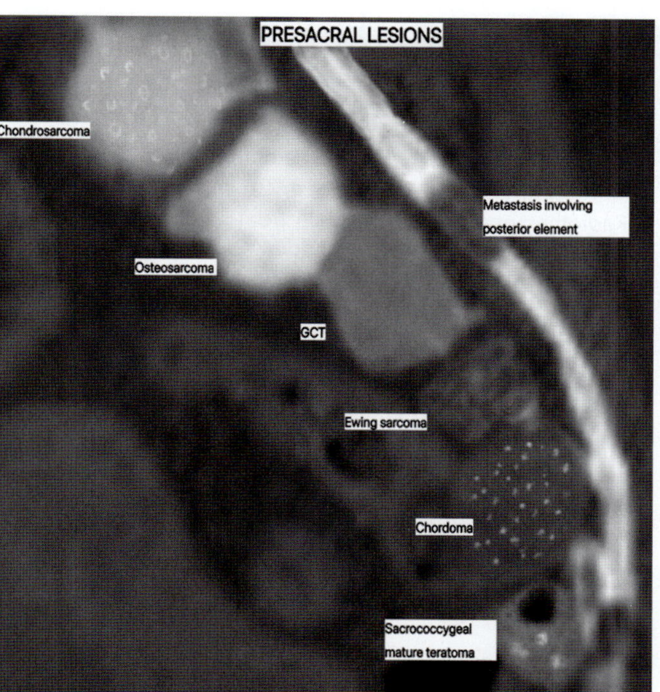

Fig. 4.56.10: Sacral bone lesions

Table 4.56.2: Approach to sacral/presacral lesions
Intrasacral cystic lesions
Tarlov cyst or perineural cyst
Dural Ectasia
Meningocele
Spinal synovial cyst
Cystic nerve sheath tumor
Spinal metastasis
Sacral masses with presacral extension
Giant cell tumor
Aneurysmal bone cyst
Chordoma
Osteogenic sarcoma
Ewing sarcoma
Pure cystic and mixed presacral masses with bony involvement
Sacrococcygeal teratoma
Anterior sacral meningocele
Dermoid cyst
Neuroblastoma
Benign schwannoma, osteomyelitis with prevertebral abscess
Pure cystic and mixed presacral masses without bony involvement
Enteric cyst
Cystic lymphatic malformation
Pelvic abscess
Lymphoma

Further Management

Investigations: Radiography of pelvis may show scimitar sign of sacral bone. Bone CT to demonstrate characteristic osseous findings that permit specific diagnosis. MRI aids in treatment planning.

Treatment

Surgical resection is curative—open posterior trans-sacral approach, patching of meningocele-dural sac connection, anterior approach is reserved for large lesion. Endoscopic approach for smaller lesions.

Discussion

Anterior sacral meningocele is a uni or multilocular protrusion of dura or arachnoid out of sacral canal into the retroperitoneum and infra-peritoneal space. It may protrude anteriorly through the body of sacrum or anterolaterally through enlarged vertebral foramina. It is a form of caudal dysgenesis. Present at birth and becomes symptomatic at a later age. Male: female ratio is 1: 4. Manifests at 2nd-3rd decade during childbearing years in women. It has an autosomal dominant inheritance and is a part of Currarino triad: It consists of anorectal anomalies, caudal regression syndrome/scimitar sacrum and presacral mass (anterior sacral meningocele/ sacrococcygeal teratoma/dermoid/epidermoid cyst). It is associated with neurofibromatosis and Marfan's syndrome.

Presacral space widening—is defined as widening of retrorectal/presacral soft tissue space at S3–S5 level is more than 1.5 cm.

Table 4.56.3: Causes of pre-sacral widening

Normal variation—40% of cases and these are mostly large or obese individuals.			
Inflammatory	*Neoplastic*	*Retro-rectal developmental cysts*	*Others*
1. Ulcerative colitis* 2. Crohn's disease* 3. Radiotherapy 4. Diverticulitis 5. Abscess	1. Carcinoma of the rectum. 2. Metastases to the rectum—especially from prostate, ovary and bladder. 3. Sacral tumors–metastases, plasmacytoma, chordoma.	1. Epidermoid—benign, unilocular. 2. Dermoid. 3. Enteric cyst—lined with intestinal mucosa a. Tailgut cyst (may be multiloculated). b. Duplication cyst.	1. Anterior sacral meningocele 2. Pelvic lipomatosis 3. Abscess 4. Pseudomyxoma retroperitonei

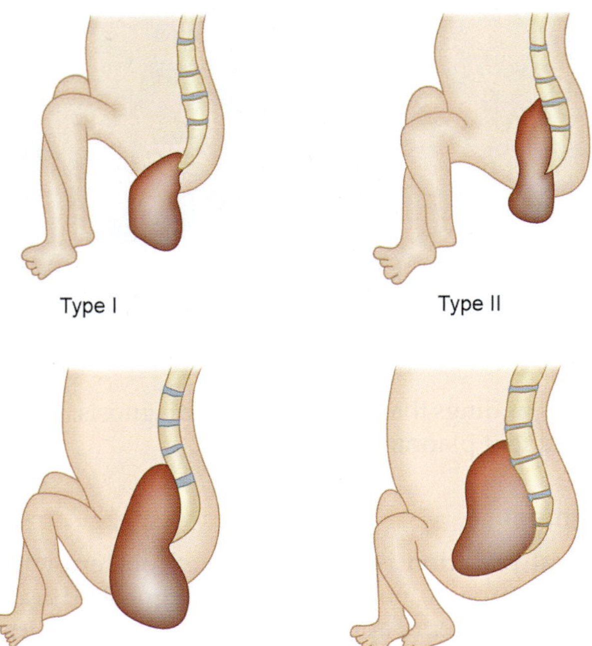

Fig. 4.56.11: Altman classification of sacrococcygeal mass

Altman classification of sacrococcygeal mass:

Type I: Predominantly external mass with a small presacral component.

Type II: External mass with a significant intrapelvic component.

Type III: External mass with a pelvic and abdominal component.

Type IV: Internal mass with an intrapelvic and abdominal location.

Anatomy of Presacral Space

The presacral space is an extraperitoneal potential space between the upper two-thirds of the rectum and the sacrum.

Boundaries: The retrorectal/presacral space is bounded anteriorly by the rectum and mesorectal fascia, superiorly by the peritoneal reflection of the recto-sigmoid colon, inferiorly by the rectosacral/Waldeyer's fascia, levator ani, posteriorly by the sacrum, coccyx and presacral fascia and laterally by the iliac vessels and ureters.

Division: The retrorectal space can be further divided into the anterior retrorectal and posterior presacral space, divided by the presacral fascia.

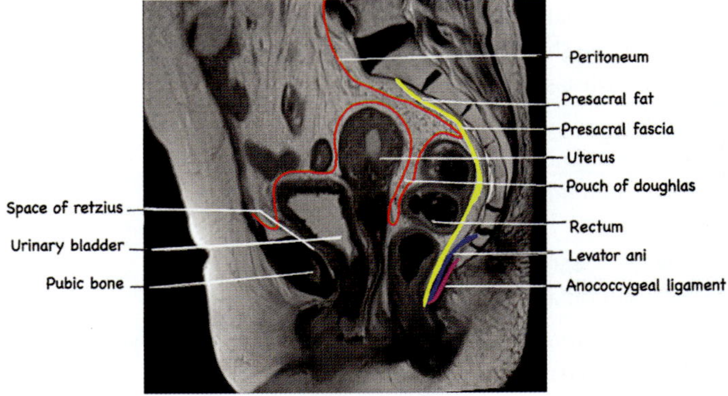

Fig. 4.56.12: Presacral space and pelvic peritoneum

4.57 SPINE

Case No. 57

Clinical history: 31 years old male with complaints of severe backache.

Radiological technique: Figures 4.57.1 to 4.57.3 are myelogram, MR spine T1 coronal, T2 sagittal images of lumbosacral spine respectively.

Observations: A well-defined lobulated intramedullary lesion, spanning over 5 vertebral segments and causing focal cord expansion is noted in the conus of spinal cord at D12–L4 level. The lesion appears T1 isointense. T2WI shows that the lesion is hyperintense and causing mild scalloping of the posterior vertebral bodies. Evidence of T2 hyperintensity noted in the dorsal spinal cord above the lesion, suggestive of cord edema. Myleogram shows loss of signal intensity in the involved segments. Flow voids noted within the lesion.

The vertebral bodies, laminae, pedicles, transverse and spinous process appear normal with normal MR signal pattern. Bony spinal canal dimensions are within normal limits. The intervertebral discs show normal morphology and signal intensity. The pre- and paraspinal regions appear normal.

Interpretation: A: 31 years old male, lumbosacral spine B: A well-defined lobulated intramedullary lesion causing focal cord expansion which is T1 isointense, T2 hyperintense. C: Mild scalloping of the posterior vertebral bodies and cord edema, D: Myxopapillary ependymoma.

Principal diagnosis: Myxopapillary ependymoma.

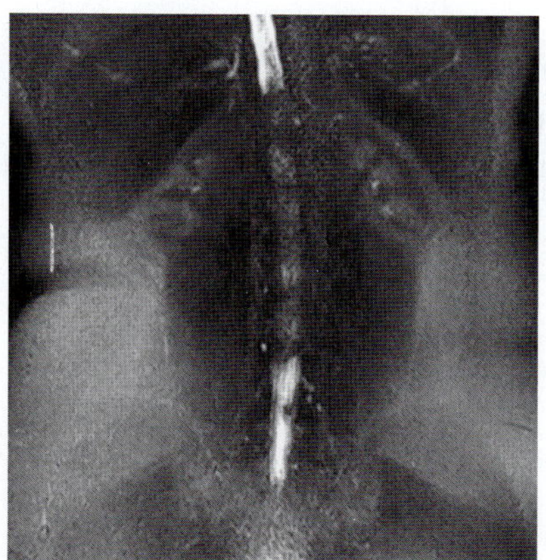

Fig. 4.57.1

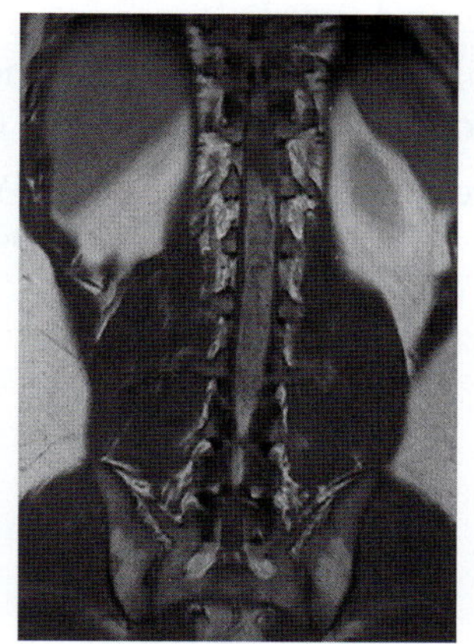

Fig. 4.57.2

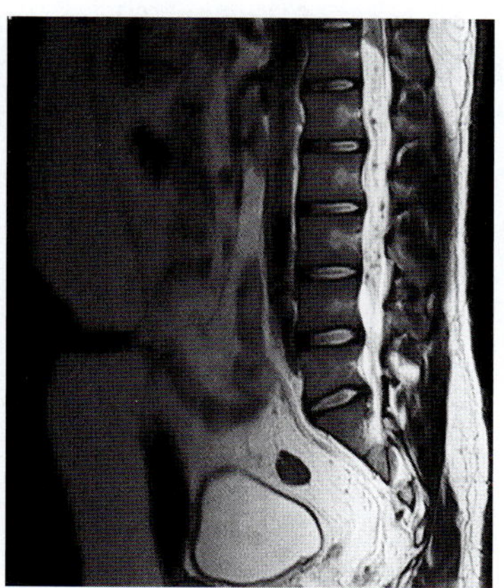

Fig. 4.57.3

Differential diagnosis for conus lesions:

Paraganglioma	*Nerve sheath tumor*	*Neurofibromatosis-1*	*(Epi) dermoid cyst*	*Hemangioblastoma*
Intradural extramedullary lesion, hypervascular intensely enhancing lesion, prominent flow voids due to enlarged draining veins with positivity in I-131 MIBG scan.	Intradural extramedullary lesion associated with nerve root extending through neural foramina, haemorrhage less common and shows heterogenous enhancement with contrast.	Plexiform neurofibroma seen in NF-1, often affect lumbosacral plexus, bilateral, multilevel, multinodular nerve enlargement, interdigitating with surrounding soft tissue.	Typically, small with no enhancement. Shows diffusion restriction. May be associated with dorsal dermal sinus.	Small nodular enhancing lesion with arterial feeder and extensive edema.
Fig. 4.57.4: Paraganglioma	**Fig. 4.57.5:** Nerve sheath tumor	**Fig. 4.57.6:** Neurofibromatosis-1	**Fig. 4.57.7:** Epidermoid cyst	**Fig. 4.57.8:** Hemangioblastoma

Other differentials include: Lipoma with tethered cord, granulomas, infections like schistosomiasis, intraspinal abscess secondary to dorsal dermal sinus and metastases.

Further Investigations

Myelography: Well-demarcated lobular mass in conus with nerve roots draping around the mass. Meniscus of contrast delineates intradural extramedullary lesions.

Management: Resection with adjuvant radiotherapy as myxopapillary ependymomas are radiosensitive.

Brief discussion: **Myxopapillary ependymoma:** WHO grade I neoplasm arising from ependymal cells of conus.

Very bright on T2, sometimes difficult to differentiate from CSF.

M/c primary spinal cord tumor in adults: Cord ependymoma most commonly cervical, cellular type.

M/c tumor of conus, filum terminale and cauda equina: Myxopapillary ependymoma (90%).

MP ependymomas: 30% of all ependymomas.

Age: Peak—30 to 40 years with slight male predominance. M:F = 2:1

Presentation

- Backpain, paraparesis and radiculopathy.
- Bladder and bowel dysfunction 20–25%.

Complications

- Acute non-aneurysmal subarachnoid haemorrhage
- Superficial siderosis
- No malignant degeneration.

Table 4.57.1: Presentation of myxopapillary ependymoma in adults and children

Adults	*Children*
Excellent prognosis	More aggressive
Less and late recurrence	Higher rate of local recurrence
CSF dissemination rare	Higher rate of dissemination
Distant metastases uncommon	Relatively more common

Subcutaneous sacrococcygeal myxopapillary ependymoma:

- Extremely rare tumor.
- Arises from coccygeal medullary vestige.
- Ependymal lined cavity of caudal neural tube at postanal pit.

4.58 SPINE

Case No. 58

Clinical history: 30 years old gentleman with complaints of backache with weakness of bilateral lower limb for 10 months.

Imaging technique and observation: Figures 4.58.1 to 4.58.6 are MRI limited sections of T1, T2, T1 post-contrast sagittal images with T1, T2, T1 post-contrast axial images respectively showing T1-isointense/T2-hyperintense ill-defined homogeneously enhancing, eccentric located fusiform expansile intramedullary long segment solid mass lesion noted from D7 to D10 vertebral level with minimal adjacent edema. No evidence of intra-lesional cystic changes/hemorrhage. No evidence of syrinx. No evidence of intra-lesional flow voids. No evidence of marrow changes in adjacent vertebra.

Interpretation: A: 30 years old male, dorsal spine, B: Ill-defined homogeneously enhancing eccentric expansile intramedullary fusiform long segment solid mass, C: Minimal adjacent edema. No evidence of intra-lesional cystic changes/hemorrhage/syrinx/intra-lesional flow voids/marrow changes in adjacent vertebra/drop metastasis, D: Spinal astrocytoma.

Principal diagnosis: Spinal astrocytoma.

Differential diagnosis:

Ependymoma Hemangioblastoma Metastasis	Cystic intramedullary lesions Demyelination: Transverse myelitis, neuromyelitis optica, multiple sclerosis. Tuberculoma, cavernoma, lipoma, hematoma.

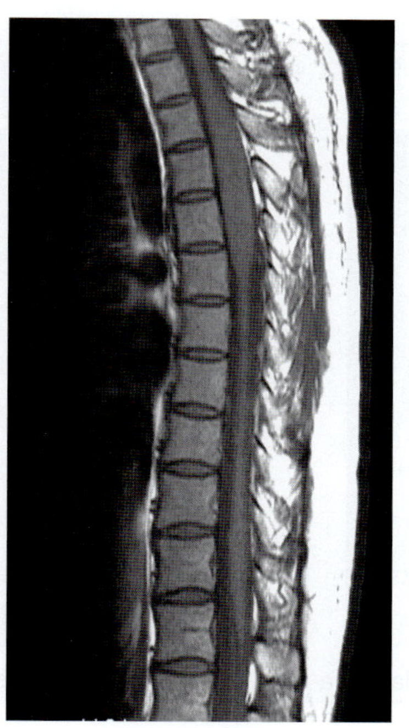

Fig. 4.58.1

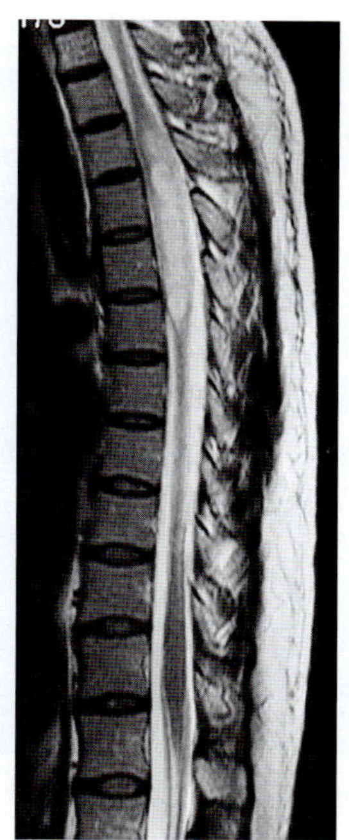

Fig. 4.58.2

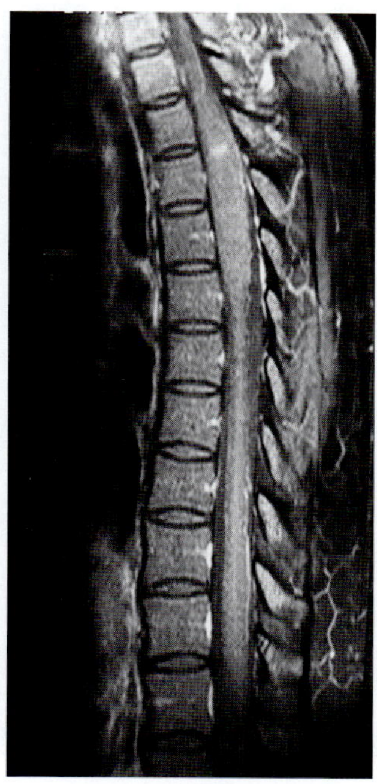

Fig. 4.58.3

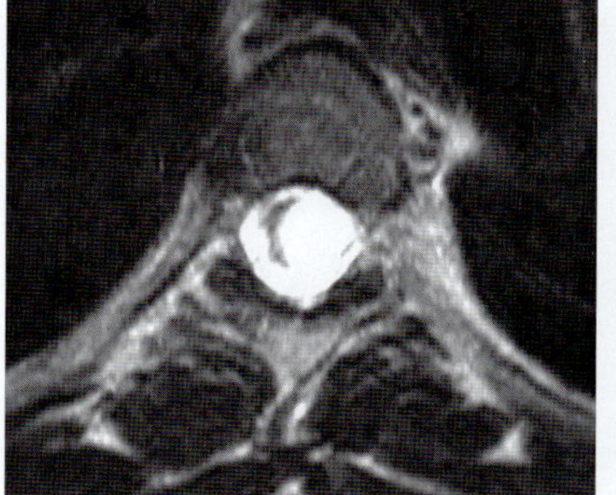

Fig. 4.58.4

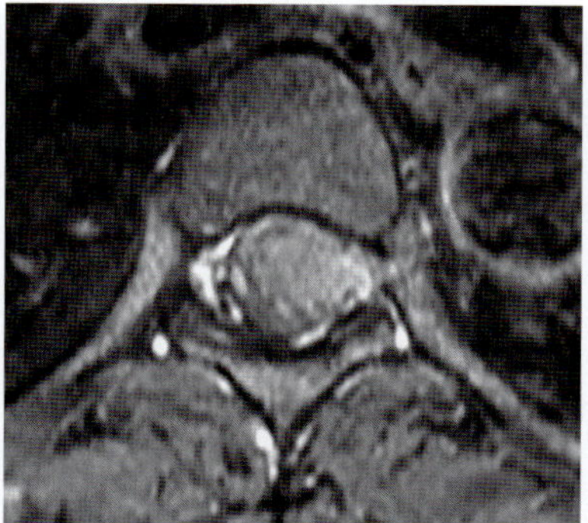

Fig. 4.58.5

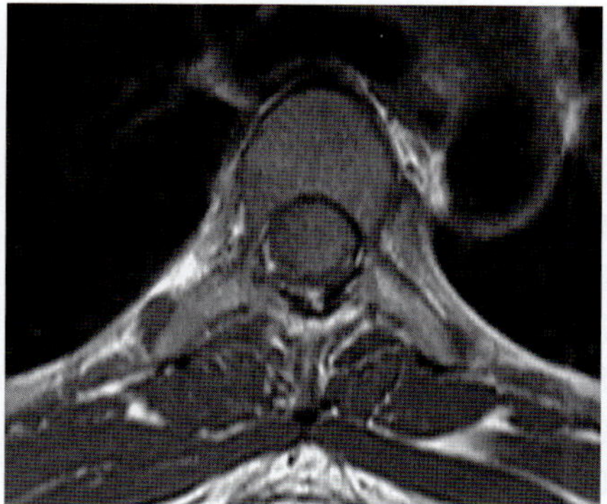

Fig. 4.58.6

Further mangement:
Surgery—total resection for low grade tumors.

Radiotherapy for infiltrative high grade tumors, subtotal resection and recurrent disease.

Prognosis: Less preoperative neurologic deficit at presentation, better postoperative outcome.

Table 4.58.1: Difference between spinal astrocytoma and ependymoma

Spinal astrocytoma	*Ependymoma*
Commoly seen in pediatric age group and young adults as intramedullary spinal cord tumor.	Most common primary spinal cord tumor in adults.
Average age of onset is 30 years.	Fourth to fifth decade of life.
Astrocytomas are more commonly located in the cervico-thoracic or thoracic segments.	**The cervical spinal cord (cellular type)** is the most common location, followed by the thoracic and the **conus medullaris (myxopapillary ependymoma)**.
Long segment involvement compared to ependymoma	Shorter segment involvement
CT and radiographs: Bone remodeling less common	Scoliosis and nonaggressive bone remodeling.
Site: More in eccentric	Site: More in central
Syrinx and hemorrhage: Less common	Hemorrhage more common, cap sign +, cap cyst seen.
Contrast: Ill-defined homogeneous enhancement	Well-defined with intense enhancement
DTI: Destruction of tracts	Displacement of tracts, since it arises from the lining of central part of cord.

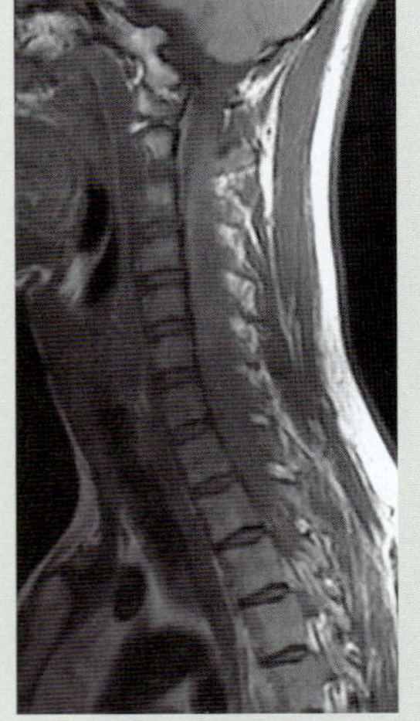
Fig. 4.58.7: Ependymoma

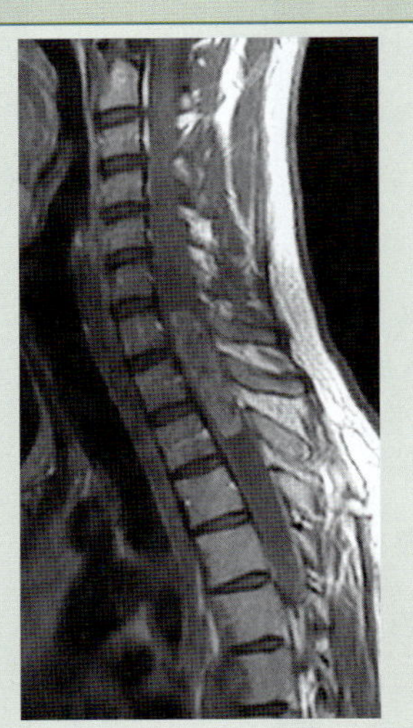
Fig. 4.58.8: Ependymoma

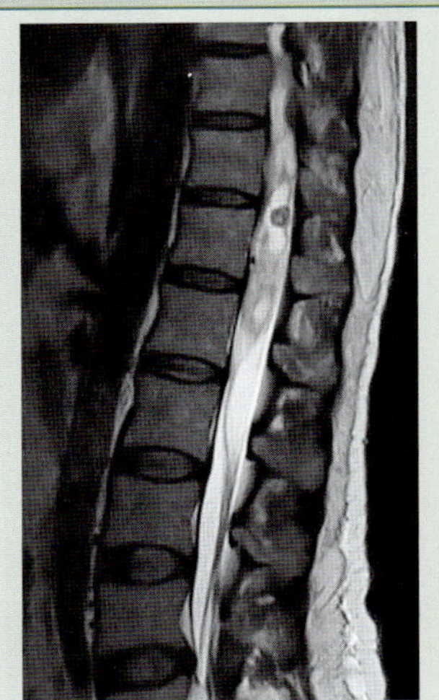
Fig.4.58.9: Hemangioblastoma

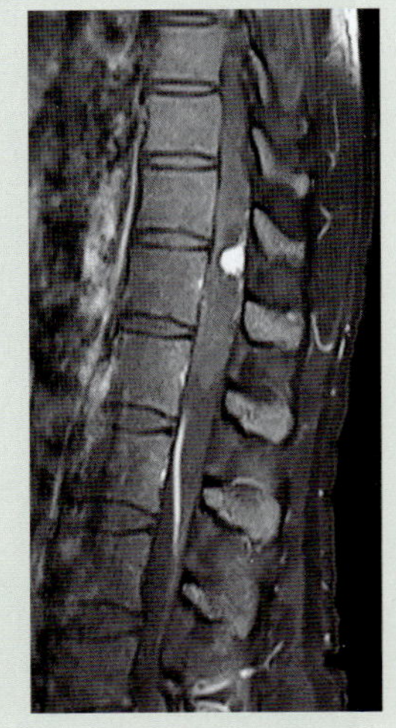
Fig. 4.58.10: Hemangioblastoma

Spinal cord lesions associated with hemorrhage:
- Ependymoma (cap sign)
- Haemangioblastoma
- Paraganglioma
- Hemorrhagic metastasis (thyroid, melanoma)
- Cavernoma
- Cord contusions

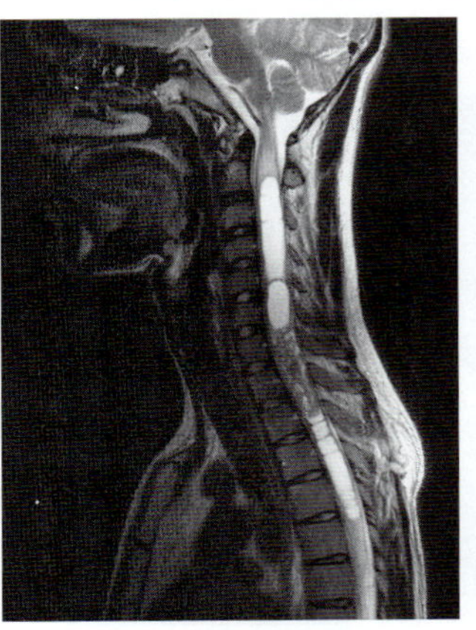
Fig. 4.58.11: Ependymoma—cap sign

Table 4.58.2: Differential diagnosis for intramedullary spinal tumors

Intramedullary spinal metastasis Most common age at presentation 5th to 6th decades. Most common clinical presentation is motor weakness. 1/3rd of patients had simultaneous cerebral metastasis.	Usually involve the cervical cord. The most common primary tumors include lung (small cell), breast, brain, thyroid, urinary bladder colon, lymphoma and kidney. **Rim sign:** Intense, thin rim of peripheral enhancement around enhancing lesion. **Flame sign:** Ill-defined, flame-shaped region of enhancement at superior/inferior margins.	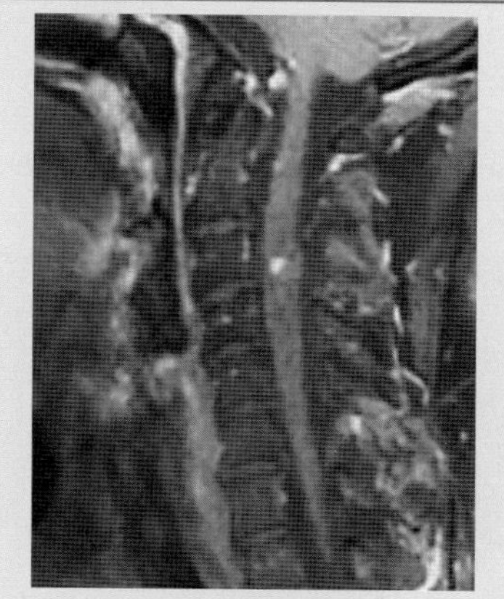 **Fig. 4.58.12:** Intramedullary spinal metastasis
Tuberculoma Rare in spinal cord. Mostly due to hematogenous spread / CSF infection.	The thoracic cord is the most common site. T2 hypointense lesion with T1 post-contrast **ring enhancement.** In case of caseation development of T2WI shows central hypointense peripheral hyperintense **Target sign.**	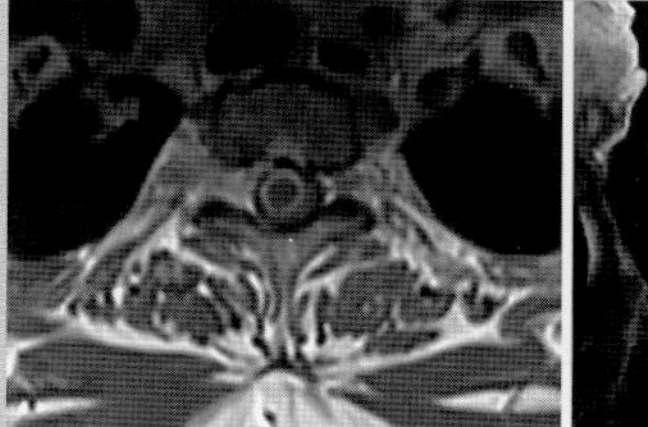 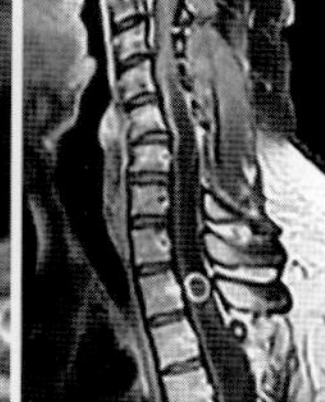 **Fig. 4.58.13:** Tuberculoma
Demyelination (e.g. transverse myelitis, NMO, MS) Most common in young females in 2nd to 3rd decade of age.	Characteristic features of transverse myelitis include involvement of 3 to 4 vertebral body length, central lesion, central enhancement, more than two-thirds cross-sectional area of spinal cord, and most common site is thoracic cord. Acute demyelination shows focal enlargement of cord and follow-up image shows reduction in size.	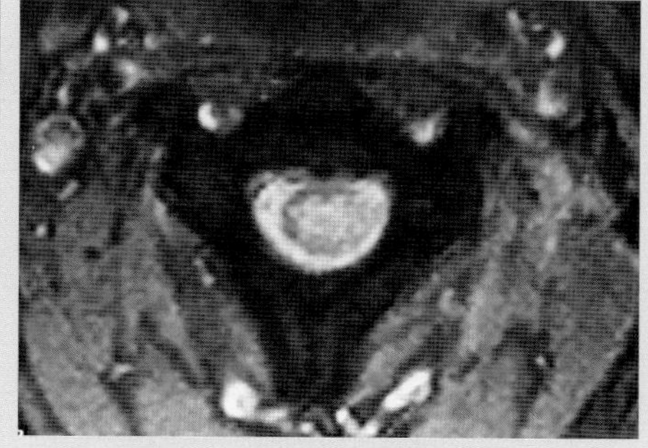 **Fig. 4.58.14:** Transverse myelitis
Cavernoma Common in females in 4th decade. It can be either discrete episodes of neurological deficit or slow progression or acute illness or acute onset of mild symptoms with gradual decline.	Vascular lesion with lobulated, thin sinusoidal vascular channels and no interspersed neural tissue. Heterogeneous mass (locules of blood with "popcorn" appearance) surrounded by dark rim (hemosiderin).	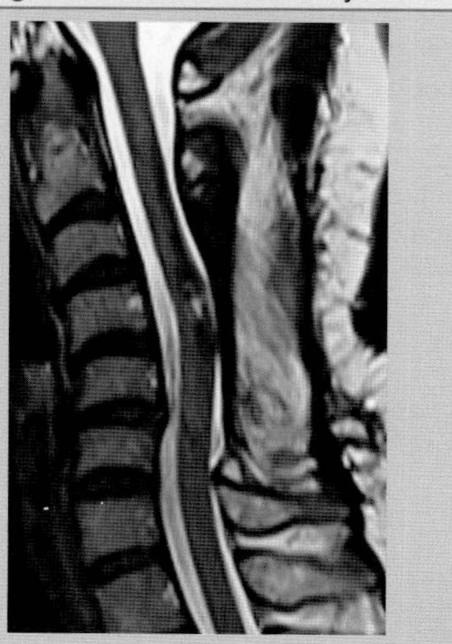 **Fig. 4.58.15:** Cavernoma

(Contd.)

Table 4.58.2: Differential diagnosis for intramedullary spinal tumors *(Contd.)*

<table>
<tr><td>Arteriovenous malformation
Age of presentation between 20–60 years. It can present as progressive myelopathy or catastrophic spinal subarachnoid hemorrhage
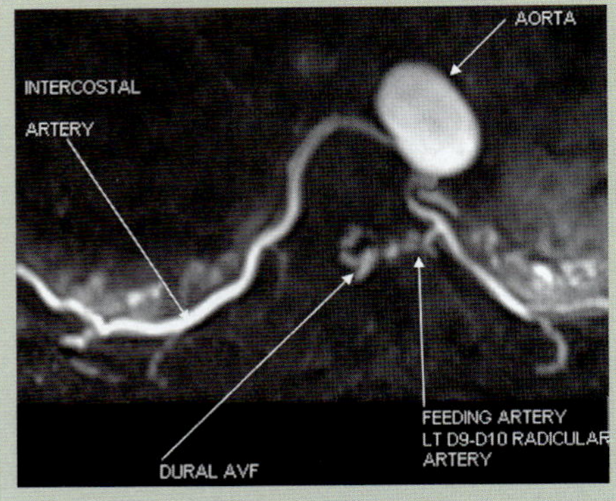

Fig. 4.58.16: Spinal dural AVF</td><td>Spinal arteriovenous malformations contain a true arteriovenous capillary nidus fed by an enlarged feeding artery and drained via an enlarged venous plexus on the cord surface and most commonly occur within the cervical or thoracic cord.</td><td>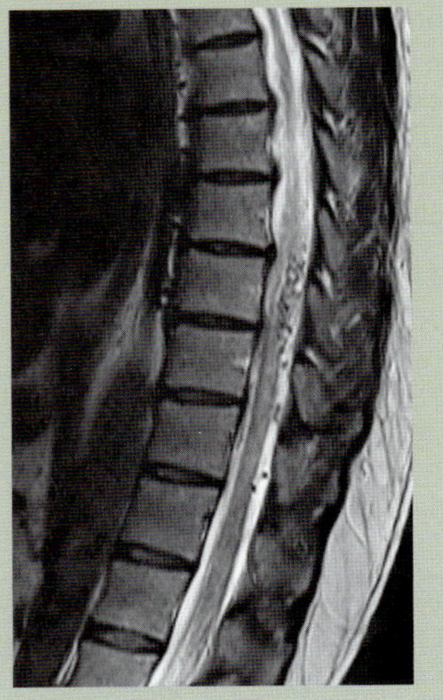
Fig. 4.58.17: Spinal dural AVF</td></tr>
</table>

Table 4.58.3: Approach to spinal cord tumors

Neoplastic lesion	*Age group*	*Location*	*Length and segment distribution*	*Enhancement*
Astrocytoma	Children and young adults	Thoracic> cervical	4–7 vertebral bodies	Heterogeneous
Ependymoma	30–45 years	Cellular ependymoma: Cervical > thoracic. Myxopapillary ependymoma: Conus medullaris	4 vertebral bodies	Solid heterogeneous
Hemangioblastoma	30 years	Thoracic> cervical Eccentric or exophytic	Short segment	Nodular, feeding vessel
Primary melanocytic neoplasm	45 years	Cervical > thoracic	Holocord involvement	Patchy enhancement, no enhancement within tumor center
Metastasis (lung, breast, thyroid, brain)	>50 years	Cervical > thoracic > lumbar	Multiple level segments	Small compared to extent of edema

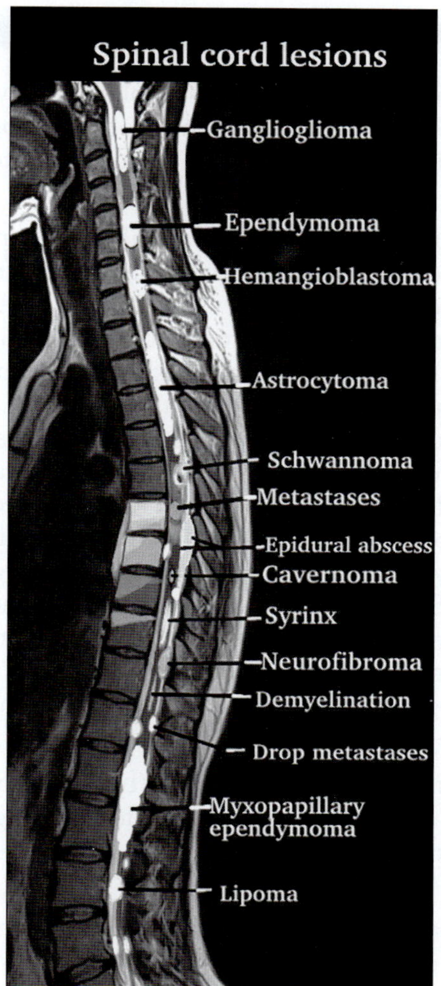

Fig. 4.58.18: Spinal cord lesions

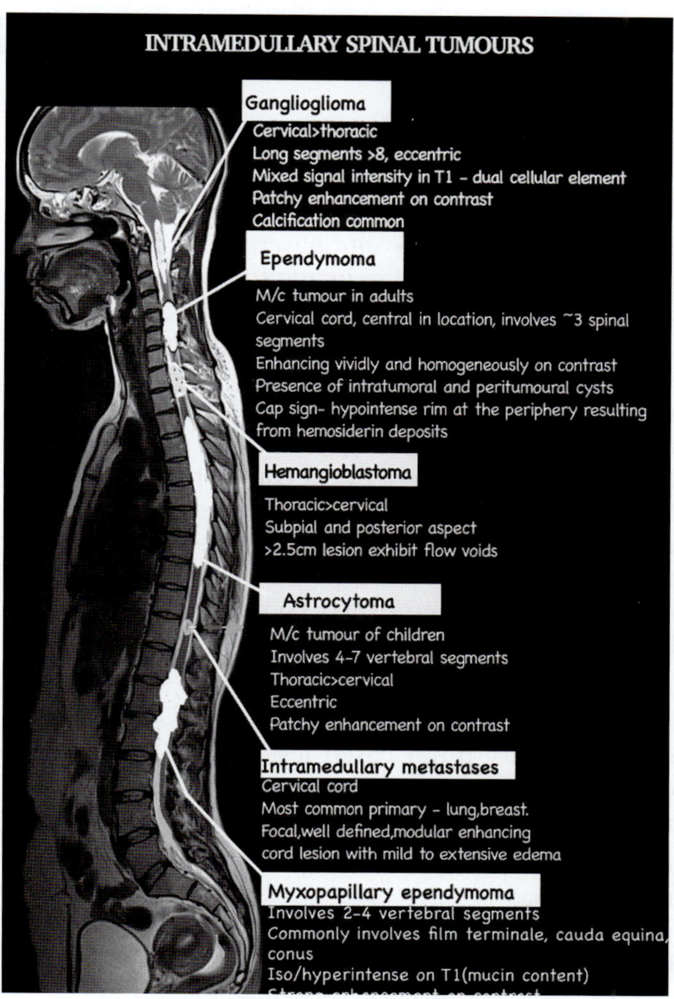

Fig. 4.58.19: Intramedullary spinal tumors

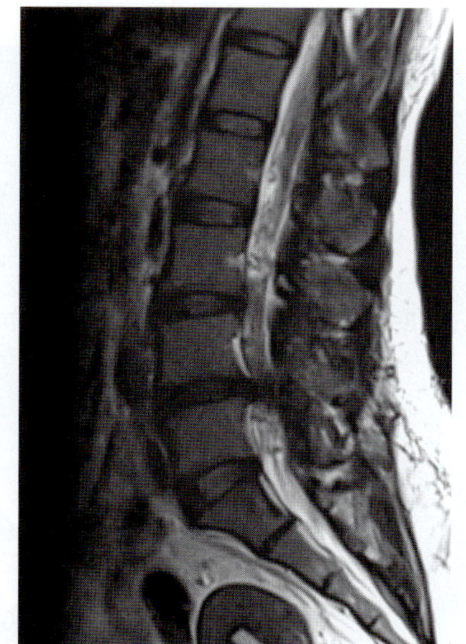

Fig. 4.58.20: Sequestered disc with altered CSF signal intensity and prominent vessels

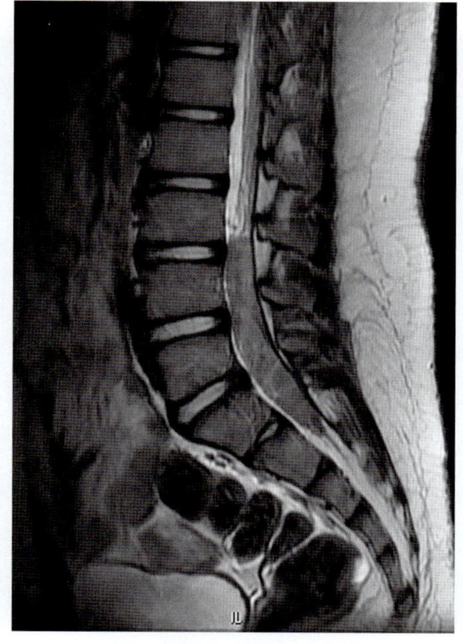

Fig. 4.58.21: Metastasis

4.59 SPINE

Case No. 59

Clinical information: A 66-year-old female with complaints of backache and radicular pain.

Radiological technique and observation: Figure 4.59.1 is MRI T2 sagittal section image showing a solid well-defined T2 hypointense dural-based lesion measuring approximately 8 × 12 × 17 mm at the level of D8-D9 vertebra in the posterolateral aspect, significantly narrowing the dorsal spinal canal. Figure 4.59.2 is MR myelogram image showing focal loss of signal intensity. Figure 4.59.3 is sagittal T1 post-contrast image showing homogeneous enhancement of the lesion with broad dural attachment. Figure 4.59.4 is axial sections show that the cord is displaced to the right with focal cord edema superior to the level of compression. No evident bone remodelling noted.

Interpretation: A—66-years-old female, dorsal spine, B—solid well-defined T2 hypointense intradural extramedullary dural based lesion with homogenous enhancement, C—focal cord edema and no bony remodelling, D—intradural extramedullary meningioma

Principal diagnosis: Intradural extramedullary meningioma.

Further Investigations

Myelogram—meniscus sign—sharp meniscus of contrast seen to be capping the lesion, ipsilateral widening of subarachnoid space, cord roots displaced away from the mass. May result in myelographic block, **Angiography**—early capillary blush-vascular stain well into venous phase.

Discussion: Intradural extramedullary meningioma is a slow-growing benign tumor originating from dura mater. Thoracic (80%)> cervical (16%) > lumbar (4%). Size frequency is roughly proportional to the surface area of dura in spine. Broad dural attachment is characteristic (more of ventral or ventrolateral) associated dural tail may be seen. Multiple meningiomas associated with NF2 radiography may show a focal intraspinal opacity if calcified. May be occult on NECT. Calcification (1–5%) hyperostosis is not a feature of spinal meningiomas. Rare bony remodelling with foraminal enlargement is possible. Strong homogenous contrast enhancement is seen. Isointense to spinal cord on T1W, majority lesion isointense to cord on T2W, hypointense if calcified. Cystic degeneration in 2–4%. Vascular meningiomas may have flow voids. >95% WHO grade 1.

Treatment: Surgical resection (best outcome with Simpson 1 resection). Radiosurgical management—short-term benefits.

Dumbell tumors or tumors extending along neural foramen into spinal canal: Neurofibroma, neuroblastoma, ganglioneuroblastoma, lymphoma, IgG4 disease, metastasis, meningocele/pseudomeningocele, perineural cyst.

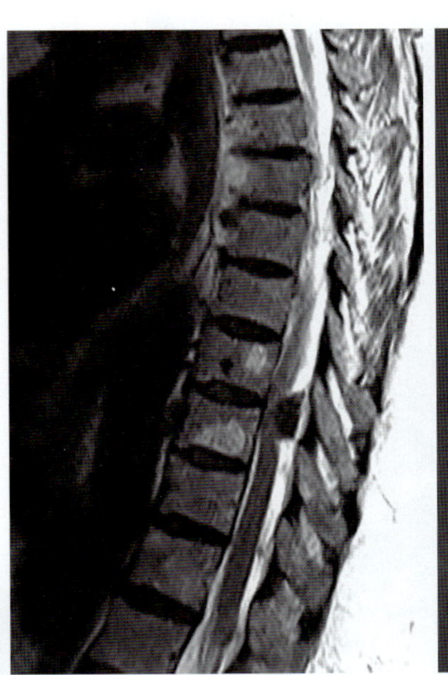
Fig. 4.59.1

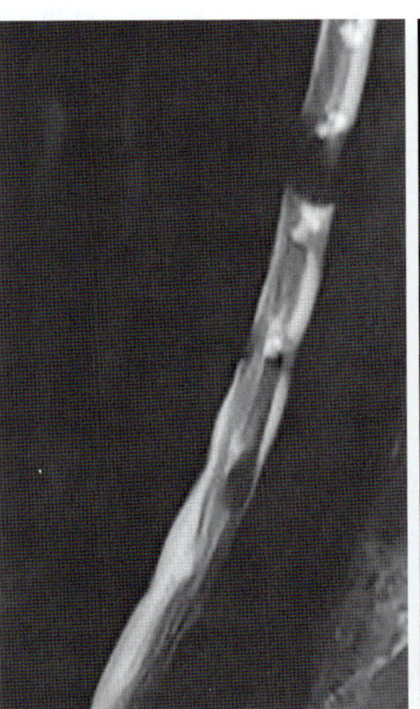
Fig. 4.59.2

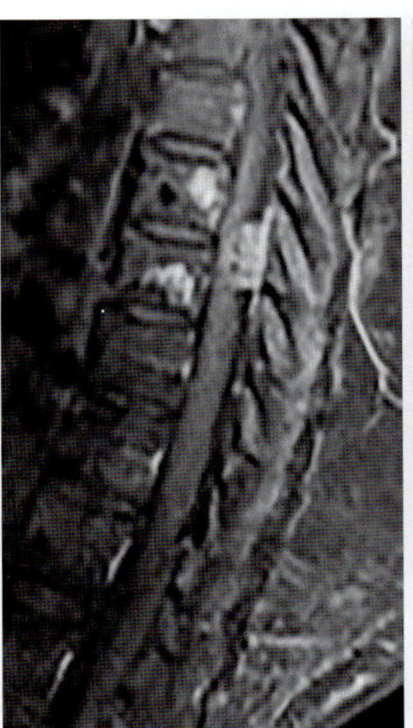
Fig. 4.59.3

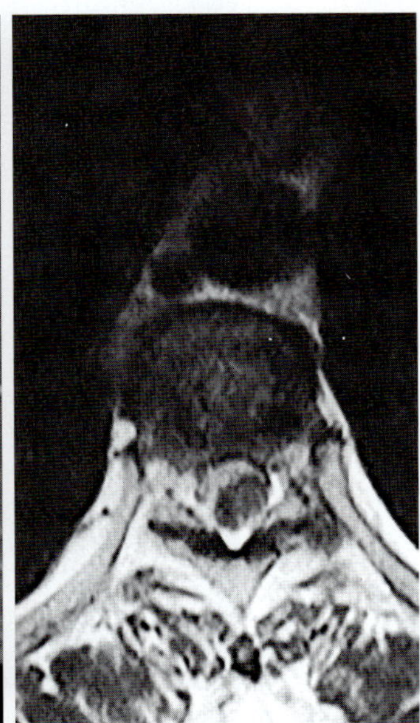
Fig. 4.59.4

Differential diagnosis of spinal lesions		
Schwannoma Age 30–60 years. 30% of primary spine tumors. Total surgical resection. Highly conformal radiosurgery for symptomatic relief with preserved functions 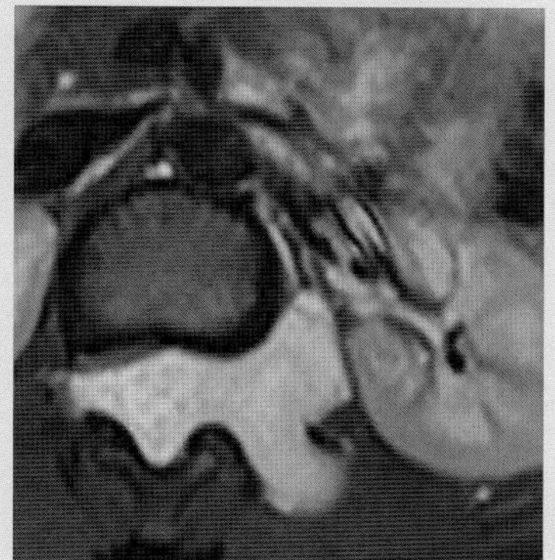 **Fig. 4.59.5:** Schwannoma	Most common intradural extramedullary lesion. 15% extradural, 15% dumbbell-shaped transforaminal. Variable enhancement, heterogeneous, Not dural based, higher signal on T2 with target appearance, cystic changes and bone remodelling + tumor located dorsal to cord is likely to be meningioma, not schwannoma as nerve roots are anterolaterally located. 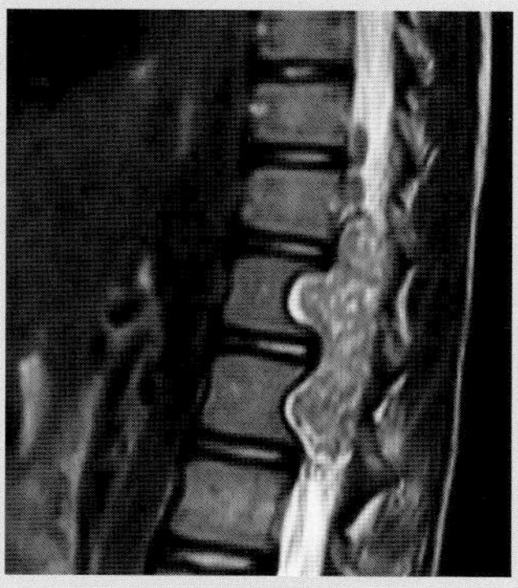 **Fig. 4.59.6:** Schwannoma	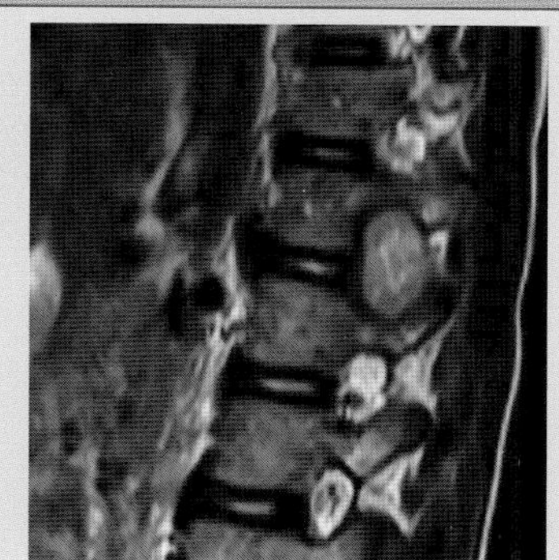 **Fig. 4.59.7:** Schwannoma
Myxopapillary ependymoma All ages, peak 30–40 years. Resection with radiotherapy. Adjuvant therapy for multifocal lesions.	Highly enhancing mass in lumbar canal, not dural based, haemorrhage/hemosiderin cap. Spans 2–4 vertebral segments. Ovoid, lobular-shaped. May cause osseous canal expansion. T2 almost always hyperintense. Intense contrast enhancement.	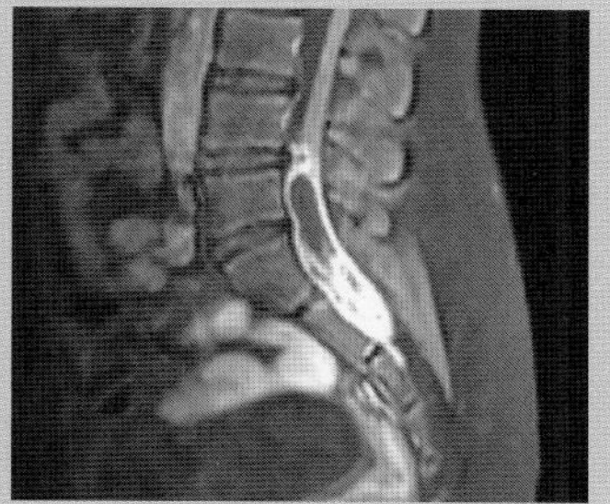 **Fig. 4.59.8:** Myxopapillary ependymoma
(Epi)dermoid cysts Common in children. Mostly acquired. Although present since birth, most congenital epidermoids present at 2nd-4th decade. Males commonly affected	Low T1 signal, similar or mildly increased signal relative to CSF. Lumbar canal/cauda equina common location. Spinal canal widening seen. 40% cases are intramedullary, 60% are extramedullary epidermoids. Acquired epidermoid almost always occurs at cauda equina.	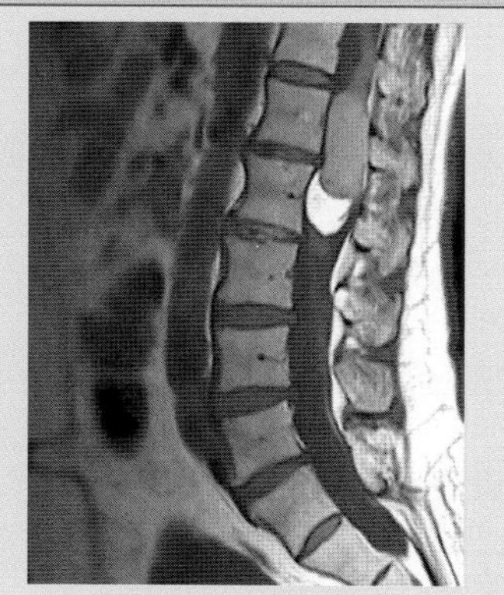 **Fig. 4.59.9:** Epidermoid cyst

Intradural metastasis Age >50 years Steroids, chemotherapy and radiotherapy. Surgery for solitary lesion,	Focal enhancing cord lesions, often multiple, typically <1.5 cm. Enlarged cord on T1. Focal high signal representing edema on T2 STIR. May have hemorrhagic components. Diffuse Leptomeningeal enhancement with sugar coating/ zuckerguss appearance may be seen.	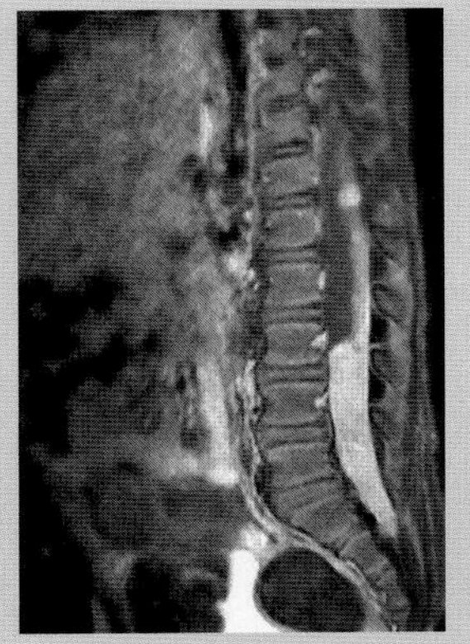 **Fig. 4.59.10:** Intradural mets
Lymphoma Peak 4th–7th decade. Male predominance radiotherapy, chemotherapy and surgical management	Enhancing epidural mass +/– vertebral involvement. Smooth or nodular pial enhancement in lymphomatous leptomeningitis. Intramedullary lymphoma–poorly defined enhancing masses. Extradural > Intradural > Intramedullary. Poor prognosis in CNS lymphoma. Best prognosis with primary osseous lymphoma.	
Subdural effusion/abscess Seen in all age group. Intravenous dexamethasone, percutaneous image-guided catheter drainage or surgery.	Most common in thoracolumbar region. Mass effect on cord and obliteration of subarachnoid space, increased subdural density on CT. T2W hyperintense and T1 hypointense. Rim enhancing fluid collection. Axial sequences to confirm dural location.	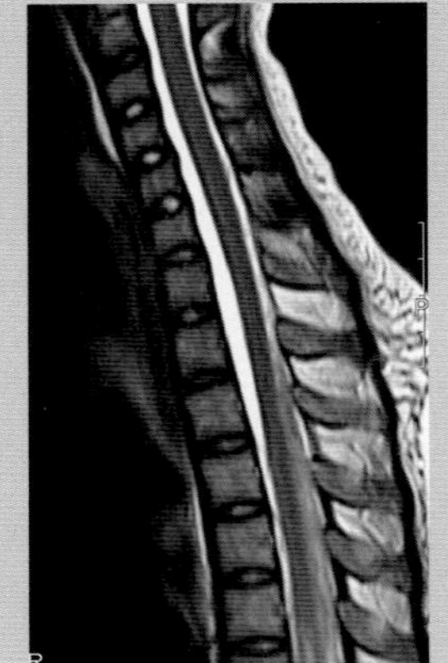 **Fig. 4.59.11:** Subdural effusion

Table 4.59.1: Difference between intramedullary lesions, intradural extramedullary and extradural spine lesions

Intramedullary lesions	*Intradural extramedullary*	*Extradural (predominantly bony pathology)*
Astrocytoma	Schwannoma	Metastasis
Cellular ependymoma	Meningioma	Haemangioma
Hemangioblastoma	Neurofibroma/malignant nerve sheath tumor	Osteoblastoma /osteoid osteoma
Melanocytoma		
Spinal cord metastasis	Hemangiopericytoma	Osteochondroma/chondrosarcoma
Ganglioglioma	Paraganglioma	Aneurysmal bone cyst
Infarct	Subdural effusion/empyema	Osteosarcoma/Ewing sarcoma
Demyelination	Metastasis	Chordoma
Granuloma		Lymphoma, leukemia, multiple myeloma
Intramedullary cystic lesions—epidermoid, neurenteric cyst, etc.		LCH Prolapsed disc Abscess Arachnoid cyst
Lipoma		Angiolipoma, extradural lipomatosis
Hematoma		Neuroblastoma
Edema		IgG4 disease, extradural haemorrhage, prominent veins, neurofibroma

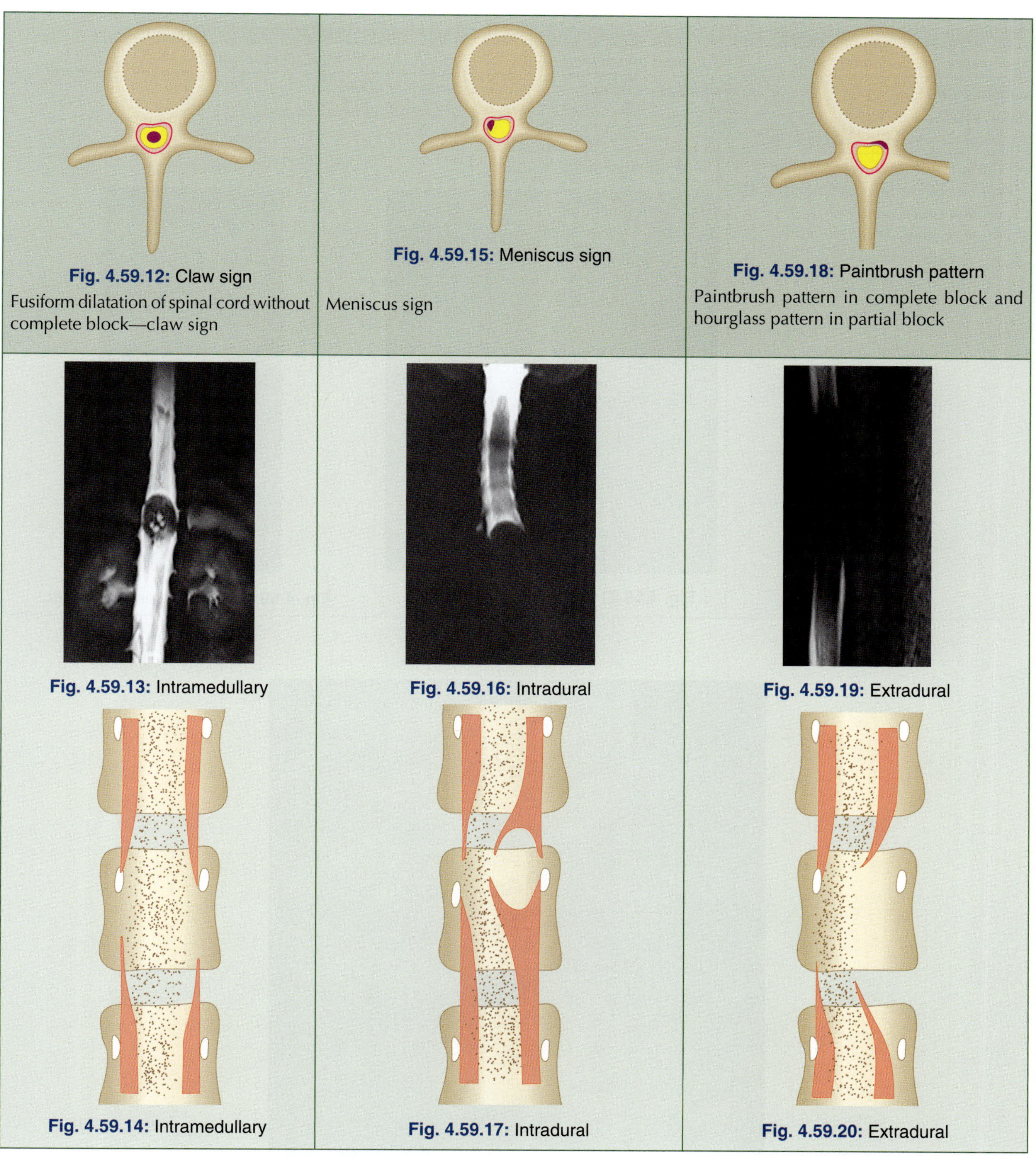

Fig. 4.59.12: Claw sign

Fusiform dilatation of spinal cord without complete block—claw sign

Fig. 4.59.15: Meniscus sign

Meniscus sign

Fig. 4.59.18: Paintbrush pattern

Paintbrush pattern in complete block and hourglass pattern in partial block

Fig. 4.59.13: Intramedullary

Fig. 4.59.16: Intradural

Fig. 4.59.19: Extradural

Fig. 4.59.14: Intramedullary

Fig. 4.59.17: Intradural

Fig. 4.59.20: Extradural

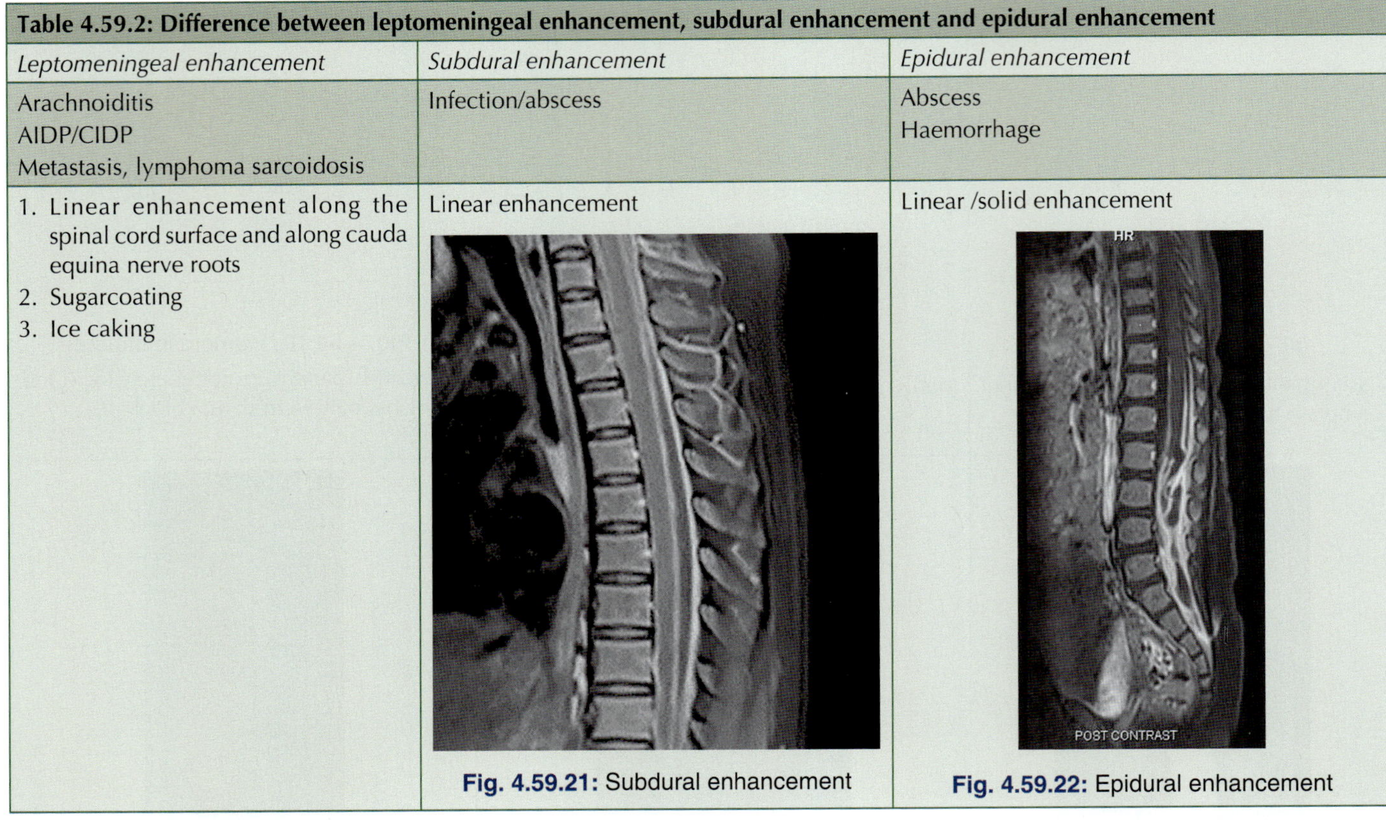

Table 4.59.2: Difference between leptomeningeal enhancement, subdural enhancement and epidural enhancement

Leptomeningeal enhancement	*Subdural enhancement*	*Epidural enhancement*
Arachnoiditis AIDP/CIDP Metastasis, lymphoma sarcoidosis	Infection/abscess	Abscess Haemorrhage
1. Linear enhancement along the spinal cord surface and along cauda equina nerve roots 2. Sugarcoating 3. Ice caking	Linear enhancement **Fig. 4.59.21:** Subdural enhancement	Linear /solid enhancement HR POST CONTRAST **Fig. 4.59.22:** Epidural enhancement

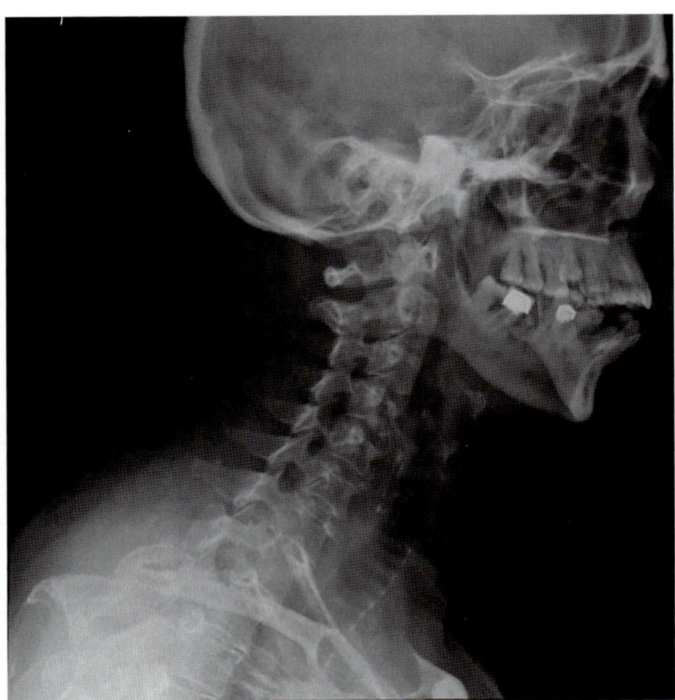

Fig. 4.59.23: Image showing cervical spine radiograph in the oblique view with widening of the C5 neural foramen

Plain X-ray signs of intraspinal tumor: Neural foramen widening on oblique images, scalloping, interpedicular distance widening.

4.60 SPINE

Case No. 60

Clinical history: 45 years old female with complaints of low back ache for 6 months.

Radiological techniques and observations: Figures 4.60.1 to 4.60.4 are MRI dorsolumbar spine with T1, T2 and STIR sagittal images, myelogram showing T1 hypointensity (to muscle) T2 STIR hyperintensity noted in the D12 and L2 vertebral bodies, with involvement of the posterior elements of L2 vertebra. A severe compression fracture of D12 vertebral body is seen, with a fluid cleft and posterior bulging of the posterior cortex of the vertebral body causing compression of the anterior thecal sac and mild narrowing of spinal canal, with no T2 cord hyperintensity. Prevertebral and paravertebral soft tissues appear normal in the visualised images. There is also a small fracture of the inferior vertebral plate of L2 vertebra. MR myelogram shows **"paintbrush"** appearance. Figure 4.60.5 is **sodium fluoride PET scan** showing increased tracer uptake at D12 and L2 vertebra. Tracer uptake in the right wrist may be due to injection site. Tracer uptake in the rest of the sites is physiological.

Interpretation: A: 45 years old female lumbosacral spine, B: T1 hypointense T2 STIR hyperintense lesion in vertebral bodies, which show increased tracer uptake in sodium fluoride PET scan, C: Fluid cleft and posterior bulging of the posterior cortex of the vertebral body causing compression of the anterior thecal sac and mild narrowing of spinal canal, D: Vertebral metastases.

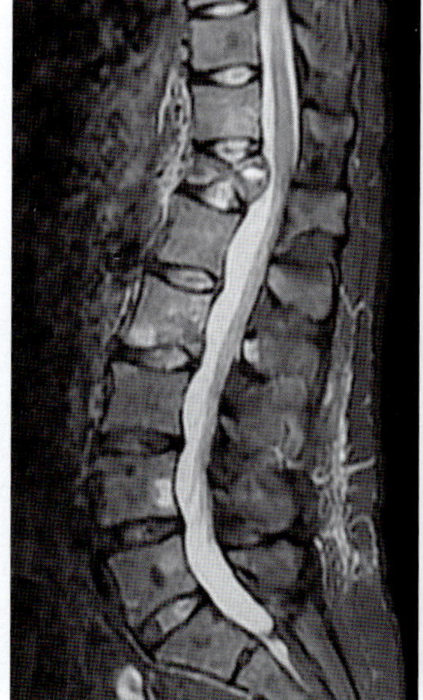

Fig. 4.60.3

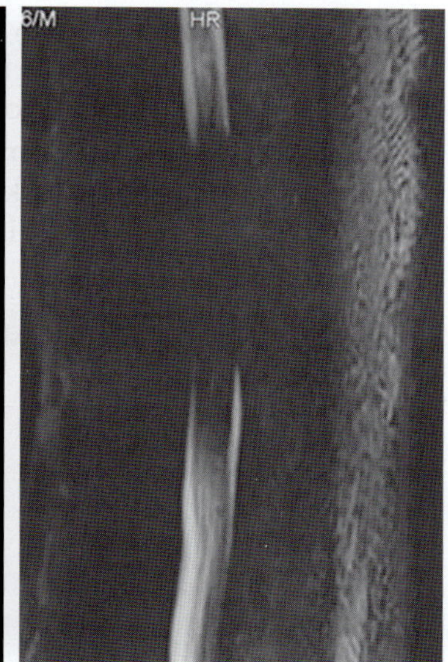

Fig. 4.60.4

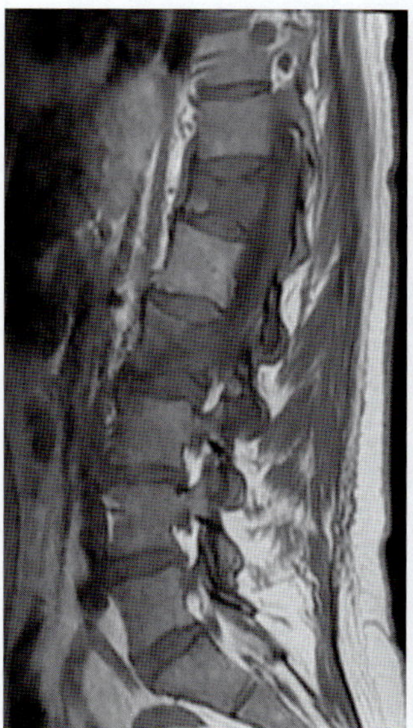

Fig. 4.60.1

Fig. 4.60.2

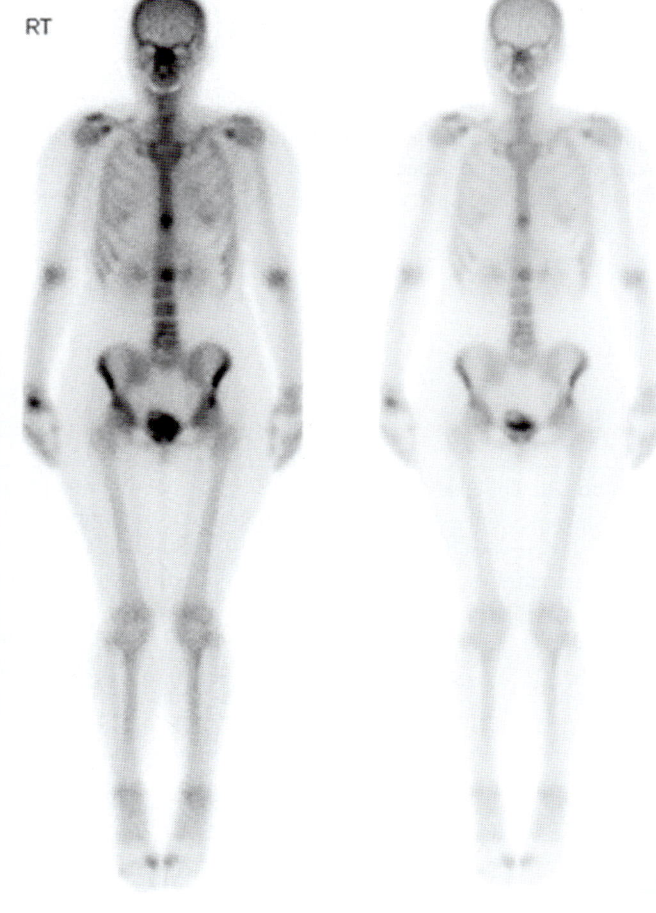

Fig. 4.60.5

Principal diagnosis: Vertebral metastases.

Differential diagnosis:

1. **Hematopoietic malignancy:** Diffuse marrow involvement more common than in metastasis. (a) Plasmacytoma, (b) Multiple myeloma (MM), (c) Lymphoma
2. **Benign (osteoporotic) compression fracture** 1/3 of fractures in patients with known primary tumor are benign. 1/4 of fractures in apparently osteopenic patients are from malignant disease. **The fluid cleft sign although pathognomic of a benign collapse may sometimes occur in a malignant collapse of vertebral body too.**
   Marrow signal with late subacute/chronic benign fractures similar to normal marrow (suppresses on STIR).
3. **Invasive haemangioma.**
4. **Schmorl's node.**

Table 4.60.1: Differential diagnosis for extradural spine lesion

Diffferential diagnosis	*Imaging findings*	*Image*
Plasmacytoma Mean age is 55 years (younger than patients with multiple myeloma) Gender: M > F (2:1) Spine is most common site. 20% have solitary lesions in rib, sternum, clavicle and scapula.	Radiography can be normal in early period. Lytic, multicystic-appearing lesion ± vertical dense striations. CT shows lytic, destructive vertebral body lesion. Compression fracture ± associated soft tissue mass. Pathologic compression fracture common. "Mini brain" appearance due to thick cortical struts in expanded vertebral body. Posterior elements involved in most cases ± associated soft tissue mass (paraspinous or epidural with "draped curtain" sign).	**Fig. 4.60.6:** Plasmacytoma
Lymphoma Occurs in adults, peak at 4th–7th decade. Slight male predominance. Most common presenting symptom is back pain.	Long bones > spine. Extradural > intradural > intramedullary. Epidural lymphoma: Thoracic > lumbar > cervical; enhancing epidural mass ± vertebral involvement. T1 post-contrast shows diffuse uniform enhancement. 67Ga scintigraphy has high sensitivity and specificity for diagnosis.	**Fig. 4.60.7:** Lymphoma
Osteoporotic collapse Increasing incidence with increasing age, **M < < F**. Progressive disease, with continual loss of bone marrow density (BMD).	May be difficult to distinguish acute osteoporotic compression fracture—DWI may be helpful. MR is extremely useful for detection of incomplete fragility or insufficiency fractures. MRI and bone scintigraphy help decide the age of the fracture, when radiograph is equivocal. Dual energy X-ray absorptiometry (DEXA) is the preferred modality to determine BMD.	**Fig. 4.60.8:** Osteoporotic collapse

(Contd.)

Table 4.60.1: Differential diagnosis for extradural spine lesion (*Contd.*)

Diffferential diagnosis	*Imaging findings*	*Image*
Invasive hemangioma Rare form of vertebral hemangioma with significant vertebral expansion, extra-osseous component with epidural extension.	Can cause disturbance of blood flow, and occasionally compression fractures can be present causing spinal cord and/or nerve root compression. **Thickened trabeculae appear as low signal areas in both T1 and T2 images.** The extraosseous component typically follows usual hemangioma signal intensity in all sequences with **high T1 and T2 signals** as well as uniform post-contrast enhancement.	**Fig. 4.60.9 and 4.60.10:** Invasive hemangioma
Schmorl node Adolescents and young adults. **M >> F**, up to **9:1** ratio. Seen in up to 75% of all normal spines. Can occur with single traumatic episode.	**Plain films:** Contour defect within endplate, extending from disc space into vertebral body spongiosa with well-corticated margins. **CT:** Island of low density surrounded by condensed bone on axial slice through vertebral body. **MR:** Focal defect in endplate filled by disc ± adjacent marrow edema, fatty marrow conversion. Acute Schmorl's nodes have been reported to be FDG-PET avid.	**Fig. 4.60.11:** Schmorl node

Management: **Patient's findings to be immediately communicated to the oncology department for further evaluation and to be posted for tumor board discussion for a multimodality approach.** 1. Cross sectional imaging to look for the morphology of the lesion. 2. To do biopsy to confirm the diagnosis by histopathology. 3. Search for the primary tumor. Surgical decompression, stabilization is done. Radiation therapy may also be choice. Pain managed with NSAIDS or opioid analgesics.

Brief discussion about the condition: **Osteolytic metastasis:** Spine is the most common site of osseous metastases. Lesion distribution proportional to red marrow (lumbar > thoracic > cervical). **MRI scan:** T1 hypointense, replacing normal T1 hyperintense marrow (discs "brighter" than bone) ± compression fracture. Paravertebral and epidural soft tissue—**"Curtain" sign**. Intervertebral discs are generally spared. T2 hypointense → hyperintense to normal marrow. **Tc99m bone scan:** Tracer avidity in regions of bone production at margins of tumor, and not directly by lytic tumor. False-negatives are seen with aggressive lytic tumor and very small lesions.

PET: FDG PET has better specificity but lower sensitivity for detecting malignant bone metastases when compared with bone scan. FDG PET/CT has better specificity for detection of malignant involvement of spine than does FDG PET alone.

Radiograph lumbosacral spine AP view shows lytic lesion in the L1 vertebra, with destruction of the left pedicle. Right pedicle appears normal.

Differential diagnosis for erosion of a pedicle (winking owl sign):

1. Metastasis
2. Multiple myeloma
3. Neurofibroma—often causes erosion of adjacent pedicle or pedicles. Chronic intramedullary tumours, typically ependymoma, cause flattening of both pedicles at affected levels, with a widened inter-pedicular distance.
4. TB—uncommonly, especially with a large paravertebral abscess.
5. Osteomyelitis
6. Benign bone tumour—aneurysmal bone cyst or giant cell tumor.
7. Congenital absence— ± sclerosis of the contralateral pedicle.

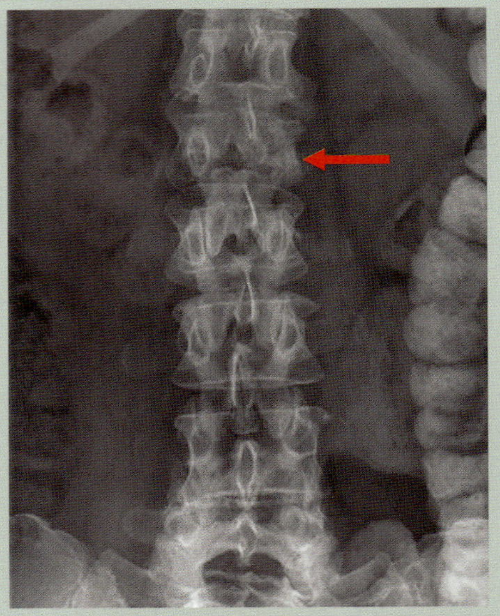

Fig. 4.60.12: Winking owl sign

Table 4.60.2: Difference between lytic bone metastasis and sclerotic bone metastasis

Lytic bone metastasis	*Sclerotic bone metastasis*
Primary: Renal, lung, breast, thyroid, GI tract, urothelial, ovarian, melanoma and paraganglioma. **Expansile lytic lesion:** 1. Giant cell tumor 2. Aneurysmal bone cyst 3. Enchondroma 4. Non-ossifying fibroma 5. Chondromyxoid fibroma	**Primary in adults:** Prostate, breast, lung, carcinoid, bladder, nasopharynx, pancreas **Primary in children:** Medulloblastoma, neuroblastoma, Ewing sarcoma
Differential diagnosis: 1. Hematopoietic malignancy 2. Benign (osteoporotic) compression fracture 3. Schmorl's node 4. Normal heterogeneous marrow 5. Spondylodiscitis 6. Osteosarcoma 7. Discogenic sclerosis	**Differential diagnosis:** 1. Treated metastases 2. Paget disease 3. Hemangioma

Table 4.60.3: Skeletal metastases: Tracer uptake patterns pn Tc-99m bone scan

Hot lesions	*Cold lesions*	*Isointense lesions*
Breast cancer	Renal cell carcinoma	Renal cell carcinoma
Lung cancer	Thyroid carcinoma	Thyroid carcinoma
Prostate cancer	Anaplastic neoplasms	Anaplastic neoplasms
Transitional cell carcinoma	Neuroblastoma	Neuroblastoma
Colorectal cancer		Multiple myeloma
Medulloblastoma		Reticulum cell sarcoma
Osteosarcoma		Histiocytosis
Neuroendocrine tumors (carcinoid)		Leukemia, lymphoma
Lymphoma		

4

Table 4.60.4: Difference between NaF PET scan and Tc99m bone scan

	NaF PET scan	*Tc-99m bone scan*
Agent used	18F sodium fluoride	Tc-99m MDP (Medronate) and Tc-99m HDP (TechneScan)
Mechanism	The mechanism of uptake is incorporation of fluoride ions into the bone matrix in sites of newly mineralizing bone, such as during growth, infection, malignancy (primary or secondary), after trauma, or during inflammation.	Both (Tc-99m MDP and Tc-99m HDP) are bone-seeking agents that undergo physicochemical adsorption (chemisorption) to the hydroxyapatite structure of bone tissue. Therefore, more uptake is seen in bone-forming pathology or growth regions of immature bone in the presence of osteoblasts.
Resolution	Greater sensitivity and better spatial resolution	Lesser compared to NaF
Pharmacokinetics	Better, with 2x greater bone uptake and faster blood clearance, making total exam time shorter	Inferior compared to NaF, and total exam time is longer
Radiation exposure to the patient	68% greater than Tc-99m scan	Lesser when compared to NaF PET scan

18F NaF PET scan	*18F FDG PET scan*
Detects osteoblastic tumors, infections, trauma and inflammation, as it is a bone seeking agent (action on the bone matrix)	Poor sensitivity for osteoblastic lesions
Greater sensitivity and better spatial resolution than bone scan in detecting osteoblastic lesions	More sensitive and specific for osteolytic lesions (round cell tumors, lymphoma)
False negative scan: Tumors confined to marrow may have no significant cortical remodelling and may not be visualized (more common in Tc-99m bone scan)	Detects marrow lesions in F18 FDG avid disease prior to cortical involvement (often before bone scan becomes positive)

CT guided vertebral biopsy: Figure 4.60.13 with the patient laying prone, CT scan is taken for planning purpose. A suitable skin site is identified and marked. The patient is prepared and draped for aseptic precaution. Skin and periosteal local anesthesia with lignocaine 1% given. Light intravenous sedation may be needed in a few. CT-guided biopsy is performed through the lytic lesion on the left aspect of D11. Sample is placed in formalin and sent for histopathology.

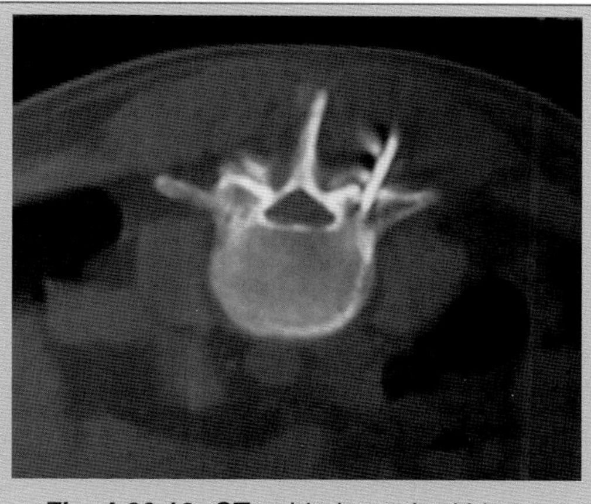

Fig. 4.60.13: CT guided vertebral biopsy

Table 4.60.5: Differential diagnosis for epidural lesions

Epidural lesions		
Bony		*Non-bony*
Primary tumors	Lymphoma	Epidural lipomatosis
Hemangioma	Myeloma	Epidural abscess
Osteoid osteoma	Plasmacytoma	Epidural metastases
Osteoblastoma	LCH	Epidural lymphoma
Aneurysmal bone cyst	Angiolipoma	IgG4-related disease/hypertrophic Pachymeningitis
Giant cell tumor	**Secondary:** Metastases	Prominent venous plexus
Osteochondroma	**Infections**	Epidural hematoma
Chondrosarcoma		Epidural haemangioma
Osteosarcoma		Disc extrusion/sequestration
Chordoma		Ossification of ligaments (PLL)

4.61 SPINE

Case No. 61

Clinical history: 20-year female with back pain for 2 months and lower limb weakness

Radiological techniques and observations: Figure 4.61.1 is frontal chest radiograph showing trachea in midline, bilateral bronchi appear normal, bilateral lungs appear clear. There is focal widening of left para spinal line with expansile lytic lesion involving the left pedicle of D10 vertebra—absent pedicle sign (winking owl sign). There is destruction of lateral border of the vertebra with preserved disc space. Both diaphragms appear normal. Rest of the visualised vertebrae appears normal.

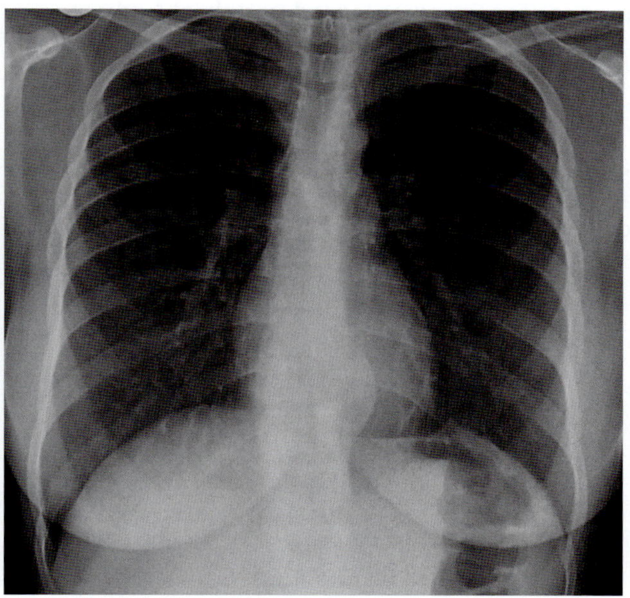

Fig. 4.61.1

With these findings, the differential diagnosis includes:

- Spondylitis with paravertebral abscess, metastasis,
- Osteoblastoma, aneurysmal bone cyst, giant cell tumor.
- Plasmacytoma, congenital absent pedicle (less likely due to soft tissue component). Further cross sectional imaging is required.

Figures 4.61.2 and 4.61.3 are CT axial, coronal and sagittal reformatted images showing an expansile lytic lesion with sclerotic margins involving the vertebral body extending to pedicle with lobulated margins and thin septations in the periphery, narrowing the spinal canal, with narrow zone of transition, focal cortical destruction. Adjacent pre-vertebral and para-vertebral extraosseous extension of the lesion in the left lateral aspect. No evidence of adjacent periosteal reaction/osteoid/chondroid matrix noted.

With these findings, a focal benign vertebral lesion could be considered as the principal diagnosis.

Figures 4.61.4 and 4.61.5 are T1 axial and T2 axial MRI images showing the expansile bone lesion with lobulated margins (blown out appearance) with thin septa, cortical thinning (egg shell), involving the vertebral body predominantly expanding in the left lateral aspect, extending to left pedicle with multiple fluid-fluid levels with haemorrhagic products. No evidence of any cortical breach. No extraosseous soft tissue component.

Interpretation: A—20-years-old female, body and left pedicle of D10 vertebra. B—expansile lytic lesion with lobulated margins and fluid-fluid levels, C—no evidence of any periosteal reaction/cortical breach/extraosseous soft tissue component, D—aneurysmal bone cyst.

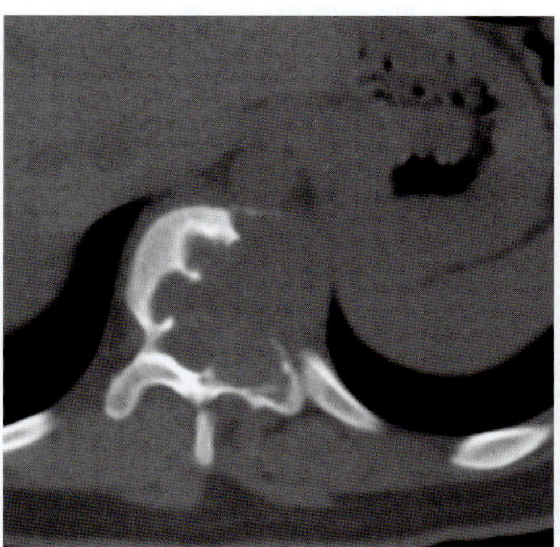

Fig. 4.61.2

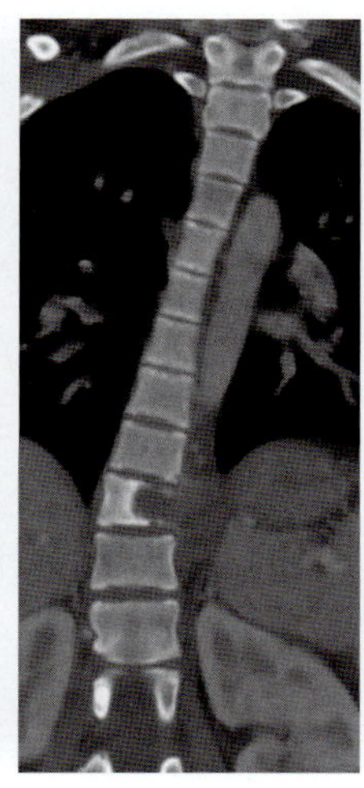

Fig. 4.61.3

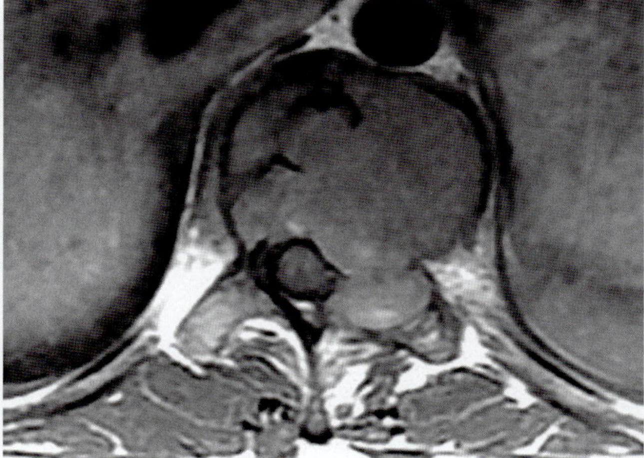

Fig. 4.61.4

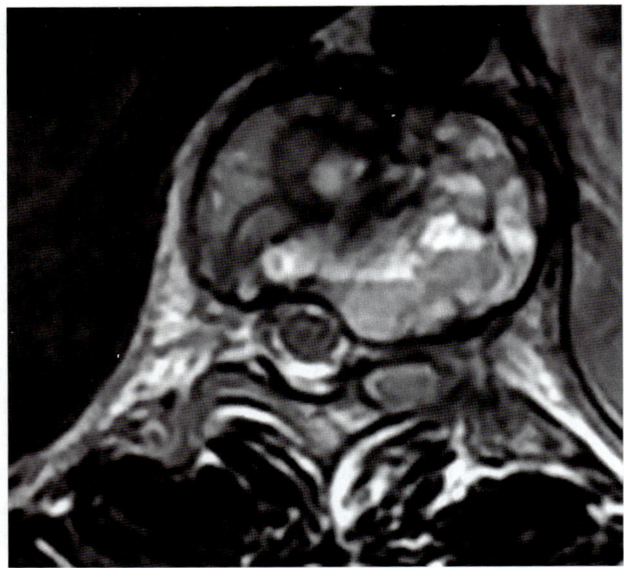

Fig. 4.61.5

Principal diagnosis: Aneurysmal bone cyst

Bone lesions with fluid-fluid levels:

1. Aneurysmal bone cyst
2. Telangiectatic osteosarcoma
3. Chondroblastoma
4. Simple bone cyst
5. Giant cell tumor
6. Osteoblastoma
7. Fibroxanthoma

Causes for secondary ABC

1. Giant cell tumor
2. Chondroblastoma
3. Fibrous dysplasia
4. Non-ossifying fibroma

Other causes for an enlarged vertebral body.

Table 4.61.1: Differential diagnosis for aneurysmal bone cyst		
Osteoblastoma 2nd–3rd decades	Expansile lesion of neural arch with bone matrix visible on plain films or CT. May be associated with ABC Sclerotic lesion more than 2 cm	Fig. 4.61.6: Osteoblastoma
Metastasis Older patients	Involves vertebral body and neural arch. Destructive lesion with associated soft tissue mass. Rare: Vascular metastasis can have fluid-fluid levels	Fig. 4.61.7: Metastasis

Contd...

Table 4.61.1: Differential diagnosis for aneurysmal bone cyst *(Contd...)*

Plasmacytoma Older patients, usually over 40 years old	Involves vertebral body, usually spares neural arch. May expand vertebral body without destruction of cortex: Mini brain appearance—cerebriform pattern	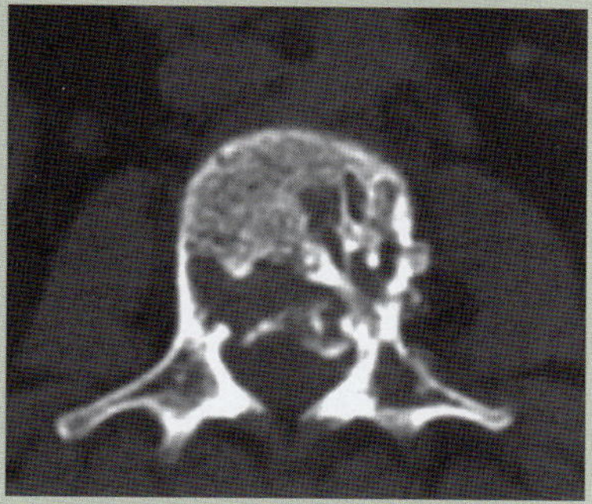 **Fig. 4.61.8:** Plasmacytoma
Aggressive hemangioma Can occur at any age with peak prevalence in young adults	T1/T2 hyperintensity with soft tissue component which may extend to spinal canal CT-polka dot sign, corduroy sign	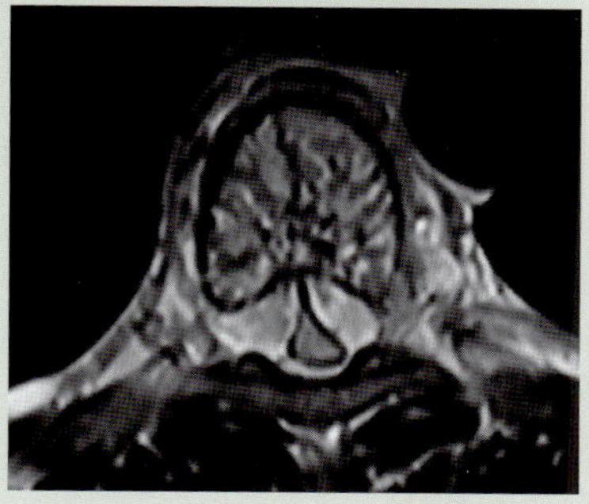 **Fig. 4.61.9:** Aggressive hemangioma
Spondylitis with abscess	T1 hypointensity with T2 hyperintensity with soft tissue component, subligamentous spread, disc involvement, contrast enhancement	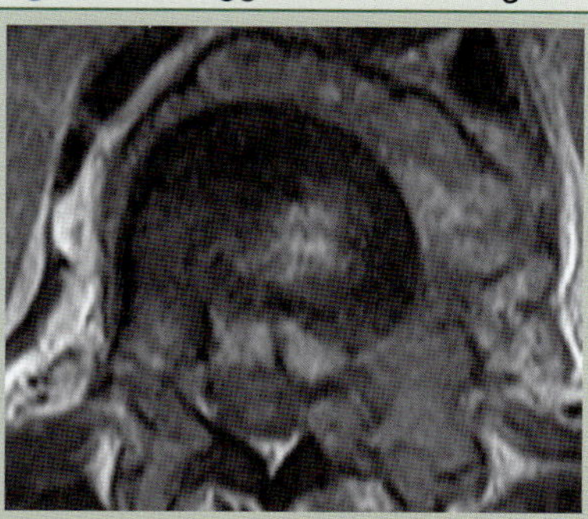 **Fig. 4.61.10:** TB spondylitis with abscess
Giant cell tumor Slightly older patients 3rd, 4th decade	Originates in vertebral body rather than neural arch. Expansile lytic lesion with soft tissue mass. May be associated with ABC.	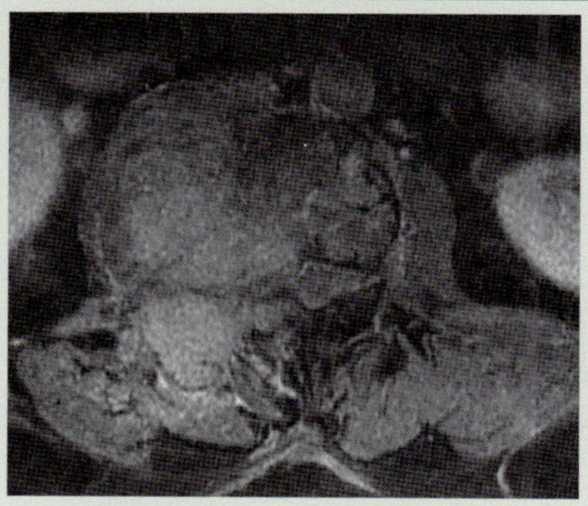 **Fig. 4.61.11:** GCT
Telangiectatic osteosarcoma	Involves vertebral body and neural arch with fluid-fluid levels, usually destroys the bone cortex rather than expanding it, permeative bone destruction with wider zone of transition, infiltrates surrounding soft tissues	

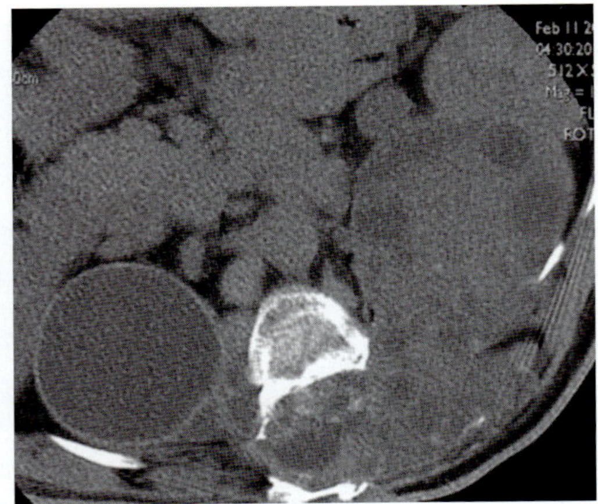

Fig. 4.61.12: Spine hydatid

Generalised enlargement: Gigantism, acromegaly.

Local (single/multiple vertebrae) enlargement: Paget's disease, fibrous dysplasia, hydatid cyst (image showing intramuscular-osseous hydatidosis with involvement of posterior elements).

ABC Age—less than 20 years, 10–30% occur in spine and sacrum.

Table 4.61.2: Classification of spinal bone tumors

Benign	*Malignant*
Osteoid osteoma	*Focal:*
Aneurysmal bone cyst	Osteosarcoma
Osteoblastoma	Ewing sarcoma
Osteochondroma	Chondrosarcoma
Giant cell tumor	Chordoma
Chondroblastoma	Plasmacytoma
Hemangioma	*Multiple:*
Eosinophilic granuloma (in children)	Metastasis
	Lymphoma/leukaemia
	Multiple myeloma

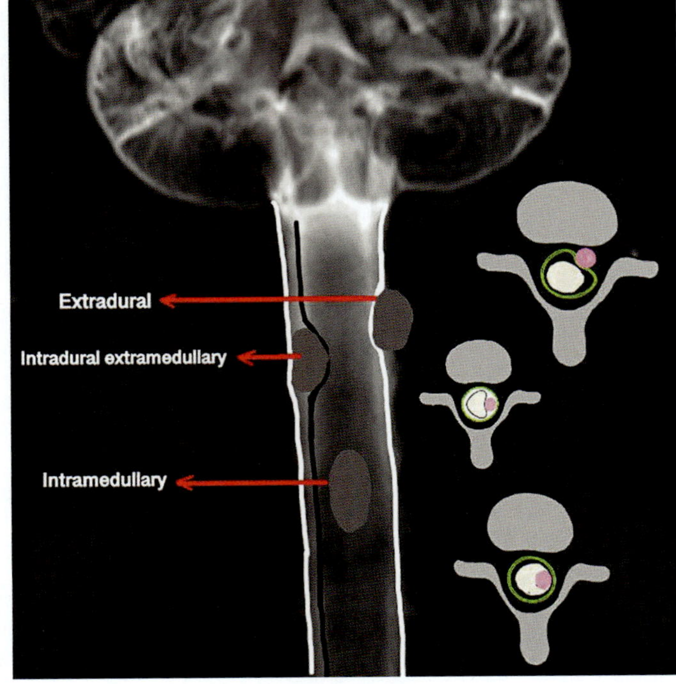

Fig. 4.61.13

Arise in neural arch and 70–90% extend into vertebral body.

Types: Primary and secondary (GCT and osteoblastoma).

Angiography: Hypervascular with vessels prominent at the periphery, drape around the lesions.

Nuclear medicine: May have rim of activity with central photopenic region—doughnut sign

Management: Referral to orthopaedic surgeon. Embolization followed by surgical excision and curettage with bone grafting. May require instrumentation for stabilisation of spine.

4.62 SPINE

Case No. 62

Clinical information: 9 months child with dyspnoea, cough.

Radiological technique and observation: Figure 4.62.1 frontal radiograph shows a well-defined lesion in the right upper zone causing mild mediastinal shift to the opposite side. The lesion extends above the level of clavicle. Remaining lung appears normal. Inferior border forms a convex margin with the lung (not a straight line to suggest consolidation), medial border of the lesion is not seen, it forms an obtuse angle with the mediastinum. No evidence of calcification/fat/air bronchogram. No evidence of lung collapse. No obvious evidence of adjacent rib changes in X-ray.

Figure 4.62.2 is CT axial sections at cervical level image showing a midline vertebral cleft and segmentation anomaly of the lower cervical vertebra. The cord also shows anterior cleft at that level. Figures 4.62.3 to 4.62.5 are MRI axial and sagittal sections showing well-circumscribed T2 hyperintense lesion predominantly from the posterior mediastinum extending to the middle mediastinum extending to the spinal canal through the posterior spinal defect.

Interpretation: A–9 months old, posterior mediastinum B–well-defined T2 hyperintense lesion predominantly from the posterior mediastinum extending to the middle mediastinum extending to the spinal canal through the posterior spinal defect, C–mediastinal shift, no calcification/fat/air bronchogram, D–**neurenteric cyst.**

Principal diagnosis: Neurenteric cyst.

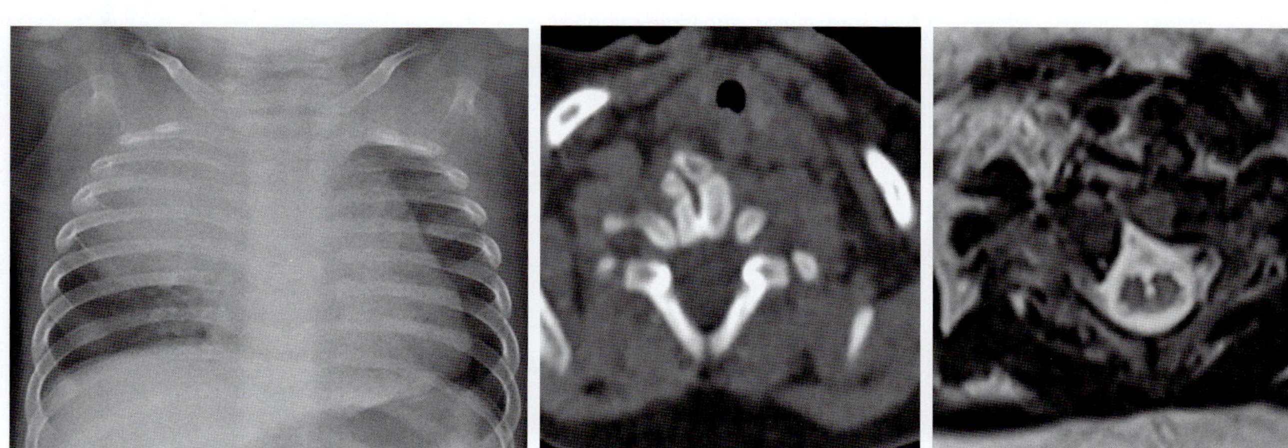

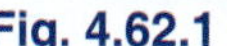

Fig. 4.62.1 Fig. 4.62.2 Fig. 4.62.3

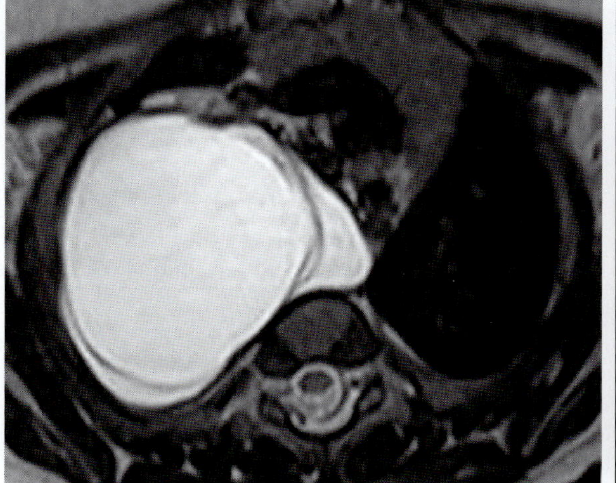

Fig. 4.62.4

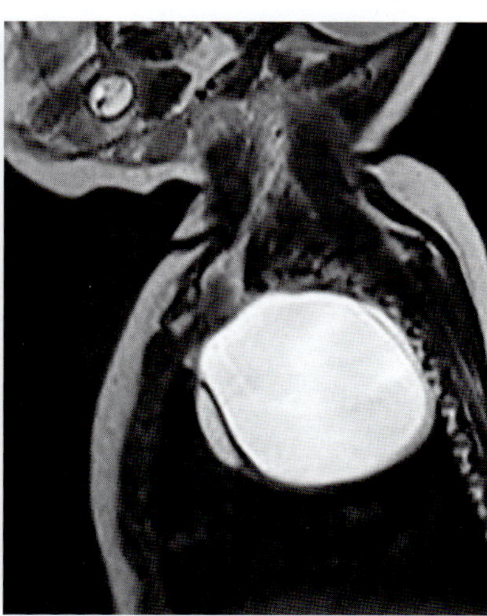

Fig. 4.62.5

Table 4.62.1: Differential diagnosis for cystic spinal cord lesions		
Arachnoid cyst Conservative management for asymptomatic cyst Percutaneous cyst aspiration and surgery after laminectomy for symptomatic cyst	CSF density/intensity on all sequences, seen more commonly in dorsal > ventral spinal canal. Extradural/ intradural extramedullary. Vertebral anomalies uncommon. No evidence of diffusion restriction. Imperceptible cyst wall. 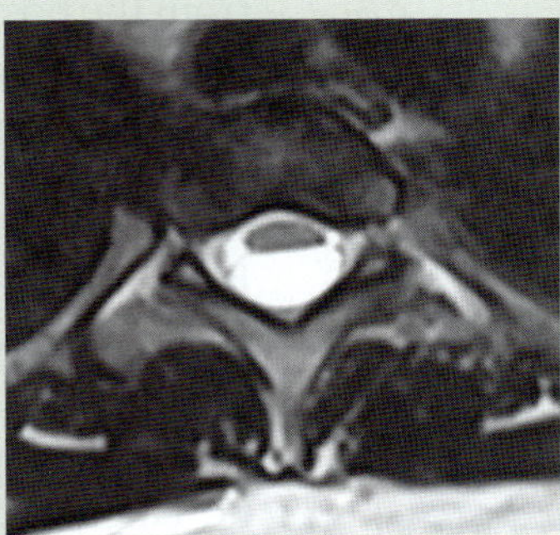 **Fig. 4.62.6:** Arachnoid cyst	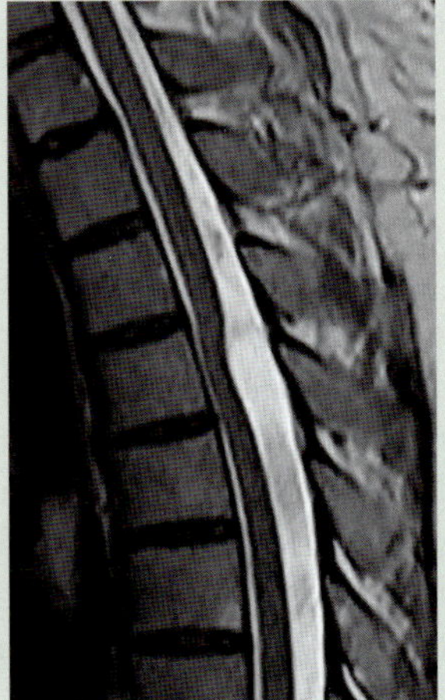 **Fig. 4.62.7:** Arachnoid cyst
Secondary arachnoid cyst/CSF loculation	CSF-filled sacs with or without communication with the subarachnoid space may form due to surgery, trauma, inflammation, haemorrhage or iatrogenic injury	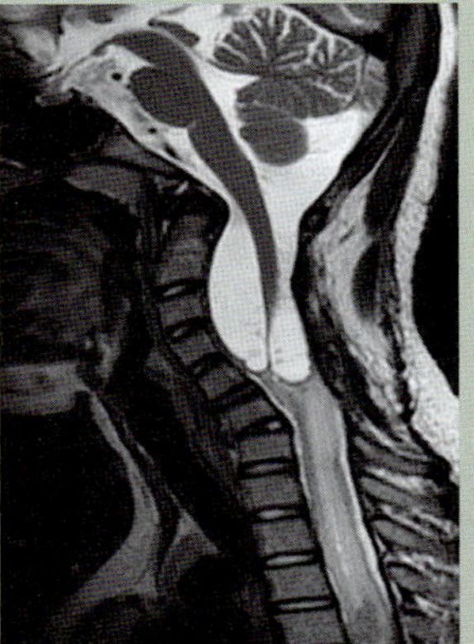 **Fig. 4.62.8:** Secondary arachnoid cyst
(Epi)dermoid cyst Common in children. Mostly acquired. Although present since birth, most congenital epidermoids present at 2nd–4th decade. Males commonly affected	Most common at cauda equina/conus level. Uncommon at the level of craniovertebral junction. May be associated with sinus tract, skin dimple and cord tethering.	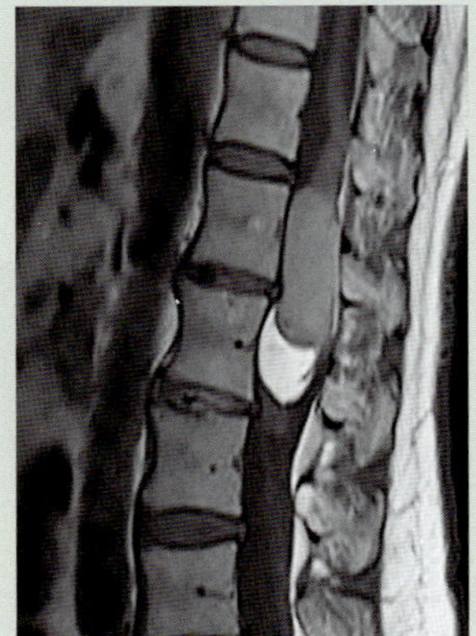 **Fig. 4.62.9:** Epidermoid cyst
Anterior thoracic meningocele Surgical resection of dural sac neck and resection of meningocele.	Anterior and dumbbell-shaped, contiguous with dural sac. Associated with ventral osseous defect. Solitary CSF intensity lesion. In sacral location—may be associated with Currarino's triad—anorectal malformation. And a scimitar sacrum	

(Contd.)

Table 4.62.1: Differential diagnosis for cystic spinal cord lesions (*Contd.*)		
Syrinx Surgery reserved for those with progressive neurological symptoms. Shunting associated with long term complications.	Syrinx refers to both hydromyelia and CSF-filled chambers in the spinal cord. Ependyma may or may not line the CSF-filled space within the spinal cord. Hydromyelia is a cystic dissection of the ependymal lining of the central canal, and the lesion is bordered with ependyma. Ependyma does not line a CSF accumulation within the cord parenchyma. On all sequences, the syrinx follows the CSF signal characteristics.	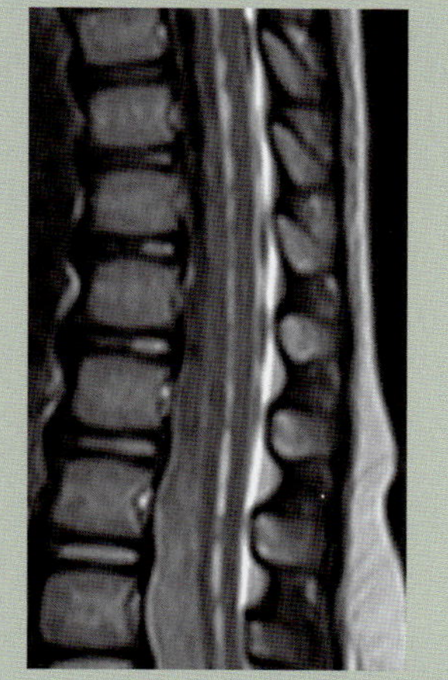 **Fig. 4.62.10:** Syrinx
Post-traumatic cyst/Syrinx Untethering of cord, duraplasty, spine realignment, cordectomy for patients with complete cord lesion.	Spinal cord swelling and edema, focal cord enlargement increased T2 signal at the level of trauma. Blooming on T2* sequences—intramedullary haemorrhage Spinal cord transection is best seen on sagittal sequences. DTI images show disruption of white matter tracts	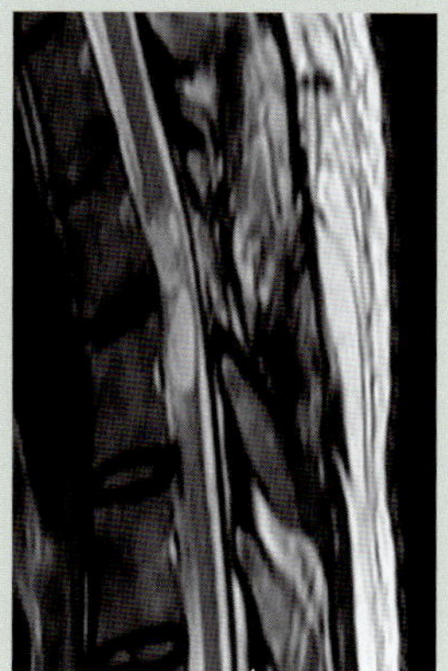 **Fig. 4.62.11:** Post-traumatic cyst 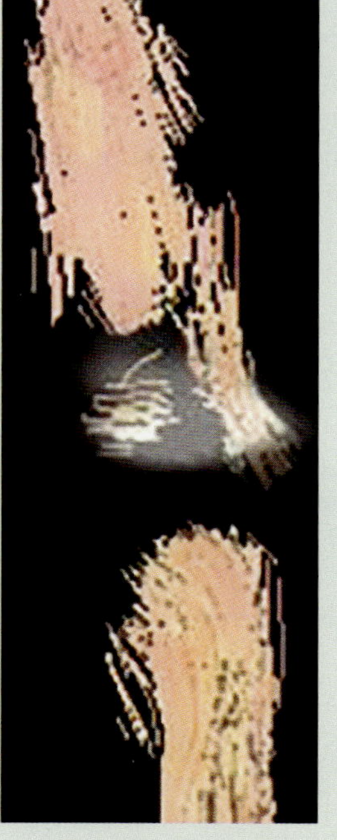 **Fig. 4.62.12:** Post-traumatic cyst

(Contd.)

Table 4.62.1: Differential diagnosis for cystic spinal cord lesions (*Contd.*)		
Non-neoplastic tumor associated cysts—refer to trapped CSF spaces as the tumor grows	Smooth well-demarcated cyst extra-axial TACs are more common than intra-axial, e.g. meningioma, craniopharyngioma, vestibular schwannoma, can be single or multiple abuts the tumor directly, vary from small to very large size. enhancement: Absent or minimal	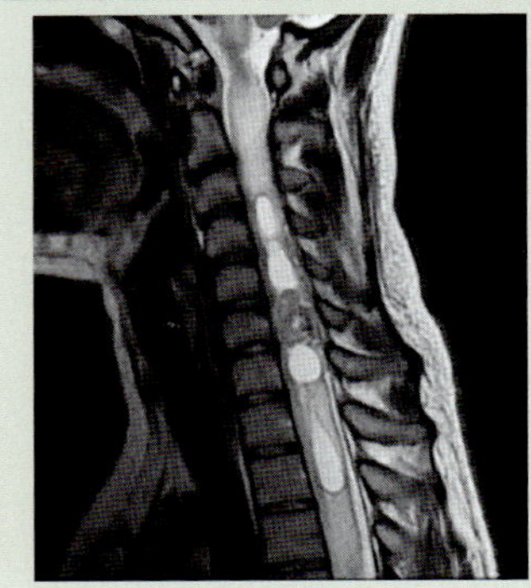 **Fig. 4.62.13:** Non-neoplastic tumor associated cysts
Ventriculus terminalis Seen in newborn at tip of conus. Transverse diameter of 2–4 mm extending for 8–10 mm.	Also known as the **5th ventricle,** and has ependymal lining; it is a fusiform dilatation of the terminal central canal, located at the transition from the tip of the conus to the commencement of the filum terminale 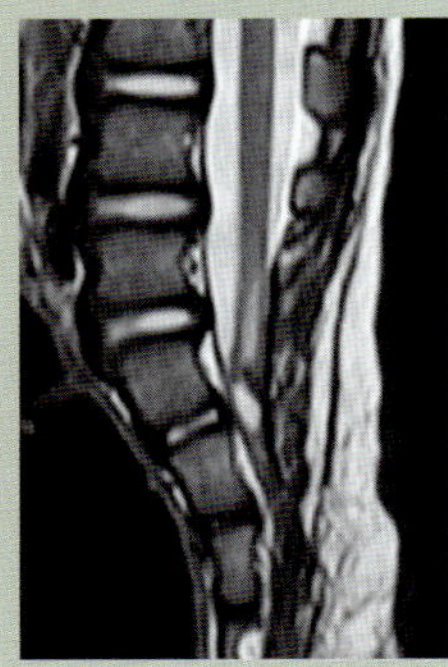 **Fig. 4.62.14:** Ventriculus terminalis	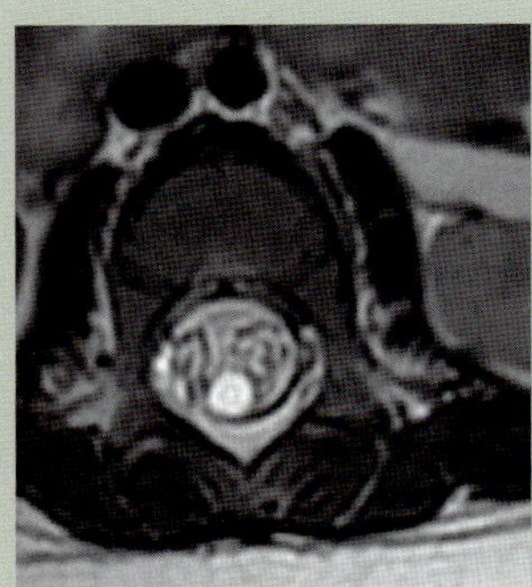 **Fig. 4.62.15:** Ventriculus terminalis
Tarlov cyst Symptomatic cysts aspirated under CT guidance using two-needle technique and fibrin injected to seal/surgical resection	Also called **perineural cysts**, are CSF-filled dilatations of the nerve sheaths at the DRG (dorsal root ganglion). Most Tarlov cysts are asymptomatic, but in some individuals can lead to neurological dysfunction and pain. This has been termed sacral symptomatic Tarlov cysts	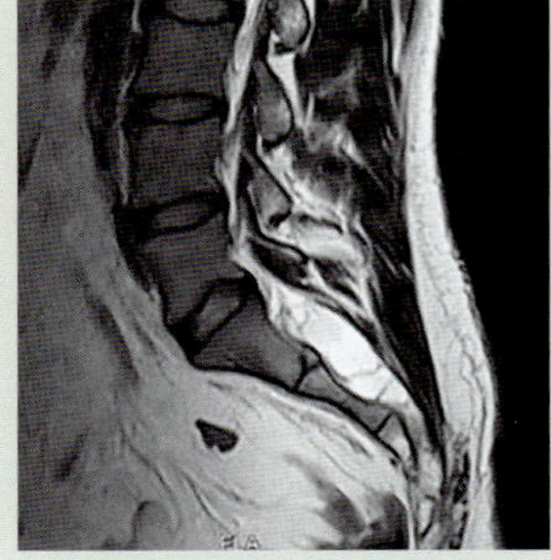 **Fig. 4.62.16:** Tarlov cyst
Filar cyst Incidental finding in neonatal lumbar sonography. It is considered a normal variant. Incidence is inversely related to age.	Longitudinally oriented, elongated, anechoic, cyst-like structure caudal to conus medullaris within the midline filum terminale.	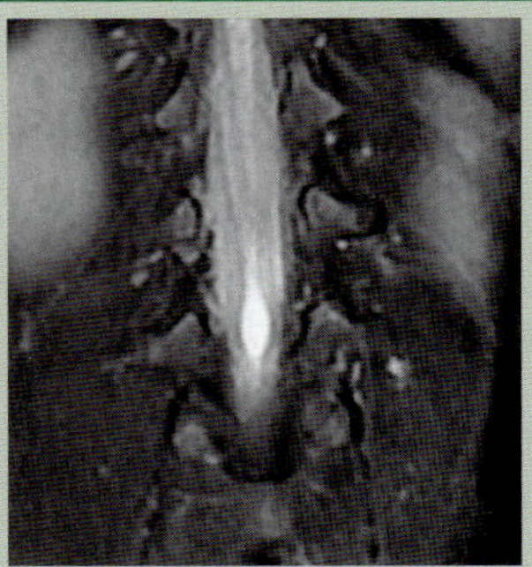 **Fig. 4.62.17:** Filar cyst

Table 4.62.2: Difference between intramedullary cysts and extramedullary cysts

Intramedullary cysts	*Extramedullary cysts*
Syrinx	Arachnoid cyst
Ventriculus terminalis	Neurenteric cyst
Tumoral cap cysts	Arachnoid web
Non-neoplastic tumor associated cysts	Hirayama's—prominent veins—mimic cysts
Post-traumatic cysts	Filar cysts
Ependymal cyst/neuroglial cyst	

DD for anterior displacement of cord

1. **Spinal cord herniation via dural defect results in focal anterior displacement of the cord with expansion of the dorsal subarachnoid space appearing similar to a dorsal arachnoid cyst.** However, an arachnoid cyst does not produce an abrupt cord deformity as in the case of herniation. Arachnoid cyst may also accompany herniation due to adhesions.
2. **Arachnoid web/arachnoid cyst**
3. **Prominent extradural space**
4. **Intracranial hypotension**
5. **Artefact**
6. **Kyphosis**

Discussion:

- Neurenteric cyst is also known as spinal enteric cyst/ dorsal enteric cyst/spinal enterogenous cyst.
- Intraspinal cyst + vertebral abnormalities (persistent canal of Kovalevsky, segmentation and fusion anomalies).
- **Location:** Thoracic (42%) > cervical (32%) >> lumbar spine, intracranial/basilar cisterns (rare).
- **Clinical symptoms:** Back/radicular pain., paraparesis, paraesthesia, gait disturbance. Children can present with cutaneous markers and spinal dysraphism. Can rarely present with meningitis due to either rupture of CSF contents into subarcahnoid space or seeding by enteric organisms.

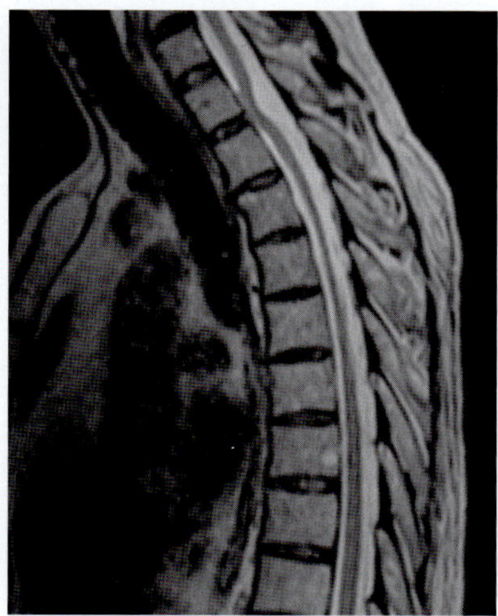

Fig. 4.62.18: Dorsal arachnoid web

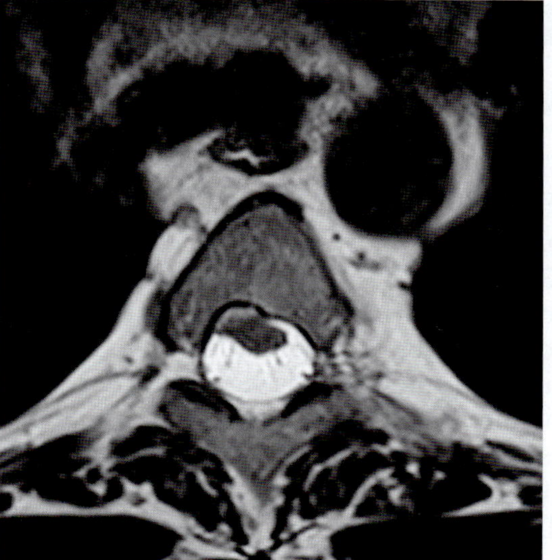

Fig. 4.62.19: Transdural dorsal cord herniation

- **Radiographic findings:** Enlarged spinal canal, widening of interpedicular distance ± vertebral segmentation/fusion anomalies, midline vertebral defect (canal of Kovalevsky).
- **CECT:** Hypodense cyst with minimal to no enhancement. The focal osseous canal enlargement, widening of interpedicular distance. Vertebral anomalies (50%, usually paediatric patient); vertebral clefts, butterfly vertebra, segmentation anomalies.
- **MR findings:** T1WI: Well-circumscribed, fluid intensity lesion ± vertebral anomalies. Iso- → hyperintense (to CSF) depending on protein/mucin content T2WI: Well-circumscribed, fluid intensity cystic lesion. Hypo- → isointense (to CSF) depending on protein/mucin content ± cord myeloschisis, focal cord atrophy due to compression.
- **Ultrasonographic findings:** Hypoechoic intraspinal cyst.
- **Myelography:**
  - Focal spinal canal enlargement, contrast filling defect.
  - Invaginating cyst mimics intramedullary lesion
- **Nuclear medicine findings:** Tc-99m pertechnetate cyst uptake (gastric mucosa) confirms diagnosis.
- **Treatment:** Complete surgical excision. Drainage/ partial resection is considered if complete excision is not possible. Reporting should **include degree of cord compression, size of cyst and severity of associated anomalies** to plan treatment and determine prognosis.

4.63 SPINE

Case No. 63

Clinical history: A 51 years old male with chronic low back pain for 6 months.

Radiological techniques and observation: Figures 4.63.1 to 4.63.4 are MRI T2WI, T1WI and STIR sagittal images respectively showing linear hypointensity representing transdiscal fracture with fluid intensity, facet joint fracture and interspinous ligament tear at D11–D12 level with narrowing of spinal canal. No altered signal intensity in spinal cord. No evidence of epidural hematoma noted.

STIR sagittal images show edema in the end plate corners representing osteitis (shiny corners). Anterior longitudinal ligament appears thickened.

Sagittal T1WI shows tear of interspinous ligament as low signal intensity in interspinous area.

Coronal T2 shows symmetrical subchondral bone marrow edema present along the bilateral sacroiliac joints, with joint space widening and erosion indicative of sacroiliitis. Visualized spine including disc also shows degenerative changes.

Interpretation: A: 51 years, dorsolumbar spine with bilateral sacroiliac joint, B: Edema in the end plate corners and bilateral symmetrical sacroiliitis. C: Transdiscal fracture, facet joint fracture and interspinous ligament tear, D: Ankylosing spondylitis.

Principal Diagnosis—Ankylosing Spondylitis

Management: The report needs to be highlighted to the referring clinician for further management including NSAIDs and brace immobilization and follow-up.

Discussion: Ankylosing spondylitis (less commonly known as Marie-Strümpell disease) is a seronegative spondyloarthritis, resulting in ankylosis of the spine and SI joints. Unknown etiology, strong genetic influence, with HLA B27 antigen. More common in young males (age 15–35 years) than in females with a ratio of 4:1 to 10:1. HLA-B27 is found in 88% of patients with ankylosing spondylitis. The chance that an HLA-B27 person will develop spondyloarthritis or eye disease is 1 in 4.

Conventional radiography: Sacroiliac joints: Sacroiliitis is usually the first manifestation and is symmetrical and bilateral. The sacroiliac joint first widen before they narrow. Subchondral erosion, sclerosis and proliferation on the iliac side of SI joints. The SI joint has lower ventral part which is cartilaginous and upper dorsal part which is fibrous joint. In the seronegative spondyloarthropathy related sacroiliitis predominantly involves the lower and posterior part of the joint (as it is has higher

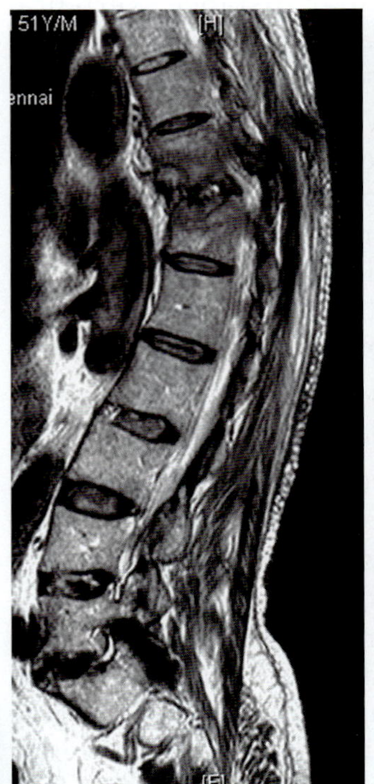

Fig. 4.63.1

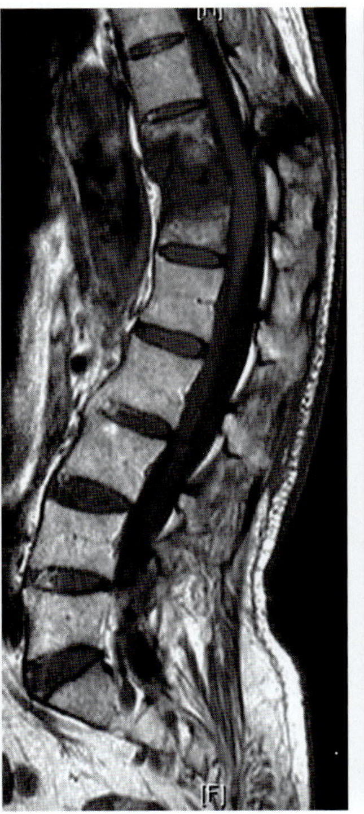

Fig. 4.63.2

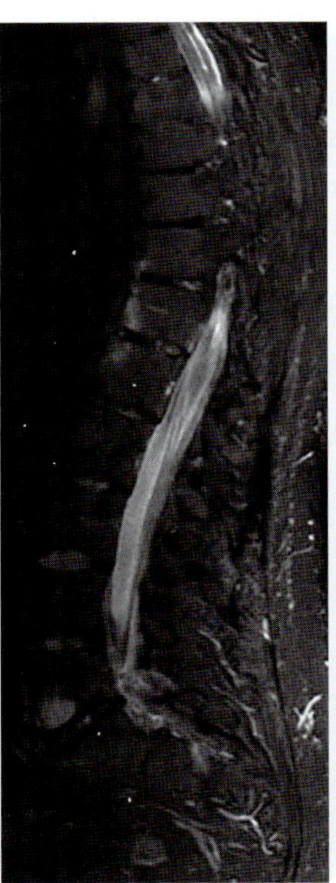
Fig. 4.63.3

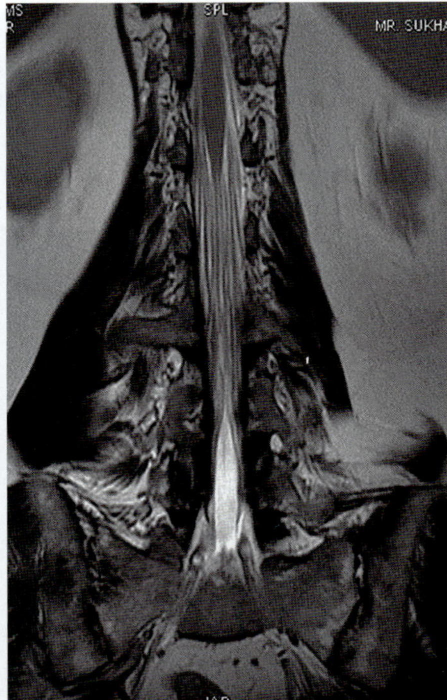

Fig. 4.63.4

Table 4.63.1: Differential diagnosis for ankylosing spondylitis		
Condition	*Radiological feature*	*Image*
Osteoporotic spinal compression fractures: Weakened vertebrae due to osteoporosis. Clinically seen in patients with pain and loss of mobility	The anterior, middle, or posterior dimensions of the vertebral body have lost more than 20% of their height. Cortical breakage or trabeculae impaction are acute fracture indicators; Fractures are chronic if we do not see these signs.	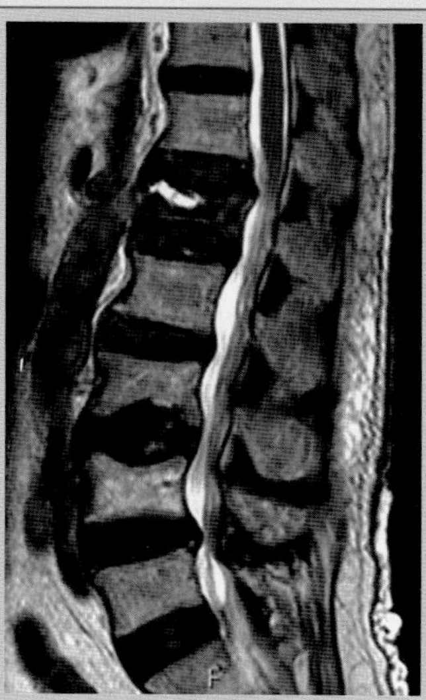 **Fig. 4.63.5:** Osteoporotic spinal compression fractures
Inflammatory bowel disease arthritis: A type of seronegative spondyloarthropathy. GIT manifestations are also associated with arthritis.	Spondylitis identical to ankylosing spondylitis, Peripheral joint arthritis, Sacroiliitis.	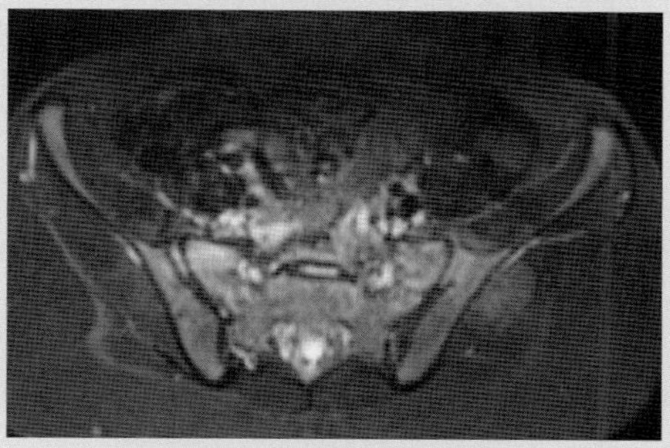 **Fig. 4.63.6:** Inflammatory bowel disease arthritis
Osteoarthritis or degenerative joint disease (DJD), spondylosis deformans is the most common form of arthritis. Primary osteoarthritis—strong genetic component with the disease primarily affecting middle-aged women. Secondary osteoarthritis is more common, caused by abnormal mechanical forces	Symmetrical joint space narrowing Sclerotic changes occur at joint margins Development of osteophytes Joints may exhibit degenerative erosions Subchondral cyst.	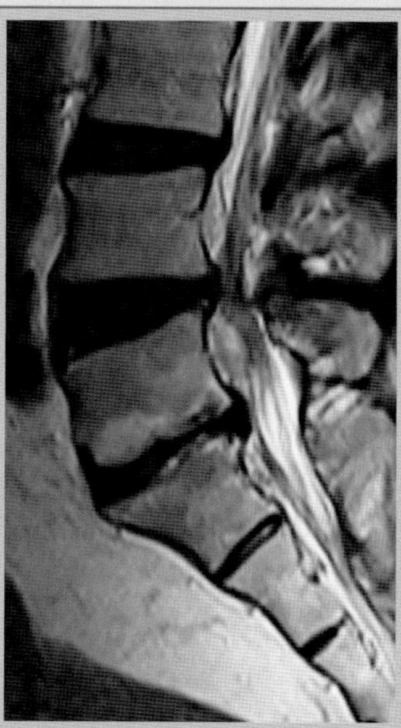 **Fig. 4.63.7:** Degenerative joint disease

(*Contd.*)

Table 4.63.1: Differential diagnosis for ankylosing spondylitis *(Contd.)*		
Condition	*Radiological feature*	*Image*
DISH (diffuse idiopathic skeletal hyperostosis): Enthesopathy and flowing ossification of the anterior longitudinal ligament involving the thoracic spine (at the iliac crest, ischial tuberosities, and greater trochanters). The sacroiliac synovial joints do not appear to be involved. Age >50 years. Treatment: Injection of glucocorticoids. Surgical resection for pain and dysphagia.	Anterior flowing ossification of ligaments rather than formation of syndesmophytes No involvement of facet joints or costovertebral joint No true sacroiliitis, ossification of non-synovial superior portion of SI joint Normal bone density. Normal intervertebral disc space.	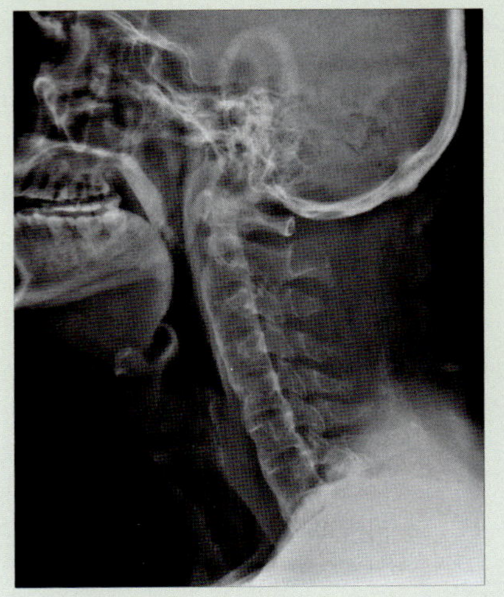 **Fig. 4.63.8** Diffuse idiopathic skeletal hyperostosis
Psoriatic spondyloarthropathy: Enthesitis and marginal bone erosions; "pencil in cup" deformities are common. Sausage digits, arthritis mutilans, ivory phalanx, asymmetric sacroiliitis, asymmetric paravertebral ossifications and relative sparing of the facet joints.	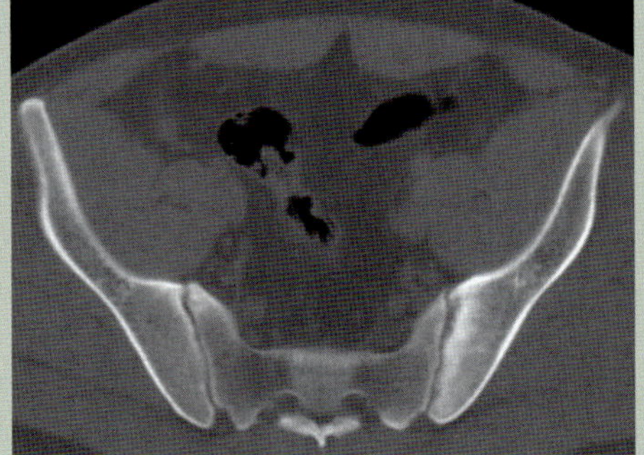 **Fig. 4.63.9:** Psoriatic spondyloarthropathy	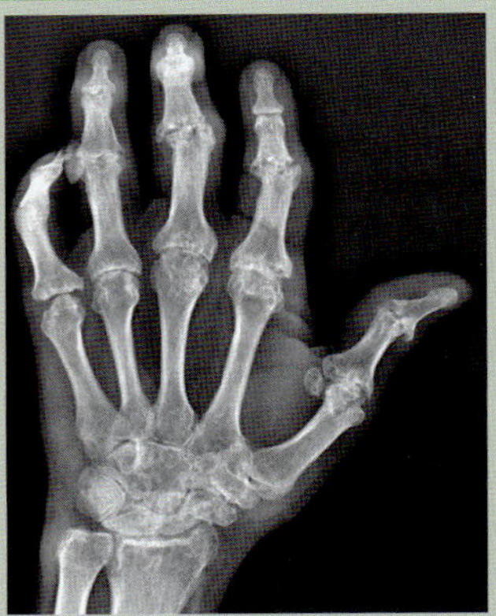 **Fig. 4.63.10:** Psoriatic spondyloarthropathy
TB spondylodiscitis: The spine is the most common location of musculoskeletal TB. Spine is involved due to hematogenous spread via Batson plexus. There is usually slow collapse of one or more vertebral bodies which spread underneath the longitudinal ligament resulting in acute kyphotic or gibbus deformity.	**Plain radiograph:** A reduction in vertebral height is often seen with the irregularity of the anterosuperior end plate being relatively early and subtle sign. Due to the subligamentous extension, there may be some irregularity of the anterior vertebral margin. **MRI:** T1 hypointense marrow in adjacent vertebrae, T2 hyperintense marrow, disc, soft tissue infection, T1C+ marrow, subligamentous, discal, dural enhancement.	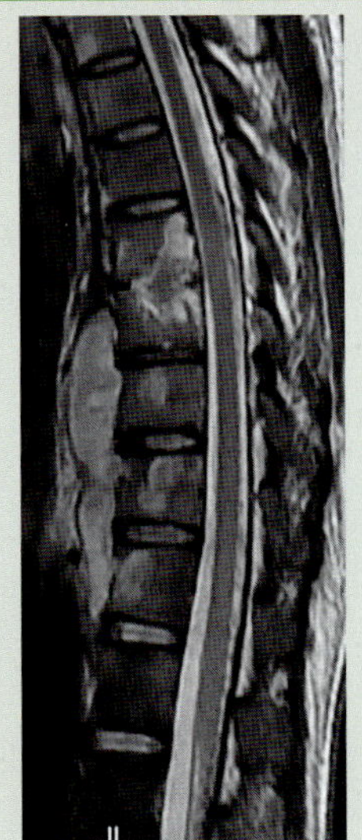 **Fig. 4.63.11:** TB spondylodiscitis
Chance fracture	Fracture involving all three vertebral columns, unstable injury occurring due to flexion	

Table 4.63.2: Bony outgrowths in ankylosing spondylitis

Dagger spine	*Syndesmophytes*	*With fracture*

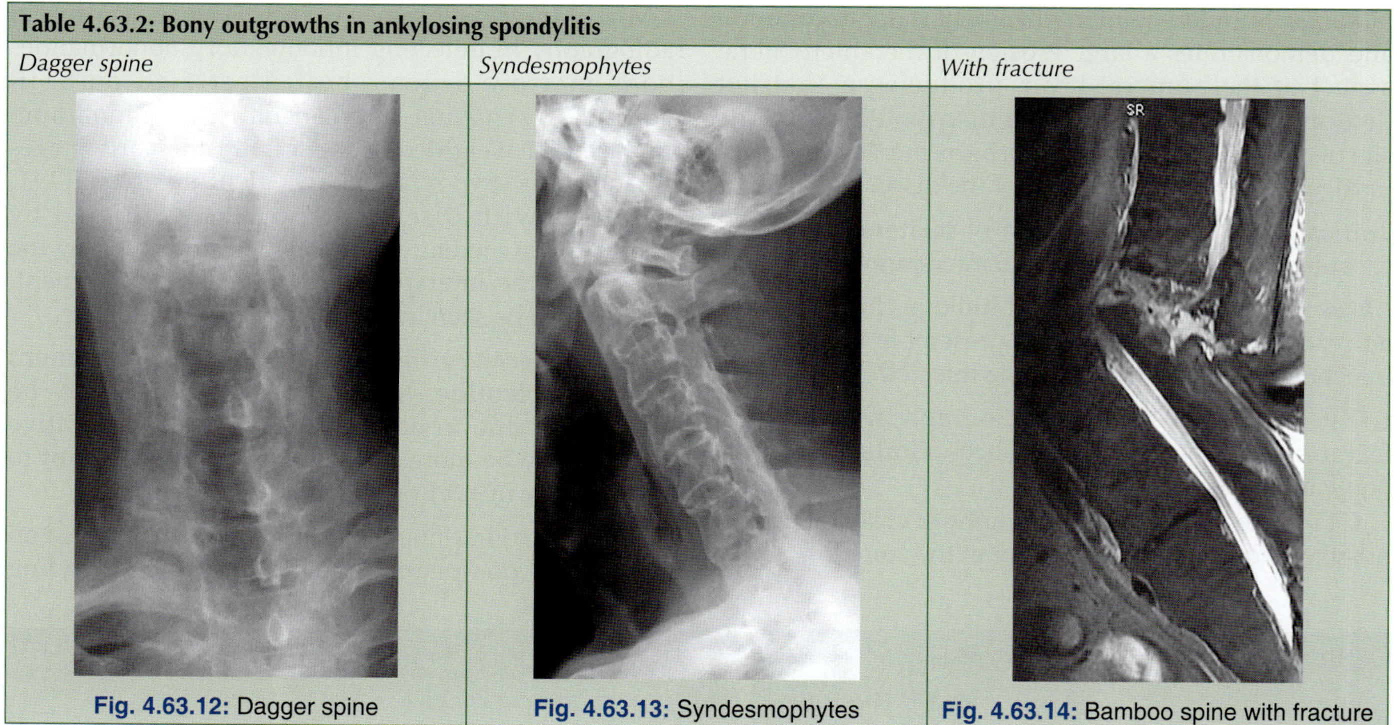

Fig. 4.63.12: Dagger spine

Fig. 4.63.13: Syndesmophytes

Fig. 4.63.14: Bamboo spine with fracture

preference for the axial skeleton with synovial joints and fibrocartilaginous).

Sacroiliitis grading: (New York criteria) grade 0: Normal; grade I: Some blurring of the joint margins—suspicious; grade II: Minimal sclerosis with some erosion; grade III: definite sclerosis on both sides of joint, severe erosions with widening of joint space with or without ankylosis; grade IV: Complete ankylosis.

Spine: Early spondylitis is characterized by small erosion at the corners with reactive sclerosis, Romanus lesion of spine (shiny corner sign). This is caused by combination of corner erosion with new periosteal bone formation along the anterior aspect of the vertebral bodies. Spinal involvement occurs at the corners of the vertebral bodies which are attachment sites of outermost portion of annulus fibrosus known as Sharpey's fibres.

Squaring of vertebral bodies: Syndesmophytes (bony spur): Hallmark of spinal diseases in AS. They appear as thin, vertically-oriented bony projections. Outer fibers of the annulus fibrosis will be ossified (Sharpey's fibres) leads to bridging of the corners of one vertebrae to another.

Posterior interspinous ligament: Ossification combined with linking of the spinous process, produce an appearance of solid midline, vertical, dense line on frontal radiograph—the **"dagger spine"** appearance.

Vertebral fusion: Progressive growth of syndesmophytes will bridge the intervertebral disc causing ankylosis and extensive bone formation produce a smooth, undulating spinal contour—the "bamboo spine". Calcification of the disc may occur at single or multiple levels.

Inflammation of costotransverse joint is typical of ankylosing spondylitis.

Fractures usually occur at the thoracolumbar and cervicothoracic junctions. Fractures typically are transverse, extend from anterior to posterior and frequently pass through the ossified disc. These are termed **'chalk stick fractures'** or **'carrot stick fractures'**.

Ghost joint: In late stages, increasing joint destruction with partial or complete fusion (ankylosis) of the joints, which can appear as "ghost joints" (ankylosis with visible joint contour).

Pseudoarthrosis is radiographically depicted as disco-vertebral destruction with adjacent sclerosis. The change referred to as **"Anderson lesion"** may resemble infection of the disc. Therefore, an important imaging feature is involvement of the posterior element, seen as linear, hypodense area with sclerotic borders. Long standing ankylosing spondylitis of cervical spine can cause osseous fusion, basilar impression and atlantoaxial subluxation.

Hip: It is involved generally bilateral and symmetric, with uniform joint space narrowing, axial migration of the femoral head (protrusio acetabuli).

Shoulder: Shoulder joint involvement is not uncommon and demonstrates a large erosion of the anterolateral aspect of the humeral head, producing a "hatchet deformity". Acromion process marrow edema at the site of deltoid muscle origin has been characterised as a particularly specific symptom of the disease.

Trolley track sign: Ossification of bilateral facet joint capsule, ligamentum flavum and interspinous ligament.

Chest: Progressive fibrosis and bullous changes at the apices (1%). These lesions may resemble tuberculosis infection and bullae may become infected.

CT: It is Superior to plain radiograph in identifying features such as joint erosion, subchondral sclerosis and bony ankylosis.

CT supplements bone scintigraphy in evaluating areas of increased uptake, particularly in the spine.

MRI is more sensitive than CT or conventional radiography in detecting inflammatory abnormalities (bone marrow oedema best illustrated on STIR sequences), synovitis, and capsulitis (on gadolinium enhanced T1 weighted sequences) in the early stages of sacroiliitis. Synovial enhancement areas on T1+C correlates with disease activity as evaluated by inflammatory mediators. Enthesitis is indicated by the increase of the interspinous ligaments enhancement. Erosions can be seen in T1 fat-sat coronal sequence.

Bone scintigraphy: Because qualitative assessment of radionucleotide deposition in SI joints may be challenging due to normal absorption, quantitative analysis may be more informative. Ratio of SI joint to sacral uptake of 1.3:1 or higher is abnormal.

Management: First-line therapy is primarily focused on NSAIDs and non-pharmacological measures including

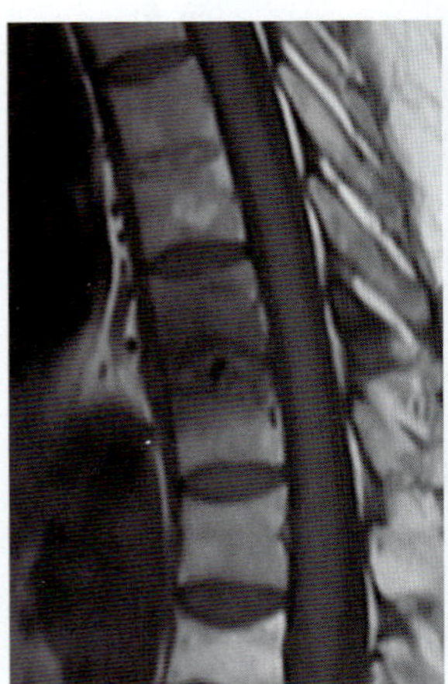

Fig. 4.63.15: Anderson lesion

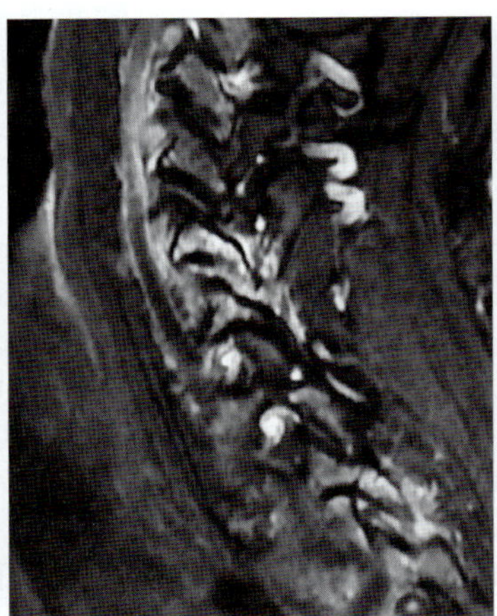

Fig. 4.63.16: Facetal arthrosis

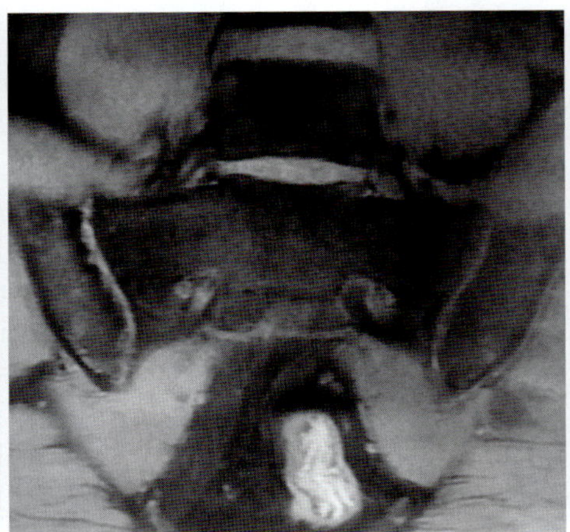

Fig. 4.63.17: T1 sequences can clearly delineate sacroiliac articular erosions, equivalent to a CT

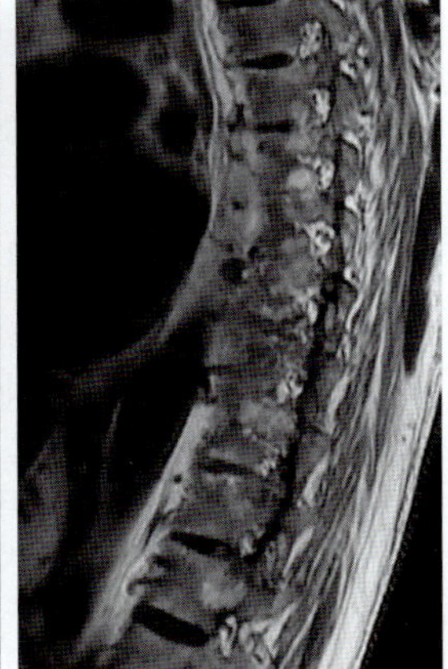

Fig. 4.63.18: Costotransverse joint involvement

Table 4.63.3: Difference between ochronosis, osteoarthritis/spondylosis deformans and ankylosing spondylitis

	Ochronosis	*Osteoarthritis/spondylosis deformans*	*Ankylosing spondylitis*
Joint involved	Spine +++ Knees+++ Hips++ Shoulders+	Spine+++ Knees++ Hips++ Hands+++	Spine+++ Knees+ Hips+
Distinguishing spine features			
Sacroiliac joints	Spared	Spared	Involved
Osteophytosis	Sparse	Prominent	None
Disc Calcification	**Dense/wafer-like**	Mild-moderate	Mild-moderate
Multiple vacuum disc	Common	Rare	Rare
Syndesmophytes	Broad	None	Thin + vertical
Apophyseal facet joint disease	Mild	Mild-severe	Severe
Ligamentous ossification	**Prominent**	Scarce	Scarce

Table 4.63.4: Approach to sacroiliitis

Bilateral symmetrical	*Bilateral asymmetrical*	*Unilateral*
Ankylosing spondylitis Inflammatory bowel disease—ulcerative colitis, Crohn's disease and Whipple's disease Psoriatic arthropathy Osteitis condensans ilii Hyperparathyroidism Paraplegia	Reiter's syndrome Psoriatic arthropathy Rheumatoid arthritis Gouty arthritis Osteoarthritis	Infection

Table 4.63.5: Differnence between ankylosing spondylitis, diffuse idiopathic skeletal hyperostosis and ossification of posterior longitudinal ligament

	Ankylosing spondylitis	*Diffuse idiopathic skeletal hyperostosis (DISH)*	*Ossification of posterior longitudinal ligament (OPLL)*
Ligaments Involved	Both anterior and posterior longitudinal ligaments	Anterior longitudinal ligament 50% DISH also have OPLL	Posterior longitudinal ligament Common in midcervical spine predisposing patient to severe cord damage with minor injuries
Shape	Thin calcification contiguous with syndesmophytes "bamboo spine"	Prominent "flowing" Anterior and lateral osteophytes involving >4 levels, bulky and undulating .	Thin or thick linear sheet of ossification, may be discontinuous in a few cases
Location	Diffuse	Most common in lower thoracic spine (T7–T11) Preferentially affects the right side of spine due to aortic pulsations on the left.	Most common in cervical or upper thoracic spine
Associated degenerative changes	Often yes—inflammatory	No loss of disc height. No apophyseal or costovertebral joint fusion. DISH is seen in adults >50 years.	Often yes—associated with disc degeneration.
	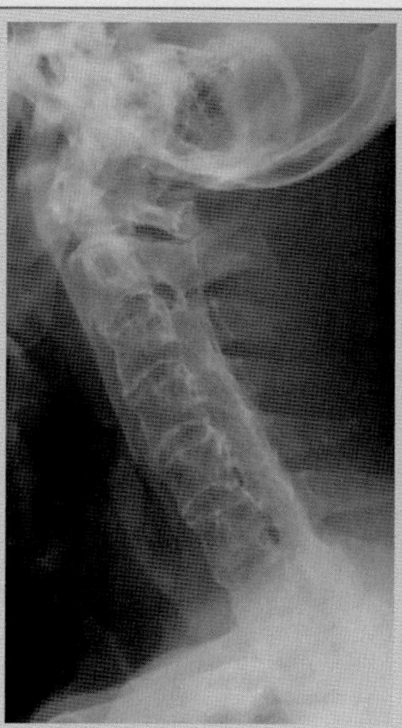 **Fig. 4.63.19:** Ankylosing spondylitis	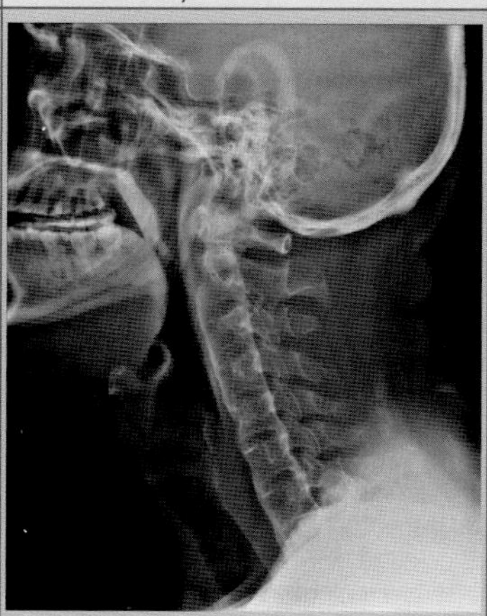 **Fig. 4.63.20:** Diffuse idiopathic skeletal hyperostosis	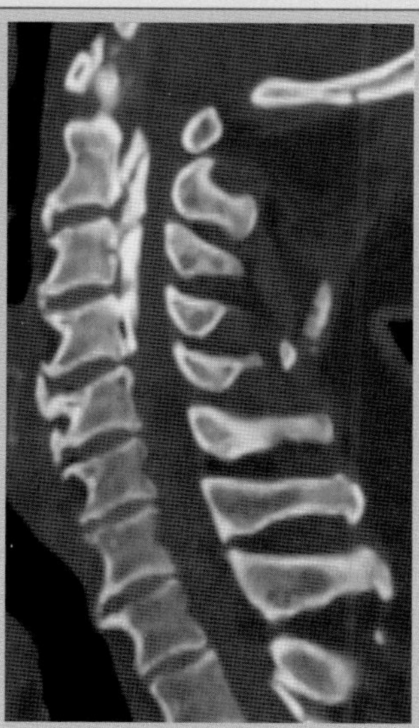 **Fig. 4.63.21:** Ossification of posterior longitudinal ligament

Table 4.63.6: Difference between osteitis condensans ilii and sacroiliitis

Osteitis condensans ilii	*Sacroiliitis*
Sclerosis of iliac side of sacroiliac joint, typically bilateral, symmetrical and triangular in shape. Lack of sacral involvement / erosion or joint space narrowing is considered diagnostic. Common in parous women	Sclerosis of endplates particularly on the iliac side, irregular joint end plates, widening of joint spaces
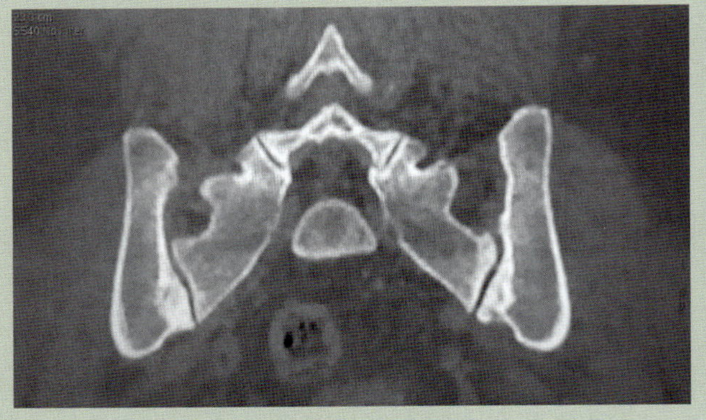 **Fig. 4.63.22:** Osteitis condensans ilii	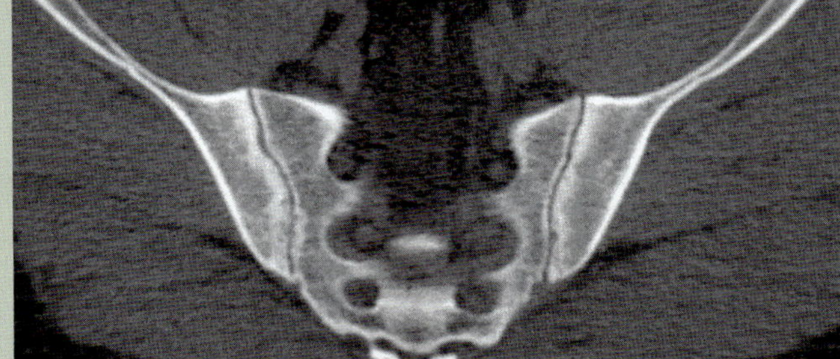 **Fig. 4.63.23:** Sacroiliitis

Table 4.63.7: Summary of bony outgrowths of spine

Syndesmophytes—ossification of annulus fibrosus 1. Ankylosing spondylitis 2. Alkaptonuria	Paravertebral ossification—ossification of paravertebral connective tissue which is separated from edge of vertebral body. 1. Reiter syndrome 2. Psoriatic arthropathy	Claw osteophytes—arising from vertebral margin with no gap and having claw appearance 1. Stress response
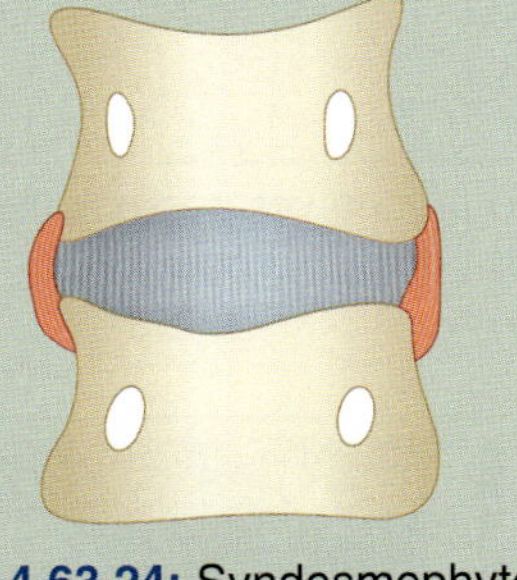 **Fig. 4.63.24:** Syndesmophytes	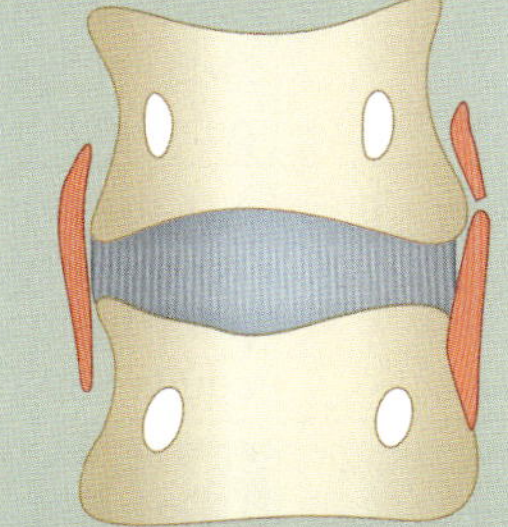 **Fig. 4.63.25:** Paravertebral ossification	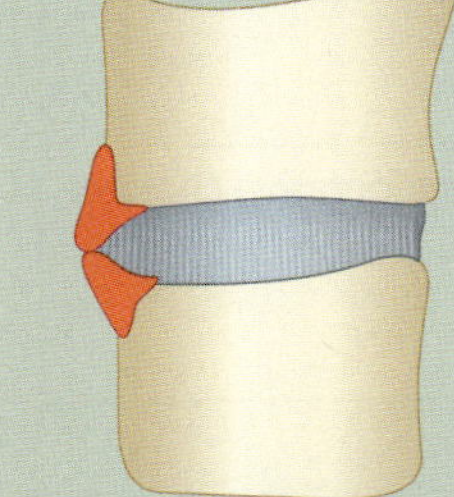 **Fig. 4.63.26:** Claw osteophytes

Traction spurs—Osteophytes having gaps between the endplate and the base, and a tip shows no protrusion beyond the horizontal vertebral endplate plane. Shear stresses across the disc	Undulating anterior ossification—undulating ossification of anterior longitudinal ligament, intervertebral disc and paravertebral connective tissue. DISH
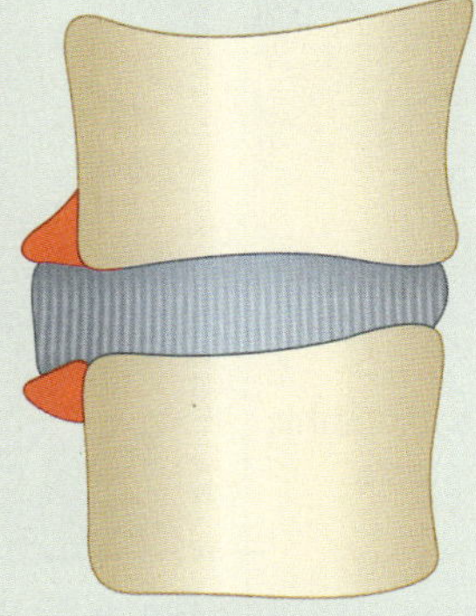 **Fig. 4.63.27:** Traction spurs	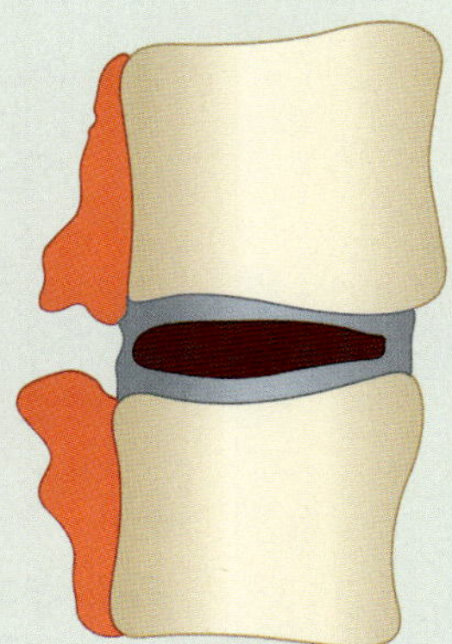 **Fig. 4.63.28:** Undulating anterior ossification

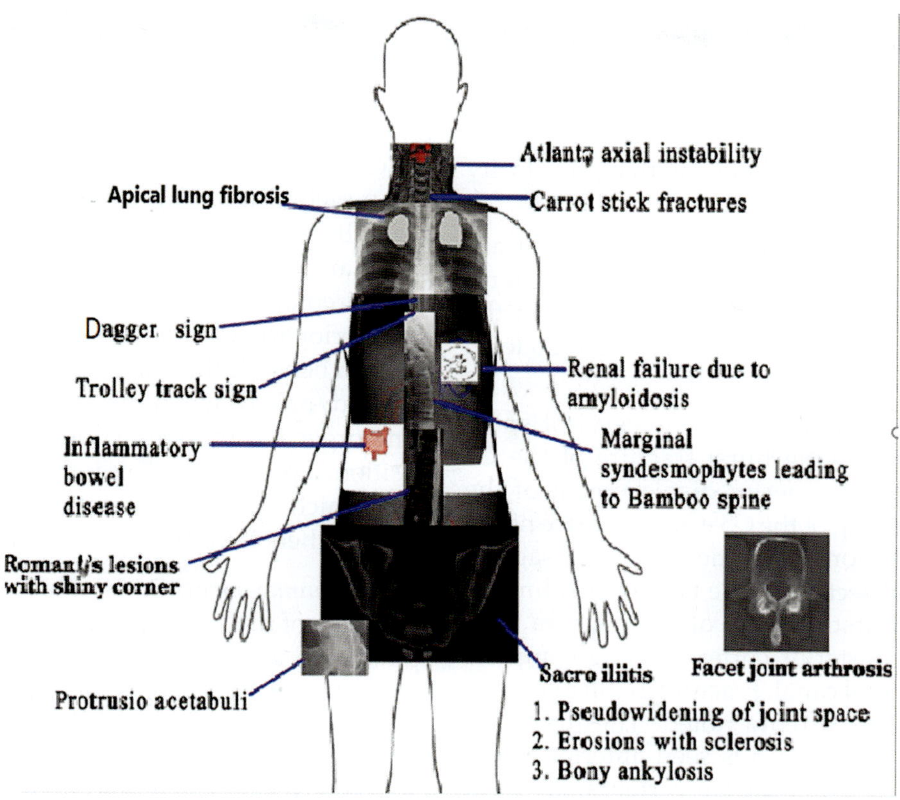

Fig. 4.63.29: Whole body illustration of ankylosing spondylitis manifestations

education, exercise, physiotherapy. Second-line therapy includes TNF-alpha blockers.

Intervertebral disc calcification (chondrocalcinosis): The differential diagnosis includes degenerative spondylosis–in the nucleus pulposus. Usually confined to the dorsal region; Alkaptonuria calcium pyrophosphate dihydrate deposition disease. Ankylosing spondylitis. Juvenile idiopathic arthritis. Haemochromatosis. Diffuse idiopathic skeletal hyperostosis (DISH)—may mimic ankylosing spondylitis. Gout. Idiopathic as a temporary condition that affects youngsters in cervical spine commonly. Although it is clinically linked to neck pain and fever, it can also be asymptomatic.

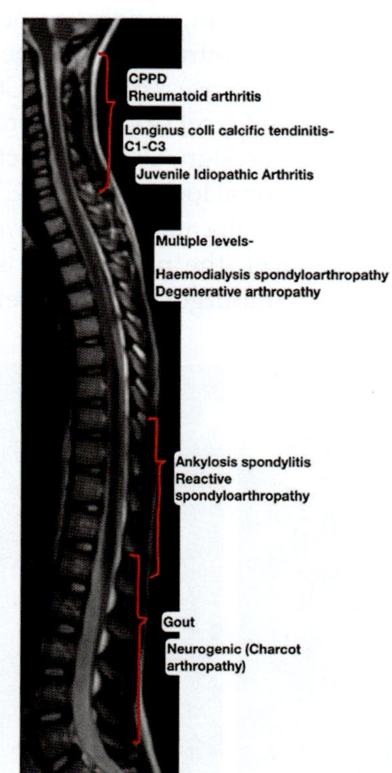

Fig. 4.63.30: Spectrum of inflammatory disorders manifesting in spine

4.64 SPINE

Case No. 64

Clinical history: A 38 years old male with high velocity road traffic injury.

Radiological technique: Figures 4.64.1 to 4.64.4 are plain radiograph of the cervical spine in the lateral view, sagittal CT sections of the cervical spine in the bone algorithm and an axial section at the C5–C6 level respectively.

Observations: Plain radiograph of the cervical spine in the lateral view showing burst fracture of the C6 vertebra with posterior superior displacement of the vertebral body. Widening of the C5–C6 joint space noted along with slight anterior subluxation of C5. CT sagittal sections and an axial section in the bone algorithm are provided showing burst fracture of C6 vertebra with retropulsion of the posterior cortex causing complete obliteration of the spinal canal. Fracture in thb e spinous process of C5 and C6 vertebra noted. The tip of the inferior articular process of C5 is seen anterior to the superior articular process of the C6 vertebra, i.e. **right unilateral locked facet** of C5 vertebra over C6 with the reverse hamburger sign demonstrated. Congenital C3–C4 block vertebra noted.

Interpretation: A: 38 years old, cervical spine, B: Burst fracture of C6 vertebra with retropulsion of the posterior cortex. Fracture of spinous process of C5 and C6 vertebra and right unilateral locked facet of C5 vertebra over C6, C: Reverse hamburger bun sign, D: Burst fracture of C6 vertebra with right unilateral locked facet of C5 over C6. When the facet joint is dislocated, most commonly in situations of locked facet, the naked facet sign (also known as the reverse hamburger bun sign) refers to the CT appearance of an uncovered vertebral articular facet. Extensive ligamentous disruption and spinal instability, which is typical of a flexion-distraction injury are seen. The vertebral facet (apophyseal) joint space looks like a hamburger on an axial CT will show the superior articular process of the vertebra below produces the semi-circular "bun" on top of the "meat patty," while the inferior articular process of the vertebra above forms the bun beneath the patty. The articular facets become exposed/naked, when the facet joint is displaced. The hamburger's top bun (the superior articular facet) is now positioned posteriorly. This is the reverse hamburger bun sign, which can be unilateral or bilateral depending on whether there is a unilateral or bilateral facet dislocation.

Further management: Cervical brace for stabilisation and restriction of movements followed by an MRI to look for spinal cord and ligamentous injury. Unilateral cervical locked facets dislocation should be treated immediately with posterior open reduction and instrumentation. Bilateral cervical locked facets dislocation can be reduced by rapid skull traction firstly and anterior cervical discectomy and interbody fusion later. For the treatment of traumatic cervical facet dislocation, the choice of anterior, posterior, or mixed cervical approaches is critical. Although satisfactory surgical outcomes can be achieved using any approach, there are several occasions where one technique may be preferred over the other. The optimal technique should be chosen depending on the location of spinal cord compression, the presence of additional bone fracture and the surgeon preference/expertise, according to some writers. A preoperative MRI is recommended when a posterior cervical approach is planned to evaluate a relevant disc herniation and anterior cord compression.

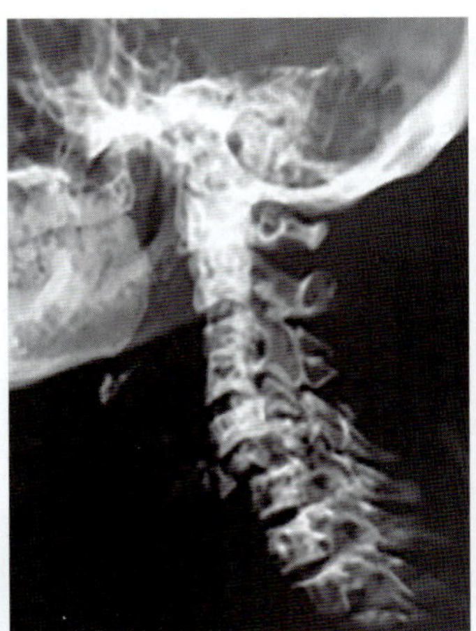
Fig. 4.64.1

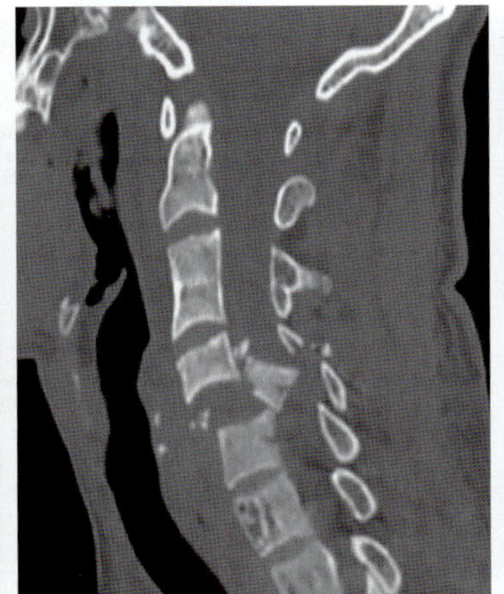
Fig. 4.64.2

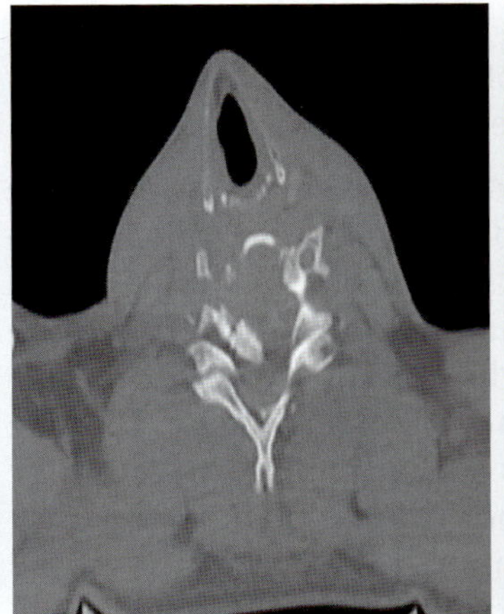
Fig. 4.64.3

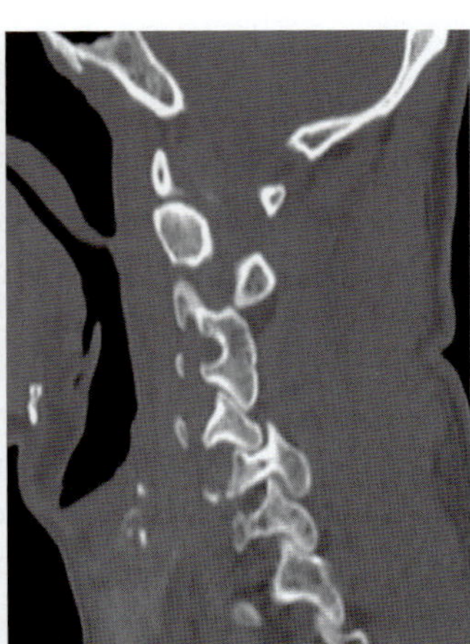
Fig. 4.64.4

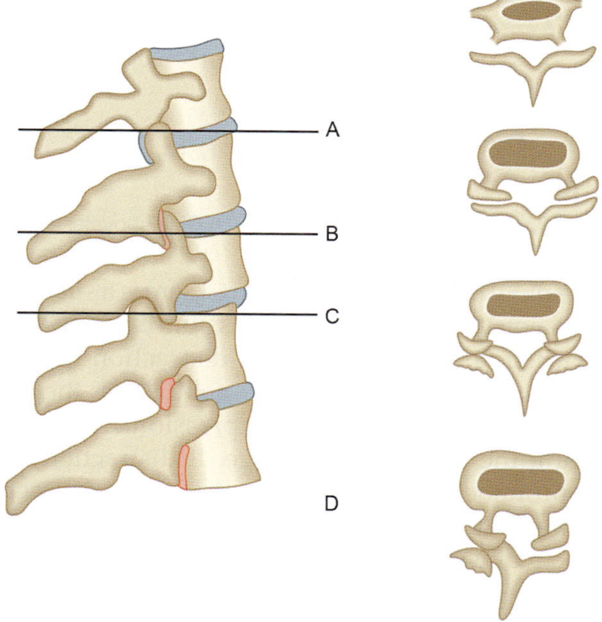

Fig. 4.64.5: Facet dislocation in trauma: (A) Perched facet, (B) normal, (C) reverse hamburger, bilateral locked fact, (D) unilateral locked facet

Table 4.64.1: Difference between the types of locked facets

Unilateral locked facet—stable	*Bilateral locked facet—unstable*
Mechanism: Flexion distraction injury	Severe flexion injury
Only 30% associated with neurologic defect	Quadriplegia frequently develops
Most often occurs at C4–5 and C5–6	Lower cervical spine usually
One vertebral body on the one below has a slight anterior subluxation **(usually less than 25% of the width)**.	A greater number of superior vertebrae subluxes forward by 50% or more of the body below. At the lesion site, both anterior and posterior ligamentous structures are damaged. If a fracture occurs via the posterior elements, there is a lower risk of neurologic damage because the cord can decompress.

Facet dislocation refers to anterior displacement of one vertebral body on another. Without a fracture, the only way anterior displacement can occur is by dislocation of the facets.

Table 4.64.2: Facet dislocation can occur to varying degrees

Subluxed facets	**Subluxed facet joint** is the mildest form in which the ligamentous injury leads to partial uncovering of facet joint. This results in mild anterior displacement of one vertebral body on another—anterolisthesis.	
Perched facets	A facet joint, whose inferior articular process appears to sit 'perched' on the ipsilateral superior articular process of the vertebra below. Any further anterior subluxation will result in dislocation, with one facet "jumping" over the other and becoming locked in this position. Hyperflexion + extreme rotational force	**Fig. 4.64.6:** Perched facets
Locked facet joint: Radiological features are widening of interspinous distance on AP view. Spinous processes are in the midline in AP view in bilateral locked facet but are displaced towards the affected side in unilateral locked facet. Narrowing of disc space at injured level. Intervertebral foramen appears enlarged on oblique projection. Spondylolisthesis. Dislocation or fracture of superior and inferior articular facets	Results from jumping of the inferior articular process over the superior articular process of the vertebra below, which becomes locked in that position. It can be unilateral or bilateral. Unilateral locked facets are stable while bilateral locked facets are unstable	**Fig. 4.64.7:** Bilateral locked facet joint
Congenital absence of cervical spine pedicle	In the case of trauma, an unintentional discovery can be mistaken as a true subluxation or dislocation. Other congenital defects, such as spina bifida, may be present. Pseudo-enlargement of neural foramina, dysplastic ipsilateral articular pillar and lamina, and transverse process are all symptoms of a missing pedicle. The superior articular facet of the vertebra above is located dorsal to the inferior articular facet. Management is done conservatively.	

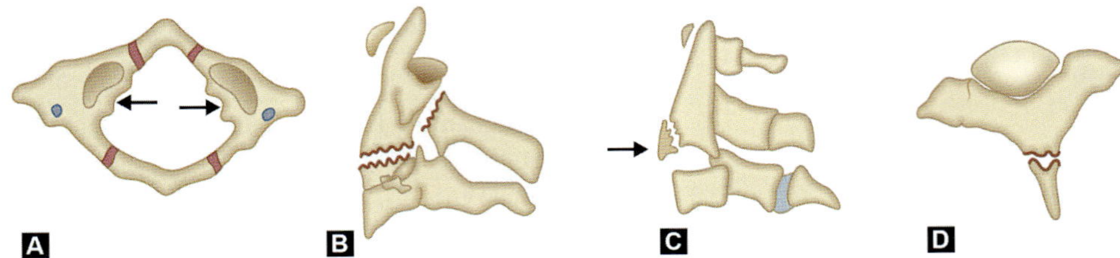

Fig. 4.64.8: Named spinal fractures: (A) Jefferson's fractures, (B) Hangman's fracture, (C) Teardrop fracture, (D) Clay-shoveler's fracture

Fat C2 sign: The fracture lines (fragment separation) may not be evident on lateral radiographs if a fracture runs obliquely through the body of the axis. However, if the fracture fragments are displaced, the body of C2 will appear bulky with respect to C3.

Unstable cervical spine fractures/injuries (Jefferson Owes Hangman A Teddy Bear):

- Jefferson's fracture
- Odontoid type 2
- Hangman's fracture
- Atlanto-occipital dislocation or subluxation
- Tear drop fracture
- Bilateral facet dislocation

Role of MRI: Can show ligamentous injuries apart from the dislocation.

Thoracolumbar injury classification and severity score (TLICS): Refer to OSCE.

Mechanisms of spinal injury:

Distraction: The separating or pulling apart of two neighbouring vertebrae is known as a distraction injury. When the osseous and ligamentous supporting tissues of the spinal cord are pushed apart, there is a substantial risk of cord damage. A compression fracture on the anterior side can result from a distraction injury on the posterior side. So we should not dismiss the injury by focusing solely on the compression fracture and ignoring the distraction damage. If distraction is the most prominent aspect, the morphology is distraction, which equals 4 points. The PLC is always involved in these circumstances, resulting in a total of 7 points for the TLICS-score. If compression is the most prominent aspect, the morphology is burst, which equals 2 points plus the PLC injury for a total of 5 points.

All fractures caused by displacement in the horizontal plane, such as left-to-right or anterior-to-posterior side-to-side motions; side-to-side rotating motion of one vertebral body with regard to another, are classified as **translation-rotation fractures**. In rotational fractures, unilateral or bilateral facet dislocation is common. PLC is almost always present in severe injuries.

Simple compression: The most frequent type of damage is a simple compression fracture, which occurs in 90% of cases. Either the anterior section of the vertebral body loses height or the vertebral endplate is disrupted. The vertebral body's posterior cortex must be intact, which distinguishes a simple compression fracture from a more serious burst fracture. In a simple compression fracture, the posterior cortex may expand somewhat posteriorly. **It is a wedge compression fracture, not a burst fracture,**

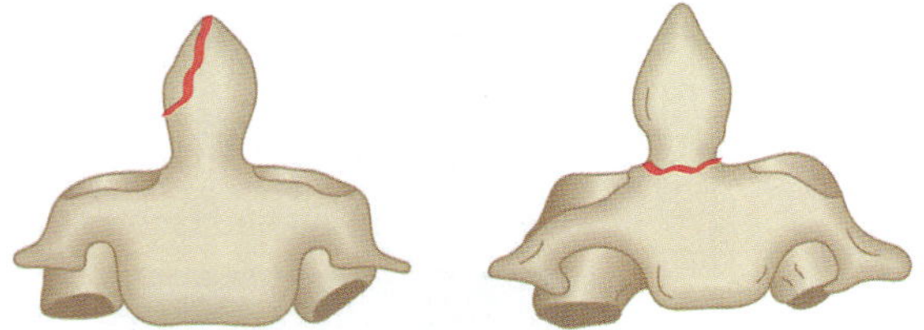

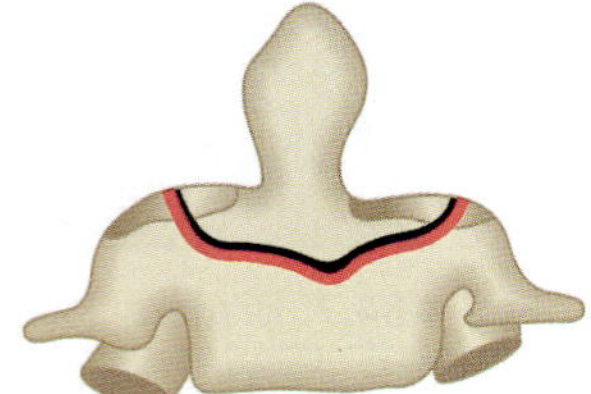

Fig. 4.64.9: Anderson and D'Alonzo classification of odontoid fractures

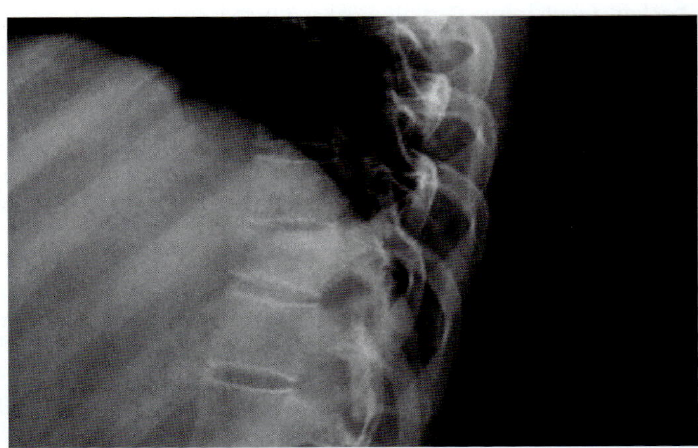

Fig. 4.64.10: Wedge compression of the D11 vertebra

as long as there is no free fragment with posterior displacement.

Burst fracture: This is a more severe type of compression fracture that has a higher risk of neurologic impairments. The name comes from the common fracture that occurs when someone falls from a great height and lands on their feet. In the TLICS, a burst fracture receives two points for morphology. PLC integrity should be established during MR imaging in the absence of a neurologic deficit, especially if cautious care of a burst fracture is anticipated. A burst fracture is classified as a two-column injury in the Denis classification, making it unstable and necessitating surgical stabilisation.

Chance fracture (3-column injury): A chance fracture is a type of flexion injury to the spine that involves compression of the anterior column and transverse fracture of the posterior parts. GQ chance was the first to describe it in 1948.

Table 4.64.3: Summary of spinal cord injuries

Spinal cord injuries are of two types:	
High signal on MR without hemorrhage due to edema	*Low signal intensity areas within the area of edema due to hemorrhage*
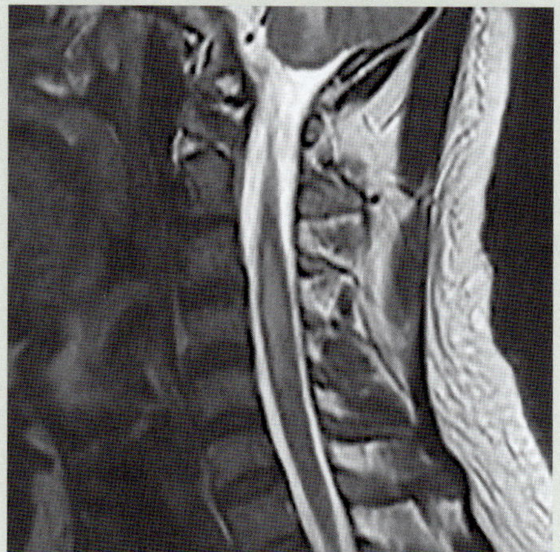 **Fig. 4.64.11:** High signal on MR without hemorrhage due to edema	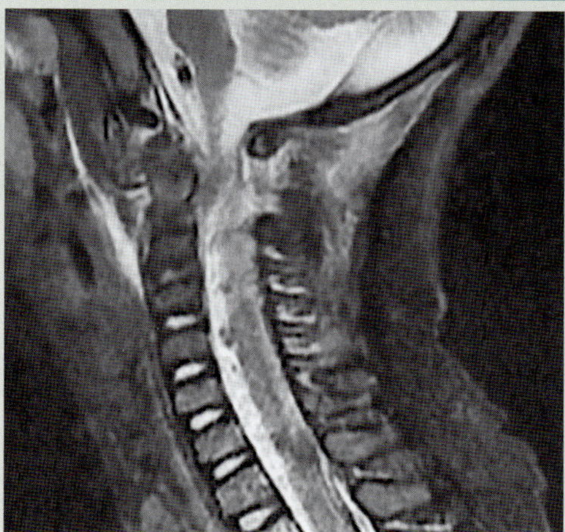 **Fig. 4.64.12:** Low signal intensity areas within the area of edema due to hemorrhage
SCIWORA—spinal cord injury without radiological abnormality. It is a pre MRI term presenting with clinical symptoms of traumatic myelopathy and shows no radiographic or computed tomographic features of spinal fracture or instability, accounting for 6 to 19% of spinal injuries in children, 9 to 14% of spinal injuries in adults. **Indicators of increasing risk of SCI as a result of** a minimal trauma: Congenital spinal canal stenosis, pre-existing spondylosis, prolapse of intervertebral disc. **MRI T1WI:** Ligamentous disruption, intervertebral disc herniation, paraspinal muscle injury, shearing of vertebral end plate sub-epiphyseal growth zone. **T2WI:** Illustration demonstrates various traumatic cord injuries. Same as T1; edema more conspicuous than on T1WI; (better seen with fat saturation) spinal cord injury (ranging from edema to transection). **STIR:** Most sensitive for spinal cord, soft tissue and ligamentous injury. Illustration demonstrates various traumatic cord injuries.	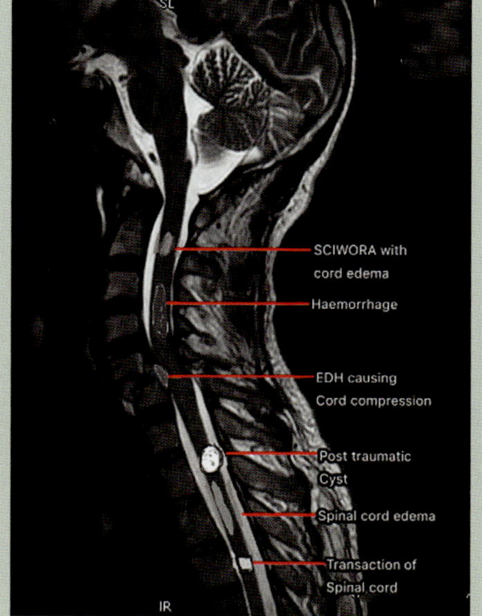 **Fig. 4.64.13:** Imaging findings in spinal cord trauma

(Contd.)

Table 4.64.3: Summary of spinal cord injuries (*Contd.*)	
Spinal cord injuries are of two types:	
High signal on MR without hemorrhage due to edema	*Low signal intensity areas within the area of edema due to hemorrhage*
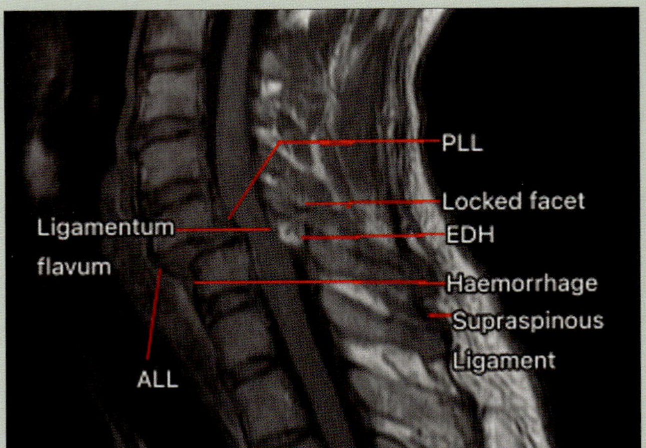 **Fig. 4.64.14:** Injuries to spinal ligaments	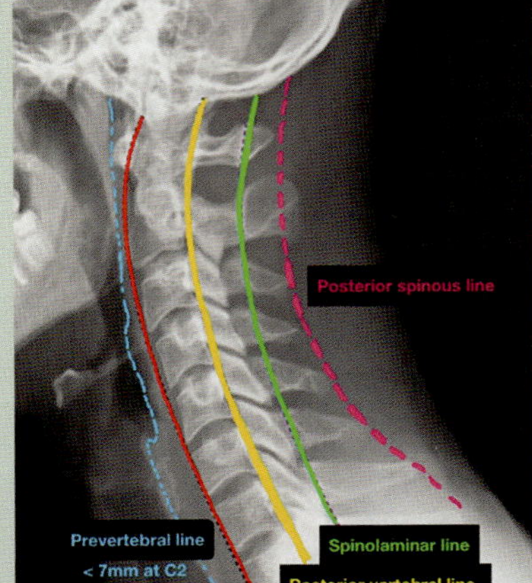 **Fig. 4.64.15:** Normal lines to be looks for in suspected case of cervical trauma
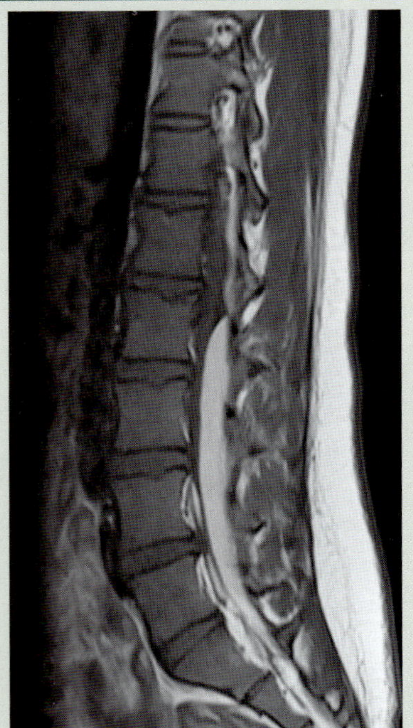 **Fig. 4.64.16:** Subdural haematoma in the lumbar region demonstrated with T1 sequences in the sagittal plane. Note the anterior displacement of the cord and cauda equina hinting at the subdural collection.	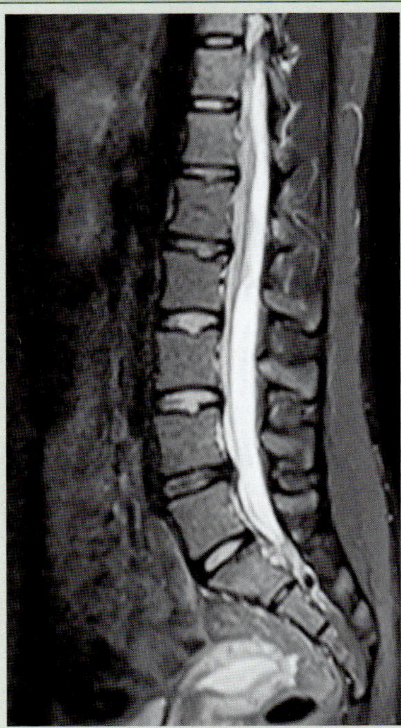 **Fig. 4.64.17:** Subdural haematoma in the lumbar region demonstrated with T2 fat saturated sequences in the sagittal plane. Note the anterior displacement of the cord and cauda equina hinting at the subdural collection.

4.65 SPINE

Case No. 65

Clinical history: A 20-years-old male patient with independent cranio-vertebral junction anomalies.

Radiological technique and observations: Figures 4.65.1 to 4.65.7 are limited sections of CT cervical spine in sagittal and coronal sections, MR Myelogram and MR sagittal showing increased Welcher basal angle, platybasia, occipitalization of C1 vertebrae, block vertebrae of C2–C3. Cervical spine and upper thoracic myelogram show loss of signal intensity at level of C1 vertebrae. Limited T2 sagittal sections has been provided shows platybasia, basilar invagination, reduction in spinal canal diameter. Odontoid hypoplasia noted. There is compression of upper cervical cord at level of C1 against the dens noted.

Interpretation: A—20 years old male, craniovertebral junction shows, B—platybasia, occipitalization of atlas,

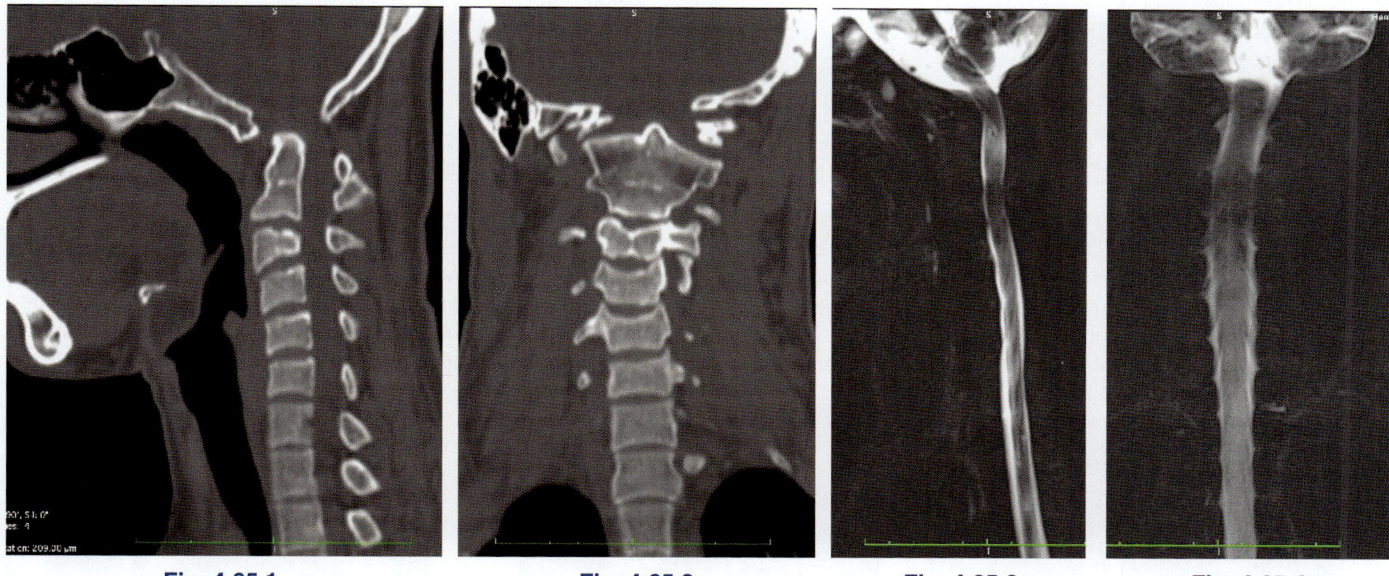

Fig. 4.65.1 Fig. 4.65.2 Fig. 4.65.3 Fig. 4.65.4

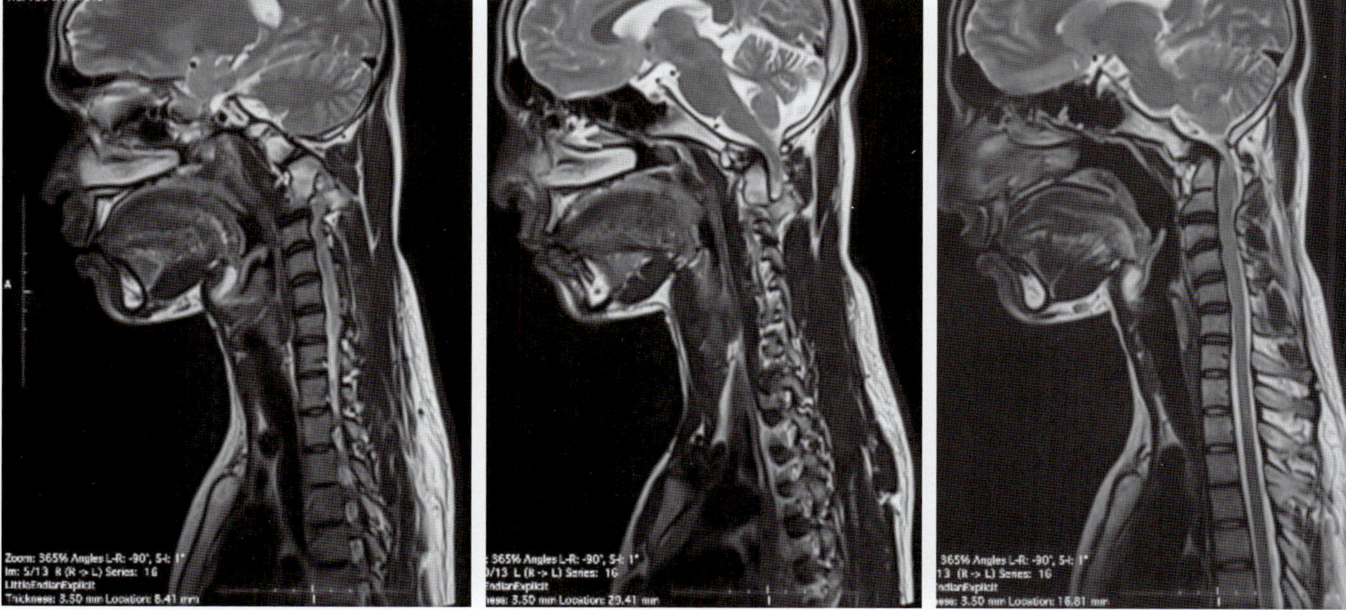

Fig. 4.65.5 Fig. 4.65.6 Fig. 4.65.7

Table 4.65.1: Classification of CVJ anomalies

Congenital	*Acquired*
Malformation of the occipital bone • Assimilation of the atlas • Atlas variants • Basilar invagination • Condylar hypoplasia • Clivus segmentation • Dens segmentation anomalies • Foramen magnum remnants *Malformations of the atlas* • Assimilation of the atlas • Atlantoaxial fusion • Aplasia of atlas arch *Malformations of the axis* • Irregular atlantoaxial segmentation • Dens dysplasias/hypoplasia/aplasia • Ossiculum terminals persistent	Abnormalities at foramen magnum • Secondary basilar invaginations (Paget's disease, rheumatoid arthritis) • Foraminal stenosis (e.g. achondroplasia) *Atlantoaxial instability* • Errors of metabolism • Down's syndrome • Infections (Grisel's syndrome) • Inflammatory (RA) • Traumatic • Tumors—neurofibromatosis • Miscellaneous: Syringomyelia, fetal warfarin syndrome, Conradi's syndrome

Table 4.65.2: Crucial lines and angles for diagnosing CVJ anomalies

Chamberlain's line: Line extend between posterior pole of the hard palate and opisthion. Tip of dens commonly lies below or just tangent to the line or may normally project 2.5 mm above this line. 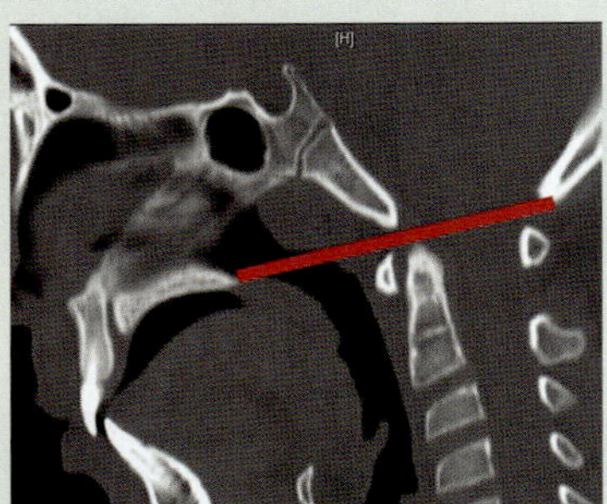 **Fig. 4.65.8:** Chamberlain's line	**McGregor line:** Line between the posterior pole of the hard palate to the lowest portion of the occipito squamosal surface. Tip of the dens should be 5 mm above this line. 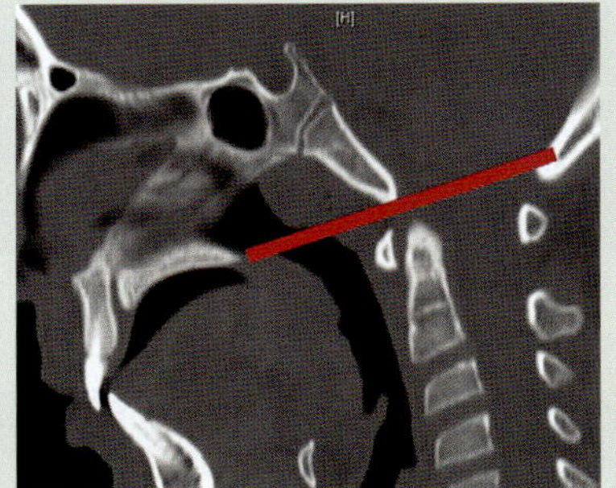 **Fig. 4.65.9:** McGregor line	**McRae's line:** Line between the basion and opisthion, tip of the dens should be below this line, if above this line s/o basilar invagination. 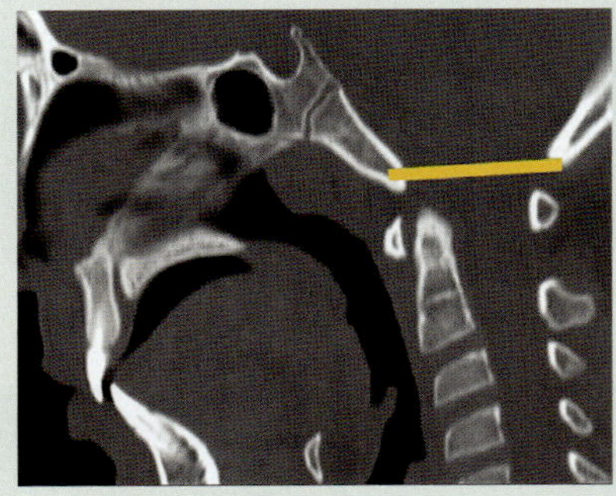 **Fig. 4.65.10:** McRae's line
Wackenheim's line (basilar line/clival canal line): It is the line along the clivus which is tangential to posterior aspect of the dens. Line should fall tangential to posterior aspect of the dens; if not s/o basilar invagination. 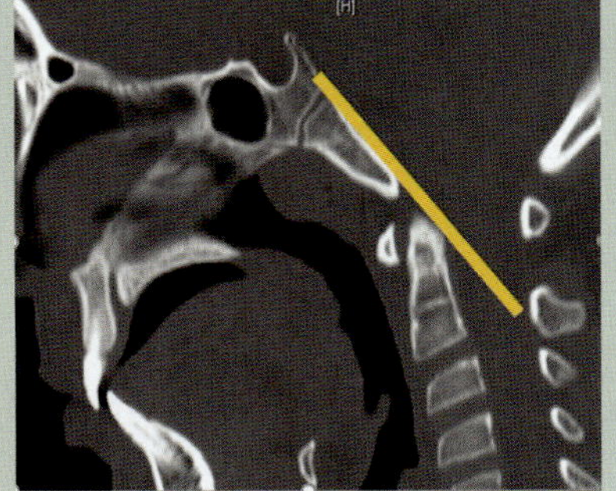 **Fig. 4.65.11:** Wackenheim's line	**Clivus canal angle:** Angle formed at the intersection of the Wackenheim's clivus baseline with a line constructed along the posterior surface of the axis body and dens. Clivus canal angle should range between 150–180 degree. 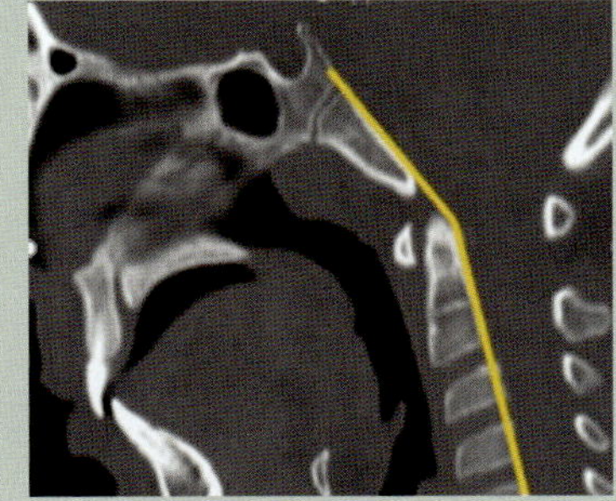 **Fig. 4.65.12:** Clivus canal angle	**Welcher basal angle:** Angle formed by intersection of the nasion-tuberculum line and tuberculum basion line. It should be less than 140 degree. 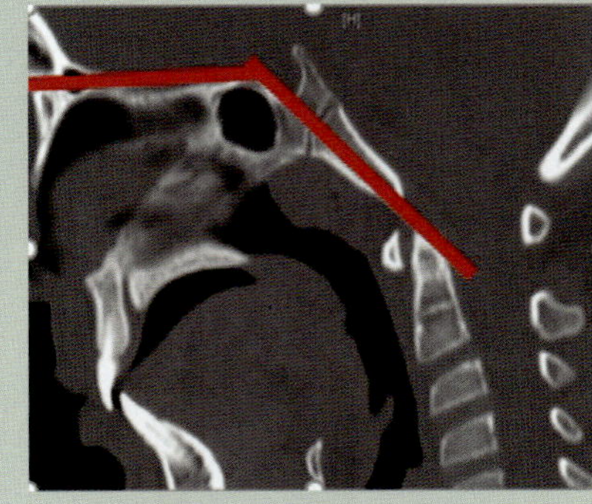 **Fig. 4.65.13:** Welcher basal angle

Contd...

<table>
<tr><th colspan="6">Table 4.65.2: Crucial lines and angles for diagnosing CVJ anomalies (Contd...)</th></tr>
<tr>
<td colspan="3">Atlanto-occipital joint axis angle (Schmidt-Fisher angle): Angle formed by line drawn parallel to both atlanto-occipital joints which typically intersects at the centre of the dens when condyles are symmetric. Average angle is 125 degree (124–127 degree) and becomes obtuse in condylar hypoplasia.
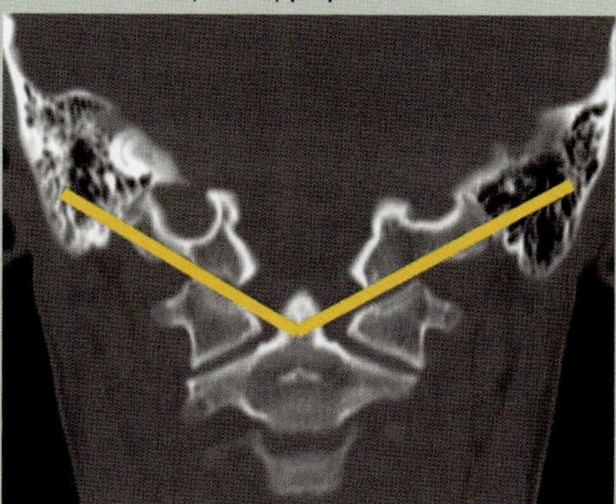
Fig. 4.65.14: Schmidt-Fisher angle</td>
<td colspan="3">Basion odontoid index (Whooley's index)
Joins basion to the tip of odontoid process. 5 mm in adults 10 mm in children (in neutral position). Measurements are altered in flexion and extension.
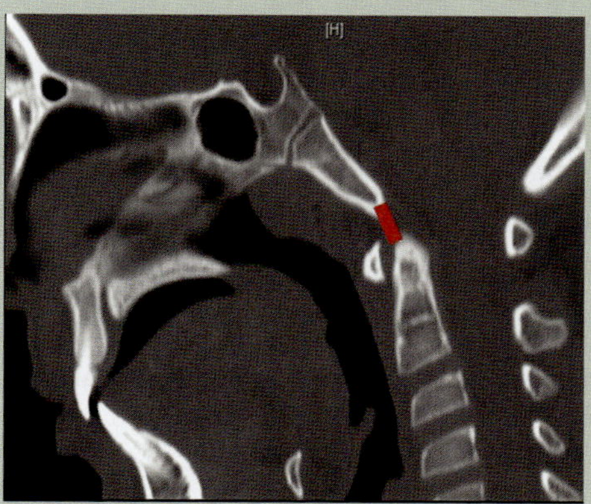
Fig. 4.65.15: Whooley's index</td>
</tr>
<tr>
<td colspan="2">Klaus index: Distance between tip of dens and tuberculum torcula line cruciate line. Normal: 40–41mm. Basilar invagination <30 mm.
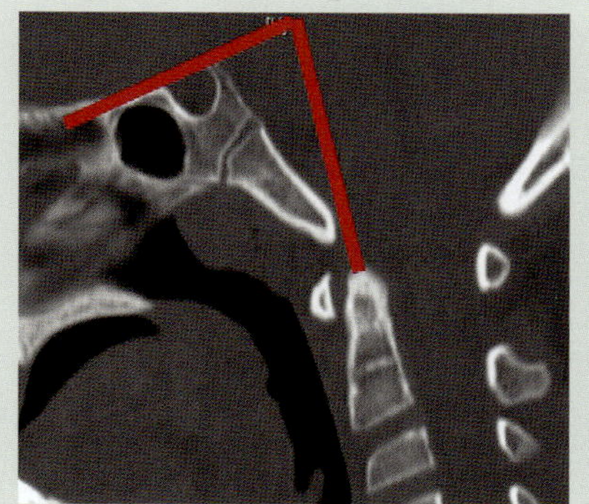
Fig. 4.65.16: Klaus index</td>
<td colspan="2">Bull's angle: Angle formed by joining the hard palate post and the line joining the midpoints of anterior and posterior arches of atlas.
<10 degrees are normal.
>13 degrees in basilar invagination.
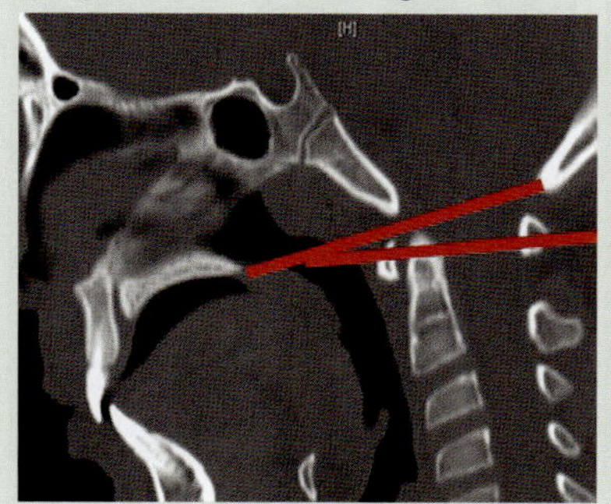
Fig. 4.65.17: Bull's angle</td>
<td colspan="2">Boogard's angle: Angle between McRae's line and the line drawn from dorsum sellae to basion along plane of clivus.
122 degree is normal. >135 degree is basilar invagination.
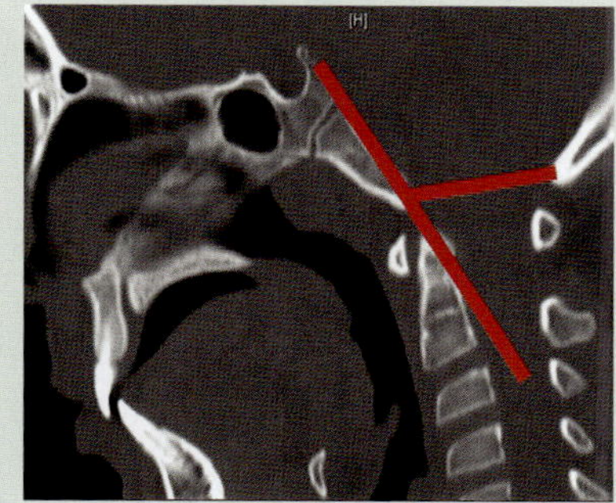
Fig. 4.65.18: Boogard's angle</td>
</tr>
<tr>
<td colspan="2">All three lines–McRae (yellow), Chamberlain's line and McGregor line in a single diagram. All three lines are called Z line.
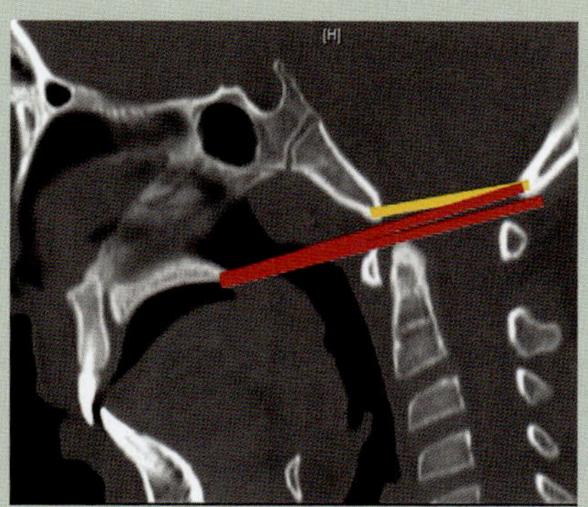
Fig. 4.65.19: Z line</td>
<td colspan="2">Powers ratio: Measurement of relationship of foramen magnum to atlas in midsagittal plane. It is used in diagnosis of atlantoaxial dissociation injuries.
Basion(A) and spinolaminar line of atlas (B), opisthion(C), anterior arch of atlas (D).
Powers ratio: AB/CD.
Normal value :<0.9–1</td>
<td colspan="2">Atlantoaxial distance (atlantodental): Normal <3 mm in adults, <4–5 mm in children.
Post-dens spinal canal diameter <10 mm indicates spinal canal stenosis.</td>
</tr>
</table>

Contd...

Table 4.65.2: Crucial lines and angles for diagnosing CVJ anomalies *(Contd...)*

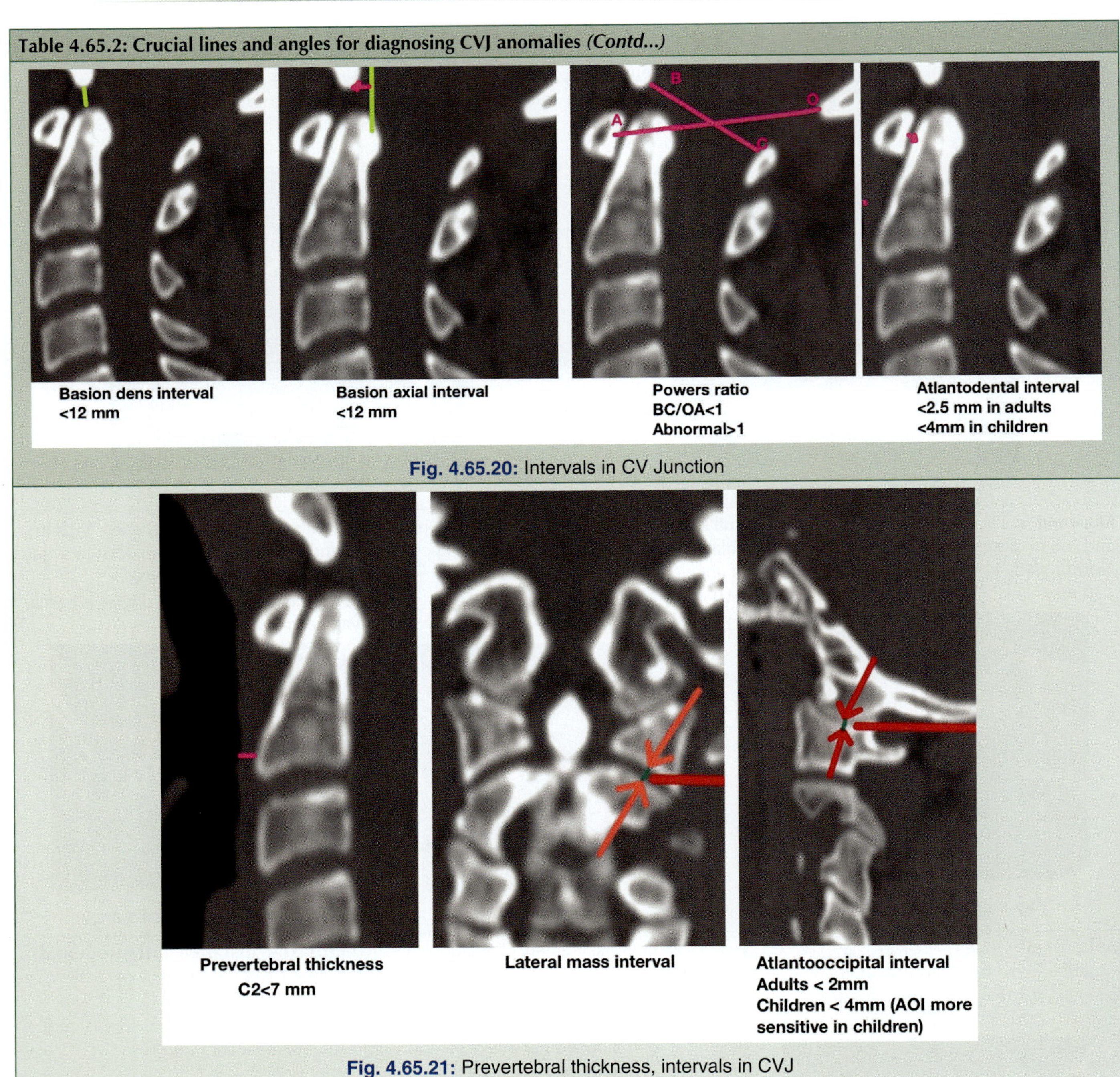

Fig. 4.65.20: Intervals in CV Junction

Fig. 4.65.21: Prevertebral thickness, intervals in CVJ

Table 4.65.3: Causes of platybasia

Congenital	*Acquired*
Achondroplasia	Paget disease
Down syndrome	Osteomalacia
Chiari malformations	Rickets
Craniocleidodysostosis	Trauma
Craniofacial anomalies	Fibrous dysplasia
Osteogenesis imperfecta	Hyperparathyroidism
	Hypoparathyroidism

basilar invagination, C—compression of upper cervical spinal cord, D—CVJ anomaly.

Principal diagnosis: Craniovertebral junction anomalies of congenital variety.

Craniovertebral junction: Craniovertebral junction comprises the occiput, occipital condyle (C0), atlas (C1), axis (C2), articulations and connecting ligaments.

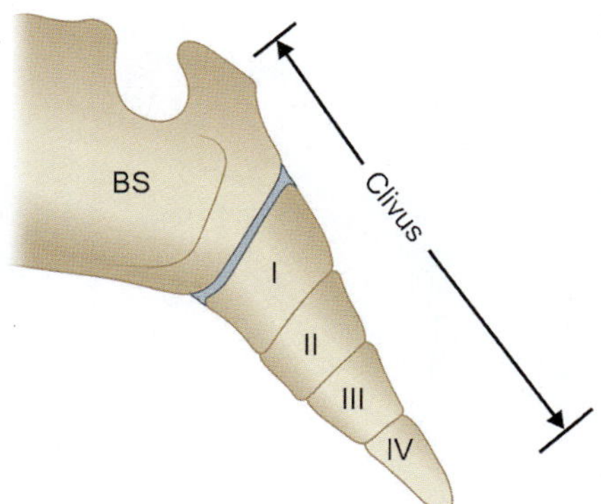

Fig. 4.65.22: Normal craniovertebral junction

Craniovertebral junction—embryology: Craniovertebral junction develops from 4 occipital somites and 2 cervical somites. It includes first 2 occipital somites form the basi occiput, 3rd somite forms the jugular tubercle, 4th somite forms the pro-atlas, the hypo centrum of the first spinal sclerotome forms the anterior arch, the centrum forms the dens, the neural arch forms the posterior arch.

Basilar invagination: It refers to a primary developmental anomaly in which the vertebral column is abnormally high and prolapsed into the skull base. Because the anomaly may be due to a number of causes (basi occiput hypoplasia, occipital condyle hypoplasia, various atlanto-occipital assimilations), it might be best to think of basilar invagination as a radiographic finding and not a diagnosis in and of itself. If at all possible, one should attempt to define the underlying abnormality responsible for the basilar invagination. There is an increased prevalence of neural dysgenesis associated with basilar invagination, such as the Chiari malformation or syringomyelia.

Basilar impression: The term 'basilar impression' should be reserved for the secondary or acquired form of basilar invagination. It results from softening of the skull base and is uncommon, mainly seen in association with Paget disease and osteomalacia. Other conditions that have been described in association with basilar impression

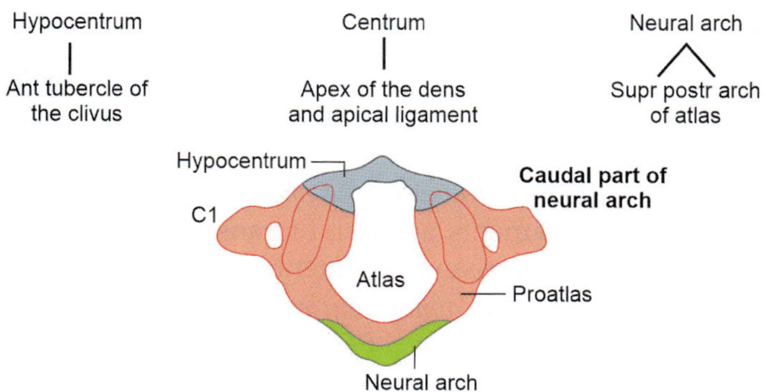

Fig. 4.65.23: Embryology of craniovertebral junction

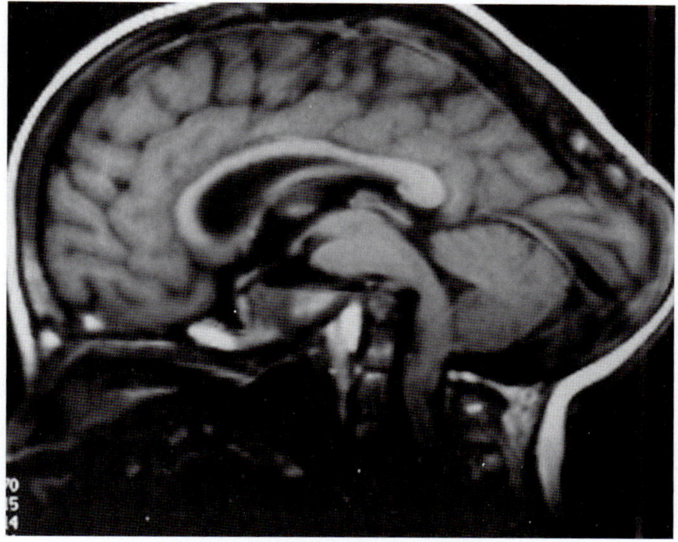
Fig. 4.65.24: Basilar invagination

include hyperparathyroidism, osteogenesis imperfecta, Hurler syndrome, rickets, and skull base infection. The term "cranial settling' is typically applied to the CVJ changes associated with rheumatoid arthritis. To say "basilar invagination or impression"—at least 2 lines should be violated.

Platybasia: Platybasia is an anthropometric term that refers to flattening of the skull base, manifested by an increase in the Welcher basal angle (>140 degree). Platybasia may occasionally be an isolated finding without associated basilar invagination.

Copper beaten skull: Copper beaten skull, also known as beaten silver skull or beaten brass skull, refers to the prominence of convolutional markings (gyral

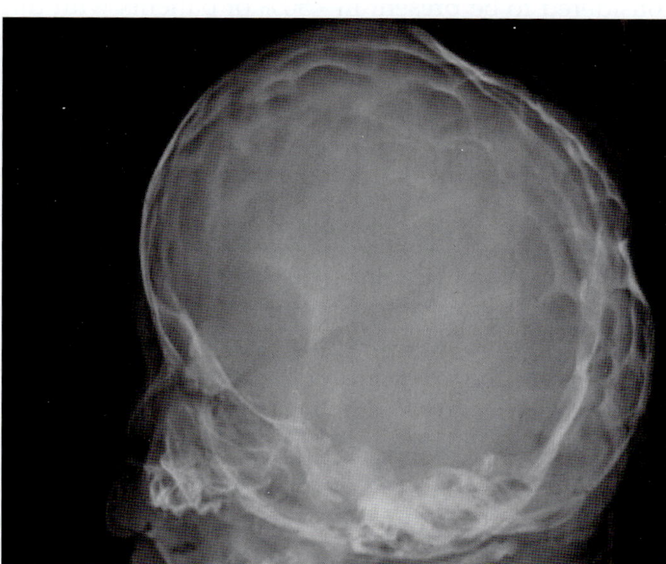
Fig. 4.65.25: Lückenschädel skull

impressions on the inner table of the skull) seen throughout the vault. The appearance of a copper beaten skull is associated with raised intracranial pressure in children. Hence, a pathology that causes raised intracranial pressure may be the primary cause of copper beaten skull; these include: craniosynostosis, obstructive hydrocephalus, hypophosphatasia, intracranial masses.

Abnormal posterior fossa in Chiari 1 malformation.

All—patients with Chiari malformation 1 demonstrate abnormal geometry of the bony posterior fossa ("normal-sized hindbrain housed in a too small bony envelope"). Various combinations of congenitally reduced clival length, shortened basi occiput, and craniovertebral junction (CVJ) fusion anomalies involving occipitalization of atlas may all result in diminished posterior cranial fossa depth and/or an abnormally small posterior fossa volume.

Lacunar skull Lückenschädel skull, also known as **lacunar skull** or **craniolacunae**, is a dysplasia of the membranous skull vault and is associated with Chiari II malformations (seen in up to 80% of such cases).

The inner table is more affected than the outer, with regions of apparent thinning (corresponding to unossified fibrous bone) of the skull vault. If particularly severe, with the individual lacunae joining into larger defects the term craniofenestrae is used.

Lückenschädel skull is characterized by groups of rounds, oval or finger-shaped pits on the inner surface of the vault (membranous part), separated by ridges of bone. They lie in the thickest part of the frontal, parietal, and upper occipital bones.

Klippel-Feil syndrome: The classic clinical triad of a short neck, low hairline, and restricted neck motion is considered to be present in <50% of patients with this syndrome. Three types grouped depending on the extent and location of vertebral fusion as well as associated vertebral abnormalities: Type I: Fusion of many cervical and upper thoracic vertebrae. Type II: Fusion of two or three vertebrae with associated hemivertebrae, occipito-atlantal fusion or other cervical spine abnormalities. Type III: Cervical fusion with lower thoracic or lumbar vertebral fusion. Vertebral fusion—fused facets and spinous processes, anteroposterior narrowing of the vertebral bodies (wasp-waist sign), hemivertebrae, omovertebral bone, spina bifida, associated scoliosis, Sprengel deformity, anomalies of the aortic arch and branching vessels, e.g. carotid, subclavian arteries, renal abnormalities, e.g. unilateral renal agenesis.

Signs of inrcreased intracranial pressure: Various mechanisms have been proposed to explain its pathogenesis, including decreased CSF absorption, increased CSF production, increased intravascular volume, increased intracranial venous pressure and hormonal changes. **Radigraphic findings:** Erosion of anterior and posterior clinoid process. Diffuse, silver beaten-copper pattern is an indicator of chronic elevated ICP, which is more common in patients with craniosynostosis. Additional findings associated with a chronic increase in ICP include macrocrania, splitting of the sutures, skull demineralization and erosion or enlargement of the sella turcica. **CT and MRI:** It follows from the Monro-Kellie doctrine that as the CSF pressure inside the skull increases, the brain and blood volume have to accommodate this, resulting in the phenomenon of mass-effect, explaining the findings of raised intracranial pressure on cross-sectional brain imaging: Effacement of the ventricles, basal cisterns and other CSF spaces, brain herniation, loss of grey-white matter differentiation, papilledema, slit like lateral ventricles.

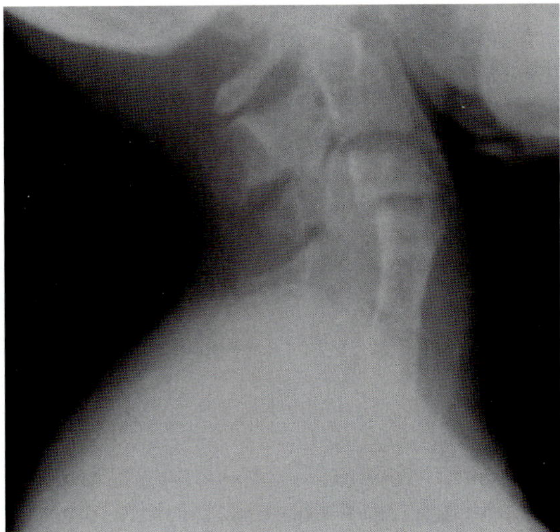

Fig. 4.65.26: Klippel-Feil syndrome

CVJ anomalies in Down syndrome: Associated CVJ anomalies (can occur isolated or in clusters)

1. *Atlanto-occipital instability:* AP translation of occiput over atlas >1 mm from flexion to extension. Post-subluxation of atlas.
2. *Atlantoaxial instability:* Atlantodental distance is >7 to 9 mm (depending on age), hypoplasia of transverse ligaments, agenesis of transverse ligaments and laxity of transverse ligaments.
3. *Abnormalities of transverse ligaments:* Hypoplasia of transverse ligaments, agenesis of transverse ligaments and laxity of transverse ligaments.
4. *Atlas and odontoid abnormalities:* Hypoplastic atlas, decreased AP diameter of C1 bony ring, non-union of posterior arch and odontoid anomalies (ossiculum terminale persistens, os odontoideum, agenesis).

Table 4.65.4: Individual CVJ anomalies

Occipitalisation of atlas: It is a congenital synostosis of the atlas to the occiput caused by a failure of segmentation and separation of the most caudal occipital sclerotome during 1st few weeks of fetal life. Complete fusion—fusion of anterior and posterior arches with the occiput as well as bilateral atlanto-occipital joint fusion. Incomplete fusion can be of many types 1) Anterior arch fusions to occiput with absence of transverse process 2) Anterior arch fusion to occiput with post-arch fusion to axis 3) Posterior arch fusion to occiput. 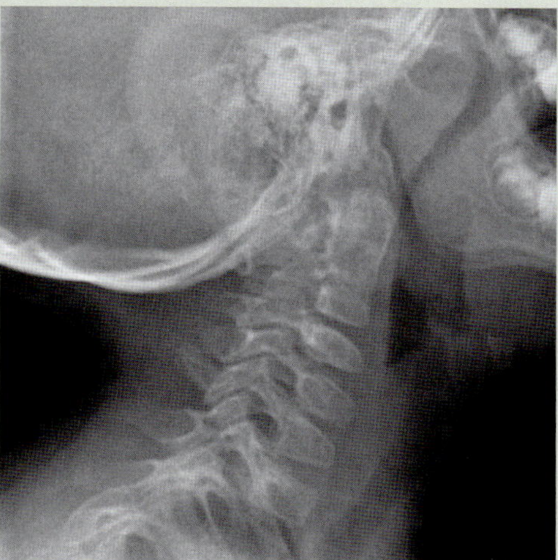 **Fig. 4.65.27:** Occipitalisation of atlas	**Occipital vertebrae:** Occipital bone is formed from union of 4 to 5 somites, which normally fuse together to encircle the foramen magnum but sometimes the last occipital somite or proatlas may fail to fully incorporate into the occiput resulting in occipital or proatlas vertebrae. 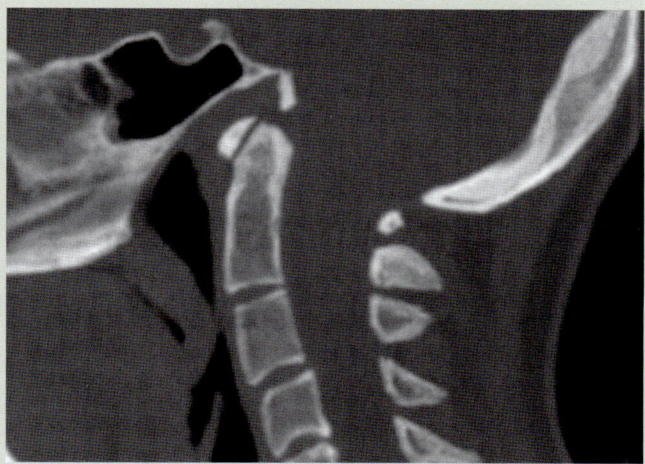 **Fig. 4.65.28:** Occipital vertebrae
3rd condyle: Most common form of occipital vertebrae. Anterior midline bony process located between 2 occipital condyles and continues with the anterior foramen magnum and extends a variable distance caudally. It occasionally articulates with the apex of odontoid process or ant arch of atlas.	**Paracondylar, paramastoid and epitransverse process:** All the above 3 are variations of bony bars that extend between occiput and transverse process of atlas May be unilateral or bilateral. Slightly rotated open mouth AP view and fine section CT are required to visualise them.
Accessory atlanto-occipital ossicles: A variety of bony fragments may develop in the atlanto-occipital interspace. May be single or multiple. Position may be anterior, posterior or lateral. Accessory ossicles may be confused with fracture of foramen magnum or atlas.	**Ponticles of atlas:** Calcification or ossification along the margins of normally occurring foramina in the atlanto-occipital ligament is referred to as ponticles also known as ponticulus posticus, arcuate foramen, Kimmerle's anomaly 1. Posterior–ossification or calcification of the oblique portion of atlanto-occipital membrane that bridges the post-lateral mass and the post-arch 2. Lateral–ossification in the oblique occipital membrane as it passes laterally from the superolateral aspect of the lateral mass to the transverse process of atlas.
Ossiculum terminale persistens (of Bergmann): Secondary apical ossification centre at the tip of dens normally appears at 2 years of age and unites to the dens at the age of 12 years. Failure of union to the dens produces an isolated ossicle at the tip that is not typically linked to neck pain syndromes. X-ray—ossicle appears as a 3 to 5 mm, discrete, ovoid or diamond-shaped ossicle visible at the most cephalic portion of the dens. Requires thin CT sections and MRI to diagnose it and exclude fractures or Down's syndrome.	**OS odontoideum:** Nonunion of the dens with the axis body. Familial incidence present. Associated conditions–Down's syndrome, occipitalization, atlas hypoplasia, block vertebra, Klippel-Feil syndrome, skeletal dysplasia and Morquio syndrome **OS odontoideum will have a corticated margin with enlarged sclerosed anterior arch of atlas.** No edema seen in MRI helps in differentiating from fracture. **Types: Orthotopic**—normal position with wide gap between C2 and os odontoideum **Dystopic**—displaced C2 (os avis)
Os odontoideum with atlantoaxial subluxation	

4

Contd...

Table 4.65.4: Individual CVJ anomalies *(Contd...)*

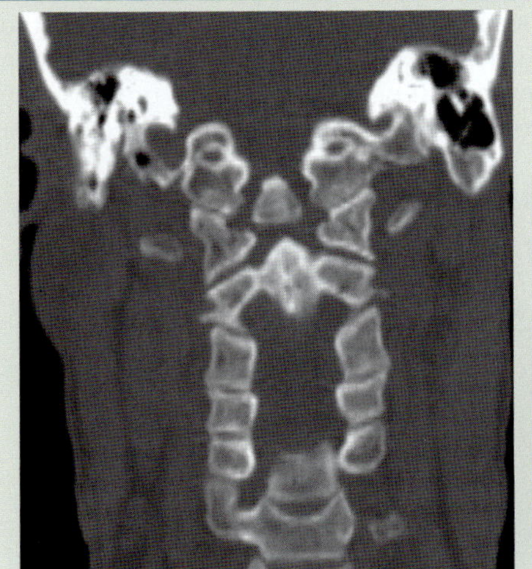

Fig. 4.65.29: Os odontoideum with atlantoaxial subluxation

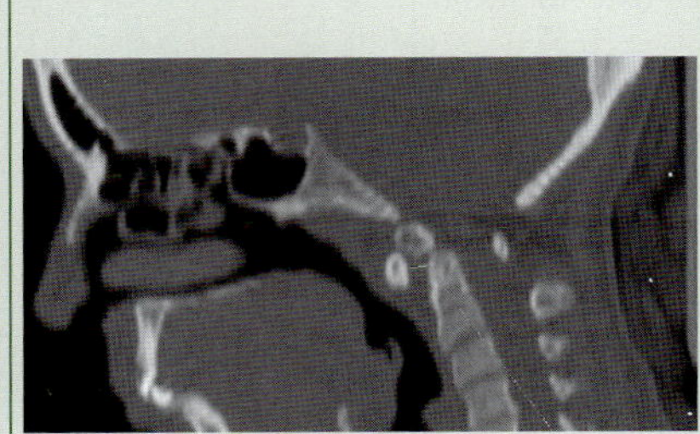

Fig. 4.65.30: Os odontoideum with atlantoaxial subluxation

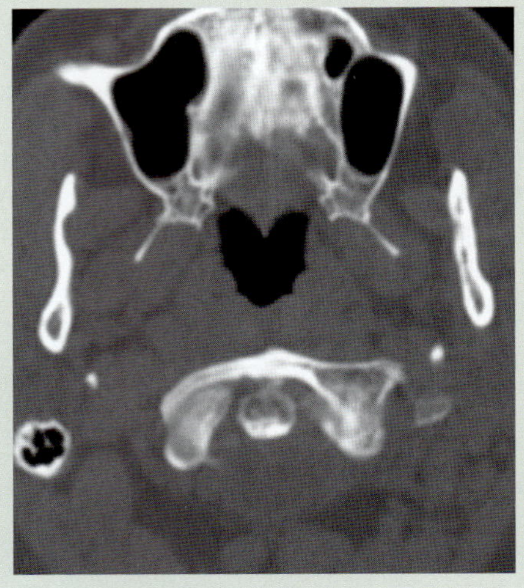

Fig. 4.65.31: Os odontoideum with atlantoaxial subluxation

Absent C1 fusion of C0 And C2 with basilar invagination

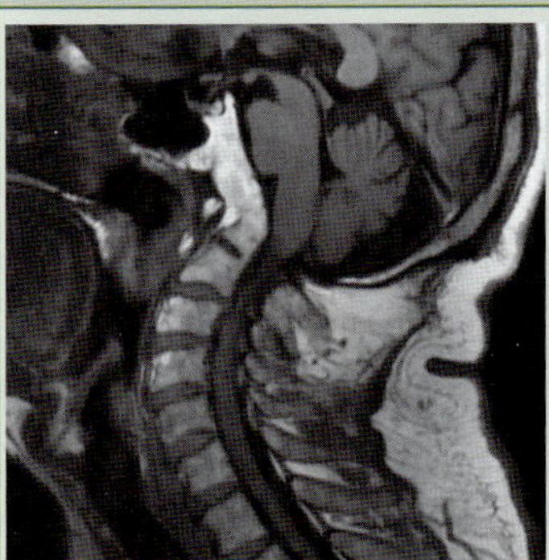

Fig. 4.65.32: Absent C1 fusion of C0 and C2 with basilar invagination

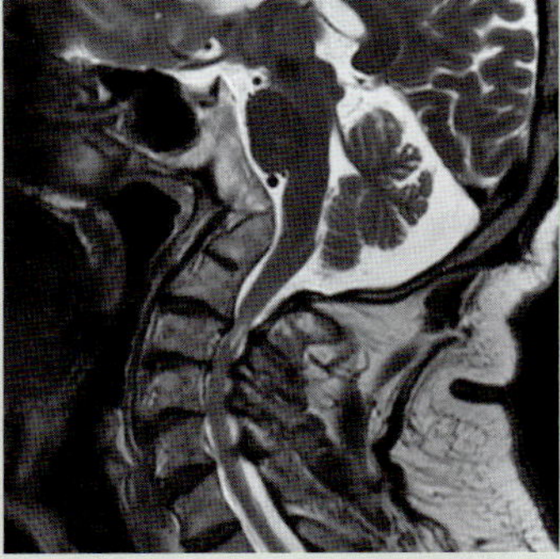

Fig. 4.65.33: Absent C1 fusion of C0 and C2 with basilar invagination

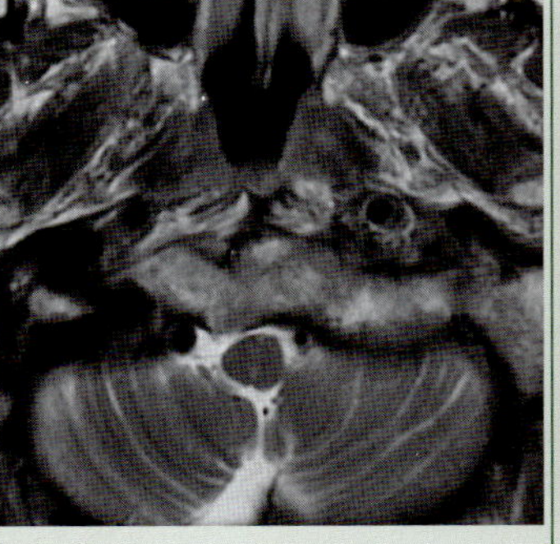

Fig. 4.65.34: Absent C1 fusion of C0 and C2 with basilar invagination

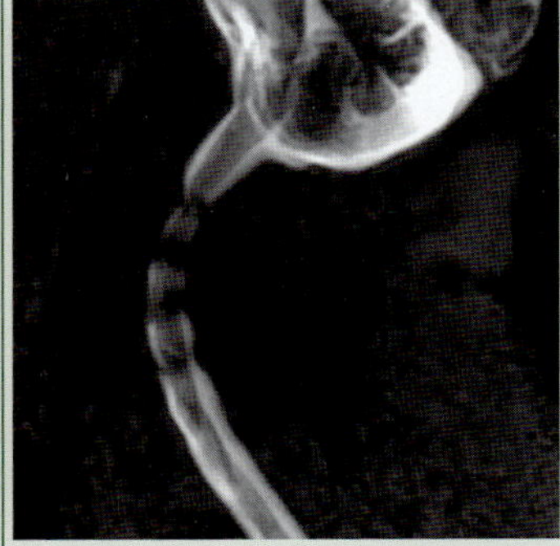

Fig. 4.65.35: Absent C1 fusion of C0 and C2 with basilar invagination

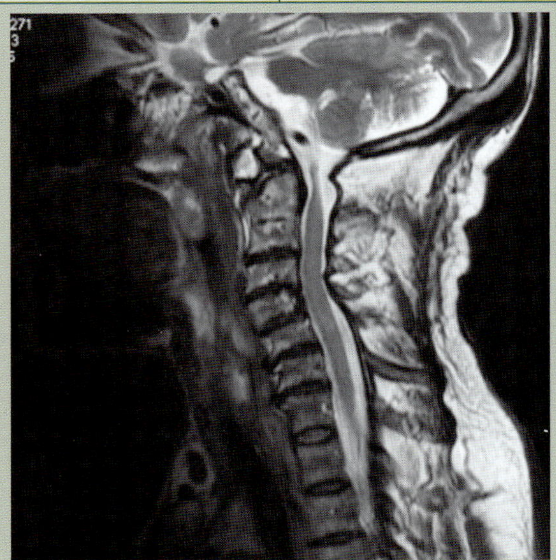

Fig. 4.65.36: Absent C1 posterior arch

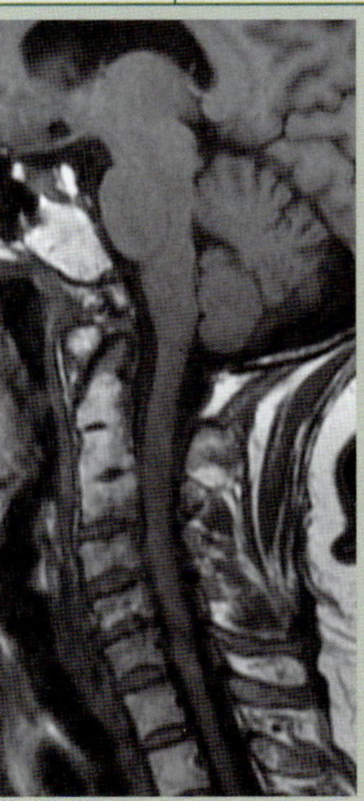

Fig. 4.65.37: Fusion of C2, C3; absent post-arch of C1

Contd...

Table 4.65.4: Individual CVJ anomalies *(Contd...)*

<table>
<tr><td colspan="2">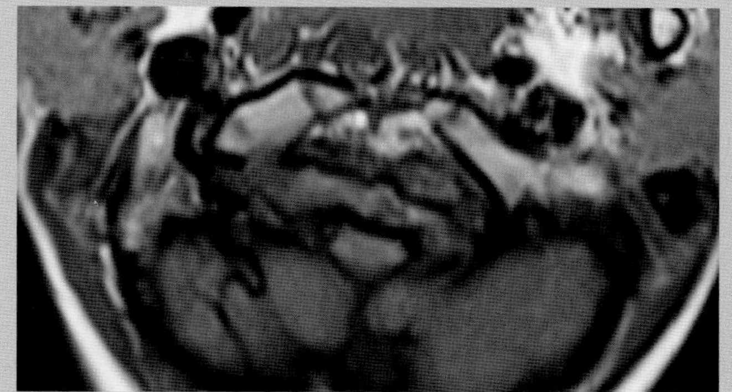
Fig. 4.65.38: Basilar invagination with atlantoaxial subluxation</td><td>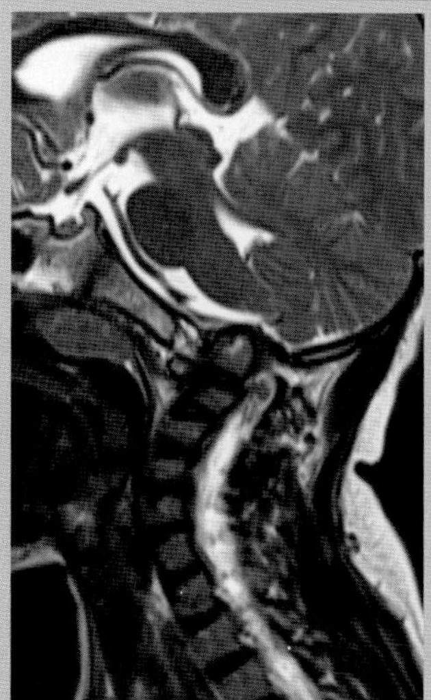
Fig. 4.65.39: Basilar invagination with atlantoaxial subluxation</td></tr>
<tr><td colspan="3">Klippel-Feil with Sprengel shoulder</td></tr>
<tr><td>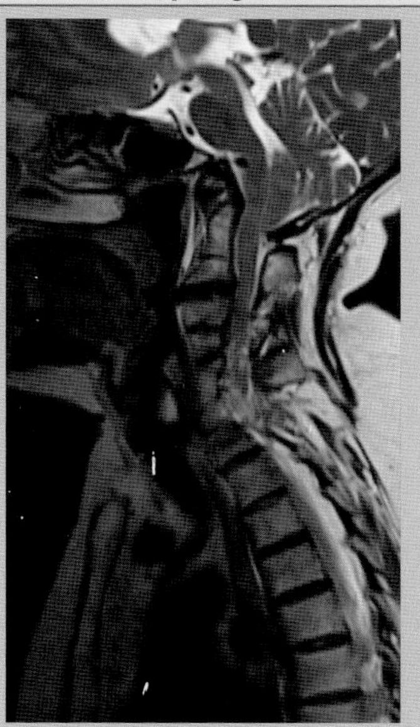
Fig. 4.65.40: Klippel-Feil with Sprengel shoulder</td><td>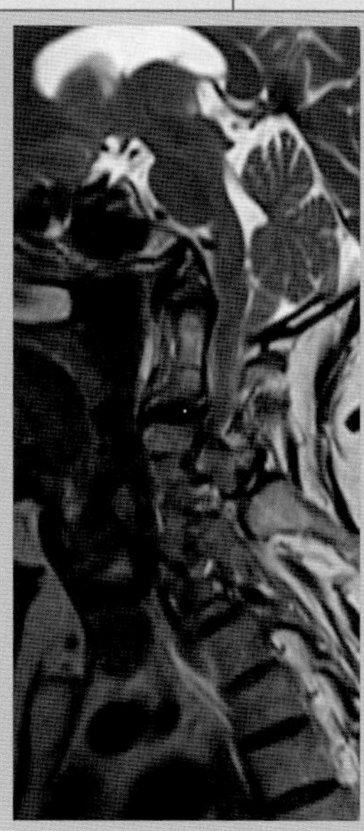
Fig. 4.65.41: Klippel-Feil with Sprengel shoulder</td><td>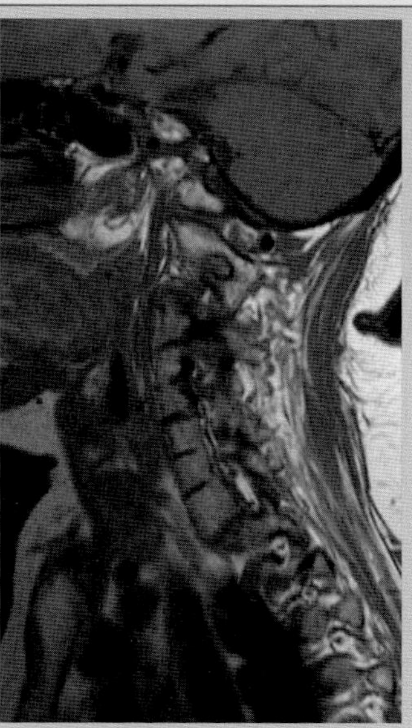
Fig. 4.65.42: Klippel-Feil with Sprengel shoulder</td></tr>
<tr><td colspan="3">Occipital vertebrae</td></tr>
<tr><td colspan="2">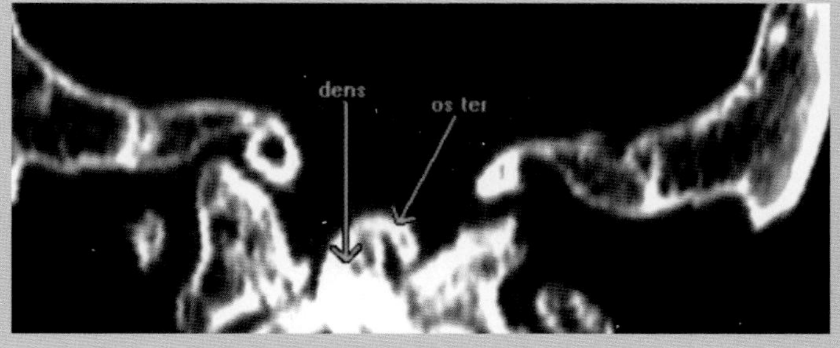

Fig. 4.65.43: Os terminale</td><td>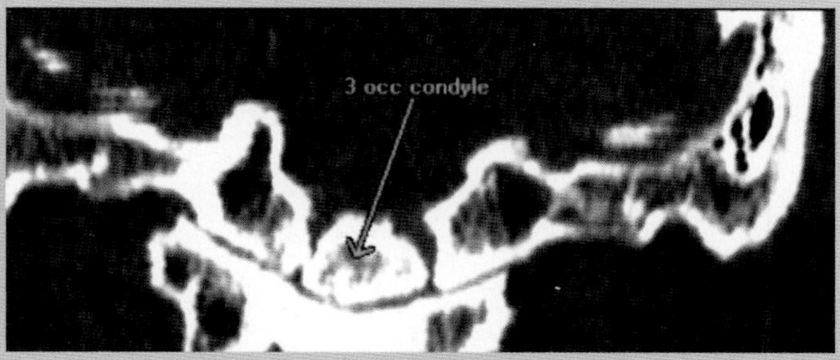

Fig. 4.65.44: Occipital condyle</td></tr>
</table>

Contd...

Table 4.65.4: Individual CVJ anomalies *(Contd...)*

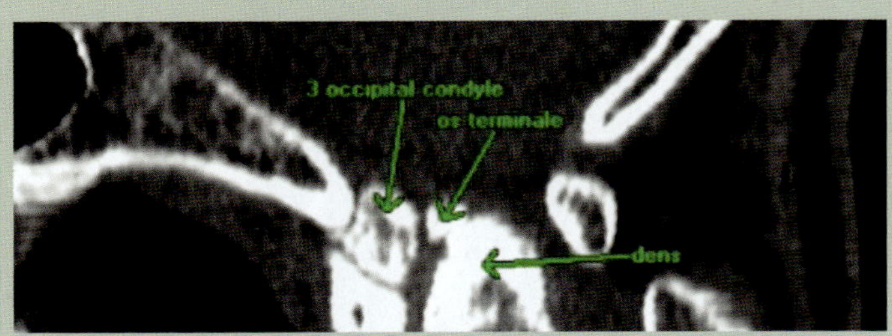

Fig. 4.65.45: Occipital condyle

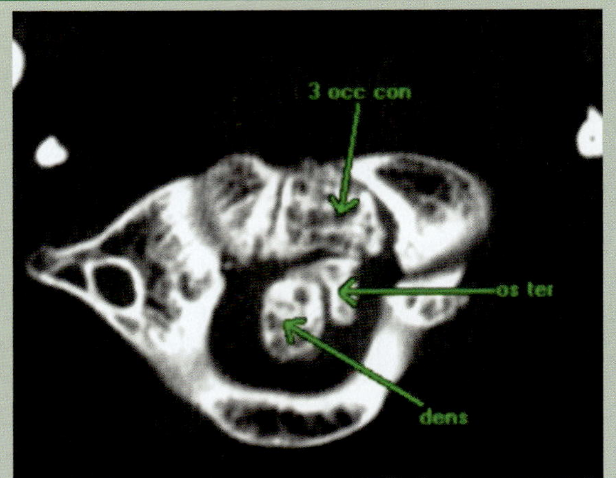

Fig. 4.65.46: Occipital condyle

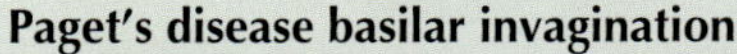

Paget's disease basilar invagination

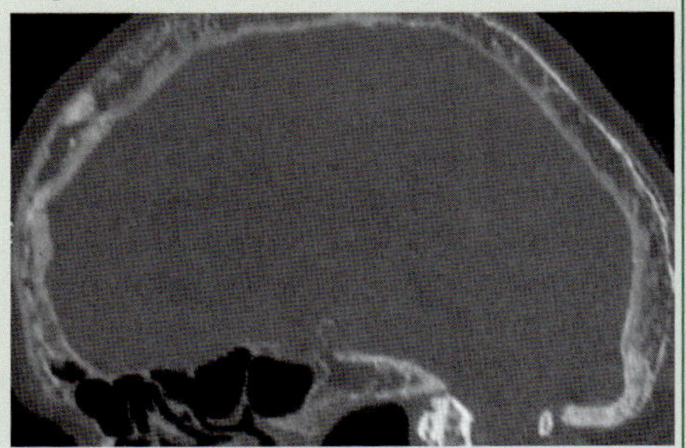

Fig. 4.65.47: Paget's disease basilar invagination

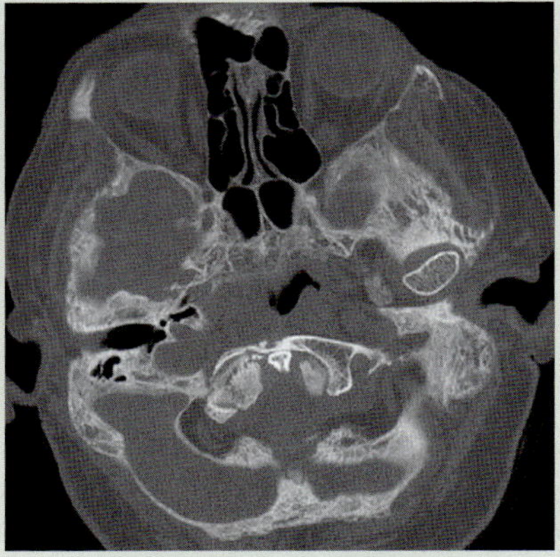

Fig. 4.65.48: Paget's disease basilar invagination

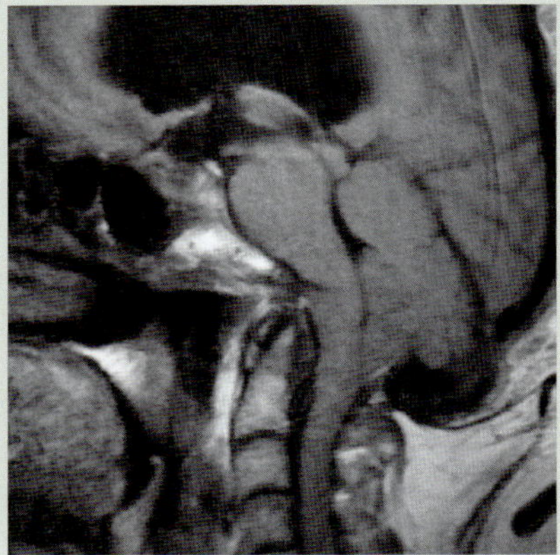

Fig. 4.65.49: Paget's disease basilar invagination

4.66 HEAD AND NECK

Case No. 66

Clinical history: A two-year-old child complaining of fever and throat pain and neck stiffness for 3 days.

Radiological technique and observation: Figures 4.66.1 to 4.66.3 are MRI neck T2 sagittal, T2 axial and DWI images showing ill defined heterointense collection, measuring maximum depth of 1.5 cm at the level of C2–C3 vertebra located posterior and to left of pharynx extending from base of skull to C5 vertebral level, displacing the oropharynx anteriorly and to the right. Enlarged medial retropharyngeal lymph node and necrotic left lateral retropharyngeal lymph node, showing diffusion restriction. Adjacent soft tissue edema noted. No evidence of epidural collection. No evidence of any bony involvement.

Interpretation: A—two years old child, lesion in retropharyngeal space, C—well-defined heterointense collection, B—shows diffusion restriction, D—retropharyngeal abscess

Principal diagnosis: Heterointense collection in clinical background of fever, neck pain suggests possibility of **suppurative adenopathy of retropharyngeal abscess**.

Differential diagnosis: The differential diagnosis of increased prevertebral soft tissues should include—retropharyngeal/prevertebral abscess, post-traumatic hematoma, and neoplasm from the adjacent bone and soft tissue structures.

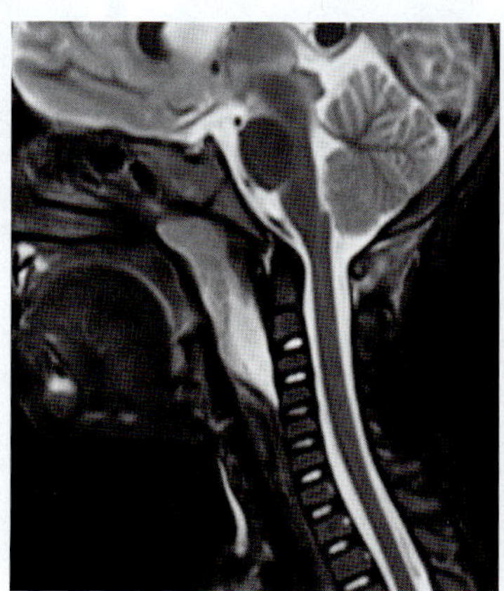

Fig. 4.66.1

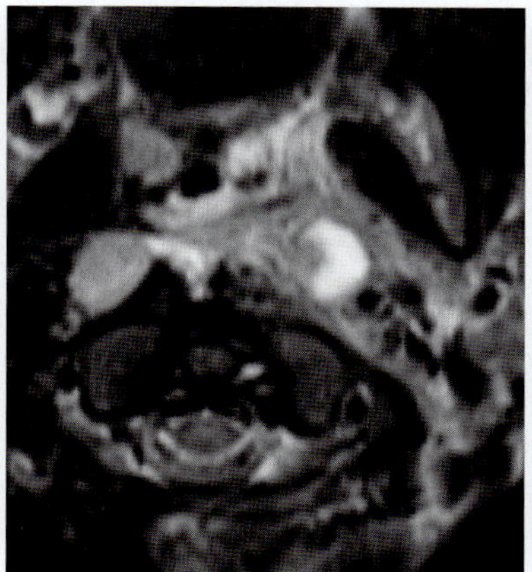

Fig. 4.66.2

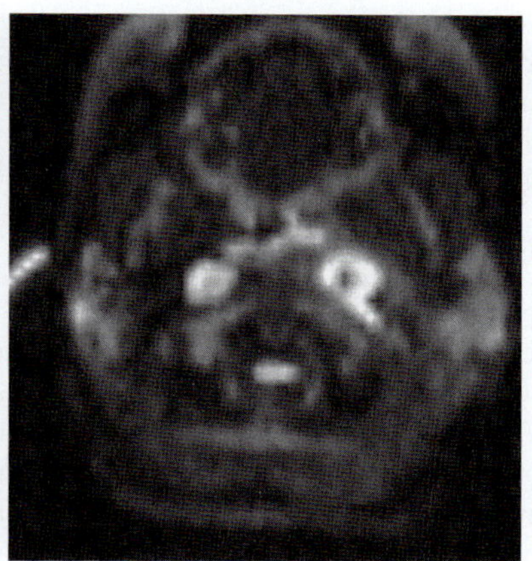

Fig. 4.66.3

Table 4.66.1: Prevertebral soft tissues normogram

	Level	Flexion (mm)	Neutral (mm)	Extension (mm)
	C1	11	10	8
Retropharyngeal interspace (RPI)	C2	6	5	6
	C3	7	7	6
Retrolaryngeal interspace (RLI)	C4	7	7	8
	C5	22	20	20
Retrotracheal interspace (RTI)	C6	20	20	19
	C7	20	20	21

If the patient's neck is flexed and/or if the radiograph is obtained during end-expiration, the prevertebral soft tissues may appear falsely widened and thus give the false impression of a possible retropharyngeal infection (RPI).

Table 4.66.2: Difference between retropharyngeal abscess and prevertebral space lesions

Retropharyngeal abscess	*Prevertebral space lesions*
Flattening of prevertebral muscles posteriorly	Anterior displacement of prevertebral muscles
Normal vertebra and discs	Vertebra ± disc destruction
Most commonly from necrotizing lymphadenitis/tonsillitis.	Most commonly from vertebral pathology

Retropharyngeal space: Midline space posterior to pharyngeal mucosa and cervical esophagus from skull base to T3 vertebral level in mediastinum.

<table>
<tr><th colspan="3">Table 4.66.3: Differential diagnosis for retropharyngeal space pathologies</th></tr>
<tr><td>Suppurative adenopathy of retropharyngeal space—lateral RPS nodes: Nodes of Rouvière</td><td colspan="2">Intranodal abscess
CT findings: NECT—prevertebral soft tissue fullness—node may be difficult to identify
CECT: Low density within enlarged node with peripheral enhancement
MR findings: T2WI—diffuse or focal central high intensity in RPS node with increased signal intensity of surrounding soft tissues
DWI—restricted diffusion in suppurative node
T1WI C+—peripheral node and adjacent soft tissue enhancement</td></tr>
<tr><td>Retropharyngeal space abscess
Midline RPS fluid collection with mass effect in toxic patient
Complications:
• Airway compromise
• Internal carotid artery (ICA) frequently narrowed
• ICA pseudoaneurysm suggests methicillin resistant Staphylococcus aureus (MRSA)
• Internal jugular vein (IJV) thrombosis
• Mediastinal extension</td><td>Extranodal purulent fluid collection in RPS.
Lateral plain radiograph.
In children: Must perform during inspiration and with neck extension
Widened prevertebral soft tissue thickness
CECT: RPS markedly distended by fluid collection with enhancing wall
MR: May aid in differentiating danger space from RPS collection (danger space is posterior to RPS, extends into mediastinum), rarely utilized in septic patient</td><td>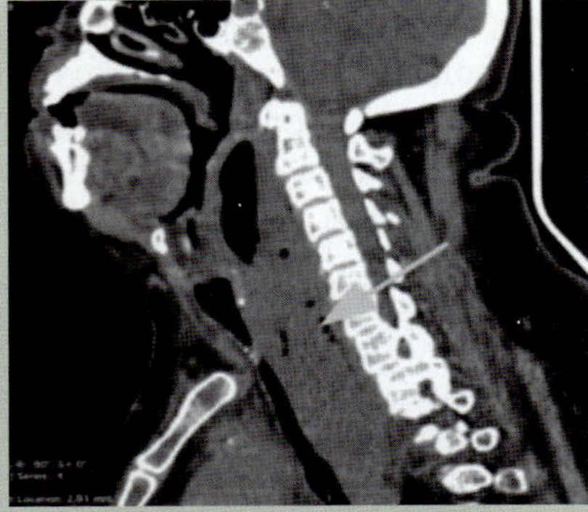
Fig. 4.66.4: Retropharyngeal space abscess</td></tr>
<tr><td colspan="3">Nodal squamous cell carcinoma of RPS: From nasopharyngeal or posterior wall oropharyngeal primary squamous cell carcinoma. CECT—round/oval, mildly enhancing soft tissue density mass in RPS. Necrosis appears as central low density with variably thick, irregular enhancing wall. Ill-defined margins ± standing of surrounding fat are features of extracapsular spread.
MR: T1WI—nodes isointense to muscle. T2WI—nodes hyperintense. T1WI C+—enhancing lateral or medial RPS node. If nodal necrosis, central low intensity with peripheral wall enhancement
Nuclear medicine findings: PET—PET has role in staging and follow-up of head and neck SCC. Cystic/necrotic nodes may be PET (–). Increased metabolic activity may diagnose metastatic SCC in small, non-necrotic RPS node.</td></tr>
<tr><td colspan="3">Nodal non-Hodgkin lymphoma in retropharyngeal space. Oval—round, solid mass >0.8 cm (axial) in RPS, typically associated with other neck adenopathy. PET—useful in staging and follow-up of most types of NHL, because of FDG avidity.</td></tr>
<tr><td colspan="3">Prevertebral abscess</td></tr>
<tr><td>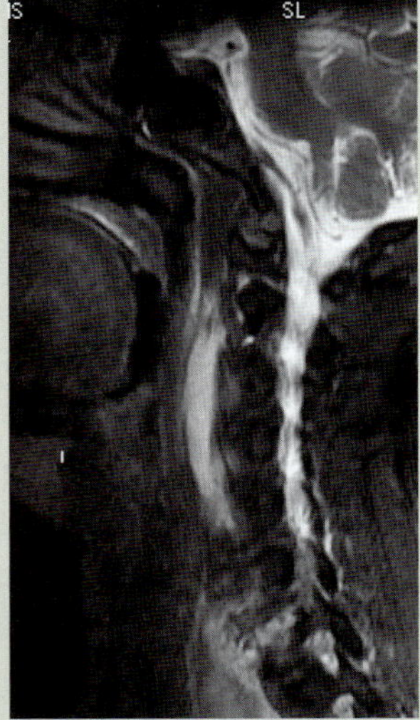
Fig. 4.66.5: Prevertebral abscess</td><td colspan="2">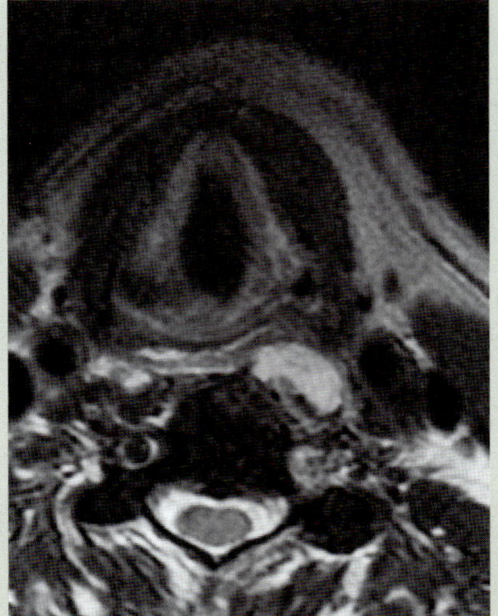
Fig. 4.66.6: Prevertebral abscess</td></tr>
</table>

(Contd.)

<table>
<tr><th colspan="3">Table 4.66.3: Differential diagnosis for retropharyngeal space pathologies (Contd.)</th></tr>
<tr><td>Suppurative adenitis
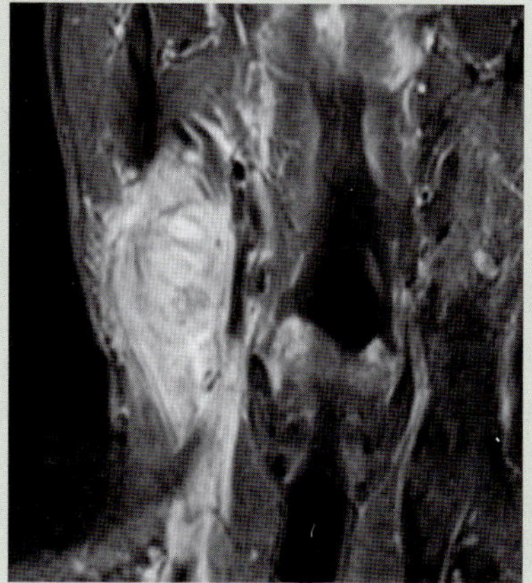
Fig. 4.66.7: Suppurative adenitis</td><td colspan="2">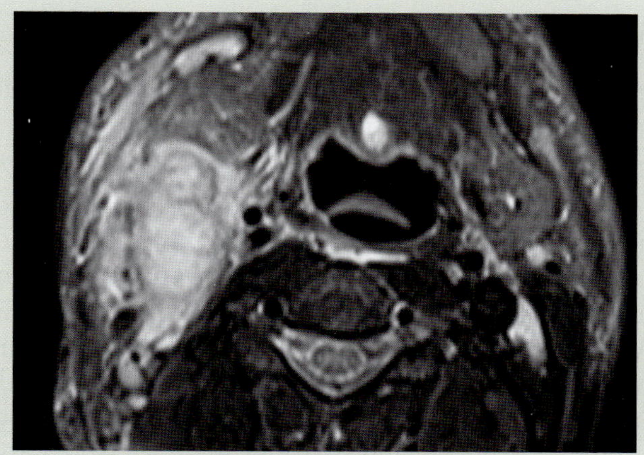
Fig. 4.66.8: Suppurative adenitis</td></tr>
<tr><td>Other differential diagnoses are foreign body (fish bone) with abscess, Thornwaldt cyst</td><td>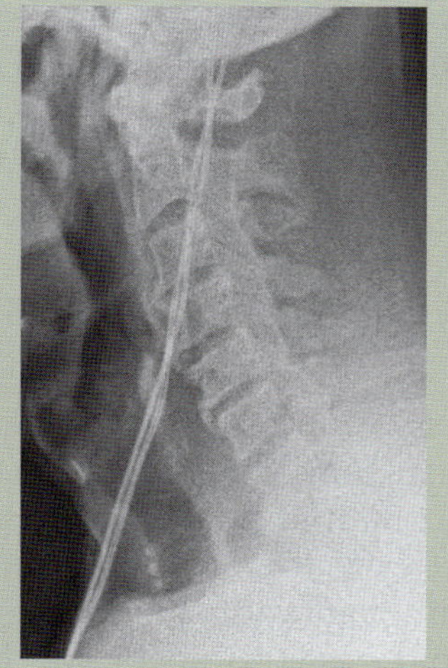
Fig. 4.66.9: Fish bone in retropharyngeal space in X-ray cervical spine</td><td>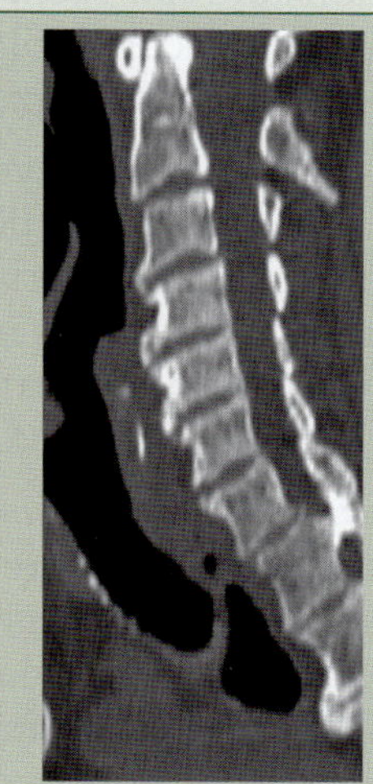
Fig. 4.66.10: CT showing fish bone in retropharyngeal space</td></tr>
</table>

Further investigations and management: Treatment is similar in principle to that of other infected collections usually requiring both surgical drainage and intravenous antibiotics. In some instances, antibiotics alone may suffice when collections are small.

<table>
<tr><th colspan="2">Table 4.66.4: Torticollis</th></tr>
<tr><td colspan="2">Torticollis (wry neck): It is a congenital or acquired deformity characterized by rotational deformity of the cervical spine with secondary tilting of the head</td></tr>
<tr><td>Congenital torticollis</td><td>Acquired torticollis</td></tr>
<tr><td>Muscles—congenital muscular torticollis, congenital absence of sternocleidomastoid
Skin—pterygium coli
Bone—occipitoaxial fusion, segmentation anomalies of axis/atlas (including Klippel-Feil syndrome, CVJ anomalies), syringomyelia, ocular abnormalities, ligamentous laxity—Down's syndrome, achondroplasia, osteogenesis imperfecta</td><td>Fibromatosis coli (sternocleidomastoid tumor)
Head and neck infections— osteomyelitis, retropharyngeal abscess, epidural abscess, lymphadenitis.
Fracture/dislocation in occipital condyle/unilateral facet dislocation.
Ligament laxity—minor trauma, Down syndrome, Arnold-Chiari, osteogenesis imperfecta and metabolic syndromes.
Idiopathic osteoarthritis, rheumatoid arthritis
Muscle spasm
Neoplasm—CNS, bone tumors, metastasis</td></tr>
</table>

4.67 HEAD AND NECK

Case No. 67

Clinical history: A 29-year-old female patient, came with complaint of a swelling in the neck.

Radiological techniques and observation: Figures 4.67.1 to 4.67.3 are T2 weighted, T1 weighted, and fat suppressed axial and sagittal MR images showing well-defined lobulated mass in the left side of the upper neck behind the region of the angle of the mandible. The lesion shows T2W high signal intensity and T1W intermediate signal intensity. There appear to be multiple tiny flow voids. There is no evidence of phleboliths (low intensity foci) or calcification within and surrounding the lesion. Large septations are not seen. There is no peri-lesion edema which is evidence of infiltration. The surrounding tissues are normal. The visualized brain parenchyma is normal.

Interpretation: A—29-year-old female, mass in the left side of the upper neck behind the region of the angle of the mandible, C—hyperintense on fat-suppressed images indicating that there is no involution and fatty change, B—homogeneous in intensity without any fluid-fluid levels, D—hemangioma.

The principal diagnosis is hemangioma: The possible differential diagnoses are: Hemangioma, lymphangioma, developmental venous malformation mixed venous malformation, branchial cleft cyst, thyroglossal duct cyst (it is usually midline), plunging ranula (no deeper extension seen here), dermoid cyst (no fat or solid component), abscess (no surrounding inflammation), rhabdomyosarcoma.

Discussion: Classification of vascular anomalies (ISSVA-2018). Can be classified as: Vascular tumors (infantile hemangioma), vascular malformation.

According to flow dynamics, vascular malformation can be further classified into high flow (AVM), lower flow (venous, lymphatic, mixed veno lymphatic, capillary).

Infantile hemangioma: They are the most common vascular lesions and are considered as a **vascular tumor**, not a vascular malformation. They are not present at birth and usually first present after 3 months of age. They have a proliferative phase and an involuting phase.

Proliferative hemangioma: Refers to the rapidly growing phase during the first few months. It is a high flow phase with bruit, pulsatility and warmth. On imaging, they show high signal intensity on T2 weighted images and intermediate signal intensity on T1 imaging. Flow voids may be present.

Involuting hemangioma: Infantile hemangiomas have a proliferating phase in the 1st few months, a slow but constant regression (involuting phase) can be seen, with the process usually being completed by 7–10 years of age. During that time, the hemangioma changes colour to greyish dark red, loses its toughness, and alters in shape, developing into a fibrofatty residuum. Imaging features: Appearances are more varied and heterogeneous. As increasing amounts of fat replace the tumor, foci of increased signal intensity are noted in the lesion on T1-weighted images and less avid enhancement is seen.

Capillary hemangioma: This is a cutaneous lesion which occurs at birth. It grows proportionately to the child without regression. It is a skin thickness lesion and does not show any characteristic imaging feature. It is associated with syndromes such as Sturge-Weber.

Congenital hemangioma: Unlike the infantile form, congenital hemangiomas are fully formed lesions at birth. They are classified as rapidly involuting congenital hemangioma (RICH), which **involutes at 1 year of age** and non-involuting congenital hemangioma (NICH) which grows proportionately with the body.

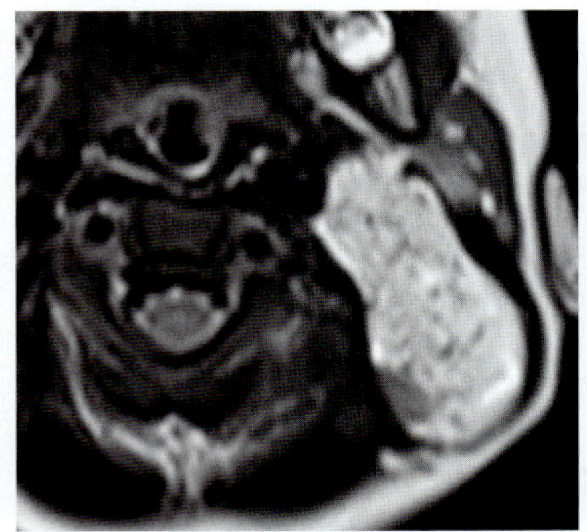

Fig. 4.67.1

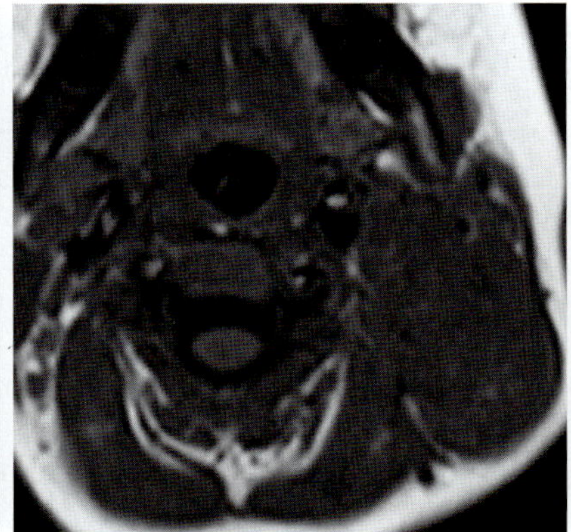

Fig. 4.67.2

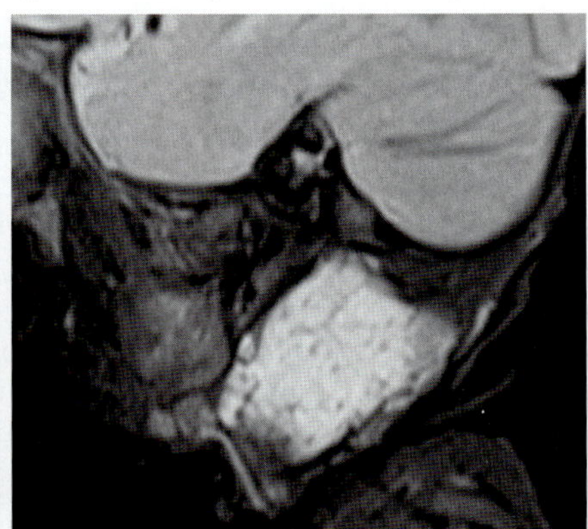

Fig. 4.67.3

Table 4.67.1: Classification of vascular anomalies (ISSVA-2018)			
Vascular anomalies	*Clinical features*	*MR imaging features*	*Treatment*
Vascular tumors			
Infantile hemangioma	Occurs in first few weeks of life, pink, pulsatile, rapidly growing, later involutes and regresses by 7–10 years	Well-defined, lobulated, low T1 and high T2 SI, flow voids and early homogeneous enhancement. Fatty replacement in involution	None
Vascular malformations—low flow			
Venous	Occurs in childhood/ early adulthood, blue, soft compressible, proportional growth without regression	Septated lobulated mass, phleboliths +, fluid-fluid levels, no flow voids, perilesional edema and infiltration +, diffuse delayed enhancement	Percutaneous sclerotherapy
Lymphatic malformation (cystic hygroma or lymphangioma)	Childhood, smooth, non-compressible, rubbery mass, grows proportionally without regression.	Septated lobulated mass, fluid-fluid levels, no flow voids, infiltrative, macrocystic—rim and septal enhancement Microcystic—no / slight enhancement	Percutaneous sclerotherapy
Mixed venolymphatic malformation			
Capillary	Occurs at birth, cutaneous, red, grows proportionally without regression	Skin thickness lesion	None
Vascular malformations—high flow			
Arteriovenous malformation (AVM) and AV Fistula	Childhood/early adulthood, red, pulsatile, thrill +, grows proportionally without regression.	No well-defined mass, enlarged feeding arteries and draining veins, flow voids +, infiltrative, early enhancement of feeding arteries and nidus with shunting to the draining veins	Transarterial embolization

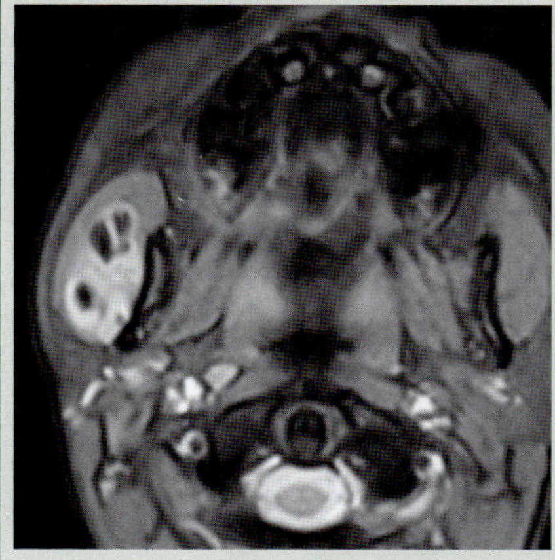

Fig. 4.67.4: Venous malformation in right side of the neck

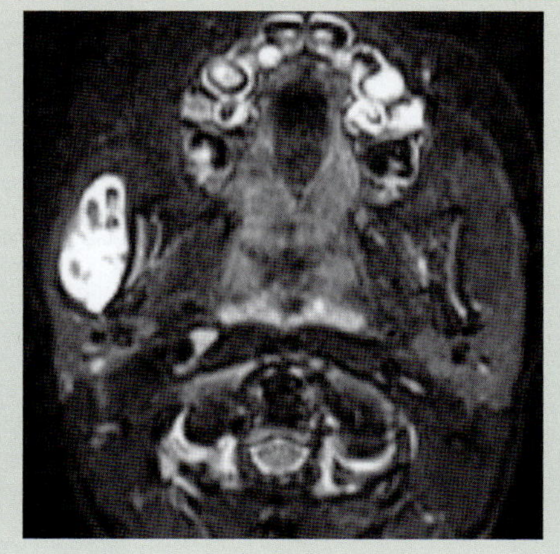

Fig. 4.67.5: Venous malformation in right side of the neck

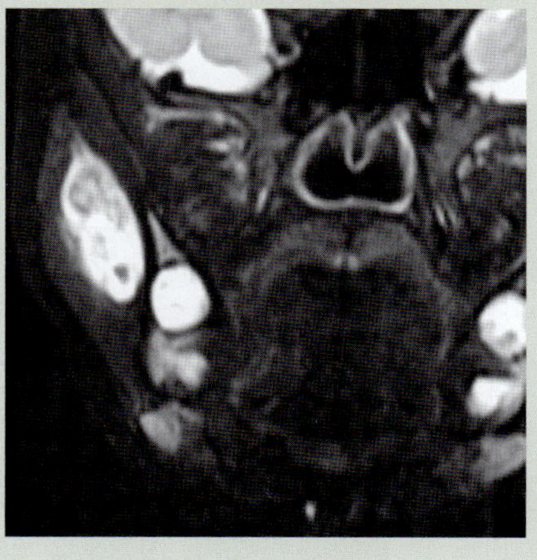

Fig. 4.67.6: Venous malformation in right side of the neck

(*Contd.*)

Table 4.67.1: Classification of vascular anomalies (ISSVA-2018) (*Contd.*)

Vascular anomalies	*Clinical features*	*MR imaging features*	*Treatment*

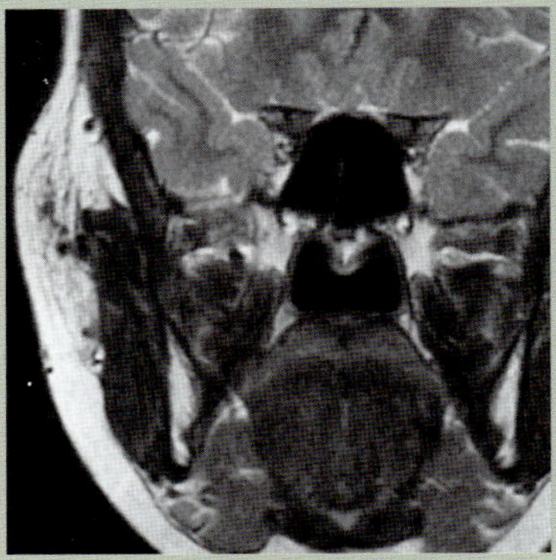

Fig. 4.67.7: AVM of cheek

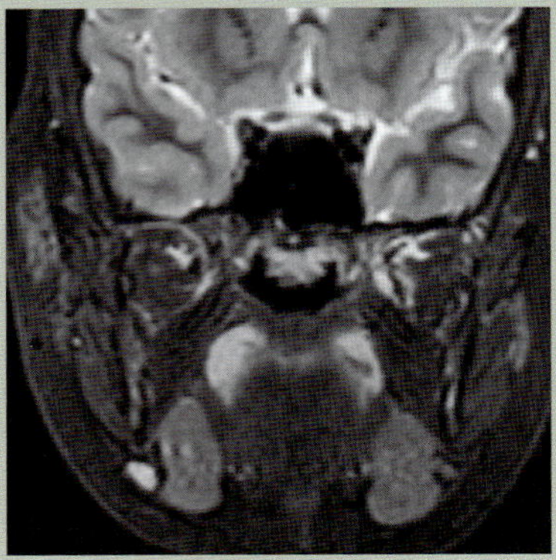

Fig. 4.67.8: AVM of cheek

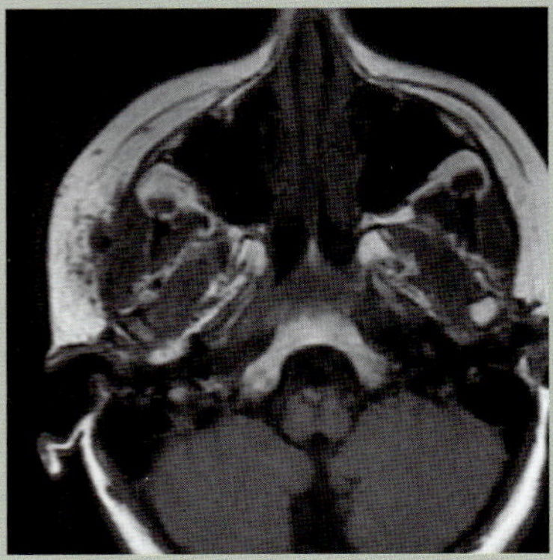

Fig. 4.67.9: AVM of cheek

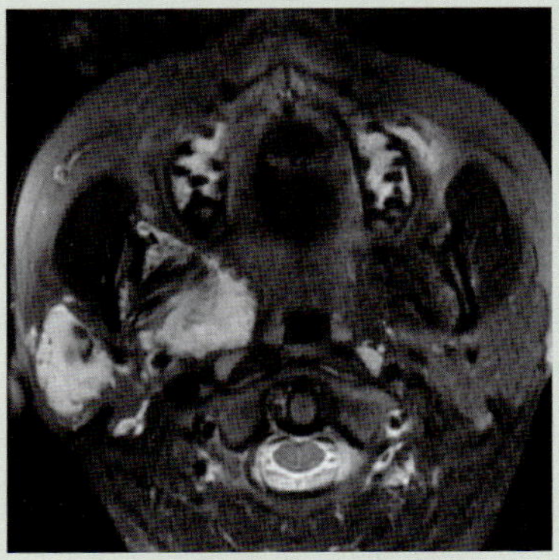

Fig. 4.67.10: Neck hemangioma

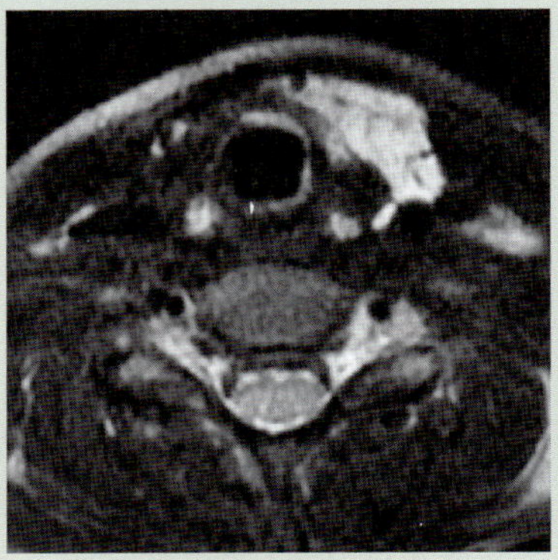

Fig. 4.67.11: Neck hemangioma

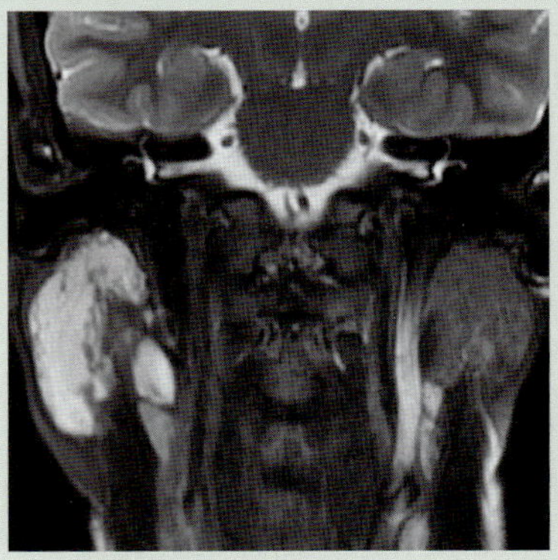

Fig. 4.67.12: Neck hemangioma

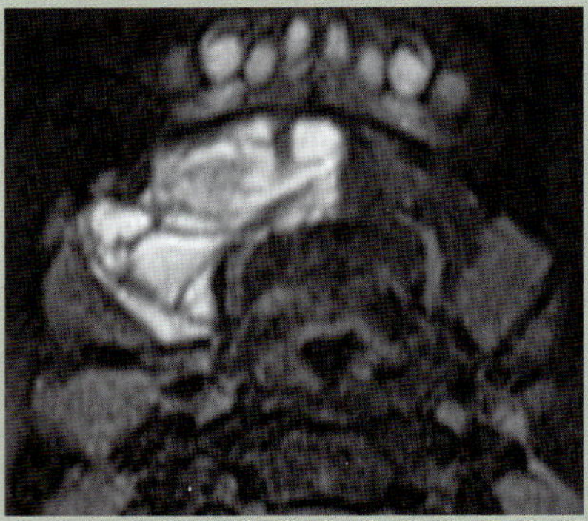

Fig. 4.67.13: Cystic lymphangioma

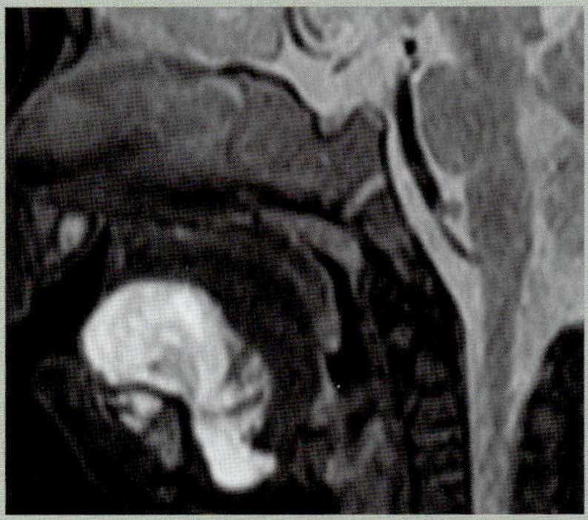

Fig. 4.67.14: Cystic lymphangioma

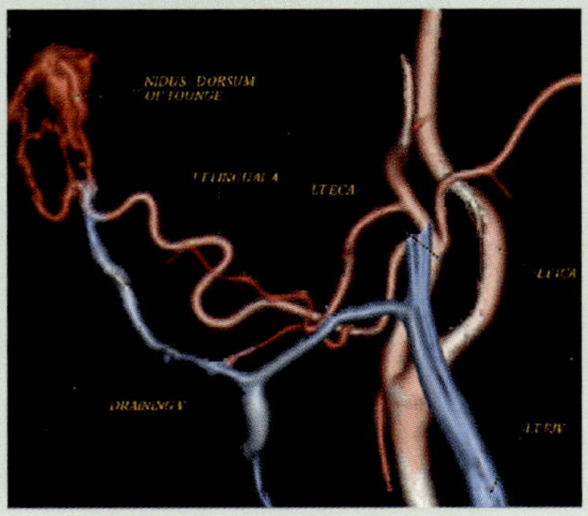

Fig. 4.67.15: AVM

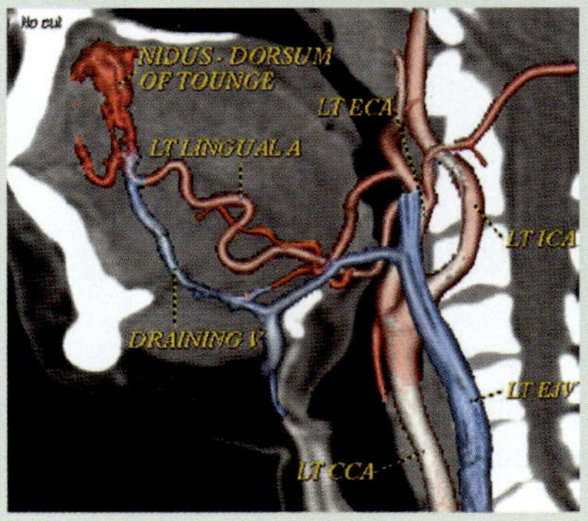

Fig. 4.67.16: AVM

Table 4.67.2: Difference between infantile hemangioma, lymphangioma and developmental venous malformation

Characteristics	*Infantile hemangioma*	*Lymphangioma*	*Developmental venous malformation*
Appearance	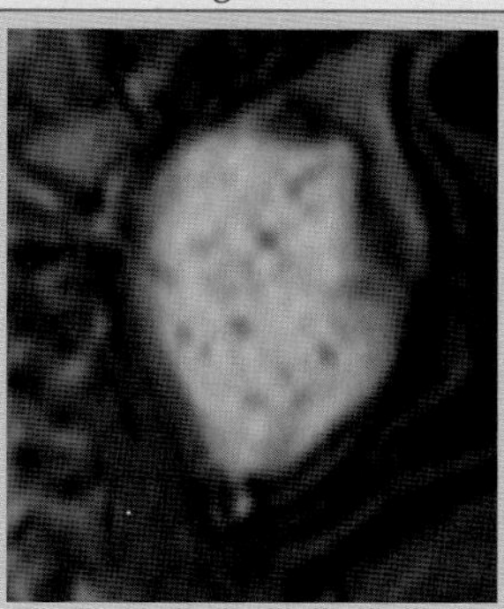 **Fig. 4.67.17:** Infantile hemangioma	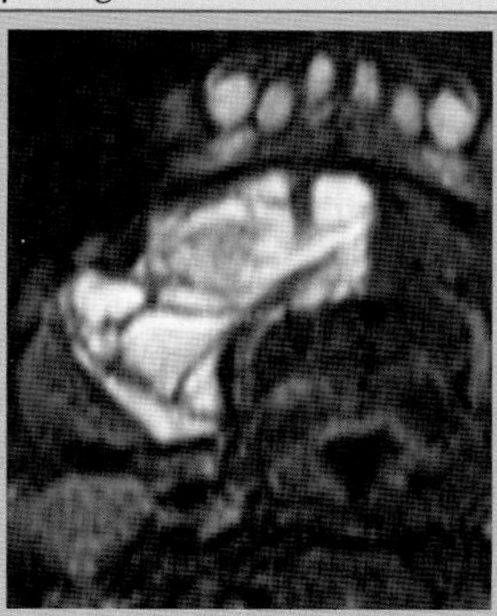 **Fig. 4.67.18:** Multiseptated multi-spatial cystic lesion	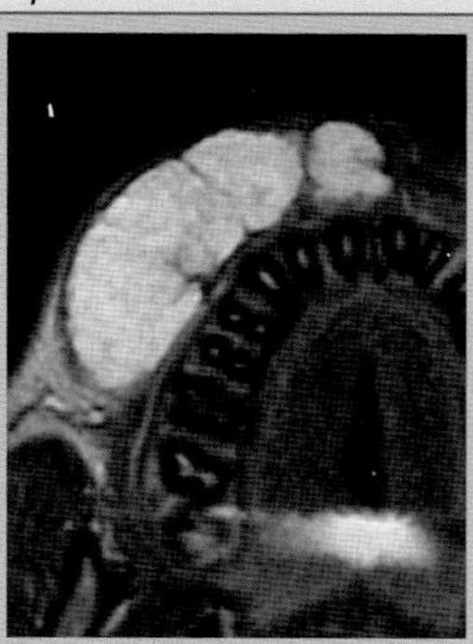 **Fig. 4.67.19:** Developmental venous malformation
Nature	Vascular tumor	Lymphatic malformation	Venous malformation
Age	1st few weeks, not visible at birth	First 2 years of life	Presents in late childhood/early adulthood.
Occurrence	Most common vascular anomaly	Second most common vascular malformation (after venous)	Most common vascular malformation
Sex	1:3–5 female predominance	—	—
Location	Face and neck (most common), trunk, extremities	Neck in posterior cervical triangle, axillary region.	Head and neck (40%), extremities (40%), trunk (20%)
Inspection	Bluish red subcutaneous masses	Smooth, translucent multiple masses under normal skin. Microcystic type is permeated.	Faint blue, soft, masses. Enlarge with Valsalva and in dependent positions and decompress with extremity elevation and local compression.
Palpation	Pulsatile, warm, bruit +	Smooth soft and rubbery consistency. Non-compressible.	Soft, easily compressible.
MR signal	T1 hypo/isointense, T2 hyperintense	T1 hypo/isointense, T2 hyperintense	Intermediate to decreased signal on T1 and T2 / STIR hyperintense
Perilesional edema	Absent	May be present	May be present
Septae	Usually absent	Present	May be present
Infiltration/multi-spatial	Absent	Present. Permeates fat planes	May be present
Fluid-fluid levels	Absent	May be present	Absent.
Flow voids	May be present	Absent	Absent
Feeding arteries/ draining veins	Present	Absent	Absent
AV shunting	Absent	Absent	Absent
Phleboliths	Absent	Absent	Present
Enhancement	Early intense and uniform enhancement	None or faint diffuse enhancement (microcystic), rim and septal enhancement (macrocystic)	Delayed images show diffuse enhancement of the slow flowing venous channels
Clinical course	Involutes and regresses at 7–10 years	Grows proportionally without regression	Grows proportionally without regression
Involution phase	Increasing fat within the lesion, less avid and heterogeneous enhancement	—	—
Treatment	None (spontaneous involution). Propranolol for aesthetic concerns	Sclerotherapy (sac drained completely, then around 50% volume of sclerosant (usually doxycycline) is administered	Sclerotherapy, usually with ethanol

4.68 HEAD AND NECK

Case No. 68

Clinical history: 40-year-old male presents with swelling over the right side of neck for 6 months, not associated with pain, soft in consistency, no warmth/ tenderness.

Radiological techniques and observation: Figures 4.68.1 and 4.68.2 are ultrasound of the submandibular region shows a well-defined anechoic thin-walled cystic lesion with posterior acoustic enhancement, the lesion is anterior to the sternocleidomastoid and posterior to the submandibular gland. No evidence of internal septations. No evidence of any solid component/calcification. No flow noted in the cystic lesion on Doppler.

Figures 4.68.3 and 4.68.7 are contrast enhanced CT scan of the neck in a 40 years old patient showing a well-defined thin walled hypodense cystic lesion with minimal wall enhancement located anterior to SCM, posterior to submandibular gland with displacement of the carotid vessels medially and compression of IJV. No evidence of internal septation/hemorrhage. No evidence of solid component/calcification within the cyst. No trans spatial extension into the adjacent neck spaces. Submandibular gland appears normal.

Figures 4.68.4, 4.68.5 are plain MRI of neck in T2 and T1 axial views at the level of submandibular gland shows a well-defined T2 hyperintense. Figure 4.68.6 shows T1 hypointense cystic lesion with minimal wall enhancement on T1 post-contrast images, located anterior to SCM and posterior to submandibular gland. No evidence of internal septation or solid component. No evidence of calcification or hemorrhage noted within the cyst.

Interpretation: A—40 years old male patient, located posterior to the submandibular gland and anterior to the sternocleidomastoid, a well-defined cystic lesion, hypointense on T1 and hyperintense on T2 with enhancement of the wall on post-contrast T1 images, B—displacing the carotid vessels medially and compressing the IJV, D—second branchial cyst.

Principal diagnosis: Second branchial cyst

Treatment: Complete surgical resection if symptomatic.

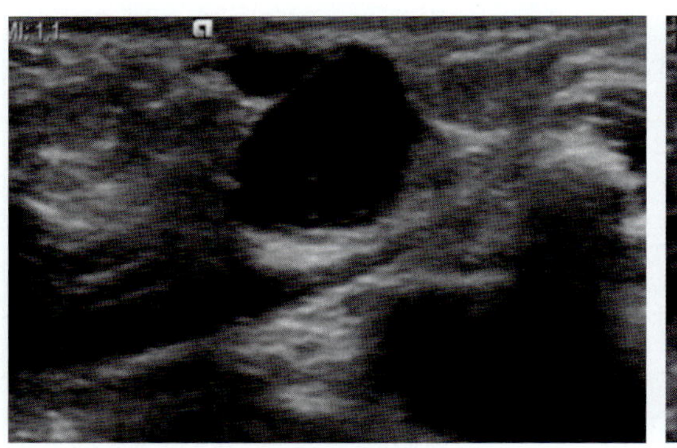

Fig. 4.68.1

Fig. 4.68.2

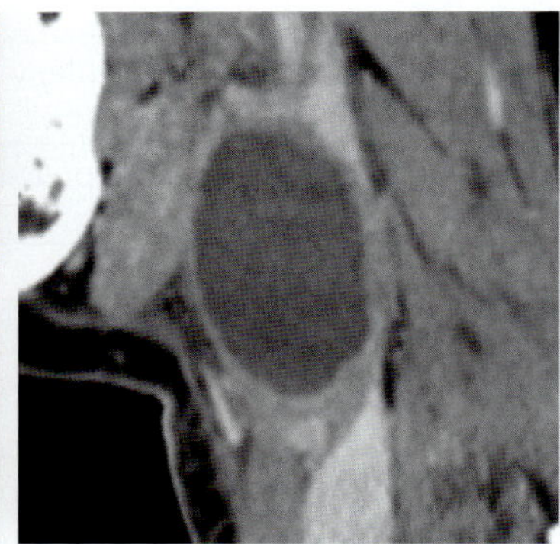

Fig. 4.68.3

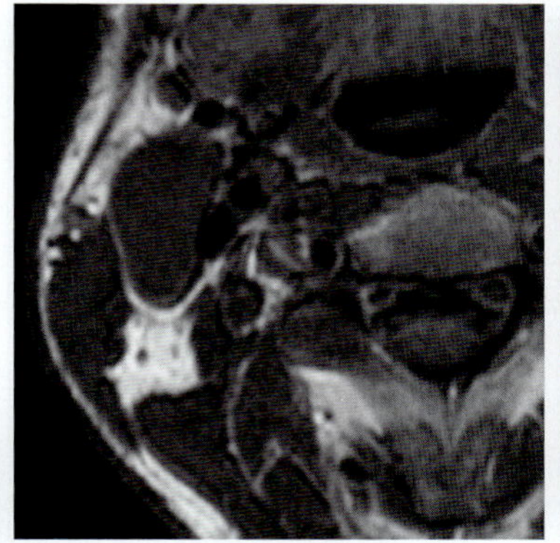

Fig. 4.68.4

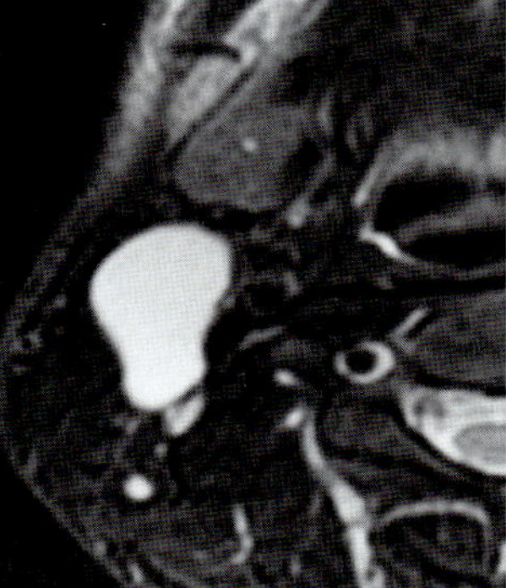

Fig. 4.68.5

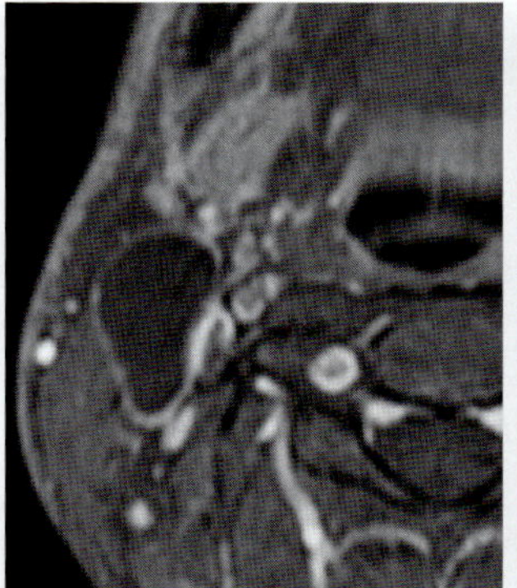

Fig. 4.68.6

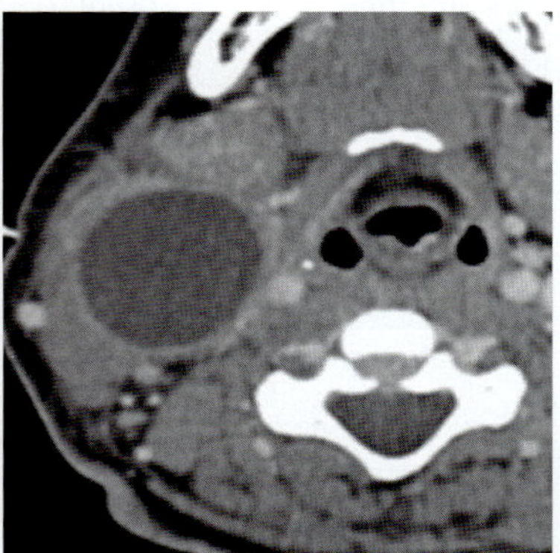

Fig. 4.68.7

Table 4.68.1: Differential diagnosis for branchial cleft cyst

Condition	*Radiological features*	*Image*
Lymphatic malformation A benign lesion of vascular origin which shows lymphatic differentiation. Also known as lymphatic hemangioma/lymphangioma Can occur in any age group most common <2 years	Well-defined unilocular/multilocular, frequently trans spatial (multi compartment) involvement USG–well-defined cystic lesion with thin septations and no flow on Doppler. MRI–T1 hyper with fluid-fluid levels if intralesional hemorrhage is present. T2 hyperlesion	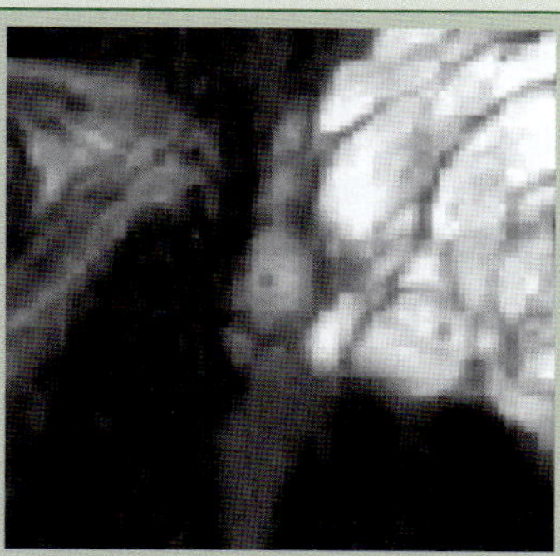 **Fig. 4.68.8:** Lymphatic malformation
Thymic cyst: Cystic remnant along the course of thymopharyngeal duct from pyriform sinus to anterior mediastinum and hence occurs in the neck, left > right	**USG**–anechoic cyst with absent flow on Doppler. **CT** non-enhancing low attenuation cystic lesion in close association with carotid sheath **MRI** thin-walled hypointense cyst with/without tiny enhancing solid isointense nodule.	
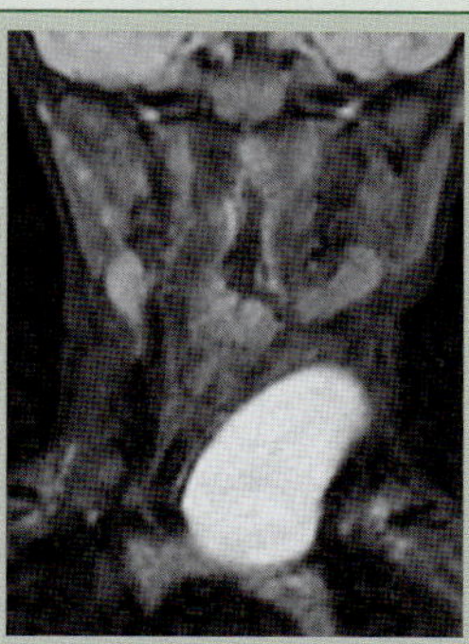 **Fig. 4.68.9:** Thymic cyst	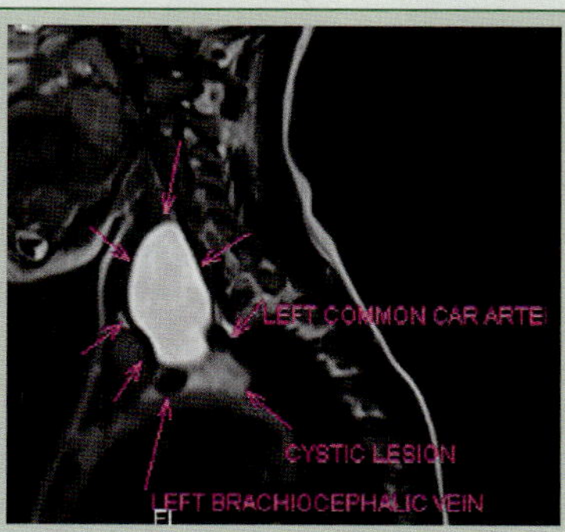 **Fig. 4.68.10:** Thymic cyst	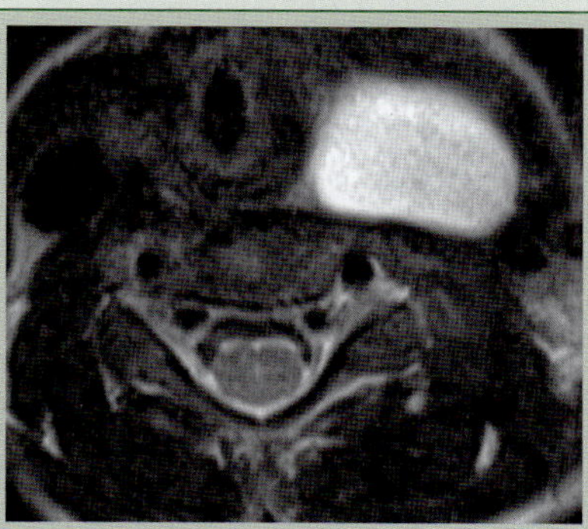 **Fig. 4.68.11:** Thymic cyst
Cystic lymph nodes 1. Papillary CA thyroid 2. Treated lymphoma 3. Squamous cell carcinoma 4. Viral lymphadenitis: HSV 5. Bacterial lymphadenitis 6. Tuberculous adenitis 7. Leukemia	**USG:** Well-defined hypo- to anechoic cystic lesions with post-acoustic enhancement, no flow on Doppler **CT:** Non-enhancing hypodense lesions in the region of lymph nodes **MRI:** T1 hypo and T2 hyperintense lesion	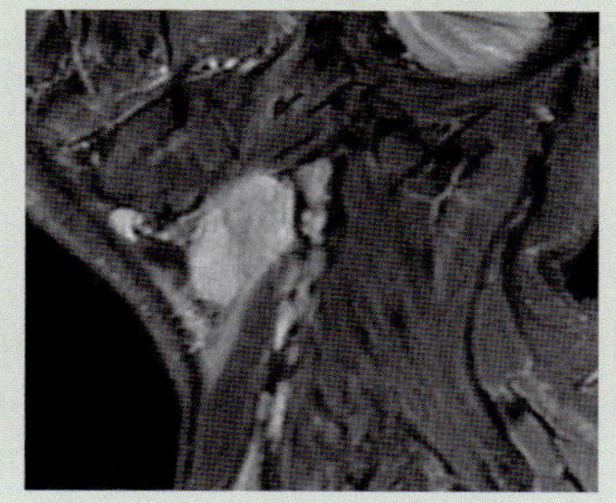 **Fig. 4.68.12:** Cystic lymph nodes
Dermoid cyst: Ectodermal in origin–contains squamous epithelium, dermal appendages—hair, fat, sebaceous glands, sweat glands, calcification. Site: Orbit, neck-suprasternal notch.	**USG:** Inhomogeneous echogenicity with fat and calcification **CECT:** Subtle rim enhancement of wall with internal fluid, fat and calcification **MRI:** Heterointense lesion with fluid and fat, fat component suppresses on the fat saturated images. Dermoid cyst in neck is seen superficial to strap muscles.	
Epidermoid cyst Common type of cutaneous cyst that has an epithelial lining. Does not have sebaceous glands on microscopic examination	**USG:** Gives a pseudo-solid appearance with cystic and solid components—sac of marbles appearance. **CT:** Well-defined low density cystic mass with or without rim enhancement of the cyst wall. **MRI:** T1, T2 hyper with diffusion restriction.	

Contd...

Table 4.68.1: Differential diagnosis for branchial cleft cyst (*Contd.*)

Condition	*Radiological features*	*Image*
Thyroglossal duct cyst suprahyoid: 20–25% at the level of hyoid bone: ~15–50%, infra-hyoid: ~25–65%). Solid component with calcification indicates papillary carcinoma transformation.	Cysts can develop at any point along the thyroglossal duct's path from the foramen caecum to the thyroid gland. No communication with the larynx.	
Laryngocele Dilatation of the saccule of laryngeal ventricle, fluid (when infected) or air-filled cystic lesions in the paraglottic space.	Internal (or simple): The dilated ventricular saccule is confined to the paralaryngeal space within the thyrohyoid membrane (~40%) External: The saccule herniates through the thyrohyoid membrane, with dilatation of the superficial portion Mixed: With dilated internal and external components (~45%) (given image)	
Ranula: Retention cyst of the sublingual salivary gland or minor salivary gland in sublingual space. can extend into floor of mouth.	Simple ranula—true cyst in sublingual gland Plunging/diving ranula—ruptured cyst extending to the submandibular space USG, CT and MRI show features of cystic lesion in the sub lingual space off midline	
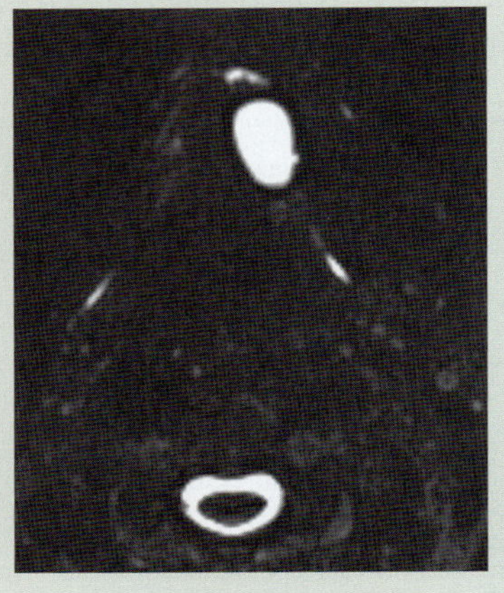 **Fig. 4.68.13:** Ranula	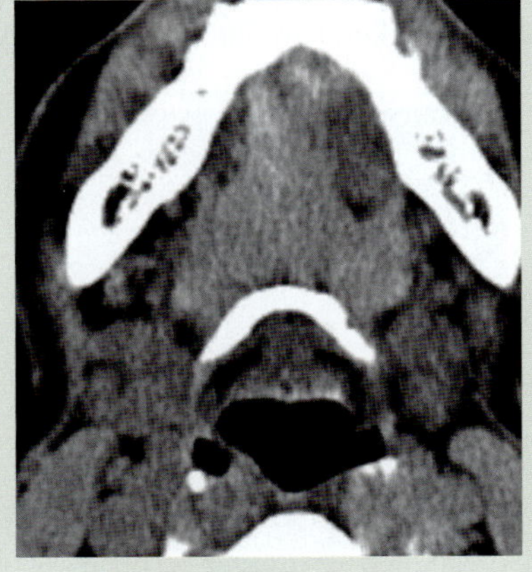 **Fig. 4.68.14:** Ranula	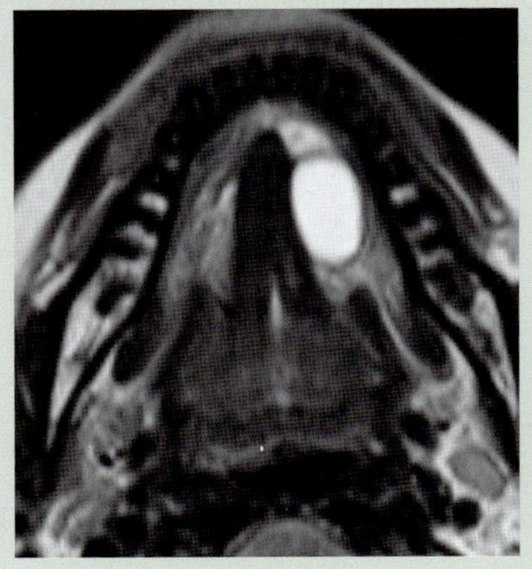 **Fig. 4.68.15:** Ranula
Vallecular cyst: Cystic mass in vallecula of child with stridor. Affects the neonates, presenting with inspiratory stridor, laryngomalacia, failure to thrive.	USG, CT and MRI show the typical features of a cystic lesion. Best diagnostic tool—direct laryngoscopy	

Differential diagnosis: 1. Lymphatic malformation, 2. thymic cyst, 3. cystic lymph nodes, 4. thyroglossal duct cyst (off midline), 5. suppurative lymph nodes, 6. epidermoid.

Discussion: Second branchial cleft cyst: A cystic dilatation of the remnants of the 2nd branchial cyst is known as a second branchial cleft cyst. The fifth cleft do not give rise to the cervical sinus, which is one of the reasons why no fifth branchial cleft defects exist.

1st branchial sinus tract opens near parotid gland, EAC, parapharyngeal space, or anterior triangle of neck.

2nd branchial sinus: Usually communicates externally along anterior margin of sternocleidomastoid muscle (SCM), rarely communicates internally to tonsillar fossa.

2nd branchial fistula: Communicates externally and internally secondary to persistence of both branchial cleft and pharyngeal pouch remnant.

3rd branchial fistula would exit base of pyriform sinus, course superior to superior laryngeal and hypoglossal nerves, and inferior to glossopharyngeal nerve.

4th branchial sinus tract: 1 opening-to-skin surface, external auditory canal, pharynx or hypopharynx.

4th branchial fistula: 2 openings; skin and lumen of foregut, arises as epithelial-lined tract left behind when there is persistence of both branchial cleft and its corresponding pharyngeal pouch.

Sonographic Features of Normal Lymph Node

1. Size—short axis is measured. Upper neck nodes are larger than lower neck nodes. Cut-off of 7 mm for level 1 and 8 mm for all other cervical nodes.
2. Shape—metastatic, lymphomatous (Hodgkin/NHL) and tuberculous nodes are rounded. Normal or reactive nodes are usually oval or flat. However,

Table 4.68.2: Imaging features in branchial cleft cysts

First branchial cleft cyst Rarest (7%), asymptomatic, seen within/ superficial to parotid	Type I: Inferior and posteromedial to the pinna Type II: The external auditory canal and the angle of the jaw Type III: Periparotid region The residual embryonic tract starts in the submandibular triangle, ascends through the parotid gland, and ends at the cartilaginous + bony external auditory canal junction.	
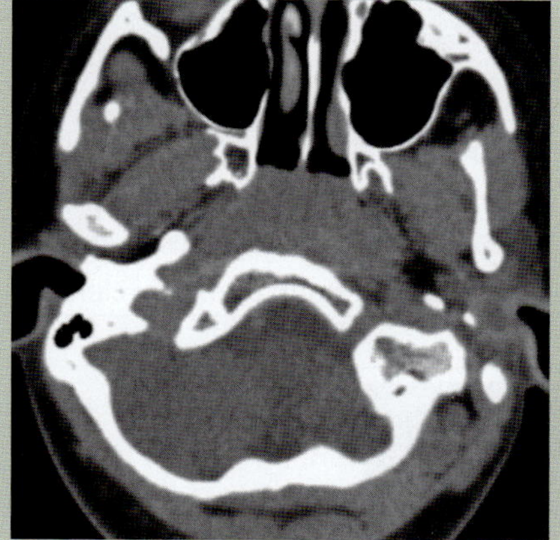 **Fig. 4.68.16:** First branchial cleft cyst	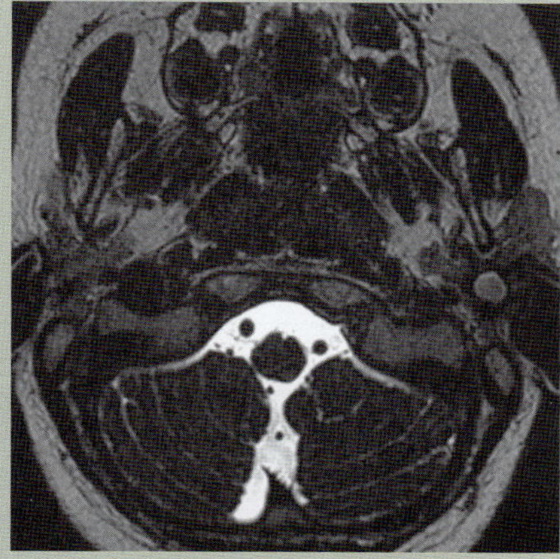 **Fig. 4.68.17:** First branchial cleft cyst	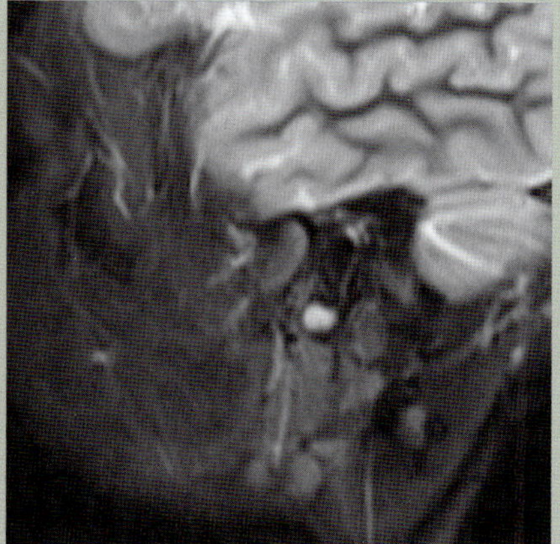 **Fig. 4.68.18:** First branchial cleft cyst
Second branchial cleft cyst Commonest, anywhere along the course of 2nd branchial arch from the pharyngeal wall to skin (laterally and inferiorly), B/W ECA and ICA, common—angle of mandible 2nd branchial fistula has an internal opening in the tonsillar fossa	**Bailey classification:** I–deep to platysma II–anterior to SCM and posterior to sub-mandibular gland III–beak sign curved rim of tissue pointing medially between internal + external carotid arteries (pathognomonic) IV–adjacent to lateral pharyngeal wall in parapharyngeal space, opens in pharynx	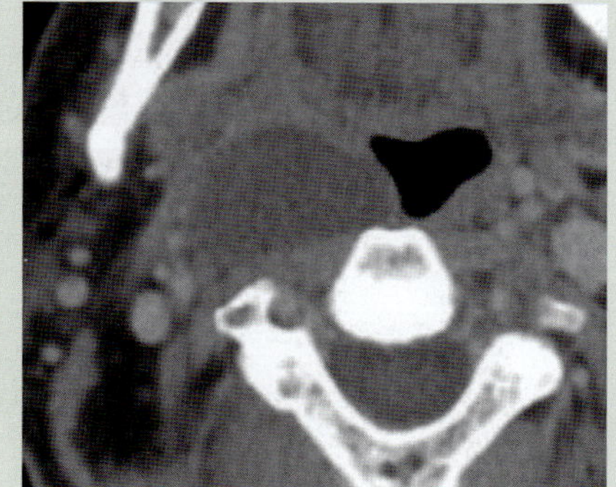 **Fig. 4.68.19:** Second branchial cleft cyst
Third branchial cleft cyst 2nd most common lesion in the posterior cervical space, next to cystic hygroma.	In the posterior cervical space, posterior to SCM, above superior laryngeal nerve The 3rd branchial cyst has internal opening in the tip of pyriform fossa.	
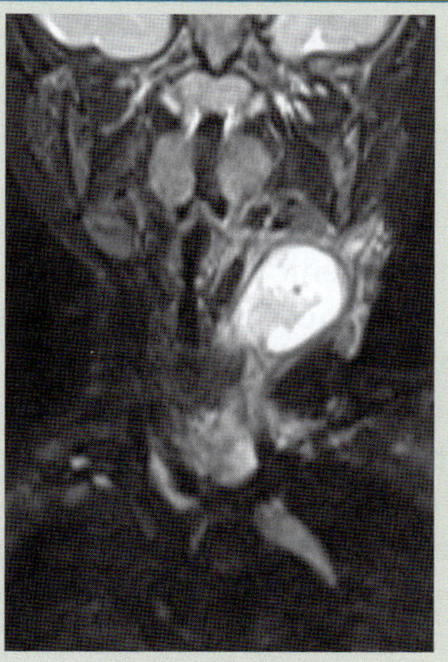 **Fig. 4.68.20:** Third branchial cleft cyst	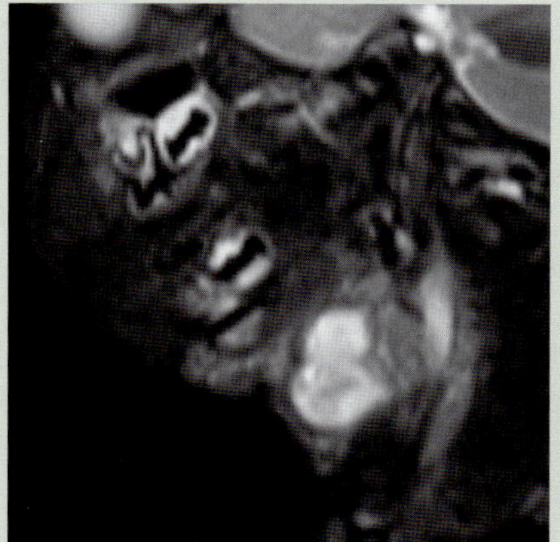 **Fig. 4.68.21:** Third branchial cleft cyst	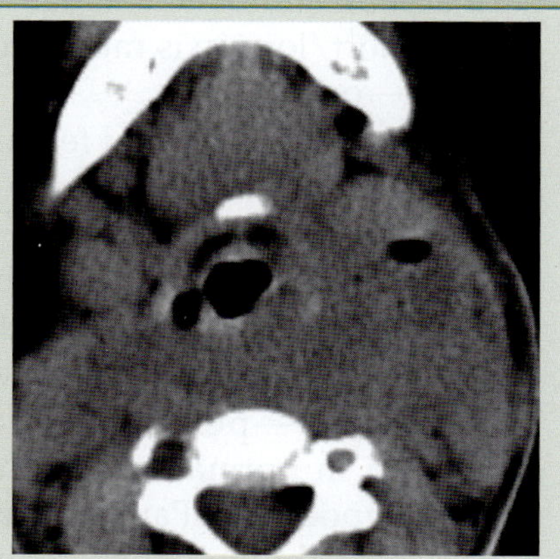 **Fig. 4.68.22:** Third branchial cleft cyst

Contd...

Table 4.68.2: Imaging features in branchial cleft cysts *(Contd...)*

Fourth branchial cleft cyst Left side most common. Most common anomalies are actually sinus tracts than cysts. Clinically presents with recurrent Suppurative thyroiditis and neck abscesses. DD: Parathyroid cyst, thyroid cyst, lymphatic malformation and thymic cyst.	Barium swallow—sinus tract extending from apex of pyriform sinus to upper aspect of left thyroid lobe. CECT—abscess in or adjacent to anterior left thyroid lobe. MRI—phlegmon or abscess in left anterior neck with deep neck inflammation extending to pyriform sinus.	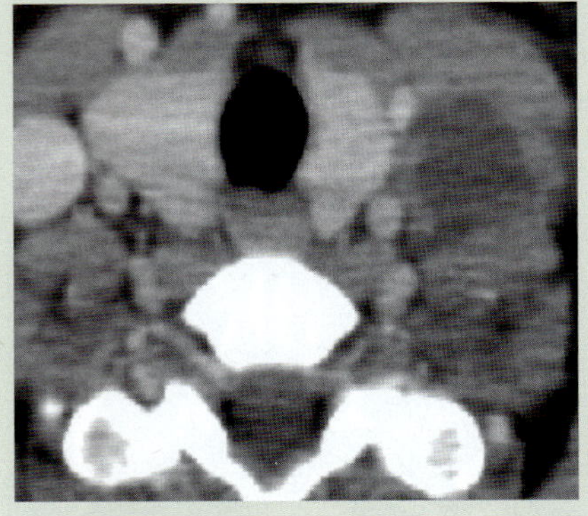 **Fig. 4.68.23:** Fourth branchial cleft cyst
Branchial fistula		
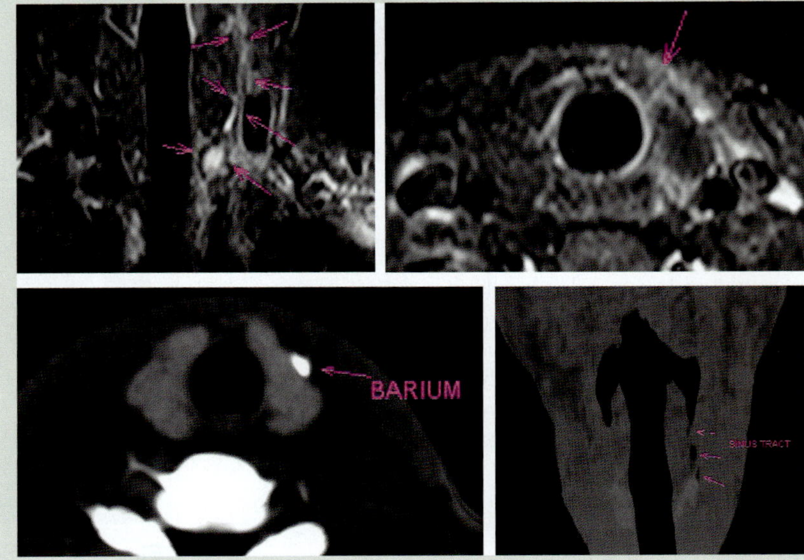 **Fig. 4.68.24:** Fourth branchial fistula		

normal submandibular and parotid nodes are usually round. Short/long axis ratio can be measured: <0.5–oval; 0.5–round.

3. Echogenic hilum—normal feature. May be absent in metastatic, lymphomatous and tuberculous nodes, but not always.
4. Nodal border—in proven malignant nodes, irregular ill-defined borders and hypoechoic change around lymph nodes indicate extra nodal extension.
5. Echogenicity—peripheral echogenicity (halo sign) seen in normal nodes, metastatic nodes are usually hypoechoic. Papillary cancer metastases are hyperechoic (thyroglobulin deposition). Tuberculous nodes are hypoechoic. Lymphomatous nodes are hypoechoic (often markedly) with posterior acoustic enhancement ± intranodal reticulation/micronodular pattern.
6. Calcification—common in metastases from papillary (fine and peripheral) and medullary (coarse) thyroid carcinomas. Calcification may be seen in other metastatic LNs after radiotherapy or rarely after chemotherapy.
7. Intranodal necrosis—late event in tumor invasion, may appear cystic or echogenic (coagulative necrosis). Cystic necrosis is common in SCC metastases (p16+ve), papillary thyroid carcinoma and TB.
8. Vascular pattern—normal and reactive nodes tend to show hilar vascularity or appear avascular. Metastatic nodes tend to have peripheral vascularity with high resistant waveform (RI >0.8, PI >1.5). Mixed vascularity is also common in lymphomatous nodes.
9. Ancillary features—matting (TB) and adjacent soft-tissue edema (may be seen around metastatic, suppurative or tuberculous nodes).

Table 4.68.3: Differential diagnosis for midline, upper neck parasagittal and lower neck parasagittal masses

Midline	*Upper neck parasagittal*	*Lower neck parasagittal*
Suprahyoid thyroglossal cyst (Epi)dermoid cyst, vallecular cyst, Thornwaldt cyst, Delphian nodes	Infrahyoid thyroglossal cyst **(deep to strap muscle)**, epidermoid (superficial to the strap muscles), laryngocele (deep to muscle and communicates with the laryngeal ventricle), necrotic lymph node, lymphatic malformation, mixed venolymphatic malformation, minor salivary gland cyst, ectatic jugular bulb, ranula, branchial cleft cyst I and II	Branchial cleft cyst (type III and IV), thymic cyst, thyroid cyst Parathyroid cyst, cystic/necrotic nodes, cystic schwannoma

Retropharyngeal abscess

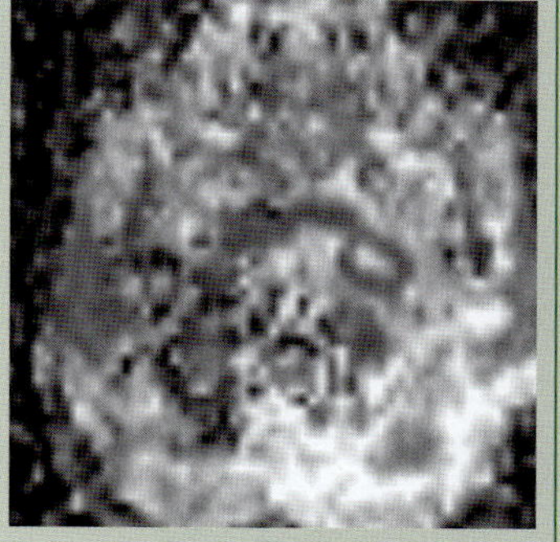

Fig. 4.68.25: Retropharyngeal abscess

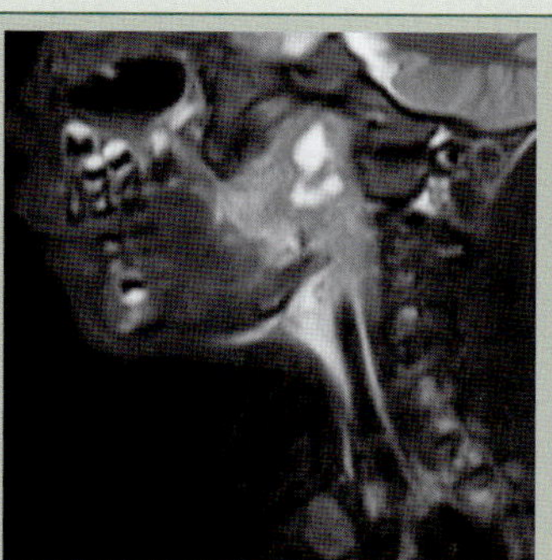

Fig. 4.68.26: Retropharyngeal abscess

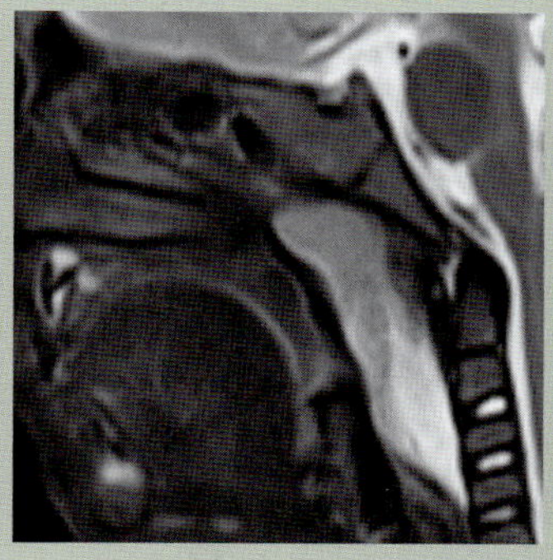

Fig. 4.68.27: Retropharyngeal abscess

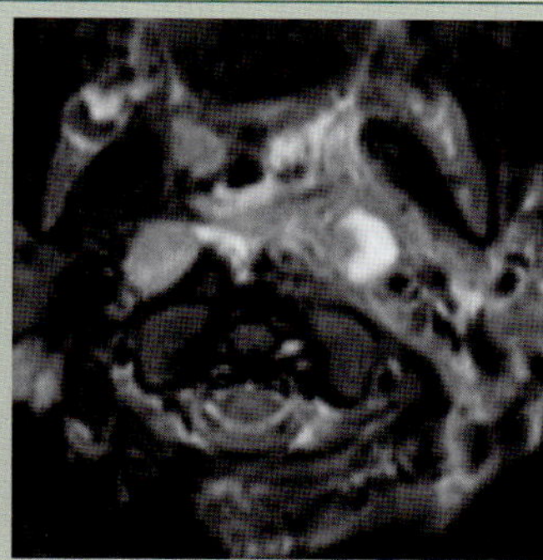

Fig. 4.68.28: Retropharyngeal abscess

Sublingual abscess

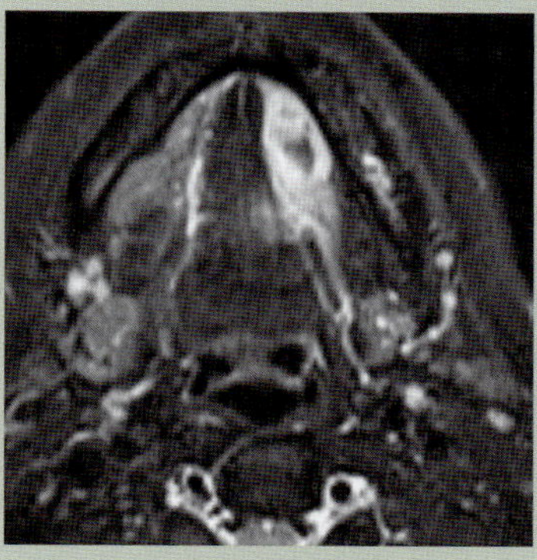

Fig. 4.68.29: Sublingual abscess

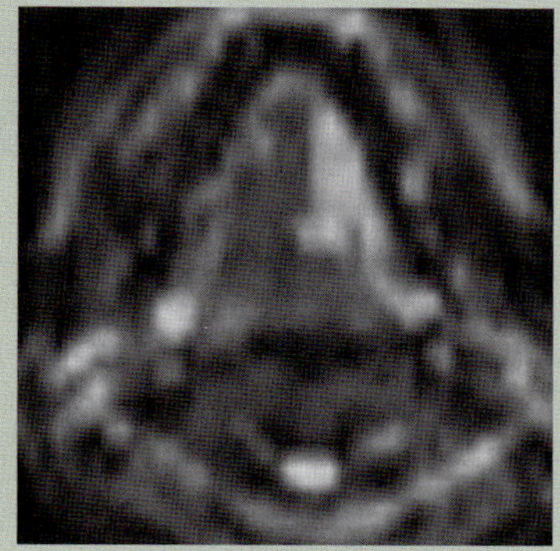

Fig. 4.68.30: Sublingual abscess

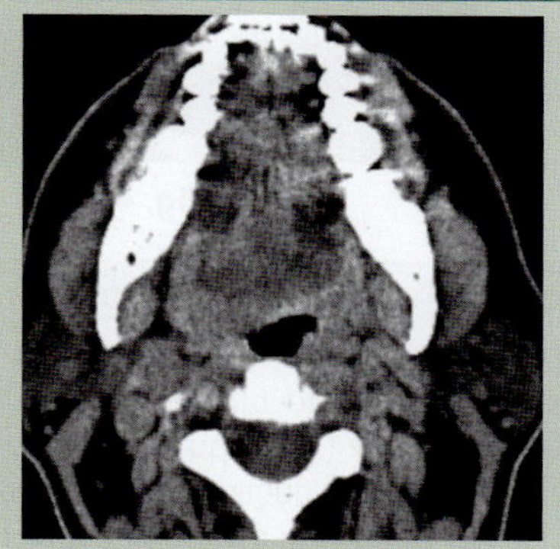

Fig. 4.68.31: Sublingual abscess

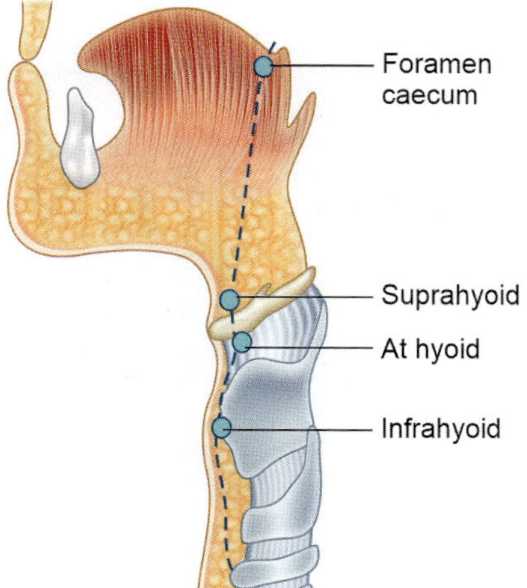

Fig. 4.68.32: Ectopic thyroid/thyroglossal cyst location with description of descent of thyroid gland

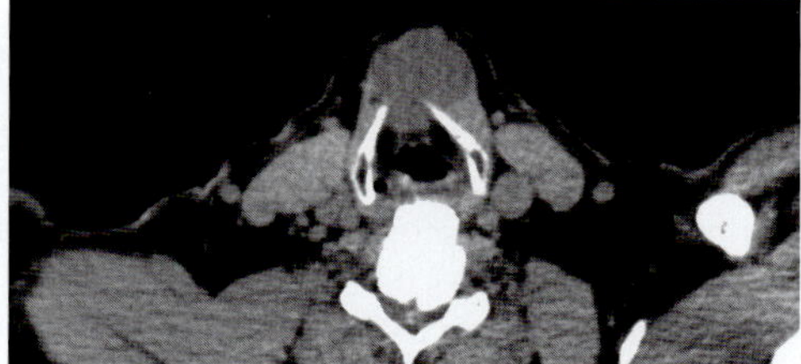

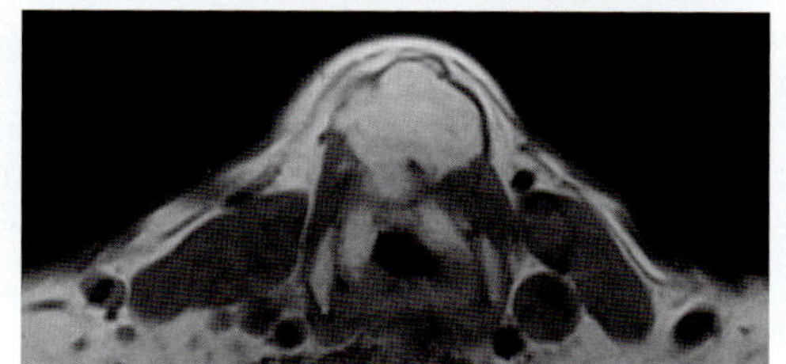

Fig. 4.68.33a and b: Thyroglossal duct cyst

4.69 HEAD AND NECK

Case No. 69

Clinical history: A 54-year-old female presented with swelling near right alar base.

Radiological techniques and observation: Figure 4.69.1 is sagittal T1-weighted image showing the well-circumscribed lesion with a homogeneous isointensity in the anterior nasal fold and expansion of the lesion toward the posterior of the nasal cavity. Figure 4.69.2 is axial T2-weighted image showing the well-circumscribed lesion with a homogeneous hyperintensity. No evidence of hemorrhage. No evidence of bone changes.

Interpretation: A—54-year-old female, lateral to pyriform lateral nasal wall beneath the alar base, C—well-circumscribed hyperintensity lesion, B—homogeneous, D—nasolabial cyst.

Principal diagnosis: Nasal labial cyst.

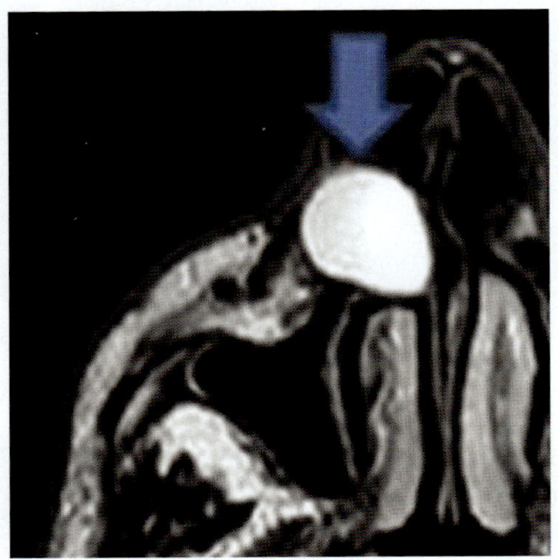

Fig. 4.69.1

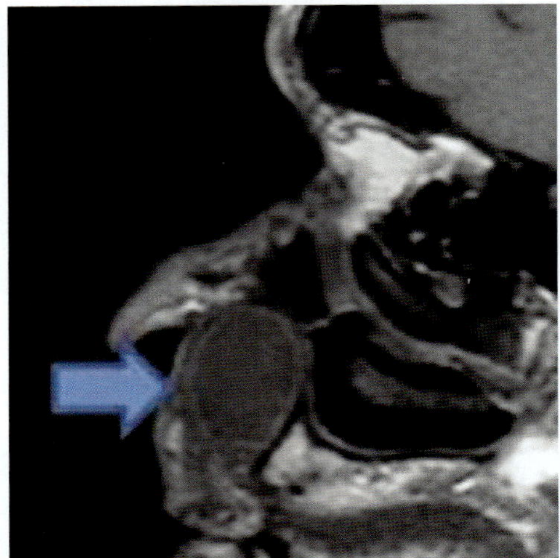

Fig. 4.69.2

Table 4.69.1: Differential diagnosis for nasolabial cyst		
Cysts of the nasopalatine duct within the incisive canal 4th to 6th decade, male > females, affects 1% population. During prenatal life, these ducts normally regress. The development of a cyst is caused by the persistence of the ductal epithelium. Enucleation is curative, and recurrence is uncommon.	They are non-neoplastic cysts that develop as a result of nasopalatine duct degeneration. They appear as a solitary well-defined oval or circular unilocular radiolucency >0.6 cm in diameter between the central incisors. There can be root resorption and tooth displacement. A strongly marginated cystic area in the vicinity of the incisive canal is frequently seen on CT through the hard palate. Although most cysts of the craniofacial regions display low to intermediate signal intensity on T1, MRI usually indicates uniform high signal intensity on both T1 and T2.	
Periapical cyst 3rd to 6th decades The most prevalent kind of odontogenic cysts. A periapical inflammatory disease (granuloma, cyst, or abscess) has eroded the bone; a careful inspection of the neighbouring teeth and testing their vitality can help rule this out. As a result, these cysts are located on the tip of the tooth and are typically small, measuring less than one centimetre in diameter. The entire cyst as well as the accompanying tooth are removed after treatment.	The radiolucency of a non-vital tooth will be visible on an OPG. CT scan and plain radiograph. They are 1 cm diameter and have a thin cortical bone rim around them. Caries manifests itself as deterioration of the related tooth's enamel/crown. MRI: Although periapical cysts appear as a non-enhancing lesion near the apex of a tooth, MRI is not the first-line imaging modality. These cysts usually have a low T1 signal and a high T2.	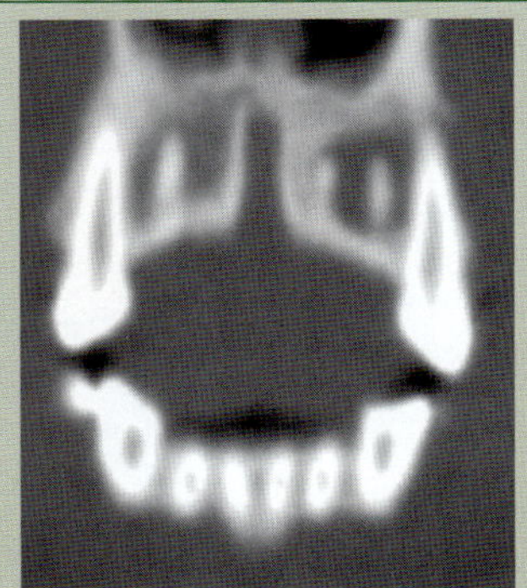 Fig. 4.69.3: Periapical cyst
Dentigerous cyst: Refer to case 80		
Keratocystic odontogenic tumors: Refer to case 80		

Management: Complete surgical excision of the nasolabial cysts utilising an open technique (sublabial incision) is the best treatment for nasolabial cysts since it allows for histological analysis.

Discussion: **Nasoalveolar cyst or Klestadt's cyst or nasolabial cyst**

- Rare developmental cyst resulting from epithelial cells remaining in the mesenchyme after foetal union of the lateral and medial nasal processes, as well as the maxillary prominence, or epithelial remnants from the nasolacrimal duct, usually unilateral but 10% bilateral.
- M: F—1:3. Occurs in age > 40 years.
- Well-circumscribed soft mass occurring beneath the alar base should raise the possibility of nasolabial cyst.

CT: A well-demarcated, rounded, homogeneous, low-density soft tissue lesion at the nasolabial region. Evidence of scalloping and bone remodeling may be depicted.

MRI: Variable intensities on T1W images owing to different viscosities of intracystic fluid.

The lesion could be diagnosed as nasolabial cyst based on its location and appearances on MR images rather than on the MR appearance of the cyst contents.

4.70 HEAD AND NECK

Case No. 70

Clinical history: A 7-month-old male child, presenting with history of not responding to auditory stimulus.

Radiological techniques and observation: Figures 4.70.1 to 4.70.2 are MR images in T2 axial and CISS axial sections showing bilobed enlarged T2 hyperintense cochlear cavity. The modiolus turns are not visualized and the vestibule is dilated. The IAC also appears dilated and the VIII nerve is not clearly visualized. The cribriform interface between the cochlea and the middle ear is not clearly defined. The visualized brain parenchyma is normal. The visualized sections of the brainstem are normal. The mastoid, external auditory canal and the VII nerve (not shown) are normal.

Interpretation: A—7-month-old male child, pathology in cochlea and vestibule, C—cystic cochlea and vestibule are however partially separated, and the modiolus is present but hypoplastic. Size of the IAC is wide but smaller than the size of the cavity. The turns of the cochlea are not visualized, B—cystic featureless cochlea described as a "snow man shape/figure of 8 appearance", D—cystic cochleovestibular malformation.

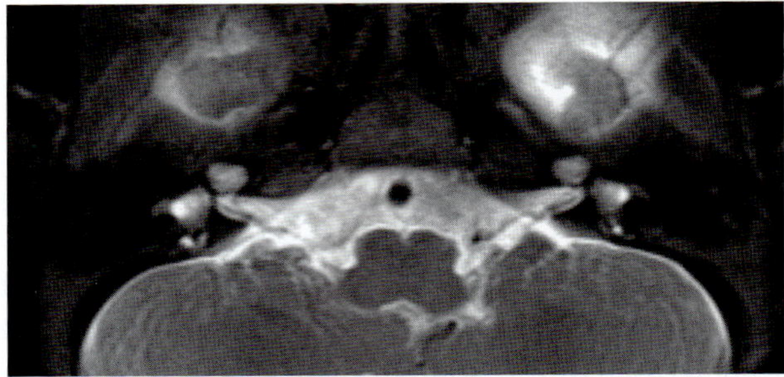

Fig. 4.70.1

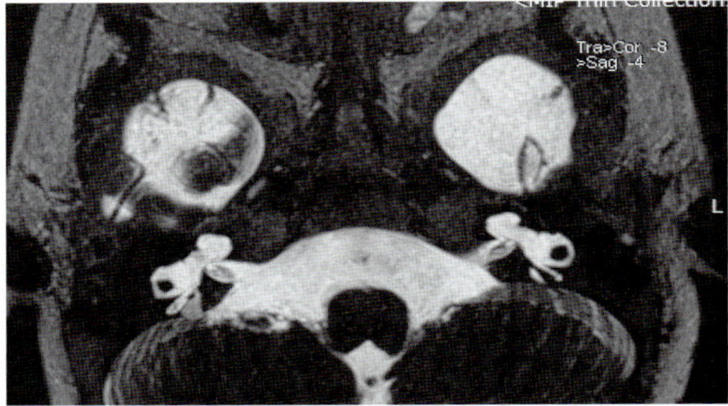

Fig. 4.70.2

Provisional diagnosis: Incomplete partition of the cochlea-cystic cochleovestibular malformation type 1.

Differential diagnosis

Diagnosis	*Imaging features*	*Image*
Complete aplasia (Michel) At the third week, the otic vesicles fail to form. Anomalies of the skull base, hypoplastic petrous apex, and aberrant ICA are all possible causes.	All inner ear structures (cochlea, vestibule, semicircular canals) are absent. Absence of cochlear promontory differentiates it from labyrinthitis ossificans.	**Fig. 4.70.3:** Complete labyrinthine aplasia
Fig. 4.70.4: Left complete aplasia (Michel)	**Fig. 4.70.5:** Left complete aplasia (Michel)	**Fig. 4.70.6:** Left complete aplasia (Michel)

(Contd.)

Diagnosis	*Imaging features*	*Image*
Cochlear aplasia Developmental arrest in the late 3rd week of GA. DDX: Labyrinthitis ossificans (no loss of convexity of medial **wall of middle ear**)	Cochlea aplastic, flat medial wall of medial ear (underdeveloped horizontal SCC). **Dysplasia of vestibule** = enlargement of SCC, hypoplasia of IAC, small cochlear nerve abnormal facial nerve course.	
Common cavity Developmental arrest at 4th week of GA. The typical separation between the cochlea and the vestibule is gone, replaced with a cystic common cavity structure.	Size of IAC corresponds to the size of cavity. Fundus defective—IAC enters the centre of cavity. In a cystic cavity of varying size with no internal architecture, the cochlea, vestibule, and horizontal semicircular canal come together. The cavity's width is usually bigger than its height, with a vertical diameter of 7 mm and a horizontal diameter of 10 mm on average. The inferior and superior semicircular canals are either missing or deformed. Vestibulocochlear nerve components will be minimal/absent. The facial canal will take an unusual path. The stapes can be normal or abnormal, and the oval window can be stenotic; the vestibular aqueduct will not be dilated, and it may be nonexistent.	
Semicircular canal dysplasia Lateral semicircular canal forms last during embryogenesis, Hence, it is most commonly affected. It is associated with CHARGE syndrome	Central bony island in LSCC is normally 3.7 mm; <3.3 mm is dysplasia. The lateral semicircular canal is widening and shortening with large vestibule	**Fig. 4.70.7:** Semicircular canal dysplasia
Large vestibular aqueduct Associated with Pendred syndrome Dilated endolymphatic sac = endolymphatic sac dilated more than the size of posterior semicircular canal	Aqueduct measuring greater than 1.5 mm is considered significant. Associated sensorineural hearing loss must be present.	**Fig. 4.70.8:** Large vestibular aqueduct
Mondini dysplasia Also called incomplete separation, type 2. Occurs during the 7th gestational week.	Absence of the modiolus with a cystic cochlear apex, dilatation of vestibular aqueduct and vestibule	

Other lesions of the temporal bone

External auditory canal	*Middle ear and mastoid*
Congenital—atresia Benign tumors • Exostosis • Osteoma Malignant tumors • SCCA • BCCA • Salivary gland tumors Cholesteatoma Keratosis obturans	Infectious • Otitis media • Mastoiditis Paraganglioma • Glomus tympanicum • Glomus jugulare Cholesteatoma • Congenital • Acquired

Diagnosis	*Imaging features*
EAC atresia Although frequently isolated a number of syndromes are associated with external auditory canal atresia: Crouzon syndrome, Treacher Collins syndrome, Goldenhar syndrome, Pierre Robin syndrome	• Small dysmorphic pinna, bony/soft tissue/mixed stenosis of EAC including membranous and bony portions, Small middle ear, fusion and rotation of malleus and incus • Congenital cholesteatoma behind the atretic plate (10%) • Aberrant course of tympanic and mastoid portions of facial nerve
Exostosis/swimmers/surfer's ear: Location • Frequently bilateral • Medial to isthmus of EAC—arises near the tympanic annulus, at the TS and TM suture lines	• Broad base, multilobulated, circumferential mass • Cortex intact • Associated with prolonged cold-water exposure
EAC osteoma: Location • Unilateral • Arise anywhere lateral to EAC isthmus • Cortex intact	Radiographic appearance • Solitary pedunculated narrow based bony mass • No association with cold water exposure
Cholesteatoma of the EAC: Location • Typically posterior EAC just lateral to the TM	Radiographic appearance • Soft tissue mass • Destruction and remodeling of adjacent bone

Diagnosis	*Imaging features*	*Image*
Otitis media Location • Middle ear and mastoid Offending organisms commonly *S. pneumoniae, M. catarrhalis, H. influenzae.* Otomastoiditis can occur with or without cholesteatoma	• Soft tissue density in middle ear with possible extension into mastoid cavity • Bony septa intact • Mastoid cortex intact • Air/fluid interface may be seen	**Fig. 4.70.9:** Otitis media
Mastoiditis Location • Mastoid, middle ear, possible extension to adjacent tissues Complications: • Bezold's abscess, dural sinus thrombosis, meningitis abscess	• Soft tissue density in mastoid cavity • Destruction of bony septae • Destruction of overlying bony cortex	**Fig. 4.70.10:** Mastoiditis

(Contd.)

Otosclerosis (otospongiosis) Spongy vascular Haversian bone in the ivory like endochondral bone of the otic capsule. Bilateral in up to 90 percent of patients. It is of two types: Cochlear and fenestral.	HRCT—**radiolucent** foci in a pericochlear distribution. In severe cases there is a hypodense ring surrounding the cochlea giving a **"double ring sign"**. MR—a ring of intermediate signal intensities in the peri cochlear and perilabyrinthine regions on T1WI. T1+C may reveal enhancing pericochlear foci which represent active lesions	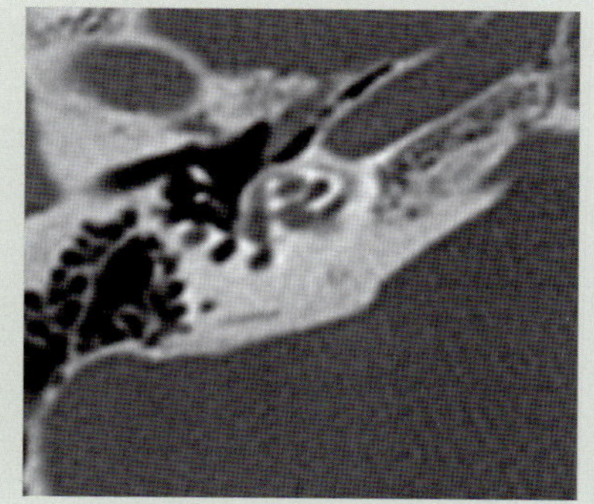 **Fig. 4.70.11:** Otospongiosis
Labyrinthitis ossificans It is most commonly connected with significant sensorineural hearing loss, but it can also cause dizziness and vertigo.	Unlike otosclerosis, which causes erosions around the labyrinth, here, bony invasion of the membrane labyrinths with progressive loss of the fluid-filled gaps of the labyrinth is seen.	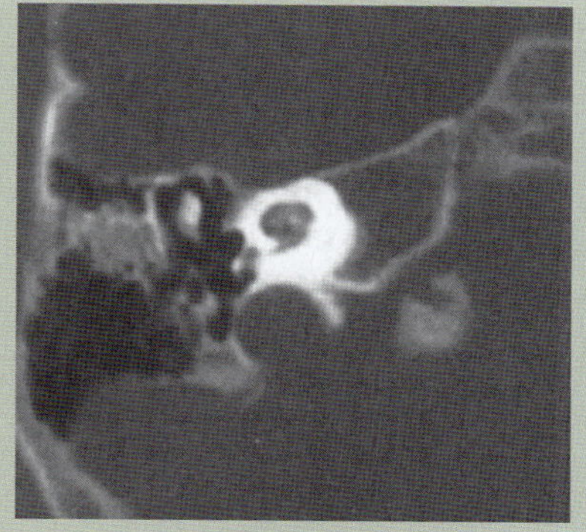 **Fig. 4.70.12:** Labyrinthitis ossificans

Some common lesions seen in temporal bone imaging		
Seventh, eighth cranial aplasia: Cystic cochleovestibular anomaly		
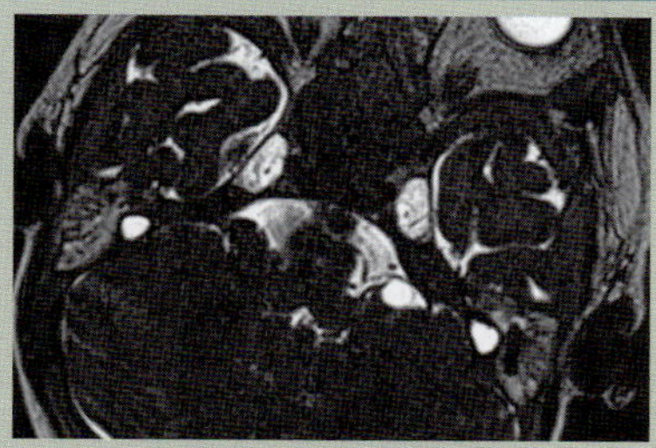 **Fig. 4.70.13:** Seventh, eighth cranial aplasia—cystic cochleo-vestibular anomaly	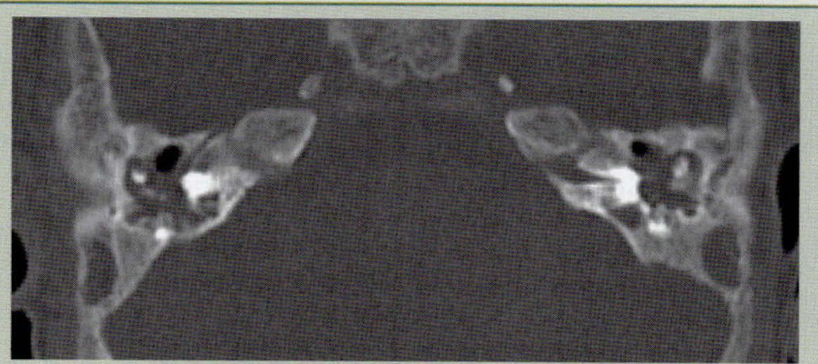 **Fig. 4.70.14:** Seventh, eighth cranial aplasia—cystic cochleo-vestibular anomaly	
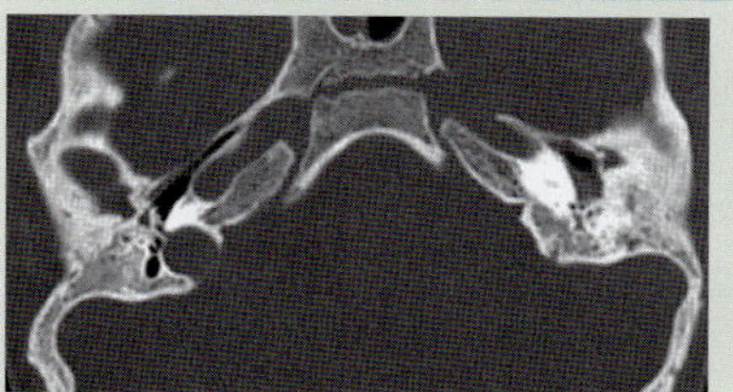 **Fig. 4.70.15:** Right bony EAC atresia	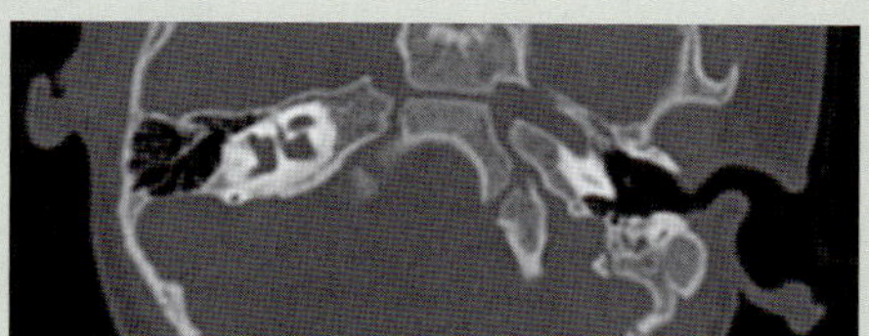 **Fig. 4.70.16:** Right bony EAC atresia	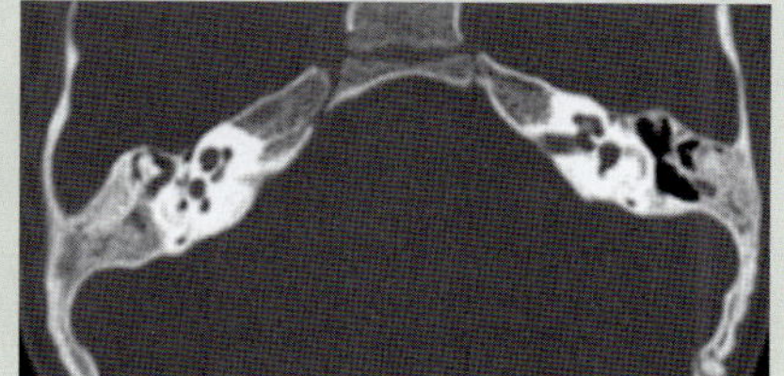 **Fig. 4.70.17:** Right bony EAC atresia

(Contd.)

Some common lesions seen in temporal bone imaging (*Contd.*)

Cholesteatoma

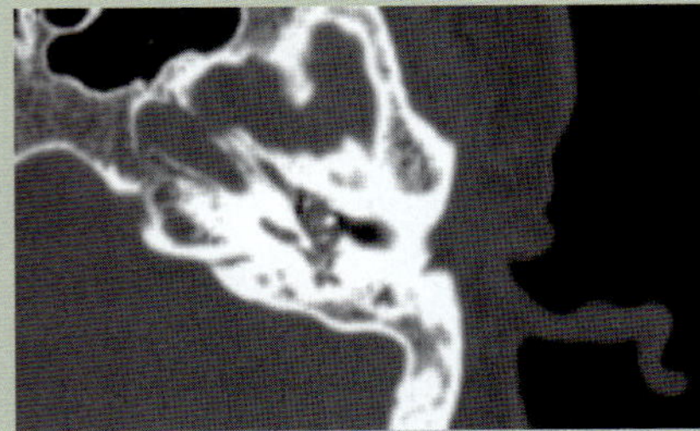

Fig. 4.70.18: Cholesteatoma

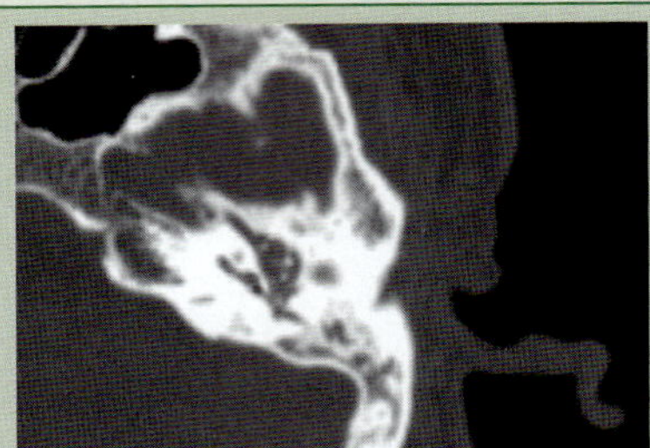

Fig. 4.70.19: Cholesteatoma

Cholesteatoma with ossicular erosion

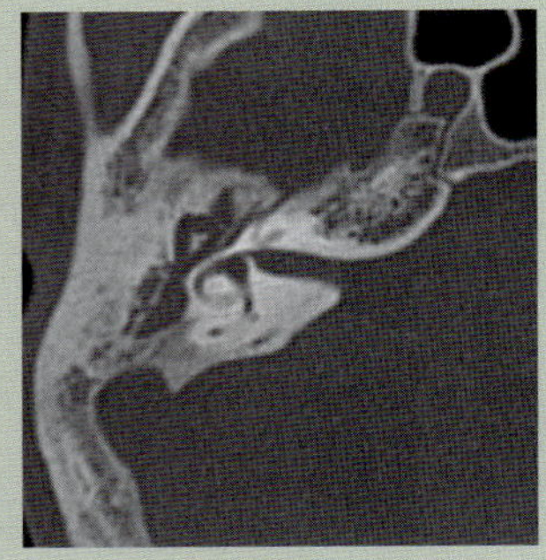

Fig. 4.70.20: Cholesteatoma with ossicular erosion

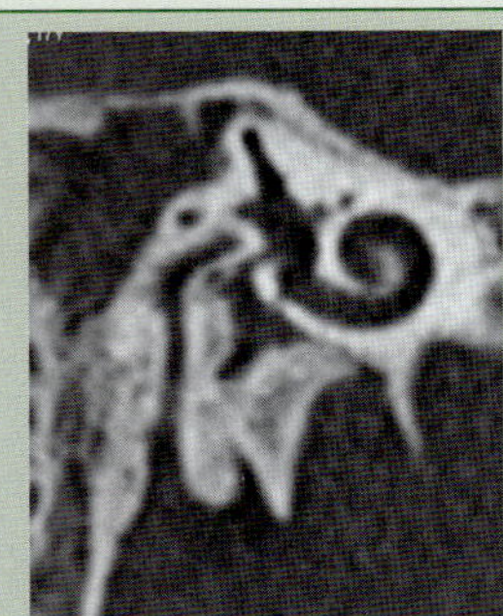

Fig. 4.70.21: Cholesteatoma with ossicular erosion

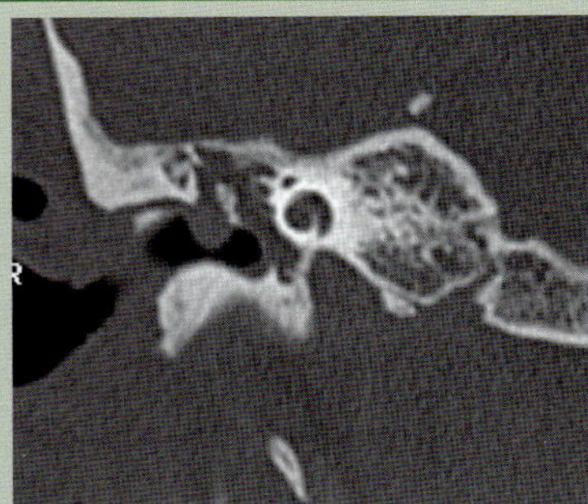

Fig. 4.70.22: Cholesteatoma with ossicular erosion

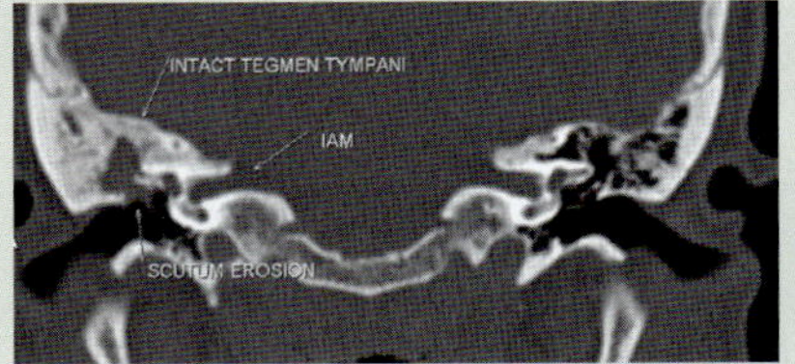

Fig. 4.70.23: Chronic otitis media with lateral SCC fistula

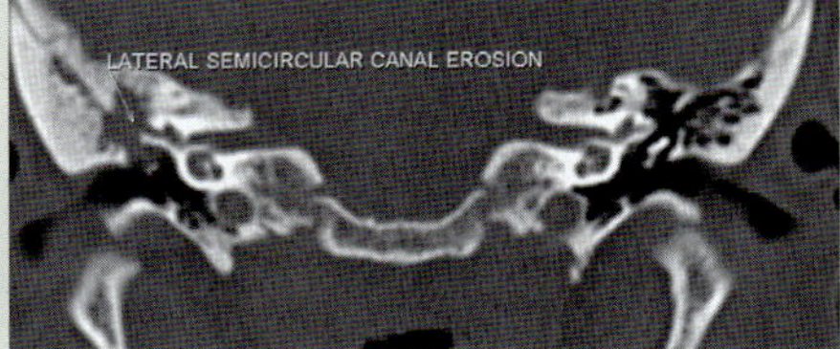

Fig. 4.70.24: Chronic otitis media with lateral SCC fistula

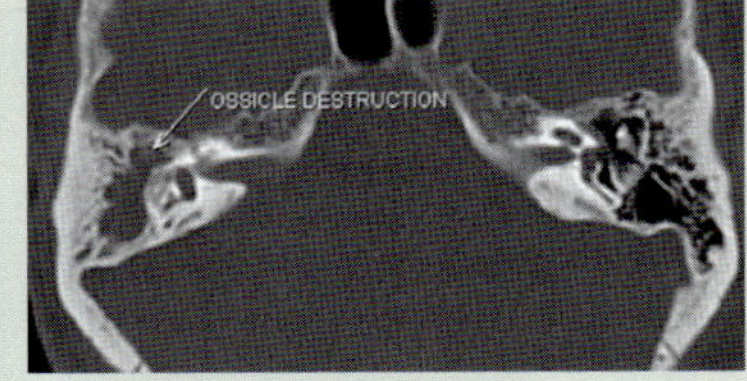

Fig. 4.70.25: Chronic otitis media with lateral SCC fistula

Chronic otomastoiditis

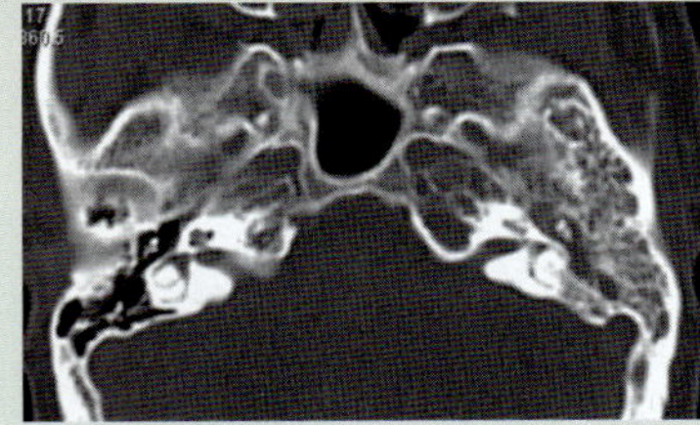

Fig. 4.70.26: Chronic otomastoiditis

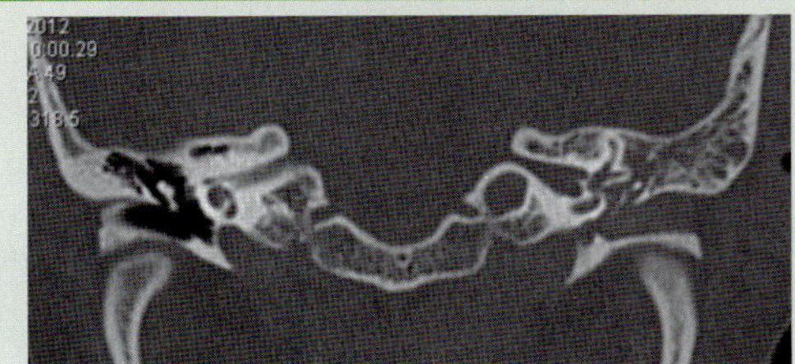

Fig. 4.70.27: Chronic otomastoiditis

Cochlear aplasia

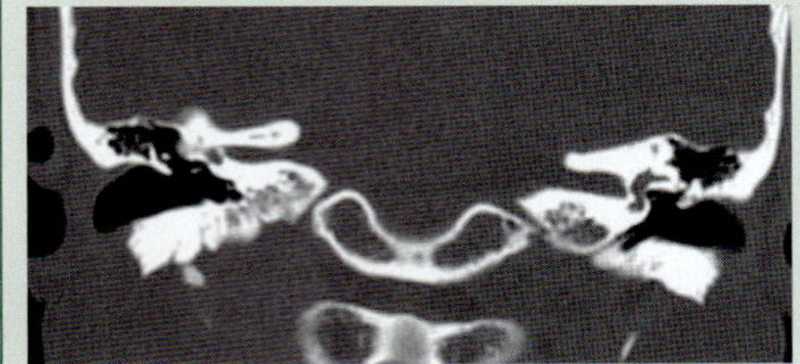

Fig. 4.70.28: Cochlear aplasia

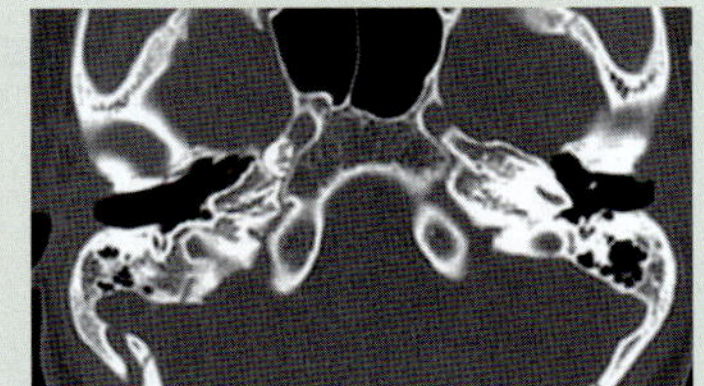

Fig. 4.70.29: Cochlear aplasia

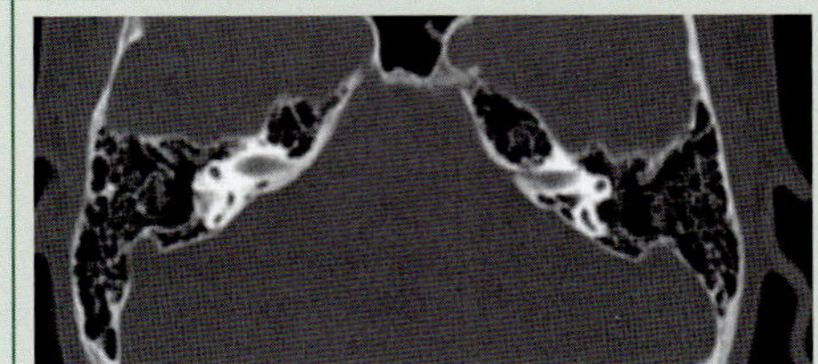

Fig. 4.70.30: Cochlear aplasia

(*Contd.*)

Some common lesions seen in temporal bone imaging (*Contd.*)

CSOM with sigmoid thrombus

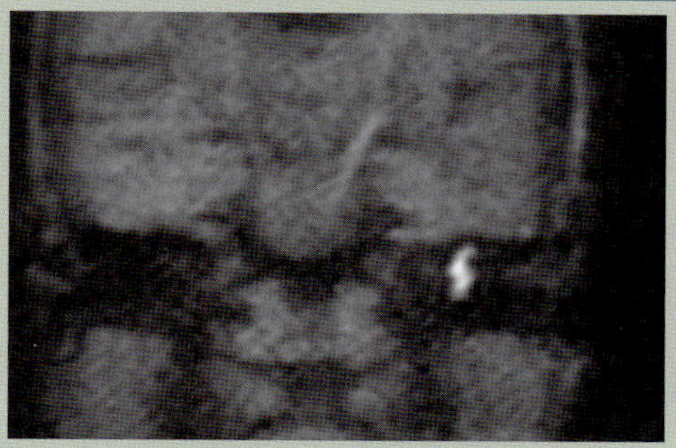

Fig. 4.70.31: Non-EPI DWI showing diffusion restriction in cholesteatoma

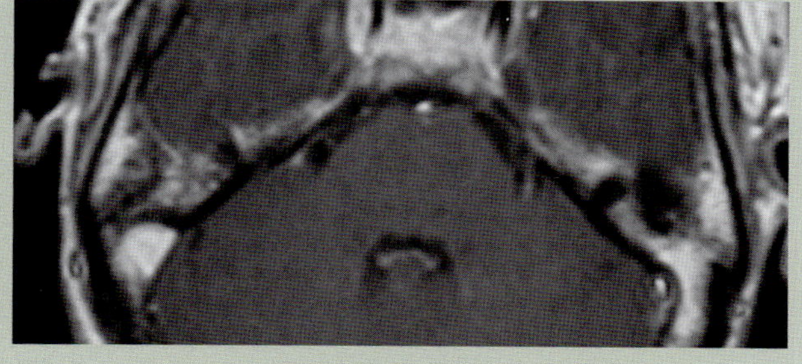

Fig. 4.70.32: Chronic otomastoiditis with sigmoid sinus thrombosis

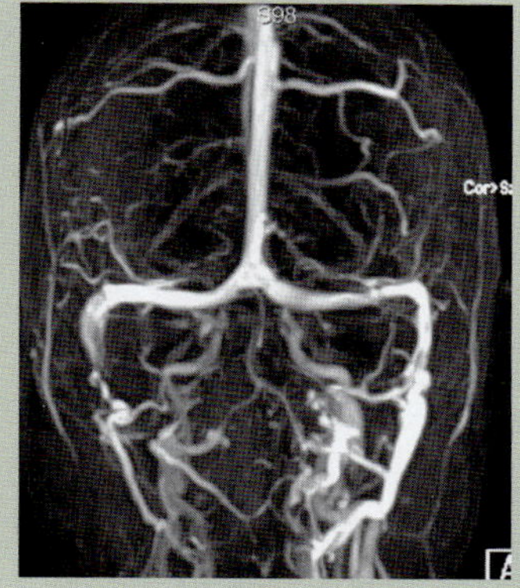

Fig. 4.70.33: Chronic otomastoiditis with sigmoid sinus thrombosis

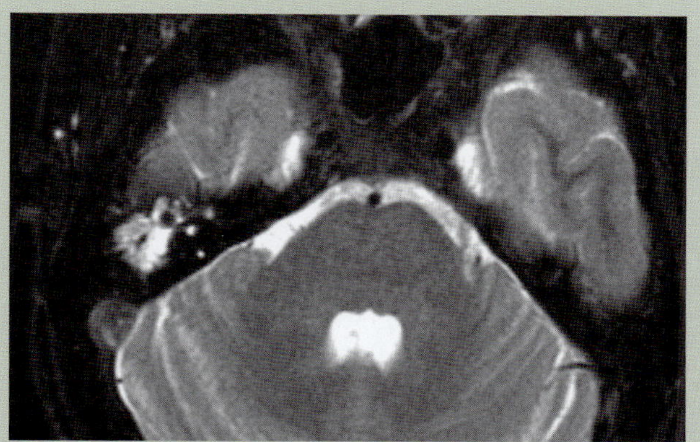

Fig. 4.70.34: Chronic otomastoiditis with sigmoid sinus thrombosis

Endolymphatic sac tumor

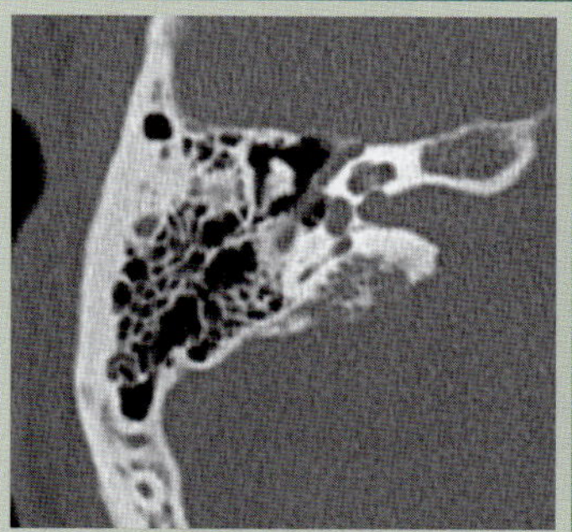

Fig. 4.70.35: Endolymphatic sac tumor

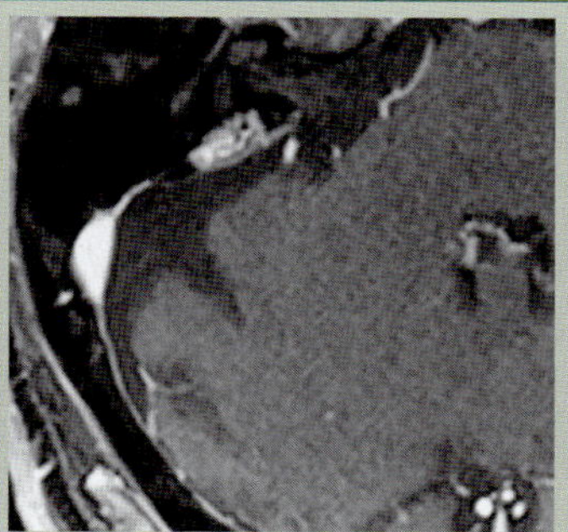

Fig. 4.70.36: Endolymphatic sac tumor

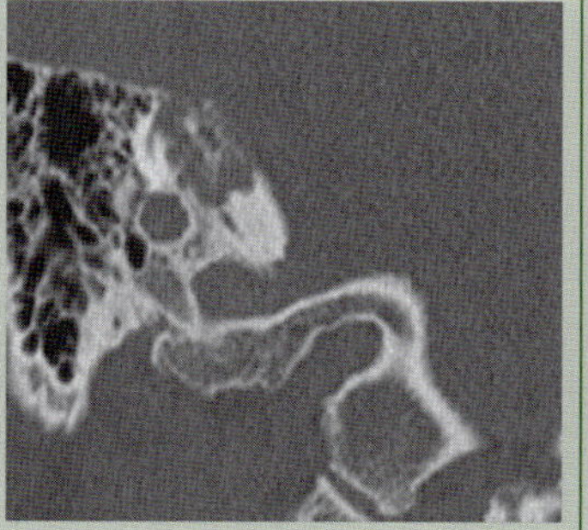

Fig. 4.70.37: Endolymphatic sac tumor

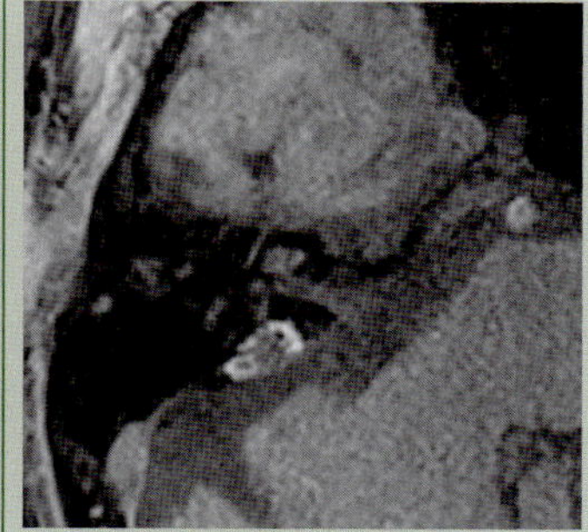

Fig. 4.70.38: Endolymphatic sac tumor

Lateral SCC dysplasia

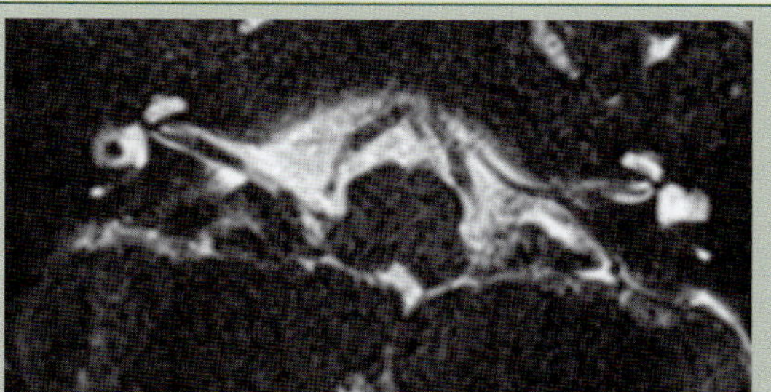

Fig. 4.70.39: Lateral SCC dysplasia

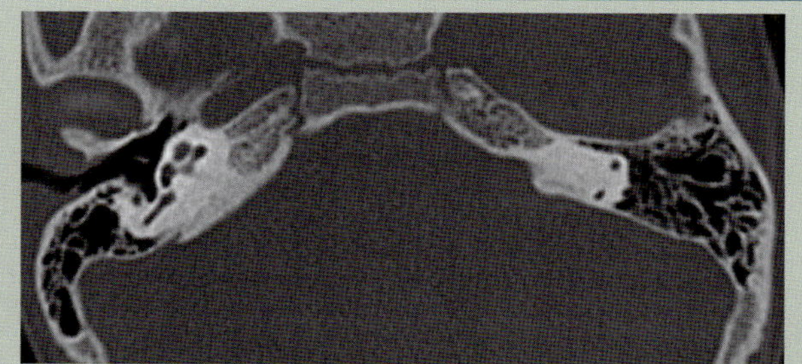

Fig. 4.70.40: Lateral SCC dysplasia

(*Contd.*)

Some common lesions seen in temporal bone imaging (*Contd.*)

Longitudinal fracture with hemotympanum

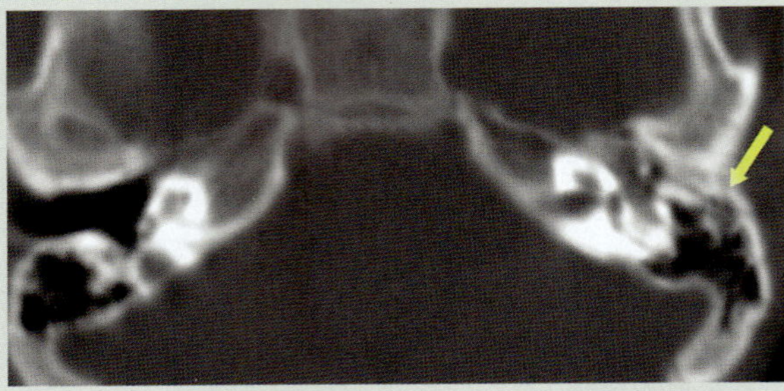

Fig. 4.70.41: Longitudinal fracture with hemotympanum

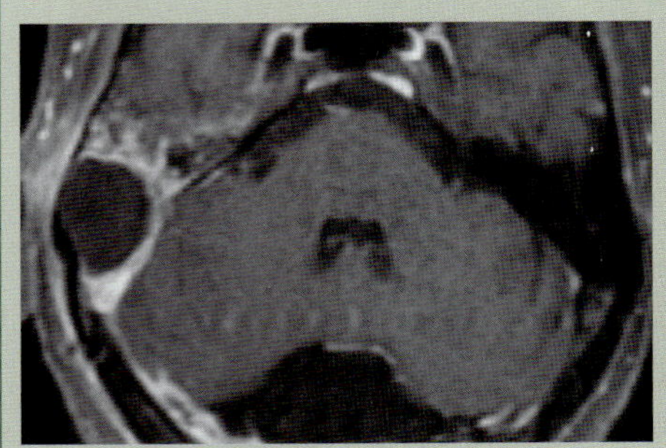

Fig. 4.70.42: Mastoid abscess

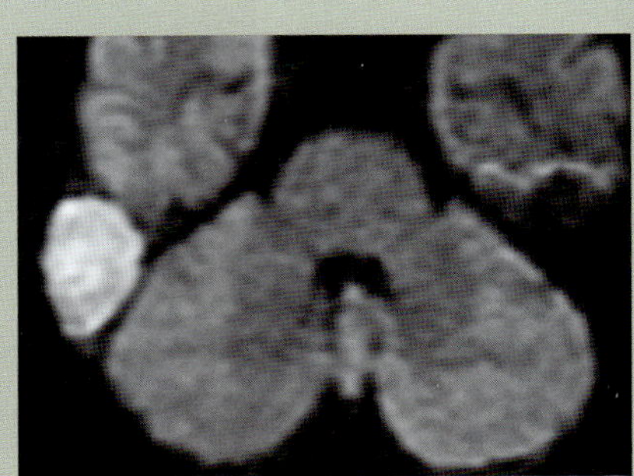

Fig. 4.70.43: Mastoid abscess

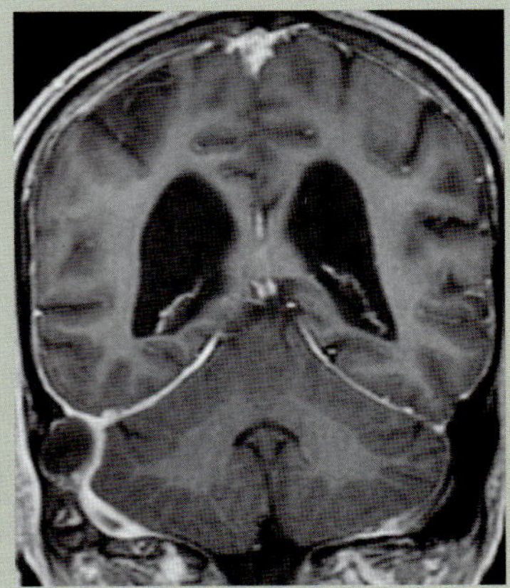

Fig. 4.70.44: Mastoid abscess with meninges involvement

Otitis media with petrous apicitis retropharyngeal abscess

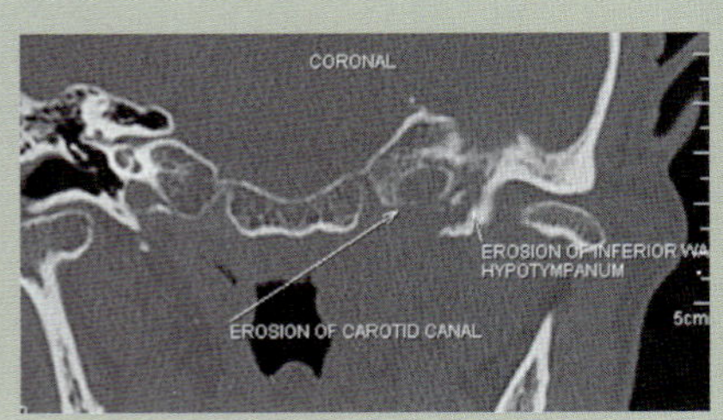

Fig. 4.70.45: Otitis media with petrous apicitis and retropharyngeal abscess

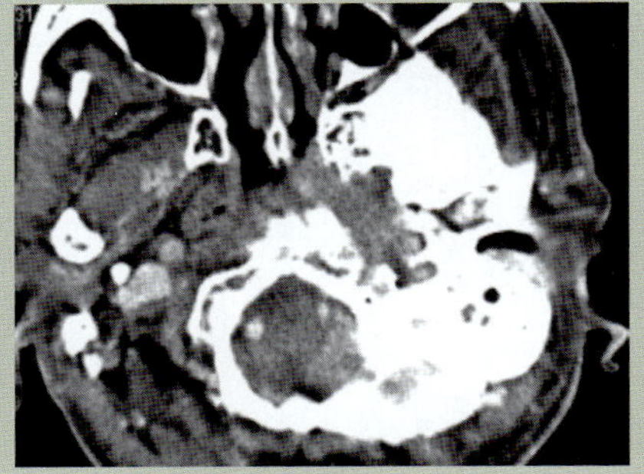

Fig. 4.70.46: Otitis media with petrous apicitis and retropharyngeal abscess

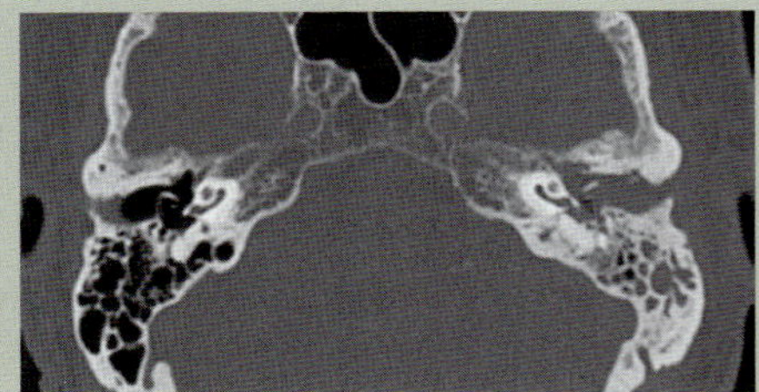

Fig. 4.70.47: Otitis media with petrous apicitis and retropharyngeal abscess

Vestibular schwannoma

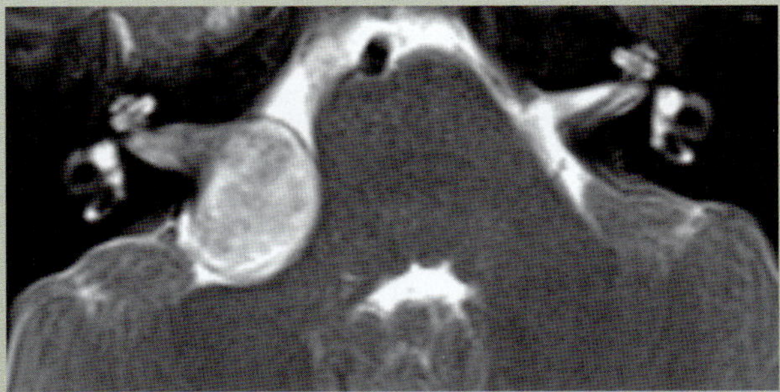

Fig. 4.70.48: Vestibular schwannoma

4.71 HEAD AND NECK

Case No. 71

Clinical history: A 30-year-old female with a 4-month history of left-sided nasal obstruction, rhinorrhea, and epistaxis.

Radiological techniques and observations: Figures 4.71.1 to 4.71.3 are MRI brain T2 axial/FLAIR coronal/T1 post-contrast axial sections revealing well-defined T2/FLAIR hyperintense solid soft tissue intracranial extra-axial mass lesion with areas of haemorrhage noted arising from left olfactory bulb region with erosion of cribriform plate of ethmoid bone with extension to nasal cavity. Cystic component of the lesion noted in the posterior aspect (peritumoral cyst). Vasogenic oedema noted in left frontal lobe probably due to lesion infiltrating the brain parenchyma. On T1 post-contrast solid soft tissue intracranial extra-axial component of the lesion shows avid enhancement. Lesion causes mass effect over the frontal horn of left lateral ventricle with midline shift to the right and dilatation of contralateral lateral ventricle. Rest of brain parenchyma appears to be normal. No evidence of any intraorbital extension. Visualised paranasal sinus appears to be normal.

Interpretations: A—30-year-old female, soft tissue intracranial extra-axial mass lesion in left olfactory bulb region, C—well-defined enhancing T2 hyperintense extra-axial lesion, B—erosion of cribriform plate with intracranial extension and peritumoral cysts, D—esthesioneuroblastoma

Principal diagnosis: Esthesioneuroblastoma (olfactory nerve neuroblastoma) (Kadish stage C)

Differential diagnosis (for T2 hypointense skull base lesions): 1. Sinonasal squamous cell carcinoma and adenocarcinomas—more common in maxillary antrum with extensive bony destruction. 2. Anterior skull base meningioma—hyperostosis of adjacent bone. 3. Non-Hodgkin's lymphoma—rarely breaches skull base/associated with cervical lymphadenopathy/hyperdense in NECT/shows diffusion restriction in MR.

Management: Craniofacial resection and radiotherapy is the treatment of choice. Radiotherapy offers better local control since negative resection margins are difficult to achieve. Chemotherapy is reserved for larger/high grade lesions.

Discussion—esthesioneuroblastoma: Age—bimodal distribution in 2nd and 6th decades, slight male preponderance. Other diseases with bimodal distribution include lymphoma, craniopharyngioma, neurosarcoid, nasopharyngeal carcinoma, breast cancer and inflammatory bowel disorders.

Paraneoplastic syndromes: Cushing syndrome due to adrenocorticotrophic hormone secretion. Hyponatremia due to antidiuretic hormone secretion.

Kadish Classification

Stage A—confined to nasal cavity. Stage B—localised to nasal cavity and sinuses. Stage C—orbital and

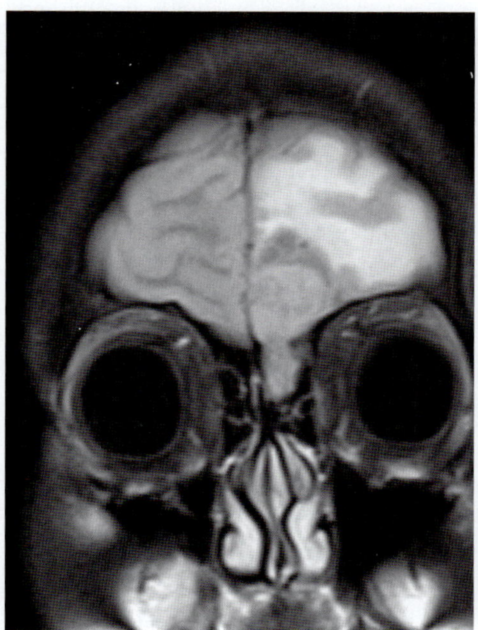

Fig. 4.71.1

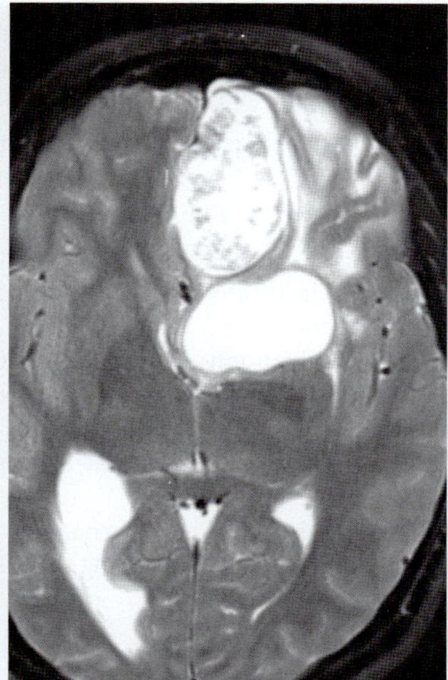

Fig. 4.71.2

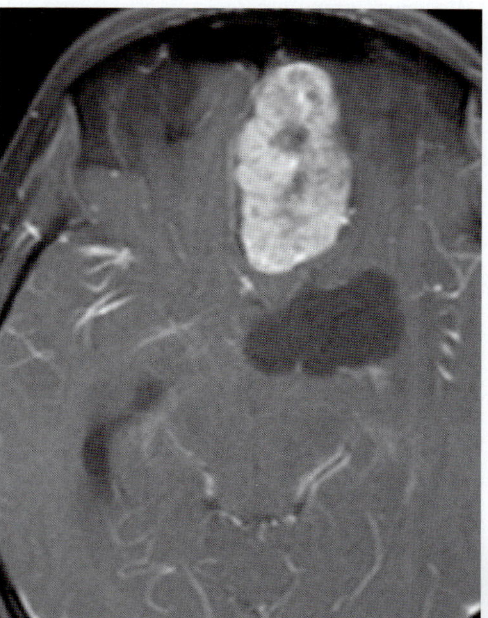

Fig. 4.71.3

Table 4.71.1: Other T2 hypointense lesions in anterior skull base

Sinonasal squamous cell carcinoma	*Anterior skull base meningioma*	*Non-Hodgkin's lymphoma*
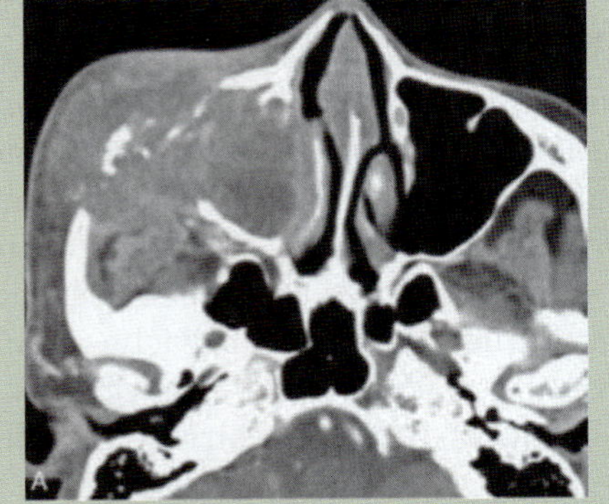 **Fig. 4.71.4:** Soft tissue mass within right maxillary sinus with adjacent bony erosions	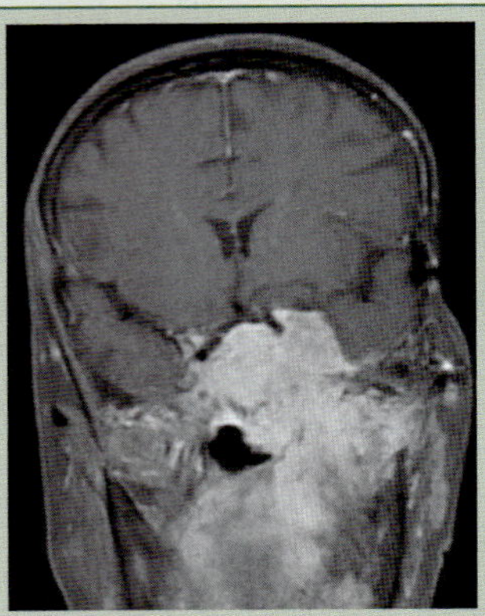 **Fig. 4.71.5:** T1 post-contrast image showing tumor extending to ethmoidal and sphenoid sinus, pituitary fossa and encasing left intracranial ICA	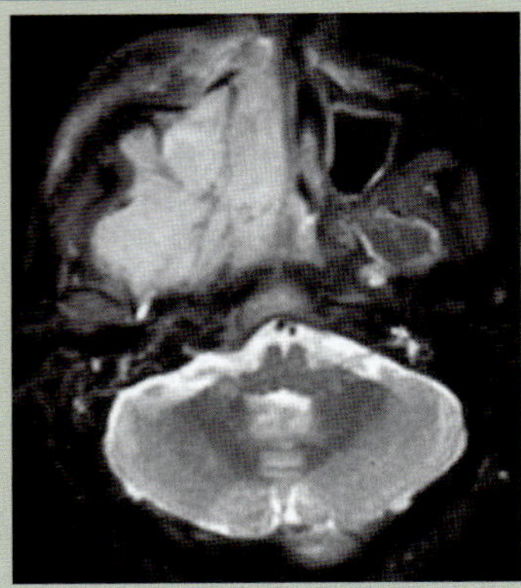 **Fig. 4.71.6:** Sinonasal lymphoma diffusely infiltrating lesion along walls of paranasal sinuses and nasal cavities or as discrete sinonasal soft tissue masses

Table 4.71.2: Anterior skull base T2 hypointense lesions

Fungal sinusitis Allergic fungal sinusitis—allergic response to fungi, eosinophilic mucin with non-invasive fungal hyphae Sinus mycetoma—chronic non-invasive form. **Acute invasive fungal sinusitis (AIFRS)**—Rapidly progressive with vascular and bone invasion.	**CT**—sinus opacification with central areas of high density and adjacent bone erosions. MRI–characteristic finding –T2-hypointense signal centrally due to dense fungal concretions. AIFRS—perimaxillary fat infiltration is seen—T1 is the best sequence to evaluate it.	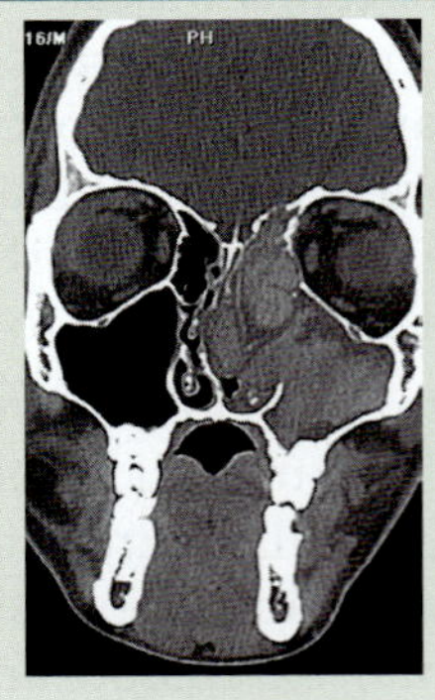 **Fig. 4.71.7:** Fungal sinusitis
Wegener's granulomatosis: Its necrotising granulomatous vasculitis that involves upper and lower respiratory tracts, kidney, skin and joints. Septal and non-septal cartilaginous and bone destruction.	**NECT**–chronic rhinosinusitis with localised mucosal nodularity and masses centred in nasal cavity. Osseous or cartilaginous erosion occurs and causes perforation. **MRI**—T1-low to intermediate signal nodular mass. T2—**decreased** signal nodular mass. Orbital involvement enhancing infiltrating mass within orbit. Orbital invasion is the most common extra Sinonasal head and neck site. **Location**—septum>turbinates>sinuses	
Skull base osteomyelitis Seen in immunocompromised and diabetic patients. Typical SBO: Infection spreads from necrotizing external otitis, temporal bone is the first to involve Pathogen: Pseudomonas Atypical SBO: Occurs secondary to invasive sinusitis or deep face infections Pathogen: Bacterial or fungal	Ill-defined and infiltrative with osseous and extraosseous abnormalities. CT: Osteolysis and erosions with swollen EAC in typical SBO and sphenoid sinus opacification in atypical SBO MR-T1: Low signal replaces normal T1 hyper-marrow fat. T1 post-contrast: Abnormal marrow enhancement and infiltrative extraosseous enhancing soft tissue.	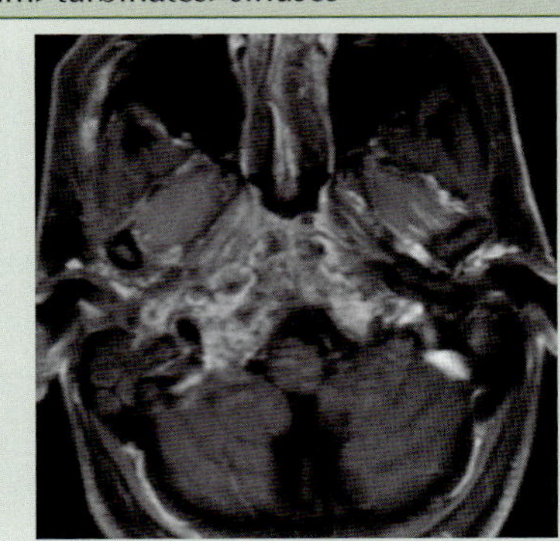 **Fig. 4.71.8:** Skull base osteomyelitis

(Contd.)

Table 4.71.2: Anterior skull base T2 hypointense lesions (*Contd.*)

Pseudotumor (idiopathic myo-fibroblastic tumor) Nonspecific inflammation not due to any known etiology or systemic disease. Types of orbital pseudotumor—myositic-extraocular muscle. Lacrimal-Lacrimal glands Anterior-Globe/retrobulbar orbit. Diffuse-Multifocal intraconal and extraconal Apical-Orbital apex with intracranial extension. Tolosa-Hunt extension of pseudotumor into cavernous sinus through fissures.	NECT: Multifocal or infiltrative soft tissue lesion CECT: Moderate enhancement. **Erosion of bone is a rare finding.** MR-T1-hypointense T2: Hypointense (abscess and tumors are T2 hyperintense). Pseudotumor of skull base can cause cavernous sinus involvement or meningeal dural thickening. Tolosa-Hunt syndrome: Enhancement and fullness of anterior cavernous sinus and orbital fissures.	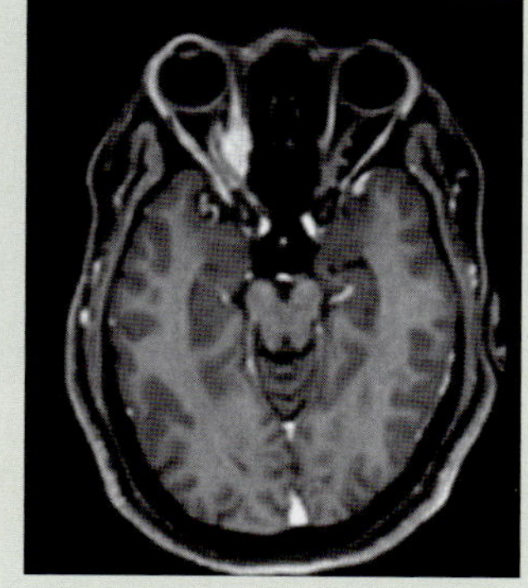 **Fig. 4.71.9:** Idiopathic myofibroblastic tumor
Frontoethmoid (sincipital) cephalocele: Midline inferior herniation of CSF with brain into nasal cavity. It is a congenital lesion. Recurrent meningitis is a presenting feature.	**NECT:** CSF attenuation mass protruding into nasopharynx. Bone CT: Osseous defects in skull base. **MR:** Mass with variable signal intensity protruding into nasopharynx, oropharynx or orbit. Presence of enhancement suggests infection or inflammation.	

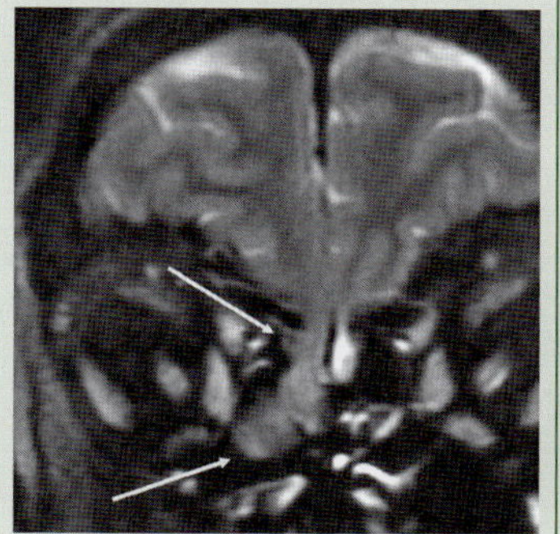

Fig. 4.71.10: Sincipital cephalocele

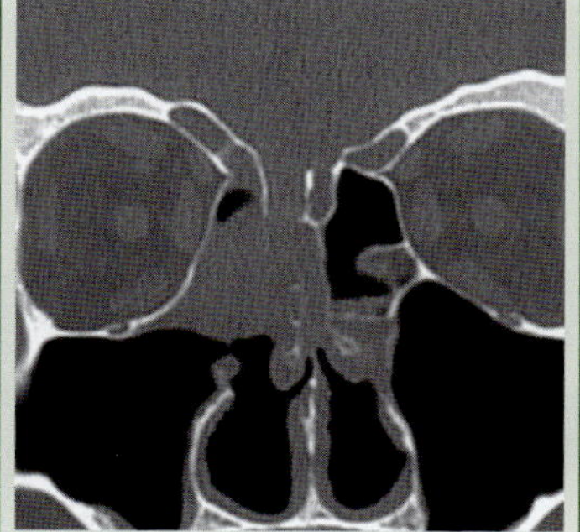

Fig. 4.71.11: Sincipital cephalocele

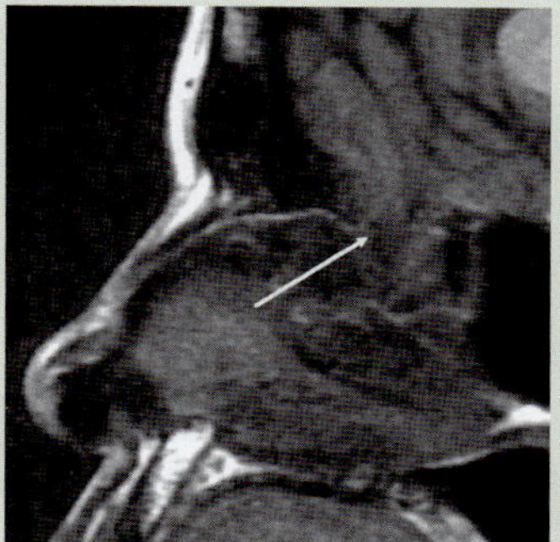

Fig. 4.71.12: Sincipital cephalocele

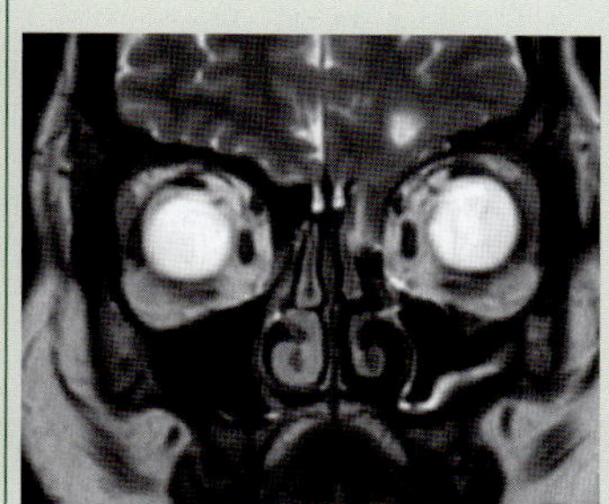

Fig. 4.71.13: Sincipital cephalocele

Table 4.71.3: Imaging features in esthesioneuroblastoma

Dumbbell shaped mass with upper portion in anterior cranial fossa, lower portion in upper nasal cavity and waist at level of cribriform plate. Cervical nodes metastasis is common. **NECT**: Bone remodelling with enlargement of nasal cavity with bony erosions especially near cribriform plate area. **CECT:** Homogeneously enhancing mass. **MRI**: T1 hypo /T2 hyperintense lesion with **T2 hyperintense cysts** at tumour brain interface which is highly specific for the lesion. Post-contrast lesions show **avid homogeneous enhancement**. **Nuclear medicine:** FDG PET positive

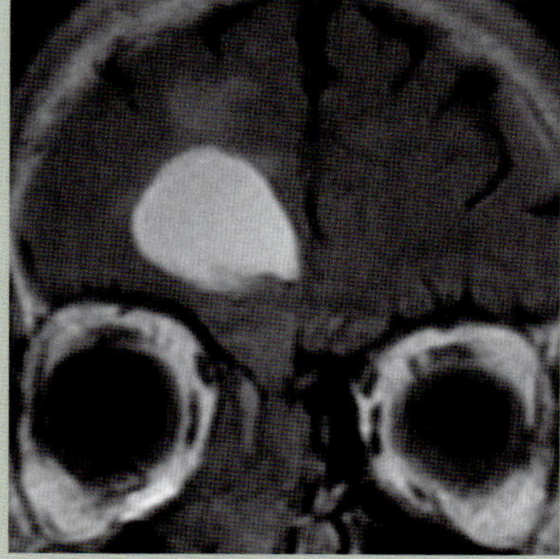

Fig.4.71.14: Esthesioneuroblastoma

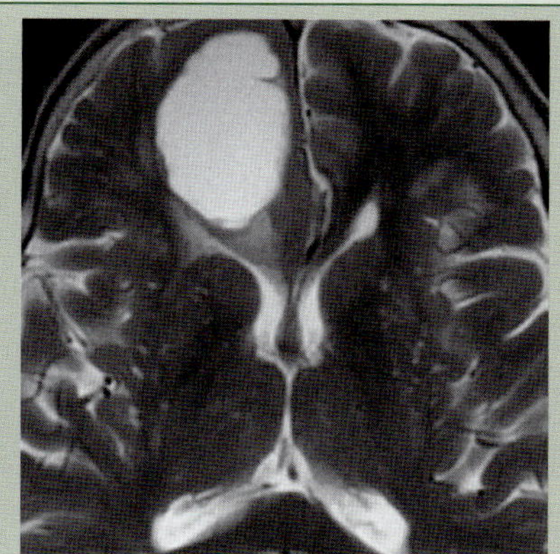

Fig. 4.71.15: Esthesioneuroblastoma

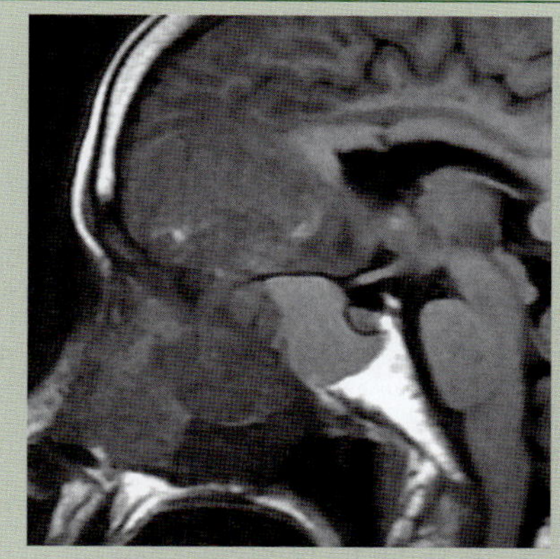

Fig. 4.71.16: Esthesioneuroblastoma

Table 4.71.4: Spectrum of findings in rhinocerebral orbital mucormycosis

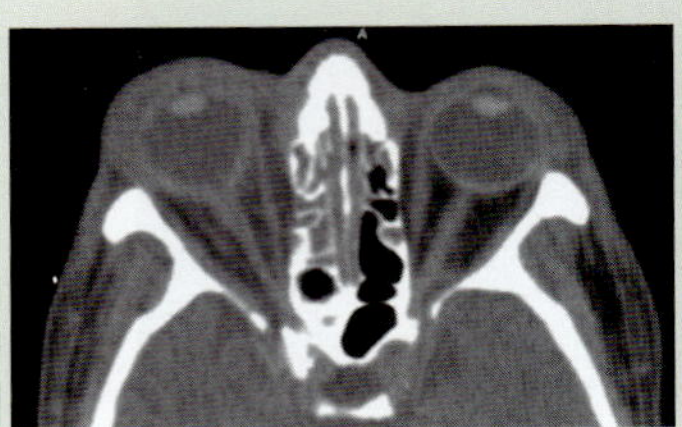
Fig. 4.71.17: Right rhino-orbital-cerebral mucormycosis

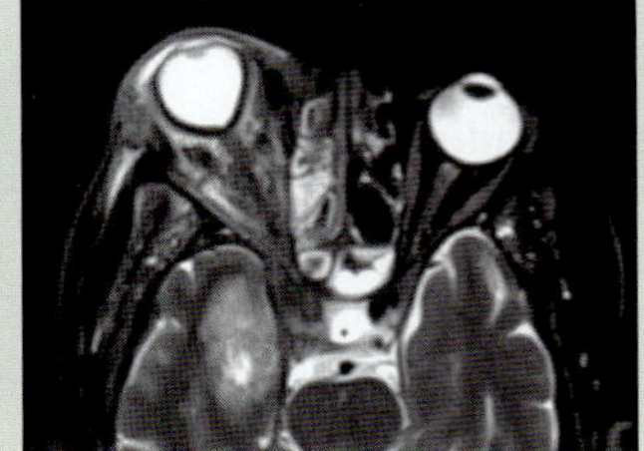
Fig. 4.71.18: Right rhino-orbital-cerebral mucormycosis

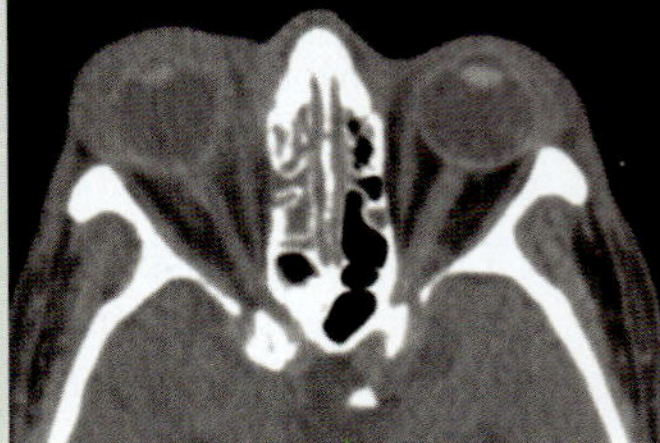
Fig. 4.71.19: Right rhino-orbital-cerebral mucormycosis

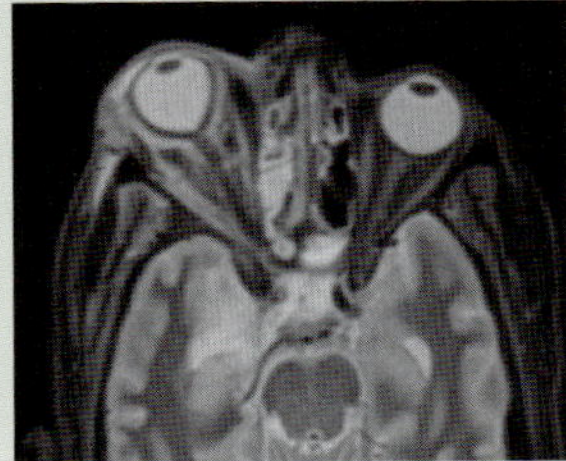
Fig. 4.71.20: Right rhino-orbital-cerebral mucormycosis

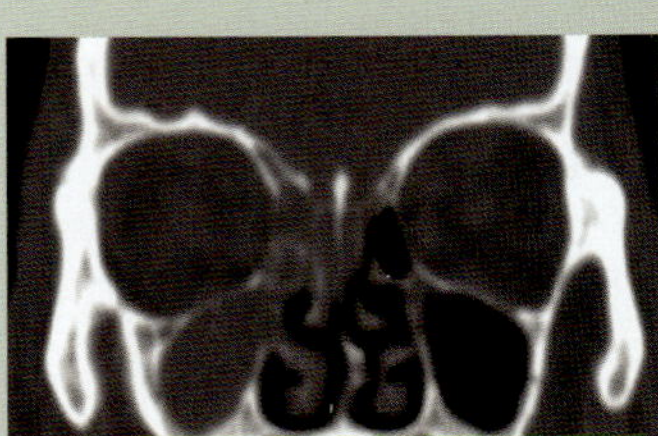
Fig. 4.71.21: Right mucormycosis with right temporal lobe and hardpalate involvement

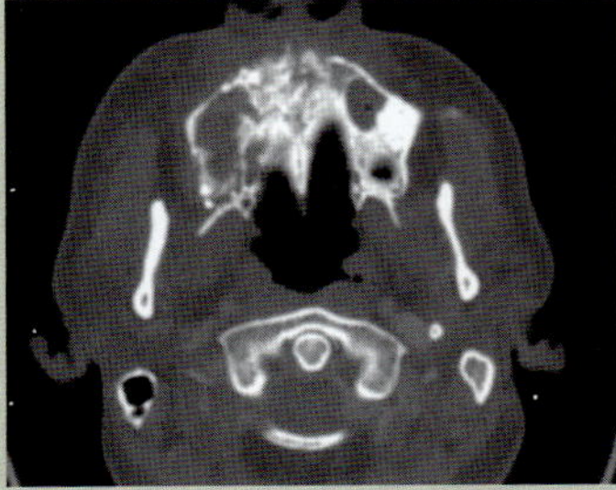
Fig. 4.71.22: Right mucormycosis with right temporal lobe and hardpalate involvement

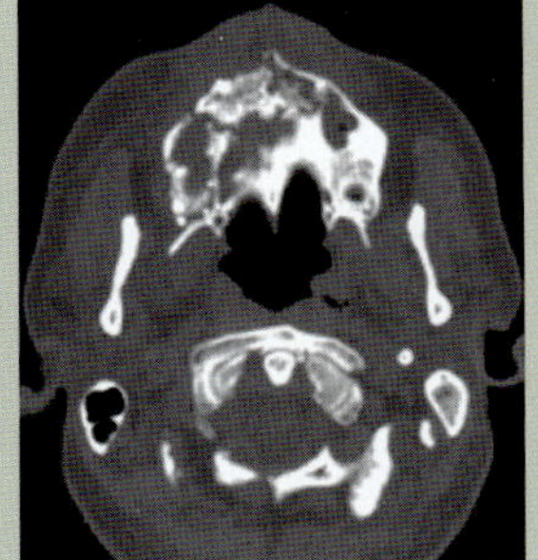
Fig. 4.71.23: Right mucormycosis with right temporal lobe and hardpalate involvement

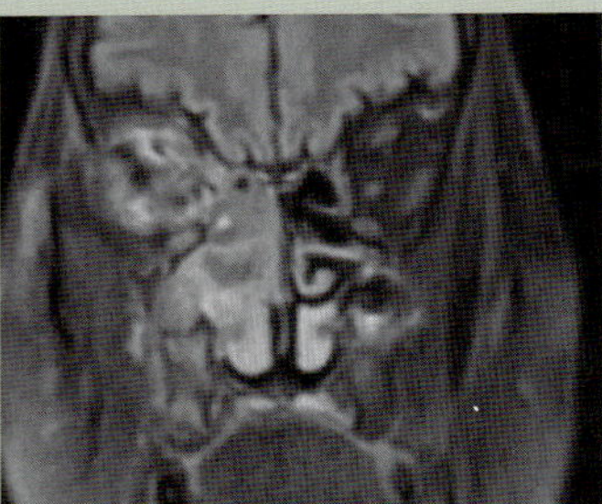
Fig. 4.71.24: Right mucormycosis with right temporal lobe and hardpalate involvement

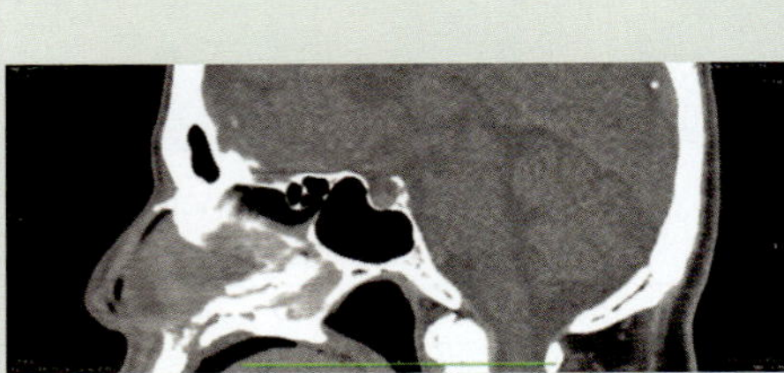
Fig. 4.71.25: Bilateral sinonasal and orbital mucormycosis with hardpalate erosion

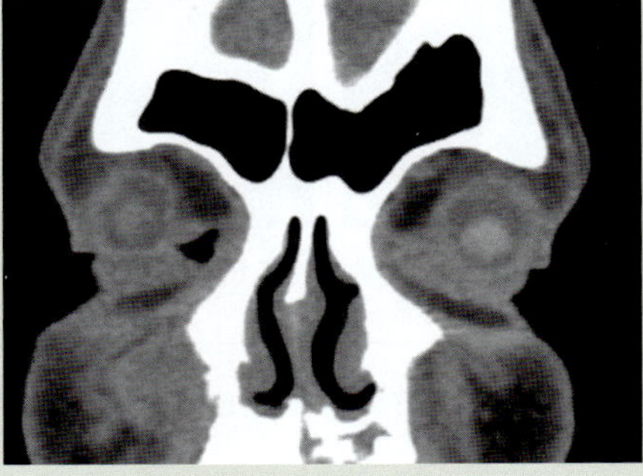
Fig. 4.71.26: Bilateral sinonasal and orbital mucormycosis with hardpalate erosion

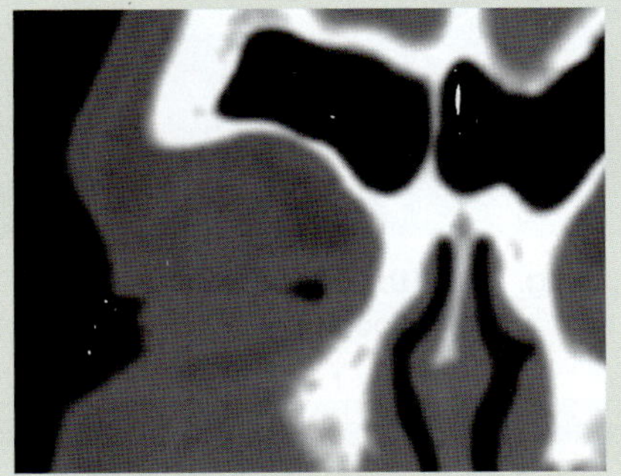
Fig. 4.71.27: Bilateral sinonasal and orbital mucormycosis with hardpalate erosion

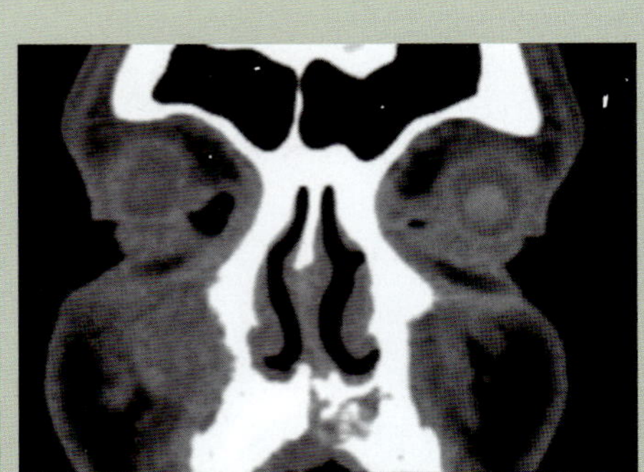
Fig. 4.71.28: Bilateral sinonasal and orbital mucormycosis with hardpalate erosion

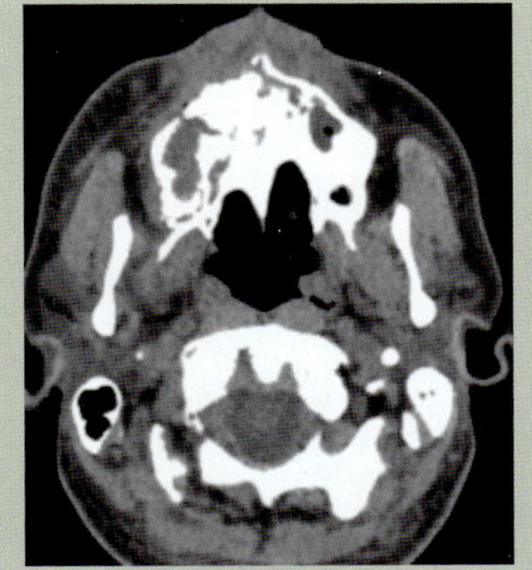
Fig. 4.71.29: Bilateral sinonasal and orbital mucormycosis with hardpalate erosion

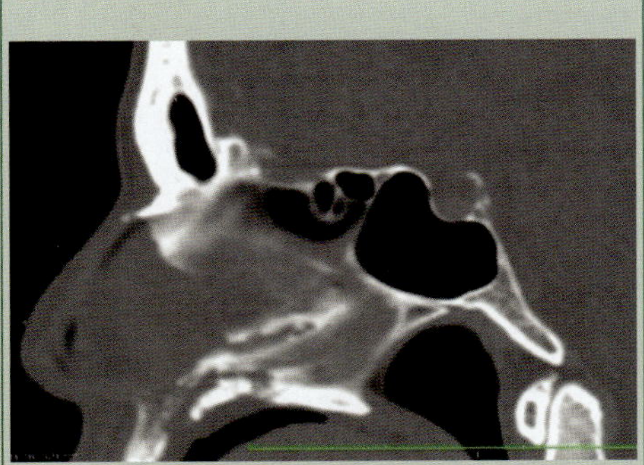
Fig. 4.71.30: Bilateral sinonasal and orbital mucormycosis with hardpalate erosion

Contd...

Table 4.71.4: Spectrum of findings in rhinocerebral orbital mucormycosis *(Contd...)*

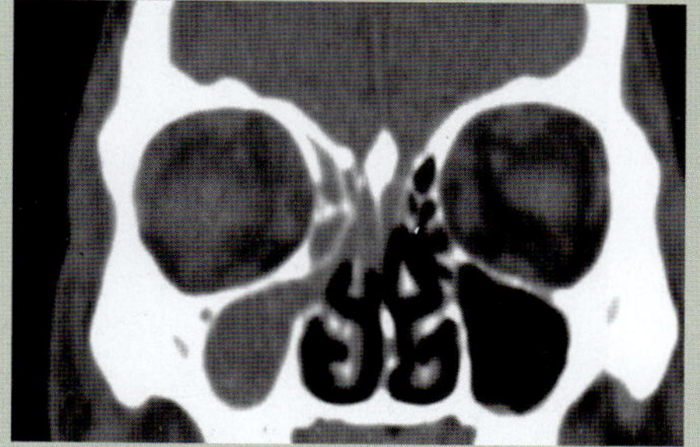

Fig. 4.71.31: Right sinonasal mucormycosis with right orbital involvement

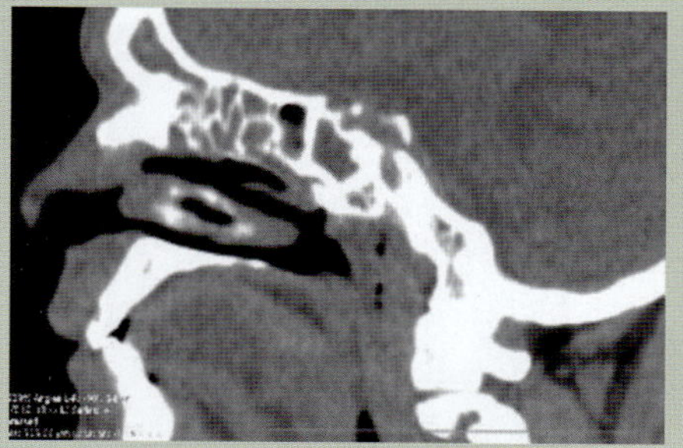

Fig. 4.71.32: Right sinonasal mucormycosis with right orbital involvement

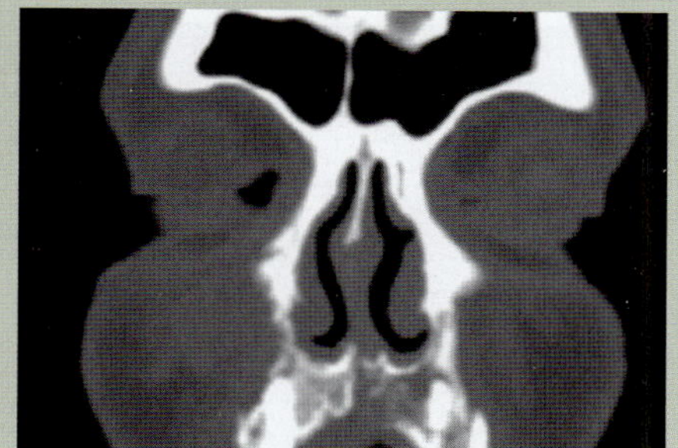

Fig. 4.71.33: Right sinonasal mucormycosis with right orbital involvement

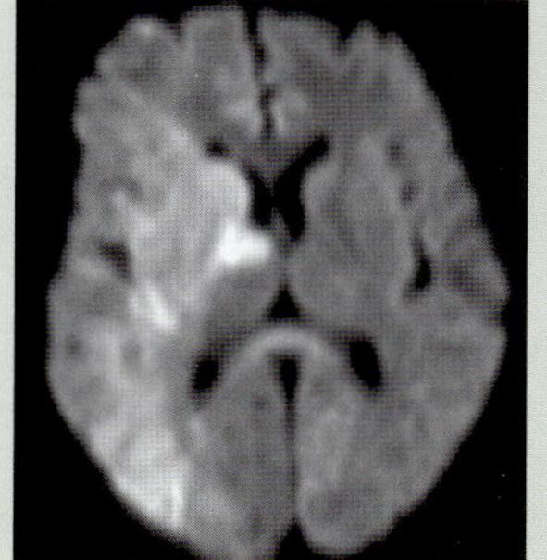

Fig. 4.71.34: Right sinonasal mucormycosis causing right MCA infarct

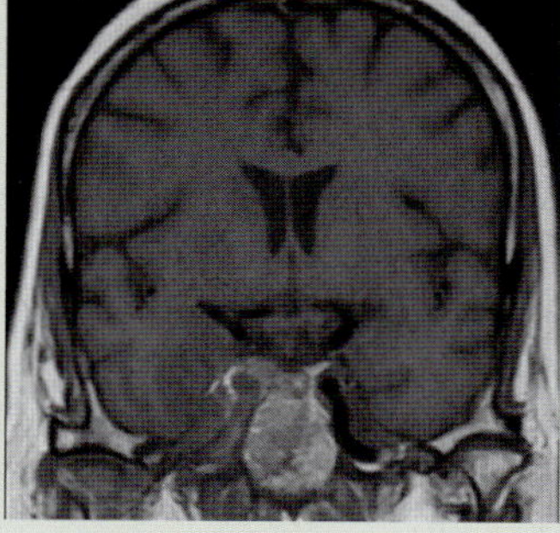

Fig. 4.71.35: Right sinonasal mucormycosis causing right MCA infarct

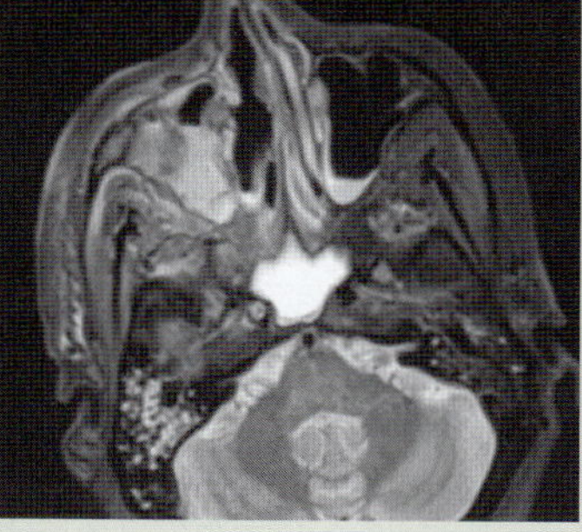

Fig. 4.71.36: Right sinonasal mucormycosis causing right MCA infarct

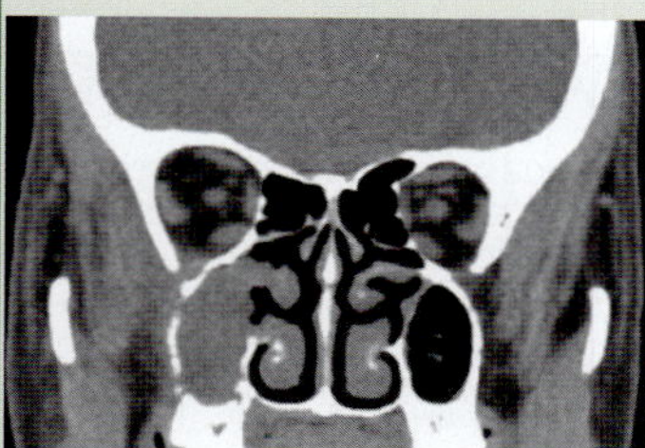

Fig. 4.71.37: Right sinonasal mucormycosis causing right MCA infarct

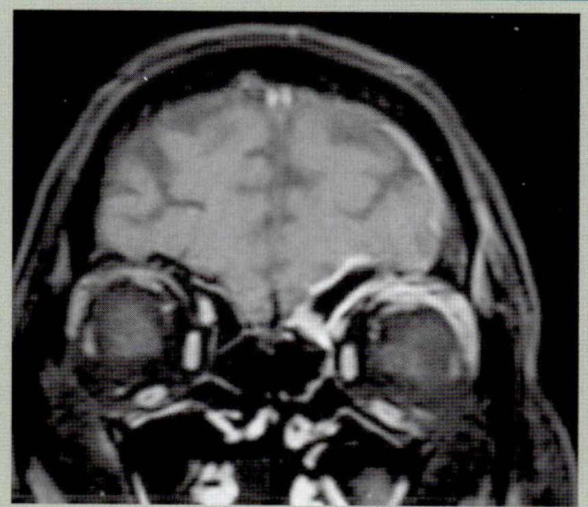

Fig. 4.71.38: Orbital mucormycosis with frontal lobe involvement

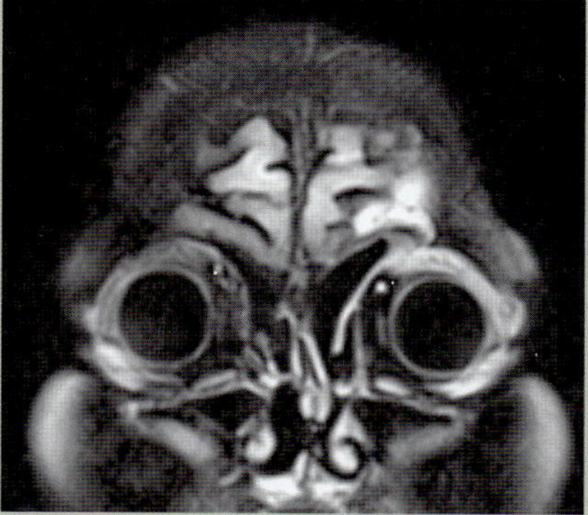

Fig. 4.71.39: Orbital mucormycosis with frontal lobe involvement

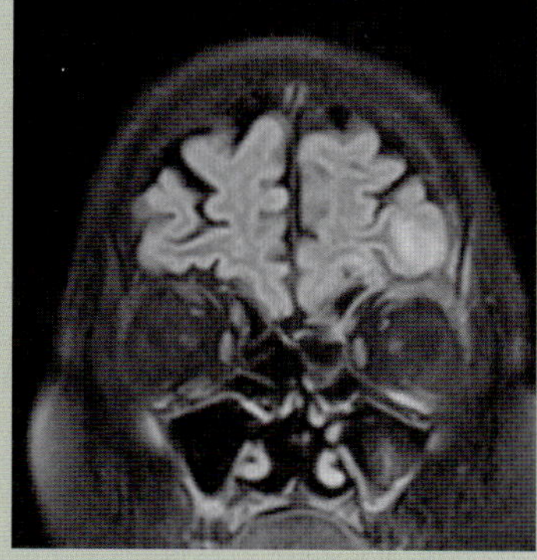

Fig. 4.71.40: Orbital mucormycosis with frontal lobe involvement

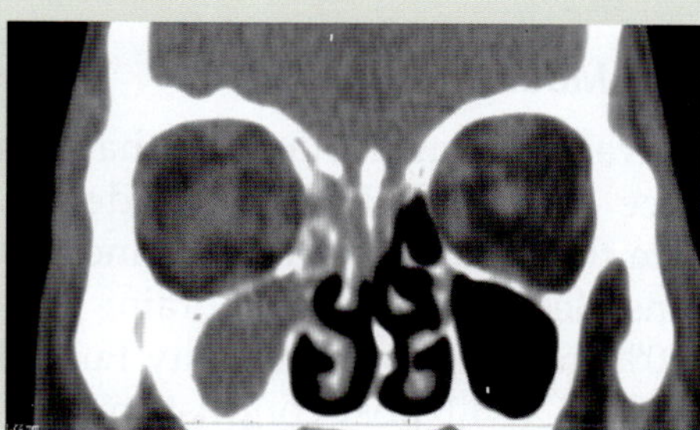

Fig. 4.71.41: Right sinonasal mucormycosis with right orbital, right MCA and right temporal lobe invasion

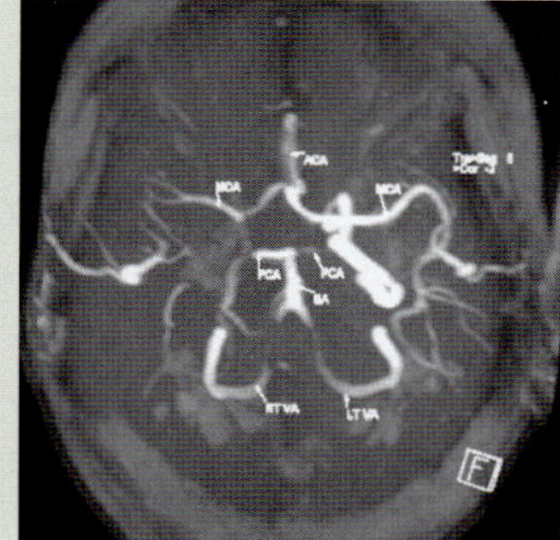

Fig. 4.71.42: Right sinonasal mucormycosis with right orbital, right MCA and right temporal lobe invasion

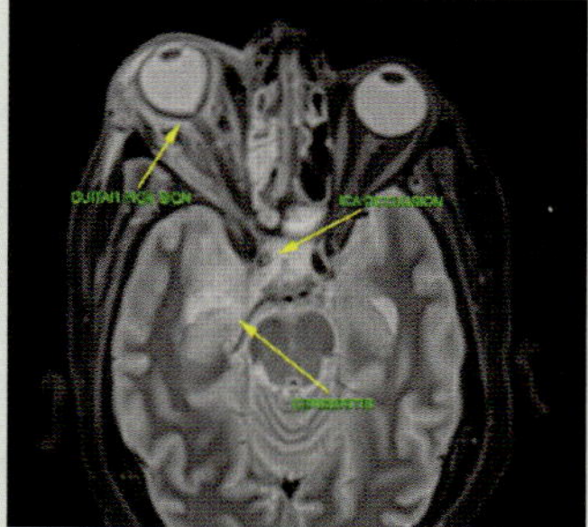

Fig. 4.71.43: Right sinonasal mucormycosis with right orbital, right MCA and right temporal lobe invasion

Contd...

Table 4.71.4: Spectrum of findings in rhinocerebralorbital mucormycosis *(Contd...)*

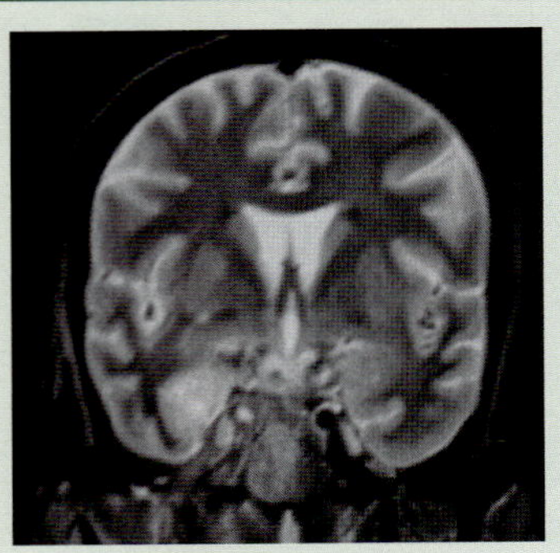 **Fig. 4.71.44:** Right sinonasal mucormycosis with right orbital, right MCA and right temporal lobe invasion	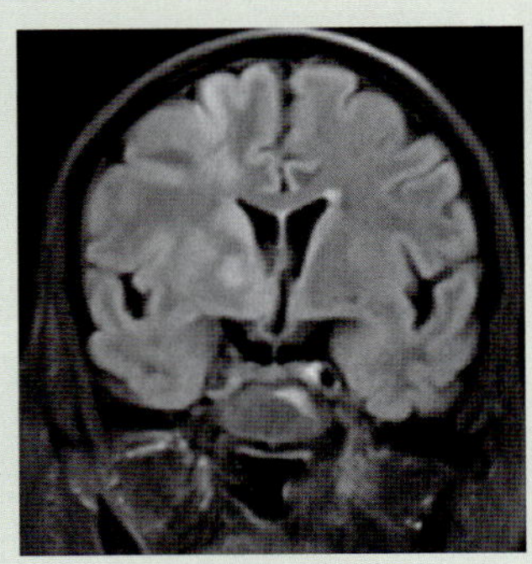 **Fig. 4.71.45:** Right sinonasal mucormycosis with right orbital, right MCA and right temporal lobe invasion	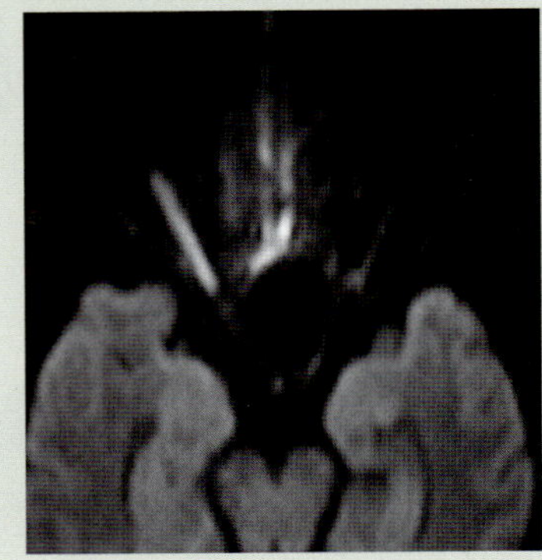 **Fig. 4.71.46:** Ischemic optic neuritis in rhino-orbital mucormycosis

Table 4.71.5: Checklist for interpretation of findings on CT/MR in acute invasive fungal rhinosinusitis/mucormycosis

Sinonasal and neck spaces	*Orbit*	*Intracranial*
Nasal cavity • Emphysematous/ulcerated mucosal thickening—especially unilateral • Nasal septum ulceration/abscess • Necrotic turbinate/black turbinate sign/lack of enhancement. **Paranasal sinuses and their drainage pathways** • Mucosal thickening—ethmoid/maxillary/sphenoid/frontal • Bony erosion **Soft tissue infiltration** • Peri-antral fat pads (anterior premaxillary and posterior retroantral) • Pterygopalatine fossa • Infratemporal fat, zygoma • Masticator space, buccal space, parapharyngeal space • Nasopharynx and prevertebral muscles **Nasolacrimal duct and nasolacrimal sac** **Hard palate, floor or maxillary sinus/alveolar process of maxilla, mandible and oral cavity** Other bone dehiscence/destruction including skull base	• Bony orbit • Preseptal oedema • Extraconal fat involvement, subperiosteal abscess • Orbital muscle cone involvement, proptosis • Intraconal fat involvement • Subperiosteal collection • Orbital apex involvement, superior and inferior orbital fissure • Globe involvement • Optic nerve involvement • Superior ophthalmic vein thrombosis	• Skull base involvement—clivus, frontal, ethmoid, sphenoid and basi occiput • Skull base foramen and perineural extension, pterygoid plates • Meningitis • Cortical edema—focal cerebritis (frontal, anteromedial temporal lobe) • Intracranial granulomas/abscess • Extra-axial/parenchymal collection • Infarct/hemorrhage • Cranial nerve/Meckel's cave involvement **Vascular complications** • Cavernous sinus thrombosis • Internal carotid artery narrowing/thrombosis/pseudoaneurysm

intracranial extension. Stage D—cervical and distant metastases.

Involvement	*Esthesioneuroblastoma*	*Sacrococcygeal teratoma*
Inner	Nasal site alone–10–33%	Intrapelvic-purely presacral–10%
Both sides	Intranasal and intracranial (dumbbell) 67–90%	Both sides (sacral bone involvement)–43%
Outer side	Purely intracranial-zero percentage	Gluteal side-exterior–47%

Rhinocerebral Orbital Mucormycosis

Uncommon acute invasive fungal infection that has increased prevalence during COVID-19 pandemic. CT helps to delineate the bone erosion. MRI findings include T1—isointense lesions relative to brain; T2—heterointense with 20% showing hyperintensity. Fungal have low signal on T2. On T1 post-contrast images, devitalised mucosa appears on contrast-enhanced MR imaging as contiguous foci of non-enhancing tissue, leading to the black turbinate sign. DWI: Increased signal intensity can be seen.

4.72 HEAD AND NECK

Case No. 72

Clinical history: 16 years old boy presented with right-sided nasal obstruction and recurrent epistasis.

Radiological imaging techniques and observation: Figure 4.72.1 is plain radiograph skull waters projection showing opacification of right nasal cavity with haziness of right maxillary and anterior ethmoid and frontal sinuses. Left maxillary, ethmoidal and frontal sinus appear normal. No evidence of lytic lesion in facial bones. No evidence of obvious fractures in visualised facial bones.

Figures 4.72.2 to 4.72.5 are plain CT PNS axial and coronal images showing a large hyperdense mass arising with epicenter from right sphenopalatine foramen extending into the posterior right nasopharynx posteriorly with osseous destruction to occupy a majority of the sphenoid sinus. There is a tiny bone defect adjacent to the mass on the superolateral margin of the right sphenoid sinus, but no indication of intracranial spread. The tumor extends into the right pterygopalatine fossa, filling it and expanding it. It spreads laterally into the masticator area through the pterygomaxillary fissure. The right orbit's medial wall is bowing, and the mass is eroding portions of the right maxillary sinus's posterior and medial walls. Left side spheno-palatine fossa, nasopharynx and nasal cavity appear normal.

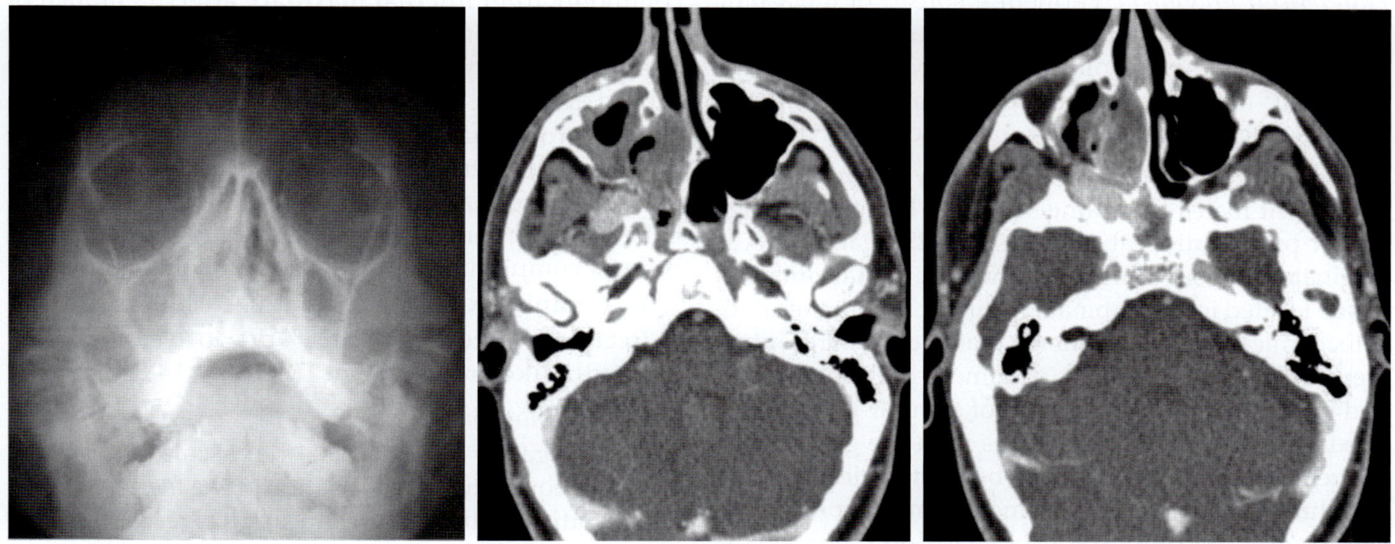

Fig. 4.72.1 Fig. 4.72.2 Fig. 4.72.3

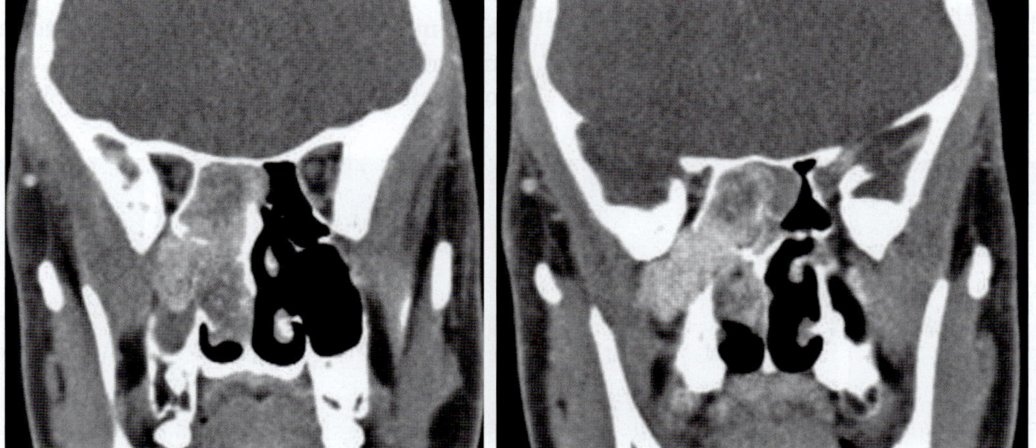

Fig. 4.72.4 Fig. 4.72.5

Figures 4.72.6 to 4.72.9 are MRI brain T1, T2 axial and T1 post-contrast coronal images showing T1 isointense/ T2 heterointense mass lesion with intense enhancement spreading from the right posterior nasopharynx to the sphenoid sinus. It widens the right pterygopalatine fossa, fills the right retroantral fat pad, and spreads laterally into the subjacent masticator area through the pterygomaxillary fissure. There is no evidence of intracranial or orbital extension.

Interpretation: A—16 years old boy, lesion in right nasopharynx, C—hypervascular mass lesion originating at sphenopalatine foramen (SPF), B—in adolescent male extending into right posterior nasopharynx, the sphenoid sinus, pterygopalatine fossa and pterygomaxillary fissure, D—JNA.

Principal diagnosis: Juvenile nasopharyngeal angiofibroma.

Differential diagnosis: Perineural spread of metastatic tumor, angiomatous polyp, sinonasal hemangioma, nasopharyngeal carcinoma, nasopharyngeal teratoma, nasopharyngeal lymphoma, esthesioneuroblastoma, sinonasal nerve sheath tumor, antrochonal polyp.

Discussion: JNA is almost exclusively encountered in adolescent males **(hormone sensitive tumor)**. Average age of presentation at 15 years (10–25 years). JNA is originate from **sex steroid–stimulated hamartomatous tissue** located in the turbinate cartilage. Recent immunocytochemical techniques shown that **androgen receptors** are present in at least 75% of tumors both in vascular and stromal elements. The rate of tumour growth and maximum development matches with the growth rate of erectile tissue in the penis, both of which grow in size throughout puberty. The most common presenting symptom is painless nasal obstruction or epistaxis; however, depending on the size and extent of the tumour mass, other symptoms may arise. These lesions are highly vascular and biopsy is contraindicated due to the risk of hemorrhage. CT or MRI have important roles in assessing the tumor mass and extension and assist with treatment planning.

Extension of JNA: Despite its benign nature, JNA is aggressive and spreads locally. The tumour grows medially from its origin to the nasopharynx, where it usually becomes symptomatic. Some tumors extend laterally to the pterygopalatine fossa and then to the infratemporal fossa as they grew larger. JNAs with extensive lateral extension in the infratemporal fossa and cheek but medial dissemination to the nasopharynx is extremely uncommon. An expanding tumour may also grow along the base of the skull posterior to the pterygoid process, potentially including the parapharyngeal region. This type of lateral growth should be diagnosed as a posterior lateral extension, as opposed to the anterior lateral extension in the pterygopalatine fossa, which is more prevalent and easier to recognise after surgery. Extra nasopharyngeal extensions of JNA include the nasal cavity, paranasal sinuses, the orbit and in advanced cases also the cranium. **Blood supply to JNA:** Most commonly from **internal maxillary artery**, a branch of external carotid artery. Other contributors are ascending pharyngeal artery, internal carotid artery and common carotid artery.

Dangerous anastomosis is between branches of the external and internal carotid artery may cause serious blindness, stroke and even death if embolization done—balloon protection of the internal carotid artery done to prevent complications during JNA embolization.

Intracranial extension seen in 10–20% of cases.

Recurrence rate as high as 50% due to overexpression of insulin like growth factor II.

Further management:

DSA: It elegantly demonstrates the vascular supply and allows preoperative embolization of the feeder vessels. **Preoperative embolization and surgical resection is the treatment of choice.** Procedure to be planned 72 hours (ideal is **24–48 hours**) before surgery in order to minimize the risk of revascularization.

Commonly used embolization materials: Particulate materials—polyvinyl alcohol (PVA), Gelfoam, Pfizer and microfibrillar collagen. Liquid embolization agents are

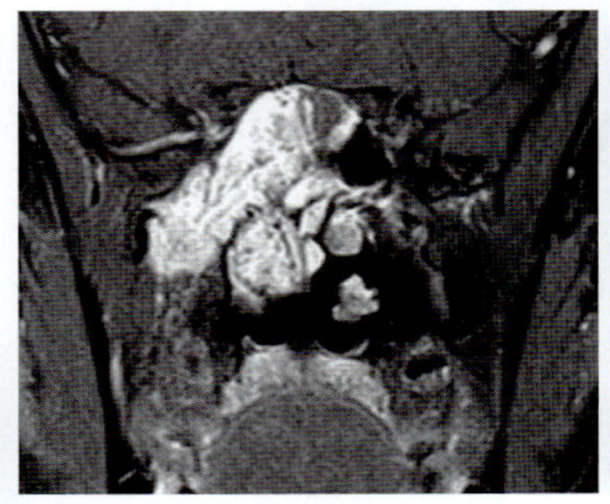
Fig. 4.72.6

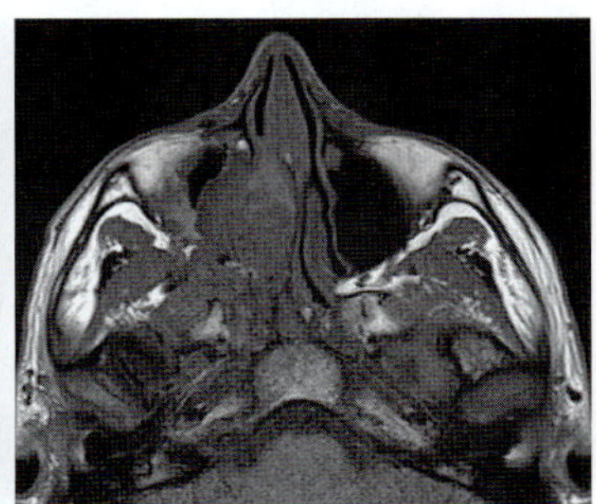
Fig. 4.72.7

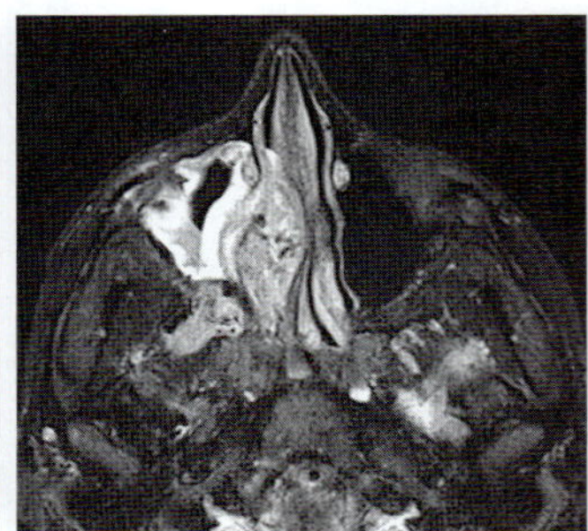
Fig. 4.72.8

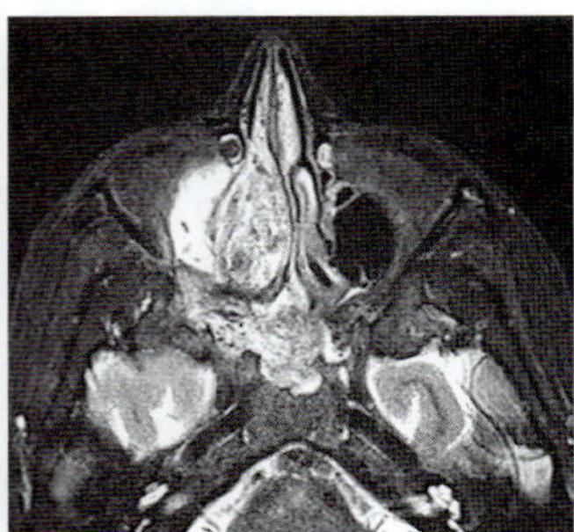
Fig. 4.72.9

onyx and ethanol. Occlusion of large vessels may require use of either pushable or detachable coils.

Left internal maxillary artery angiography showing pre- and postembolisation of JNA with non-detachable balloon and onyx cast.

Blood loss: According to Ardehali et al. the mean intraoperative blood loss in patients with embolized tumor was **770 ml** compared with **1403.6 ml** in patients with non-embolized tumors.

Procedure: A non-detachable balloon placed in the cavernous segment of the internal carotid artery protected the orbital and cerebral arteries from the potential, inadvertent migration of onyx into the cerebral arteries. Finally, the use of the dual-lumen balloon catheter enabled excellent control of bleeding during the repeated punctures of the tumor as well as very rapid and effective occlusion of the distal maxillary or sphenopalatine arteries.

The posterior wall of the maxillary sinus will show anterior bowing as observed on a lateral skull radiograph or cross-sectional imaging is known as the **Holman-Miller sign or antral sign** in juvenile nasopharyngeal angiofibroma.

Nasal cavity tumors: Nasal dermal sinus cyst/tract/fistula, anterior cephalocele, polyp, nasolabial cyst, septal abscess, septal hemangioma, septal hematoma, JNA, ABC, infantile hemangioma, nasopharyngeal carcinoma, esthesioneuroblastoma.

Table 4.72.1: Differential diagnosis for JNA		
Angiomatous polyp Nasopharyngeal polyp that becomes hyper-vascular due to repeated injury. Common presentation is nasal mass with epistaxis	Homogeneous soft tissue dense mass with avid enhancement for contrast. Does not involve SPF or PPF Less hypervascular than JAF. MRI useful assess the extension and nature of polyp.	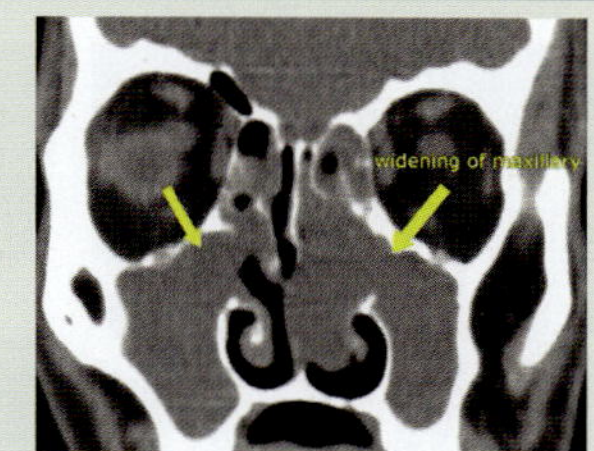 **Fig. 4.72.10:** Angiomatous polyp
Rhabdomyosarcoma Most common childhood soft tissue sarcoma 70% under 12 years, 40% under 5 years of age. Treatment: Surgical debulking, chemo-therapy ± radiation therapy	Homogeneous mass ± bone destruction. Not necessarily centered in posterolateral nasal cavity. Rarely penetrates SPF into PPF. Adjacent metastatic lymphadenopathy Frequently with calcifications	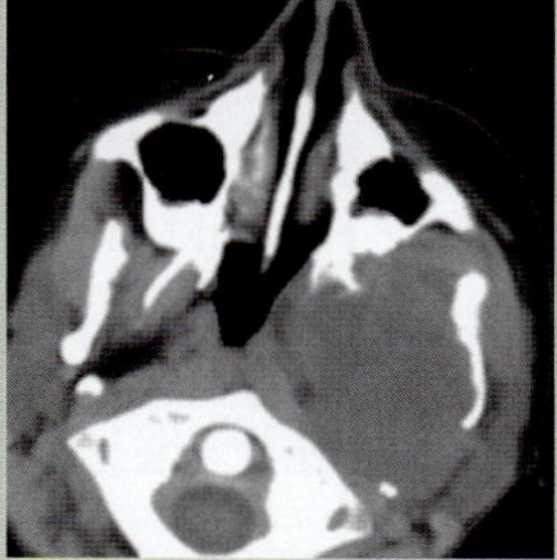 **Fig. 4.72.11:** Rhabdomyosarcoma
Nasopharyngeal carcinoma Primary mucosal malignancy arising in nasopharynx, most strongly associated with EBV infection.	Heterogeneously enhancing large mass lesion with adjacent bony remodelling and dsetruction of clivus. Metastatic nodes often large, ± necrosis. Retropharyngeal nodes often subtle on imaging, as they appear isodense to muscle.	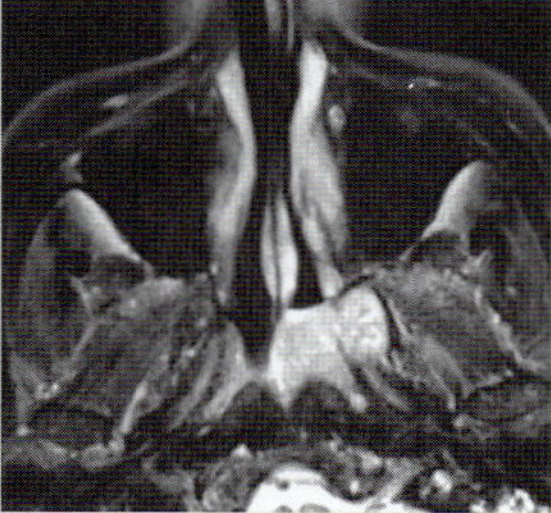 **Fig. 4.72.12:** Nasopharyngeal carcinoma
Sinonasal nerve sheath tumor: Slow-growing, benign tumors arising from nerve sheath (schwannoma) or peripheral nerve tissue (neurofibroma). Well-defined, expansile soft tissue mass arising in nasoethmoid region with adjacent bone remodeling. Schwannoma: Whorled pattern of enhancement. NECT best shows benign osseous remodeling		
Sinonasal hemangioma: Benign capillary proliferation showing distinct lobular architecture affecting skin and mucous membranes of oral cavity, nose. avidly enhancing well-defined nasal cavity mass arising from anterior septum or turbinates.		
Esthesioneuroblastoma: Refer to case 71		

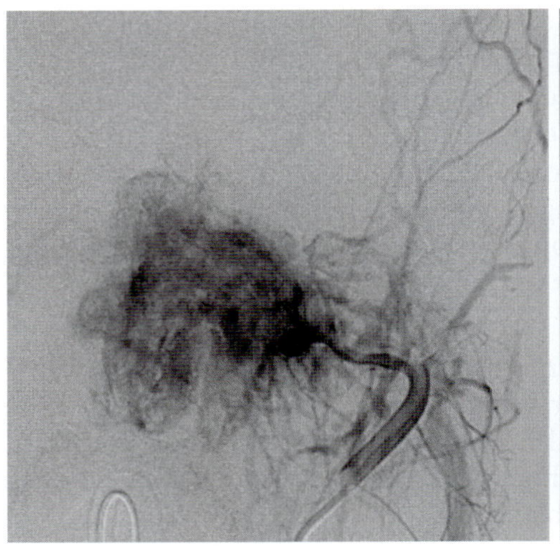

Fig. 4.72.13: Pre-embolisation selective left internal maxillary artery angiogram in JNA

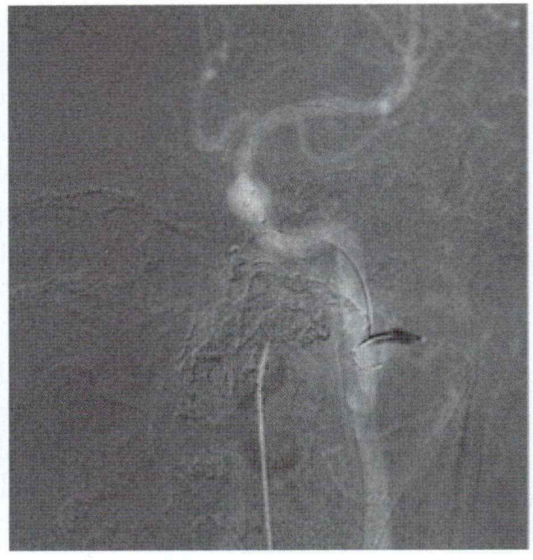

Fig. 4.72.14: DSA during injection of gel foam into left internal maxillary artery

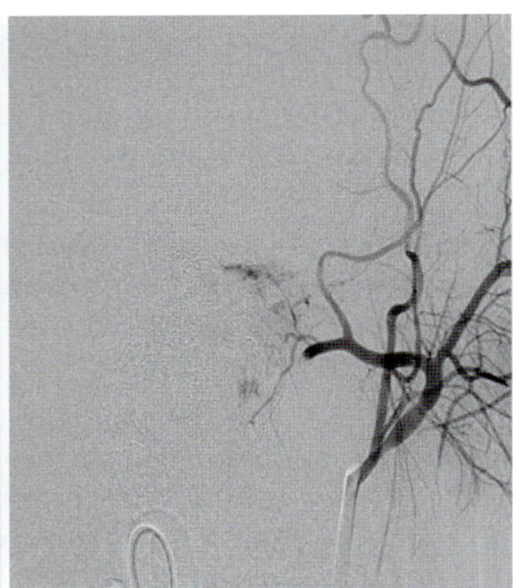

Fig. 4.72.15: Post-embolisation angiogram in JNA

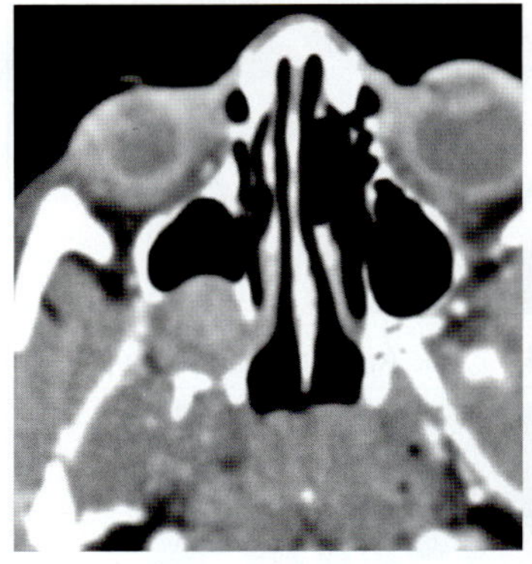

Fig. 4.72.16: Holman-Miller sign

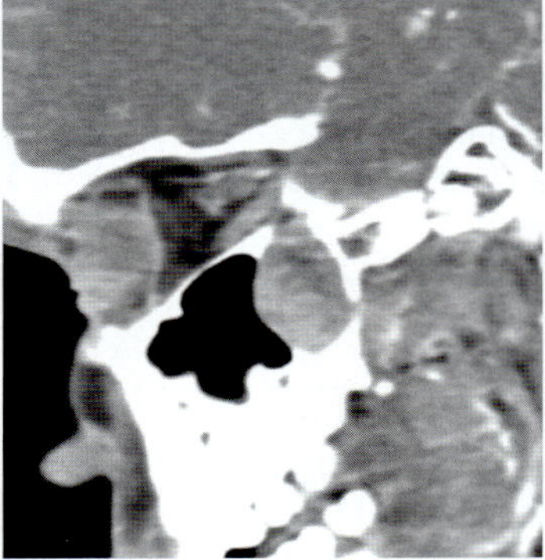

Fig. 4.72.17: Right JNA

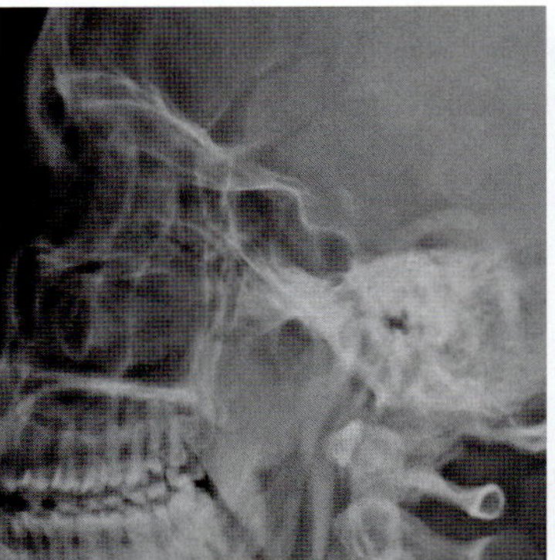

Fig. 4.72.18: Left JNA

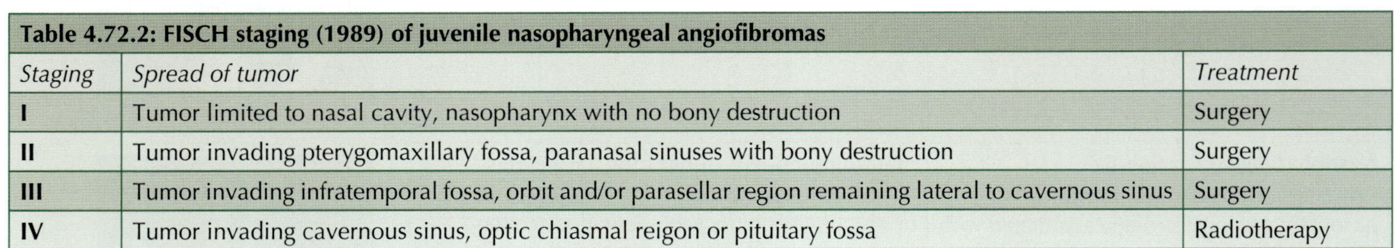

Table 4.72.2: FISCH staging (1989) of juvenile nasopharyngeal angiofibromas

Staging	*Spread of tumor*	*Treatment*
I	Tumor limited to nasal cavity, nasopharynx with no bony destruction	Surgery
II	Tumor invading pterygomaxillary fossa, paranasal sinuses with bony destruction	Surgery
III	Tumor invading infratemporal fossa, orbit and/or parasellar region remaining lateral to cavernous sinus	Surgery
IV	Tumor invading cavernous sinus, optic chiasmal reigon or pituitary fossa	Radiotherapy

4.73 HEAD AND NECK

Case No. 73

Clinical history: The 32-year-old female patient had come with the complaints of chronic headache which was insidious in onset and diffuse in nature. Patient gave history of repeated cold.

Radiological techniques and observation: Figure 4.73.1 is **X-ray PNS (Waters view)** showing enlarged right maxillary sinus with increased radio-opacity noted in the right maxillary sinus showing a **'ground-glass' appearance** and indistinct margins. 'Bubbly' appearance of right mandible. Thickened and sclerotic left temporal bone and there is suspicious thickening of the temporal bone on the right side. Visualized bilateral nasal cavity, bilateral frontal sinus, sphenoid sinus and bilateral mastoid air cells appears normal. The above findings suggest diagnosis of polyostotic craniofacial fibrous dysplasia. For further characterization CT is needed—to look for the extent of involvement/the pathological fractures/to delineate the mass effects over adjacent structures.

Figures 4.73.2 to 4.73.6 are **CT in bone window of the paranasal sinuses** showing predominantly homogeneous bony expansion with **ground-glass opacity** involving bilateral maxillary sinus, bilateral pterygoid plates, right parieto-occipital bone, bilateral greater wing of sphenoid.

Interpretation: A—32-year-old female, lesion involving bilateral maxillary sinus, bilateral pterygoid plates, right parieto-occipital bone, bilateral greater wing of sphenoid. C—showing homogeneous bony expansion, ill-defined borders with, B—ground-glass opacity and 'Bubbly' appearance of right mandible, D—polyostotic craniofacial fibrous dysplasia.

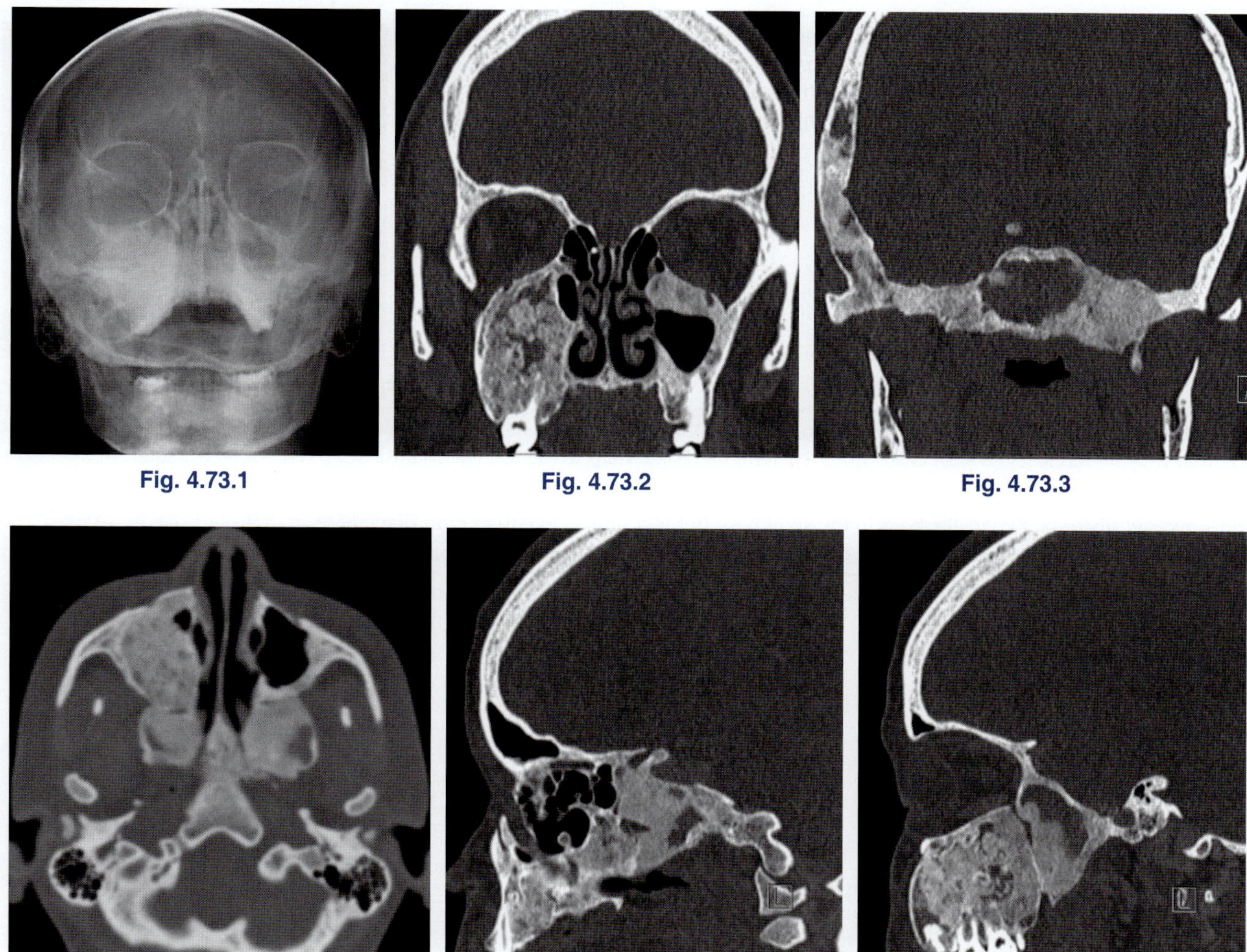

Fig. 4.73.1 Fig. 4.73.2 Fig. 4.73.3

Fig. 4.73.4 Fig. 4.73.5 Fig. 4.73.6

Table 4.73.1: Differential diagnosis for fibrous dysplasia

Cementifying fibroma/ossifying fibroma: Age: 40 years. Cemento-ossifying fibroma (COF) is rare, benign neoplasms that usually arise from mandible/maxilla. They most often arise from the tooth bearing areas of these bones.	Cemento-ossifying fibromas are usually **well-circumscribed masses** which expand the underlying bone. They are usually small but can become large. This is particularly the case when they arise from the maxilla or paranasal sinuses because there is more room to expand. They are initially lucent on X-ray with soft tissue attenuation on CT. As they **mature, they gradually develop increasing amounts of calcification/ossification.** They usually expand the bone without cortical breach	
Paget's disease: It is relatively common and can affect up to 4% of individuals over 40 and up to 11% over the age of 80. There may be a slight male predilection	Bilateral. Older patients. The degree of osseous thickening is not the same as in FD. There are three classically described stages, which are part of a continuous spectrum: **Early destructive stage** (incipient active, lytic): Predominated by osteoclastic activity; **Intermediate stage** (active, mixed); **Late stage** (inactive, sclerotic/blastic)	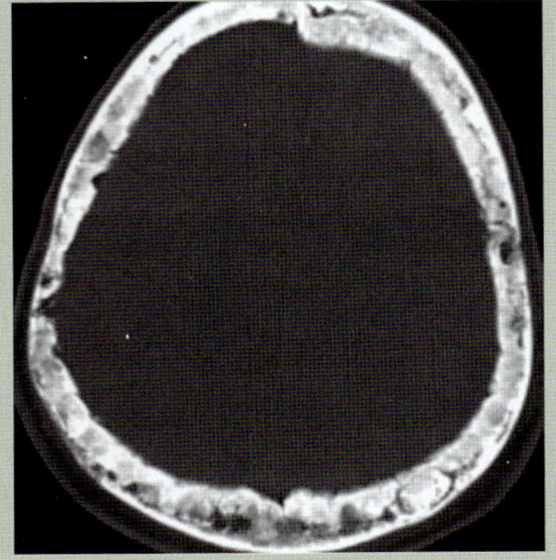 **Fig. 4.73.7:** Paget's disease
Hyperparathyroidism: Increased levels of the parathyroid hormone lead to increased osteoclastic activity. The resultant bone resorption produces cortical thinning (subperiosteal resorption) and osteopenia.	Sclerotic bone with ground-glass appearance **(salt and pepper appearance)**. Skeletal manifestations are evident symmetrically along with the systemic hypercalcaemia	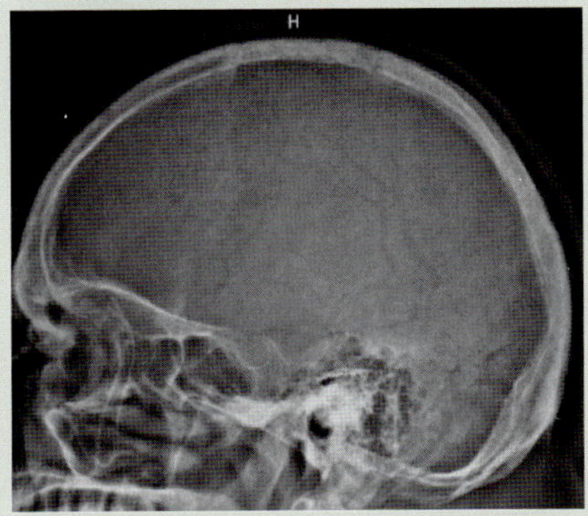 **Fig. 4.73.8:** Salt and pepper appearance
Sclerotic metastasis: Primary tumors most frequently encountered as metastases to the skull include breast cancer, lung cancer, melanoma, prostate cancer. 90% of cases other skeletal metastases are evident. Lytic metastases most common, sclerotic metastases can particularly occur from breast and prostate cancers mixed lytic and sclerotic metastases		
Chondromyxoid fibroma: Expansile mass in the skull base but less destructive than craniofacial FD. Lobulated outline with sharp margins, and has sclerotic rim and approximately 13% of tumors show some discrete areas of calcification.		
Chondrosarcoma	Bony erosion and destruction of posterior nasal septum with epicenter at the septum with ring and arc calcification	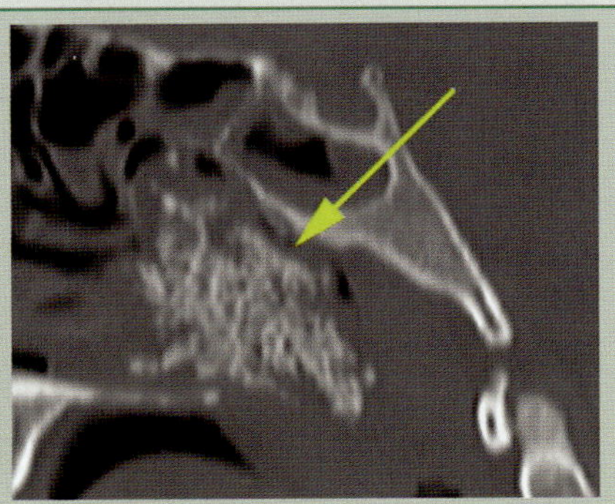 **Fig. 4.73.9:** Chondrosarcoma

(Contd.)

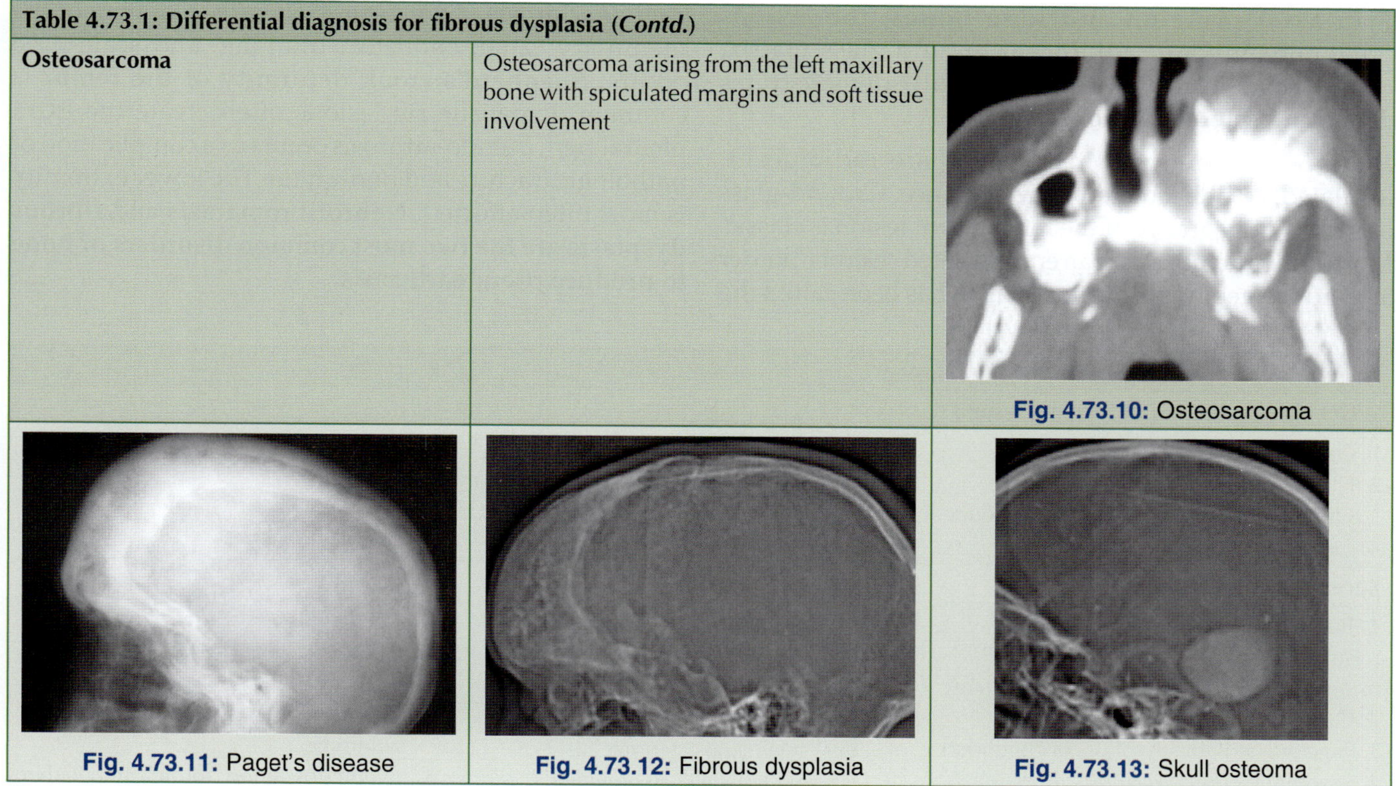

Table 4.73.1: Differential diagnosis for fibrous dysplasia (*Contd.*)		
Osteosarcoma	Osteosarcoma arising from the left maxillary bone with spiculated margins and soft tissue involvement	**Fig. 4.73.10:** Osteosarcoma
Fig. 4.73.11: Paget's disease	**Fig. 4.73.12:** Fibrous dysplasia	**Fig. 4.73.13:** Skull osteoma

Principal diagnosis: Polyostotic craniofacial fibrous dysplasia.

Further management: Usually, no treatment is required, if a mass effect is severe, then surgical decompression may be considered.

Complications: Pathological fractures, Sarcomatous dedifferentiation (osteosarcoma [most common], fibrosarcoma, malignant fibrous histiocytoma, or rarely chondrosarcoma) is occasionally seen (<1%).

Discussion—fibrous dysplasia: Age of presentation varies from **8 to 14 years**. An even sex distribution, except for the associated McCune-Albright syndrome, which is almost exclusively found in females. Most lesions are asymptomatic. Bowing deformities and pathologic fracture are the most common causes of symptoms (i.e. **shepherd's crook deformity**). **Café-au-lait spots**—chestnut-pigmented, non-elevated macules, present in 30% of patients with polyostotic fibrous dysplasia. The serrated irregular margins have been referred to as **the coast of Maine appearance**. Also found in neurofibromatosis, but these margins are smooth and are referred to as the coast of California appearance.

Types: **Monostotic fibrous dysplasia** (solitary lesion) is most commonly found in the ribs, femur (proximal), tibia (anterior cortex), and skull (75% of cases).

Polyostotic fibrous dysplasia (multiple bones) is most commonly found in the femur, skull, tibia, humerus, ribs, fibula, radius, and ulna. Vertebral involvement is rare; when present, it affects the vertebral body rather than the arch and is found usually in the polyostotic form of the disease. **McCune-Albright syndrome** represents polyostotic fibrous dysplasia associated with **skin pigmentation and precocious sexual development. Mazabraud syndrome:** Polyostotic fibrous dysplasia with soft-tissue myxomas (rare); **Cherubism** represents a familial fibrous dysplasia of the jaws.

Pathology: Represents an abnormality in which normal bone undergoes physiologic resorption and replacement with abnormal proliferation of fibrous tissue. The fibrous lesion often creates widening of the medullary canal, thinning of the cortex, and endosteal scalloping; scalloping of the endosteum is a sign seen in lesions of fibrous and cartilaginous matrix. The fundamental lesion of fibrous dysplasia is that of a fibrous-based matrix with scattered bony spicules intermixed. This renders an increase in radiopacity to the existing radiolucent lesion and has been called the **ground-glass appearance**. Sarcomatous transformation is rare (0.5%). The femur and skull are the target sites, with **fibrosarcoma and osteosarcoma** being the most common complicating tumor types.

Three patterns of fibrous dysplasia: Lytic, sclerotic and mixed type.

In **axial skeleton and long bones,** the lesions predominantly are **radiolucent ground-glass matrix, craniofacial fibrous dysplasia (skull)** demonstrates **dense and sclerotic lesions.**

Radiologic features: Most lesions are radiolucent, loculated, or trabeculated in appearance. Ground-glass or smoky appearance of the radiolucent lesion is classic. Most lesions demonstrate an encapsulated sclerotic border around the geographic lesion, which has been called **the rind of sclerosis.** Bone expansion with widening of the medullary canal, endosteal thinning, and scalloping occurs. **Shepherd's crook deformity of the femur** is common. Expansile rib lesions often create the extra pleural sign. Pseudo-arthrosis occurs as a complication of pathologic fracture and non-union. The lower extremity is most often affected. **Neurofibromatosis and fibrous dysplasia are the two most common disorders of bone to produce pseudoarthrosis.**

Table 4.73.2: Classification of fibrosseous lesions

WHO classification of fibrosseous lesions		
1. Ossifying fibroma 2. Fibrous dysplasia 3. Osseous dysplasia—periapical/florid/focal 4. Cental giant cell granuloma	5. Cherubism 6. Aneurysmal bone cyst 7. Solitary bone cyst	
Recent (Eversole classification 2008)		
1. Bone dysplasia I. Fibrous dysplasia: A. Monostotic, B. Polyostotic, C. Polyostotic with endocrinopathy 2. Osteitis deformans 3. Pagetoid heritable dysplasia of childhood 4. Segemntal odontomaxillary dysplasia	**2. Cemento-osseous dysplasia** 1. Focal 2. Florid **3. Inflammatory** 1. Focal sclerosing osteomyelitis 2. Diffuse sclerosing osteomyelitis 3. Proliferative periostitis	**4. Metabolic:** Hyperparathyroidism **5. Neoplastic** 1. Ossifying fibroma 2. Hyperparathyroidism jaw lesion syndrome 3. Juvenile ossifying fibroma trabecular/psammomatoid types 4. Gigantiform cementoma

Table 4.73.3: Difference between ossifying fibroma and fibrous dysplasia

Characteristics	*Ossifying fibroma*	*Fibrous dysplasia*
Disease	Neoplasm	Bone disease
Type	Normal and juvenile type	Monostotic and polyostotic type
Matrix	Vascular matrix	Cellular/fibrous matrix
Bone	Single	Multiple, adjacent bone
Hormone relation	Hormone related	Not
Age	40 years (juvenile 10 years)	10 years
Margin	Well-defined margin	Blended margins
Serum ALP	Normal	Mildly raised
Treatment	Local excision	Recontour
Images	**Fig. 4.73.14:** Ossifying fibroma	**Fig. 4.73.15:** Fibrous dysplasia

4.74 HEAD AND NECK

Case No. 74

Clinical history: 47-year-old male presented with complaints of painless swelling in left cheek for 2 years.

Radiological technique and observation: MRI neck—T1WI, T2 fat sat axial and coronal, DWI section (Figs 4.74.1 to 4.74.4) shows a well-defined mass involving right parotid gland which appears hypointense on T1 and slightly hyperintense on T2 and bright on diffusion. No evidence of cervical lymph node enlargement seen. No evidence of nerve/vessel involvement. Visualized pharynx and rest of other organs appear normal.

Interpretations: A—47 years old male, right parotid gland, Lesion that is T1 hypo/T2 hyperintense and diffusion bright, B—no evidence of perineural extension, C—pleomorphic adenoma of right parotid gland.

Principal diagnosis: Pleomorphic adenoma of right parotid gland.

Differential diagnosis of mass lesion of parotid: Warthin tumor, mucoepidermoid carcinoma, adenoid cystic carcinoma, parotid nodal metastasis, parotid non-Hodgkin lymphoma.

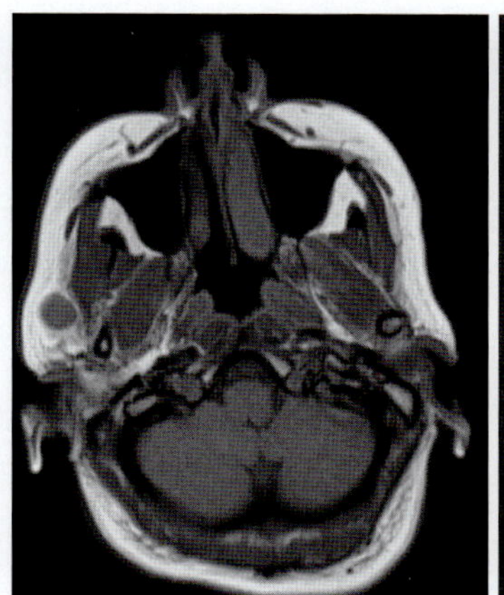

Fig. 4.74.1

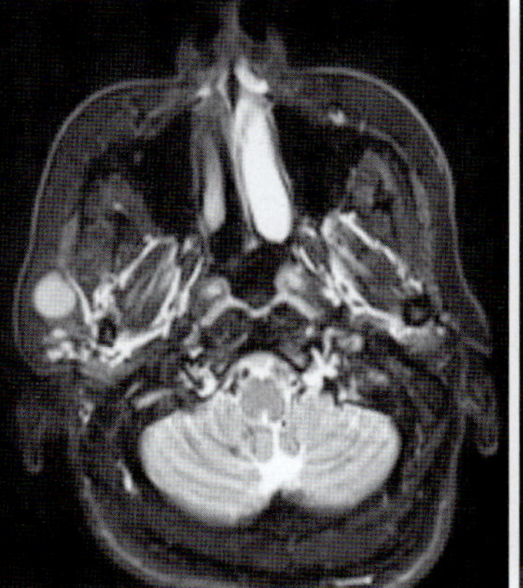

Fig. 4.74.2

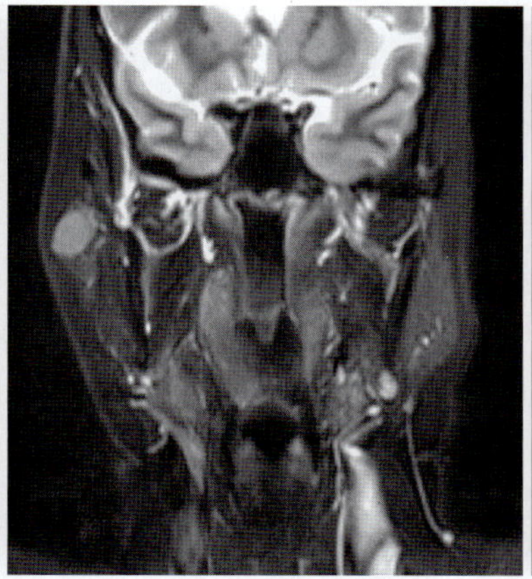

Fig. 4.74.3

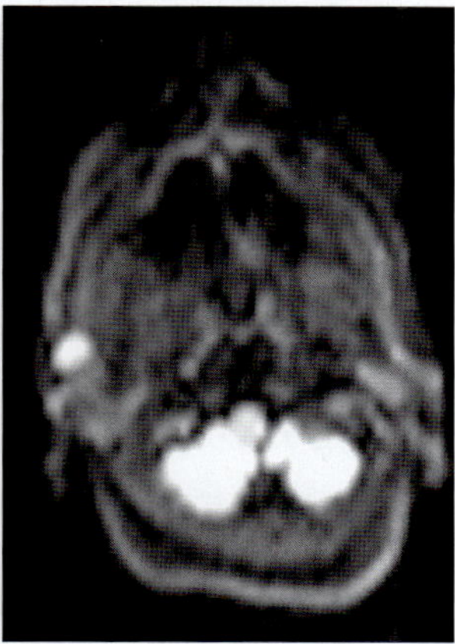

Fig. 4.74.4

Table 4.74.1: Differential diagnosis of mass lesion of parotid

Condition	*Radiological feature*	*Image*
Warthin tumor: (Lymphomatous papillary cystadenomas) 2nd most common benign parotid tumor. Bilateral in 10%, 5th–6th decade, M > F, associated with smoking and irradiation.	Classic appearance is a well-defined heterogeneous **solid cystic lesion** within the superficial lobe of parotid/**parotid tail**. Cyst containing cholesterol components appears T1 bright. No calcification, usually moderate contrast enhancement, **presence of mural nodule is strongly suggestive of Warthin tumor,** can be often seen bilaterally. Increased uptake in Tc99.	
Mucoepidermoid carcinoma Most prevalent malignant salivary gland tumor in pediatric group. Low-grade cancers resemble benign mixed tumors in appearance. To check for perineural spread, fat saturated post-contrast T1 sequences must be used to evaluate the cranial nerves.	Low-grade tumors present as well-circumscribed masses with cystic components in the majority of cases. The solid components enhance, and calcification is sometimes seen. The margins of high-grade tumours are poorly defined, they infiltrate locally, and they appear solid. On T1, the tumor appears hypointense; on T2, it is hyper-intense.	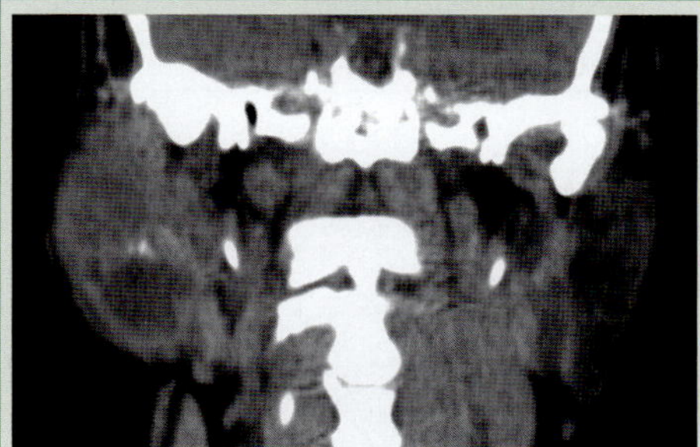 Fig. 4.74.5: Mucoepidermoid carcinoma

(Contd.)

Table 4.74.1: Differntial diagnosis of mass lesion of parotid (*Contd.*)

Condition	*Radiological feature*	*Image*
Adenoid cystic carcinoma (ACC) (Cylindroma): Locally aggressive with a tendency for perineural spread. Arise typically in the minor salivary glands. Perineural spread (through cranial nerve VII) is typically seen in adenoid cystic carcinomas, which can be shown on MRI. Lung, cervical lymph node, bone, liver, and brain metastasis	Low-grade tumors tend to be well-defined, in contradistinction to high-grade tumors, which appear infiltrative. However, both subtypes are usually homogeneously enhancing after contrast administration. T1: Hypo- to isointense T2: Slightly hyperintense, with higher grades being much more so. T1C+: Homogeneous enhancement	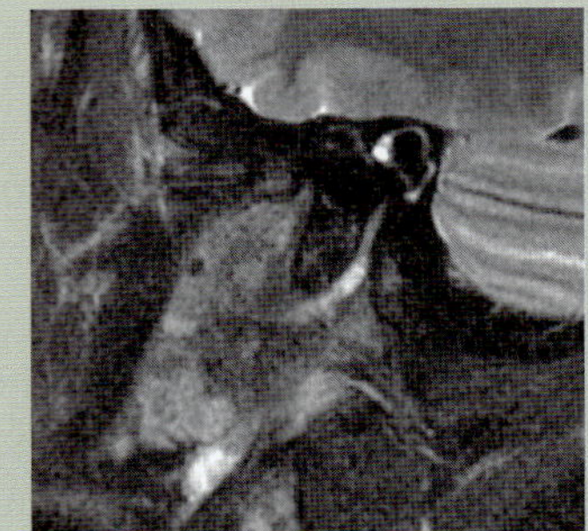 **Fig. 4.74.6:** Perineural spread (via cranial nerve VII)

Right maxillary sinus carcinoma with perineural spread involving pterygomaxillary fissure, sphenopalatine foramen, inferior orbital fissure, extending up to cavernous sinus

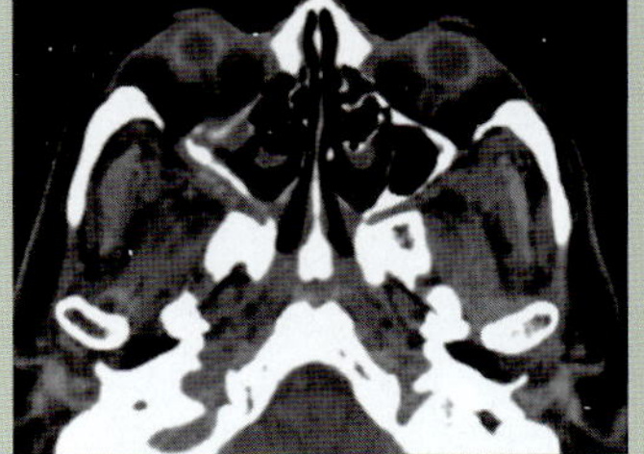 **Fig. 4.74.7:** Right maxillary sinus carcinoma	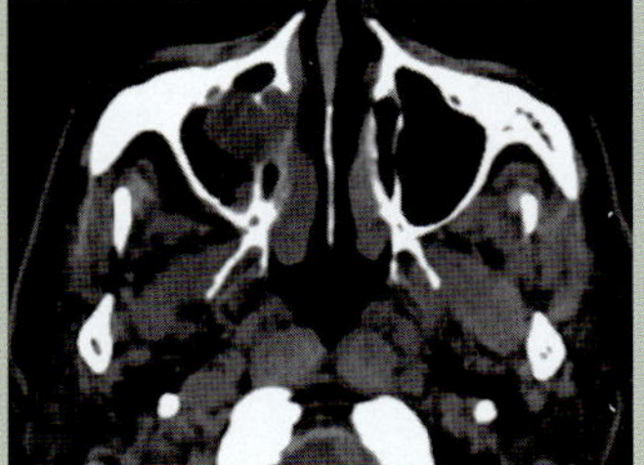 **Fig. 4.74.8:** Right maxillary sinus carcinoma	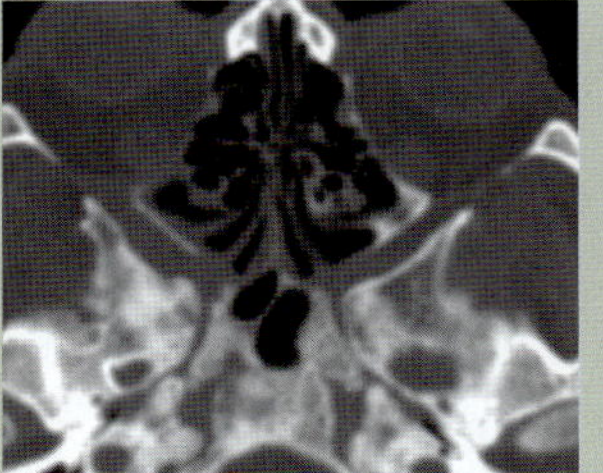 **Fig. 4.74.9:** Right maxillary sinus carcinoma	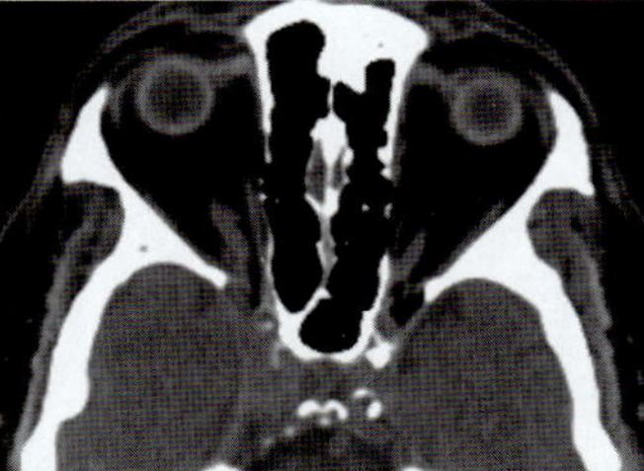 **Fig. 4.74.10:** Right maxillary sinus carcinoma

Perineural invasion of squamous cell carcinoma along auriculotemporal nerve and left infraorbital nerves

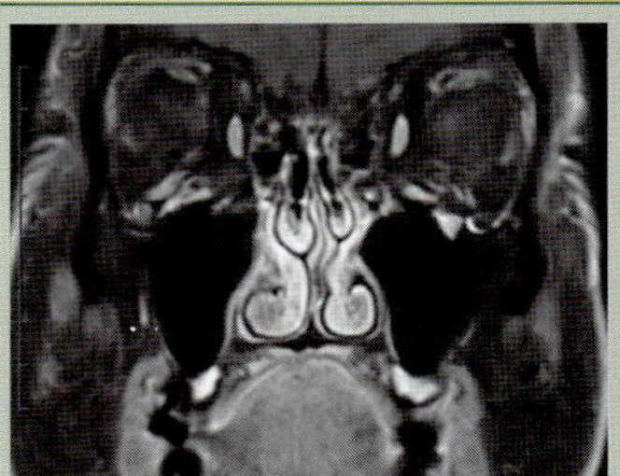 **Fig. 4.74.11:** Perineural invasion of squamous cell carcinoma along left infraorbital nerve	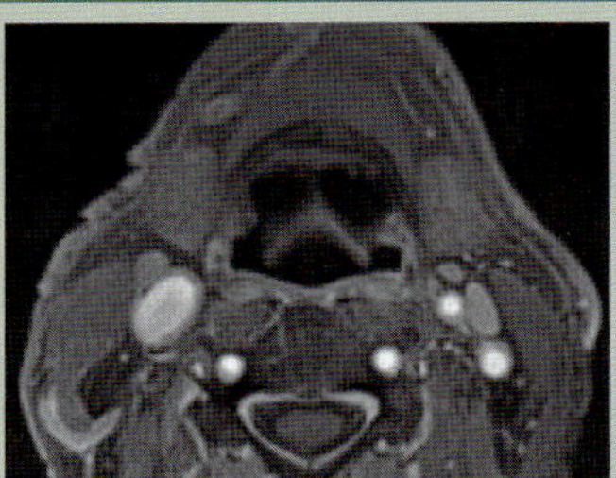 **Fig. 4.74.12:** Perineural invasion of squamous cell carcinoma along auriculotemporal nerve	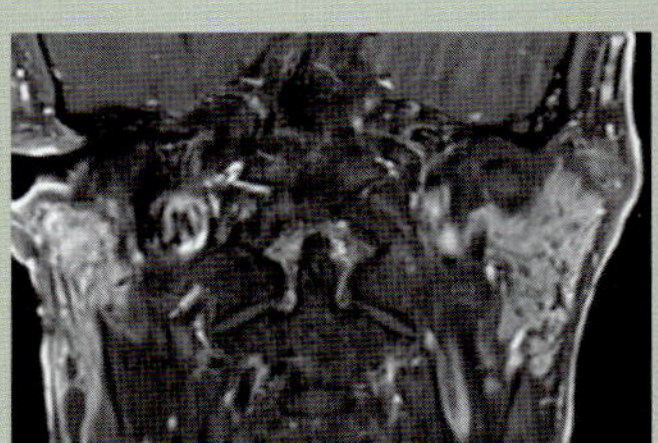 **Fig. 4.74.13:** Perineural invasion of squamous cell carcinoma along auriculotemporal nerve	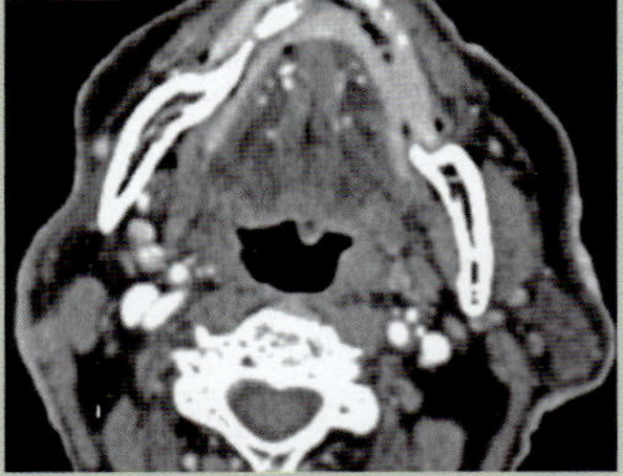 **Fig. 4.74.14:** Perineural invasion of squamous cell carcinoma along auriculotemporal nerve

Pleomorphic adenoma

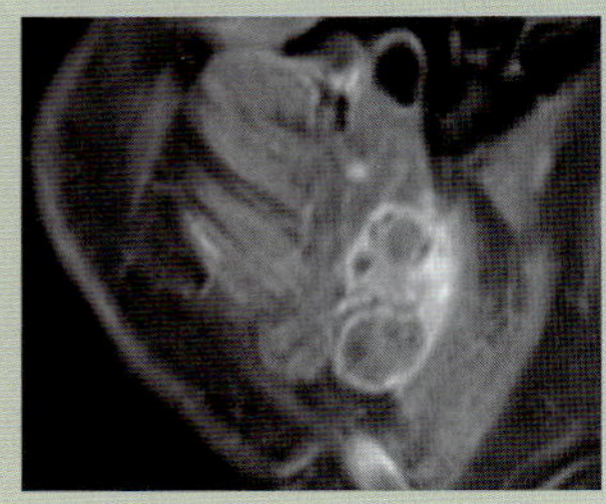 **Fig. 4.74.15:** Pleomorphic adenoma	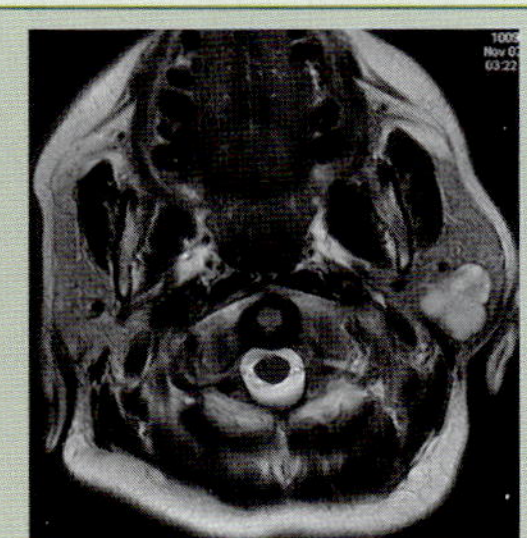 **Fig. 4.74.16:** Left parotid gland pleomorphic adenoma	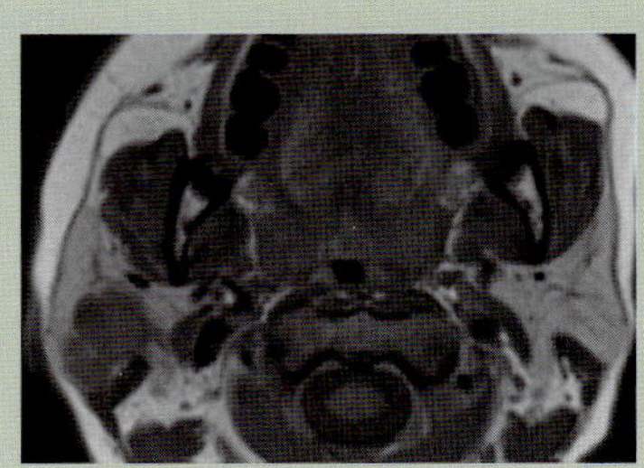 **Fig. 4.74.17:** Pleomorphic adenoma

(Contd.)

Table 4.74.1: Differential diagnosis of mass lesion of parotid (*Contd.*)

Condition	*Radiological feature*	*Image*	
Pleomorphic adenocystic carcinoma			
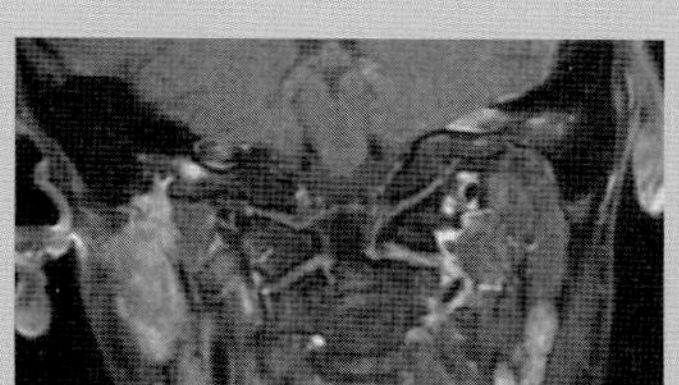 Fig. 4.74.18: Adenoid cystic carcinoma	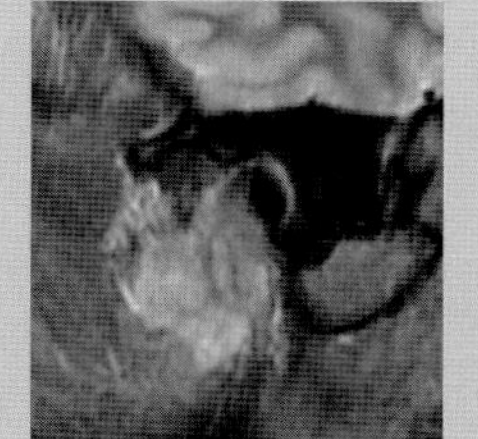 Fig. 4.74.19: Adenoid cystic carcinoma	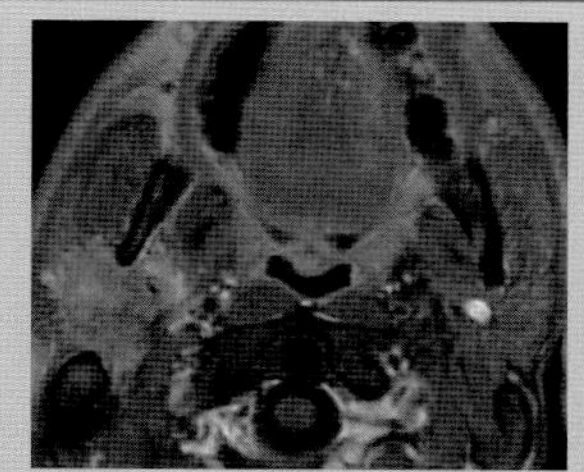 Fig. 4.74.20: Adenoid cystic carcinoma	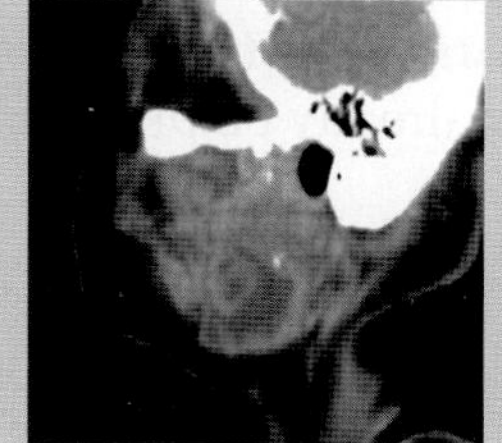 Fig. 4.74.21: Mucoepidermoid carcinoma
Parotid cyst			
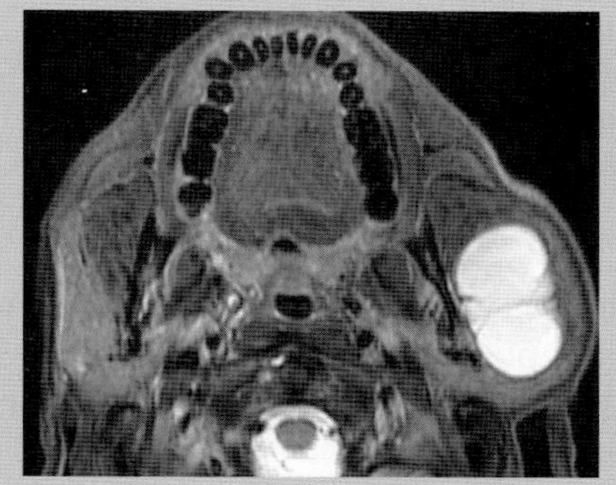 Fig. 4.74.22: Parotid cyst	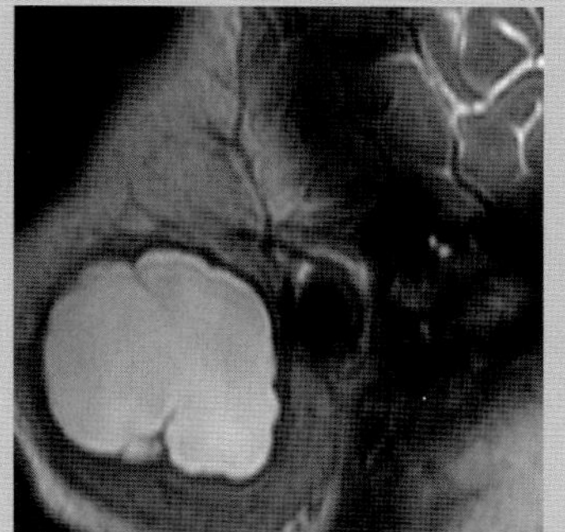 Fig. 4.74.23: Parotid cyst	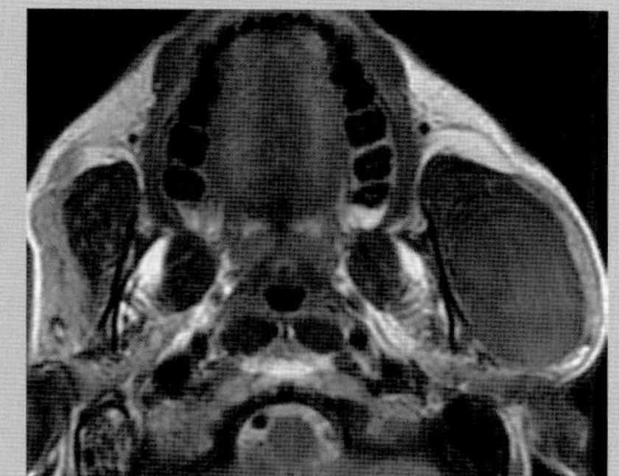 Fig. 4.74.24: Parotid cyst	
Parotiditis			
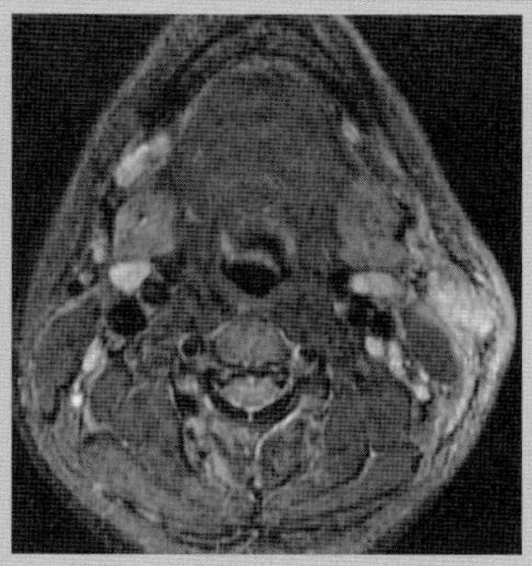 Fig. 4.74.25: Parotitis	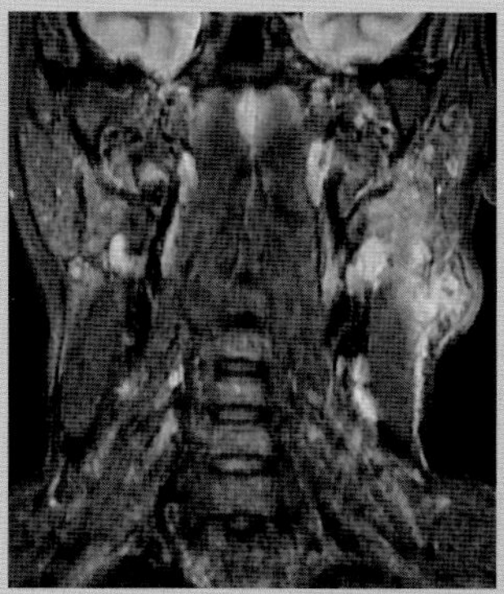 Fig. 4.74.26: Parotitis	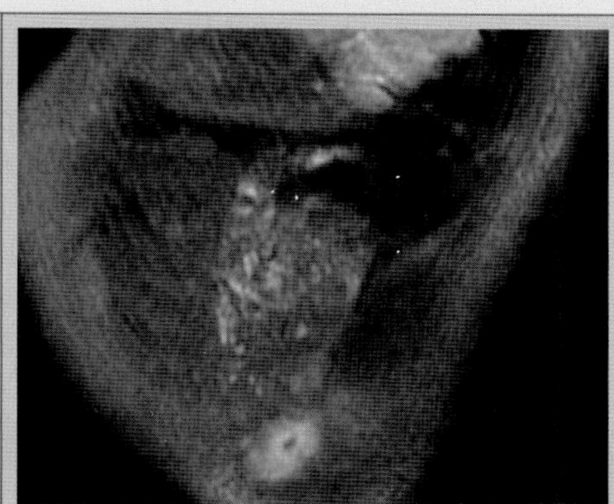 Fig. 4.74.27: Parotitis	
Lymphangioma			
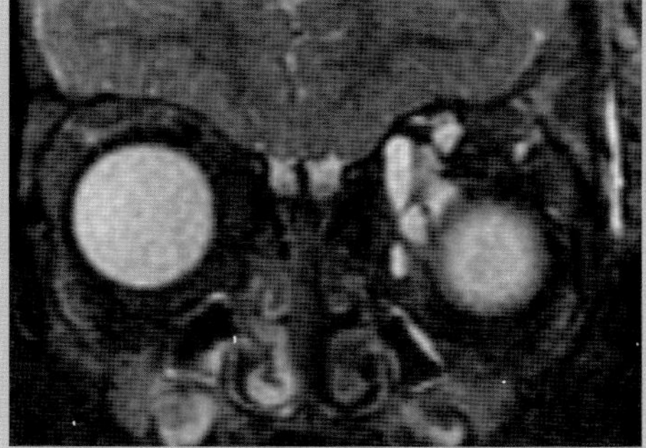 Fig. 4.74.28: Lymphangioma	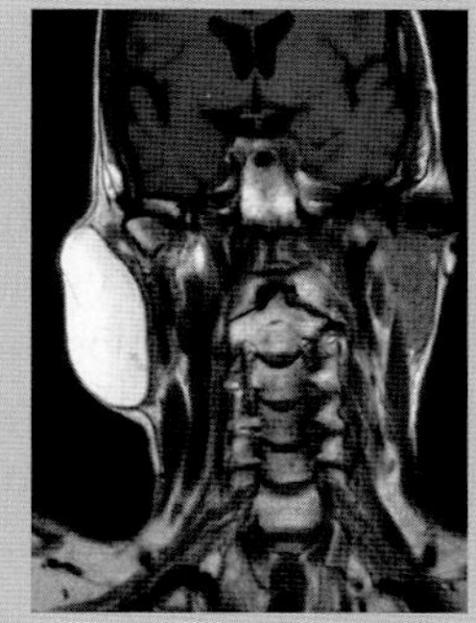 Fig. 4.74.29: Lymphangioma	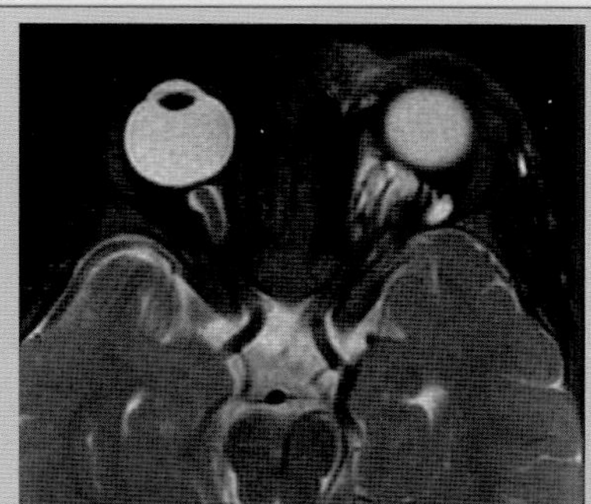 Fig. 4.74.30: Lymphangioma	

Parotid nodal metastasis: Intra-parotid nodes may be site of systemic nodal metastasis.

Known **primary periauricular skin malignancy,** single or multiple nodes seen.

Parotid non-Hodgkin lymphoma: Chronic systemic NHL may already be present.

Solitary, multiple or bilateral solid masses of parotid gland.

Further investigation and management: Next line of investigation will be USG and confirmation of diagnosis by USG guided FNAC/biopsy followed by surgical excision.

Parotid gland tumors				
Benign tumors		*Malignant tumors*	*Cystic parotid lesions*	
Epithelial	*Non-epithelial*		*Unilateral*	*Bilateral*
Pleomorphic adenoma Warthin's tumor Oncocytoma Myoepithelioma Intraductal papilloma	Hemangioma Lipoma Lymphangioma	Mucoepidermoid carcinoma Adenoid cystic carcinoma Squamous cell carcinoma Adenocarcinoma Lymphoma Malignant mixed carcinoma	Warthin tumor Sialocele First branchial cleft cyst Parotid lymphangioma Benign lymphoepithelial cyst Necrotic lymph node (squamous cell carcinoma) Infected lymph node(s)	Warthin tumor Benign lymphoepithelial Lesions of HIV Sjögren syndrome Sialocele

Hypoechoic lesion with post-acoustic enhancement: Pleomorphic adenoma, fibroadenoma—breast and lymphoma.

Hyperechoic lesion with post-acoustic enhancement: Hemangioma.

Pleomorphic adenomas of the salivary glands/benign mixed tumors: The most frequent salivary gland tumors are pleomorphic adenomas, which are also known as benign mixed tumors. A smooth, painless, growing lump is the most common symptom. These tumors often present as spherical masses with well-defined "bosselated" or "poly lobulated" boundaries on all modalities (many small undulations, not truly lobulated). The parotid gland—superficial lobe is where they are most usually found. Ultrasound reveals posterior enhancement and is hypoechoic.

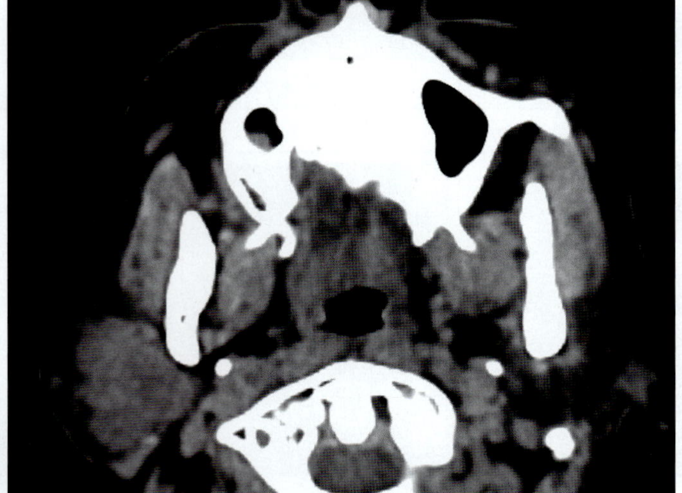

Fig. 4.74.31: Pleomorphic adenomas of the salivary glands

Homogeneous attenuation and significant enhancement on computed tomography.

T1 shows usually low intensity, T2 shows are typically very high intensity (particularly myxoid type), and T2-W features a ring of decreasing signal intensity depicting the surrounding fibrous capsule. T1 C+ (Gd): shows homogeneous enhancement.

Core biopsy: It is more invasive and requires added care in procedural planning to avoid threatening the **facial nerve**. Core biopsy may be considered when FNA has been non-diagnostic, a lymphoproliferative lesion is suspected or where tumor classification and grading will influence management.

Perineural pathway of tumor spread

Facial nerve: Look for evidence of abnormal thickening or enhancement of facial nerve or effacement of perineural fat in the stylomastoid notch.

Auriculotemporal nerve: Provides a route of communication between CNVII and CNV3. The auriculotemporal nerve travels posteroinferiorly from its origin below foramen ovale via the medial aspect of the lateral pterygoid muscle. It penetrates the parotid capsule and wraps around the posterior border of the mandible just above the ECA terminal bifurcation. Within the parotid it communicates with CNVII and ramifies extensively.

Treatment: Complete surgical resection of encapsulated mass within adequate margin of surrounding parotid gland tissue to avoid cellular spilling and seedling.

Table 4.74.2: Diagnostic pearls of pleomorphic adenoma
Most common salivary gland tumor, hypoechoic lesion with posterior acoustic enhancement, single lesion, no perineural spread
Rule of 80% for benign salivary lesions: 80% of salivary gland masses are benign, 80% are found within the parotid gland, 80% lie within the superficial lobe, 80% are pleomorphic adenomas

Perineural spread in head and neck tumors: **Direct imaging features:**

Post-contrast nerve full enhancement: Infiltration of carcinomatous cells into the nerve enables accumulation of contrast agent in entire circumference of affected nerve.

Symmetrical peripheral nerve enhancement could be seen at foraminal segments of trigeminal branches and semilunar ganglion because of perineural venous plexus and is considered as normal finding.

Nerve enlargement

Foraminal fat planes obliterations: Thickened nerve supersedes surrounding fat, best seen at extracranial foraminal openings, pterygopalatine fossa and superior orbital fissure.

Foraminal enlargement or destruction can developed secondary due to increasing pressure of advanced nerve enlargement.

Intracranial spread is detected after further centripetal spread through the nerves´ foramina in skull base: Cavernous sinus enlargement, bulging of its lateral wall and enhancement of trigeminal ganglion or cisternal nerve segments can be seen. Adjacent dura could be thickened.

Indirect imaging feature: Denervation atrophy is most commonly seen in masticatory or ipsilateral tongue muscles when motoric branch of V3 and hypoglossal nerve are affected, respectively. Facial muscle atrophy is rarely seen. In acute or subacute phase muscle oedema develops, with typical hyperintense signal on T2 weighted MR images and increased contrast enhancement. After four weeks, in chronic phase, muscle atrophy with fatty infiltration takes place. Hyperintense signal on T1 and T2—weighted sequences are seen.

Denervation atrophy must be distinguished from direct tumor infiltration of muscles, where muscle volume is usually increased. Signal changes are also less generalized and less intense than in denervation atrophy. Hypoglossal denervation causes ipsilateral tongue muscles atrophy, which results in tongue displacement more posteriorly. This may simulate tongue enlargement on axial images.

Table 4.74.3: Early detected signs of perineural spread in head and neck tumor

Fat pad or muscle sign/cranial nerves involved	
Anterior fat pad to the superior orbital rim	V1
Fat superior to the levator palpebrae muscle	V1
Preantral and post-antral fat pads	V2
Fat in pterygopalatine fossa	V2
Fat pad anterior to the mental foramen	V3
Mandibular bone marrow fat—after red bone marrow has changed to fatty bone marrow in older adults	V3
Fat pad at mandibular foramen	V3
Muscle of mastication	V3
Fat pad at stylomastoid foramen	VII

Perineural tumor (PNT) spread and their pathway

Tumors with perineural spread: 1. Adenoid cystic carcinoma, 2. Squamous cell carcinoma (skin, palate, nasopharynx and oral cavity), 3. Mucoepidermoid carcinoma, 4. Melanoma, 5. Lymphoma.

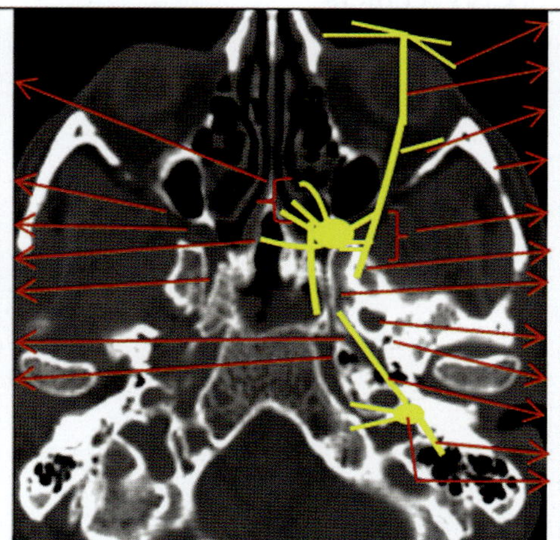

Fig. 4.74.32: Routes of perineural spread in malignancy in pterygopalatine fossa

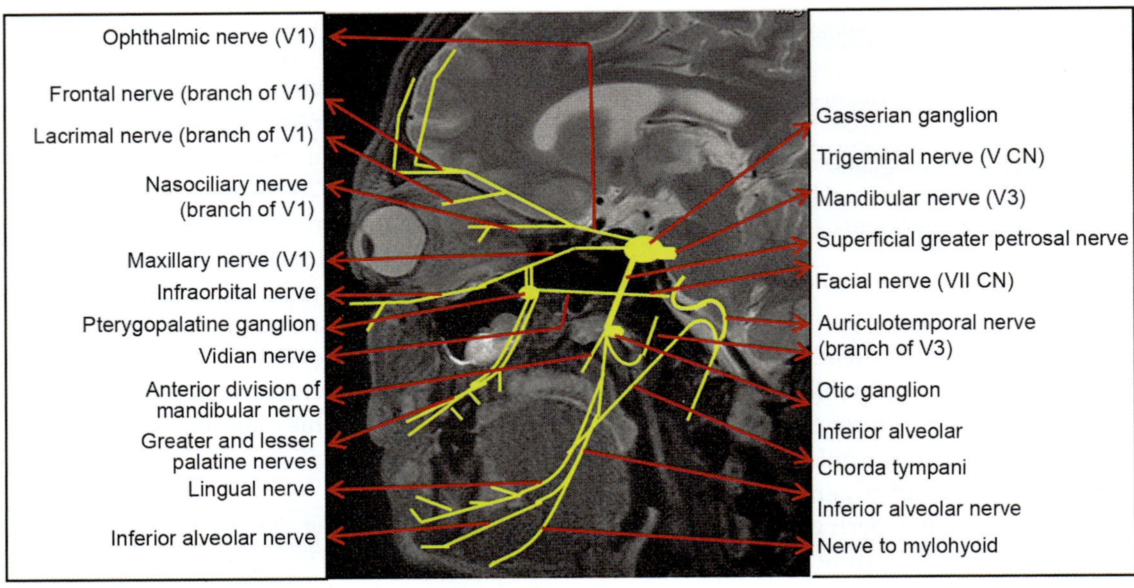

Fig. 4.74.33: Perineural spread pathways available for oral carcinoma and salivary gland tumors

Adenoid cystic carcinoma has highest propensity for perineural tumor spread. **Squamous cell carcinoma** is the most common source since it is the most common head and neck tumor. **PNT spread is a poor prognostic sign** indicating increased incidence of local recurrence. Presence of PNT may preclude primary surgical therapy.

Most common pathways of perineural tumor spread (Figs 4.74 32 and 4.74.33) **include:**

CN V2: Maxillary division → PPF: (1) Infraorbital nerve: Cheek or maxillary sinus tumors; (2) Greater and lesser palatine nerves: Minor salivary gland tumors.

CN V3: Mandibular division → foramen ovale → Meckel cave.

Mental nerve: Lip or cutaneous SCC. Inferior alveolar nerve: Mucosal oral cavity SCC.

Auriculotemporal nerve (ATN) branch of CNV3: Enters parotid, and its anterior and posterior communicating rami interface with CNVII. Mandibular main trunk: Masticator space 1 or 2 malignancy.

CN V1: Ophthalmic division → cavernous sinus: Rare; most often forehead SCC, melanoma

CNVII: Facial nerve: Intraparotid branches → intratemporal CNVII → internal auditory canal

Greater superficial petrosal nerve (GSPN): From geniculate ganglion, joins deep petrosal nerve at foramen lacerum → vidian nerve → PPF

Direct through sphenopalatine foramen → PPF: Nasopharynx cancer, nasal malignancies

From PPF, tumor may access multiple sites

1. Through inferior orbital fissure to orbital apex
2. Along vidian canal to CNVII geniculate ganglion
3. Foramen rotundum → cavernous sinus or to Meckel cave.

4.75 HEAD AND NECK

Case No. 75

Clinical history: A 58-year-old female patient came with swelling in left side of neck for 3 years, which gradually progressed to present size. No H/o trauma/pain.

Radiological technique and observations: Figures 4.75.1 and 4.75.2 are CT, coronal sections and axial sections of neck showing a large homogeneous soft tissue density dense lesion (similar to muscle) noted involving the left para-pharyngeal space. The para-pharyngeal fat pad is displaced antero-medially by the lesion. No cystic component, calcification, necrosis and hemorrhage noted within the lesion. No evidence of adjacent bone destruction.

Figures 4.75.3 to 4.75.5 are plain contrast enhanced CT, axial sections and reformatted coronal sections of neck, volume rendered images respectively. A multilobulated, ovoid, heterogeneous intensely enhancing soft tissue density mass involving the left carotid space. The lesion causes splaying of left internal and external carotid artery giving the appearance of classical **"Lyre sign"**. Anterior displacement of para-pharyngeal fat and medial displacement of the left pharyngeal wall show the location of lesion. No evidence of lesion in the contralateral side. No evidence of lymphadenopathy. Visualized lung sections appear normal.

Interpretation: A—58-year-old female patient, multilobulated, ovoid, heterogeneous intensely enhancing soft tissue density mass involving the left carotid space, B—splaying of left internal and external carotid artery giving the appearance of classical **"Lyre sign"**, C—carotid body tumor (carotid body chemodectoma).

Principal diagnosis: Carotid body tumor (carotid body chemodectoma).

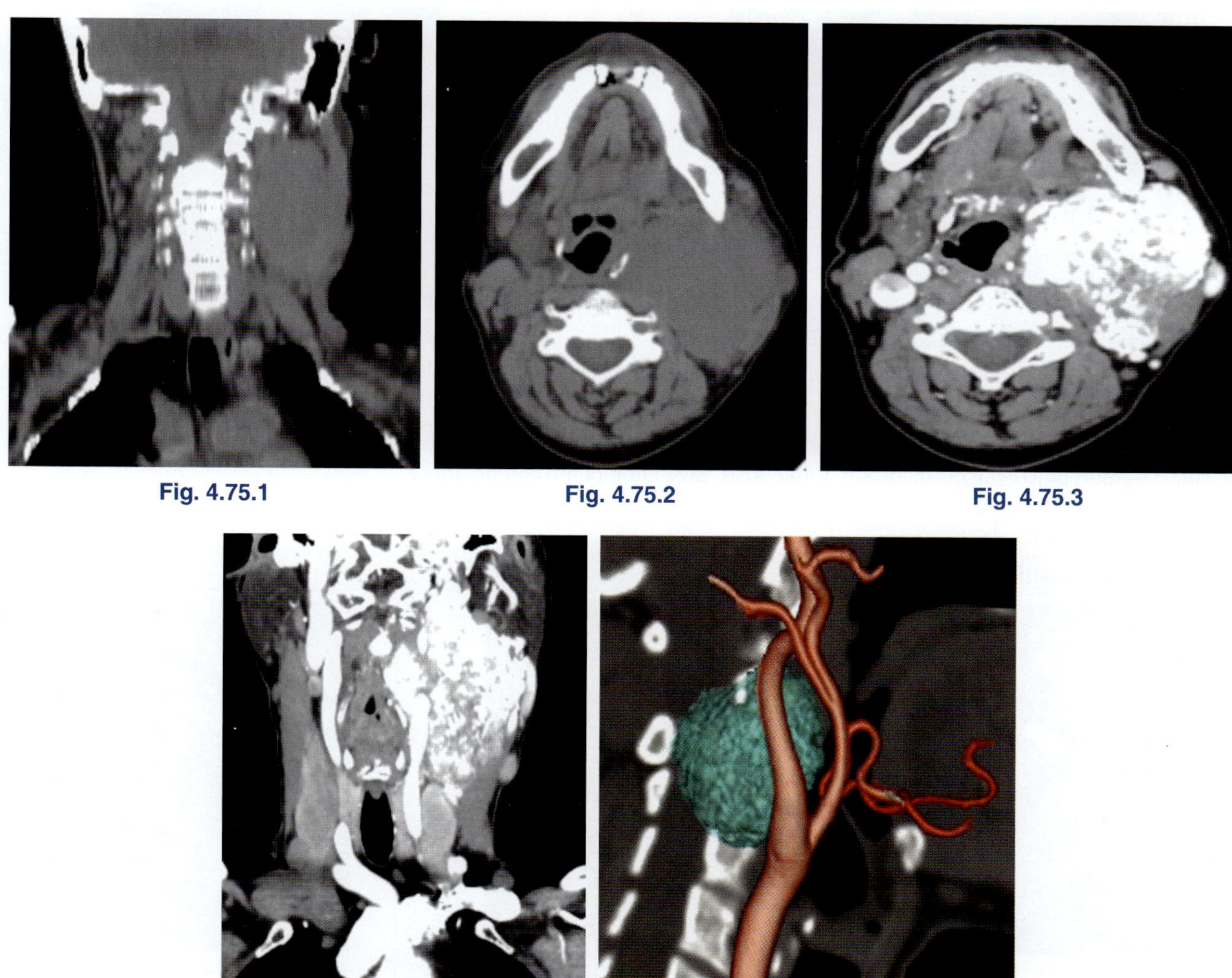

Fig. 4.75.1 Fig. 4.75.2 Fig. 4.75.3

Fig. 4.75.4 Fig. 4.75.5

Differential diagnosis

<table>
<tr><th colspan="6">Table 4.75.1: Displacements of carotid space lesions</th></tr>
<tr><td colspan="3">Vagal schwannoma: "Displace carotid anteriorly and internal jugular vein posteriorly"</td><td colspan="3">Glomus vagale: "Displace carotid anteriorly and internal jugular vein posteriorly". Usually 2 cm away from the jugular foramen</td></tr>
<tr><td colspan="3">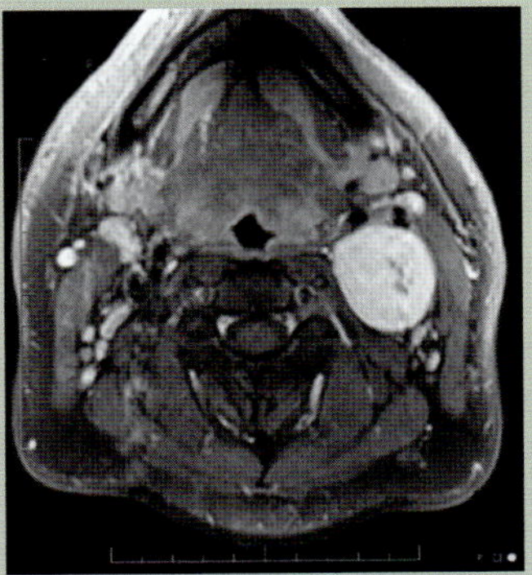
Fig. 4.75.6: Vagal schwannoma</td><td colspan="3">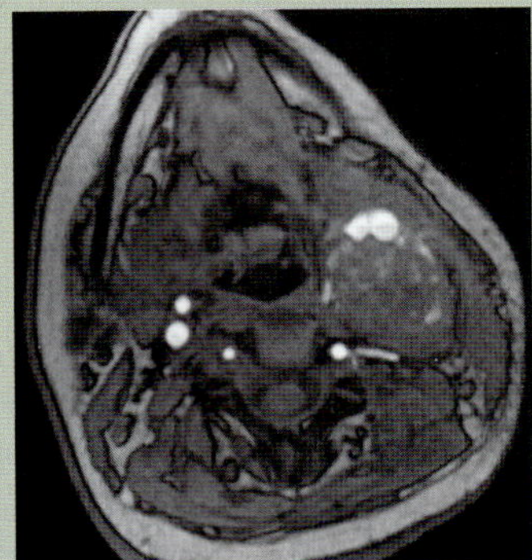
Fig. 4.75.7: Glomus vagale</td></tr>
<tr><td colspan="3">Sympathetic chain schwannoma
"Displacement of carotid and internal jugular vein anterolaterally rather than splaying"</td><td colspan="3">Carotid body tumor
"Splaying of carotid vessels"</td></tr>
<tr><td colspan="3">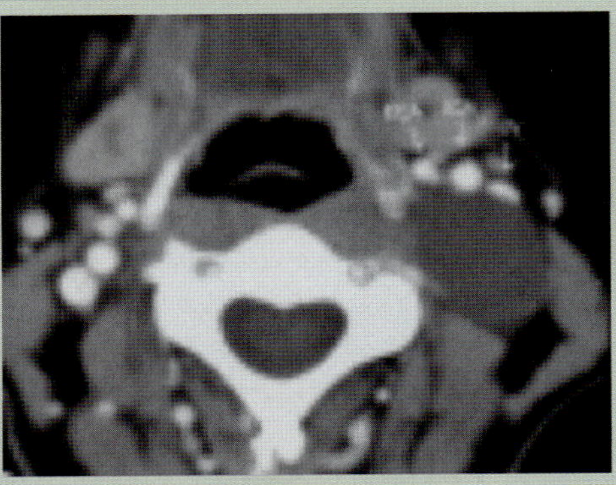
Fig. 4.75.8: Sympathetic chain schwannoma</td><td colspan="3">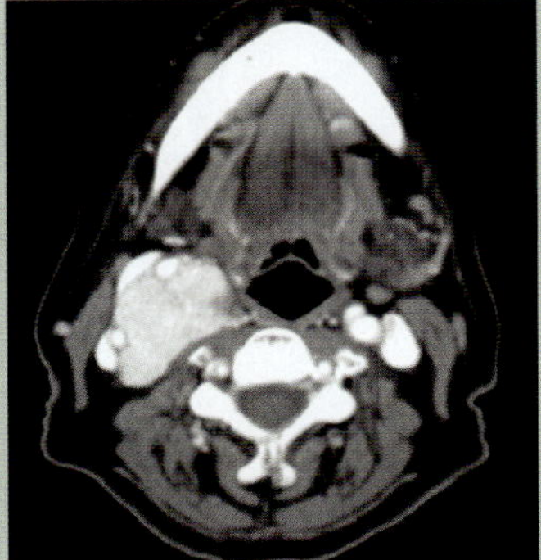
Fig. 4.75.9: Carotid body tumor</td></tr>
<tr><td colspan="6">Other differentials
• Lymph node mass: May look similar if hypervascular (lymphoma/castleman disease—calcification also).
• Vascular: Carotid bulb ectasia, aneurysm, thrombosis, dissection of the carotid artery.
• Thrombosis, thrombophlebitis of the internal jugular vein.
• Second branchial cleft cyst.</td></tr>
<tr><th colspan="6">Glomus jugular mass with AVF</th></tr>
<tr><td colspan="2">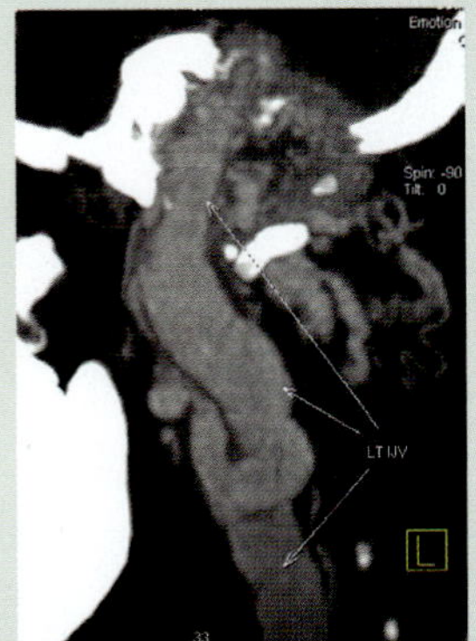

Fig. 4.75.10: Glomus jugulare</td><td colspan="2">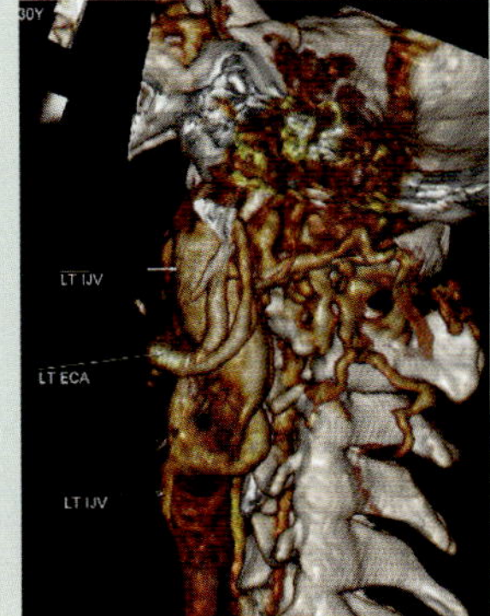

Fig. 4.75.11: Glomus jugulare</td><td colspan="2">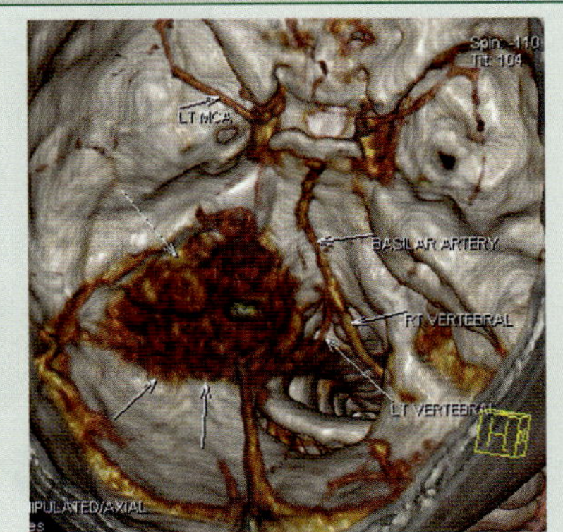

Fig. 4.75.12: Glomus jugulare</td></tr>
</table>

(Contd.)

Table 4.75.1: Displacements of carotid space lesions (*Contd.*)		
Glomus jugulotympanicum		
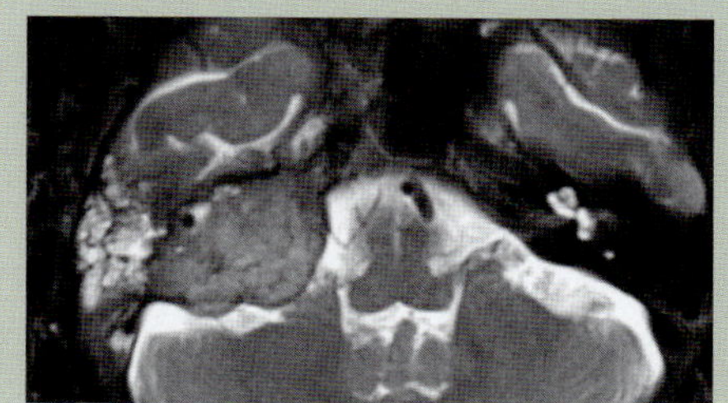 **Fig. 4.75.13:** Glomus jugulotympanicum	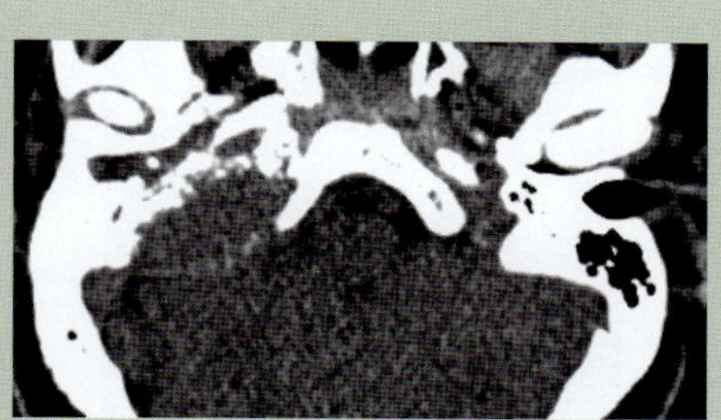 **Fig. 4.75.14:** Glomus jugulotympanicum	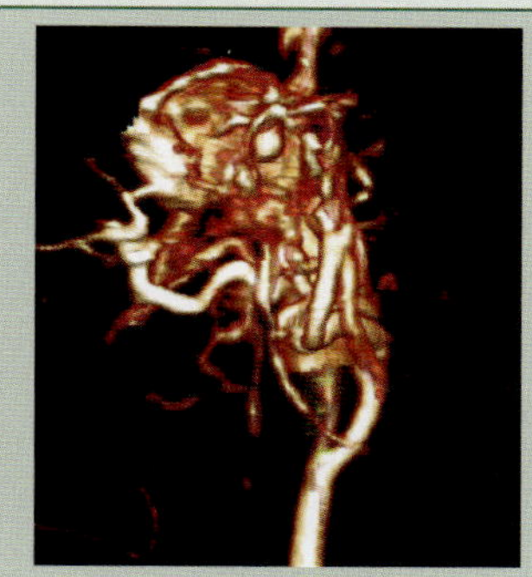 **Fig. 4.75.15:** Glomus jugulotympanicum
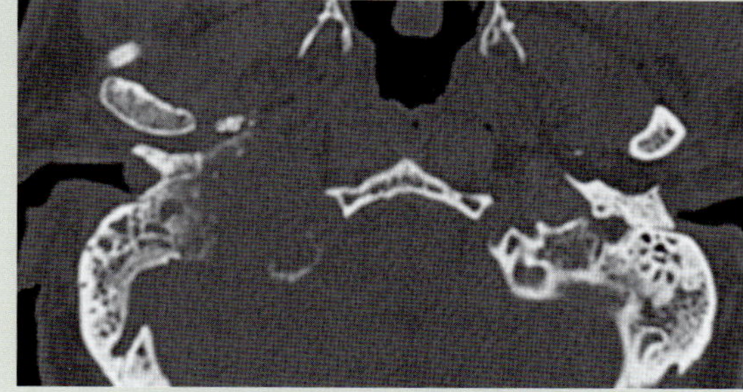 **Fig. 4.75.16:** Glomus jugulotympanicum	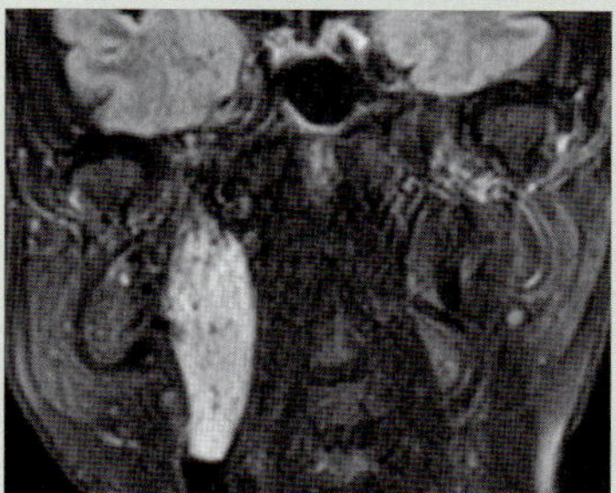 **Fig. 4.75.17:** Glomus jugulotympanicum	
Glomus vagale		
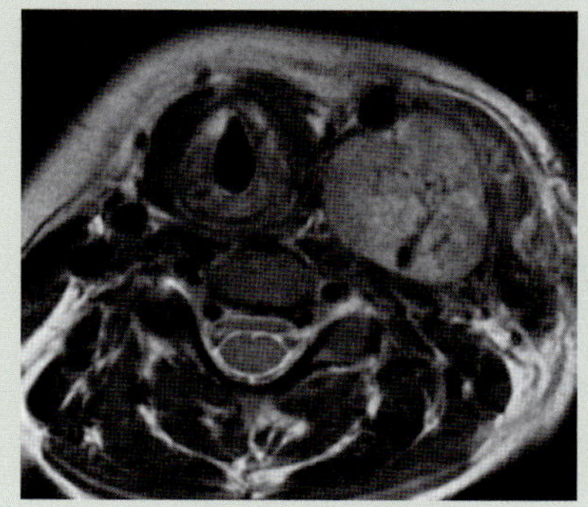 **Fig. 4.75.18:** Glomus vagale	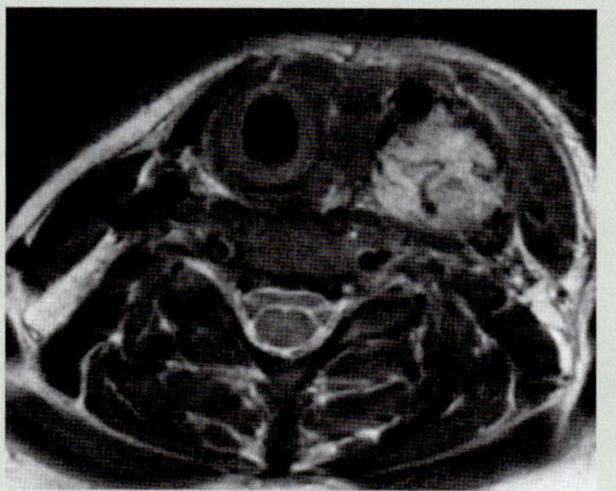 **Fig. 4.75.19:** Glomus vagale	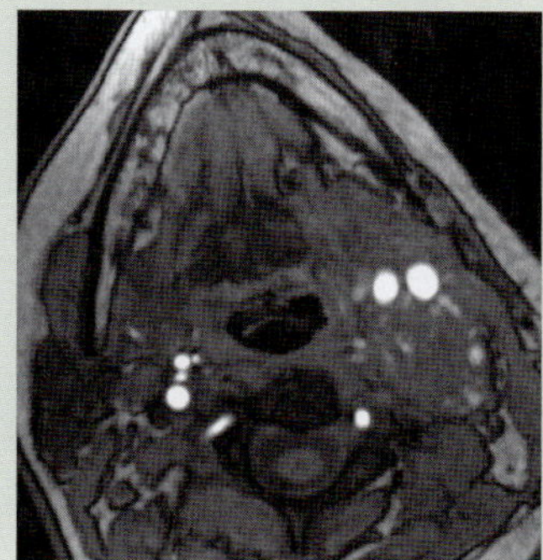 **Fig. 4.75.20:** Glomus vagale
Glomus vagale schwannoma		
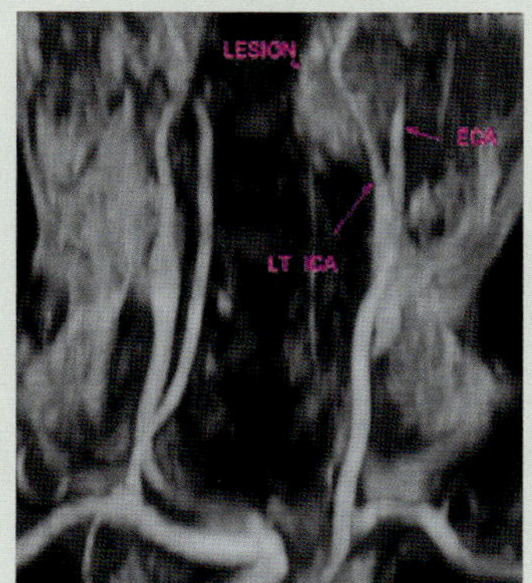 **Fig. 4.75.21** Glomus vagale schwannoma	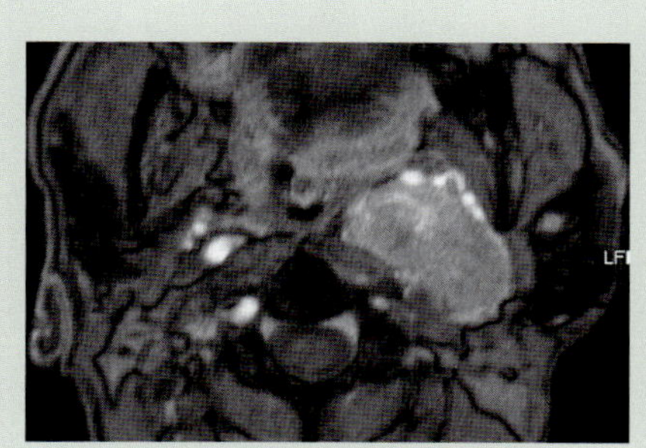 **Fig. 4.75.22** Glomus vagale schwannoma	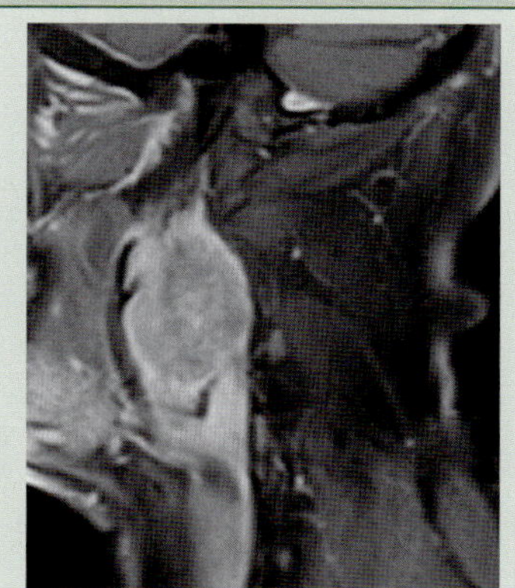 **Fig. 4.75.23** Glomus vagale schwannoma

(*Contd.*)

Table 4.75.1: Displacements of carotid space lesions (*Contd.*)

<table>
<tr><td colspan="3">Chemodectoma</td></tr>
<tr><td>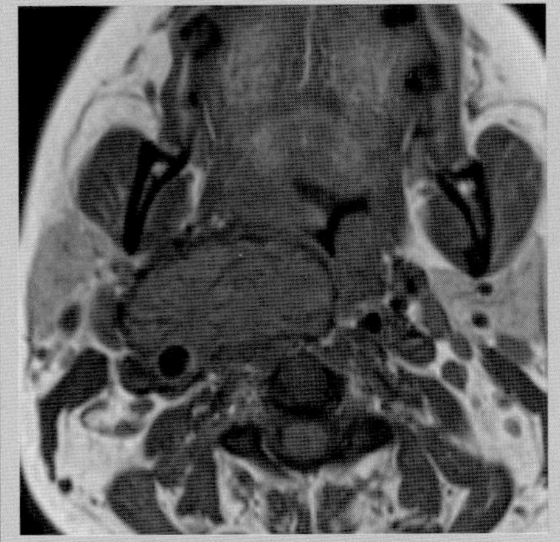
Fig. 4.75.24: Chemodectoma</td><td>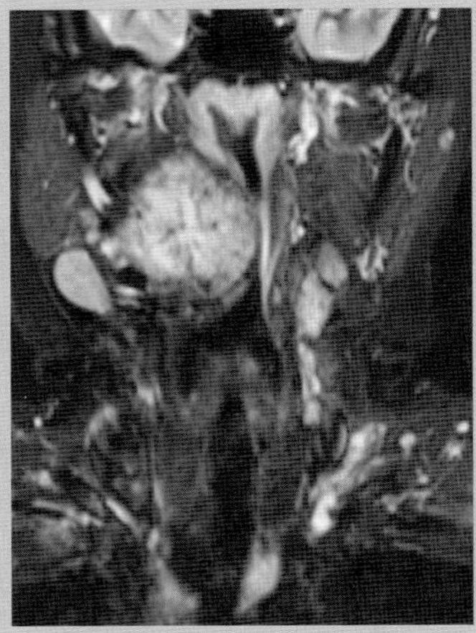
Fig. 4.75.25: Chemodectoma</td><td>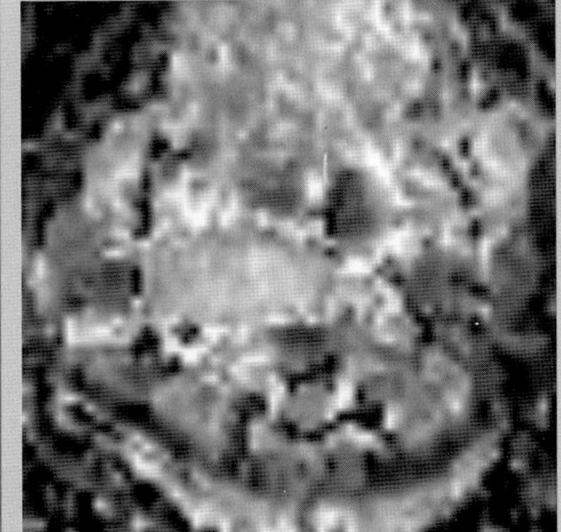
Fig. 4.75.26: Chemodectoma</td></tr>
<tr><td colspan="3">Vagal schwannoma</td></tr>
<tr><td>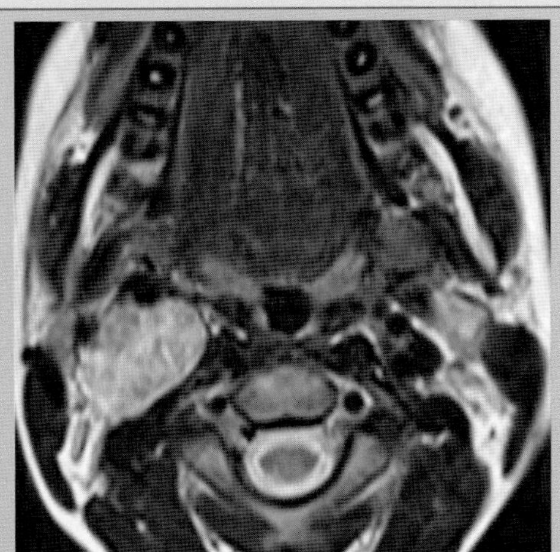
Fig. 4.75.27: Vagal schwannoma</td><td colspan="2">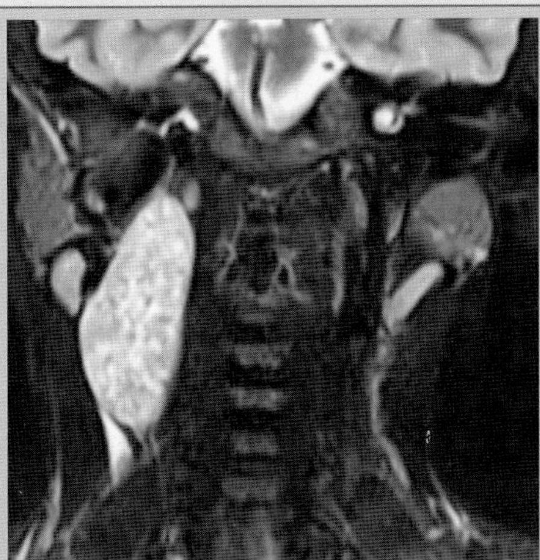
Fig. 4.75.28: Vagal schwannoma</td></tr>
<tr><td colspan="3">12th cranial nerve schwannoma</td></tr>
<tr><td>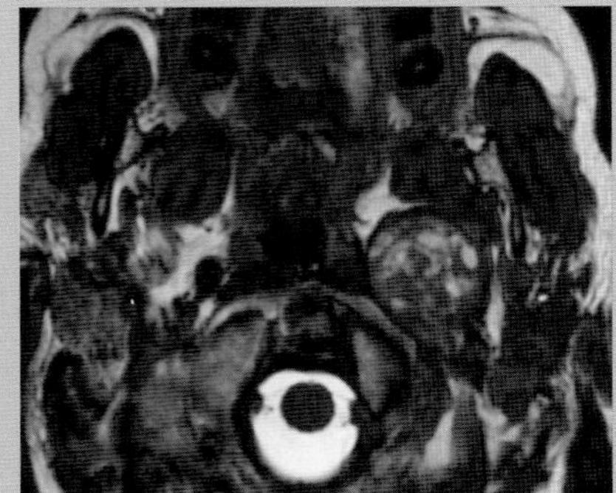
Fig. 4.75.29: 12th cranial nerve schwannoma</td><td>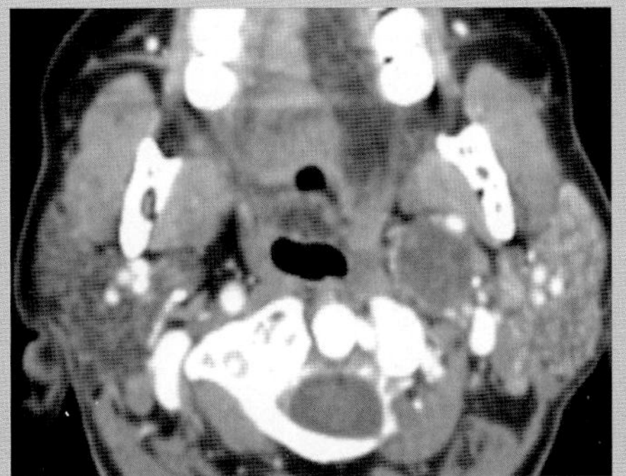
Fig. 4.75.30: 12th cranial nerve schwannoma</td><td>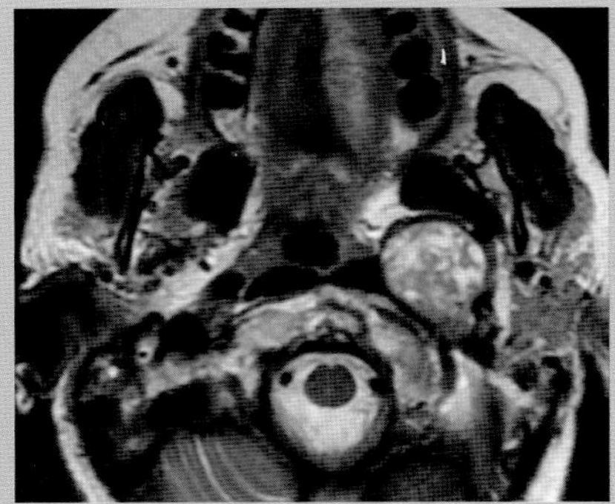
Fig. 4.75.31: 12th cranial nerve schwannoma</td></tr>
</table>

(Contd.)

Table 4.75.1: Displacements of carotid space lesions (*Contd.*)

Mandibular neurofibroma

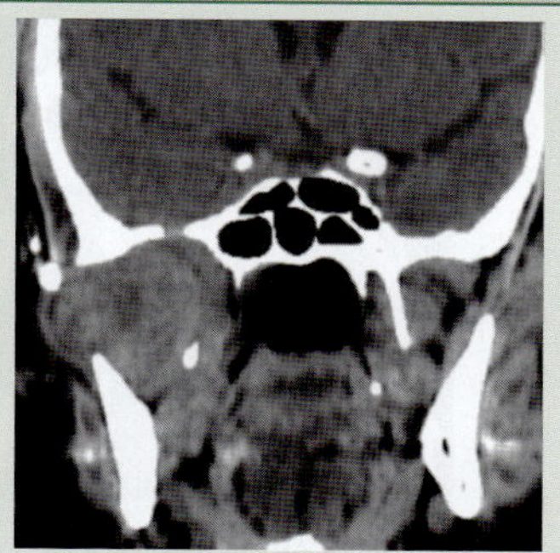

Fig. 4.75.32: Mandibular neurofibroma

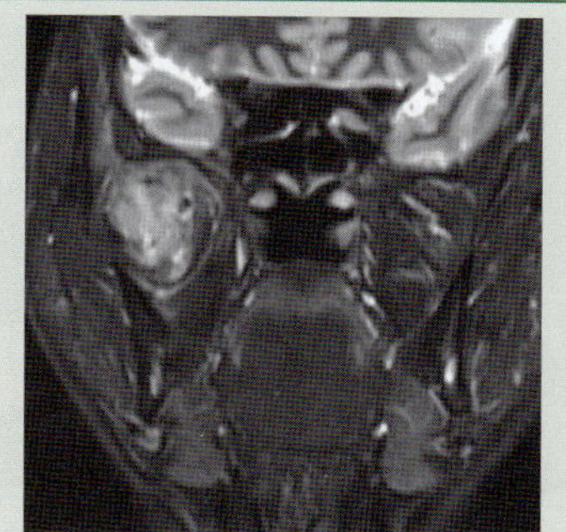

Fig. 4.75.33: Mandibular neurofibroma

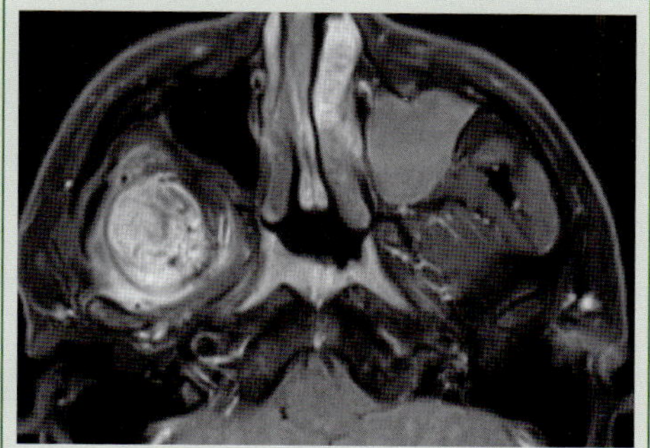

Fig. 4.75.34: Mandibular neurofibroma

Mandibular schwannoma

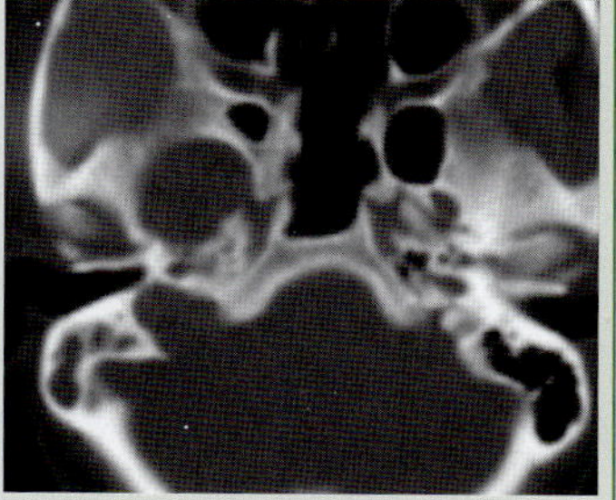

Fig. 4.75.35: Mandibular schwannoma

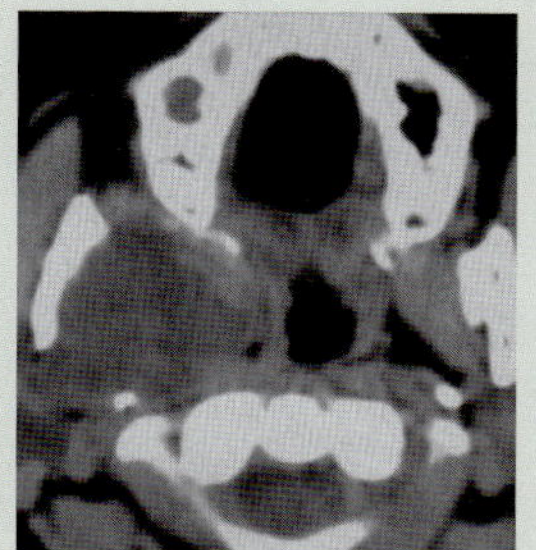

Fig. 4.75.36: Mandibular schwannoma

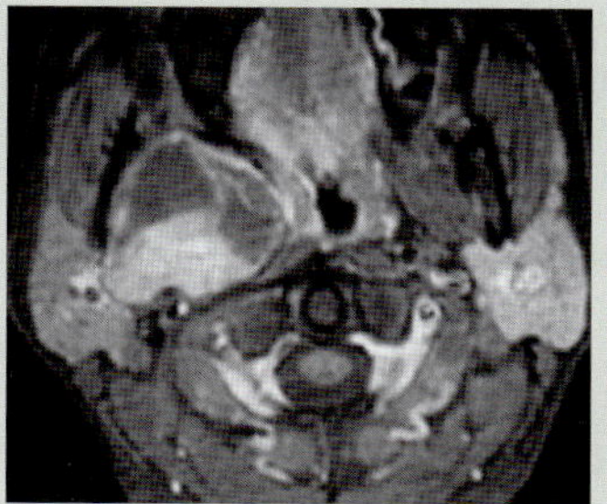

Fig. 4.75.37: Mandibular schwannoma

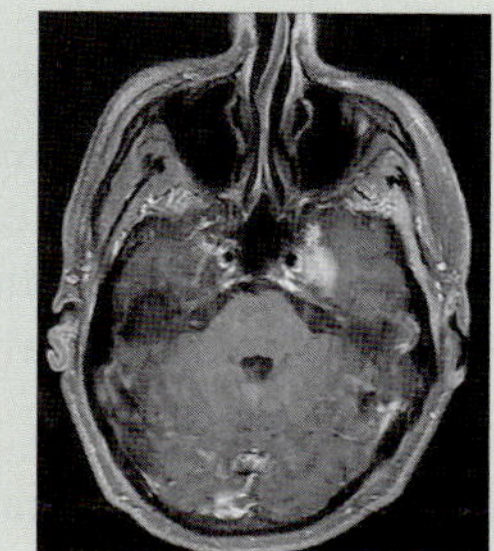

Fig. 4.75.38: Mandibular schwannoma

Nasopharyngeal carcinoma

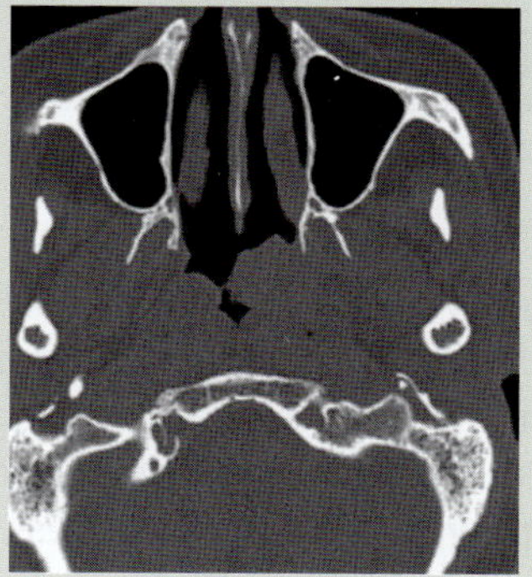

Fig. 4.75.39: Nasopharyngeal carcinoma

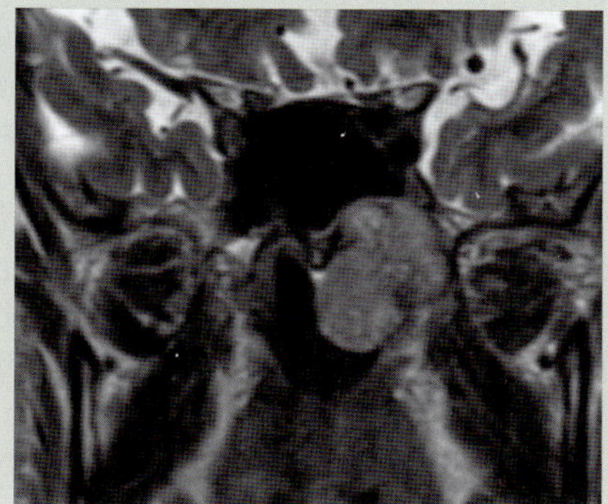

Fig. 4.75.40: Nasopharyngeal carcinoma

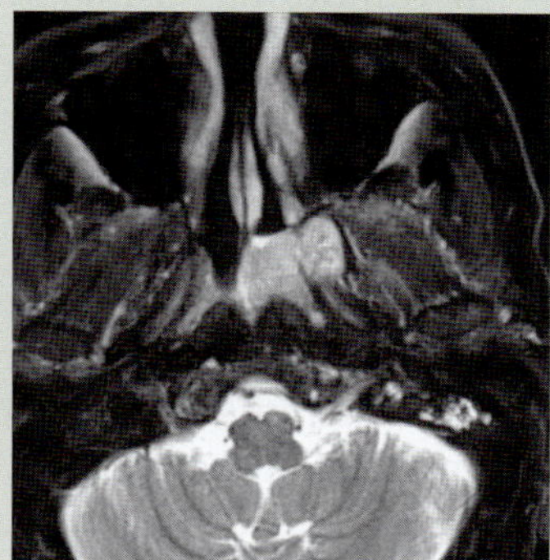

Fig. 4.75.41: Nasopharyngeal carcinoma

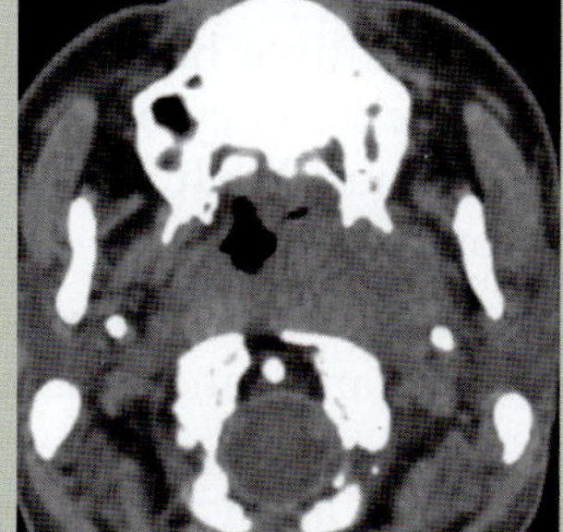

Fig. 4.75.42: Parapharyngeal mass lesion

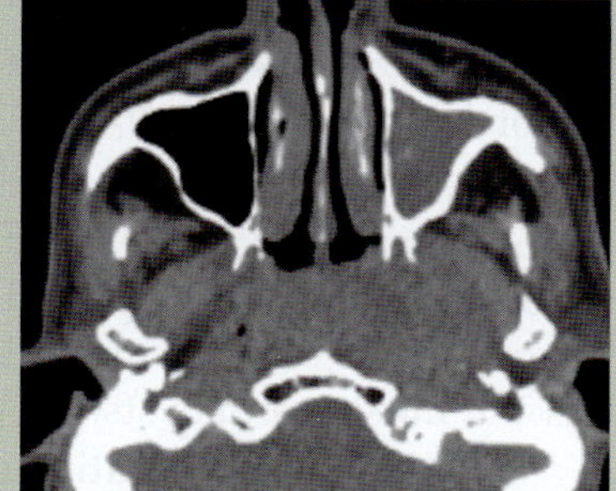

Fig. 4.75.43: Parapharyngeal mass lesion

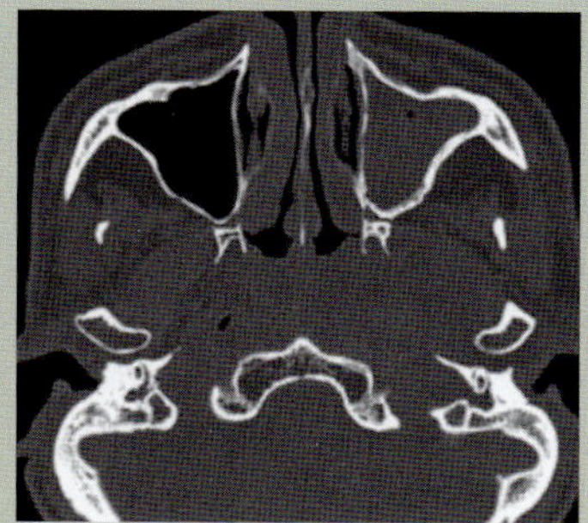

Fig. 4.75.44: Parapharyngeal mass lesion

(*Contd.*)

Table 4.75.1: Displacements of carotid space lesions (*Contd.*)

Rhabdomyosarcoma			
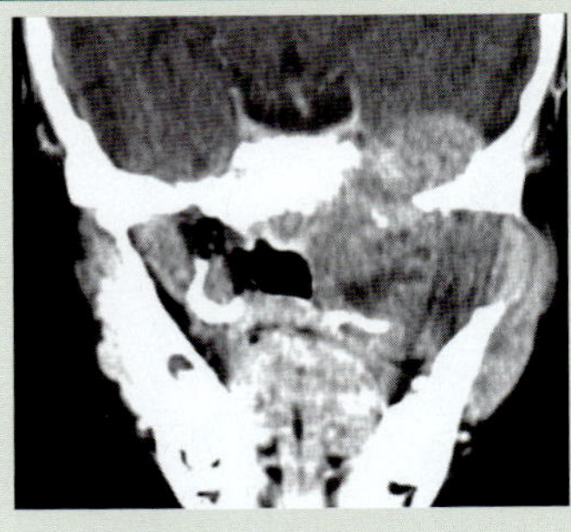	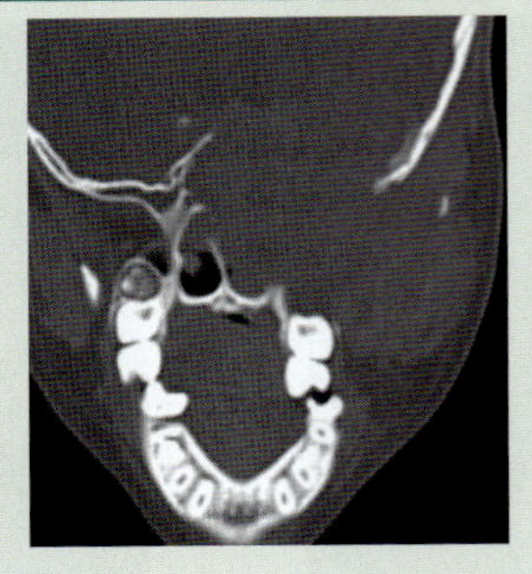	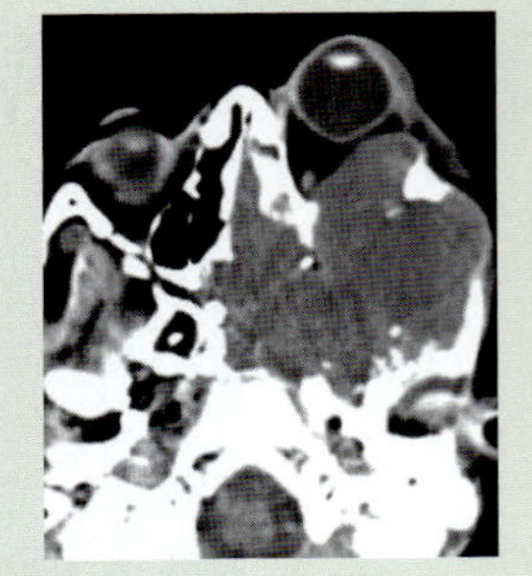	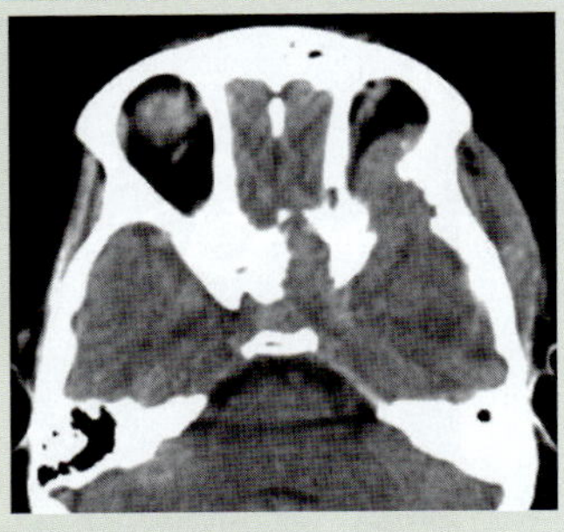
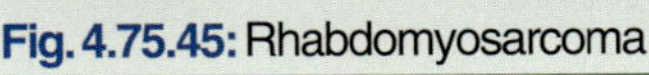 **Fig. 4.75.45:** Rhabdomyosarcoma	**Fig. 4.75.46:** Rhabdomyosarcoma	**Fig. 4.75.47:** Rhabdomyosarcoma	**Fig. 4.75.48:** Rhabdomyosarcoma

Further investigations and management: The next line of investigation for this patient is digital subtraction angiography. Surgical excision is treatment of choice. Follow smaller lesions with "wait and scan" approach. Preoperative embolization of larger lesions may reduce blood loss (500–700 ml) and operation time. Radiotherapy in poor surgical candidates.

Discussion

Shamblin grading for carotid body tumors:

- The type I tumor has an ICA maximum circumference of contact less than or equal to 180°,
- Type II tumors has more than 180° and less than 270°,
- Type III tumors has a maximum circumference of contact of 270° of more.

Carotid body tumor: Glomus caroticum/chemodectoma/nonchromaffin paraganglioma. Most common in 4th and 5th decade. Can occur in children.

CECT: Avidly enhancing mass at bifurcation between ECA and ICA. Extends cephalad from carotid bifurcation. Dynamic enhancement is rapid compared to nerve sheath tumors and other masses.

CTA: Oblique sagittal reconstruction shows enhancing tumor in "Y" of carotid bifurcation.

MRI:

T1 → Salt and pepper appearance in larger lesions.

"Salt" is due to secondary to subacute hemorrhage. Uncommon finding of limited diagnostic value.

"Pepper": Hypointense serpentine or punctate vascular channels show flow void. Expected finding in tumors > 2 cm. May be seen on tumor margin or within fibrous matrix of tumor parenchyma. This is the **most specific finding**.

T2WI → Mildly hyperintense compared to muscle. Multiple flow voids appear as **"salt"** combined with hyperintense areas appearing as **"pepper"** giving the **"salt-and-pepper"** appearance in tumor.

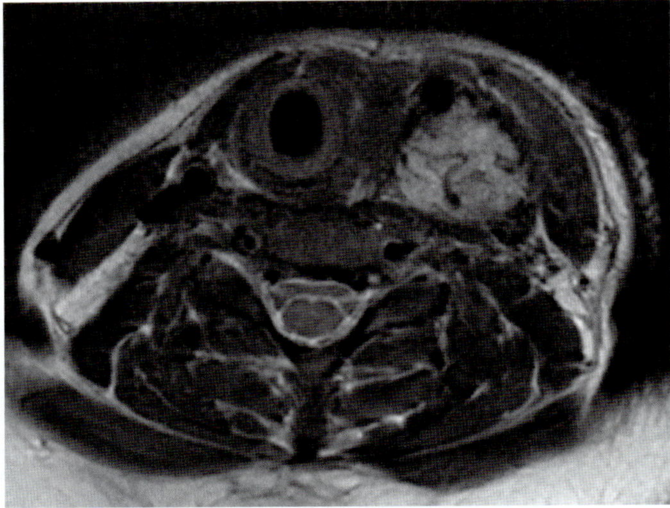

Fig. 4.75.49: Paraganglioma

Angiographic findings: Splaying of ICA and ECA on early arterial images is known as "Lyre sign". Prolonged, intense tumor blush is seen. Arteriovenous shunting creates "early vein" phenomenon. Ascending pharyngeal artery is typical arterial feeder. Angle of bifurcation predicts resectability—splaying >90° indicates less easily resected.

Associated abnormalities:

Paraganglioma syndromes: Multiple head and neck paragangliomas. Adrenal pheochromocytoma in some subtypes. MEN type 2 syndromes: Medullary thyroid carcinoma adrenal pheochromocytoma

von Hippel-Lindau syndrome: Hemangioblastoma, endolymphatic sac tumor. Renal and pancreatic tumors and cysts.

Preoperative embolization: Used as an adjunct tool, in surgical management for tumors >3 cm. Classified as multi-compartment/mono-compartment vascularity. PVA particle size (140–250 mm), Gelfoam is used as embolization materials. Surgery is done, 1–2 days post-

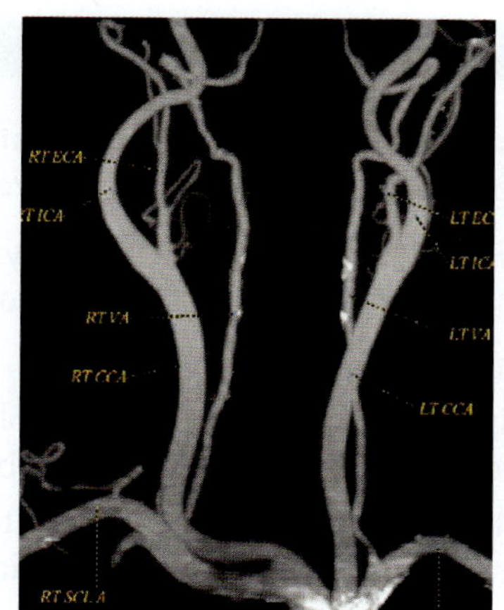

Fig. 4.75.50: Lyre sign on right side

embolization and no longer than 2 weeks, so blood loss can be reduced to 500–750 ml. Ear pain, cerebral ischemia and cranial nerve palsies are complications.

Table 4.75.2: Differential diagnosis based on appearance

Splaying of ICA and ECA	Separation between IJV and ICA	Displacement of both IJV and ICA antero-laterally	Displacement of both IJV and ICA medially
Carotid body tumor Lymph node enlargement	Glomus vagale Vagal schwannoma Lymph node enlargement	Sympathetic schwannoma Lymph node enlargement	XIth cranial nerve Schwannoma

Table 4.75.3: 90% and 10% tumors

Craniopharyngioma 90% Children 90% Calcify 90% Cystic changes 90% Enhancing solid component 90% Adamantinomatous type 90% Adults show visual symptoms	**Warthins' tumor** 10% Multifocal 10% Bilateral 10% of all parotid tumors	**Wilms' tumor** 10% Unfavorable histology 10% Vascular invasion 10% Pulmonary metastasis 10% calcification 10% Associated with syndromes 10% Bilateral
Insulioma 90% Benign 90% Solitary 90% Intrapancreatic site 90% Less than 2 cm	**Carotid body tumor** 10% Malignant 10% Bilateral 10% associated with MEN2/VHL	**Pheochromocytoma** 10% Extra adrenal, 10% bilateral 10% Malignant 10% Familial 10% Children 10% Calcification 10% No hypertension

4.76 HEAD AND NECK

Case No. 76

Clinical history: A 50 years old male with symptoms of dysphagia.

Radiologic technique and observation: Figures 4.76.1 and 4.76.2 are axial T2/T1W MRI images respectively showing well-defined isointense mass lesion in right parapharyngeal space with hyperintense foci due to hemorrhage within the mass. Figure 4.76.3 showing mass of homogeneous contrast enhancement. Right parapharyngeal fat is displaced anteromedially (hence the possibility of lesion arising from deep lobe of parotid/masticator space cannot be ruled out).

Interpretation: A—50 years old male, lesion in right parapharyngeal space, C—T1 well-defined isointense mass lesion with homogeneous contrast enhancement and internal hemorrhagic foci, B—parapharyngeal fat is displaced anteromedially, D—right parapharyngeal space pleomorphic adenoma (minor salivary glands).

Principal diagnosis: Right parapharyngeal space pleomorphic adenoma (minor salivary glands).

Differential diagnosis

- Benign mixed tumor, parotid deep lobe—identical appearance but within parotid deep lobe
- Pterygoid venous plexus asymmetry—tubular enhancing structures in PPS or medial masticator space
- Neurogenic tumor—well-defined, oval mass. Intermediate T2, homogeneous contrast enhancement if small.
- 2nd branchial cleft cyst—Type IV branchial cleft cyst lies within PPS. Cystic mass abutting lateral pharyngeal wall.

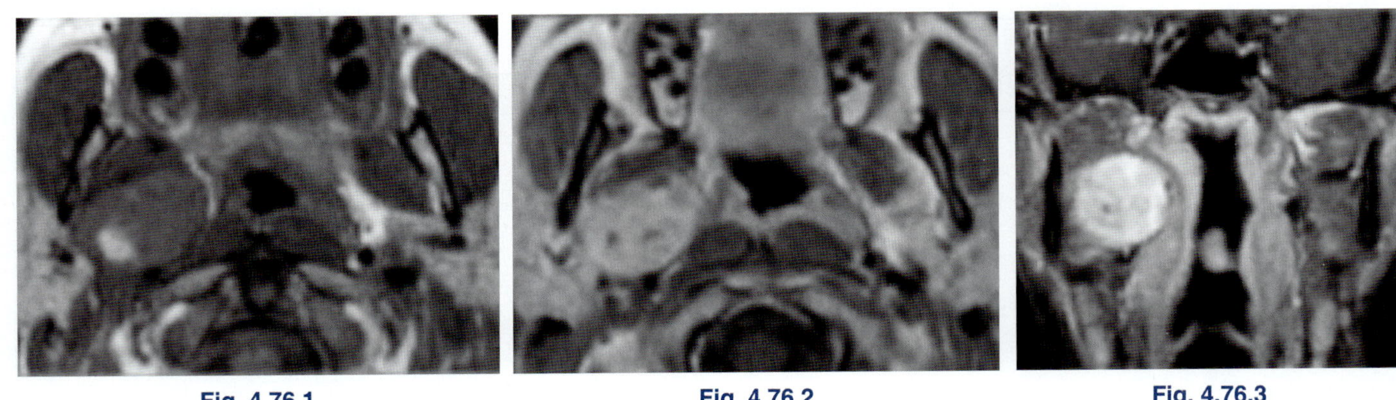

Fig. 4.76.1 **Fig. 4.76.2** **Fig. 4.76.3**

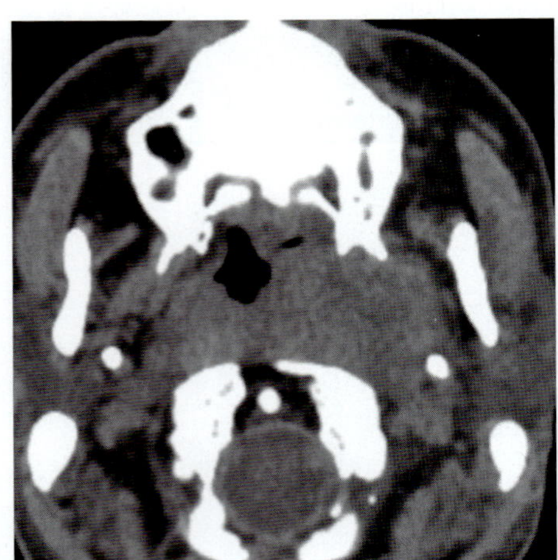

Fig. 4.76.4: Parapharyngeal space mass lesion

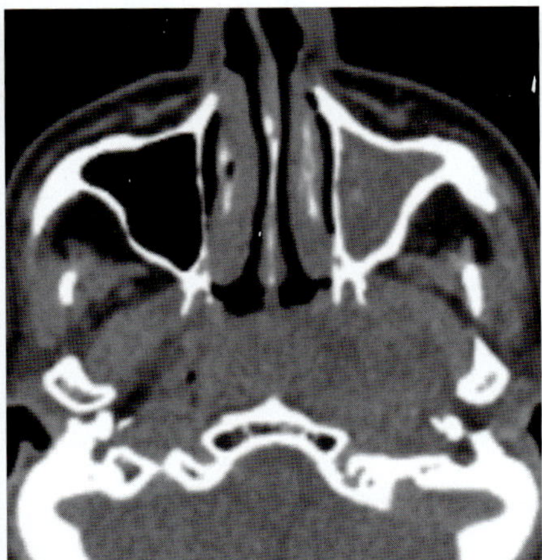
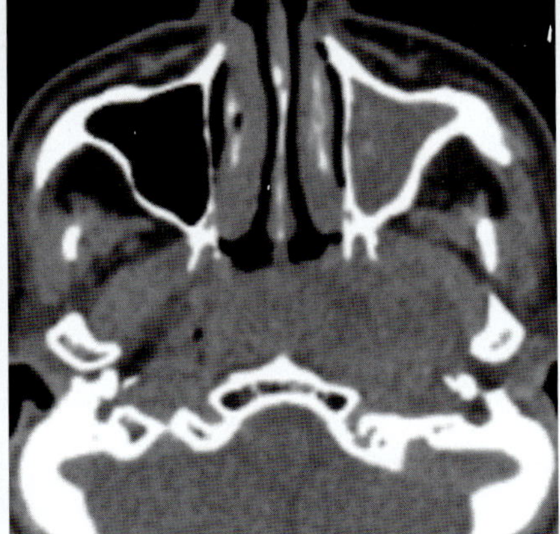

Fig. 4.76.5: Parapharyngeal space mass lesion

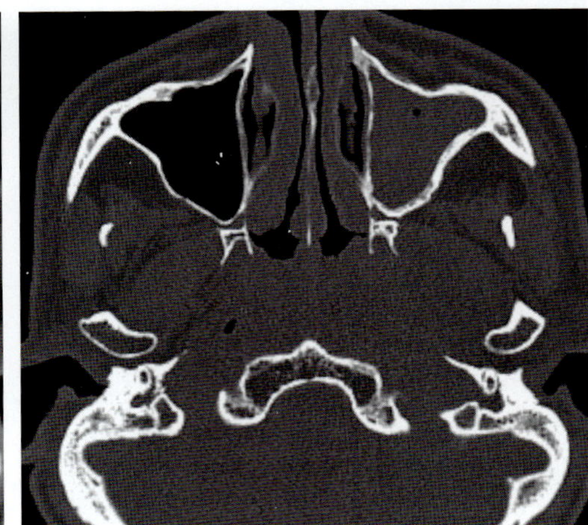

Fig. 4.76.6 Parapharyngeal space mass lesion

Table 4.76.1: Neck spaces applied anatomy			
Neck spaces applied anatomy	*Boundaries*	*Content*	*Pathologies*
Buccal space 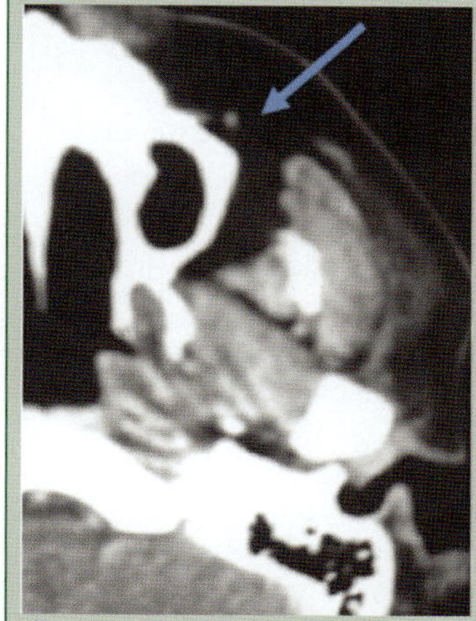 Fig. 4.76.7: Buccal space	Bordered by buccinator medially Masticator space posteriorly Depressor anguli oris muscle and the deep fascia attaching to the mandible inferiorly Platysma muscle and subcutaneous tissues laterally	Fat, minor salivary gland, LN, parotid duct, buccal branch of Cr N V3 and V2	• SCC • Minor salivary • Hemangioma • Lipoma • Accessory parotid, dilated duct • Abscess
Masticator space 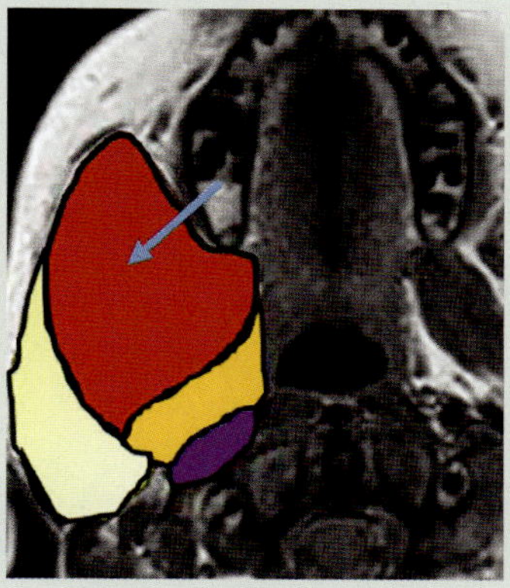 Fig. 4.76.8: Masticator space	Lateral to parapharyngeal space, superficial layer of deep cervical fascia encloses muscles of mastication	Masseter, temporalis, medial and lateral pterygoid muscles. Ramus and body of mandible. Cranial nerve V3	• Squamous cell carcinoma • Salivary gland tumors • Lymphoma • Hemangioma • Abscess • Rhabdomyosarcoma
Pharyngeal mucosal space 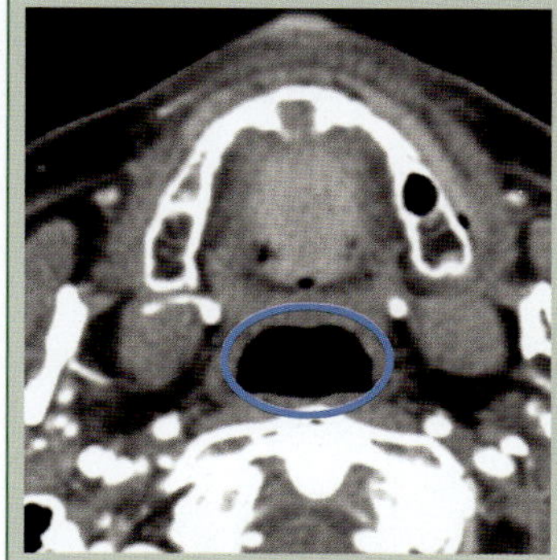 Fig. 4.76.9: Pharyngeal mucosal space	Torus tubarius anteroinferiorly and fossa of Rosenmüller posterosuperiorly	Waldeyer's ring: Tonsils, adenoids, superior and middle constrictor muscles, salpingopharyngeal, levator palatini, lymphoid tissue, minor salivary glands	• Squamous cell carcinoma • Adenoid cystic carcinoma • Lymphoma • Juvenile nasal angiofibroma • Thornwaldt's cyst

Contd...

Table 4.76.1: Neck spaces applied anatomy *(Contd...)*

Parapharyngeal space (fat) **Fig. 4.76.10:** Parapharyngeal space	Middle layer of deep cervical fascia medially, superficial layer of deep cervical fascia laterally, carotid sheath posteriorly.	**Prestyloid (parapharyngeal)** Contains fat, connective tissue, nodes **Poststyloid (carotid space)** Carotid sheath Cranial nerves IX, X, XII Prestyloid (parapharyngeal)	**Prestyloid pathologies** • Intrinsic—very rare! (<0.5% H&N NPL) • Minor (ectopic) salivary gland tumors • Trigeminal nerve tumors • Vascular malformations • Branchiogenic cysts • 2. extrinsic—mainly from parotid space • Parotid tumors—deep lobe origin (>80%)
Retropharyngeal space **Fig. 4.76.11:** Retropharyngeal space	Extending from skull to T4, anterior to prevertebral space and posterior to pharyngeal mucosal space. Mid + deep layers of cervical fascia, alar fascia laterally.	Fat, medial and lateral retropharyngeal nodes **Danger space:** Contains very loose areolar tissue offering little resistance	• Infection • Tumor spread • Lymph node
Prevertebral space **Fig. 4.76.12:** Prevertebral space	Skull base to T4 posterior to retropharyngeal space. Boundaries anterior cervical fascia from one transverse process to anteriorly in front of longus colli muscle. Posterior compartment from transverse process posteriorly to spinous process	Longus colli, scalene muscles, Vertebral artery and vein, brachial plexus, phrenic nerve	• Vertebral body mass • Infection • Degenerative osteophyte

Contd...

Table 4.76.1: Neck spaces applied anatomy *(Contd...)*

Carotid space (poststyloid parapharyngeal space) 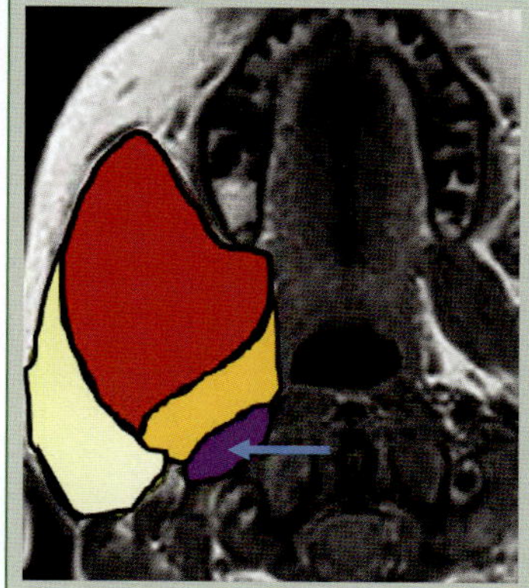 **Fig. 4.76.13:** Carotid space	From skull to aortic arch	**Below hyoid bone:** Common carotid, internal jugular vein, vagus nerve and cervical sympathetic plexus. At the level of nasopharynx: internal carotid artery, internal jugular vein, nodes, cranial nerves 9–12.	• Intrinsic • Neurogenic tumors (25% of all PPS lesions) • Paragangliomas (10–15% of all PPS lesions) • Vascular anomalies • Extrinsic • Pharyngeal mucosal space, retropharyngeal space, prevertebral space, trans-spatial lesions
Parotid space 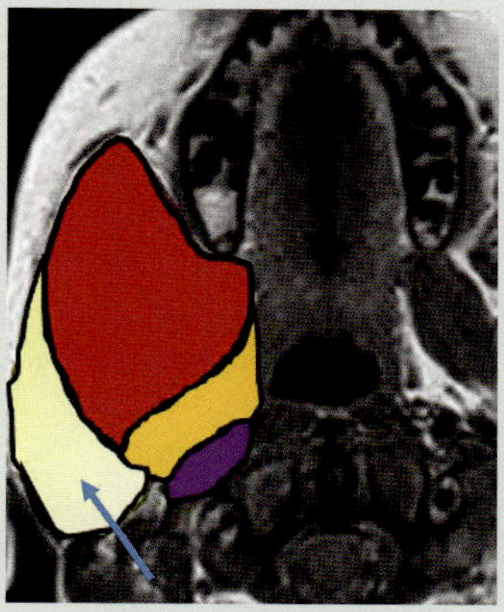 **Fig. 4.76.14:** Parotid space	Superficial layer of deep fascia Dense septa from capsule into gland	Parotid gland with duct, intraparotid nodes, external carotid artery, retromandibular vein and facial nerve	• Abscess, • tumor, • duct calculus, • sialectasis, • facial nerve lesions.
Submandibular space 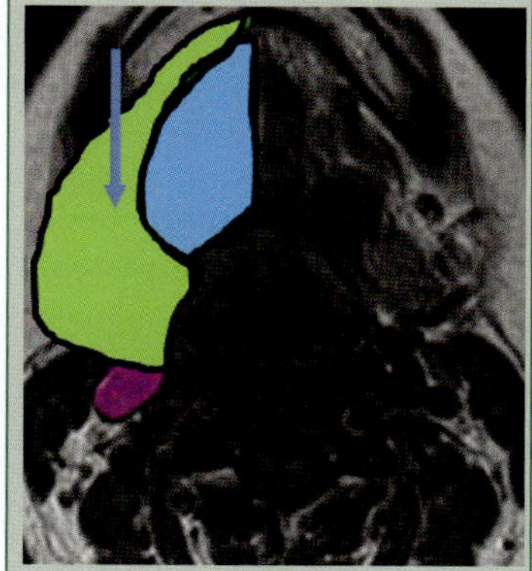 **Fig. 4.76.15:** Submandibular space		Submandibular gland with Wharton's duct, facial artery and vein, CN 12	• Supramylohyoid portion (sublingual space) • Sublingual gland • Hypoglossal and lingual • Nerves • Portion of submandibular gland • Inframylohyoid portion (submaxillary) • Submandibular gland • Wharton's duct • Anterior bellies of digastric

Contd...

Management: Resection of the tumor is the treatment of choice.

Discussion: Pleomorphic adenoma/benign mixed tumor: Benign tumor arising from aberrant minor salivary gland rests in parapharyngeal space. Rounded, well-defined lesion within PPS, distinct from parotid deep lobe. Age—adults; peak in 5th decade with slight female predominance. CT findings: CECT—heterogeneous,

Table 4.76.1: Neck spaces applied anatomy *(Contd...)*			
Posterior cervical space **Fig. 4.76.16:** Posterior cervical space	Complex fascial margins; comprises tissues posterior to visceral space and separate from perivertebral, carotid, and retropharyngeal spaces.	**Contents:** Fat, lymph nodes, nerves (including accessory CN XI). Common masses: Adenopathy (infection or tumor), nerve sheath tumors, cystic hygroma	• Lipoma, • Schwannoma • Lymphoma • Cystic hygroma • Third branchial cyst • 11th nerve schwannoma
Visceral space 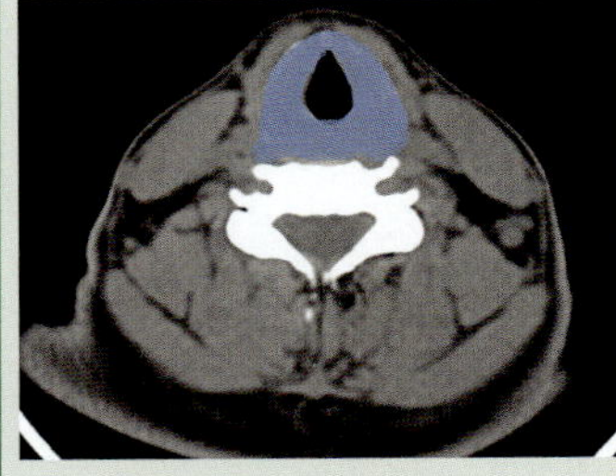 **Fig. 4.76.17:** Visceral space	Extends from hyoid bone to mediastinum.	Thyroid, parathyroid, larynx, trachea, esophagus, lymph nodes, recurrent laryngeal nerves. Common masses: Thyroid tumors, nodal disease, esophageal tumors, laryngeal SCCA.	• Laryngocele • Zenker's diverticulum • Carcinoma stenosis of trachea • Goitre, colloid cyst Hashimoto's thyroiditis, CA thyroid • Adenoma parathyroid, thyroglossal duct cyst • 3rd branchial cyst, metastasis, lymphoma

Table 4.76.2: Localizing neck lesion
Localizing neck lesions can be done based on 1. Symmetry, 2. Localization specific lesion site, 3. **Displacement patterns of PPS fat**—the parapharyngeal space (PPS) is surrounded by four key spaces parapharyngeal mucosal space (PMS), retropharyngeal space (RPS), masticator space (MS), parotid space (PS) in suprahyoid neck (SHN). The displacement direction of the PPS by a mass lesion from the surrounding space can be a crucial findings in pinpointing its origin space. PPS is pushed anteromedially by a PS mass lesion. PPS is pushed posteromedially by an MS mass lesion. PPS is pushed laterally by a PMS mass lesion. PPS is pushed anterolaterally by RPS mass. Prestyloid PPS is pushed anteriorly by retrostyloid PPS lesion.; 4. **Anterior displacement of styloid:** Carotid space lesions/stylomandibular foramen widening: Deep lobe of parotid, parapharyngeal space lesions/**displacement of great vessels:** Splaying of carotid—carotid body chemodectoma/ IJV and ICA displacement: Vagal schwannoma/distal changes—tongue atrophy is 12th nerve palsy, vocal cord palsy with 10th nerve involvement. 5. **Flow voids (T1 pepper)**—paraganglioma. 6. **Solid/cystic lesions** 7. **Signs:** Example: Tail sign, split fat sign, target sign—indicating neurofibroma. 8. **Perineural spread and nerve enhancement** 9. **Lymph node calcification**: Calcification with enhancement, e.g.: Castleman's disease. 10. **Enhancement pattern:** Homogeneous, heterogeneous, peripheral or non-enhancing.

well-defined mass within PPS fat with occasional focal ossification or calcification. MR findings—T1WI: Well-circumscribed rounded lesion within PPS fat. T2WI FS—marked hyperintensity similar to CSF. T1WI C+ FS–heterogeneous enhancement especially when large. Natural history and prognosis—slow growing; may be asymptomatic even when large. Uncommonly degenerates to malignant mixed tumor (carcinoma ex pleomorphic adenoma). Treatment—resection for definitive pathological diagnosis or if large and symptomatic.

Table 4.76.3: Retropharyngeal space, masticator space and prevertebral space

Retropharyngeal space	*Masticator space*	*Prevertebral space*
Contents 1. Fat 2. Lymph nodes a. Lateral retropharyngeal (of Rouvière) b. Medial retropharyngeal	**Contents** 1. Mandible (ramus + posterior body) 2. Muscles of mastication: Lateral pterygoid/ Medial pterygoid/masseter. 3. Temporalis 4. Inferior alveolar and lingual nerve (branch of mandibular division of trigeminal nerve)	**Contents** 1. Prevertebral muscles. 2. Scalene muscles. 3. Vertebral arteries and veins. 4. Brachial plexus. 5. Phrenic nerve
Lesions • Pseudomass 1. Tortuous internal carotid artery 2. Edema fluid or lymph spilling into RPS secondary to venous or lymphatic obstruction. • Congenital 1. Hemangioma 2. Lymphangioma • Inflammatory 1. Reactive adenopathy 2. Suppurative adenopathy (intra-nodal abscess) 3. Cellulitis/abscess. • Benign tumour 1. Lipoma • Malignant tumor 1. Nodal metastases a. SCC of head and neck(M/C nasopharynx) b. Melanoma c. Thyroid carcinoma 2. Nodal non-Hodgkin's lymphoma. Direct invasion from primary SCC (especially posterior wall lesions.)	**Lesions** • Pseudomass 1. Accessoy parotid gland. 2. Benign masseter hypertrophy (unilateral/bilateral) 3. Mandibular nerve denervation atrophy. • Congenital 1. Hemangioma 2. Lymphangioma. • Inflammatory 1. Odontogenic abscess (especially lower 2nd and 3rd molars) 2. Mandibular osteomyelitis. • Benign tumor 1. Osteoblastoma 2. Leimyoma 3. Nerve sheath tumor (schwannoma, neurofibroma). • Malignant tumor 1. Sarcoma, chondrosarcoma, osteosarcoma, soft tissue sarcoma. 2. Malignant schwannoma. 3. Non-Hodgkin's lymphoma 4. Infiltrating SCC from oropharynx, retromolar trigone. 5. Rhabdomyosarcoma.	**Lesions** 1. Pseudomass a. Vertebral body osteophytes. b. Anterior disc herniation. 2. Inflammatory. a. Vertebral body osteomyelitis (pyogenic/ TB) b. Cellulitis/abscess 3. Vascular a. Vertebral artery dissection, aneurysm, pseudoaneurysm. 4. Benign tumors. a. Schwannoma/ neurofibroma (cervical nerve roots/ brachial plexus) b. Vertebral body benign bony tumors. 5. Malignant a. Primary—chordoma. b. Non-Hodgkin's lymphoma. c. Vertebral body primary malignancy. 6. Metastasis. 7. Direct invasion of SCC

Table 4.76.4: Difference between pharyngeal mucosal space and reterostyloid PPS and carotid space

Pharyngeal mucosal space	*Retrostyloid pps and carotid space*
Contents—Mucosa; submucosa containing minor salivary glands, lymphoid tissue (adenoids, palatine, and lingual tonsil), pharyngeal fascia; superior and middle constrictor muscles; buccopharyngeal fascia (enclosing layer)	**Contents**—Internal carotid artery, internal jugular vein, lower 4 cranial nerves, sympathetic chain and lymph nodes (deep cervical chain)
Lesions • Pseudomass—asymmetric fossae of Rosenmüller; pharyngitis—post-irradiation/infectious • Congenital—Thornwaldt's cyst. • Inflammatory—adenoid and tonsillar hypertrophy/abscess/ inflammation • Post-inflammatory—dystrophic calcification, retention cyst. • Benign tumor—juvenile angiofibroma, pleomorphic adenoma (benign mixed tumor) of minor salivary glands. • Malignant tumor—SCC, non-Hodgkin's lymphoma, minor salivary gland. Malignancy, rhabdomyosarcoma	**Lesions** • Pseudomass—ectatic internal carotid artery; asymmetrical internal jugular veins. • Inflammatory—carotid space cellulitis or abscess that spread from adjacent spaces/breakdown of infected internal jugular lymph node. • Vascular—internal jugular vein thrombosis or thrombophlebitis; Internal carotid artery thrombosis, mural thrombus, aneurysm, pseudoaneurysm or dissection. • Benign tumor—paraganglioma glomus jugulare/ glomus vagale/ carotid body tumor; nerve sheath tumour—schwannoma/neuro-fibroma/meningioma (of jugular foramen) • Malignant tumors

4.77 HEAD AND NECK

Case No. 77

Clinical history: 13 years old female presenting with hoarseness of voice for 6 months duration and Grade II tonsillitis.

Radiological technique: Radiograph, plain CT, contrast enhanced CT neck and MRI brain.

Observations: Figure 4.77.1 is modified submento vertical view showing widening of right jugular foramen with ill-defined margins and soft tissue opacity over it.

Figure 4.77.7 is bone window shows widening of right jugular foramen with irregular erosion of the foraminal wall probably due to an expansile jugular foramen mass lesion.

Figure 4.77.5 is soft tissue window of the axial plain CT neck shows enlarged right pyriform sinus with medialization and thickening of right aryepiglottic fold—right vocal cord palsy. Figures 4.77.3 to 4.77.6 are axial sections of CECT neck shows a lesion with homogenous intense vascular enhancement causing bony erosion and widening of the right jugular foramen. Erosion of carotico-jugular spine **"Phelp's sign"** noted. The lesion is seen infiltrating the right jugular bulb and extending inferiorly into the right parapharyngeal space. Also, it extends superiorly into the right CP angle cistern indenting the brain stem. Prominent nasopharyngeal mass possibly enlarged adenoids seen (younger age).

Figures 4.77.8 and 4.77.9 are T1/T2W MRI images showing T1 and T2 heterointense lesion arising from the right jugular foramen with a CSF cleft between parenchyma and the lesion. Characteristic T1 and T2 flow voids with salt and pepper appearance, salt-haemorrhage or slow flow and pepper-flow voids. But T1 salt and pepper appearance is more specific and seen in lesions >2 cm. Compression of pons and adjacent cerebellar hemispheres noted. Right mastoid effusion noted possibly secondary to eustachian tube occlusion.

Interpretation: A—13 years old female, lesion in right jugular foramen, C—T1 and T2 flow voids with salt and pepper appearance, B—T1 and T2 heterointense intensely enhancing lesion arising from the right jugular foramen causing irregular bone erosion, compression of pons and adjacent cerebellar hemispheres, D—right glomus jugulare tumor.

Principal diagnosis: Right glomus jugulare tumor.

Next line of investigation: Digital subtraction angiography—to evaluate the patency of jugular vein, identify the feeding vessel and plan for pre-operative embolization 48 hours before surgery.

Management: Surgical excision/stereotactic radiosurgery. Pre-op embolization 1–2 days prior to surgery with ethyl vinyl alcohol (Onyx) is done.

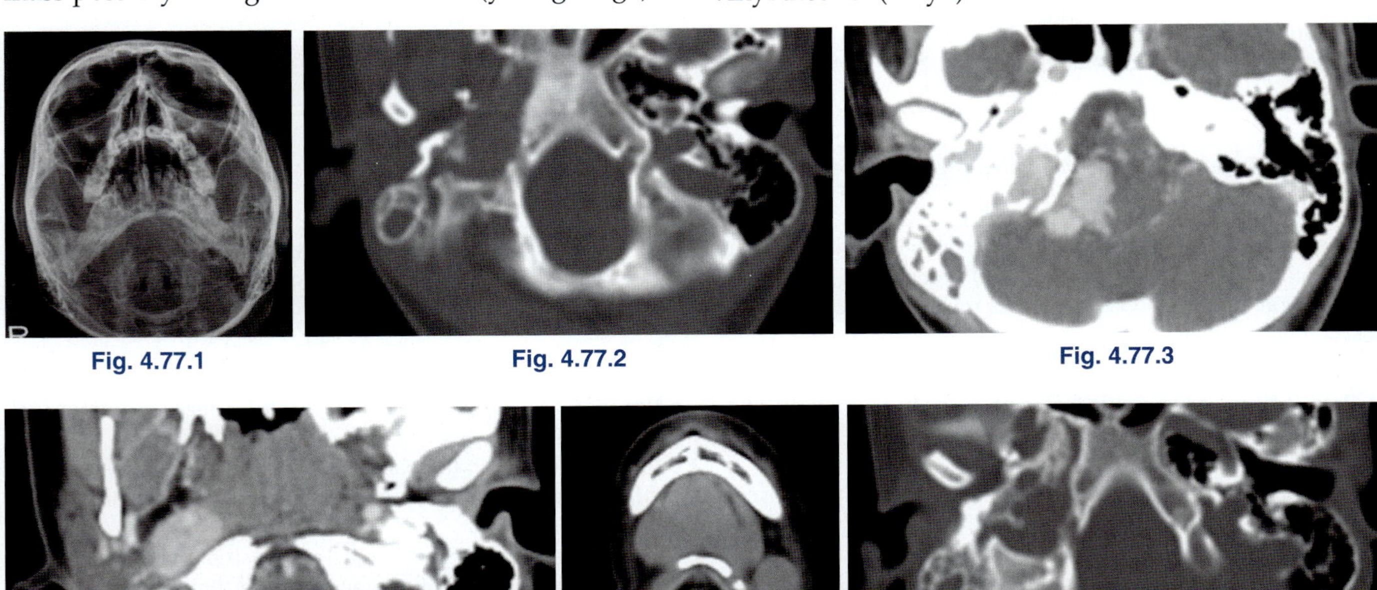

Fig. 4.77.1 Fig. 4.77.2 Fig. 4.77.3

Fig. 4.77.4 Fig. 4.77.5 Fig. 4.77.6

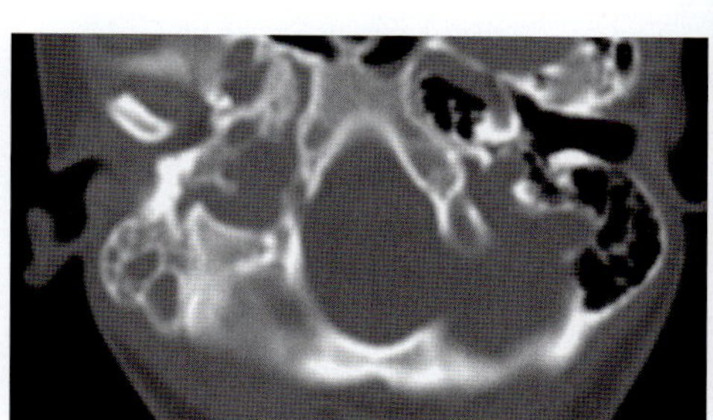

Fig. 4.77.7

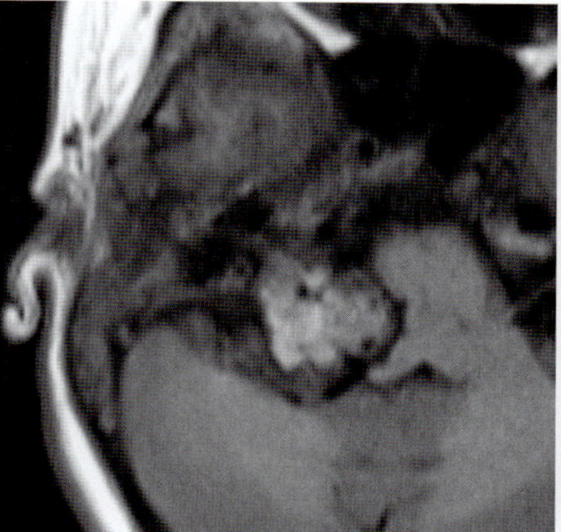

Fig. 4.77.8

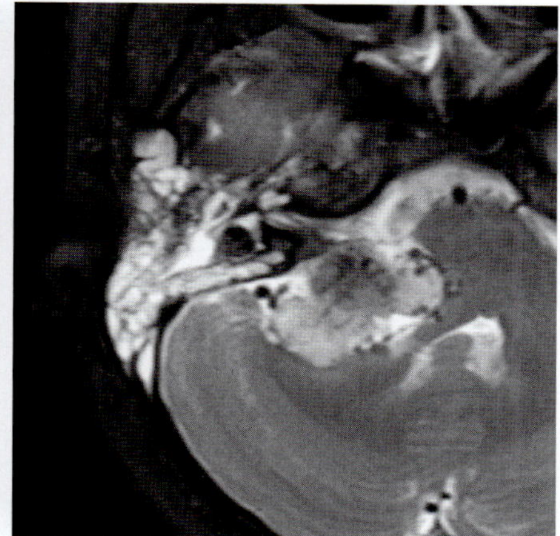

Fig. 4.77.9

Table 4.77.1: Differential diagnosis for glomus jugulare

<table>
<tr><td>1. Glomus Jugulare
Irregular permeative bone erosion "moth eaten" pattern, Intense enhancement, with vector of extension superolateral towards the sigmoid sinus/ inferior petrosal sinus, salt and pepper with characteristic T1 flow voids.
DCE: Early intensely enhancing mass with rapid washout after 150s.
Indium 111 octreotide: Shows uptake.</td><td>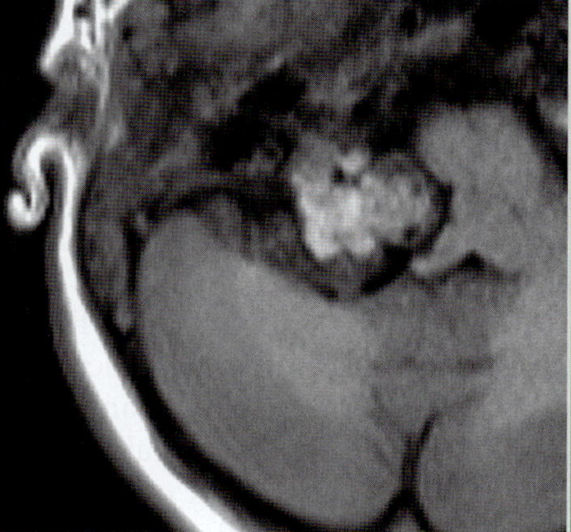
Fig. 4.77.10: Glomus jugulare</td><td>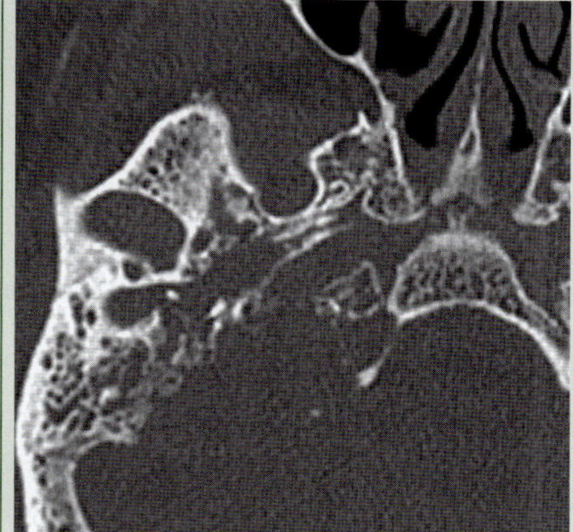
Fig. 4.77.11: Glomus jugulare</td></tr>
<tr><td>2. Schwannoma
Smooth sclerotic scalloping of Jugular foramen, encapsulated, typically avascular on angiography, it spreads superiomedially towards the brain stem. Towards the brain stem, secondary changes like vocal cord palsy, hemiatrophy of tongue and T2 target appearance with heterogeneous enhancement.
DCE: Early non-enhancement with delayed enhancement.
Indium 111 octreotide: No uptake.</td><td>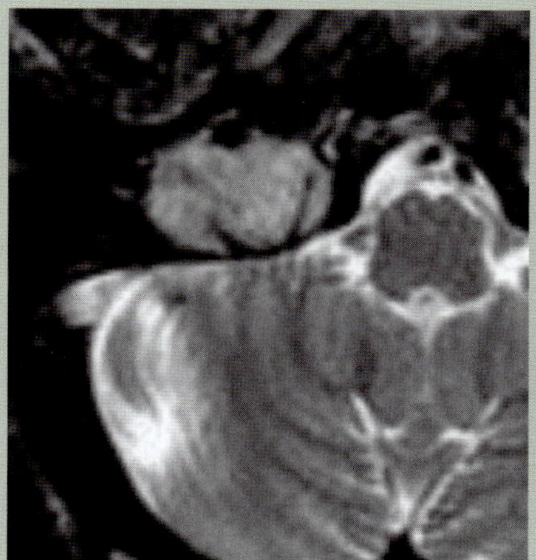
Fig. 4.77.12: Schwannoma</td><td>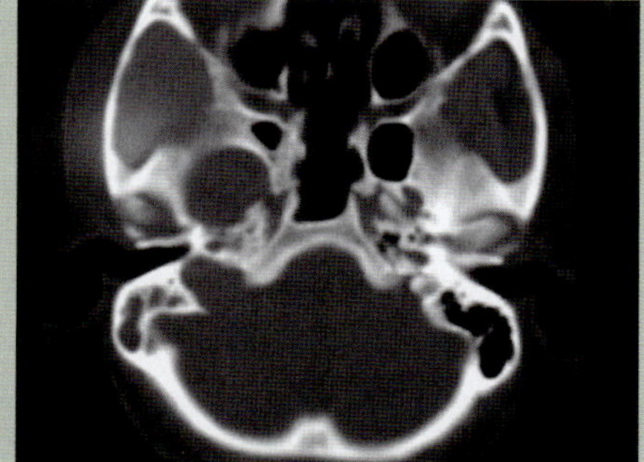
Fig. 4.77.13: Multiple schwanoma in jugular foramen and foramen ovale</td></tr>
<tr><td colspan="3">3. Meningioma causes sclerosis of adjacent bone, prominent dural thickening, vector of spread along the dura/calvarium, T2–ISO to hypointense with homogenous enhancement.</td></tr>
<tr><td colspan="3">4. Metastases irregular lysis of adjacent bone with adjacent infiltration. Hypervascular metastases from RCC and thyroid.</td></tr>
</table>

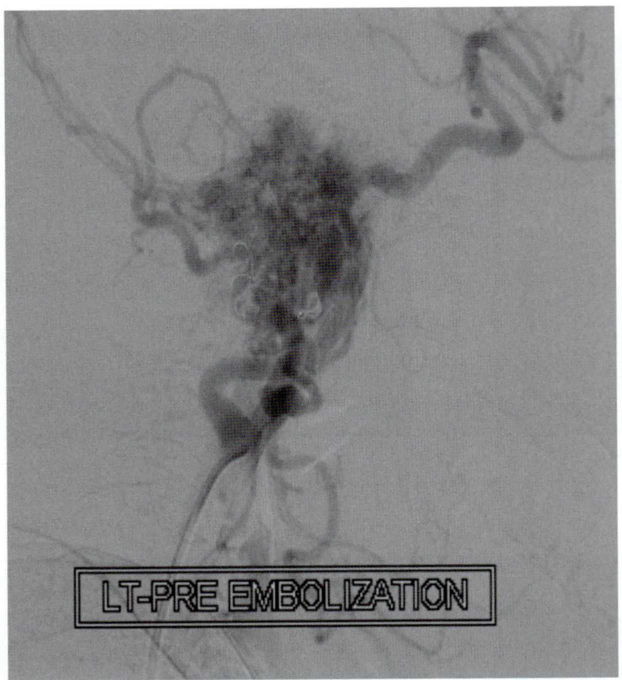

Fig. 4.77.14: Pre-embolization in glomus jugulare

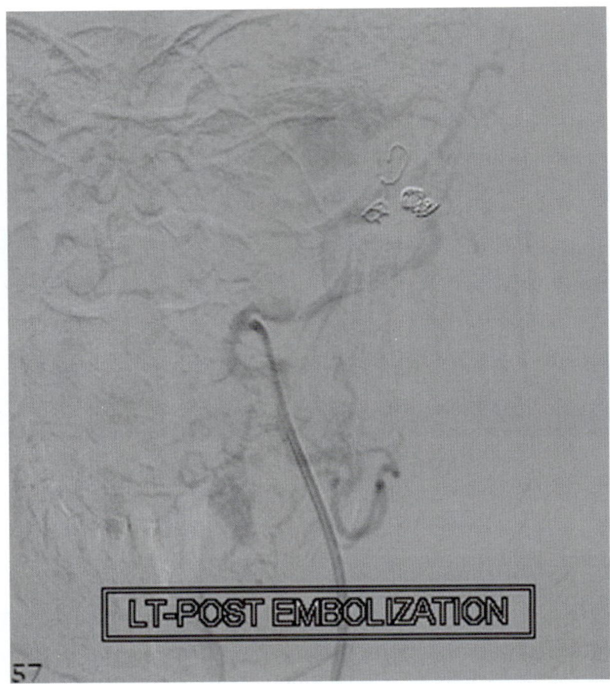

Fig. 4.77.15: Post-embolization in glomus jugulare

Glomus jugulare also called chemodectomas/glomus jugulare.

Most common tumor in jugular fossa with intracranial extension.

Arise from paraganglionic tissue in the adventitia of jugular vein or along Arnold's or Jacobson's nerve. Histologically—zellballen nests are seen.

CECT: Permeative lytic bone destruction in jugular foramen (usually within 2 cm) with significant enhancement. Enhances strongly after contrast administration.

- Destruction of posteroinferior petrous pyramid
- Corticojugular spine of jugular foramen
- Destruction of ossicles (usually incus), otic capsule, posteromedial surface of petrous bone.

Extension into middle ear cavity is called glomus jugulare tympanicum (glomus vagale/carotid body chemodectoma: >2 cm from jugular foramen).

Table 4.77.2: Differential diagnosis for jugular fossa lesions

Vascular	*Infections*
Asymmetrically enlarged Jugular foramen Jugular ectasia Jugular thrombosis (Lemierre's syndrome) Jugular diverticulum AV malformation High riding jugular bulb	Abscess Cholesteatoma **Tumors** Glomus jugulare Schwannoma Meningioma Metastasis

MRI—T1-hypointense and T2-hyperintense, a speckled "salt and pepper appearance" can be seen in both TI and T2. T1 salt- Foci of haemorrhage or slow flow. T1 pepper: Flow voids. T2 salt: Foci of haemorrhage. T2 pepper- Flow voids. But T1 pepper appearance is more specific and seen in lesions >2 cm. Tumor extends in a predictable pattern through least ways of resistance, most commonly to hypotympanum, mastoid cells or adjacent carotid artery.

Glenner classification of extra adrenal paragangliomas: (a) Branchiomeric distribution associated with great vessels of chest + neck including carotid body, glomus jugulare, glomus tympanicum (b) Parasympathetic distribution associated with vagal nerve, associated with aorticosympathetic chain in thoracolumbar region from aortic arch to urinary bladder, including organ of Zuckerkandl, Associated with visceral organs

Multiple paragangliomas in up to 20%, particularly in hereditary disorders (multiple endocrine neoplasia syndromes, neuroectodermal syndromes). Functioning paragangliomas: (a) Adrenal medulla (>80%) (b) extra adrenal intra-abdominal (8–16%) (c) extra adrenal in head and neck (2–4%). Four primary sites in head and neck and chest: 1. Carotid body, 2. Jugular foramen (glomus jugulare), 3. Path of vagus nerve (glomus vagale), 4. Middle ear hypotympanum (glomus tympanicum).

Less common sites in head and neck: Sella turcica, pineal gland, cavernous sinus, larynx (laryngeal branches of vagus nerve), orbit (ciliary ganglion of the eye), thyroid gland, nasopharynx, mandible, soft palate, face, cheek.

Arterial supply of glomus jugulare

Tympanic branch of ascending pharyngeal artery supplies inferomedial compartment.

Others: Anterior tympanic artery—anterior compartment and posterior auricular artery via stylomastoid branch—posterolateral compartment, meningeal branch of occipital artery, caroticotympanic branches of internal carotid artery, internal maxillary artery.

"Artery of paraganglioma"—ascending pharyngeal artery.

Complications: Malignant transformation with metastases to regional lymph nodes (in 2–4%).

Glomus tympanicum: Most common neoplasm of middle ear. Enhancing mass with flat base on promontory of cochlea found along inferior tympanic nerve (Jacobson's nerve). Large lesions fill middle ear space with permeative destruction of bones, medial wall and ossicles. Floor of middle ear cavity intact (if dehiscent to consider glomus jugulare).

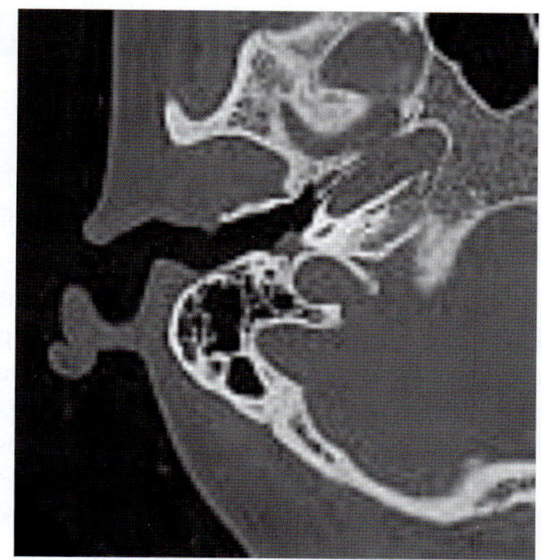

Fig. 4.77.16: Glomus tympanicum

Table 4.77.3: Glasscock-Jackson classification

Stage	*Glomus jugulare*	*Glomus tympanicum*	
I	Tumor involving jugular bulb, middle ear and mastoid process.	Small tumor confined to promontory	Glomus tympanicum; Glomus jugulare; Glomus vagale; Carotid body tumor — **Fig. 4.77.17:** Sites of paraganglioma
II	Tumor extending under IAC, may have intracranial extension.	Tumor completely filling middle ear space.	
III	Tumor extending into petrous apex, may have intracranial extension.	Tumor filling middle ear and extending into mastoid process.	
IV	Tumor extending beyond petrous apex into clivus or infratemporal fossa.	Tumor filling middle ear extending into mastoid process or through TM to fill EAC, may extend anterior to IAC	

Table 4.77.4: Approach to jugular fossa lesions

CT bone changes	*Moth eaten*	*Glomus tumor*
	Smooth scalloping	Schwannoma
	Sclerotic	Meningioma
	Lytic/ destructive	Metastasis
MRI T1/T2	T1/T2 salt and pepper (T1 pepper)	Paraganglioma
	T1/T2 isointense	Meningioma
	Target lesions	Neurofibroma
Contrast enhanced MRI	Intense heterogeneous enhancement	Glomus/paraganglioma
	Peripheral	Schwannoma
	Intense with dural tail	Meningioma
Direction of spread	Along brain stem	Nerve sheath tumors
	Along the dura	Meningioma
	Towards sigmoid sinus	Glomus tumor
	External mass	Metastasis

4.78 HEAD AND NECK

Case No. 78

Clinical history: A 75-year-old male with left-sided sensorineural hearing loss, vertigo tinnitus and headache for past 6 months.

Radiological techniques and observation: Figures 4.78.1 to 4.78.4 are MRI T1 plain sagittal, CISS, magnitude axial and T1 post-contrast coronal images respectively showing the lesion to be hyperintense in T1 (possibly due to haemorrhage) with epicentre around vestibular aqueduct which shows avid contrast enhancement. Bilateral internal auditory canal, cochlea appears to be normal. Visualised brain parenchyma appears to be normal. Visualised vessels appear to be normal. No abnormal meningeal enhancement.

Interpretation: A—75 years old right temporal bone, C—T1 hyperintense avidly enhancing moth eaten lytic lesion in posterior/retrolabyrinthine aspect of left petrous bone with involvement of right vestibular aqueduct, B—No extension of lesion into semicircular canals/brain parenchyma, D—Heffner's tumor.

Principal diagnosis: Endolymphatic sac tumour (Heffner's tumor).

Management: Complete surgical resection is the treatment/pre-operative embolization for larger lesions.

Brief discussion about the condition [Endolymphatic Sac Tumor (ELST)]: Size of endolymphatic sac is 1.5 mm. Increase in size when more than 2 mm is seen in ELST.

Clinical features: Hearing loss and tinnitus in 90 percent cases. Vertigo and tinnitus. Aural fullness. ELST can occur on its own or in association with von Hippel–Lindau (VHL) syndrome. Bilateral cases are seen associated with VHL, in general, sporadic cases are more common than cases associated with VHL.

Imaging: Imaging hallmark of ELST is a retrolabyrinthine mass associated with osseous erosion. Bone CT shows infiltrative poorly circumscribed lytic lesion with central bone spicules. Petrous bone erosion by endolymphatic sac tumor is typically described as "moth eaten".

Location between internal auditory canal and sigmoid sinus is characteristic for ELST.

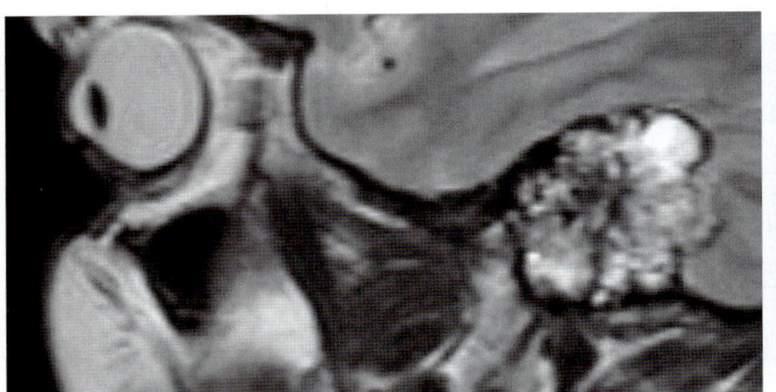

Fig. 4.78.1

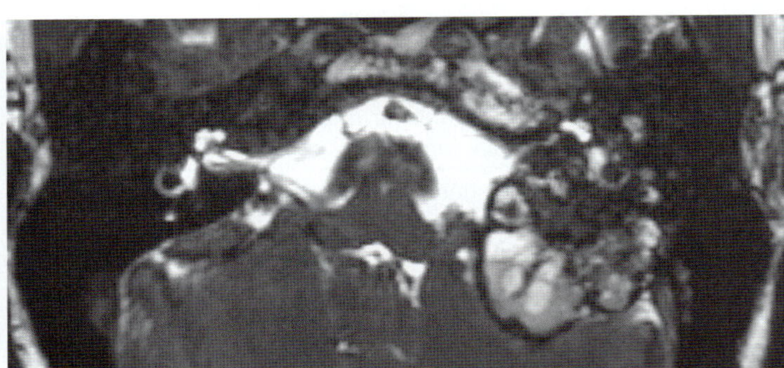

Fig. 4.78.2

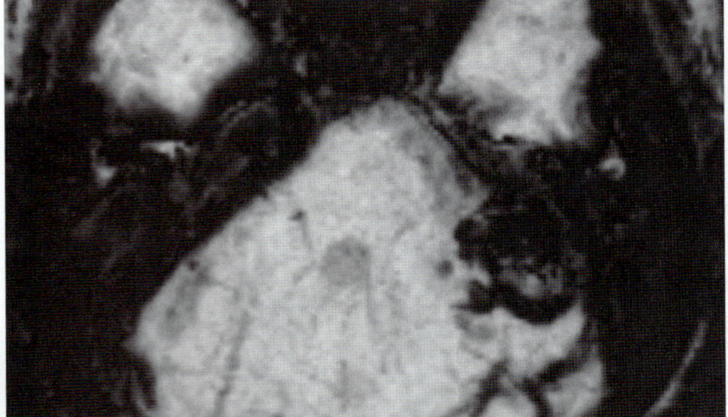

Fig. 4.78.3

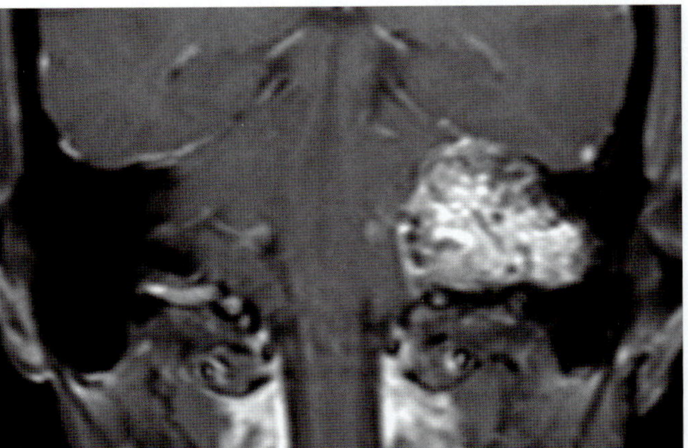

Fig. 4.78.4

Table 4.78.1: Differential diagnosis

Glomus jugulotympanicum Glomus jugulare extending into middle ear cavity (hypotympanum). They arise from Jacobson nerve at the cochlear promontory. Age—40 to 60 years M: F—1:4 Pulsatile tinnitus is the most common clinical manifestation. O/E—red pulsatile retrotympanic mass	**CT**-permeative destructive bone invasion without spicules.MR-salt and pepper appearance in both T1 and T2 weighted images. **T1 salt and pepper is characteristic. T1 salt represents hemorrhage and pepper represents flow voids.** Centre of the lesion at jugular bulb rather than vestibular aqueduct.	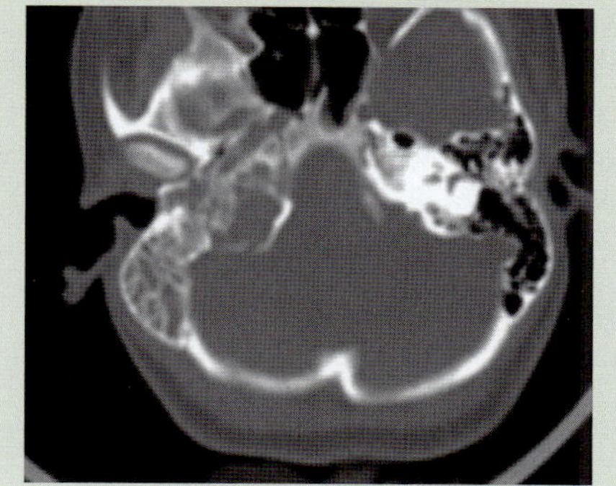 **Fig. 4.78.5:** Glomus jugulotympanicum
Lymphoma of temporal bone Seen in elderly. Second most common malignant tumor in head and neck region. Most lymphomas of head and neck region are NHL facial nerve palsy is rare because nerve sheath is resistant to tumor invasion. Second most common malignancy in head and neck is non-Hodgkin's lymphoma (first is squamous cell carcinoma)	**Radiograph:** Most common is permeative lytic pattern. **CT:** Permeative lytic lesions of temporal bone indistinguishable from other pathologies. **MR:** Identify leptomeningeal spread and brain invasion. **CE-MRI**: To look for perineural spread. **PET**: Staging, pathology in any other sites and response to therapy.	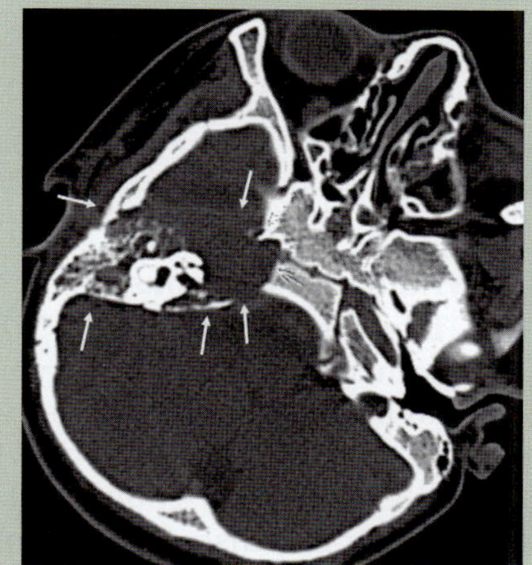 **Fig. 4.78.6:** Lymphoma of temporal bone
Plasmacytoma Rare cause of lytic lesion of temporal bone. It presents with headache, swelling and other vague complaints. Localised radiotherapy is treatment of choice. HPE-positive for CD 138. CT may demonstrate subtle lytic lesion or small soft tissue masses that are not visible on radiography.	Punched out lytic mass with **non-sclerotic margins.** CT—locally destructive lesion involving temporal bone with erosion of adjacent affected bones and a soft tissue component. Lesion will show homogeneous contrast enhancement on CE MRI.	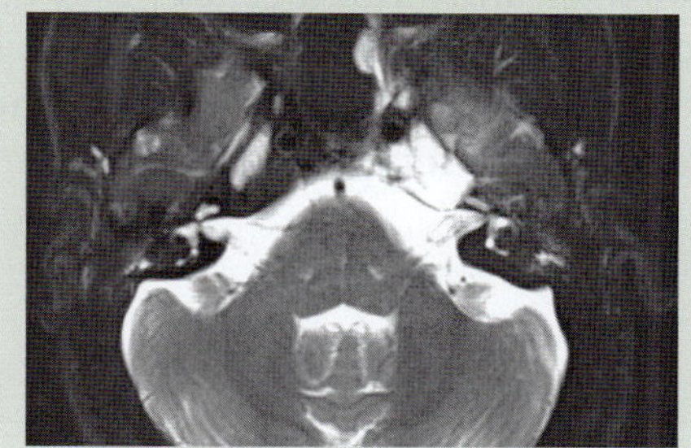 **Fig. 4.78.7:** Plasmacytoma
Complicated mastoiditis Suppurative infection of mastoid air cells. Complication or chronicity leads to subsequent osteoclasia and decalcification which creates bone loss. Most vulnerable ossicle is incus.	**CT-bone window:** Loss of equal to sign of ossicles. Non-visualisation of **ice-cream cone** appearance of ossicles. Vertical segment of **ossicular right angle** missing. Erosive changes in adjacent bones.	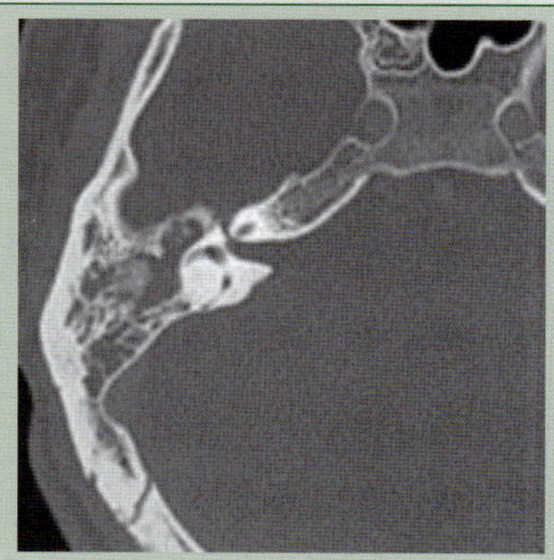 **Fig. 4.78.8:** Complicated mastoiditis

(Contd..)

Table 4.78.1: Differential diagnosis *(Contd..)*

Metastases Most common site—petrous apex. Most common primary is lung cancer. Other causes include haematological malignancies, breast, prostate and renal cancers.	Enhancing marrow space mass with or without extraosseous extension. Lesions can be lytic or sclerotic. MRI T1: **Hypointense marrow lesion replaces high signal fat**	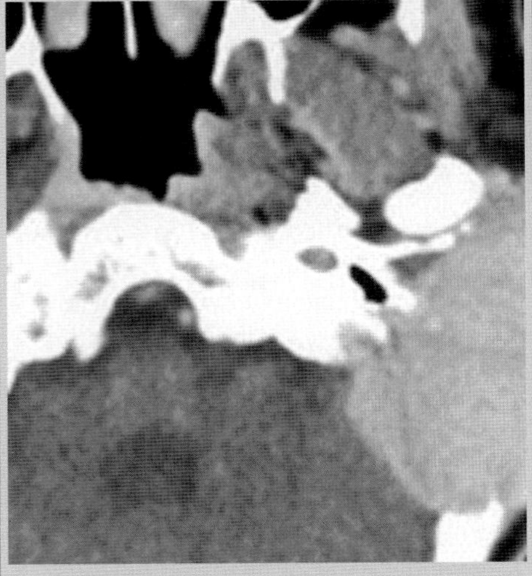 **Fig. 4.78.9:** Metastasis

Labyrinthine is a petrous part of temporal bone.

CECT-intense enhancement. **MRI**-T1 hyperintense in 80 percent cases. T2 is mixed hypo and hyperintense. ESLTs can be heterogeneous mass with a hyperintense foci in T1 and T2 sequences due to blood products, proteinaceous cysts or cholesterol clefts. Vessels and calcifications can also show signal voids. Contrast enhancement reveals the tumor's hypervascular character, and inhomogeneity may be related to the solid portion's enhancement.

Grading of endolymphatic sac tumor. Grade I: Confined to temporal bone and middle ear with or without EAC involvement. Grade II: Posterior cranial fossa extension. Grade III: Posterior and middle cranial fossa extension. Grade IV: Clival extension

Bilateral endolymphatic sac tumor—think of von Hippel-Lindau disease.

Tullio phenomenon is the precipitation of vertigo and nystagmus on hearing loud noise occurring in superior semicircular canal dehiscence syndrome, Ménière's syndrome, perilymphatic fistula, congenital syphilis, post-fenestration surgery (if the footplate is mobile).

4.79 HEAD AND NECK

Case No. 79

Clinical history: A 35-year-old male patient with headache and dizziness for 1 year.

Radiological techniques and observations: Figures 4.79.1 and 4.79.2 are axial and coronal non-contrast CT of head showing well-defined, expansile lytic lesion of left petrous apex with thin rim of cortex. No evidence of calcification/hemorrhage/air-fluid level noted inside the lesion. There is no specific matrix within the lesion. Bilateral mastoid air cells appear pneumatized without any fluid density. Visualized portion of middle ear appears normal. Further imaging work-up with MRI is essential to characterize the lesion.

Figures 4.79.3 to 4.79.6 are axial T2WI, coronal FLAIR, axial T1 fat sat, T1+C MR images respectively. Well-defined homogeneous T2/FLAIR hyperintense lesion in left petrous apex region. The lesion is hyperintense on T1. Post-contrast T1WI image demonstrates no appreciable internal enhancement. There is no adjacent otic capsule and carotid canal involvement. The mastoid air cells appear normal without any hyperintensity on T2WI. The visualized cerebellum and brainstem appear normal. There is no flow void within the lesion. There is no dural tail seen post-contrast.

Interpretation: A—35 years old male left petrous apex, C— well-defined homogeneous T1 fat sat hyperintense lesion (possibly due to hemorrhage with lesion), B—no dural tail, no diffusion restriction, mastoid air cells appear normal, D—cholesterol granuloma.

Principal diagnosis: **Cholesterol granuloma of right petrous apex.**

Differential diagnosis: Petrous apex congenital cholesteatoma, apical petrositis with abscess formation, petrous apex meningioma, petrous apex cephalocele.

Management: Referral to head and neck surgeon. asymptomatic patients can be safely followed with imaging. Traditional surgical treatment—drainage and stent placement to re-establish petrous apex aeration via transtemporal approach—fluid described "crankcase oil". Reported recurrence rate is about 60%. Extended middle cranial fossa approach. Selective trans-sphenoidal endoscopic drainage.

Brief discussion on cholesterol granuloma: **Clinical features:** Cholesterol granulomas occur in young to middle-age adults and presents as an incidental, asymptomatic lesion. Facial pain, hearing loss, or diplopia can occur if CNV-VIII involved. Audiometric exam: Sensorineural hearing loss or mixed pattern.

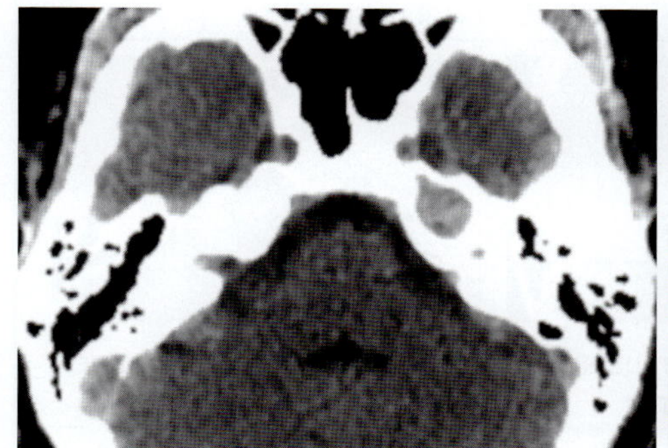

Fig. 4.79.1

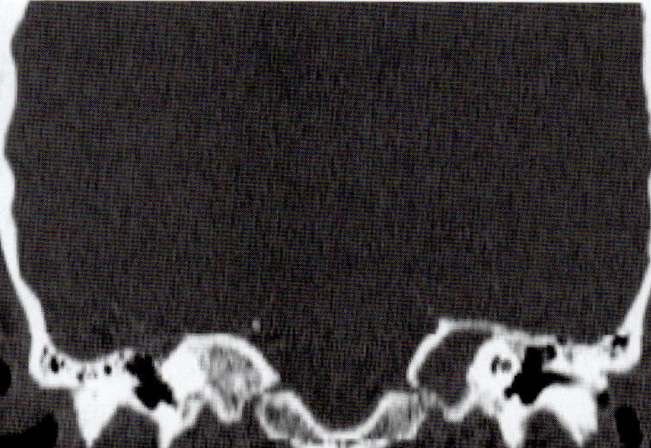

Fig. 4.79.2

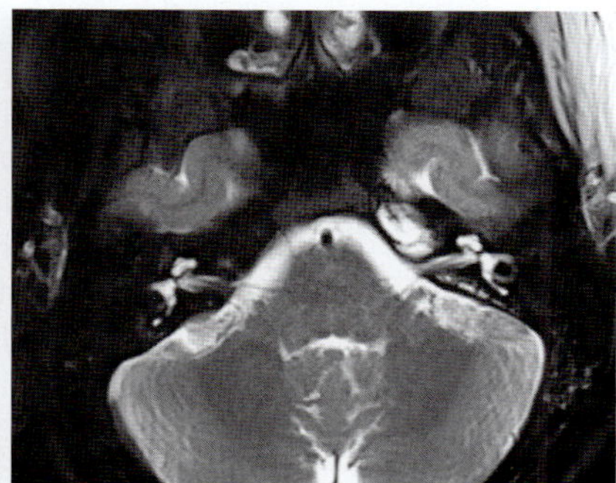

Fig. 4.79.3

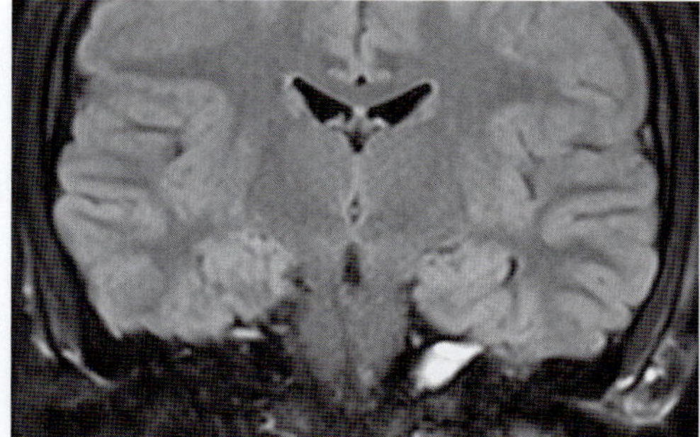

Fig. 4.79.4

Fig. 4.79.5

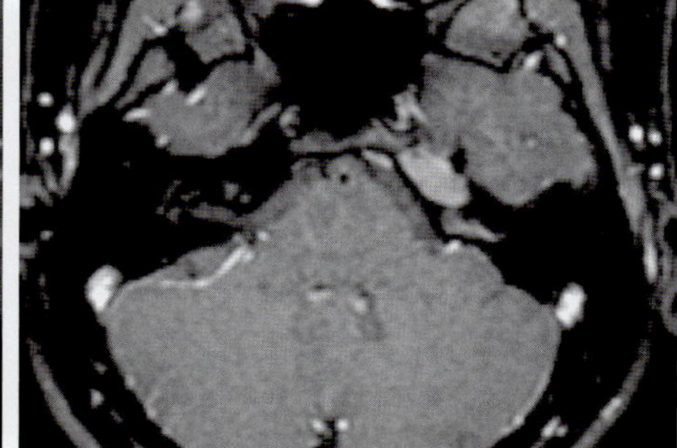

Fig. 4.79.6

Discussion:

Table 4.79.1: Differential diagnosis for petrous apex lesion

Petrous apex congenital cholesteatoma/epidermoid cyst: Rests of epithelial tissue of embryonal origin. Locations—middle ear > CPA > mastoid > petrous apex > facial nerve canal	CT: Smooth, expansile margins T1 MR: Low to intermediate signal; T2 MR: Intermediate to high signal. DWI: Restricted diffusion (high signal).	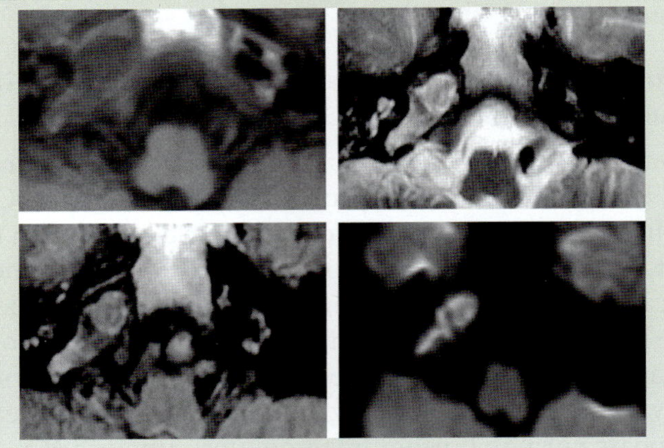 **Fig. 4.79.7:** Epidermoid cyst
Apical petrositis: Extension of middle ear-mastoid infection into pneumatized petrous apex with resulting suppuration.	CT: Permeative, destructive changes of bone; T1 MR: Low signal; T2 MR: High signal; T1 C+ MR: Thick, enhancing rim around fluid; enhancing right mastoid air cells. DWI: Shows restriction. It is associated with ear discharge **sixth nerve palsy** at **Dorello's canal,** causing retro-orbital pain and V2 division at Meckel's cave **(Gradenigo syndrome).**	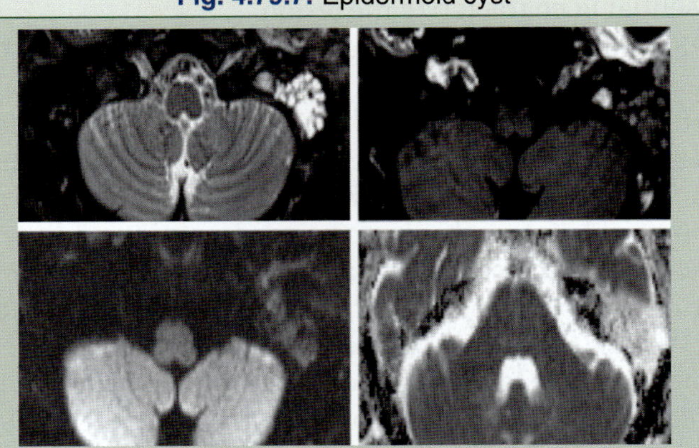 **Fig. 4.79.8:** Apical petrositis
Petrous apex meningioma: Most common extra-axial tumor. M : F = 1:2 to 1:4. Petrous apex is a less common location.	NECT shows a hyperdense lesion noted in the left petrous apex with a few calcifications and hypodensity in the adjacent pons. Contrast-enhanced MR image will show avid enhancement. Dural tail with associated hyperostosis may be seen.	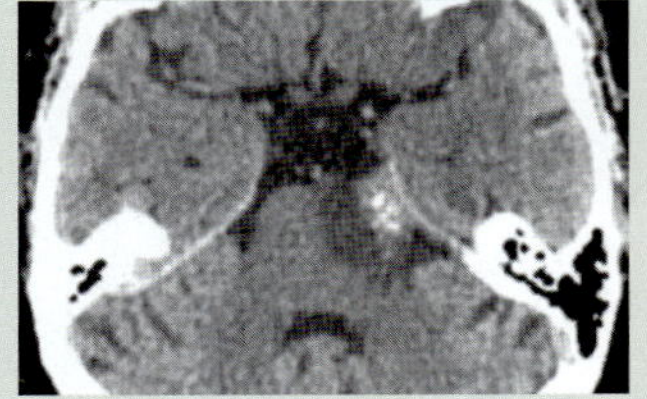 **Fig. 4.79.9:** Petrous apex meningioma 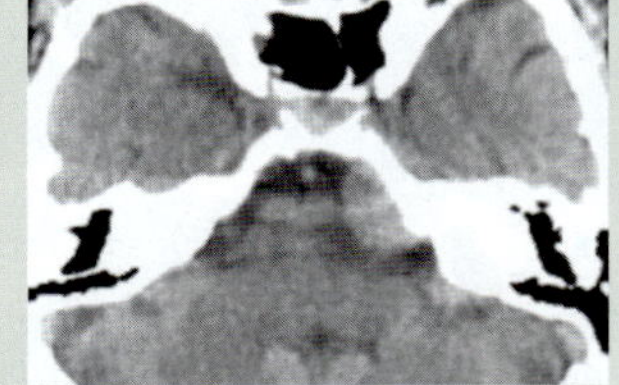 **Fig. 4.79.10:** Petrous apex meningioma
Petrous apex cephalocele/petrous apex arachnoid cyst/trapped CSF: Congenital or acquired herniation of posterolateral wall of Meckel cave (MC) into petrous apex. **CT:** Homogeneously low-density area is noted in the petrous apex with sharply defined margins. **MR:** The signal intensities follow that of CSF, **T2:** Hyperintense, **FLAIR:** Typical CSF suppression.		
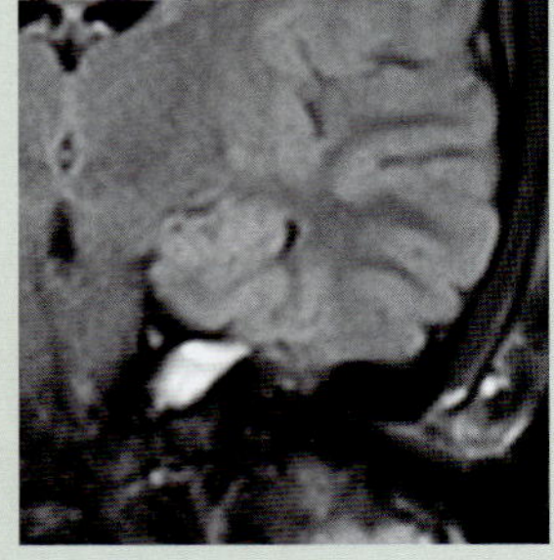 **Fig. 4.79.11:** Petrous apex cephalocele	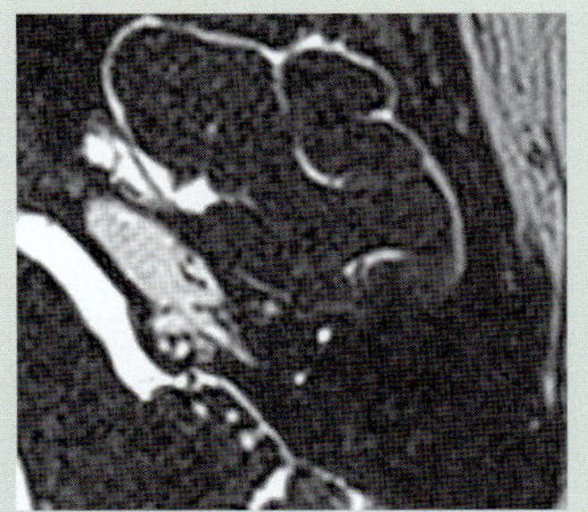 **Fig. 4.79.12:** Petrous apex cephalocele	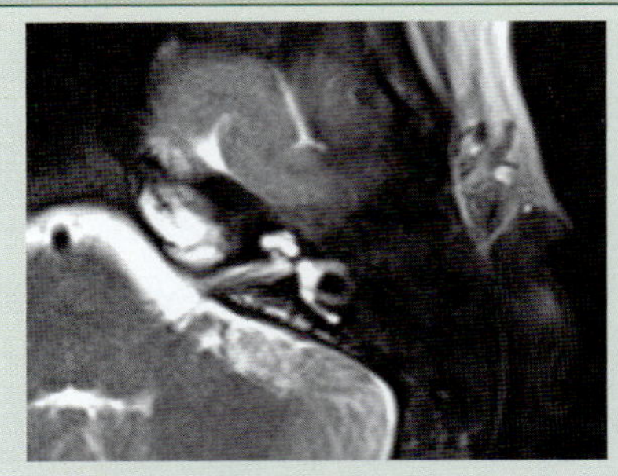 **Fig. 4.79.13:** Petrous apex cephalocele

(Contd.)

Table 4.79.1: Differential diagnosis for petrous apex lesion (*Contd.*)		
Schwannoma seen in petrous apex		
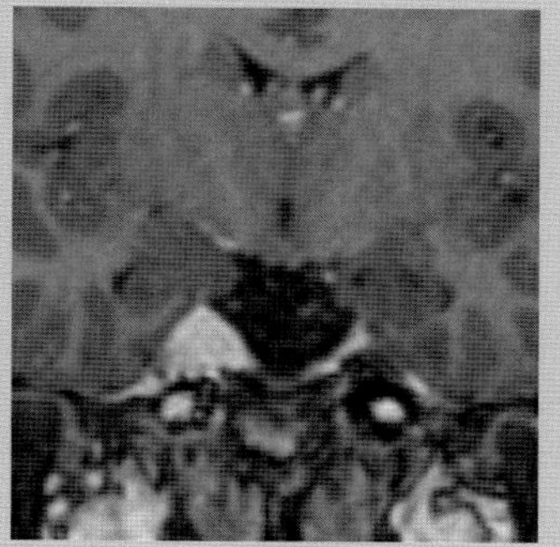 Fig. 4.79.14: Schwannoma seen in petrous apex	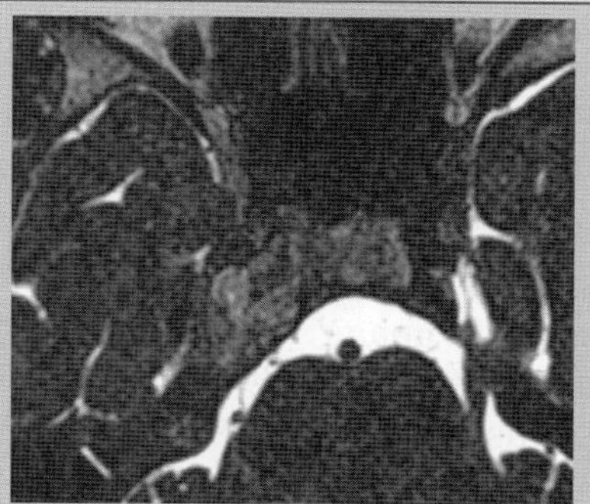 Fig. 4.79.15: Schwannoma seen in petrous apex	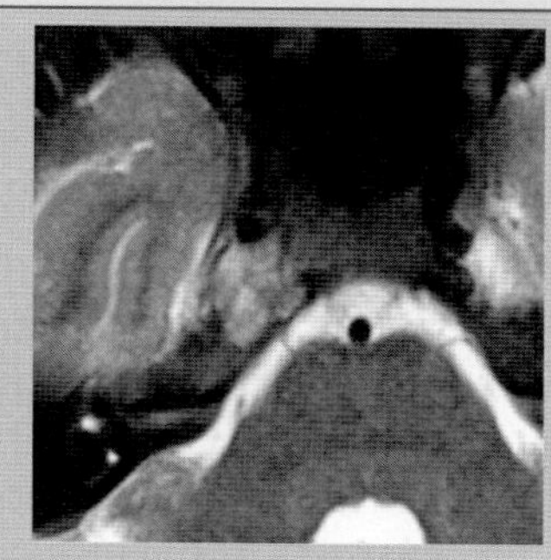 Fig. 4.79.16: Schwannoma seen in petrous apex

Table 4.79.2: Imaging features of petrous apex lesions

Petrous apex lesions	*Imaging characteristics*
Developmental lesions	
Cholesteatoma	Restricted diffusion in DWI
Inflammatory lesions	
Cholesterol granuloma	Increased signal intensity on both T1WI and T2WI
Petrous apicitis	Fluid in petrous apex, enhancing rim on contrast
Osteomyelitis	Bone erosion
Benign tumors	
Meningioma	Dural based, avidly enhancing, hyperostosis
Trigeminal schwannoma	Smooth expansile remodelling of bone
Paraganglioma	Salt-and-pepper appearance at MR imaging, permeative bone changes
Chondroma	Chondroid matrix, calcification
Malignant tumors	
Chondrosarcoma	Chondroid matrix, calcification, destruction Honeycomb enhancement
Chordoma	Bone destruction
Metastasis	Lytic lesion with non-sclerotic margin;
Plasmacytoma	T1 hypo/T2 intermediate or hyperintense
LCH	Lytic lesion
Vascular lesions	
Petrous carotid aneurysm	Continuity with ICA in CTA/MRA with flow voids +/– mural thrombus
Intraosseous dural arteriovenous fistula	Multiple intraosseous flow voids
Osseous dysplasias	
Fibrous dysplasia	Ground-glass matrix calcification
Paget disease	Diffuse bone thickening with lysis (early), sclerosis(late) or mixed density
Pseudo-lesions	
Asymmetric marrow	Fat signal intensity with all sequences
Trapped fluid/effusion	T2 hyperintense, T1 variable based on protein content
Cephalocele	CSF signal intensity with all sequences

Pathogenesis: Obstruction—vacuum theory—otitis media creates mucosal obstruction of pneumatized petrous apex causing development of vacuum which leads to rupture of blood vessels and hemorrhage in petrous apex air cells. Anaerobic degradation of red blood cells forms cholesterol crystals, which incite foreign body granuloma.

Imaging: On non-contrast CT, the lesions are well defined and smoothly expansile. Faint peripheral enhancement may be present on CECT. Bony destruction and involvement of the otic capsule and carotid canal can be evaluated using a CT scan. Cholesterol granulomas are distinguished from cholesteatomas by their brilliant appearance on all spin-echo sequences. MRA helps in surgical planning, such as determining if the petrous ICA should be encased. When it comes to detecting recurrence, MR is more sensitive than CT. T1 signal increases in the post-operative petrous apex, indicating recurrence.

Table 4.79.3: Diagnostic pearls for petrous apex lesions

Fluid within petrous apex	Apical petrositis/cephalocele
Bony erosion + restricted diffusion	Congenital cholesteatoma
No diffusion restriction + T1 hyperintense	Cholesterol granuloma
Dural tail + intense enhancement	Meningioma
Well-circumscribed lytic lesion in a child	Eosinophilic granuloma
Aggressive appearing, irregular	Metastasis/myeloma
Aggressive appearing with calcification, T2 hyperintense	Chondrosarcoma/chordoma

4.80 HEAD AND NECK

Case No. 80

Clinical history: A 29-year-old female with history of swelling in the preauricular region for 7 months.

Radiological techniques and observations: Figure 4.80.1 is orthopantogram and Figures 4.80.2 to 4.80.4 are CT axial, coronal images of mandible. OPG image showing well-defined large (>3 cm) lobulated expansile lytic lesion in the posterior body and ramus of right mandible. Margins of the lesion is smooth, not sclerotic. Focal discontinuity in the superior aspect of the lesion. No evidence of any periosteal reaction, extension into surrounding soft tissues. No evidence of any soft tissue calcification, septations. No evidence of impacted tooth. The lesion is not related to crown of unerupted tooth.

Axial bone algorithm and coronal reformatted image in bone and soft tissue algorithm shows well-circumscribed, expansile-buccolingual expansion, lytic lesion without septations in the posterior body and ramus of right side of mandible. Significant cortical thinning and remodelling are seen in lingual cortex. There are cortical defects on both buccal and lingual aspects of right-side mandible.

No soft tissue component/calcifications noted.

Interpretation: A—29 years old female, lesion in posterior body and ramus of right side of mandible, C—lobulated lytic lesion with, B—buccolingual expansion, cortical thinning and defects, D—unicystic ameloblastoma

Principal diagnosis: Unicystic ameloblastoma.

Further investigation and management: Biopsy and histopathological examination to confirm the diagnosis.

Treatment: surgical en-bloc resection. Local curettage has high rate of local recurrence (up to 90%).

Discussion: Ameloblastomas have a mixed solid and cystic pattern on MRI, with a thick uneven wall and solid papillary features protruding into the lesion. These components tend to show intense enhancement making it easy to distinguish them from other lucent mandibular tumors. Multicystic ameloblastomas account for 80–90 percent of cases with well-defined borders and no matrix calcification, which are characteristic expansile soap bubble lesions with well-defined boundaries and no matrix calcification. Resorption of neighbouring teeth and "root blunting" are common occurrences. It may also erode through the cortex and into neighbouring soft tissues as it grows larger. Unicystic ameloblastomas are well-defined unilocular tumors that are frequently found pericoronally. These are most typically found in the back of the mandible, especially near the molars. On CT, they are indistinguishable from cysts, ameloblastic keratocysts, and odontogenic keratocysts, which are all unilocular pericoronal lesions. MRI: Ameloblastomas have a mixed solid and cystic pattern on MRI.

Approach to jaw lesions unilocular well-defined lesion—benign slow growing, multilocular well-defined lesions—benign, but more aggressive, ill-defined lesions—malignant/inflammatory, cortical expansion and bowing–benign, Widened inferior alveolar canal with preserved cortical margin—benign, displacement of teeth–benign, resorption of teeth—benign and malignant; malignant process is indicated by cortical destruction periosteal reaction, associated soft tissue involvement, widening and destruction of lamina dura.

The name lamina dura (or alveolus) is applied to the thin layer of dense cortical bone (the so–called cribriform plate or alveolar bone proper) which lines the normal tooth socket. Lamina dura erosion causes A) focal erosion–inflammatory peri-apical disease, peri-apical granuloma, radicular cyst, simple bone cyst, peri-apical cemental dysplasia, osteomyelitis, B) Generalised—idiopathic, Paget disease of bone, leukemia, metastasis (breast CA).

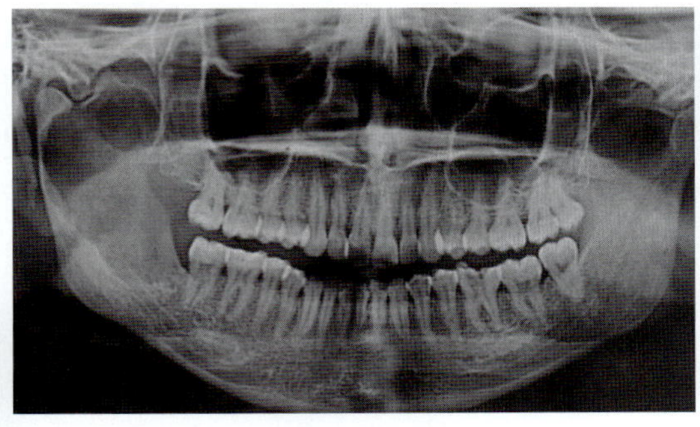

Fig. 4.80.1

Fig. 4.80.2

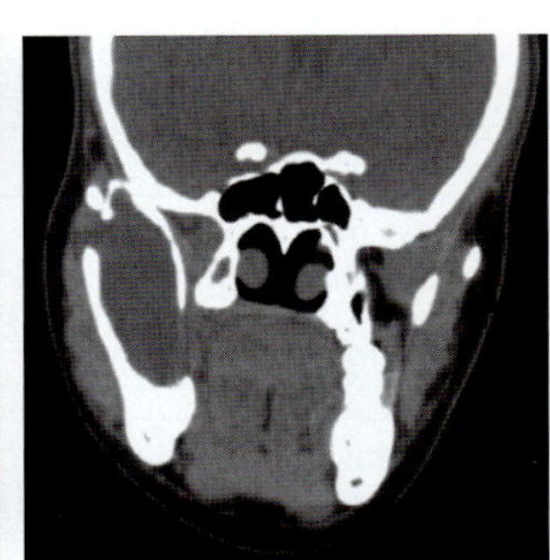

Fig. 4.80.3

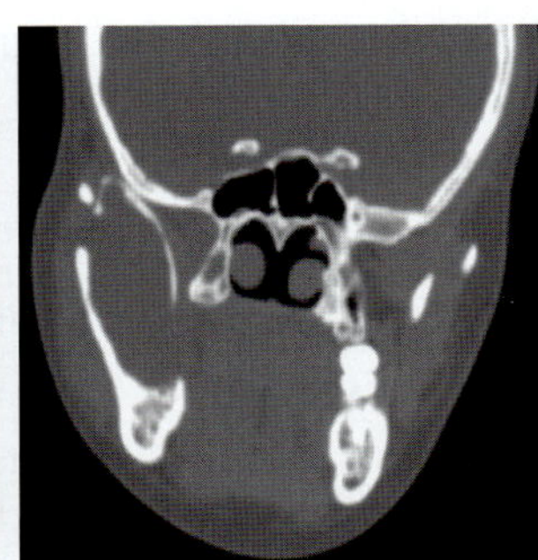

Fig. 4.80.4

Table 4.80.1: Differential diagnosis for mandibular unilocular cystic/lytic lesions

Condition	*Imaging features*	
Odontogenic keratocyst Benign cystic lesions arising from dental lamina common in younger patients (2nd–3rd decades) and may be seen in either the body/ramus of the mandible (~70%) presents as jaw swelling and painful. Treatment marsupialisation/enucleation/excision. High recurrence rate up to 60%, so follow-up should be done. Gorlin syndrome characterized by multiple odontogenic keratocyst and basal cell carcinoma.	**OPG and CT** (axial image bone algorithm): Single, radiolucent, unilocular expansile lesion with smooth, corticated borders, typically scalloped around tooth roots. The posterior mandible accounts for three-quarters of all lesions, which normally extend down the length of the bone with buccolingual growth. They grow into the maxillary sinus in the maxilla. They are about 3 cm usually.	**T1W—hyperintense** due to cholesterol and keratin contents **T2W:** Heterogeneous **DWI:** Diffusion restriction (due to keratin content) **T1+ C:** Peripheral enhancement and no enhancing components within. 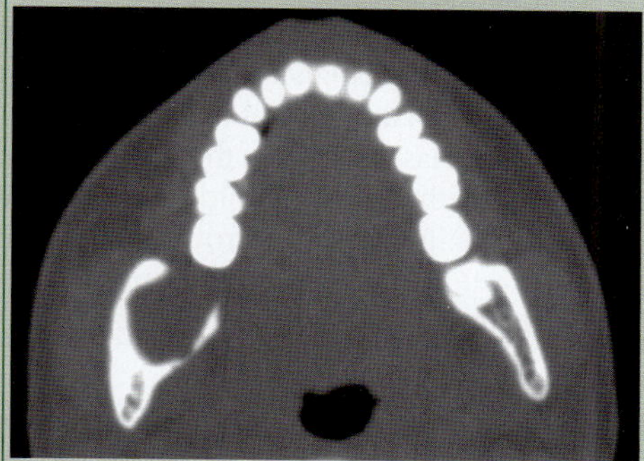 **Fig. 4.80.5:** Odontogenic keratocyst
Dentigerous cyst Second most common odontogenic cysts. Present 10 to 40 years of age as painless lesion. They exclusively occur in secondary dentition Treatment: Removal of the entire cyst/marsupialisation	OPG and CT (axial image bone algorithm) A cystic expansile pericoronal lesion containing the crown of an impacted tooth projecting into cystic cavity is considered pathognomonic and often no further imaging is required MRI T1: Low signal, similar to water/CSF T2: High signal, similar to water/CSF; T1 C+ (Gd): no solid component or enhancement, except for potentially a thin peripheral rim of enhancement	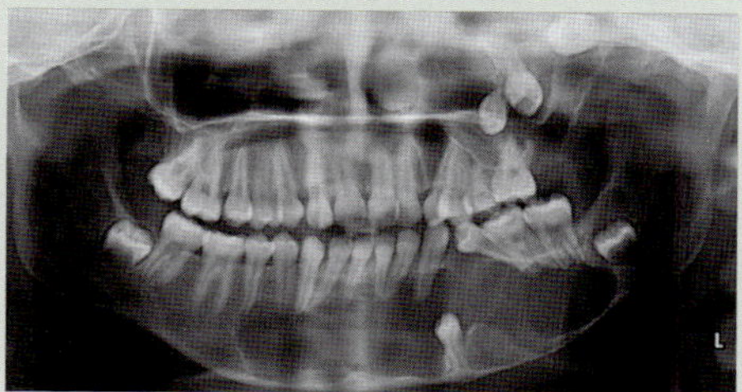 **Fig. 4.80.6:** Dentigerous cyst
Radicular cysts Most frequent lesions and result from infection of tooth. Common in Middle to older age group Enucleation and curettage is the treatment.	OPG and CT (axial image bone algorithm) Most round- or pear-shaped, unilocular, lucent lesions in the periapical region. They are <1 cm in diameter with thin cortical bone rim. The linked tooth has carious lesion or a deep restoration. Caries manifests itself as deterioration of the related tooth's enamel/crown. Although periapical cysts appear as a non-enhancing lesion near the apex of a tooth, MRI is not the first-line imaging modality. These cysts usually have a low T1 signal and a high T2.	
Odontogenic myxomas Typically seen in the 10 to 30 years of age (earlier than ameloblastomas). They are usually not painful. Arises from mesenchymal odontogenic tissue. Treatment and prognosis Wide marginal excision	The radiographic appearance is remarkably similar to that of an ameloblastoma: A lytic septated cystic lesion of the mandible/maxilla that has soap bubble appearance. When compared to ameloblastoma, myxomatous matrix resulted in higher HU on CT and low T2 signal intensity.	
Floating tooth are teeth that have lost their alveolar bone support due to a destructive process involving the mandible or maxillary alveolar ridge. Causes include severe periodontal disease, hyperparathyroidism, metastases, multiple myeloma, ameloblastoma, osteomyelitis, lymphoma, eosinophilic granuloma, cherubism, Gorham disease, LCH.	Loss of alveolar bone, lamina dura loss, and, in the event of unerupted teeth, loss of the dental follicle are all radiographic manifestations. Resorption of the root tips of the affected teeth is a possible. The tooth will eventually be lifted and displaced from neighbouring teeth, giving it the appearance of dangling or floating in soft tissue with no bone support on radiography. A single tooth, a group of teeth, or the entire dental arch, including erupted or non-erupted deciduous or permanent teeth, may be destroyed.	

Table 4.80.2: Key points about ameloblastoma

Ameloblastoma is the second most frequent odontogenic tumor and most common lucent lesion (odontoma is the overall most common odontogenic tumor), accounting for up to 1/3rd of all cases. They are slow-growing and appear in the third to fifth decades of life, with no sex predilection. They are hard, painless lesions that usually appear in the angle of the jaw, near the 3rd molar tooth, however, they can occur anywhere along the alveolus of the mandible (80%) and maxilla (20 percent). The tumor is found in the premolar region of the maxilla and can expand up into the maxillary sinus when the maxilla is affected. It is a locally aggressive neoplasm. Despite being benign, it has higher reoccurrence rate. Dentigerous cysts and unerupted teeth are present in around 20% of patients. Pathology ameloblastomas are tumors that develop from ameloblasts, which are cells in the odontogenic epithelium that produce enamel and eventually form the crown. Unicystic, solid (multicystic), desmoplastic, and peripheral forms (extraosseous) have all been documented in the literature.	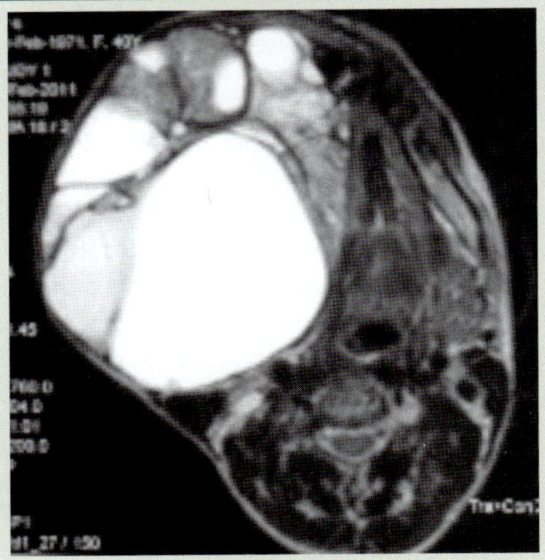 Fig. 4.80.7: Ameloblastoma

Table 4.80.3: Cystic lesions of mandible

Odontogenic	*Nonodontogenic*
Inflammatory • Periapical cyst and granuloma development • Primordial cyst • Dentigerous cyst • Lateral periodontal cyst • Odontogenic keratocyst • Calcifying odontogenic cyst	• Nasopalatine or incisive canal cyst • Globulomaxillary cyst • Traumatic bone cyst • Stafne cyst • Hematopoietic bone marrow defect

Table 4.80.4: Approach to jaw lesion

Well-circumscribed radiolucent	*Poorly-circumscribed radiolucent*	*Radiopaque/sclerotic*	*Mixed density*
Periapical cyst	Acute osteomyelitis	Odontoma	Fibrous dysplasia
Dentigerous cyst	Primary bone neoplasm	Torus	Ossifying fibroma
Odontogenic keratocyst	Direct tumor extension	Osteoma cementoma	Osseous dysplasia
Ameloblastoma	Lytic metastasis	Osteochondroma	Chronic osteomyelitis
Simple bone cyst		Cementoblastoma	Osteosarcoma
Incisive canal cyst		Fibrous dysplasia (late)	Metastasis
Central giant cell granuloma			

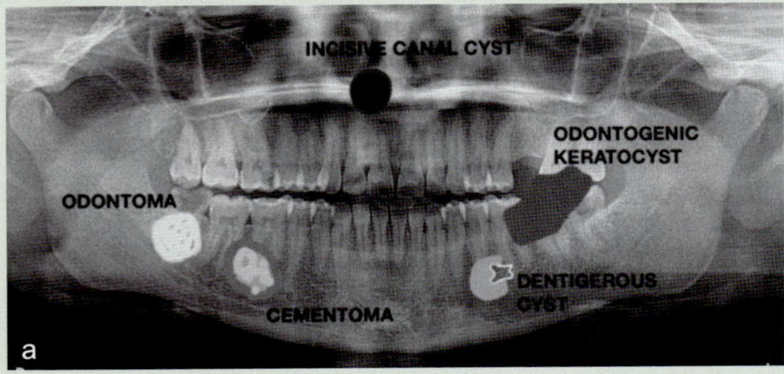

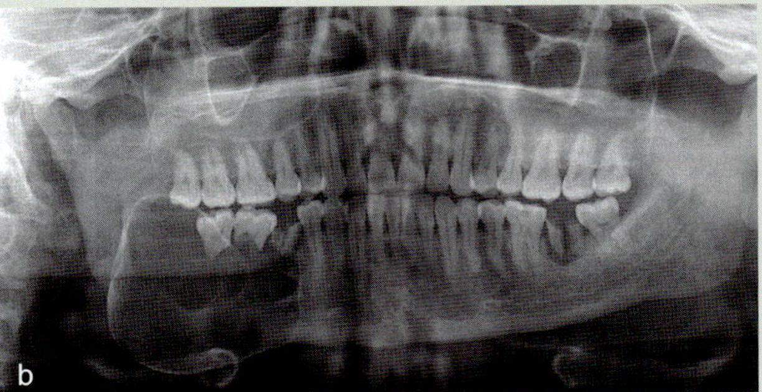

Fig. 4.80.8: a. Approach to jaw lesions on OPG; b. Ameloblastoma

Table 4.80.5: Identification of radiolucent jaw lesions by location

Unilocular	*Multilocular*
Midline of maxilla superior to central	**Anterior to 1st and 2nd molar**
Incisors—incisive canal cyst	Central giant cell granuloma
Between maxillary lateral incisor and cuspid—globulomaxillary cyst	Aneurysmal bone cyst
Mid-palatal area—Mid -palatal fissural cyst	Simple bone cyst
Apex of non-vital teeth—periapical granuloma, periapical cyst	Brown tumor
Apex of vital teeth—immature cementoma	**Posterior involving ramus**
Crown of impacted teeth—dentigerous cyst	Ameloblastoma
Overlying mandibular canal—neurofibroma, neurilemmoma	Pindborg tumor
Inferior to mandibular canal in 2nd molar area—Stafne cyst	Odontogenic myxoma
Focal or noncontiguous multiple—myeloma, LCH, metastasis	Cherubism
	No site predilection
	Fibrous dysplasia
	Central hemangioma
	Odontogenic keratocyst of basal cell naevus syndrome

Table 4.80.6: Sclerotic lesions of the mandible

Type	*Lesion*
Tooth related	
Periapical	Cementoblastoma, cemento-osseous dysplasia, Condensing osteitis
Pericoronal	Odontoma
Nontooth related	
Nonexpansile	Idiopathic osteosclerosis
Expansile	Osteoma
Exophytic	Exostosis, tori

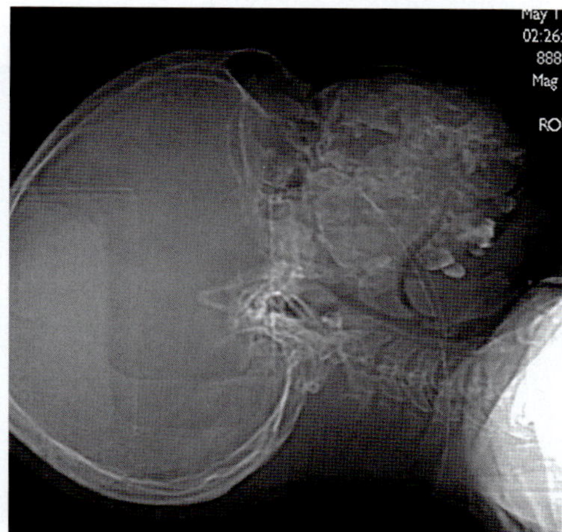

Fig. 4.80.10: Cherubism

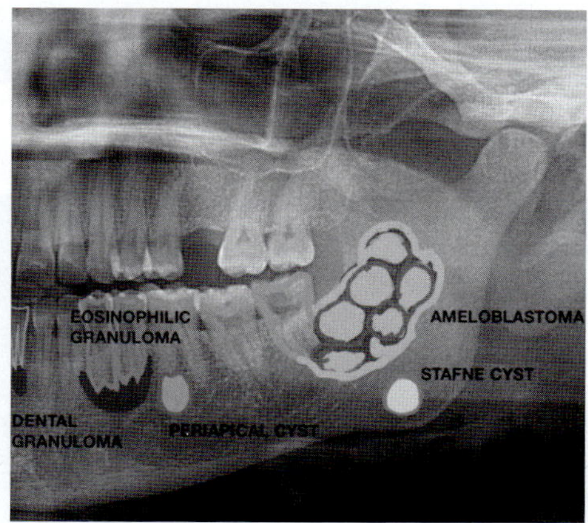

Fig. 4.80.9: Approach to jaw lesions on lateral mandible radiograph

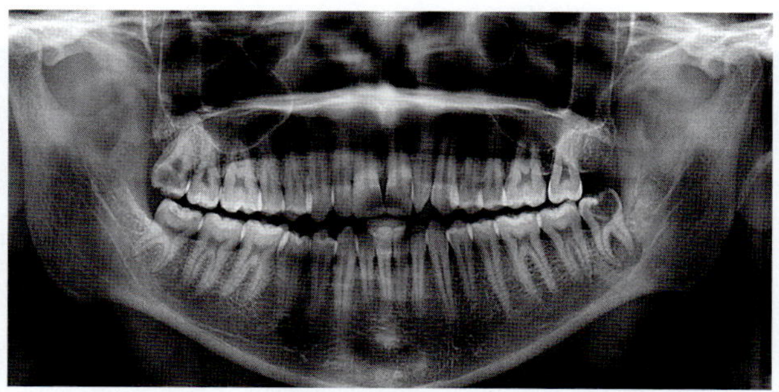

Fig. 4.80.11: Periapical cyst

4.81 HEAD AND NECK

Case No. 81

Clinical history: A 45-year-old male, with c/o right side facial pain

Radiological techniques and observations: Figures 4.81.1 to 4.81.9 are MRI PNS T1 axial and T1 post-gadolinium contrast axial and coronal images showing an ill-defined T1 isointense (to muscle) soft tissue mass lesion in the right nasopharyngeal cavity, which shows heterogeneous contrast enhancement. Tumor extends from the right nasopharyngeal cavity to the right pterygopalatine fossa. The tumor extends into the posterior right orbit via the right inferior orbital fissure. Visualised sections of bilateral frontal and temporal lobes and cerebellum appear normal, with no evidence of intracranial extension. Right mastoiditis noted. Bilateral maxillary sinuses appear normal. Retropharyngeal, parapharyngeal lymph nodes could not be visualised in the given images.

Interpretation: A—45 years old male, lesion in right nasopharyngeal cavity, C—ill-defined T1 isointense (to muscle) heterogeneous enhancing soft tissue mass lesion, B—extends to right pterygopalatine fossa, intraorbital extension, no intracranial extension, D—nasopharyngeal carcinoma.

Principal diagnosis: Nasopharyngeal carcinoma with intraorbital extension through inferior orbital fissure—perineural spread via infraorbital nerve—TNM staging IV-A.

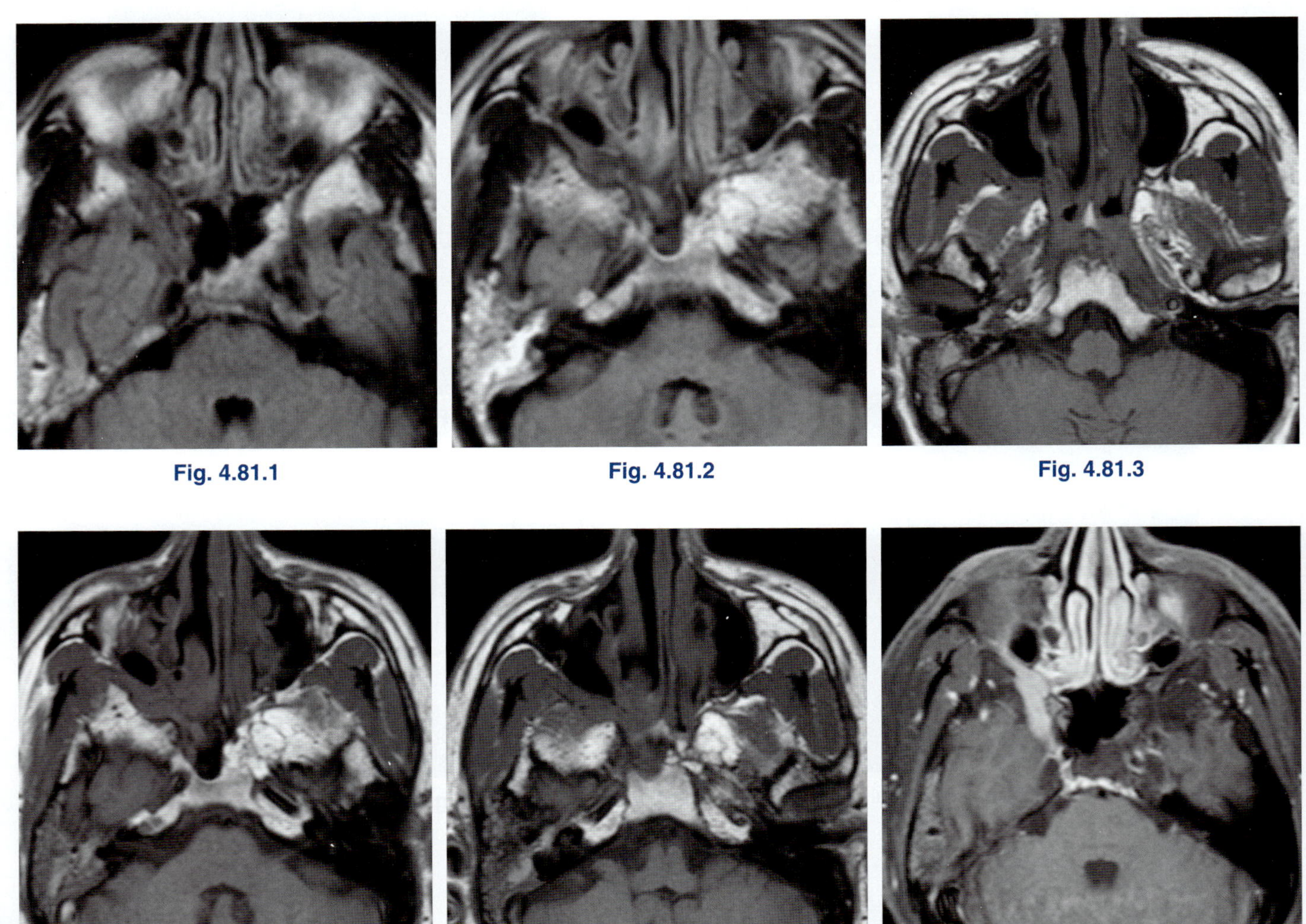

Fig. 4.81.1

Fig. 4.81.2

Fig. 4.81.3

Fig. 4.81.4

Fig. 4.81.5

Fig. 4.81.6

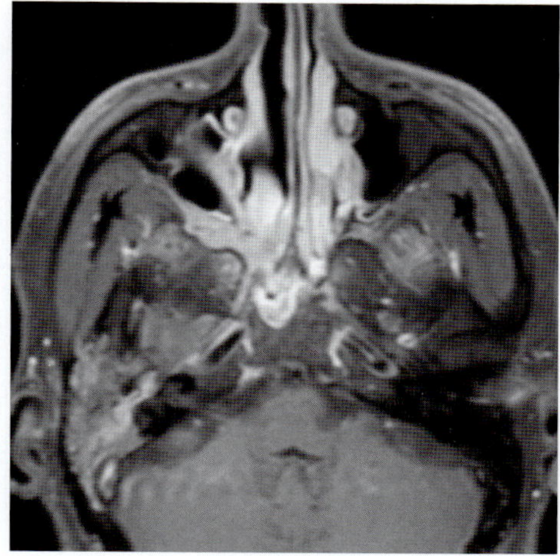
Fig. 4.81.7

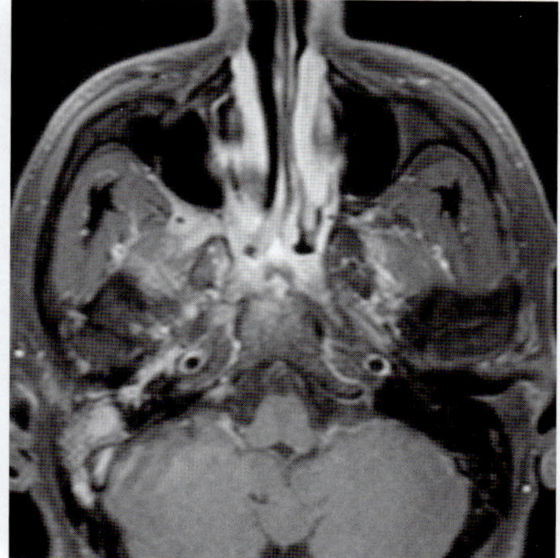
Fig. 4.81.8

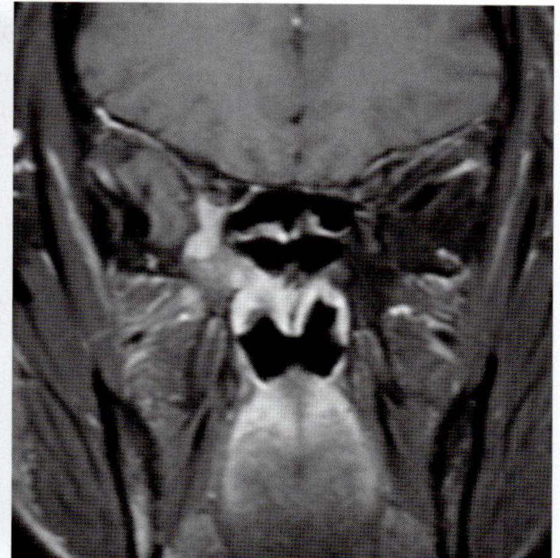
Fig. 4.81.9

Table 4.81.1: Differential diagnosis for nasopharyngeal mass		
Adenoid cystic carcinoma Malignant salivary type of adenocarcinoma. They have a notable tendency for **perineural spread**. They have a wide distribution and mainly occur in relation to the airways, lacrimal glands and breasts. Maxillary > nasal cavity.	Low grade: Solid enhancing, well-defined soft tissue mass. High grade: Poorly defined, heterogeneous + bone destruction ± perineural tumor spread (PNTS). On CT **chondroid matrix calcification** is seen. MRI with contrast and fat suppression is recommended.	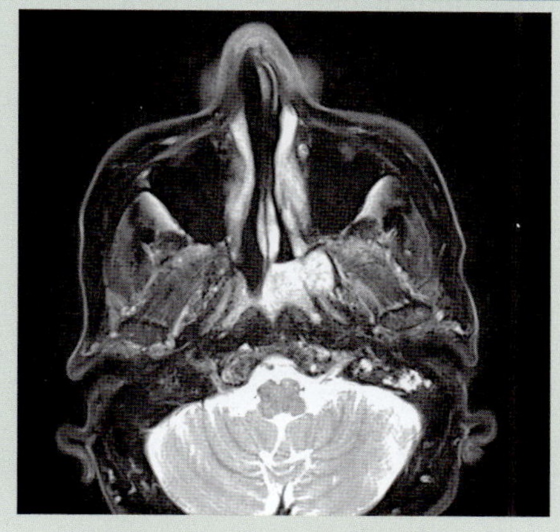 Fig. 4.81.10: Adenoid cystic carcinoma
Sinonasal lymphoma B-cell (Western) type: 6th decade T-cell (Asian) type: 7th decade Western form: M = F Asian form: M > F **B-cell type** can have slow, indolent course if left untreated Prognosis generally good with > 50% 5-year survival **Asian (T-cell) type** has much worse prognosis; can be rapidly fatal. Predilection for nasal cavity > sinuses.	Appearance can mimic variety of neoplasms and aggressive inflammatory disorders. CT shows homogeneous mass ± bone remodeling or destruction. Imaging modality of choice is MR with T1 C+ FS. Lesion is hypointense on T2, shows restricted diffusion due to high cellularity. PET for initial staging and treatment response.	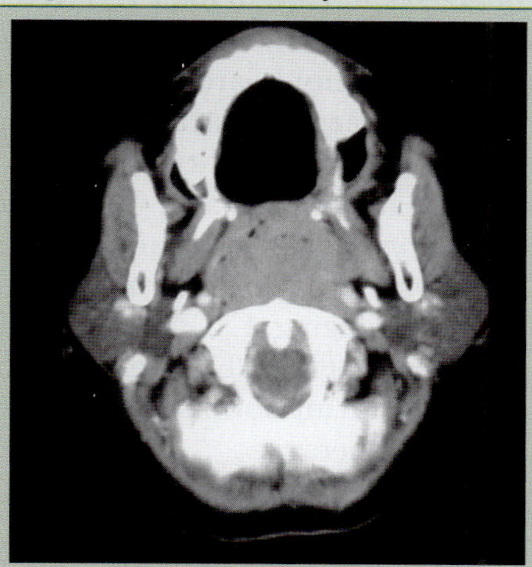 Fig. 4.81.11: Nasopharyngeal lymphoma
Juvenile nasopharyngeal angiofibroma: Refer to case 72		
Skull base osteomyelitis (SBO): Refer to case 71		

(Contd.)

Table 4.81.1: Differential diagnosis for nasopharyngeal mass (*Contd.*)

<table>
<tr><td>Inflammatory myofibroblastic tumor (IMT), Tolosa-Hunt syndrome (THS), and idiopathic hypertrophic pachymeningitis (IHP)-IMT/THS/IHP spectrum
Can occur at any age.
No gender predilection.
A trial of steroids may cause the mass to shrink and eliminate the need for a biopsy or surgery.</td><td>Irregular infiltrative mass-like lesion in the right parapharyngeal and carotid space. Lesion is hypo on T1, T2 and STIR. Leptomeningeal enhancement. Diffuse, linear, continuous, non-nodular continuous pachymeningeal thickening and enhancement in the right side of posterior fossa, tentorium.</td><td>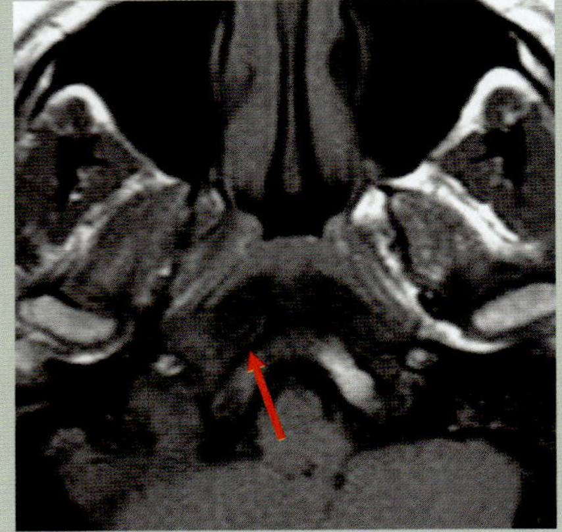
Fig. 4.81.12: Inflammatory myofibroblastic tumor</td></tr>
<tr><td colspan="3">Inverted papillomas are a type of Schneiderian papilloma, representing an uncommon non-cancerous sinonasal tumor that mostly affects middle-aged men. They occasionally undergo malignant transformation. On imaging, they classically demonstrate a convoluted cerebriform pattern seen on both T2 and contrast-enhanced T1 weighted MRI images.</td></tr>
<tr><td>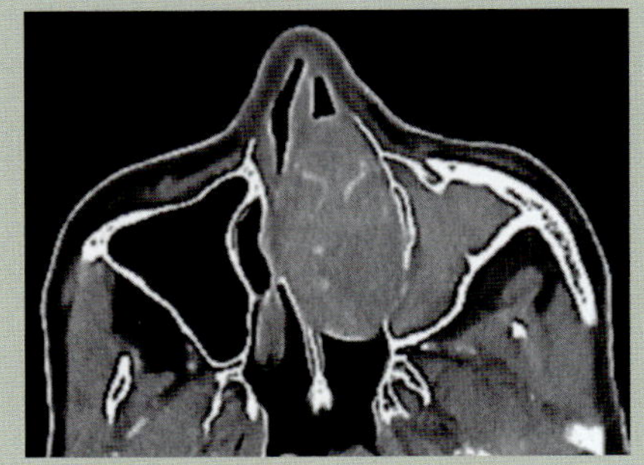
Fig. 4.81.13: Inverted papillomas</td><td>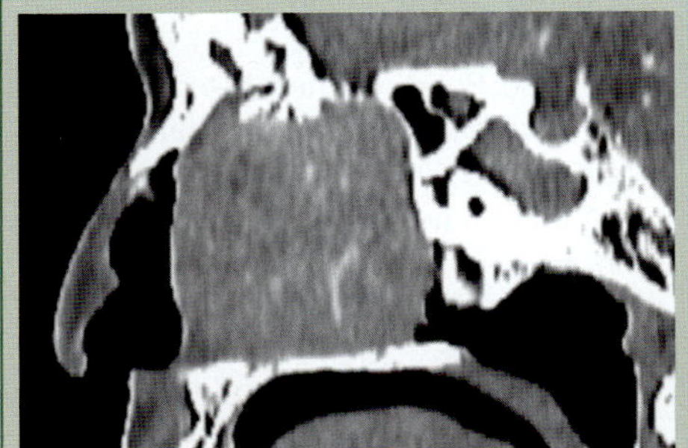
Fig. 4.81.14: Inverted papillomas</td><td>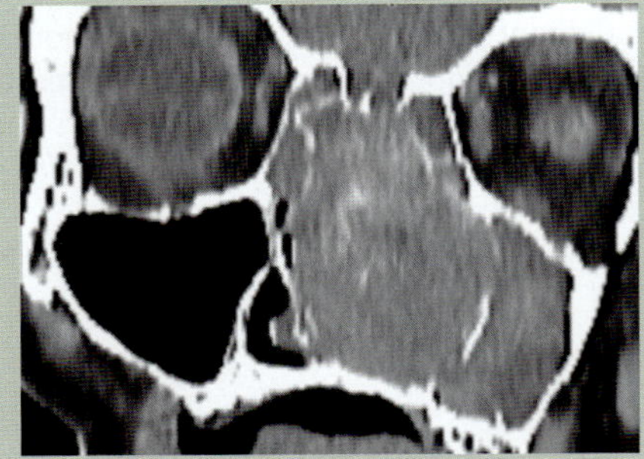
Fig. 4.81.15: Inverted papillomas</td></tr>
</table>

Management: **Patient to be referred immediately to the oncology department for further evaluation and to be posted for tumor board discussion for a multimodality approach based on the tumor staging**. MR with contrast is the imaging modality of choice and the following are to be looked for, as it determines the staging, viz. parapharyngeal fat infiltration (T2), skull base invasion (T3), intracranial or cranial nerve involvement (T4) and nodal staging. CT PNS to look for bony erosion or sclerosis. F-18 FDG-PET is sensitive for nodal metastases. Our case with intraorbital extension needs radiotherapy and chemotherapy.

Brief discussion about the condition: **Nasopharyngeal carcinoma** appear as soft tissue masses most commonly centred at the **fossa of Rosenmuller**. The pharyngobasilar fascia confines small lesions to the nasopharynx, making them unrecognisable from large adenoidal tissue and causing them to show as unknown secondary nodes. In cases of unilateral serous otitis media/mastoiditis, suspect it. Larger/aggressive tumors can erode the base of the skull and migrate through the Eustachian tube, foramen lacerum, or foramen ovale, or directly through the bone into the clivus, cavernous sinus, and temporal bone. The bone exhibits uneven borders where it has been damaged in some situations, which is typical of aggressive processes.

Because MRI is more sensitive to perineural dissemination and early identification of infiltration alterations in the bone marrow, a contrast MRI is required. On MRI, post-radiotherapy fibrosis can be separated from a recurring or persistent tumor. On T2, fibrotic scarring has a modest signal intensity and does not show amplification in these situations. Early fibrotic change is difficult to identify from a residual/recurrent tumor because both are hyperintense on T2 and show enhancement.

4.82 HEAD AND NECK

Case No. 82

Clinical history: A 7-year-old female child, with the history of swelling in the left upper eyelid.

Radiological techniques and observation: Figures 4.82.1 and 4.82.2 are frontal and lateral radiographs of skull show an **ill-defined lytic** lesion in the **superolateral margin of left orbit** extending to adjacent frontal bone. The lesion shows **narrow margin of transition**. No marginal sclerosis, no soft tissue component, no obvious bevelled margins in the skull, no specific periosteal reaction (sunburst), sella appears normal. **Rest of the skull appears normal**. Further imaging workup with USG ORBIT, CT ORBIT, MRI brain is essential to characterize the lesion, extension and intracranial spread.

Figures 4.82.3 and 4.82.4 are ultrasound images shows an ill-defined **heteroechoic lesion** noted in the superolateral region of left orbit with multiple internal hyperechoic areas possibly bony spicules/calcification and associated soft tissue component.

Figures 4.82.5 and 4.82.6 are CT orbit in bone and soft tissue window showing a lytic lesion noted involving the orbital plate of frontal bone forming the roof and zygomatic bone forming the lateral wall of orbit. The left lacrimal gland is not visualized separately and is replaced by an **ill-defined preseptal and extraconal soft tissue component**. Visualised globe appears normal.

Figure 4.82.7 **is MR T2 axial** image showing relatively heterointense lesion in the superolateral extraconal compartment in the lacrimal fossa **with extradural component** and **no intradural/intraparenchymal extension.** The brain parenchyma appears normal.

Interpretation: A—7-year-old female, superolateral margin of left orbit, B—extraconal and extradural soft tissue component, C—ill-defined lytic lesion, D—embryonal rhabdomyosarcoma.

Principal diagnosis: With these imaging findings possibilities include lacrimal gland tumor with bone involvement or primary bony lesion with extraconal soft tissue component. **Embryonal rhabdomyosarcoma**

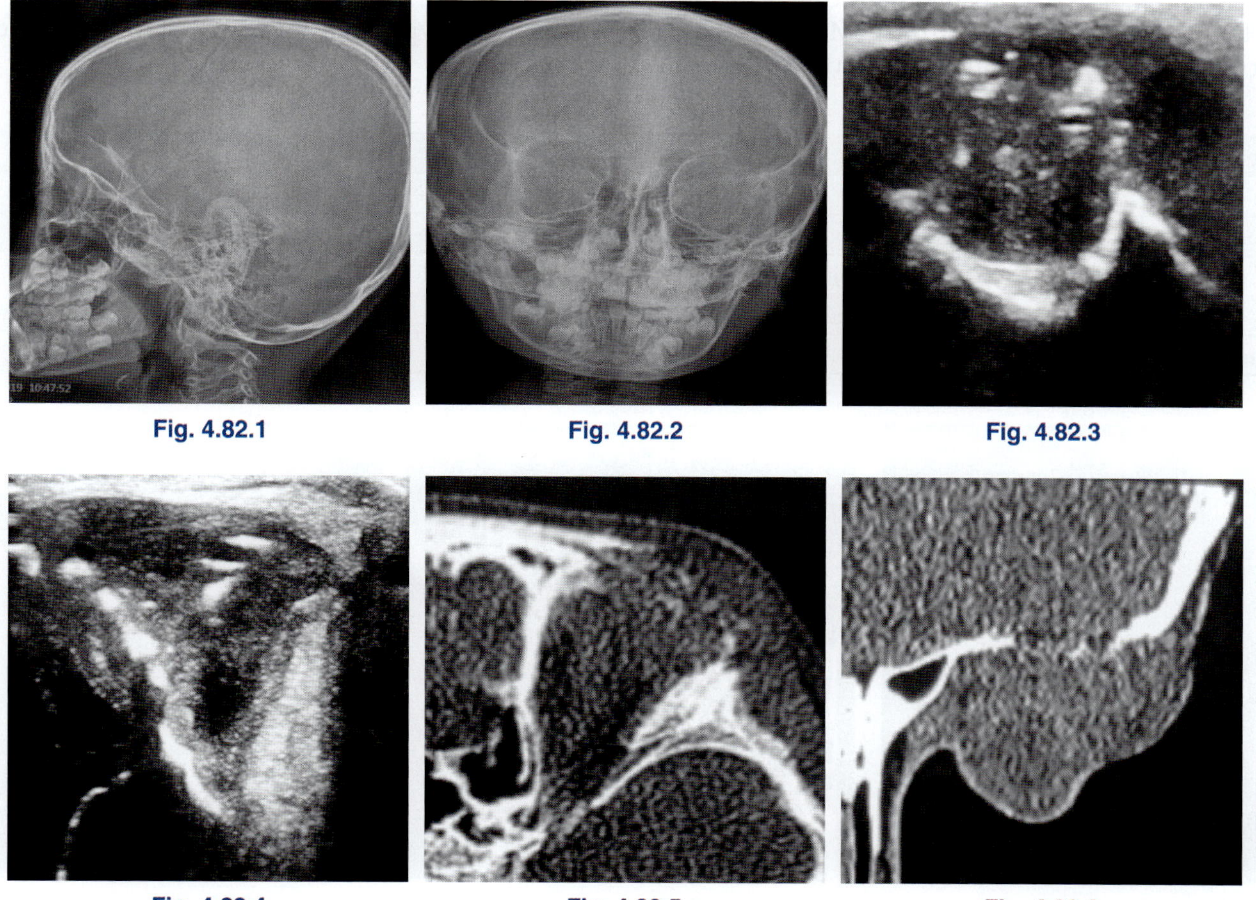

Fig. 4.82.1 Fig. 4.82.2 Fig. 4.82.3

Fig. 4.82.4 Fig. 4.82.5 Fig. 4.82.6

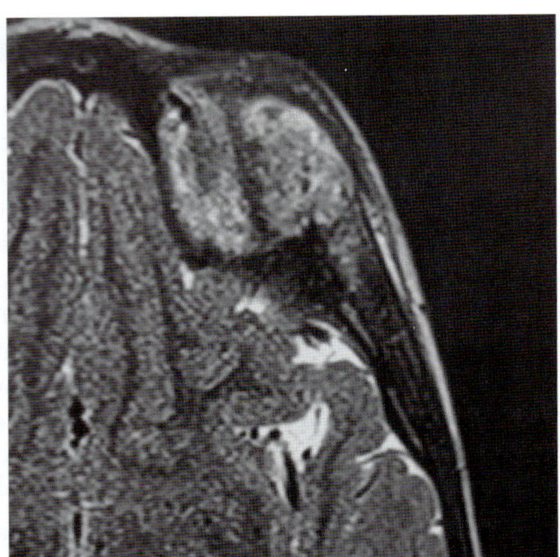

Fig. 4.82.7

could be the principal diagnosis (though common location is superomedial orbit). Malignant epithelial tumour of lacrimal gland will be the principal diagnosis in view of extensive bone destruction to be considered as a first possibility in adults with similar imaging findings.

Differential diagnosis: (1) Langerhans cell histiocytosis (LCH), (2) Neoplastic (children): Metastasis from neuroblastoma/leukemia/medulloblastoma/rhabdomyosarcoma/osteosarcoma/Ewing's sarcoma/retinoblastoma/hepatoma/clear cell sarcoma of kidney, (3) Benign: Epidermoid, dermoid, fibrous dysplasia, hemangioma, meningocele, (4) Traumatic: Leptomeningeal cysts, burr hole, (5) Normal: Venous lakes, vascular channels, pacchionian granulation, anterior and posterior fontanelles, prominent normal markings, (6) Infective: Complication of sinusitis, mastoiditis, TB, hydatid, syphilis (moth eaten), osteomyelitis.

Adults neoplastic (adult): Myeloma, mets (breast, lung, RCC, leukemia, prostate, thyroid), intra-diploic meningioma, lymphoma, sarcoma secondary to Paget's disease.

Management: USG guided biopsy was advised to decide on the course of management. Patient referred to general surgeon.

Discussion: **Orbital rhabdomyosarcoma:** Most common childhood soft tissue sarcoma, up to **40%** occurs in head and neck and **7%** of head and neck rhabdomyosarcoma occurs in temporal bone. Male predominance. Typically, in children **below 15 years** of age.

CECT: Variable contrast enhancement. MRI: T1: Low to intermediate intensity, isointense to adjacent muscle, T2: Usually hyperintense, T1+C: Shows considerable enhancement.

Table 4.82.1: Types of rhabdomyosarcoma

Type	Embryonal	Alveolar	Pleomorphic
Occurrence	Most common	2nd most common	Least common
Age	Younger children	15–25 years	40–60 years
Site	Head and neck, pelvis	Extremities	Extremities
Prognosis	Good	Worst	Poor

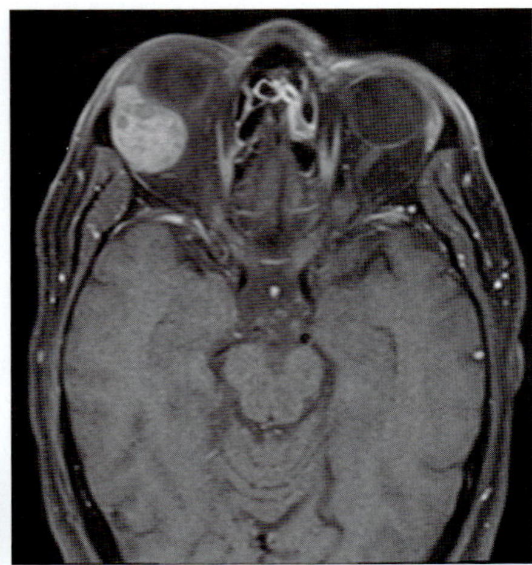

Fig. 4.82.8: Pleomorphic adenoma

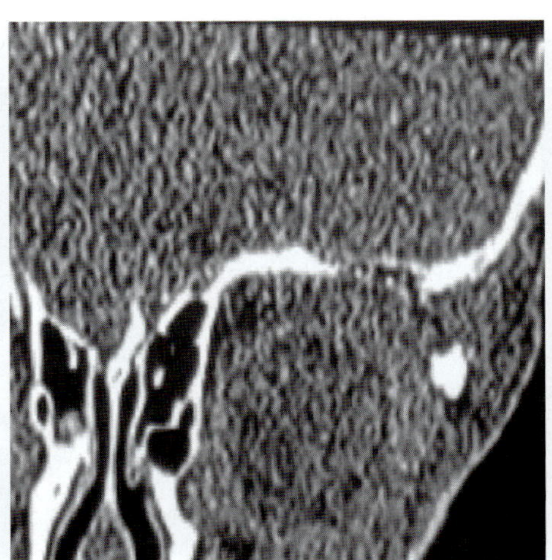

Fig. 4.82.9: Rhabdomyosarcoma

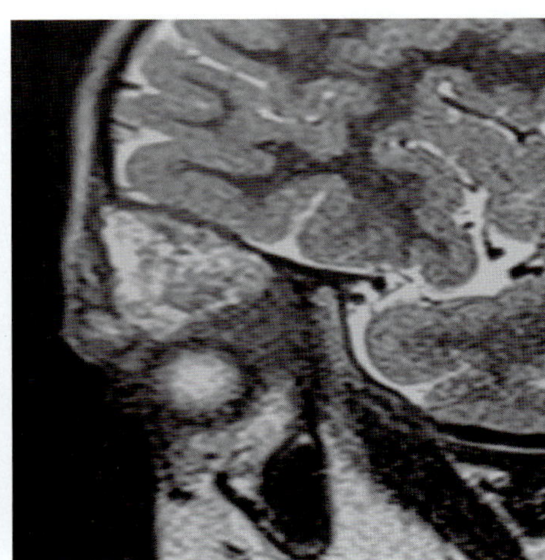

Fig. 4.82.10: Rhabdomyosarcoma

Table 4.82.2: Differential diagnosis for lacrimal gland lesions	
1. Metastasis: Unlike primary orbital tumors which most frequently present with proptosis and/or visual loss, orbital metastases most commonly present with diplopia. Pain is also frequently present. **Superior lateral extraconal quadrant is most frequently involved site.** Treatment is primarily with radiotherapy, typically with a total dose of 30–40 Gy. Depending on the tumor histology, chemotherapy may also be useful.	In most instances, soft tissue attenuating material is identified, located in the **extraconal compartment**. In general, enhancement is present. Bony destruction may also sometimes be seen. MRI-T1: Isointense to muscles. T2: Hyperintense to muscle, hypointense to fat. T1 C+ (Gd): Enhancement present but variable.
2. Mucoepidermoid CA: The **most common malignant salivary gland tumor of childhood.** In the parotid gland they are the most common malignant primary neoplasm. A slight female predilection has been described, and radiation has been implicated as a risk factor.	**Infiltrative lesion with bony scalloping** or destruction and occasional invasion into adjacent structures. Distant **metastases to the brain have been reported.** Low grade treated with wide local excision. High grade treated by excision and adjuvant radiotherapy.
3. Pleomorphic adenoma is the **most common benign epithelial tumor of the lacrimal gland.** Patients usually present between 20 and 40 years old with **unilateral and painless proptosis.** Treatment consists of complete surgical removal without rupture of the tumor capsule.	Slow growth of a pleomorphic adenoma often results in **smooth bony scalloping. Moderate contrast enhancement** is common, but calcification within the tumor is rare. On MRI, a pleomorphic adenoma appears as a unilateral orbital lobe mass that has low to intermediate signal compared with muscle on T1-weighted imaging and intermediate signal compared with brain cortex on T2-weighted imaging.
4. Adenoid cystic carcinoma: The **most common malignant lacrimal gland tumor** and it accounts for 50% of malignant tumors of lacrimal gland and 25% of all lacrimal gland tumors. Adenoid cystic carcinomas are generally considered low grade. The tumors have a notable tendency for perineural spread. The other sites that can be involved are: Salivary glands, nasopharynx, larynx, hard palate, eyelid, bronchial tree, trachea, lung, breast, cervix, Bartholin glands.	On CT, adenoid cystic carcinoma appears as a well-defined, homogeneous, and unilateral solid mass involving the **orbital lobe of the lacrimal gland**. There is typically associated bone destruction, and there may be calcifications within the lesion. The tumor may extend along **perineural pathways** (cranial nerve branches of V1 and V2) through the superior orbital fissure into the cavernous sinus. After contrast administration, the tumor usually shows diffuse enhancement. The combination of chemotherapy and radiation therapy is considered experimental.
5. Lymphoma: Primary lymphoma of the orbit is one of the commonest orbital tumors and accounts for as much as half of all orbital malignancies. Typically, patients are between 50 and 70 years of age, with no recognized gender predilection. It is a B-cell non-Hodgkin lymphoma, and in most cases arises from mucosa-associated lymphoid tissue (MALT).	Lymphoma is **isodense to muscle** and shows mild enhancement after contrast administration. There is **typically no infiltrative bone destruction**, although bone remodelling and/or sclerosis may be present. Surgical biopsy/resection, radiotherapy and chemotherapy have all been used.
6. Dacryoadenitis: It is infection of the lacrimal gland results in diffuse homogeneous enlargement, which can sometimes compress the globe. Most common organisms are ***Staphylococcus aureus***, mumps, infectious mononucleosis, and influenza virus. Treatment varies by etiology, as follows: Viral (most common)—self-limiting, supportive measures like warm compresses, oral nonsteroidal anti-inflammatories. Bacterial—initiate with first-generation cephalosporins.	On CT, there is unilateral involvement with diffuse enlargement of the lacrimal gland that affects both the orbital and palpebral lobes. There is **avid contrast enhancement in the acute phase** of disease representing hyperemia, often with periglandular inflammatory changes and occasionally complicated by abscess formation. MRI shows similar unilateral diffuse enlargement and hyperenhancement of the lacrimal gland, with surrounding inflammatory changes but no bone involvement. Acute infectious dacryoadenitis responds well to antibiotic therapy.

Rhinogenic proptosis: Proptosis arising from complicated ethmoid sinusitis presenting with subperiosteal abscess in the medial wall of the orbit and secondary to sinonasal malignancies.

Causes for bilateral lacrimal gland enlargement: Idiopathic orbital inflammation, lymphoid tumors, sarcoidosis, Rosai-Dorfman disease, Erdheim-Chester disease and Sjögren's disease.

Causes of dilatation of superior ophthalmic vein: Carotid—cavernous sinus fistula, cavernous sinus thrombosis, venous varix, Graves' disease, normal variant.

Mass in superolateral quadrant of orbit: Lacrimal gland tumor, dermoid cyst, metastasis (breast, prostate, lung), lymphoma, leukemic infiltration of lacrimal gland, sarcoidosis, Wegener granulomatosis, pseudotumor, frontal sinus mucocele.

Table 4.82.3: Differential diagnosis for globe lesions		
Lesions of globe		
Ocular lesions		*Preseptal space lesions*
Pediatric	*Adults*	Cellulitis Hematoma Infantile hemangioma
Tumors Retinoblastoma Metastasis Choroidal hemangioma Medulloepithelioma	**Tumors** Uveal melanoma Intra-ocular primary malignant melanoma Retinal hemangioblastoma	
Non-tumors Mitochondrial myopathy—Kearns-Sayre syndrome, MELAS Congenital cataract Coats disease Retrolental fibroplasia PHPV—persistent hyperplastic primary vitreous	**Non-tumors** Hyphema Detachments	**Extraconal-extra orbital lesion** A. From sinus: Maxillary, sphenoid sinuses are rare locations of origin 1. Tumor: Squamous cell carcinoma (80%), lymphoma, adeno-carcinoma, adenoid cystic carcinoma, 2. Mucocele, 3. Paranasal sinusitis (most common cause of orbital infection) Origin: from ethmoid sinuses (in children), from frontal sinus (in adolescence) Complication: (1) Epidural abscess, (2) subdural empyema, (3) cavernous sinus thrombosis, (4) meningitis, (5) cerebritis, (6) brain abscess B. From skin orbital cellulitis, C. From lacrimal gland—mass arising from superolateral aspect of orbit
Intraconal compartment		**Conal lesions (extraocular muscular compartment)**
With optic nerve/sheath involvement **Tumors** Optic nerve glioma Optic nerve sheath meningioma (10% of orbital neoplasm) Intraorbital lymphoma Optic neuritis Inflammatory pseudotumor (may surround optic nerve) Sarcoidosis	**Without optic nerve involvement** **Tumors** Lymphangioma Neurilemmoma **Non-tumors** Cavernous hemangioma Orbital varix Carotid-cavernous fistula Arteriovenous malformation Hematoma	**A. Endocrine:** 1. Graves' disease (50%), 2. Acromegaly **B. Inflammation:** Myositis, orbital cellulitis, Sjögren disease, Wegener granulomatosis, lethal midline granuloma, SLE, sarcoidosis, foreign-body reaction **C. Tumor:** Pseudotumor, rhabdomyosarcoma, metastasis, lymphoma, leukemia **D. Vascular:** Spontaneous I traumatic hematoma, arteriovenous malformation, carotid-cavernous sinus fistula
Intraorbital extraconal lesions: Dermoid cyst—most common lesion in pediatrics, dacryocystocele, capillary hemangioma and cavernous hemangioma, plexiform neurofibroma, orbital pseudotumor, Langerhans cell histiocytosis, rhabdomyosarcoma of the orbits, lymphoma/leukemia.		

4.83 HEAD AND NECK

Case No. 83

Clinical history: A 9 years old female child presented with gradual loss of vision in right eye.

Radiological techniques and observation: Figure 4.83.1 is CT brain plain image showing fusiform enlargement of the right optic nerve and widening of the optic canal. No evidence of calcification. Figure 4.83.2 is axial contrast enhanced CT showing well-defined low-density enlarged optic nerve with peripheral enhancement, extending up to orbital apex. Figure 4.83.3 is sagittal non-contrast T1 weighted MRI shows enlargement intra-orbital part of optic nerve with widening of the optic canal and intracranial extension. Optic chiasma appears normal. Rest of the intraconal compartment appears normal. Extraconal compartment appears normal. Eyeball appears normal. No evidence of calcification, cystic components, blood vessel encasement.

Interpretation: A—9 years old female child, C—peripherally enhancing fusiform-shaped enlarged right optic nerve with intraorbital involvement, B—widening of the optic canal and intracranial extension, D—optic nerve glioma

Table 4.83.1: Treatment of optic nerve glioma

Good vision	No treatment
No growth	
No cosmetic deformity	
Unilateral optic nerve glioma	Follow-up examination at regular intervals
Rapid intra-orbital tumor growth	Surgical excision
Unresectable tumors	Radiation therapy
Most spontaneous regression	NF-1 cases

Principal diagnosis: Optic nerve glioma.

Differential diagnosis (thickened optic nerve sheath complex)

Optic nerve sheath meningioma, peri-optic neuritis, intracranial hypertension, lymphomatous/leukemic infiltration, sarcoidosis, infectious etiologies (measles, mumps, syphilis), metastases, Erdheim-Chester disease.

Treatment of optic nerve glioma: Since optic nerve glioma is typically a low-grade tumor and do not metastasize, they may even spontaneously regress. Non-progressive tumors are usually monitored conservatively. Treatment is deferred until unless there is evidence of progression. Ophthalmic examination is performed at least every 3 months with or without serial neuro-imaging with gradually increasing the intervals, if the visual function is stable.

Surgery alone is rarely curative, since tumor often extends beyond what the MRI findings suggest and surgery has significant side-effects, causing complete loss of vison of the affected eye.

Chemotherapy: It is considered as the first line of treatment regimen (carboplatin and vincristine) given weekly is shown to effective in newly diagnosed. It is subsequently found to improve the visual outcome in patients with NF-1. If there is still progression of the disease, next step is to change the chemotherapeutic regimen.

Radiotherapy: It was previously a common treatment for optic nerve glioma in children, however, long-term follow-up revealed patient had a significant risk of developing severe complications like secondary CNS tumors and occlusive cerebral vasculopathy. Therefore, radiotherapy is rarely treatment of choice. Even with treatment including high-dose radiotherapy and

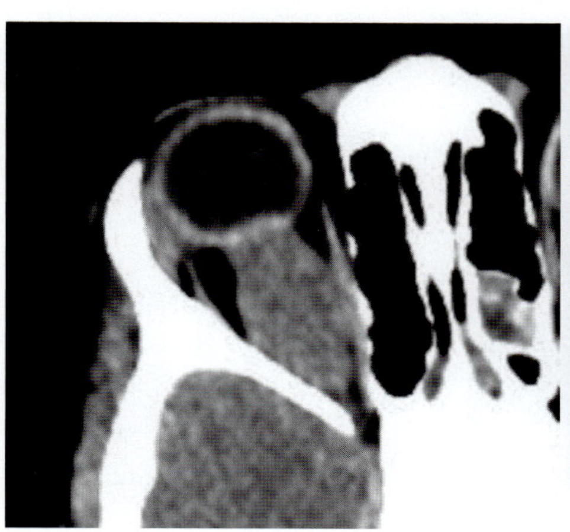

Fig. 4.83.1

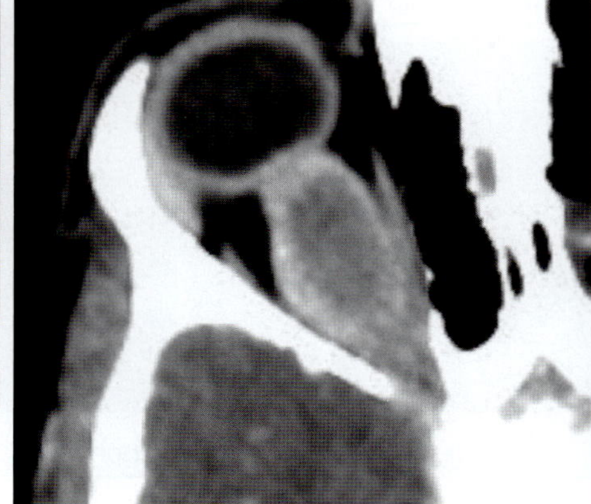

Fig. 4.83.2

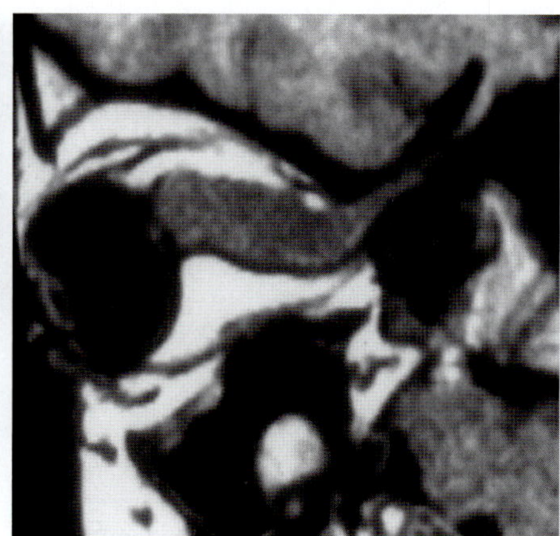

Fig. 4.83.3

Table 4.83.2: Differential diagnosis for optic nerve glioma

Perioptic neuritis MC—predominantly young adults M: F – 1: 3 Unilateral >> Bilateral Treatment: Self-limiting High dose corticosteroids	Retrobulbar intra-orbital segment of left optic nerve, appears swollen, with a high T2 signal. Loss of normal target appearance. High T2 signal persists and may be permanent. Chronically the nerve will appear atrophied rather than swollen.	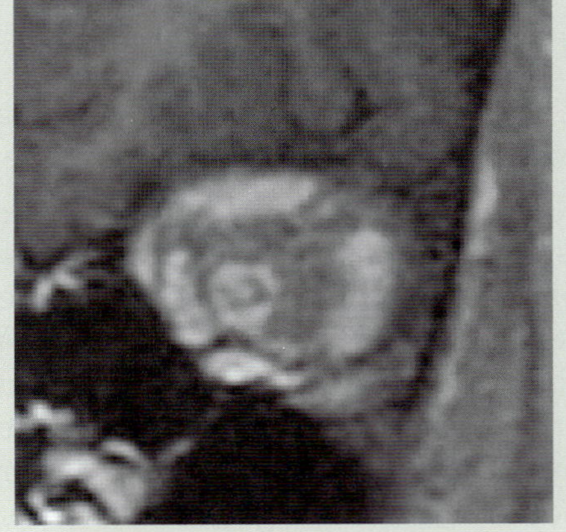 **Fig. 4.83.4:** Perioptic neuritis
Intracranial hypertension also called pseudotumor cerebri MC—affects middle-aged obese females	Prominent subarachnoid space around the optic nerves, causing flattening of posterior sclera and vertical tortuosity of the optic nerves, papilledema intraocular protrusion of the optic nerve head. Enhancement of the prelaminar (intra-ocular) optic nerves. Treatment involves diuretics, CSF drainage, CSF shunting. Decompressive craniectomy is the treatment.	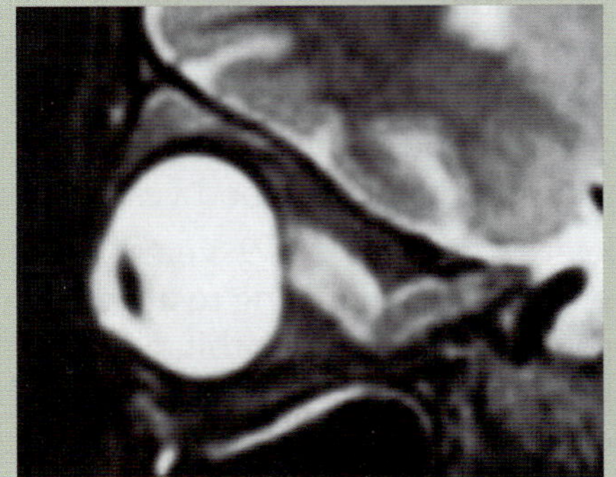 **Fig. 4.83.5:** Intracranial hypertension
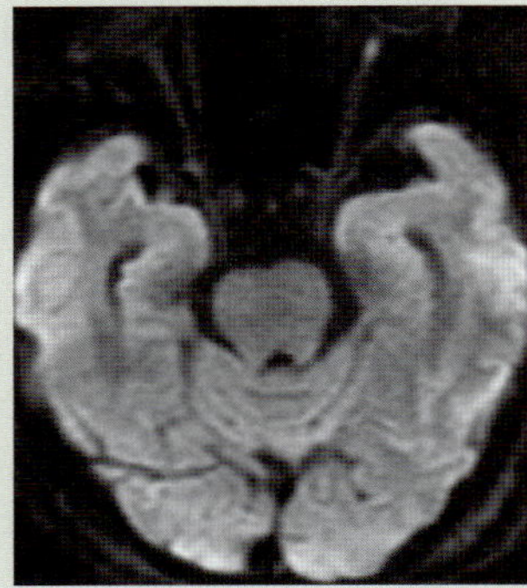 **Fig. 4.83.6:** Infarct causing ischemic optic neuritis	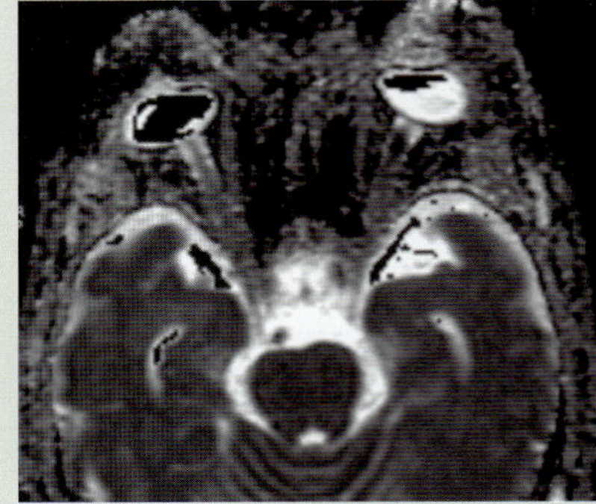 **Fig. 4.83.7:** Infarct causing ischemic optic neuritis	
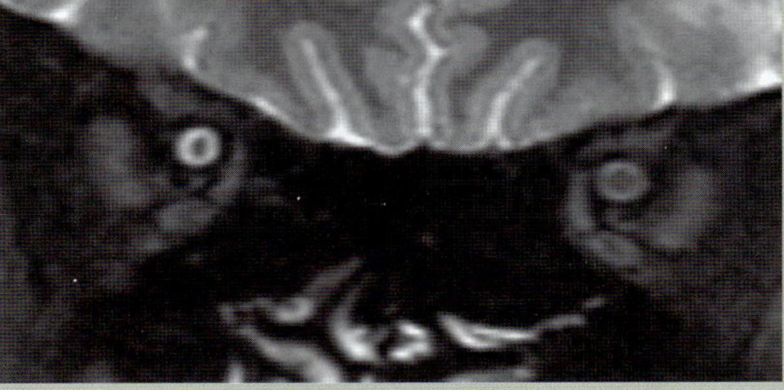 **Fig. 4.83.8:** Right optic atrophy		

Contd...

Table 4.83.2: Differential diagnosis for optic nerve glioma *(Contd...)*		
Fig. 4.83.9: Optic nerve sheath meningioma	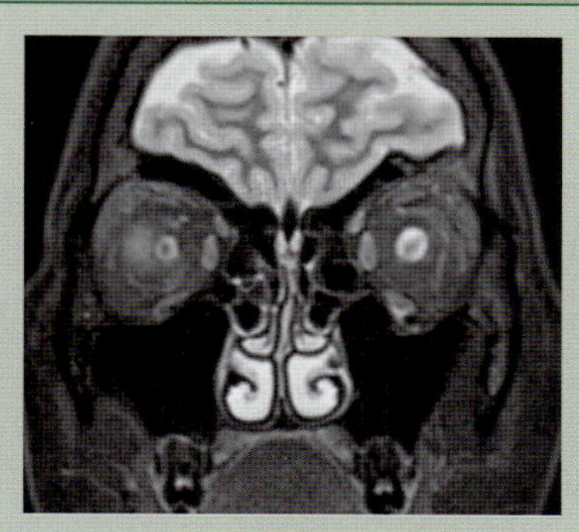 **Fig. 4.83.10:** Optic nerve sheath meningioma	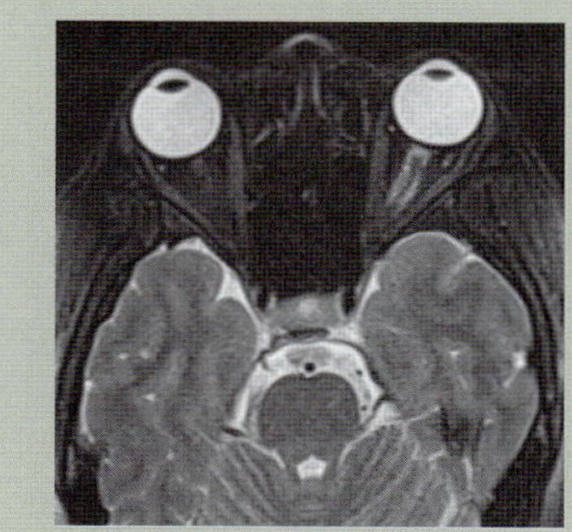 **Fig. 4.83.11:** Optic nerve sheath meningioma
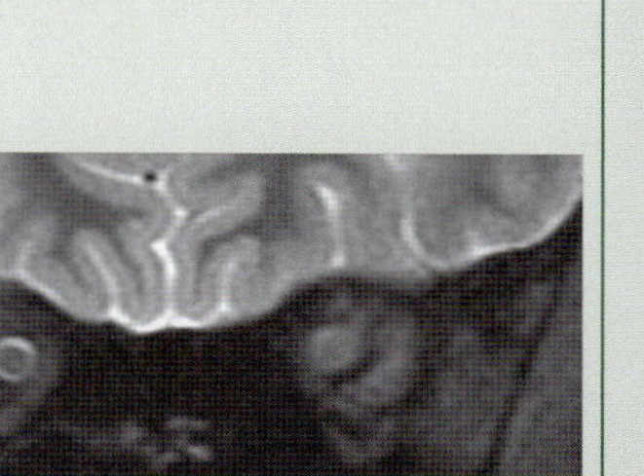 **Fig. 4.83.12:** Left optic neuritis	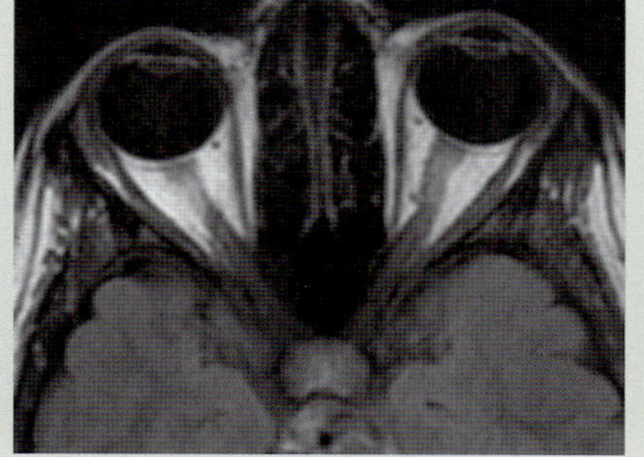 **Fig. 4.83.13:** Left optic neuritis	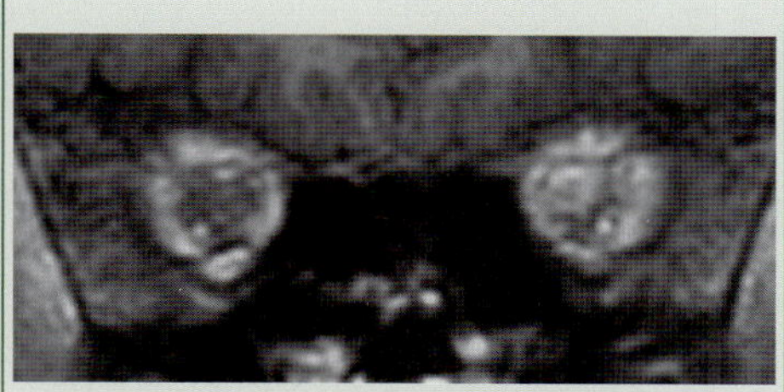 **Fig. 4.83.14:** Left optic neuritis
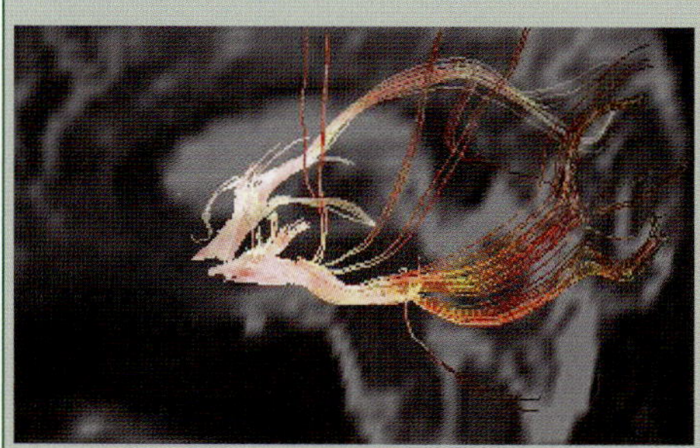 **Fig. 4.83.15:** Normal DTI optic pathway	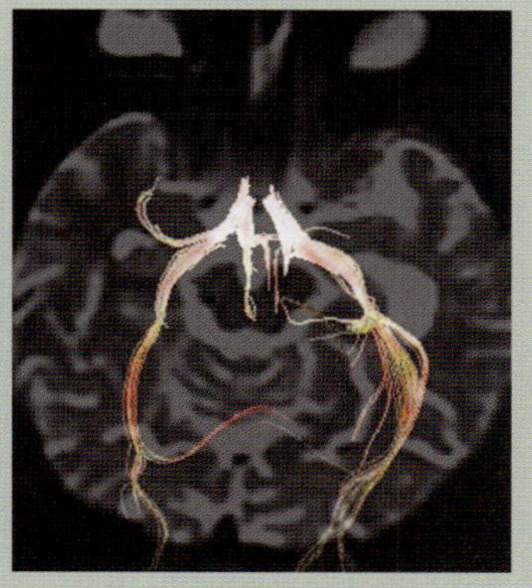 **Fig. 4.83.16:** Normal DTI optic pathway	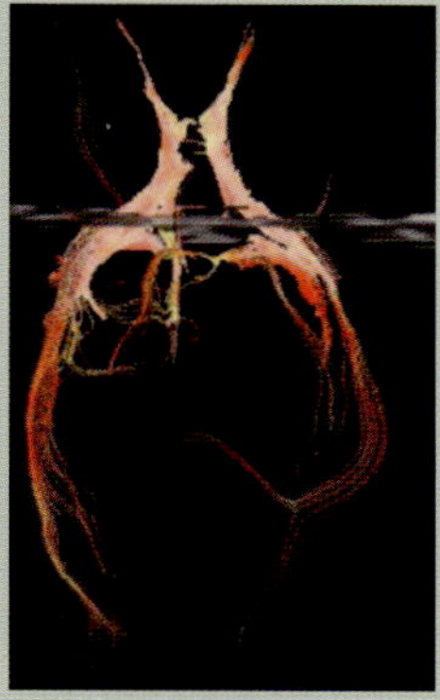 **Fig. 4.83.17:** Normal DTI optic pathway
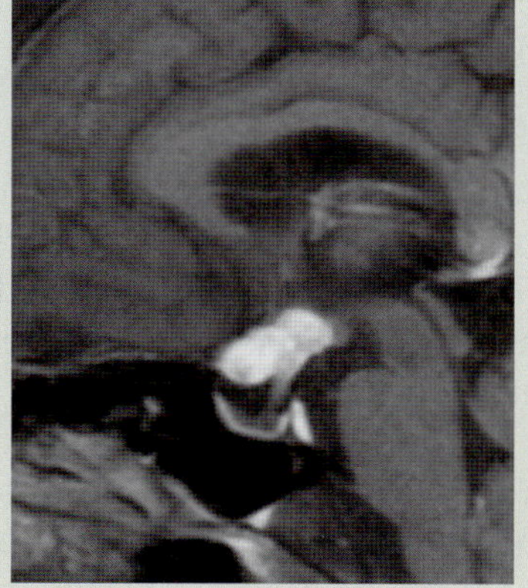 **Fig. 4.83.18:** Optic chiasm glioma	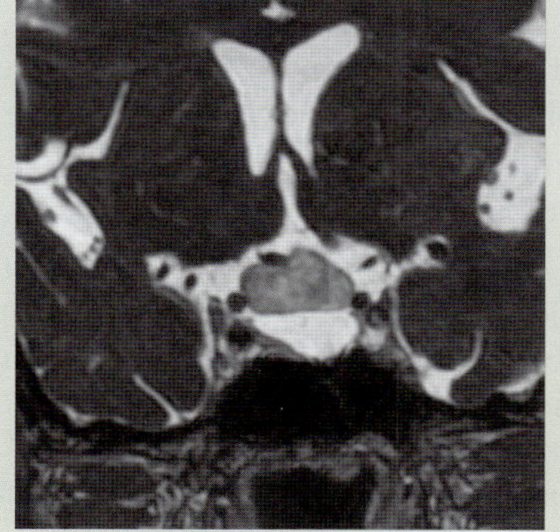 **Fig. 4.83.19:** Optic chiasm glioma	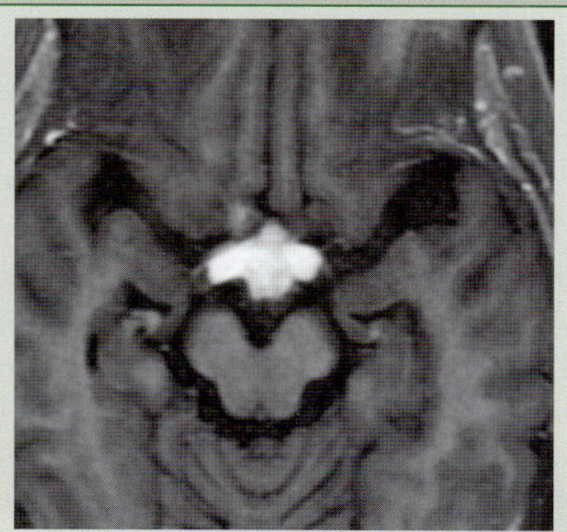 **Fig. 4.83.20:** Optic chiasm glioma

Contd...

Table 4.83.2: Differential diagnosis for optic nerve glioma *(Contd...)*

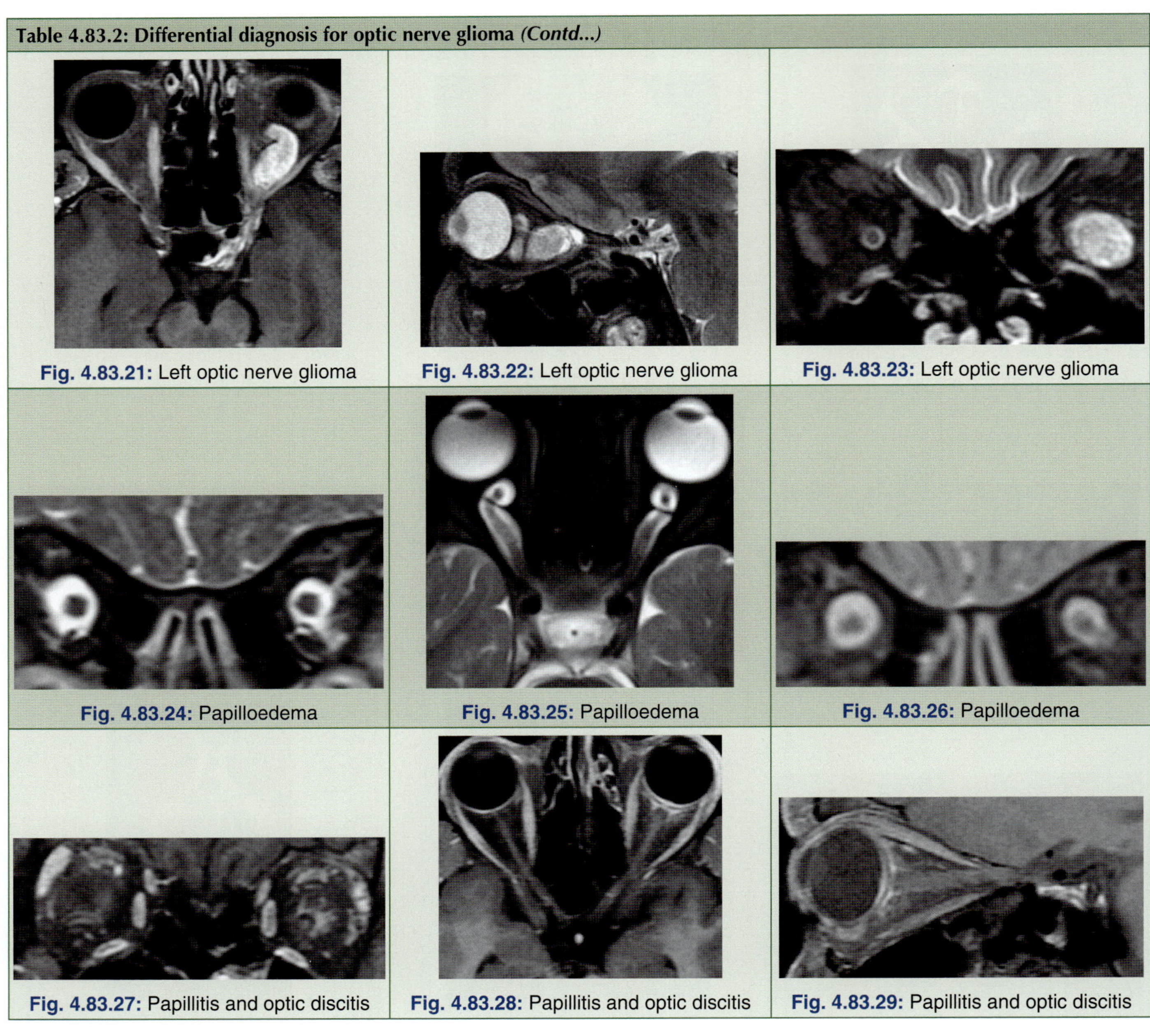

Fig. 4.83.21: Left optic nerve glioma

Fig. 4.83.22: Left optic nerve glioma

Fig. 4.83.23: Left optic nerve glioma

Fig. 4.83.24: Papilloedema

Fig. 4.83.25: Papilloedema

Fig. 4.83.26: Papilloedema

Fig. 4.83.27: Papillitis and optic discitis

Fig. 4.83.28: Papillitis and optic discitis

Fig. 4.83.29: Papillitis and optic discitis

chemotherapy, these tumors usually result in death within 6–12 months in malignant gliomas (glioblastomas).

Optic nerve gliomas are associated with NF-1; hence MRI brain and clinical examination should be done.

Discussion: **Optic nerve glioma**–MC cause of optic nerve enlargement–low grade pilocytic astrocytoma. It has strong relationship with neurofibromatosis 1 (if bilateral). Common in children rare in adults (75% first decade of life). Female > male. Asymmetric widening of optic canal on radiographs. CT 1) Reveals widening of the optic canal. 2) In patients with associated NF1, there is typically a fusiform enlargement of the optic nerve with a clear-cut margin produced by intact dural sheath. 3) In patients without NF1 the nerve may be more irregular and have some low-density areas.

MRI: 1) Detects intracanalicular, intracranial extension. 2) MRI often reveals enlargement, kinking, and buckling of the optic nerve. 3) The nerve becomes enlarged and fusiform in shape because of attachment of the investing dura to the periosteum of the optic canal. 4) T2W hyperintense and may seem heterogeneous due to cystic degeneration. Glioma can enhance heterogeneously or show no enhancement, if there is cystic degeneration. 5) Intracranial extension can be seen, 6) T1WI—hypointense. 7) T2WI—hyperintense. 8) T1WI + C—enhance with gadolinium.

Table 4.83.3: Difference between optic nerve glioma and optic nerve sheath meningioma	
Optic nerve glioma	*Optic nerve sheath meningioma*
50% <5 years of age	Usually middle-aged women
Can be bilateral	Usually unilateral
Slowly progressive, painless loss of vision; central scotoma. Childhood tumors may remain quiescent for years, particularly in the presence of NF. Adult tumors are aggressive.	Slowly progressive, painless loss of vision; proptosis
NF1in 25%; bilateral disease strongly suggests neurofibromatosis	NF1/2 in 4–6%; Bilateral disease may occur with or without NF
No orbital hyperostosis	Hyperostosis
Widened optic canal is seen in 90% cases but intracranial extension is unusual	Widened optic canal in 10%
Kinking and buckling of the optic nerve is common. Smooth outline.	Straight optic nerve, but tumor may be eccentric
Well-defined margins	More infiltrative.
Calcifications rare without prior radiotherapy.	Calcifications (linear/plaque-like/granular) are more common—tram-track appearance
T1W Isointense; T2W hyperintense	Similar signal to optic nerve on most unenhanced MR pulse sequences.
Variable contrast enhancement with mottled lucencies due to mucinous degeneration	Diffuse homogeneous enhancement+/- serrated margins
----------	Negative image of optic nerve within the tumor (tram-track sign).
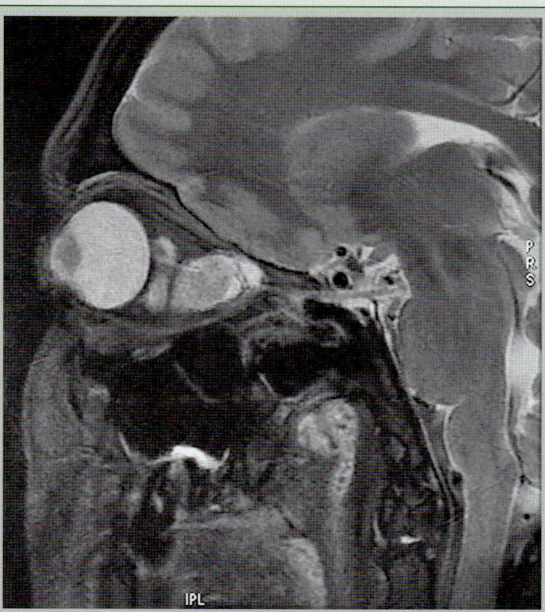 **Fig. 4.83.30:** Optic nerve glioma	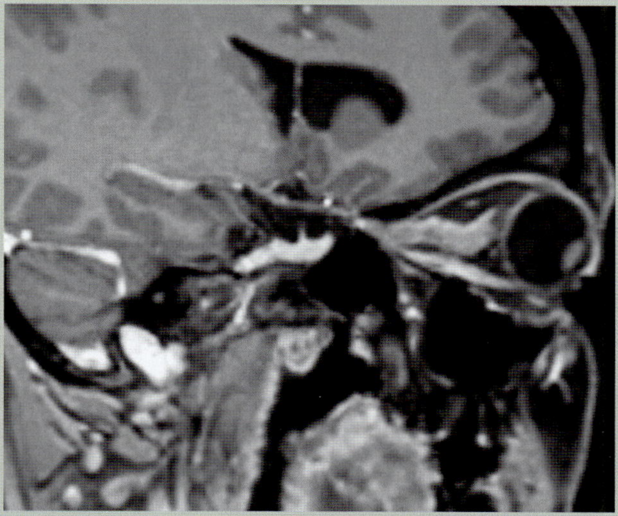 **Fig. 4.83.31:** Optic nerve sheath meningioma

Histologically, optic nerve glioma is characterized as juvenile pilocytic astrocytoma characterized by cells with prominent eosinophilic processes called Rosenthal fibers.

Cavernous hemangioma	*Lymphangioma*
Young to middle-aged adults.	Infancy through the first decade.
Well encapsulated with distinct margin	Intraconal or extraconal compartment.
Usually intraconal, grow slowly.	Usually lobulated, with ill-defined borders. Multilocular or cystic blood collections common
CT: Well-marginated soft tissue mass Mild to heterogeneous enhancement	May contain septation. Varying degrees of contrast enhancement. Lesions commonly haemorrhagic.
MRI: Isointense to slightly increased signal on T1 and marked signal intensity on T2	MRI increased signal on T1 and marked signal intensity on T2 indirect involvement of the orbit and optic pathways
Fig. 4.83.32: Cavernous hemangioma	**Fig. 4.83.33:** Cavernous hemangioma
Fig. 4.83.34: Cavernous hemangioma	**Fig 4.83.35:** IgG4 disease (pseudotumour)
Fig. 4.83.36: Lymphangioma	**Fig 4.83.37:** Lymphangioma

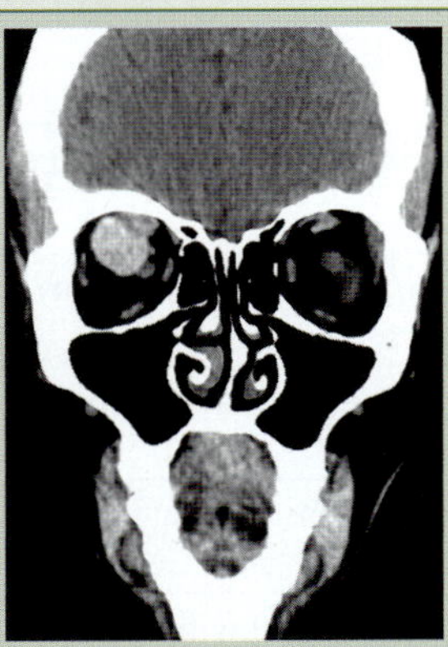

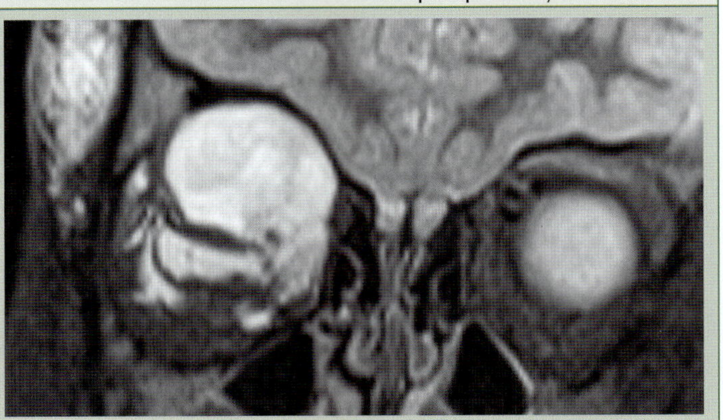

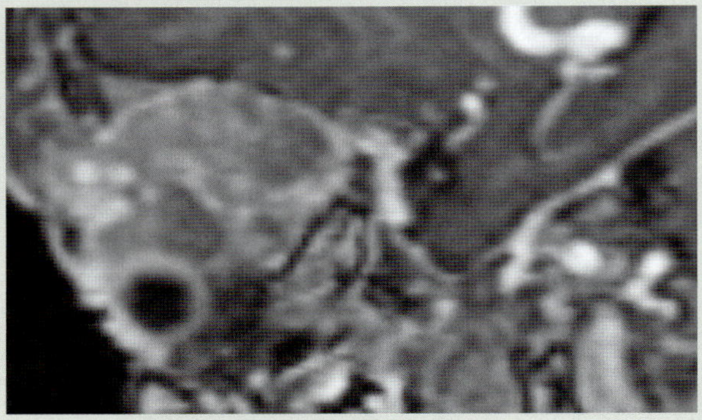

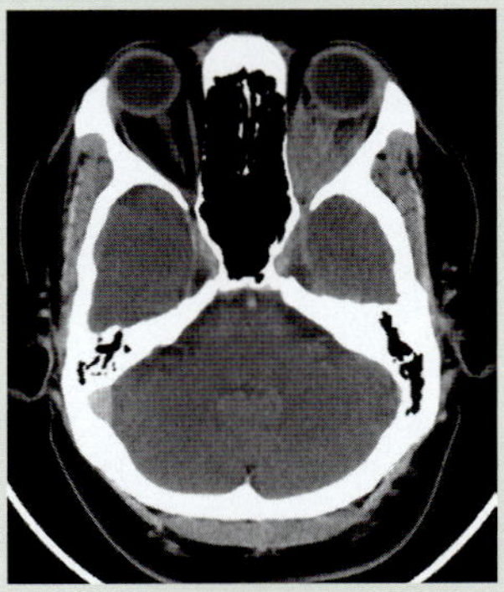

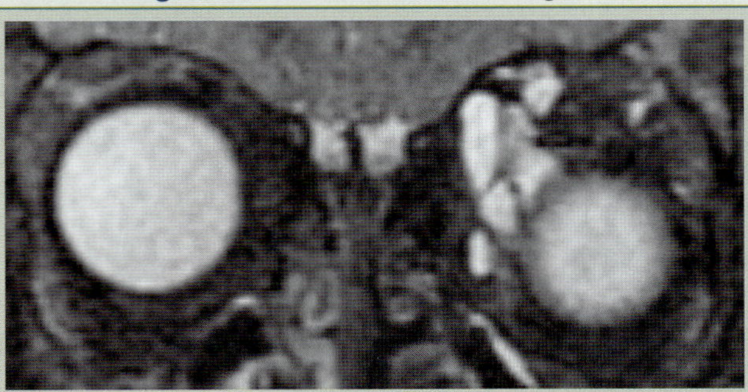

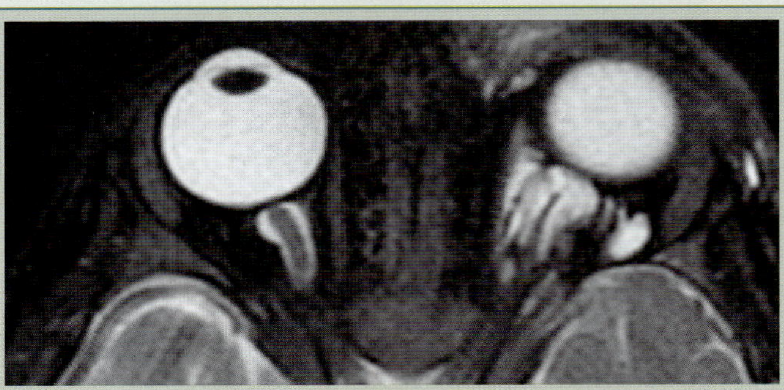

4.84 HEAD AND NECK

Case No. 84

Clinical history: 40-year-old female patient presenting with proptosis, headache and redness of eye.

Radiographic techniques and observation: **MRI brain–plain with contrast:** Figures 4.84.1 and 4.84.2 are T2-axial images showing hyperintensity in the orbit involving left lateral rectus and left orbit apex. Figure 4.84.3 is FLAIR coronal image showing hyperintense left orbital apex. Figure 4.84.4 is T1 axial image showing thickened left lateral rectus. Right orbit and orbital apex appear normal. Figures 4.84.5 and 4.84.6 are post-contrast coronal T1 weighted fat sat images showing enhancement in the left orbit apex involving optic nerve, lateral rectus. There is thrombosis of left ICA, cavernous sinus with enhancement of adjacent meninges.

Interpretation: A—40-year-old female, left orbital apex, left lateral rectus, C—thickening and enhancement of the left lateral rectus, optic nerve, orbital apex, B—thrombosis of left ICA, cavernous sinus with enhancement of adjacent meninges. D—left orbital pseudotumor.

Principal diagnosis: Left orbital pseudotumor.

Management: Steroids.

Orbital pseudotumor/inflammatory myofibroblastic tumor/idiopathic orbital syndrome: It is an idiopathic nongranulomatous inflammatory process affecting all intraorbital soft tissue. 2nd most common cause of exophthalmos (25% of all unilateral exophthalmos). 3rd most common primary tumor of the orbit in adults. **Occurs alone or in combination with maxillary sinus pseudotumor. Clinical features:** Sudden acute onset of unilateral eye pain with ophthalmoplegia (= impaired ocular movement) + diplopia/decreased visual acuity, proptosis; eyelid swelling, chemosis. **Spectrum—orbital pseudotumor, Tolosa-Hunt syndrome, hypertrophic**

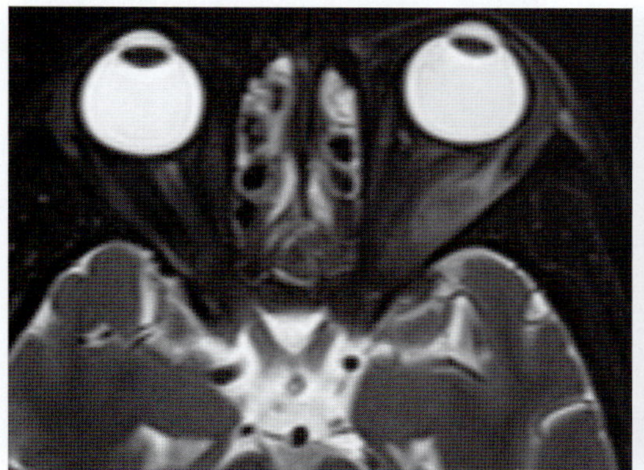

Fig. 4.84.1

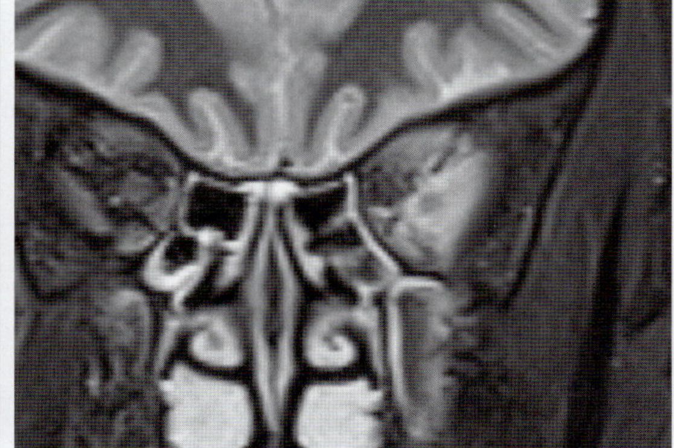

Fig. 4.84.2

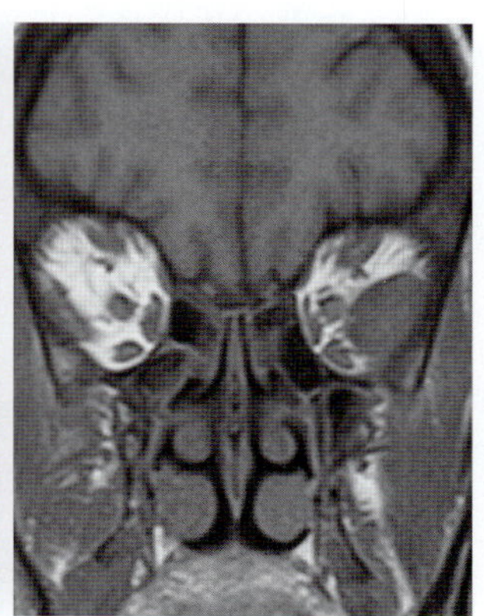

Fig. 4.84.3

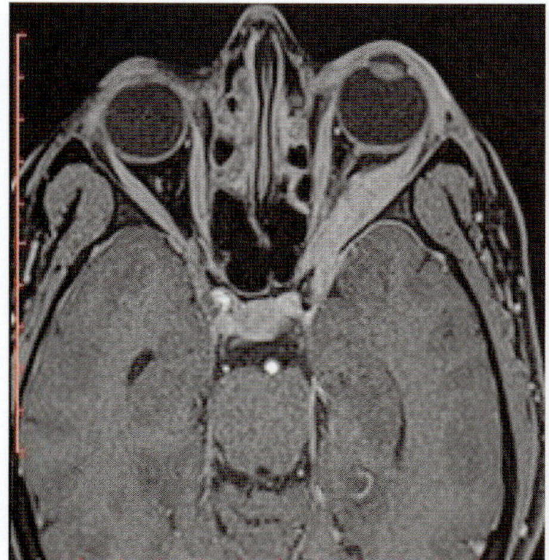

Fig. 4.84.4

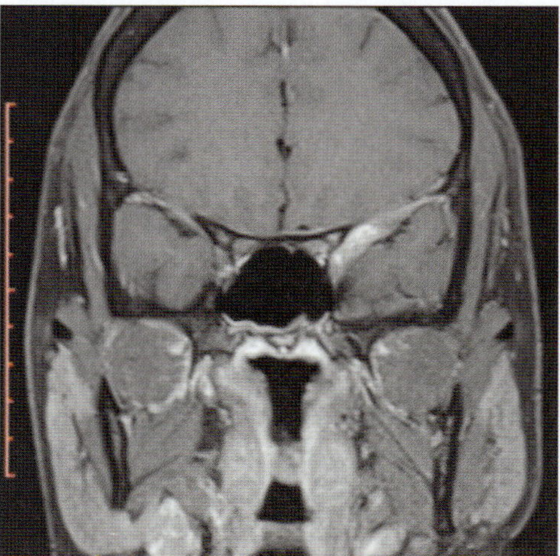

Fig. 4.84.5

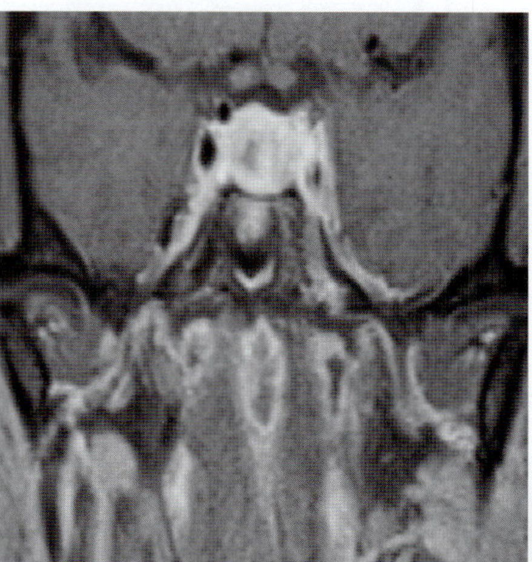

Fig. 4.84.6

Differential diagnosis (for conal lesions)

Tolosa-Hunt syndrome: Variant of orbital pseudotumor Painful ophthalmoplegia, characterised by inflammation of orbital apex and cavernous sinus	**Inflammatory soft-tissue enhancing mass around orbital apex + occlusion of cavernous sinus with or without superior ophthalmic vein**	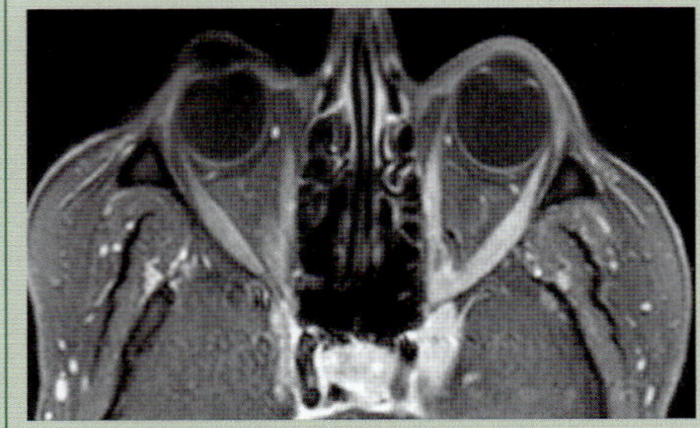 **Fig. 4.84.7:** Tolosa-Hunt syndrome
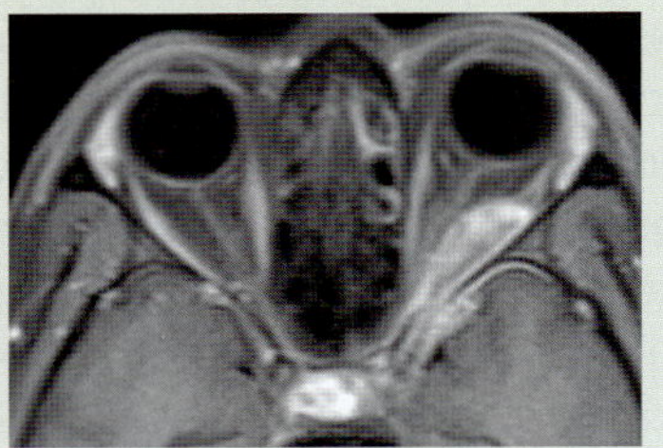 **Fig. 4.84.8:** Tolosa-Hunt syndrome	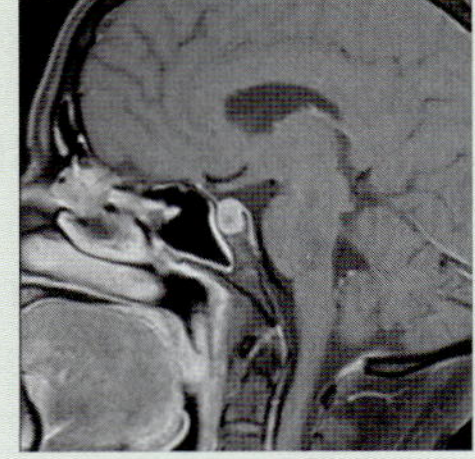 **Fig. 4.84.9:** Tolosa-Hunt syndrome	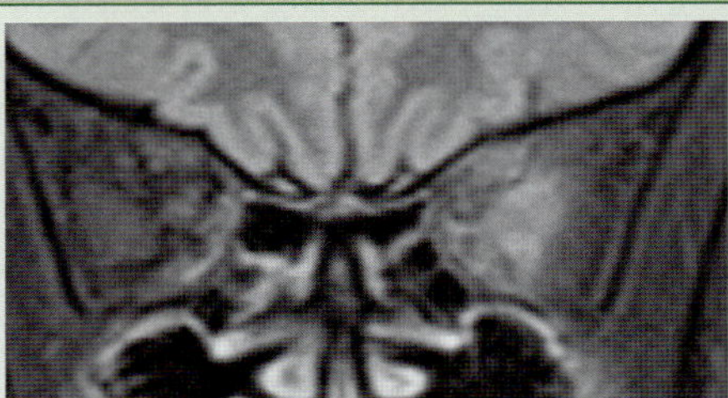 **Fig. 4.84.10:** Tolosa-Hunt syndrome
Orbital cellulitis	Inflammation involving extracoronal and intraconal orbital compartments with/without extension into cavernous sinus. Diffuse edema in preseptal and periorbital region. Associated sinusitis present in most of the cases	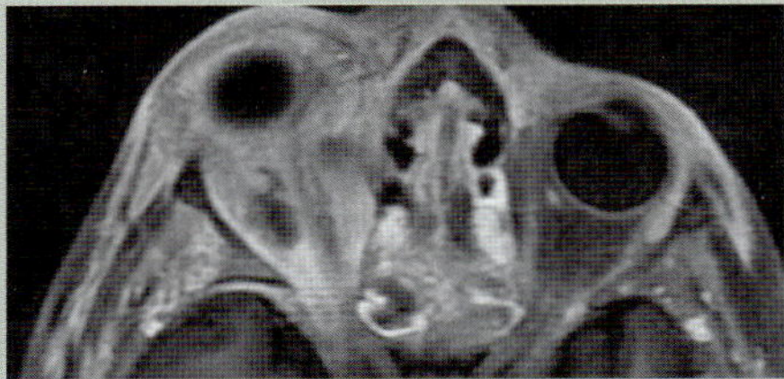 **Fig. 4.84.11:** Orbital cellulitis
Orbital abscess		
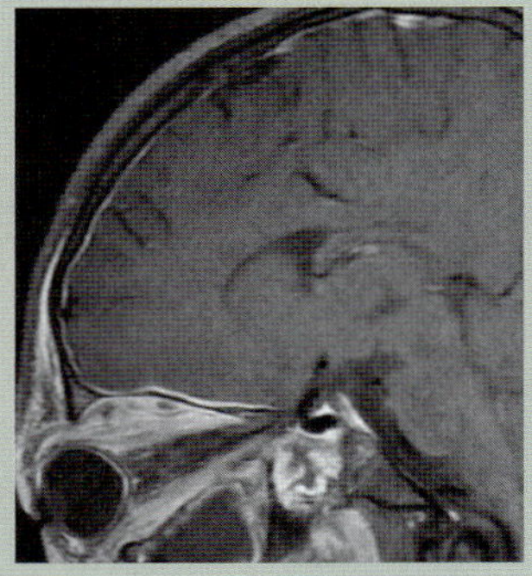 **Fig. 4.84.12:** Orbital abscess	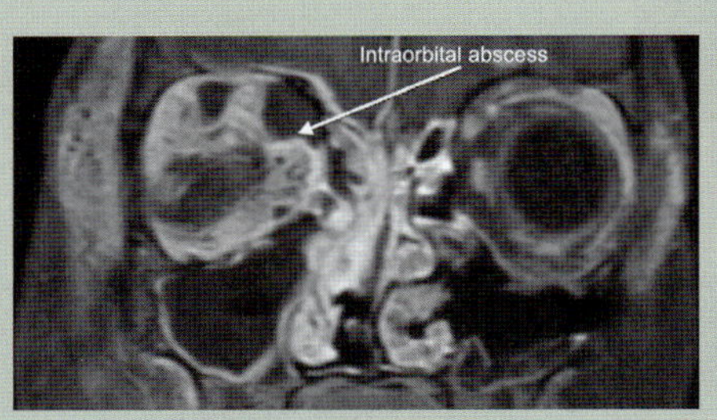 **Fig. 4.84.13:** Orbital abscess	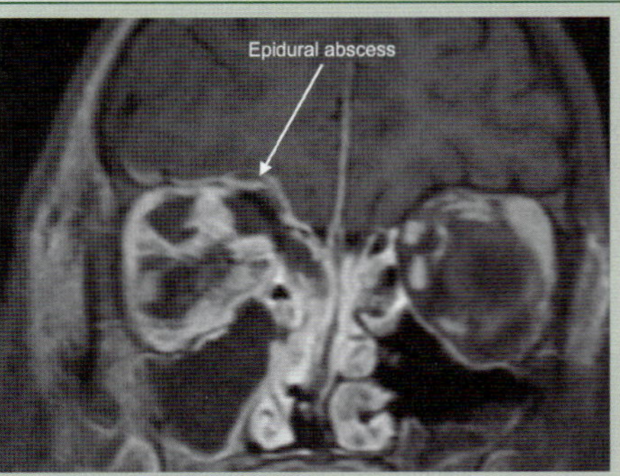 **Fig. 4.84.14:** Orbital abscess
Thyroid orbitopathy Immune-mediated disorder, which most commonly presents in association with hyperthyroidism in Graves' disease middle-aged females	**Bilateral involvement** is the most frequent presentation. Classic imaging appearance is **fusiform muscle enlargement with sparing of the muscular tendon—coke bottle appearance.**	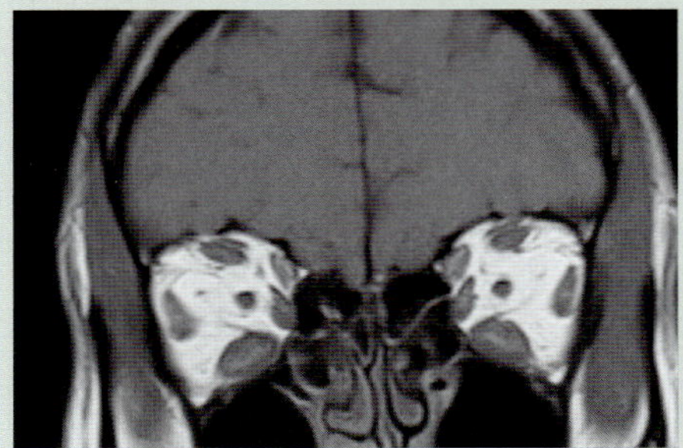 **Fig. 4.84.15:** Thyroid orbitopathy

(Contd.)

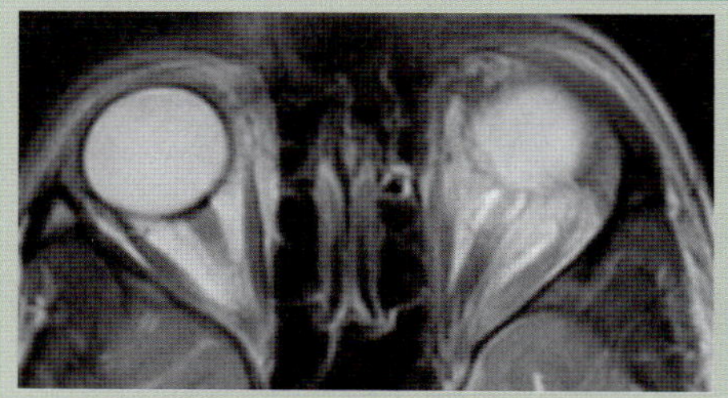 **Fig. 4.84.16:** Thyroid orbitopathy	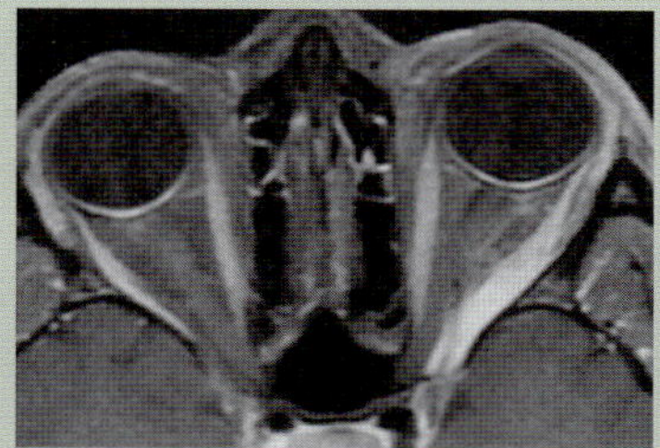 **Fig. 4.84.17:** Thyroid orbitopathy	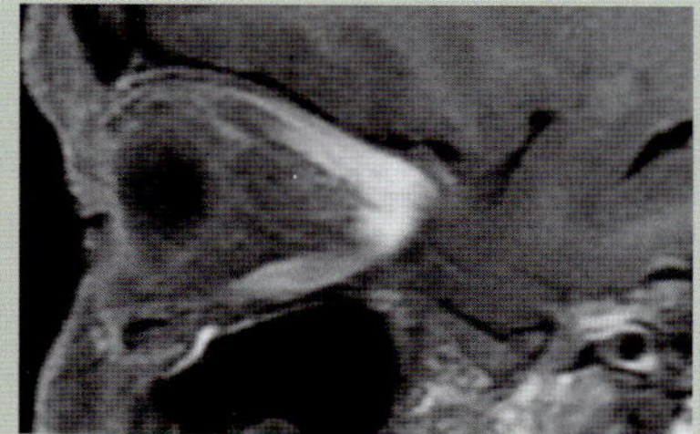 **Fig. 4.84.18:** Thyroid orbitopathy
Orbital lymphoma Most commonly non-Hodgkin lymphoma Common in old age (50 years)	Extraocular muscles surrounded by mass which appears isodense to hyperdense on CT, with involvement of lacrimal gland. MRI-T1 HYPO/T2 hyper/homogeneous enhancement	
Orbital hemangioma	Soft tissue mass in the intraconal compartment which enhances with contrast	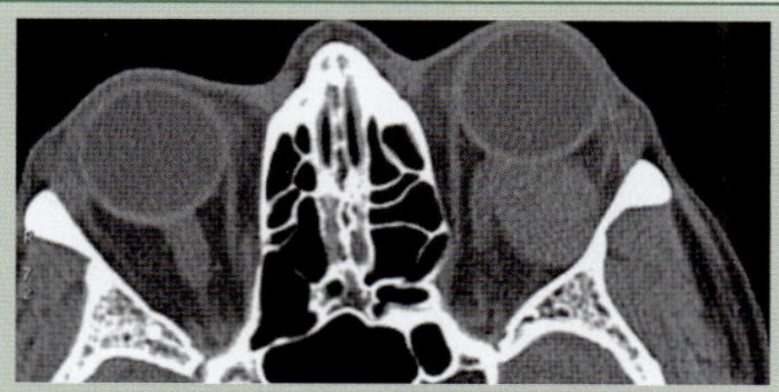 **Fig. 4.84.19:** Orbital hemangioma
Idiopathic intracranial hypertension (pseudotumor cerebri /benign intracranial hypertension)	Young, moderately obese female, presenting with headache empty sella. Bilateral prominent perioptic CSF space with vertical tortuosity of optic nerves. Flattening of posterior aspect of eyeball	
Carotico-cavernous fistula—Refer to case 35		
Proptosis 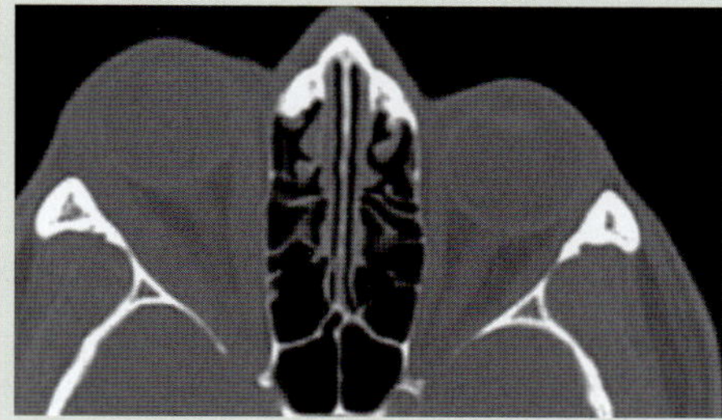 **Fig. 4.84.20:** Proptosis in case of carotico-cavernous fistula	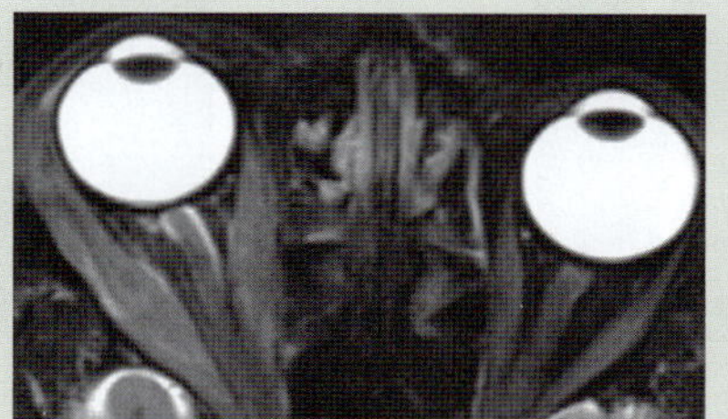 **Fig. 4.84.21:** Enlarged superior ophthalmic vein and extraocular muscles in case of carotico-cavernous fistula	**Neurofibroma** 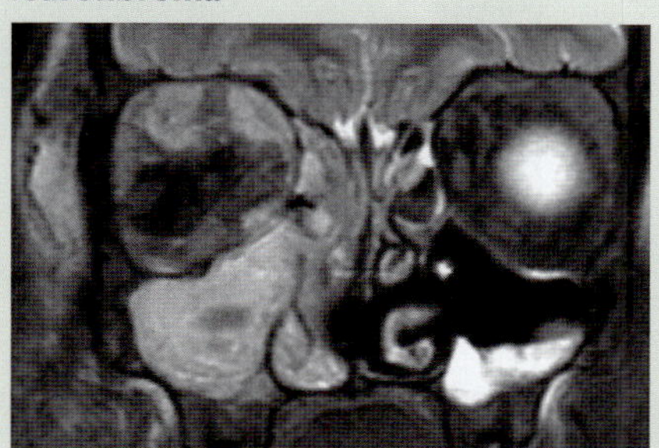 **Fig. 4.84.22:** Neurofibromatosis
Intraconal NCC		
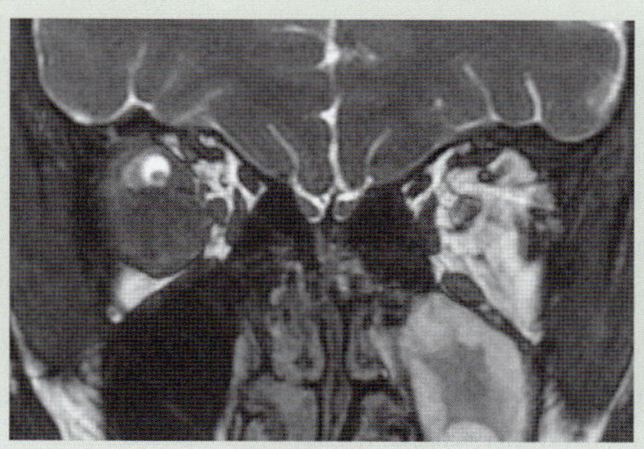 **Fig. 4.84.23:** Intraconal NCC	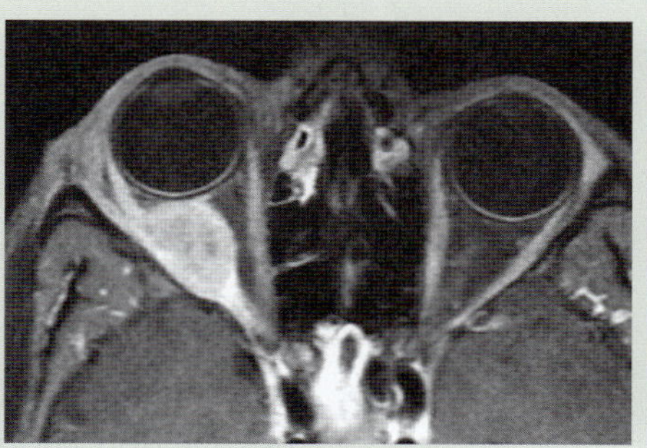 **Fig. 4.84.24:** Intraconal NCC	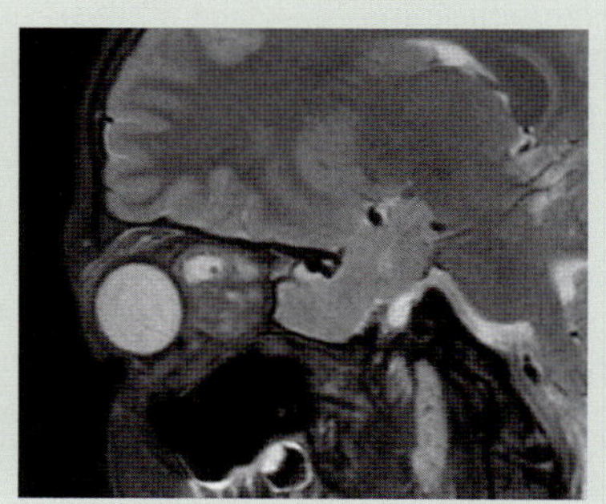 **Fig. 4.84.25:** Intraconal NCC

(Contd.)

Intraconal cyst

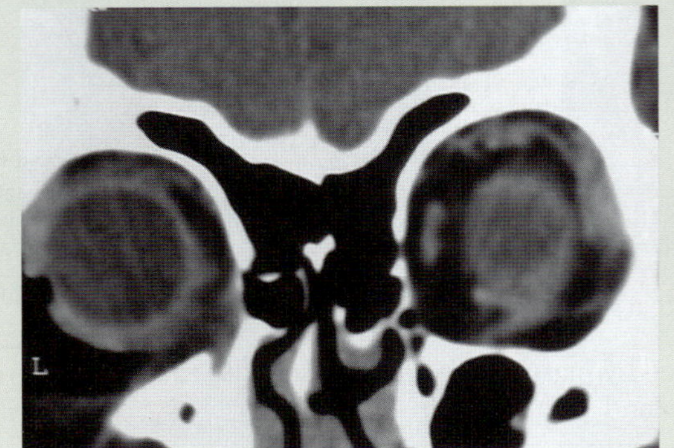

Fig. 4.84.26: Intraconal cyst

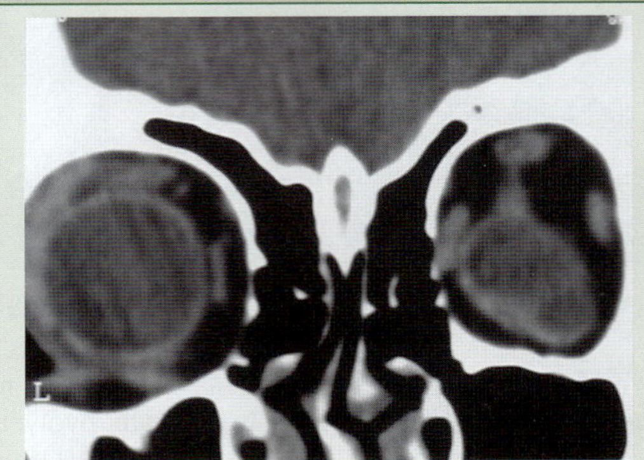

Fig. 4.84.27: Intraconal cyst

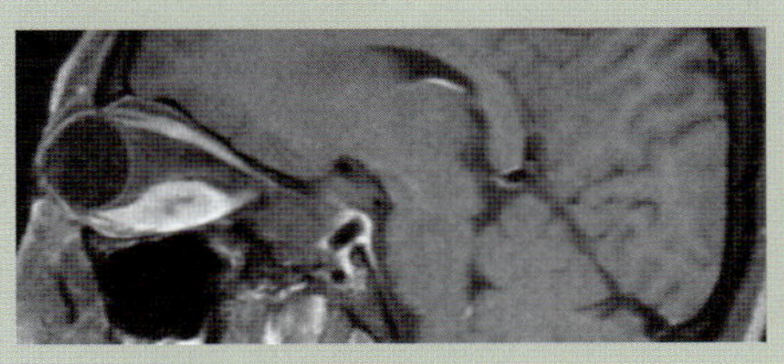
Fig. 4.84.28: Intraconal cyst

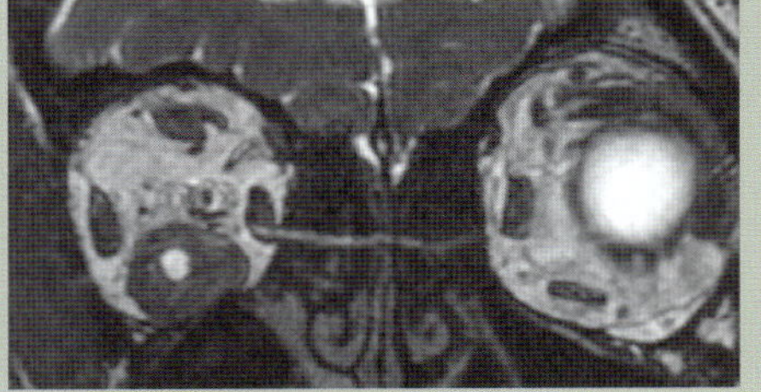
Fig. 4.84.29: Intraconal cyst

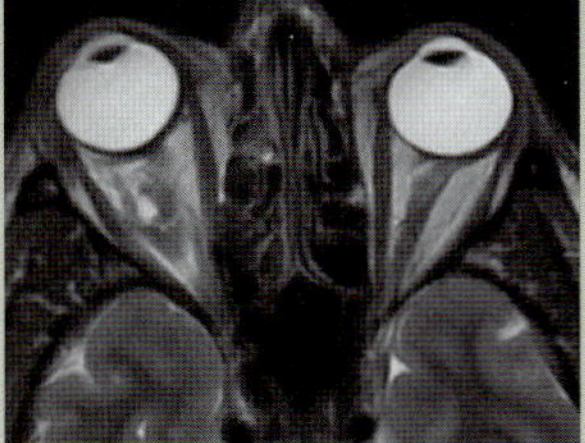
Fig. 4.84.30: Intraconal cyst

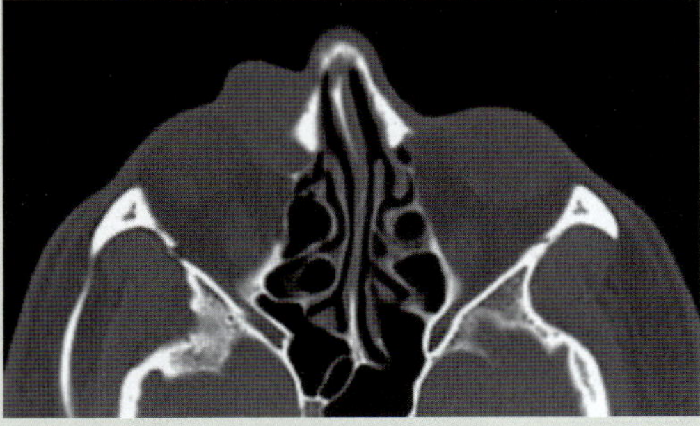
Fig. 4.84.31: Dacrocystocele

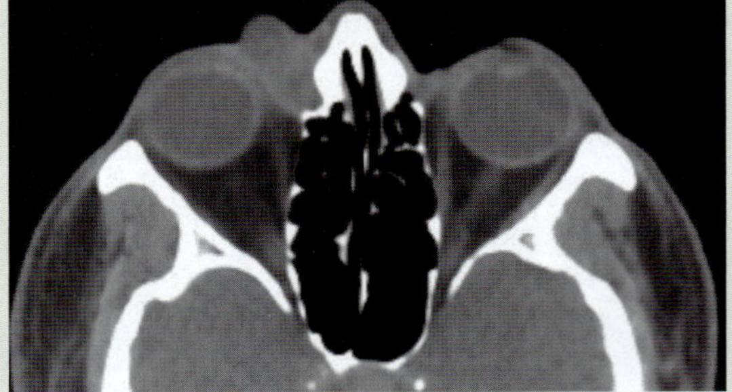
Fig. 4.84.32: Dacrocystocele

Table 4.84.1: Differential diagnosis for T1 hyperintense orbital masses

Tumor	Other
• Melanotic melanoma • Retinoblastoma • Choroidal metastases • Hemangioma **Detachment** • Coats disease • Persistent hyperplastic primary vitreous • Trauma	• Hemorrhage • Phthisis bulbi • Intravitreal oil treatment for detachment • Orbital varix (worsened by Valsalva maneuver) • Hemorrhage into cavernous hemangioma • CCF • Hemorrhage into lymphangioma • Thrombosis of superior orbital vein

pachymeningitis. Types—myositic type (most common)—affects extraocular muscle—muscles and tendon insertions, **dacryoadenitis-related form**—affects lacrimal gland, **neuritis-associated form**—affects optic nerve sheath, **apical form**—affects orbital apex, **episcleral form**—affects anterior orbit with sclera and preseptal soft tissues, **diffuse form**—affects entire orbit.

Imaging findings: **Fibrous encasement with multicompartment extension involving extra-ocular muscle, orbital apex, meninges.** Uveoscleral thickening with enhancement (sclera near Tenon capsule). Orbital muscle thickening due to myositis, enhancement of optic nerve sheath, enlarged inflamed lacrimal gland, bone destruction and intracranial extension.

Management: Steroids.

Table 4.84.2: Difference between inflammatory orbital pseudotumor and thyroid orbitopathy

Inflammatory orbital pseudotumor	*Thyroid orbitopathy*
Rare disease Idiopathic granulomatous disorder Usually unilateral Acute onset Severe pain and congestion Any extraocular muscle affected **Diffuse enlargement of muscles and tendon** **Adjacent fat, lacrimal gland, optic nerve and intra-cranial involvement** Ptosis may be seen Dramatic response to steroids	Autoimmune disorder Usually bilateral Chronic disease No pain/mild discomfort Inferior rectus followed by medial rectus affected Order of involvement—**I'M SLow** (inferior, medial, superior, lateral) **Central enlargement with sparing of tendons—coke bottle appearance** Exophthalmos noted Moderate response to steroids

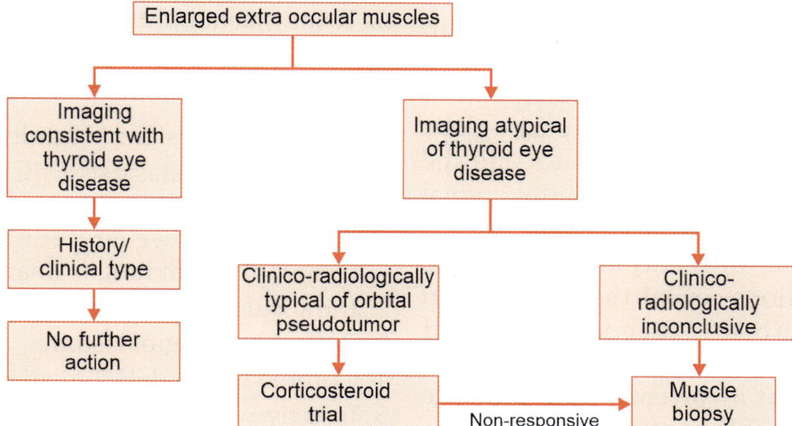

Fig. 4.84.33: Approach to extraocular muscle pathologies

4.85 HEAD AND NECK

Case No. 85

Clinical history: 18 months old male infant with complaints of leukocoria and defective vision.

Radiological techniques and observation: Figure 4.85.1 is CT with post-contrast study of the orbit revealing bilateral ill-defined lobulated retrolental mass with calcification and post-contrast-enhancement. A dense vitreous probably due to haemorrhage is also seen. No evidence of extra ocular lesion. The possible differentials for intra-ocular mass with calcifications are Drusen wherein 1% of population seen at optic disc (benign)—hyaline bodies are a relatively common entity usually found incidentally on CT; retinoblastoma—more in early childhood; retinal astrocytic hamartomas seen in tuberous sclerosis; retrolental fibroplasia (retinopathy of prematurity); coats disease (exudative retinitis)—globe is hyperdense due to proteinaceous exudates and the vitreous space may be obliterated due to extensive retinal detachment; chorioretinitis, choroidal osteoma.

Figures 4.85.2 to 4.85.4 are MRI study in CISS sequence in axial and lateral sections reveal the lesions is in posterior aspect of globe in both eyes appears ill-defined lobulated and T2 hypointense compared to the vitreous. No evidence of extra ocular involvement. No evidence of abnormal enhancement of the optic nerve.

Interpretation: A—18 years old male, bilateral intra-ocular mass in posterior aspect probably arising from retina, C—with calcifications which has intense post-contrast enhancement, B—without extra ocular extension. D—bilateral retinoblastoma.

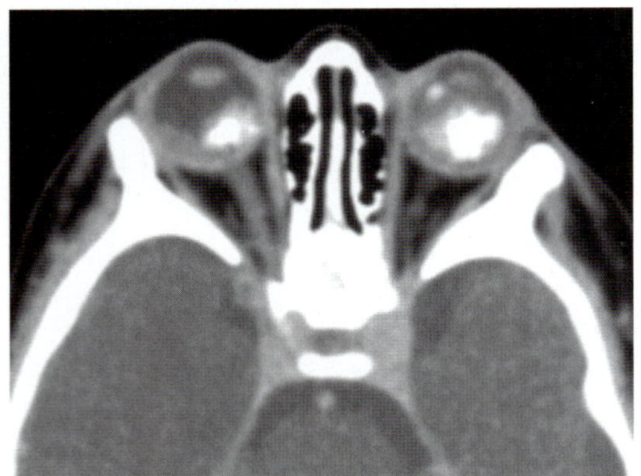

Fig. 4.85.1

Principal diagnosis: Bilateral retinoblastoma

Differential diagnosis: For intra-ocular lesions in paediatrics,

1. Persistent hyperplastic primary vitreous (unilateral >bilateral 3:1).
2. Coats' disease (90% unilateral, bilateral when syndromic) with retinal detachment.
3. Norrie's disease (bilateral) (retinal dysplasia)
4. Retinal astrocytic hamartomas of tuberous sclerosis
5. Toxocara endophthalmitis (unilateral)
6. Retinopathy of prematurity (bilateral)
7. Medulloepithelioma (unilateral)

For intraocular lesions in adults,

1. Intraocular metastasis (MC breast). Most common cause for intraocular metastasis is from breast carcinoma, however, retinal metastases are most commonly from lung primary.
2. Intraocular primary malignant melanoma.
3. Retinal hemangioblastoma.
4. Chronic retinal detachment
5. Infective endophthalmitis

Mnemonic for childhood orbital masses: "LO VISON:"

- **L**eukemia
- **O**ptic nerve glioma
- **V**ascular malformation (hemangioma, lymphangioma)
- **I**nflammation
- **S**arcoma, rhabdomyosarcoma
- **O**phthalmopathy, orbital pseudotumor
- **N**euroblastoma

Further management: Treatment is best determined by a multidisciplinary team at an experienced cancer center. Historically, enucleation has been the mainstay of treatment for retinoblastoma. Other more conservative methods include cryoablation, laser photocoagulation, and chemotherapy.

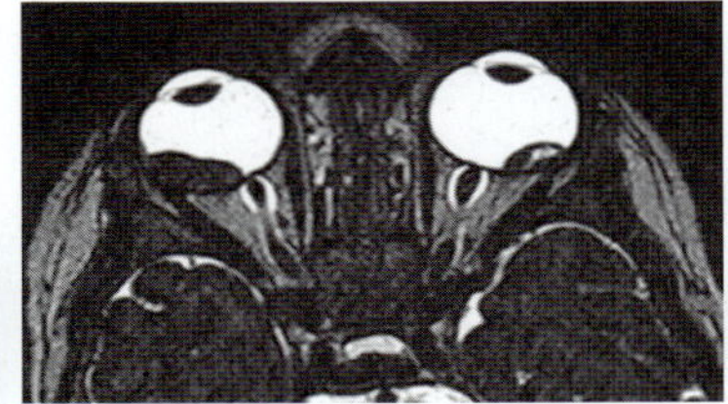

Fig. 4.85.2

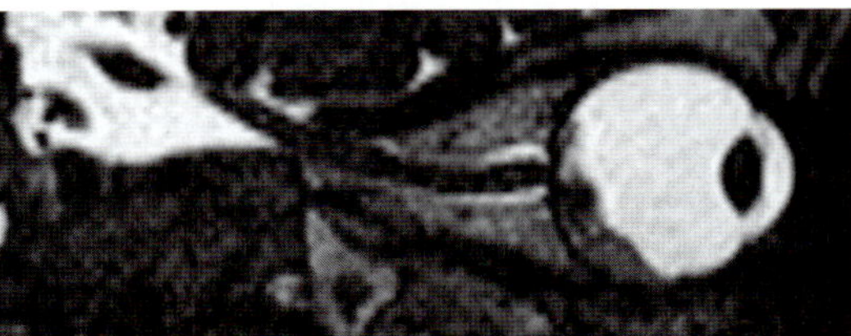

Fig. 4.85.3

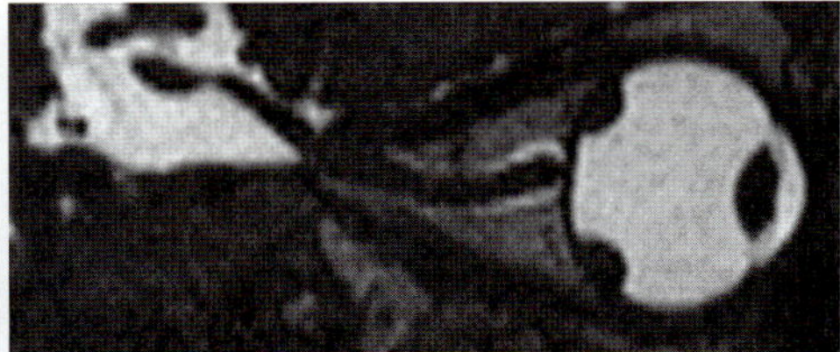

Fig. 4.85.4

Table 4.85.1: Differential diagnosis of intraocular lesions		
Condition	*Imaging*	
Persistent hyperplastic primary vitreous also known as the persistent fetal vasculature, a rare congenital developmental malformation of the eye. Failure of normal regression of the embryonic hyaloid vascular system Clinically, manifests as unilateral > bilateral leukocoria. Patients may also have poor vision, small eye (microphthalmia) and strabismus. Treatment is vitrectomy.	In USG echogenic band extending from posterior surface of lens to optic disc which shows arterial flow in color Doppler. CT-**Small globe, hyperdense vitreous**. Calcification rare. Hyperdense **hemorrhagic retinal detachment** common. MRI-retrolental tissue stalk is hypointense on T2WI, post-contrast **"martini glass shape"** of enhancing triangular retrolental vascular tuft of tissue.	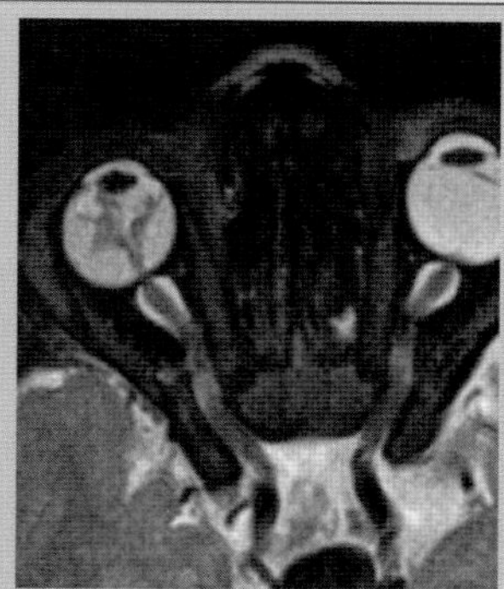 **Fig. 4.85.5:** Persistent fetal vasculature
Coats disease: Exudative retinitis, also known as retinal telangiectasis. Predominantly in young males, presenting in the first decade (3–9 years). Associated with VACTERL. Abnormal retinal capillary development leading to subretinal accumulation of exudate with retinal detachment.	Normal-size globe, CT-hyperdense; Enhancement may be seen at the margins of the exudate and may have a **V-shaped pattern similar to retinal detachment**, no Ca^{++}. MRI-Hyperintense on T1WI and T2WI due to protein exudates. Post-contrast detached retina enhances. Unilateral in 90%. Calcifications rare treatment is laser photocoagulation, cryotherapy and surgical repair of retinal detachment	
Retinopathy of prematurity: Old term Retrolental fibroplasia due to traction retinal detachment as a result of abnormal of the neovascularization in retinal vessels secondary to the prolonged oxygen therapy in premature delivery, low birth weight, and/or prolonged ventilatory support. It often occurs bilaterally.	**Small globe, in CT it appears hyperdense, bilateral involvement.** Calcification is seen in advanced cases. **Retinal detachment with sub-retinal fluid is seen.** MRI appears T2 hyperintense with post-contrast enhancement. The **sub-retinal fluid appears hyperintense in both T1 and T2.** Treatment is laser photocoagulation.	
Intraocular toxocariasis, also called ocular larva migrans, and scalarising endophthalmitis is a granulomatous nematode infection. Mean age 8 years, Male >Female. Loss of visual acuity and leukocoria is seen clinically.	CT-**enhancing nodule posteriorly** in eye, mostly unilateral. No calcification seen. Vitreal hyperdensity due to retinal detachment. MRI-**T2 hypointense, post-T1 contrast enhancement**. USG-**echogenic nodular granuloma**, vitreous membranes and retinal folds. Treatment is albendazole /steroids, surgical vitrectomy and photocoagulation	
Retinal astrocytoma: Low grade neoplasm arising from the nerve fiber layer of retina and optic nerve, childhood presentation with 50% seen associated with tuberous sclerosis and 14% in NF1. Leukocoria is seen asymptomatic slow progressive loss of vision.	CT demonstrates **soft tissue mass** or **multiple fine nodules** called **mulberry lesions** in posterior retina. Post-contrast enhancement is seen. Occasionally calcification can occur. Necrosis and hemorrhage is absent.	
Ocular primary malignant melanoma: Malignant tumor that usually originates in the uveal layers. Can extend posteriorly to the rest of the orbit.	MRI—intraorbital extent of melanoma, metastatic disease. **Melanin shortens T1 and T2, increased signal on T1-weighted images and decreased signal on T2**-weighted with hemorrhage detachments distinguished Gadolinium enhancement. Nonpigmented melanomas cannot be reliably differentiated	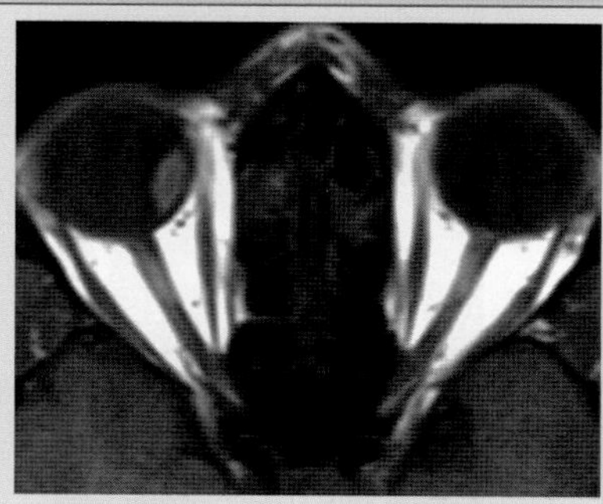 **Fig. 4.85.6:** Ocular primary malignant melanoma

Contd...

Table 4.85.1: Differential diagnosis of intraocular lesions *(Contd...)*

Intraocular metastases accounts for over 80% of all ocular pathology. The choroid is the most common ocular structure affected by metastases. Most common primary from breast, thyroid, testicular, lung carcinoma and neuroblastoma. Uveal metastases can be bilateral (up to 25%). Treatment is radiotherapy and enucleation. Extraocular metastasis can also infiltrate globe.	Appears to be echogenic in B mode USG and reflective in A mode. MRI often shows a well-demarcated choroidal mass that appears isointense on T1-weighted images and hypointense on T2-weighted images.	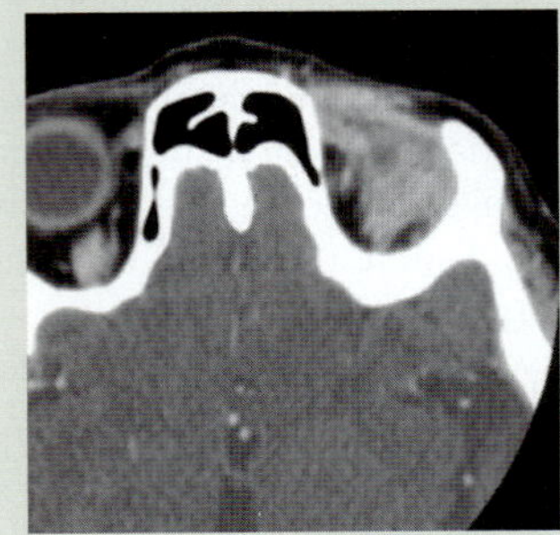 **Fig. 4.85.7:** Intraocular metastases
Medulloepithelioma: Intraocular malignant tumor usually occurs in the first decade of life. This non-pigmented, vascular mass is different in location compared with retinoblastoma; it arises from the ciliary body. It is associated with superficial cystic elements, vision loss, a lens notch, and pain due to subluxation of the lens.	**Ultrasound demonstrates a solid mass with cystic components,** usually arising from the ciliary body. T1 iso to hyperintense, T2 hypointense and the solid component enhances markedly on post-contrast administration, distant metastasis and is rare. Associated retinal detachment is common. Patients may show secondary neovascular glaucoma, dystrophic calcifications. Histopathology shows folded cords and sheets (resembling a fisherman's net, "diktyoma" pattern). Iridocyclectomy may be followed by local recurrence requiring enucleation	
Retinal hemangioblastoma: Also called retinal angiomas or capillary hemangiomas, may develop in 45–60% of VHL cases. The mean age of onset is 25 years (range, 1–68 years). Bilateral involvement may manifest in 50% of cases. Occasionally, these may be the sole manifestation of VHL.	Magnetic resonance imaging of the brain or orbit may show a tiny T2 hyperintense retinal nodule, with or without retinal detachment. Treatment is argon laser photocoagulation, cryotherapy, photodynamic therapy, proton-beam radiation therapy and surgical excision	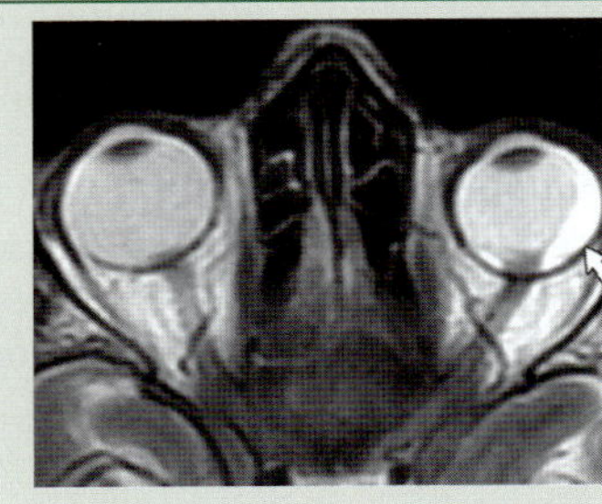 **Fig. 4.85.8:** Retinal hemangioblastoma
Infective endophthalmitis potentially sight-threatening condition that involves intraocular inflammation. Eye pain and discomfort with blurred vision. Ocular surgery penetrating injury spread of periocular infection. Treatment is intravitreal antibiotics and vitrectomy with debridement in severe cases.	CT shows proptosis intraorbital fat stranding, scleral thickening, choroidal enhancement post-contrast often in early disease, hyperdensity of the vitreous. MRI shows FLAIR hyperintensity in the vitreous. T1iso intensity or hyperintensity of the vitreous depending on the proteinaceous content restricted diffusion on DWI similarly to an abscess, this is virtually diagnostic of endophthalmitis.	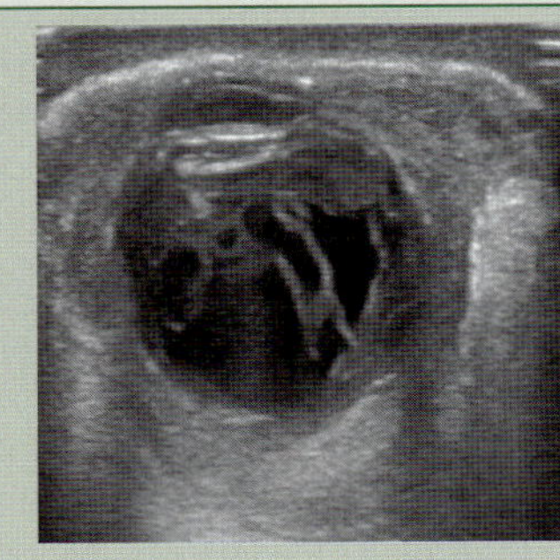 **Fig. 4.85.9:** Infective endophthalmitis
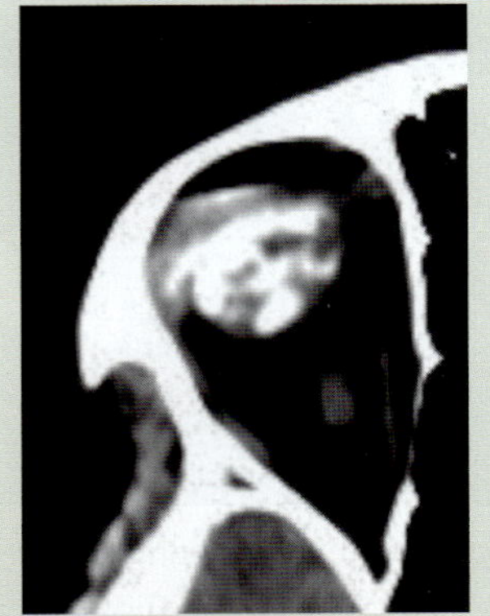 **Fig. 4.85.10:** Retinal calcification	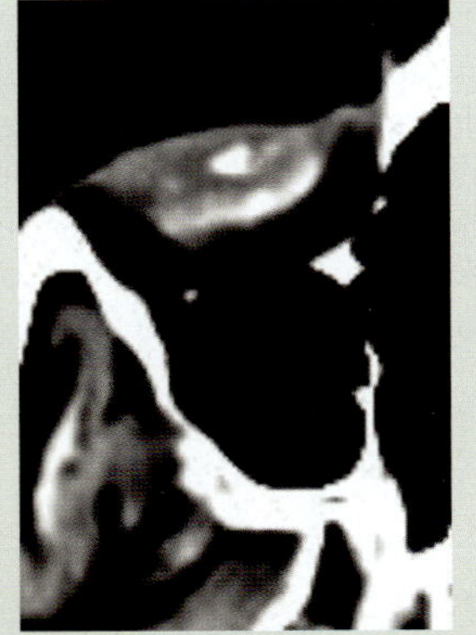 **Fig. 4.85.11:** Retinal calcification	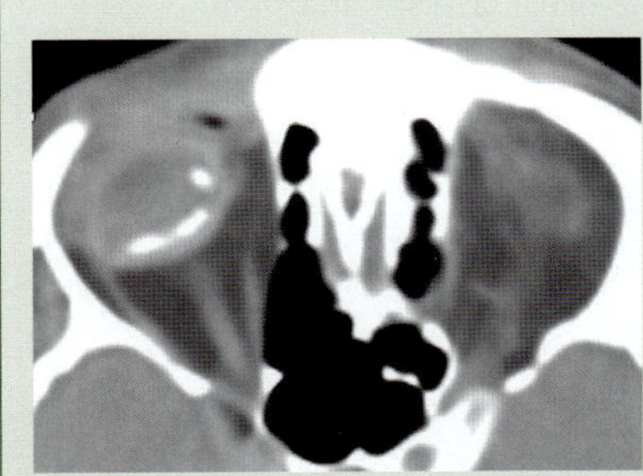 **Fig. 4.85.12:** Eyeball calcification

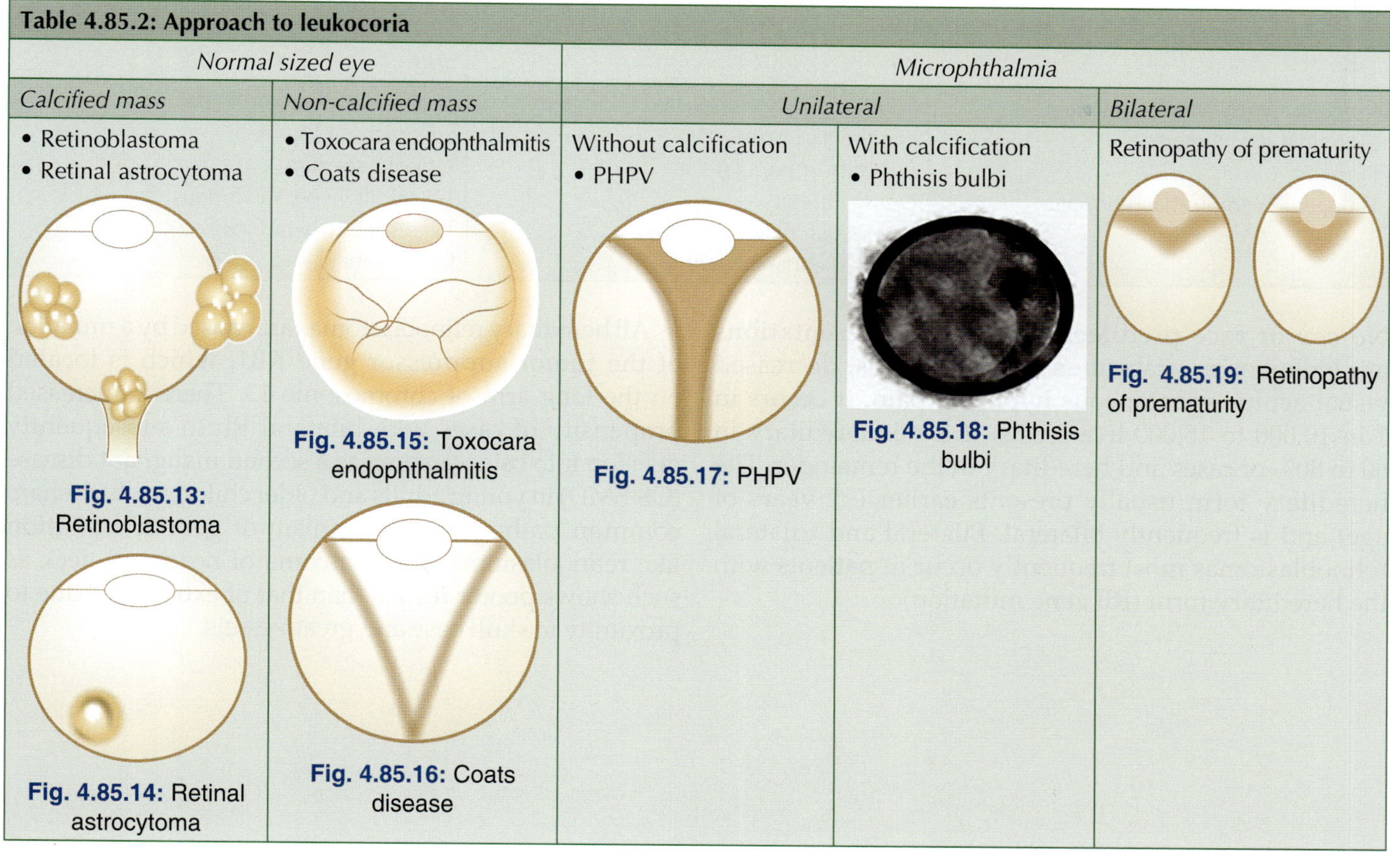

Table 4.85.2: Approach to leukocoria

Normal sized eye		*Microphthalmia*		
Calcified mass	*Non-calcified mass*	*Unilateral*		*Bilateral*
• Retinoblastoma • Retinal astrocytoma	• Toxocara endophthalmitis • Coats disease	Without calcification • PHPV	With calcification • Phthisis bulbi	Retinopathy of prematurity
Fig. 4.85.13: Retinoblastoma **Fig. 4.85.14:** Retinal astrocytoma	**Fig. 4.85.15:** Toxocara endophthalmitis **Fig. 4.85.16:** Coats disease	**Fig. 4.85.17:** PHPV	**Fig. 4.85.18:** Phthisis bulbi	**Fig. 4.85.19:** Retinopathy of prematurity

Optic nerve involvement is an important port for dissemination of tumor cells into the sub-arachnoid space. If enucleation is performed, resection of a long segment of the optic nerve is attempted to reduce the risk for tumor spread to the subarachnoid space. If the optic nerve is unaffected, the overall mortality rate is less than 10%. Hematogeneous metastasis to lungs and bones can occur it has poor prognosis. The tumor shows restricted diffusion on DWI at high b values. It exhibits low ADC values in contrast to the high intensity of the vitreous in the ADC maps.

ADC map can be used to differentiate viable and necrotic tumor. DWI is valuable in evaluating the response to eye-preservation treatment.

Brief Discussion about the Condition: Trilateral Retinoblastoma

Trilateral retinoblastoma refers to a primary midline intracranial tumor (usually pineoblastoma) in the presence of unilateral or bilateral retinoblastoma. The presence of a second midline tumor in the suprasellar or parasellar region is referred to as quadrilateral retinoblastoma.

Retinoblastoma is neuroepithelioma of retina arising from primitive photoreceptor cells of retina. Leukocoria (60%) followed by strabismus (20%). In 25–33% patients the disease is bilateral and represents autosomal dominant. Three growth patterns are described: (a) Endophytic anterior tumor growth from retina into vitreous cavity (simulating endophthalmitis), (b) Exophytic tumor into subretinal space, producing secondary retinal detachment (simulating Coats' disease) (c) Diffuse tumor growth along the retina appearing as a placoid mass. The detection of calcification is an important diagnostic criterion. Optic nerve involvement increases mortality rate. Involvement of optic nerve or choroid infiltration is an important predictor of metastases in retinoblastoma.

International classification of retinoblastoma staging,

Stage 0: Patients treated conservatively
Stage I: Eye enucleated, completely resected histologically
Stage II: Eye enucleated, microscopic residual tumor
Stage III: Regional extension A: Overt orbital disease; B: Preauricular or cervical lymph node extension
Stage IV: Metastatic disease A: Haematogeneous metastasis without CNS involvement single lesion, multiple lesions; B: CNS metastatic involvement, prechiasmatic lesion, CNS mass, leptomeningeal disease

Clinical: Most common intraocular neoplasm in childhood. Mean age is 18 months, 95% in <5 years.

Table 4.85.3: Imaging features of retinoblastoma		
USG	*CT*	*MRI*
Irregular hyperechoic solid mass 20 retinal detachment Fine Ca^{++} Echogenic vitreous haemorrhage	Solid smoothly marginated lobulated Hyperdense mass Punctate or nodular Ca^{++} Dense vitreous Extraocular extension–25% Contrast enhancement–25%	Assess extent into optic pathway Subarachnoid space Vitreous seeding T1–Mildly hyper to vitreous T2–distinctly hypointense Enhancement ++

No sex or race predilection. Clinical presentations are leukokoria, strabismus, rubeosis iridis, decreased visual acuity, spontaneous hyphema pain. It occurs in 1 in 10,000 to 15,000 live births. It is nonhereditary in 60 to 80% of cases and hereditary in the remainder. The hereditary form usually presents earlier (<2 years of age) and is frequently bilateral. Bilateral and trilateral retinoblastomas most frequently occur in patients with the hereditary form (RB gene mutation).

All hereditary retinoblastomas are caused by a mutation of the tumor suppressor gene RB1, which is located on the long arm of chromosome 13. There is increased propensity of cases with bilateral Rb to subsequently develop into osteosarcoma as a second malignant disease (OS-SMD) in young adults and older children which share common pathogenic mechanism of genetic mutation like retinoblastoma. Osteosarcoma of head and neck as such shows poorer results than that of extremities due to proximity to skull base and great vessels.

4.86 HEAD AND NECK

Case No. 86

Clinical history: A 75-year-old man with painless and progressive visual field loss for the past 20 days was examined.

Radiological techniques and observation: Figures 4.86.1 to 4.86.4 are axial T1/T2-weighted image with FLAIR/ T2W coronal images showing well-defined hyper-intense signal intensity mass in the right sub-retinal region with retinal detachment. Considering the age of patient enhancing mass in this location most likely to be malignant lesion. Figure 4.86.5 is axial contrast-enhanced T1W with fat sat showing intense homogeneous enhancement.

Principal diagnosis: A—71 years. old male, lesion in right retina, C—T1 hyperintense mass lesion arising from the right subretinal region, B—showing intense enhancement, D—right choroidal melanoma.

Management: Further work up – FDG PET uptake study for systemic staging and local metabolic activity.

Further screening of axial skeleton, lung, should be done to rule out distant metastasis.

Treatment: Treatment for uveal malignant melanoma depends on tumor size and clinician's preference. Options include photocoagulation, transpupillary thermotherapy (TTT), brachytherapy, local excision, or enucleation.

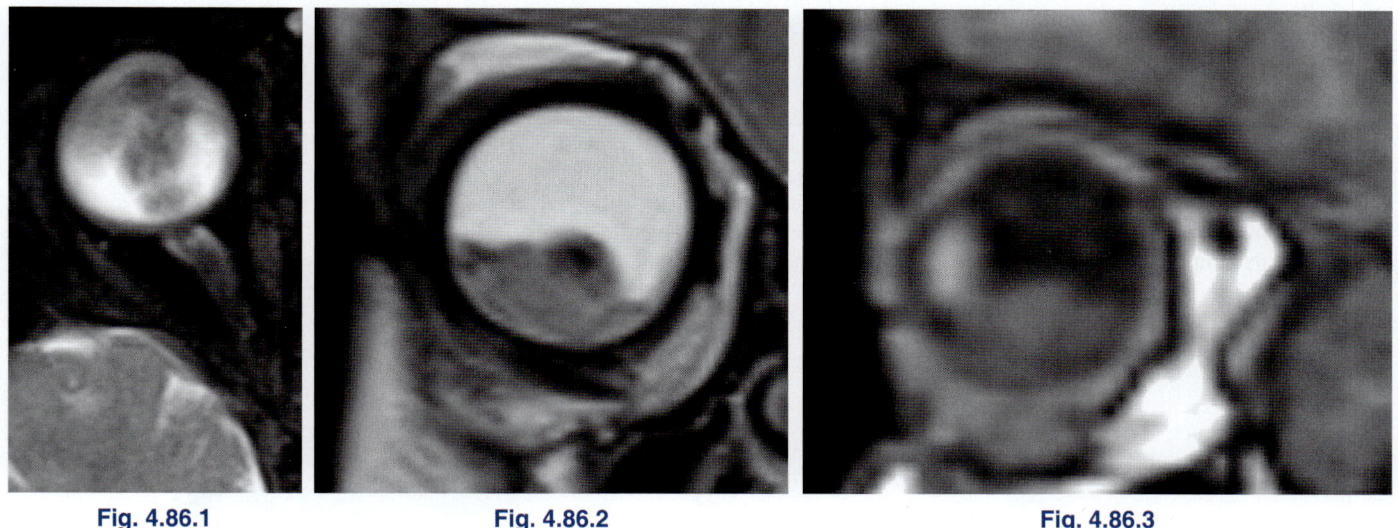

Fig. 4.86.1 Fig. 4.86.2 Fig. 4.86.3

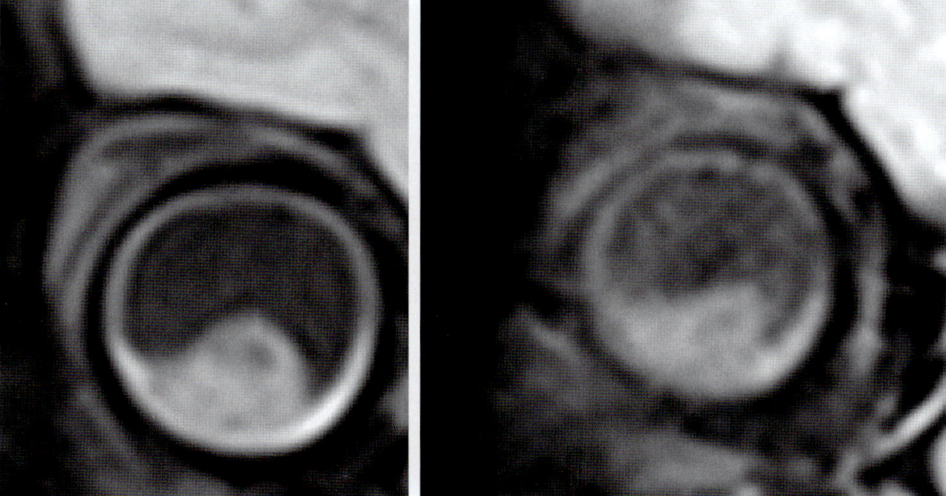

Fig. 4.86.4 Fig. 4.86.5

Table 4.86.1: Differential diagnosis for choroidal melanoma	
Sinonasal undifferentiated carcinoma with orbital invasion. Seen from 4th to 6th decade. Male to female ratio of 3:1.	**CECT:** Tumors tend to enhance in varying degrees. **MRI:** Most lesions show intermediate signal intensity on T1-W MR images and slight hypointense signal intensity on T2-W images with associated bone destruction.
Orbital lymphoma (B cell lymphomas): Most common primary orbital tumor in older adults (≥60 years of age). The majority of lesions are unilateral (76%) and often they are extraconal. Treatment is chemoradiotherapy.	Bulky, homogeneous, T1/T2W intermediate signal intensity and shows moderate enhancement. The lacrimal gland is involved in nearly 40% of cases.
Metastatic breast cancer has higher predilection to metastasis into the orbit, followed by metastatic prostate carcinoma, melanoma and lung cancer. Treatment: Concurrent chemo radiotherapy.	On T2-W MR images, metastasis from hemorrhagic tumors and mucinous adenocarcinoma of the colon can appear as hypointense signal intensity lesions, while the absence of a primary tumor and the presence of homogeneous enhancement can also suggest primary melanoma. Breast cancer will localize to orbital fat and muscle, prostate cancer will spread to bony orbit, lung CA has predilection to choroid, and melanoma has strong preference for muscle.
Orbital hemangioma: Seen in 30 to 50 years age group with female predominance. Conservative treatment for asymptomatic cases and surgical excision in symptomatic cases.	**CT:** Well-marginated soft tissue mass showing mild or heterogeneous enhancement. **MRI:** Isointense to slightly increased signal on T1 and marked signal intensity on T2. **DSA:** Hemangiomas are occult as enhancement occurs only in a delayed fashion.
Choroidal hemorrhage leading to choroidal detachment: It mostly occurs between 55 and 70 years. No sex predilection. Mostly after trauma/surgery. Other causes are medications, spontaneous, hypertension and ocular malignancy. Treatment for trauma cases is done with tamponade procedures and for non-trauma cases, underlying cause is treated.	**CT:** Choroidal hemorrhage classically appears as a hyperdense lentiform lesion. **MRI:** Will show haemoglobin products throughout the sequences, typically with a high T1 signal. 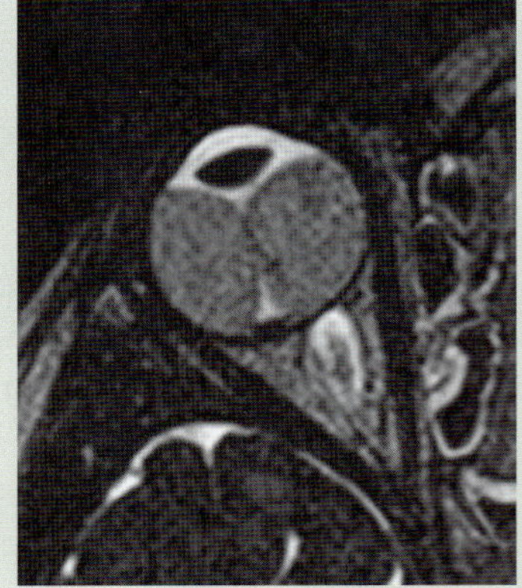 Fig. 4.86.6: Choroidal detachment
Vitreous hemorrhage leading to vitreous detachment is male predominant, occurring between 40 and 60 years. Extravasation/blood leakage in vitreous humor of the eye. Treatment is posterior vitrectomy.	**Ultrasound:** Acute vitreous hemorrhage is seen as scattered, ill-defined collections of slightly echogenic opacities. **CT:** Hemorrhage usually demonstrates hyperattenuation, which may be either homogeneous or heterogeneous, in the vitreous chamber.
Endophthalmitis: No age or sex predilection. It is severe form of ocular inflammation due to intraocular infection cavity that can lead to irreversible vision loss unless treated on time. Intravitreal antibiotics are used for treatment.	**MRI:** T1 isointensity or hyperintensity of the vitreous with DWI restriction, intraocular edema and high FLAIR signal.
Coats disease unilateral retinal telangiectasias in young adults (6 to 9 years) with male sex predilection causing subretinal exudative deposits and retinal detachment without retrolental mass.	**CT** enhancement may be seen at the margins of the exudate and may be similar to retinal detachment. **MRI T1:** High signal due to proteinaceous nature of the exudates. **T2:** High signal due to proteinaceous nature of the exudates.

(Contd.)

Table 4.86.1: Differential diagnosis for choroidal melanoma (*Contd.*)

Retinal detachment: More common in 6th to 7th decade with male predilection. It can be treated using scleral buckling, pneumatic retinopexy, pars plana vitrectomy or injection of intraocular silicone oil.	**CT:** Subretinal fluid appears hyperdense **MRI** T1-hyperintense T2-hypointense **T1 C+ (Gd)**-enhancement of the detached retina may be visible.	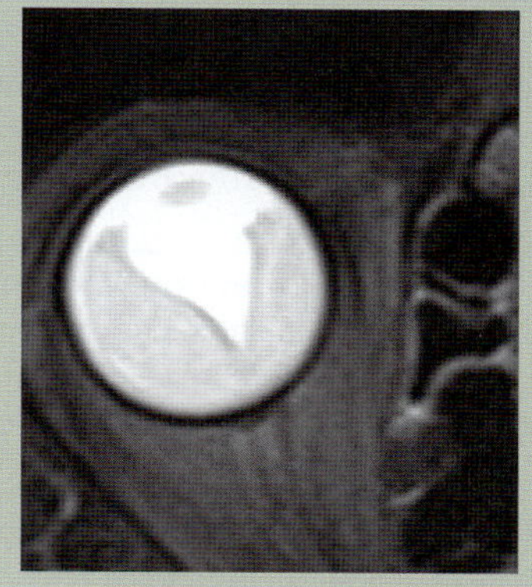 **Fig. 4.86.7:** Retinal detachment
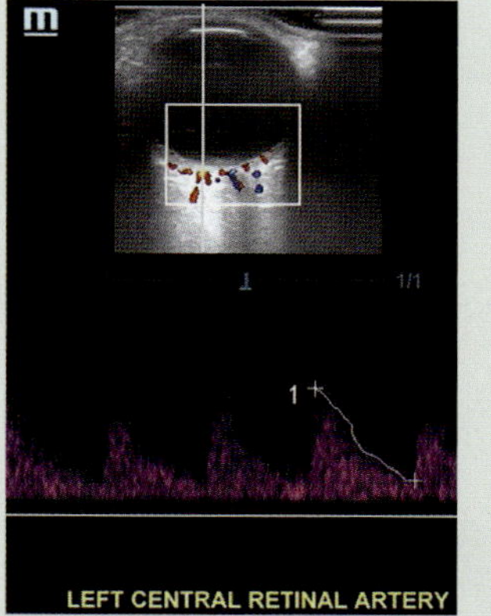 **Fig. 4.86.8:** Normal left retinal artery	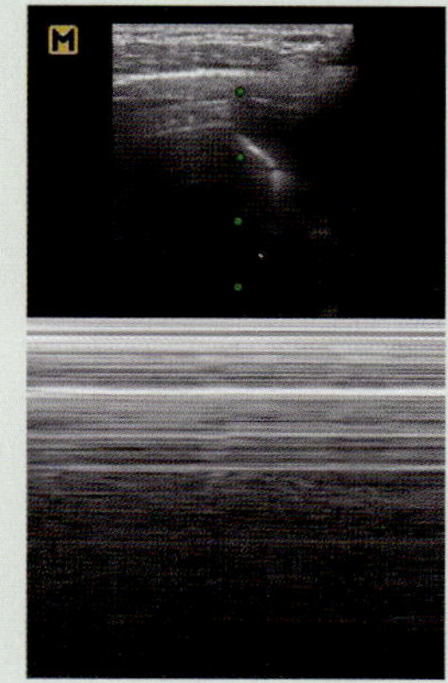 **Fig. 4.86.9:** Retinal detachment	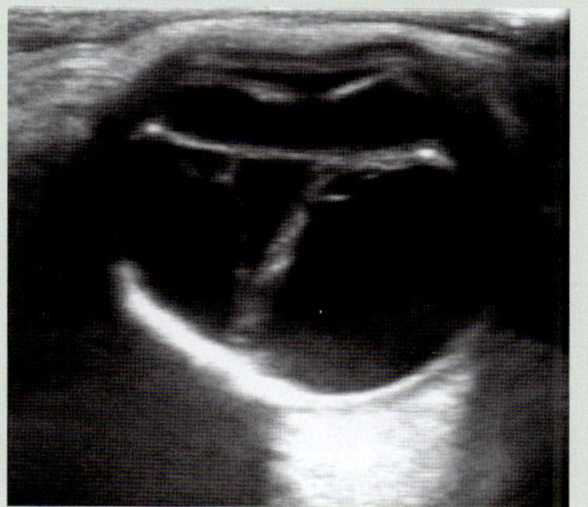 **Fig. 4.86.10:** Retinal detachment
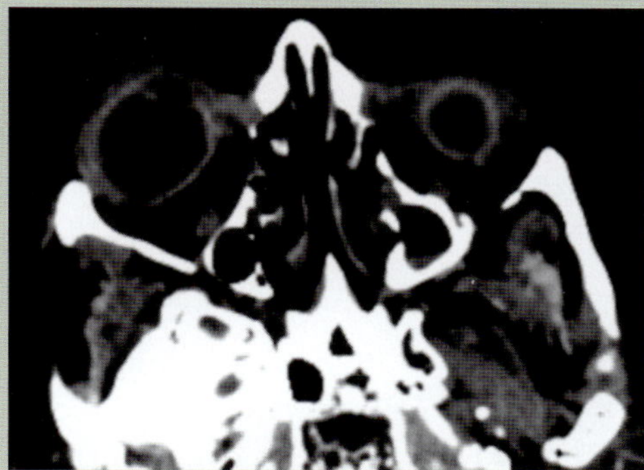 **Fig. 4.86.11:** Coloboma	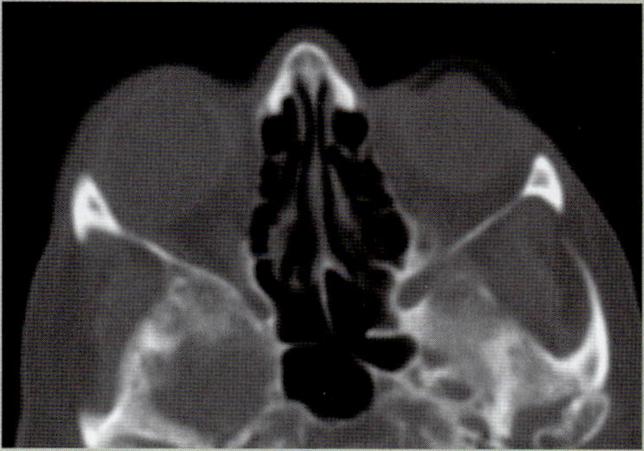 **Fig. 4.86.12:** Coloboma	
Lens dislocation		
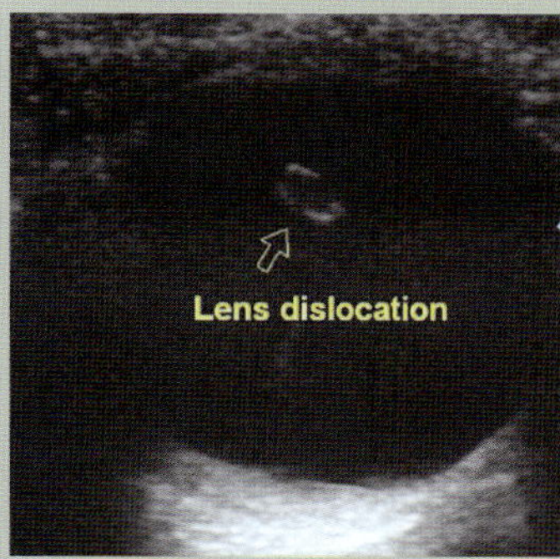 **Fig. 4.86.13:** Lens dislocation	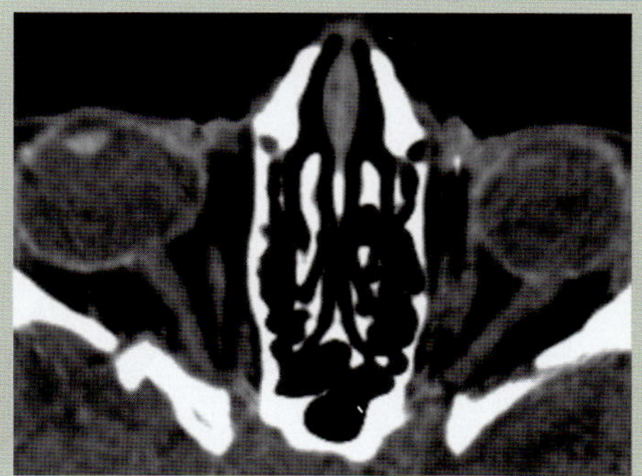 **Fig. 4.86.14:** Lens dislocation	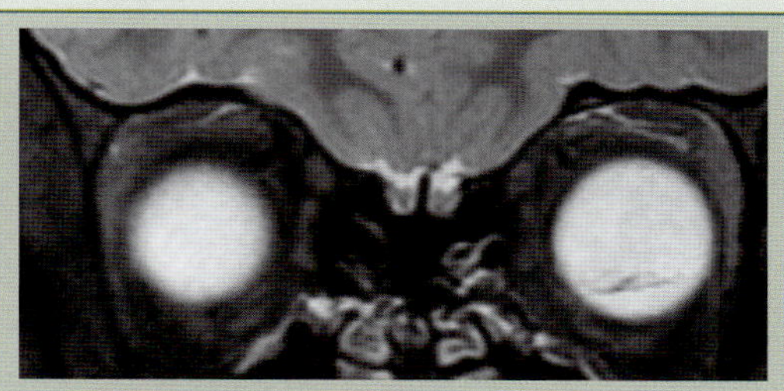 **Fig. 4.86.15:** Lens dislocation

Table 4.86.2: Difference between retinal, choroidal and vitreous detachment		
Retinal detachment	*Choroidal detachment*	*Vitreous detachment*
Accumulation of blood or fluid in subretinal space between 2 layers of retina, inner sensory layer and outer pigmentary epithelium.	Accumulation of blood or fluid in suprachoroidal space between choroid and sclera, so collection extend circumferentially along the entire suprachoroidal space.	When the retinal layer and vitreous body/ posterior hyaloid membrane dissociate, with an intervening fluid collection forming in the subhyaloid space.
Configuration of collection **crescent shaped/V shaped** on axial sections, limbs of V represent detached leaves of retina converging towards optic disc represent apex of V.	Configuration of collection is **lentiform shaped** along medial as well as lateral wall of globe, choroid bulging medially on either side giving so **kissing choroid sign**.	Don't have any pathognomonic shapes. They are **more hypointense on T2-weighted** images than are melanomas and do not show enhancement.
Collection anteriorly extend up to ora serrata represent anterior limit due to normal anterior attachment of retina.	Collection anteriorly extend up to ciliary bodies and posterior limit formed by anchoring effect of short posterior ciliary arteries and nerves that prevent convergence of detached choroidal leaves to single point.	Collection noted within the vitreous humor.

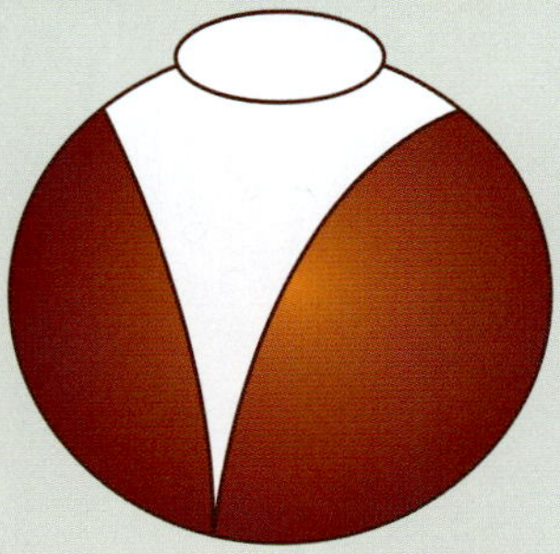

Fig. 4.86.16: Retinal detachment

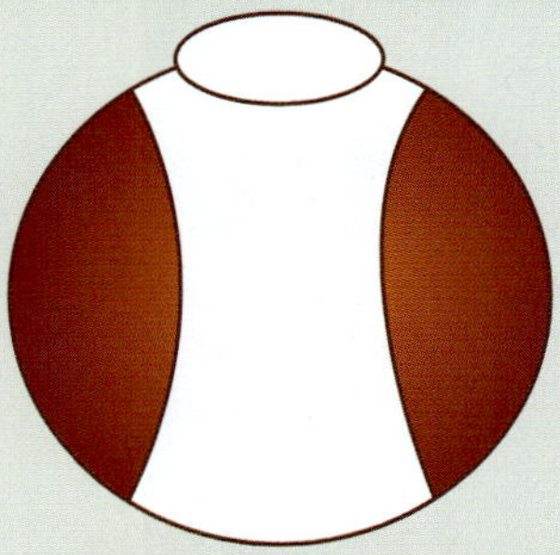

Fig. 4.86.18 Choroidal detachment

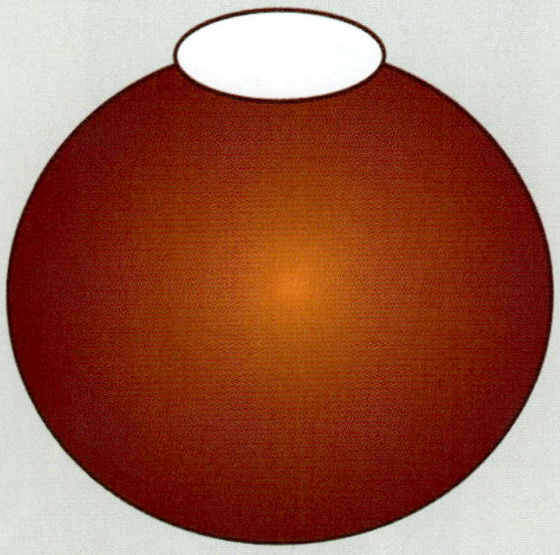

Fig. 4.86.20: Vitreous detachment

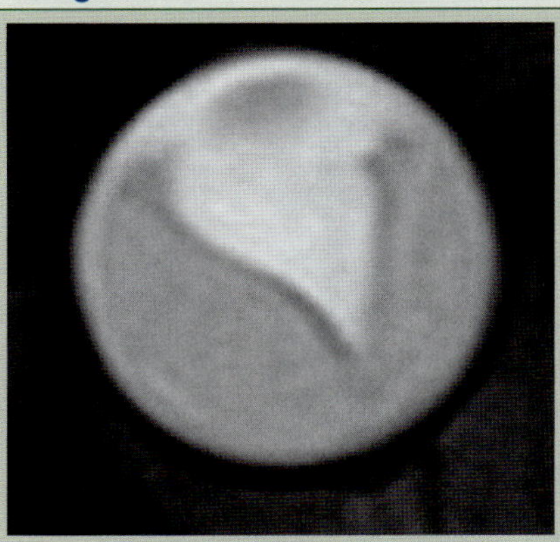

Fig. 4.86.17: Retinal detachment

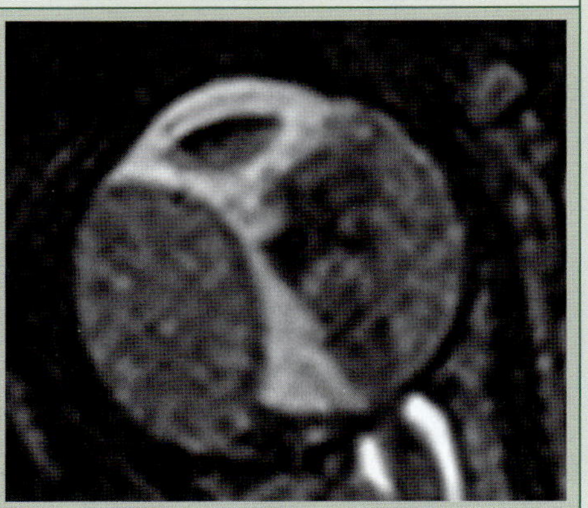

Fig. 4.86.19: Choroidal detachment

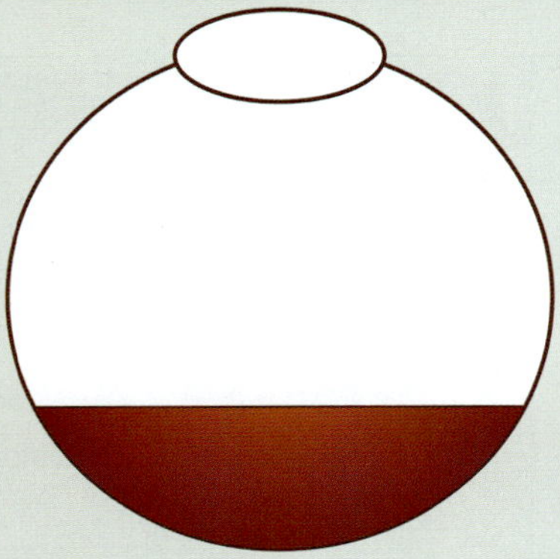

Fig. 4.86.21: Posterior hyaloid detachment

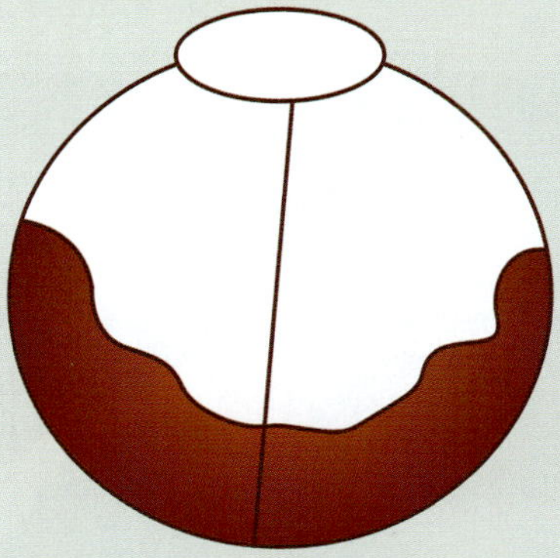

Fig. 4.86.22: Persistent hyperplastic primary vitreous with RD

Table 4.86.3: Causes of orbital calcification

Extraocular calcifications	*Post-therapeutic orbital changes*	*Intraocular calcifications*
Trochlear calcifications (age-related normal variant/young diabetics) Limbus calcifications	• Lens implant • Scleral band • Intraocular silicon gel injections • Pneumatic retinopexy • Globe prosthesis	• Retinoblastoma • Astrocytic hamartoma • Choroidal osteoma • Optic drusen • Phthisis bulbi • Calcified cataract • Retrolental hyperplasia • Scleral calcifications

Prognosis: WHO grading of head and neck tumours–grade IV tumor, poor prognosis

Discussion: Malignant, invasive, highly cellular tumor, WHO grade—IV tumor.

Age group—50 to 80 years. There is no evidence of sex predominance. The incidence is higher amongst fair-skinned pale-eyed individuals. Melanoma is due to proliferation of melanocytes, which derive from the neural crest and subsequently migrate into the nasal mucosal surfaces with an ectodermal origin. The etiology of choroidal melanoma is still unknown at present. It is a malignant tumor that usually originates in the uveal layers and can extend posteriorly to the rest of the orbit. They are T1 hyperintense and T2 hypointense tumor. The free radical found in melanin or in paramagnetic metals bound to melanin is thought to be responsible for this paramagnetic feature. The signal intensities are determined by the amount of melanin in the tumor and its distribution. When it comes to determining episcleral extension, MRI is the method of choice. With haemorrhage, the differential diagnosis includes retinal and choroid detachments. Detachments are distinguished on gadolinium enhancement. Non-pigmented melanomas cannot be reliably differentiated.

4.87 HEAD AND NECK

Case No. 87

Clinical history: Nine months old male child presenting with large head with mild developmental delay.

Radiological technique and observation: Figure 4.87.1 is **X-ray skull AP view** showing large head with midface hypoplasia. Bilateral orbits appear prominent. Coronal and sagittal sutures appear to be fused. Prominent convolutional markings noted in the skull. Figure 4.87.2 is **X-ray hand AP view** showing fusion of distal phalanges of second and third finger and fusion of middle and distal phalanges of second finger.

Interpretation: A—Nine months old male child, skull and hand shows, C—macrocephaly with syndactyly, B—craniosynostosis, D—Apert syndrome.

Principal diagnosis: Acrocephalosyndactyly—Apert syndrome.

Discussion: **Acrocephalosyndactyly** = syndrome characterized by craniosynostosis, syndactyly of fingers/toes. If associated with multiple fingers—acrocephalopolysyndactyly.

Craniosynostosis: Premature closure of sutures (closing normally at about 30 years of age).

Age: Often present at birth; M: F = 4:1.

Types: Sagittal suture most commonly affected followed by coronal suture: 1. Scaphocephaly = Dolichocephaly (55%): premature closure of sagittal suture (long skull), 2. Brachycephaly = premature closure of coronal/ lambdoid sutures (short tall skull), 3. Plagiocephaly (7%): unilateral early fusion of coronal + lambdoidal suture (lopsided skull), 4. Trigonocephaly: Premature closure of metopic suture (forward pointing skull), 5. Oxycephaly=Acrocephaly = Turricepahly: Premature closure of coronal, sagittal, lambdoid sutures (conical skull); most severe form of craniosynostosis, 6. Cloverleaf skull = Kleeblattschädel—intrauterine premature closure of sagittal, coronal, lambdoid sutures may be associated with thanatophoric dysplasia.

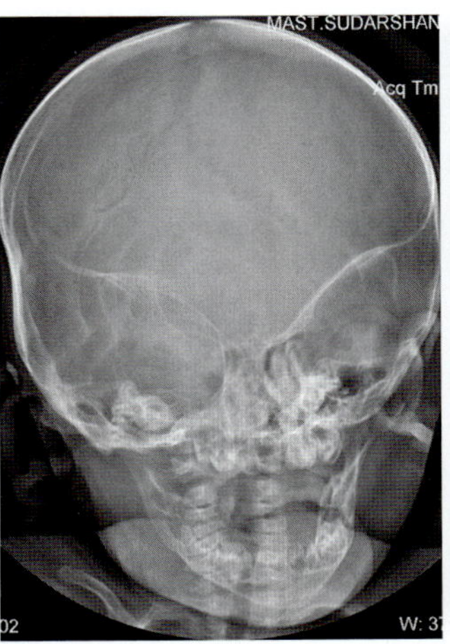

Fig. 4.87.1

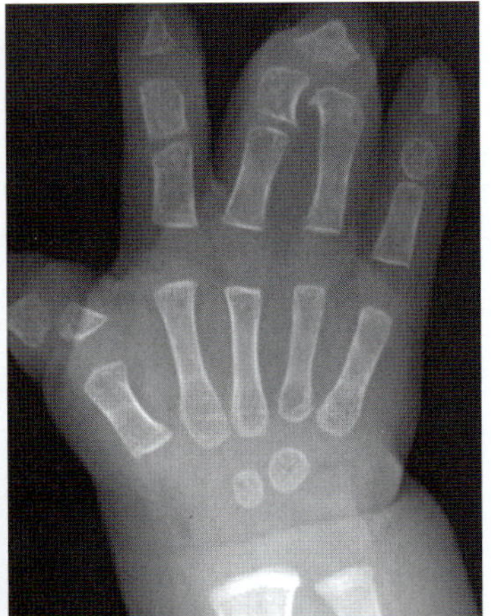

Fig. 4.87.2

Types of Acrocephalosyndactyly and Acrocephalopolysyndactyly

Table 4.87.1: Types of acrocephalosyndactyly

Types of acrocephalo-syndactyly	*Syndrome*
1	Apert syndrome
2	Crouzon syndrome
3	Saethre–Chotzen syndrome
4	Waardenburg type
5	Pfeiffer syndrome

Table 4.87.2: Types of acrocephalopolysyndactyly

Types of acrocephalo-polysyndactyly	*Syndrome*
1	Noack syndrome
2	Carpenter syndrome
3	Sakati-Nyhan-Tisdale syndrome
4	Goodman syndrome
5	Pfeiffer syndrome

Apert syndrome: Apert syndrome is a rare type I acrocephalosyndactyly syndrome which presents with craniosynostosis, syndactyly of the hands and feet, and dysmorphic features of the face.

Autosomal dominant disorder with the locus of a mutation of FGFR2 on chromosome 10q.

Imaging findings: Brachycephalic skull (← coronal craniosynostosis) + flat occiput, hypertelorism, shallow orbits with proptosis, underdeveloped paranasal sinuses, underdeveloped maxilla with prognathism, enlargement of sella, stylohyoid ligament calcification, cervical spine fusion (in up to 71%), commonly of 5th and 6th vertebrae, choanal stenosis, severe symmetric syndactyly = fusion of distal portions of phalanges, metacarpals, carpals (most often of 2nd, 3rd + 4th digit), absence of middle phalanges, missing/supernumerary carpal/tarsal bone/pseudarthroses, cryptorchidism, hydronephrosis, polycystic kidneys (rare) bicornuate uterus (rare).

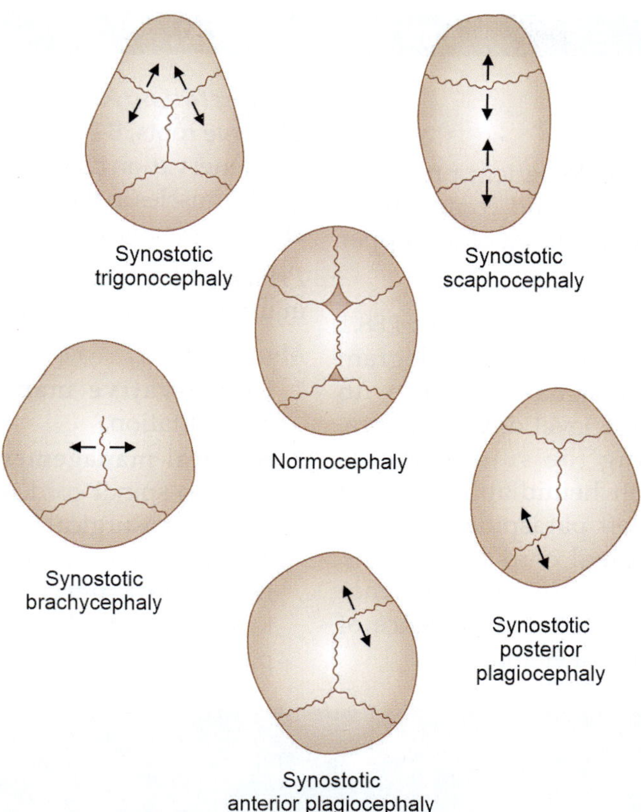

Fig. 4.87.3: Types of craniosynostosis

Crouzon syndrome: AD inheritance.

Imaging findings: Skull + cranial base deformities characterized by craniosynostosis, maxillary hypoplasia; Chiari I malformation, hydrocephalus, agenesis of corpus callosum; Shallow orbits, ocular proptosis, bifid uvula, cleft palate; Stylohyoid ligament calcification; Elbow malformation (18%); Minor hand deformities (10%); Visceral anomalies (7%); Musculoskeletal deformities (7%) but no limb anomaly.

Pfeiffer syndrome: Acrocephalosyndactyly type 5.

Imaging findings: Craniosynostosis, hypertelorism, proptosis; maxillary hypoplasia; brachydactyly/ syndactyly; broad thumbs + toes; mild soft-tissue syndactyly.

4.88 HEAD AND NECK

Case No. 88

Clinical history: A 28-year-old male patient presented with history of road traffic accident and complains of breathlessness, weakness and paresthesia of left upper limb.

Radiological techniques and observations: Figures 4.88.1 to 4.88.3 are STIR coronal, T2 axial, MR myelogram images showing abnormal CSF signal intensity with empty thecal diverticulum at the level of C8 vertebra, denervation edema involving the supraspinatus and infraspinatus, elevated left hemidiaphragm and hyperintensity involving the left paraspinal muscles. No evidence of transdural spinal cord herniation/ altered signal intensity in the cord. No obvious evidence of vascular injury/hematoma noted. No evidence of fracture noted in the surrounding skeleton.

Interpretation: A—28 years old male with lesion in C5 to T1 nerve roots, B—presence of pseudomeningocele with C—denervation changes in the paraspinal and shoulder girdle muscles in the setting of trauma, D—preganglionic brachial plexus avulsion injury.

Principal diagnosis: C5–T1 total brachial plexus avulsion injury (preganglionic) with distal denervation changes.

Management:

1. **Conservative management:** Physical therapy, rehabilitation.
2. **Surgical management:** Reanastomosis of avulsed roots to spinal cord is not generally advocated, but new microsurgical techniques are prompting review. Nerve bypass or graft, reconstruction with neurolysis, nerve graft, nerve transfer, functioning muscle/ tendon transfer. Dorsal root entry zone (DREZ) lesion palliation for intractable pain.

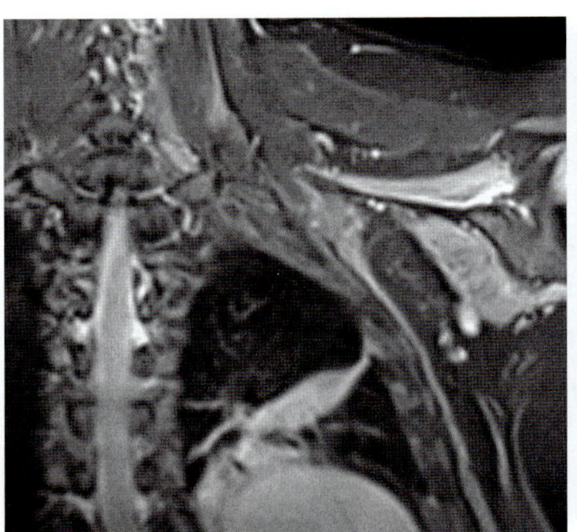

Fig. 4.88.1

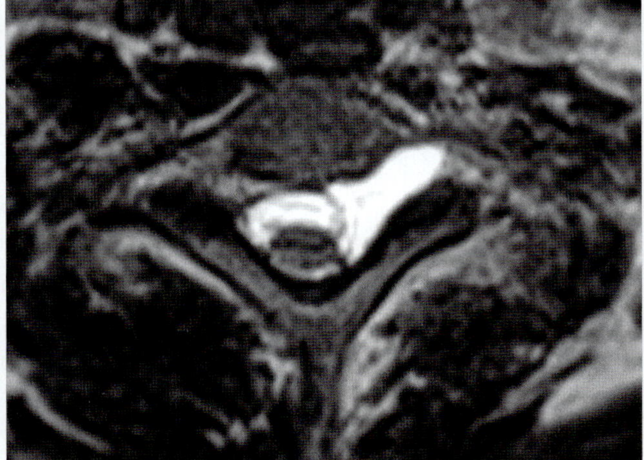

Fig. 4.88.2

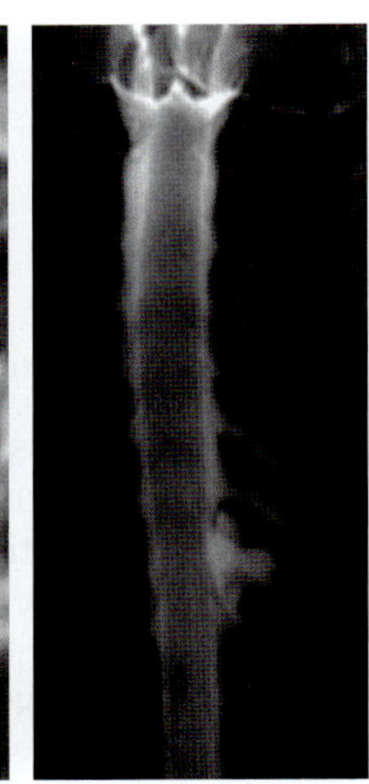

Fig. 4.88.3

Table 4.88.1: Differential diagnosis for brachial plexus lesion		
Brachial plexus lesion	*Imaging findings*	*Image*
Brachial plexus stretch injury Enlargement or attenuation of stretched (but contiguous) plexus elements seen in patients with history of trauma.	Enlargement with T1 hypo/T2 hyperintense signal of neural elements, without any discontinuity.	Fig. 4.88.4: Brachial plexus stretch injury

(Contd.)

Table 4.88.1: Differential diagnosis for brachial plexus lesion (*Contd.*)		
Brachial plexus lesion	*Imaging findings*	*Image*
Superior sulcus tumor/pancoast tumor Benign or malignant neoplasm extending to superior thoracic inlet with severe shoulder/arm pain along C8, T1, T2 nerve trunks, Horner syndrome, weakness + atrophy of intrinsic hand muscles (Pancoast syndrome). Non-small cell lung carcinoma (NSCLC)—most frequent etiology.	T2 hyperintense apical lung mass with chest wall/paravertebral extension. Post-contrast T1 imaging shows variably enhancing mass. Fat suppression improves detection of epidural/foraminal extension	
Brachial plexus neuritis Also known as **Parsonage-Turner syndrome.** Immune-mediated neuropathy of brachial plexus. Often associated with bacterial/viral infection/post-vaccination. Any muscle innervated by brachial plexus can be involved, but most commonly involved are Rotator cuff, deltoid, biceps, triceps.	In brachial plexus—affected nerves high signal intensity on T2WI, STIR and nerves show mild enhancement with gadolinium. In affected muscles—denervation edema with diffuse, homogeneous high signal on T2WI, STIR throughout affected muscle without disruption of muscle fibres. Fatty atrophy seen in chronic denervation.	**Fig. 4.88.5:** Brachial plexus neuritis
Radiation-induced fibrosis (RIF) Upper brachial plexus (BP) (C5–C7) > lower BP (C8, T1) following radiation therapy (XRT) for breast and lung cancer, lymphoma. Potentiated by chemotherapy.	Smooth, diffuse T2 hyperintensity ± enhancement of multiple plexus elements. **More focal and nodular enhancing lesions involving the lower roots are suggestive of malignant infiltration.** Pain often relatively mild compared to malignant plexopathy.	
Thoracic outlet syndrome Neural, venous, and/or arterial compressive syndrome at thoracic outlet. Involving interscalene, costoclavicular space, retro pectoralis minor space (subcoracoid tunnel).	T2WI may show **focal abnormal brachial plexus T2 hyperintensity in thoracic outlet** with or without brachial plexus compression or distortion, scalene muscle inflammation or fibrosis, abnormal vascular flow voids. Positional occlusion or narrowing of SCA with arm hyperabduction, external rotation seen in angiographic imaging. Congenital bony/fibromuscular anomalies, trauma, phenotype, and posture contribute to compression or elongation of neurovascular bundle as it passes through these compartments.	
Nerve sheath tumor Plexiform neurofibroma (NF1), solitary nerve sheath tumor mimics root avulsion. Clinical signs of NF-1 stigmata are characteristic.	T2 hyperintense lesion along the course of the nerve showing tumoral enhancement on post-contrast imaging. **Tail sign, split fat sign seen.**	**Fig. 4.88.6:** Neurofibroma

(Contd.)

Table 4.88.1: Differential diagnosis for brachial plexus lesion (*Contd.*)

Brachial plexus lesion	*Imaging findings*	*Image*
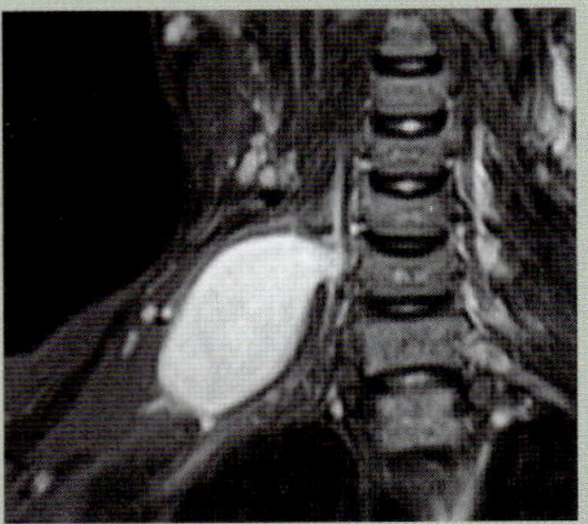 **Fig. 4.88.7:** Neurofibroma	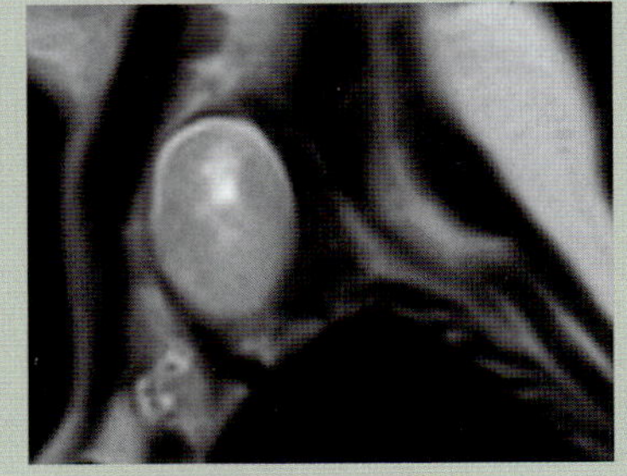 **Fig. 4.88.8:** Neurofibroma	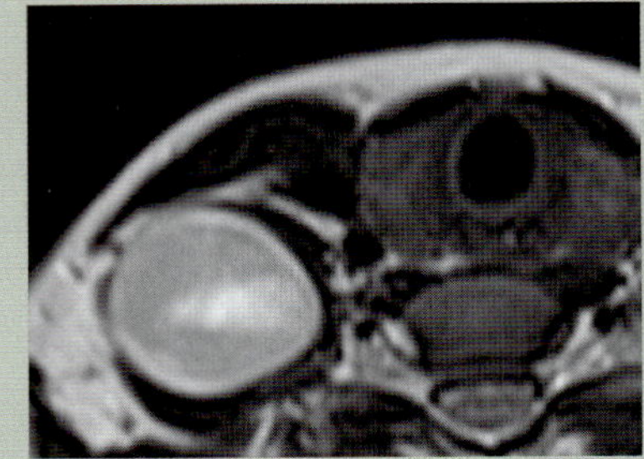 **Fig. 4.88.9:** Neurofibroma
Lateral meningocele It is comprised by a protrusion of the arachnoid and dura through the foramina and represent the most severe and extreme end of the dural ectasia spectrum.	Lateral meningocele mimics pseudomeningocele (T2 hyperintense thecal diverticulum), **but contains neural elements.** Seen in Marfan syndrome, Ehlers-Danlos syndrome, NF1.	
Nerve root sleeve cyst Perineural cysts are CSF-filled dilatations of the nerve root sheath at the dorsal root ganglion (posterior nerve root sheath). No history of trauma.	T2 hyperintense thin-walled cystic structures. Intact nerve root peripherally displaced by cyst. Foraminal widening may be seen. **Associated with risk of sudden rupture and consequent idiopathic intracranial hypotension.**	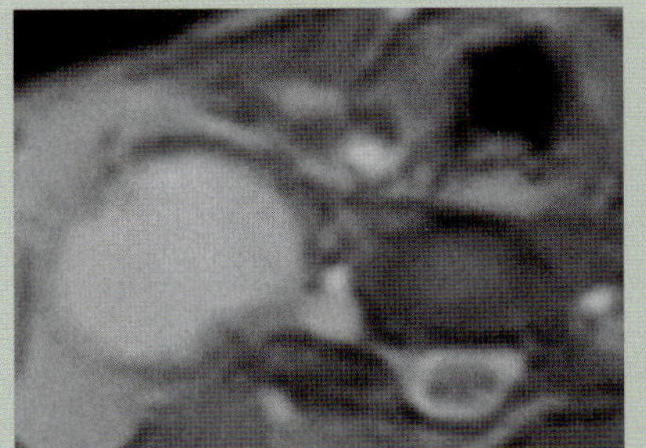 **Fig. 4.88.10:** Perineural cysts
Brachial plexus metastasis		
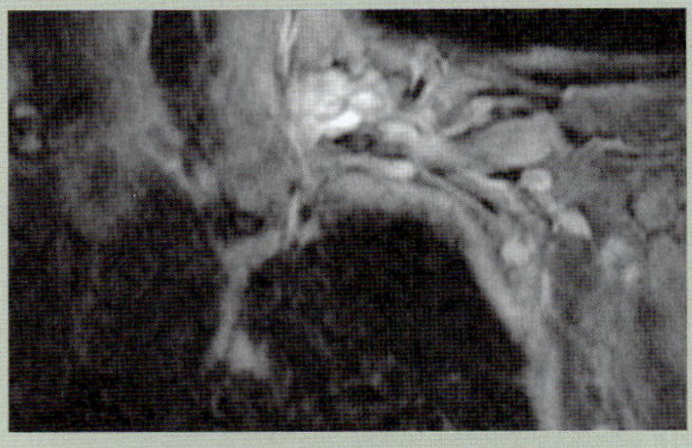 **Fig. 4.88.11:** Brachial plexus metastasis	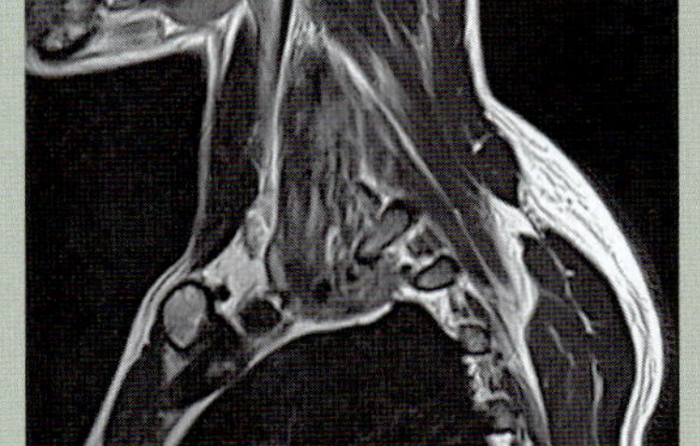 **Fig. 4.88.12:** Inflammatory myofibroblastic tumour	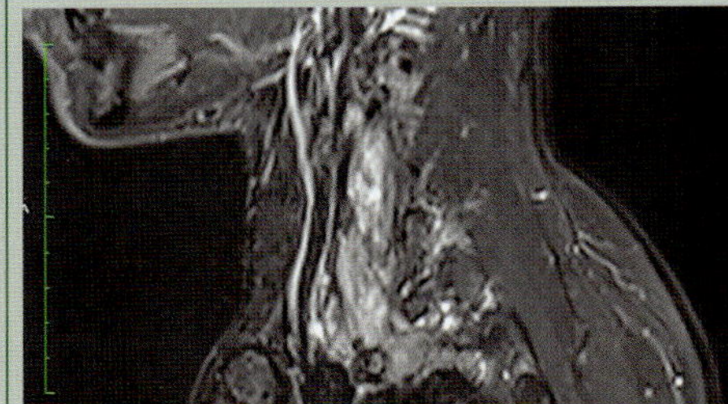 **Fig. 4.88.13:** Inflammatory myofibroblastic tumour
Brachial cyst		
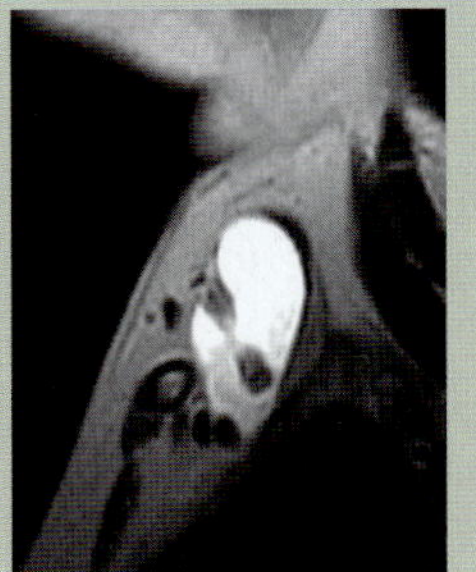 **Fig. 4.88.14:** Brachial cyst	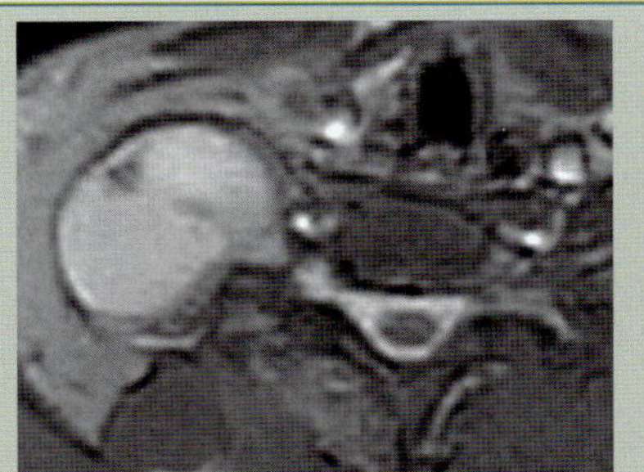 **Fig. 4.88.15:** Brachial cyst	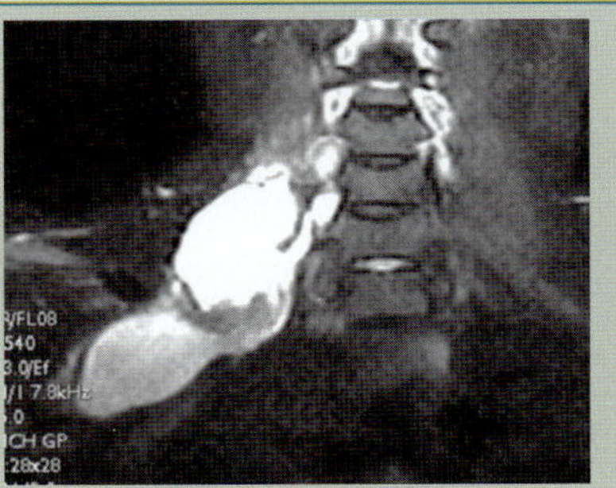 **Fig. 4.88.16:** Brachial cyst

(*Contd.*)

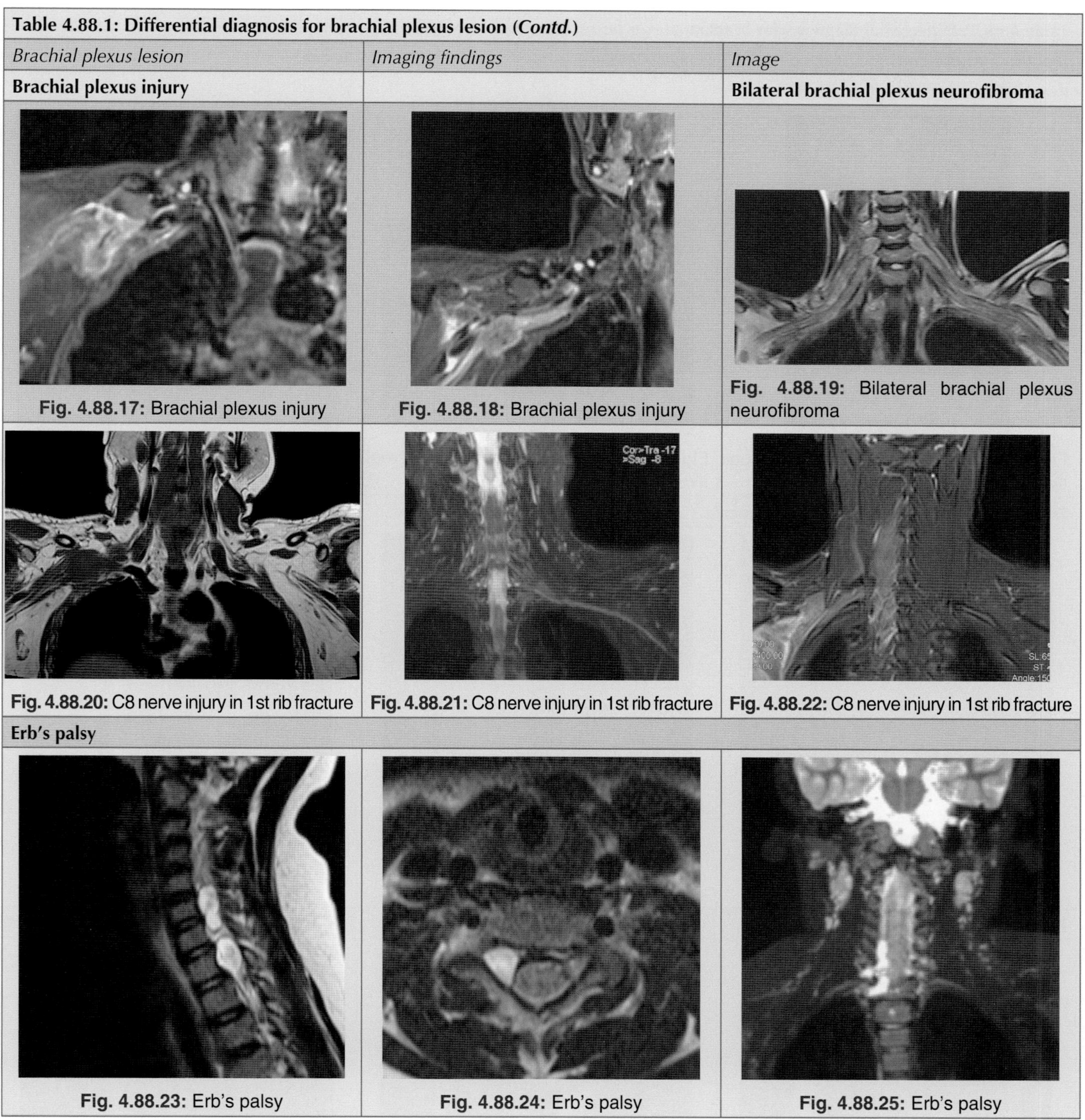

Table 4.88.1: Differential diagnosis for brachial plexus lesion (*Contd.*)

Brachial plexus lesion	*Imaging findings*	*Image*
Brachial plexus injury		**Bilateral brachial plexus neurofibroma**
Fig. 4.88.17: Brachial plexus injury	**Fig. 4.88.18:** Brachial plexus injury	**Fig. 4.88.19:** Bilateral brachial plexus neurofibroma
Fig. 4.88.20: C8 nerve injury in 1st rib fracture	**Fig. 4.88.21:** C8 nerve injury in 1st rib fracture	**Fig. 4.88.22:** C8 nerve injury in 1st rib fracture
Erb's palsy		
Fig. 4.88.23: Erb's palsy	**Fig. 4.88.24:** Erb's palsy	**Fig. 4.88.25:** Erb's palsy

(Contd.)

Table 4.88.1: Differential diagnosis for brachial plexus lesion (*Contd.*)

Brachial plexus lesion	*Imaging findings*	*Image*
Preganglionic nerve root avulsion		
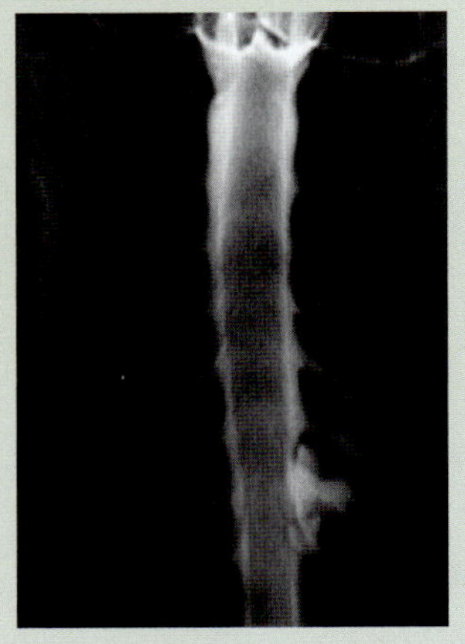 **Fig. 4.88.26:** Preganglionic nerve root avulsion	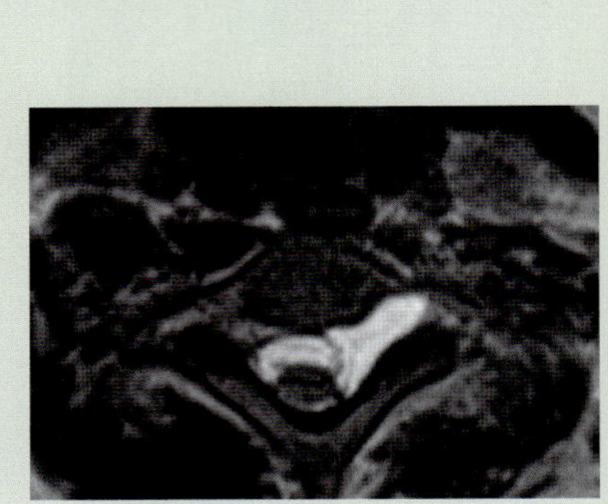 **Fig. 4.88.27:** Preganglionic nerve root avulsion	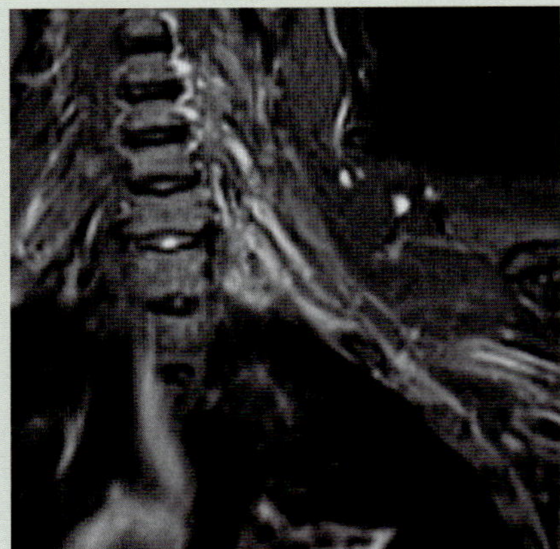 **Fig. 4.88.28:** Preganglionic nerve root avulsion
Retraction wall avulsion pseudomeningocele		
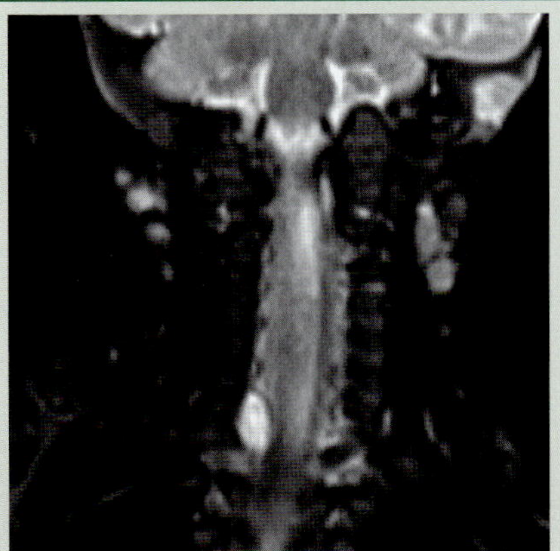 **Fig. 4.88.29:** Retraction wall avulsion pseudomeningocele	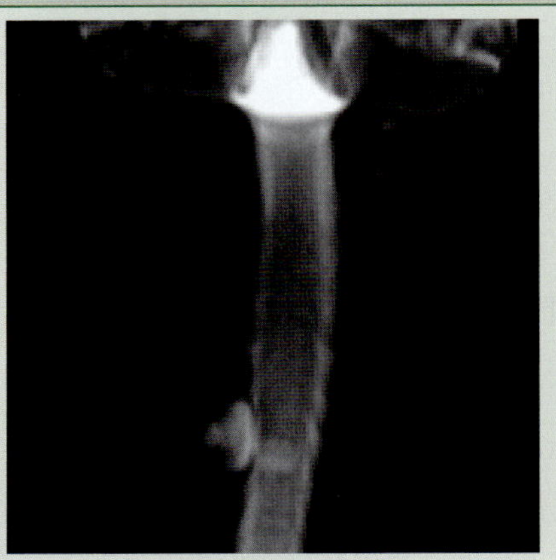 **Fig. 4.88.30:** Retraction wall avulsion pseudomeningocele	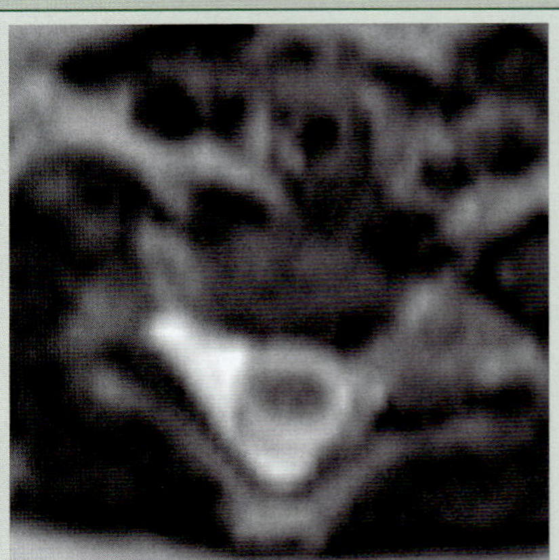 **Fig. 4.88.31:** Retraction wall avulsion pseudomeningocele
Root avulsion with pseudomeningocele		
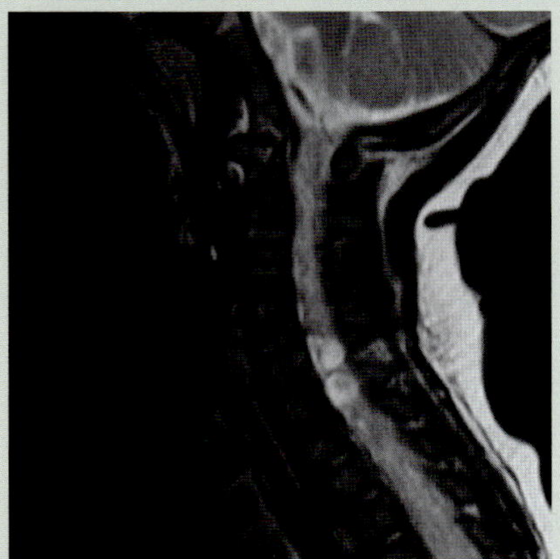 **Fig. 4.88.32:** Root avulsion with pseudomeningocele	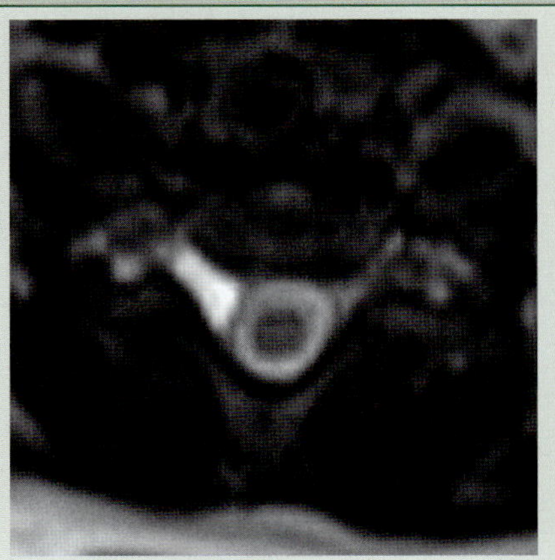 **Fig. 4.88.33:** Root avulsion with pseudomeningocele	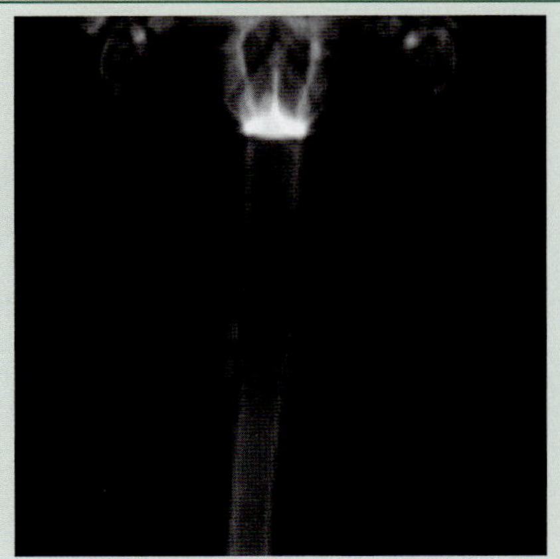 **Fig. 4.88.34:** Root avulsion with pseudomeningocele

(*Contd.*)

Table 4.88.1: Differential diagnosis for brachial plexus lesion (*Contd.*)		
Brachial plexus lesion	*Imaging findings*	*Image*
Stretch injury		

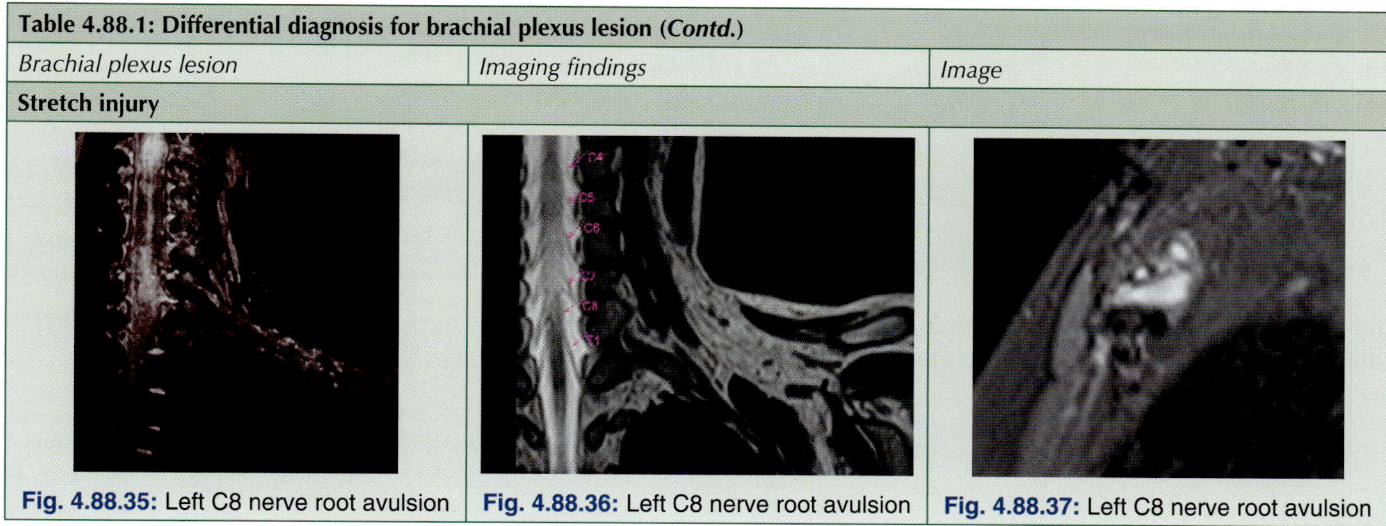

Fig. 4.88.35: Left C8 nerve root avulsion

Fig. 4.88.36: Left C8 nerve root avulsion

Fig. 4.88.37: Left C8 nerve root avulsion

Discussion: The brachial plexus (BP) provides sensory and motor innervation to the ipsilateral shoulder, chest, arm, and hand. Arising from the C5-T1 ventral rami of the spinal cord, the brachial plexus is divided anatomically into roots, trunks, divisions and cords.

The goal of imaging the BP is to visualize the entire course of the neural network from its preganglionic segments like nerve rootlets and intra-foraminal nerve segments and the postganglionic segments from dorsal root ganglion to the terminal branches. Focused multiplanar, multisequence MRI is required to completely image the brachial plexus and offers superior contrast resolution compared to computed tomography (CT).

Presenting symptoms referable to the BP can range from vague and nonspecific like regional shoulder pain, upper extremity weakness, or altered upper extremity/ shoulder sensorium to symptoms with specific nerve distribution like pain or motor/sensory deficit.

The acutely abnormal nerve demonstrates one or more of the following findings: Segmental nerve enlargement, disruption of nerve anatomic continuity, T2 signal intensity approaching that of regional blood vessels on

Table 4.88.2: Difference between preganglionic injury and postganglionic injury	
Preganglionic injury	*Postganglionic injury*
Injury proximal to the dorsal nerve root ganglion (DRG)	Injury distal to DRG
Motor deficit, sensory intact	Both motor and sensory deficits
Avulsion injury, paraspinal hematoma +/–	Stretch injury of the plexus
Altered signal intensity in the cord	Cord appears normal
Paraspinal muscles show denervation changes and atrophy	Paraspinal muscles intact
Elevation of diaphragm may be seen	Diaphragm appears normal
Treatment involves nerve transfer. Tendon transfer and arthrodesis may be needed.	Treated with nerve repair and rehabilitation
Worse prognosis	Better prognosis

Table 4.88.3: Difference between avulsion injury and stretch injury	
Avulsion injury	*Stretch injury*
Discontinuity of nerve elements noted	Enlarged or attenuated, but contiguous nerve elements noted
Pseudomeningocele with absent nerve roots and distal retraction ball seen	T2 hyperintense enlarged nerve roots. No evidence of pseudo-meningocele/retraction ball
Associated with preganglionic injury	Associated with post-ganglionic injury
Type of nerve injury: Neurotmesis	Neuropraxia or axonotmesis

Table 4.88.4: Types of nerve injury			
Seddon type	*Neuropraxia*	*Axonotmesis*	*Neurotmesis*
Myelin intact	No	No	No
Axon intact	Yes	No	No
Endoneurium intact	Yes	Variable	No
Wallerian degeneration	No	Yes	Yes
Reversibility	Yes	Variable	No

fat-saturated T2WI or STIR sequences, or disruption or distortion of normal fascicular architecture. Entrapped or scarred nerves may show abrupt change in caliber or course.

4.89 CHEST

Case No. 89

Clinical history: A 45 years old female with increasing shortness of breath and right side chest pain.

Radiological techniques and observation: Figure 4.89.1 is chest X-ray image showing whiteout right side hemithorax. Trachea and mediastinum shifted to left. Radiodense lesion seen involving the right side chest wall probably breast. Left side breast and lung appears normal. Visualised spine, clavicle, ribs and scapula appear normal. Cardiac and mediastinal shadows are normal.

Figures 4.89.2 to 4.89.4 are CECT chest coronal and axial images showing non-enhancing fluid density seen involving the right-side pleural cavity with collapse of right lung and trachea, mediastinum and heart shifted to left. Soft tissue dense lesion with retracted nipple seen involving the right-side breast. Fat plane between the lesion and right pectoralis major muscle is lost. The suspicious loss of fat plane between the chest wall–external intercostal muscle and the lesion. Visualised left lung, left breast and vertebrae appear normal.

Interpretation: A—45 years old female, right hemithorax, C—white out right hemithorax with tracheal and mediastinal shift to left, B—non-enhancing fluid density involving the right pleural cavity causing collapse of right lung with tracheal and mediastinal shift to left, D—malignant right pleural effusion.

Diagnosis: Malignant right-sided pleural effusion.

Management: Pleural analysis and therapeutic pleural drainage.

Differential diagnosis: Depends upon the tracheal shift divides into: 1. Trachea pulled toward the opacified side, 2. Trachea remains central in position, 3. Trachea pushed away from the opacified side.

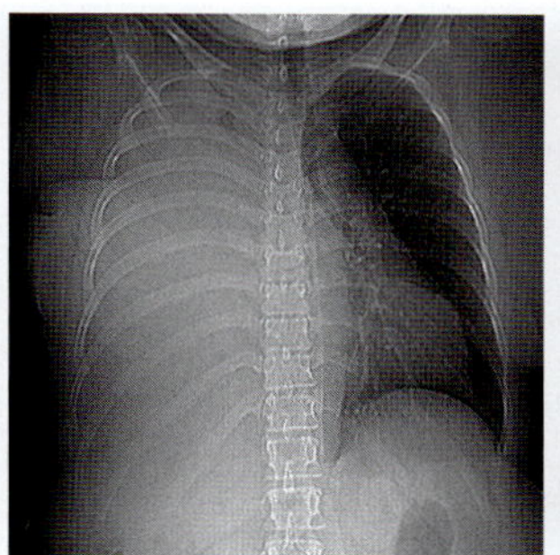

Fig. 4.89.1

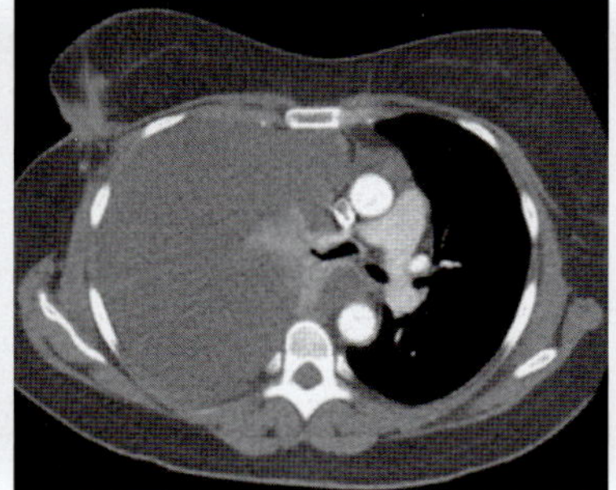

Fig. 4.89.2

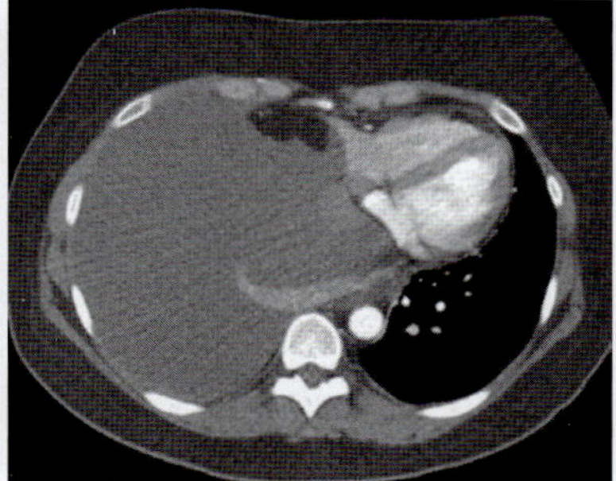

Fig. 4.89.3

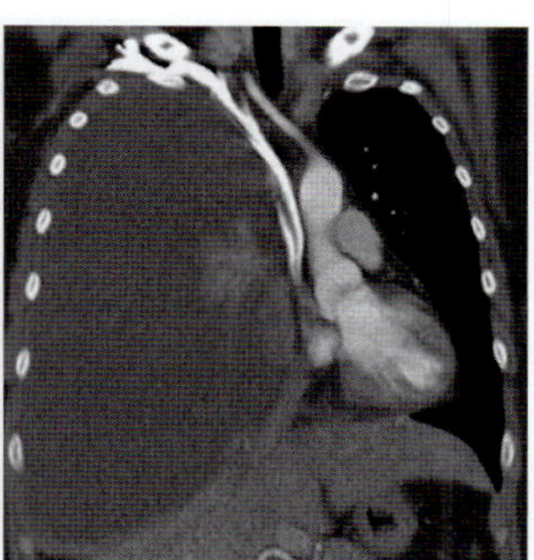

Fig. 4.89.4

Table 4.89.1: Tracheal position and their expected imaging findings

Tracheal position	*Findings*
Trachea pulled toward the opacified side Pneumonectomy, Total lung collapse, e.g. endobronchial intubation Pulmonary agenesis and Pulmonary hypoplasia	Right side lung collapse, trachea and mediastinum shifted to right side, left lung field may appear hyperexpanded.
Trachea remains central in position Consolidation/airway opacification (pulmonary edema/ARDS) Pleural mass, e.g. mesothelioma Chest wall mass, e.g. Askin/Ewing sarcoma	Bilateral massive pulmonary oedema, trachea in midline, bilateral perihilar opacity with lower lobe predominance, normal heart size
Trachea pushed away from the opacified side Pleural effusion Diaphragmatic hernia Large pulmonary mass and diaphragmatic rupture	Right diaphragmatic hernia appears opaque than left side diaphragmatic hernia because of air within herniated bowel loops. But in early neonatal period, left diaphragmatic hernia also appears opaque when air has not yet had time to reach herniated bowel.

Contd.

Table 4.89.1: Tracheal position and their expected imaging findings (*Contd.*)	
Tracheal position	*Findings*
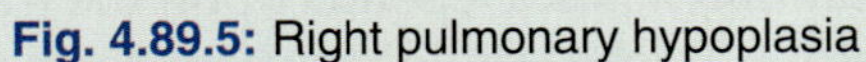 **Fig. 4.89.5:** Right pulmonary hypoplasia	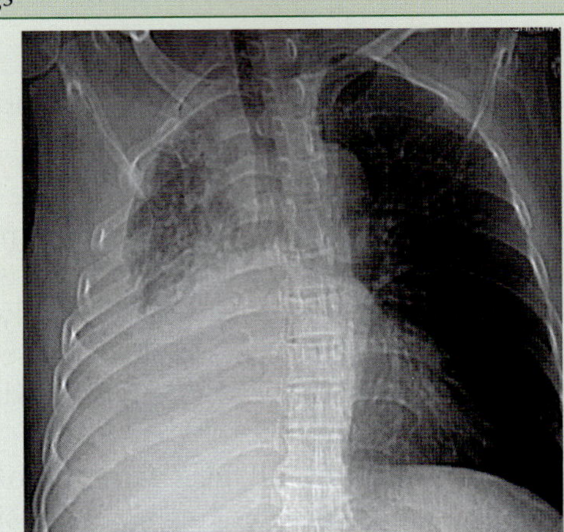 **Fig. 4.89.6:** Bronchogenic carcinoma
Note: Large pleural effusion without mediastinal shift indicates significant lung collapse or relative fixation of mediastinum by malignant cells (e.g., malignant pleural mesothelioma)	

Table 4.89.2: Difference between benign and malignant pleural effusion	
Malignant pleural effusion	*Benign pleural effusion*
Circumferential pleural thickening	Usually not seen
Nodular pleural thickening	Smooth pleural thickening
Parietal pleural thickening >1 cm	Parietal pleural thickening <1 cm
Mediastinal pleural involvement seen	Mediastinal pleural involvement usually not seen
Pleural calcification uncommon	Calcification favours benign etiology
No mediastinal shift due to infiltration and fixing of pleura	Mediastinal shift to opposite side

4.90 CHEST

Case No. 90

Clinical history: 40 years old female, known case of carcinoma breast—post-surgical status.

Radiographic technique and observation: Figure 4.90.1 is chest X-ray PA view image showing hypertranslucency of left hemithorax and absent left breast shadow. Lung parenchyma appears normal. Bones appear normal.

Next line of investigation—CT chest: Figure 4.90.2 is CECT chest section image confirms the absence of left breast. Contralateral right breast appears normal.

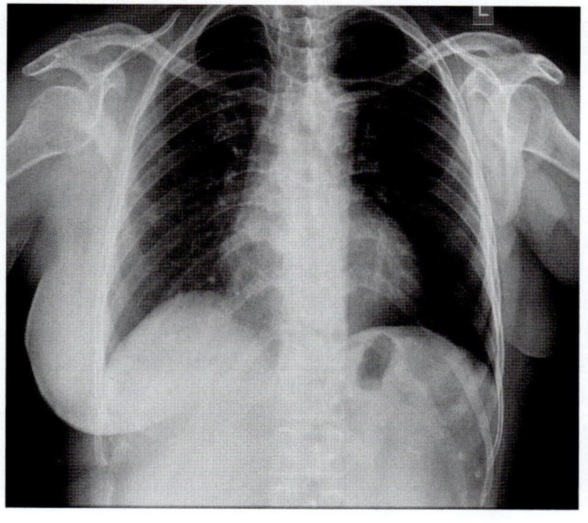

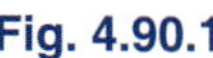

Fig. 4.90.1

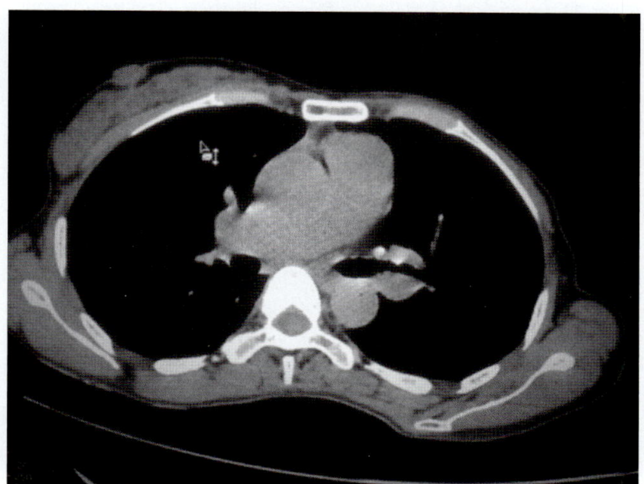

Fig. 4.90.2

Table 4.90.1: Differential diagnosis for unilateral hypertranslucent hemithorax

	Pediatrics		*Adults*
Technical	Rotation		Rotation
Chest wall	Poliomyelitis, Poland syndrome		Post-mastectomy status
Pleura	Pneumothorax		Pneumothorax
Lung	Bronchial atresia Congenital lobar emphysema Congenital pulmonary emphysema Bronchial foreign body (obstructive emphysema) Congenital pulmonary airway malformation.	Congenital diaphragmatic hernia Pneumatocele Pleuropulmonaryblastoma compensatory hyperinflation in contralateral pulmonary aplasia/hypoplasia Interstitial emphysema	Post-lobectomy with compensatory hyperexpansion. Bullae.
Pulmonary vessels	Swyer-James syndrome		Pulmonary embolism
1. Pneumothorax Accumulation of air in the pleural cavity. Causes: Traumatic > spontaneous (most common cause ruptured bullae).	Signs in chest X-ray—visceral pleural sign/deep sulcus sign/double diaphragm sign/absent vascular markings USG sign—barcode sign		Fig. 4.90.3: Pneumothorax

Contd...

Table 4.90.1: Differential diagnosis for unilateral hypertranslucent hemithorax *(Contd...)*

	Pediatrics	*Adults*
Pneumothorax size: Average interpleural distance (AID) = (A + B + C) ÷ 3 [in cm] and convert to percentage of pneumothorax. PA view of chest *Aid* / *Erect(%)* / *Supine(%)* 0.5 / 10 / 15 1 / 15 / 20 1.5 / 20 / 25 2 / 25 / 30 2.5 / 30 / 35 3 / 35 / 40 3.5 / 40 / 45 4 / 45 / 50 4.5 / 50 / 55		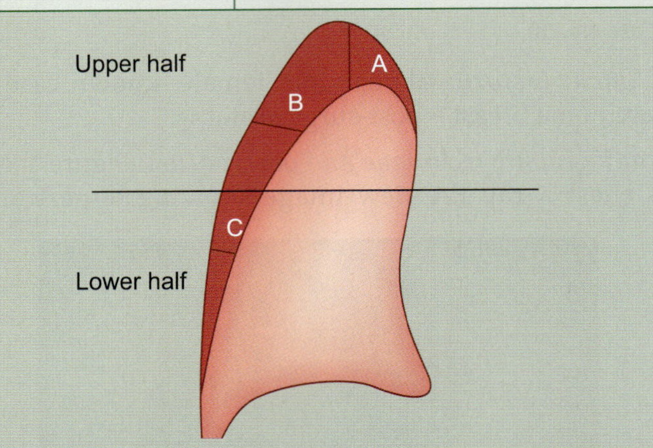 **Fig. 4.90.4:** Quantification of pneumothorax. A—maximum apical interpleural distance, B—interpleural distance at midpoint of upper half of lung, C—interpleural distance at midpoint of lower half of lung. If A = 2, B = 3, C = 1. A + B + C = 6, A + B + C/3 = 2. If patient is in + supine–30%, pneumothorax, if patient on erect–25%, pneumothorax
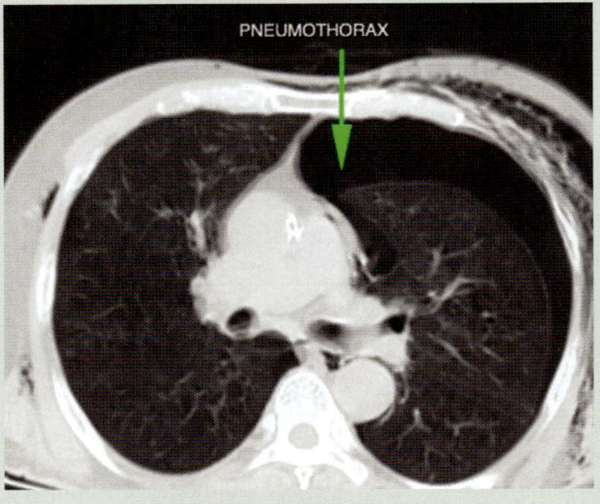 **Fig. 4.90.5:** Pneumothorax		
Tension pneumothorax is defined as when intrapleural air accumulates progressively in such a way as to exert positive pressure on mediastinal and intrathoracic structures. Treatment is needle thoracostomy.		
2. Swyer-James syndrome: Post-infectious bronchiolitis obliterans (BO) secondary to adenovirus infection in childhood.	**Imaging findings** • Small lung with hyperlucency of all or part of a lung • Diminished arterial flow with hypogenesis of pulmonary arteries • Overexpansion of the contralateral lung.	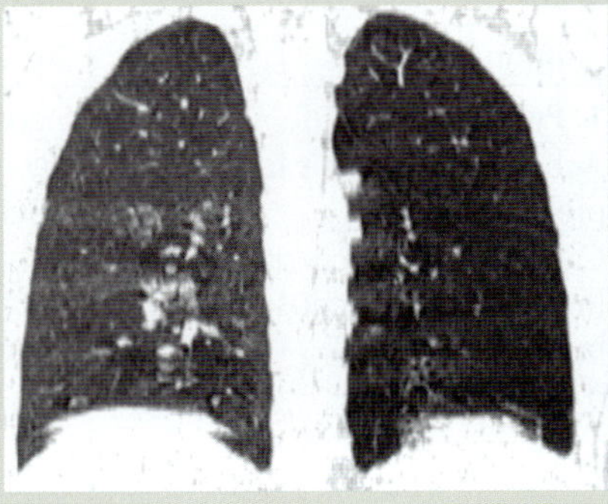 **Fig. 4.90.6:** Swyer-James syndrome

Contd...

Table 4.90.1: Differential diagnosis for unilateral hypertranslucent hemithorax *(Contd...)*

	Pediatrics	*Adults*
3. Poland syndrome: Congenital absence of pectoralis major muscle and breast shadow	Hyperlucent unilateral chest Rarely associated with dextrocardia and syndactyly	
4. Congenital diaphragmatic hernia—refer to case 91		
5. Obstructive emphysema—refer to case 91		
Congenital lobar emphysema: More common in males (M: F = 3:1)	Hyperlucent lung with mass effect and contralateral mediastinal shift. Associated with VSD, PDA, TOF.	**Fig. 4.90.7:** Congenital lobar emphysema
Bronchial atresia Anomaly resulting from focal obliteration of a segmental, sub-segmental or lobar bronchus with air trapping Common in left upper lobe > right UL > right ML Atretic bronchus with bronchocele—finger in glove appearance Distal lung—hyperinflation, hypovascularity, increased in volume	**Fig. 4.90.8:** Bronchial atresia	**Fig. 4.90.9:** Bronchial atresia
Pulmonary embolism	Earlier change in X-ray—nil **Westermark sign**—focal oligemia. **Hampton hump sign**—peripheral wedge-shaped density above diaphragm. **Fleischner sign**—enlarged proximal occluded pulmonary artery. **Palla sign**—enlarged right descending pulmonary artery.	
Langerhans cell histiocytosis Lung involvement in 40%; may be an isolated abnormality 90% of adult patients are smokers	Granulomas in early stages Lung cysts late in course Cysts irregular in shape Upper lobe predominance Spare costophrenic angles Nodules or cavitary nodules	**Fig. 4.90.10:** LCH

Contd...

Table 4.90.1: Differential diagnosis for unilateral hypertranslucent hemithorax *(Contd...)*

	Pediatrics	*Adults*
Lymphangiomyomatosis Women of childbearing age Identical to the lung disease seen in tuberous sclerosis	Lung cysts, round in shape, diffuse distribution Involve the costophrenic angles, nodules occasionally seen Cystic lung destruction Chylous effusions Renal angiomyolipoma are present in 15%	
Oligemic lung fields in cyanotic congenital heart disease: Decreased pulmonary vascularity • TOF • Tricuspid atresia • Pulmonary stenosis	Bilateral translucent thorax Cardiomegaly not seen in TOF while present in tricuspid atresia and pulmonary stenosis	**Fig. 4.90.11:** TOF

Table 4.90.2: Bilateral translucent hemithorax causes

With over-expansion of lungs	*With normal or small lungs*
1. Emphysema 2. Asthma 3. Acute bronchiolitis 4. Tracheal/laryngeal/bilateral bronchial stenosis 5. Cystic lung diseases (LAM, LCH)	1. CHD with oligemia—right to left shunts 2. Pulmonary artery stenosis 3. Multiple pulmonary emboli 4. Idiopathic pulmonary hypertension 5. Metastatic trophoblastic tumor 6. Schistosomiasis 7. Bronchiectasis 8. Interstitial lung disease

Interpretation: A—40 years old female, C—absence of left breast, D—left post-mastectomy status.

Principal diagnosis: Left post-mastectomy status.

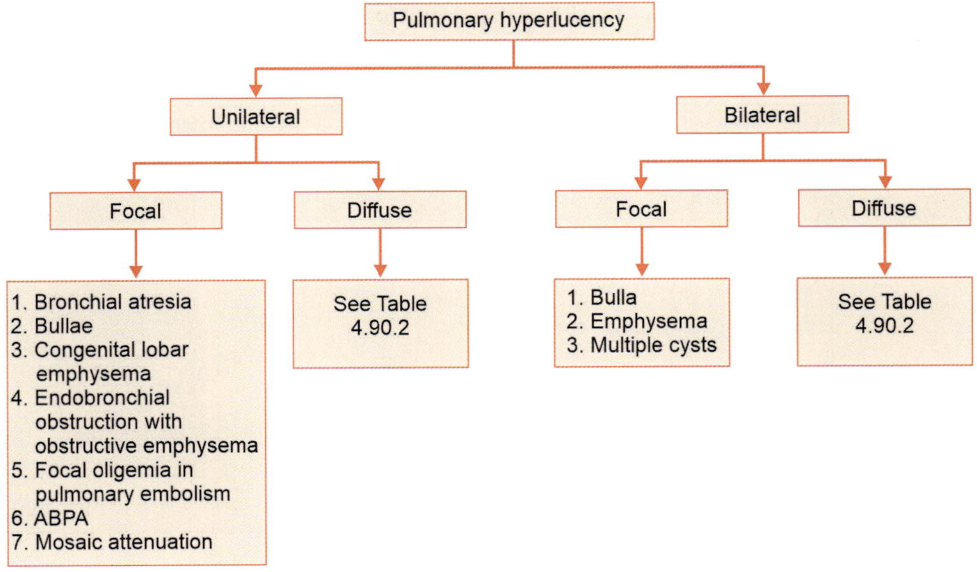

Fig. 4.90.12: Approach to pulmonary hypertranslucency

Emphysema: Defined as the "permanent abnormal enlargement of the airspaces distal to the terminal bronchioles accompanied by destruction of the alveolar wall and without obvious fibrosis". Types—centrilobular/paraseptal/panlobular emphysema.

Centrilobular emphysema: Focal areas of lucency without visible walls, usually with upper lobe predominance.

Panlobular emphysema: Large areas of low attenuation, usually diffuse and associated with decreased vessel size.

Paraseptal emphysema: Subpleural lucencies marginated by interlobular septa or subpleural bullae, usually with an upper lobe predominance.

Radiologic signs of hyperinflation: Chest X-ray-PA view: Lung height—more than 29.9 cm. Flattening of the right hemidiaphragm, with highest level of dome of right hemidiaphragm less than 1.5 cm above a perpendicular line drawn between the costophrenic angle laterally.

Chest X-ray lateral view: Flattening of the right hemidiaphragm, with height of less than 2.7 cm measured from anterior to posterior costophrenic angles. Increased retrosternal air space, measuring more than 4.4 cm at a level 3 cm below the manubrial sternal junction.

4.91 CHEST

Case No. 91

Clinical history: Newborn with progressive respiratory distress.

Radiological technique and observation: Figure 4.91.1 is chest radiography in frontal view showing a large multiseptated cystic lesion in right upper and lower zones with mediastinal shift to left. Right cardiac border is not visible. The lesion is extending up to diaphragmatic surface inferiorly. (Possibilities include congenital diaphragmatic hernia, CPAM, pneumatocele, congenital lobar emphysema.) Figures 4.91.2 and 4.91.3 are axial, coronal CT sections showing a large multiloculated cystic lesion centered in the superior segment of right lower lobe. Minimal wall thickening noted in periphery of lesion which raises the possibility of secondary inflammation or infection. Hyperinflation of the basal medial and lateral basal segment is noted. The lesion displaces the posterior right upper lobe superiorly and displaces the hilar and the right middle lobe anteriorly. The left lung fields appears normal. The diaphragm appears intact.

Interpretation: A—newborn, right lung field, C—multicystic pulmonary mass lesion causing mediastinal shift, B—periphery of the lesion shows some wall thickening which raises the possibility of secondary inflammation or infection, D—CPAM

Principal diagnosis: Congenital cystic adenomatoid malformation (also known as congenital pulmonary airways malformation) difficult to differentiate from pleuropulmonary blastoma.

Discussion: Congenital pulmonary airway malformations (CPAM) are multicystic masses of segmental lung tissue showing abnormal bronchial proliferation. CPAMs are part of the spectrum of bronchopulmonary foregut malformations. The estimated incidence is 1:1500–4000 live births and there is slight male predominance. Previously known as CCAM (congenital cystic adenomatoid malformation). It receives normal blood supply from pulmonary artery and vein.

Five subtypes are currently classified, mainly depending on cyst size:

Type I Macrocystic: Most common: 70% of cases, large cysts, one or more dominant cysts: 2–10 cm in size, may be surrounded by smaller cysts.

Type II Microcystic: 15–20% of cases, cysts are <2 cm in diameter associated with other abnormalities like renal agenesis or dysgenesis, pulmonary sequestration, congenital cardiac anomalies.

Type III Mixed: ~10% of cases, microcysts: <5 mm in diameter typically involves an entire lobe has a poorer prognosis.

Type IV: Unlined cyst typically affects a single lobe indistinguishable from type I on imaging.

Type 0 very rare, lethal postnatally, acinar dysgenesis or dysplasia, represents global arrest of lung development.

Antenatal ultrasound: Intrathoracic isolated cystic or solid mass. A solid intrathoracic mass is usually indicative of a type III CPAM and is usually hyperechoic. Hydrops and polyhydramnios may develop and may be detected on ultrasound as ancillary sonographic features.

Plain radiograph: Type I and II CPAMs may demonstrate a multicystic (air-filled) lesion. Large lesions may cause a mass effect with resultant mediastinal shift, depression, and even inversion of the diaphragm. Lesions may change in size on interval imaging (expand from

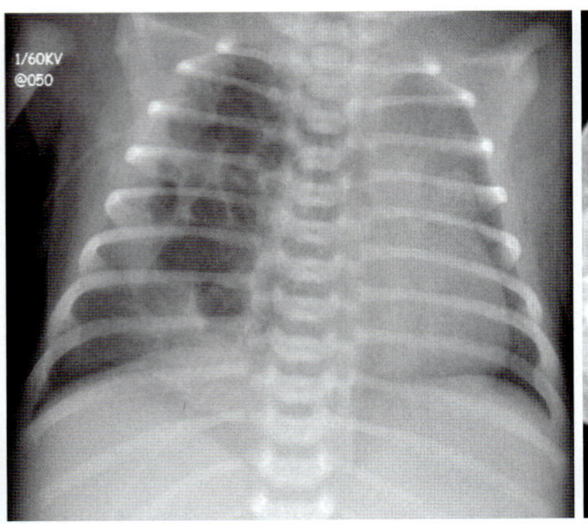

Fig. 4.91.1

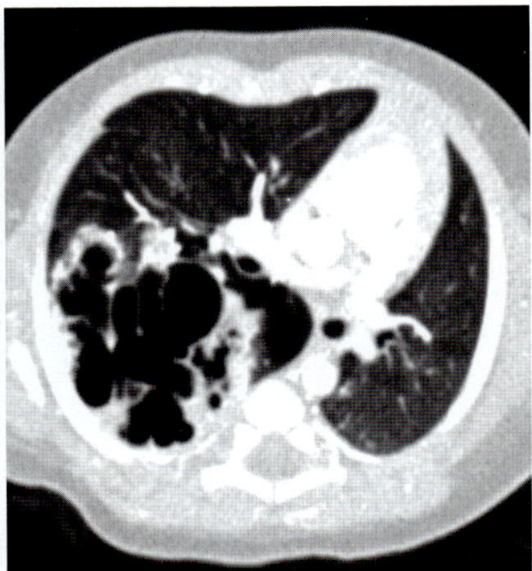

Fig. 4.91.2

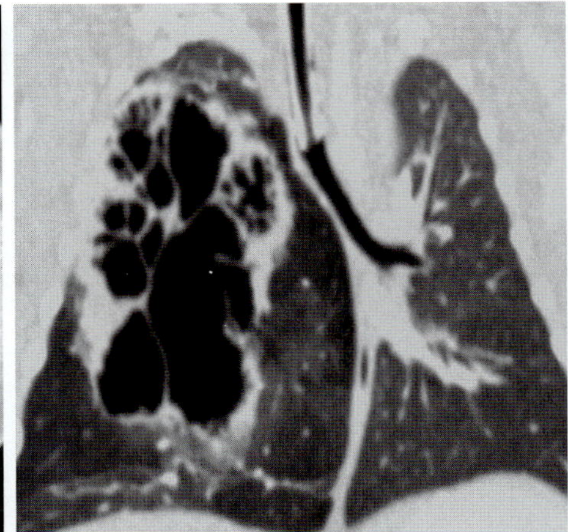

Fig. 4.91.3

Table 4.91.1: Differential diagnosis of focal air-filled cystic lesions of lung

Pleuropulmonary blastoma: Rare childhood primary intrathoracic malignancy. Age group: Within 1st year of life. Complete surgical resection is treatment of choice. Type 1 can mimic type 4 CPAM	Air-filled single cyst or multicystic lesion (type 1 pleuropulmonary blastoma)can mimic CPAM appearance. Large cyst with solid soft tissue component, multilobar and bilateral involvement and DICER 1 gene mutation with concurrent cystic nephroma make the diagnosis more likely.	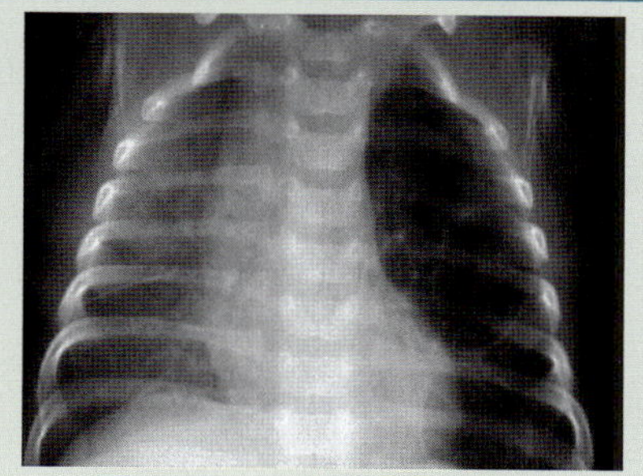 **Fig. 4.91.4:** Pleuropulmonary blastoma—on left side
Congenital diaphragmatic hernia Right anterior—Morgagni (R-A-M) Left posterior—Bochdalek 1 in 2000–4000 live births. 84% left sided. Management: Surgery/fetal tracheal occlusion therapy.	Radiologically appears as multicystic air containing mass, cysts uniform in size and morphology. Altered course of nasogastric tube (Ryles tube J sign) with stomach herniation and umbilical venous catheter with liver herniation. Paucity of abdominal bowel gas and scaphoid abdomen.	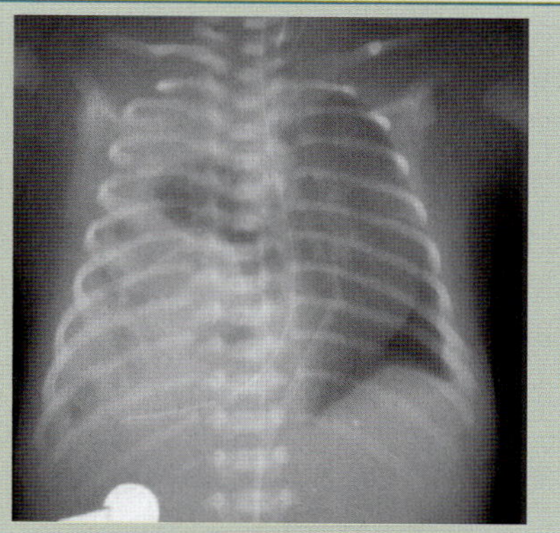 **Fig. 4.91.5:** Morgagni hernia
Bronchopulmonary sequestration Male predilection M: F~4:1 Extra lobar sequestration more common in neonates with respiratory distress	Left > Right lower lobes. Solid appearing, becomes airfilled after infection. Systemic arterial supply on fetal USG/MRI or CT angio. Mixed CPAM/ sequestration hybrid lesions common and more likely to have discrete cysts.	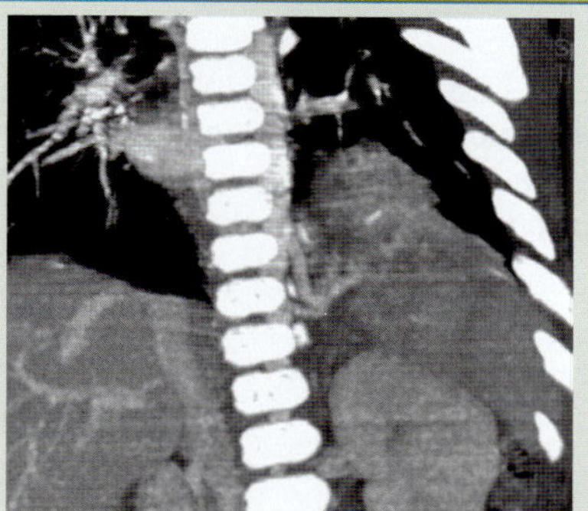 **Fig. 4.91.6:** Bronchopulmonary sequestration
Cavitary necrosis/abscess complicating pneumonia—Most commonly caused by *Streptococcus pneumoniae*.	Typically surrounded by consolidated lung. Lesion progressing during illness, resolution after illness and previous normal chest radiographs suggest diagnosis.	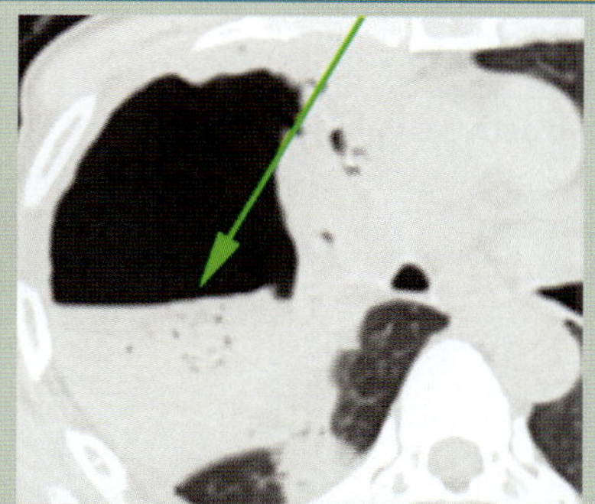 **Fig. 4.91.7:** Abscess complicating pneumonia

(Contd...)

Table 4.91.1: Differential diagnosis of focal air-filled cystic lesions of lung *(Contd...)*		
Congenital lobar over inflation: More common in males 3:1. Most common within 6 months of life. **Management:** Elective intubation of opposite lung. Surgical lobectomy. Conservative treatment for minimal symptoms.	Progressive lobar expansion in foetus/ neonates. Preserved pulmonary markings without discrete cyst wall. Rarely occurs in lower lobes.	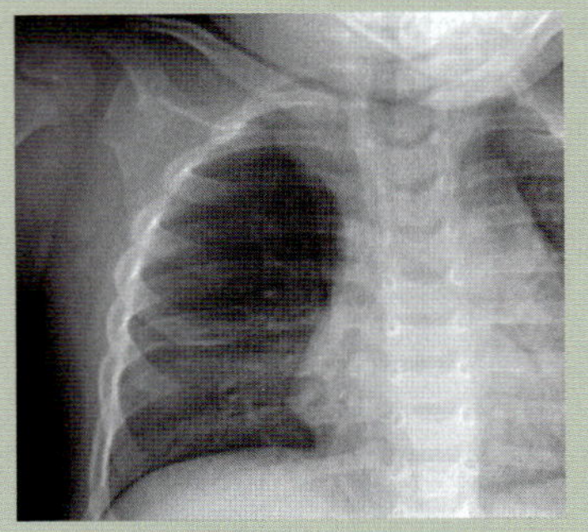 **Fig. 4.91.8:** Congenital lobar overinflation
Persistent pulmonary interstitial emphysema: Highest frequency in low birth weight infants. High frequency ventilation, selective bronchial intubation, lobectomy.	Regional small bubbly interstitial lucencies in background of granular airspace opacities of surfactant deficiency.	
Congenital cystic bronchiectasis	Now referred to as Williams-Campbell syndrome, and is the result of a deficiency of cartilage in the bronchial wall.	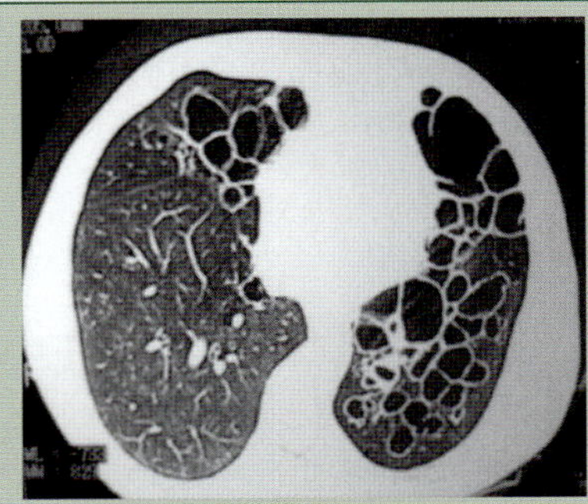 **Fig. 4.91.9:** Congenital cystic bronchiectasis
Pneumatocele: Post-infectious spontaneously resolve. Surgical intervention in symptomatic or ruptured pneumatocele.	Appears during 1st week on infection resolves during 6th week. Smooth inner margins. Fluid levels, thin regular wall. Tend to persist despite absence of symptoms	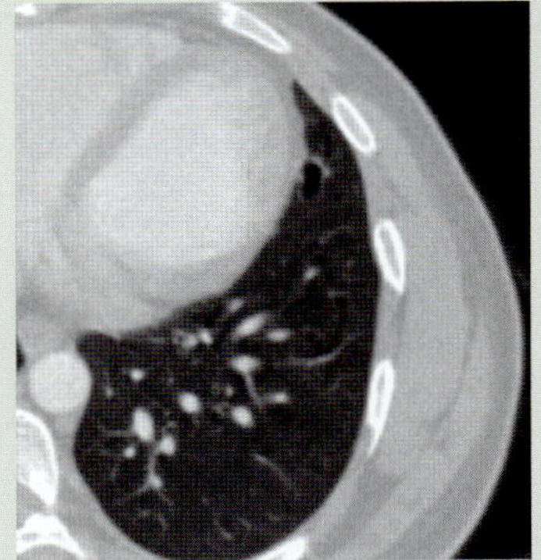 **Fig. 4.91.10:** Pneumatocele
Obstructive emphysema <4 years increased risk of foreign body aspiration.	Affected lung appears overinflated and hyperlucent with concomitant rib flaring. Interrupted bronchus sign. CT used to assess missed or retained foreign body. Male predominance. Predilection for right tracheobronchial tree	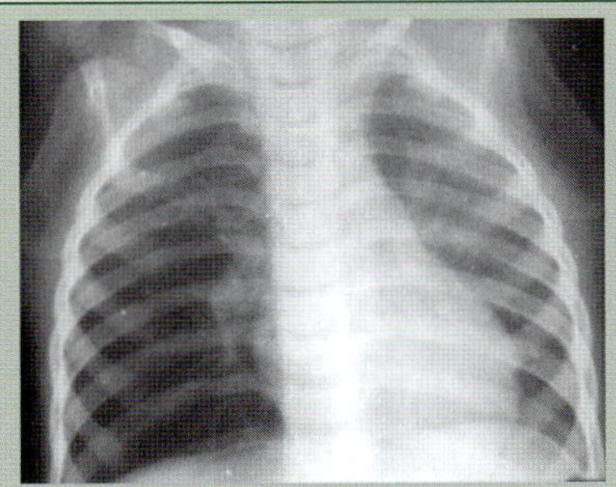 **Fig. 4.91.11:** Right obstructive emphysema

(Contd...)

Table 4.91.1: Differential diagnosis of focal air-filled cystic lesions of lung *(Contd...)*		
Contralateral lung aplasia/hypoplasia More common in cases with premature rupture of membrane.	Increased radiolucency with decreased vascular and hilar markings with contralateral lung hypoplasia. Deviation of mediastinum towards the side of hypoplasia. Antenatal USG may show associated oligohydramnios.	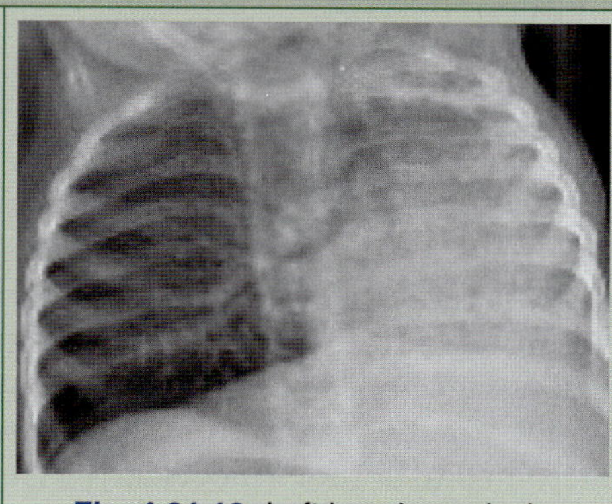 **Fig. 4.91.12:** Left lung hypoplasia

collateral ventilation via pores of Kohn). Type III lesions appear solid.

CT: Firstly, it more accurately delineates the location and extent of the lesion. Secondly, and most important in surgical candidates, CT angiography is able to identify systemic arterial supply, if present.

Appearance reflects the underlying type, and a type III lesion can appear as a consolidation.

Treatment: In symptomatic patients, surgery (elective lobectomy) is the treatment of choice, both for those who come early with respiratory compromise and for those who present later with recurring infections. There have been reports of spontaneous regression, especially in those who have been serially monitored with prenatal ultrasound.

Complications

- Recurrent pneumothorax
- Hemopneumothorax
- Pyopneumothorax
- Possible incidence of certain malignancies, which include:
  - Bronchoalveolar carcinoma
  - Bronchogenic carcinoma
  - Pleuropulmonary blastoma
  - Rhabdomyosarcoma
  - Potential *in utero* complications include: Hydrops may rarely develop when there is severe compression of the fetal heart or great vessels. Compression of the normal fetal lung can also rarely cause pulmonary hypoplasia.

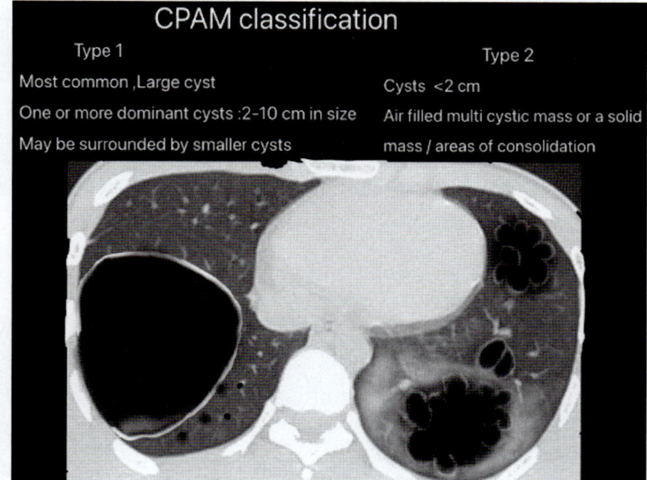

Fig. 4.91.13: CPAM type 1 and 2

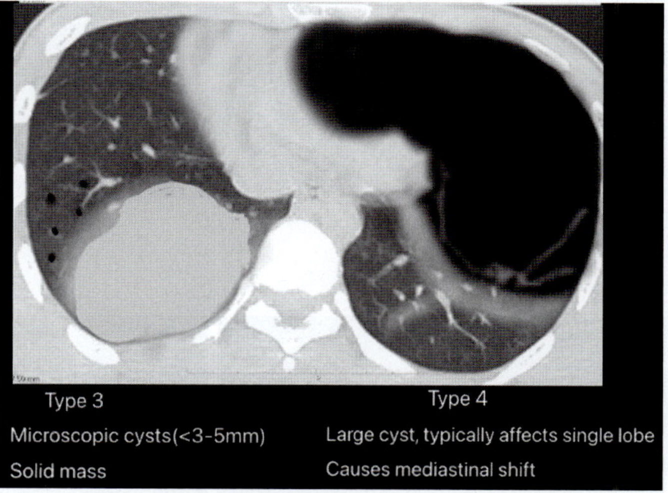

Fig. 4.91.14: CPAM type 3 and 4

4.92 CHEST

Case No. 92

Clinical history: 16 years old female presented with the complaints of recurrent cough with expectoration.

Radiological techniques and observation: Figure 4.92.1 is chest radiograph PA view showing well-defined near rounded radio-opaque lesion in the retrocardiac region. Figures 4.92.2 and 4.92.3 show superior, lateral borders of the lesion are clearly visualized, whereas inferomedial border is not clearly visualized. The lesion makes acute angle with the mediastinum. There is no evidence of calcification/air fluid level seen inside the lesion.Visualized ribs and soft tissues appear normal. Heterodense lesion in the posterior basal segment of left lower lobe of the lung. Figures 4.92.4 to 4.92.6 are post-contrast lesion showing heterogeneous enhancement, receiving supply from the aorta. There is no evidence of intrabronchial lesion. Surrounding lung parenchyma appears normal.

Interpretation: A: 16 years old female, lesion in the right lower lobe, C: Heterogeneously enhancing lesion in the left lower lobe of the lung, B: On contrast enhancement images vessel arising from the aorta and supplying the area of hyperdensity in the lesion, D: Pulmonary sequestration.

Principal diagnosis: Pulmonary sequestration (intralobar).

Differential diagnosis: Necrotizing pneumonia/pulmonary AVM/infected bronchogenic cyst/anomalous systemic arterial supply to normal lung (is an anatomical variant where a portion of the lung—usually a basal segment gets supplied by a systemic vessel without a distinct pulmonary sequestration). Spectrum of the scimitar syndrome.

Management: Traditionally treatment has been surgical resection. Extralobar sequestrations with their separate pleural investments can usually be removed sparing normal lung tissue, although, with an intralobar type, segmental resection or even lobectomy will be necessary.

Brief discussion about the condition: Pulmonary sequestration, also called accessory lung, refers to the aberrant formation of segmental lung tissue that has no connection with the bronchial tree or pulmonary arteries. It is a bronchopulmonary foregut malformation (BPFM). There are two types: Intralobar sequestration (ILS) and extralobar sequestration (ELS)—extralobar intrathoracic and extralobar subdiaphragmatic.

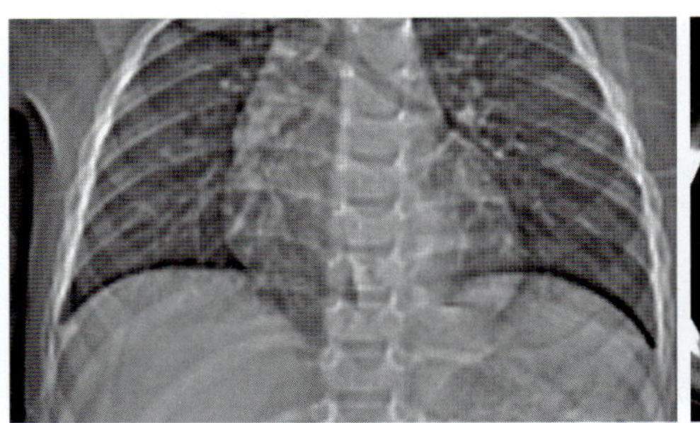

Fig. 4.92.1

Fig. 4.92.2

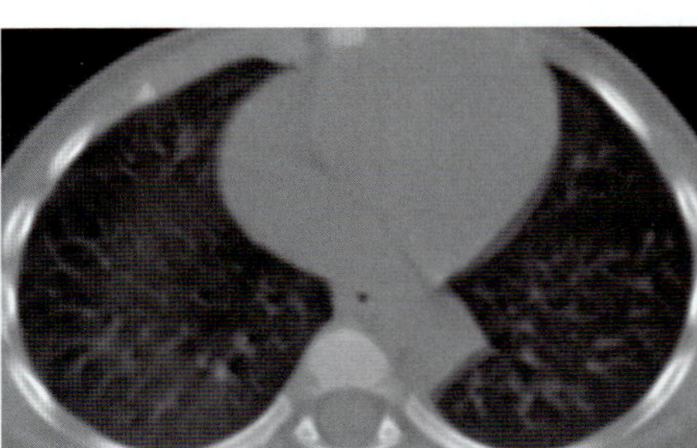

Fig. 4.92.3

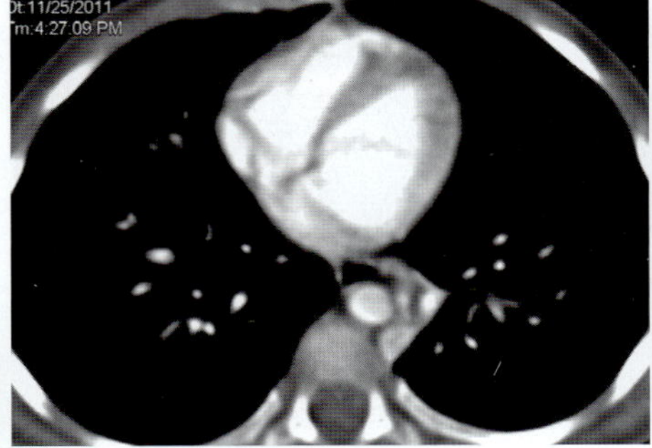

Fig. 4.92.4

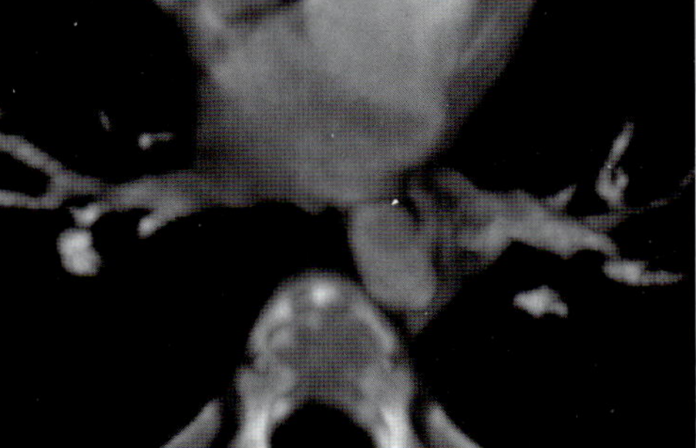

Fig. 4.92.5

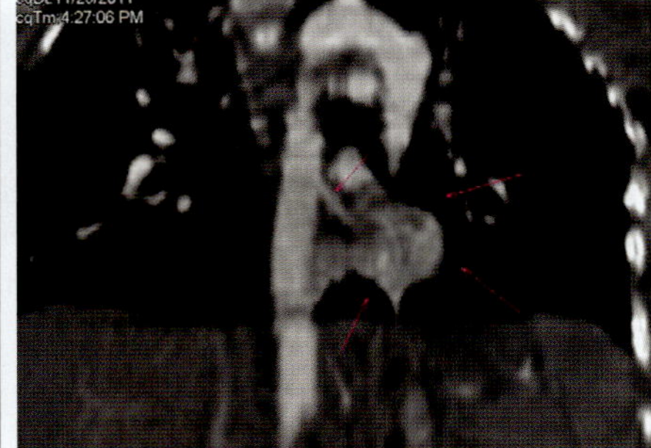

Fig. 4.92.6

Table 4.92.1: Differential diagnosis for pulmonary sequestration

1. CPAM TYPE III Failure of normal bronchoalveolar development with a hamartomatous proliferation of terminal respiratory units in a gland-like pattern (adenomatoid) without proper alveolar formation	Five types. CPAM appears as an isolated cystic or solid mass. A solid thoracic mass is usually indicative of a type III CPAM and is typically hyperechoic. There can be a mass effect over mediastinal structures.	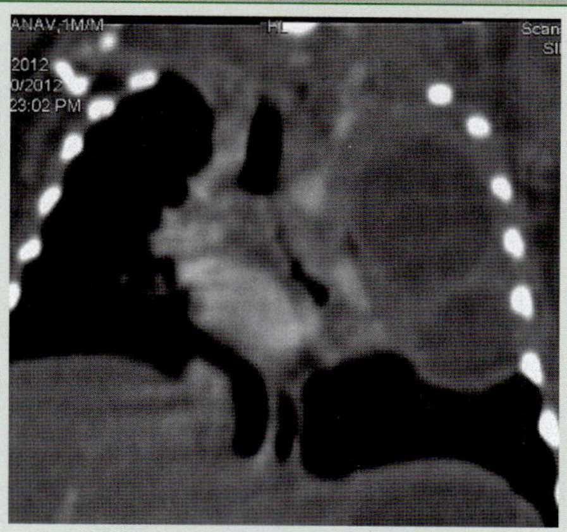 **Fig. 4.92.7:** CPAM type III
2. Necrotizing pneumonia Development of the necrosis within infected lung tissue.	CT imaging may show distinct areas of low attenuation with decreased parenchymal enhancement (representing liquefaction 4) in all or parts of the affected area of infection (consolidation)	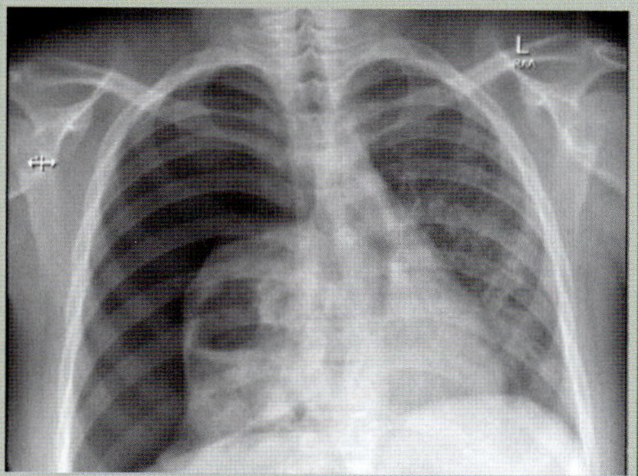 **Fig. 4.92.8:** Necrotizing pneumonia in right side
3. Pulmonary AVM Direct high flow, low-resistance fistulous connections between the pulmonary arteries and veins. CT shows well-circumscribed, non-calcified nodule up to several centimeters in diameter or the presence of a serpiginous mass connected with blood vessels.		Occasionally associated phleboliths may be seen as calcifications. Contrast injection demonstrates enhancement of the feeding artery, the aneurysmal part, and the draining vein on early-phase sequences.
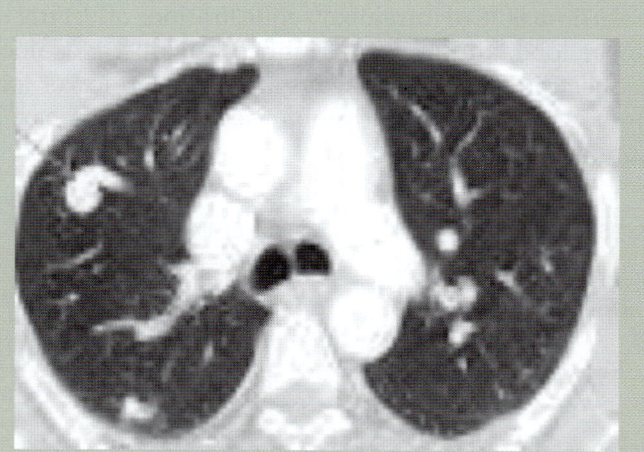 **Fig. 4.92.9:** Pulmonary AVM	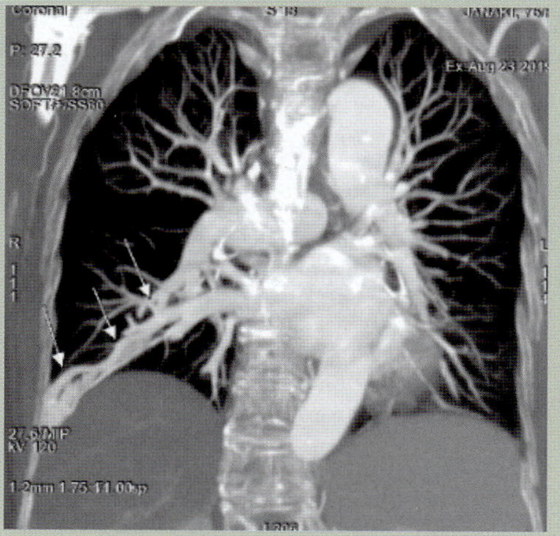 **Fig. 4.92.10:** Pulmonary AVM	
4. Anomalous systemic arterial supply to normal lung	An anatomical variant in which a portion of the lung (usually a basal segment) is supplied by a systemic vessel without a distinct pulmonary sequestration	
5. Scimitar's syndrome—Systemic arteries can supply lung. Refer to case 93		

Table 4.92.2: Difference between intralobar and extralobar sequestration

Characteristics	*Intralobar*	*Extralobar*
Incidence	Adult/older child	Infant/child
Prevalence	75%	25%
Location	60% of intralobar sequestrations affect the left lower lobe, and 40% the right lower lobe	Left lower lobe, however, ~10% of extralobar sequestrations can be subdiaphragmatic
Pleural investment	Visceral pleura	Own pleura
Arterial supply	Thoracic aorta	Abdominal aorta
Venous drainage	Pulmonary veins	Systemic veins
Symptomatic	Adulthood	First 6 months
Etiology	Acquired	Developmental
Congenital anomalies	15%	50%
Complications	Massive spontaneous non-traumatic pleural hemorrhage, chronic inflammation, fibrosis	Infection (in cases of communication with bronchus/GI tract)
Treatment	Lobectomy	Resection
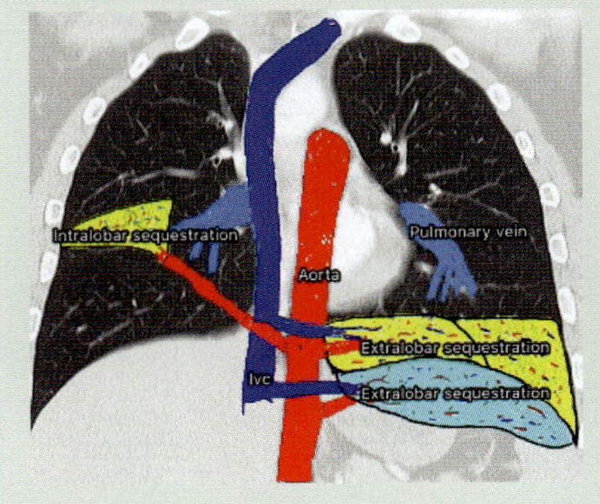 **Fig. 4.92.11:** Extralobar and intralobar sequestration	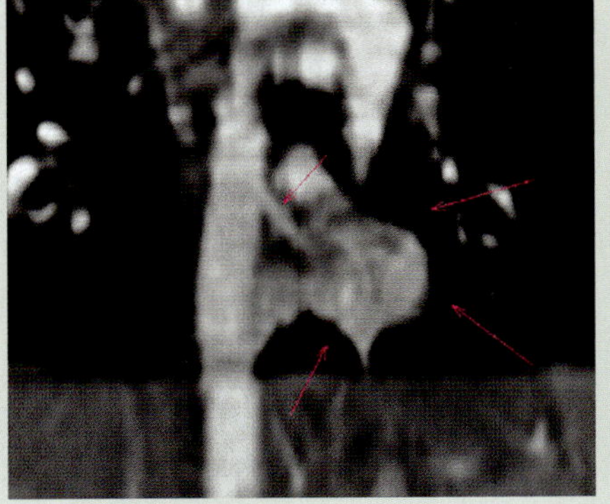 **Fig. 4.92.12:** Intralobar sequestration	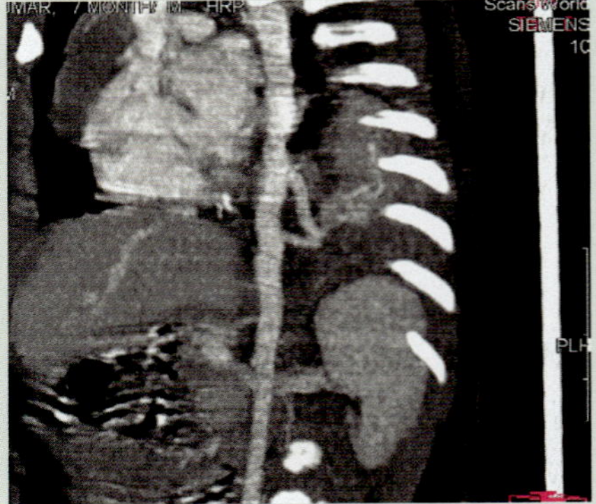 **Fig. 4.92.13:** Extralobar sequestration

Intralobar sequestrations: Venous drainage commonly occurs via the pulmonary veins, but can occur through the azygous-hemiazygous system, portal vein, right atrium or inferior vena cava, closely connected to the adjacent normal lung and do not have a separate pleura.

Extralobar sequestrations: Venous drainage most commonly through the systemic veins into the right atrium (but is variable). Separated from any surrounding lung by its own pleura.

Location: 60% of intralobar sequestrations affect the left lower lobe, and 40% the right lower lobe. Extralobar sequestrations almost always affect the left lower lobe, however, ~10% of extralobar sequestrations can be subdiaphragmatic.

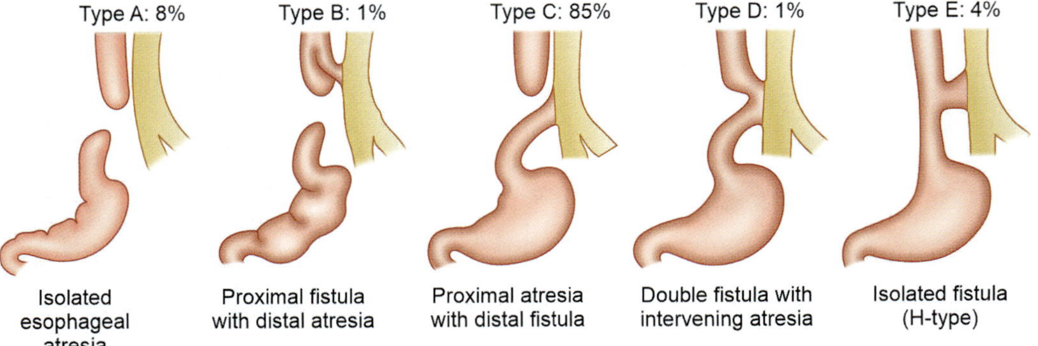

Fig. 4.92.14: Types of tracheoesophageal fistula

Air bronchogram: Refers to the occurrence whereby the opacification of surrounding alveoli (grey/white) makes air-filled bronchi (black) apparent. A pathologic airspace/alveolar process, in which something other than air fills the alveoli, is usually often the reason. If the bronchi themselves are opacified (e.g., by fluid), air bronchograms will not be visible, indicating patent proximal airways.

Air bronchograms *seen with several processes:* Pulmonary consolidation, pulmonary edema especially with alveolar edema, non-obstructive atelectasis, severe interstitial lung disease, *Neoplasms:* Bronchoalveolar carcinoma; pulmonary lymphoma, pulmonary infarct, pulmonary hemorrhage, normal expiration.

Non-resolving pneumonia: Absence of clinical response even after 10 days of antibiotic treatment, and radiological abnormalities persist even after 12 weeks.

Causes: Bacterial pneumonia, bronchogenic carcinoma, Wegner's granulomatosis, tuberculosis, pulmonary sequestration.

4.93 CHEST

Case No. 93

Clinical history: 15 years old female with cough with expectoration for 3 days.

Radiological techniques and observations: Chest radiograph PA view and contrast enhanced CT.

Figure 4.93.1 is PA radiograph of chest shows mild volume loss in the right lung with dextroposition of heart. Suspicious ill-defined non-tapering tubular radio-opacity along the right heart border extending across the right dome of diaphragm. Figures 4.93.2 to 4.93.6 are CT chest showing abnormal right pulmonary vein communicating with the inferior vena cava. Mild hypoplasia of the right lung with mild hypoplasia of right pulmonary artery noted.

Interpretation: A: 15 years old female, right lung and right pulmonary artery, C: Abnormal drainage of right pulmonary vein into IVC, B: mild hypoplasia of right lung and right pulmonary artery, D: Scimitar syndrome.

Principal diagnosis: Scimitar syndrome.

Management: Surgical correction should be considered in the presence of significant left to right shunting and pulmonary hypertension. Creation of a inter atrial baffle to redirect the pulmonary venous return into the left atrium. The anomalous vein can be re-implanted directly into the left atrium.

Discussion: Scimitar syndrome (congenital pulmonary venolobar syndrome or hypogenetic lung syndrome)

Rare congenital anomaly occurring in 1–3/100000 population.

Form of partial anomalous pulmonary venous connection.

Always in the right side.

Cause: Early lung bud developmental anomaly

Scimitar sign: Characteristics curvilinear vein that extends from the right lung to the drain into suprahepatic IVC.

Components: Lung hypoplasia, dextroposition of heart, partial anomalous pulmonary venous connection, abnormal lobation and bronchial anatomy, right pulmonary artery hypoplasia, systemic arterial supply, heart defects—ASD/PDA/VSD, congenital diaphragmatic hernia, horseshoe lung.

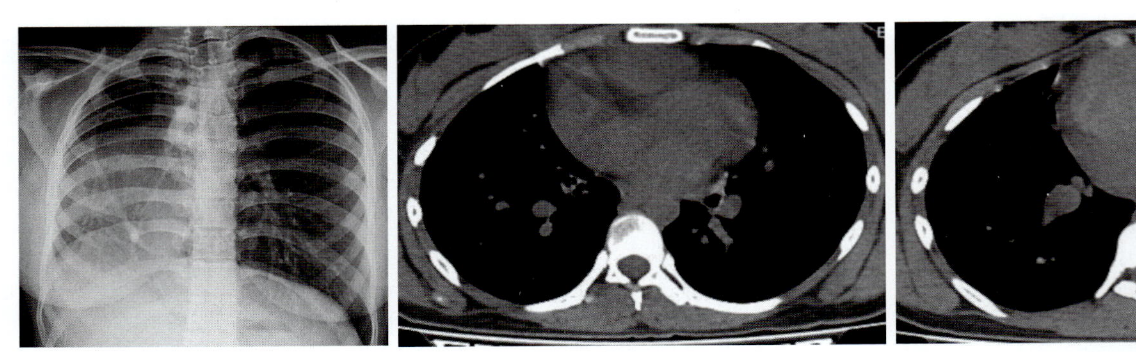

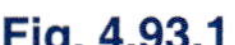

Fig. 4.93.1 Fig. 4.93.2 Fig. 4.93.3

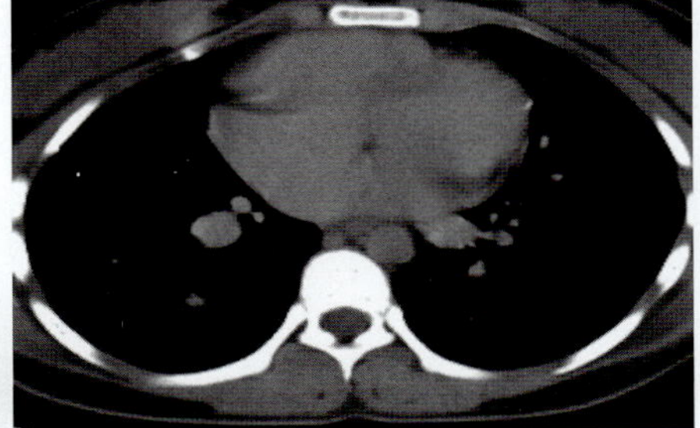

Fig. 4.93.4

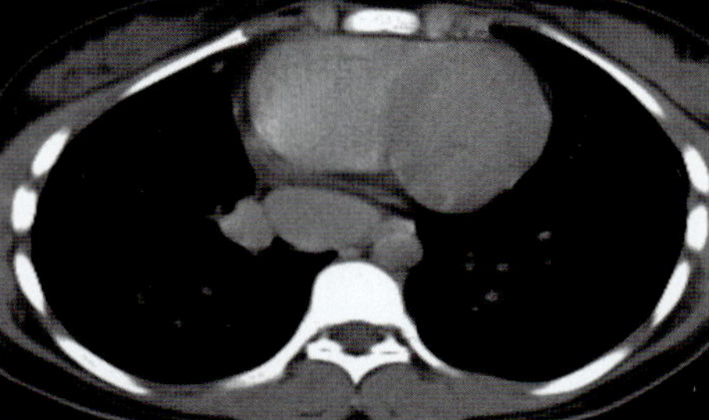

Fig. 4.93.5

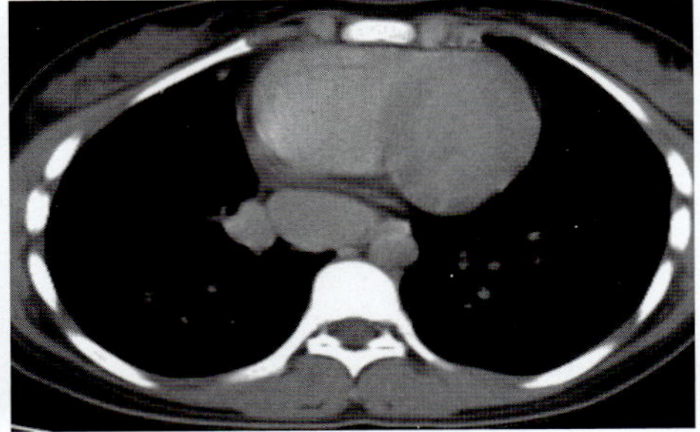

Fig. 4.93.6

Table 4.93.1: In a chest radiograph, for a linear opacity extending along right heart border up to or below the right dome of diaphragm, possible differentials include		
Bronchial atresia Most common location—apico-posterior location of left upper lobe	Developmental anomaly characterised by focal obliteration of the proximal segment of a bronchus. The bronchi distal to the atresia become filled with mucus and may form a mucocele. The distal lung develops normally but is overinflated due to air trapping.	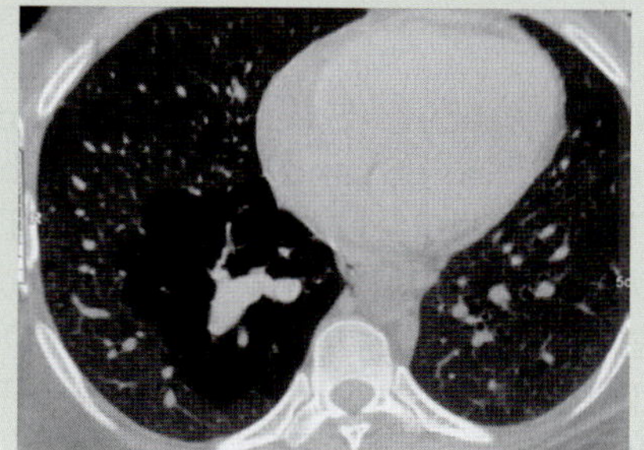 **Fig. 4.93.7:** Bronchial atresia
Allergic broncho-pulmonary aspergillosis Seen in patients with asthma	Central upper lobe saccular bronchiectasis involving segmental and sub-segmental bronchi is characteristic. Mucoid impaction results in bronchocele with "finger in glove" appearance. Fleeting pulmonary alveolar opacities common.	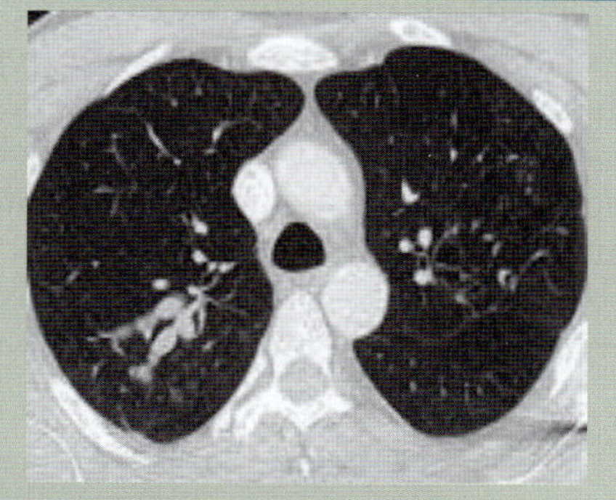 **Fig. 4.93.8:** ABPA
Arteriovenous malformation or venous varix—refer to Case 92		

Table 4.93.2: Types of scimitar syndrome	
Infantile	*Childhood/ adult onset*
First few months of life Associated with CHD	Lung hypoplasia Asymptomatic
Complicated by CCF, PHT	Recurrent LRI
Infantile	*Adult*
CCF/PHT/gypoxemia/cyanosis	RVH/RBBB Pulmonary—hemoptysis/ recurrent LRI

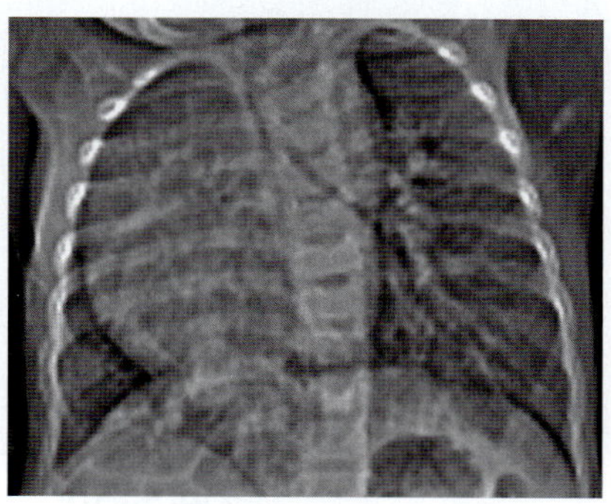

Fig. 4.93.9: Scimitar syndrome

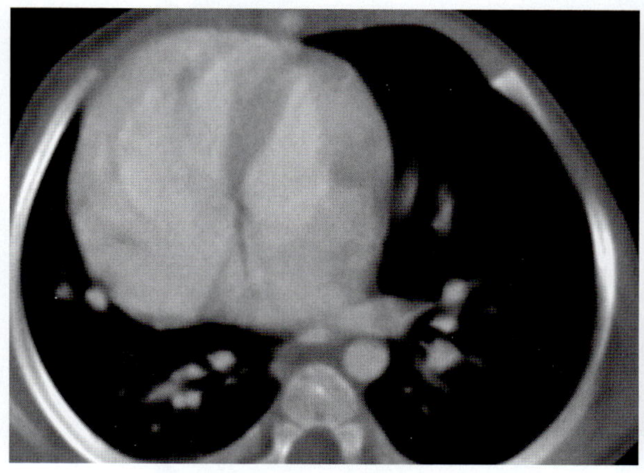

Fig. 4.93.10: Scimitar syndrome

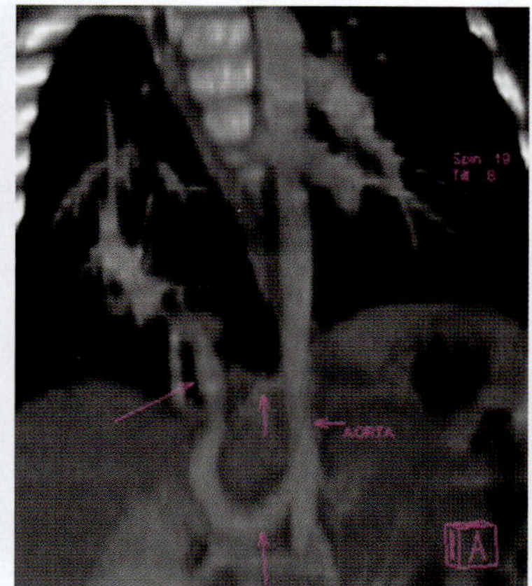

Fig. 4.93.11: Scimitar syndrome

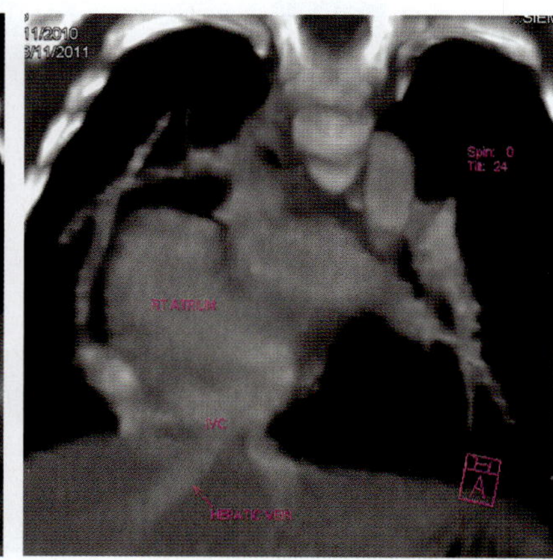

Fig. 4.93.12: Scimitar syndrome

4.94 CHEST

Case No. 94

Clinical history: 85 years old gentlemen with complaints of chronic cough and shortness of breath.

Figures 4.94.1 to 4.94.4 are CT chest mediastinal window coronal and axial sections, lung window axial sections showing bilateral lower posterior costal pleura appears thickened with calcification. Calcification and thickening of left diaphragmatic pleura noted with sparing of costophrenic angles. A few linear regions of fibrotic strands noted extending from these pleural thickening into lung parenchyma, representing calcified pleural plaques. Interlobular septal thickening with honeycombing and traction bronchiectasis involving the bilateral basal lung fields noted. No suspicious pulmonary nodule or mass. No focal consolidation or lobar collapse. No pleural effusion. No enlarged thoracic lymph node. No evidence of esophageal dilatation. No evidence of cardiomegaly. No evidence of lytic lesion in visualized thoracic vertebra/ribs.

Interpretation: A—85 years old male, bilateral lung fields, C—calcified pleural plaques, B—interlobular septal thickening, honeycombing and traction bronchiectasis predominantly involving the lung bases, D—asbestosis.

Principal diagnosis: Asbestosis

Differential diagnosis:
- Connective tissue disorder
- Idiopathic pulmonary fibrosis
- Drug toxicity
- Radiation fibrosis
- Chronic hypersensitivity pneumonitis
- Familial pulmonary fibrosis

Management: Pulmonary function test and oximetry, bronchoalveolar lavage, bronchoscopy, biopsy.

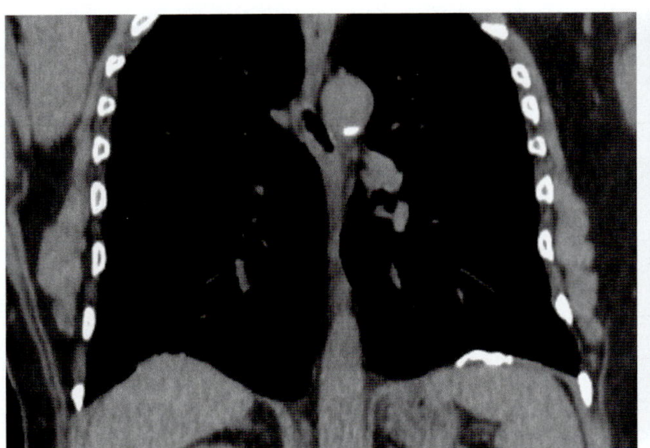

Fig. 4.94.1

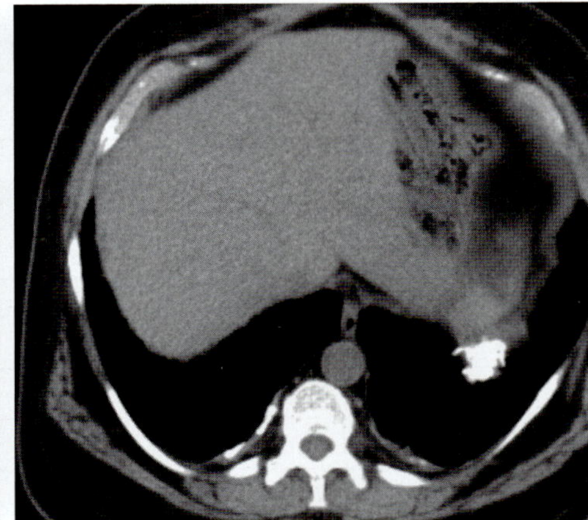

Fig. 4.94.2

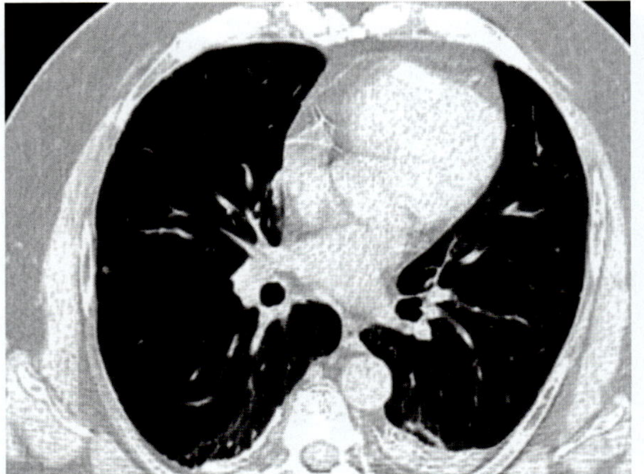

Fig. 4.94.3

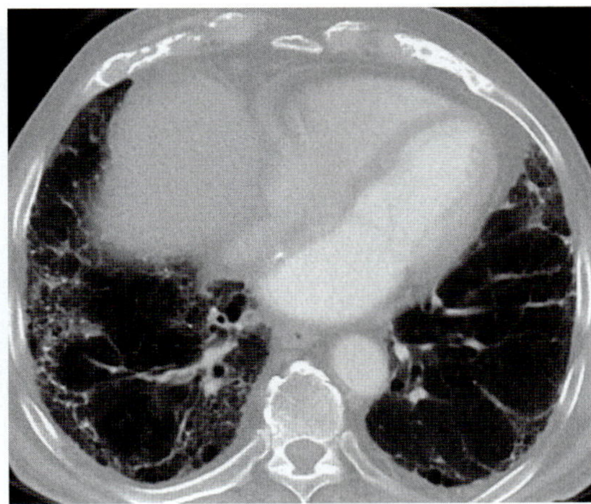

Fig. 4.94.4

Table 4.94.1: Differential diagnosis for asbestosis

Idiopathic pulmonary fibrosis	Exclusion of other known causes of infiltrative lung disease such as exposures, drugs, and connective tissue disease. HRCT findings of bibasilar reticulation with minimal groundglass opacity—UIP pattern.	**Fig. 4.94.5:** Idiopathic pulmonary fibrosis
Connective tissue disorder	The two most common conditions associated with lung disease are rheumatoid arthritis (RA) and scleroderma (progressive systemic sclerosis. HRCT findings are bibasilar reticulation with minimal ground-glass opacity—UIP.	
Chronic hypersensitivity pneumonitis	Chronic HP most often shows fibrosis involving mid-lung or lower lung zone predominance with relative sparing of the lung bases.	**Fig. 4.94.6:** Chronic hypersensitivity pneumonitis

Table 4.94.2: Causes of fibrosis

Causes of upper zone fibrosis (mnemonic—APICES)	*Causes of lower zone fibrosis (mnemonic—CIA)*
• Ankylosing spondylosis • Pulmonary TB, pneumoconiosis • Irradiation • Cystic fibrosis • Extrinsic allergic alveolitis • Sarcoidosis	• Connective tissue disorder • Idiopathic • Asbestosis

Table 4.94.3: Types of asbestos fibers

Amphibole	*Serpentine*
Subtypes: Crocidolite, amosite, and tremolite. Crocidolite is more common.	Subtype: Chrysotile
Most common cause of asbestos-related disease	Less likely to result in disease than amphiboles.

Causes of death in asbestosis: Respiratory failure, cor pulmonale, asbestosis related malignancies, especially bronchogenic carcinoma and mesothelioma.

Table 4.94.4: Asbestos related benign pleural and parenchymal diseases

Lung disease in asbestos exposure	*Asbestos-related pleural disease*
Asbestosis Rounded atelectasis	• Pleural plaques • Visceral pleural thickening—usually along the lateral pleural surface of the lower lobes. • Benign exudative pleural effusion • Diffuse pleural thickening • Pleural calcification
Legally eligible to get compensation	Not eligible to get compensation

Chronic diffuse infiltrative lung disease with reduced lung volume due to fibrotic process: Systemic lupus erythematosus, collagen vascular disease (e.g., scleroderma, dermatomyositis, polymyositis), idiopathic pulmonary fibrosis, chronic interstitial pneumonias, asbestosis.

Chronic diffuse infiltrative lung disease with pleural thickening: Asbestosis, collagen vascular disease.

Table 4.94.5: Asbestos-related pleural diseases	
Pleural plaque	*Diffuse pleural thickening*
• Localized areas of pleural thickening (2–10 mm in thickness), bilateral, multifocal • Nearly always involve parietal pleura. • Posterolateral thorax and on the diaphragm • Spare the apices and costophrenic angles • May calcify (10–15% in X-ray,15–20% in CT) • Characteristic discrete elevated lesions with thickened, nodular and rolled edges (holly leaf appearance)	Continuous sheet of pleural thickening with >3 mm thick, >5 cm width and >8 cm craniocaudal extent with edges will be tapered. May involve costophrenic angles and apices.

Table 4.94.6: Diagnostic pearls of mesothelioma		
Diagnostic pearls of mesothelioma: Commonly related to asbestos exposure, incidence up to 5% in heavily exposed subjects, latency period of 2Q-40 years, arises in relation to the parietal pleura Types: Epithelial (50%), sarcomatous (25%), or mixed (25%) cell types, pleural effusion, concentric and lobulated pleural thickening, frozen mediastinum sign, involvement of fissure, chest wall invasion or distant metastases and poor prognosis		
Causes of pleural calcification: A. Infection: 1. Healed empyema, 2. tuberculosis, histoplasmosis. B. Trauma 1. Healed hemothorax = Fibrothorax, 2. Radiation therapy; C. Pneumoconiosis: 1. Asbestos-related pleural disease, 2. Talcosis, 3. Bakelite, 4. Muscovite mica D. Hypercalcemia: 1. Pancreatitis 2. Chronic renal failure E. Miscellaneous: 1. Mineral oil aspiration, 2. Pulmonary infarction		
Frozen mediastinum sign: Seen in malignant pleural effusion (e.g. mesothelioma), because of pleural thickening and mediastinal infiltration, the involved hemithorax may be normal in volume, without mediastinal shift, despite the presence of a large effusion.		
CT features of malignant pleural disease: 1. Nodular pleural thickening, 2. Circumferential pleural thickening, 3. Parietal pleural thickening greater than 1 cm, 4. Mediastinal pleural thickening		
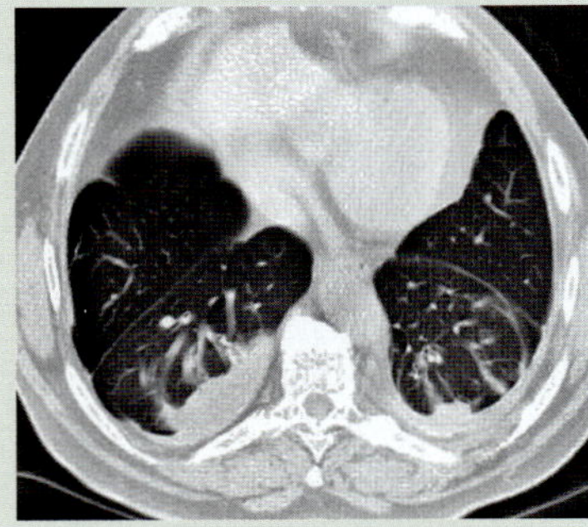 **Fig. 4.94.7:** Round atelectasis	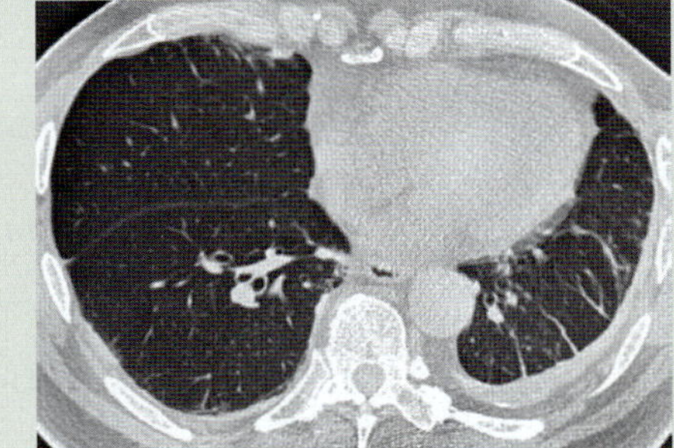 **Fig. 4.94.8:** Pleural thickening	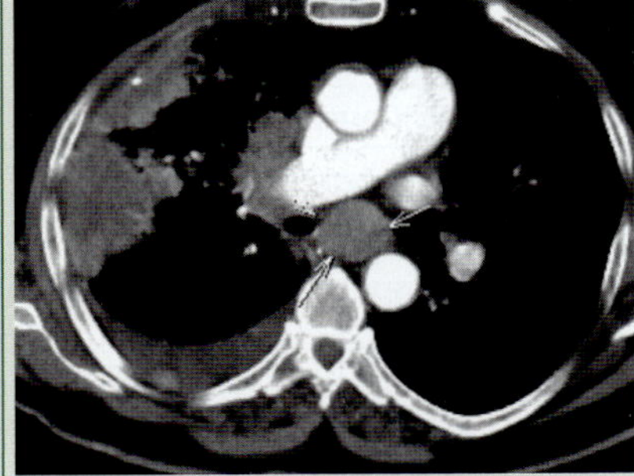 **Fig. 4.94.9:** Mesothelioma

Asbestos-related Disease

Asbestos-related malignant diseases: Bronchogenic carcinoma, mesothelioma (pleural or extra pleural (peritoneal mesothelioma). Rarely renal cell cancer and laryngeal cancer.

Asbestos-related parenchymal lung disease

1. *Asbestosis:* It is an interstitial lung fibrosis due to asbestos exposure, 20–30 years after start of exposure; Appearance may mimic idiopathic pulmonary fibrosis. Associated pleural disease differentiates asbestosis from idiopathic pulmonary fibrosis. Coarse linear opacities extending to abnormal pleural surface is known as parenchymal bands, when grouped together, they resemble crow's foot.
2. *Rounded atelectasis:* The term rounded atelectasis refers to the presence of focal rounded lung collapse which is commonly associated with asbestos exposure. (Other causes include empyema, pleural effusion of any cause like tuberculous effusion.)
   - Round or elliptical, posterior location.
   - Peripheral in location with significant contact with abnormal pleural surface.
   - Associated with ipsilateral pleural abnormality (effusion/thickening)

4

Table 4.94.7: International labour office (ILO) classification of pneumoconioses

Opacity type	*Perfusion (of small opacities)*
Small rounded opacities (diameter) p <1.5 mm, q >1.5–3 mm, r >3–10 mm Small irregular opacities (thickness) s <1.5 mm, t >1.5–3 mm, u >3–10 mm Large opacities (diameter) A: One or a cluster of several opacities >10 mm to 5 cm, B: Larger or more numerous than A, not larger than the right upper lobe, C: Larger than B	0—Absent or less profuse than 1 1—Definitely present but few in number (normal lung markings are still visible) 2—Numerous small opacities (normal lung markings partially obscured) 3—Very numerous small opacities (normal lung markings usually obscured)

- Associated with volume loss in affected lung
- Associated with curving of pulmonary vessels and bronchi into the edge of lesion (comet tail sign)

Atypical presentations like irregular surface, no comet tail sign, anterior location can happen with asbestos exposure, should be differentiated from lung carcinoma.

Hairy pleural plaques seen in plaques arise from the visceral pleura, typically from an interlobar fissure. The hairiness stems from short radially-oriented linear regions of fibrosis extending from the plaque into the adjacent lung parenchyma.

Pleural calcification is hallmark of asbestos exposure. Bilateral diaphragmatic calcification with clear costophrenic angles are pathognomonic.

4.95 CHEST

Case No. 95

Clinical history: 41-year-old male, presented with complaints of dry cough and breathlessness for 1 month.

Radiological techniques and observations: Plain radiograph chest frontal view (Fig. 4.95.1) shows ill-defined confluent radio-opacities in the upper zone of bilateral lung fields. Bilateral perihilar radio-opacities are seen. A few suspicious foci of intralesional calcifications noted. No evidence of intralesional cavity, fat, air bronchogram or air fluid level noted. Trachea is mildly shifted to the right. Bilateral costophrenic and cardiophrenic angles are free. Cardiac silhouette appears normal. Visualized bones and soft tissue appear normal.

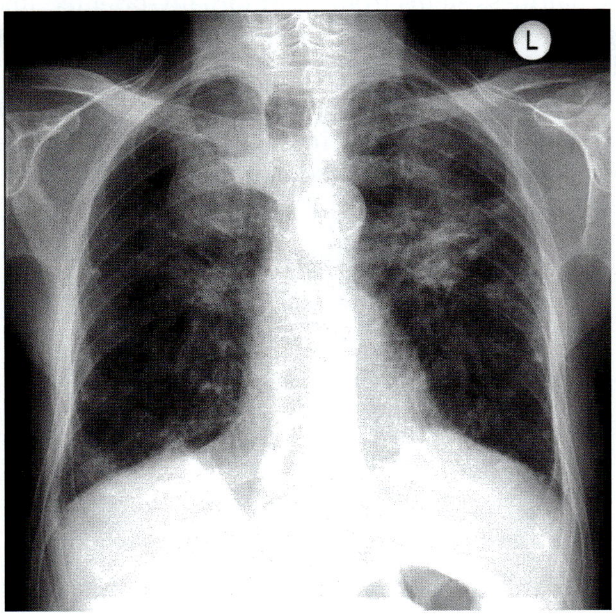

Fig. 4.95.1

Non-enhanced CT chest axial and coronal reformatted sections (Fig. 4.95.2) in lung and mediastinal window given. Spiculated mass with irregular borders and fibrosis in bilateral upper lobes (left side more than right) and in the bilateral perihilar region, with adjacent multiple pulmonary blebs. A few foci of dense calcification noted within the mass. A few nodules noted adjacent to the mass. Volume loss noted in bilateral upper lobes. No evidence of intralesional cavity, fat, air bronchogram, air fluid level or necrosis. Adjacent pleural thickening noted on either side. Tracheal and mediastinal shift to the right noted. Left lower paratracheal and left hilar lymph node enlargement with calcifications noted. There is left mild pleural effusion. Visualized bones and soft tissues appear normal.

Interpretation: A: 41-year-old male, bilateral upper lobe, C: Spiculated mass with irregular border and fibrosis, foci of calcification, nodules B: Pleural thickening on either side, lymph node enlargement with calcification D: Silicosis with progressive massive fibrosis.

Principal diagnosis: Silicosis with progressive massive fibrosis (PMF).

Differential diagnoses

1. **Pulmonary tuberculosis**
2. **Silicotuberculosis**
3. **Sarcoidosis:** Large opacities are conglomerations of small opacities.

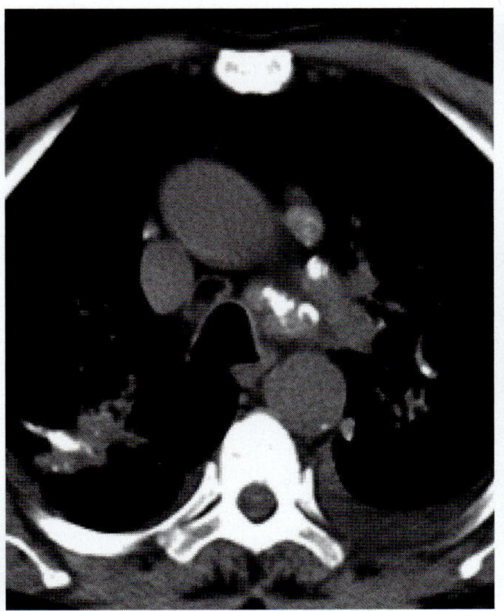
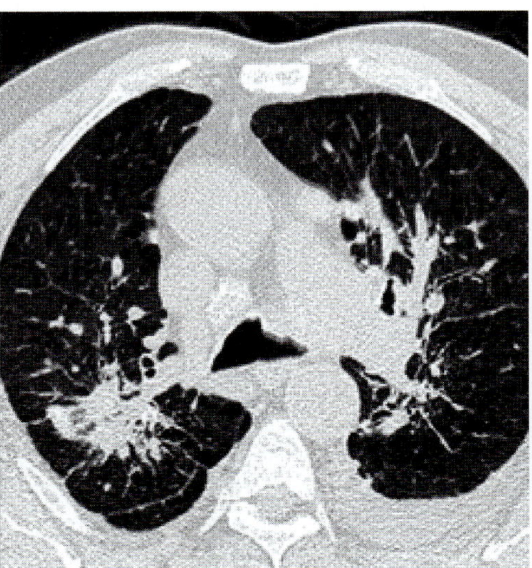
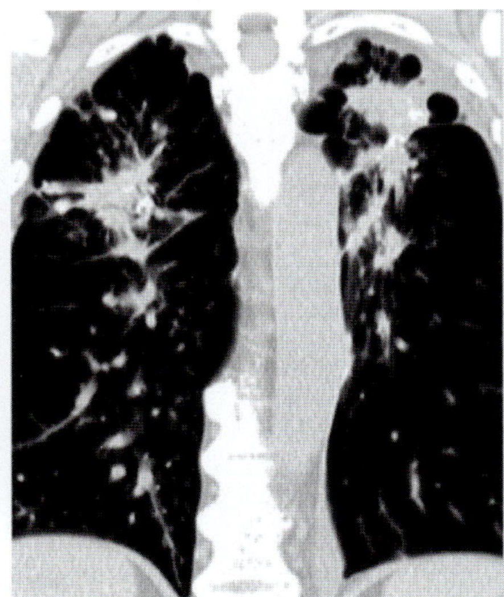

Fig. 4.95.2

Table 4.95.1: Differential diagnosis for silicosis		
1. Primary pulmonary **Tuberculosis:** Pulmonary tuberculosis is reported to be higher in those patients with silicosis. Clinical history, asymmetric involvement, upper lobe predominance differentiate TB from silicosis.	Imaging findings include asymmetric centrilobular nodules or consolidation, cavitation progressing to fibrosis and traction bronchiectasis with upper lobe predominance.	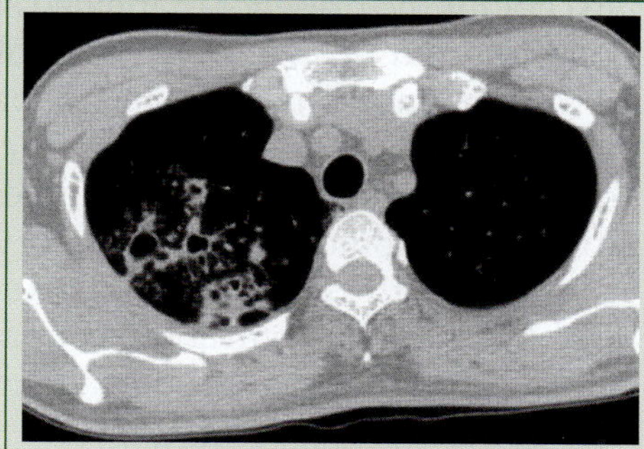 **Fig. 4.95.3:** Primary pulmonary tuberculosis
2. Sarcoidosis–refer to case 102.		
3. Berylliosis: Commonly seen in workers in the ceramics industry, fluorescent lamp manufacturing, nuclear weapons production, and aerospace manufacturing.		
4. Siderosis: Refers to iron deposition within the lung. Two types: **1. Primary pulmonary hemosiderosis** (associated with Goodpasture syndrome) or idiopathic **2. Secondary pulmonary hemosiderosis,** often due to mitral stenosis.	Multiple small and poorly defined centrilobular nodules in the upper lobe of both lungs, with areas of ground-glass attenuation.	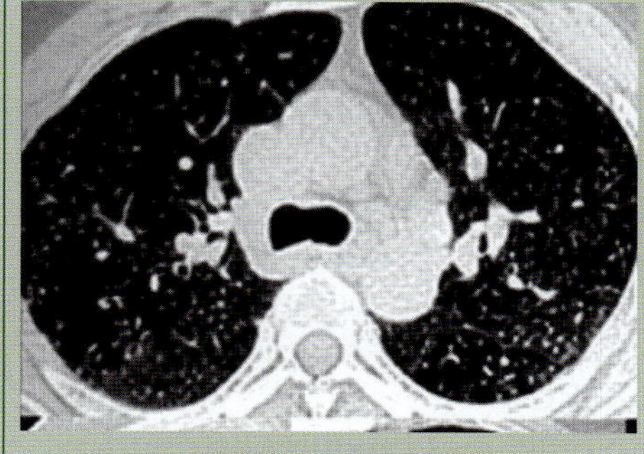 **Fig. 4.95.4:** Siderosis

4. **Occupational disorders** like berylliosis, siderosis, talcosis.
5. **Caplan's syndrome:** Consists of large necrobiotic nodules (rheumatoid nodules) superimposed on silicosis or coal worker's pneumoconiosis (CWP). More common with CWP. Scleroderma, rheumatoid arthritis and SLE are associated with silicosis.
6. Miliary TB, miliary fungal infection, miliary metastasis (differential for simple silicosis)
7. **Malignant mass** (very unlikely due to age group and bilateral involvement)

Management: Patient to be referred to pulmonology department for further evaluation and multimodality approach required for vocational rehabilitation regarding the occupation. The diagnosis of silicosis requires the combination of an appropriate history of silica exposure and characteristic findings on the chest radiograph. The presence of silica in the bronchoalveolar lavage (BAL) confirms the diagnosis (especially in acute silicosis). Whole lung lavage (WLL) appears to be a feasible means of removing dust, cytokines, and dust-laden cells that may reflect differential disease activity and allow modification of the progressive fibrosis that is associated with silica exposure.

Brief Discussion about the Condition

Pneumoconiosis: Refers to presence of lung disease related to dust inhalation. Pneumoconiosis may be clinicopathologically classified as fibrotic (involving focal nodular or diffuse fibrosis) or nonfibrotic (involving particle-laden macrophages, with minimal or no fibrosis).

Silicosis, coal worker pneumoconiosis, asbestosis, berylliosis, and talcosis are fibrotic forms of pneumoconiosis. Siderosis (from iron oxide), stannosis (from tin oxide), and barytosis (from barium sulfate) are nonfibrotic forms of the disease. Silicosis and coal worker pneumoconiosis (CWP) are pathologically distinct entities with differing histology, resulting from the inhalation of different inorganic dusts. The radiographic and HRCT appearances of these diseases, however, may not be distinguishable from each other.

Silicosis is a fibrotic pneumoconiosis caused by the inhalation of fine particles of crystalline silicon dioxide (silica). Occupations such as mining, quarrying, and tunneling are associated with silicosis. It usually becomes evident 10 to 20 years after the onset of exposure. Two forms of silicosis are as follows.

1. **Acute silicosis:** A unique manifestation of acute exposure to large amounts of silica (e.g. in sand

blasting) is termed acute silicosis or silicoproteinosis. Except for the presence of inhaled silica which could be found out during bronchoalveolar lavage (BAL), it is indistinguishable from idiopathic pulmonary alveolar proteinosis. In acute silicosis, the clinical course is usually progressive and ends in death due to cor pulmonale and respiratory failure despite therapy with corticosteroids. Imaging findings include bilateral centrilobular opacities, multifocal patchy ground-glass opacities and consolidation with occasional crazy paving.

2. **Classic silicosis** which manifests as a chronic interstitial reticulonodular disease. The classic form is common than the acute form and can be classified as simple or complicated, according to the radiographic findings.

Simple/uncomplicated silicosis:

1. Small well-defined nodules of 2–5 mm in diameter in both lungs.
2. Nodules may be diffuse and symmetrical with upper lobe and posterior lung zone predominance
3. Nodules may be calcified
4. Centrilobular, subpleural distribution of nodules on HRCT
5. Sometimes random distribution
6. Often hilar and mediastinal lymph nodes enlargement. Calcification of lymph nodes is common and typically occurs at the periphery of the node. The so-called eggshell calcification pattern is highly suggestive of silicosis.

Subpleural nodules have a rounded or triangular configuration, and if they are confluent, they may resemble pleural plaques, termed pseudoplaques/ candlewax lesions.

Complicated silicosis has large conglomerate opacities—progressive massive fibrosis. Appearance of large opacities (>1 cm), also known as conglomerate masses, indicate the presence of complicated silicosis (progressive massive fibrosis). These large opacities result from nodule coalescence and are observed commonly in the middle lung zone, peripheral one-third of the lung on axial chest images and in the upper lung zone on longitudinal images. The large opacities gradually migrate toward the hilum, leaving emphysematous lung tissue between the fibrotic tissue and the pleural surface.

1. Worsening symptoms in patient with silicosis
2. Large symmetric bilateral opacities with an irregular margin (in midzone) on CXR.
3. Focal conglomerate soft tissue masses, often with irregular or ill-defined margins with a background of small nodules on HRCT. Upper lobe nodules may decrease in number.
4. Soft tissue masses may cavitate (due to ischemia, tuberculosis, bacterial infection)
5. Calcification common
6. Adjacent emphysema may be present.

The risk of silicosis is dose related. Progression of disease both radiographically and clinically may occur for years after exposure has ended.

Silicosis complications: 1. Predisposes to tuberculosis (cavitation within fibrotic mass may suggest the presence of silicotuberculosis) 2. Carcinoma (enhancing mass lesion with high signal intensity on T2-weighted MR images highly suggestive of lung cancer and histo-pathologic analysis should be performed for diagnosis, whereas PMF shows hypointensity on T2-weighted MR images and peripheral enhancement on post-contrast images).

Table 4.95.2: Silicosis and coal workers pneumoconiosis

Silicosis-progressive massive fibrosis	*Coal workers pneumoconiosis*
Numerous aggregated nodules associated with dense fibrous tissue.	Amorphous black mass of dust surrounded by some fibrous tissue.

Table 4.95.3: Differential diagnosis for upper lobe lesions and multiple hyperdense pulmonary micronodules

Upper lobe lesions (APICES)	*Multiple hyperdense pulmonary micronodules (0.5–2 mm)*
1. Ankylosing spondylitis 2. Pulmonary tuberculosis, pneumoconiosis 3. Irradiation 4. Cystic fibrosis 5. Eosinophilic pneumonia 6. Hypersensitivity pneumonitis 7. Sarcoidosis 8. Silicosis	1. Hemosiderosis—smaller than miliary tuberculosis 2. Silicosis—relative sparing of bases and apices. 3. Siderosis—lower density than silica. Widely disseminated. 4. Stannosis 5. Barytosis

Table 4.95.4: Causes of hilar enlargement

Unilateral	*Bilateral*
Infection: TB, viral, bacterial Tumour: Lung carcinoma, lymphoma and metastasis Vascular: Pulmonary artery aneurysm/ stenosis, pulmonary embolism	Sarcoidosis/silicosis Infection: TB, viral, bacterial, histoplasmosis Tumour: Lymphoma and metastasis Vascular: Pulmonary artery hypertension

Diffuse or multiple calcifications in lung DD: Infections

- Tuberculosis—healed miliary, histoplasmosis and varicella, chronic pulmonary venous hypertension.
- Silicosis—in up to 20% of those showing nodular opacities, metastases, alveolar microlithiasis—often familial, metastatic due to hypercalcemia—chronic renal failure, secondary hyperparathyroidism and multiple myeloma. Lymphoma following radiotherapy.

Egg Shell Calcification: Criteria

1. Shell-like calcifications up to 2 mm thick must be present in the peripheral zone of at least two lymph nodes
2. The calcifications may be solid or broken
3. In at least one of the lymph nodes, the ring-like shadow must be complete
4. The central part of the lymph node shows additional calcifications
5. One of the lymph nodes must be at least 1 cm in its greatest diameter

DD: 1. Silicosis: 5% patients, 2. Treated lymphoma (post-irradiation, Hodgkin disease): Usually 1–9 years following treatment, 3. Coal workers' pneumoconiosis (CWP): 1% patients, 4. Sarcoidosis: Calcification is uncommon (only 5% of patients) and occurs late in the disease; only rarely does it have an eggshell configuration, 5. Scleroderma, 6. Amyloidosis (rare), 7. Tuberculosis, blastomycosis and histoplasmosis (rare).

Table 4.95.5: Difference between pulmonary tuberculosis and progressive massive fibrosis

Findings	*Pulmonary tuberculosis*	*Progressive massive fibrosis*
Pathology	Liquefaction of caseous necrosis, formation of cavities with progressive fibrosis and lung destruction. Pleural adhesions, and formation of traction bronchiectasis.	Large conglomerate masses in patients with long standing silicosis. Conglomeration of small interstitial nodules in combination with a variable degree of fibrosis.
Location	Apicoposterior lung segments and to a lesser degree in the apical segments of the lower lobes.	Usually in the upper or mid-lung, are distinct from the hila and are separated from the peripheral pleural surface.
Bilateral	Less common	Bilateral and symmetrical
Cavity	Seen in 40%. Air-fluid levels in the cavity occur in 10% of cases.	Rare
Pleural exudates	+	–
Pleural effusion	++	+/–
Calcification	+/-	++ Egg shell calcification of hilar lymph nodes

4.96 CHEST

Case No. 96

Clinical history: 35 years old young man presents with fever.

Radiological techniques and observation: Figure 4.96.1 is frontal radiograph of chest showing multiple small cavitating lesions in the right mid and lower zone and left lung lower zone. There is no obvious hilar or paratracheal lymph node enlargement, but there is mild blunting of right costophrenic angle which may be due to right-sided pleural effusion. Lesions projected over right diaphragm also appears cavitatory. Left lateral chest wall shows soft tissue thickening with a vertical line of gas.

Figures 4.96.2 to 4.96.4 are axial CT images demonstrate multiple thin-walled cavities of roughly similar size in right upper lobe posterior segment, right lower lobe superior segment. Centrilobular nodules noted in right lower lobe superior segment. Basal consolidation with minimal effusion noted in right lower lobe basal segments. There is collection with air pockets in left lateral chest wall representing abscess.

Interpretation: A—35 years old male, bilateral lung fields show, C—multiple cavitating nodules with right pleural effusion, B—with evidence of infection in left chest wall, D—septic emboli.

Principal diagnosis: Septic emboli due to infection.

Differential diagnosis for multiple lung cavities: Septic emboli, in an immunocompromised or neutropenic patient, these appearances may be caused by angioinvasive aspergillosis during the phase of neutrophil recovery; Wegener's granulomatosis, rheumatoid nodules; cavitating pneumonia,tuberculosis; pneumatocele; cystic bronchiectasis; Langerhans cell histiocytosis predominantly cystic changes with increased lung volume; metastases from a primary squamous cancer (head and neck, lung), GIT adenocarcinoma, sarcoma may lead to this appearance, but in a young man, this diagnosis is less likely; cavitating primary malignancy—bronchogenic carcinoma, lymphoma.

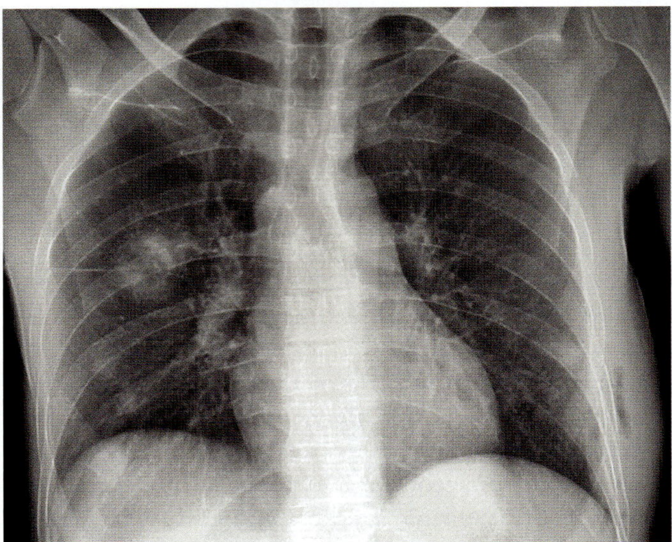

Fig. 4.96.1

Table 4.96.1: Imaging features of benign and malignant cavities

Benign cavity	*Malignant cavity*
Wall thickness, 7 mm benign, 8–24 mm mixed	>24 mm—malignant
Smooth walls	Irregular internal walls—in malignant cavity
Location—anywhere	More common in upper lobe
Surrounding consolidation, satellite nodules, bronchial wall thickening—more common in benign cavities	Less common

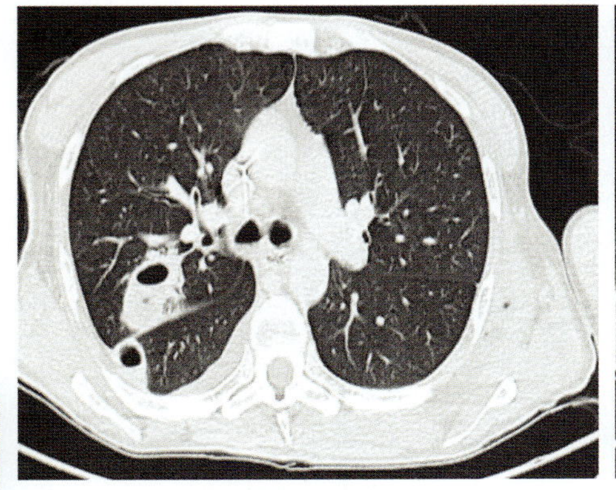

Fig. 4.96.2

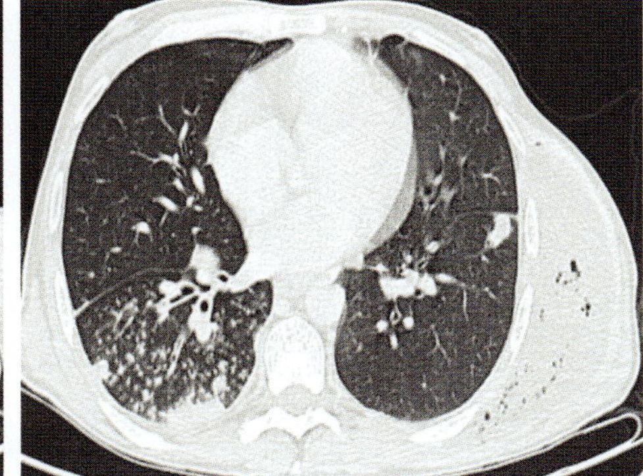

Fig. 4.96.3

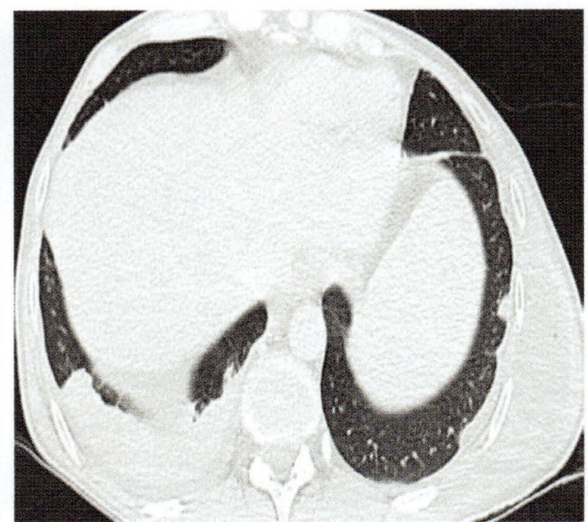

Fig. 4.96.4

4

Table 4.96.2: Mimics of cavities: Cystic lung disease

Cystic bronchiectasis	Clustered or perihilar distribution; air-fluid levels may be present and patchy distribution helps in differentiating from diffuse cystic lung disease.signet ring sign—dilated artery	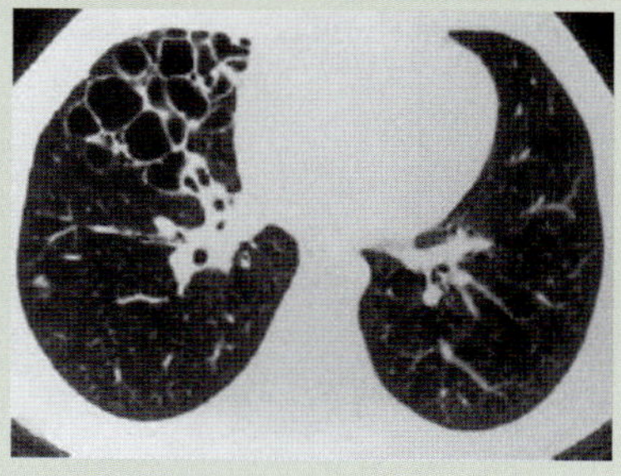 Fig. 4.96.5: Cystic bronchiectasis
Wegener granulomatosis Associated sinusitis and laryngeal involvement seen	Multiple nodules with cavitation in random distribution with associated bronchial wall thickening. Peribronchovascular nodules/centrilobular nodules seen	
PCP: Pneumocystis pneumonia Immunocompromised	Patchy bilateral ground-glass opacities, thick or thin walled irregular septated cysts, may have pneumothorax	
LAM (Lymphangioleiomyomatosis): Almost exclusively in women of childbearing age; associated with tuberous sclerosis.	Cysts usually round and relatively uniform in size and shape; diffuse lung involvement	
LCH: Langerhans cell histiocytosis smoking related (80–90%)	Cysts have unusual shapes; larger and more numerous in lung apices; thick or thin walled; costophrenic angles usually spared; small nodules and cavitary nodules may be present	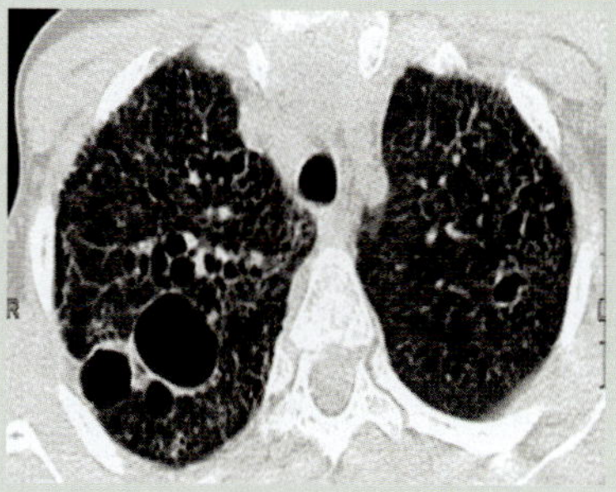 Fig. 4.96.6: Langerhans cell histiocytosis
LIP: Lymphoid interstitial pneumonia associated with Sjögren syndrome, collagen-vascular diseases, immunosuppression	Less numerous cysts than in LAM or histiocytosis; vessels may be seen in relation to the walls of cysts, lower lobe predominant; thickening of bronchovascular bundles and interstitial thickening along the lymph channels	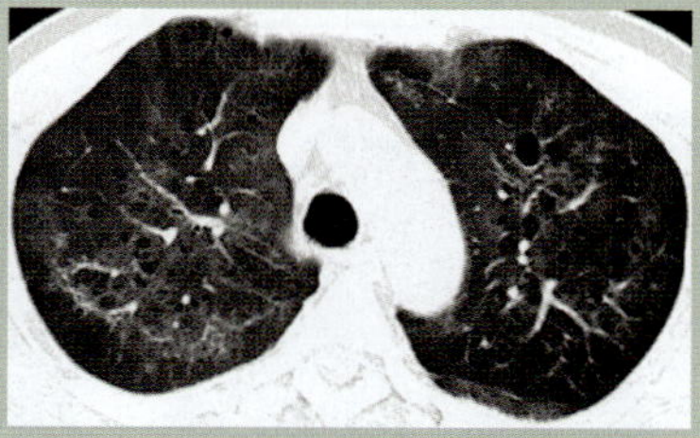 Fig. 4.96.7: Lymphoid interstitial pneumonia
Tracheobronchial papillomatosis related to human papillomavirus Juvenile and adult form	Thin walled cysts and adjacent nodules; posterior predilection due to gravity. Laryngeal or tracheal lesions consistent with papillomas	
Paraseptal emphysema	Air-filled cysts without perceptible wall in subpleural location with a peripheral distribution within secondary pulmonary lobule	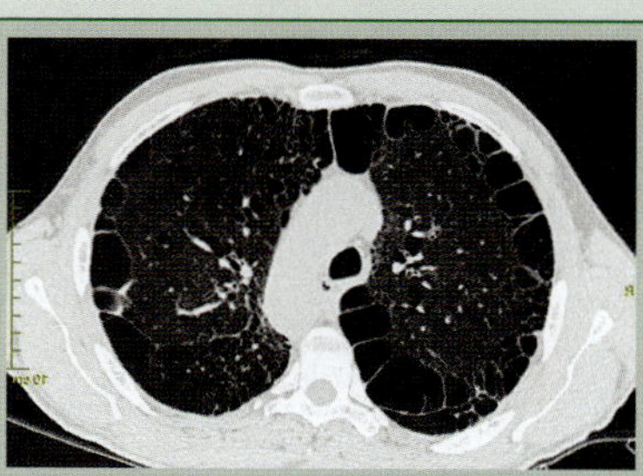 Fig. 4.96.8: Paraseptal emphysema

(Contd.)

Table 4.96.2: Mimics of cavities: Cystic lung disease (*Contd.*)		
Honeycombing in ILD	Clusters lustered cystic air spaces (between 3–10 mm in diameter, but occasionally as large as 2.5 cm) that are usually subpleural and basal in distribution. Wall thickness 1–3 mm	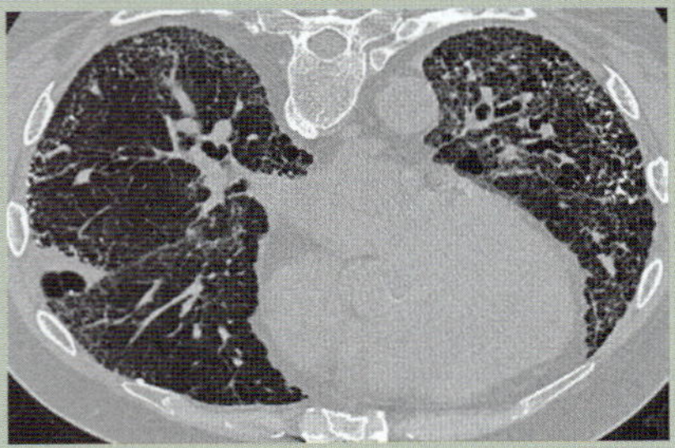 Fig. 4.96.9: Honeycombing in ILD
Amyloidosis and light-chain deposition disease	Associated with Sjögren syndrome; nodules may be present Appearance may be indistinguishable from LIP	
Birt-Hogg-Dubé syndrome	Associated with fibrofolliculomas distributed over the face, neck, and upper trunk and renal tumors Cysts often thin-walled and subpleural or related to fissures; may be lenticular; larger than in LAM, LCH, LIP	
Other causes of lung cysts	**Benign metastasizing leiomyoma. Desquamative interstitial pneumonia, hypersensitivity pneumonitis, bullae, pneumatoceles, bronchiectasis**	

Table 4.96.3: Differential diagnosis of cysts and cavity in lung	
Cavity—wall >3 mm	*Cysts—wall <3 mm*
Infection • Staphylococcus • Gram negative bacteria • Anaerobe in aspiration • TB, fungal (aspergillosis) Neoplasm: Lung ca—squamous, BAC Vascular: Lung infarction	Congenital • Bronchogenic cyst • CPAM Bulla Pneumatocele • Post-traumatic

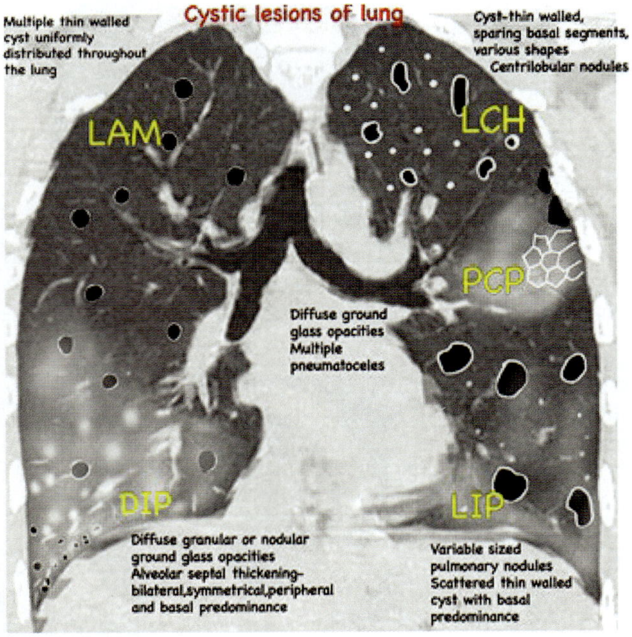

Fig. 4.96.10: Cystic lesions of lung illustration showing LAM, LCH, DIP and LIP

Focal regions of emphysema with no discernible wall <1 or 2 cm –bleb; >1 or 2 cm–bulla.

Cysts in lung

Focal cysts: Chronic bronchial cysts, interstitial cyst, cystic lung disease, emphysema.

Diffuse cysts cause: Pulmonary Langerhans cell histiocytosis, lymphocytic interstitial pneumonitis, lymphangioleiomyomatosis with or without tuberous sclerosis; tracheobronchial papillomatosis, desquamative interstitial pneumonia, Sjögren syndrome, neurofibromatosis type 1, Birt-Hogg-Dubé syndrome, pulmonary mesenchymal cystic hamartoma.

Focal cysts: Bronchogenic cyst, cystic adenomatoid malformation, bulla, pneumatocele (post-traumatic).

Discussion

Sources of septic emboli: Right-sided infective endocarditis, particularly tricuspid valve; Infection elsewhere in the body (e.g. soft tissue/bone infection) with associated septal defects; infected deep venous thrombosis; immunologic deficiencies; infected catheters/lines; venous lines/central venous catheters, pacemaker wires, post-anginal septicemia, periodontal disease.

The distribution of cavitating lesions: Predominantly upper zone distribution may be seen in tuberculosis; peripheral cavities may suggest that the lesions are infarcts; sparing of the tips of the middle and/or lingula lobe and the extreme lung bases seen in Langerhans' cell histiocytosis.

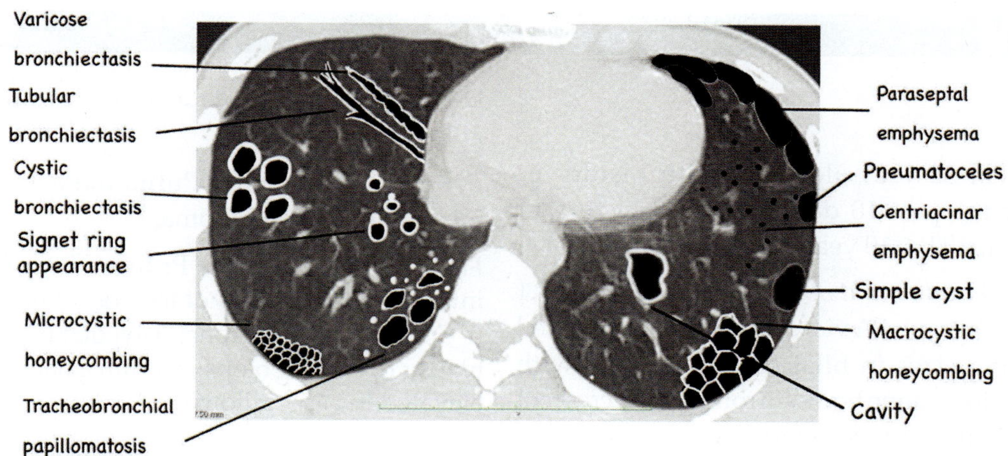

Fig. 4.96.11: Cystic lung lesions

Ancillary features: Look for destructive bone (i.e. vertebral/rib) lesions, which may suggest that the cavities are metastatic, indwelling catheters (septic emboli), associated nodules (Langerhans' cell histiocytosis), enlarged intrathoracic nodes lymph nodes, "vegetations" on the heart valves (septic emboli).

Treatment: Parenteral antibiotics.

Complications: Pyothorax, empyema, pneumothorax.

4.97 CHEST

Case No. 97

Clinical history: 35-year-old male with history of hemoptysis for the past 10 days with past history of treated pulmonary TB—10 years back.

Radiological techniques and observation: Figure 4.97.1 is plain chest radiograph PA view showing thick -walled cavity of varying sizes in bilateral upper zone with intracavitory radio-opaque body surrounded by crescent of air **(air crescent sign)**. No evidence of calcification noted in the cavity. Trachea appears to be slightly pulled to the right. Mediastinum, thoracic cage and diaphragm appear normal. No evidence of cardiomegaly. Visualised mid and lower zone shows no similar lesions. Contrast enhanced chest CT is required to further characterise the lesion.

Figures 4.97.2 and 4.97.3 are axial contrast enhanced CT showing thick-walled cavity of varying sizes noted in bilateral upper lobe with intracavitatory body of soft tissue attenuation which appears to fill the cavity and has reticular appearance with multiple irregular air pockets surrounded by crescent of air. Multiple fibrotic strands appear to extend from the wall of cavity to the pleural surface on both side. A few centrilobular nodules in tree in bud pattern noted in the anterior segment of right upper lobe. No evidence of contrast enhancing areas within the intracavitatory body. No evidence of rib/ vertebral body erosion.

Interpretation: A—35-year-old male, bilateral upper lobes show, C—thick walled cavity in bilateral upper lobe with intracavitatory body surrounded by crescent of air, B—a few centrilobular nodules in tree in bud pattern noted in the anterior segment of right upper lobe, D—pulmonary TB sequelae with intracavitary aspergilloma.

Principal diagnosis: Pulmonary TB sequelae with intracavitary aspergilloma.

Further investigation: Prone CT to demonstrate the intracavitary mobility of aspergilloma.

Sputum culture, bronchoalveolar lavage, transthoracic biopsy, open lung biopsy/serum galactomannan levels—elevated in aspergilloma.

Treatment: Aspergilloma—oral itraconazole and intracavitary amphotericin B.

- Invasive and semi-invasive aspergillosis—voriconazole is the treatment of choice.
- Hemoptysis may require bronchial artery embolisation or surgical resection.

Discussion: Aspergillosis is a mycotic disease caused by usually *A. fumigatus*. The manifestations of pulmonary aspergillosis are determined by the number and virulence of the organism and the patient's immune response.

Pulmonary aspergillosis is subdivided into five categories. **Lung scar carcinoma (LSC)** was first described in 1939 by Friedrich as a form of lung cancer that originates from peripheral scars in the lung. These, in turn, may arise from infection, injury, intrinsic pulmonary disease, or recurrent episodes of tumor necrosis and healing. The most common etiologic factor for the development of LSC is scarring secondary to tuberculosis, but it is also known to occur in the setting of pneumonia, pulmonary abscess, bronchiectasis, and pulmonary infarction. SC is most commonly subpleural adenocarcinoma. It is hypothesized that impedance of lymphatic drainage by scar tissue can lead to accumulation of malignant cells with subsequent accelerated vascular and/or lymphatic spread of LSC.

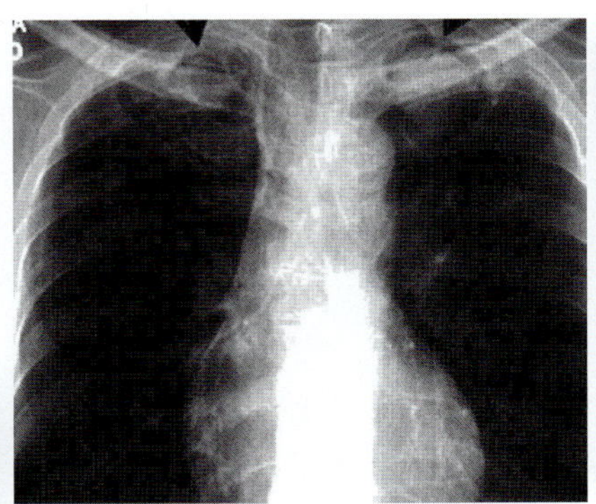
Fig. 4.97.1

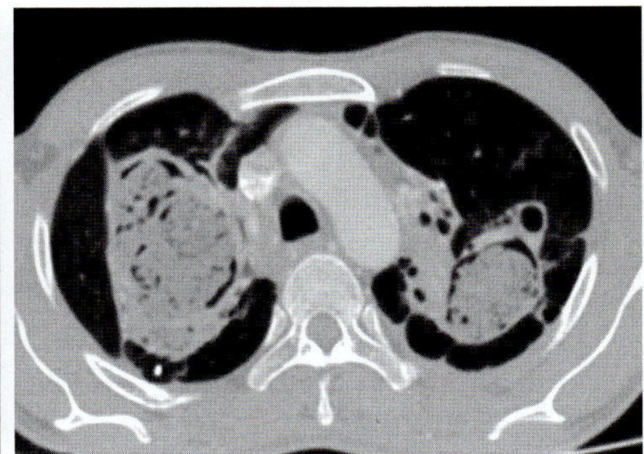
Fig. 4.97.2

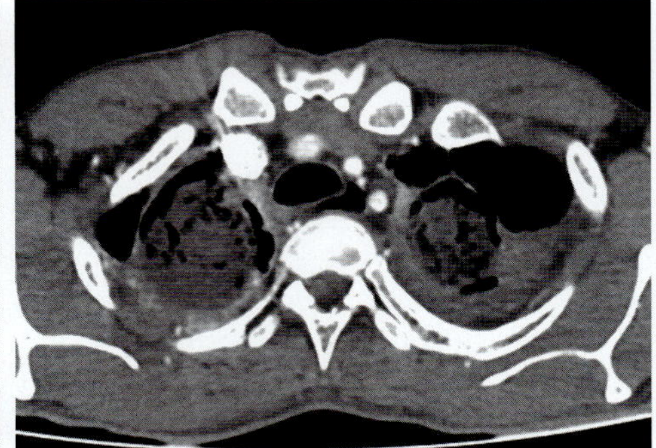
Fig. 4.97.3

Table 4.97.1: Differential diagnosis for intracavitary bodies	
1. Clot	Soft tissue dense/slightly **hyperdense** nodules within the cavity surrounding by crescent of air which **changes position with supine and prone images. Does not show contrast enhancement.**
2. Rasmussen's aneurysm **Pulmonary artery** pseudoaneurysm secondary to pulmonary tuberculosis. Granulation tissue in the vessel wall is replaced by fibrosis with subsequent thinning of the wall and pseudoaneurysm formation. Definitive management is endovascular embolisation.	Soft tissue dense/slightly hyperdense nodules within the cavity surrounding by crescent of air which **does not change position with supine and prone images**—fixed to the cavity wall and the **nodule shows intense contrast enhancement.**
3. Malignant mass: Nonsmall cell lung cancer.	Soft tissue dense nodules with areas of central necrosis within the cavity surrounding by crescent of air which does not change position with supine and prone images—fixed to the cavity wall and the nodule shows **variable contrast enhancement with areas of necrosis.**

Table 4.97.2: Types of pulmonary aspergillosis		
1. Saprophytic aspergillosis (aspergilloma) Most common clinical symptom—hemoptysis and the most common underlying causes are tuberculosis and sarcoidosis. Others include—bronchogenic cyst, pulmonary sequestration, pneumatoceles secondary to PCP pneumonia in AIDS patients.	It shows solid , round or oval mass with soft tissue opacity within a thick-walled lung cavity. Adjacent pleural thickening noted. **"Air crescent"** sign **is seen.** **Differential diagnosis for air crescent sign:** Angioinvasive aspergillosis, echinococcal cyst, tuberculosis. Rasmussen aneurysm in a tuberculous cavity, cavitatory carcinoma, bronchogenic carcinoma arising in a cyst, papillomatosis, hematoma, *P. carinii* pneumonia	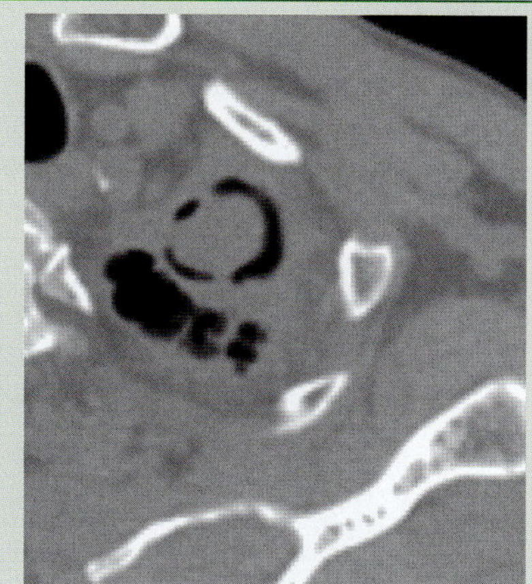 **Fig. 4.97.4:** Aspergilloma
2.Hypersensitivity reaction (allergic bronchopulmonary aspergillosis) Most common in patients with long standing **bronchial asthma.** A complex type I and III hypersensitivity reaction with resultant bronchial wall damage and bronchiectasis. Clinical symptoms—recurrent sneezing with cough and sputum production. Laboratory findings: **Elevated IgE and eosinophilia.**	**Fitting and fleeting** homogeneous, tubular, **finger in glove areas of increased opacity** in a bronchial distribution, predominantly or exclusively involving upper lobes with **mucoid impaction and central bronchiectasis.** In 30% cases, the impacted mucus will have **high attenuation** or shows calcification on CT. **Differential diagnosis for mucoid impaction** 1. Endobronchial lesions 2. Bronchial atresia 3. Bronchiectasis 4. ABPA **(high attenuation mucus)**	
3. Semi-invasive (chronic necrotizing) aspergillosis Chronic form more common in patients with diabetes mellitus, chronic obstructive pulmonary disease and prolonged cortico-steroid therapy. Definitive diagnosis is based on the bronchoscopic findings and chest radiography consistent with tissue invasion.	Unilateral or bilateral patchy consolidation with or without cavitation, adjacent pleural thickening and multiple nodules of increased opacity. Rarely, circumferential bronchial wall thickening and bronchial obstruction may be seen.	

(Contd.)

Table 4.97.2: Types of pulmonary aspergillosis (*Contd.*)

4. Airway invasive aspergillosis Manifestation includes acute tracheobronchiolitis, bronchiolitis, bronchopneumonia, obstructing bronchopulmonary aspergillosis—characterized by intraluminal growth of *Aspergillus fumigatus* in patients with AIDS. **Clinical presentation:** Cough with sputum production (fungal cast of bronchi) in immunocompromised cases. Obstructing bronchopulmonary aspergillosis mimics allergic bronchopulmonary aspergillosis.	Aspergillus bronchopneumonia have predominant peribronchial areas of consolidation. Bronchiolitis will produce centrilobular nodules in "tree in bud "pattern. **Differential diagnosis for centrilobular nodules in "tree in bud" pattern:** Endobronchial spread of infection. Mucus plugging (asthma), aspiration, invasive mucinus adenocarcinoma, cystic fibrosis, lymphangitis carcinomatosis, eosinophilic granuloma, intravascular metastasis.	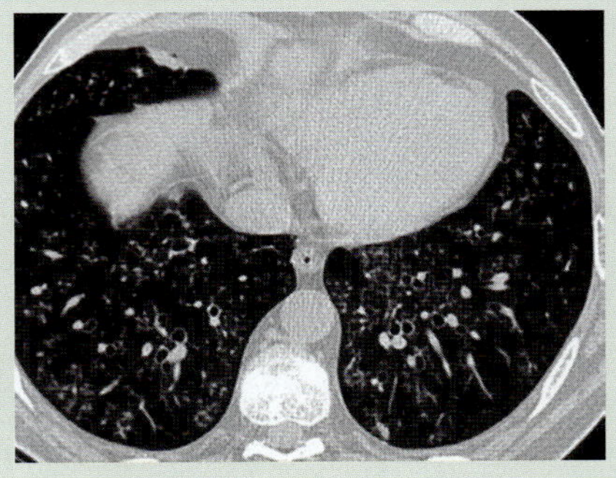 **Fig. 4.97.5:** Airway invasive aspergillosis
5. Angioinvasive aspergillosis Occurs in immunocompromised with severe neutropenia and in patients undergoing intensive chemotherapy for myeloma, resistant leukemia, solid tumors, difficult to treat lymphoma. Histology: Occlusion of small to medium-sized pulmonary arteries by fungal hyphae. **Differential diagnosis for "reverse halo sign/atoll sign":** Tuberculosis, pulmonary zygomycosis, adenocarcinoma lung, cryptogenic organising pneumonia, sarcoidosis, lipoid pneumonia, post-radiation therapy.	Nodules surrounded by a halo of ground-glass opacity—**"halo sign"**. Pleural based, wedge-shaped areas of consolidation—hemorrhagic infarcts. **Differential diagnosis for "halo sign":** 1. Infection (candida, herpes simplex and cytomegalovirus) 2. Wegener's granulomatosis 3. Kaposi sarcoma 4. Hemorrhagic metastasis 5. Postbiopsy pseudonodule	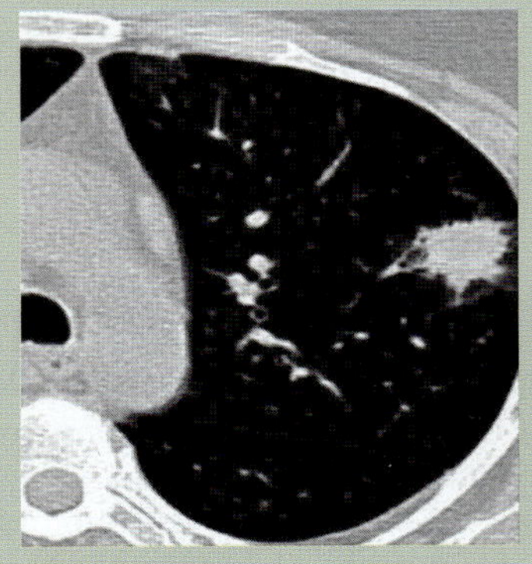 **Fig. 4.97.6:** Angioinvasive aspergillosis
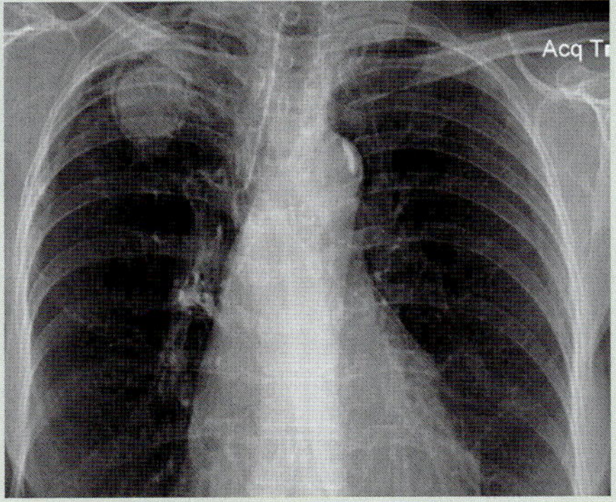 **Fig. 4.97.7:** Fungal ball	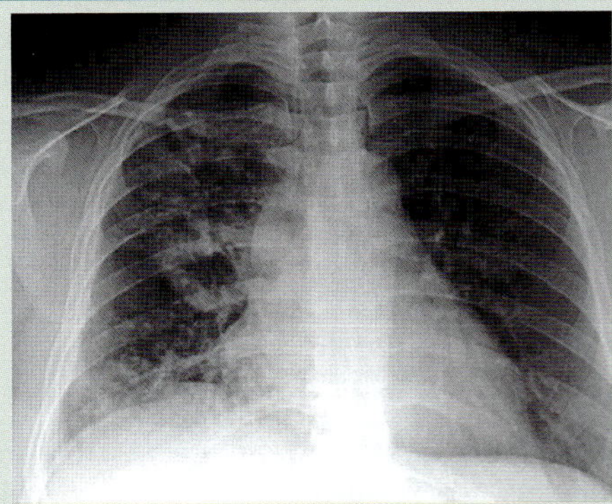 **Fig. 4.97.8:** Finger in glove in ABPA	

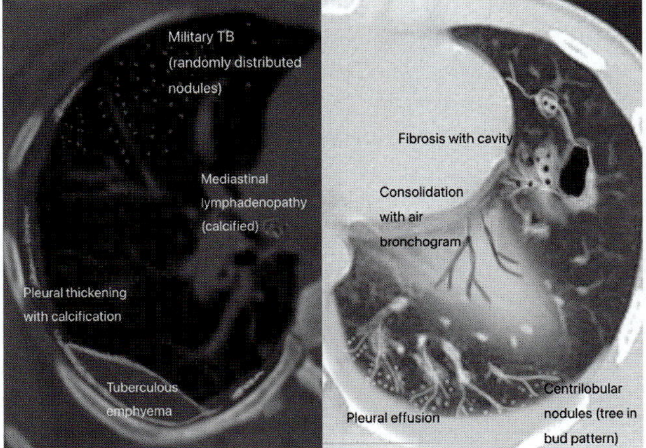

Fig. 4.97.9: Tuberculosis manifestations in thorax

4.98 CHEST

Case No. 98

Clinical history: 50-year-old female, complaints of several-week history of progressive shortness of breath.

Radiological techniques and observation: Figure 4.98.1 is plain radiograph of chest showing **subpleural reticular or reticulonodular opacity in a basal predominant distribution.** No evidence of bilateral hilar lymphadenopathy. Cardiac silhouette appears to be normal. Bilateral costophrenic and cardiophrenic angles are free. No evidence of dilated pulmonary arteries. No evidence of soft tissue calcification/superior rib notching/lateral end of clavicle erosion. Figure 4.98.2 is coronal reformatted image of HRCT thorax in lung window, showing mild volume loss. **Increased ground-glass opacity (GGO), reticular interstitial thickening** that is more predominant in the lung bases. Mild traction bronchiolectasis is noted. Mild visceral pleural thickening is noted. In soft tissue window, **dilated esophagus** can be seen.

Interpretation: A—50-year-old female, bilateral lower lobe basal segments, C—shows increased ground-glass opacity (GGO) and reticular interstitial thickening, B—dilated esophagus, D—scleroderma with NSIP.

Principal diagnosis: With this imaging findings, the principal diagnosis is **scleroderma with interstitial lung disease—NSIP pattern.** Biopsy will be done to confirm the diagnosis.

Differential diagnosis: Includes other interstitial lung disease.

Table 4.98.1: Current treatment options for SSc-ILD

Drug in use	*Mechanism of action*
Cyclophosphamide	Alkylating agent, crosslinks DNA, decreasing DNA synthesis and preventing cell division
Mycophenolate mofetil	Inhibits inosine monophosphate dehydrogenase, inhibits *de novo* guanosine nucleotide synthesis, prevents T and B proliferation
Azathioprine	Metabolites incorporated into replicating DNA, blocks the pathway for purine synthesis
Lung transplant	

Table 4.98.2: Investigational treatments for SSc-ILD

Drug under trial	*Mechanism of Action*
Rituximab	Monoclonal antibody against CD20 on B lymphocytes
Bosentan	Endothelin-1 receptor antagonist
Imatinib	Tyrosine kinase inhibitor
Pirfenidone	Anti-fibrotic and anti-inflammatory effects
Hematopoietic stem cell transplant: Lymphocyte ablation	

Brief discussion about the condition:

SCLERODERMA (PROGRESSIVE SYSTEMIC SCLEROSIS)

A relatively rare **autoimmune connective tissue disorder** characterized by microvascular injury and deposition of **collagen and extracellular matrix**. The most obvious clinical manifestation of the disease is induration and thickening of the skin. However, **Raynaud's**

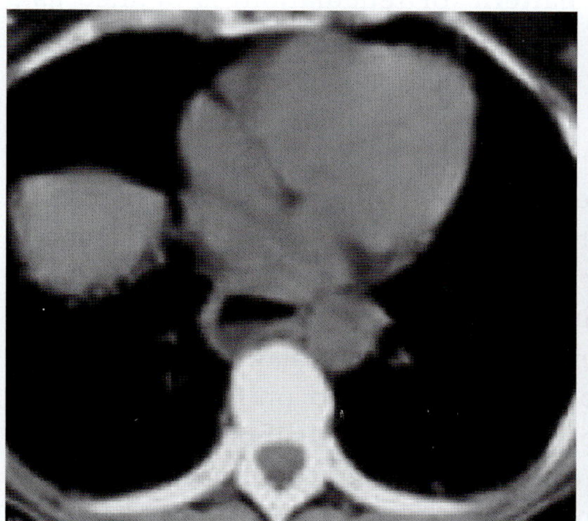

Fig. 4.98.1

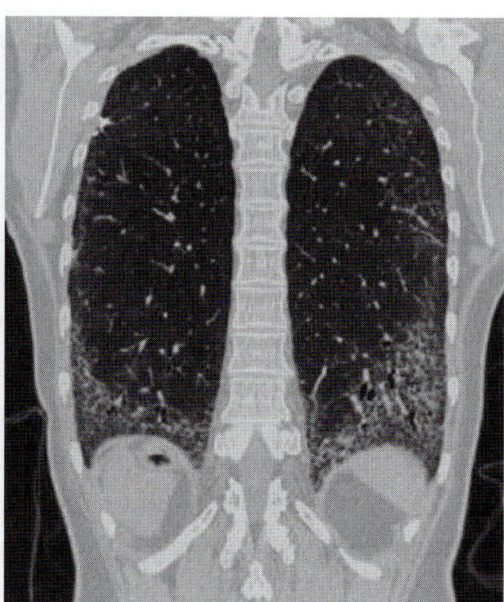

Fig. 4.98.2

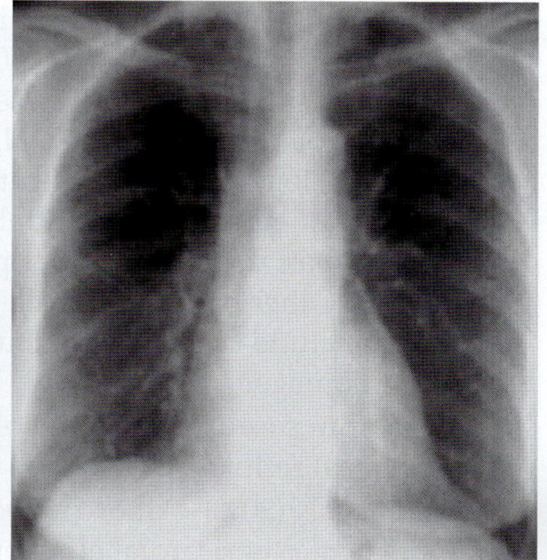

Fig. 4.98.3

phenomenon (plus other vascular manifestations) and involvement of other organ systems (typically, lungs, heart, renal and gastrointestinal) are not uncommon. **Anti-Sc170 (antitopoisomerase 1) antibody.**

Skin:
1. Thickening, tightness and **non-pitting induration**—extent of skin disease defines two important clinical subsets:
   - **Limited** cutaneous scleroderma (lcSSc; skin involvement distal to the elbows) and
   - **Diffuse** cutaneous scleroderma (dcSSc).
2. Raynaud's phenomenon—occurs in over 80% of patients and can precede skin changes by years.
3. Hyperpigmentation, hypopigmentation and depigmentation.
4. Telangiectasia.
5. **Digital pitting scars.**
6. Loss of soft-tissue substance from finger pads.

Joints:
1. Eventually **50%** of patients have articular involvement. Fingers, wrists and ankles are commonly affected.
2. Terminal phalangeal resorption is associated with soft-tissue atrophy.
3. Erosions at the distal interphalangeal, first carpometacarpal, metacarpophalangeal and metatarsophalangeal joints.

Mandible: Thickening of the periodontal membrane ± loss of the lamina dura.

Ribs: Symmetrical erosions on the superior surfaces which predominate along the posterior aspects of the third to sixth ribs.

Cardiopulmonary:
1. **Lung disease most common cause of death** (due to pulmonary hypertension and/or interstitial fibrosis). Prevalence between 40 and 80% (but crucially dependent on method of detection) and more common in patients with **anti-DNA-topoisomerase 1 antibodies.** Fibrosis more prevalent than in rheumatoid arthritis. Non-specific interstitial pneumonia more prevalent than usual interstitial pneumonia pattern of fibrosis. Other patterns of lung disease in systemic sclerosis include organizing pneumonia and diffuse alveolar damage.
2. Aspiration pneumonia—secondary to gastro-oesophageal reflux.
3. Cardiomegaly (30%)— due to myocardial ± pericardial involvement ± pericardial effusion.
4. Cor pulmonale.

Gastrointestinal system:
1. Oesophageal abnormalities **(50%)**—dilatation, atonicity, poor or absent peristalsis and free gastro-oesophageal reflux through a widely open gastro-oesophageal junction.
2. Small bowel (75%)—dilated, atonic mucosal folds and pseudosacculation (hide bound bowel sign—narrow separation between the valvulae conniventes which are of normal thickness despite dilatation of bowel lumen).
3. Colon (75%)—atonic with pseudosacculations on the antimesenteric border.

There are a few roles of imaging in scleroderma interstitial lung disease:
1. Detection of lung involvement,
2. Identification of patients likely to respond to treatment,
3. Assessment of treatment efficacy, and
4. Exclusion of other diseases like cardiac and esophageal abnormalities.

Interstitial Lung Disease

Pulmonary lobules are the **smallest lung units** bounded by interlobular septa. Each lobule is supplied by a lobular airway and arterial branch. The interlobular septa contain lymphatics, venous radicals and interstitium. Any pathological process involving the lymphatics, veins or interstitium might render interlobular septa visible. On chest radiography abnormal thickening of interlobular septa is seen in the costophrenic angles, but thickened interlobular septa are more readily visible on CT. (A few normal interlobular septa are commonly seen on CT.)

Reticular pattern (with or without honeycombing): A **reticular pattern** (or reticulation) is defined as a lacework of innumerable small linear opacities which on CXR become summated and produce an appearance resembling a **'net'**. The characteristics of a reticular pattern are better appreciated on CT. A reticular pattern generally indicates interstitial lung disease. (A reticular pattern may also be caused by thickening of interlobular septa, perilobular infiltration or another cause of parenchymal destruction which spares the septa; *see* below.) There may or may not be associated honeycombing (characterized on CT by clustered cystic air spaces usually in the subpleural lung). The distribution of a reticular pattern (i.e. upper zone versus lower zone or central versus peripheral) is of diagnostic value.

Reticular Pattern—Diffuse Interstitial Lung Diseases

1. **Idiopathic pulmonary fibrosis (IPF)**—most common idiopathic interstitial pneumonia. Associated with the histological/radiological pattern of UIP. Typical patient is male, aged 50–60 years and complaining of progressive dyspnoea. On CXR there is a reticular pattern in mid/lower zones. Predominant basal and subpleural reticular pattern with honeycombing is the characteristic finding on CT. Ancillary findings include ground-glass opacification (less extensive than reticular pattern), traction bronchiectasis/bronchiolectasis and mediastinal lymph node enlargement. Atypical HRCT findings in around 30–50%. Coexistent emphysema in upper zones (associated with preserved lung volumes). Increased incidence of lung cancer.
2. **Connective tissue diseases (CTDs)**—fibrotic lung disease is common and most frequent cause of death. Variable patterns of interstitial lung disease including UIP, NSIP, lymphoid interstitial pneumonia (LIP) and diffuse alveolar damage. Variable prevalence in different CTDs: UIP pattern more prevalent than NSIP in rheumatoid arthritis; NSIP pattern more prevalent in systemic sclerosis and polymyositis/dermatomyositis; LIP most prevalent in rheumatoid arthritis and Sjögren's syndrome.
3. **Occupational lung disease**
   a. **Asbestosis**—basal and subpleural fibrosis, almost indistinguishable from IPF on histopathology and radiology although fibrosis may be coarser in asbestosis than IPF and pleural abnormalities absent in IPF. Long latency period (>20 years) following exposure.
   b. **Hard metal pneumoconiosis**—exposure to alloys of tungsten, carbon and cobalt ± other metals.
   c. **Paraquat poisoning**—late phase of poisoning associated with pulmonary fibrosis.
4. **Sarcoidosis**—archetypal granulomatous fibrotic diffuse interstitial lung disease. Typically associated with symmetrical, bronchocentric reticular pattern in upper zones. Calcified mediastinal and hilar lymph nodes.
5. **Chronic hypersensitivity pneumonitis**—secondary to repeated exposure to a potentially wide variety of particulate (1–5 μm diameter) organic antigens originating from animals, plants, drugs or bacteria/fungi. A reticular pattern ± honeycombing, ground-glass opacification ± traction bronchiectasis/bronchiolectasis and lobular areas of apparently 'spared' lung are characteristic on CT.
6. **Cystic lung diseases**—because of the effects of anatomical superimposition on chest radiographs, the multiple cysts in disorders such as Langerhans' cell histiocytosis, lymphangioleiomyomatosis and tuberous sclerosis can manifest as a reticular pattern. **Relative preservation of lung volumes**.
7. **Drug-induced lung disease**, e.g. caused by nitrofurantoin, busulphan, cyclophosphamide, bleomycin and melphalan.
8. **Bone marrow transplantation**—airways disease (constrictive obliterative bronchiolitis) and upper zone fibrosis associated with recurrent small pneumothoraces.
9. **Miscellaneous causes of diffuse lung disease**—(a) Alveolar proteinosis, (b) Idiopathic pulmonary haemosiderosis, (c) Amyloidosis.

Pulmonary venous engorgement: Left ventricular failure, mitral stenosis, pulmonary veno-occlusive disease.

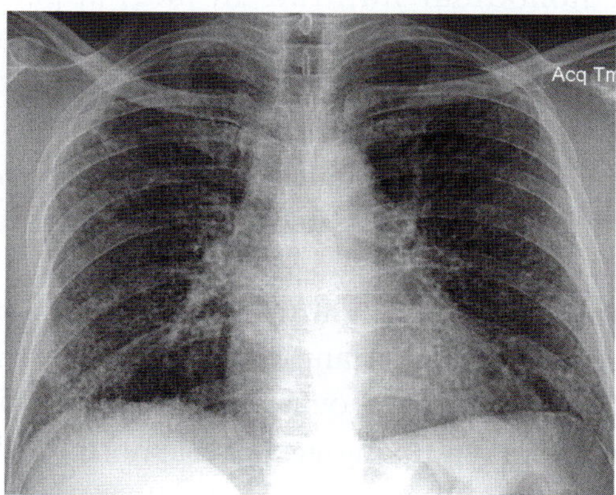

Fig. 4.98.4: ILD showing reticular pattern—caused by thickened interlobular septa

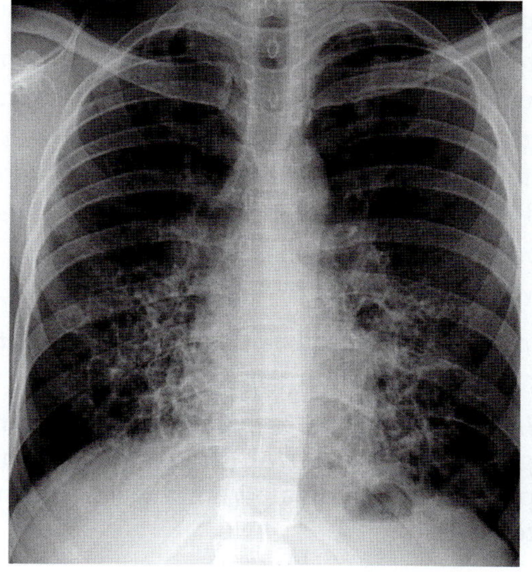

Fig. 4.98.5: Bronchiectasis

Lymphatic/Interstitial Infiltration

1. **Lymphangitis carcinomatosa/lymphomatosa**—most often caused by lymphatic infiltration in patients with cancer of the lung, breast, stomach and pancreas or lymphoma. Nodular thickening (typically bilateral) of interlobular septa is the characteristic finding on CT.
2. **Pneumoconioses**—surrounding tissues may contain a heavy metal, e.g. tin, which contributes to the density.
3. **Sarcoidosis**—septal lines are uncommon.
4. **Idiopathic bronchiectasis**—thickened interlobular septa are a feature in around one-third of patients.
5. **Erdheim–Chester disease**—infiltration of pulmonary interstitium by histiocytes of non-Langerhans' type. Primarily a bone disorder but extraskeletal involvement in around 50%. Lung involvement in around one-third of patients. On chest radiography, reticulonodular infiltrate in mid/upper zones. On CT, smooth thickening of interlobular septa is characteristic, associated with ground-glass opacification and centrilobular nodules.
6. **Diffuse pulmonary haemorrhage**—with recurrent episodes of bleeding, thickened interlobular septa may be seen on CT.
7. **Diffuse pulmonary lymphangiomatosis**—proliferation of lymphatic channels in pleura, interlobular septa and peribronchovascular connective tissue.
8. **Congenital lymphangiectasia**—abnormal dilatation of lymphatic vessels. (NB: No increase in number of lymphatics; lymphangiomatosis.) May be associated with extrathoracic congenital anomalies (e.g. renal, cardiac). Usually fatal.
9. **Alveolar proteinosis**—smooth thickening of interlobular (and intralobular) septa in geographical areas of ground-glass infiltration (i.e. the 'crazy-paving' pattern). Infiltration of air spaces and interstitium and air spaces by PAS-positive macrophages.
10. **Alveolar microlithiasis.**
11. **Amyloidosis.**

Reticular pattern: **Caused by perilobular infiltration**—a variant pattern seen in organizing pneumonia.

Reticular pattern: **Due to parenchymal destruction leaving 'remnant' interlobular septa**—Seen in α_1-antitrypsin deficiency-related emphysema; seen in the lower zones.

Table 4.98.3: Distribution patterns in ILD

Distribution	
1. Upper lobes **("CASSET P" or APICES)** • Cystic fibrosis (not an interstitial disease) • Ankylosing spondylitis • Silicosis • Sarcoid • Eosinophilic pneumonia (sparing of costophrenic angles) • Tuberculosis • *Pneumocystis carinii* **2. Lower lobes** **("BADAS or CIA")** • Bronchiectasis (not an interstitial disease) • Aspiration • Drugs, DIP • Asbestosis • Scleroderma, other collagen vascular diseases **3. Acute ("HELP")** • Hypersensitivity (allergic alveolitis) • Edema • Lymphoproliferative • Pneumonitis, viral	**4. Chronic ("LIFE")** • Lymphangitic spread • Inflammation, infection • Fibrosis Edema **5. Lung volume** **Increased** • Cystic fibrosis (associated with this pattern but not an interstitial disease) • Eosinophilic granuloma (pneumothorax, 20%) • Lymphangioleiomyomatosis (pneumothorax) **Decreased** • Idiopathic pulmonary fibrosis • Scleroderma **Lymph nodes** **6. Enlarged** **7. Calcified**—silicosis
Pleural disease • Pleural plaques—asbestosis • Pleural effusion—CHF, lymphangitic carcinomatosis, rheumatoid disease • Malignant adenopathy • TB, fungus • Sarcoid	**Rheumatoid arthritis—UIP pattern** **SLE—NSIP pattern** **Sjögren's syndrome—LIP pattern**

Biopsy to confirm ILD: Should be taken from, ground-glass opacity, active disease/treatable/no complications when taken from cyst. It should be avoided in chronic disease/end stage disease/complications like pneumothorax.

Table 4.98.4: Diagnostic pearls in SR-ILD

Smoking related interstitial lung disease (SR- ILD)	ILD–X-ray findings
• Respiratory bronchiolitis • Respiratory bronchiolitis ILD • Desquamative interstitial pneumonitis • Pulmonary Langerhans cell histiocytosis • Acute eosinophilic pneumonia • Combined pulmonary fibrosis and emphysema All except desquamative interstitial pneumonitis affect upper lobe.	Linear opacities, reticular shadows Reticulonodular shadows, lung volume, hilar lymph nodes—for sarcoidosis, cardiomegaly—for cardiac failure, pleural effusion Dilated oesophagus, dilatation of pulmonary artery, soft tissue calcification, superior rib notching Lateral end of clavicle erosion—for rheumatoid arthritis. 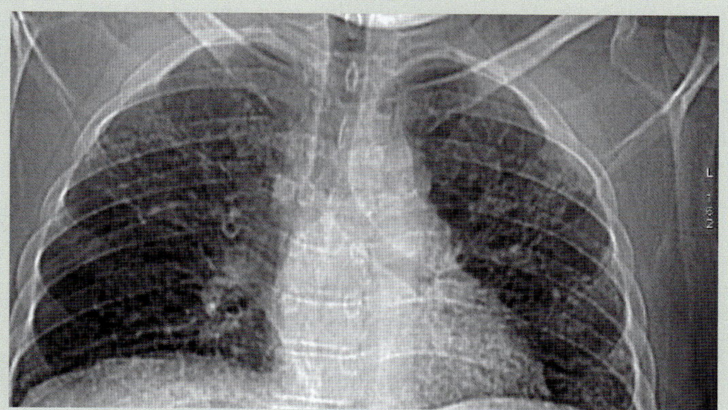 **Fig. 4.98.6:** Smoking-related interstitial lung disease

Diagnosing idiopathic pulmonary fibrosis according to updated 2018 diagnostic criteria guidelines: Fleischner Society White Paper Consensus Statement and ATS/ERS/JRS/ALAT Guideline.

HRCT Diagnostic Categories of UIP Pattern

Regarding the HRCT diagnostic criteria, both documents incorporate four diagnostic criteria of UIP, instead of the three previous 2011 categories:

1. "Usual interstitial pneumonia (UIP) pattern",
2. "Probable UIP pattern",
3. "Indeterminate for UIP" pattern and
4. "Alternative diagnosis"/"most consistent with non-IPF diagnosis".

Both documents have removed the previous "possible usual interstitial pneumonia (UIP)" and two new patterns have been described: "probable UIP" and "Indeterminate for UIP pattern". They included a fourth category with features indicative of an "alternative diagnosis"/"most consistent with non-IPF diagnosis".

Table 4.98.5: ILD pattern of involvement

The UIP pattern is the radiographic hallmark of **IPF**. A typical UIP pattern is sufficient to ensure a diagnosis of IPF without performing a surgical lung biopsy or other invasive interventions. The presence of honeycombing is mandatory in the UIP pattern. The UIP pattern is characterized by honeycombing and reticular opacities, usually associated with traction bronchiectasis. GGO superimposed on the other features can be present. The typical distribution of UIP is subpleural with basal predominance, although upper lobe involvement is common. Asymmetric disease may occur in a quarter of the cases.	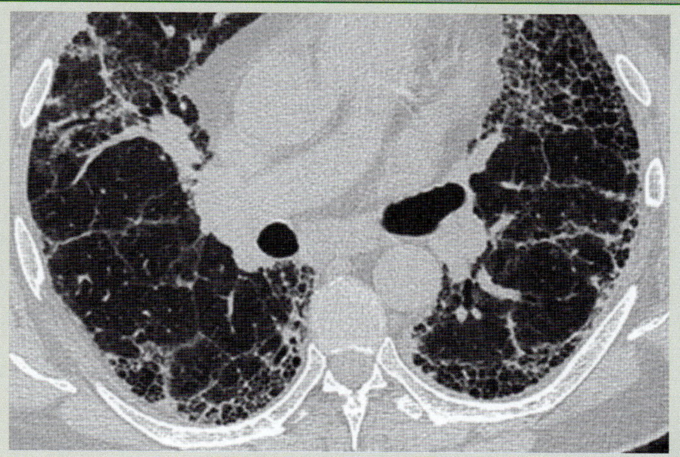 **Fig. 4.98.7:** UIP pattern

(Contd.)

Table 4.98.5: ILD pattern of involvement (*Contd.*)

Probable UIP pattern Subpleural, basal predominant reticular abnormalities with peripheral traction bronchiectasis or bronchiolectasis but without honeycombing is regarded as a "probable UIP" pattern. On the basis that some studies have shown that the **absence of honeycombing** should not exclude a diagnosis of UIP if all other features of UIP are present, particularly subpleural and basal predominance and traction bronchiectasis, Fleischner Guideline recommend that in a consistent clinical context of IPF, a lung biopsy is not necessary for the diagnosis of IPF. While the ATS guideline recommends as a conditional recommendation to perform a surgical lung biopsy in a patient with a probable UIP pattern on CT.	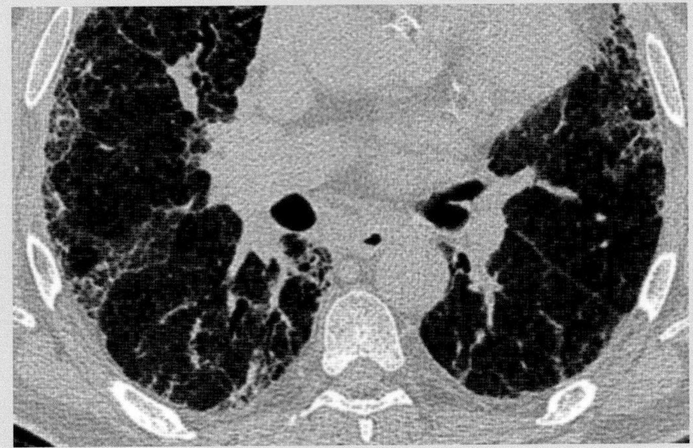 **Fig. 4.98.8:** Probable UIP pattern
Indeterminate for UIP pattern This pattern includes subtle subpleural and basilar predominant reticulation with or without mild ground-glass opacities or architectural distortion. It demonstrates features of fibrosis but without UIP or probable UIP criteria and does not explicitly suggest an alternative diagnosis. A UIP pattern can still be found on histological testing of patient who do not have typical or probable UIP patterns.	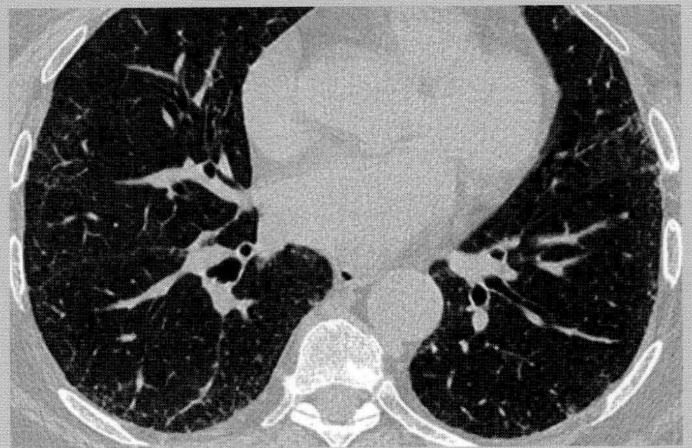 **Fig. 4.98.9:** Indeterminate for UIP pattern
Alternative diagnosis/most consistent with non-IPF diagnosis In this category, there are **atypical** radiographic features suggesting an alternative diagnosis, including upper lobe bronchocentric fibrosis, air trapping, and extensive ground-glass opacification with subpleural sparing. The presence of **ancillary** findings suggesting an alternative diagnosis, even in the presence of UIP, probable UIP, or indeterminate pattern, should reconsider an alternative diagnosis to IPF.	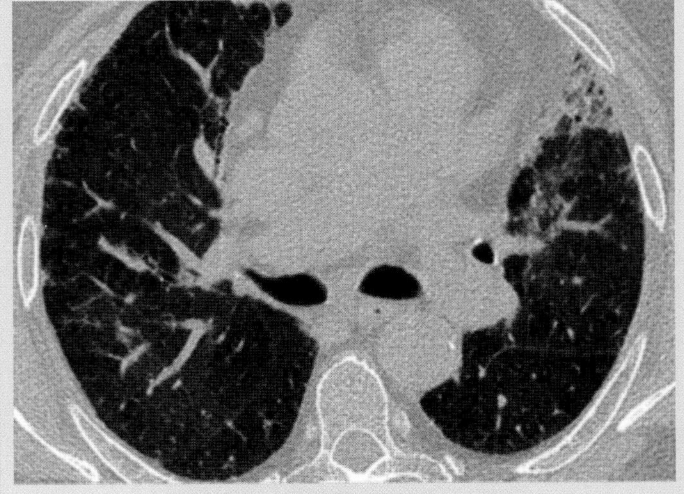 **Fig. 4.98.10:** Non-IPF diagnosis

Honeycombing: Honeycombing is a CT imaging descriptor referring to clustered cystic air spaces (between **3–10 mm in diameter**, that are usually subpleural and basal in distribution. The walls of the cysts are well-defined and often thick **(1–3 mm)**. They represent an irreversible finding commonly seen in diffuse pulmonary fibrosis (usual interstitial pneumonia—UIP).

They can be subdivided into:

1. **Microcystic honeycombing:** An imaging descriptor on thoracic HRCT/CT which is typically given to denote extremely small cysts typically occurring in a subpleural location on a background of interstitial lung disease. It is typically described in association with non-specific interstitial pneumonitis (NSIP). The size of cysts should be under 4 mm in order to be classified as microcystic honeycombing.
2. **Macrocystic honeycombing:** Refers to a morphological subtype of honeycombing.The individual lung cysts greater than 4 mm in diameter to be classified into this category. This form is considered to be more commonly associated with UIP.

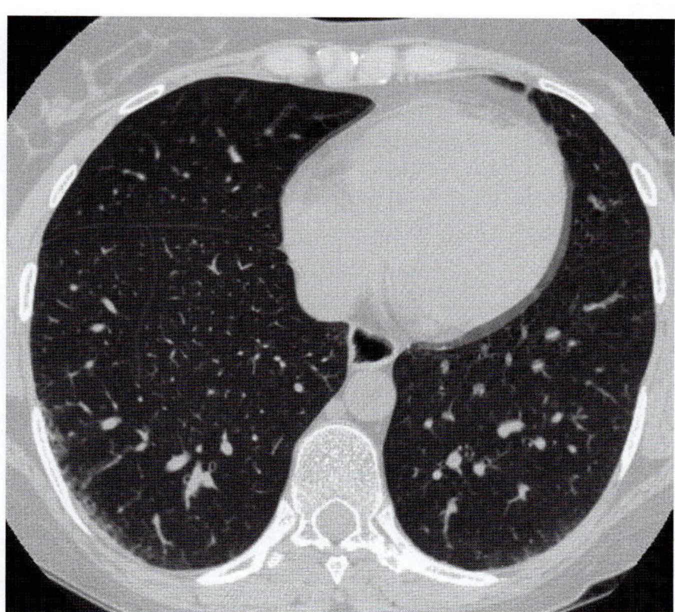

Fig. 4.98.11: Microcystic honeycombing

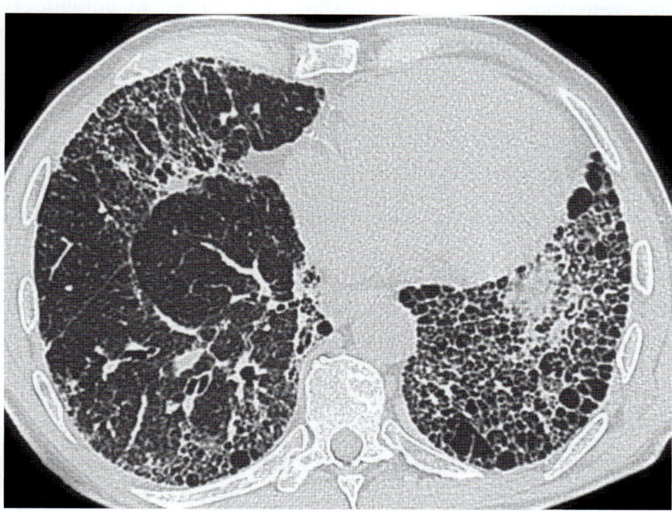

Fig. 4.98.12: Macrocystic honeycombing

Distinguishing Honeycombing and Paraseptal Emphysema

Distinguishing between honeycombing and paraseptal emphysema may be difficult, especially when coexisting on a single scan. As compared with honeycombing, which may present as multiple layers of cysts stacked upon one another, **emphysema presents as a single layer of holes without stacking.** Furthermore, emphysematous holes are typically not hexagonal; therefore, the shape of the cysts and their propensity to stack can help to distinguish one from the other.

A number of features are helpful in diagnosing bronchiectasis: Bronchus visualized within 1 cm of pleural surface, especially lung adjacent to costal pleura (most helpful sign for early cylindrical change) Lack of tapering **Increased bronchoarterial ratio:** Diameter of a bronchus should measure approximately 0.65–1.0 times that of the adjacent pulmonary artery branch. Between 1 and 1.5 may be seen in normal individuals, especially those living at high altitude. **Greater than 1.5 indicates bronchiectasis** **A number of ancillary findings are also recognized:** Bronchial wall thickening: Normally wall of bronchus should be less than half the width of the accompanying pulmonary artery branch. Mucoid impaction. Air-trapping and mosaic perfusion **Signs described on CT include:** Tram-track sign/signet ring sign/ string of pearls sign/cluster of grapes sign	**Traction bronchiectasis** refers to an etiological subtype of bronchiectasis where there is **irreversible** dilatation of bronchi and bronchioles within areas of pulmonary fibrosis or distorted lung parenchymal architecture. **Preserved bronchoarterial ratio.** **Pathology** It can arise from a number of underlying causes which result in lung fibrosis. The bronchus is pulled apart by the traction of surrounding parenchymal fibrosis. **Distribution** There may be a predilection for the **upper** lobes where there is less supporting cartilage.

HYPERSENSITIVITY PNEUMONITIS SYNDROME

Farmer's lung (antigen: Thermophilic actinomycetes) in moist hay, **bird fancier's lung** (antigen: Bird proteins) **mushroom worker's lung** (antigen: Thermophilic actinomycetes) **malt worker's lung** (antigen: Aspergillus species) **maple-bark disease** (Cryptostroma species) **bagassosis** (thermophilic actinomycetes in sugarcane fibers) building-associated HP, **Hot-tub lung**

(mycobacteria). Reduced incidence of HP in tobacco smokers. Radiographic and pathologic abnormalities occurring in patients with HP are similar regardless of the organic antigen.

Table 4.98.6: Types of hypersensitivity pneumonitis

Acute hypersensitivity pneumonitis Exposure to large amounts of antigen Acute dyspnea Acute lung injury with diffuse alveolar damage, edema, or hemorrhage. Air-space consolidation on radiographs and HRCT	**Subacute hypersensitivity pneumonitis** Ongoing or recurrent exposure to antigen Interstitial infiltrates, poorly defined granulomas, cellular bronchiolitis **HRCT** Patchy ground-glass opacity Centrilobular nodules Mosaic perfusion **"Headcheese"** sign Air trapping Lung cysts May progress to fibrosis
Chronic hypersensitivity pneumonitis Fibrosis **HRCT** Irregular reticular opacities Traction bronchiectasis Honeycombing Often appears **patchy and parahilar rather than subpleural**	

Table 4.98.7: Classification of eosinophilic lung disease

Idiopathic eosinophilic lung disease Simple pulmonary eosinophilia Chronic eosinophilic pneumonia Acute eosinophilic pneumonia Hypereosinophilic syndrome Churg-Strauss syndrome Bronchocentric granulomatosis	**Idiopathic eosinophilic lung disease and angiitis** Wegener's granulomatosis Polyarteritis Collagen-vascular diseases **Eosinophilic lung disease with a known cause** Drugs, fungi, parasitic disease and tropical pulmonary eosinophilia, bronchocentric granulomatosis
Simple pulmonary eosinophilia (Loeffler's syndrome) History of asthma or atopy often present. Focal consolidation, usually transient or **fleeting**. May be self-limited	**Hypereosinophilic syndrome** **Multiorgan** infiltration by eosinophils. Pulmonary and pleural involvement in 40%. Ground-glass opacity or areas of consolidation. **Cardiac involvement:** Cardiomegaly, pulmonary edema, pleural effusion, poor prognosis
Acute eosinophilic pneumonia Eosinophilia on bronchoalveolar lavage. Rapidly progressing respiratory failure. Radiographic findings resemble pulmonary edema	**Chronic eosinophilic pneumonia** **Patchy peripheral consolidation**, often persistent patchy ground-glass opacity. Mimics organizing pneumonia/bronchiolitis obliterans organizing pneumonia, but usually shows an **upper** lobe predominance. Rapid resolution with steroids.
Churg-Strauss syndrome: Three phases • **Allergic phase:** With rhinitis, sinusitis and asthma • **Eosinophilic phase:** Blood and tissue eosinophilia. Findings of simple pulmonary eosinophilia or chronic eosinophilic pneumonia • **Systemic or small vessel vasculitis phase:** Heart, kidney, musculoskeletal and nervous systems involved. Nodules or masses; may cavitate. Responds well to steroids.	

Acute respiratory distress syndrome (ARDS) is a form of acute lung injury (ALI) and occurs as a result of a severe pulmonary injury that causes alveolar damage heterogeneously throughout the lung. It can either result from a direct pulmonary source or as a response to systemic injury.

Early phase pulmonary opacification: Often demonstrates an anteroposterior density gradient within the lung, with dense consolidation in the most dependent regions, merging into a background of widespread ground-glass attenuation and then normal or hyperexpanded lung in the non-dependent regions.

Late phase and appearances in long-term survivors:

Complete resolution: May occur in some.

Coarse reticular pattern and ground-glass opacification in the anterior (non-dependent) part of the lungs: Considered more typical.

Collagen Vascular Diseases with Pulmonary Involvement

Pulmonary manifestations: Interstitial pneumonia and fibrosis, pleural effusion or pleural thickening, organizing pneumonia (OP), bronchiectasis, bronchiolitis obliterans pulmonary hypertension.

Caplan's syndrome: Rheumatoid arthritis with pneumoconiosis or silicosis.

CREST syndrome: Variant of scleroderma—calcification (subcutaneous)/Raynaud's phenomenon/esophageal dysmotility/sclerodactyly/telangiectasia.

"Shrinking lung" syndrome:
- Common manifestation of SLE.
- Etiology is unclear.
- May be due to diaphragmatic dysfunction or pleuritic chest pain with restriction of respiration.
- Radiographs show progressive loss of volume in the lower lobes.

Clinical triad of Sjögren's syndrome:
- Keratoconjunctivitis sicca
- Xerostomia
- Recurrent swelling of the parotid gland.

Table 4.98.8: Approach to interstitial lung disease

Histologic pattern	*Idiopathic clinical syndrome*	*Differential diagnosis of the histologic pattern*	*Key HRCT findings*	*Distribution*
Usual interstitial pneumonia (UIP)	Idiopathic pulmonary fibrosis (IPF)	Collagen vascular disease, asbestosis, drug toxicity, radiation, chronic hypersensitivity pneumonitis, familial pulmonary	Subpleural, fibrosis basal **honeycombing**	Peripheral, basal, subpleural, patchy
Nonspecific interstitial pneumonia (NSIP)	Nonspecific interstitial pneumonia (NSIP)	Collagen vascular disease, hypersensitivity pneumonitis, drug toxicity, infection, immunodeficiency	Concentric subpleural ground-glass opacity without honeycombing	Peripheral, basal, subpleural, concentric
Organizing pneumonia (OP)	Cryptogenic organizing pneumonia (COP)	Infection, bronchial obstruction, aspiration, drug reactions, collagen vascular disease, toxic-fume inhalation, radiation pneumonitis, hypersensitivity pneumonitis	Patchy subpleural and peribronchial consolidation or nodules. Atoll sign migrate, even without treatment.	Basal, subpleural, peribronchovascular
Diffuse alveolar damage (DAD)	Acute interstitial pneumonia (AIP)	Acute respiratory distress syndrome **(ARDS)** of known cause (e.g. sepsis, shock, infection, drug toxicity, toxic inhalations, trauma)	Typical findings of ARDS	Diffuse, lower lobe predominance
Respiratory bronchiolitis (RB)	Respiratory bronchiolitis–interstitial lung disease (RB-ILD)	Smoking (usually), inhalations	**Centrilobular nodules** of ground-glass opacity	Diffuse, upper lobe predominance
Desquamative interstitial pneumonia (DIP)	Desquamative interstitial pneumonia (DIP)	**Smoking** (usually), inhalations	Diffuse ground-glass opacity	Peripheral, lower lobe predominance
Lymphoid interstitial pneumonia (LIP)	Lymphoid interstitial pneumonia (LIP)	Collagen-vascular diseases (particularly Sjögren's syndrome, rheumatoid arthritis, and lupus), immunologic disorders, autoimmune, hemolytic anemia, myasthenia gravis, pernicious anemia, immunodeficiency (e.g. AIDS), drug toxicity	**Ground-glass opacity or air-filled cysts**	Diffuse

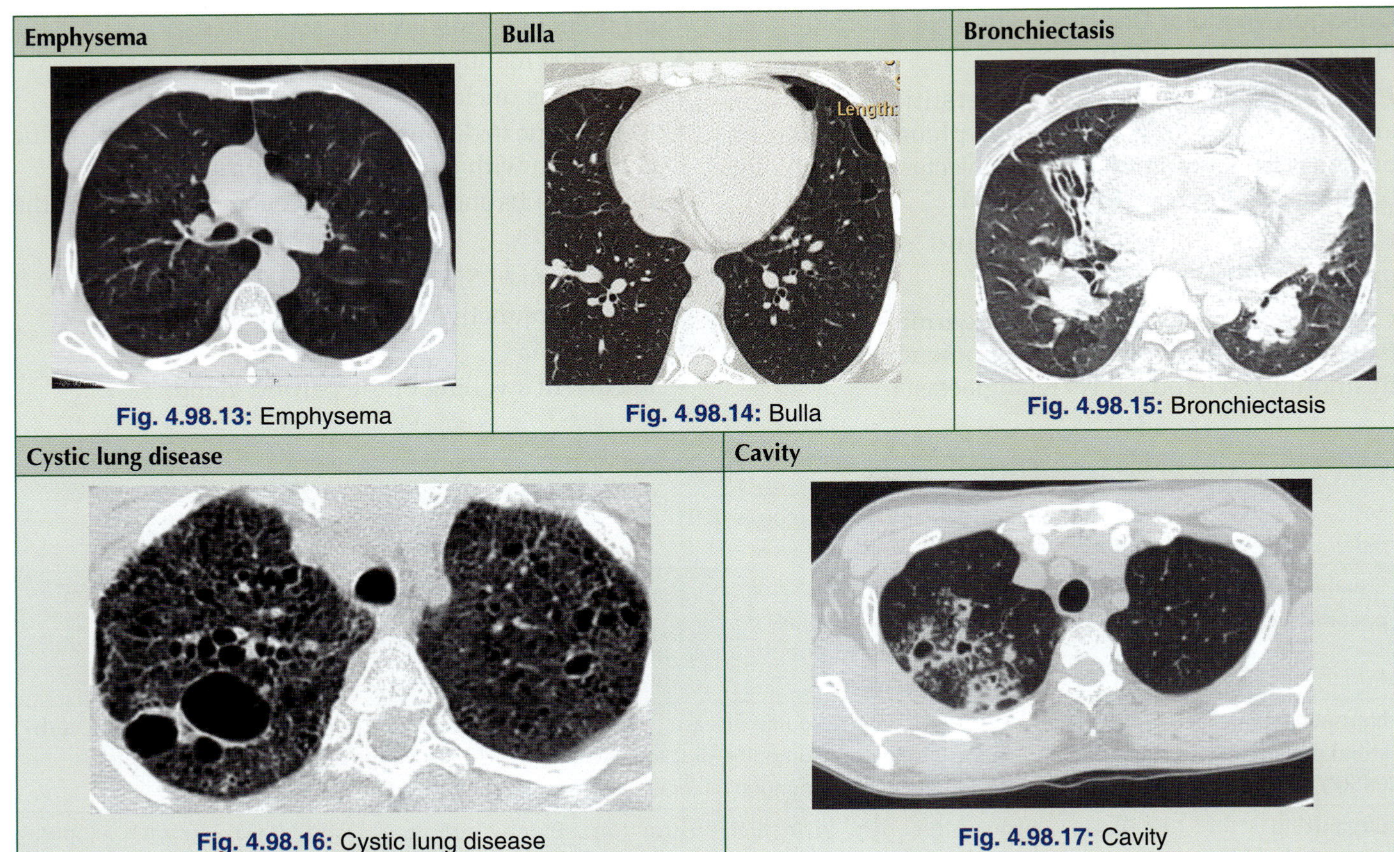

Fig. 4.98.13: Emphysema

Fig. 4.98.14: Bulla

Fig. 4.98.15: Bronchiectasis

Fig. 4.98.16: Cystic lung disease

Fig. 4.98.17: Cavity

Table 4.98.9: Four radiological patterns of diffuse lung disease

Pattern 1 *Ground-glass and consolidation*	*Pattern 2* *Fibrosis*	*Pattern 3* *Nodules*	*Pattern 4* *Mosaic patterns/cysts*
Oedema Infection Aspiration hypersensitivity pneumonitis (extrinsic allergic alveolitis) Drug reactions (toxic and hypersensitivity) Fumes and toxin injury related to rheumatic disease **Idiopathic interstitial pneumonias** • Non-specific interstitial pneumonia • Lymphoid interstitial pneumonia • Desquamative interstitial pneumonia **Respiratory bronchiolitis—associated interstitial lung disease** Lymphangitic tumours Wegener granulomatosis (haemorrhage variant) Alveolar proteinosis Amyloidosis	Pneumoconioses Chronic granulomatous infection Usual interstitial pneumonia Chronic hypersensitivity pneumonitis Related to rheumatic disease Chronic drug reactions sarcoidosis **Lymphoid interstitial pneumonia** **Fibrotic non-specific interstitial pneumonia** Chronic aspiration chronic radiation injury Advanced Langerhans cell histiocytosis Hermansky–Pudlak syndrome Erdheim–Chester disease (non-Langerhans cell histiocytosis)	Carcinomas and sarcomas Lymphoproliferative diseases Miliary granulomatous infections Aspiration bronchiolitis Hypersensitivity pneumonitis Pulmonary Langerhans cell histiocytosis sarcoidosis Wegener granulomatosis Necrotising sarcoidosis Silicosis and silicate disease	Small airways disease with constrictive bronchiolitis Vasculopathic diseases lymphangioleiomyomatosis Langerhans cell histiocytosis

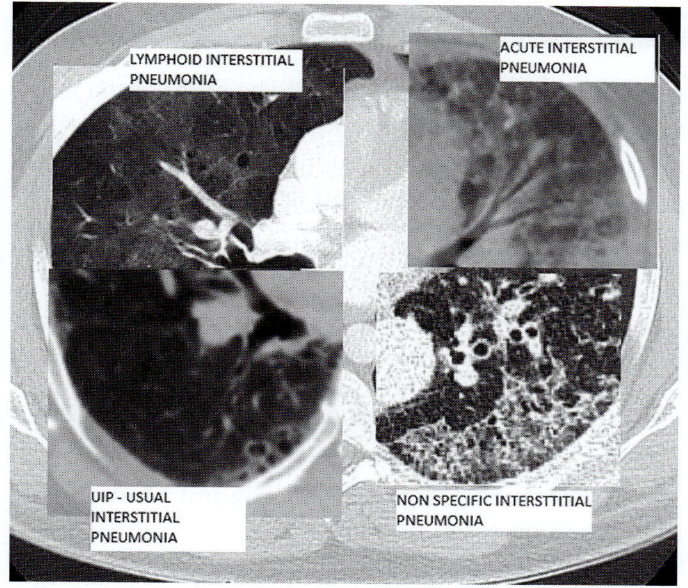

Fig. 4.98.18: ILD patterns—1

Fig. 4.98.19: ILD patterns—2

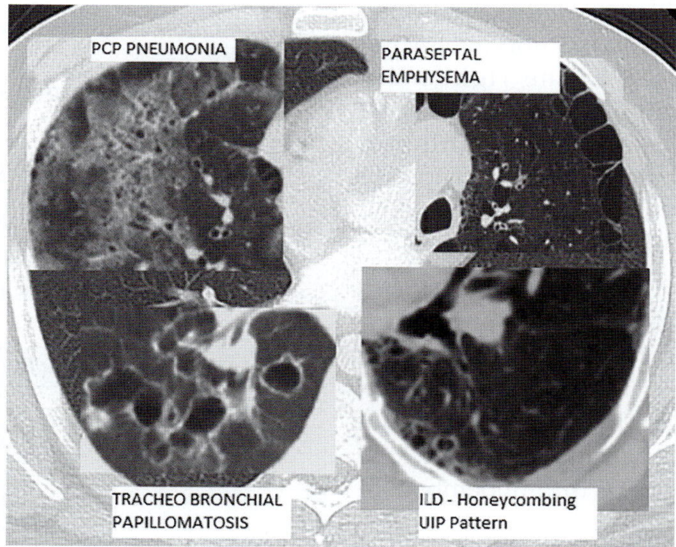

Fig. 4.98.20: ILD patterns—3

4.99 CHEST

Case No. 99

Clinical features: A 43-year-old male patient came to the emergency department with complaints of sudden onset breathlessness and chest pain.

Radiological imaging techniques and observations: Figure 4.99.1 is frontal chest X-ray showing focal oligemia of left lung upper and middle zone with decreased visualization of pulmonary vessels and a dilated prominent left pulmonary artery. No peripheral wedge-shaped opacity visualized. No evidence of pneumothorax. Rest of the lung fields, heart and other visualized structures appear normal.

Figures 4.99.2 and 4.99.3 are CT pulmonary angiography images showing hypoattenuated nonenhancing intraluminal thrombus measuring 6.1 × 1.7 cm in the left main pulmonary artery extending from the bifurcation of the pulmonary trunk to the lower lobar segmental branches. The thrombus is resulting in subtotal (>80–85%) luminal obstruction. Hypoattenuated non-enhancing intraluminal thrombus noted in the right main pulmonary artery also extending to right lower lobe segmental branches. The thrombus is resulting in subtotal (>80–85%) luminal obstruction. Patchy opacity noted in the left upper lobe in the mediastinal window suggests pulmonary infarct. There is incidental left vetricular hypertrophy.

Interpretation: A—43-year-old male, main pulmonary vein, C—hypoattenuated non-enhancing thrombus in the bifurcation of main pulmonary trunk, right and left main pulmonary arteries, B—bilateral lower lobe segmental branches with a patchy opacity in the left upper lobe suggesting infarct, D—pulmonary thromboembolism with pulmonary infarct.

Principal diagnosis: Pulmonary thromboembolism with pulmonary infarct.

Management: The report needs to be highlighted to the referring clinical team urgently.

Investigations: D-dimer levels in the blood is to be tested and look for ECG changes: S1Q3T3 pattern.

Treatment: Thrombolysis/mechanical thrombectomy.

Triple rule out in CT angiography in acute chest pain: 1. Aortic dissection, 2. Pulmonary thromboembolism, 3. Coronary artery thrombosis.

Imaging Findings in Pulmonary Thromboembolism

Chest X-ray signs:

A. ***Westermark's sign:*** Focal oligemia beyond an occluded vessel.
B. ***Hampton hump:*** Circumscribed, subpleural opacity with a rounded or truncated convex medial border facing toward the pulmonary hilum.
C. ***Palla's sign:*** Enlarged right descending pulmonary artery.
D. ***Fleischner's sign:*** Enlarged thrombosed pulmonary artery.
E. ***Chang sign:*** Enlarged right descending artery with abrupt cut off.
F. ***Knuckle sign:*** Abrupt tapering/cut-off of a pulmonary artery secondary to an embolus.
G. ***Melting ice cube sign:*** When there is pulmonary infarction following PE, typical wedge-shaped, pleural-based opacification resolves from periphery to central.

Table 4.99.1: Difference between consolidation and lung infarct

Lung consolidation	*Lung infarct*
Patchy opacity	Peripheral pleural-based wedge-shaped opacity with apex towards the hilum
Resolves from central to periphery	Resolves from periphery to central

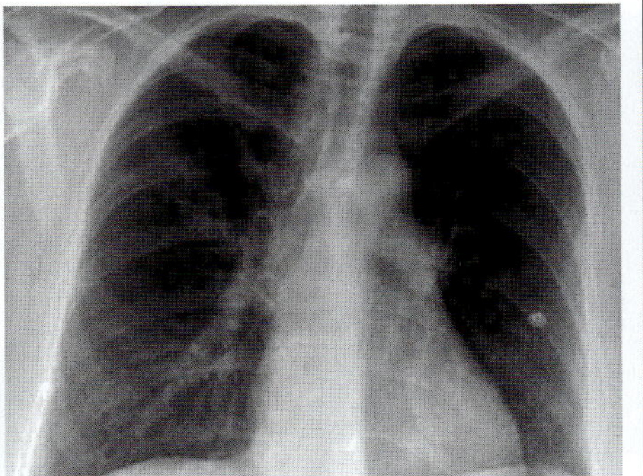

Fig. 4.99.1

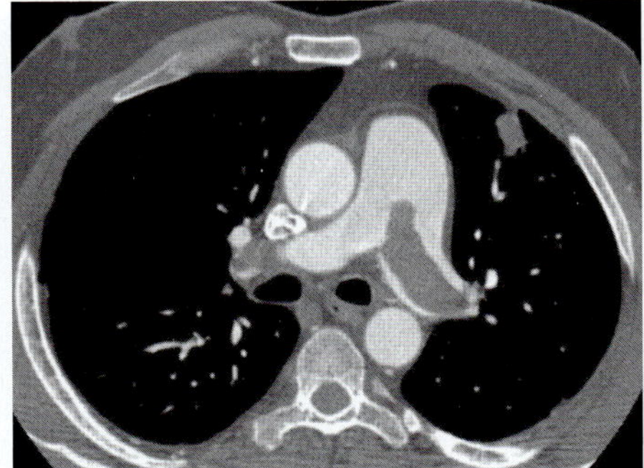

Fig. 4.99.2

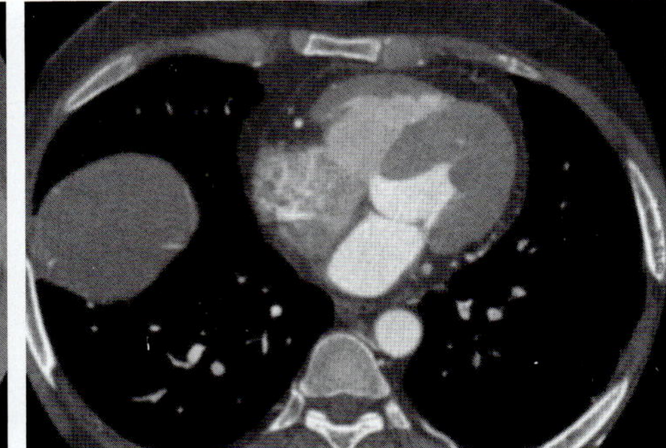

Fig. 4.99.3

Stripe sign: If peripheral segment of lung is spared in perfusion scan, then there is low probability of pulmonary embolism.

Pulmonary thromboembolism:

- Pulmonary embolism (PE) is blockage of the pulmonary artery or one of its branches by a substance that has travelled from elsewhere in the body through the bloodstream (embolism).
- PE mostly results from deep vein thrombosis that breaks off and migrates to the lung, a process called as venous thromboembolism (VTE).
- A small percentage of cases are caused by the embolization of air, fat, or talc in drugs of intravenous drug abusers.

Diagnosis of pulmonary embolism:

- Clinicals: In accurate (dyspnea, chest pain, hemoptysis)

CT pulmonary angiography (gold standard) signs:

- **Polo mint sign**
- **Tram-track sign:** Peripheral intraluminal filling defect with acute angles
- Lung opacity: Infarct
- RV enlargement
- IVC thrombosis

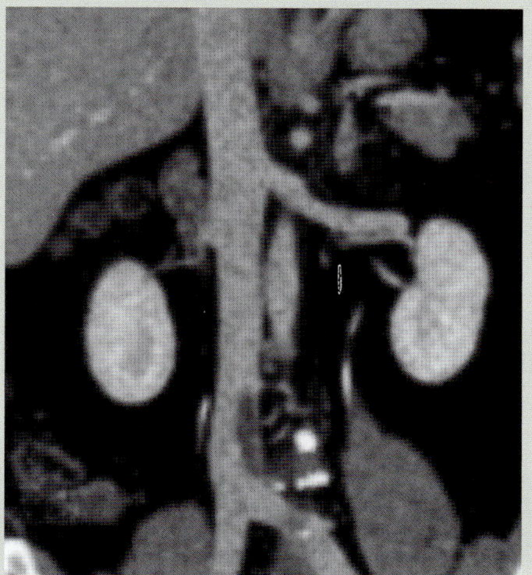

Fig. 4.99.4: IVC thrombosis

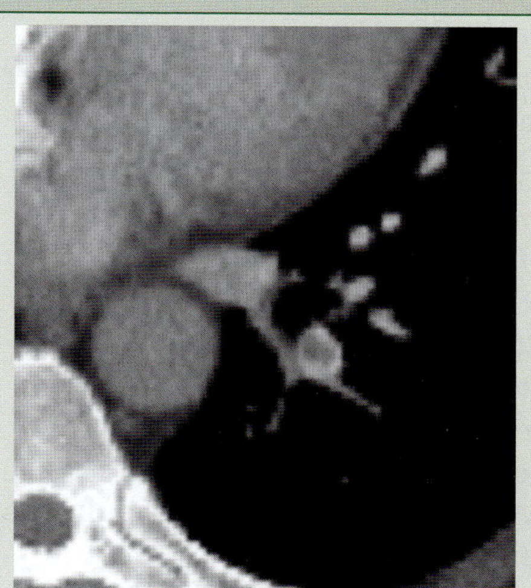

Fig. 4.99.5: Polo mint sign

Table 4.99.2: Lower limb Doppler findings in deep venous thrombosis

Normal	Deep venous thrombosis
Thin smooth wall	Wall thickening in chronic thrombosis
Anechoic lumen **with complete filling of colour flow**	Hypoechoic lumen with dilated vein (acute) Hyperechoic lumen with small calibre (chronic)
Compressible	Non-compressible
Spontaneous flow with phasic variation present	No spontaneous flow and phasic variation absent
Augmentation reflux present	Augmentation reflux absent

Table 4.99.3: Varicose veins in Doppler study

Veins	*Normal*	*Incompetent*
Peforator diameter	<3 mm	>4 mm
GSV diameter	<5 mm at the level of femoral condyle	>6 mm
SSV diameter	<3 mm	>5 mm
Reflux time	<0.5 sec	>0.5 sec

Table 4.99.4: Ventilation–perfusion scan interpretation			
	Ventilation (V)	*Perfusion (Q)*	*Causes*
Normal	No defect	No defect	
V/Q mismatch	Normal	Defect	Pulmonary thromboembolism Vasculitis Pulmonary vascular anormalies
V/Q mismatch	Defect	Normal	Airway abnormalities
Matched defect	Defect	Defect	Pleural effusion Pulmonary trauma Mucous plug Bronchogenic CA
Triple match	Matching ventilation, perfusion and CXR abnormality		Very low probability of PE

- Lab tests: D-dimer
- Arterial blood gases: Hypoxemia, A-A gradient
- ECG: Classic S1Q3T3 pattern
- CXR: Normal or mild abnormal (rule out other diseases)
- V/Q lung scan: V/Q mismatched defects
- CTPA (CT pulmonary arteriography): Gold standard

CT pulmonary angiography protocol:

Position of the patient: Supine with their arms above their head.

Scannogram: Apices to diaphragm.

Scan extent: Apices to diaphragm

Scan direction: Caudocranial

Region of interest: Below the carina at the level of the pulmonary trunk with an ROI on the pulmonary artery.

Threshold: 100 HU.

Volume: 60 ml of non-ionic contrast with 100 ml saline chaser at 4.5/5 ml/s

Scan delay: Minimal scan delay.

Respiration phase: Inspiration.

CT venography: Can be obtained at the same time of CTPA—limiting the need for additional time consuming studies up to the level of knee. CTV obtained following CTPA is called indirect venography.

Lower limb ultrasound: It is an important step in diagnosis of venous thromboembolism.

Widespread availability, lack of radiation low cost are the advantageous components of US.

Inferior vena cava filter: It is an endovascular device which is typically placed in infrarenal IVC with apex of the filter at or just below the level of the renal veins to prevent pulmonary embolism. Filters can be inserted by femoral or jugular veins. Retrieval is via the jugular route.

Suprarenal positioning: May be necessary when IVC thrombosis extends above the renal veins or there is renal vein thrombosis.

Table 4.99.5: IVC filter in pulmonary thromboembolism	
Indications	**Contraindications**
1. Contraindications to anticoagulation 2. Pulmonary embolism despite anticoagulation 3. Large iliocaval/floating IVC thrombus (widow maker thrombus)	1. Complete vena cava thrombosis 2. Septic thromboembolism 3. Vena cava is too small/ too large to safely admit a filter
When to remove IVC filter? IVC filters may be left in permanently/ can be retrieved after a period of time which varies depending on the individual filter.	

Table 4.99.6: Catheter directed therapy in pulmonary thromboembolism	
Indications	**Absolute contraindications**
• Patients with massive or submassive PE • Failed systemic thrombolysis • Multiple comorbidities and poor surgical candidates • Patients benefit from catheter-directed therapies that aim to reduce clot burden rapidly and restore hemodynamic stability • Patients with submassive PE benefit from catheter directed therapies by preventing clot progression to massive PE, which can result in RV failure and pulmonary hypertension	• Active internal bleeding • Absolute contraindication to anticoagulation • Contraindications to thrombolytic drugs • Recent neurosurgery • Stroke or intracranial trauma within 3 months

Catheter-directed therapies

Mechanical thrombus disruption—Suction—Fragmentation

- **Catheter-directed thrombolysis:** Pharmacologic techniques result in lower doses of thrombolytics when compared to systemic thrombolysis—lower risk of bleeding events since thrombolytic directly delivered into pulmonary arteries (PAs).

- **US-assisted catheter-directed thrombolysis** (pharmacomechanical technique) in both massive and submassive PE has shown significant reduction in RV/left ventricular diameter ratio, mean PA peak systolic pressure, and PA angiographic obstruction over 48 hours.

Combination of mechanical disruption to expose more surface area of thrombus and direct thrombolytic infusion is currently thought to be most efficacious technique.

Well's scoring: Clinical scoring method used.

Table 4.99.7: Perfusion lung scan and ventilation lung scan

Perfusion lung scan	Ventilation lung scan
• Tracer: Tc-99m MAA, particle size = 10–30 um • Biological $T_{1/2}$ in the lungs = 2–4 hr → RE system Number of particles: Minimum = 100,000 optimum = 200,000–600,000	Tracers Aerosol* (0.5 u): ^{99m}Tc-DTPA/ phytate Technegas: Tc-99m aerosol particle size: 0.02–0.2 um Inert gas: ^{133}Xe, ^{127}Xe, ^{81m}Kr

Typical Scintigraphic findings for PE: Mismatched V/Q Defects

Interpretation:

"The prospective investigation of pulmonary embolism diagnosis" (PIOPED)

- **High probability:** >80%
  - Two large segmental perfusion defects without corresponding ventilation or roentgenographic abnormalities or substantially larger than either matching ventilation or CXR abnormality.
  - Two moderate segmental perfusion defects without corresponding ventilation or roentgenographic abnormalities and 1 large mismatched segmental defect.
  - Four moderate segmental perfusion defects without ventilation or CXR abnormalities.

Flowchart 4.99.1: Diagnostic algorithm in suspected pulmonary embolism

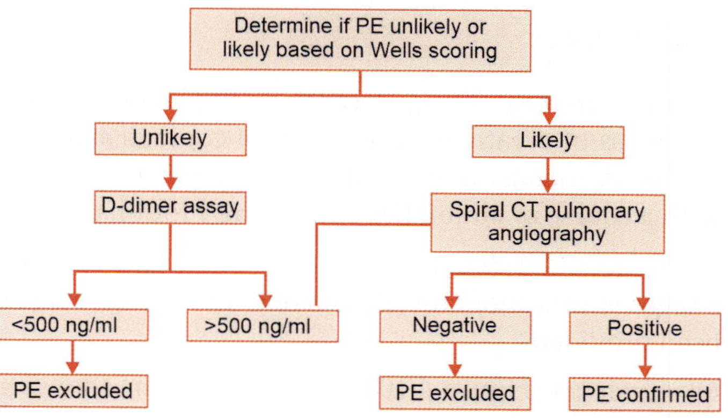

- **Intermediate probability (indeterminate):** 20–80%
  - Not falling into normal, very low-, low-, or high-probability categories.
  - Borderline high or borderline low.
  - Difficult to categorize as low or high.
- **Low probability:** <20%
  - Nonsegmental perfusion defects
  - Single moderate mismatched segmental perfusion defect with normal CXR
  - Any perfusion defect with a substantially larger CXR abnormality.
  - Large or moderate segmental perfusion defects involving no more than 4 segments in 1 lung and no more than 3 segments in 1 lung region with matching ventilation defects either equal to or larger in size and chest roentgenogram either normal or with abnormalities substantially smaller than perfusion defects.
  - >3 small segmental perfusion defects with a normal CXR
- **Very low probability:** <10%
  - <3 small segmental perfusion with a normal CXR.
  - Normal: <5%.

4.100.1 CHEST

Case No. 100.1

Clinical history: 53 years old female presented with shortness of breath, expectoration of copious amounts of mucus, malaise and weight loss. Patient was treated with a course of antibiotics and referred for imaging.

Radiological techniques: CT chest plain and contrast images with scanogram taken at one-month interval has been provided.

Observation: Figure 4.100.1.1 is scanogram showing trachea in midline, ill-defined radio-opacity with air bronchogram noted in the middle and lower zone of right lung with obliteration of right costophrenic angle and loss of silhouette of right heart border and right dome of diaphragm noted. No evidence of calcification, fat density or fluid-fluid levels multiple focal areas of lucencies noted within the opacities more along the lower medial aspect. Rest of visualized lung field appears normal. Left costophrenic angle appears free. Visualized skeleton appears normal. Superior mediastinum appears widened.

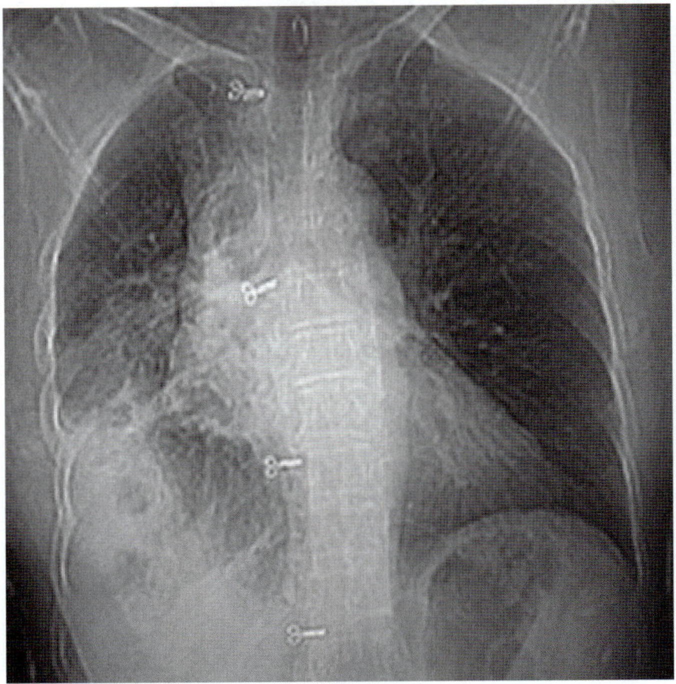

Fig. 4.100.1.1

Figures 4.100.1.2 to 4.100.1.4 are contrast enhanced CT chest taken after a course of antibiotics **(one month interval)** showing heterogeneously enhancing 50 (HU) ill-defined patchy consolidation with air bronchogram and CT angiogram sign in the middle lobe and superior segment of right lower lobe with a few centrilobular nodules representing lepidic spread. No evidence of lung cavitation and pleural effusion noted. Visualized ribs and thoracic vertebra appear normal. No evidence of cardiomegaly.

Interpretations: A—53 years old female, middle lobe and superior segment of right lower lobe, C—heterogeneously enhancing ill-defined patchy consolidation with air bronchogram and a few centrilobular nodules representing the lepidic spread, B—interval imaging after a month shows no change in the findings, D—broncho-alveolar carcinoma.

Principal diagnosis: Invasive adenocarcinoma **(broncho-alveolar carcinoma).**

Differential diagnosis:

1 Lobar consolidation
2. Pulmonary edema (unilateral less likely)
3. Diffuse pulmonary haemorrhage

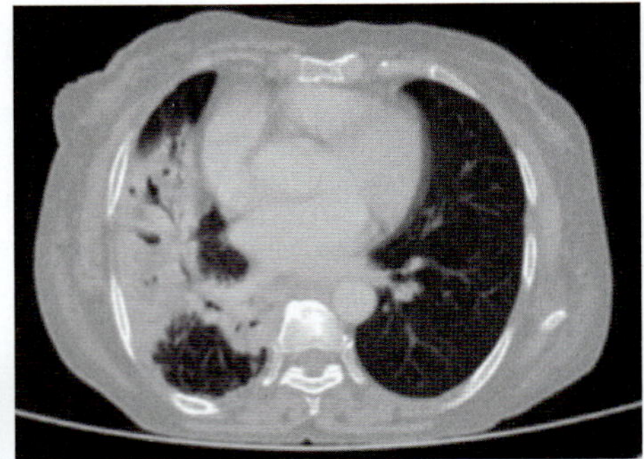

Fig. 4.100.1.2

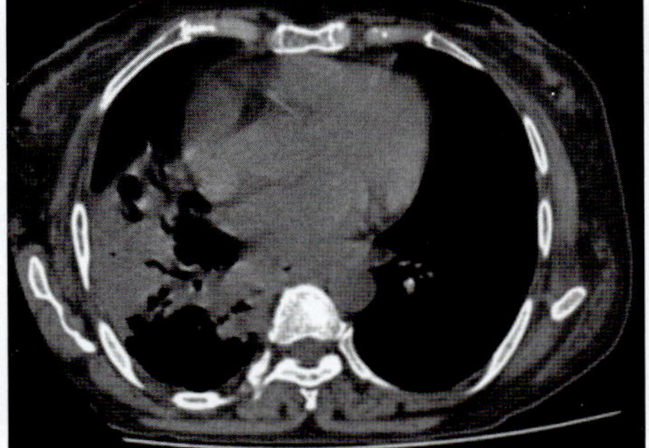

Fig. 4.100.1.3

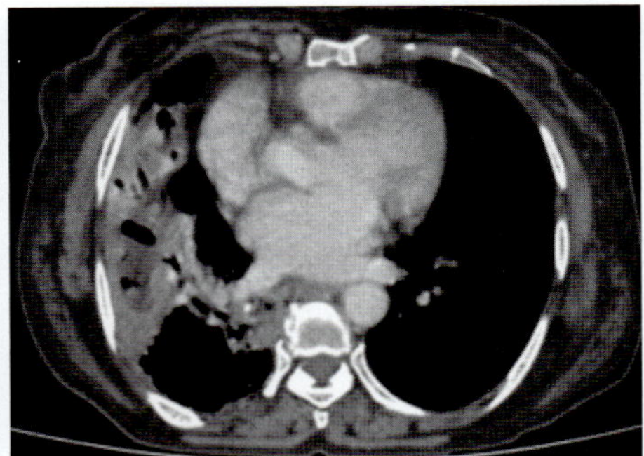

Fig. 4.100.1.4

Table 4.100.1.1: Differential diagnosis for consolidation

Differential diagnosis	*Radiological features*	*Imaging*
1. Lobar pneumonia: Also known as non-segmental pneumonia is a radiological pattern associated with homogeneous and fibrino suppurative consolidation of one or more lobes of a lung in response to bacterial pneumonia. *Streptococcus pneumoniae* is the most common cause.	Appears as a focal dense opacification of the majority of an entire lobe with relative sparing of the large airways. There may be additional areas of ground-glass opacity in a lobar or segmental pattern, likely representing areas of partial involvement or simply atelectasis. In about 30% of patients radiological resolution takes about 10 days and in 70% findings reslove within a month, however, patient's age, underlying comorbidities and micro-organism to be considered	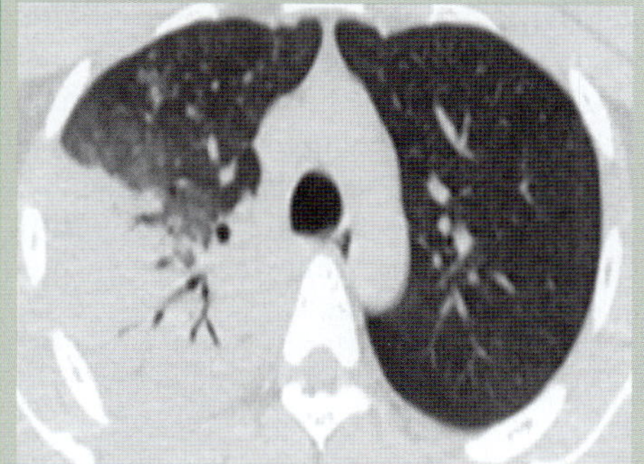 **Fig. 4.100.1.5:** Lobar pneumonia
2. Pulmonary edema, is a broad descriptive term and is usually defined as an abnormal accumulation of fluid in the extravascular compartments of the lung. **CT chest:** Patchy area of consolidation are seen on CT. The fluffy margins are due to variable involvement of alveoli at the edges.	**Plain radiograph:** Increased cardiothoracic ratio/cardiac silhouette size. **Features of pulmonary interstitial edema:** Peribronchial cuffing and perihilar haze, septal lines/Kerley lines, thickening of interlobar fissures. **Features of pulmonary alveolar edema:** Air space opacification classically in a batwing distribution, may have air bronchograms, pleural effusions and fluid in interlobar fissures.	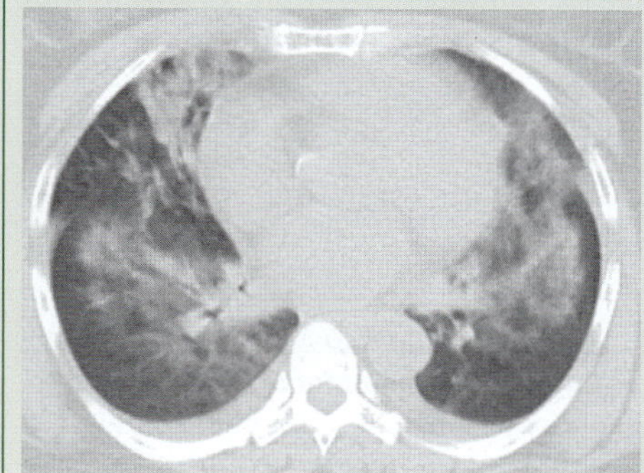 **Fig. 4.100.1.6:** Pulmonary edema
3. COVID-19 pneumonitis: Infectious disease caused by severe acute respiratory syndrome corona virus 2(SARS-CoV-2), a strain of coronavirus. **CT finding:** Ground-glass opacities in bilateral, subpleural peripheral predominance, crazy paving appearance, air space consolidation, traction bronchiectasis. 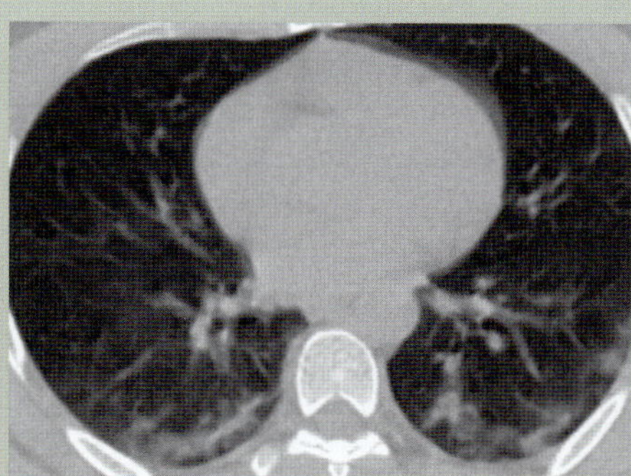 **Fig. 4.100.1.7:** COVID-19 pneumonitis	Ground-glass opacities in early imaging. 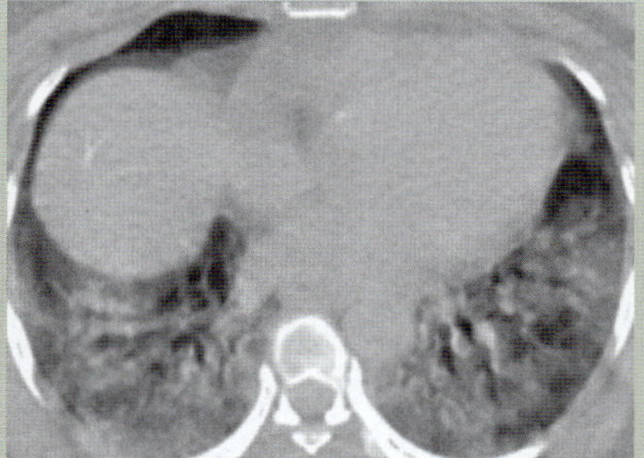 **Fig. 4.100.1.8:** COVID-19 pneumonitis	Four days later imaging shows progression of ground-glass opacities to consolidation. 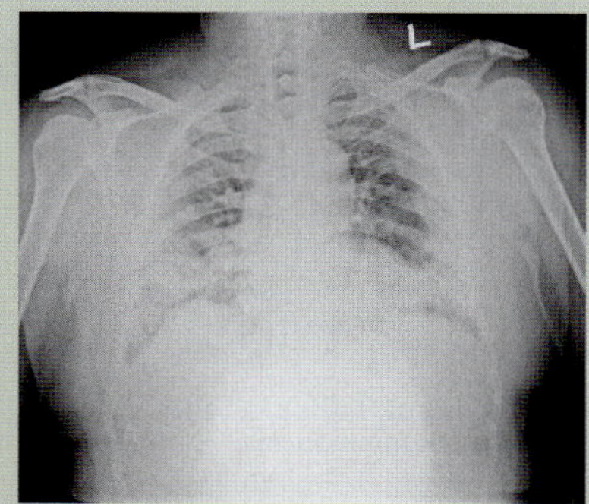 **Fig. 4.100.1.9:** COVID-19 pneumonitis

(Contd.)

Table 4.100.1.1: Differential diagnosis for consolidation (*Contd.*)

Differential diagnosis	*Radiological features*	*Imaging*
4. Diffuse pulmonary haemorrhage: Idiopathic pulmonary haemosiderosis, anti-glomerular basement disease, microscopic polyangiitis, systemic lupus erythematous, Behçet syndrome, Wegener's granulomatosis, contusion, bleeding diatheses, Goodpasture's syndrome, pulmonary infarction.	**HRCT:** Shows areas of widespread ground-glass opacification +/– crazy paving pattern +/– areas of consolidation. In the subacute phase HRCT may show fine diffuse nodular densities. In later stage interlobular septal thickening due to intralymphatic accumulation of hemosiderin	**Fig. 4.100.1.10:** Diffuse pulmonary haemorrhage
5. Eosinophilic lung disease: Heterogeneous group of disorders that are characterized by excess infiltration of eosinophil within the lung interstitium and alveoli	Air space opacification seen characteristically non-segmental, in the upper zones and paralleling the chest wall.	**Fig. 4.100.1.11:** Eosinophilic lung disease
6. Organizing pneumonia: May be cryptogenic or as a response to other 'insult' (e.g. infection, drug toxicity, connective tissue disease).	Multifocal air-space opacities in periphery of mid/lower zones. Occasionally a single focus may be present. Another pattern is the so-called 'reverse halo' or Atoll sign (a ring of consolidation surrounding central ground-glass opacification)	**Fig. 4.100.1.12:** Organizing pneumonia

Further management: CT findings are discussed with chest physician and suggested CT guided biopsy for tissue diagnosis and PET scan to rule out distant metastasis.

Staging: Based on CT findings staging is T2bN0M0 according to TNM staging, 8th edition

Brief discussion about consolidation: There are multiple differential diagnoses for consolidation.

Table 4.100.1.2: The characteristic radiographic and CT findings of consolidation and atelectasis

Consolidation	*Atelectasis*
• Homogeneous opacity obscuring vessels • Air bronchograms • Ill-defined or fluffy opacities • "Air alveolograms" • Patchy opacities • "Acinar" or air-space nodules • Preserved lung volume • Extension to pleural surface • "CT angiogram" sign	Direct sign: Due to lobar volume loss • Displacement of fissures • Crowding of vessels Indirect signs: Secondary to volume loss • Diaphragmatic elevation • Mediastinal shift • Compensatory over inflation of normal lung • Hilar displacement • Reorientation of the hilum or bronchi • Approximation of the ribs • Increased lung opacity • Absence of air bronchogram • Shifting granuloma sign

Table 4.100.1.3: Based on the duration consolidation classified into acute and chronic to narrow down the differential diagnosis acute last for less than three weeks	
Acute consolidation	*Chronic consolidation*
Pulmonary edema	Bronchioalveolar carcinoma
Pneumonia	Eosinophilic pneumonia
Aspiration	Sarcoidosis
Hemorrhage/contusion	Radiation pneumonitis
Infarction	Organizing pneumonia

Table 4.100.4: Pneumonia—spectrum of findings		
Type	*Pathogen*	*Imaging*
Lobar pneumonia	*S. pneumoniae, K. pneumoniae* Others: *S. aureus* and *H. influenzae*	Air bronchogram,consolidation (no volume loss), lobar distribution
Bronchopneumonia	*S. aureus* Gram negatives Others: *H. influenzae* and Mycoplasma	• Patchy consolidation in segmental distribution
Nodules	Fungal • Histoplasma • Aspergillus • Cryptococcus • Coccidioides Bacterial • Legionella • Nocardia	
Cavitatory lesions	Pneumatoceles (*S. aureus*) Anaerobes Fungal TB	
Diffuse opacities	Viral TB PCP	Reticulonodular pattern: viral Alveolar location: PCP Miliary pattern: Hematogenous spread of TB

Table 4.100.1.5: Based on the pattern of involvement consolidation can be divided into diffuse consolidation and lobar consolidation	
Lobar consolidation	*Diffuse consolidation*
Lobar pneumonia: • *Streptococcus pneumoniae* • Klebsiella • TB • Aspiration **Neoplasm:** • Lung with obstructive pneumonia • BAC • Lymphoma **Hemorrhage:** • Contusion • Infraction **Others:** • Organizing pneumonia • Eosinophilic pneumonia • Sarcoidosis • Sequestration • Mitral regurgitation with RUL edema	**Edema:** • Heart failure • Volume overload • ARDS • Low albumin • Renal failure • Transfusion reaction **Hemorrhage:** • SLE • Henoch-Schönlein purpura • Wegener • Goodpasture **Bronchopneumonia:** • *Staph. aureus* • Gram negative • PCP • Viral-fungal **Others:** • BAC • Lymphoma • Organizing pneumonia • Eosinophilic and hypersensitivity pneumonia

Perihilar consolidation: It shows central consolidation with sparing of the lung periphery giving **"bat-wing"** appearance. Sparing of the lung periphery has been attributed to better lymphatic clearance of fluid in this region.

Peripheral or subpleural consolidation: Consolidation is seen adjacent to the chest wall, with sparing of the perihilar regions, giving reverse bat-wing pattern.

Table 4.100.1.6: Causes of bat-wing and reverse bat-wing appearance on CT

Perihilar consolidation (bat-wing)	*Peripheral or subpleural (reverse bat-wing)*
Pulmonary edema Bronchopneumonia PCP Viral pneumonia	Bronchoalveolar carcinoma Organizing pneumonia (COP) COVID pneumonitis Chronic eosinophilic pneumonia

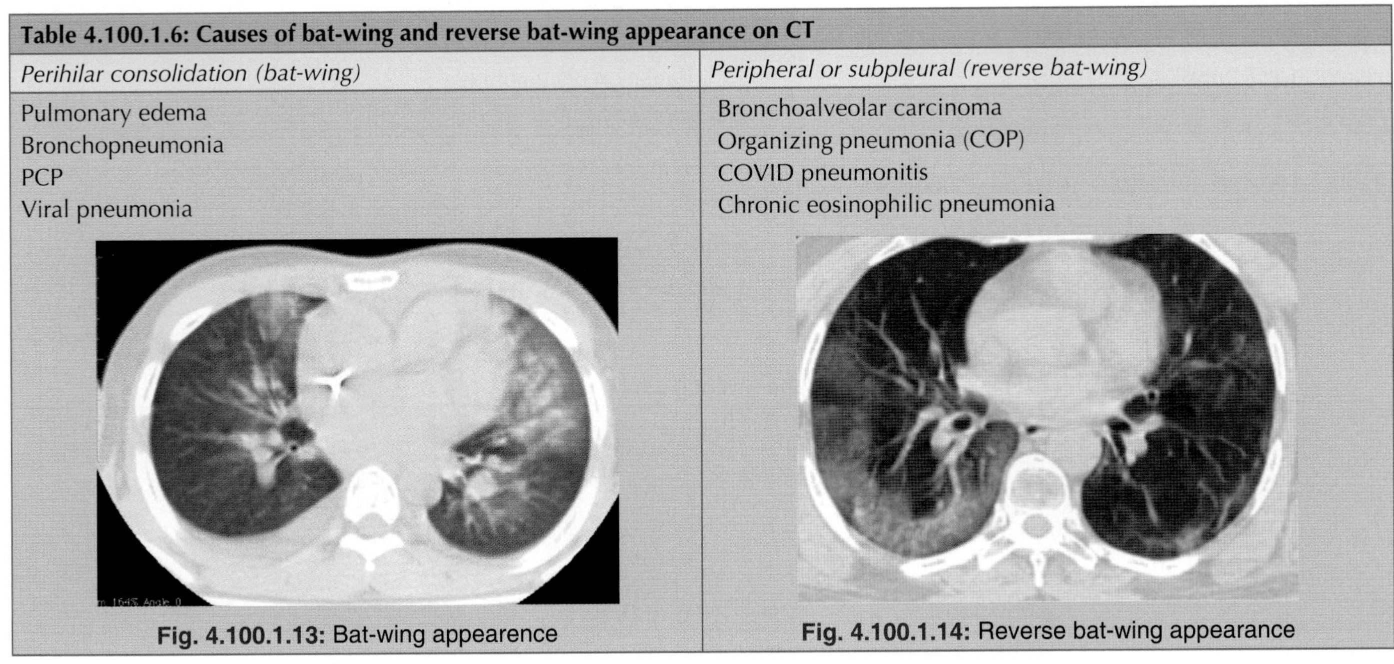

Fig. 4.100.1.13: Bat-wing appearence

Fig. 4.100.1.14: Reverse bat-wing appearance

Table 4.100.1.7: Difference between lung abscess and empyema in CT

Lung abscess	*Empyema*
Round shape	Lenticular
Thick irregular wall	Regular well-defined thin wall
Vessels not displaced	Lung and vessels displaced
Acute angle with chest wall	Obtuse angle
—	Split pleura sign—separated pleural layers seen

Primary signs of malignancy:

- Mass (>3 cm) or nodule (<3 cm) or with speculated, irregular borders.
- Unilateral enlargement of hilum, mediastinal widening, hilar prominence.
- Cavitation: Most common in upper lobes or superior segments of lower lobes
- Wall thickness is indicative of malignancy
  - <4 mm: 95% of cavitated lesions are benign
  - >15 mm: 85% of cavitated lesions are malignant.

  Cavitations most common in SC.
- Certain tumors may present as chronic airspace disease: Bronchoalveolar carcinoma, lymphoma.
- Some air bronchograms are commonly seen by HRCT in adenocarcinoma.

Secondary signs of malignancy:

- Atelectasis (golden interval "s" sign in RUL collapse.
- Obstructive pneumonia
- Pleural effusion
- Interstitial patterns: Lymphangitic tumor spread
- Hilar and mediastinal adenopathy
- Metastases to ipsilateral, contralateral lung.

Invasive mucinous adenocarcinoma: It is a subtype of invasive adenocarcinoma of the lung, formerly known as mucinous bronchoalveolar carcinoma (BAC). IMA is a tumor consisting of malignant cells having goblet or columnar cell morphology with abundant intracytoplasmic mucin. IMA may show a heterogeneous mixture of lepidic, acinar, papillary, micropapillary, and solid tumor growth. These tumors have a strong correlation with KRAS mutation and a lack of EGFR mutations. IMAs have a propensity for multicentric, multilobar, and bilateral lung involvement, likely as the result of aerogenous metastasis (metastatic spread via airways). Diffuse or multifocal lung involvement may have the appearance of lung consolidation or multiple ill-defined nodules, which are solid or of GGO.

Clinical features: Often symptomatic with insidious onset, pleuritic chest pain, cough (35–60%), hemoptysis (11%), bronchorrhea (abundant white mucoid/watery expectoration) can produce hypovoluemia with electrolyte depletion, shortness of breath, weight loss and fever.

Investigation:
- Chest radiograph shows nodules or consolidation due to the mucin produced from the tumor that do not resolve over time.
- CT chest: Consolidations, air bronchogram, multifocal and sometimes multilobar solid and subsolid nodules or masses, which tend to be centrilobular or bronchiectatic. Lower lobe predominance is common for both localized and multifocal form of the disease. The bubble-like lucency of pseudocavitation formation in the consolidation or nodule is also a major finding, "CT angiogram" sign = low-attenuation consolidation does not obscure vessels.
- PET and SPECT imaging can be used to assess the involvement of lymph nodes and distant metastasis which helps in TNM staging and planning for further management
- CT guided biopsy can be done for histopathological examination.

Cardiogenic pulmonary edema without cardiomegaly causes: Acute event, constrictive pericarditis, restrictive cardiomyopathy.

Air bronchogram causes: Pulmonary consolidation, pulmonary edema, non-obstructive atelectasis, severe interstitial lung disease, bronchoalveolar carcinoma; pulmonary lymphoma, pulmonary infarct, pulmonary hemorrhage, normal expiration.

Fluid bronchogram causes: Foreign body aspiration (children), tumors, infection (including aspergillus), mucus plugging.

CT angiogram sign causes: Bronchoalveolar carcinoma, pulmonary lymphoma, infectious and post-obstructive pneumonia.

Feeding vessel sign—causes: Pulmonary infarction, angioinvasive pulmonary aspergillosis, pulmonary vasculitis, pulmonary embolism, pulmonary arterio-venous malformation, pulmonary metastases, septic pulmonary emboli.

Open bronchus sign: The **positive bronchus sign** is seen on CT chest, and refers to the presence of a bronchus leading directly to a peripheral lung lesion.

Fallen lung sign: The appearance of collapsed lung away from the mediastinum encountered with tracheo-bronchial injury (in particular those >2 cm away from the carina).

Round pneumonia: Round pneumonia is a type of pneumonia usually only seen in pediatric patients. They are well defined, rounded opacities that represent regions of infected consolidation

Lipoid pneumonia: Form of pneumonia associated with oily or lipid components within the pneumonitis component. Causes include aspiration of oily substances (exogeneous lipoid pneumonia) or endogeneous accumulation of lipid substances in the alveoli (endogenous lipoid pneumonia).

Table 4.100.1.8: Spectrum of adenocarcinoma of lung

Spectrum of adenocarcinoma of lung (formerly bronchioloalveolar carcinoma 2011)		
Term	*Pathology*	*CT*
Adenocarcinoma *in situ* (AIS)	Noninvasive ≤3 cm mass, purely lepidic growth	Nonsolid mass +/– small scattered sites of low attenuation <3 cm, pseudocavitation
Minimally invasive adenocarcinoma (MIA)	Invasive ≤3 cm mass with lepidic growth (depth of invasion ≤5 mm)	Partly solid mass <5 mm central solid component
Lepedic adenocarcinoma	Invasive nonmucinous adenocarcinoma with predominantly lepidic growth	Partly solid mass + bubble-like component
Acinar/papillary/micropapillary/solid adeno-carcinoma	Invasive nonmucinous adenocarcinoma + small proportion of lepidic growth	Usually solid mass ± small nonsolid component
Invasive mucinous adenocarcinoma	Invasive mucinous adenocarcinoma + lepidic growth as predominant component	Solid/mostly solid /partly solid/nonsolid mass

Table 4.100.1.9: TNM staging of lung carcinoma, 8th edition

T	*N*	*M*
TNM 8th: Primary tumor characteristics **Tx:** Tumor in sputum/bronchial washings but not be assessed in imaging or bronchoscopy. To: No evidence of tumor **Tis:** Carcinoma *in situ* **T1:** <3 cm which is surrounded by lung/visceral pleura, not involving main bronchus T1a(mi): Minimally invasive carcinoma T1a: 1 cm or less in greater dimension T1b: >1 to <2 cm T1c: > 2 to <3 cm **T2:** >3 to 5 cm or Involvement of main bronchus without carina, regardless of distance from carina or invasion visceral pleural or atelectasis or post-obstructive pneumonitis extending to hilum. T2a: >3 to 4 cm T2b: >4 to 5 cm **T3:** >5 to 7 cm in greatest dimension or tumor of any size that involves chest wall, pericardium, phrenic nerve or satellite nodules in the same lobe. **T4:** >7 cm in greatest dimension or Any tumor with invasion of mediastinum, diaphragm, heart, great vessels, recurrent laryngeal nerve, carina, trachea, oesophagus, spine or separate tumor in different lobe of ipsilateral lung.	**1.** Ipsilateral peribronchial and/or hilar nodes and intrapulmonary nodes **2.** Ipsilateral mediastinal and/or subcarinal nodes **3.** Contralateral mediastinal or hilar; ipsilateral/contralateral scalene/supraclavicular	**M1:** Distant metastasis **M1a:** Tumor in contralateral lung or pleural/pericardial nodule/malignant effusion **M1b:** Single extrathoracic metastasis, including single non-regional lymph node **M1c:** Multiple extrathoracic metastases in one or more organs

Table 4.100.1.10: Lung cancer staging groups (TNM8)

	N0	*N1*	*N2*	*N3*
T1	IA	IIB	IIIA	IIIB
T2a	IB	IIB	IIIA	IIIB
T2b	IIA	IIB	IIIA	IIIB
T3	IIB	IIIA	IIIB	IIIC
T4	IIIA	IIIA	IIIB	IIIC
M1a	IVA	IVA	IVA	IVA
M1b	IVA	IVA	IVA	IVA
M1c	IVB	IVB	IVB	IVB

Table 4.100.1.11: Lung cancer treatment related to stage

Stage	Common treatment
I	Resection
II	Resection
IIIA	Radiation or chemotherapy followed by resection
IIIB	Radiation and/or chemotherapy
IV	Chemotherapy

4.100.2 CHEST

Case No. 100.2

Clinical details: 40 years old male presented with c/o fever and breathlessness for 2 days.

Radiographic technique and observation: Chest X-ray PA view (Figures 4.100.2.1 and 4.100.2.2) showing patchy opacities in bilateral mid and lower zone. Bilateral costophrenic and cardiophrenic angles appear free. Trachea appears to be in midline. Cardiac shadow appears normal.

Visualized skeleton and soft tissues appear normal. CT chest axial section in lung window shows patchy ground-glass opacities noted in bilateral lung fields with peripheral predominance. A few of them going for consolidatory changes, no significant mediastinal lymphadenopathy/pleural effusion.

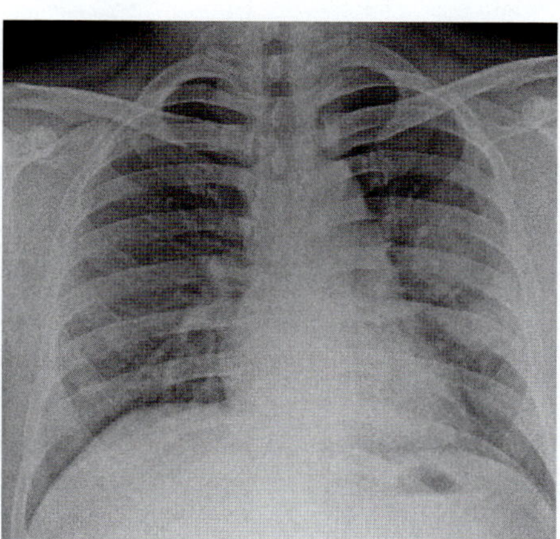

Fig. 4.100.2.1

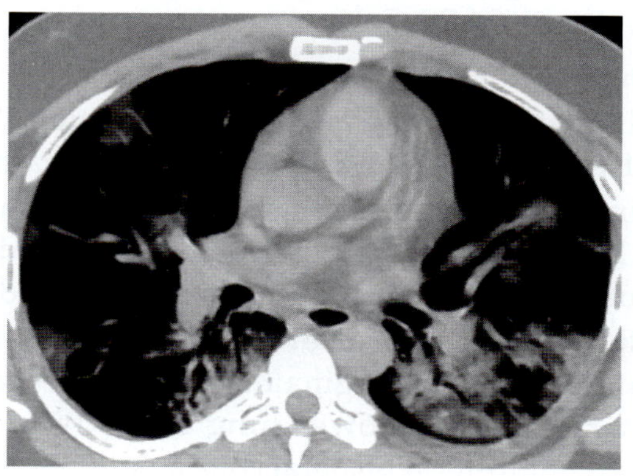

Fig. 4.100.2.2

Interpretation: A—bilateral lung fields, C—patchy ground-glass opacities with peripheral predominance (reverse bat-wing pattern), B—no significant lymphadenopathy/pleural effusion, D—COVID-19 pneumonia

Principal diagnosis: CORADS-5, COVID-19 pneumonia (CT severity index—10/25, moderate disease).

Differential diagnosis for reverse bat-wing pattern of pneumonia:

1. Organizing pneumonia (COP)
2. COVID pneumonitis
3. Chronic eosinophilic pneumonia
4. Bronchoalveolar carcinoma

Table 4.100.2.1: Differential diagnosis for reverse bat-wing pattern of pneumonia

1. Eosinophilic lung disease: Heterogeneous group of disorders that are characterized by excess infiltration of eosinophil within the lung interstitium and alveoli	Air space opacification seen characteristically non-segmental, in the upper zones and paralleling the chest wall.	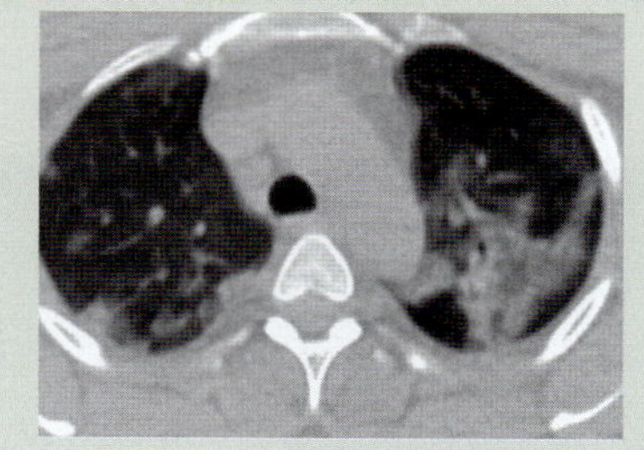 Fig. 4.100.2.3: Eosinophilic lung disease
2. Organizing pneumonia: May be cryptogenic or as a response to other 'insult' (e.g. infection, drug toxicity, connective tissue disease).	Multifocal air-space opacities in periphery of mid/lower zones. Occasionally a single focus may be present. Another pattern is the so-called 'reverse halo' or atoll sign (a ring of consolidation surrounding central ground-glass opacification)	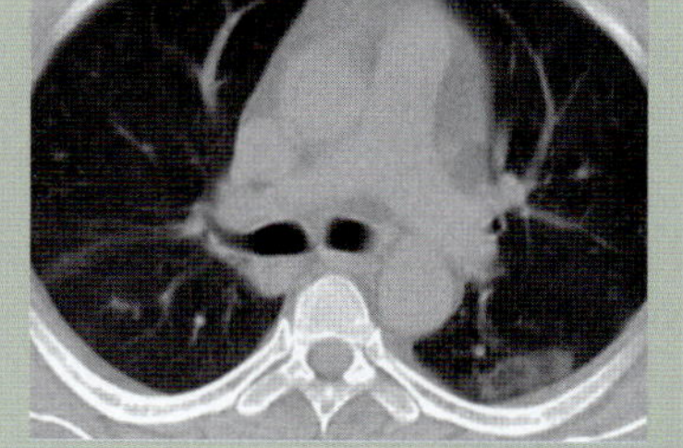 Fig. 4.100.2.4: Organizing pneumonia
3. Bronchoalveolar carcinoma—refer to case 100		

Discussion: Coronavirus disease 2019 (COVID-19) is a disease caused by the severe acute respiratory syndrome coronavirus 2 (SARS-CoV)

Imaging modalities:

A. Plain chest radiography. B. High resolution CT scan (HRCT lungs). C. POCUS (Point-of-care ultrasound)

Plain chest radiography used as 1. Initial base line study, 2. For monitoring rapid progression of disease, 3. For monitoring the progression of COVID-19 disease.

CXR findings typical of COVID-19 pneumonia is bilateral poorly marginated opacities especially peripheral mid and lower lung zones (sometimes rounded), multi-focal bilateral consolidations.

Diffuse air space disease/ARDS.

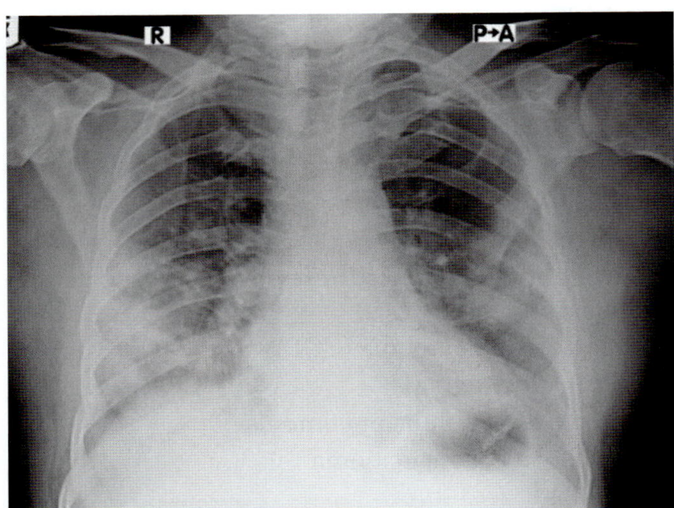

Fig. 4.100.2.5: Typical COVID-19

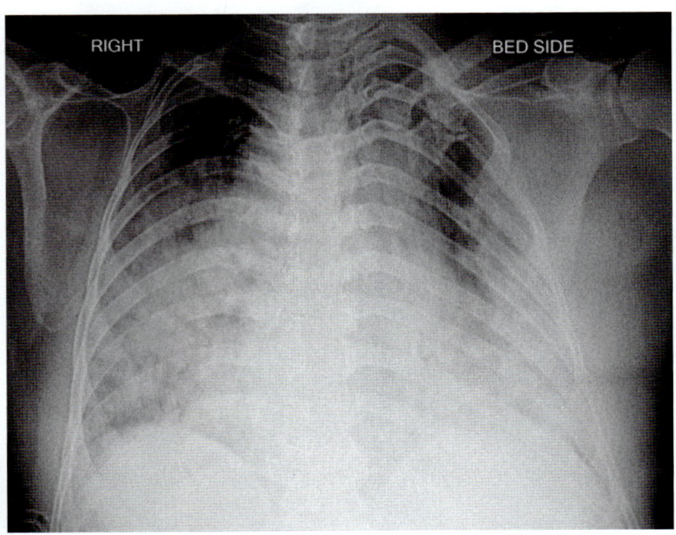

Fig. 4.100.2.6: ARDS in COVID-19

Spectrum of imaging findings in HRCT—chest in a patient with COVID-19 pneumonia.

Common imaging findings:

1. Ground-glass opacities:

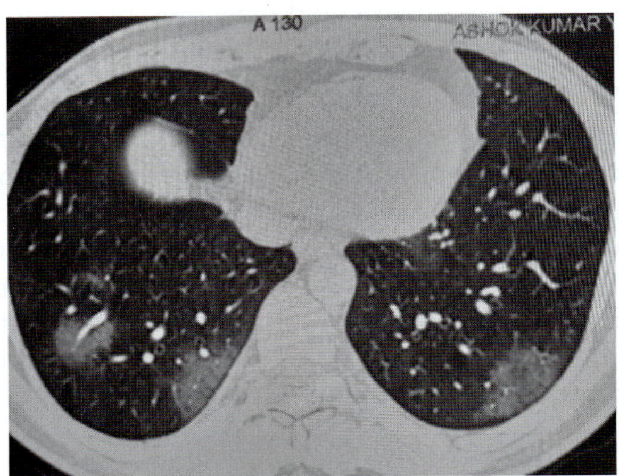

Fig. 4.100.2.7: Ground-glass opacities in COVID-19

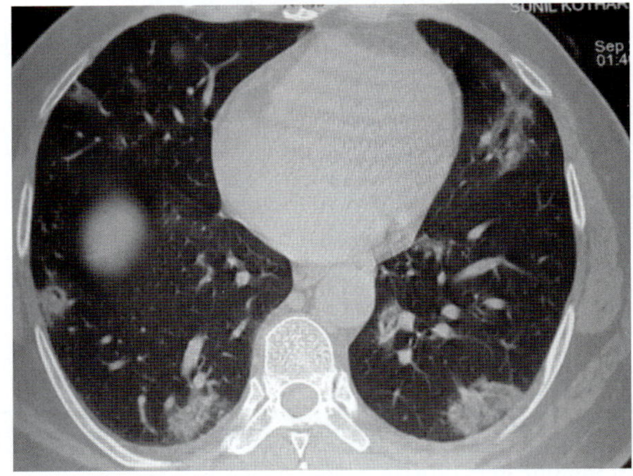

Fig. 4.100.2.8: Ground-glass opacities in COVID-19

2. Consolidation:

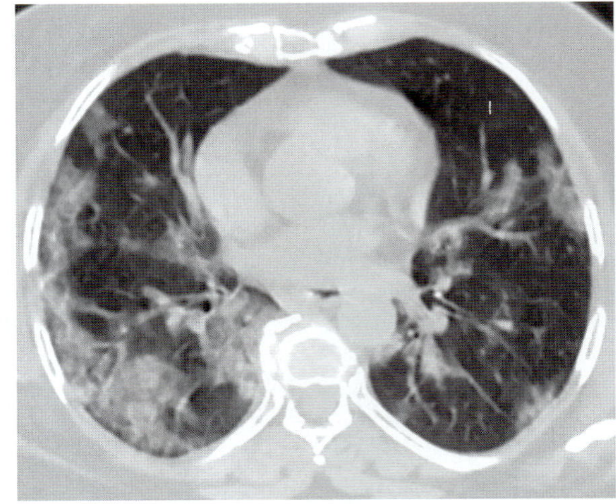

Fig. 4.100.2.9: Consolidation in COVID-19

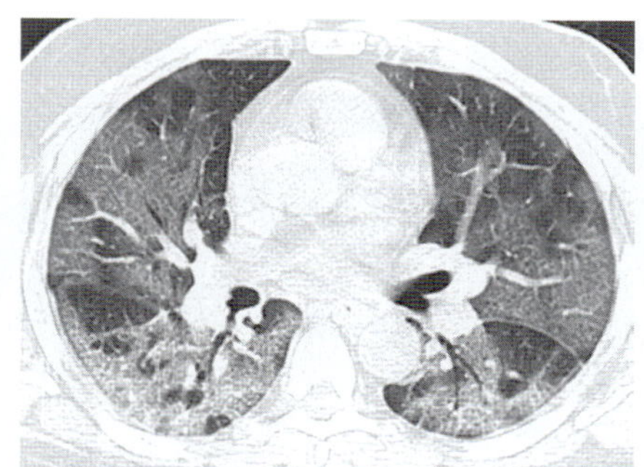

Fig. 4.100.2.10: Crazy pavement pattern in COVID-19

3. Crazy paving: Ground-glass opacity with superimposed interlobular septal thickening. This indicates interstitial inflammation and alveolar damage and may progress to consolidation.

4. Air bronchogram and airway changes: Air-filled low attenuation bronchi on a background of opaque lung. There may be associated bronchial mucus plugging or bronchiolectasis.

5. Vascular enlargement: Represents hypertrophy of the sub-segmental pulmonary vessels. This is an important imaging finding in COVID pneumonia (non-COVID-19 pneumonias do not show this finding).

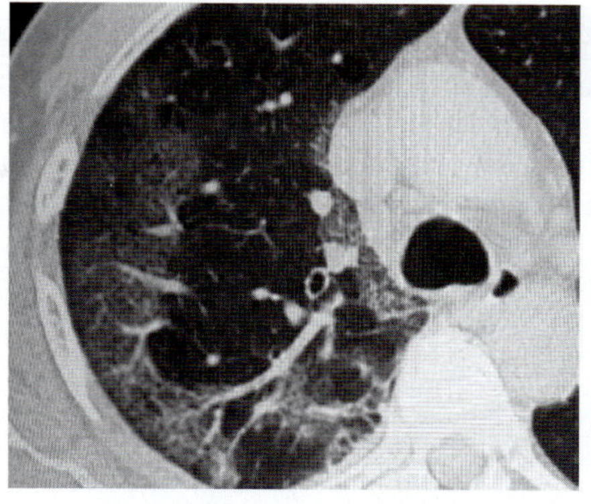

Fig. 4.100.2.12: Crazy paving pattern in COVID-19

6. Reticular pattern and linear opacities: Represents involvement of the pulmonary interstitial secondary to interlobular septal thickening and prominent intralobular lines; this is seen in patients with longer disease course. Cured patients with COVID-19 pneumonia may continue to show reticular opacities.

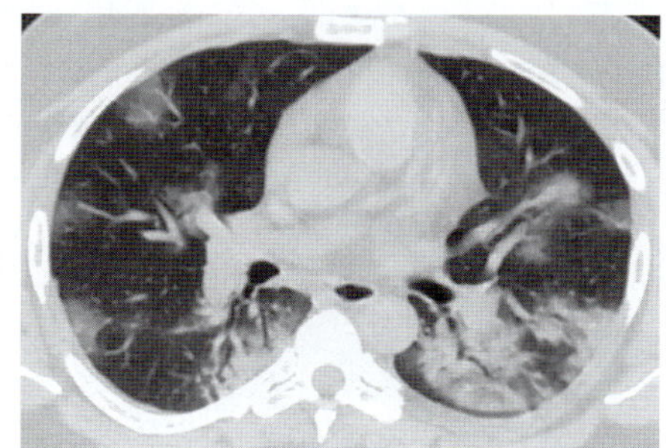

Fig. 4.100.2.11: Air bronchogram and airway changes in COVID-19

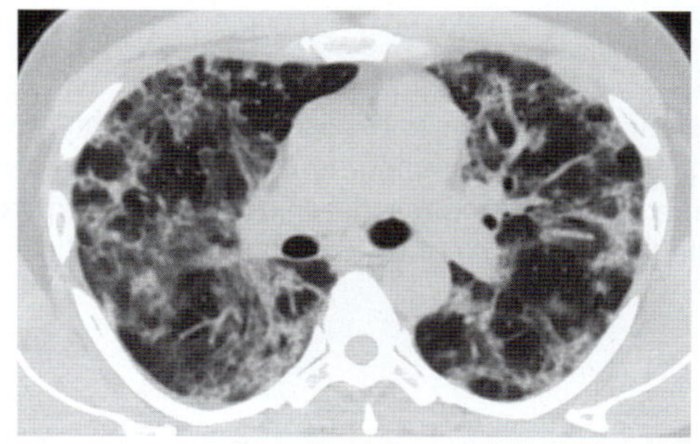

Fig. 4.100.2.13: Reticular pattern and linear opacities in COVID-19

Table 4.100.2.2: Less common or unusual findings	
Less common or unusual findings	
1. Pneumomediastinum/pneumothorax/subcutaneous emphysema: Uncommonly seen with high CT severity scores. These are thought to represent air leaks secondary to high intraalveolar pressure with subsequent spread of air along the bronchovascular bundles.	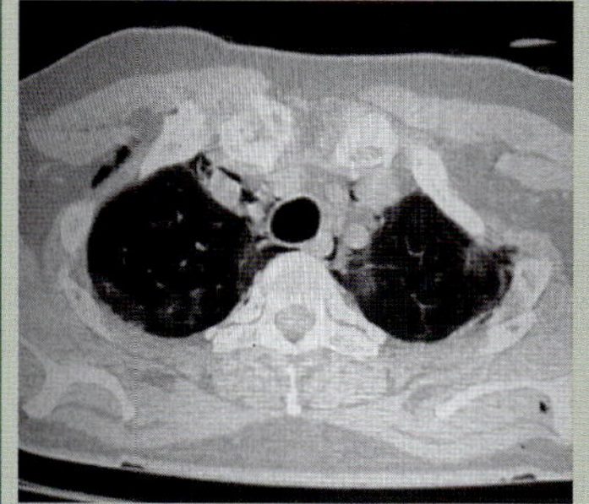 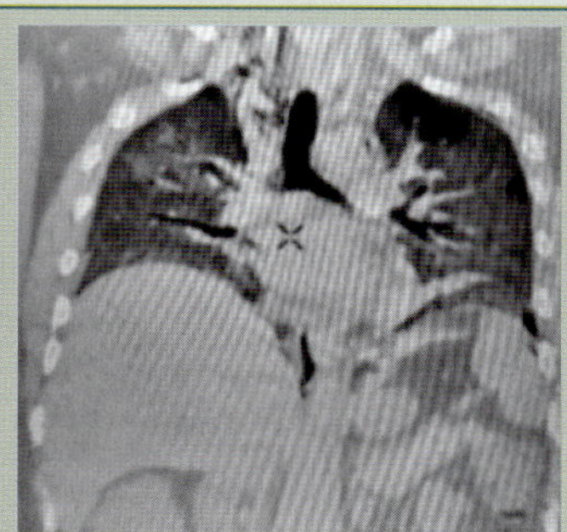 **Figs 4.100.2.14 and 15:** Pneumomediastinum
2. Pleural effusion/thickening: Uncommonly seen; usually in later phase of disease. The presence of pleural effusion is a sign of poor prognosis in COVID-19 pneumonia	

(*Contd.*)

Table 4.100.2.2: Less common or unusual findings (*Contd.*)

3. Nodules: Denote focal air space opacities of less than 3 cm size; although tree-in-bud opacities can be seen in COVID-19 pneumonia, the presence of nodules is suspicious of secondary bacterial infection or aspiration	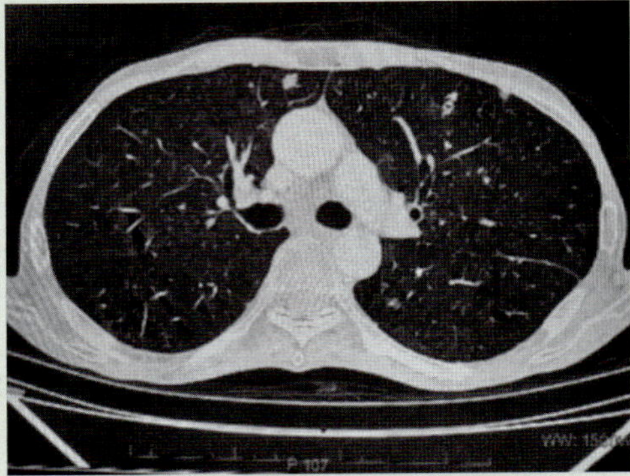 **Fig. 4.100.2.16:** Focal air space nodules in COVID-19
4. Mediastinal adenopathy: Seen infrequently in COVID-19 patients. Its presence is a risk factor for progressive disease. When present with pleural effusion, tree in bud micronodules suggests possibility of a bacterial superinfection	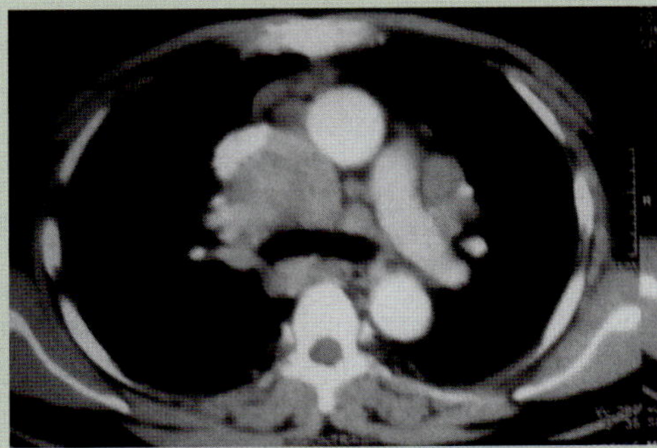 **Fig. 4.100.2.17:** Mediastinal adenopathy
5. Atoll sign: Also known as reverse halo sign which is described in cryptogenic organizing pneumonia (COP). It represents an area of central ground-glass opacity (seen as relatively reduced density) surrounded by a ring of consolidation	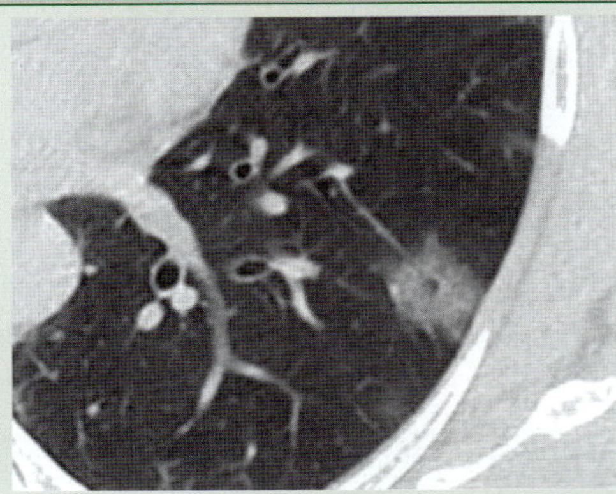 **Fig. 4.100.2.18:** Atoll sign 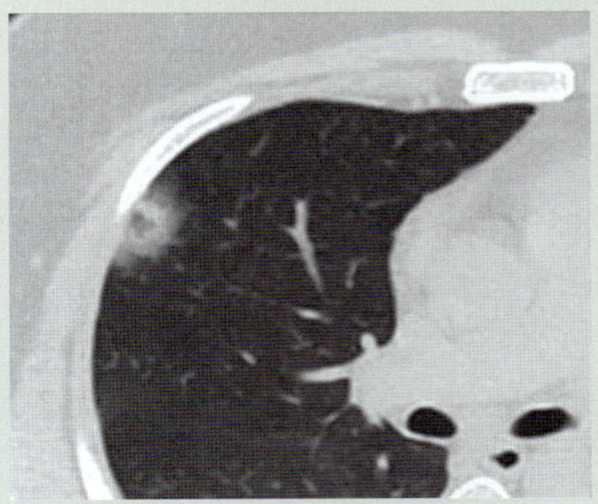 **Fig. 4.100.2.19:** Atoll sign

Table 4.100.2.3: Imaging findings in COVID-19 pneumonia	
Common imaging findings	*Less common or unusual imaging findings*
Bilateral peripheral ground-glass patches	Central and peripheral ground-glass patches
Multilobar affection	Single lobar affection
Consolidation	Pneumomediastinum/pneumothorax/subcutaneous emphysema
Crazy paving	Pleural effusion/pericardial effusion
Air bronchograms or airway changes	Nodules including tree-in-bud opacities
Vascular enlargement	Mediastinal lymphadenopathy
Reticular pattern or linear opacities	Halo sign, reverse halo sign or atoll sign
Pulmonary thromboembolism	Air bubble sign
	Sub-pleural atelectasis
	Cavitation or cavity within a consolidation, mass or nodule
	Bronchiectasis

CT severity score: A CT severity score is assigned to an individual study to decide upon the aggressiveness of the treatment. The system is a visual based scoring which assigns a score of 0–5 to each of the 5 lobes based on the extent of involvement (no involvement—score of 0, <5% involvement—score of 1; between 5–25% involvement—score of 2, between 26–50%—score of 3; between 51–75%—score of 4 and over 75%—score of 5). The total scoring is out of 25.

Table 4.100.2.4: COVID CT severity score		
Lung lobes	*CT severity score*	*Lung lobe involvement and score*
Right upper lobe		Score 0: 0% involvement
Right middle lobe		Score 1: <5% involvement
Right lower lobe		Score 2: 5–25% involvement
Left upper lobe		Score 3: 26–50% involvement Score 4: 51–75% involvement
Left lower lobe		Score 5: >76% involvement
Total CT severity score (25)	/25	
(Score <8: Mild, 9–17: Moderate, >18: Severe)		

Table 4.100.2.5: COVID-19 pneumonia			
COVID-19 pneumonia—coinfections and secondary infections—imaging features			
Gram negative bacteria	*Coronavirus disease-associated mucormycosis (CAM)*	*Influenza-associated pulmonary aspergillosis (IAPA)*	*COVID-19-associated pulmonary aspergillosis (CAPA)*
Bilateral recent onset consolidation with or without necrosis	Mass like consolidation, crosses the fissures. Multiple nodular ground-glass opacity/consolidation.	Wedge-shaped lobar or segmental consolidation with air bronchogram cavity formation, tree-in-bud pattern	May exhibit non-specific CT findings, such as bilateral areas of ground-glass opacity or crazy paving, extensive consolidations associated with peripheral traction bronchiectasis
Multiple cavitating nodules/ abscess	Cavity—birds nest formation/ reverse halo sign is seen.	Nodules with halo signs	Peribronchial consolidation
Unilateral pleural effusion	Pleural effusion	Bronchial wall thickening seen	Bronchial wall thickening seen
	Concomitant sinusitis	Tracheobronchitis with tracheal and bronchial ulceration	Pseudoaneurysm
	Voriconazole prophylaxis +		Serum galactomannan antigen test positive

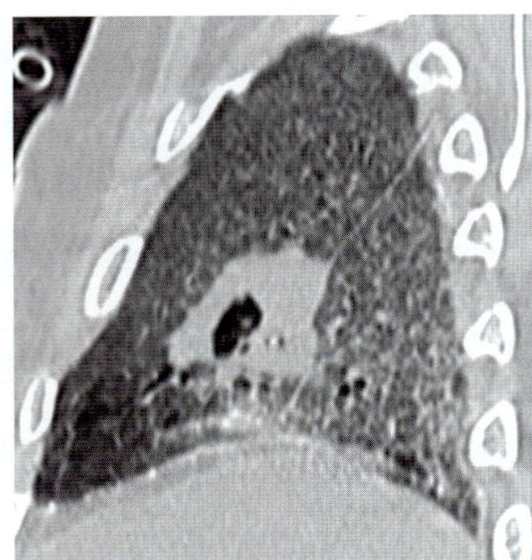

Fig. 4.100.2.20: Coronavirus disease associated mucormycosis; left upper lobe cavitating consolidation as noted on sagittal image. Note the ground-glass changes elsewhere, consistent with COVID infection.

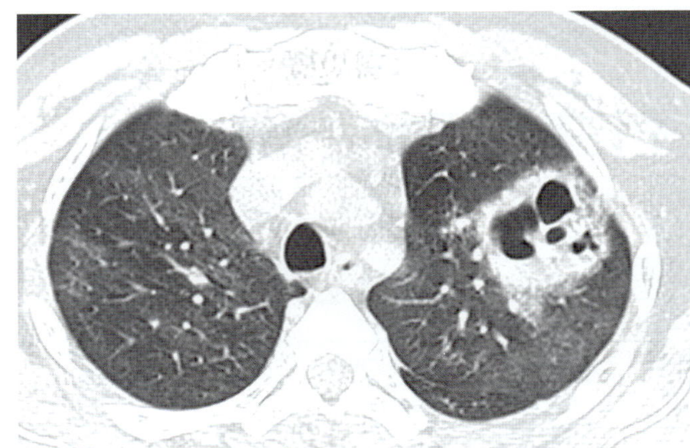

Fig. 4.100.2.21: Coronavirus disease associated mucormycosis; left upper lobe cavitating consolidation as noted on axial images; note the ground-glass changes elsewhere, consistent with COVID infection.

Stages of COVID-19 Pneumonia and Lung Changes

In patients recovering from COVID-19 various stages of lung involvement are defined on CT scans as shown in Table 4.100.2.6. Initial lung findings are small subpleural ground glass opacities which may be uni or bilateral with usually a lower lobe distribution that grow larger with crazy paving and consolidation. Lung involvement progress to dense consolidation up to two weeks from onset of initial symptoms. Subsequently the lesions are gradually absorbed leaving behind ground-glass opacities and linear subpleural parenchymal bands. Most of the lesions resolve completely.

Table 4.100.2.6 Stages of COVID-19 pneumonia and lung changes

Day of symptoms	*Phase*	*Imaging findings*
0–5 days Early stage 1	Exudative stage (leakage of fluid into interstitium)	Normal. Presence of unilateral/bilateral ground-glass opacities predominantly in lower lobe, usually posteriorly distributed with the predilection for subpleural and peripheral involvement
5–9 days Progressive Stage 2	Inflammatory stage (alveolar leak of protein/fluid resulting in diffuse alveolar opacities, increasing exudation-consolidation, progression to white out lungs–ARDS)	Diffuse GGO/crazy paving, mixed GGO and consolidation pattern, multilobar distribution
9–13 days Peak Stage 3	Interstitial changes due to septal congestion, edema, cellular infiltration, inflammation, hemorrhage and early fibrosis	Bilateral multilobe distribution, complex evolution into dense consolidation. Interstitial changes manifests as crazy paving, subpleural bands/linear opacities at this stage.
>14 days Absorption Stage 4	Stage of resolution/organising pneumonia/post-COVID fibrotic like changes	Gradual resorption of consolidation (crazy paving no longer seen) Parenchymal bands /atelectasis/ fibrosis in bilateral subpleural lung fields Increased area of GGO involvement but density of GGO decreased (tinted sign/ melting sugar) GGO and fibrotic strips GGO completely resolved (in a median period of two weeks in many patients)
Up to 6 months	Delayed absorption/post-COVID fibrotic-like changes	GGO and interstial thickening Traction bronchiectasis, parenchymal bands, and/or honeycombing Some may show complete resolution from scarring.
>6 months	Probable post-COVID fibrosis	Traction bronchiectasis, parenchymal bands, and/or honeycombing. Few areas of GGO/reticulation may present.

Table 4.100.2.7: Other system manifestations of coronavirus disease
I. Neurological manifestations: • Thromboembolic infarcts—the commonly observed patterns of acute cerebral thromboembolic disease are large vessel occlusion with territorial infarcts, branch vessel occlusion, small vessel occlusion, small vessel infarcts, watershed infarcts, and extensive bilateral multivessel infarcts • Hemorrhage • Leukoencephalopathy—symmetrical confluent white matter T2 hyperintensity and diffusion restriction sparing the juxtacortical and infratentorial white matter • PRES • Global hypoxic injury—predominant involvement of the basal ganglia, thalami, hippocampi and cortex • Meningitis and encephalitis • Cytotoxic lesions of corpus callosum • Olfactory bulb involvement—edema in the olfactory bulb and track with increased T2 signal intensity in the gyrus rectus • Cranial nerve enhancement—optic neuritis, oculomotor nerve enhancement and Miller Fisher syndrome • Mucormycosis—manifestations include skull base osteomyelitis, pachymeningeal enhancement, leptomeningeal enhancement, cerebritis progressing to abscess, cranial nerve infiltration, infarcts, cavernous sinus thrombosis, mycotic pseudoaneurysm, subarachnoid hemorrhage and intraparenchymal hemorrhage
II. Spinal manifestations: Guillain-Barré syndrome is seen in association with COVID-19 characterized by T2 hyperintensity in the distal cord and enhancement of the caudal nerve roots.
III. Abdominal manifestations: 1. Bowel wall thickening (small and large bowel) in 15–31% associated with hyperaemia and mesenteric thickening. 2. Fluid-filled colon (homogeneous fluid attenuation contents in the lumen of colon without formed stool) without wall thickening or pericolonic stranding. 3. Mesenteric ischemia (enteritis accompanied by ischemia) 4. Pneumatosis intestinalis or portal venous gas in approximately 10% 5. Acute pancreatitis 6. Solid organ infarctions or vascular thromboses (18%) 7. Mesenteric stranding 8. Ascites 9. Gallbladder sludge, newly found hepatosteatosis, hepatitis, acute liver injury 10. Enlarged kidneys, bilateral renal infarcts and other abnormalities of the urinary tract (12%): Cystitis, pyelonephritis, renal abscess 11. Ileocolic intussusception (in paediatric population) 12. Nonspecific: Gastritis, equivocal findings of appendicitis, perforated marginal ulcer at the gastrojejunal anastomosis in a gastric bypass patient, stercoral colitis, and concurrent stercoral colitis and diverticulitis, liver abscess, progression of hepatic metastases
IV. Multisystem inflammatory disorder: MIS-C is a syndrome associated with COVID-19 disease. Unlike typical COVID-19 disease, which presents with respiratory symptoms and pneumonia, MIS-C associated with COVID-19 typically presents with multiorgan injury, mainly cardiovascular manifestations. Pulmonary manifestations are uncommon. In the abdomen, the common imaging findings are ascites, hepatomegaly, and echogenic kidneys, indicating multiorgan inflammatory disease. Due to nonspecific clinical presentation of MIS-C associated with COVID-19 disease, imaging is crucial in establishing the diagnosis. Radiologists should be aware of the constellation of these imaging findings, that, although nonspecific, when combined with the clinical presentation and a history of exposure to SARS-CoV-2, should suggest the diagnosis of MIS-C associated with COVID-19, because patients may rapidly deteriorate. Although most patients with MIS-C who are admitted to the hospital are severely ill and require admission to the PICU, most improve clinically with appropriate management after accurate diagnosis. Nevertheless, the long-term outcome of MIS-C is yet to be determined. Most common thoracic imaging findings were cardiomegaly, congestive heart failure or cardiogenic pulmonary edema, and pleural effusions. Pneumonia, although reported with high incidence in pediatric and adult patients with COVID-19, is uncommon in MIS-C associated with COVID-19. Abdominal imaging findings were notable for ascites, hepatomegaly, and echogenic kidneys in approximately one-third of the patients and for other findings in several patients, including thickened gallbladder, bowel, and urinary bladder walls and bowel distention, reflecting an underlying multisystemic inflammatory process. MIS-C is a syndrome of multisystemic inflammation in which patients present with a high fever and gastrointestinal and mucocutaneous symptoms with rapid progression to cardiogenic shock and multisystem injury. Hepatic injury based on blood chemistry results was present in the majority of patients, and one-third of patients developed acute kidney injury. Imaging findings of hepatomegaly and echogenic kidneys reflected parenchymal injury to these organs in one-third of the patients. Ascites and bowel wall thickening, gallbladder, and urinary bladder thickening were also identified and may have reflected inflammation or low serum albumin levels.
V. Rhinocerebral mucormycosis: Refer to case 4.71

4.101 CHEST

Case No. 101

Clinical history: A 65-year-old male with history of weight loss.

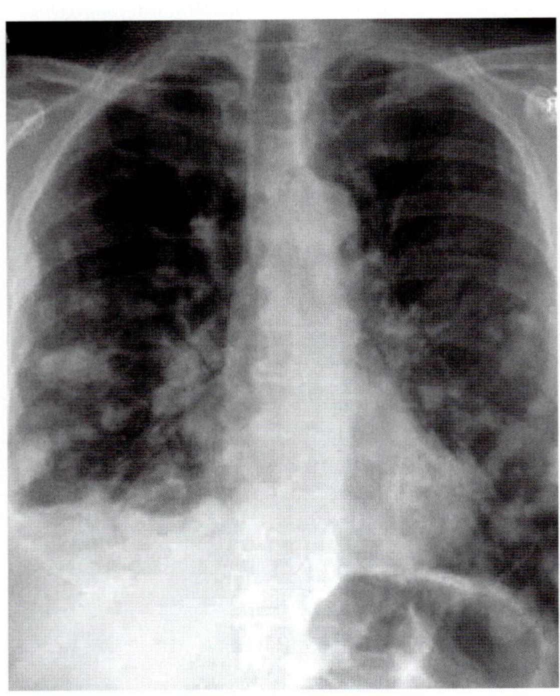

Fig. 4.101.1

Radiological technique and observation: Frontal chest radiograph (Fig. 4.101.1) shows multiple pulmonary nodules of varying sizes (10–20 mm) in random distribution.

The trachea appears to be in midline. Cardiac shadow appears normal.

The visualized bones appear normal.

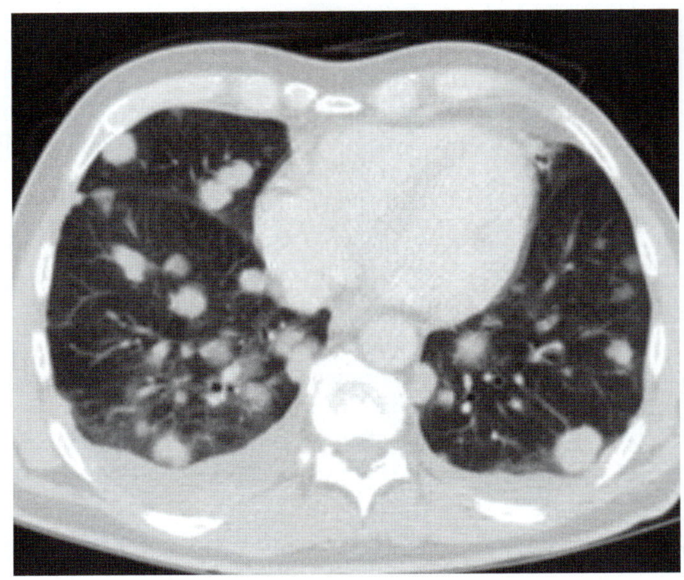

Fig. 4.101.2

Table 4.101.1: Differential diagnosis for multiple pulmonary nodules based on size	
Multiple pulmonary nodules (>5 mm)	
Metastases	Most commonly from breast, thyroid, kidney, gastrointestinal tract and testes. In children, Wilms' tumor, Ewing's sarcoma, neuroblastoma and osteosarcoma. Predilection for lower lobes and more common peripherally. Lesions can be well defined or ill-defined, ill-defined lesions suggest metastasis from prostate, breast or stomach. Hilar lymphadenopathy and effusions are uncommon
Lymphoma	One manifestation of secondary lymphoma is multiple nodules, which often have fuzzy outlines and are most numerous in the lower lobes. This appearance is usually associated with mediastinal and hilar lymph node enlargement
Bronchoalveolar carcinoma	Multiple discrete small nodules, either randomly distributed or primarily centrilobular, BAC may mimic hematogenous metastases. A more common appearance of this condition is diffuse, patchy, or multifocal areas of consolidation that are peribronchovascular and contain air bronchograms or air-filled cystic spaces
Kaposi sarcoma	Irregular (flamed-shaped) and ill-defined peribronchovascular nodules combined with peribronchovascular and interlobular septal thickening, pleural effusions, and lymphadenopathy may develop in patients with Kaposi sarcoma.
Infections Abscesses	Widespread distribution but asymmetrical. Commonly *Staphylococcus aureus*. Cavitation common. No calcification
Coccidioidomycosis	In endemic areas. Well-defined with a predilection for the upper lobes. 0.5–3 cm. Calcification and cavitation may be present.

(Contd...)

4

Table 4.101.1: Differential diagnosis for multiple pulmonary nodules based on size *(Contd...)*	
Histoplasmosis	In endemic areas. Round, well-defined and a few in number. Sometimes calcify. Usually unchanged for many years
Hydatid	More common on the right side and in the lower zones. Well-defined unless there is surrounding pneumonia. Often 10 cm or more. 'water lily' sign may be seen.
Immunological Wegener's granulomatosis	Bilateral nodules or masses (± cavitation in 30–50% of cases) or unifocal/multifocal consolidation. Widespread distribution. Round and well-defined. No calcification.
Rheumatoid nodules	Peripheral and more common in the lower zones. Round and well-defined. No calcification. Cavitation common.
Caplan's syndrome	Well-defined nodules. Develop rapidly in crops, later coalesce to form large granuloma. Calcification and cavitation occur. Background stippling of pneumoconiosis.
Silicosis	Silicosis typically appears as fine nodular opacifications (1–10 mm) that are diffusely scattered throughout both lungs in a centrilobular and subpleural location. The nodules calcify in about 3% of cases, and chains of subpleural nodules may produce pseudoplaques
Sarcoidosis	Sarcoidosis typically presents as irregular micronodules (1–5 mm) with interstitial thickening that extends along the bronchovascular bundles from the hilum to the periphery, predominantly in the upper lung zones. Alveolar sarcoid is an atypical pulmonary manifestation. Appears as large areas of opacification 1–4 cm. Typically found along bronchovascular bundles or in subpleural location. **Galaxy sign:** Conglomerate of these opacities are accompanied by multiple surrounding nodules, representing granulomas
Organizing pneumonia Amyloidosis	Multiple nodules of varying size (calcified in up to 50%). Multiple nodules may cavitate and show calcification or ossification.
Hypersensitivity pneumonitis	Appears acutely as small, ill-defined centrilobular nodules and bilateral airspace consolidation. In the subacute stage, there are patchy ground-glass opacities with ill-defined centrilobular nodules.
Vascular Arteriovenous malformations	33% are multiple. Well-defined. Lobulated. Tomography may show feeding or draining vessels. Calcification is rare.
Multiple Small ('pin-point') Micronodules	
Post-lymphangiography	Iodized oil emboli. Contrast medium may be visible at the site of termination of the thoracic duct
Stannosis	Inhalation of tin oxide. Even distribution throughout the lungs. With Kerley A and B lines
Barytosis	Inhalation of barytes. Very dense, opacities which are discrete. Generalized distribution although bases and apices usually spared.
Alveolar microlithiasis	Familial disorder. Lung detail obscured by miliary calcifications. A few symptoms but it may progress to cor pulmonale. Pleura, heart and diaphragm seen as 'negative' shadows.
Multiple Micronodules (0.5–2 mm)	
Soft-tissue or ground-glass attenuation Miliary tuberculosis	Widespread and secondary to haematogenous dissemination. Uniform size. Indistinct margins but discrete. No septal lines.
Fungal infection	Histoplasmosis, coccidioidomycosis, blastomycosis and cryptococcus (torulosis). Similar appearance to miliary tuberculosis.
Coal miner's pneumoconiosis	Predominantly mid zones with sparing of the extreme bases and apices. Ill-defined and may be arranged in a circle or rosette. Septal lines.
Sarcoidosis	Predominantly upper/mid zones and strikingly bronchocentric (causing 'bronchovascular beading') enlarged hilar lymph nodes.
Greater than soft-tissue density Haemosiderosis	Secondary to chronic raised venous pressure (seen in 10–15% of patients with mitral stenosis), repeated pulmonary haemorrhage (e.g. Goodpasture's disease) or idiopathic. Septal lines. Smaller than miliary tuberculosis.
Silicosis	Relative sparing of bases and apices. Very well-defined and dense when due to inhalation of pure silica: Ill-defined and of lower density when due to mixed dusts. Septal lines.
Siderosis	Lower density than silica. Widely disseminated

Right costophrenic angle appears blunted.

A few nodules noted along the subpleural location. CT thorax single axial image in lung window provided (Fig. 4.101.2). It shows multiple randomly distributed round nodules of varying sizes in both lungs. There are also small bilateral pleural effusions, right > left. Heart, visualized bones, chest wall, esophagus appear normal.

Interpretation: A—65 years old male, bilateral lung fields show, B—multiple randomly distributed round nodules, C—of varying sizes, D—metastasis

Principal diagnosis: Bilateral pulmonary metastasis.

Differential diagnosis: Miliary nodules: <2 mm, pulmonary micronodule: 2–7 mm, pulmonary macronodule: 7–30 mm, pulmonary mass: >30 mm

The initial evaluation of multiple nodules usually is based on history, clinical studies, and assessment of radiographic findings. Percutaneous biopsy may be needed for eventual diagnosis.

A nodule is a well- or ill-defined, roughly rounded opacity measuring up to 3 cm in diameter. Nodules <3 mm are called 'micronodules', whereas those >3 cm in diameter are termed 'masses'. Further characterization of nodules (solid versus pure ground-glass versus part-solid, centrilobular versus random distribution) is possible with CT.

Size: There is a tendency for multiple nodular metastases to vary in size, whereas benign processes result in nodules of similar size.

Table 4.101.2: Common primaries causing lung metastases

Adults	*Children*
Breast carcinoma Colorectal carcinoma Renal cell carcinoma Uterine leiomyosarcoma Head and neck squamous cell carcinoma	Rhabdomyosarcoma Osteosarcoma Wilms tumor Ewing sarcoma Neuroblastoma

Number: Multinodular metastases may be few in number or innumerable, but a large number of nodules suggest this diagnosis. Most infectious and inflammatory diseases result in less than a dozen nodules.

Location: Metastases, infarction, and septic emboli have a predilection for the lung periphery and the lung bases. Abscesses related to aspiration often are posterior or basal in distribution.

Metastases tend to have a peripheral and basal predominance.

Edge appearance: Metastases are usually sharply marginated as are nodules in amyloidosis, rheumatoid nodules, AVMs, hematomas, and Caplan's syndrome. Infectious lesions, invasive mucinous adenocarcinoma, lymphoma, conglomerate masses and progressive massive fibrosis, and granulomatosis with polyangiitis (GPA; Wegener's granulomatosis) are often ill defined. An increase in sharpness of the edge of a lesion with time suggests the resolution of a benign inflammatory process.

Table 4.101.3: Differential diagnosis for multiple pulmonary nodules based on appearance

Based on appearance	
Miliary nodules	Miliary tuberculosis Silicosis Pulmonary sarcoidosis Diffuse pulmonary metastases Diffuse panbronchiolitis
Cavitatory nodules	Septic pulmonary emboli Cavitating Metastases—squamous cell neoplasms (also adenocarcinomas of the large bowel and sarcomas) Multiple cavitating infection
Calcific nodules	Tuberculosis Silicosis Calcifying metastases–sarcomas—osteosarcoma, chondrosarcoma, synovial sarcoma. mucinous type carcinomas—carcinomas of the colon, ovarian cancers, breast cancer, medullary thyroid carcinoma, treated metastatic choriocarcinoma, giant cell tumor of the bone.
Based on lobar involvement	
Upper and middle lobes	Silicosis
Upper lobe	Sarcoidosis, respiratory bronchiolitis
Peripheral	Infection
Peripheral and lung bases	Metastases

Attenuation: Metastases are usually of soft tissue attenuation, but invasive mucinous adenocarcinoma may result in multiple nodules of GGO. Infection and diffuse inflammatory lung diseases such as hypersensitivity pneumonitis may result in multiple GGO nodules; organizing pneumonia may result in multiple nodules, either solid or of GGO. Some diseases, particularly granulomatous infections, sarcoidosis, and amyloidosis, result in multiple nodules, which may be calcified.

Cavitation: Thick-walled cavities are consistent with malignancy, but thick walls may be seen with inflammatory, nonmalignant lesions as well. Very thin-walled cavities usually are benign, although metastatic tumors, particularly squamous cell carcinoma of the head and neck or sarcomas and tracheobronchial papillomatosis, may be associated with thin-walled lesions. An air-fluid level tends to predict benign disease.

Growth: Rapid growth with an increase in size over a period of a few days suggests infection (e.g., bacterial infection or fungus or TB in an immunosuppressed patient). Progression over a period of a few weeks is typical of indolent infections (e.g., TB or fungus in an immunocompetent patient), noninfectious inflammatory disease, or rapidly progressing malignancy. Nodules that appear stable over a period of weeks or show slow growth during a few months are likely to be either malignant or due to indolent inflammatory conditions (e.g., rheumatoid nodules).

Resolution of lesions with or without treatment suggests benign disease. Slow resolution is typical of hematoma and infarction. Rapid resolution is typical of treated infections.

Phantom tumor: It is caused by a loculated pleural effusion (pleural pseudotumor) trapped in the pleural fissures.

4.102 CHEST

Case No. 102

Clinical history: 40-year-old female with complaints of fever.

Radiological techniques and observation: Dual energy chest radiographs (Figs 4.102.1 and 4.102.2) with soft tissue window are provided. The film is overpenetrated, mildly rotated showing mediastinal widening with bilateral hilar and right paratracheal adenopathy. Enlarged hilum is not tapered along branches of the pulmonary arteries and the pulmonary convergence is negative (not enlarged pulmonary artery). Suspicious linear shadows in bilateral lower zones. Trachea in midline. No cardiac enlargement. Bilateral costophrenic angles appear free. Pleura/chest wall/abdomen and diaphragm appear normal. CT lung window (Fig. 4.102.3) showing multiple well-defined micronodules in perilymphatic distribution with fissural thickening and bilateral hilar enlargement. No evidence of calcification/cavitation/fibrosis/honeycombing.

Interpretation: A: 40 years old female, mediastinal lymph nodes, C: Bilateral perihilar and right paratracheal lymphadenopathy, B: Perilymphatic micronodules with upper lobe predominance, D: Sarcoidosis stage II.

Principal diagnosis: Sarcoidosis stage II

Management: Serum ACE, calcium and other biochemical test to confirm diagnosis. Corticosteroid therapy can be given.

Differential diagnosis based on stage of disease:

Stage 1: Adenopathy alone—symmetrical bilateral hilar and right paratracheal (75–90%) ("1-2-3 sign"/ "Pawnbroker sign"/"Garland sign") other nodes–aortopulmonary and intrapulmonary nodes (12–14 station). The nodes are well defined, discrete, homogeneous with intact perinodal fat without any intranodal necrosis. Egg shell calcification in long standing cases. Presence of intrapulmonary nodes are very specific for sarcoidosis.

Atypical patterns (more common in >50 years of age): Unilateral, isolated, anterior and posterior mediastinal lymphadenopathy.

DD

1. Metastastic lymphadenopathy (presence of necrosis, mass effect on adjacent vascular structures),
2. Mediastinal lymphoma (conglomerate nodes, encasing vascular structures, abutment of the cardiac silhouette)
3. Infective etiology (tuberculosis-necrotic nodes, diffusely calcified lymph nodes),
4. Castleman's disease
5. Silicosis, scleroderma (symmetrical hilar lymphadenopathy, uniformly enhancing nodes, no mass effect on adjacent vascular structures, do not abut the cardiac silhouette. Cluster of black pearls sign—presence of multiple tiny round nodules (1–2 mm) distributed uniformly within whole or part of a homogeneously enhancing lymph node, Dark lymph nodes sign (presence of internal hypo-intensity with peripheral thin rim of hyperintensity on T2W MRI) differentiate sarcoidosis from other conditions).

Differential diagnosis for bilateral hilar lymphadenopathy: Sarcoidosis, tuberculosis, histoplasmosis, lymphoma, silicosis, berylliosis.

Stage 2/3: Parenchymal lung disease

Nodular pattern: Small nodules in a perilymphatic distribution. These nodules are found most often in the subpleural peribronchovascular interstitium and less often in the interlobular septa. Always look for small nodules along the fissures, because this is a very specific and typical sign of sarcoidosis. These nodules are bilateral, symmetrical and upper and

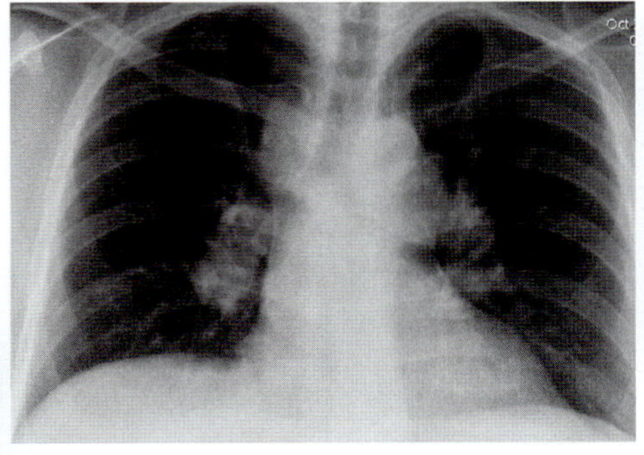

Fig. 4.102.1

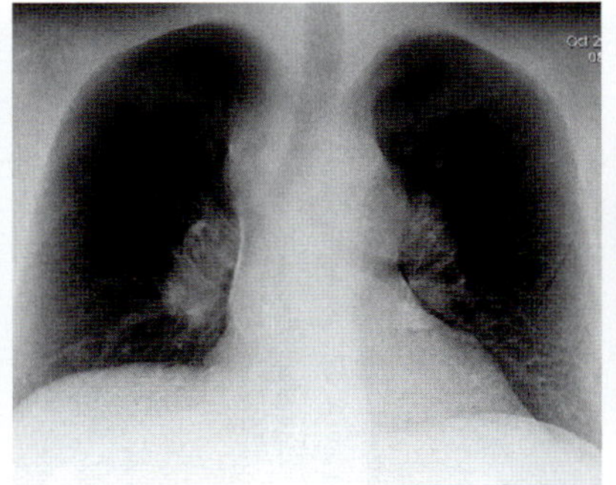

Fig. 4.102.2

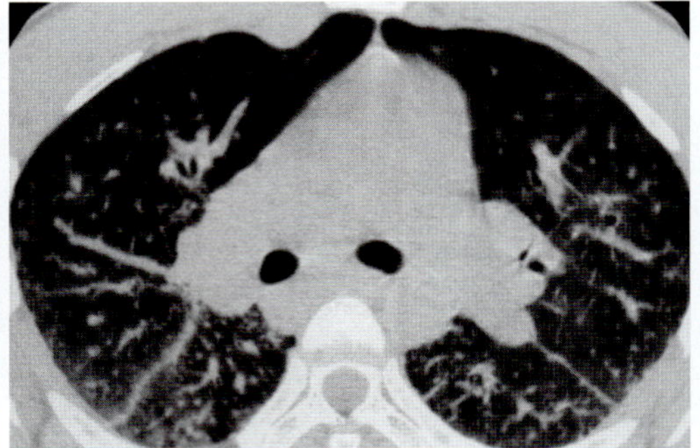

Fig. 4.102.3

Table 4.102.1: Differential diagnosis for sarcoidosis		
1. Lymphangitic carcinomatosis: Usually secondary to adenocarcinoma (breast ca most common).	Irregular nodular interlobular septal thickening, reticulonodular pattern, thickening of bronchovascular interstitium pleural effusion, hilar and mediastinal lymphadenopathy	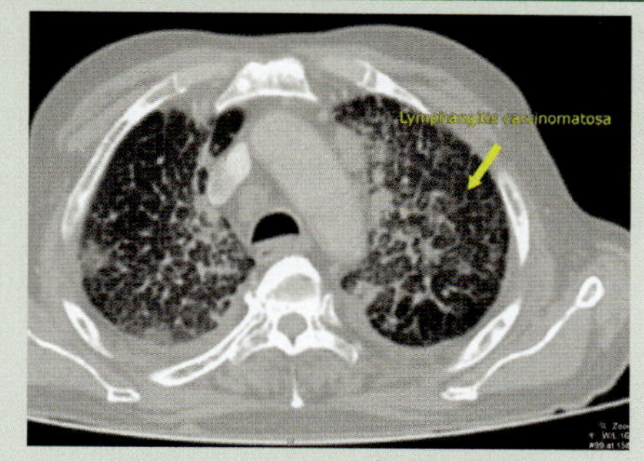 **Fig. 4.102.4:** Lymphangitic carcinomatosis
2. Silicosis (uncomplicated)–refer to case 95		
Lymphoma: 60% of all Hodgkin lymphoma and 20% of non-Hodgkin lymphoma involve the mediastinum at presentation. Mediastinal widening, retrosternal space obliterated. Pleural effusion, pericardial effusion, chest wall invasion, egg shell calcification seen following therapy.	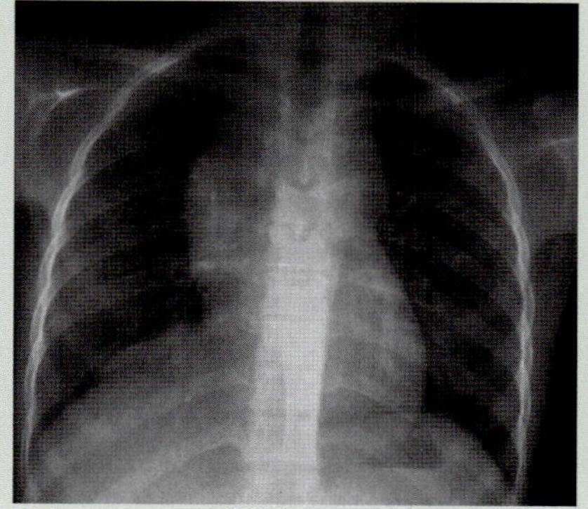 **Fig. 4.102.5:** Lymphoma	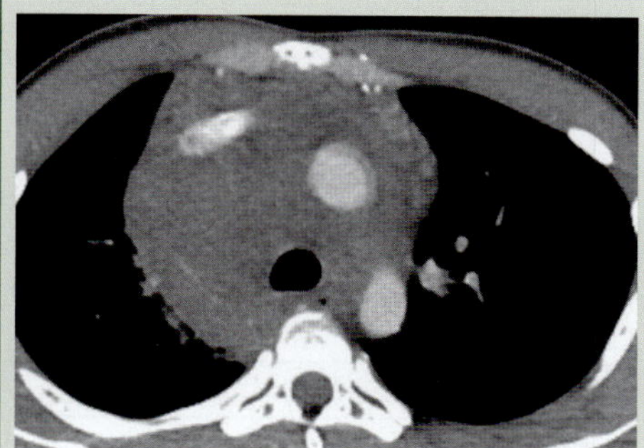 **Fig. 4.102.6:** Lymphoma
Cryptogenic organizing pneumonia: Idiopathic form of organizing pneumonia is called cryptogenic organizing pneumonia (COP)	**Plain radiograph:** Peripheral, subpleural, peribronchovascular unilateral or bilateral patchy areas affecting all zones. **CT:** Patchy consolidation, small or large nodules, bronchial wall thickening, interlobular septal thickening, crazy paving pattern, reverse halo sign .	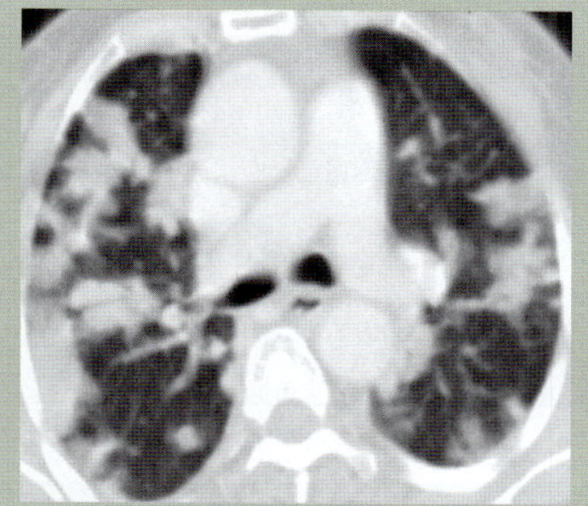 **Fig. 4.102.7:** Cryptogenic organizing pneumonia
Extrinsic allergic alveolitis. An inflammatory reaction to inhalation of an allergen that can lead to lung fibrosis	Homogeneous ground-glass opacity, numerous round centrilobular nodules, mosaic attenuation pattern, head cheese sign, small mediastinal lymphadenopathy	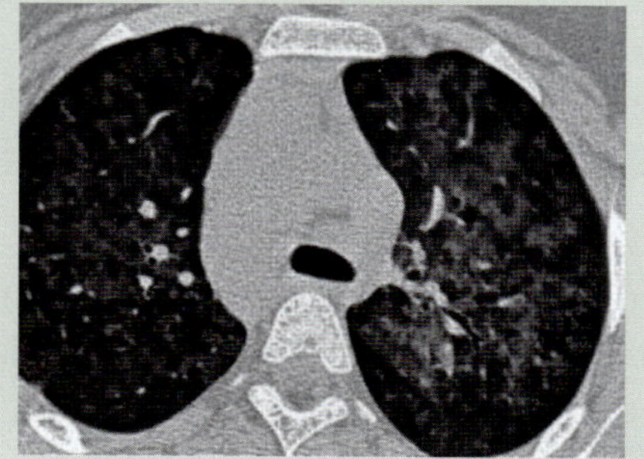 **Fig. 4.102.8:** Hypersensitivity pneumonitis

Contd...

Table 4.102.1: Differential diagnosis for sarcoidosis *(Contd...)*		
Congestive cardiac failure: a. Low output heart failure b. Heart failure with preserved ejection fraction (diastolic heart failure) c. High output heart failure.	**Plain radiograph:** In left-sided failure, there is pulmonary venous congestion, cephalization of pulmonary veins, pulmonary interstitial edema, pulmonary alveolar edema, cardiomegaly, pleural effusion. Mediastinal lymph nodes may be seen.	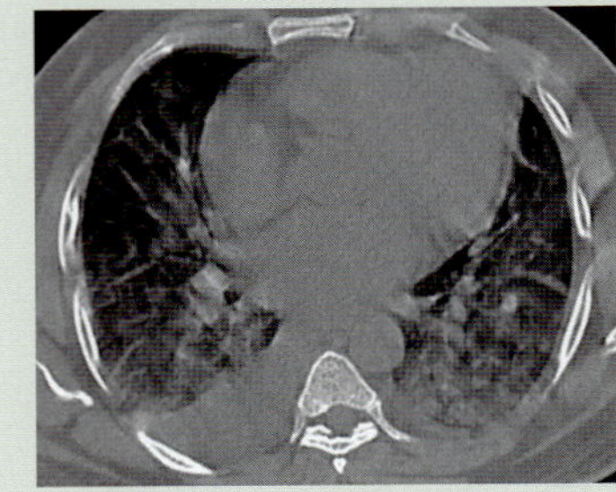 **Fig. 4.102.9:** Congestive cardiac failure

Table 4.102.2: Difference between sarcoidosis and tuberculosis		
Lymph node features	*Sarcoidosis*	*Tuberculosis*
Distribution Nodal sites Unilateral/bilateral	Hilar, right paratracheal Usually bilateral, symmetrical	Right paratracheal, hilar, subcarinal, mediastinal Usually unilateral
Morphology Margin Enhancement pattern Calcification	Sharp and discrete Homogeneous, "Cluster of Black Pearls" Focal, bilateral hilar lymph node calcification.	Conglomerate, obscured perinodal fat. Heterogeneous, rim enhancement Complete, unilateral hilar lymph node calcification
Diffusion weighted MRI	ADC value in lymphoma lower than sarcoidosis. No discriminatory pattern between sarcoid and tuberculosis	
Lymphoma: Bulky non-necrotic lymph nodes with homogeneous enhancement showing increased uptake in PET CT.		

Table 4.102.3: Difference between sarcoidosis and lymphangitis carcinomatosa	
Sarcoidosis	*Lymphangitis carcinomatosis*
• Nodules are subpleural and along the peribronchovascular interstitium • Less often in the interlobular septa • Septal thickening is not extensive	• Nodules are predominantly along the interlobular septa and also subpleural, along the peribronchovascular interstitium • Septal thickening is more prominent and extensive out of proportion to presence of nodules. • Older age group, symptomatic patient, H/O malignancy, presence of associated pleural effusion favors lymphangitis than sarcoidosis

Table 4.102.4: Difference between sarcoidosis and silicosis	
Sarcoidosis	*Simple/uncomplicated silicosis*
• Predominantly perilymphatic • Nodules are smaller • Nodular septal thickening, fissural thickening is common • No occupational history	• Predominantly centrilobular along with perilymphatic • Nodules are somewhat larger than sarcoidosis • Fissures, interlobular septum are relatively spared • Occupational history +

middle zone predominance. Sarcoid granulomas frequently cause nodular or irregular thickening of the peribronchovascular interstitium, however, it is not extensive.

DD: Silicosis, berylliosis, coal worker's pneumoconiosis, lymphangitis carcinomatosis.

4

Chronic air space opacities

- Micronodules are also known to group in the periphery of lung–sarcoid cluster sign.
- Micronodules coalesce over time, forming larger lesions (macronodules and masses)—appear as peripheral or parahilar confluent masses appear as consolidation which radiate from hilum to periphery

with or without air bronchogram. These masses surrounded by smaller satellite micronodules which is known as sarcoid galaxy sign.

- *Atypical presentations:* Patchy air space consolidation (acinar or alveolar sarcoidosis), patchy ground-glass opacities.

DD: Cryptogenic organizing pneumonia, hypersensitivity pneumonitis, eosinophilic pneumonia.

Stage 4: Pulmonary fibrosis—linear opacities, traction bronchiectasis, and architectural distortion (displacement of fissures and bronchovascular bundles, elevation of hila), these abnormalities are bilateral, symmetrical perihilar (follows larger airways), predominantly involving the upper and middle lung zones. Rarely associated with cavitation. Formation of confluent fibrotic masses with irregular margin more than 1 cm is known as progressive massive fibrosis. Atypical presentations like fibrocystic changes can also happen which include fibrotic cysts, bulla, paracicatricial emphysema, honeycomb like cyst in subpleural location involving upper and mid-lung zone.

DD: Silicosis, tuberculosis (unilateral, asymmetrical), coal worker's pneumoconiosis, talcosis, berylliosis, usual interstitial pneumonia (basal and peripheral predominance, honeycombing), chronic hypersensitivity pneumonitis (midzone fibrosis with mosaic pattern, careful analysis of patient history and prior exposure is important).

Other Pulmonary Manifestations

Airway abnormalities: Endobronchial granulomas, nodular bronchial wall thickening, air trapping and mosaic attenuation, and may have atelectasis.

Pleural abnormalities: Rare (approximately 1%), usually manifests as pleural effusion or pleural thickening.

Role of Imaging in Sarcoidosis

1. *CXR:* First imaging investigation

- Useful in follow-up imaging in parenchymal and nodal changes
- Sensitivity is low for detection of parenchymal nodules
- To assess the prognosis (depends on stage of disease)
- Signs in sarcoidosis: Garland sign/pawnbroker sign, cluster of black pearls sign/dark lymph node sign, sarcoid galaxy sign/sarcoid cluster sign and lambda sign/panda sign

2. *HRCT*

- Better efficacy for nodules, faint GGO and alveolar opacities
- To differentiate active inflammation vs fibrotic disease
- Unusual clinical and radiographic presentation
- For the detection of pulmonary complication
- Selection of biopsy site

3. *PET/CT:* PET/CT may be useful for identification of occult sites of disease, suitable target for diagnostic biopsy, gauging active inflammatory disease in patients with prolonged symptoms, assessing response to treatment.

4. *Scintigraphy:* Gallium-67 scintigraphy usually shows high uptake in active sarcoidosis and is useful for assessing disease activity and response to treatment, although as it is a non-specific marker of inflammation. It has a role also in detecting extra-thoracic involvement. The gallium equivalent of 1-2-3 sign or Garland triad is known as the lambda sign. The **panda sign of sarcoidosis** is a gallium-67 citrate scan finding. It is due to bilateral involvement of parotid and lacrimal glands in sarcoidosis, superimposed on the normal uptake in the nasopharyngeal mucosa.

Biomarkers include—elevated ACE, hypercalcemia, hypercalciuria. Positive **Kveim-Siltzbach skin test** confirms the diagnosis.

Complications of Sarcoidosis

- Pulmonary fibrosis (stage IV)
- Pulmonary arterial hypertension and cor pulmonale
- Aspergilloma

Discussion: Sarcoidosis is a non-caseating granulomatous multisystem disease. Typically affects adults less than 40 years of age with peak incidence in 3rd decade, slightly more common in female.

Clinical presentation: 50% asymptomatic, symptoms include dyspnea, cough, fatigue, night sweats, weight

Table 4.102.5: Difference between pulmonary massive fibrosis caused by sarcoidosis and silicosis

PMF—silicosis	*PMF–sarcoidosis*
• Confluent masses tend to form in periphery moves towards hila. • Lateral margin of masses parallel to chest wall • Paracicatricial emphysema laterally • Cavitation is common (ischemic necrosis or TB)	• Confluent masses tend to form in perihilar region moves towards periphery • Lateral margin of masses not parallel to chest wall • Cavitations are rare

4

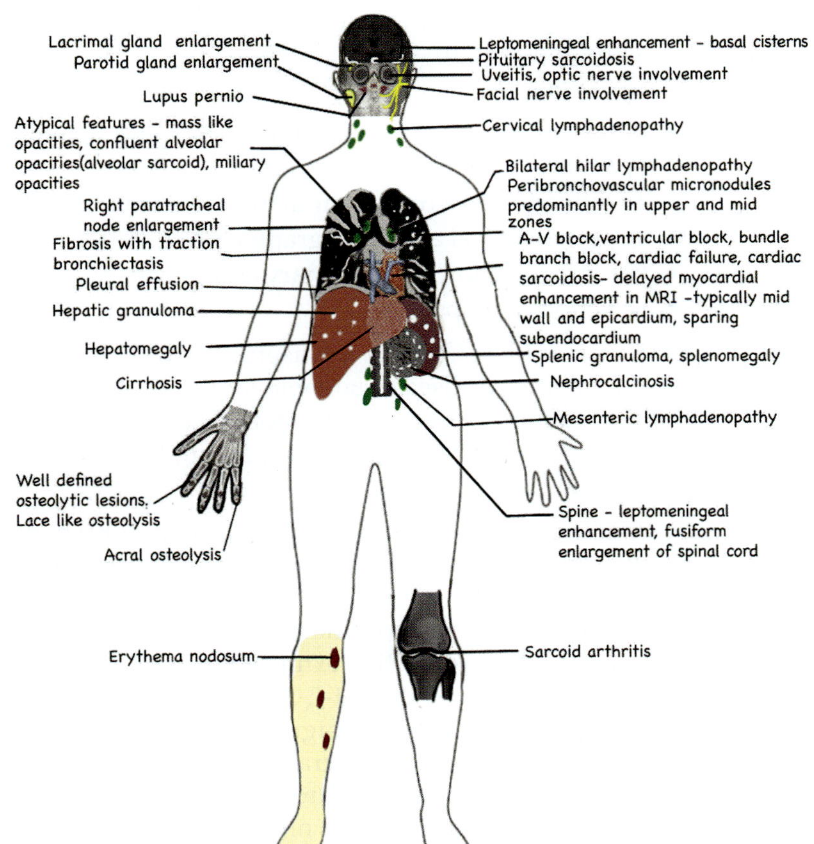

Fig. 4.102.10: Whole body illustration showing manifestations of sarcoidosis

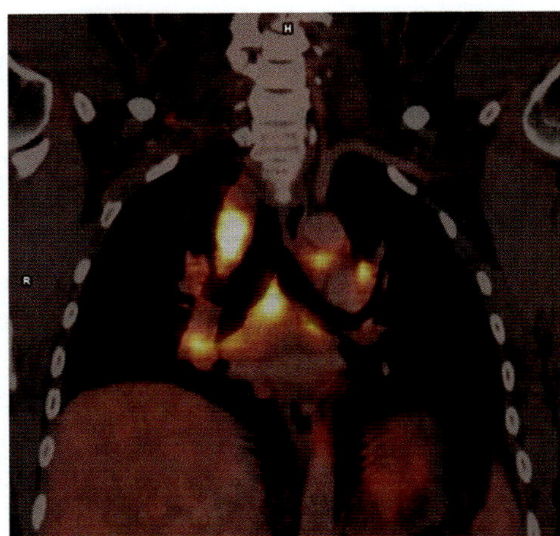

Fig. 4.102.11

Table 4.102.6: Siltzbach classification on sarcoidosis

The Siltzbach classification based on the chest radiograph findings defines five stages	*Chance of spontaneous remission*
Stage 0: Normal appearance at chest radiography (5–10% at presentation)	
Stage 1: Lymphadenopathy (50%)	60–90%
Stage 2: Lymphadenopathy and parenchymal lung disease (25–30%)	40–70%
Stage 3: Parenchymal lung disease (10–12%)	10–20%
Stage 4: Pulmonary fibrosis (5% at presentation, up to 25% during course of disease)	0%

loss, erythema nodosum. Pulmonary disease present in 90% of patients.

IgG4 disease: Systemic disease that is characterized by fibroinflammatory infiltration of various organs, by plasma cells that express IgG4. **Central nervous system:** IgG4-related hypertrophic pachymeningitis, IgG4-related hypophysitis, chronic subdural hemorrhage. **Head and neck:** Sialadenitis/chronic sclerosing sialadenitis (Küttner tumor), Riedel thyroiditis, IgG4-related orbital disease, pansinusitis. **Thoracic:** Interstitial pneumonia/IgG4-related lung disease, IgG4-related cardiovascular disease. **Abdominopelvic**-autoimmune pancreatitis, sclerosing cholangitis, sclerosing mesenteritis, cholecystitis, IgG4-related renal diseases, tubulointerstitial nephritis, retroperitoneal fibrosis, inflammatory aortic aneurysm, prostatitis, multisystem-inflammatory pseudotumors (e.g. presenting as paravertebral masses), lymphadenopathy.

Criteria for mediastinal widening: Mediastinal widening is present when the mediastinum measures greater than 8 cm at the aortic arch in adults or the mediastinum: Chest width ratio is greater than 0.25 in children.

Lofgren syndrome: An uncommon but specific acute presentation of sarcoidosis with a better prognosis.

Heerfordt syndrome: An uncommon variant of sarcoidosis comprising of fever, parotid enlargement facial palsy, and anterior uveitis.

Table 4.102.7: Difference between smooth and nodular septal thickening

Smooth interlobular septal thickening	*Nodular interlobular septal thickening*
• Pulmonary edema • Lymphangitic spread of carcinoma/lymphoma • Alveolar proteinosis • Amyloidosis, LIP, lymphangiomatosis, Erdheim-Chester disease	• Lymphangitic spread of carcinoma/lymphoma • Silicosis • Sarcoidosis

Table 4.102.8: Multisystem manifestations in sarcoidosis

I. Neurosarcoidosis 1. Solitary or multiple enhancing T2 hyperintense periventricular and deep white matter lesions. 2. Diffuse or nodular leptomeningeal enhancement with thickening (sarcoid meningitis) 3. Enhancing plaque-like or nodular thickening in the infundibular stalk and optic chiasm 4. Hydrocephalus 5. Cranial neuropathy—abnormal enhancement and enlargement of cranial nerve (most common facial nerve)
II. Spinal cord involvement: Leptomeningeal enhancement, fusiform spinal cord enlargement, focal or diffuse intramedullary disease, intradural extra medullary lesions, extradural lesions, and spinal cord atrophy. Typically, the lesions are T1 hypointense and T2 hyperintense and show patchy enhancement
III. Head and neck sarcoidosis 1. Anterior uveitis 2. Nodular thickening and enhancement of optic nerve 3. Enlarged and enhancing lacrimal gland and parotid gland 4. Nodular thickening and enhancement of nasal septum, turbinates and rarely laryngeal structures 5. Cervical lymphadenopathy
IV. Abdominal sarcoidosis 1. Liver: Hepatomegaly, Heterogeneous liver parenchyma, and increased liver echogenicity, hypoechoic, hypodense and T1/T2 hypointense sarcoid nodules. Sarcoidosis also can involve the intrahepatic and extrahepatic bile ducts, resulting in biliary dilatation and bile duct strictures. 2. Spleen–splenomegaly with sarcoid nodules 3. Stomach can be involved with nodular thickening of gastric mucosa 4. Lymphadenopathy
V. Urogenital: Hypercalcemia induced nephrocalcinois is the commonest renal manifestation. Direct granulomatous involvement of kidney can cause glomerulonephritis and interstitial nephritis with latter demonstrated as striated nephrogram on contrast enhanced CT. Single or multiple hypoechoic testicular nodules may be seen on ultrasound which demonstrate T2 hypointensity on MRI and enhancement on T1 following contrast administration.
VI. Cardiac sarcoidosis 1. Ventricular arrhythmia, heart block, dilated cardiomyopathy, congestive heart failure and sudden cardiac death 2. Cardiac sarcoidosis usually is associated with patchy and multifocal late gadolinium enhancement in the basal segments, particularly of the septum and the lateral wall, and tends to affect the mid-myocardium and epicardium, sparing the subendocardium
VII. Musculoskeletal sarcoidosis 1. Any bone in axial and appendicular skeleton can be involved. But most common is small bones of the hand (in particular, the distal and middle phalanges of the second and third digits). Bone radiograph demonstrates reticular, lacy pattern with multiple lytic lesion. Resorption of distal phalanges (acro-osteolysis) secondary to granulomatous inflammation has a punched out appearance. Sausage like dactylitis seen. No associated periosteal reaction. 2. Polyarthritis or oligoarthritis is much more common than monoarthritis. The ankles, knees, wrists, proximal interphalangeal joints, metacarpophalangeal joints, and elbows are the most commonly affected joints. 3. Nodular sarcoid myopathy can manifest as single or multifocal soft-tissue masses, often involving the lower extremities. In nodular sarcoid myopathy, lesions may have a star-shaped area of low signal intensity in the center and high signal intensity in the periphery on T2-weighted images (i.e., the "dark star" appearance)
VIII. Cutaneous sarcoidosis: Lupus pernio, the most characteristic specific cutaneous manifestation of sarcoidosis, appears as reddish-purple plaques associated with prominent telangiectasia and typically are seen in the nose, ear, cheek, and hand.

4.103 CHEST

Case No. 103

Clinical details: A 30-year-old male with complains of fever and cough.

Radiological techniques and observations: Plain radiograph chest PA view Fig. 4.103.1 reveals large well-defined round homogeneous single radio-opacity in right lower and middle zones. All the borders are well demarcated suggestive of parenchymal lesion. Right heart border and right diaphragm is not obscured. Pulmonary artery and right hilum is seen through the lesion. Surrounding lung parenchyma appears to be normal. No evidence of intralesional calcification, air fluid level, air bronchogram or any fat density within the lesion. Bilateral cardiophrenic and costophrenic angles appear to be normal. Visualised skeleton and soft tissue appear to be normal. Visualised abdomen appears to be normal. CECT axial sections in mediastinal window Fig. 4.103.2 reveals single well-defined non-enhancing smooth walled hypodense cystic lesion noted in right lower lobe without any evidence of calcification/septations or any adjacent lung parenchymal changes. No evidence of any pleural effusion or mediastinal shift or any other similar lesions in lung fields. Visualised skeleton and soft tissue appears to be normal.

Interpretations: A—30 years old male, lesion in right lower lobe, C—smooth walled cystic lesion, B—without any evidence of calcifications/septations, D—hydatid cyst of lung.

Principal diagnosis: Hydatid cyst of lung.

Differential diagnosis: Lung abscess, congenital cysts (intrapulmonary bronchogenic cysts/CPAM), lung laceration with pneumatocele, cystic bronchiectasis, diaphragmatic hernia.

Cystic pulmonary metastases, granulomatosis with polyangitis.

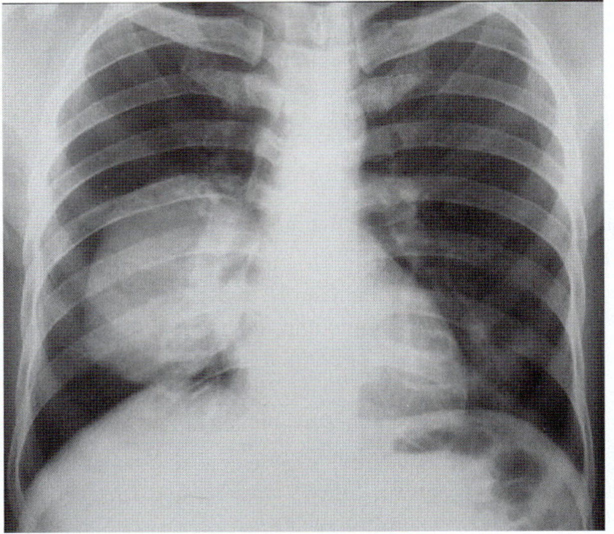

Fig. 4.103.1

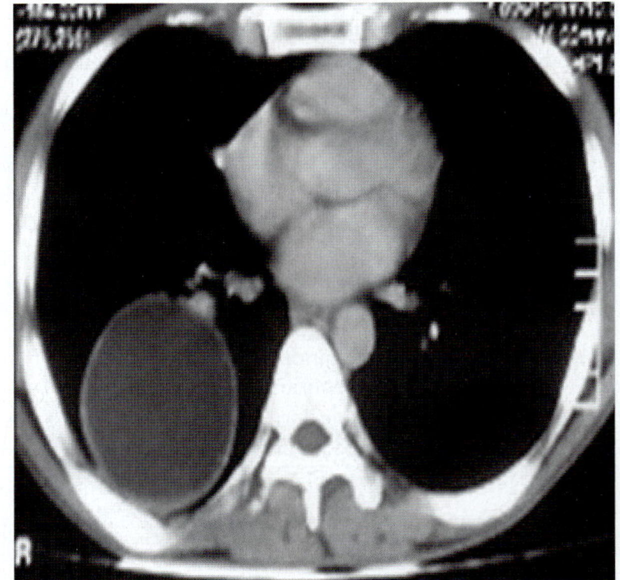

Fig. 4.103.2

Table 4.103.1: Differential diagnosis for cystic lung lesions

Lung abscess: Cavitatory lung lesions produced by infectious agents. They are most commonly caused by aspiration.	Abscess vary in size, generally round in shape. They may contain only fluid or can have air fluid level. Surrounding consolidation will be seen. It is usually thick walled and luminal surface is irregular. CT is helpful in differentiating abscess from empyema.	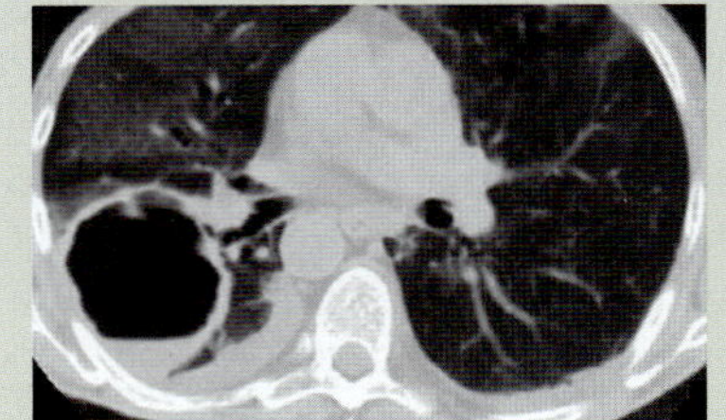 Fig. 4.103.3: Lung abscess

(Contd.)

Table 4.103.1: Differential diagnosis for cystic lung lesions (*Contd.*)		
Lung laceration with pneumatocele (traumatic lung cyst or traumatic pseudocyst).	Cavitation associated with post-contusion pneumonia can develop days after initial trauma, whereas lacerations are seen at initial time of imaging. Observation is the only management required. It will heal by itself within weeks to months. Lung contusion characteristically clear rapidly within 48 hours.	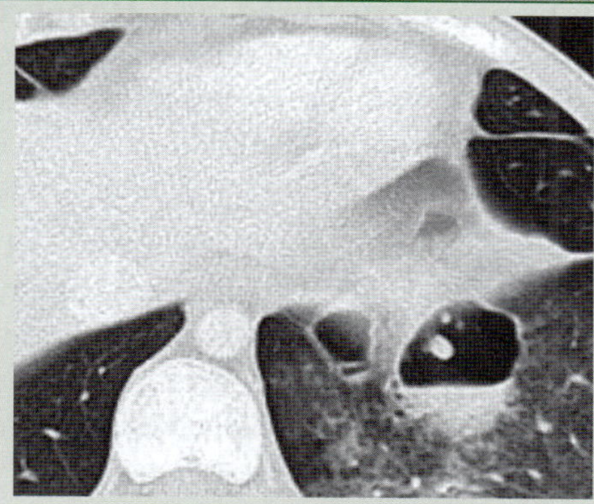 **Fig. 4.103.4:** Lung laceration with pneumatocele
Hiatus hernia—many cases are asymptomatic. It is considered to have an association with gastroesophageal reflux disease.	Herniation of abdominal contents through oesophageal hiatus of diaphragm into thoracic cavity. CT reveals omentum and other contents herniating through phrenico oesophageal ligament into thorax. There are 2 main types of hiatus hernia—sliding (>90%) and rolling (paraoesophageal—less than 10%)	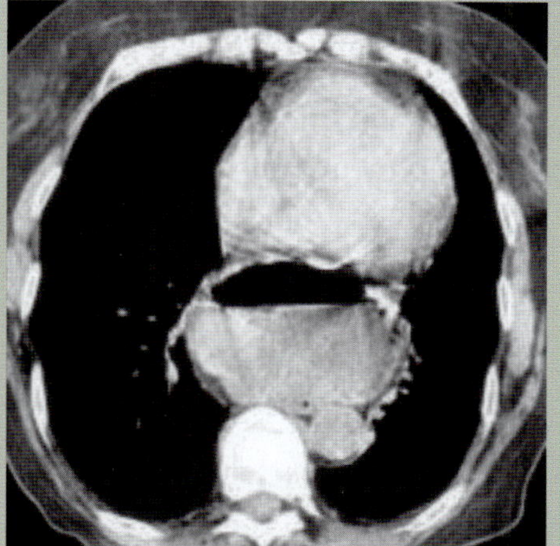 **Fig. 4.103.5:** Hiatus hernia
Cystic/cavitating pulmonary metastases	70% caused by squamous cell carcinoma of lung/head or neck, carcinoma cervix, endometrial carcinoima, all sarcomas, urothelial carcinoma. One of the complications that can occur with cystic lung metastases is development of pneumothoraces.	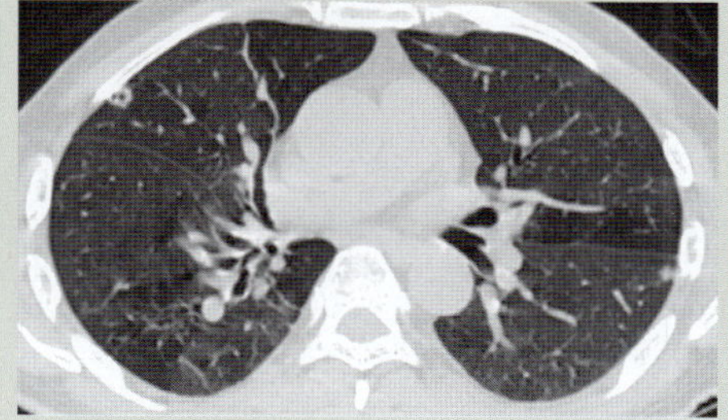 **Fig. 4.103.6:** Cystic lung metastasis

Brief discussion about the condition: Most common site of secondary involvement in children. Hematogeneous spread from liver lesion.

Clinical features: Asymptomatic/eosinophilia (<25%)/sudden cough attacks, hemoptysis, chest pain, fever/expectoration of cyst fluid, membranes and scolices/positive Casoni skin test in 60%/hypersensitivity reaction (if cyst rupture occurs).

Location: Lower lobe in 70% cases. Solitary in 75% cases. Multiple in 30% cases/spherical and ovoid masses.

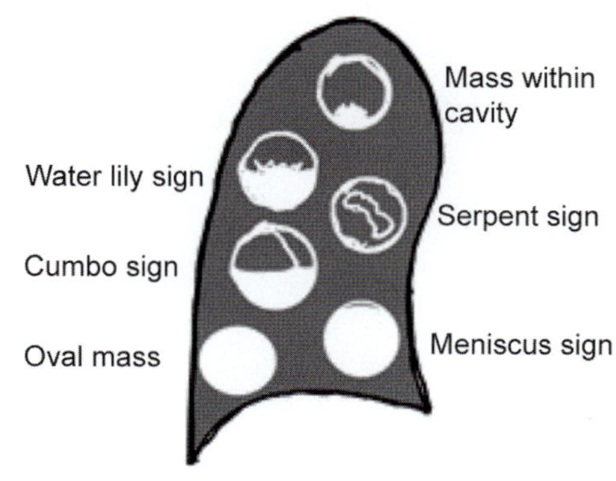

Fig. 4.103.7: Radiological signs of hydatid disease

Radiological signs of lung hydatid (Fig. 4.103.7).

Signs of non-ruptured cyst: Honeycomb sign—multi-vesicular mother cyst with daughter cysts separated by radiating septate representing cyst walls and hydatid sand. **Double line sign**—unilocular cyst with double layered wall representing pericyst and laminated cyst membrane.

Signs of partial rupture: Crescent sign—when the hydatid cyst erodes adjacent bronchus or bronchiole, trapped air between pericyst and laminated membrane of endocyst give a cresecent-shaped rim of air around the cysts. **Inverted cresecent sign**—crescent-shaped rim of air at the lower edge of cyst.

Signs of complete rupture: Cumbo sign (double air sac sign)—air-fluid level inside endocyst, air between pericyst and endocyst with an onion peel appearance. **Water lily sign**—completely collapsed crumpled cyst membrane floating on the cyst fluid. **Empty cyst sign**—empty cavity with thin walls after complete evacuation of hydatid membrane.

Other signs: Meniscus sign—thin radiolucent crescent in uppermost part of cyst (due to rupture of pericyst with air dissecting between pericyst and laminated membrane). Air-fluid level due to rupture of all cyst walls with air entering the endocyst. **Serpent sign**—collapsed membranes inside cyst outlined by air (after expectoration of cyst contents). **Mass within cavity**—crumpled membranes fall to most dependent portion of cavity after complete expectoration of cyst fluid. **Whirl sign**—floating detached membranes in cystic cavity with minimal pleural effusion. **Sign of detachment**—if air enters the potential space between pericyst and ectocyst, local detachment of parasitic membranes from pericyst occurs. **Four treatment options are currently available:** Surgical excision, PAIR (puncture, aspiration, injection of protoscolicidal agent and reaspiration), chemotherapy with an anti-helminthic agent (albendazole, mebendazole), watch and wait for inactive and silent cysts.

4.104 CHEST

Case No. 104

Clinical details: A 59-year-old male patient, who came to the master health checkup for screening chest X-ray.

Radiological techniques and observation: A frontal radiograph (Fig. 4.104.1) of a skeletally mature 59-year-old male. There is a well-defined small opacity in the left upper zone. All borders of the lesion can be visualized and appear rounded. The trachea is in midline and cardiac borders appear normal. The bones, soft tissues of the chest wall appear normal.

The imaging finding is a **solitary pulmonary nodule** in the left upper lobe.

Further imaging: **Serial axial sections** (Figs 4.104.2 and 4.104.3) **of non-contrast and contrast CT thorax images in lung and mediastinal windows have been provided.**

The well-defined, soft tissue dense lesion is present in the left upper lobe and is completely surrounded by normal lung parenchyma. The size is around 1 cm. The margins appear spiculated. There is no internal calcification or fat density. There is no air bronchogram. There is no feeding artery. There is no surrounding ground-glass opacity. On contrast, the lesion shows enhancement with a HU value greater than 15 HU.

Interpretation: A—59-year-old male, lesion is present in the left upper lobe, C—well-defined, soft tissue dense lesion, completely surrounded by normal lung parenchyma. The size is around 1 cm. The margins appear spiculated. B—surrounding lung parenchyma appears normal. There is no evidence of any similar lesions in the opposite lung. There is no calcification or air or internal fat density within the lesion on X-ray (ruling out hamartoma). There is no evidence of a fluid level (abscess). No evidence of cavitation. No evidence of air crescent (aspergilloma). No evidence of any air bronchogram (consolidation). No evidence of mediastinal or hilar enlargement, D—solitary pulmonary nodule.

The principal diagnosis is a possibly malignant solitary nodule of the left upper lobe of lung.

Discussion: **A solitary pulmonary nodule** is as a discrete, well-magrinated, rounded opacity less than or equal to 3 cm in diameter that is completely surrounded by lung parenchyma, does not touch the hilum or mediastinum, and is not associated with adenopathy, atelectasis, or pleural effusion.

- **Mass** is >3 cm
- **Micronodule:** Rounded opacity measuring <3 mm
- **Pseudonodule:** Radiographic nodule mimics—nipple, rib/skin/pleural lesion, artifact, summation of markings.

Role of PET/CT

- PET—positive lung nodules detected in patients over 60 years of age have a 90% likelihood of malignancy.
- Inflammatory nodules may yield false-positive results, indolent and low-grade malignancies such as some adenocarcinomas and carcinoid tumors may yield false-negative results. Lung nodules < 1 cm may also yield false-negative results.
- In general, FDG activity higher than background in a SPN <1.5 cm and SUV >2.5 in any nodule are highly suspicious features for malignancy.

Fleischner 2017 guideline for pulmonary nodule: High risk factors include smoking, exposure to asbestos or radium, family history of lung cancer, older age,

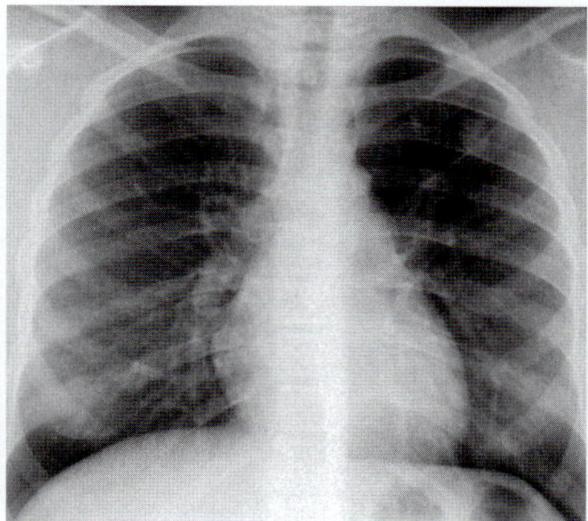

Fig. 4.104.1

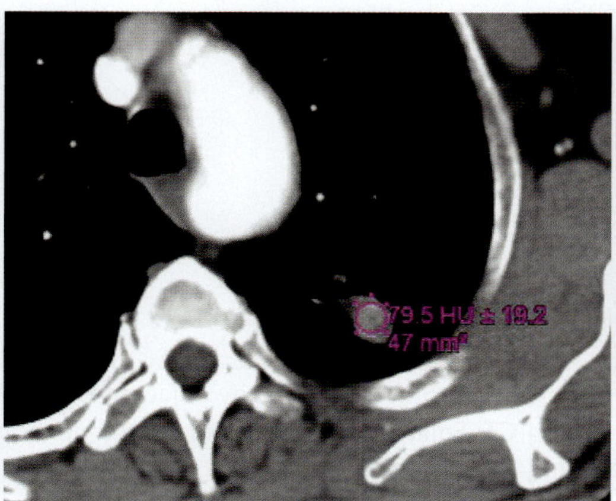

Fig. 4.104.2

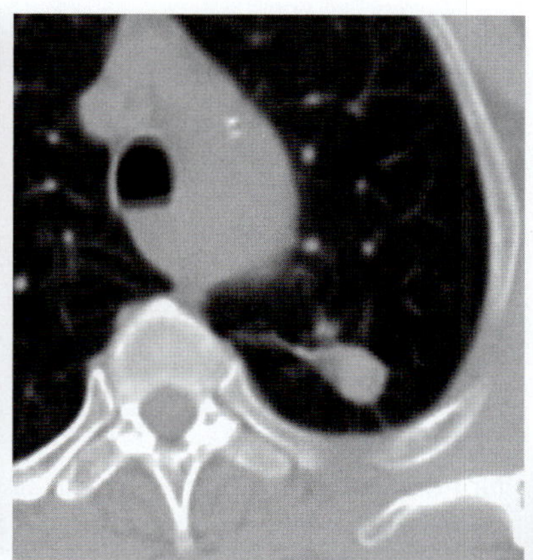

Fig. 4.104.3

Table 4.104.1: Differential diagnoses for solitary pulmonary nodule

Bronchial atresia Congenital focal atresia of usually segmental bronchus	Rounded, tubular, or branching, non-enhancing, low-attenuation mucocele with surrounding wedge-shaped hyperlucent lung (expiratory air trapping). Obstructing central lesion must be ruled out.	
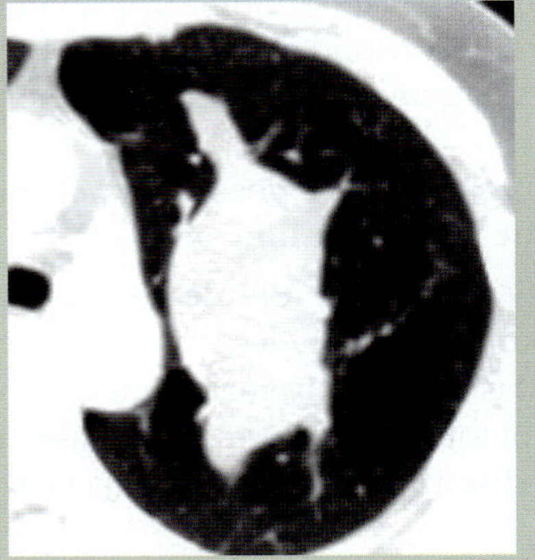 **Fig. 4.104.4:** Bronchial atresia	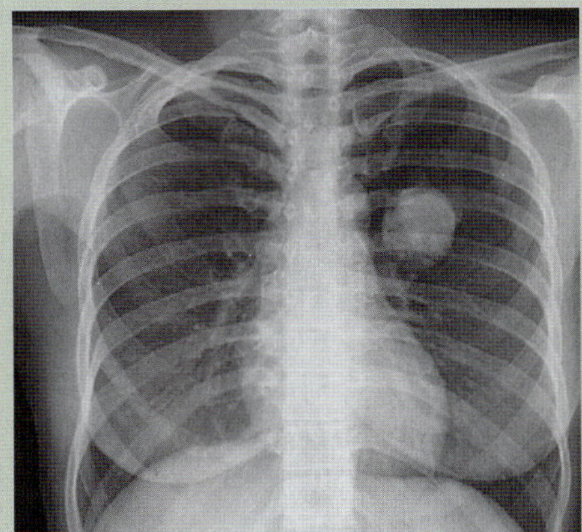 **Fig. 4.104.5:** Bronchial atresia	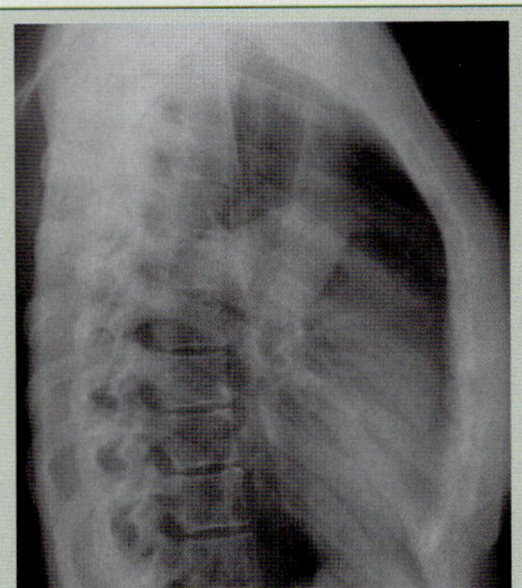 **Fig. 4.104.6:** Bronchial atresia
Hamartoma Benign pulmonary neoplasm containing varying amounts of cartilage, fat, connective tissue, muscle	Solitary nodule or mass, smooth or lobular borders. Calcification more common in larger hamartomas ("popcorn"). Fat attenuation present in 60%. Heterogeneous enhancement with enhancing internal septations. Up to 20% show FDG uptake.	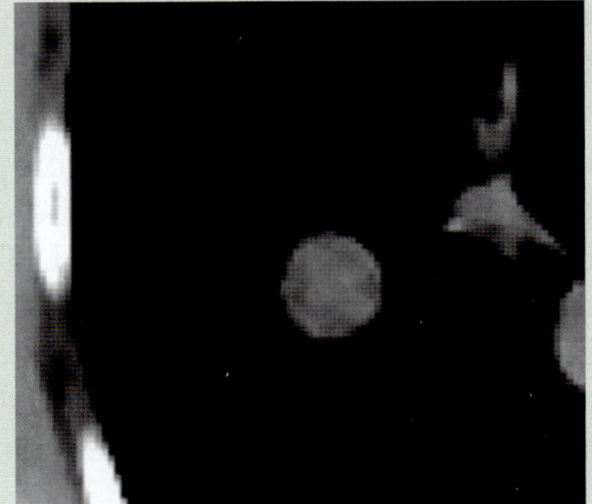 **Fig. 4.104.7:** Hamartoma
Arteriovenous malformation Abnormal direct communication between PA and PVs (right-to-left shunt)	X ray—nodule with feeding vessel, CT—sharply defined round or oval nodule with feeding artery/arteries and draining vein(s). Enhancement equal to vessels on contrast. Tc-99m MAA—to assess size of right to left shunt.	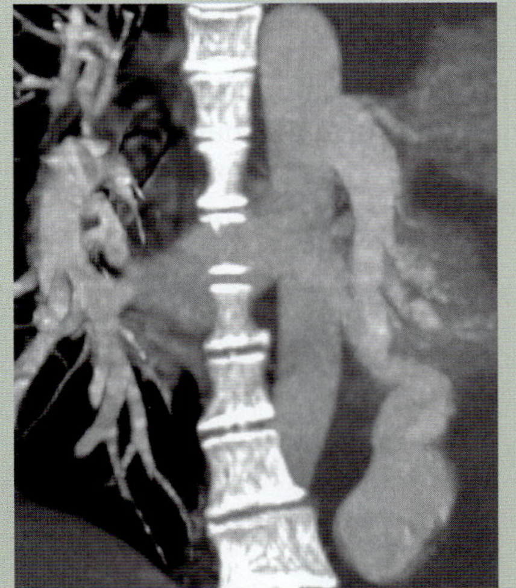 **Fig. 4.104.8:** Arteriovenous malformation
Venous varix Nonobstructive dilatation of 1 or more pulmonary veins at insertion into left atrium	**X-ray:** Soft tissue opacity adjacent to left atrium **CT:** Enlarged confluence of dilated pulmonary vein with maximum enhancement during pulmonary venous phase	

(*Contd.*)

Table 4.104.1: Differential diagnoses for solitary pulmonary nodule (*Contd.*)		
Aspergilloma Occur in individuals with normal immunity but structural abnormalities of lung (cavities)	Well-formed cavity with a central soft tissue rounded mass surrounded by a crescent of air. The mass is spherical or ovoid. On different positioning of the patient, the mass is mobile. Calcification is common. The adjacent pleura may well be thickened. 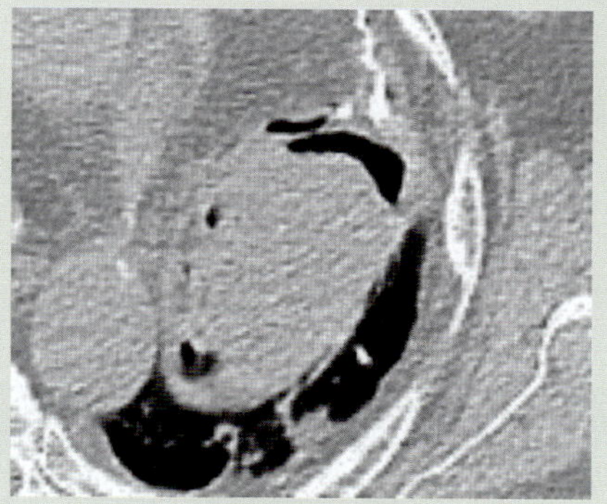 **Fig. 4.104.9:** Aspergilloma	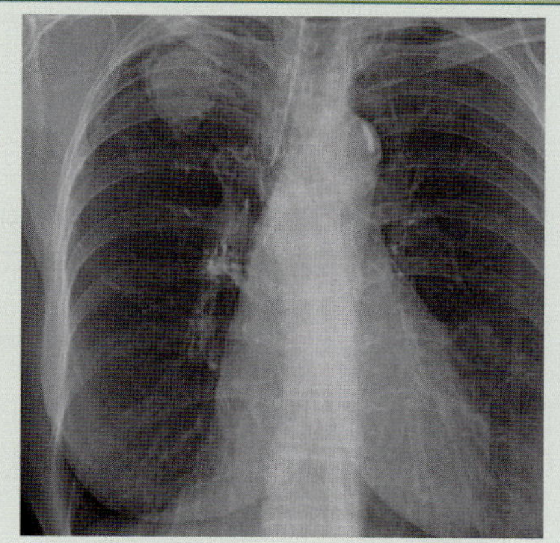 **Fig. 4.104.10:** Aspergilloma

marginal spiculation, upper lobe location, emphysema and pulmonary fibrosis.

Subsolid nodule: Subsolid nodules can be ground glass or part solid. Ground-glass nodules do not obscure the underlying pulmonary vasculature on imaging. Whereas part solid nodule has solid components which may obscure the underlying pulmonary vasculature.

Table 4.104.2: Causes of solitary pulmonary nodules		
Most common	**Uncommon and rare**	Wegener's granuloma
Granuloma	Mucoid impaction	Carcinoid
Less common	Abscess	Sarcoid granuloma
Bronchial carcinoma	Infected bulla	AV malformation
Metastasis	Infarction	Intrapulmonary lipoma
Organizing pneumonia	Hematoma	Intrapulmonary lymph node
Hamartoma	Rheumatoid nodule	Hydatid cyst

Table 4.104.3: Causes of multiple nodules in lung			
Multiple nodules			
• Metastases – Renal – GI – Melanoma – Uterus – Testis – Sarcoma • Uncommon Bronchoalveolar cell CA Lymphoma Kaposi sarcoma	**Infection** • TB • Fungal – Histoplasmosis – Coccidiodomycosis – Invasive aspergillosis • Septic emboli	**Inflammation** • Sarcoid • RA nodules • Wegener's granulomas • Organizing pneumonia **Vascular** • Osler-Weber-Rendu syndrome • Pulmonary infarcts	**Inhalation** • Mucoid impaction (ABPA) • Silicosis **Congenital** • Lung cyst • Bronchial atresia • AVM

Flowchart 4.104.1: Approach to solitary pulmonary nodule

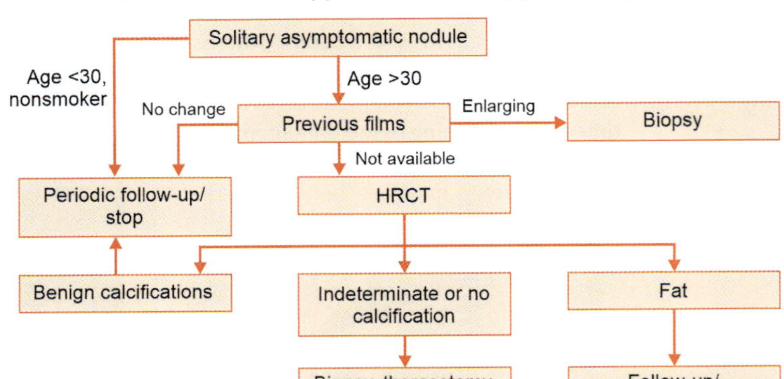

Table 4.104.4: Difference between benign and malignant lung nodule

	Benign	*Malignant*
Shape	Round	Irregular
Size	<3 cm	>3 cm
Spiculations	No	Yes
Edge	Well defined	Ill defined
Satellite lesions	Yes	No
Cavitation	No	Yes
Doubling time (volume)	<1 month or >2 years	>1 month or <2 years
Contrast uptake	Less than 15 HU enhancement	More than 15 HU enhancement
FDG uptake	May be present	Yes

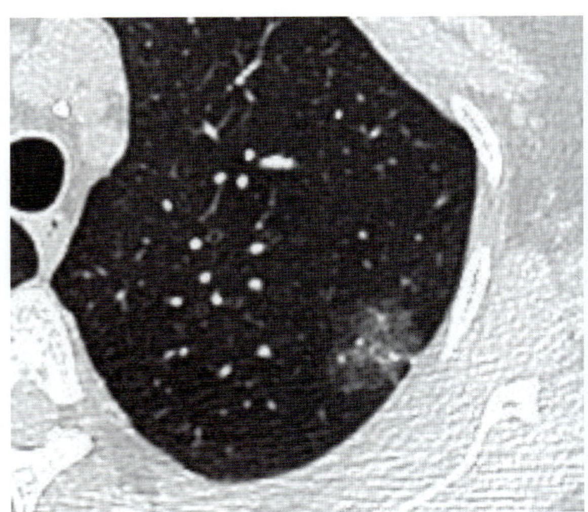

Fig. 4.104.11: Subsolid nodule

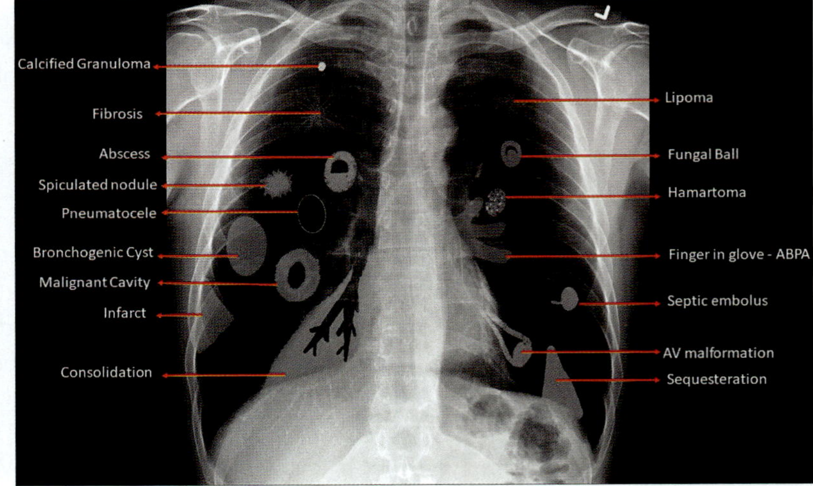

Fig. 4.104.12: Radiological appearances of solitary pulmonary nodules

4.105 CHEST

Case No. 105

Clinical history: A 64 years old female with complaints of chronic cough associated with hemoptysis also new onset partial seizures for 2 months with back pain.

Radiological techniques and observation: The scanogram of the chest. Figure 4.105.1 shows an ill-defined radio-opacity in the left upper zone of the lung. The lesion is surrounded by lung parenchyma and medial border is clearly seen. The left costophrenic angle and cardiophrenic angle is obliterated, with linear opacity in lower zone representing fissural thickening and mild elevation of the left hemidiaphragm. No evidence of rib destruction. No evidence of hilar nodes.

CT chest plain in lung window (Figures 4.105.2 to 4.105.5) shows ill-defined solitary pulmonary mass with spiculated margins and pleural tail in the left upper lobe anterior segment with bronchial cut-off at segmental bronchus, adjacent fissural thickening, fat plane between the mass and mediastinum is lost and pleural tail sign seen. Associated left pleural effusion. The coronal reformatted images of the abdomen and chest in soft tissue window (Figs 4.105.4 and 4.105.5) show the ill-defined lesion with soft tissue density in left

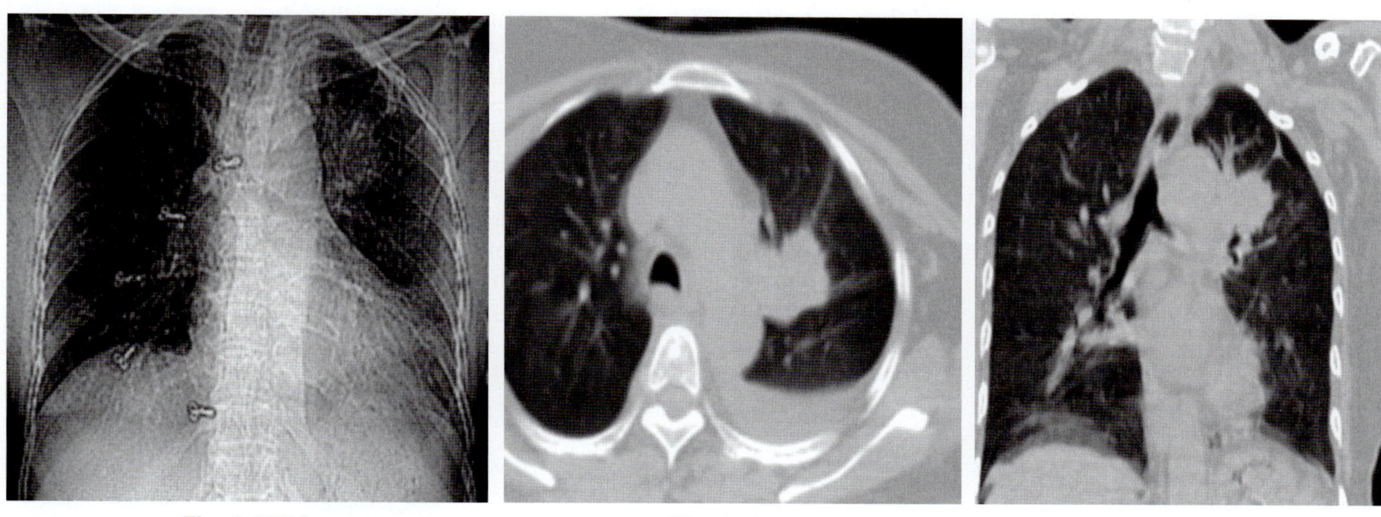

Fig. 4.105.1 Fig. 4.105.2 Fig. 4.105.3

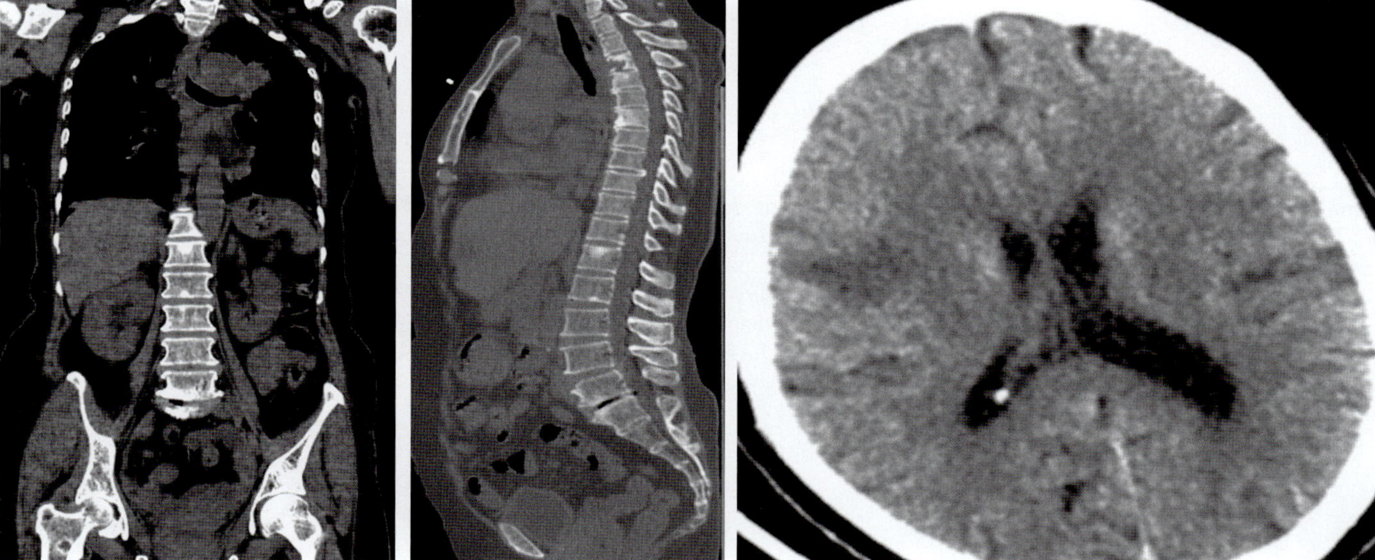

Fig. 4.105.4 Fig. 4.105.5 Fig. 4.105.6

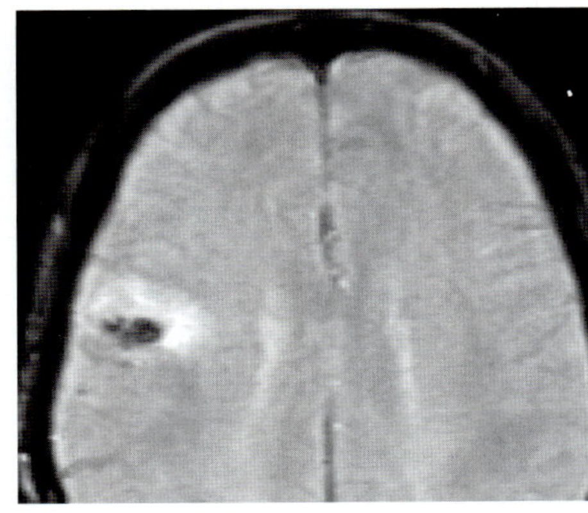

Fig. 4.105.7

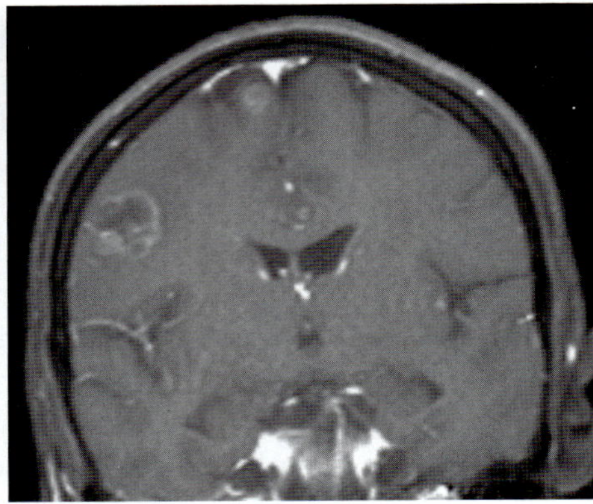

Fig. 4.105.8

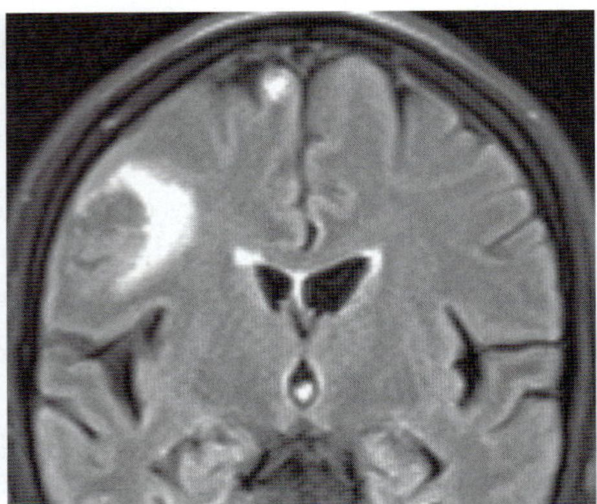

Fig. 4.105.9

Table 4.105.1: Differential diagnosis for lung mass with metastasis

Squamous cell carcinoma of lung These are 20% of the primary lung cancers. Strongly associated with cigarette smoking. Common presentation after 6th decade and in males. Metastasis occurs late. Relatively good prognosis (non-small cell lung carcinoma). Chemotheraphy is mainstay of treatment. Cetuximab given in EGFR positive cases.	HRCT findings are 65% arise in main, lobar or segmental bronchi presents as, endobronchial mass with bronchial obstruction and/or infiltration of bronchial wall with local invasion. Hilar region is the common site. Atelectasis and consolidation common. 30% mass presents as solitary mass or nodule. Pleural effusion may be seen. Cavitation relatively common. Thick walled nodular cavity with thickness of cavity greater than 15 mm is highy suspicious of malignant lesion.	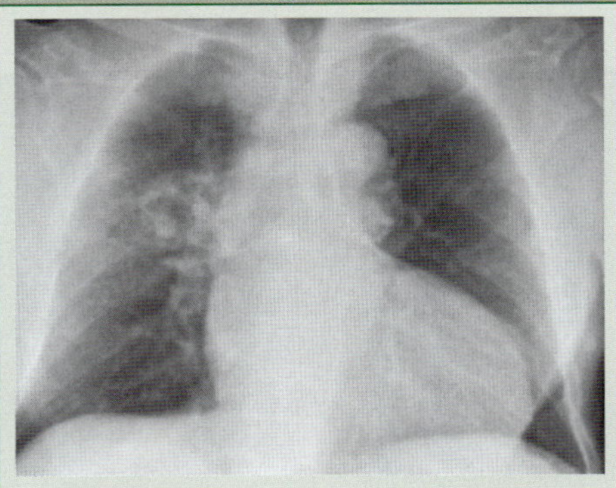 **Fig. 4.105.10:** Squamous cell carcinoma of lung 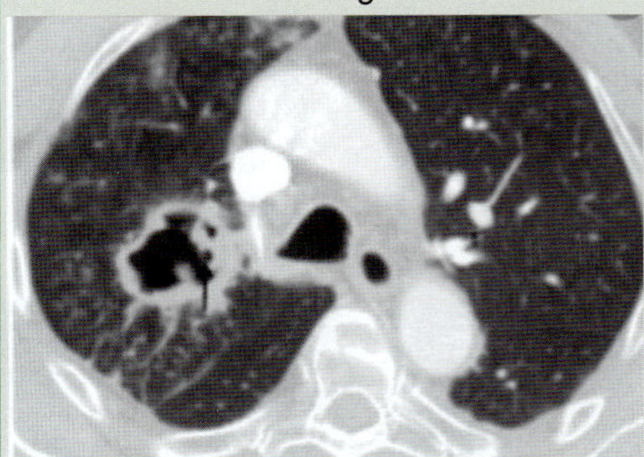 **Fig. 4.105.11:** Squamous cell carcinoma of lung
Small cell carcinoma of lung: 15–20% of lung cancers. Strongly associated with smoking. Typical age group are 60 years and common in males. Paraneoplastic syndrome commonly associated. Treatment is radio and chemotherapy.	In HRCT findings most occur in main or lobar bronchi, extensive peribronchial invasion. Large hilar or parahilar mass. Bronchial narrowing. Lymp node enlargement. Metastases at diagnosis in >90%. Prognosis very poor. FDG-PET will show increased uptake.	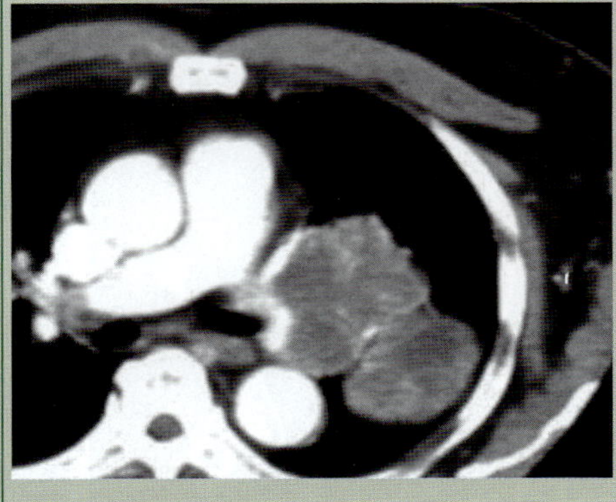 **Fig. 4.105.12:** Small cell carcinoma of lung

Table 4.105.2: Difference between adenocarcinoma, squamous cell carcinoma and small cell lung carcinoma

	Adenocarcinoma	*Squamous cell carcinoma*	*Small cell lung carcinoma*
Prevalance	40–50% of lung cancer cases	20% of lung cancer cases	15–20% of lung cancers
Association with smoking	Weak	Strong	Strong
Location	Upper lobe	Main, lobar and segmental bronchi. Hilar mass	Main and lobar bronchi
Initial CT finding	75% present as peripheral lung nodule.	Endobronchial mass with bronchial obstruction. 30% present as solitary nodule or mass	Large hilar and parahilar mass
Consistency	Solid/part solid and GGO	Mostly solid mass	Solid/part solid mass
CT appearance	Often spiculated. Part solid with surrounding GGO. Lepidic spread. Irregular spiculated mass with pleural tail.	Hilar mass with consolidation and atelectasis. Cavitation common	Extensive peribronchial invasion, large hilar or parahilar mass. Bronchial narrowing. Mediastinal nodes common.
Metastasis	Early metastasis common	Late metastasis	Early, >90% at the time of diagnosis
Prognosis	Relatively good depends on staging	Relatively good	Bad prognosis
Subtypes	Mucinous and non-mucinous subtypes	Keratinizing, non-keratinizing and basaloid	
Specific drug treatment	EGFR and ALK targeted therapy	P40, P63 and negative TTF1 based targeted therapy	It is a neuroendocrine tumor a/w paraneoplastic syndrome

upper lobe and bronchial cut-off. Sagittal reformatted images in bone window show multiple mixed lytic and sclerotic lesions in the visualised dorsolumbar spine. No evidence of focal/multiple liver lesions, no evidence of similar lesions in lung, no evidence of lymphangitic spread. CT brain plain (Fig. 4.105.6) shows heterodense lesion with surrounding edema noted in the right frontoparietal region.

In MRI plain and contrast study (Figs 4.105.7 to 4.105.9) shows T1 hypointense lesion in right fronto-parietal region which appears heterointense on T2/FLAIR and shows blooming on SWI sequence with surrounding edema, also there was a similar lesion in the right para-sagittal ragion. On post-T1 contrast the lesion shows irregular complete ring enhancement. On coronal reformatted images there is a similar lesion seen in the right parasagittal region.

Interpretation: A: 64 years old female, lesion in left upper lobe and brain, C: Ill-defined soft tissue dense mass lesion in the left upper lobe with spiculated margins and pleural tail causing bronchial cut-off of upper lobe bronchus. B: Multiple lytic and sclerotic lesions in multiple veretebral bodies likely to be metastases. T2 hyperintense lesion with surrounding edema and irregular ring enhancement in the right parietal lobe favours brain metastasis. D: Primary lung carcinoma with lymphangitic spread with brain and skeletal metastasis.

Principal diagnosis: Primary lung carcinoma with lymphangitic spread (bronchial cutt-off + fissural thickening + pleural effusion) with brain and skeletal metastasis.

Considering early metastasis, location and morphology of the lesion possibly adenocarcinoma of the lung could be the possible type.

The differential diagnosis are other types of primary lung carcinoma like squamous cell carcinoma, small cell carcinoma, large cell carcinoma, adenosquamous, papillomatous, pecomas, salivary gland type intra-pulmonary tumor, intrapulmonary thymoma, germ cell tumor; solitary lung metastasis—primary from colorectal ca, malignant melanoma, skeletal sarcoma; lymphoma, pulmonary tuberculosis with multifocal extra pulmonary tuberculosis; benign tumors like carcinoid and pulmonary hamartoma mimicking lung mass.

The differential diagnosis for multiple skeletal mixed lytic and sclerotic lesions are multifocal osteomyelitis, myeloma, metastasis.

Causes of Hand Pain in Bronchogenic Carcinoma

- Acral metastasis
- Brachial plexus involvement
- Hypertrophic pulmonary osteoarthropathy

Causes for unilateral elevation of the hemidiaphragm are, **above the diaphragm:** Decreased lung volume, atelectasis/collapse, lobectomy/pneumonectomy, pulmonary hypoplasia, lung mass with phrenic nerve involvement. **Diaphragm:** Phrenic nerve palsy, diaphragmatic eventration, contralateral stroke: Usually middle cerebral artery distribution. **Below the diaphragm:** Hepatomegaly due to liver metastases or primary malignancy, subphrenic abscess, subpulmonic effusion, distended stomach or colon.

Percentage of metastasis to various organs in primary lung cancer: Lung cancer most commonly spread through bloodstream to the liver (34.3%) and adrenal glands (32.6%), followed by bones (14.9%) and other organs involved are central nervous system (CNS) (12%), kidney (10.9%), myocardium (9.1%), pancreas (5.1%), spleen (4%), stomach (2.3%) and small or large intestines (3.4%), thyroid gland (1.7%), and the ovary (0.6%).

Lung lesions causing paraneoplastic syndrome.

- Small cell carcinoma (ACTH)—Cushing's syndrome
- Squamous cell carcinoma (PTH)—hyperparathyroidism
- Carcinoid tumor (serotonin)—serotonin syndrome
- Large cell neuroendocrine carcinoma
- Atypical carcinoid
- DIPNECH (diffuse intraparencymal neuroendocrine hyperplasia).

Large cell carcinoma of lung: It is a high grade neuroendocrine carcinoma. It is round or oval-shaped mass commonly locate in periphery of lung. Size usually ranges from 1 to 9 cm. In CT typically lobulated and sharply marginated. Post-contrast in homogeneous enhancement. Better prognosis than SCLC.

Lymphoma: It can be broadly divided as primary or secondary lymphoma: Primary pulmonary lymphoma is confined to the lung associaed with or without mediastinal lymphadenopathy and without evidence of extrathoracic disease for at least three months after the first diagnosis. Low-grade B-cell lymphoma (MALToma)—commonest of primary lymphoma.

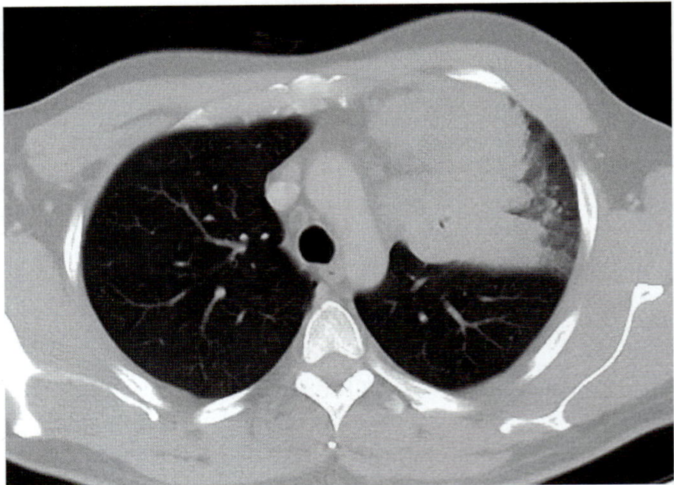

Fig. 4.105.13: Large cell carcinoma of lung

Two additional categories have been described which include:

- PTLD-lymphoma in patients with post-transplant lymphoproliferative disorders
- AIDS-related pulmonary lymphoma (ARL/ARPL)

HRCT findings in lymphoma:

- A mass or mass-like consolidation greater than 1 cm with or without cavitations or bronchograms
- Masses of pleural origin
- Nodules <1 cm
- Alveolar or interstitial infiltrates
- Peribronchial or perivascular thickening with or without atelectasis
- Pleural effusions
- Hilar or mediastinal lymphadenopathy

Solitary metastasis: It accounts for 3–5% of asymptomatic nodules. 25% of pulmonary metastases may be solitary. Most likely primary tumors are breast, sarcoma, seminoma and renal cell carcinoma. Predilection for the lung periphery. Calcification is rare but when present suggests metastatic osteosarcoma, or chondrosarcoma.

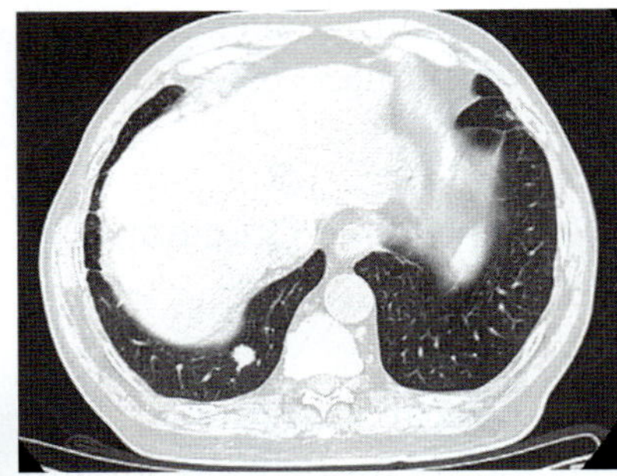

Fig. 4.105.14: Solitary pulmonary metastasis

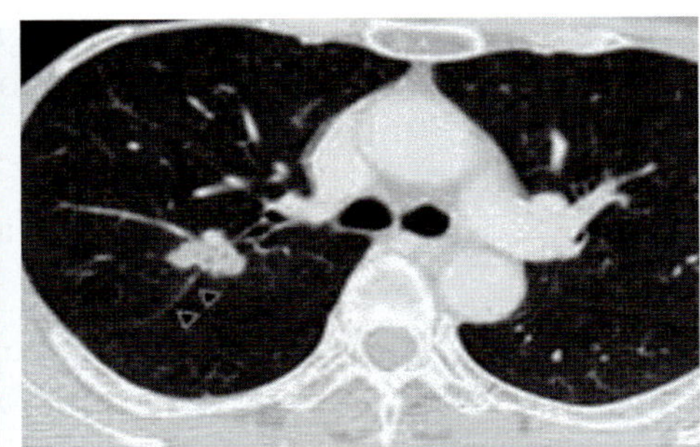

Fig. 4.105.15: Sarcoidosis

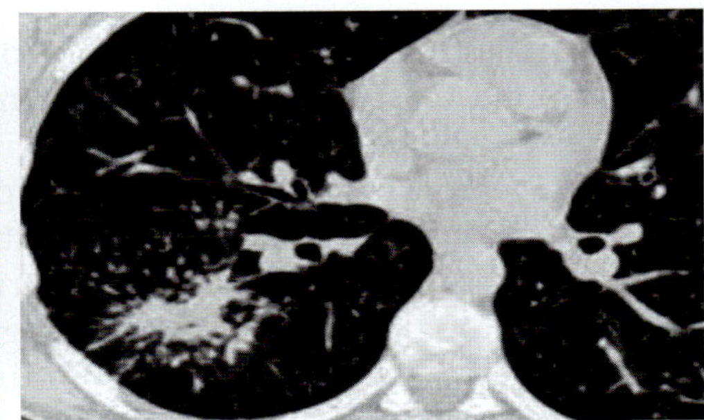

Fig. 4.105.16: Granulomatous lesion

Granulomatous lesion mimicking carcinoma, tuberculoma—more common in upper lobes and on right side. Well defined (0.5 to 4 cm in size). 25% lobulated. 80% have satellite lesions.

Sarcoidosis: Solitary mass simulating malignancy.Galaxy sign is seen in CT. Associated hilar and para tracheal lymphadenpathy with egg shell calcifications are seen.

Wegener's granulomatosis: Solitary nodules in up to one-third of patients.

Histoplasma: More frequent in lower lobes. Well defined (<3 cm). Target calcification.

Benign tumors:

Carcinoid tumor: Typical carcionoid are major accounts for 90% of cases, tend to benign and central in location. May be associated with ectpoic ACTH production.

Hamartoma: 96% occurs over the age of 40 years. 90% intra-pulmonary usually, 2 cm from the pleura. Well-defined <4 cm. Popcorn calcifications (calcifications in 30% cases, 75% if >5 cm).

Further management: Further HPE and PET-CT to be done for staging and molecular subtyping of the lesion. Also immunohistochemistry is done prior to treatment.

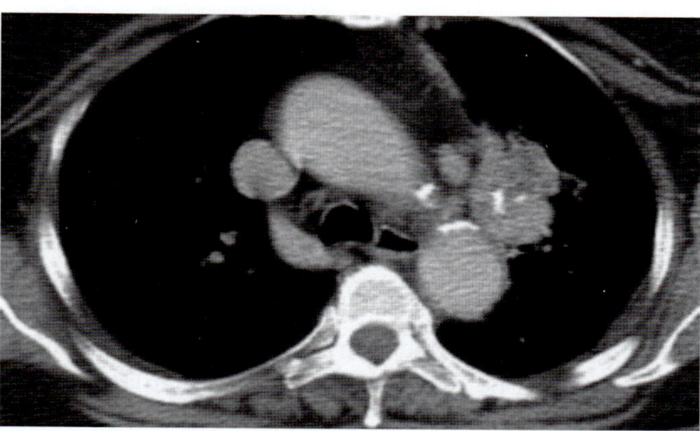

Fig. 4.105.17: Carcinoid tumor

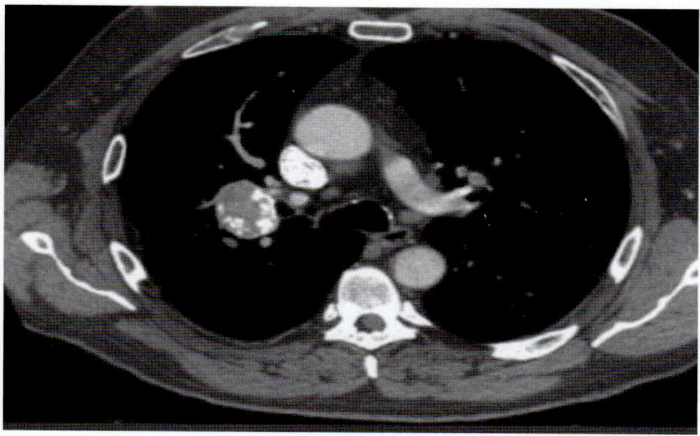

Fig. 4.105.18: Hamartoma

Treatment and prognosis vary not only with stage but also with cell type. In general, surgery, chemotherapy, and radiotherapy are offered according to the stage, resectability, operability, and functional status.

PET-CT plays an important role in the evaluation of solitary nodules.

When performing PET-CT, have to realize the following: PET has a very high sensitivity 95%, but a lesser specificity of only 81%. PET is false positive in granulomatous disease. PET is usually false negative in small lesions. With these specificity numbers, there will be false positives in about 20%, depending on the background prevalence of granulomatous disease.

Treatment

- Operable disease (stage I to IIIA): Surgery
- Unresectable disease: Neoadjuvant chemotherapy, radiotherapy
- Advanced disease: Palliative combined chemotherapy
- Prognosis (5-year survival rates)
- Local (stage I): 55–67%
- Locally advanced (stages II–IIIA): 23–40%
- Advanced (stages IIIB and IV): 1–3%

Small-cell carcinoma treatment

- Limited disease: Chemoradiotherapy
- Extensive disease: Palliative combined chemotherapy prognosis is poor. In limited the 5-year survival rate 15–25% and in extensive it is 2-year survival rate 20% (with palliative combined chemotherapy and supportive care).

TNM staging, The IASLC (International Association for the Study of Lung Cancer), 8th edition, lung cancer staging system

Stage 0—TNM equivalent: Tis, N0, M0

Stage Ia—TNM equivalent: T1, N0, M0 (5-year survival: up to 92%)

Stage Ib—TNM equivalent: T2a, N0, M0 (5-year survival: 68%)

Stage IIa—TNM equivalent: T2b, N0, M0 (5-year survival: 60%)

Stage IIb—TNM equivalent: T1/T2, N1, M0 or T3, N0, M0 (5-year survival: 53%)

Stage IIIa—TNM equivalent: T1/T2, N2, M0 or T3/T4, N1, M0 or T4, N0, M0 (5-year survival: 36%)

Stage IIIb—TNM equivalent: T1/T2, N3, M0 or T3/T4, N2, M0 (5-year survival: 26%)

Stage IIIc—TNM equivalent: T3/T4, N3, M0 (5-year survival: 13%)

Table 4.105.3: T-staging for lung carcinoma
T1—<= 3 cm
T2—>3 <5 cm hilar and visceral pleura
T3—>5 <7 cm-parietal, pericardial, chest wall and phrenic nerve infiltration
T4—>7 cm with mediastinum and diaphragm infiltration
No—no regional nodes
N1—ipsilateral regional, hilar (10) nodes
N2—ipsilateral mediastinal and subcarinal nodes (7)
N3—contralateral hilar, mediastinal and ipsilateral supraclavicular
M0—no metastasis
M1a—opposite lung, pleura and pericardium
M1b—single extra thoracic metastasis
M1c—multiple extra thoracic metastasis

Stage IVa—TNM equivalent: Any T, any N with M1a/M1b (5-year survival: 10%)
Stage IVb—TNM equivalent: Any T, any N with M1c (5-year survival: 0%)

Brief discussion about the condition: Primary lung carcinoma.

Primary signs of malignancy

- Mass (>3 cm) or nodule (<3 cm) with spiculated and irregular borders
- Unilateral enlargement of hilum: Mediastinal widening or hilar prominence
- Associated with cavitation: Most common in upper lobes or superior segments of lower lobes.
- Wall thickness is indicative of malignancy.
- <4 mm: 95% of cavitated lesions are mostly benign lesions.
- >15 mm: 85% of cavitated lesions are mostly malignant lesions.
- Cavitation is common in SCC.

Table 4.105.4: Types of carcinoma and their location

Tumor	*Frequency*	*Location*	*Comments*
Adenocarcinoma	40%	Peripheral	Scar carcinoma
Squamous carcinoma	20%	Central, peripheral	cavitation
Small cell carcinoma	15%	Central, peripheral	Endocrine activity
Large carcinoma	1%	Central, peripheral	Large mass

Certain tumors may present as chronic airspace disease: Bronchoalveolar carcinoma, lymphoma. Sometime air bronchograms are commonly seen by HRCT in adenocarcinoma.

Secondary signs of malignancy

- Atelectasis (Golden inverted "S" sign in RUL collapse)
- Obstructive pneumonia
- Pleural effusion
- Interstitial patterns: Lymphangitic tumor spread
- Hilar and mediastinal adenopathy
- Metastases to ipsilateral, contralateral lung

Malignant solitary nodules are usually >2 cm. Accounts for less than 15% of all solitary nodules at 40 years, almost 100% at 80 years. However, up to 38% of small (< 1 cm) nodules identified by CT may be primary lung cancer. Radiological appearances suggesting malignancy include recent appearance or rapid growth (review previous CXRs), size greater than 4 cm, the lesion crosses a fissure (although some fungal infections may also do so), ill-defined margins, umbilicated or notched margin (if present it indicates malignancy in 80%), corona radiata (spiculation) (but also seen in PMF and granulomas), peripheral line

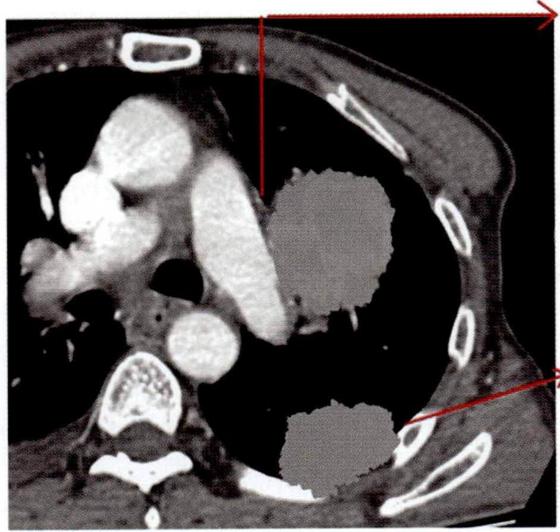

Fig. 4.105.19: Criteria for mediastinal invasion in lung carcinoma

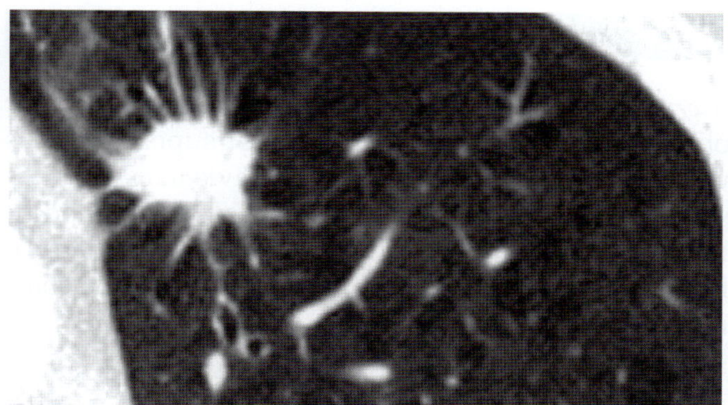

Fig. 4.105.20: Corona radiata sign in malignant lesion

shadows. Calcification is rare (but seen in up to 10% at CT). Most lung cancers appear 'solid'on CT although foci of low (fluid) attenuation, denoting necrosis, may be present. Recent evidence points to significance of pure ground-glass/part-solid ground-glass nodules larger than 5 mm diameter and indicates that these may represent premalignant lesions, adenocarcinoma *in situ* or malignant adenocarcinoma.

CT criterion for abnormal nodes: Short-axis diameter of lymph node more than 1 cm (60–70%).

Chest wall invasion: Accuracy for detection of chest wall invasion by CT is 40–60%.

Radiographic features: Soft tissue mass in chest wall, Bone destruction, obtuse angle at contact between tumor and pleura, >3 cm of contact between tumor and pleura, pleural thickening, increased density of extrapleural fat.

Mediastinal invasion: CT findings regarded as indicating "definite" or "gross" mediastinal invasion and unresectability are extensive replacement of mediastinal fat by soft-tissue mass, mass surrounding mediastinal vessels, trachea, or esophagus, mass resulting in obvious invasion of one of these structures.

Additional CT findings: Tumor contact of more than 3 cm with the mediastinum, tumor contact with more than one-fourth (90°) of the circumference of the aorta or other mediastinal structures, obliteration of the fat planes that are normally seen adjacent to the aorta or other mediastinal structures, compression of mediastinal structures by a mass and mediastinal pleural or pericardial thickening.

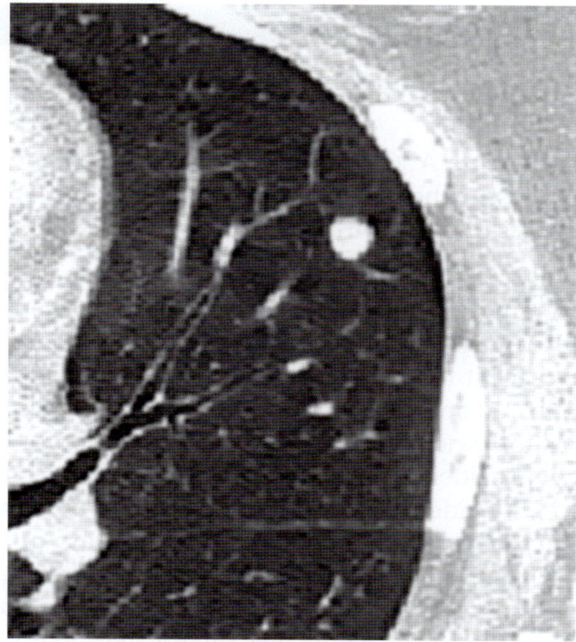

Fig. 4.105.21: Smooth margin in benign lesion

Margin: Corona radiata sign—highly suggestive of malignancy, lobulated or scalloped margins—intermediate probability. Smooth margins—more likely benign unless metastatic in origin.

Air bronchogram sign: It is commonly seen in adenocarcinoma.

Solid and ground-glass components: Another result from screening studies is that nodules containing a ground-glass component are mostly malignant. Part solid lesions with ground-glass areas had a malignancy rate of 63%. Nonsolid-only ground-glass lesions has a malignancy rate of 18%. Lesions with only solid components had a malignancy rate of only 7%.

4.106 CHEST

Case No. 106

Clinical details: A 56-year-old man presented with cough, sensory loss in the region of right ulnar distribution and hoarseness of voice for last 2 months.

Radiological imaging technique and observation: Scanogram (Fig. 4.106.1) shows a homogenous opacity in the apex of the left lobe and upper zone of left lung with adjacent 1st and 2nd rib destruction. Left superior mediastinal margin is obscured by lesion causing mediastinal widening. Mild tracheal deviation to right noted. No evidence of air bronchogram/air alveologram noted. No evidence of elevated hemidiaphragm/juxta phrenic peak. Right and left heart borders appear normal. Cardiophrenic and costophrenic angles appear normal. Rest of the lung fields appear normal. CT plain and contrast serial axial images (Figs 4.106.2 to 4.106.6) at the level of thoracic inlet shows ill-defined soft tissue mass measuring approximately 8.4 × 8.2 × 8 cm extending laterally into left costoclavicular space and causing erosion of the 1st and 2nd ribs. The lesion has chest wall contact for length of approximately 8 cm, it also has mediastinal contact for length of 2.5 cm. There is no elevation of hemidiaphragm (elevation indicates the phrenic nerve palsy due to infiltration). Loculated pleural effusion is seen on the right side.

Interpretation: A—56 year old male, lesion in right upper lobe, C—ill defined soft tissue mass (superior sulcus tumor) extending laterally into costoclavicular space, B—eroding the 1st and 2nd ribs and dorsal vertebral body, transverse process and pedicle. There is asymmetrical thickening of the apical pleura in left side, D—pancoast tumor

Principal diagnosis: Pancoast tumor (superior sulcus tumour) with TNM staging of T4N1M0.

Further management: Refer urgently to chest physician. MRI to assess the brachial plexus involvement, spinal canal extension local staging of soft tissue mass, and antomy. Biopsy to confirm the diagnosis, PET scan for systemic staging and Multi-disciplinary Tumor Board for management.

Elevated Ipsilateral Dome of Diaphragm in Lung Mass

- Pulmonary collapse
- Phrenic nerve palsy
- Hepatic metastasis
- Subpulmonic effusion (pseudodiaphragm)

Golden S sign: Chest radiograph shows in right upper lobe collapse created by central mass obstructing the upper lobe bronchus and should raise suspicion of bronchogenic carcinoma. It is also seen in the following

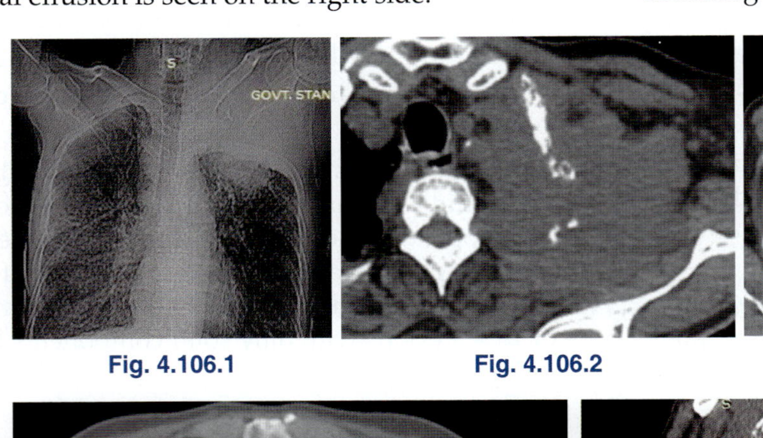

Fig. 4.106.1 Fig. 4.106.2

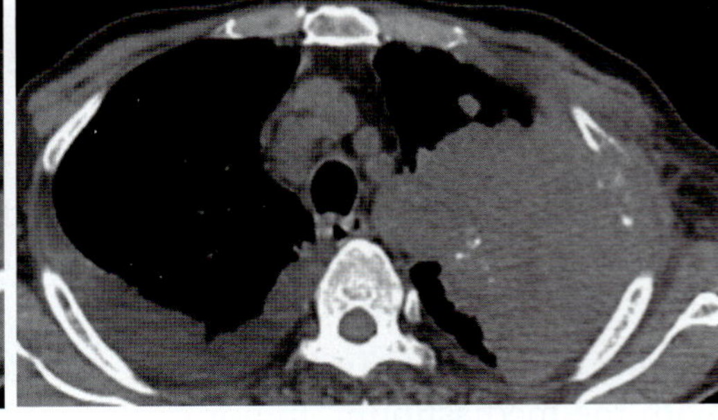

Fig. 4.106.3

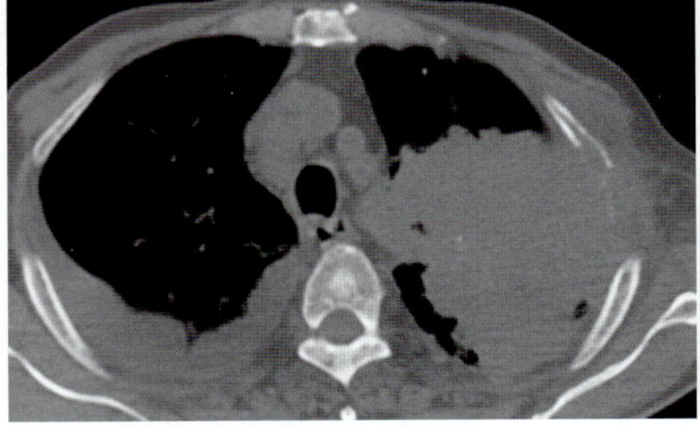

Fig. 4.106.4

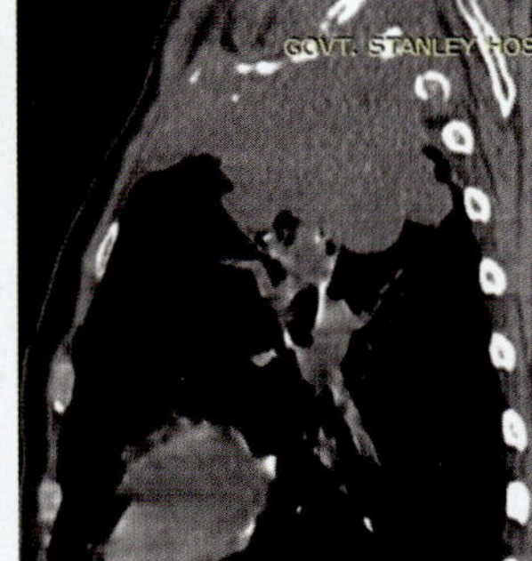

Fig. 4.106.5

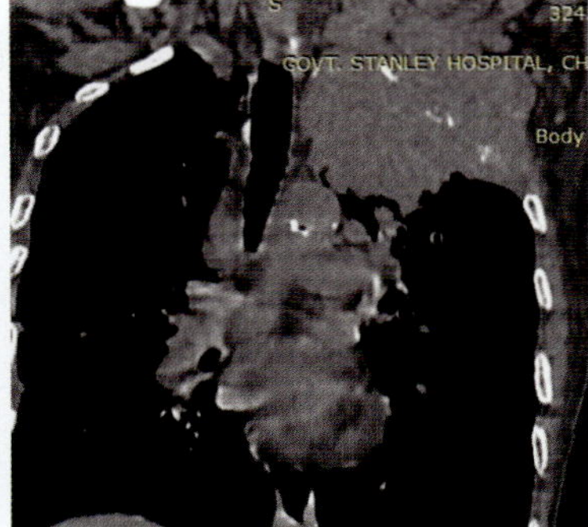

Fig. 4.106.6

<table>
<tr><th colspan="3">Table 4.106.1: Differential diagnosis for apical cap: Apical cap is asymmetrical apical pleural thickening more than 5 mm</th></tr>
<tr><td colspan="3">Normal apical cap: Unilateral or bilateral apical caps. usually <5 mm in thickeness seen in 10% normal chest radiograph</td></tr>
<tr><td>Extrapleural fat : Extrapleural fat deposition causes smooth, symmetrical apical cap seen in normal, obese, cushing and patient on steroid treatment.</td><td colspan="2">On plain radiograph seen as soft tissue shadow may confuse with pleural thickening or pleural plaques. It occurs from inward displacement of extrapleural fat by extrapleural mass or extrapleural hematoma.</td></tr>
<tr><td>Inflammatory disease(tuberculosis): It is rare and associated with upper lobe fibrosis, volume loss and lung destruction. The cap appears as irregular due to adjacent lung abnormality.</td><td colspan="2">On radiograph extensive cavitating nodular opacities in the right upper lobe. Focal pleural thickening visualized in the upper lobe . Post primary TB shows consolidation predominantly apex and upper lung zone, nodules and cavitation.</td></tr>
<tr><td>Mesothelioma: It can be benign or malignant pleural mesothelioma. Benign mesothelioma <5% of all pleural tumors not associated with asbestos exposure. Mean age 50–60 years. Excision is the curative treatment. On progression causes malignant degeneration.</td><td colspan="2">Radiograph well-defined spherical or ovoid lobular mass making obtuse angle towards chest. Ipsilateral pleural effusion CT: Cirucmferential and nodular irregular pleural thickening (>1 cm) and homogenous mass with intermediate to high attenuation with calcifications and hemorrhage, also mediastinal pleural is involved. Frozen mediastinum sign is seen. Shows heterogeneous enhancement of conrast. MRI: T1 hypo- and T2 hyperintensity. Malignant mesothelioma associated with asbestos exposure most common primary tumor of pleura. Mean age 50–70 years</td></tr>
<tr><td>Radiation fibrosis: Radiation therapy can cause apical fibrosis mimicking an apical cap. It is commonly associated with head, neck and supraclavicular nodes radiation.</td><td colspan="2">On plain radiograph: Hazy opacity progressively becoming more reticular or linear with volume loss, architectural distortion, mediastinal shift, hemidiaphragm elevation. CT post-contrast does not demonstrate enhancement, useful in differentiating from recurrence. Treatment: Once fibrosis established, no treatment, only follow-up for assessment of tumor recurrence.</td></tr>
<tr><td>Plasmacytoma: Discrete solitary tumor of neoplastic monoclonal plasma cell in bone or soft tissue. There are two types: (1) Solitary bone plasmacytoma, (2) extramedullary plasmacytoma. Pain at the site of skeletal lesion due to bone destruction by infiltrating plasma cell tumor. Treatment consists of radiotherapy alone or surgery alone or combination of two depending on location and resectibility of plasmacytoma.</td><td>Radiograph shows well defined "punched out" lytic lesion with associated extra-osseous soft tissue masses. In advanced plasmacytoma marked erosion, expansion, destruction of the bone cortex, with thick ridging around the periphery giving "soap bubble" appearance. On CT lytic lesion or small soft tissue masses are visualized. It has high rate of progression to multiple myeloma.</td><td>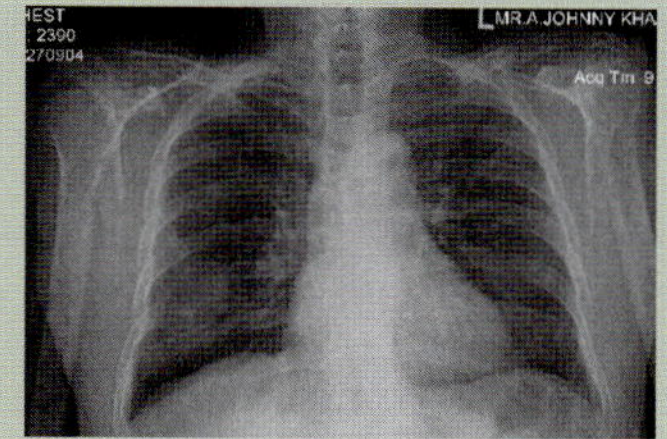
Fig. 4.106.7: Plasmacytoma rib</td></tr>
<tr><td colspan="3">Subclavian artery aneurysm: Extremely rare condition.</td></tr>
<tr><td colspan="3">Ankylosing spondylitis: Chronic multisystem inflammatory disorder, present with articular and extra-articular features. Affect the tracheobronchial tree and the lung parenchyma, and respiratory complications include chest wall restriction, apical fibrobullous disease. Bilateral upper lobe fibrosis can occur.</td></tr>
<tr><td>Chronic hypersensitivity pneumonitis: Indicates the end-stage of repeated or persistent pneumonitis.
HRCT—shows centrilobular peribronchiolar nodular opacities–micronodules of varying numbers.
It shows ground-glass opacity, mosaic perfusion, pulmonary fibrosis and honey-combing.</td><td>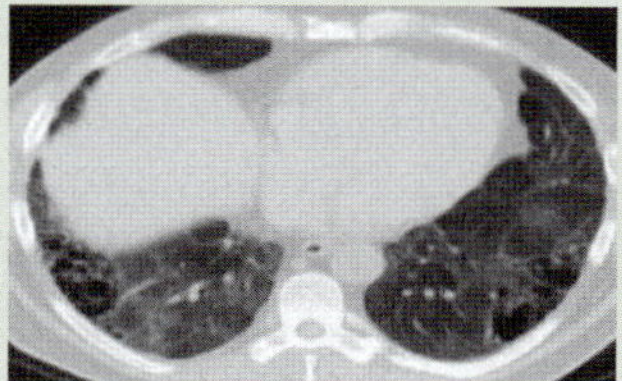
Fig. 4.106.8a: Chronic hypersensitivity pneumonitis</td><td>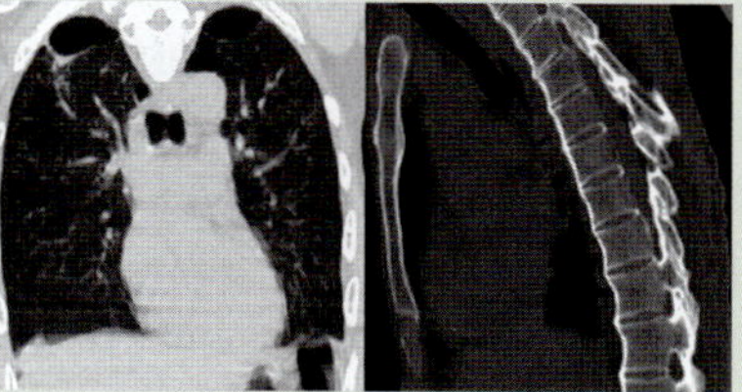
Fig. 4.106.8b: Ankylosing spondylitis with upper lobe fibrosis</td></tr>
<tr><td colspan="3">Cystic schwannoma: Can mimic a upper lobe mass.</td></tr>
<tr><td>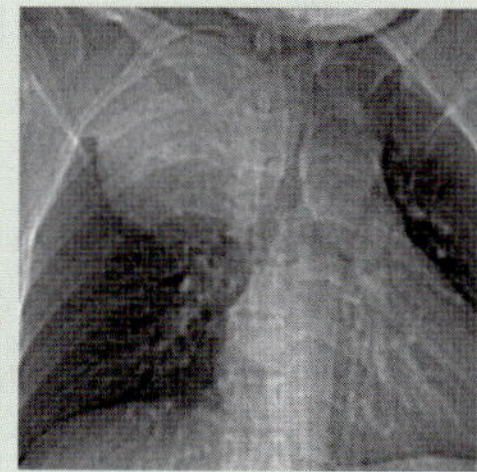
Fig. 4.106.9: Cystic schwannoma mimicking an upper lobe mass</td><td>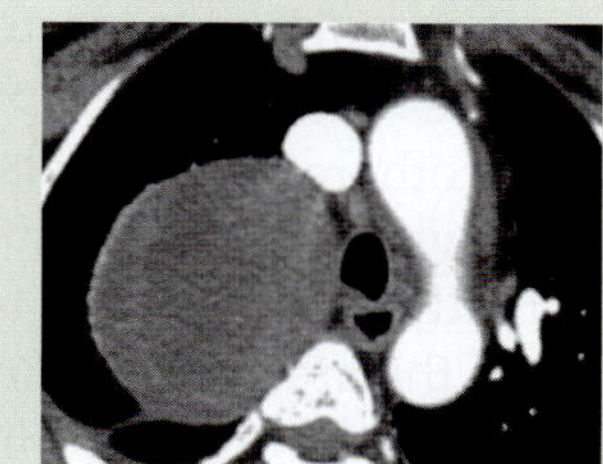
Fig. 4.106.10: Cystic schwannoma mimicking an upper lobe mass</td><td>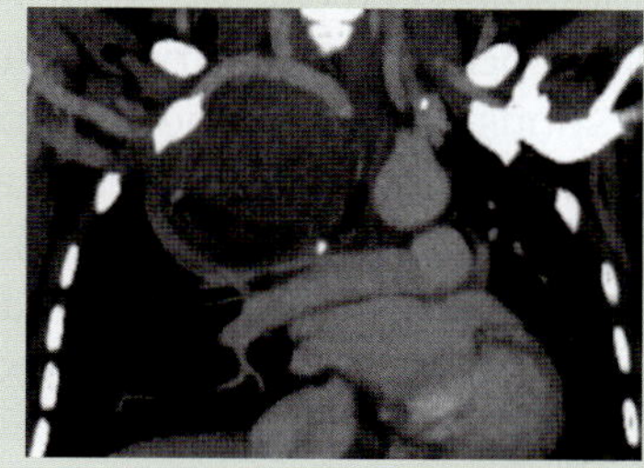
Fig. 4.106.11: Cystic schwannoma mimicking an upper lobe mass</td></tr>
</table>

Table 4.106.2: Differentials for lytic rib lesion with lung infiltration

Metastasis: Metastasis usually from thyroid, breast, esophagus, renal cell carcinoma and prostate cancer, but commonly breast cancer can cause Pancoast syndrome. In children neuroblastoma can present as chest wall mass.	CT will help to know extent of bony involvement and lung infiltration. MRI gives an idea about bone marrow status. Primary lesion in breast and axillary lymph nodes help in differentiating from other tumor causing Pancoast tumor
Lymphoma: Occurs in <5% in all bone tumor and 5% of extranodal lymphoma. Non-Hodgkin's lymphoma with diffuse large B cell lymphoma is common (80%). Median age 36–52 years. Local swelling and palpable mass. Treatment is radiation and chemotheraphy following staging and extraskeletal involvement.	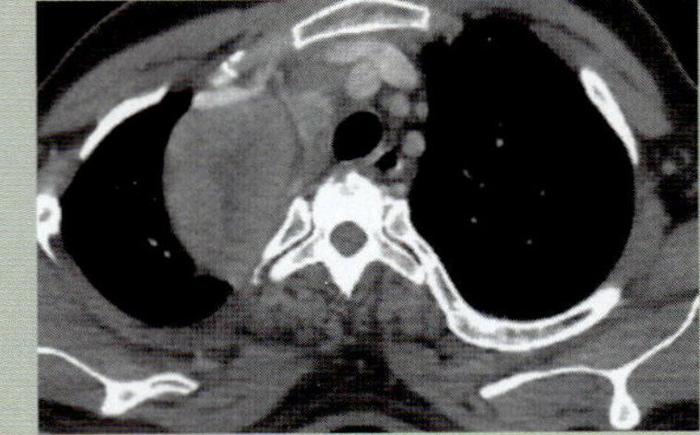 **Fig. 4.106.12:** Lymphoma
Chondrosarcoma/fibrosarcoma: It can be primary or secondary and classified into central, peripheral, clear cell, synovial and extraskeletal chondrosarcoma. Mean age of chondrosarcoma occurring in rib is 45 years. Treatment wide resection.	CT-expansile lesion with chondroid matrix with ring and arcs/ floculent/stippled pattern of calcification. CT helps in identifying extension into soft tissue and lung parenchyma MRI: T1hypo and T2 hyperintense but calcified portions appears hypointense in T2. Bone scan shows increased uptake.
Ewing sarcoma: It is also called a skin tumor/PNET. Mean age of presentation is 14.5 years. Chest wall mass with/without pain. Large tumor involving chest wall and pleura with high vascularity causing rib destruction (25–63%) associated with lung parenchymal extension (25%) and calcifications (10%). Often large pleural effusion is seen.	CT: Large heterogenous chest wall mass with intra and extrathoracic component. Pleural, vertebral, pericardial extension can be seen. MR: Intermediate signal intensity on T1 and hyperintense on T2. Nuclear medicine. Increased uptake in pentreotide111 + TC^{99}-MIBI scan.

conditions like metastasis, primary mediastinal tumor, enlarged lymph nodes.

Signs of lung collapse: *Direct sign*—displacement of interlobar fissures, crowding of pulmonary vessels, loss of aeration. *Indirect sign*—elevation of the ipsilateral hemidiaphragm with or without juxtaphrenic peak sign, crowding of ipsilateral ribs, mediastinal shift towards the side of atelectasis, compensatory hyperinflation of normal lobes, hilar displacement towards the collapse and shifting granuloma sign.

Brief Discussion about the condition: Pancoast tumor described by Henry Pancoast in 1932. Also known as superior sulcus tumor, thoracic inlet carcinoma, or simply apical carcinoma. The cancer arises from apex of the lung and invading the surrounding soft tissue. It is non-small cell cancer. Approximately 3 to 5% of lung cancers occur in the superior sulcus; any cell type may be responsible, but adenocarcinoma predominates. These tumor causes invasion of brachial plexus, cervicothoracic sympathetic ganglia, subclavian artery and vein and vertebral column. The abnormality on chest radiograph may be easily missed as it is located in one of the areas known as "blind spot". Pancoast syndrome from involvement of the brachial plexus and sympathetic ganglia and consists of the combination of:

1. Pain in the shoulder.
2. Radicular pain along the distribution of the eighth cervical and first and second thoracic nerves, sometimes associated with wasting of the small muscles of the hand.
3. Horner's syndrome, consisting of ptosis, miosis, and hemifacial anhidrosis.

Radiographic finding: An apical mass (60%), unilateral or asymmetrical apical pleural thickening ("apical cap," 40%), and bone destruction (25%). Asymmetry pleural thickness of an apical >5 mm is highly suggestive of Pancoast tumor. Treatment is a combination of pre- or postoperative radiation, chemotherapy, and en bloc resection of the tumor and adjacent chest wall; 5-year survival rates as high as 30 to 50% have been reported using this approach. Contraindications to this therapy include: (1) Tumor involvement of the great vessels above the lung apex, principally the subclavian artery or vein; (2) extensive brachial plexus invasion; (3) extensive vertebral body or spinal canal invasion; (4) clinical evidence of recurrent laryngeal nerve or phrenic nerve involvement; (5) involvement of the mediastinum, including the trachea or esophagus; and (6) distant metastases.

4.107 CHEST

Case No. 107

Clinical history: 70 years old male with presenting complaints of cough.

Radiological techniques and observation: Frontal and lateral views of chest radiograph (Figs 4.107.1 and 4.107.2) show a lobulated well-defined opacity in the region of right hilum with **broad base towards the mediastinum** obscuring the right upper cardiac silhouette. Hilum is seen through the lesion **(hilum overlay sign—positive)**. Pulmonary vessels seen through the lesion and not converging at the periphery of the lesion. No evidence of calcification/compression of the right main bronchus/ collapse of lung segments/ elevated dome of diaphragm. Bilateral lung fields appear normal. No cardiomegaly. Trachea appears to be in midline. No mediastinal shift. No destructive bone lesions noted. The lesion corresponds to anterior mediastinal soft tissue opacity on the lateral projection by **obliteration of retrosternal clear space**.

Limited axial sections of contrast enhanced CT chest in lung and mediastinal window (Figs 4.107.3 to 4.107.5) show: Lobulated soft tissue dense lesion showing homogenous enhancement, abutting great vessels and major veins. Fat plane between the great vessels and the mass lesion is not maintained. The lesion is encircling ascending aorta for about 100° to 120°. Prominent vessels within and around the mass. No pulmonary or pleural masses. No hilar, axillary or upper abdominal lymphadenopathy. No destructive bone lesions noted.

Interpretation: A: 70 years old male, anterior mediastinal mass, C: Lobulated homogeneously enhancing lesion, B: Abutting great vessels and major veins with no intervening fat plane in between, no lymphadenopathy, D: Thymic carcinoma.

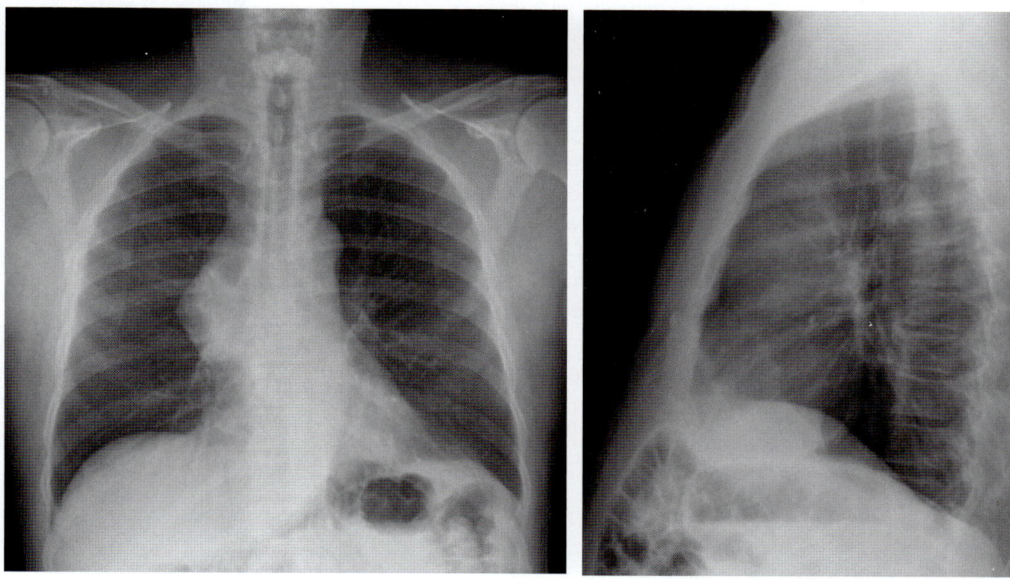

Fig. 4.107.1 Fig. 4.107.2

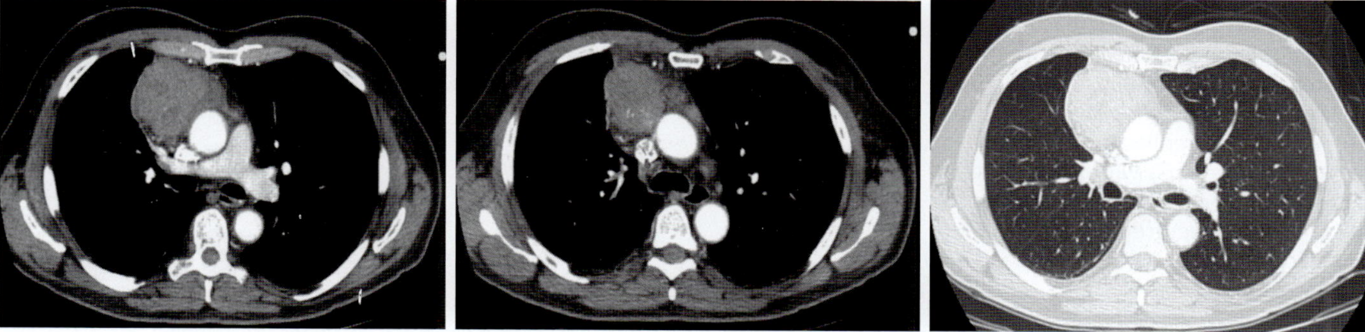

Fig. 4.107.3 Fig. 4.107.4 Fig. 4.107.5

Table 4.107.1: Differential diagnosis for thymoma		
Condition	*Radiological features*	*Images*
Lymphoma (Terrible lymphoma) Mediastinal lymphomas arise from either the thymus or lymph nodes,accounting for their predilection for the anterior and middle mediastinum. Treatment of disease depends on the type of lymphoma and the stage of disease, but requires chemotherapy with or without radiotherapy.	CT demonstrates a soft tissue dense mass, with **smooth or lobulated margins** which conform to surrounding structures. Both gallium-67 scintigraphy and FDG-PET are better for assessing tumor viability following treatment than CT.	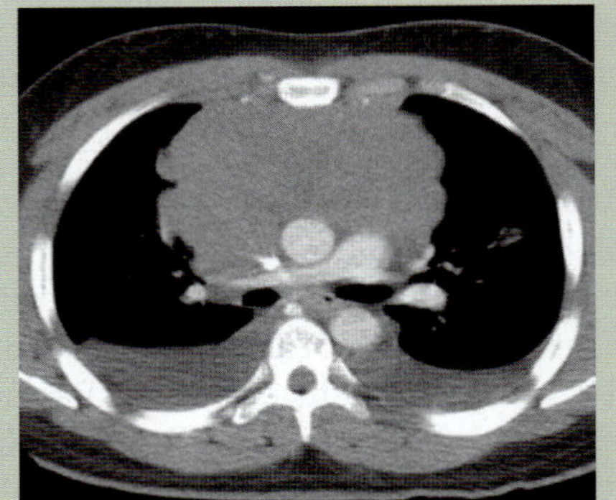 **Fig. 4.107.6:** Lymphoma
Teratoma They account for 15% of anterior mediastinal masses in adults and 25% in children. They are by far the most common mediastinal germ cell tumor. Treatment depends on whether the teratoma is mature or immature. In the former, surgical resection is curative. In the later management depends on alpha-FP levels. If these are elevated, then postoperative chemotherapy is usually employed.	Usually cystic: 90%, may be uni- or multiloculated with septal/rim contrast enhancement. Variable attenuation, consistent with different tissues fat, water density cystic spaces, fat-fluid levels (specific), homogeneous soft-tissue density, calcification: 26%, identifiable teeth or bone is seen in up to 8% of cases.	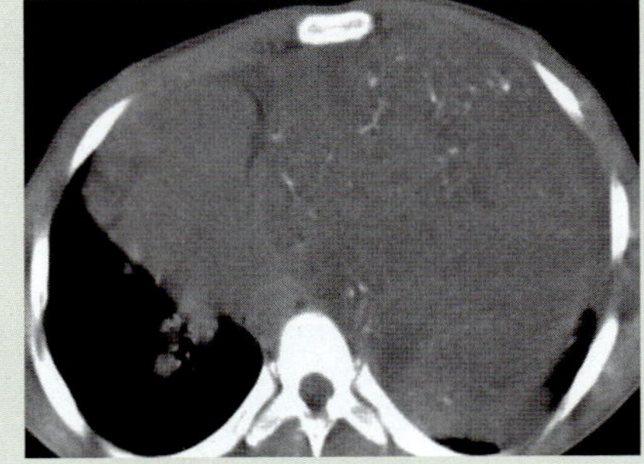 **Fig. 4.107.7:** Teratoma
Thoracic aortic aneurysm Ascending aortic aneurysms represent 60% of thoracic aortic aneurysms. The patient is uually asymptomatic. Ascending aortic aneurysms are defined as a permanent dilatation of the ascending aorta diameter ≥5 cm. Mild to moderate aneurysm treated conservatively. When the diameter reaches 5–6 cm intervention is usually considered as the risk of rupture is significantly elevated.	Ascending aortic aneurysms may manifest as a widening of the aortic or mediastinal silhouettes. The ascending aorta usually does not form part of the right cardiomediastinal margin in the first five decades. If it does, suspect dilatation or aneurysm formation. Treatment options include: Open repair, elephant graft repair, endovascular repair.	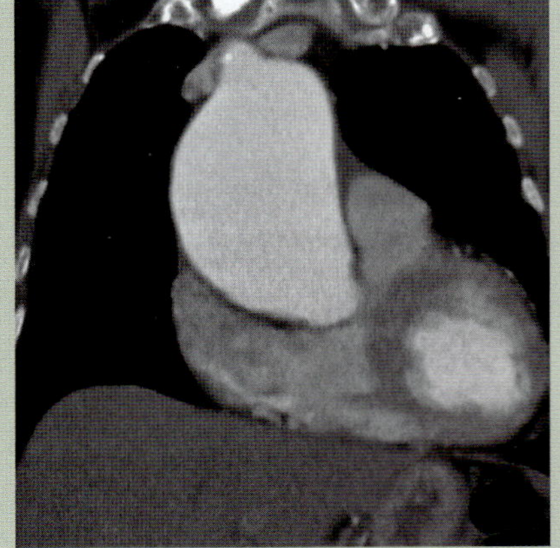 **Fig. 4.107.8:** Thoracic aortic aneurysm
Thymolipoma Rare, benign anterior mediastinal mass of thymic origin, containing both thymic and mature adipose tissue. Thymolipomas comprise ~5% of all thymic neoplasms. There is no sex predilection and age range between 3–56 years, with a mean age of 22 years. Surgically local resection curative, no reports of recurrence, metastasis or mortality.	On CT thymolipomas typically appears almost entirely fatty with some areas of inhomogeneous soft tissue density that represent thymic tissue. MRI: Thymolipomas have fat and soft tissue signal characteristics: T1: Typically the adipose tissue within the tumor returns high T1 signal and thymic component a more intermediate T1 signal.	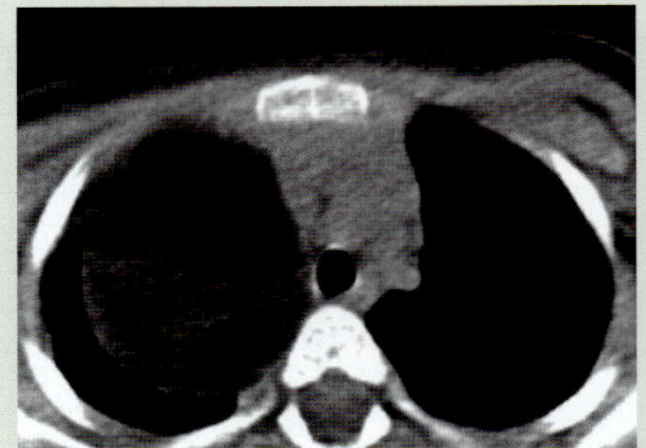 **Fig. 4.107.9:** Thymolipoma

(Contd...)

Table 4.107.1: Differential diagnosis for thymoma *(Contd...)*

Condition	*Radiological features*	*Images*
Substernal thyroid is a goiter which requires mediastinal exploration and dissection for complete removal or an intrathoracic component extending more than 3 cm in the thoracic inlet. Most anterior substernal thyroid goitres are approched via a transcervical approach. In complicated cases partial upper sternotomy and clavicular head resection or mini-thoracotomy for adequate exposure.	On chest X-ray **superior mediastinal radiopacity which causing the deviation of trachea to the opposite site.** The superior margin of the radiopacity is usually untraceable (positive cervicothoracic sign).	**Fig. 4.107.10:** Substernal thyroid

Principal diagnosis: With this imaging findings the anterior mediastinal mass is a thymic carcinoma. Differentiating thymoma from thymic carcinoma is only readily done when there is evidence of local invasion or metastatic disease.

Differential diagnosis: 5Ts of anterior mediastinal mass lesion: Thymoma/thymic carcinoma, **T**errible Lymphoma, **T**eratoma (Germ cell tumor, with the latter unlikely given the patient's age), **T**horacic aortic aneurysm, Ascending aorta aneurysm, post-surgical

Table 4.107.2: Classification of mediastinal lesions based on content

Mediastinum	*Solid*	*Cystic*	*Fat*	*Calcification*
Anterior	Goitre, thymic hyperplasia, thymoma, thymic carcinoma, thymic carcinoids, lymphoma, germ cell tumors	Cystic hygroma, pericardial cyst, thymic cyst, germ cell tumors, ascending aortic aneurysms.	Germ cell tumors (teratoma), thymolipoma, prominent fat pad	Goiter, germ cell tumors (teratoma), treated lymphoma.
Middle	Lymphadenopathy Mesenchymal masses Tracheal masses Hemangioma Esophageal masses	Foregut duplication cysts, pleuropericardial cyst, lymphangioma, necrotic nodes, pericardial recess, hiatus hernia Retroperitoneal lesion (pancreatic pseudocyst) extension. **Vascular:** Esophageal varies. Aortic arch anomaly Dilated azygous and hemi-azygous veins	Lipoma, lipoblastoma, esophageal lipoma, esophageal fibrovascular polyps.	Aortitis with calcification.
Posterior	Nerve sheath tumors, sympathetic ganglion tumors, thoracic spine abnormalities, paraganglioma.	Neuroenteric cyst, bronchogenic cyst, esophageal duplication cyst, pseudocyst, hydatid cyst, Pott spine with paravertebral abscess, cystic schwannoma, hiatus hernia, Bochdalek hernia, lymphangioma, lateral thoracic meningocele. **Vascular:** Descending thoracic aortic aneurysms	Extramedullary hematopoiesis	Chondrosarcoma, chordoma
More than one compartment		Lymphangioma, mediastinitis	Liposarcoma	

Table 4.107.3: Signs in plain radiograph to localise mediastinal lesions		
Anterior mediastinal mass lesion	*Middle mediastinal mass lesion*	*Posterior mediastinal mass lesion*
Displaced anterior junctional line. Obliterated cardiophrenic angles. Obliterated retrosternal clear space. Hilum overlay sign. Effacement/dense ascending aorta. Hilum overlay sign (anterior and posterior). Anterior rib changes.	Widened paratracheal stripes. AP window mass. Obliterated left SCA reflection. Displaced azygoesophageal recess on the right. Pseudoparavertebral line on the left. Lateral indentation of trachea and oesophagus. Posterior indentation of trachea and anterior indentation of oesophagus (tracheoesophageal groove). Lateral view—doughnut sign. Cervicothoracic sign with non-visualization of superior margin of lesion (thyroid lesions and vascular). Hilum convergence sign.	Cervicothoracic sign with superior margin of lesion seen clearly. Widening of paravertebral stripes. Posterior rib changes. Vertebral changes. Descending thoracic aorta and aortic knuckle changes. Hilum overlay sign.

pseudoaneurysm of aorta, Thyroid and parathyroid benign/malignant lesions.

Management: Often associated with poor prognosis. Resection and radiation therapy and follow-up CT to look for recurrence. Patient referred to cardiothoracic surgeon.

Discussion: Thymic mass lesions: Numerous histologic classification systems for thymic epithelial neoplasms developed over the years. "A widely used classification includes:

Non-invasive thymoma: Localised mass lesion without adjacent invasion.

Invasive thymoma: With contiguous pleural and pericardial invasion.

Thymic carcinoma: With distant metastasis, distal pleural and pericardial spread.

Associations: Myasthenia gravis: Most common association 10–20% of patients with myasthenia gravis have a thymoma. 30–50% of patients with a thymoma have myasthenia gravis.

Pure red cell aplasia: 50% of patients with pure red cell aplasia have a thymoma, 5% of patients with a thymoma have pure red cell aplasia.

Most of the mediastinal lesions are bicompartmental (middle and posterior mediastinum)

Cardiophrenic angle mass

- Fat pad (most common cause)
- Diaphragmatic hernia (second most common): Morgagni (anterior), Bochdalek (posterior)
- Pericardial cyst
- Cardiophrenic angle nodes (lymphoma usually recurrent, status postradiation)
- Aneurysm
- Dilated right atrium
- Anterior mediastinal mass
- Primary lung or pleural mass

4.108 CHEST

Case No. 108

Clinical history: 29 years old male presented with dyspnoea for 5 days.

Radiological techniques and observation: Frontal chest radiograph (Fig. 4.108.1) of a skeletally mature patient shows well-defined homogeneous radio-opaque lesion with broad base/obtuse angle towards the mediastinum, in right hilar region involving the subcarinal region, lateral margin of the lesion seen clearly with a sharp lung lesion interface. Medial margin could not be visualized. Pulmonary vessels are seen through the lesion (hilum overlay sign positive, thus the lesion is either anterior/posterior). SVC silhouette is seen (the lesion is not an anterior mediastinal mass). No calcification/air fluid level. No evidence of any vertebral deformity. Rest of the lung fields appear normal, bilateral costophrenic and cardiophrenic angles appear normal. Rib cage appears normal. No evidence of any soft tissue swelling. Visualized clavicle appears normal. With these findings, it is a middle or posterior mediastinal mass.

Contrast enhanced CT in limited axial section at the level of aortic arch and just below the carina (Figs 4.108.2 to 4.108.4) shows a well-defined non-enhancing hypodense cystic lesion in close proximity to trachea, right main bronchus and esophagus without any calcification/septation. No evidence of solid components/fat content in the lesion. No evidence of hemorrhage within the lesion. No evidence of neural foraminal extension of the lesion. No evidence of scalloping/lysis/defect of the adjacent vertebral body and ribs.

Interpretation: A—29 years old male, posterior mediastinal lesion, C—well-defined homogeneous radio-opaque lesion with broad base/obtuse angle towards the mediastinum, in right hilar region, lateral margin of the lesion seen clearly with a sharp lung lesion interface, B—hilum overlay sign positive (anterior/posterior) and SVC silhouette is seen (the lesion—not an anterior mediastinal mass) and enhancement of the wall of the lesion is seen, D—foregut duplication cyst.

Principal diagnosis: Foregut duplication cyst possibly bronchogenic cyst/esophageal duplication cyst.

Differential diagnosis: Cystic lesions: Neuroenteric cyst, bronchogenic cyst, esophageal duplication cyst, hydatid cyst, pseudocyst, lateral thoracic meningocele. **Neurogenic tumor:** Nerve sheath tumor, sympathetic ganglion tumors, paraganglioma. **Spine lesions:** Extramedullary hematopoiesis, thoracic spine abnormalities. **Mesenchymal lesions:** Lipomatosis, lipoma. **Nodal lesion:** Lymphoma (non-Hodgkin's), metastasis. **Others:** Esophageal masses, varices, hernia, hemangioma, lymphangioma, dilated azygos/hemiazygos vein, thymic mass/germ cell tumor.

Fat containing mediastinal lesions: Lipoma, lipoblastoma, liposarcoma, mediastinal lipomatosis, thymolipoma, diaphragmatic hernia with fat as content, benign mature teratoma, extramedullary hematopoiesis (posterior medisatinum).

Lesions between trachea and esophagus: Pulmonary sling (left pulmonary artery arising from the right pulmonary artery), esophageal tumors, tracheal tumors, thyroid masses, bronchogenic cyst/foregut cyst.

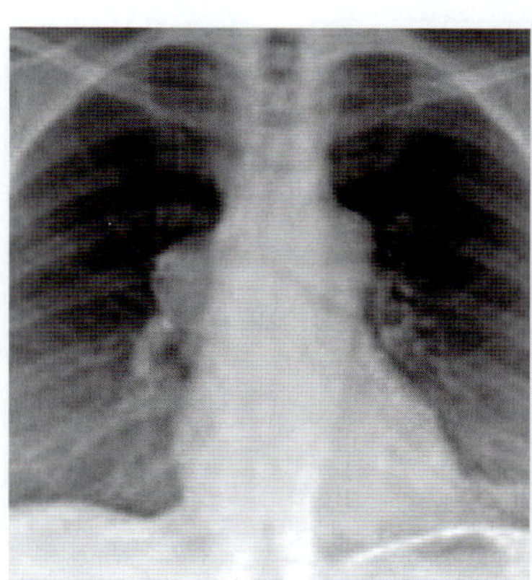

Fig. 4.108.1

Fig. 4.108.2

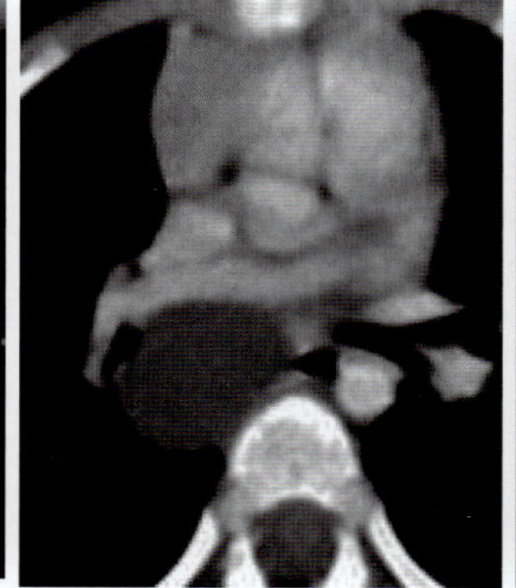

Fig. 4.108.3

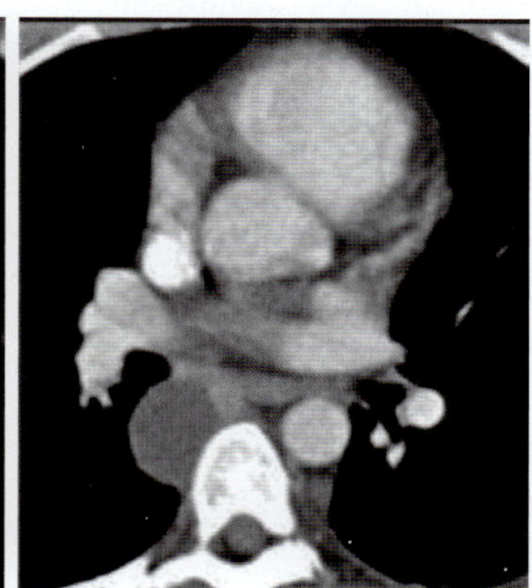

Fig. 4.108.4

Table 4.108.1: Differential diagnosis for posterior mediastinal lesions		
Bronchogenic cyst 60% of foregut duplication cyst Location subcarinal (50%), paratracheal (20%), retrocardiac (10%) Intra-parenchymal bronchogenic cyst (10%)	**X-ray:** Smooth, sharply marginated, round or elliptical mass with displacement of trachea **CECT:** Well-defined non-enhancing hypo-dense cystic lesion in close contact with trachea or bronchus. Long standing bronchogenic cyst appears hyperdense on NECT **MRI:** T1 hypo to hyper (if protein/mucin/hemorrhage +) T2 hyperintense lesion with no enhancement on contrast	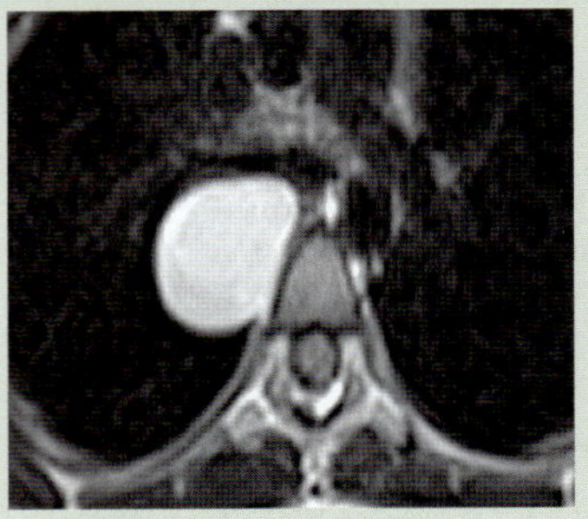 **Fig. 4.108.5:** Bronchogenic cyst
Esophageal duplication cyst Lined by GIT mucosal cells	Similar to bronchogenic cyst in X-ray, CT, MRI except that it is in close proximity to the esophagus. Common in lower and posterior mediastinum	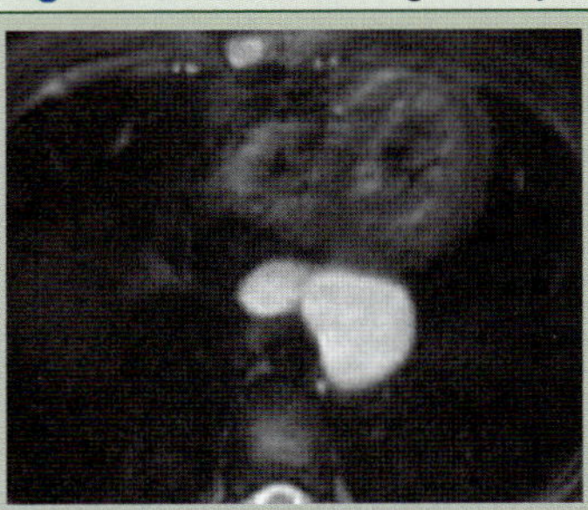 **Fig. 4.108.6:** Esophageal duplication cyst
Neuroenteric cyst Rare, posterior mediastinum, contains both **meningeal and GIT cells**, communicates with the **spinal canal** with the defect in the one or more vertebrae	The appearance of neurenteric cyst on CT is the same as that of other duplication cysts, but the presence of a vertebral abnormality can point to the diagnosis **vertebral anomalies** (e.g. **hemivertebrae or butterfly vertebrae**) or scoliosis is present in about half of cases.	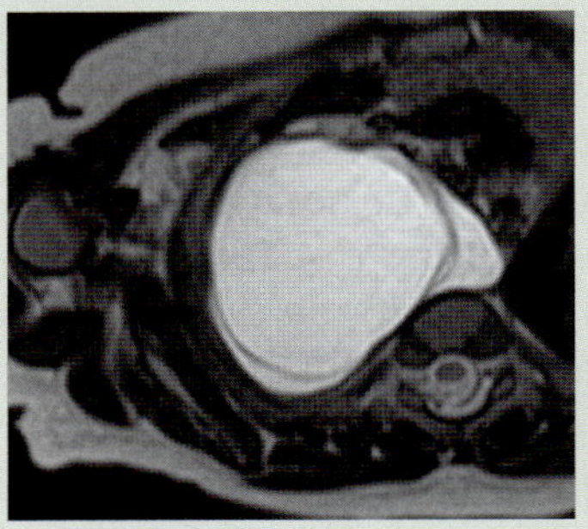 **Fig. 4.108.7:** Neuroenteric cyst
Schwannoma peripheral nerves and nerve sheath: Schwannoma, neurofibroma, Malignant nerve sheath tumor Adult → nerve sheath tumors Children → sympathetic ganglia	X-ray PA Well-defined radio dense lesion, broad base towards the mediastinum Cardiac borders seen through the lesion **Lateral X-ray** lesion lies in the posterior mediastinum **CT**—well defined cystic lesion with areas of solid components in the right paravertebral region **CECT**—enhances heterogeneously	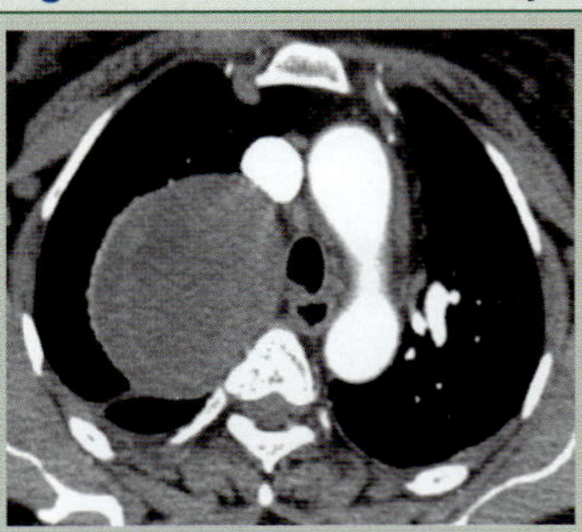 **Fig. 4.108.8:** Schwannoma
Hydatid cyst: Caused by *Echinococcus granulosus*/multilocularis. Cyst contains-pericyst, ectocyst and endocyst (germinal layer)	**X-ray:** Well-defined homogeneous radio-paque lesion with broad base to the mediastinum. **CT:** Well-defined cystic lesion with multiple daughter cysts. **On contrast:** Cyst wall enhances. **MRI:** Cyst follows fluid intensity in all sequences with hypointense walls of daughter cysts.	

4

(Contd.)

Table 4.108.1: Differential diagnosis for posterior mediastinal lesions (*Contd.*)		
Neuroblastic tumor: Tumors according to age <5 years → neuroblastoma 5–10 years → ganglioneuroblastoma 10–20 years → ganglioneuroma >30 years → neurofibroma >40 years → schwannoma	**CXR:** Well-defined radiodense with areas of punctate calcification **CT:** Well-defined paravertebral lesion with areas of necrosis and multiple specs of calcification. **T2-weighted MRI:** Shows a large mass in the posterior mediastinum extending into the spinal canal through a neural foramen, displacing the spinal cord to the right. It can be **tumors from sympathetic ganglia:** Ganglioneuroma, ganglioneuroblastoma and neuroblastoma	**Fig. 4.108.9:** Neuroblastic tumor
Pseudocyst: Extension of the pancreatic pseudocyst into the posterior mediastinum through the esophageal/aortic hiatus.	**X-ray:** Well-defined homogeneous radiopaque lesion with broad base to the mediastinum, abdomino thoracic sign positive. **CT:** Well-defined cystic lesion in the posterior mediastinum with continuity to the abdomen in the background of pancreatitis. Rarely communication with the pleura may be present. **On contrast, cyst wall enhances.** **MRI:** Cyst follows fluid intensity in all sequences, continuity with the abdomen made out. Pancreatitis +	
Pott's spine with paravertebral abscess Osteomyelitis of the vertebral body with intervertebral discitis due to TB.	**X-ray:** Decrease in the vertebral body height with paravertebral soft tissue shadow. May show gibbus deformity/vertebral collapse. **MRI:** T1 hypo, T2 hyperintense vertebral body with subligamentous spread, epidural and paravertebral spread.	**Fig. 4.108.10:** Pott's spine with paravertebral abscess

Table 4.108.2: Felson's classification of mediastinum			
Mediastinum	*Anterior*	*Middle*	*Posterior*
Extent	From the posterior surface of sternum to a line drawn along the anterior border of trachea and the posterior border of heart in the lower mediastinum	Between anterior compartment in the front and posterior compartment behind	Posterior to a line 1 cm behind the anterior margin of the vertebral column, anterior to the chest wall
Content	Thymus, heart, ascending aorta and great vessels, anterior portion of the main pulmonary artery, pericardium, fat, lymph vessels and nodes	The trachea and main bronchi superior vena cava, mid-portion of the aortic arch, azygos arch, lymph nodes, esophagus, descending aorta (sometimes)	Vertebral bodies, paravertebral tissues, descending aorta, posterior azygos vein, hemiazygos vein, lymph nodes
Corresponding plain film features	Anterior junction line, cardiophrenic angles, retrosternal stripe, retrosternal space	B/L paratracheal stripes, SVC interface, AP window, left subclavian artery interface, azygoesophageal recess, preaortic interface	Paravertebral stripes

Table 4.108.3: Anterior mediastinal masses	
Thymic masses—thymic cyst, thymolipoma, thymoma, cystic-benign (noninvasive) thymoma, malignant (invasive) thymoma, thymic carcinoma Thymic carcinoid, thymic lymphoma	Germ cell tumors (male > female) Seminoma, embryonal cell carcinoma, teratoma, choriocarcinoma Lymphadenopathy

Table 4.108.4: Superior mediastinal masses		
Thyroid masses	Lymphatic cysts, cystic hygroma	Adenopathy (primary head and neck tumors)
Lymphoma	Small cell carcinoma of the lung	Aneurysm and vascular anomalies may involve both the anterior and superior mediastinum

Table 4.108.5: Middle mediastinal masses	
Adenopathy	Congenital cysts—bronchogenic cyst, pericardial cyst
Aneurysm	Esophagus—neoplasm, diverticula Megaesophagus—achalasia, hiatal hernia, colonic interposition
Other	Mediastinal hemorrhage, mediastinal lipomatosis, bronchogenic cancer arising adjacent to mediastinum, aberrant RSA with diverticulum, varices, neurinoma from recurrent laryngeal nerve, malignancy of trachea, pancreatic pseudocyst

Table 4.108.6: Posterior mediastinal masses	
Neurogenic (90%)—**peripheral nerve**—schwannoma, neurofibroma, **sympathetic ganglia**—ganglioneuroma, neuroblastoma, **paraganglion cells**—pheochromocytoma	Thoracic spine—neoplasm, hematoma, extramedullary hematopoiesis, discitis
Vascular—aneurysm	Lesions from chest wall and ribs

Table 4.108.7: Radiographic difference between a lung and a mediastinal lesion	
Mediastinal mass	*Lung mass*
Broad base towards the mediastinum/obtuse angle with the mediastinum	Narrow base towards mediastinum/acute angle with the mediastinum/chest wall
Smooth and sharp margins	Irregular margins
No air bronchogram	Air bronchogram +/–
Bilateral possible	Unilateral
Lung lesion interface sharp	Bronchial cut-off with collapse of lung segments with hazy interface

Table 4.108.8: Summary of various classifications of mediastinum		
Anatomical classification	*Radiological classification (Felson)*	*ITMIG classification*
	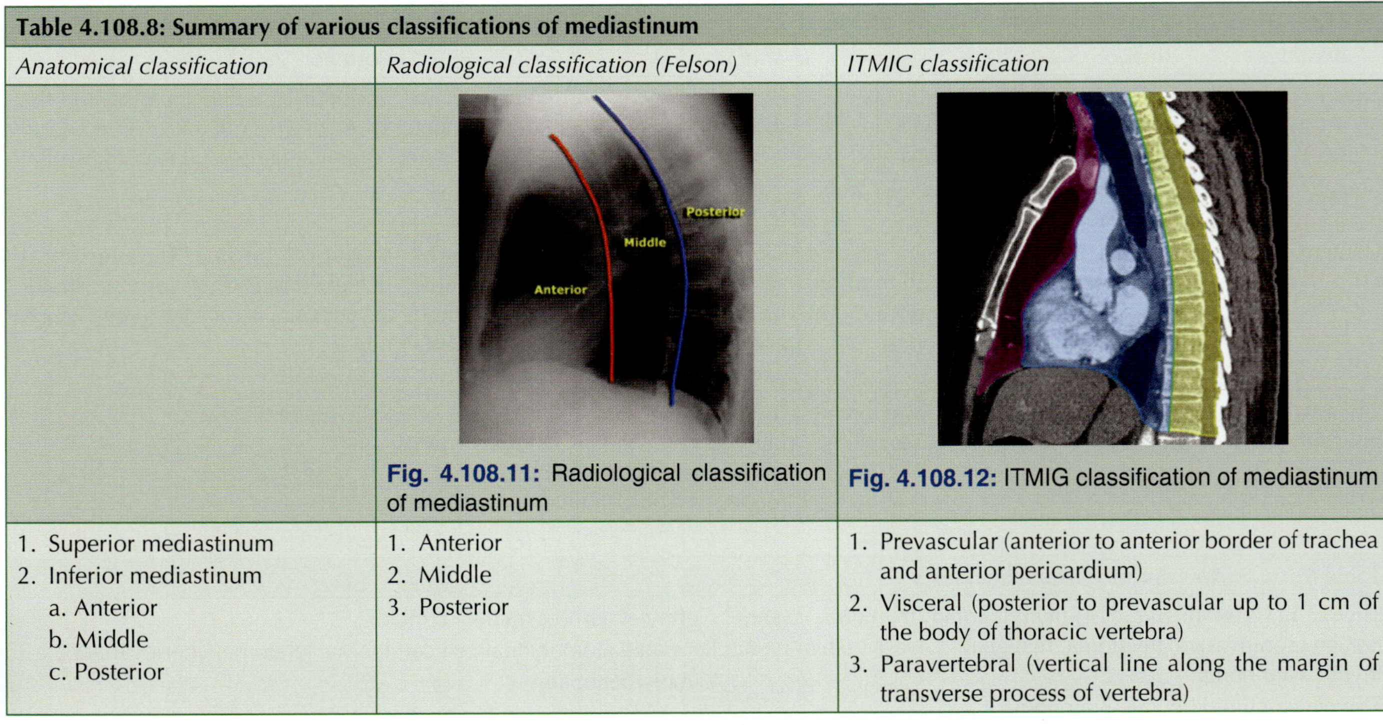 **Fig. 4.108.11:** Radiological classification of mediastinum	**Fig. 4.108.12:** ITMIG classification of mediastinum
1. Superior mediastinum 2. Inferior mediastinum a. Anterior b. Middle c. Posterior	1. Anterior 2. Middle 3. Posterior	1. Prevascular (anterior to anterior border of trachea and anterior pericardium) 2. Visceral (posterior to prevascular up to 1 cm of the body of thoracic vertebra) 3. Paravertebral (vertical line along the margin of transverse process of vertebra)

Table 4.108.9: ITMIG classification of mediastinum

Prevascular compartment	Visceral compartment	Paravertebral compartment
Boundaries	*Boundaries*	*Boundaries*
Superior: Thoracic inlet Inferior: Diaphragm Anterior: Posterior cortex of the sternum Lateral: Parietal mediastinal pleura Posterior: Anterior aspect of the pericardium	Superiorly: Thoracic inlet Inferiorly: Diaphragm Anteriorly: Posterior boundary of the prevascular compartment of mediastium Posterior: A vertical line which connecting a point on each thoracic vertebral body 1 cm posterior to its anterior margin (visceral-paravertebral compartment boundary line)	Superior: Thoracic inlet Inferior: Diaphragm Anterior: Posterior boundaries of the visceral compartment Posterolateral: Vertical line against the posterior margin of the chest wall at the lateral margin of the thoracic spine
Contents	*Contents*	*Contents*
Thymus lymph nodes Left brachiocephalic vein Fat	Trachea/carina esophagus Lymph nodes, heart Ascending aorta; aortic arch; descending thoracic aorta Superior vena cava Intrapericardial pulmonary arteries Thoracic duct	Thoracic spine and paravertebral soft tissues

Companion Case

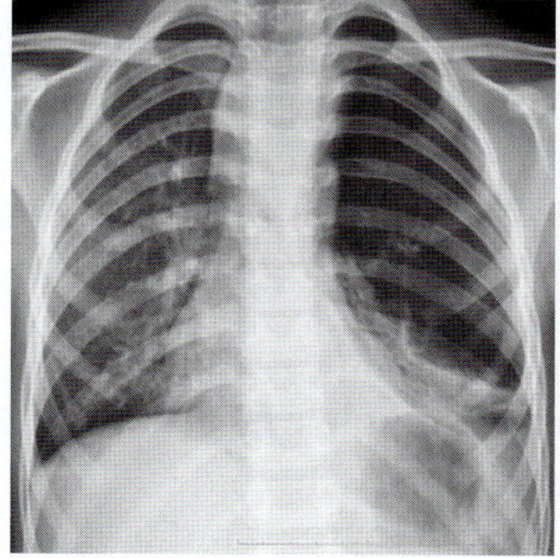

Fig. 4.108.13: Superior mediastinal widening with left lower lobe collapse

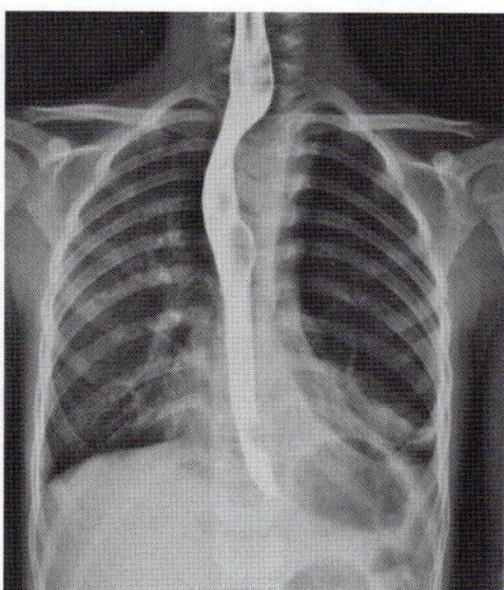

Fig. 4.108.14: Extrinsic indentation of the upper thoracic esophagus

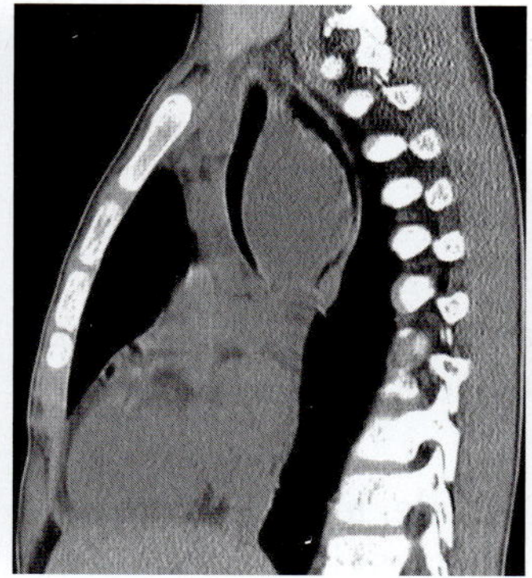

Fig. 4.108.15: Foregut duplication cyst

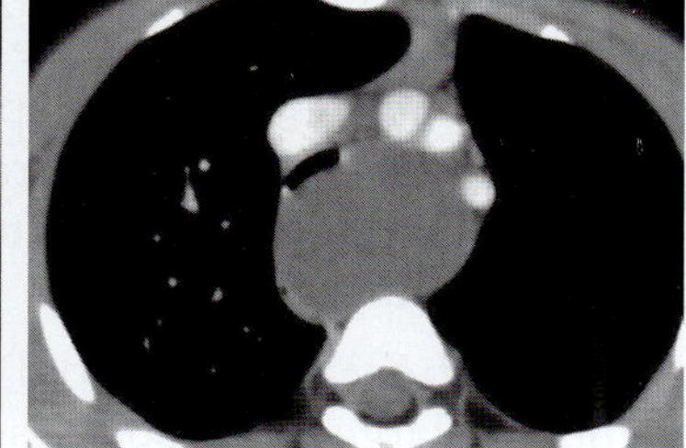

Fig. 4.108.16: Foregut duplication cyst

Plain radiograph (Fig. 4.108.13) of a 20 years old male patient in frontal view shows upper mediastinal widening in the right side, collapse of the left lower lobe with compensatory emphysematous change on the left upper lobe. Cardiac silhoutte appears normal. Elevated left hemidiaphragm noted. Right costophrenic and cardiophrenic angle appears normal. In Barium swallow (Fig. 4.108.14) there is smooth extrinsic indentation of the upper thoracic esophagus without any luminal narrowing. No evidence of mucosal irregularity.

Plain CT in sagittal view in mediastinal window (Fig. 4.108.15) shows a well-defined hypodense cystic lesion in close proximity to both trachea and esophagus. Noted between trachea and esophagus causing splaying of the two. Contrast enhance CT in axial view (Fig. 4.108.16) shows a well-defined cystic lesion without any enhancement displacing the trachea anteriorly and esophagus posteriorly—**foregut duplication cyst.**

4.109 CHEST

Case No. 109

Clinical history: 45-year-old female with progressive dysphagia and breathing difficulties.

Radiological technique and observation: AP and lateral radiograph of neck (Figs 4.109.1 and 4.109.2) demonstrates a large soft tissue opacity mass in the left side of neck, superior mediastinum and pretracheal region. The mass causes marked narrowing and displacement of cervical and thoracic trachea to the right. Inferior border of the lesion not visible clearly. The superior portion of the lesion is not outlined by air and the mass extends superiorly beyond the level of clavicle, suggestive of positive cervicothoracic sign. Superior mediastinal widening noted. No bony erosions seen. Supraclavicular extension/not outlined by air in the thoracic cavity.

Further investigation: Axial and coronal reformatted CECT neck (Figs 4.109.3 and 4.109.4) of the same patient demonstrates markedly heterogeneous lobulated enlarged appearance of bilateral lobes (more on the left) and isthmus of thyroid. Calcification and frank cysts are not evident. The trachea is displaced towards the right, despite the heterogeneity the margins of the gland is well defined and it merely displaces adjacent structures. Coronal image shows the craniocaudal extension of the lesion and retrosternal extension inferiorly into the superior mediastinum.

Interpretation: A–45-year-old female, lesion in thyroid gland, C—large soft tissue opacity mass in the neck. The outline of the mass fades out inferiorly. The superior portion of the lesion is not outlined by air, B—extends superiorly beyond the level of clavicle (positive cervicothoracic sign) heterogeneous lobulated enlarged appearance of bilateral lobes of thyroid displaces adjacent structures with retrosternal extension into the superior mediastinum, D—retrosternal goitre

Principal diagnosis: Retrosternal goitre.

Discussion

- The anterior mediastinum usually stops at the level of superior border of clavicle.
- Therefore, when a mass extends above the superior clavicle, it is located either in the middle or posterior mediastinum/great vessels and structures extending across the neck.
- When lung tissue comes in between the mass and the neck, the mass is probably from the posterior mediastinum.
- This is known as cervicothoracic sign.
- Benjamin Felson, an American radiologist, who is believed to be the first to describe this sign.
- 40% of multinodular goitre have retrosternal extension. Most common cause of anterior mediastinal mass. X-ray shows superior mediastinal widening (>8 cm or more than one-third transverse diameter of thorax) + Tracheal deviation/ narrowing. CECT is the imaging of choice to evaluate extension.
- Incidental thyroid nodules detected in CT/MRI if <35 years, USG is more than 1 cm, if >35 years, USG for >1.5 cm nodules.
- *Treatment indication:* If symptomatic/causing local mass effect. Surgery: Partial/complete resection.
- *Radioiodine occasionally used:* Dose = thyroid weight × planned radioiodine delivery to thyroid/radioiodine uptake. Ethanol injection leads to risk of recurrent laryngeal nerve injury. Hot nodules are followed clinically with USG. Cold nodules have a 20% risk of malignancy. Suggested USG guided FNAC.
- Patients with MNG are at increased risk of iodinated contrast-induced thyrotoxicosis.

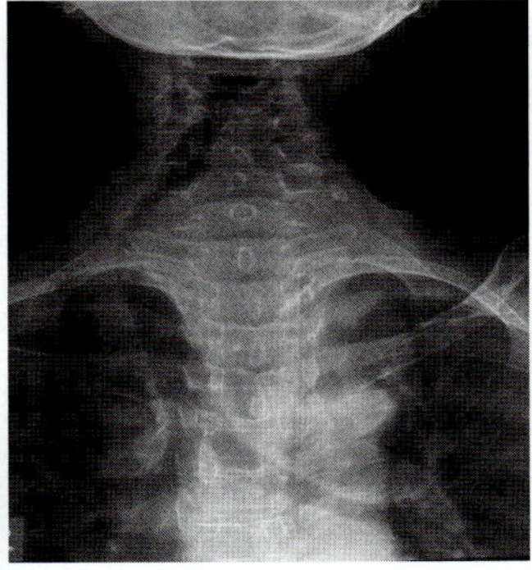
Fig. 4.109.1

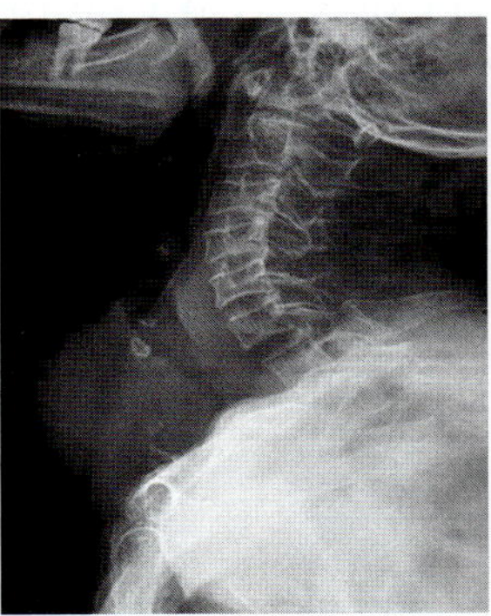
Fig. 4.109.2

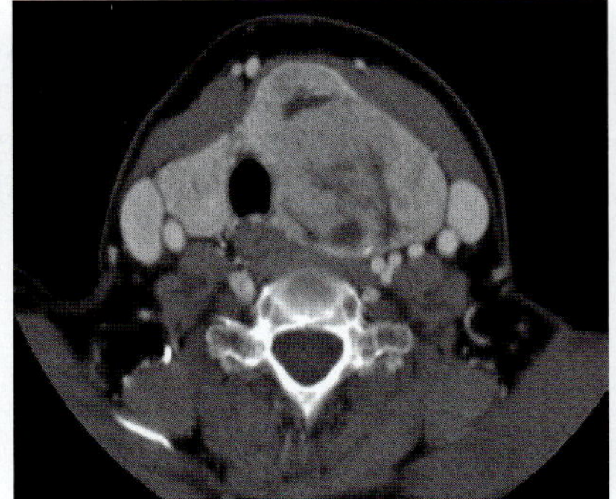
Fig. 4.109.3

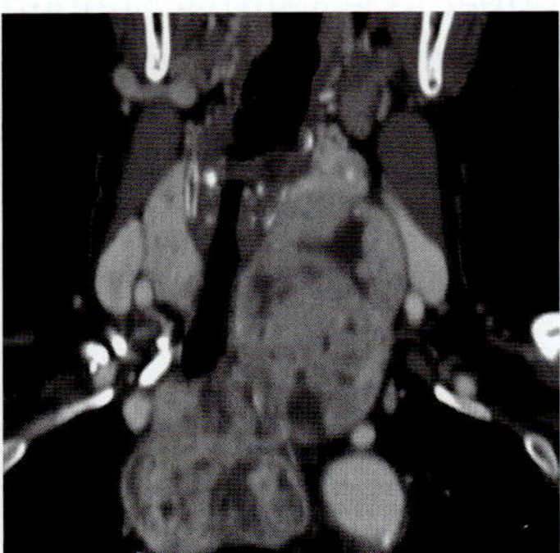
Fig. 4.109.4

TIRADS—Scoring System—Refer to OSCE, Case 44, Table 5.23 (page 1578)

Table 4.109.1: Differential diagnosis for lesions showing positive cervicothoracic sign		
Posterior mediastinal mass	Mediastinal mass extending above the level of the clavicle. Suggests the lesion is not present in the anterior mediastinum. The mass is outline superiorly by air. The lesion is not extending from the neck to thorax or vice versa.	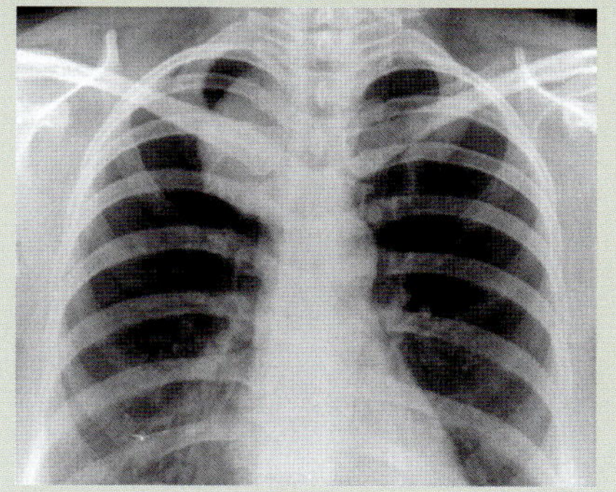 **Fig. 4.109.5:** Posterior mediastinal mass
Transthoracic shadow: Aortic aneurysm Other: Brachiocephalic, subclavian and ICA aneurysms	Exception: Anterior mediastinal lesion showing positive cervicothoracic sign. Mural calcifications may be seen in atherosclerotic causes and certain aortitis.	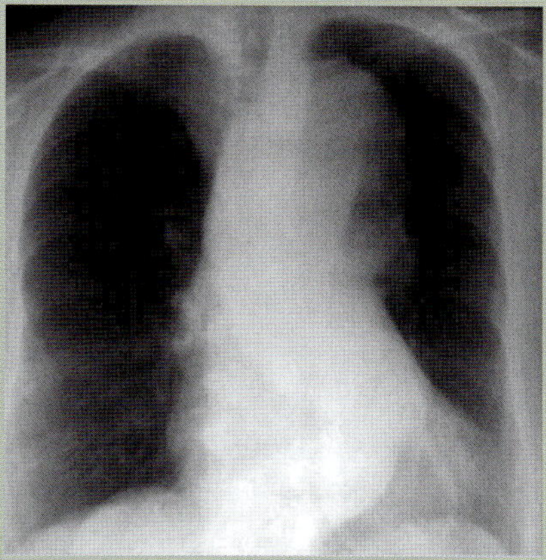 **Fig. 4.109.6:** Aortic aneurysm with brachiocephalic artery
Transthoracic shadow: Achalasia cardia	Convex opacity overlying the right mediastinum, air fluid level may be seen due to stasis. Small or absent gastric bubble. Anterior displacement or bowing of trachea on lateral. Patchy alveolar opacities bilaterally	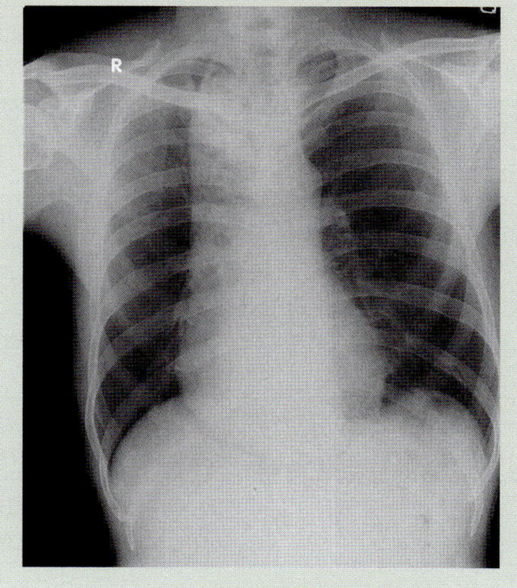 **Fig. 4.109.7:** Achalasia cardia

(Contd.)

Table 4.109.1: Differential diagnosis for lesions showing positive cervicothoracic sign (*Contd.*)		
Transthoracic shadow: Mediastinal lipomatosis	Caused by deposition of a large amount of mature adipose tissue in the mediastinum. It is a relatively common benign cause of mediastinal widening. Associated with steroid use, Cushing's and obesity	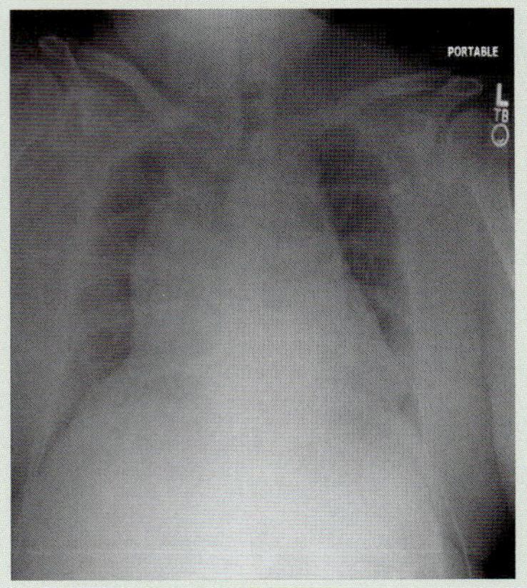 **Fig. 4.109.8:** Mediastinal lipomatosis
Cervicothoracic shadow retrosternal extension of thyroid lesion:	Exception: Retrosternal extension of MNG—anterior mediastinal lesion showing positive cervicothoracic sign	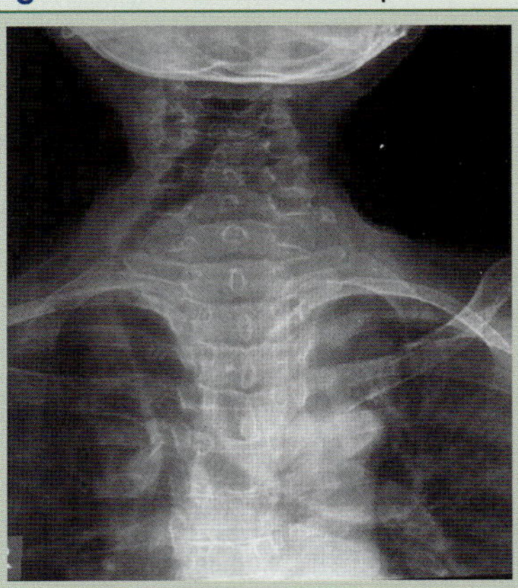 **Fig. 4.109.9:** Retrosternal extension of thyroid lesion

Table 4.109.2: Difference between benign and malignant nodule		
Imaging features	*Benign nodule*	*Malignant nodule*
USG	Anechoic, wide, well-defined smooth with or without macrocalcification	Very hypoechoic, irregular with extrathyroidal extension, tall with micro or punctate calcification. Lymphadenopathy, thick halo.
Doppler	Peripheral flow pattern with decreased resistive index	Intranodular vascularity with high resistive index (mean 0.73) and PI (1.3)
Elastography	Pattern 1 soft tissue strain and 2 presence of harder blue areas not constant on real time imaging	Pattern 3 constant hard blue areas in centre or periphery and 4 totally hard tissue compared to surrounding thyroid
CT	Peripheral calcification, well-defined margin, intact capsule. Larger in size comparatively	Completely solid, internal calcification, ill-defined margin, incomplete capsule

4.110 CHEST

Case No. 110

Clinical history: 20-year-old female presented with cough with expectoration × 2 months with evening raise of temperature, loss of weight and loss of appetite.

Radiological techniques and observation: Plain radiograph chest frontal view (Fig. 4.110.1) shows trachea in midline, no cardiomegaly, bilateral costophrenic and cardiophrenic angle appear normal. Right hilar lymphadenopathy noted. Bilateral lung fields show subtle patchy opacity in left midzone. No evidence of calcification. Soft tissues, bones and abdomen appear normal. CT thorax in lung window (Fig. 4.110.2) shows patchy areas of centrilobular nodules in left upper lobe

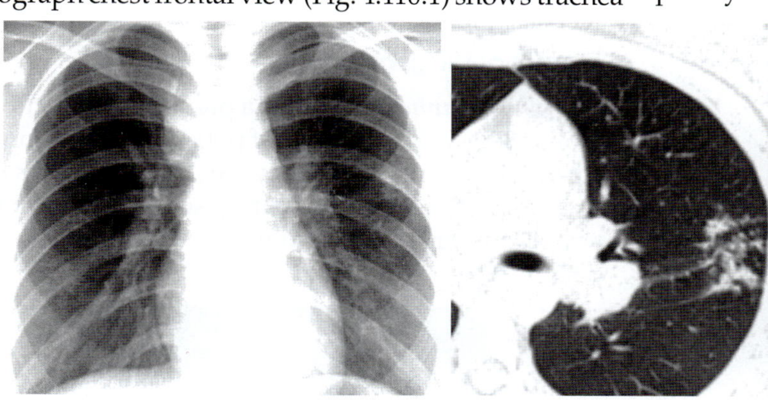

Fig. 4.110.1 **Fig. 4.110.2**

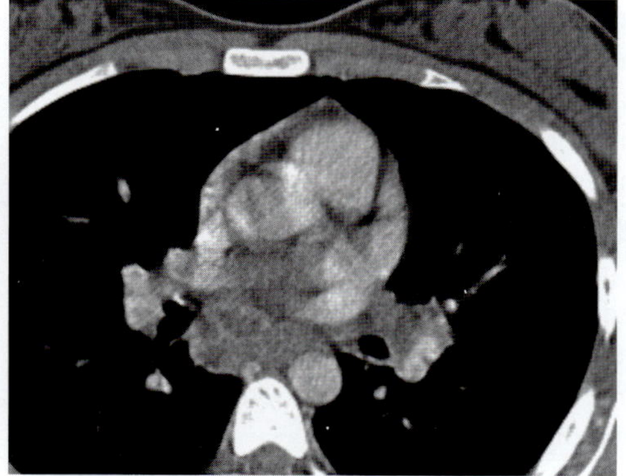

Fig. 4.110.3

Table 4.110.1: Differential diagnosis for mediastinal lymphadenopathy	
Calcified lymph nodes • Infectious granulomatous disease (tuberculosis, histoplasmosis) • Sarcoidosis • Silicosis • Hodgkin's lymphoma (following treatment) **Rare** • *P. carini* pneumonia • Metastasis (mucinous adenocarcinoma, thyroid carcinoma, osteosarcoma) • Amyloidosis • Scleroderma • Castleman's disease	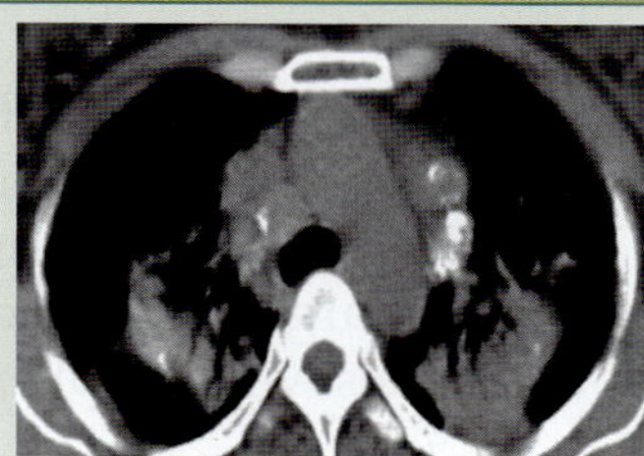 **Fig. 4.110.4:** Silicosis PMF
Low attenuation/necrotic lymph nodes: • Infectious granulomatous disease—tuberculosis, histoplasmosis • Metastasis (lung carcinoma, seminoma, ovarian, thyroid, gastric carcinoma) • Lymphoma (10–20%) • Sarcoidosis (rare)	 **Fig. 4.110.5:** Lymphoma
Enhancing lymph node • Metastasis (vascular tumors—renal cell carcinoma, papillary thyroid carcinoma, sarcoma, melanoma, lung carcinoma) • Rim enhancing (breast carcinoma) • Tuberculosis **Rare** • Castleman's disease • Sarcoidosis • Angio immunoblastic lymphadenopathy	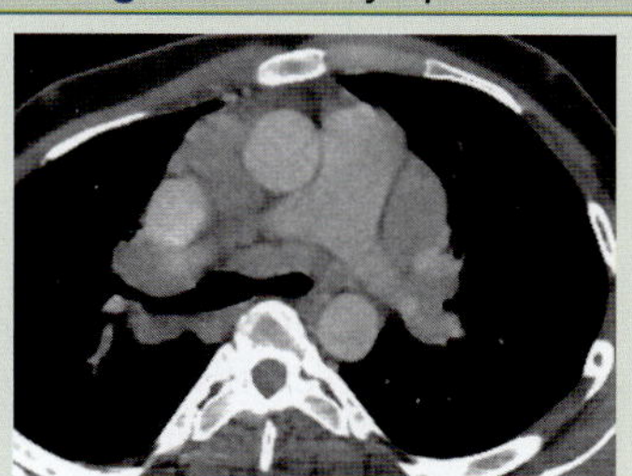 **Fig. 4.110.6:** Castleman's disease

Table 4.110.2: Different lymph node size: diameter upper limits of normal	
Different lymph node size: Diameter upper limits of normal	
Site	*Short axis (mm)*
Cervical	
All groups	8
Jugulodigastric nodes	10 (<10 with central necrosis)
Axilla	10
Mediastinum	
Subcarinal	12
Paracardiac	8
Retrocrural	6
Other sites	10
Abdomen	
Gastrohepatic ligament	8
Porta hepatis	8
Portocaval, celiac axis to renal artery	10
Renal artery to aortic bifurcation	12
Common iliac	9
Internal iliac	7
Obturator	8
External iliac, inguinal	10

anterior segment. No evidence of pleural effusion, cavitation, fibrosis, volume loss, honeycombing, bronchial cut-off. On post-contrast CT (Fig. 4.110.3) shows multiple enlarged necrotic mediastinal and perihilar lymph nodes with peripheral enhancement.

Interpretation: A—20-year-old female, lesion in left lung and mediastinal nodes, C—centrilobular nodules and multiple enlarged necrotic mediastinal and perihilar lymph nodes, B—peripheral enhancement of nodes, D—primary pulmonary tuberculosis.

Principal diagnosis: Primary pulmonary tuberculosis.

Management: Patient is referred to thoracic physician microbiological diagnosis and drug susceptibility testing to start ATT.

Differential Diagnosis

Hodgkin's lymphoma: HL has a predilection for thoracic involvement, and up to 85% of patients with HL present with mediastinal adenopathy. HL most often involves the superior mediastinal (prevascular, paratracheal, aortopulmonary) lymph nodes.

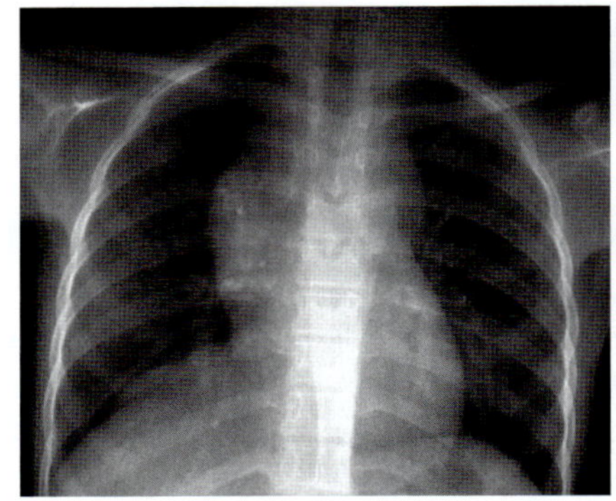

Fig. 4.110.7: Hodgkin's lymphoma

Table 4.110.3: Lymph node characteristics for clue to diagnosis		
Plain CT	HU—fat dense	Whipple's disease
	Egg shell calcification	Silicosis, sarcoidosis, coalminers pneumoconiosis, lymphoma after RT, amyloidosis, blastomycosis
	Central calcification	Tuberculosis, Castleman's disease
	Foamy calcification	Pneumocystis carini infection
Arterial, venous phase	Central necrosis	Metastasis—testicular, malignant lymphoma, tuberculosis
	Intense uniform enhancement	Lymphoma vascular tumors—renal, thyroid, melanoma, carcinoid, leiomyoma/sarcoma Castleman's disease
With lung findings	Nodules	Tuberculosis, sarcoidosis, lymphoma, silicosis
	Mass	Metastasis
Location	1-2-3 sign, Garland triad, Pawnbroker's sign—bilateral hilar nodes, right paratracheal nodes. **Node of woods**—Jugulodigastric nodes (chiefly drains the tonsil) **Delphian node**—Pretracheal node	Sarcoidosis 1-2-3-4 sign—bilateral hilar nodes, right paratracheal and aortopulmonary window lymph nodes. **Node of Rouvière**–lateral group of retropharyngeal node (sentinal node in nasopharyngeal carcinoma) **Virchow's node**—left supraclavicular node

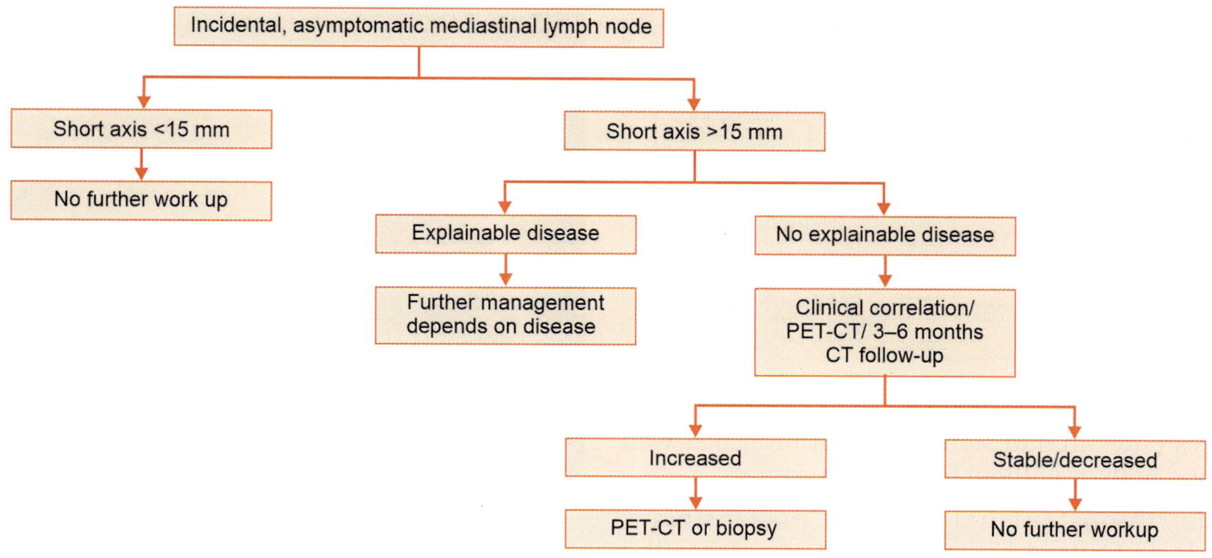

Fig. 4.110.8: Management of incidental asymptomatic mediastinal lymph node

Lymph node enlargement in malignant lymphoma and leukemia (Fig. 4.110.7).

Bilateral and asymmetrical involvement of anterior mediastinal, paratracheal, tracheobronchial and subcarinal nodes. Hilar, posterior mediastinal nodes are rare. Paracardiac nodes in recurrent disease.

Discussion: The approach to thoracic lymph node enlargement (MAGIC)

- M: Malignancy—primary lung carcinoma, metastasis, lymphoma, non-Hodgkin's lymphoma.
- A: Autoimmune diseases—systemic lupus erythematosus, rheumatoid arthritis, amyloidosis, allergic alveolitis (hypersensitivity pneumonitis)
- G: Granulomatous diseases—tuberculosis, silicosis, sarcoidosis.
- I: Infection—Histoplasmosis, pulmonary coccidioidomycosis, Epstein-Barr virus (EBV), varicella-zoster virus, hantaviruses, influenza viruses, dengue virus.
- I: Interstitial lung diseases, iatrogenic (phenytoin, methotrexate, sulfonamides, penicillin, allopurinol, aspirin, and erythromycin)
- C: Chronic heart failure

Pulmonary tuberculosis pathophysiology: Classically TB is divided into primary, common in childhood and self-limiting and post-primary, usually presenting in adults. It is caused by infection with *Mycobacterium tuberculosis*, accounting for over 95% of pulmonary infection. Following inhalation, the droplet nuclei usually implants in the bronchioles or alveoli. A delayed hypersensitivity response with macrophages results in tissue damage causing a solid caseating centre. Over time a mounted response from macrophages destroy the bacilli. However, in many cases delayed hypersensitivity reaction can cause local tissue damage, resulting in progressive enlargement of lesion.

Anatomically the right bronchus bifurcates at an angle of about 70 degrees, giving a greater volume and respiratory capacity to the right lung. Because of this reason, primary tuberculosis, with round infiltrates and consolidations, is mostly seen in the right lung, in the basal portions of the lower and middle lobe and in the anterior segment of the upper lobe.

The term post-primary tuberculosis is generally used to refer to both re-infection and reactivation of primary tuberculosis. It occurs in patients who are previously sensitised to *M. tuberculosis*. Typical are centrilobular

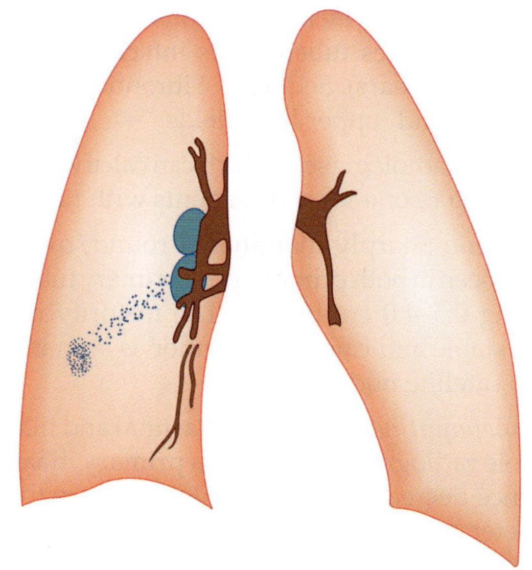

Fig. 4.110.9: Pathogenesis of primary pulmonary tuberculosis

Table 4.110.4: Comparison of primary and secondary TB		
	Primary TB	*Reinfection TB*
Location	Usually bases	Upper lobes, superior segment
Appearance	Focal	Patchy
Cavitation	No	Frequent
Only adenopathy	Common	No
Effusion	Common	Uncommon
Miliary pattern	Yes	Yes

nodules with a diameter of 2–4 mm and branched linear structures ("tree-in-bud sign"); distinct bronchial wall thickening with or without bronchiectasis.

Caverns: Important hallmark of post-primary tuberculosis Caused by attachment of a caseating consolidation to the bronchial system. In 40–45% of patients with post-primary tuberculosis, one or more cavities are detectable, important activity marker in patients with tuberculosis. They are typically thick-walled and irregularly contoured, less often thin-walled and smoothly bounded. In 9–21% of patients there is a secretion-air-level in the cavern as an indication of a bacterial/mycotic superinfection.

Consolidations: Primary tuberculosis–dense, homogeneous, Usually in middle lobe, lower lobes or anterior segment of the upper lobes, unilateral. In post-primary tuberculosis consolidation is patchy, heterogeneous, ill-defined, segmental, usually in the apical or posterior segment of the upper lobes or the superior segment of the lower lobes. 2 or more segments usually involved, bilateral—which are often indistinguishable from bacterial infection. Lymphadenopathy, lack of response to conventional antibiotics indicates tuberculosis infection. Resolution is slow (even 2 years). Sequelae: Fibronodular opacities seen on apex and upper lung fields.

Ghon focus: Radiologic scar which can calcify. It is usually present in up to one-third of patients with tuberculosis.

Tuberculoma: Sharply marginated round/oval lesions which are seen in both primary, post-primary tuberculosis, measuring 0.5–4.0 cm in size. The majority of lesions remains stable and calcify. Cavitation is seen in 10–50% of cases; satellite nodules in 80%.

Lymphadenopathy: Usually mediastinal and hilar, it can be the sole radiographic feature in primary infection. Its prevalence decreases with age. Nodes more than 2 cm in diameter are highly suggestive. Sequelae are calcified normal-sized lymph nodes; more than six months after the initial infection. With continuation of treatment, there

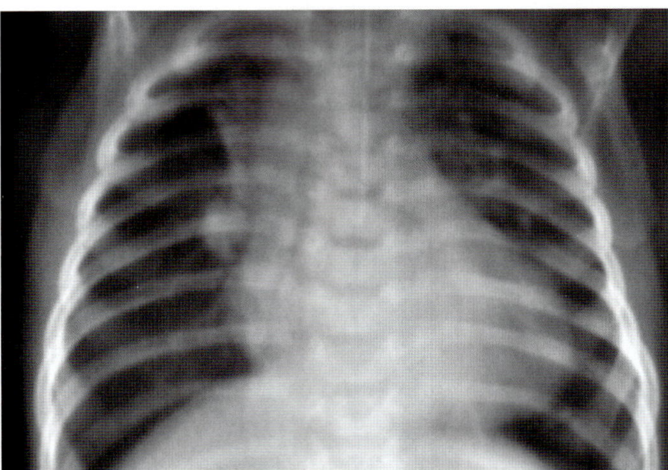

Fig. 4.110.10: Ghon complex

is a slower resolution of the lymph nodes compared to the parenchymal disease, so nodal calcification may develop **Ranke complex:** The combination of calcified hilar nodes and a Ghon focus.

Miliary tuberculosis: Haematogenous seeding of TB with acute, severe illness with high mortality. 1–7% of patients with all forms of tuberculosis. Evenly distributed diffuse 2–3 mm sized nodules, in both lungs, with a slight lower lobe predominance. Thickening of inter- and intra-lobular septa. CXR allows diagnosis in 59–69% of cases. Early in the course of the illness, CXR is normal in 25–40% of cases. Nodules usually resolve within 2–6 months with treatment, without scarring or calcification; however, they may coalesce with a "snowstorm" appearance. Complications: Acute respiratory distress syndrome, distribution of tuberculosis in other organs, pneumothorax (rare).

Pleural effusion: 25–38% of primary tuberculosis cases; 18% of post-primary tuberculosis. Increasing prevalence with age. In primary tuberculosis—unilateral, large, not loculated. On the same side as the primary focus, +/– evidence of parenchymal disease on CXR. In post-primary tuberculosis—small, loculated + parenchymal disease. Rarely the sole imaging manifestation, can remain stable for many years.

Complications: **Tuberculous empyema:** Loculated pleural fluid collection with parenchymal disease and cavitation, associated with pleural thickening, **broncho-pleural fistula:** Air-fluid level within an empyema. **Empyema necessitates:** Untreated empyema extends into the chest wall, bone erosion. Sequelae residual pleural thickening and calcification.

Cavitation: Hallmark of post-primary tuberculosis (about 50% of patients), it can occur in a minority of primary tuberculosis (29%), usually multiple within areas of consolidation. Complications: Superinfections—air-fluid levels inside cavities, pneumothorax (5%), lobar or complete lung opacification and destruction, if untreated, endobronchial spread—caseous necrosis of bronchial walls with airway communication.

Sequelae: Emphysematous changes, fibrosis/scarring, predisposition to bacterial superinfection and mycetoma formation (air crescent sign), volume loss (especially apical), atelectasis, architectural distortion or traction bronchiectasis, interstitial fibrosis.

Diagnosis: Microbiological, microscopy, culture, DNA detection (PCR), tuberculin skin test, interferon test (T-Spot). Advantage: No false positive results. Disadvantage: False negative in immunosuppression/infants.

Treatment: The preferred regimen for treating adults with TB remains a regimen consisting of an intensive phase of 2 months of isoniazid (INH), rifampicin (RIF), pyrazinamide (PZA), and ethambutol (EMB) followed by a continuation phase of 4 months of INH and RIF.

CT-guided thoracic biopsy: Usually performed for the diagnosis of suspicious lung, pleural or mediastinal lesions. Laboratory parameters—complete blood count (CBC)—platelet >50000/mm^3, coagulation profile (INR) ≤1.5–2, normal prothrombin time (PT), partial thromboplastin time (PTT).

Pre-procedure evaluation: Review the diagnostic CT and other relevant imaging first (e.g. PET/CT) to clarify the lesion that is requested to be biopsied. By considering various factors, that influence suitability and degree of risk should be reviewed, including the site and size of the nodule/mass and its relationship to surrounding structures including vessels, bleb, bullae, central bronchi, fissures. With cavitating lesions, the needle must be targeted to the periphery.

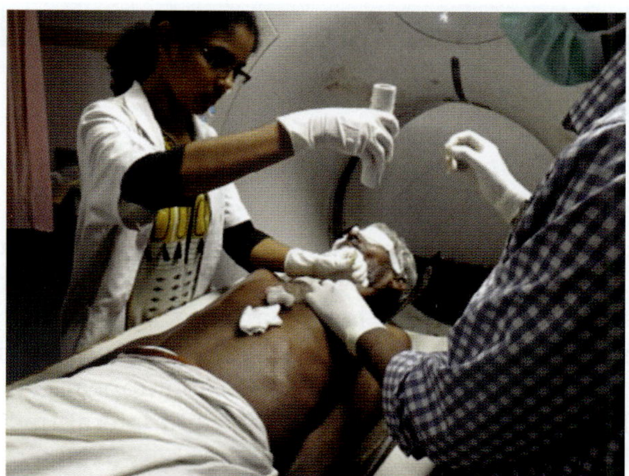

Fig. 4.110.11: Procedure of CT-guided biopsy

Positioning: The patient can be positioned prone, supine or laterally (decubitus) depending on the location of the lesion and their respiratory function.

Biopsy: A radiopaque grid or skin marker should be utilized to focus the optimal access point then, after preliminary images, this point is marked with a pen. Local anaesthesia with lidocaine is given and skin orifice is made using a scalpel blade, the biopsy needle is introduced as previous planning and activate biopsy gun (Fig. 4.110.11).

Cutting needles: These needles have a variegated tip or cutting notch on the side. In the single needle technique, a needle is directly advanced into the lesion and if multiple samples are required each time, a new pass will be made. The main advantage of the coaxial technique is that multiple needle passes may be made into a lesion without the time-consuming process of repositioning the needle within the subcutaneous tissues for each pass.

Complications: Pneumothorax (8–64%), alveolar haemorrhage ~10%, haemoptysis in 1–5%, air embolism.

4.111 CHEST

CASE No. 111

Clinical history: 5-year-old male with history of breathlessness.

Radiological techniques and observation: Scanogram Fig. 4.111.1 shows a suspicious soft tissue dense radio-opaque intraluminal lesion arising from the right lateral wall of the trachea causing significant luminal narrowing. The margins of the lesion appear regular making an obtuse angle with the right lateral tracheal wall. Noncontrast and contrast CT of chest-axial section, coronal reformation in mediastinal window and VRT images (Figs 4.111.2 to 4.111.6) demonstrate a well enhancing polypoid intraluminal mass of soft-tissue attenuation with extension through the proximal tracheal wall, at the level of D3 and D4 vertebra. The margins of the mass appear lobulated and regular. The mass is adherent to the wall of the trachea between 6 and 9 o'clock. The mass causes 90% occlusion of the tracheal lumen at this level. The longitudinal extent of the mass is greater than their axial extent and the mass involves more than 180° of the airway circumference. Bilateral lower lobe consolidation, much more pronounced on the left, keeping in with aspiration pneumonia. No significant mediastinal lymphadenopathy.

No evidence of fat component, calcification, cartilage noted within the lesion. No evidence of local mediastinal extension and lung metastasis.

Interpretation: A—44-year-old male, lesion in proximal trachea, C—irregular polypoid intraluminal mass of soft tissue attenuation with extension through the proximal tracheal wall, B—longitudinal extent of the mass is greater than axial extent, and the mass involves more than 180° of the airway circumference, D—adenoid cystic carcinoma.

Principal diagnosis: Adenoid cystic carcinoma arising from the proximal trachea.

Further investigations and management: Surgery is curative in this patient. Histopathology should be done to confirm the diagnosis.

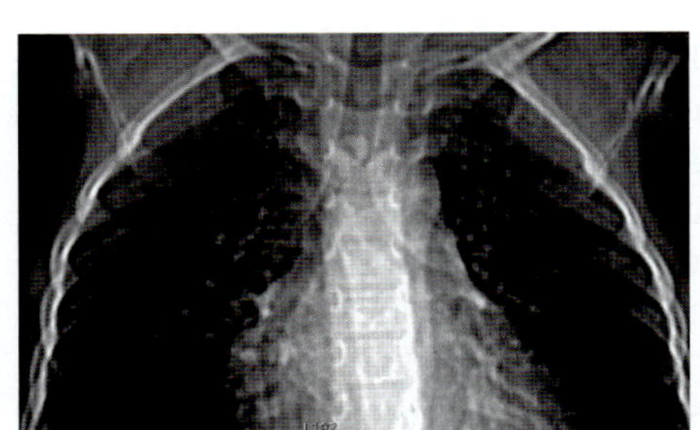

Fig. 4.111.1

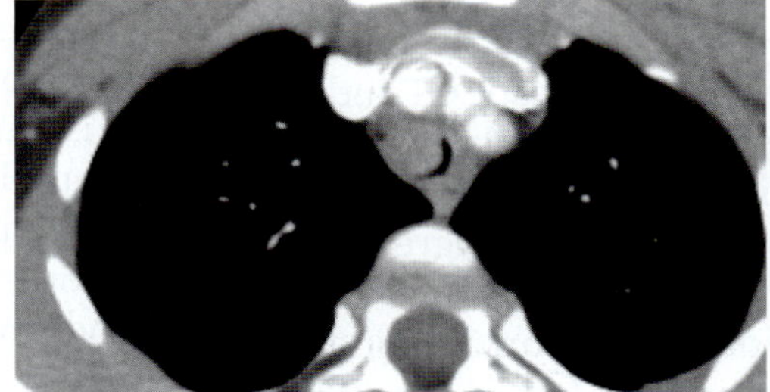

Fig. 4.111.2

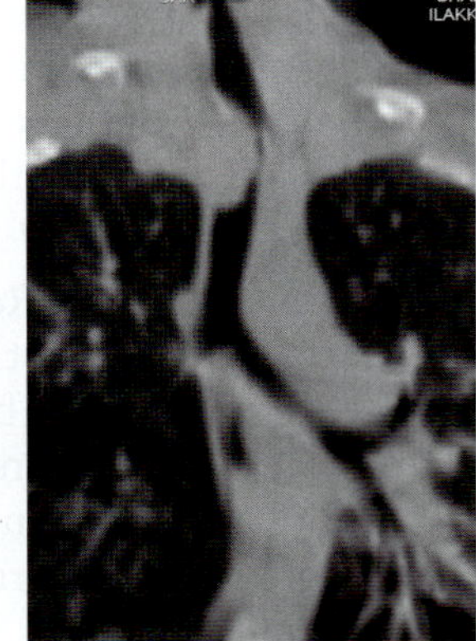

Fig. 4.111.3: Hamartoma

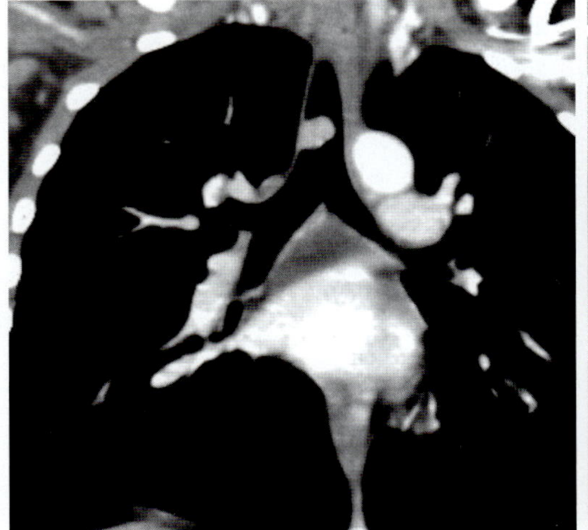

Fig. 4.111.4

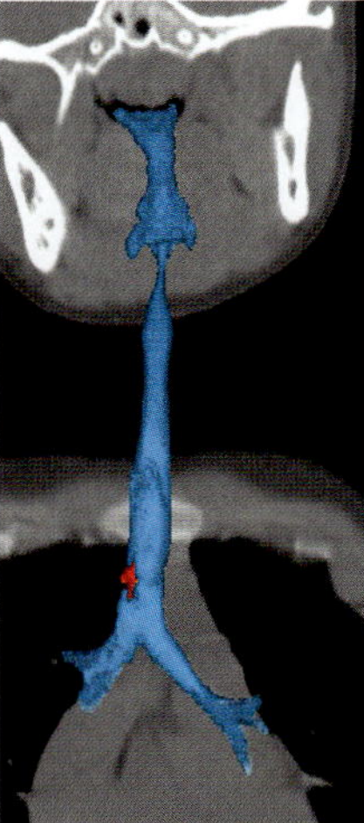

Fig. 4.111.5

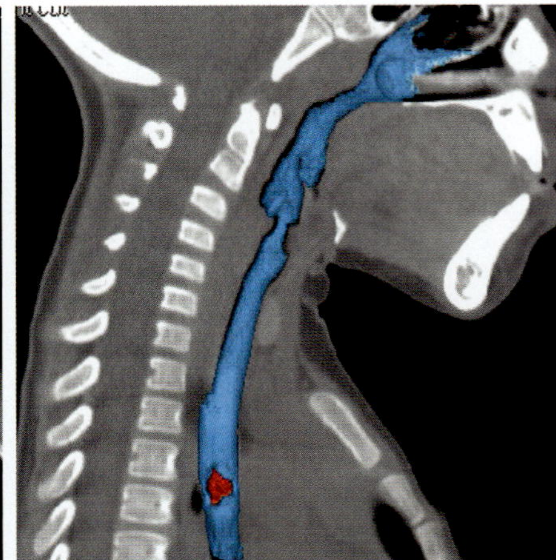

Fig. 4.111.6

Table 4.111.1: Classification of tracheobronchial tumors		
Origin of tumor	*Primary malignant tumors*	*Benign tumors*
Surface epithelium	Squamous cell carcinoma (SCC), adenocarcinoma, neuroendocrine tumors (carcinoid tumor, large cell neuroendocrine tumors, small cell carcinoma)	Squamous cell papilloma, papillomatosis
Salivary glands	Adenoid cystic carcinoma (ACC), mucoepidermoid carcinoma (MEC), epithelial-myoepithelial carcinoma (EMEC)	Pleomorphic adenoma, mucous gland adenoma, oncocytoma
Mesenchyme	Sarcoma, malignant lymphoma	Hamartoma, leiomyoma, lipoma, fibroma, neurogenic tumors
Direct invasion	Thyroid cancer, laryngeal cancer, lung cancer and esophageal cancer	
Hematogenous metastasis	Breast cancer, renal cell carcinoma, colon cancer, melanoma	

Discussion

Table 4.111.2: Malignant tracheal masses	
Squamous cell carcinoma. SCC is the most common primary tracheo-bronchial malignancy and develops mainly in the 6th and 7th decades of life.	Involve the posterior wall of the trachea in lower two-thirds. One-third of patients have either mediastinal or pulmonary metastases at diagnosis. Polypoid lesion/focal sessile lesion causing eccentric narrowing of the airway lumen, or circumferential wall thickening. Associated with habitual cigarette smoking, (M>F). High uptake at FDG PET
Adenoid cystic carcinoma ACC is the common type of lung cancer with salivary gland origin. ACC has no sex predilection and commonly occurs in the 4th and 5th decades of life	ACC usually occurs in the central airways (the trachea or main bronchus). Striking tendency toward submucosal extension which manifests with circumferential and infiltrative growth. FDG uptake can vary depending on the grade of differentiation of lesion.

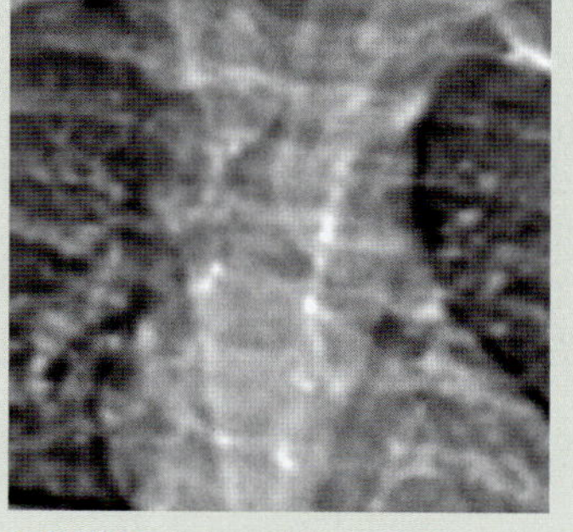

Fig. 4.111.7: Adenoid cystic carcinoma

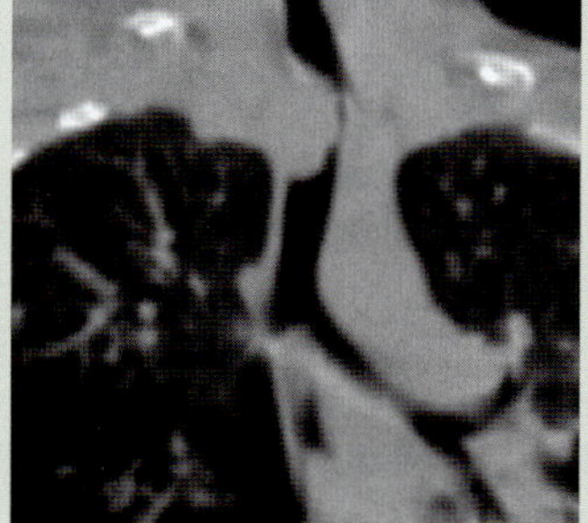

Fig. 4.111.8: Adenoid cystic carcinoma

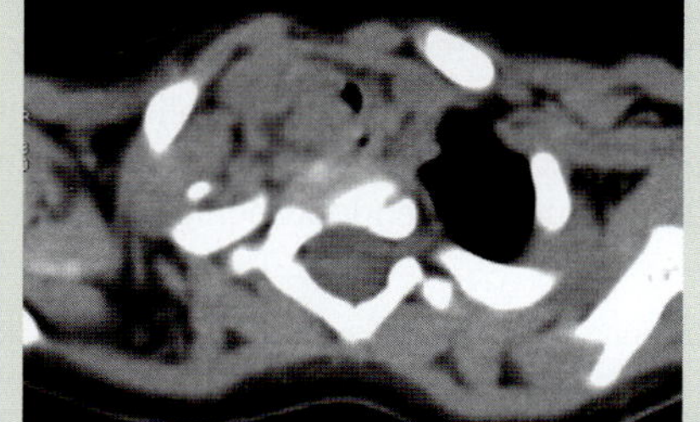

Fig. 4.111.9: Adenoid cystic carcinoma

Mucoepidermoid CA. Rare, arise from the minor salivary glands in the tracheobronchial tree. Nearly one-half of whom are under 30 years old	CT as an intraluminal nodule confined to the branching features of the airways. Avid uptake has been reported in high-grade MECs, with mild FDG uptake found in low-grade MECs
Carcinoid tumor: Pulmonary or bronchial Carcinoid tumors accounting for over 25% of all carcinoid tumors and for minority of (1–2%) of all pulmonary neoplasms. At FDG PET, carcinoid tumors usually have lower uptake.	At CT, a carcinoid tumor of the tracheobronchial tree is seen as a well-defined spheric or ovoid nodule with a slightly lobulated border. The intraluminal component is relatively small compared with the bulk of the tumor (iceberg tumor). Demonstrate intense enhancement.

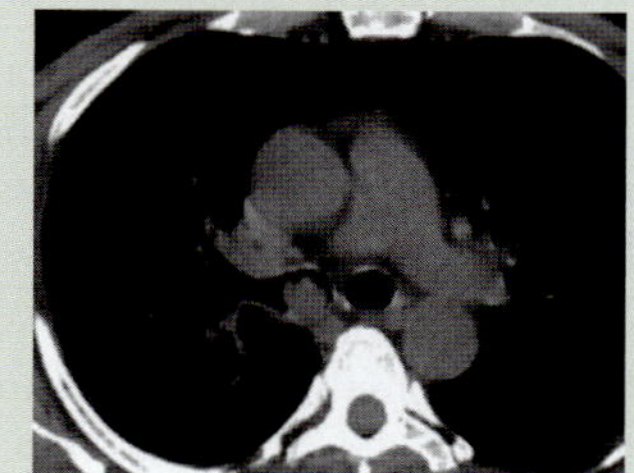

Fig. 4.111.10: Carcinoid tumor

Sarcoma. Primary thoracic sarcomas with mesenchymal origin are extremely rare	Chondrosarcoma, fibrosarcoma, and synovial sarcoma occur in the tracheobronchial tree, manifesting as an endoluminal mass. At FDG-PET, this tumor may demonstrate avid uptake depending on metabolic activity of lesion.

Table 4.111.3: Benign tracheal masses

Hamartoma: Hamartoma is defined as a benign tumor which has tissue elements that are normally present in an affected organ	Endobronchial hamartoma contains cartilage, fat, fibrous tissue, and epithelial components. Findings such as internal fat and "popcorn" calcification help distinguish hamartomas from malignancies. At FDG-PET, hamartomas may show a little or no uptake	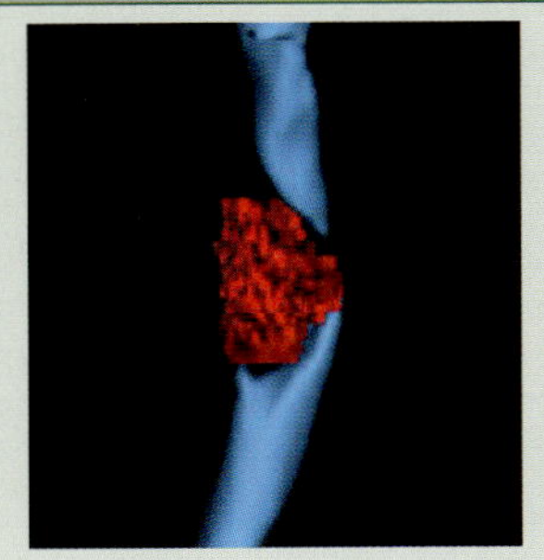 **Fig. 4.111.11:** Tracheal hamartoma
Tracheobronchial papillomatosis. Tracheobronchial papillomatosis is usually seen in young children. The larynx is most commonly affected with, extension into the trachea.	Multiple small nodules projecting into the airway/diffuse nodular thickening of the airway wall is common. Involvement of the distal airways, parenchyma can result in multiple nodules, which cavitate.They may undergo malignant transformation to SCC	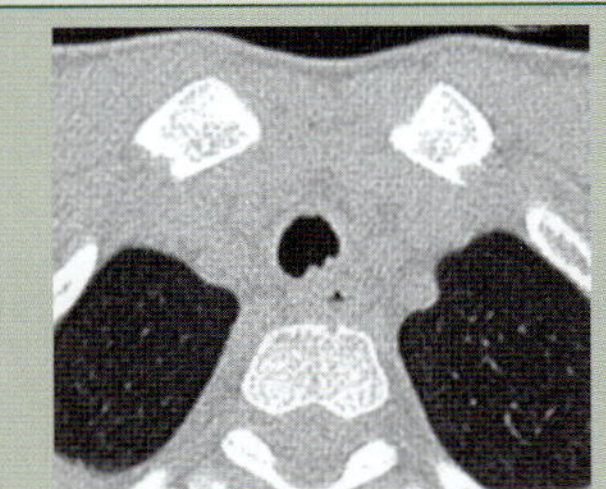 **Fig. 4.111.12:** Tracheobronchial papillomatosis
Lipoma. Lipoma is defined as a mass composed of mature fat tissue. Most intrathoracic lipomas are endobronchial. Generally occur in late-middle-aged men	CT is highly specific, sensitive in the detection of fat and can be helpful in diagnosing tracheobronchial lipomas. Endobronchial hamartoma can manifest as a fatty mass at CT	
Leiomyoma. Primary leiomyoma of the tracheobronchial tree is an uncommon tumor that affects about 2% of people. Tracheal tumors arise from the tracheal wall's smooth muscle, particularly the posterior membranous region.	Homogeneously enhancing intraluminal mass without extraluminal extension. It may show increased FDG uptake	
Neurogenic tumors. Most intrathoracic neurogenic tumors, including schwannoma and neurofibroma, occur in the posterior mediastinum. 25% tumors are endobronchial	At CT, these tumors have been described as round or lobulated homogeneous masses. Neurogenic tumors with increased FDG uptake to undergo malignant change. With use of an SUV of 2.5 as a cut-off value, they were able to differentiate between malignant and benign neurogenic tumors	

Table 4.111.4: Inflammatory tracheal disease

Inflammatory tracheal disease	*Radiological features*
Wegener's granulomatosis (WG): WG is a multisystem necrotising granulomatous vasculitis affecting arteries, capillaries and veins (small to medium-sized), with a clinical predilection for involvement of the upper airways, lungs, and kidneys.	CT examination reveals a circumferential, symmetrical soft tissue swelling in the trachea, from the most proximal subglottis area extending into the proximal trachea
Tracheobronchial amyloidosis: It is a rare occurrence, according to some accounts, with fewer than 100 documented cases at the time of writing. An elevated, tumor-like mass of amyloid material (amyloid pseudotumor /amyloidoma) is a rare symptom of the condition.	Mucosal thickening +/– calcification in trachea and bronchial segments are possible. The posterior membrane is usually affected when the trachea is compromised. The distribution of disease might be either localised or diffuse.
Relapsing polychondritis (RP): Seen in middle age and no sex predilection. Commonly affected areas are tracheobronchial tree (50%), external ear cartilages, nasal cartilages, peripheral joints and laryngeal cartilages	Increased airway wall attenuation is common, smooth anterior and lateral tracheal wall thickening. Sparing of the posterior membranous wall noted. Tracheobronchial and peripheral bronchial luminal narrowing
Tracheobronchopathia osteochondroplastica: 5th to 6th decades and there may be a male predilection.The etiology is ecchondrosis and exostosis from cartilage rings or cartilaginous and osseous metaplasia of the elastic tissue in the internal elastic fibrous membrane.	Irregular thickening and nodularity of tracheal cartilage, sparing the posterior (membranous) tracheal wall. Small discrete endophytic nodules (typically ~3–8 mm) may be cartilagenous or calcific (ossified)

4.112 CHEST

Case No. 112

Clinical history: 50 years old male presented with the complaints of cough with expectoration and wheezing.

Radiological techniques and observation: Figures 4.112.1 and 4.112.2 are chest X-ray PA view and lateral chest images showing triangular right retrocardiac opacity which shows loss of silhouette with the diaphragm. However, there is no silhoutteing of the right cardiac border. There is shift of mediastinum and trachea to the right with elevation of the right hemidiaphragm. Other visualized lung fields appears normal. Visualized bone and soft tissues appear normal. With these findings right lower collapse to be considered.

Causes of lobar collapse: **Luminal:** Aspirated foreign material, mucous plugging **mural:** Bronchogenic carcinoma, bronchial carcinoid **extrinsic:** Compression by adjacent mass. For further characterization CT is needed.

Figures 4.112.3 and 4.112.4 are Non enhanced CT chest in limited axial sections in mediastinal window showing there is a mass lesion located within the right main bronchus which is causing partial occlusion of the right main bronchus causing collapse of superior segment of right lower lobe. Figures 4.112.5 to 4.112.8 are post-contrast images showing heterogenous enhancement following administration of contrast with prominent vessel supplying from aorta. There is no evidence of hilar and mediastinal lymphadenopathy.

Interpretation: A: 50 years old male, endobronchial mass lesion in right main bronchus, C: Calcification and heterogenous enhancement, B: Prominent vascular supply from aorta, D: Central bronchial carcinoid tumor.

Principal diagnosis: Right endobronchial central bronchial carcinoid tumor.

Differential diagnosis: Bronchogenic carcinoma.

Further investigations: PET-CT–68 Ga-DOTATE—to confirm the uptake in the carcinoid. Histopathological examination.

Treatment: Resectable tumors: Those that can be treated with surgery. Unresectable tumors: Those that cannot be removed completely by surgery, chemotherapy, radiation.

Brief discussion about the condition: Neuroendocrine tumors of the lung arise from enterochromaffin cells, neuroepithelial bodies, or pluripotent bronchial epithelial stem cells that are normally present in the bronchial mucosa. Lung carcinoid tumors account for more than 25% of all carcinoid tumors in the body, as well as 1–2% of all pulmonary neoplasms.

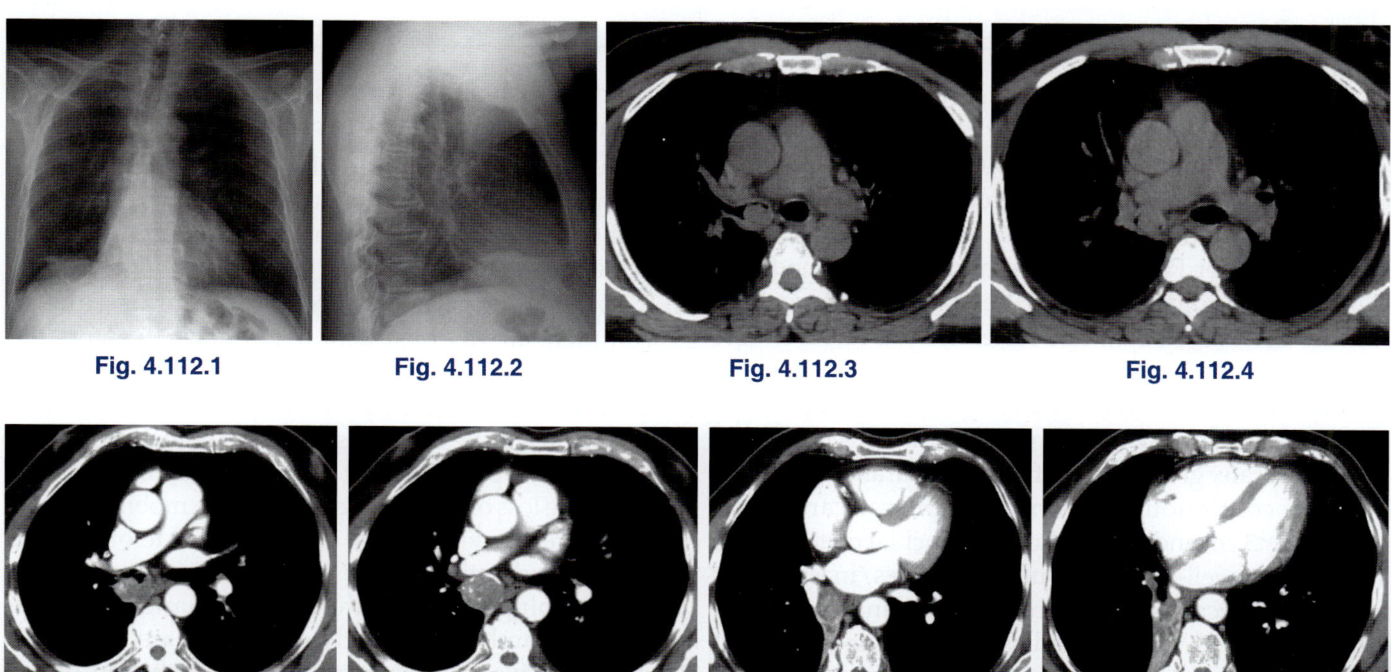

Fig. 4.112.1 Fig. 4.112.2 Fig. 4.112.3 Fig. 4.112.4

Fig. 4.112.5 Fig. 4.112.6 Fig. 4.112.7 Fig. 4.112.8

Table 4.112.1: Imaging finding in bronchogenic carcinoma

Bronchogenic carcinoma Bronchial cut-off with fluid bronchogram 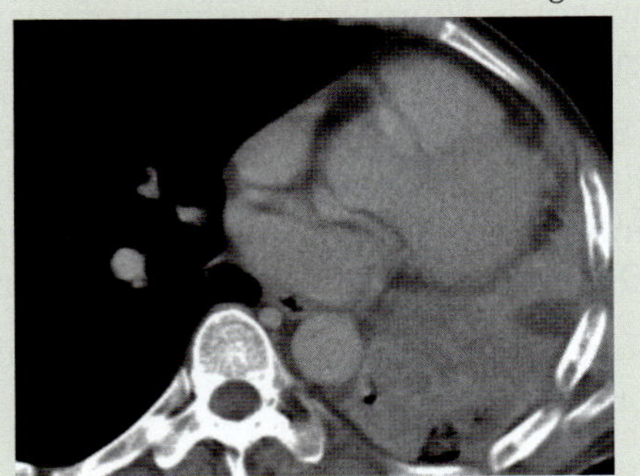 **Fig. 4.112.9:** Bronchial cut-off with fluid bronchogram	HRCT findings are 65% arise in main, lobar or segmental bronchi presents as, endobronchial mass with bronchial obstruction and/or infiltration of bronchial wall with local invasion. Hilar region is the common site. Atelectasis and consolidation common. 30% mass presents as solitary mass or nodule. Pleural effusion may be seen.Cavitation relatively common.	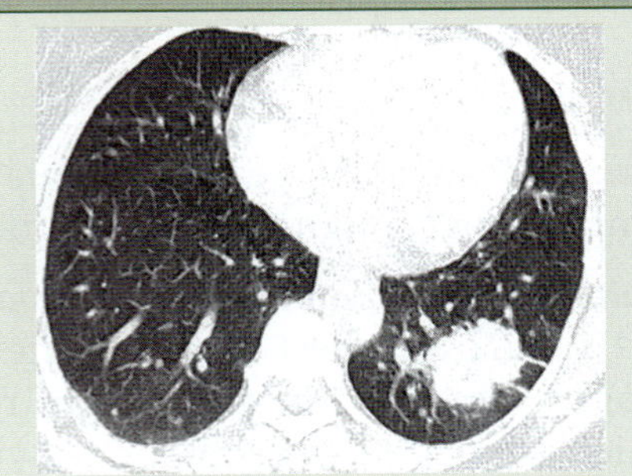 **Fig. 4.112.10:** Bronchogenic carcinoma presenting as solitary mass

Table 4.112.2: Difference between typical carcinoid, atypical carcinoid and small cell carcinoma

Features	*Typical carcinoid*	*Atypical carcinoid*	*Small cell carcinoma*
1. Mean age	45–60	60	More than 60
2. Male : Female	0.8–1	2;1	4;1
3. Smoking	Uncommon	Common	Very common
4. Symptoms	75%	50%	90%
5. Regional metastases	5–15%	40–60%	More than 90%
6. Distant metastases	Rare	20%	More than 90%
7. 5-year survival	90–95%	50–70%	5%
8. Endobronchial mass	80%	10%	20%
9. Lung nodule or mass	20%	90%	20%
10. Large hilar mass	50%	10%	80%

Centrally located bronchial carcinoids (50%) are more common and anatomically closely related to the airways. Peripheral carcinoids (40%) are seen distal to the segmental bronchi. At CT, carcinoid tumors are seen as a spherical nodule/mass with a well-defined and mild lobulated border. Rarely, they present as multiple nodules. Central carcinoids are near the tracheal bifurcation and are seen as a small nodule entirely located within the lumen of a bronchus. Calcification (30%) is more common in central carcinoids. They can also cause distal obstructive atelectasis, pneumonitis, or mucus plugging, which typically give a gloved finger appearance (multiple dilated contiguous bronchi). Peripheral carcinoids measures <3 cm and do not show a bronchial relationship, appearing as well-defined lobulated nodules/masses with or without necrosis.Intense contrast enhancement (>30 HU) is seen with hilar or mediastinal lymphadenopathy (reactive/metastatic). Metastases to the intrathoracic lymph nodes, liver, CNS, skeletal bones, adrenals, mammary glands, testis, and pancreas occur in 15% cases.

Bronchial carcinoid tumors are seen in relation to a bronchus (segmental or larger bronchus).

Collapse/atelectasis: Lung atelectasis refers to collapse/incomplete expansion of pulmonary parenchyma. Based on underlying mechanism atelectasis can be subcategorised, as follows:

1. *Resorptive atelectasis (obstructive)* occurs as due to complete airway obstruction. No new air enters the lung distal to the obstruction and already present air in bronchus is absorbed into the pulmonary capillary system, resulting in collapsed affected lung. As parietal and visceral pleura do not separate, traction is created, and if the loss of volume is considerable, mobile thoracic structures may be pulled toward the side of volume loss ("mediastinal shift"). Obstructing neoplasms, mucus plugging in asthmatics or dangerously ill patients, and foreign body aspiration are all causes of resorptive atelectasis. Complete occlusion of the right or left main bronchus might result in resorptive atelectasis of the entire lung (collapsed lung).

Table 4.112.3: Imaging findings in collapse on chest radiograph

1. Right upper lobe collapse: Increased density in the medial side of right hemithorax. Elevation of the horizontal fissure/superior bowing, loss of normal right medial cardiomediastinal shape, elevated right hilum, laterally rotated bronchus intermedius making it appear more horizontal than typical. Increased translucency of the mid and lower regions of the right lung results from hyperinflation of the right middle and lower lobes. Right juxtaphrenic peak (Kattan sign). A hilar mass is a common cause of lobar collapse. An S-shape to elevated horizontal fissure results when a right hilar mass is paired with collapse of the right upper lobe. This is referred to as the Golden S symbol.	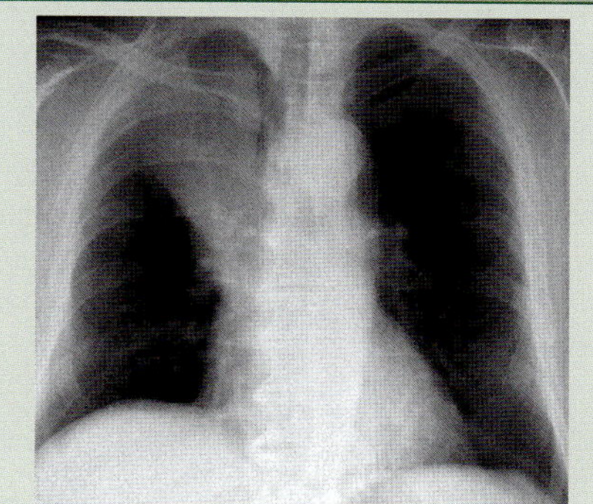 **Fig. 4.112.11:** Right upper lobe collapse
2. Right middle lobe collapse: Right mid to lower zone air space opacification (which can be subtle). The normal horizontal fissure is no longer visible (as it rotates inferiorly rendering it non-tangental to the X-ray beam). Obscuration of the right heart border.	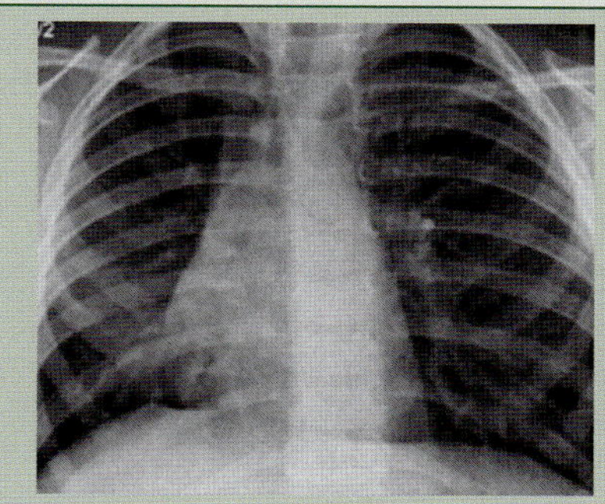 **Fig. 4.112.12:** Right middle lobe collapse
3. Right lower lobe collapse: Triangular opacity at the right lower zone (usually medially) with the apex pointing towards the right hilum is seen. Obscuration of the medial aspect of dome of right hemidiaphragm is seen. Inferior displacement of the right hilum. Descending interlobar pulmonary artery is not visible. Preservation of a clear right heart border, which is contacted by the right middle lobe (cf. obscuration seen in RML collapse or consolidation). Inferiorly displaced horizontal fissure may be seen.	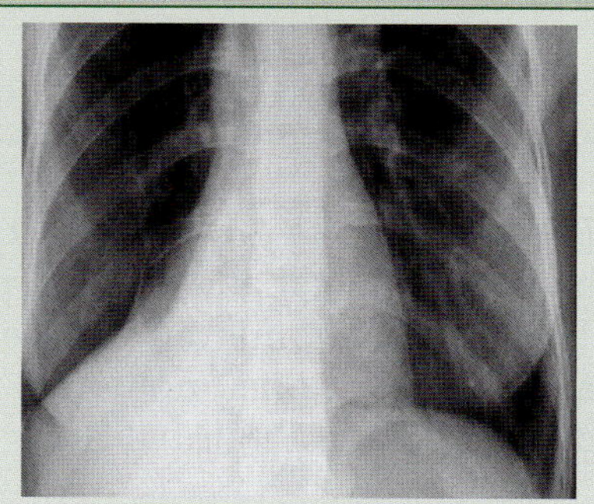 **Fig. 4.112.13:** Right lower lobe collapse
4. Left upper lobe collapse: The left upper lobe collapses anteriorly becoming a thin sheet of tissue apposed to the anterior chest wall and appears as a hazy or veiling opacity extending out from the left hilum and fading out inferiorly (Weil sign). In some cases the hyperexpanded superior segment of the left lower lobe insinuates itself between the left upper lobe and the superior mediastinum, sharply silhouetting the aortic arch and resulting in a sickle-shaped lucency medially. This is known as the luftsichel sign. The left hilum is drawn upwards, resulting in an almost horizontal course of the left main bronchus and vertical course of the left lower lobe bronchus.	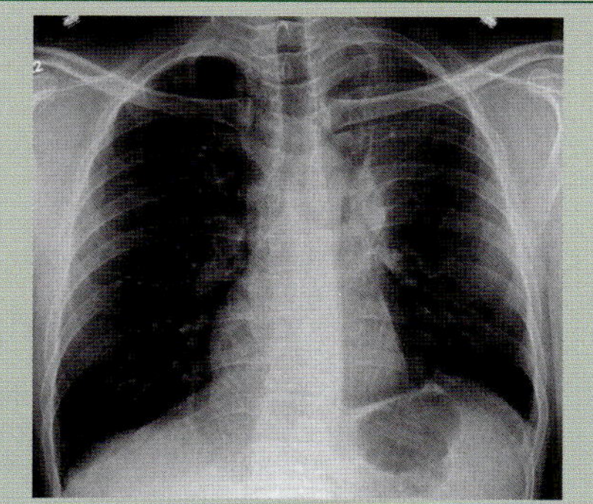 **Fig. 4.112.14:** Weil sign in left upper lobe collapse

(Contd.)

Table 4.112.3: Imaging findings in collapse on chest radiograph (*Contd.*)	
5. Left lower lobe collapse: Triangular opacity in the posteromedial aspect of the left lung (retrocardiac sail sign). Left lower zone opacification (usually medially) with the apex pointing towards the left hilum. Edge of the collapsed lung may create a 'double cardiac contour'. Inferior displacement of the left hilum. Flat waist sign: Flattening of the left heart border. Obscuration of the left hemidiaphragm. Obscuration of the descending aorta. Descending interlobar pulmonary artery is not visible. Preservation of a clear left heart border, which is contacted by the lingular segments of the left upper lobe (c.f. obscuration seen left lower lobe consolidation)	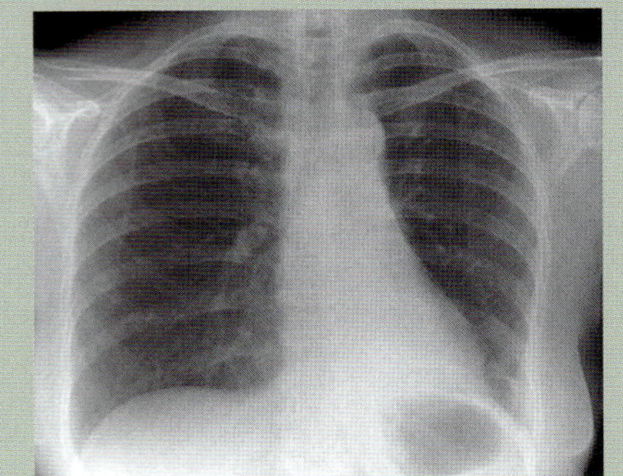 **Fig. 4.112.15:** Inferior displacement of the oblique fissure
Right middle lobe collapse: Non-homogeneity straight /concave border in lateral view wedge like outline with the base reaching the sternum absence of minor fissure. *Fissural effusion features:* • Homogeneous • Borders will be rounded • Does not reach till sternum • Minor fissure will be present	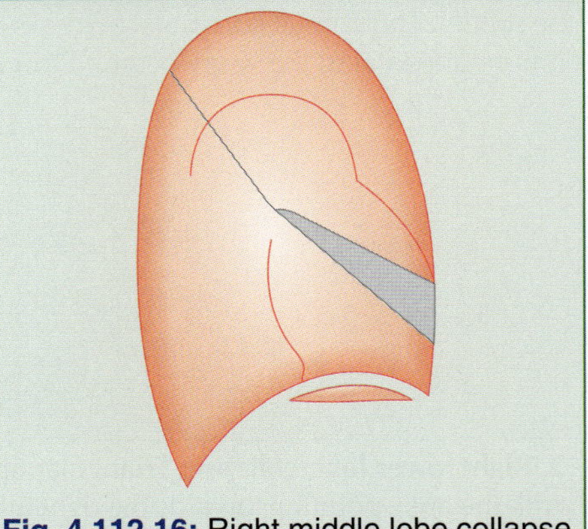 **Fig. 4.112.16:** Right middle lobe collapse

2. *Passive atelectasis (relaxation):* It occurs if the contact between parietal and visceral pleura is interrupted. The most common specific etiologies of passive atelectasis are pneumothorax, pleural effusion and diaphragmatic abnormality.
3. *Compressive atelectasis:* It occurs as a result of any thoracic space-occupying lesion compressing the lung and forcing air out of the alveoli.
4. *Cicatrisation atelectasis:* Scarring or fibrosis can cause atelectasis, which limits lung expansion.

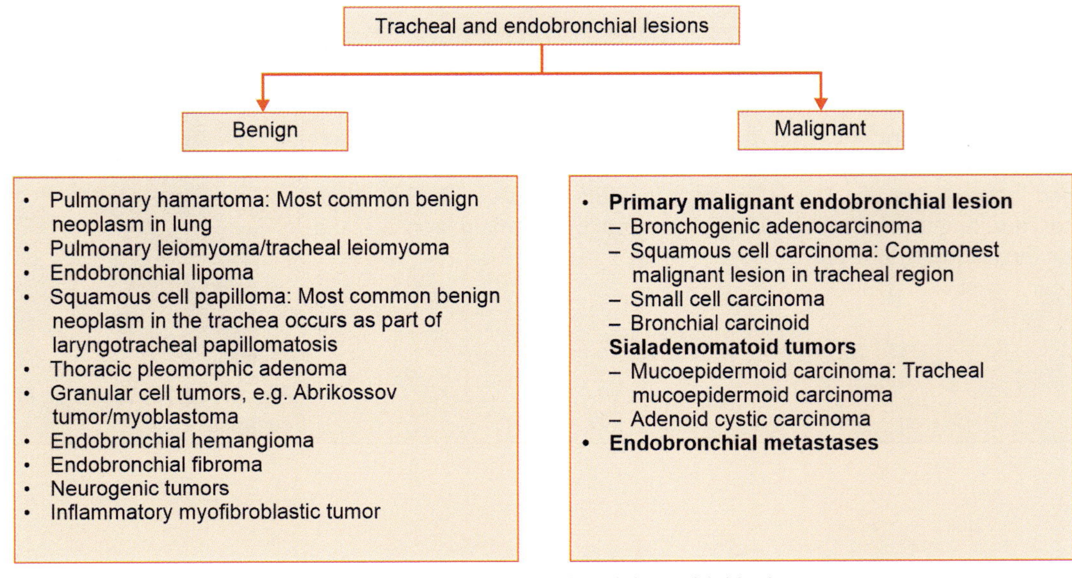

Fig. 4.112.17: Tracheal and endobronchial lesions

Granulomatous disease, necrotizing pneumonia, and radiation fibrosis are all common causes.

5. Adhesive atelectasis is caused by a lack of surfactant. This insufficiency may be diffuse throughout the lungs or localised, depending on the aetiology.
6. Gravity dependent atelectasis (dependent atelectasis) in the most dependent portions of the lungs due to the weight of the lungs

Atelectasis can also be subcategorised by morphology as follows:

1. Linear (plate, band, discoid, subsegmental) atelectasis: A minimal degree of collapse as seen in patients who are not taking deep breaths ("splinting"), such as postoperative patients or patients with rib fracture or pleuritic chest pain; this is very common
2. Lobar atelectasis is collapse of one or more lobes of a lung.
3. Segmental atelectasis is collapse of one or more individual pulmonary segments
4. Subsegmental atelectasis
5. Round atelectasis is associated with asbestos exposure.

Direct signs of atelectasis: Displacement of interlobar fissures, Crowding together of pulmonary vessels, Crowded air bronchograms (also seen in subsegmental atlectasis, usually by secretions; if the cause of the atelectasis is central bronchial obstruction, there will usually be no air bronchograms).

Indirect signs of atelectasis: Pulmonary opacification, compensatory hyperexpansion of the surrounding or contralateral lung, shifting granuloma, displacement of the heart, mediastinum, trachea, hilum, diaphragmatic elevation.

4.113 CHEST

Case No. 113

Clinical features: A 45-year-old male patient came with complaints of difficulty in swallowing (liquids> solids) for the past 6 months.

Radiological imaging techniques and observations: Figures 4.113.1 and 4.113.4 are frontal and lateral radiograph of the chest showing double contour of the right mediastinal border. A well-defined homogeneous oblong-shaped radio-opacity noted along the right heart border that is crossing the diaphragm with no evidence of calcification in the wall. On lateral view trachea is displaced anteriorly with indentation on the posterior wall of trachea. Stomach bubble seen. Possibly dilated esophagus. Differential diagnoses for transthoracic mediastinal shadow: Mediastinal lipomatosis, aortic aneurysm, achalasia, thymoma. Figures 4.113.2 and 4.113.3 are single contrast barium swallow image showing posteroanterior and right anterior oblique projection. There is a dilatation of esophagus with smooth, tapered narrowing just above the gastroesophageal junction. Close-up view shows smooth birds beak-like tapering of the distal esophagus. No evidence of shouldering. No evidence of mucosal irregularity.

Interpretation: A: 45-year-old male, C: Dilated esophagus with smooth birds beak-like narrowing of the distal esophagus, B: Without any shouldering or mucosal irregularity, D: Primary achalasia cardia.

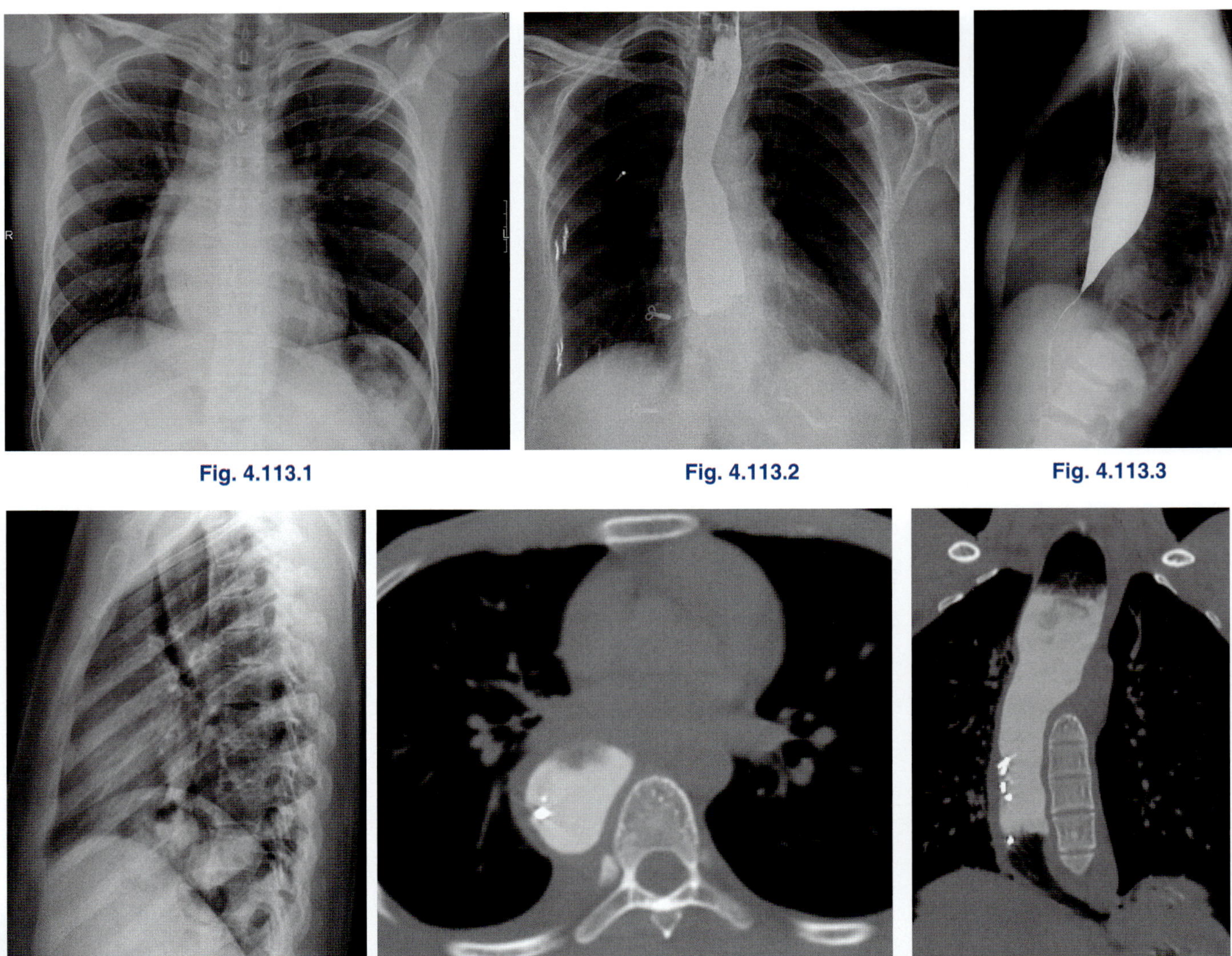

Fig. 4.113.1

Fig. 4.113.2

Fig. 4.113.3

Fig. 4.113.4

Fig. 4.113.5: Post-POEM procedure

Fig. 4.113.6: Post-POEM procedure

Table 4.113.1: Difference between primary achalasia and pseudoachalasia		
Findings	*Primary achalasia*	*Pseudoachalasia*
1. Length of abnormal segment	<One vertebral body height	>One vertebral body height
2. Maximum caliber	>One vertebral body height	<One vertebral body height
3. Tram-track appearance	Present	-
4. Shouldering	-	Present
5. Filling defects	-	Present
6. Tertiary contractions	Present	-
7. Appearance	Birds beak	Rat tail
8. Hot water/coke test	LES relaxation and emptying	-
9. Amyl nitrate inhalation	LES relaxation and emptying	-
	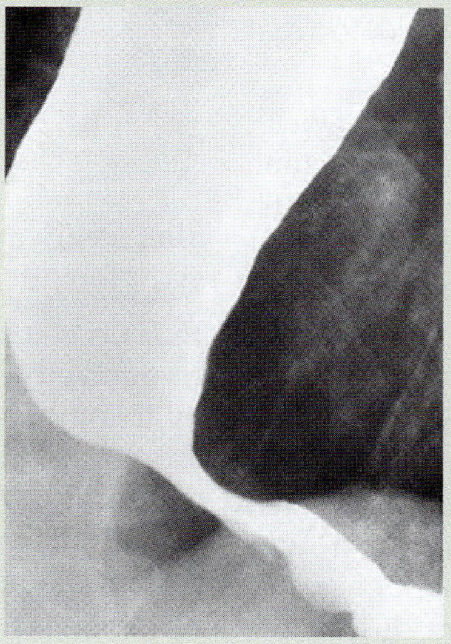 **Fig. 4.113.7:** Primary achalasia	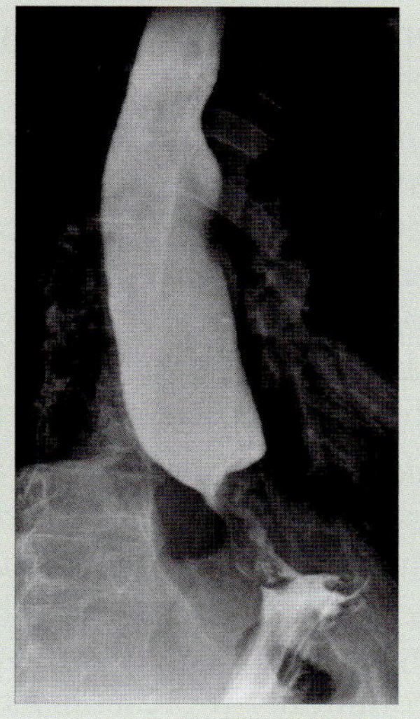 **Fig. 4.113.8:** Pseudoachalasia

Table 4.113.2: Anatomy of lower esophageal sphincter	
Anatomy of lower esophageal sphincter	
A ring	Muscular ring. Smooth, broad narrowing. Results from transient muscular contractions
	Location: They are above the B ring and occur a few centimeters proximal to the GE junction
	A rings are uncommonly symptomatic
B ring	Mucosal ring, smooth and symmetric
	Location: Less than 2 cm from the hiatal margin. Only visible when GE junction is above hiatus. Thin ledge like ring just above the mucosal junction
	Associated with hiatal hernias. Dysphagia possible if <13 m in diameter
C ring	Rare anatomic finding seen in cases of hiatal hernia caused by indentation of diaphragmatic crura.
	Location: Below the B ring
	Rarely symptomatic
Z line	Zigzag shaped squamocolumnar junction line
	Site: 1–2 cm above gastric sling fibres. Corresponds to B ring
Vestibule	Saccular dilatation of the lower esophagus with upper boundary at tubulovestibular junction and lower boundary at oesophagogastric junction.
Lower esophageal sphincter	Physiologic 2–4 cm high pressure zone correspond to esophageal vestibule

Principal diagnosis: It is primary achalasia cardia.

Differential diagnosis: Pseudoachalasia cardia.

Management: Investigations: Oesophageal manometry: Gold standard. Elevated/normal resting LES pressures, and incomplete or absent LES relaxation in response to deglutition. Fluoroscopy: Absence of primary peristalsis and incomplete or absent LES relaxation in response to deglutition, secondary and tertiary contractions.

Treatment: Younger patients with achalasia may have more effective long-term treatment of achalasia by pneumatic dilation or laparoscopic or surgical myotomy. Achalasia may be treated by botulinum toxin injection of the LES in older patients. POEM (PerOral Endoscopic Myotomy) is an endoscopic procedure used to treat achalasia.

Anatomy: Ten segments of esophagus: 1. Cervical, 2. Paratracheal, 3. Aortic, 4. Interaortic, 5. Bronchial, 6. Interbronchial, 7. Retrocardiac, 8. Epiphrenic, 9. Phrenic, 10. Subphrenic

Esophagus can also be divided into upper, middle and lower. Length of esophagus: 25 cm, length of esophagus from the level of incisor is 40 cm.

Schatzki ring: A–Schatzki ring, also called Schatzki-Gary ring, is symptomatically narrow esophageal, B–Ring occurring in the distal esophagus and usually associated with a hiatus hernia. Relatively common, lower esophageal rings are found in ~10% of oesophagograms. Most commonly it presents as intermittent dysphagia, especially to solid food.

Depending on its luminal diameter, an esophageal B–ring may be symptomatic or asymptomatic: <13 mm: almost always symptomatic, 13–20 mm: Sometimes symptomatic, >20 mm: Rarely symptomatic.

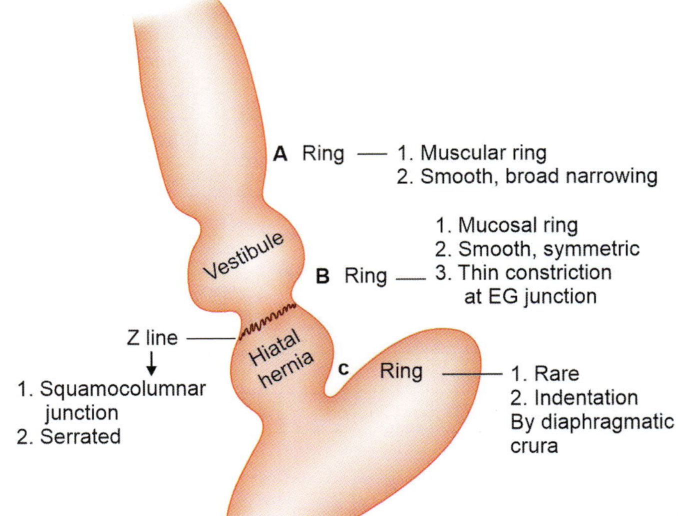

Fig. 4.113.9: Anatomy of lower esophagus

Primary achalasia cardia: Achalasia is a well-recognized esophageal motility disorder characterized by a combination of absent primary peristalsis in the esophagus and impaired LES opening in response to deglutition. Achalasia has no gender predilection and usually affects patients in the middle decades of life. Most patients complain of long-standing, slowly progressive dysphagia for solids and liquids, often associated with regurgitation of bland, undigested food and saliva.

Long-standing primary achalasia is a precursor of esophageal carcinoma. If dysphagia has a recent

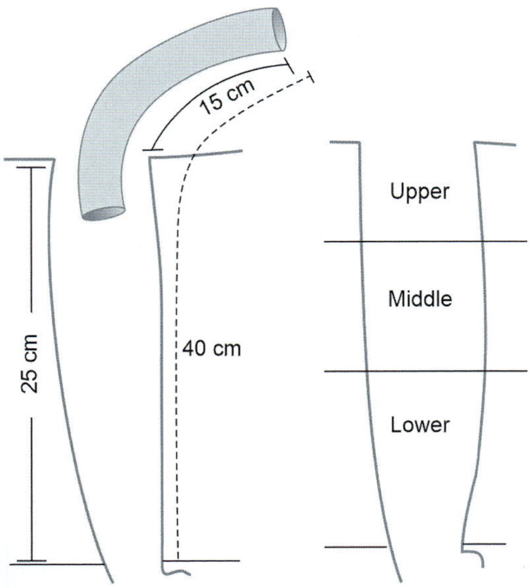

Fig. 4.113.10: Anatomy of esophagus

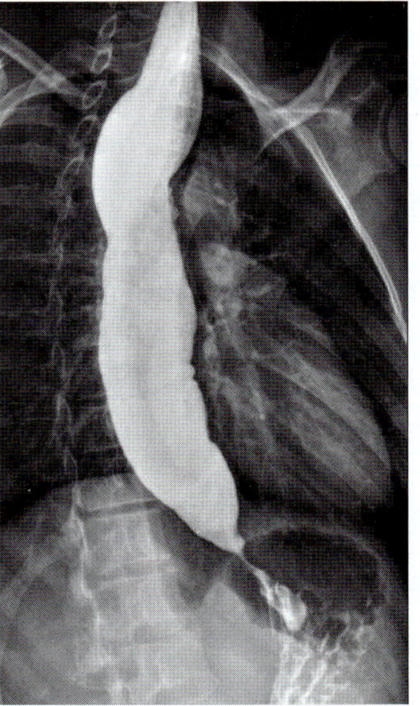

Fig. 4.113.11: Normal esophagus on barium swallow

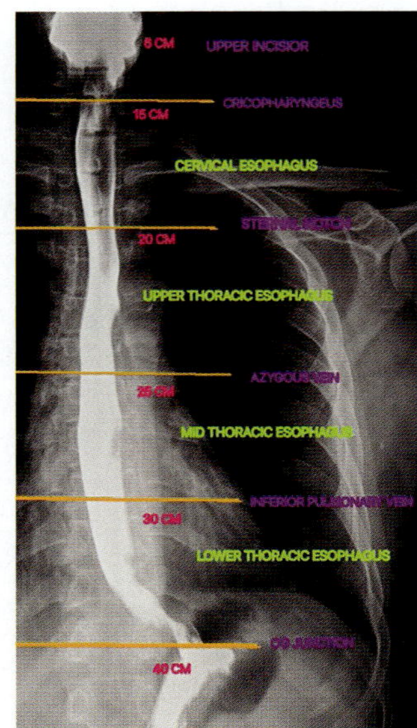

Fig. 4.113.12: Parts of esophagus on barium swallow

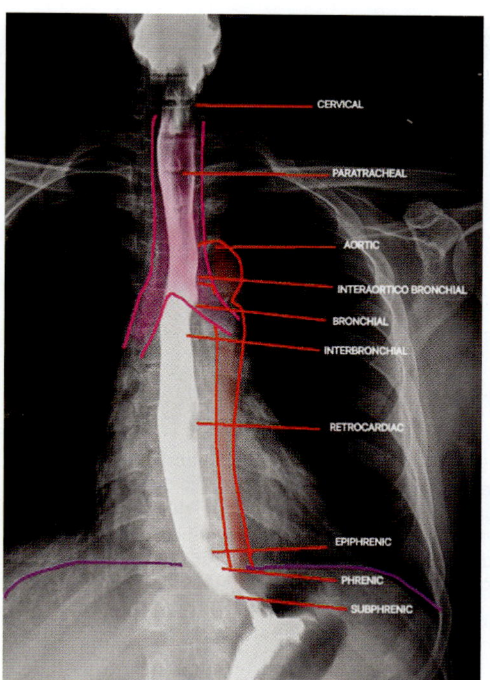

Fig. 4.113.13: Parts of esophagus on barium swallow

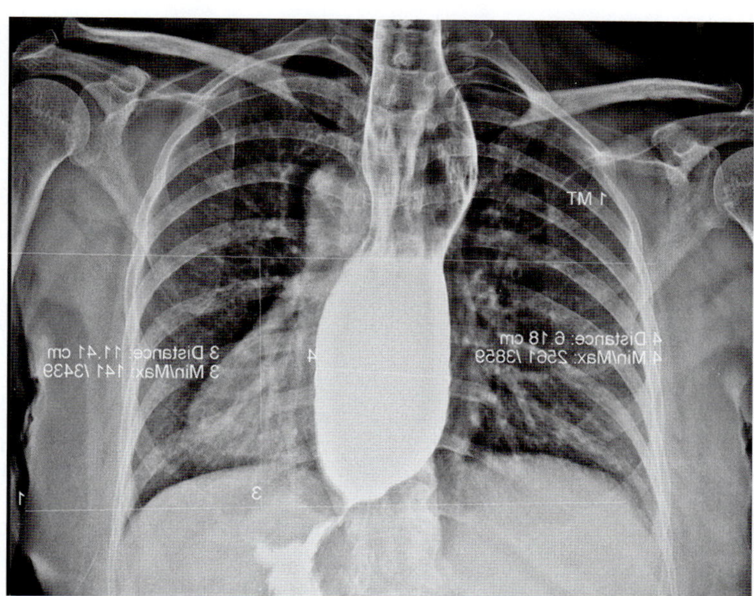

Fig. 4.113.14: Timed barium swallow at 1 min

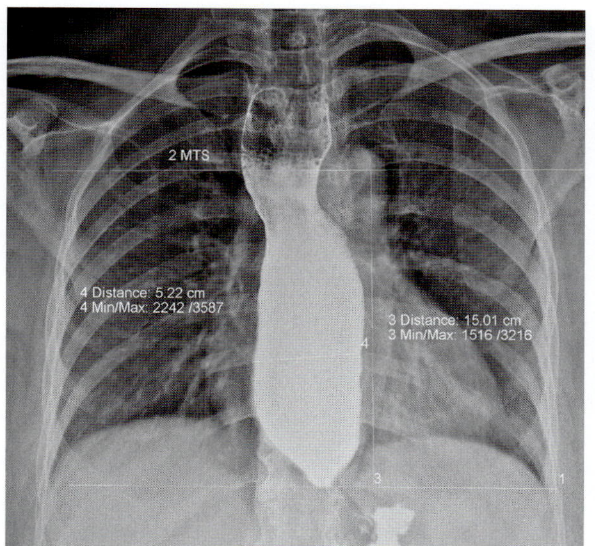

Fig. 4.113.15: Timed barium swallow at 2 min

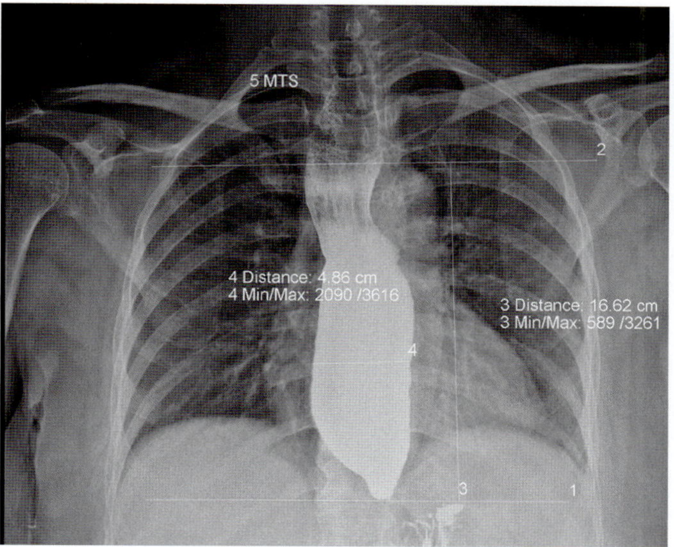

Fig. 4.113.16: Timed barium swallow at 5 min

onset and is rapidly progressive in older patients with radiographic or manometric findings of achalasia, secondary achalasia caused by malignancy should be strongly suspected.

On fluoroscopy: Absent primary and secondary esophageal peristalsis. Presence of tertiary contractions.

Hurst phenomenon: When the barium column is high enough, the hydrostatic pressure can overcome the LES pressure, allowing passage of contents.

Causes of megaesophagus: Achalasia, Chagas disease, scleroderma, malignant strictrure, benign stricture, extrinsic compression.

Timed barium swallow: Used to assess oesophageal emptying in patients with achalasia before and after therapy. The patient stands. The patient ingests 100–200 ml of low density barium (45% weight by volume) over 30–45s. Three spot films are taken at 1 min, 2 min and 5 min after ingestion with patient in left posterior oblique.

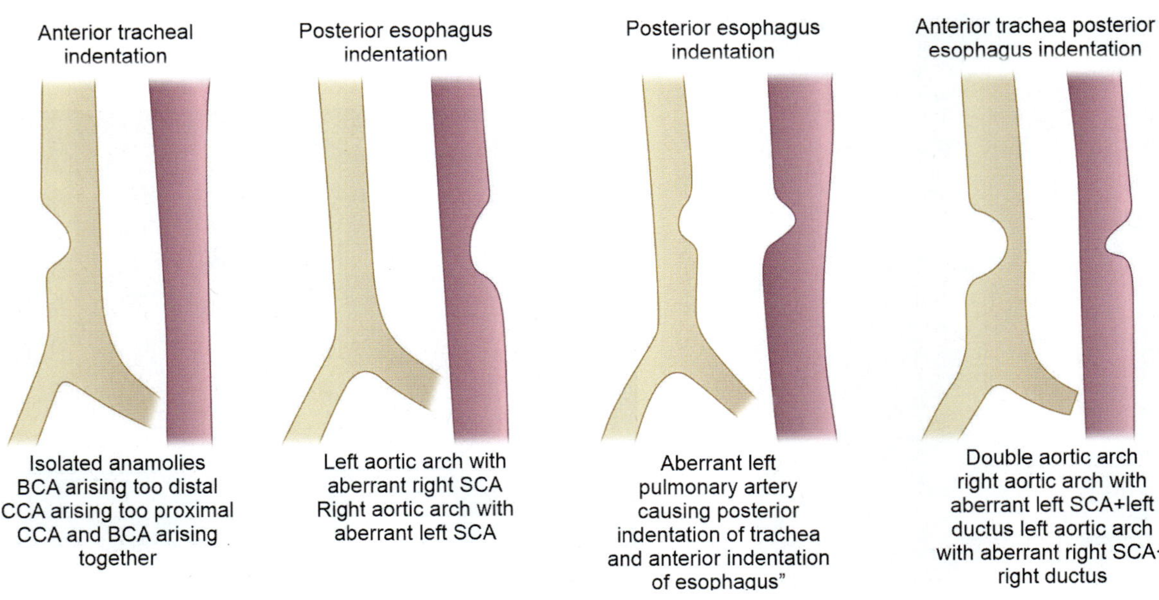

Fig. 4.113.17: Tracheal and esophagus indentation

The distane of fluoroscope carriage from the patient is kept constant. The degree of emptying is calculated by measuring width, height and change in area between 1 and 5 min films. 2 min film is optional.

4.114 CHEST

Case No. 114

Clinical history: 57-year-old male presented with complaints of dysphagia, vomiting and weight loss.

Radiological techniques and observation: Figures 4.114.1 to 4.114.6 are chest radiographs (AP and lateral), CECT chest axial, coronal and sagittal section with oral contrast and lung window axial section respectively. Chest radiographs in PA and lateral views show which right paratracheal stripe is obliterated with widening of superior mediastinum. CT of the patient shows heterogeneously enhancing circumferential irregular mural thickening of the mid and distal esophagus for the length of approximately 11 cm and maximum thickness of 17 mm with mass effect over left atrium, luminal narrowing and subsequent mild proximal esophageal dilatation. Loss of fat plane noted between thoracic aorta and esophagus with contact of less than 90 degrees. Loss of fat plane between the bronchus and esophagus at the level of tracheal bifurcation. A few enlarged lymph nodes noted in right hilar region. Visualized lung sections/ skeleton appear normal.

Interpretations: A: 57-year-old male, C: Circumferential irregular mural thickening of the distal esophagus, B: Luminal narrowing and subsequent proximal esophageal dilatation, D: Carcinoma esophagus.

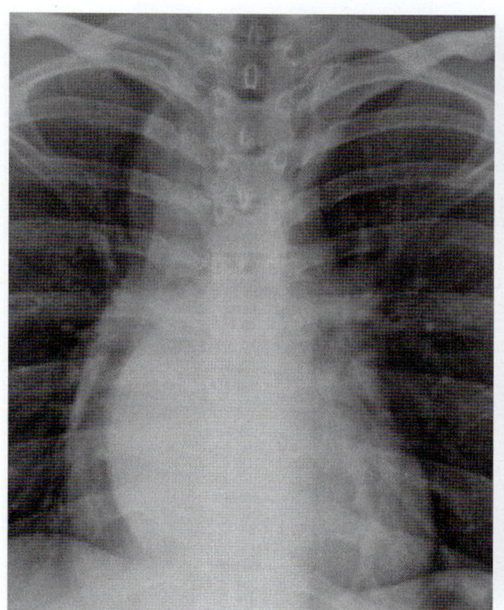

Fig. 4.114.1

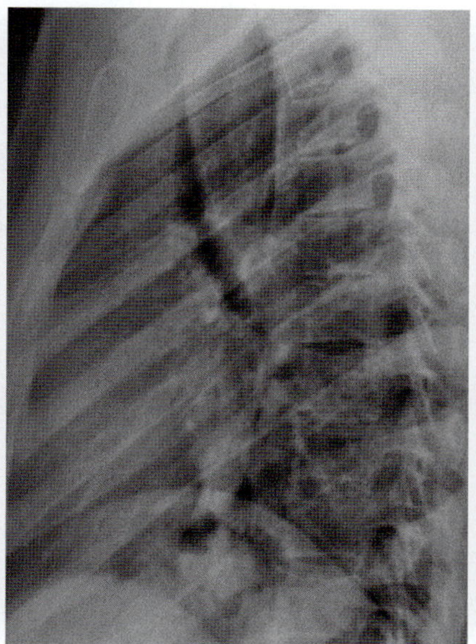

Fig. 4.114.2

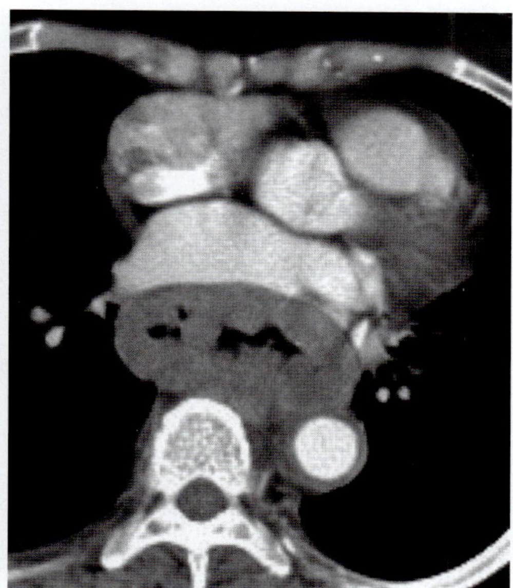

Fig. 4.114.3

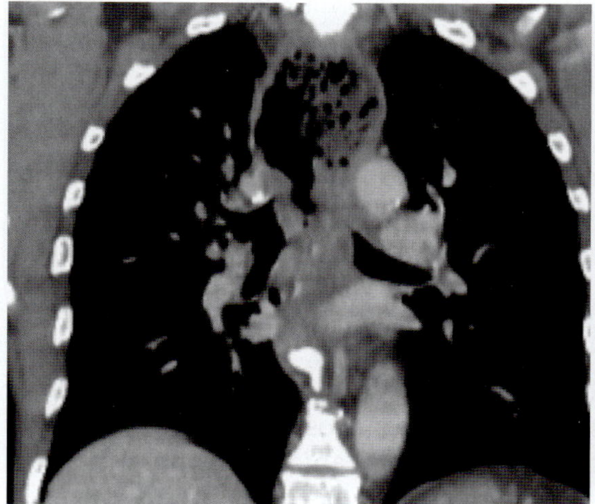

Fig. 4.114.4

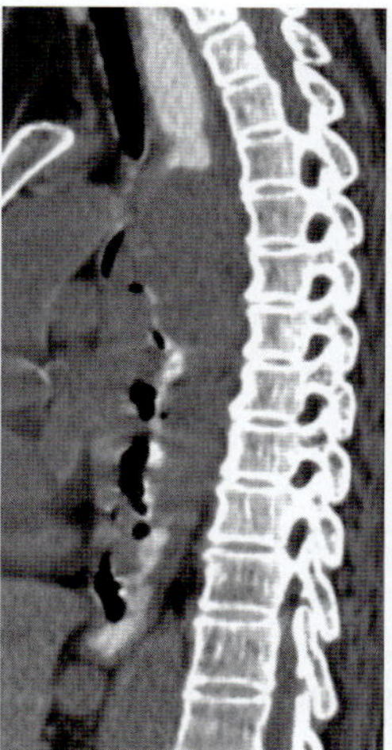

Fig. 4.114.5

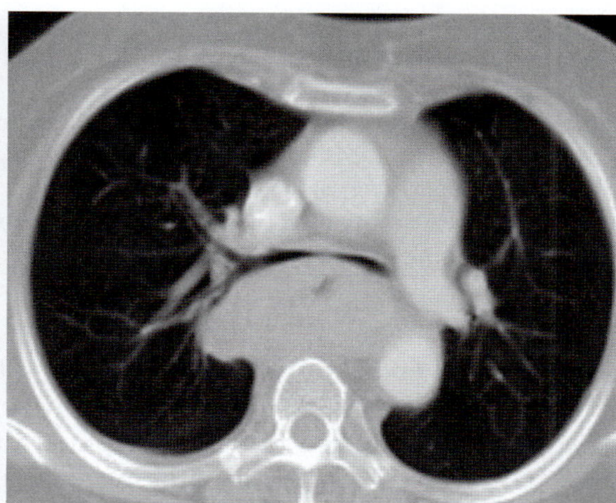

Fig. 4.114.6

Table 4.114.1: Differential diagnosis for carcinoma esophagus	
Reflux esophagitis: Inflammation of esophageal mucosa due to gastroesophageal reflux. Location: Distal third of esophagus. Double contrast esophagography: Irregular ulcerated mucosa of distal esophagus. Finely nodular or granular appearance with poorly defined radiolucencies that fade peripherally due to edema and inflammation of mucosa. Foreshortening of esophagus. Hiatal hernia in more than 95% with stricture noted.	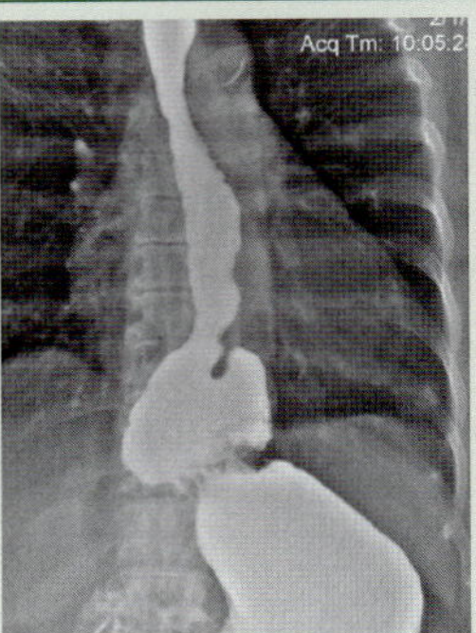 **Fig. 4.114.7:** Reflux esophagitis
Esophageal leiomyoma: It is the common benign tumor of the esophagus which originates from smooth muscles. Typically involve the mid-to-distal esophagus. On barium swallow, may be seen as a discrete ovoid mass that is well outlined by barium. Its borders form slightly obtuse angles with the esophageal wall. CT—ovoid intramural solitary mass with a smooth surface and narrowing of the esophageal lumen. The presence of calcifications is almost pathognomonic.	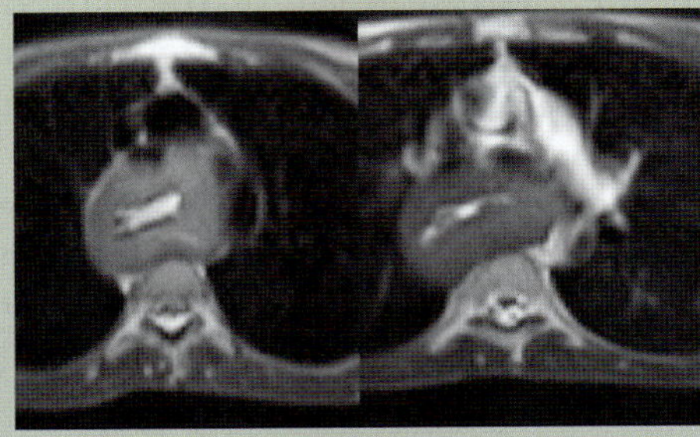 **Fig. 4.114.8:** Esophageal leiomyoma
Esophageal metastasis: Direct, lymphatic or hematogenous spread. Direct invasion most common route: Gastric and lung cancer most common primary tumors.	From gastric cancer: Ulcerated /polypoid mass of gastric cardia extending into distal esophagus. From lung cancer: Extrinsic indendation with/without luminal narrowing of upper half of esophagus.
Hiatus hernia: The gastro-esophageal junction (GEJ) is usually displaced >2 cm above the esophageal hiatus. More common in old age females. X-ray-retrocardiac opacity with air-fluid level. Fluroscopy: Numerous coarse thick gastric folds within the suprahiatal pouch Tortuous esophagus with an eccentric gastroesophageal junction. CT: Focal fat collection in the middle mediastinum, widening of esophageal hiatus.	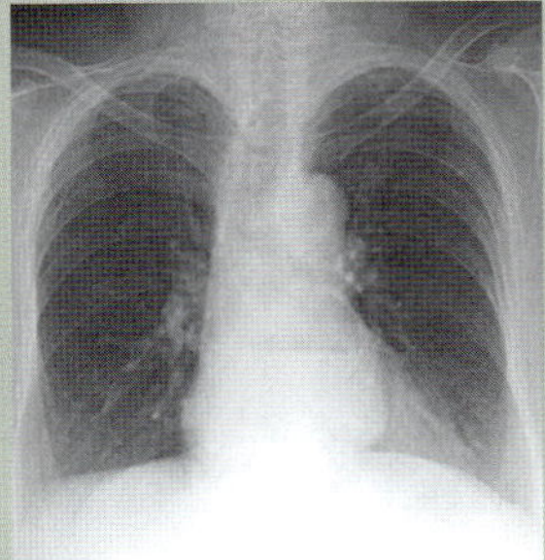 **Fig. 4.114.9:** Hiatus hernia
Esophageal varices: Dilated submucosal veins of esophagus and important portosystemic collateral pathway. a. Uphill esophageal varices: Most common form, caused by portal hypertension (m.c cirrhosis), lower third of esophagus, occurs in association with gastric varices. b. Downhill varices: Caused by superior vena cava obstruction, upper third of esophagus.	**Plain radiograph:** Non-specific appearance of mass in posterior mediastinum. **Fluoroscopy:** Barium swallow may reveal longitudinal esophageal luminal filling defect CT/MRI: Esophageal and paraesophageal varices are readily visible on contrast-enhanced cross-sectional imaging, as tortuous, enlarged, smooth enhancing tubular structures.

Principal diagnosis: Carcinoma esophagus

Management: Endoscopy, trans esophageal ultrasound and PET/CT scan are used for staging of the disease. This patient is referred to multidisciplinary team for histopathological diagnosis/staging/management. Based on the stage surgical or palliative treatment can be started.

Further Investigation and Management

A combination of endoscopy, CT, transesophageal ultrasound and PET/CT scan are used for staging of the disease. Endoscopic mucosal resection associated without or with localized ablation is an treatment option for localized (T1a) disease. These epithelial tumors are usually less than 2 cm, asymptomatic,

Table 4.114.2: Staging of AJCC (2010) for esophageal carcinoma			
Esophageal carcinoma	*Regional lymph node*	*Distant metastasis*	*Histologic grade*
TX: Primary tumor cannot be assessed	NX: Regional lymph nodes cannot be assessed	M0: No distant metastasis	GX: Grade cannot be assessed-stage grouping as G1
T0: No evidence of primary tumor	N0: No regional lymph node metastasis	M1: Distant metastasis present	G1: Well differentiated
Tis: High-grade dysplasia	N1: Metastasis in 1–2 regional lymph nodes		G2: Moderately differentiated
T1a: Invasion of lamina propria or muscularis mucosae	N2: Metastasis in 3–6 regional lymph nodes		G3: Poorly differentiated
T1b: Invasion of submucosa	N3: Metastasis in ≥7 regional lymph nodes		G4: Undifferentiated—stage group as G3 squamous
T2: Invasion of muscularis propria			
T3: Invasion of adventitia			
T4: Invasion of adjacent structures			
T4a: Resectable (pericardium, pleura, or diaphragm)			
T4b: Unresectable (other structures such as, vertebral body, aorta, trachea, vertebral body, etc)			

and noncircumferential lesions. For T1b tumors and above, surgery is limited to esophagectomy (including sometimes with palliative colonic interposition).

Benign stricture	*Malignant stricture*
Long segment (>2 cm)	Short segment (<2 cm)
Concentric and smooth tapering	Eccenteric and irregular abrupt tapering
No shouldering	Shouldering is seen
No mucosal irregularity	Associated with nodular mucosal irregularity

Discussion

Chest radiograph: Azygo-esophageal recess appear widened with convexity is seen toward right lung (in 30% of distal and mid-esophageal cancers), thickening of posterior tracheal stripe, right paratracheal stripe >4 mm (if tumor located in the upper third of esophagus), tracheal deviation/posterior tracheal indentation/mass, retrocardiac or posterior mediastinal mass lesion, esophageal air-fluid level, Lobulated mass extending into gastric bubble **(Kirklin sign)**.

Fluoroscopy/barium swallow: Irregular stricture, pre-stricture dilatation with 'hold up', shouldering of the stricture.

Endoscopic US: Most accurate imaging modality for the T staging of esophageal cancer. It shows the layers of the esophageal wall so it can differentiate T1, T2, and T3 stage of tumors. The esophagus consists of 5 layers. The first hyperechoic layer is the interface between the balloon and the superficial mucosa. Second hypoechoic layer—lamina propria, muscularis mucosae. The third hyperechoic layer indicate the submucosa. The fourth hypoechoic layer indicates the muscularis propria. The fifth layer indicates the interface between the adventitia and surrounding tissues.

CT staging (Moss): Stage 1: Intraluminal tumor/localized wall thickening of 3–5 mm (inadequate for depth of infiltration). Stage 2: Localized/circumferential wall thickening >5 mm (inadequate for depth of infiltration). Stage 3: Contiguous spread into adjacent mediastinum (trachea, thyroid, larynx, bronchi, aorta, lung, pericardium, diaphragm). Loss of fat planes (nonspecific due to cachexia, often still resectable). Mass in contact with aorta >90 arc (in 20–70% still resectable). Displacement/compression of airway (90–100% accuracy for invasion). Esophagotracheal/bronchial fistula (unresectable) pericardial thickening, pericardial effusion, loss of pericardial fat plane, indentation of heart. Stage 4: Distant metastases, enlarged abdominal lymph nodes >10 mm (12–85% accuracy). Hepatic, pulmonary, adrenal metastases. Direct erosion of vertebral body. Tumor >3 cm wide = high frequency of extraesophageal spread.

FDG PET/CT is useful for detecting esophageal primary tumors but it has limited role in assessing about the depth of tumor invasion. PET/CT is also superior

Table 4.114.3: Summary of esophageal diverticulum

Upper esophagus	*Middle esophagus*	*Lower esophagus*
Zenker diverticulum (pharyngeal pouch) Mucosal herniation through area of anatomic weakness just above cricopharyngeal muscle (Killian dehiscence). Barium filled sac posterior to cervical esophagus Neck of diverticulum with its opening into posterior hypopharyngeal wall above cricopharyngeal muscle.	**Traction diverticulum:** Acquired due to subcarinal or perihilar granulomatous lymph node pathology. Barium study shows traction diverticulum at mid esophagus, tented or triangular in shape with pointed tip, wide mouth.	**Epiphrenic diverticulum:** Pulsion diverticulum of the distal esophagus arising just above lower esophageal sphincter more frequently on right posterolateral wall. On chest X-ray appears as retrocardiac soft tissue mass with or without air-fluid level mimicking hiatus hernia.
Killian–Jamieson diverticulum: It is false diverticulum and represent an outpouching of mucosa through a muscular defect. They are located just below cricopharyngeal muscle, anteriorly and laterally. They are smaller than Zenker diverticulum usually <1.5 cm.		

to CT for identifying lymph node metastases and can show metastases in normal-sized lymph nodes which show uptake of FDG. PET/CT useful in the depiction of distant metastasis. The most distant metastatic sites at PET (but frequently missed at CT) are the bones, liver.

Complications: Fistula formation to the trachea (5–10%), bronchi or mediastinum: Can be either due to direct tumor progression or iatrogenic effects (e.g. radiation therapy). Esophageal perforation.

Treatment: Tumor staging, comorbidities and age should be taken in consideration to define the best therapy assessment. Esophagectomy remains the primary treatment for esophageal carcinoma when the tumor is easily resectable and clinical conditions permits. T1a (high grade dysplasia and intramucosal cancer which is limited to the muscularismucosa) have low risk of LN involvement, estimated between 0 to 2%, and can be managed with endoscopic therapy [endoscopic submucosal resection (EMR)], radiofrequency ablation in some cases. Indications for esophagectomy is incomplete EMR/failure of endoscopic therapy. T1b and T2 have risk of lymph node involvement compared with T1a secondary to the muscularis mucosa invasion by the lesion. Esophagectomy is advised if clinical condition permits.

Locally advanced EC are managed with combined modality treatment, which consist of definitive chemoradiation therapy (CRT) and neoadjuvant chemotherapy, radiotherapy, esophagectomy.

Surgical resection or definitive CRT is ideal to patients with complete metabolic response on PET/CT since residual microscopic tumor may not be detected.

Supportive care treatment for nonsurgical patients are esophageal stent placement/percutaneous gastrostomy/chemotherapy and radiotherapy.

Esophageal web: Thin mucosal fold narrowing esophageal lumen that lacks muscle layer. In Barium swallow appears as 1–2 mm wide, shelf-like filling defect along anterior wall of cervical esophagus. Partial obstruction suggested by Jet Phenomenon (Barium spurting through ring). Dilatation of esophagus or pharynx proximal to web.

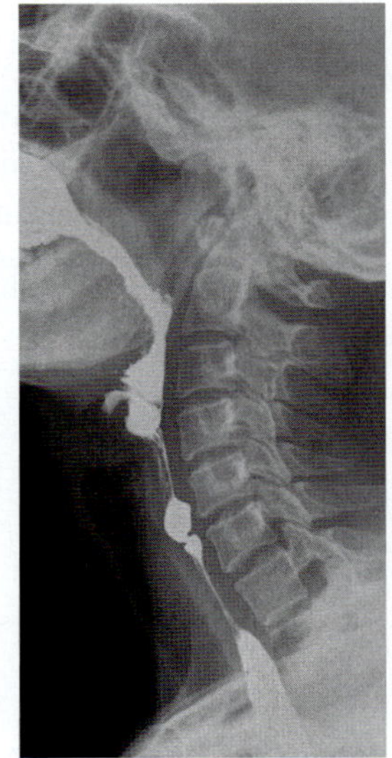

Fig. 4.114.10: Esophageal web

Cricopharyngeal achalasia: Failure of cricopharyngeal muscle (upper esophageal sphincter) relaxation due to hypertrophy or spasm. Prominent cricopharnygeus muscle at pharyngoesophageal junction (C5–C6 level) with retention of barium in pharynx on lateral view.

Schatzki ring: Annular, inflammatory, symptomatic narrowing of normal lower esophageal mucosal or B ring. Single–contrast barium esophagram shows thin (2–4 mm in height), web–like constriction at gastroesophageal junction. Margins are smooth and symmetric.

Cheap steakhouse syndrome: Due to inadequately chewed piece of meat impacted above ring.

4.115 CHEST

Case No. 115

Clinical history: 31-year-old male patient, who had a screening chest X-ray taken.

Radiological techniques and observation: Figures 4.115.1 and 4.115.2 are frontal and lateral plain radiograph of the chest of a skeletally mature patient. There are three well defined, rounded radiopaque lesions noted in the right hemithorax. The outer border of these lesions blends into the chest wall. These lesions have a broad base of contact with the chest wall and make an obtuse angle with the chest wall. The other three borders can be clearly made out. The margins of the lesions are well tapered. There is no internal calcification or internal fat tissue density. There is no lobulation of the contour. The ribs appear thinned out with suspicious inferior rib notching. Patchy fibrosis and volume loss noted in left upper lobe with tracheal deviation to left.

Figures 4.115.3 and 4.115.4 are axial CT sections in mediastinal, lung and bone windows images showing pleural based lesion with a broad region of contact and obtuse angle. There is no obvious pleural thickening. The surrounding lung parenchyma is normal. There is scalloping of the underlying ribs. There is no calcification or hemorrhage. With these imaging findings, the lesions are probably pleural in origin. In view of inferior rib

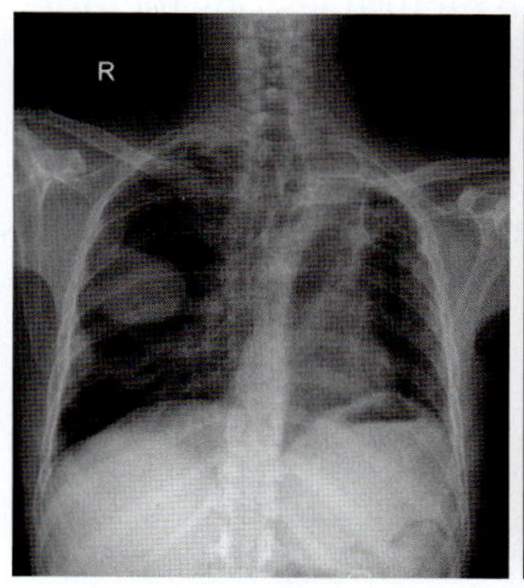

Fig. 4.115.1

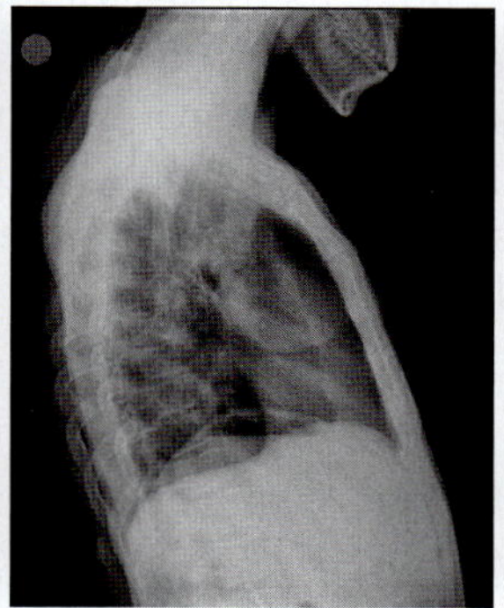

Fig. 4.115.2

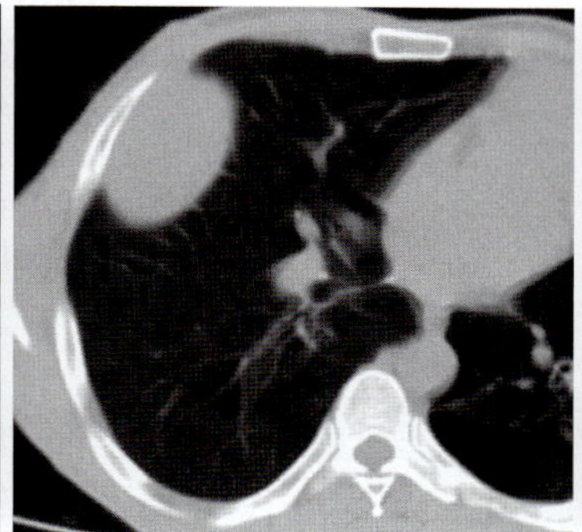

Fig. 4.115.3

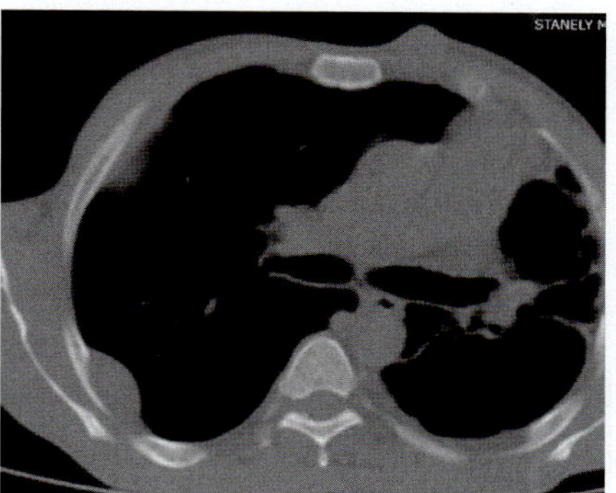

Fig. 4.115.4

Table 4.115.1: Differential diagnosis for pleural mass

Solitary fibrous tumor: Rare benign tumor, clinical presentation can be with either a cough, chest pain, or shortness of breath, but is most commonly an asymptomatic incidental finding	Calcification, rib destruction, and pleural effusions are typically not associated features. CT tends to have soft tissue attenuation and shows homogeneous intense background enhancement on contrast-enhanced scans. Non-enhancing areas may be present, corresponding to necrosis, myxoid degeneration, or hemorrhage within the tumor. MRI: Typically low to intermediate signal overall due to fibrous component.	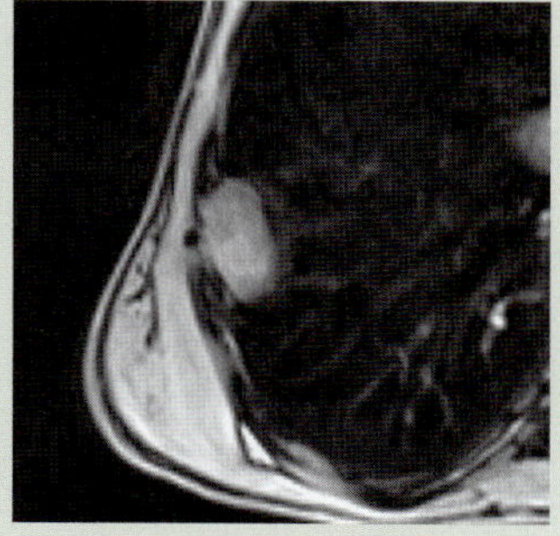 Fig. 4.115.5: Solitary fibrous tumor
Mesothelioma – refer to case no 116		
Pleural metastases: Most common malignant lesion of the pleura. Usually histologically adenocarcinoma. M/C lung > breast > ovarian, lymphoma, thymoma, etc.	Pleural effusion is often the major manifestation of metastatic disease to the pleura, other findings include pleural nodules or extensive pleural thickening. CT is ideal to show nodules not seen on chest X-ray due to pleural effusion. The pleural metastases usually manifest as enhancing nodular or lenticular masses. Other features are enlarged mediastinal lymph nodes, lung nodules, rib lesions, subcutaneous extension.	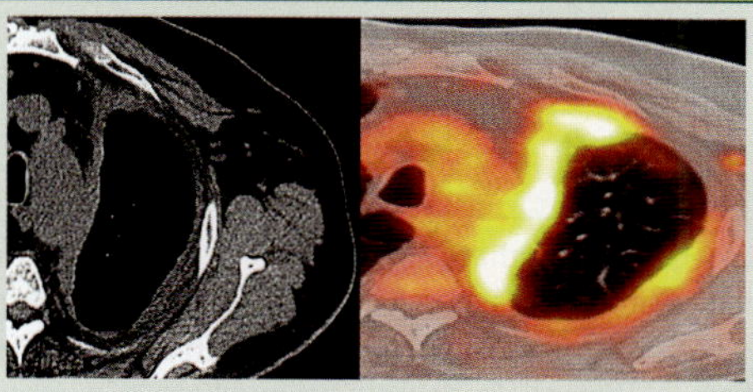 Fig. 4.115.6: Pleural metastases

notching and chest wall lesions, suggests the possibility of neural origin.

Interpretation: A: 31 years old male, pleural-based lesion, C: Focus of fibrosis in the left upper lobe causing volume loss with tracheal deviation to the left (fibrosis possibly due to old PTB sequelae), B: On lateral radiograph, the largest mass is projected over the anterior mediastinum with inferior rib notching, D: NF1

The ***principal diagnosis*** is neurofibromatosis type I.

Flowchart 4.115.1: Summary of pleural-based lesions

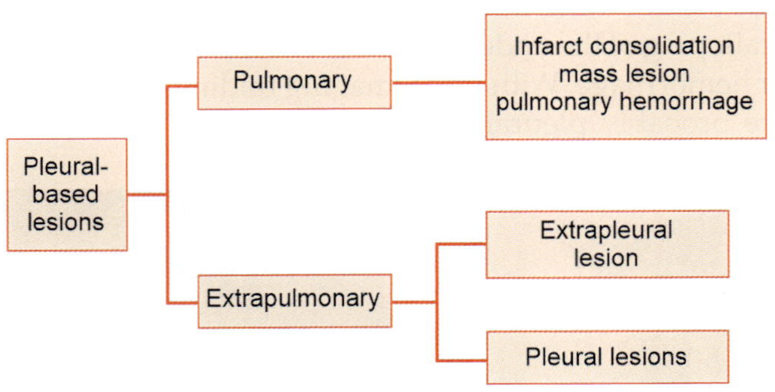

Table 4.115.2: Pleural based lesion

Pulmonary	*Pleural*	*Extrapleural*
• Infarct • Hemorrhage • Consolidation • Mass • Lymphoma	**Benign:** • Fibroma • Lipoma • Loculated empyema • Loculated hematoma **Malignant** • Mesothelioma • Metastasis • Lymphoma • Pleural synovial sarcoma	• Mesenchymal tumor • Nerve sheath tumor • Tumors from bone origin • Diaphragm, para-spinal muscles

Differential diagnoses for the pleural lesions include: Fibroma, spleniosis (but there is no history of trauma), Extrapleural hematoma (but there is no prior history of trauma/anticoagulation), lymphoma, lipoma (but not fat density), mesothelioma, pleural sarcoma, metastasis (unlikely due to age).

Table 4.115.3: Difference between pleural lesion, pulmonary lesion and mediastinal lesion

Pleural	*Pulmonary*	*Extrapleural (chest wall)*	*Mediastinal*
Obtuse angle	Acute angle	Obtuse angle	Obtuse angle
Displaces pulmonary vasculature	Engulfs pulmonary vasculature	Displaces pulmonary vasculature	Displaces pulmonary vasculature
Centered along chest wall	Centered in the lung	Centered along chest wall	Centered along the mediastinum
Tapered well-defined margins Incomplete border sign Pregnant lady in profile sign Cat under the rug sign Extrapleural sign	Non-tapered ill-defined margins	Tapered well-defined margins	Tapered well-defined margins
Changes location with respiration	-	-	Does not change location with respiration
Displaces extrapleural fat outward	-	Displaces extrapleural fat inward	-
Rib erosion unusual	Rib erosion unusual	Rib erosion common	Erosion of spine, sternum and ribs may be seen
-	-	-	Mediastinal lines (azygoesophageal recess, anterior and posterior junction lines) will be disrupted.

Superior rib notching causes: Osteogenesis imperfecta, connective tissue diseases, local pressure, abnormal osteoclastic activity (hyperparathyroidism), neurofibromatosis type 1, restrictive lung disease, poliomyelitis, progeria, abnormal muscle pull

Inferior rib notching (Roesler sign): Enlarged collateral vessels (coarctation of the aorta, interrupted aortic arch, subclavian artery obstruction, Takayasu disease, Blalock-Taussig shunt: Involves only upper two rib spaces), arteriovenous malformation (AVM) of the chest wall,pulmonary AVM, superior vena cava obstruction with enlarged venous collaterals, tetralogy of Fallot, neurogenic tumors (neurofibroma)

Calcified pleural lesion causes–calcified pleural plaques from asbestos exposure, hemothorax, infection involving the pleura like pyothorax/empyema, tuberculous pleuritis, previous surgery, extraskeletal osteosarcoma of pleura, radiation therapy

Flowchart 4.115.2: Approach to pleural lesions

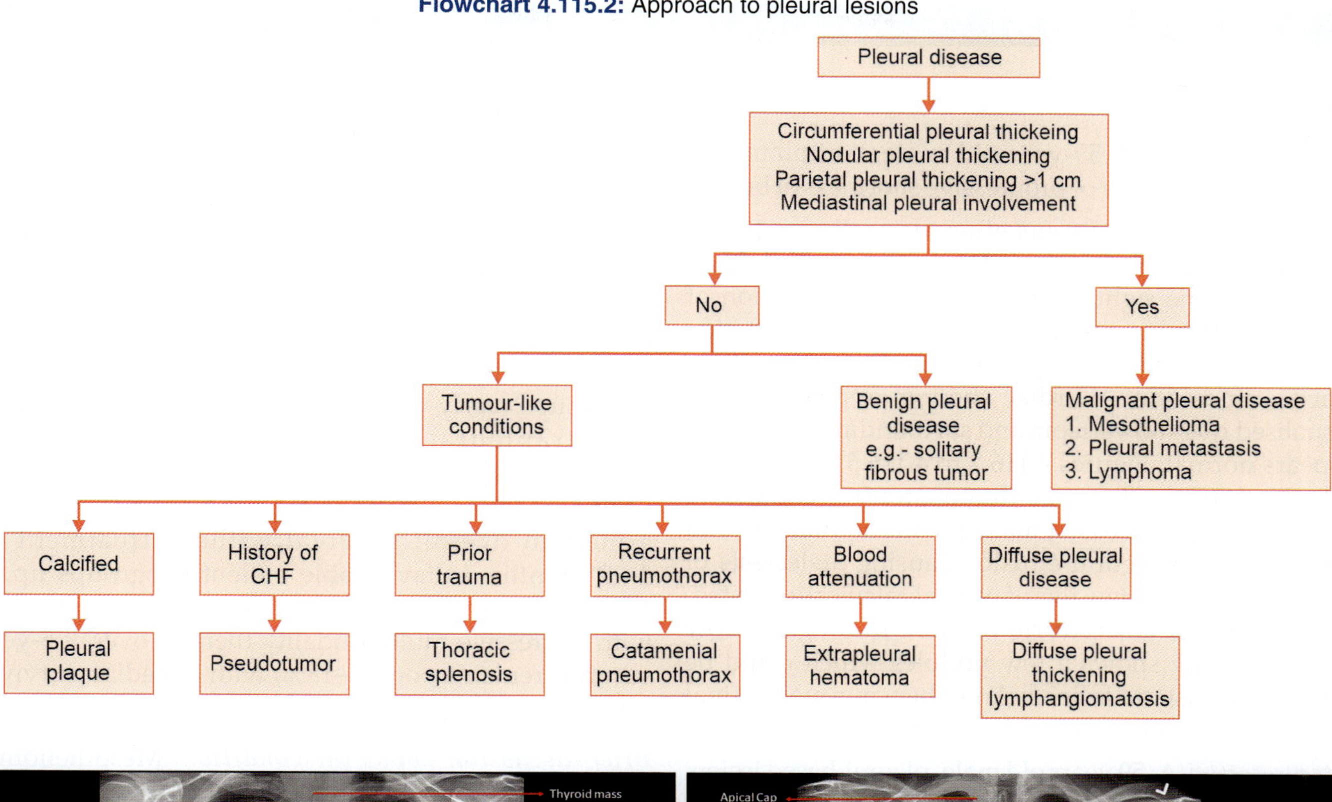

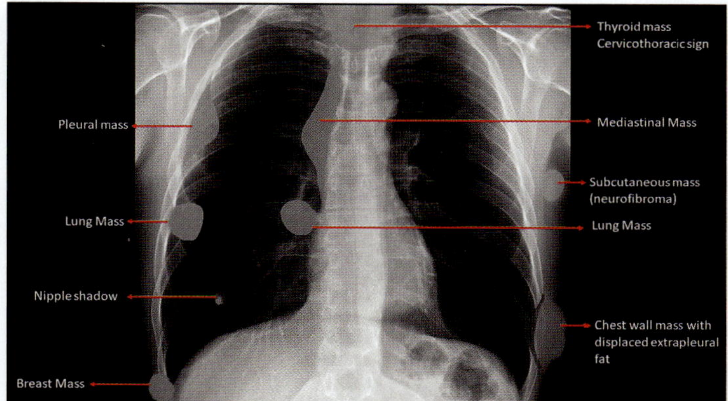

Fig. 4.115.7: Masses in chest radiograph

Apical Cap
Pleural Sarcoma
Neurofibroma
Solitary Fibrous tumour
loculated effusion
Fibrothorax (will have associated volume loss)
Lymphoma / Mesothelioma
Asbestosis
Calcified Empyema
Subpulmonic effusion

Fig. 4.115.8: Pleural-based mass

Management: The next step would be histopathological diagnosis by CT or US guided biopsy of the lesion.

Role of PET CT: Malignant mesothelioma: For staging, therapy planning, response monitoring. SUV is also a predictor of prognosis. Solitary fibrous tumor—to differentiate between benign and malignant lesions. Also in surgical planning, identifying distant metastases. Pleural lipoma/liposarcoma—lipomas show low FDG uptake, whereas liposarcoma shows high uptake. Pleural metastases—to identify pleural dissemination of lung carcinoma.

4.116 CHEST

Case No. 116

Clinical history: A 59-year-old male, complaints of several weeks history of progressive shortness of breath.

Radiological techniques and observation: Figure 4.116.1 is chest radiograph PA view showing some ill-defined opacities in the right lower zone with obliteration of right costophrenic and cardiophrenic angle. Left side costophrenic and cardiophrenic angles appear free. Trachea in midline. Cardiac shadow appear normal. Visualised ribs and vertebra and surrounding soft tissues appears normal. Figures 4.116.2 to 4.116.5 are contrast-enhanced axial CT image demonstrating enhancing right sided pleural based masses with nodular pleural thickening and pleural effusion causing atelectasis of underlying lung. A few foci of pleural calcification noted. No evidence of adjacent rib erosion. In lung window ipsilateral lung shows a few nodules which could be possibly metastatic lesions. An enhancing mediastinal lymph node noted in subcarinal region.

Interpretation: A: 59 years old male, pleural-based lesion, C: Large, ill-defined radio-opacity occupying the right lower zone, B: Nodular pleural thickening and effusion with ipsilateral right lung nodules, D: Right-sided malignant mesothelioma.

Principal diagnosis: With these imaging findings, the principal diagnosis is malignant mesothelioma of right pleura with ipsilateral lung metastasis.

Treatment: Treatment continues to be challenging and the long-term survival is poor. Single modality treatment (surgery, radiotherapy, chemotherapy, immunotherapy and even photodynamic therapy) has not been shown to improve survival. More recently multi-modality treatment has some impact on favourable subgroups (early disease, and epithelioid histology). 1. Extrapleural pneumonectomy, 2. adjuvant chemotherapy, 3. Radiotherapy.

The prognosis is poor for all tumor types with a median overall survival without treatment of 4–12 months. In favourable patient subgroups up to 45% 5-year survival may be achievable, however, even with aggressive multi-modality therapy overall 5-year survival remains poor (3–18%) with a median survival time of approximately 18 months.

Brief discussion about the condition: Mesothelioma, also known as malignant mesothelioma, is an aggressive malignant tumor of the mesothelium. Mesothelioma can arise in various locations: 1. Pleural mesothelioma (~90%), 2. Peritoneal mesothelioma (~10%),

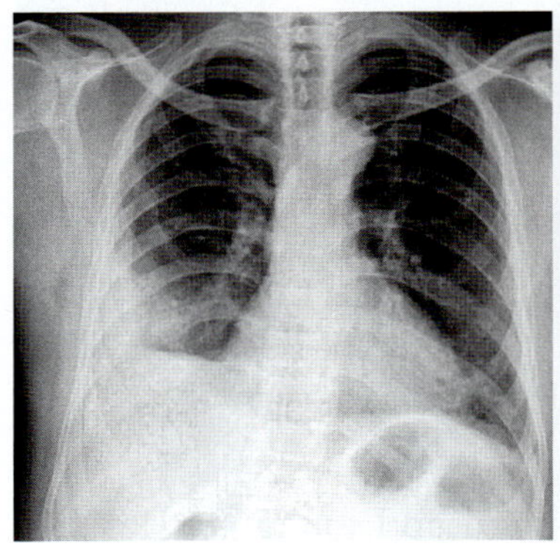

Fig. 4.116.1

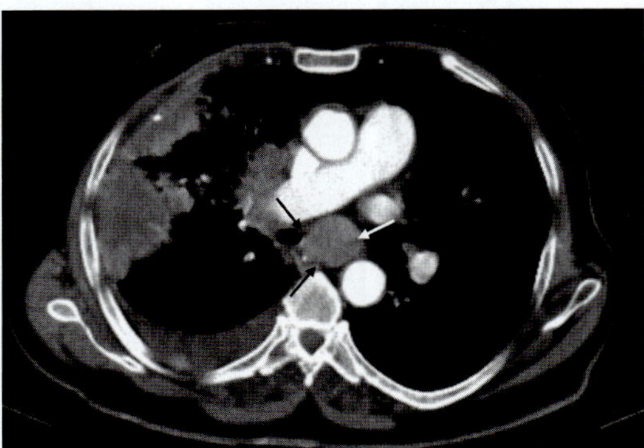

Fig. 4.116.2

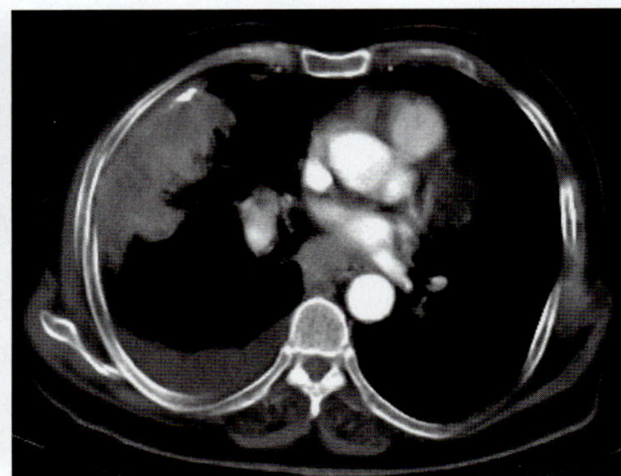

Fig. 4.116.3

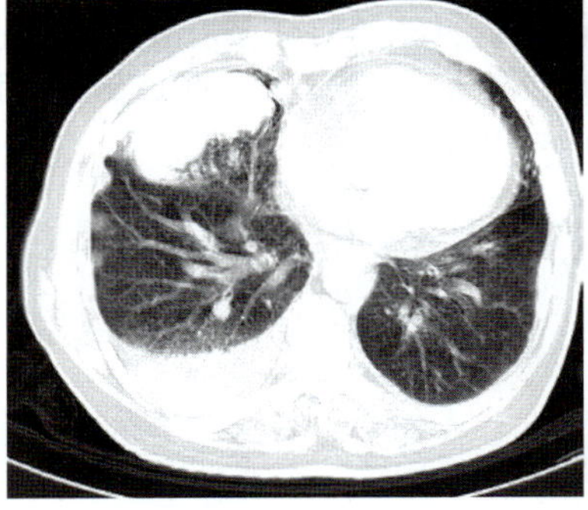

Fig. 4.116.4

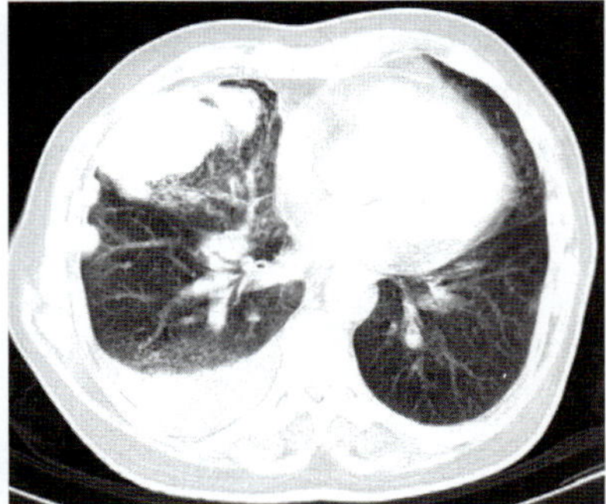

Fig. 4.116.5

Differential diagnosis		
1. Chest wall and pleural metastases—usually the most common primary tumors are themselves located in the chest: Lung cancer and breast cancer.	• Enhancing pleurally-based masses • Nodular pleural thickening • Pleural effusion (most common finding) • +/– rib destruction +/-hilar/mediastinal lymphadenopathy Hypointense on T1; variably hyperintense on T2. Metastasis is difficult to differentiate from malignant mesothelioma.	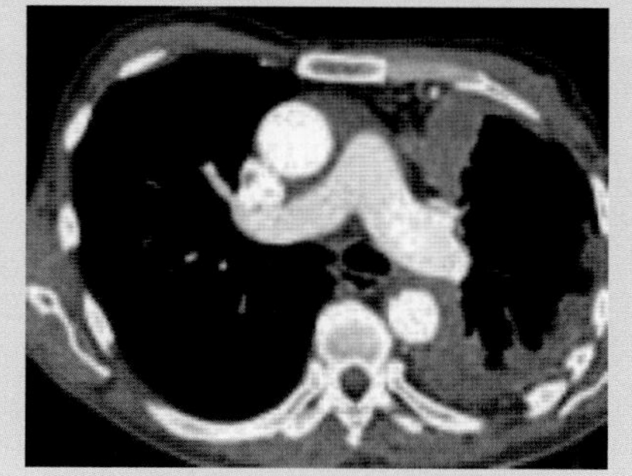 **Fig. 4.116.6:** Chest wall and pleural metastases
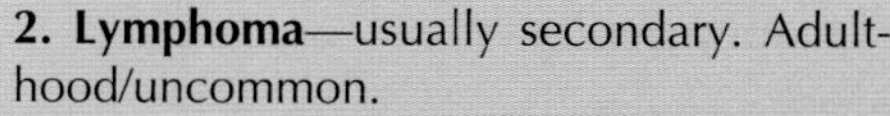 **2. Lymphoma**—usually secondary. Adulthood/uncommon. Association with AIDS, metallic implant, immunosuppression. No calcification (may be seen after radiotherapy)	• Solid pleurally-based nodule • Focal/diffuse nodular pleural thickening associated with lymphadenopathy • Pleural effusion often associated • Homogeneous, vividly enhancing chest wall mass without rib destruction.	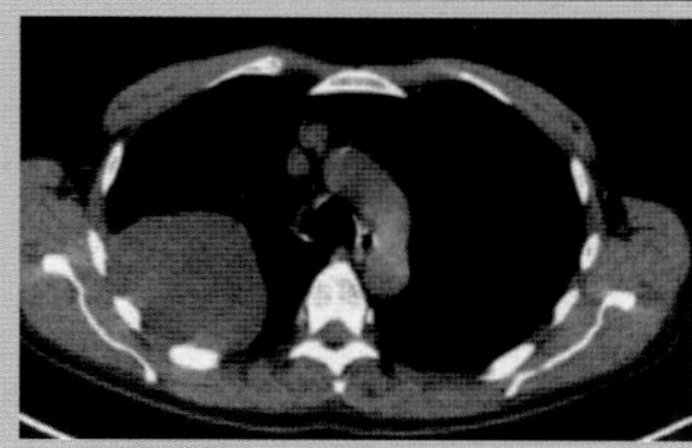 **Fig. 4.116.7:** Lymphoma
3. Solitary fibrous tumor of the pleura—(previously called pleural fibroma)–20% contain malignant elements. Arising more frequently from the visceral pleura than the parietal pleura.	Usually a solitary smooth lobular mass, 2–15 cm diameter. May change position due to pedunculation. Forms an obtuse angle with the chest wall suggesting extra pulmonary location. Patients usually over 40 years of age and asymptomatic. It is hypointense on both T1 and T2 weighted images due to fibrous content. When SFT is present, there is a high chance of hypertrophic osteoarthropathy.	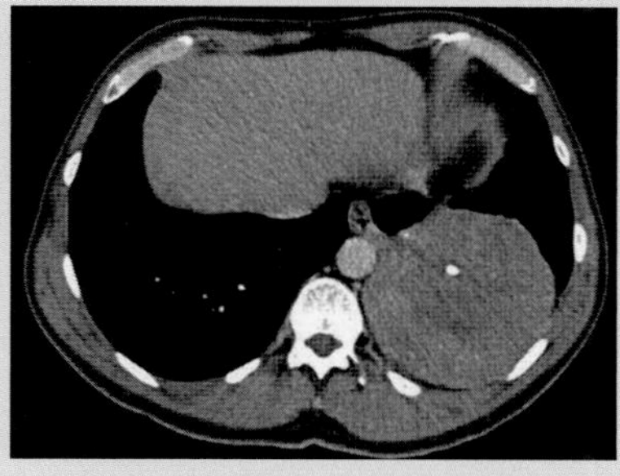 **Fig. 4.116.8:** Pleural fibroma
4. Rhabdomyosarcoma—usually indistinguishable/ thorax is a rare location. Typically occur in childhood or in the fifth to seventh decades of life with a male predominance	Heterogeneous signal intensity on both T1- and T2-weighted images; low signal intensity foci indicate necrosis in alveolar and pleomorphic subtypes; Ring-like enhancement. Ill-defined contours; rapid growth; bone invasion (in 20% of patients)	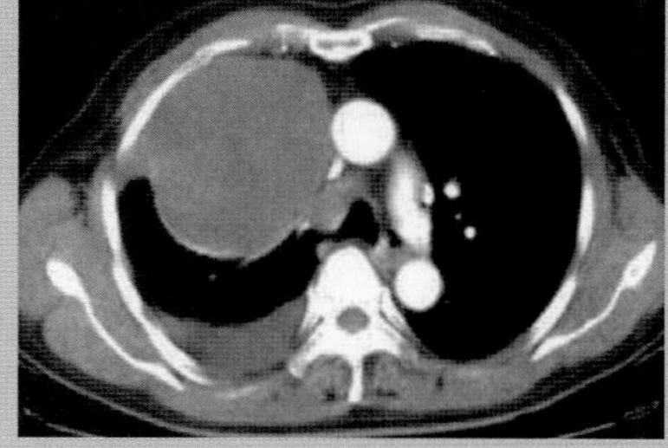 **Fig. 4.116.9:** Rhabdomyosarcoma
5. Askin tumors (Ewing sarcoma family of tumors)—are malignant tumors affecting children and young adults, originating either from the osseous structures or the soft tissues of the chest wall. Infiltration into chest wall, mediastinum and sympathetic chain is pathognomonic.	On imaging, they are usually characterized as a large extra pulmonary invasive soft tissue masses that are heterogeneous due to the presence of haemorrhage, necrosis, or cystic changes. Enhancement is intense and there is increased uptake in the nuclear medicine studies. Calcifications are uncommon and a small pleural effusion is frequently present.	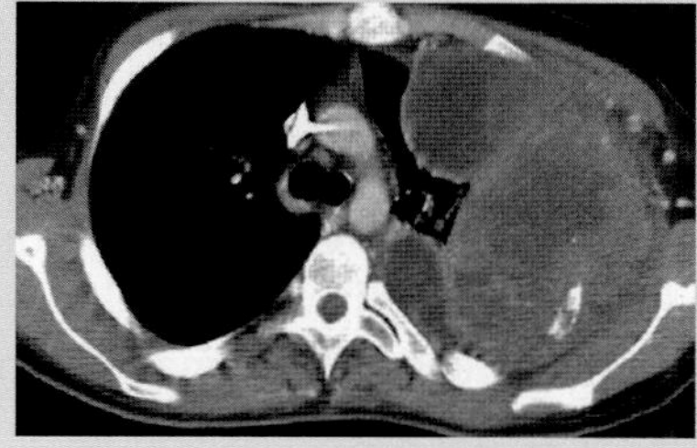 **Fig. 4.116.10:** Askin tumor

Table 4.116.1: Difference between pleural malignant mesothelioma and pleural metastasis	
Pleural malignant mesothelioma	*Pleural metastasis*
Usually unilateral	Usually bilateral
Calcific plaques might be seen	Usually not
Involvement of fissures can be seen	Less common
Volume contractures of lung without mediastinal shift	Contralateral mediastinal shift
Usually not	Pulmonary mets and septal thickening may be seen
-	PET-CT may find the primary elsewhere

3. Pericardial mesothelioma (<1%), 4. cystic/multicystic mesothelioma 5. tunica vaginalis testis mesothelioma (<1%). Mesothelioma is an uncommon entity and accounts for 5–28% of all malignancies that involve the pleura. There is a strong association with exposure to asbestos fibres (~10% risk during lifetime; 40–80% of patients have a history of asbestos exposure). Unlike other asbestos-related lung diseases, it does not appear to be dose-dependent. 60–80% of cases are encountered in males, in general, 20 to 35 years after asbestos exposure. There is also increased risk for those with household exposure (e.g. family of exposed workers).

Clinical presentation: Typically, patients present with dyspnoea and low back non-pleuritic chest pain. Pleural effusions are seen in the vast majority of patients at some stage during their disease. Up to 25% of patients have metastatic disease at the time of presentation if staged with FDG PET.

Typically, mesothelioma is thought of as a locally-aggressive disease, however distant extra nodal metastases are seen.

Etiology: Asbestos-fiber exposure: It causes majority of cases. Erionite-fiber exposure: Naturally occurring mineral used in building, particularly in Turkey. Simian virus 40 (sv40). Radiation exposure.

Histology: There are three histological types of mesothelioma: 1. Epithelial: ~60%, 2. Mixed: 25%, 3. Sarcomatoid: 15%.

Specific markers are helpful including: Calretinin/epithelial membrane antigen/cytokeratin/mesothelin (elevated in 84% of malignant mesothelioma versus <2% with other pleural diseases)

Plain radiograph: Chest radiographs are non-specific and of limited utility.

- Pleural opacity which may extend around and encase the lung
- Reduced volume of the affected hemithorax, resulting in ipsilateral shift of the mediastinum (common)
- Rib destruction or extension beyond the lateral and anterior margins of the chest wall
- +/- Mediastinal lymphadenopathy
- +/- Pleural effusion

CT: It is the most commonly used for imaging assessment of mesothelioma, and sufficient for accurate staging of disease in most patients. Pleural mass or nodular thickening of soft tissue attenuation, tends to cause "inward" contraction of the hemithorax, e.g. ipsilateral mediastinal shift. The pattern of spread is initially to adjacent pleura with involvement of pleural fissures, eventually grows toward lung encasement ('pleural rind'). Predilection for local invasion including involvement of chest wall, diaphragm, and mediastinal contents, infiltration of the extra-pleural fat plane and obvious direct extension in bone or muscle. Known to invade along prior catheter and biopsy tracks. Pericardial effusion may suggest trans pericardial extension. Frequent metastasis to local lymph nodes and contralateral lung. Calcification—seen in 20%—usually represents engulfment of calcified pleural plaques rather than true tumor calcification. Sarcomatoid variants may contain calcific osteosarcoma or chondrosarcomatous components. An uncommon variant is the solitary mediastinal malignant mesothelioma which has appearances reminiscent of a solitary fibrous tumor of the pleura. Subtypes such as multicystic/cystic mesothelioma are rarer and less aggressive.

MRI: Although not routinely used, MRI may have a role in refining the staging and better delineating the extent of the disease in surgical candidates especially concerning the chest wall and diaphragmatic invasion. T1: Iso to slightly hyperintense to muscle, T2: Iso to hyperintense to muscle, C+ (Gd): Enhancement usually present.

PET: Positron emission tomography is becoming useful in two clinical settings:

- Differentiating between benign and malignant asbestos-related pleural thickening
- Assessing for nodal metastases

Table 4.116.2: Causes of focal rib lesion	
Focal rib lesion (solitary or multiple) Neoplastic: Secondary more common than primary. Primary malignant more common than benign. 1. **Metastases:** Adult male—bronchus, kidney or prostate most commonly; Adult female—breast. 2. **Primary malignant:** Multiple myeloma/plasmacytoma, chondrosarcoma, Askin tumor–uncommon tumor of an intercostal nerve causing rib destruction. 3. **Benign:** Osteochondroma, enchondroma, Langerhans' cell histiocytosis.	**Non-neoplastic** 1. Healed rib fracture 2. Fibrous dysplasia 3. Paget's disease. 4. Brown tumor of hyperparathyroidism. 5. Osteomyelitis—bacterial, tuberculous or fungal. 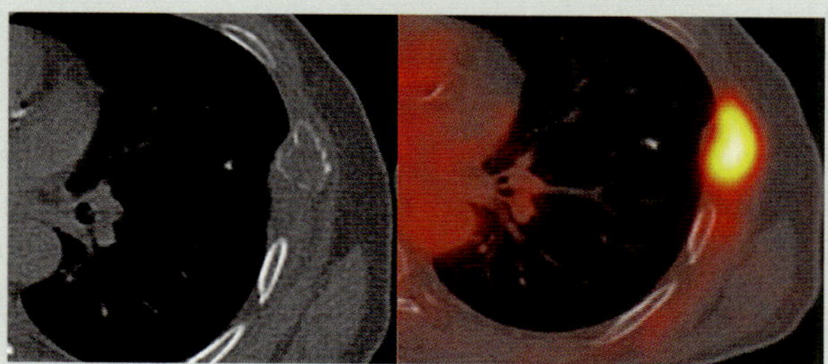 **Fig. 4.116.11:** Rib metastasis

Table 4.116.3: Rib lesion with an adjacent soft-tissue mass	
Neoplastic 1. Bronchogenic carcinoma—solitary site unless metastatic 2. Metastases—solitary or multiple 3. Multiple myeloma—classically multiple sites and bilateral 4. Mesothelioma—rib destruction occurs in 12% 5. Lymphoma 6. Fibrosarcoma—similar appearances to mesothelioma 7. Neurofibroma—rib notching 8. Chondrosarcoma	**Infective** 1. Tuberculosis osteitis—commonest inflammatory lesion of a rib but a rare manifestation of tuberculosis. Second only to malignancy as a cause of rib destruction. Clearly defined margins ± abscess. 2. Actinomycosis—usually a single rib and often associated with a lung mass due to consolidation. 3. Nocardiosis. 4. Blastomycosis—adjacent patchy or massive consolidation ± hilar lymphadenopathy.
Metabolic 1. Renal osteodystrophy 2. Cushing's syndrome—rib fractures and osteopenia associated with a subpleural haematoma. 3. Hemophilic pseudotumor	**Inflammatory** Radiation osteitis

Table 4.116.4: Chest wall lesions in children	
Congenital or developmental abnormalities Prominent costal cartilage Pectus excavatum Pectus carinatum	**Infection** Bacterial infection Fungal infection Chronic recurrent multifocal osteomyelitis
Trauma—accidental trauma and non-accidental trauma (child abuse)	
Neoplasm *Benign soft tissue tumors* Infantile haemangiomas Infantile fibrous hamartoma Inflammatory myofibroblastic tumor of the lung (inflammatory pseudotumour) *Benign osseous tumors* Osteoid osteoma Osteochondroma Fibrous dysplasia Mesenchymal hamartoma	**Malignant soft-tissue tumors** Rhabdomyosarcoma Malignant peripheral nerve sheath tumors Pleuropulmonary blastoma **Malignant osseous tumors** Ewing sarcoma family of tumors Osteosarcoma **Metastatic disease (most common)** Neuroblastoma Rhabdomyosarcoma Lymphoma or leukemia

4.117 CHEST

Case no. 117

Clinical history: A 60 years old male with vague left-sided chest pain × 2 months, right nephrectomy 6 months back, no history of trauma, no fever.

Radiological techniques and observation: Figure 4.117.1 is plain radiograph chest frontal view showing trachea in midline. Cardiac shadow appears normal. No cardiomegaly, bilateral costophrenic and cardiophrenic angle appears normal. No obvious hilar enlargement seen. Patchy opacity is seen in right lower zone without obscuring right heart border. Suspicious ill-defined lytic lesion noted in posterior aspect of left 8th rib. Bilateral diaphragm and vertebra appears normal. Figure 4.117.2 is CECT chest axial section showing ill-defined expansile lytic lesion noted in the posterior aspect of left 8th rib with soft tissue component. Bilateral lung fields show consolidation in right lower lobe superior segment consistent with infective etiology (not shown). No pleural thickening. No mediastinal lymphadenopathy.

Interpretation: A—60 years old male, rib lesion, C—ill-defined lytic lesion with soft tissue component, B—past history of nephrectomy, D—lytic metastasis.

Principal diagnosis is metastasis by considering the age of the patient and past history of right nephrectomy.

Management: This patient is further evaluated with PET-CT to look for other metastatic lesions and referred to multidisciplinary team for histopathological diagnosis, staging and further management. Based on the staging palliative treatment can be started.

Differential diagnosis: Differential diagnosis for lytic rib lesions in adults.

Metastasis: History of primary tumor, multiple lesions (polyostotic). Most common tumors to metastasize to rib are breast, lung, kidney, or thyroid carcinoma. Most common solitary rib metastasis secondary to thyroid or renal cell carcinoma.

Eosinophilic granuloma: Expansile lytic lesion, no sclerotic rim, polyostotic, ± soft tissue mass.

Lymphoma: Heterogeneous or homogeneous soft tissue mass, ± mediastinal lymphadenopathy, extrathoracic disease is common, 30% have lung involvement.

Expansile lesion of rib: Primary malignancy—plasmacytoma, secondary malignancy—metastasis. Non-malignant—fibrous dysplasia, chondrosarcoma, enchondroma, eosinophilic granuloma, neurofibromatosis.

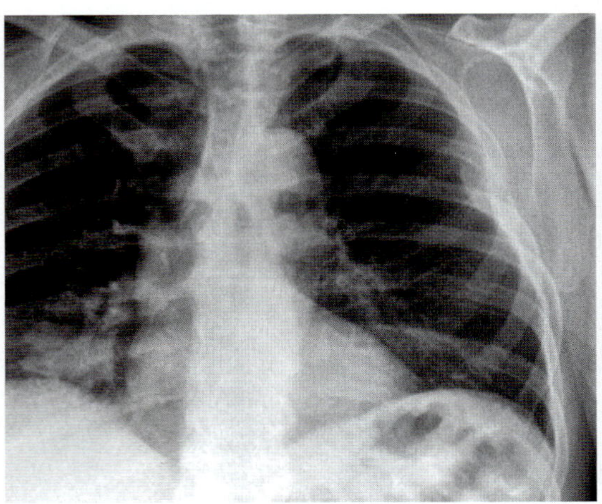

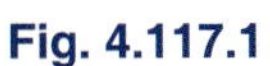

Fig. 4.117.1

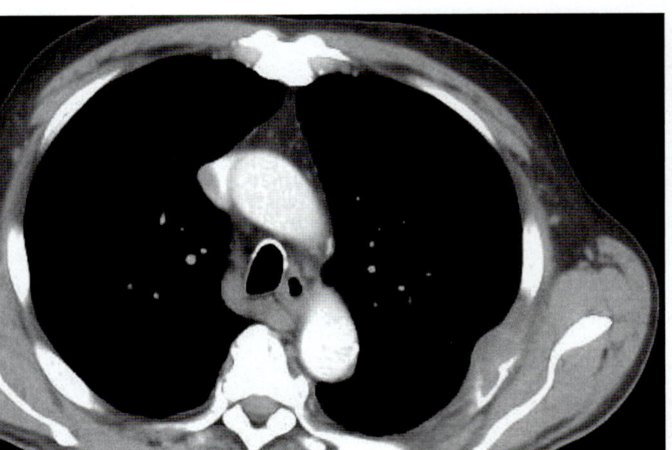

Fig. 4.117.2

Table 4.117.1: Differential diagnosis for lytic rib lesions in adults		
Multiple myeloma 2nd most common cause of rib destruction in adults. Most common bone manifestation is generalized osteopenia.	Solitary expansile lytic lesion may indicate solitary plasmacytoma. Typical lesion appears hypointense on T1 due to low fat content, on T2 FS images hyperintense due to high cellularity and high water. Rib on T2FS appears bright—white rib sign.	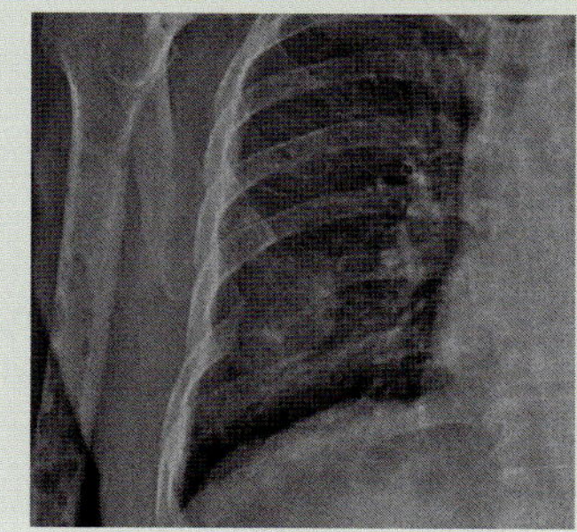 **Fig. 4.117.3:** Multiple myeloma
Bronchogenic carcinoma Pancoast tumor, Horner syndrome, syndrome of ipsilateral arm pain, and ipsilateral hand muscle wasting.	Rib destruction can indicate chest wall invasion. MR can be used for identifying neurovascular invasion. Superior sulcus tumor invades apical fat and involves brachial plexus and sympathetic ganglia	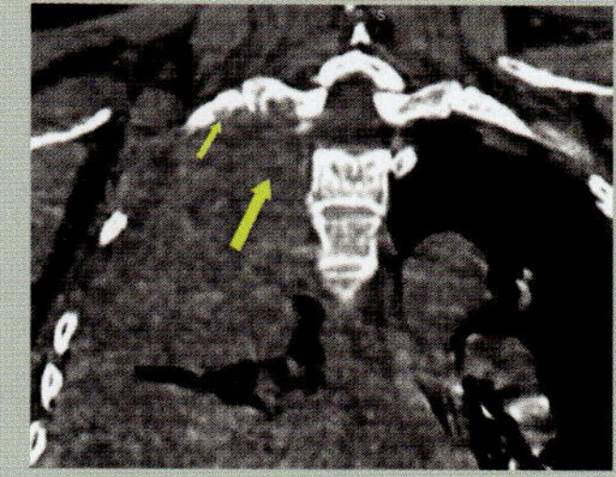 **Fig. 4.117.4:** Bronchogenic carcinoma
Fibrous dysplasia Non-neoplastic osteoblastic differentiation and maturation of normal bone does not require treatment. Bone expansion with ground-glass matrix. It shows increased radiotracer uptake on bone scan.	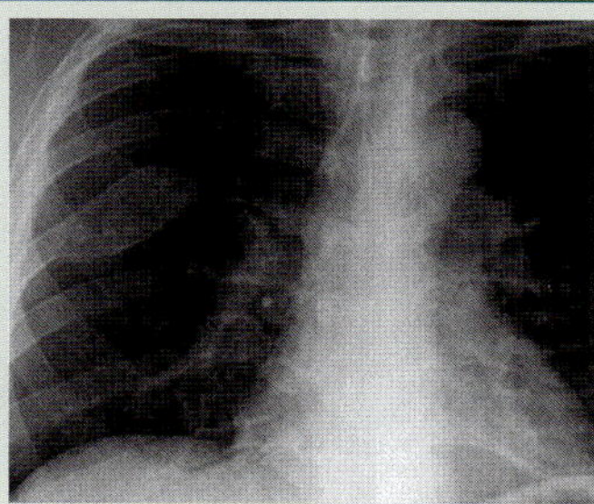 **Fig. 4.117.5:** Fibrous dysplasia	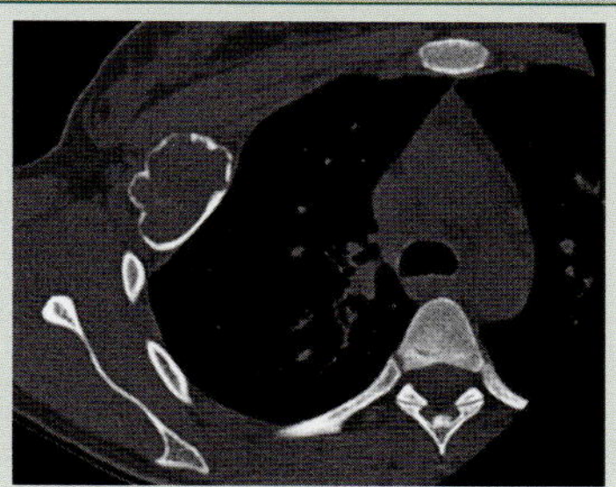 **Fig. 4.117.6:** Fibrous dysplasia
Aneurysmal bone cyst: Rapidly growing benign lesion.	Expansile, eccenteric osteolytic lesion. An aneurysmal bone cyst also contains multiple thin-walled blood-filled cavities.	
Enchondroma	Focal expansile, radiolucent lesions consisting of hyaline cartilage lobules in the medullary cavity on HPE.	
Chondrosarcoma most common primary malignant rib neoplasm, that arises in and around costochondral junction.	CT—lobulated masses containing the typical flocculent, stippled, or ring and arc like calcifications.	
Bone inflammation due to bacterial infection usually. Acute or chronic. May cause cold abscess. Commonly TB, actinomycosis and others. CT is better than MRI and plain film in showing the bony margins and identifying a sequestrum or involucrum.	MRI is most sensitive and specific method to identify soft-tissue/joint complications. Bone marrow oedema is the earliest feature of acute osteomyelitis seen on MRI as early as 1 to 2 days after the onset of infection. T1-intermediate to low signal, T2 central high signal intensity. T1 C+ enhancement of bone marrow, abscess margins, periosteum and adjacent soft tissue collections.	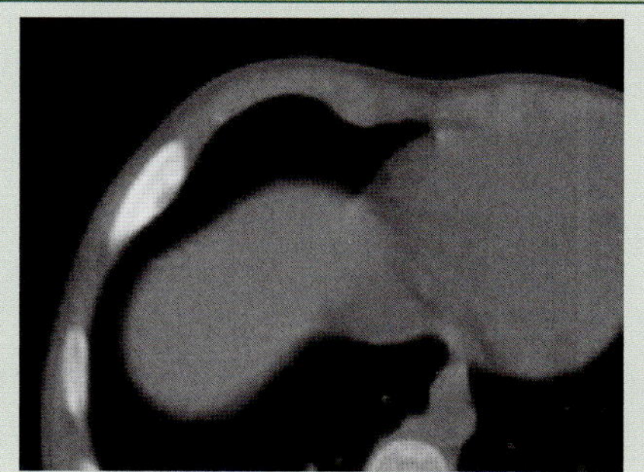 **Fig. 4.117.7:** Osteomyelitis

Table 4.117.2: Causes of focal rib lesions in adults	
Neoplastic	*Non-neoplastic*
1. Metastasis (solitary/multiple) Adult male: Bronchus, kidney, prostate Adult female: Breast 2. Primary malignant Multiple myeloma, chondrosarcoma, Askin tumor 3. Benign: Osteochondroma, enchondroma, LCH 4. Others: Lymphoma, fibrosarcoma, mesothelioma, neurofibroma (rib notching)	1. Inflammatory: Radiation osteitis 2. Metabolic: Renal osteodystrophy, Cushing's syndrome. 3. Infective–tuberculosis, actinomycosis (osteoblastic/osteolytic lesions with bone thickening + respiratory infections, nocardiosis, blastomycosis)

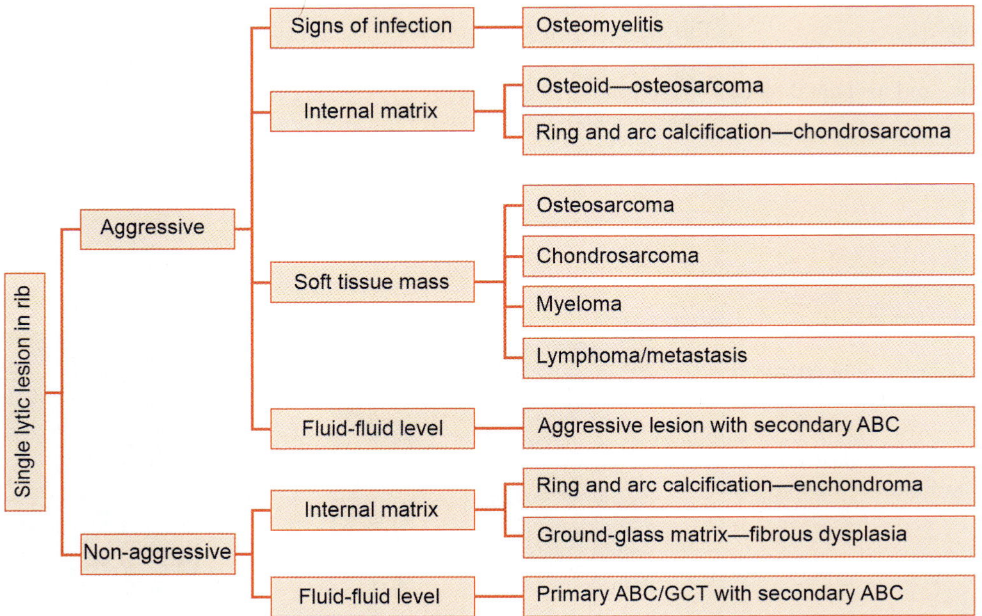

Fig. 4.117.8: Approach to rib lesions (single lesion)

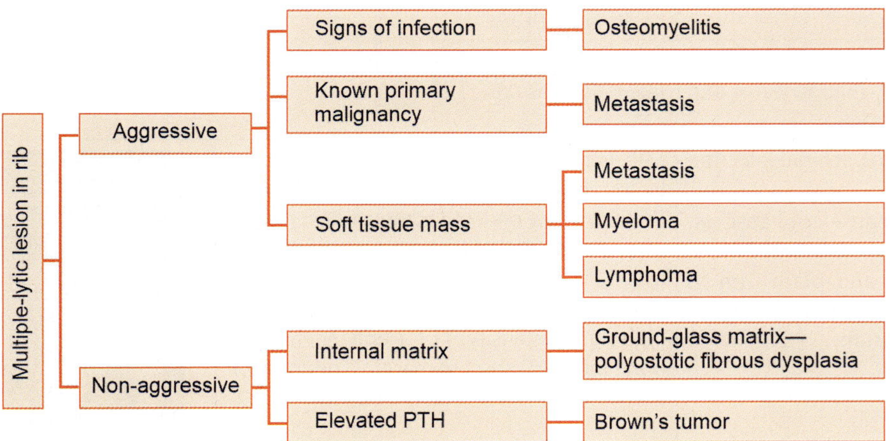

Fig. 4.117.9: Approach to multiple lytic lesions in rib

Table 4.117.3: Summary of lytic lesions in ribs—benign

Conditions	*Age group*	*Site*	*X-ray/CT*	*MRI*
Fibrous dysplasia (most common benign rib tumor)	1–3rd decade	Medullary cavity	Ground-glass matrix, sclerotic border, narrow zone of transition	Low signal on T1, high signal on T2, variable enhancement
Enchondroma (second most common benign rib tumor)	3–5th decade	Costochondral or costovertebral junction	Lucent lesion with well-demarcated margin, rings and arc calcification	High signal on T2
Aneurysmal bone cyst	Adolescent	Posterior arch	Expansile, eccentric lytic lesion with endosteal scalloping and cortical thinning	Fluid–fluid level on T2 weighted MRI
GCT	3–5th decade	Subchondral region, head or tubercle	Lucent lesion without sclerotic border	Low signal in T2/T1
Osteochondroma	Adolescent	Costochondral junction	Exophytic lesion showing corticomedullary continuity	Hyperintense cartilage cap on T2 images
Brown's tumor	Patient with hyperpara-thyroidism	Rib body	Lytic lesion. Look for other signs of HPT	-

Table 4.117.4: Summary of lytic lesions in ribs—malignant

Conditions	*Age group*	*Site*	*X-ray/CT*	*MRI*
Metastasis	Older adults	Rib body (single or multiple lesion)	Lytic or sclerotic lesion, imaging features of primary malignancy	T1-↑ SI with melanoma or haemorrhagic metastases, avid enhancement
Multiple myeloma: Ribs are the second most frequently involved site in multiple myeloma approximately (59%)	5–6th decades	Rib body (single or multiple lesion)	Lucent, well-defined lesion; soft-tissue mass	T1-↓ SI; T2-↑ SI; DWI-↑ SI
Lymphoma	6–8th decades	Rib body	Destructive or permeative osteolysis, lamellated periosteal reaction, soft-tissue mass	T1-↓ SI, T2-↑ SI homogeneous enhancement
Chondrosarcoma (most common primary rib malignancy)	4–5th decades	Costochondral or chondrovertebral junction	Calcified rings-and-arcs matrix, extra osseous soft-tissue mass (>4 cm), cortical disruption, deep endosteal scalloping	T1-↓ SI, T2-↑ SI peripheral and septal enhancement
Osteosarcoma—most common in metaphysis of long bones. Short bones and flat bones less frequently involved	Primary—2nd decade Secondary—older age	Costochondral junction	Dense ossified matrix centrally, sunburst periosteal reaction, heterogeneous internal components (secondary to haemorrhage and necrosis)	Variable signal intensity depends on mineralization and variable haemorrhage
Ewing sarcoma-common aggressive bone tumor of adolescents and young adults. Ewing's sarcoma of ribs is usually lytic. Mixed lytic sclerotic lesions do occur in case of atypical ribs. Most of the costal Ewing's sarcoma associated with disproportionate soft tissue component and approximately one-third of lesions are expansile.				
Direct involvement of ribs can be seen in Pancoast tumor and breast cancer.				

Other Chest Wall Lesions

1. Elastofibroma dorsi: Elastofibroma dorsi is located in the infrascapular regions, deep to the serratus anterior and latissimus dorsi musculature.
   USG—well-defined multi-layered pattern of hypoechoic linear areas of fat deposition intermixed with echogenic fibroelastic tissue.
   CT—poorly defined soft-tissue masses with attenuation similar to that of the adjacent skeletal muscle.
   MRI—T2-fibrous component: Isointense to muscle fatty component: High signal. Heterogeneous low level enhancement on contrast. Mild to moderate FDG uptake.
2. Lymphangioma–chest wall
3. Hemangioma chest wall

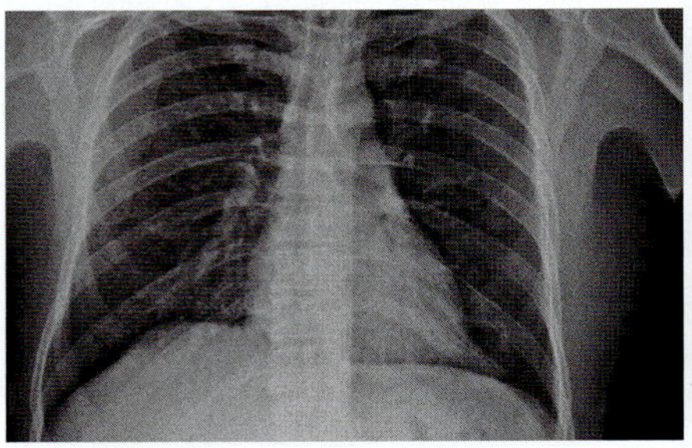

Fig. 4.117.10: Elastofibroma dorsi

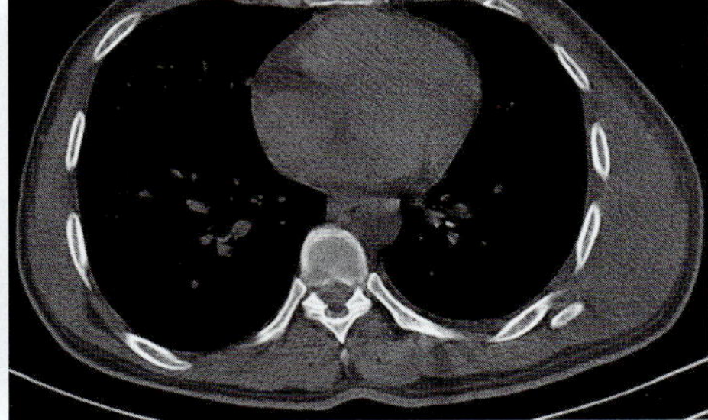

Fig. 4.117.11: Elastofibroma dorsi

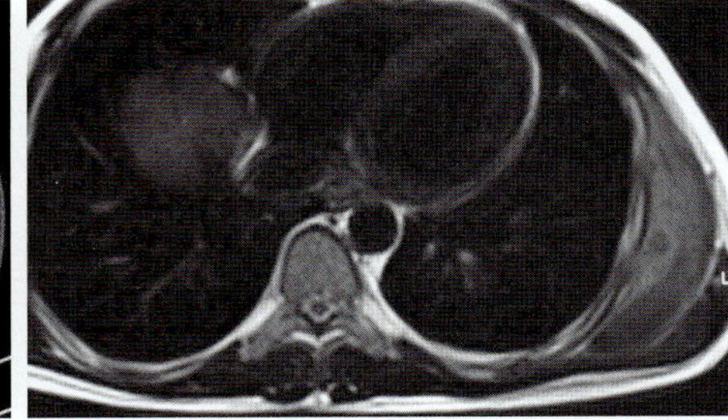

Fig. 4.117.12: Elastofibroma dorsi

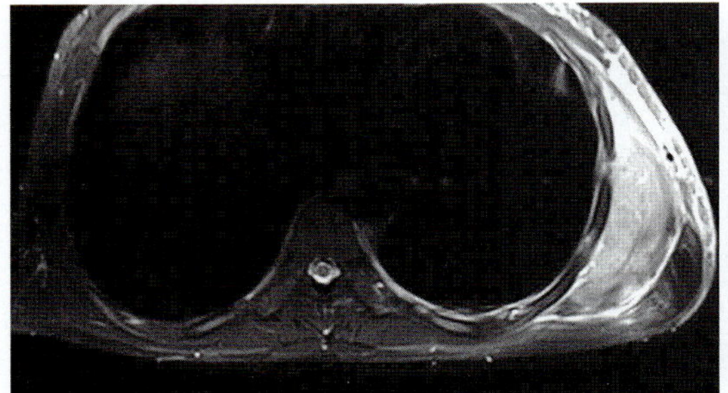

Fig. 4.117.13: Elastofibroma dorsi

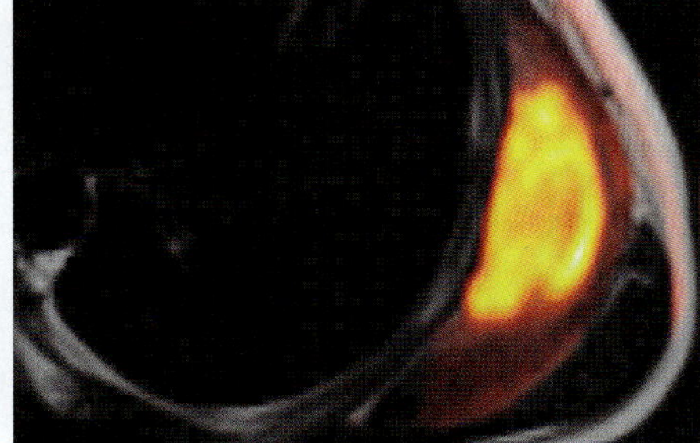

Fig. 4.117.14: Elastofibroma dorsi

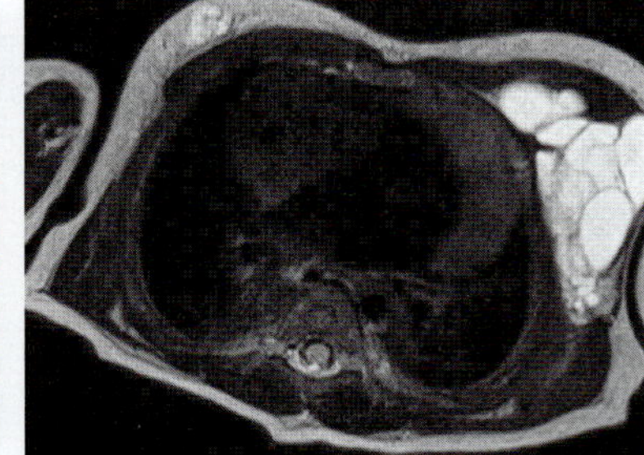

Fig. 4.117.15: Lymphangioma chest wall

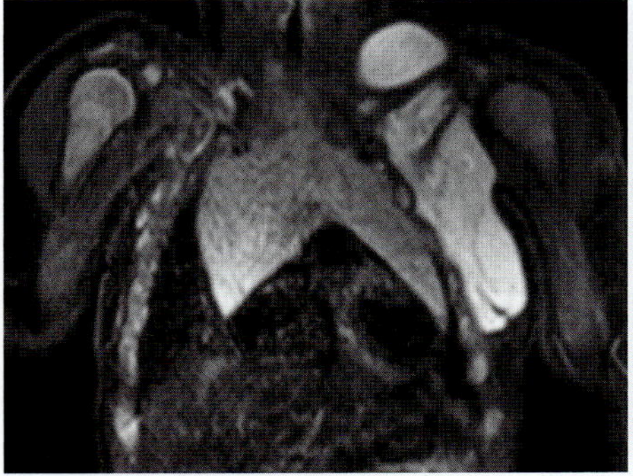

Fig. 4.117.16: Lymphangioma chest wall

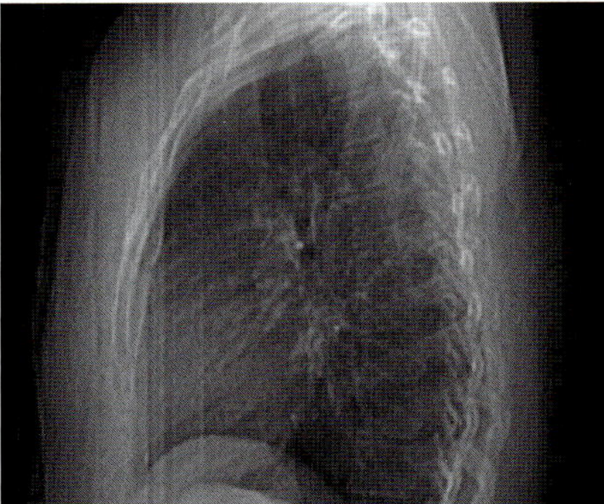

Fig. 4.117.17: Hemangioma chest wall

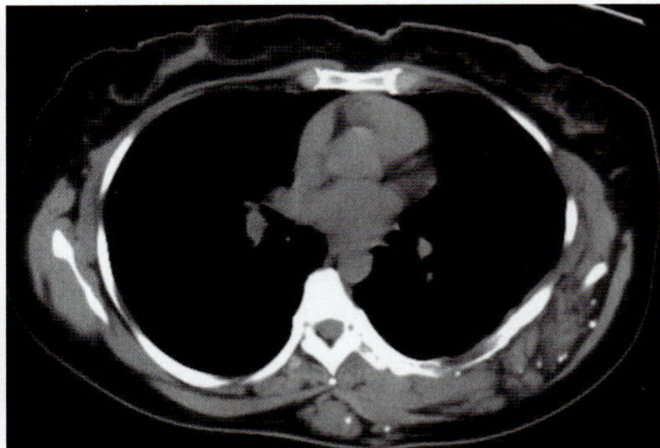

Fig. 4.117.18: Hemangioma chest wall

Table 4.117.5: Radiologic differentiation of malignant chest wall tumors	
Imaging finding Fat component	**Tumor type** Liposarcoma
Calcification **Skeletal** Rings and arcs, flocculent or stippled Centrally dense **Extra skeletal** Heterogeneous Speckled	Ring and arc, flocculent stippled—chondrosarcoma Centrally dense—osteosarcoma Heterogenous—ganglioneuroblastoma Speckled—proximal type epithelium sarcoma
Diffuse osteolytic change	Myeloma
Ill-defined mass Eccentric growth, in children and young adults	Ewing sarcoma
Fluid-fluid levels and calcification, in adolescents and adults	Synovial sarcoma
Chronic lymphedema	Angiosarcoma
Infiltrative growth	Malignant lymphoma
Nonspecific findings	Leiomyosarcoma, rhabdomyosarcoma, malignant fibrous histiocytoma, aggressive fibromatosis, malignant peripheral nerve sheath tumor, or dermatofibrosarcoma protuberans

4.118 BREAST

Case No. 118

Clinical history: 28-year-old female patient with a palpable lump in the left breast.

Radiological techniques and observation: Figures 4.118.1 and 4.118.2 mammography of the left breast MLO and CC views showing Type C breast with a well-defined, oval, lobular high-density mass without calcification in lower medial quadrant. No evidence of spiculations. No architectural distortion. No dermal changes/axillary lymphadenopathy. Nipple and areolar region appear normal.

The patient can be further evaluated by USG to narrow down the diagnosis.

Figure 4.118.3 is ultrasound showing an oval, macro lobulated sharply demarcated hypoechoic mass in the left breast at the lower and medial quadrant with a thin echogenic rim (pseudocapsule). The lesion is oriented parallelly and is wider than taller. No Doppler images has been provided to look for vascularity. And no elastogram has been provided. No architectural distortion. No ductal enlargement. No dermal changes/ axillary lymphadenopathy.

Interpretation: Site: Left breast lower inner quadrant Zone 2 Region B ~7 o'clock position. Well-defined macro lobular circumscribed lesion in lower medial quadrant of left breast. No evidence of spiculations, calcification, dermal changes or axillary lymphadenopathy noted.

Principal diagnosis: With these imaging findings the principal diagnosis would be BI-RADS 3 (typical fibroadenoma) of the left breast.

Differential diagnosis: Hamartoma, fibrocystic disease.

Management: Clinical follow-up to be advised and no need of biopsy. Patient referred to general surgeon. They are benign lesions with low risk of malignant transformation (0.0125–0.3%).

Discussion: Fibroadenoma is common benign breast lesion resulting from the excess connective tissue proliferation. Fibroadenomas contain both stromal and epithelial cells that occur in women of 10 and 40 years age and most common breast lesion in the adolescent and young women. Incidence peaks between 25 and 40, then decreases after 40 years. They have a predilection for the upper outer quadrant, but can occur anywhere. Giant fibroadenomas are fibroadenomas weighing more than 500 grams or measuring >5 cm in size. A juvenile fibroadenoma of the breast (~0.5–2% of all fibroadenomas) is a rapidly-growing fibroadenoma that cause asymmetry of the breast, distortion of the overlying skin, and stretching of the nipple seen in children or adolescents and associated with Cowden syndrome, cyclosporin use, fibroadenomas can be stimulated by oestrogen and progesterone. Some fibroadenomas have receptors for growth hormone and epidermal growth factor.

Mammography: Fibroadenomas can range in appearance from a well-circumscribed discrete oval mass that is hypo- or isodense to breast glandular tissue to a mass with macrolobulation or a partially concealed edge on mammography. Calcification may be seen in involuting fibroadenomas in older, generally postmenopausal patients, resulting in the distinctive, coarse popcorn calcification appearance (BI-RADS 2). The entire lesion may be hardened in some circumstances. Calcification might seem as broken stone or microcalcification, making it difficult to distinguish it from cancer.

Ultrasound of the breast typically reveals a well-circumscribed, spherical to ovoid, or macrolobulated mass with homogeneous hypoechogenicity. In 10% of cases,

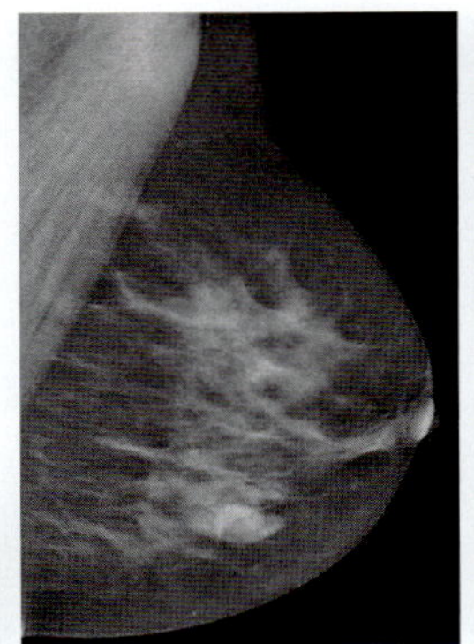

Fig. 4.118.1

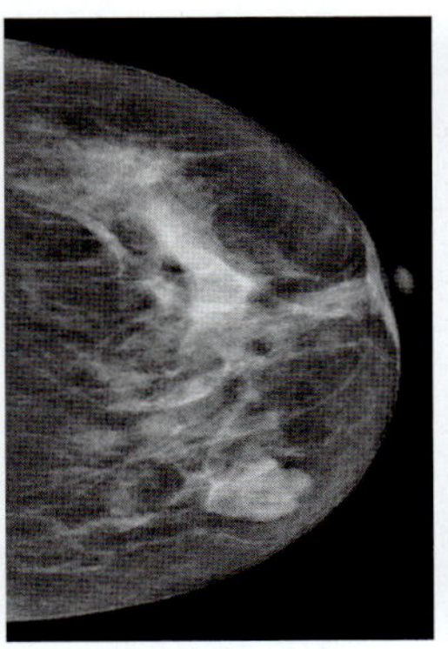

Fig. 4.118.2

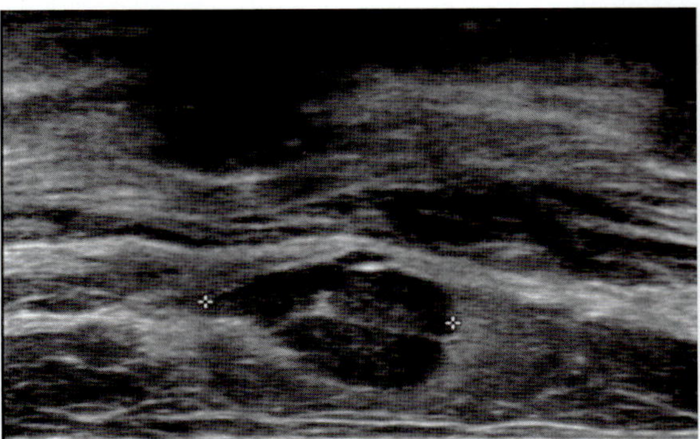

Fig. 4.118.3

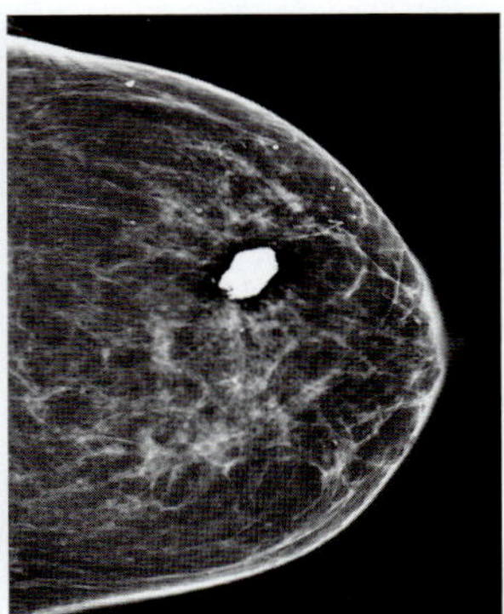

Fig. 4.118.4: BI-RADS 2

Table 4.118.1: Differential diagnosis for fibroadenoma

Condition	*Radiological features*	*Images*
Breast hamartoma (Fibroadenolipoma) Benign fibrous, glandular, and fatty tissue proliferation with thin of connective tissue capsule. They occur in women >35 years of age.	Well-circumscribed, round or oval mass surrounded by a thin capsule comprising of both fat and soft-tissue internal densities, i.e. fat component appears radiolucent, soft tissue component appears radiodense. "Breast within a breast" or a "slice of sausage" appearance. Surgical excision is the definitive treatment. Hamartomas have the same malignant potential as normal breast tissue, unless greater than 6 cm, and thus do not require any additional treatment than one would for adenoma or other benign lesions.	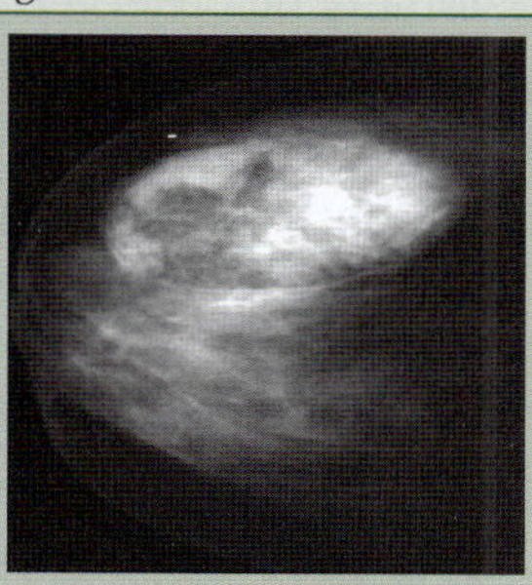 **Fig. 4.118.5:** Fibroadenolipoma
Breast lipoma: Asymptomatic seen as painless palpable breast lump which is soft and mobile. Occur in adults between 40 and 60 years of age. Lipoma enlargement is an indication for biopsy.	Seen as a radiolucent mass with no calcification. They may have a thin, peripheral, fluid density capsule. Incidentally seen on routine screening. Rarely undergo malignant transformation Not associated with an increased risk of developing breast cancer.	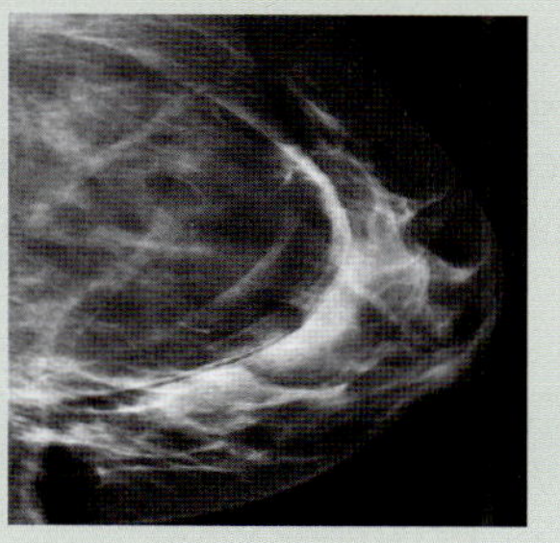 **Fig. 4.118.6:** Breast lipoma
Simple breast cyst: Breast cysts are caused by blockage of the terminal acini with resultant dilatation of ducts. Cysts may be unilateral, although they tend to be bilateral and multifocal. Symptomatic large cysts may warrant aspiration.	Cysts appear as a breast mass with the following features: Oval or round shape; High density mass with circumscribed margins. Multiple round masses in both breasts are suggestive. On USG, anechoic with posterior acoustic enhancement.	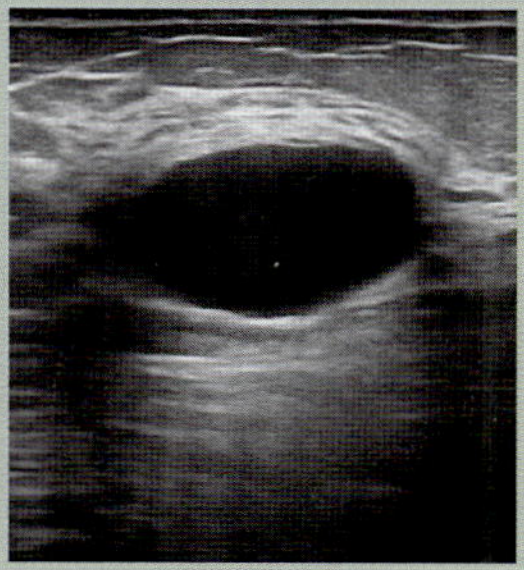 **Fig. 4.118.7:** Simple breast cyst
Oil cyst: They are benign breast lesions where an area of focal fat necrosis becomes walled off by fibrous tissue. Usually asymptomatic. Multiple intradermal oil cyst can be part of steatocystoma multiplex.	Typically radiolucent rounded mass of fat density . Wall calcification, which if present typically appears as eggshell calcification. Usually well-circumscribed. On USG, hypoechoic with smooth walls. Fat fluid levels are better characterised. Complex features include thick walls, mural nodularity and internal echoic bands. 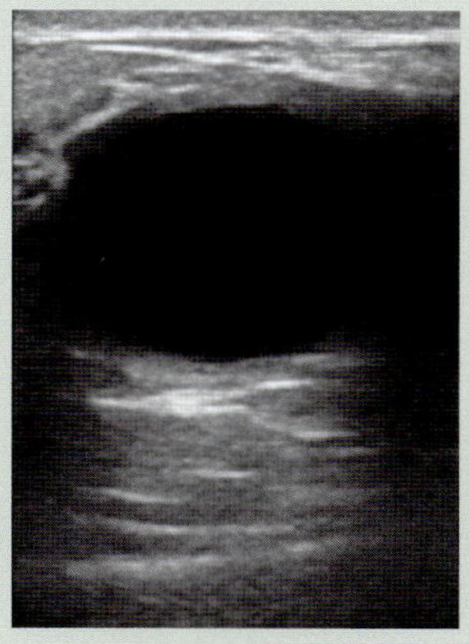 **Fig. 4.118.8:** Oil cyst	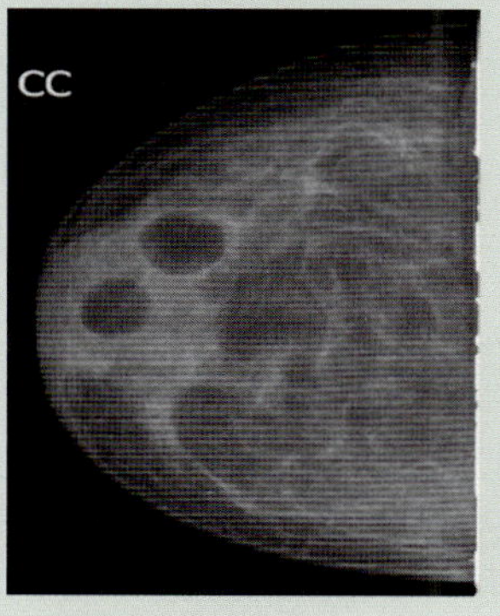 CC **Fig. 4.118.9:** Oil cyst

sonographically identifiable intralesional calcification can be found. A thin echogenic rim (pseudocapsule) can occasionally be observed sonographically.

MRI of the breasts: T1: Typically hypointense or isointense in comparison to adjacent breast tissue; T2: Can be hypo- or hyperintense; T1 C+ (Gd): Can vary, but the majority will show slow initial contrast enhancement followed by a persistent delayed phase (type I enhancement curve); non-enhancing internal septations may be visible.

Mass: Space occupying lesion that has three dimensions.

Non-mass: Enhancement occurs in an area of the fibroglandular tissue that otherwise appears normal on precontrast images without mass effect. Focal enhancing area of less than 5 mm that is too small to be further characterized. In the majority of cases, these foci will be due to a focal proliferation of the glandular tissue (so-called focal adenosis).

Mass enhancement occurs in six main patterns:

1. Homogeneous enhancement is enhancement that is uniform and consistent across the bulk.
2. Heterogeneous enhancement refers to nonuniform enhancement within a mass.
3. Rim enhancement is a type of enhancement that focuses on the periphery of the mass. High-grade invasive ductal carcinoma, fat necrosis, and inflammatory cysts are all known to have this type of augmentation.
4. Non-enhancing septations in an enhancing mass are referred to as dark internal septations. These are common in fibroadenomas, especially if the margins are smooth or lobulated.
5. Malignancy is often characterised by the increase of internal septations.

Table 4.118.2: BI-RADS staging ACR guidelines

Final assessment categories			
	Category	*Management*	*Likelihood of cancer*
0	Need additional imaging or prior examinations.	Recall for additional imaging and/or await prior examinations.	N/A
1	Negative	Routine screening	Essentially 0%
2	Benign	Routine screening	Essentially 0%
3	Probably benign	Short term interval follow-up (6 months) or continued.	> 0% but ≤ 2%
4	Suspicious	Tissue diagnosis.	4a. Low suspicion for malignancy (>2 to ≤10%) 4b. Moderate suspicion of malignancy (>10% to ≤50%) 4c. High suspicion of malignancy (>50% to <95%)
5	Highly suggestive of malignancy	Tissue diagnosis	≥95%
6	Known biopsy proven	Surgical excision when clinically appropriate	N/A

Table 4.118.3: BI-RADS—MRI lexicon

Lesion type	*Focus, mass, non-mass*
Focus	An area of enhancement <5 mm in diameter which is too small to characterize.
Mass—margin Shape Enhancement	Smooth, irregular, spiculated. Round, oval, lobular, irregular. Homogeneous, heterogeneous, rim, dark internal septations, enhancing internal septations, central enhancement.
Non-mass—type If linear Otherwise	Linear/ductal, linear/nonspecific, segmental, regional, multiple, diffuse. Smooth, irregular, clumped. Homogeneous, heterogeneous, stippled, clumped, septal/dendritic.
Visual kinetic pattern	Progressive, plateau, washout.
Final assessment	Benign, probably benign, suspicious, highly suggestive of malignancy.

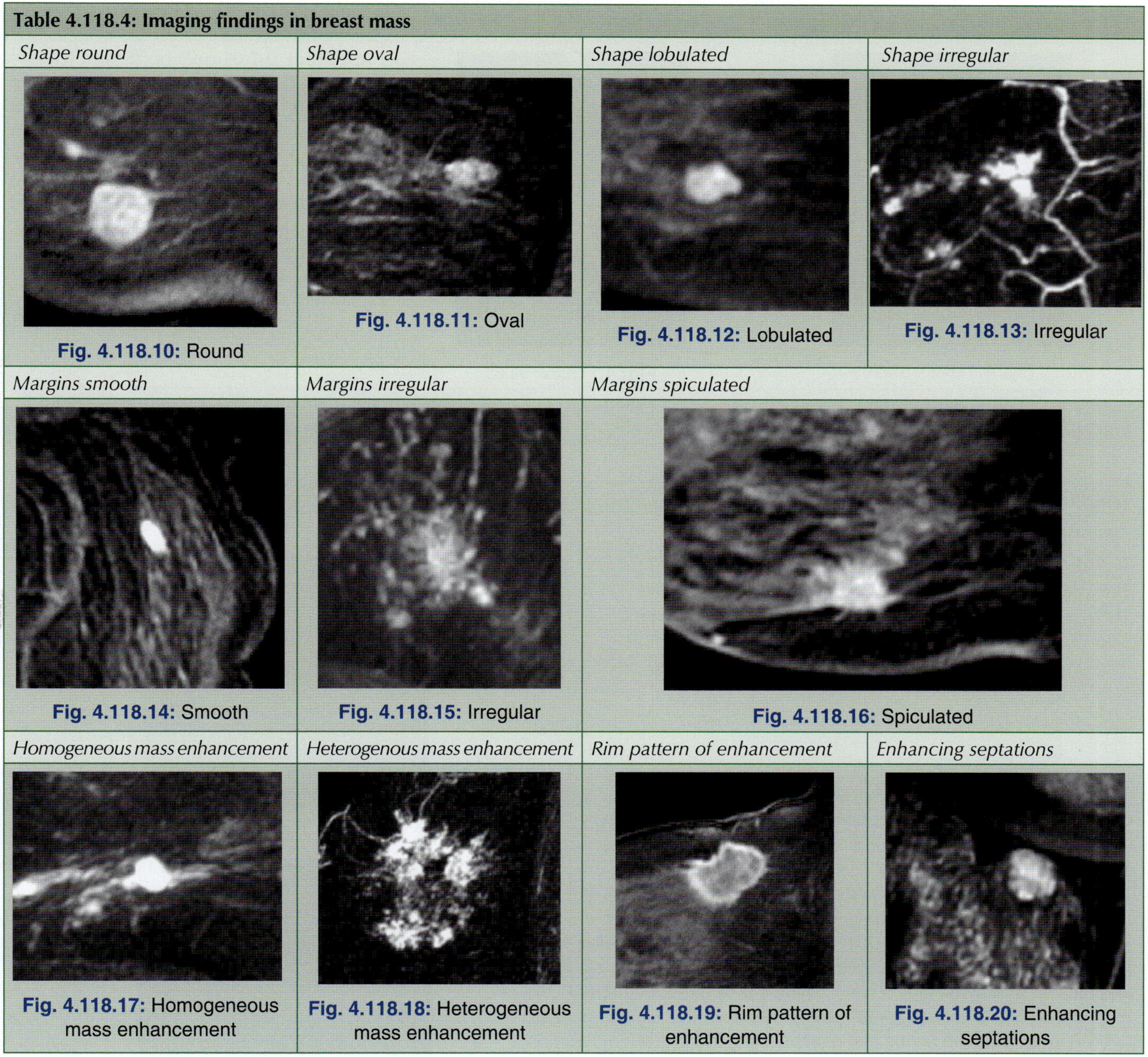

Table 4.118.4: Imaging findings in breast mass

Shape round	*Shape oval*	*Shape lobulated*	*Shape irregular*
Fig. 4.118.10: Round	**Fig. 4.118.11:** Oval	**Fig. 4.118.12:** Lobulated	**Fig. 4.118.13:** Irregular
Margins smooth	*Margins irregular*	*Margins spiculated*	
Fig. 4.118.14: Smooth	**Fig. 4.118.15:** Irregular	**Fig. 4.118.16:** Spiculated	
Homogeneous mass enhancement	*Heterogenous mass enhancement*	*Rim pattern of enhancement*	*Enhancing septations*
Fig. 4.118.17: Homogeneous mass enhancement	**Fig. 4.118.18:** Heterogeneous mass enhancement	**Fig. 4.118.19:** Rim pattern of enhancement	**Fig. 4.118.20:** Enhancing septations

6. A substantial enhancement of a nidus within an augmenting mass is known as central enhancement. High-grade ductal cancer has been linked to central enhancement.

Non-mass like enhancement in breast lesions: Intraductal (DCIS), mastocytic changes (fibroadenosis), hormonal stimulation, inflammatory changes.

MR dynamic contrast kinetic analysis (curves): First, we look at the initial upslope of the curve during the first one to two minutes.

This is either slow, medium or rapid. Rapid upstroke indicates malignancy.

Then there is the delayed phase—two minutes or more after the injection of contrast.

This part of the curve shows either an increase, plateau or washout. The kinetic analysis takes about six minutes of repetitive scanning in total and can lead to three types of curve.

MR spectroscopy in breast malignancy: For increased diagnostic confidence Presence of choline (3.22 ppm) is

Table 4.118.5: Diffusion weighted breast MR and ADC values

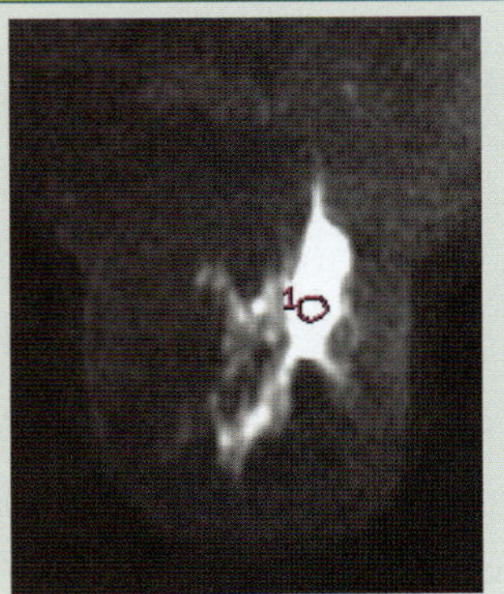 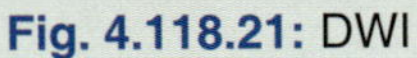 **Fig. 4.118.21:** DWI	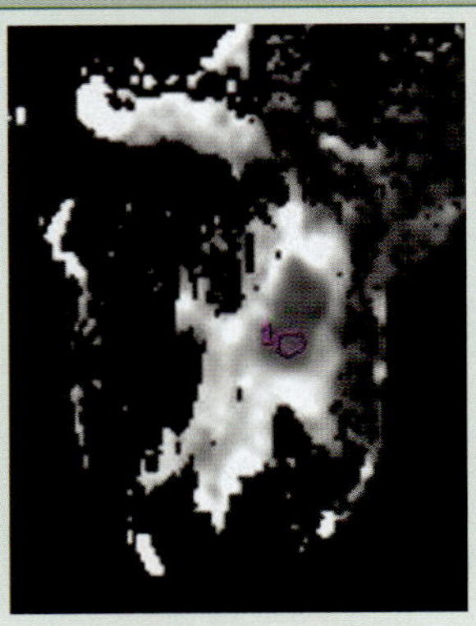 **Fig. 4.118.22:** ADC	Apparent diffusion coefficient values in DWI (b = 1000 s/mm^2) if less than 1.3×10^{-3} mm^2/s is highly suggestive of malignancy. A decrease in the apparent diffusion coefficient (ADC) provides strong evidence of malignant-type changes in the microstructure of a tissue. Restricted diffusion and decrease in ADC value shows a sensitivity of 95% and specificity of 80%.
Figures 4.118.21 and 4.118.22 are axial sections showing the breast lesion showing low ADC value 0.673×10^{-3} mm^2/s and diffusion restriction suggestive of malignancy proven by biopsy.		

Table 4.118.6: Contrast kinetic curve characteristics

Contrast kinetic curve characteristics	*Image*
Type 1 (progressive wash in curve) The image on the left is a type 1 curve. There is a slow and continued rise with time. A lesion with a type 1 curve has a chance of 6% being malignant.	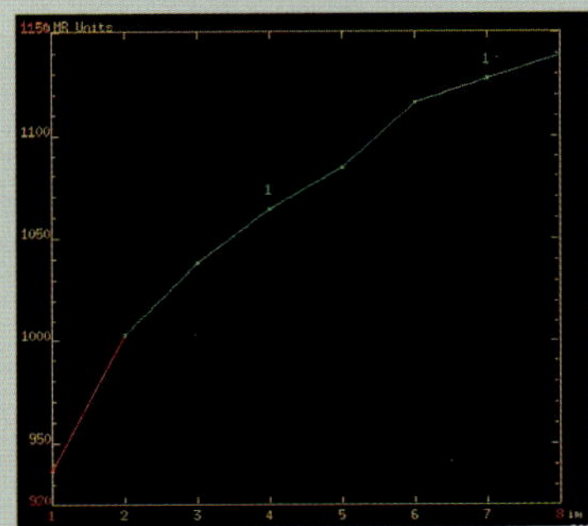 **Fig. 4.118.23:** Type 1 (progressive wash in curve)
Type 2 (plateau curve) Then there is the type 2 curve, a slow or rapid initial rise followed by a plateau in the delayed phase, which is allowed a variance of 10% up or down. The chance of a lesion with a type 2 curve being malignant lies somewhere between the 6% of the type 1 curve and the 29–77% of the type 3 curve. Many physicians will biopsy lesions with type 2 curves. For non-mass enhancement, kinetics is not very useful. If there is clumped enhancement in a breast it must be biopsied, even though there are no areas with a type 3 curve.	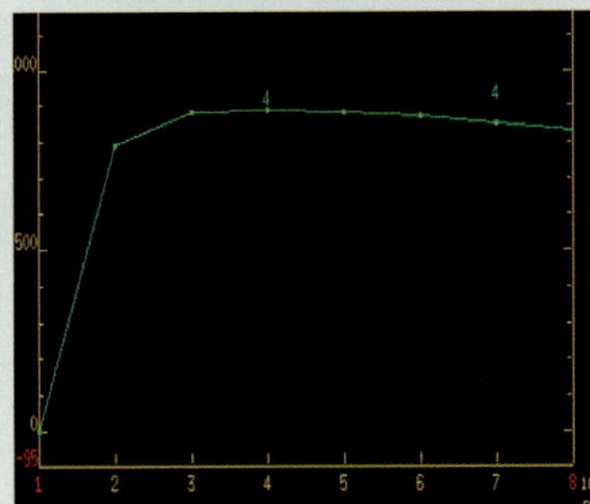 **Fig. 4.118.24:** Type 2 (plateau curve)
Type 3 (rapid wash-in and wash-out curve) The type 3 curve shows a rapid initial rise, followed by a drop-off with time (washout) in the delayed phase. A lesion with this type of curve is malignant in 29–77%.	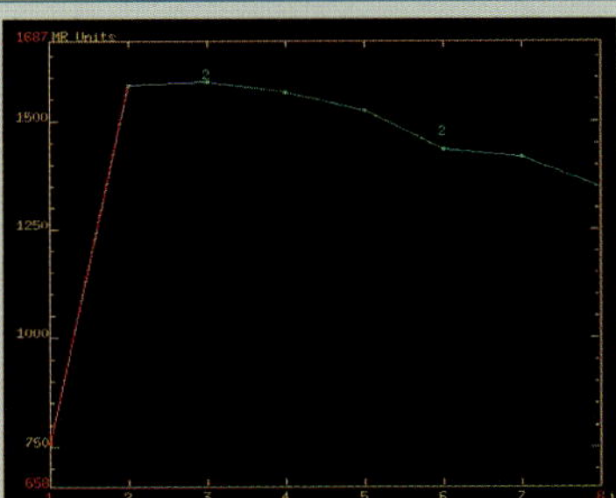 **Fig. 4.118.25:** Type 3 (rapid wash-in and wash-out curve)

indicative of malignancy with 85–100% specificity and avoids unnecessary biopsy.

Example of a breast lesion characterisation using MR imaging: A 32-year-old female with pathologically proven granulomatous mastitis in left breast—DCE MRI revealed an ill-defined area of abnormal MRI signal predominantly at upper quadrant with regional heterogeneous non-mass-like enhancement; DWI showed restricted diffusion (ADC value was 1.4×10^{-3} mm^2/s); kinetic curve showed type II plateau curve pattern; MRS was positive for choline (choline peak = 0.6 mmol/l): Figures 4.118.27 to 4.118.30.

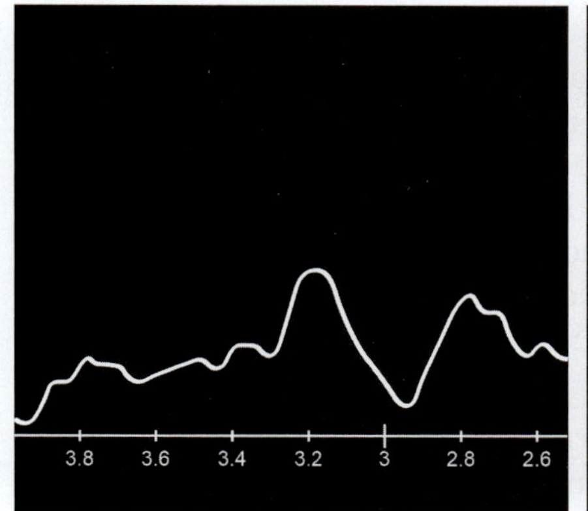

Fig. 4.118.26: MRS in a breast carcinoma showing choline peak

Fig. 4.118.27

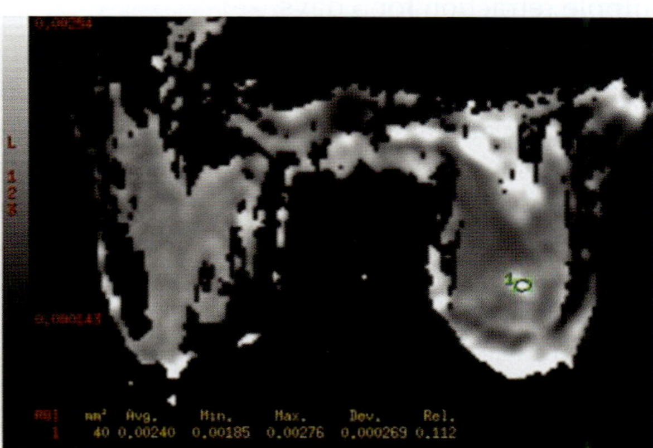

Fig. 4.118.28

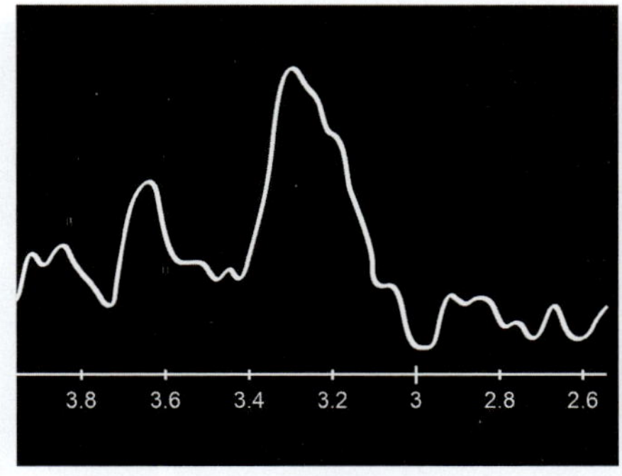

Fig. 4.118.29

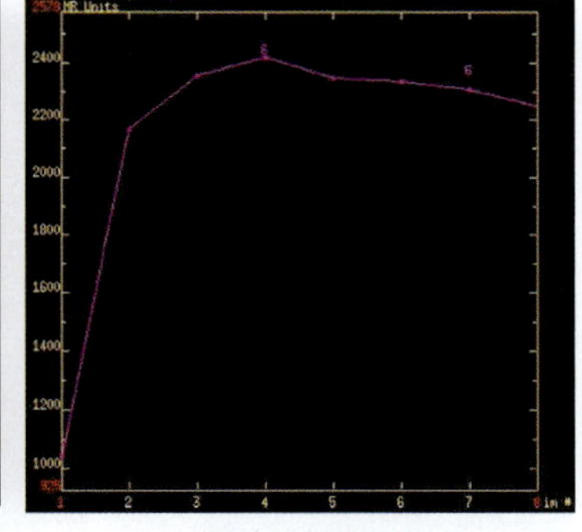

Fig. 4.118.30

Table 4.118.7: T2 fat suppressed sequence

Moderate signal	*Low signal*	*High signal*
Invasive lobular carcinoma	Invasive ductal carcinoma	Mucinous carcinoma of breast
DCIS	Sclerotic fibroadenoma	
Fibrocystic change	Scar	

4.119 BREAST

Case No. 119

Clinical history: A 44 years old female patient presented with complaints of lump in the left breast for 4 months, not associated with pain, H/o bloody discharge and nipple retraction for 3 days.

Radiological techniques and observation: Figures 4.119.1 and 4.119.2 are X-ray mammogram of the left breast in the Craniocaudal (CC) and mediolateral Oblique (MLO) view showing heterogeneously dense, type C breast. A relatively ill-defined high density lesion with spiculated margins in the lower outer quadrant. There is an enlarged axillary lymph node visible on MLO view. No evidence of adjacent skin thickening. No evidence of nipple retraction. No evidence of visible microcalcifications noted in the breast. No evidence of similar lesion noted in the rest of the breast. No evidence of breast asymmetry/ architectural distortion noted. No other suspicious lesion noted in the contralateral breast on screening.

Figures 4.119.3 and 4.119.4 are ultrasound of left breast show an ill-defined hypoechoeic lesion in the upper outer quadrant with lobulated margins, the lesion is taller than wider. The lesion shows posterior acoustic shadowing. No evidence of calcification. No evidence of adjacent inflammatory changes. No evidence of any other lesion noted in the breast.

Figures 4.119.5 and 4.119.6 shows a well-defined hyperintense lesion noted in the lower outer quadrant of left breast with type 3 kinetic curve, a rapid initial peak and a gradual wash out on delayed imaging. No evidence of any other lesion noted. Enlarged axillary lymph nodes noted. No evidence of internal mammary lymph nodes. Figure 4.119.7 is MRS image showing presence of choline peak at 3.2 ppm.

Findings and interpretation: Site: Left breast lower outer quadrant Zone 3 Region B ~4 o'clock position. Mammogram of left breast in CC and MLO view shows a predominantly fatty, type A breast, with an ill-defined

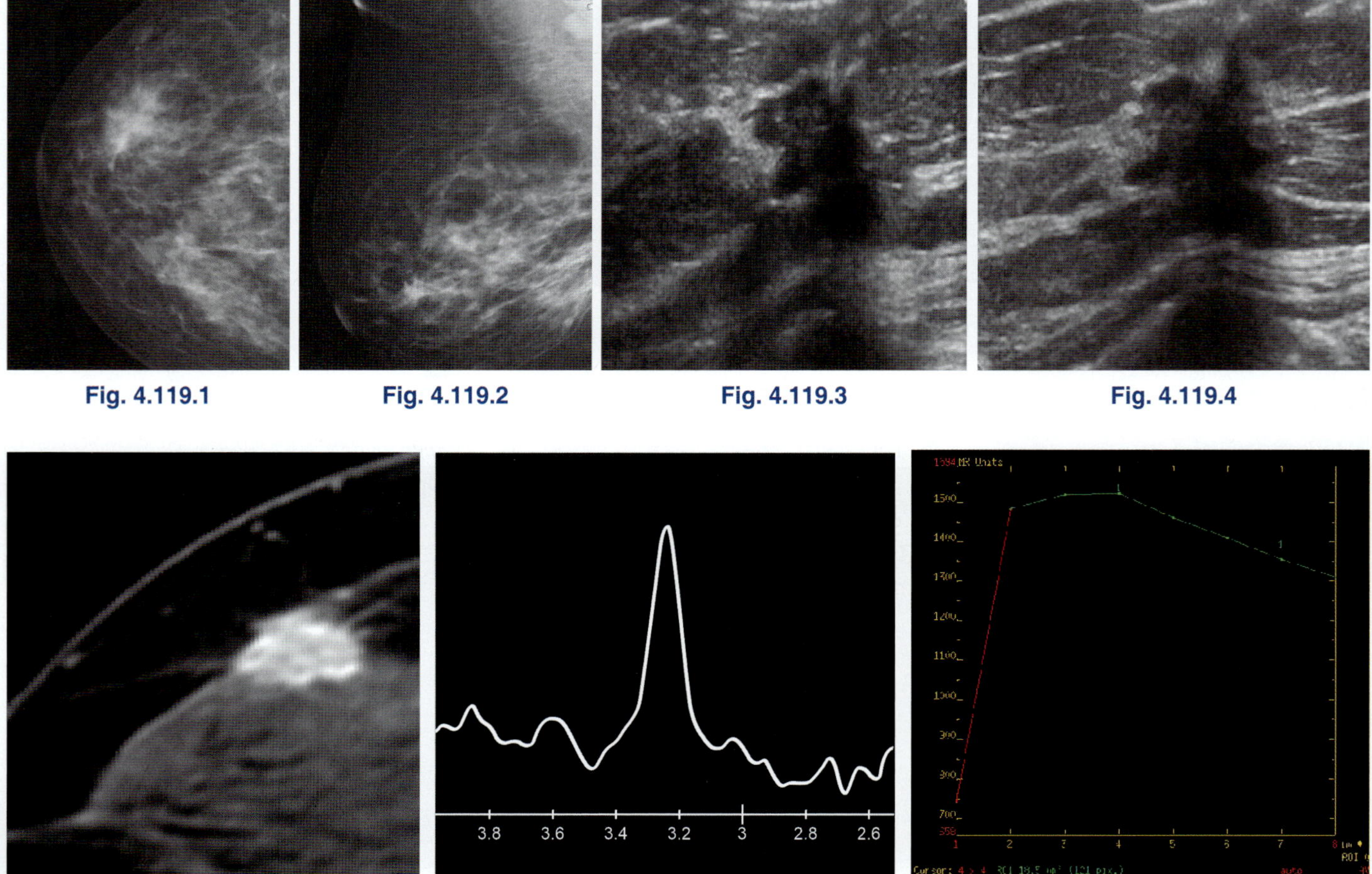

Fig. 4.119.1 Fig. 4.119.2 Fig. 4.119.3 Fig. 4.119.4

Fig. 4.119.5 Fig. 4.119.6 Fig. 4.119.7

Table 4.119.1: Standard form of reporting breast lesion in mammogram
1. Indication
2. Breast composition
3. Findings
4. Comparison with previous studies
5. Overall assessment

high density lesion with spiculated margins in the upper outer quadrant. The lesion is hypoechoeic on USG with posterior acoustic shadowing. On MRI the lesion is T2 hyperintense with type 3 contrast kinetic curve (wash-out) and MRS showing choline peak suggestive of malignancy.

Principal diagnosis: BI-RADS V

Treatment: Mastectomy (radical) with neoadjuvant chemotherapy.

Discussion: Carcinoma breast—malignant tumor arising from the epithelial cells of terminal lobular ductal unit, can be invasive—crosses basement membrane or non-invasive—contained in basement membrane. Needs USG guided biopsy for histopathological diagnosis and treatment varies depending upon the staging.

Mammography views: There are numerous mammography views that can broadly be split into two groups: Standard views and supplementary views. Bilateral craniocaudal (CC) and mediolateral oblique (MLO) views are used in screening mammography. Supplementary views such as straight lateral (SL) and rolled CC (rolled) views with additional magnification views (mag views) used for parenchymal asymmetries and calcifications. The mediolateral (ML) view used to view lateral side of the breast and it is most common place for pathological changes. The best view of the lateral side of the breast is from the middle of the chest and outward to the side (ML). On a mammography, the chest muscle (pectoral) appears as a narrow dense band on around half of the image in this view. In profile, the imaging of the nipple is also obvious. The entire breast is seen in the top-down or cranial caudal (CC) perspective. On an X-ray, the fat tissue closest to the breast muscle should appear as a dark strip. The nipple is also more clearly depicted in the CC view.

Screening mammography: In general terms, screening mammography is performed on asymptomatic women to identify malignant breast pathology at an early, potentially curable stage. Regardless of confusing statistics in lay publications, the earlier breast cancer is picked up, all other factors being equal, the better the survival rate. Screening mammography is performed on clients, not patients.

Hypoechoic lesions with postacoustic enhancement: Lymphoma, fibroadenoma and pleomorphic adenoma.

Hyperechoic lesions with post-acoustic enhancement: Hemangioma.

Anechoic lesions with post-acoustic enhancement: Cystic lesions.

Table 4.119.2: BI-RADS mammography lexicon

Breast composition	a. Entirely fatty. b. Scattered areas of fibroglandular density. c. Heterogeneously dense, which may obscure masses. d. Extremely dense, which lowers sensitivity		
Mass	Shape	Oval, round, irregular.	
	Margin	Circumscribes, obscured, microlobulated, indistinct, spiculated	
	Density	Fat, low, equal, high	
Asymmetry	Global/ focal/ developing.		
Architectural distortion	Distorted parenchyma with no visible mass		
Calcification	Morphology	Typically benign	
		Suspicious	1. Amorphous. 2. Coarse heterogeneous. 3. Fine pleomorphic 4. Fine linear or fine linear branching
	Distribution	Diffuse/regional/grouped/linear/segmental	
Associated features	Skin/nipple retraction, skin thickening (>2 mm), trabecular thickening, axillary adenopathy, architectural distortion, calcification		

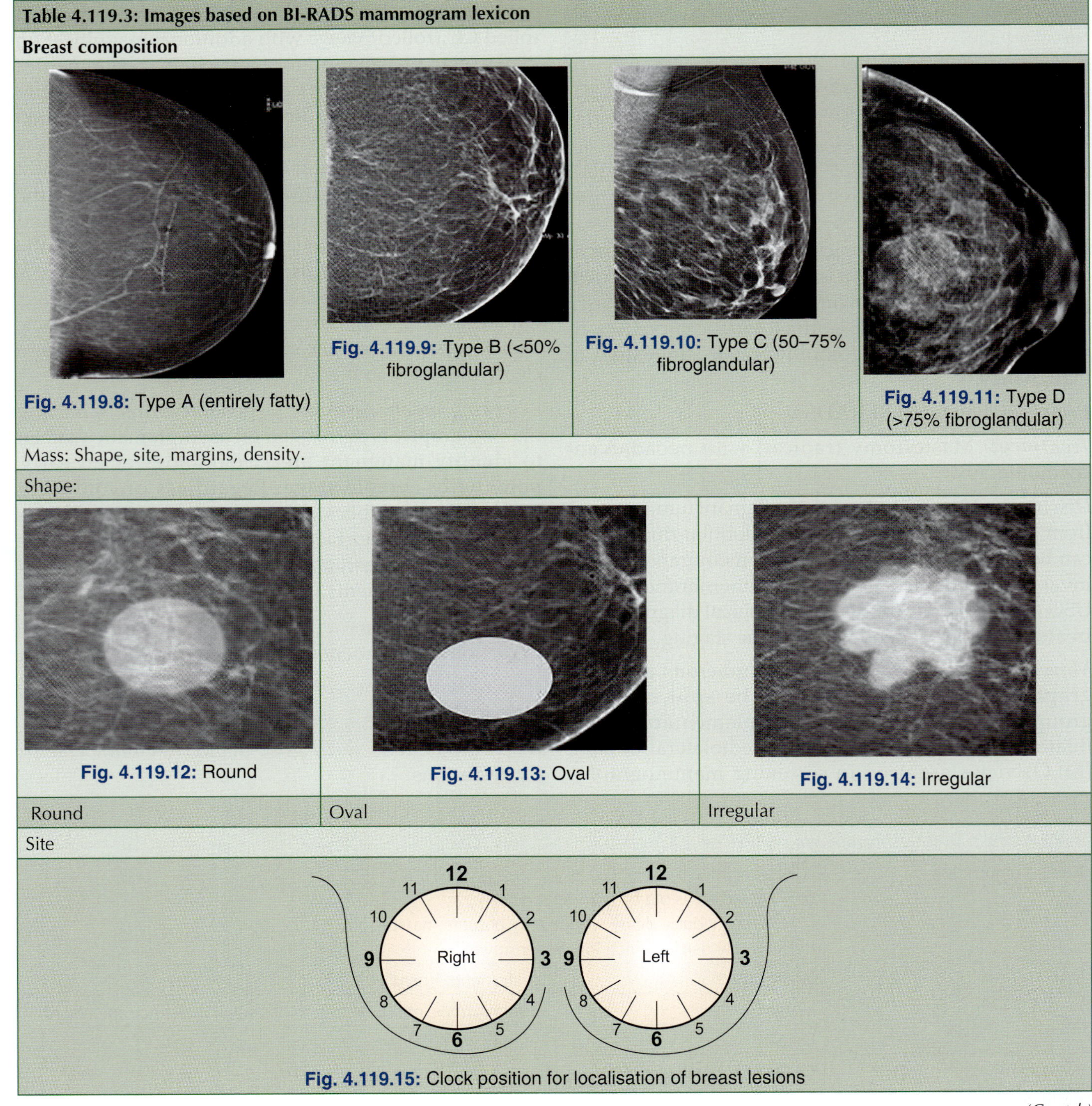

Table 4.119.3: Images based on BI-RADS mammogram lexicon			
Breast composition			
Fig. 4.119.8: Type A (entirely fatty)	Fig. 4.119.9: Type B (<50% fibroglandular)	Fig. 4.119.10: Type C (50–75% fibroglandular)	Fig. 4.119.11: Type D (>75% fibroglandular)
Mass: Shape, site, margins, density.			
Shape:			
Fig. 4.119.12: Round	Fig. 4.119.13: Oval	Fig. 4.119.14: Irregular	
Round	Oval	Irregular	
Site			

Fig. 4.119.15: Clock position for localisation of breast lesions

(Contd.)

Table 4.119.3: Images based on BI-RADS mammogram lexicon (*Contd.*)

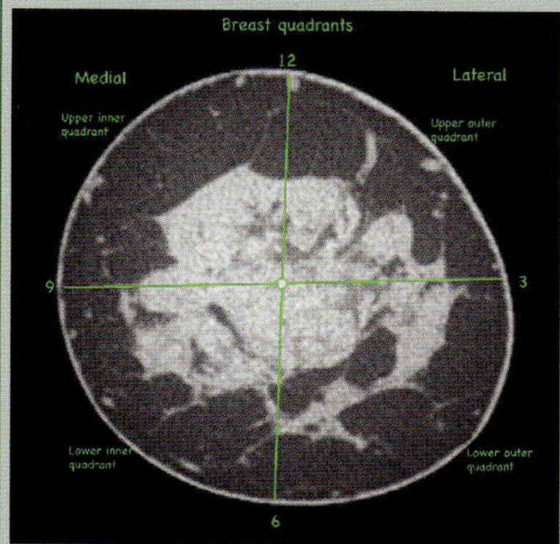 **Fig. 4.119.16:** Normal breast quadrants	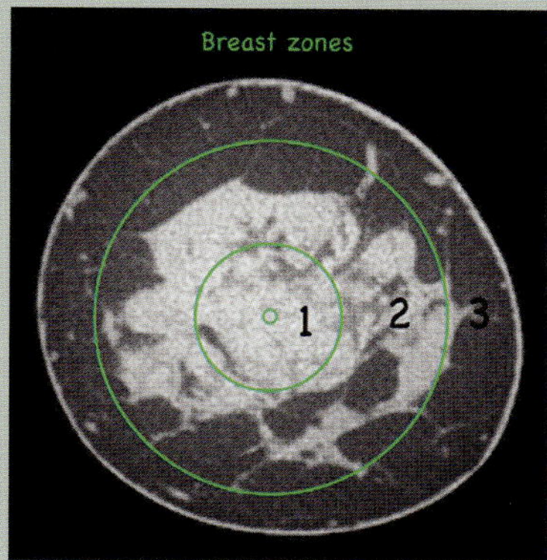 **Fig. 4.119.17:** Breast zones	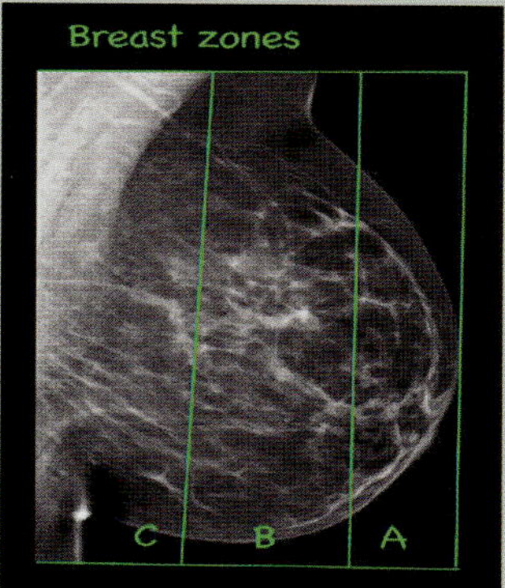 **Fig. 4.119.18:** Breast zones

Zones 1, 2 and 3 show the location in the transverse plane from the nipple to the axilla.
Zone 1: Adjacent to the nipple (includes first 1/3rd of the breast).
Zone 2: Midway from the nipple (includes 2/3rd of the breast).
Zone 3: Towards the peripheral breast.

Regions A, B and C denote the depth/distance of the lesion from nipple (equally divided into 3 parts by 2 vertical lines):
Region A: Near the surface—consists of premammary (PM) or subcutaneous fat zone containing Cooper ligaments (CL), and in some cases, a small number of peripheral ducts and lobules.
Region B: Midway between the nipple and chest wall (mammary zone) contains all of the central ducts and most of the peripheral ducts and lobules. The anterior mammary fascia (AMF) and the retromammary fascia (RMF) encase the mammary zone.
Region C: Chest wall—the retromammary zone (RM) is the deepest of the three zones and contains only fat and ligaments.

Margins

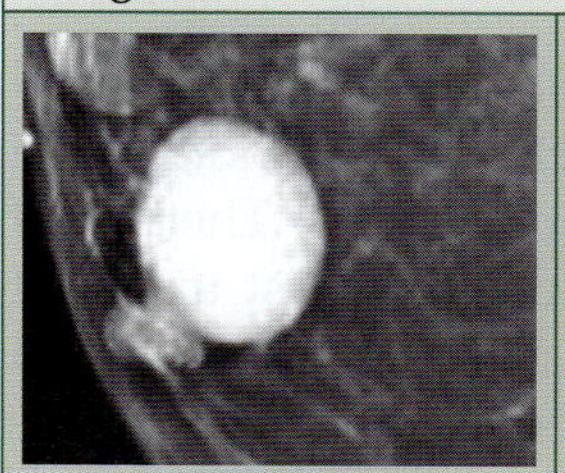 **Fig. 4.119.19:** Circumscribed	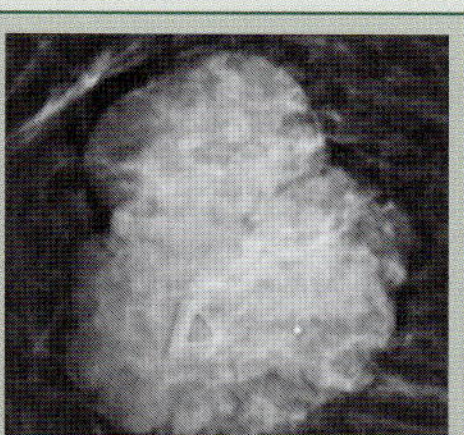 **Fig. 4.119.20:** Microlobulation	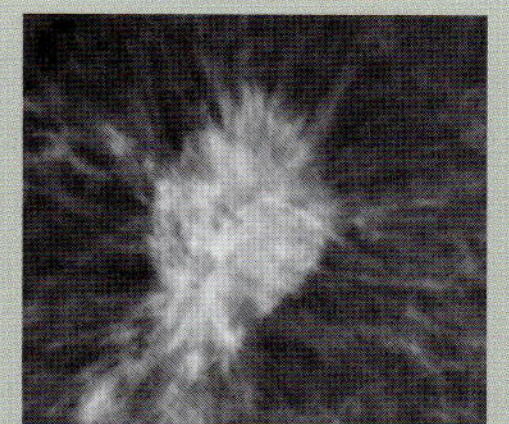 **Fig. 4.119.21:** Spiculated	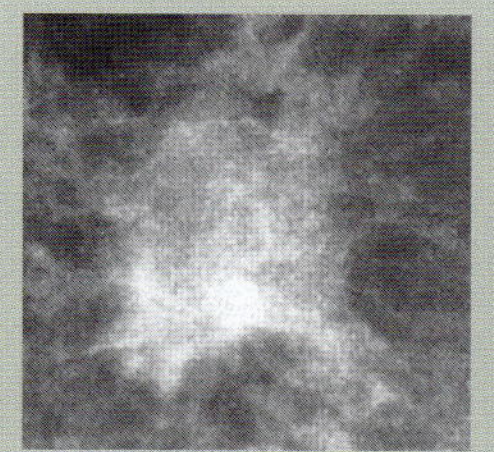 **Fig. 4.119.22:** Obscured	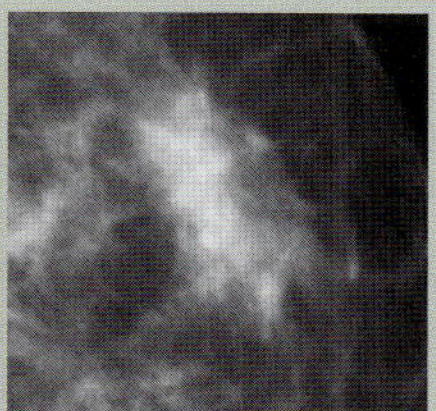 **Fig. 4.119.23:** Indistinct

Density

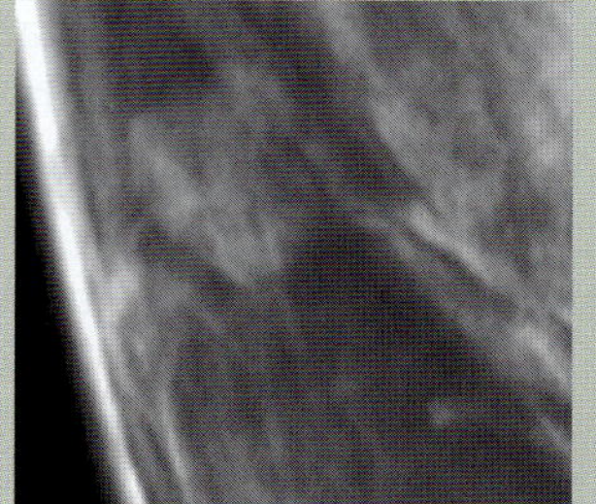 **Fig. 4.119.24:** Low density	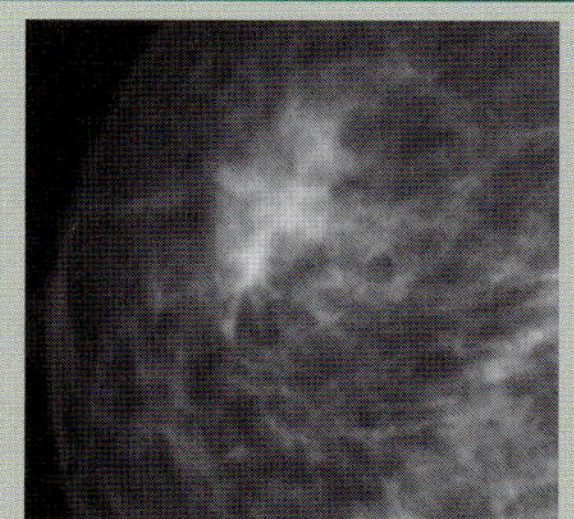 **Fig. 4.119.25:** Equal density	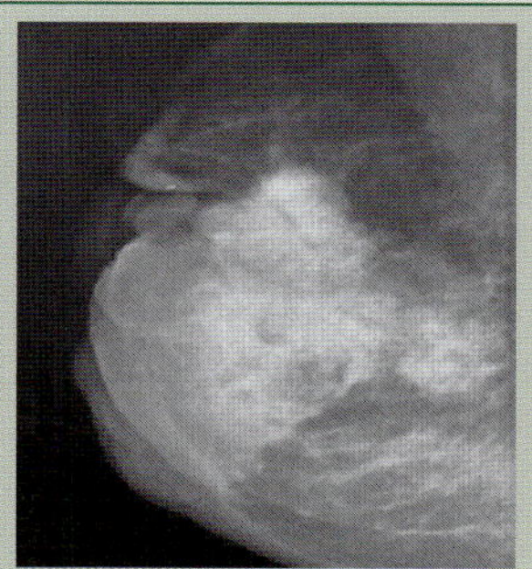 **Fig. 4.119.26:** High density	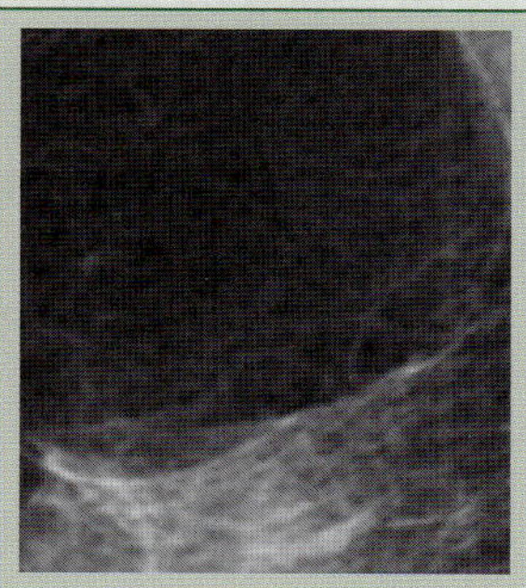 **Fig. 4.119.27:** Fat density

(Contd.)

Table 4.119.3: Images based on BI-RADS mammogram lexicon (*Contd.*)

<table>
<tr><td colspan="3">Asymmetries: Superimposition of normal breast tissue causes an area of fibroglandular tissue visible on only one mammographic projection.
Focal asymmetry: If it is visible on two projections, it is a real finding rather than a superimposition and helps to distinguish from a mass.
Global asymmetry that consists of asymmetry over at least one-fourth of the breast. It is a normal variant.
Developing asymmetry: It is new, larger, and more visible than it was on a previous examination.</td></tr>
<tr><td>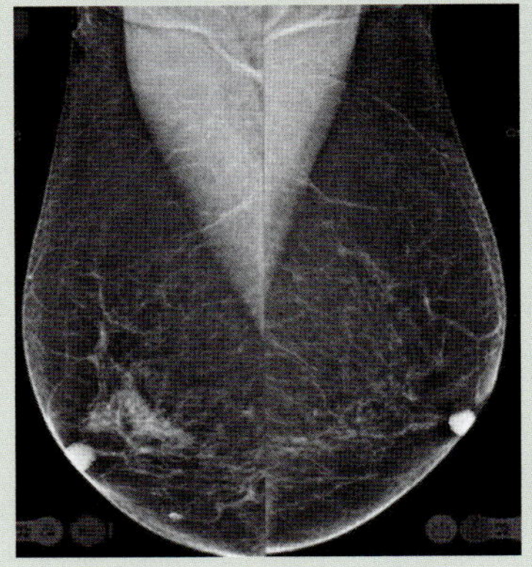
Fig. 4.119.28: Focal asymmetry seen on MLO view in retroareolar region</td><td>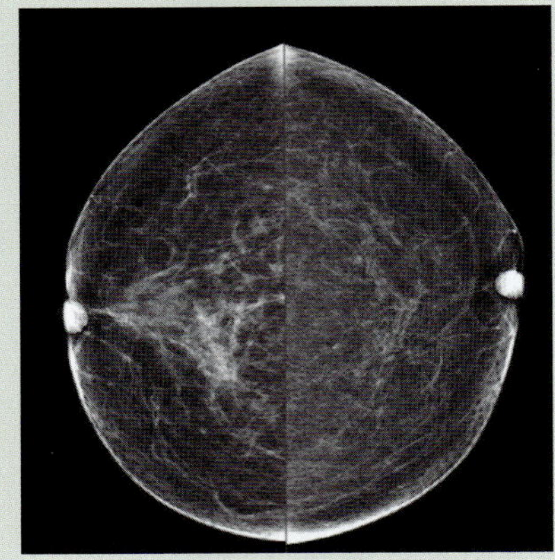
Fig. 4.119.29: Focal asymmetry seen on CC views in retroareolar region</td><td>Figures 4.119.28 and 4.119.29 are an example of a focal asymmetry seen on MLO and CC views in retroareolar region. Local compression views and USG did not show any mass.</td></tr>
<tr><td colspan="3">Architectural distortion: May be seen as a distortion of the normal architecture without any visible mass. Straight lines or spiculations radiating from a point, focal retraction, distortion or straightening at the edges of parenchyma.</td></tr>
</table>

Automated breast ultrasound (ABS): It is also known as automated 3D US breast volume scanning (ABVS). It was initiated to get a 3D view of the breast and to overcome the drawback of dense breast. It is done by acquiring volumetric data. A rigid pivoted stationary frame is manually pushed so that the transducer with gel applied in it comes in contact with breast and an optimal scan is acquired. This is analyzed and converted into thin tomographic slices. There is a facility to use a virtual probe by which multiple other scan planes can be acquired and a lesion, if visualized, can be better demonstrated with its adjacent structures. It can be combined with MRI or mammography to reproduce fusion images.

Role of CT in breast imaging involves good visualization of breast mass with adjacent dermal thickening, gives the status of axillary and internal mammary nodal involvement, chest wall and pleural invasion and for assessment of metastasis. The use of dynamic contrast-enhanced CT of the breast to detect intraductal extension of breast cancer has been found to be effective, and it is thought to be beneficial in the preoperative assessment of the extent of disease prior to breast-conserving surgery. CT can assist distinguish between benign and malignant nodes by detecting morphologic changes. On CT, tumors appear as dense lesions with early contrast enhancement, similar to what is seen on dynamic MRI. When microcalcification is the only symptom of early cancer, CT is less sensitive than mammography in detecting it.

Axial noncontrast CT sections (Figs 4.119.37 and 4.119.38) showing a large lobulated right breast mass

Table 4.119.4: Calcification in breast lesion: Based on BI-RADS 2013	
Typically benign calcification	*Suspicious malignancy*
Skin	Amorphous (4B)
Vascular	
Coarse or popcorn like	Coarse heterogeneous (4B)
Large rod-like	
Round or punctate	Fine pleomorphic (4C)
Rim calcification	
Dystrophic	Fine linear (4C)
Fat necrosis	
Milk of calcium	Fine linear branching (4C)
Suture	
Fig. 4.119.30: Amorphous	Fig. 4.119.31: Fine pleomorphic
Fig. 4.119.32: Coarse heterogeneous	Fig. 4.119.33: Fine linear
Distribution of calcification:	

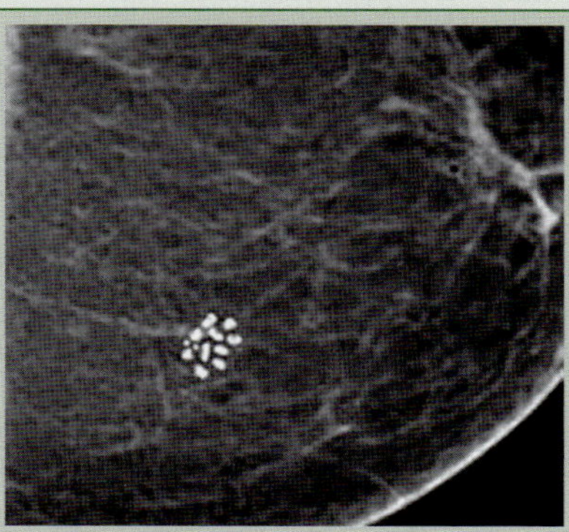

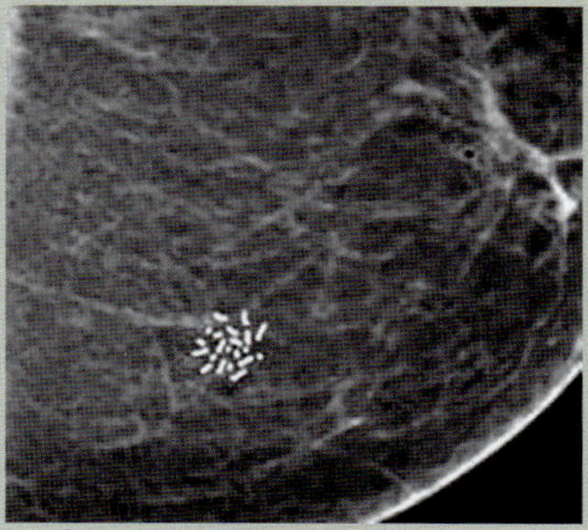

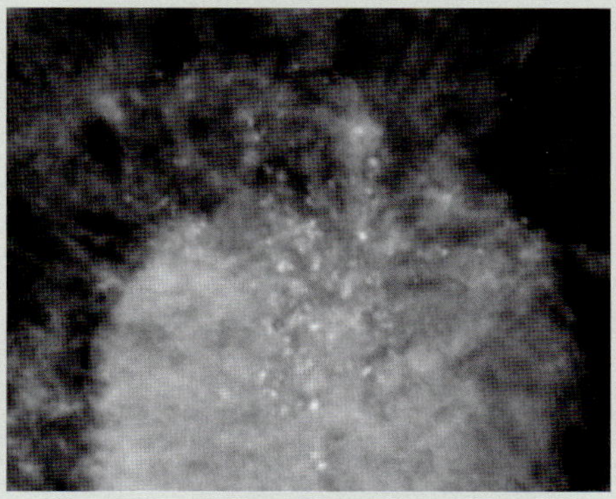

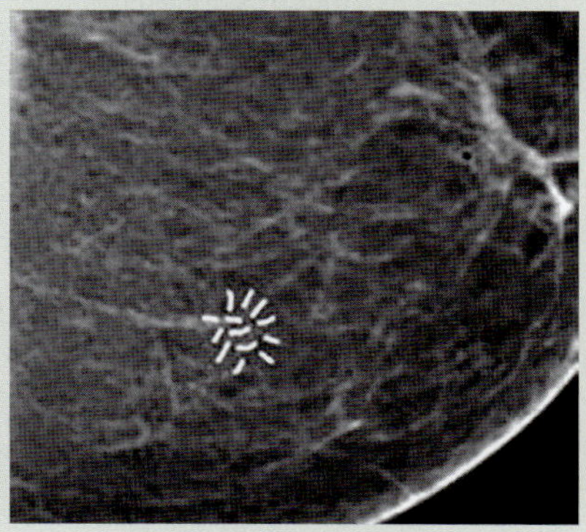

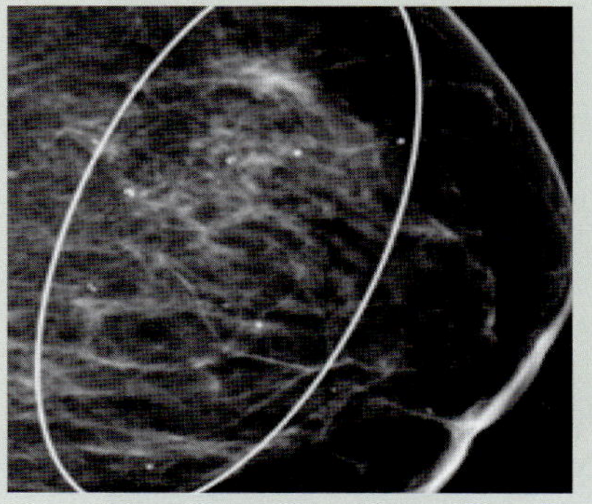

Fig. 4.119.34: Diffuse

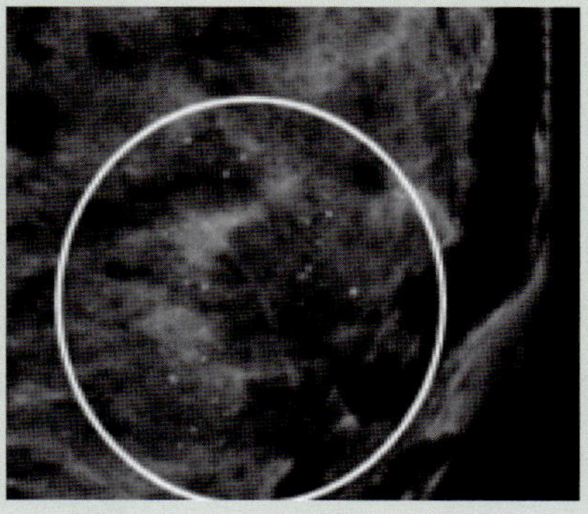

Fig. 4.119.35: Regional

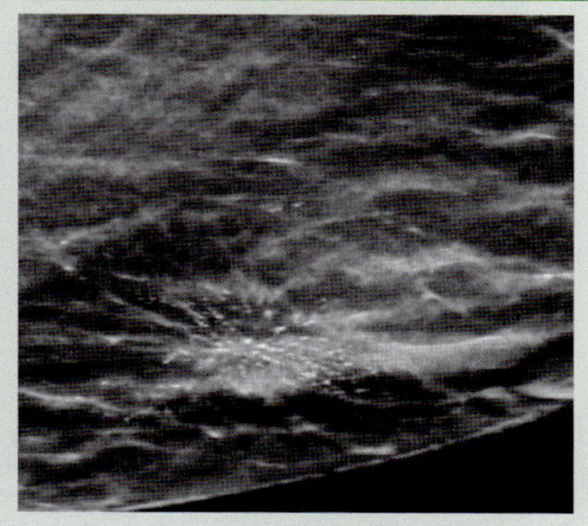

Fig. 4.119.36: Grouped

Table 4.119.5: Difference between benign and malignant microcalcifications	
Benign microcalcification	*Malignant microcalcification*
Smooth and round	5 or more in number
Calcification with lucent center	Each =/< 0.5 mm in size
Dermal calcification	Pleomorphic (size, shape and density)
Vascular calcification	Fine linear branching
Large rod-like calcification	Dot and dash pattern
Popcorn calcification	V, Y pattern of calcification

Table 4.119.6: Difference between screening mammography and diagnostic mammography	
Screening mammography	*Diagnostic mammography*
Asymptomatic	Symptomatic (include palpable finding, pain, spontaneous nipple discharge).
Purpose is detection of possible abnormalities	Call back of a patient with an abnormal screening mammogram.
	After a complete work-up, recommendations can range from normal 1-year follow-up to biopsy for histologic diagnosis.
Standard two views of each breast (mediolateral oblique and craniocaudal)	Views tailored to the patient's problem (may include spot or magnification views, additional projections, and ultrasound).
Batch read by radiologist	Usually performed in the presence of the radiologist and interpreted at the time of examination.

Table 4.119.7: BI-RADS ultrasound lexicon		
Breast composition	a. Homogeneous—fat b. Homogeneous—fibroglandular c. Heterogeneous.	
Mass	Shape	Oval/ round/ irregular
	Margin	Circumscribed/not circumscribed (indistinct/angular/microlobulated/speculated)
	Orientation	Parallel or not parallel
	Echo pattern	Anechoeic/hyperechoeic/complex cystic/hypoechoeic/isoechoeic.
	Posterior features	No features/enhancement/shadowing
Calcification	In mass/ outside mass/intraductal	
Associated features	Architectural distortion/duct changes/skin thickening/skin retraction/edema/vascularity (internal/peripheral/absent), elasticity.	
Special cases (case with a unique diagnosis)	Simple cyst/clustered microcysts/complicated cyst/mass in or on skin/foreign body/intramammary lymph node/AVM/Mondor disease/post-surgical fluid collection/ fat necrosis.	

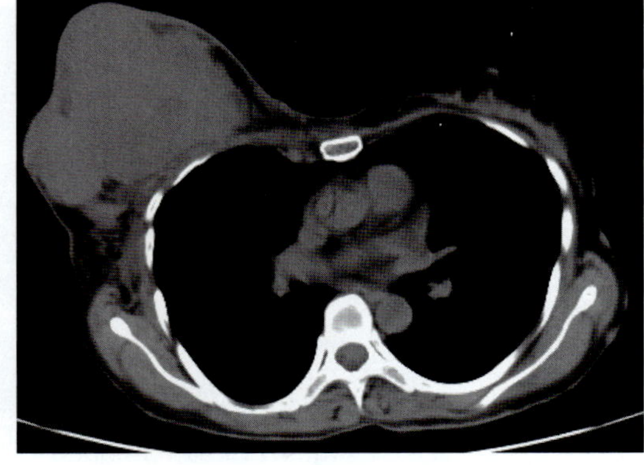

Fig. 4.119.37: Phyllodes tumor

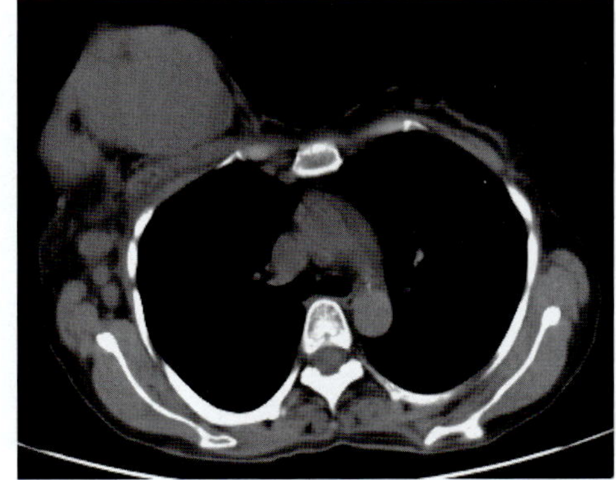

Fig. 4.119.38

Table 4.119.8: Difference between benign and malignant breast lesions		
Features	*Benign lesion*	*Malignant lesion*
Shape	Oval/ ellipsoid	Variable
Alignment	Wider than deep, parallel to tissue planes	Deeper than wide
Margins	Smooth, thin echogenic pseudocapsule with macro lobulations	Irregular/peculated/echogenic halo
Echotexture/homogenecity of internal echoes	Variable to intense hyperechogenicity with uniform internal echoes	Low to marked hypoechoic with non-uniform internal echoes
Lateral shadowing	Present	Absent
Posterior effect	Minimum attenuation/post-acoustic enhancement	Attenuation with obscured posterior margin
Others	Nil	Ca^{2+}, micro lobulation, intraductal extension
Elastogram	Soft	Hard
MRI kinetic curve	Type I	Type III
MR spectroscopy	Normal	Increased Choline peak
DWI	$>1.3 \times 10^{-3}$ except abscess	$<1.1 \times 10^{-3}$

with dermal thickening and enlarged right axillary and internal mammary lymph nodes.

Metastasis from breast carcinoma: Chest—lung metastases can have a variable appearance with mediastinal adenopathy, pleural effusions and lymphangitic spread.

Bone: Lytic and sclerotic deposits.

Liver: This is generally less common than bone or lung metastases. They are usually low attenuation lesions (CT) and can be diffuse and infiltrating and therefore difficult to detect.

Brain: This is not uncommon and can also involve the meninges and spinal cord.

Staging of Breast Cancer

T0: No evidence of primary tumor

Tis: Carcinoma *in situ*

Tis (DCIS): Ductal carcinoma *in situ*

Tis (LCIS): Lobular carcinoma *in situ* (not treated as cancer clinically)

Tis (Paget): Paget disease of nipple with no tumor

Tl: Invasive tumor ~2.0 cm in greatest dimension

Tlmic: Microinvasion ~0.1 cm in greatest dimension

Tla: Tumor >0.1 cm but ~0.5 cm in greatest dimension

Tlb: Tumor >0.5 cm but ~1 cm in greatest dimension

TIc: Tumor >1 cm but ~2 cm in greatest dimension

T2: Tumor >2 cm but ~5 cm in greatest dimension

T3: Tumor >5 cm in greatest dimension

T4: Tumor of any size with direct extension to chest wall or skin, only as described

T4a: Extension to chest wall, not including pectoralis muscle

T4b: Edema (including peau d' orange) or ulceration of the skin of the breast, or satellite skin nodules confined to the same breast

T4c: Both T4a and T4b

T4d: Inflammatory carcinoma

Regional lymph nodes (N)

NX: Regional lymph nodes cannot be assessed (e.g., previously removed)

NO: No regional lymph node metastasis

Nl: Metastasis in movable ipsilateral ALN

N2: Metastases in ipsilateral ALN fixed or matted, or in clinically apparent ipsilateral IMN in the absence of clinically evident ALN metastasis

N2a: Metastasis in ipsilateral ALN fixed to one another (matted) or to other structures

N2b: Metastasis only in clinically apparent ipsilateral IMN and in the absence of clinically evident ALN metastasis

N3: Metastasis in ipsilateral infraclavicular lymph node(s), or in clinically apparent ipsilateral IMN(s) and in the presence of clinically evident ALN metastasis; or metastasis in ipsilateral supraclavicular lymph node(s) with or without ALN or IMN involvement

N3a: Metastasis in ipsilateral infraclavicular lymph node(s) and ALN

N3b: Metastasis in ipsilateral IMN and ALN

N3c: Metastasis in ipsilateral supraclavicular lymph node(s)

Table 4.119.9: Important terms to note down—multifocal and multicentric breast carcinomas		
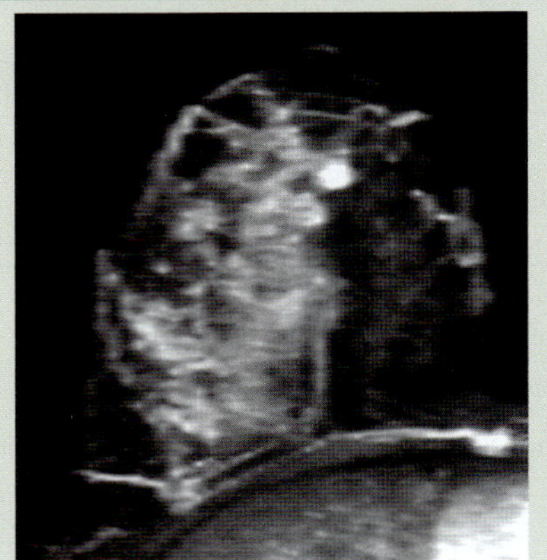 **Fig. 4.119.39:** Multifocal breast CA	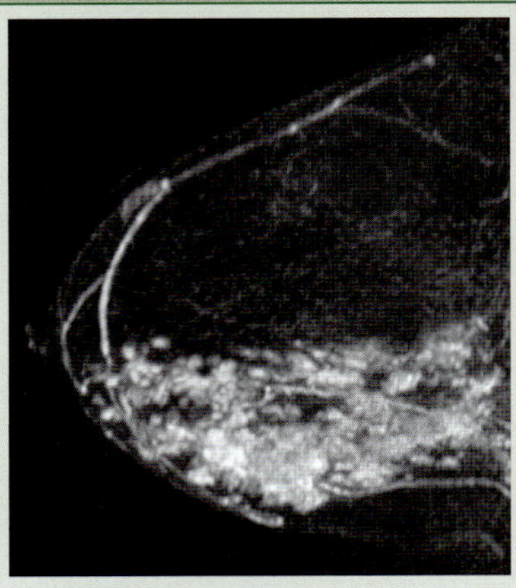 **Fig. 4.119.40:** Multifocal breast CA	**Multifocal breast CA:** Multiple malignant lesions in the same quadrant, arise from same ductal system, <5 cm apart.
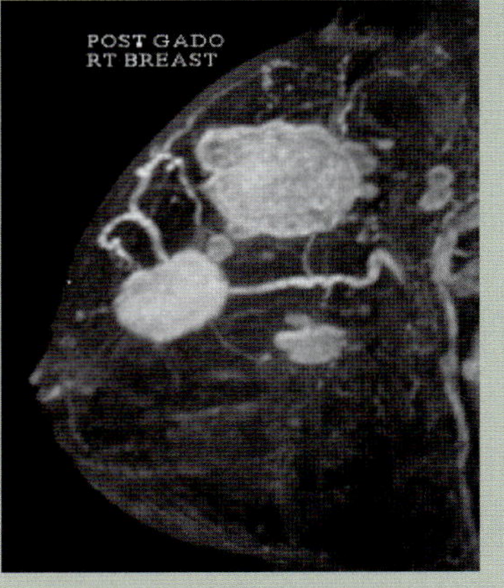 **Fig. 4.119.41:** Multicentric breast CA	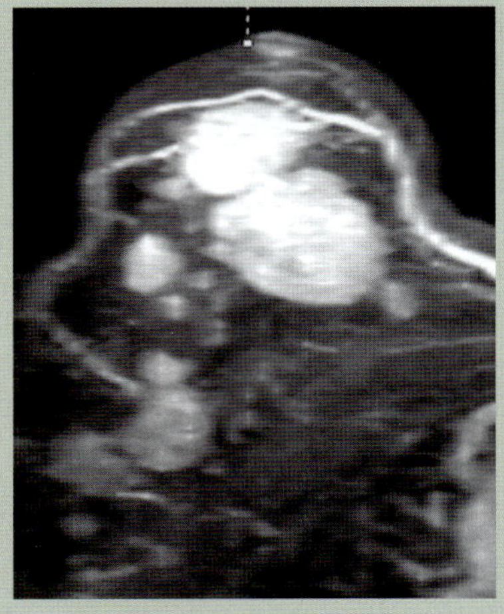 **Fig. 4.119.42:** Multicentric breast CA	**Multicentric breast CA:** Multiple lesions in different quadrants of same breast, arise from different ductal system and >5 cm apart
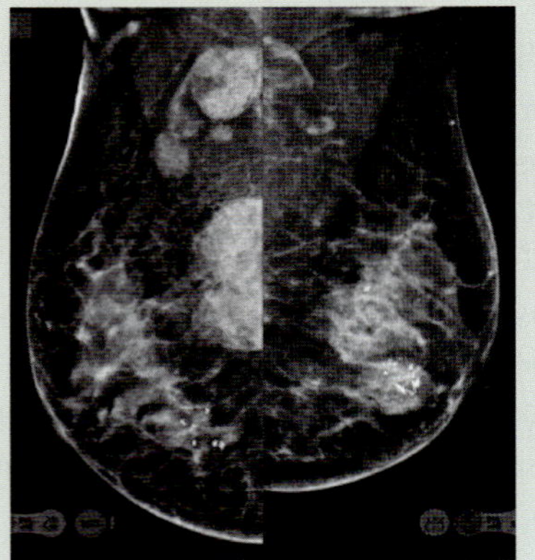 **Fig. 4.119.43:** Multicentric and bilateral breast CA	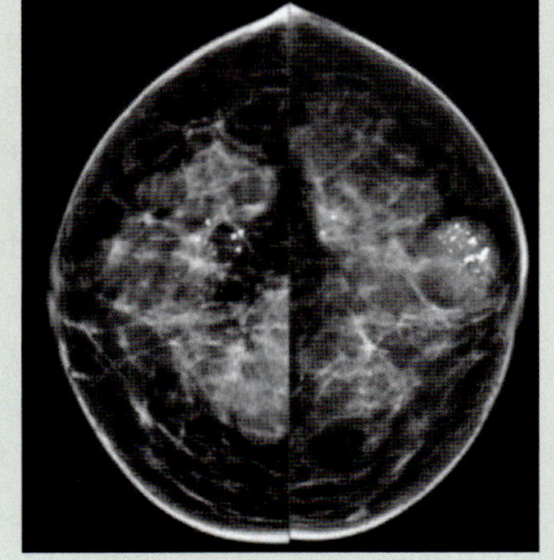 **Fig. 4.119.44:** Multicentric and bilateral breast CA	**Multicentric and bilateral breast CA:** Multicentric lesions involving both breast

Staging of Breast Ca as per AJCC

Stage 0 (TisNOMO)
Stage I (T1NOMO)
Stage IIA (TON1MO, T1N1MO, T2NOMO)
Stage II B (T2N1MO, T3NOMO)
Stage III A (TON2MO, T1N2MO, T2N2MO, T3N1 MO, T3N2MO)
Stage IIIB (T4NOMO, T4N1MO, T4N2MO)
Stage IIIc (Any T N3MO)
Stage IV (Any T Any N, M1)

Treatment:

1. Surgical—mastectomy/conservative breast surgery.
2. Hormonal therapy—tamoxifen
3. Chemotherapy—5 FU, Cisplatin

Synchronous tumors: 2nd tumor identified within 3 months of the 1st tumor.

Metachronous tumors: 2nd tumor identified >3 months of 1st tumor.

American Cancer Society Guidelines for Early Detection of Cancer: If women between the ages of 40 and 44 choose to start annual breast cancer screening with mammograms (breast X-rays), they should be able to do so. Mammograms should be done every year for women aged 45 to 54. Women age >55 years should get mammograms every two years, or yearly screening can be continued. Screening should be done as long as a woman is in excellent health and expects to live for another 10 years or more. Breast cancer screening has a number of established benefits, limitations, and potential risks that all women should be aware. High risk mammography: For women with BRCA1 or BRCA2 mutations, current guidelines recommended screening by clinical breast examination and mammography starting at age 30. For certain high-risk women, additional screening with magnetic resonance imaging (MRI) is encouraged.

WHO classification of breast tumors: The vast majority of breast cancers are adenocarcinomas (99%):The most common types are invasive carcinoma of no special type (ductal carcinoma not otherwise specified): 40–75%, ductal carcinoma *in situ*: 20–25%, invasive lobular carcinoma: 5–15%.

Categories of benign epithelial neoplasms include: Papillary and adenomatous lesions.

Nonepithelial malignancies are uncommon and include: Breast sarcomas, malignant phyllodes tumor, metastases to the breast and breast lymphoma.

Medullary carcinoma of breast: Uncommon type of breast carcinoma accounting for about 5% of total breast carcinomas. Occurs between 46 and 54 years of age, mean age being 35 years. Mammography—well-defined lesion with microlobulation, low incidence of calcification. USG—well-defined hypoechoic lesion with post-acoustic enhancement may be seen in 50% of cases. MRI—well-circumscribed T2 iso or hyperintense lesion with/without a hypointense rim surrounding the lesion which shows peripheral rim enhancement with enhancing internal septation on post-contrast imaging.

Mucinous carcinoma of breast: It is invasive ductal carcinoma subtype, also called colloid breast carcinoma. Occurs in older women. Mammography: Relatively well-defined lobular low-density mass due to mucin. USG—mixed echogenicity, distal enhancement with microlobulated margins. MRI—very high signal on T2W imaging. Low signal on DWI and increased ADC values. Post-contrast shows benign appearing kinetics. It has relatively good prognosis compared to other adenocarcinomas.

4.120 BREAST

Case No. 120

Clinical history: A 40-year-old female patient with a growing mass in the left breast over the last couple of years.

Radiological techniques and observation: Figures 4.120.1 and 4.120.2 are CC and MLO views showing type B breast showing large ovoid high-density lesion with lobulated margins occupying most of the left breast. No evidence of spiculations. No associated calcification. No dermal changes/axillary lymphadenopathy/architectural distortion. The patient can be further evaluated by USG to narrow down the diagnosis.

Figures 4.120.3 and 4.120.4 are USG showing a well-circumscribed oval heteroechoic mass lesion measuring about 13 × 10 cm in its maximum dimensions with stretching of overlying skin noted in the left breast. No associated lymphadenopathy. No associated post-acoustic shadowing/enhancement.

Interpretation: Large mass lesion noted occupying most of the left breast with well-circumscribed margin. No obvious skin infiltration. No enlarged axillary/retromammary lymph nodes noted.

Principal diagnosis: Giant left breast mass and considering the patient age and rapid growth rate, phyllodes tumor (BI-RADS 4) is more likely. Core needle biopsy was advised under USG guidance. Core biopsy was done showing biphasic fibroepithelial tumor showing proliferating spindle cells within collagenized occasionally loose stroma entangling bland epithelial component in the form of patent and focally compressed ducts. Picture impressive of a phyllodes tumor.

Differential diagnosis: Giant fibroadenoma of the breast, Primary sarcoma of the breast.

Management: It is a locally invasive tumor. Treatment is usually with surgical excision. Patient referred to general surgeon. A full mastectomy may be required if the tumor is large. Phyllodes tumors, both benign and malignant, have a tendency to recur if they are not completely removed. In 5–25% of cases, malignant degeneration can be detected (malignant phyllodes tumor). Local recurrence (up to 25%) is common after broad local excision, and up to 10% of patients can develop metastasis.

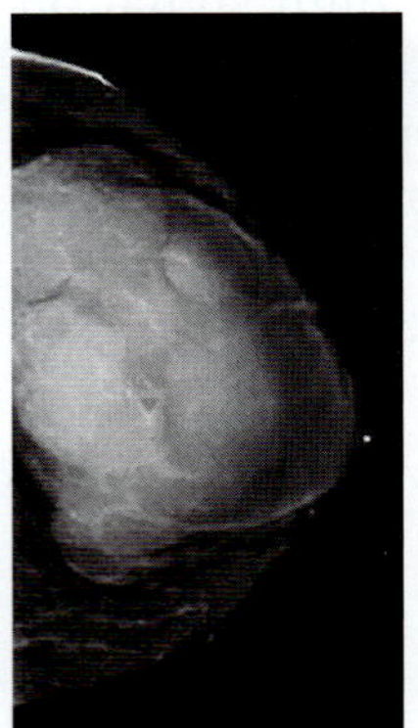

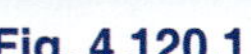

Fig. 4.120.1

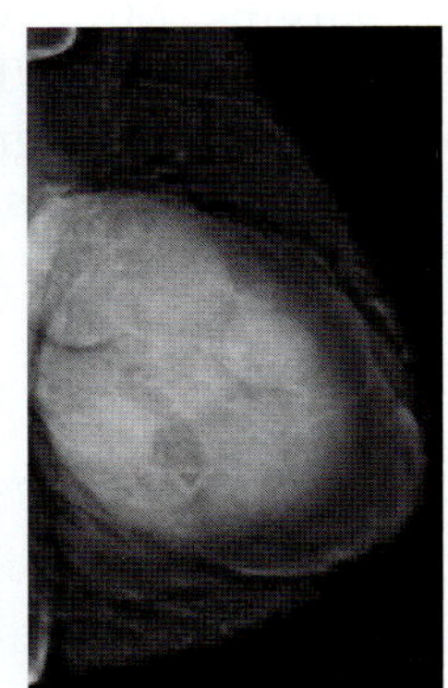

Fig. 4.120.2

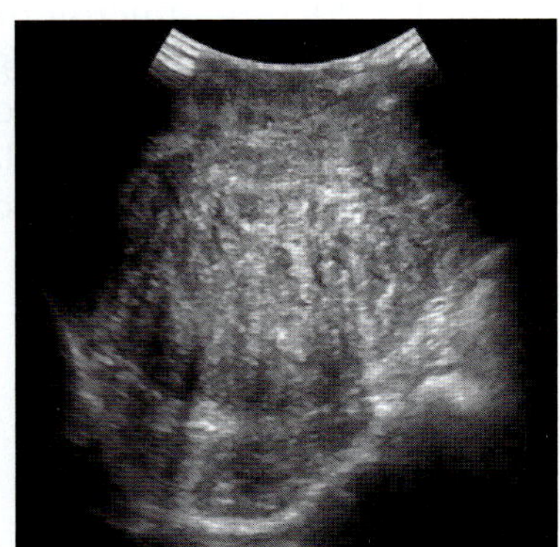

Fig. 4.120.3

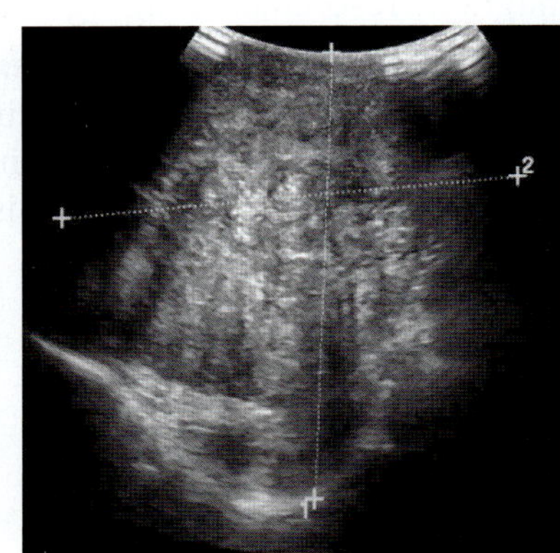

Fig. 4.120.4

Table 4.120.1: Features of giant fibroadenoma

Giant fibroadenoma These are fibroadenomas weighing more than 500 grams or measuring >5 cm in size. Treatment: Symptomatic lesion treated by surgical excision.	Well-circumscribed discrete oval mass hypo- or isodense to the breast glandular tissue. Involuting lesions can produce classic, coarse popcorn calcification appearance.	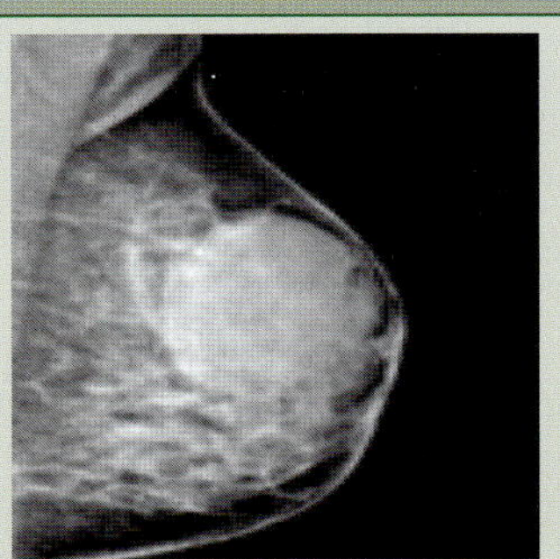 **Fig. 4.120.5:** Giant fibroadenoma

In such circumstances, haematogenous metastases are the most common.

Radiographic Features of Phyllodes Tumor

Mammography: Non-specific large rounded oval or lobulated lesions with smooth edges that are generally well confined. Radiolucent halo may be present. Calcification (usually coarse and plaque-like) can be found in a few cases. Ultrasound: Inhomogeneous, solid-appearing lesion on ultrasound. A solid mass with cystic spaces, round or cleft like, with posterior acoustic amplification strongly confirms the diagnosis of phyllodes tumor. Vascularization is more commonly found in solid components. On mammography and ultrasound, most lesions are indistinguishable from fibroadenomas in practise. This is why a fibroadenoma's interval expansion is considered a reason for a needle biopsy. Because needle biopsy may not be typical of the pathology in the entire lesion, large lesions (i.e. >4 cm) may qualify for excision out of hand.

T1: Usually low signal, T2: Can range from homogeneous low signal to high signal, T1C + (Gd): The solid components enhance following contrast administration, dynamic contrast: The kinetic curve pattern can be gradual/rapid type.

Recent Advances in Breast Imaging

Contrast enhanced mammography: Contrast-enhanced mammography is an emerging modality with many current and developing clinical applications, such as depicting abnormalities seen at screening, demonstrating disease extent, depicting response to neoadjuvant therapy, and breast cancer screening. Recent advances in breast MRI have allowed better disease evaluation. MRI is not always readily available, time consuming and is contraindicated in some patients. CEM can be an alternative to ultrasound/MRI and also be used to obtain contrast material–enhanced information and standard mammograms simultaneously. A CEM examination is less time consuming than that of MRI, and the modalities have similar rates of sensitivity to detect lesions. CEM has lesser costs than MRI.

Digital mammography: also known as full field digital mammography (FFDM). It is a mammography system with the solid-state detectors (convert X-rays into electrical signals) replaces X-ray film, creating digital image which can be manipulated to improve contrast and resolution. The sharper image aids interpretation by making dense breast tissue and tiny tumors easier to see, and it frequently reduces the need for further follow-up imaging.

Fig. 4.120.6: Craniocaudal contrast enhanced low energy showing non-mass enhancement in retroareolar region of left breast which on biopsy revealed invasive ductal carcinoma

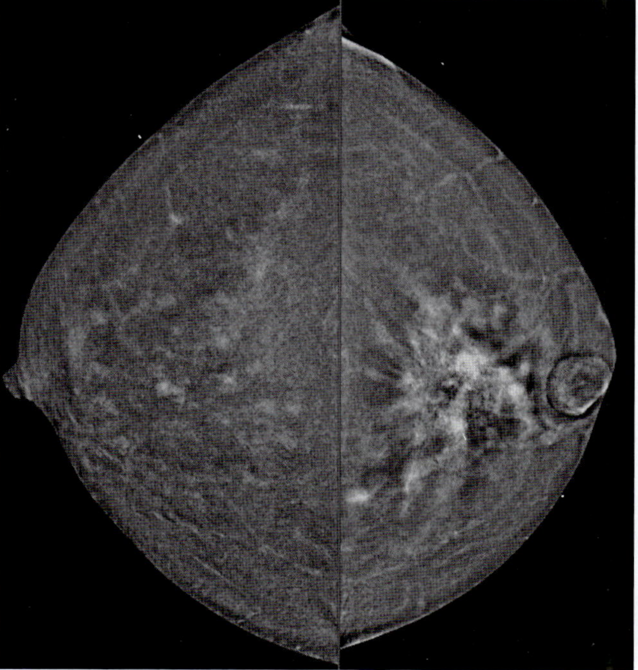

Fig. 4.120.7: Craniocaudal recombinant mammogram showing non-mass enhancement in retroareolar region of left breast which on biopsy revealed invasive ductal carcinoma

Computer-aided detection: They use digitized mammographic image obtained from either a conventional film mammogram or digitally acquired mammogram. The computer software will search for abnormal areas of density, mass, or calcification which are suspicious of breast cancer. The CAD system will highlight the suspicious areas on the images, cautioning the radiologist to the look for further analysis.

Digital breast tomosynthesis: It is an imaging technique which allow a volumetric reconstruction of the whole breast from a finite number of low-dose two-dimensional projections obtained by different X-ray tube angles, with a geometric principle very similar to that applied in stratigraphic technique. During a "3D" exam, an X-ray arm sweeps in a slight arc over your breast, taking multiple low dose X-ray images. Then, a computer produces synthetic 2D and 3D images of your breast tissue. The images include thin one millimeter slices, enabling the radiologist to scroll through images of the entire breast. The "3D" images reduce the overlap of breast tissue, and make it possible for a radiologist to better see through your breast tissue on the mammogram.

Breast elastography: Ultrasound elastography provides a non-invasive evaluation of the "stiffness" of a lesion. It increases the specificity of conventional B-mode ultrasound by more precise characterization of breast lesions. Ultrasound elastography has 86.5% sensitivity, 89.8% specificity, and 88.3% diagnostic accuracy in the differentiation of benign from malignant solid breast masses.

Stereotactic breast biopsy: Stereotactic breast biopsy refers to percutaneous sampling of breast tissue using mammographic guidance for targeting. It is the biopsy method of choice when the finding of interest is best seen on mammography, such as microcalcifications (most common), architectural distortion, or an asymmetry or mass without a sonographic correlate.